D1208907

DIAGNOSTIC NUCLEAR MEDICINE

FOURTH EDITION

MARTIN P. SANDLER, M.D., F.A.C.N.P.
*Professor and Vice Chairman
Radiology and Radiological Sciences
Vanderbilt University Medical Center
Nashville, Tennessee*

R. EDWARD COLEMAN, M.D.
*Professor and Chairman
Department of Radiology
Division of Nuclear Medicine
Duke University Medical Center
Durham, North Carolina*

JAMES A. PATTON, Ph.D.
*Professor
Radiology and Radiological Sciences
Vanderbilt University Medical Center
Nashville, Tennessee*

FRANS J. TH. WACKERS, M.D.
*Professor of Diagnostic Radiology and Medicine
Director, Cardiovascular Nuclear Imaging
Departments of Diagnostic Radiology and Medicine
Yale University School of Medicine
New Haven, Connecticut*

ALEXANDER GOTTSCHALK, M.D., F.A.C.R.
*Professor of Radiology
Department of Radiology
Michigan State University
East Lansing, Michigan*

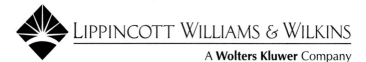

LIPPINCOTT WILLIAMS & WILKINS
A **Wolters Kluwer** Company
Philadelphia • Baltimore • New York • London
Buenos Aires • Hong Kong • Sydney • Tokyo

Acquisitions Editor: Joyce-Rachel John
Developmental Editor: Joanne Bersin
Production Editor: Allison L. Risko
Manufacturing Manager: Colin Warnock
Cover Designer: Co.Laborative Design
Compositor: Maryland Composition Company
Printer: Maple Press

© 2003 by LIPPINCOTT WILLIAMS & WILKINS
530 Walnut Street
Philadelphia, PA 19106 USA
LWW.com

Printed in the USA

First Edition, 1976
Second Edition, 1988
Third Edition, 1996

Library of Congress Cataloging-in-Publication Data

Diagnostic nuclear medicine/editors Martin P. Sandler . . . [et al.].–4th ed.
   p. ; cm
  Rev. ed. of: Diagnostic nuclear medicine / Martin P. Sandler. 3rd ed. c 1996.
  Includes bibliographic references and index.
  ISBN 0-7817-3252-2 (alk. paper)
  1. Radioisotope scanning. 2. Nuclear medicine. I. Sandler, Matin P.
  [DNLM: 1. Radionuclide Imaging. 2. Nuclear Medicine. WN 445 D53455 2003]
  RC78.7.R4D465.F86 2003
  618.9'8021—dc20
  DNLM/DLC
                                                  200203274

This text is dedicated to our families

PREFACE

The fourth edition of *Diagnostic Nuclear Medicine* has been designed by the editors to provide an encyclopedic reference for those who are mainly involved in nuclear medicine, including specialists in nuclear cardiology and the rapidly growing field of molecular oncology. The first edition of *Diagnostic Nuclear Medicine* was published in 1976, the second edition 12 years later in 1988, and the third edition 7 years later in 1995. The third edition had grown to 2 volumes, expanded to include 6 editors, 15 sections, 85 chapters, and over 150 contributors.

The fourth edition, published 7 years later, has, by design, been condensed into a single volume with 11 sections and 61 chapters. The essence of the text was to remove non-essential material, update all chapters, and expand on new developments.

Innovative advances in technology covered in the fourth edition include new coincidence detectors, crystal development, and x-ray attenuation in hybrid imaging systems for both CT/SPECT and CT/PET. The use of lymphoscintigraphy for sentinel node mapping in patients with breast cancer and melanoma has become an integral part of nuclear imaging. Similarly, PET has moved from the area of investigational research to the clinical arena in a variety of oncological indications and for the detection of hibernating myocardium. Newer investigations using PET are currently under review, including a host of malignant diseases and patients with dementia. The therapeutic use of radioisotopes has also gone from investigational studies to clinical practice in patients with lymphoma using monoclonal antibodies. Somatostatin receptor binding agents and labeled peptides are still being studied for therapy in a variety of cancers.

The next decade will involve the field of functional/molecular imaging with newer instrumentation, including micro-PET/CT, allowing us to examine smaller and smaller components of the human body. This progression from macro- to micro-imaging may lead to our ability to radiolabel minute cell structures and provide important diagnostic information from organ structures, blood, and amniotic fluid samples in animal models and to further refine these techniques before moving into the clinical environment.

Once again, it is our hope that the fourth edition of *Diagnostic Nuclear Medicine* will allow those in the field to keep abreast of new innovations and open a window into the exciting technology of functional and molecular imaging.

MARTIN P. SANDLER, M.D.
R. EDWARD COLEMAN, M.D.
FRANS J. TH. WACKERS, M.D.
JAMES A. PATTON, PH.D.
ALEXANDER GOTTSCHALK, M.D.

PREFACE TO THE FIRST EDITION

This book is designed to be useful to the practicing radiologist with a significant commitment to nuclear medicine. Many of the chapters about the current practice of nuclear radiology, such as those related to the use of cameras and scanners as well as those describing imaging of various organ systems, have a combination of useful "tricks of the trade," and a miniatlas with key illustrations available for study of reference.

It is inevitable, however, that nuclear medicine will become progressively more inclusive and therefore more complicated. As a result, several chapters have a more sophisticated bent. It is difficult, if not impossible, to take topics like collimator design; compartments, pools and spaces; and flow measurements; and couch them in terms of "2 x 2" arithmetic. In spite of this, it seems to us that these chapters are necessary both as reference material and for those instances in which the radiologist may be actually involved in utilizing the techniques or principles described. In short, this volume was written to help the radiologists practice better nuclear radiology now, and in the future.

ALEXANDER GOTTSCHALK, M.D.
E. JAMES POTCHEN, M.D.

ACKNOWLEDGMENTS

We are all extremely grateful to Paul B. Hoffer, MD, for his invaluable work in co-editing the earlier editions of *Diagnostic Nuclear Medicine*. Without his considerable efforts in helping to lay the foundations of this text, this current edition would not be possible. Our gratitude is also extended to the authors and publishers who generously granted permission to reproduce illustrations from other books and journals. Finally, we would like to thank all of the staff at Lippincott Williams & Wilkins for their tireless assistance and unwavering commitment to this text.

CONTRIBUTING AUTHORS

John Aarsvold, MD Nuclear Medicine Service, Veterans Affairs Medical Center and Division of Nuclear Medicine, Department of Radiology, School of Medicine, Emory University, Atlanta, GA

Esma A. Akin, MD Assistant Professor, Department of Radiology, George Washington University School of Medicine; Director, Division of Nuclear Medicine, George Washington University Hospital, Washington, DC

Abass Alavi, MD Professor of Radiology and Neurology, and Chief, Division of Nuclear Medicine, University of Pennsylvania Medical Center, Philadelphia, PA

Naomi Alazraki, MD Professor of Radiology, Emory University School of Medicine; Co-Director Nuclear Medicine; Chief, Nuclear Medicine, VA Medical Center, Atlanta, GA

Rachel Bar-Shalom, MD Nuclear Medicine Physician, Department of Nuclear Medicine, Rambam Medical Center, Haifa, Israel

Bruce J. Barron, MD Professor of Radiology, Department of Radiology, University of Texas Medical School-Houston, TX

Jeroen J. Bax, MD, PhD Director of Noninvasive Imaging, Department of Cardiology, Leiden University Medical Center, Leiden, The Netherlands

David V. Becker, MD Professor, Department of Radiology and Medicine, Cornell University Medical College; Director, Division of Nuclear Medicine, The New York Hospital-Cornell Medical Center, New York, NY

Lewis C. Becker, MD Professor, Department of Medicine, Johns Hopkins Medical Institutions, Baltimore, MD

Mats Bergström, MD Uppsala University PET Centre, University Hospital, Uppsala, Sweden

Daniel S. Berman, MD Co-chairman, Department of Imaging, Cedars-Sinai Medical Center; Professor of Medicine, UCLA School of Medicine, Los Angeles, CA

Glen M. Blake, PhD Consultant Physicist, Department of Nuclear Medicine, Guy's Hospital, London, United Kingdom

Eric Boersma, PhD Department of Cardiology, Leiden University Medical Center; Department of Cardiology/Epidemiology, Thorax Center, Rotterdam, The Netherlands

Robert O. Bonow, MD Goldberg Distinguished Professor, Department of Medicine; Chief, Division of Cardiology, Northwestern University Medical School and Northwestern Memorial Hospital, Chicago, IL

Frederick J. Bonte, MD Krohmer Professor and Director, Nuclear Medicine Center, Department of Radiology, The University of Texas Southwestern Medical Center at Dallas; Honorary Consultant, Parkland Memorial Hospital, Dallas, TX

James E. Bowsher, MD Department of Radiology, Duke University, Durham, NC

Robert J. Boudreau, MD, PhD Professor of Radiology, and Director, Division of Nuclear Medicine, University of Minnesota, Minneapolis, MN

Manuel L. Brown, MD Chairman, Department of Radiology, Henry Ford Hospital, Detroit, MI

Thomas F. Budinger, MD Professor, Lawrence Berkeley Laboratory, University of California at Berkeley, Berkeley, CA

Chuong Bui, MD Division of Nuclear Medicine, Department of Radiology, University of Michigan; Department of Veterans Affairs Health Systems, Ann Arbor, MI

Jerrold T. Bushberg, PhD Clinical Professor, Department of Radiology; Director of Health Physics Programs, Environmental Health & Safety, University of California Davis Medical Center, Sacramento, CA

Michelle G. Campbell, MD Department of Radiology and Radiological Sciences, Vanderbilt University Medical Center, Nashville, TN

Ana M. Catafau, MD Head of Exploratory Clinical Medicine, Clinical Pharmacology Discovery Medicine, Centre of Excellence for Drug Discovery, Psychiatry, Barcelona, Spain

Martin Charron, MD Associate Professor of Radiology, Department of Radiology, University of Pennsylvania; Director, Division of Nuclear Medicine, Radiology, Children's Hospital of Philadelphia, Philadelphia, PA

Vaseem U. Chengazi, MD, PhD Assistant Professor, Department of Radiology, Division of Nuclear Medicine, University of Rochester; Chief, Division of Nuclear Medicine, Strong Memorial Hospital, University of Rochester Medical Center, Rochester, NY

R. Edward Coleman, MD   Professor and Vice Chairman, Department of Radiology, Duke University Medical Center, Durham, NC

Simon R. Cherry, PhD   Professor, Department of Biomedical Engineering, University of California Davis, Davis, CA

Frederick L. Datz, MD   Retired, Salt Lake City, UT

Marion DeJong, MD   Department of Nuclear Medicine, University Hospital of Rotterdam, Rotterdam, The Netherlands

Dominique Delbeke, MD, PhD   Professor, Department of Radiology and Radiological Sciences; Director of Nuclear Medicine/PET, Vanderbilt University Medical Center, Nashville, TN

Michael D. Devous, Sr., PhD   Professor, Department of Radiology and Nuclear Medicine; Associate Director, Nuclear Medicine Center, Department of Radiology, The University of Texas Southwestern Medical Center, Dallas, TX

Marcelo F. DiCarli, MD   Assistant Professor of Radiology, Harvard Medical School; Director of Nuclear Cardiology, Division of Nuclear Medicine, Brigham and Women's Hospital, Boston, MA

Eva V. Dubovsky, MD, PhD   Professor, Department of Radiology, University of Alabama at Birmingham Medical Center; Staff Physician, Department of Nuclear Medicine, VA Medical Center, Birmingham, AL

Barbro Eriksson, MD   Associate Professor, Department of Medical Sciences; Head of Section for Endocrine Oncology, University Hospital, Uppsala, Sweden

Alan J. Fischman, MD, PhD   Associate Professor, Radiology, Harvard Medical School; Director, Radiology Nuclear Medicine, Massachusetts General Hospital, Boston, MA

Mathews B. Fish, MD   Nuclear Medicine Physician, Department of Nuclear Medicine, Sacred Heart General Hospital; Director and CEO, Oregon Medical Laboratory, Eugene, OR

Ignac Fogelman, MD   Professor of Nuclear Medicine, Division of Radiological Sciences, Guy's, King's and St. Thomas' Medical School, London, UK

John E. Freitas, MD   Clinical Professor of Radiology, University of Michigan Medical School; Director, Nuclear Medicine Services, Department of Radiology, St. Joseph Mercy Hospital, Ypsilanti, MI

Greg G. Gaehle, MD,   Division of Radiological Sciences, Mallinckrodt Institute of Radiology, St. Louis, MO

Michael J. Gelfand, MD   Children's Hospital Medical Center of Cincinnati; Chief, Section of Nuclear Medicine, Cincinnati, OH

Victor H. Gerbaudo, PhD   Lecturer in Radiology, Harvard Medical School; Director of Methodology and Operations, Division of Nuclear Medicine, Brigham and Women's Hospital, Boston, MA

Guido Germano, PhD, MBA   Professor, Medicine and Radiological Sciences, UCLA School of Medicine; Director, Artificial Intelligence Program, Department of Medicine, Cedars-Sinai Medical Center, Los Angeles, CA

Julian Gibbs, DDS, PhD   Professor Emeritus, Department of Radiology and Radiological Sciences, Vanderbilt University, Nashville, TN

David L. Gilday, BEE, MD   Professor of Medical Imaging, University of Toronto; Head of the Division of Nuclear Medicine, Department of Diagnostic Imaging, The Hospital For Sick Children, Toronto, Ontario, Canada

Stanley J. Goldsmith, MD   Professor, Radiology and Medicine; Director, Nuclear Medicine, New York Presbyterian Hospital–Weill Cornell Medical Center, New York, NY

Alexander Gottschalk, MD   Professor, Department of Radiology, Michigan State University, East Lansing, MI

L. Stephen Graham, PhD   Medical Physicist, VA Greater Los Angeles Healthcare System; Professor of Biological Imaging, UCLA School of Medicine, Los Angeles, CA

Sandra F. Grant, MD   Nuclear Medicine Service, Veterans Affairs Medical Center, Atlanta, GA

Milton D. Gross, MD   Professor, Department of Radiology, Division of Nuclear Medicine and Internal Medicine, University of Michigan Medical Center; Department of Veterans Affairs Health System, Nuclear Medicine, Ann Arbor, MI

Randall A. Hawkins, MD   Professor, Department of Radiology, University of California San Francisco Medical Center, San Francisco, CA

Carl K. Hoh, MD   Associate Professor, Department of Radiology, University of California San Diego, Division Chief, Nuclear Medicine, University of California San Diego Medical Center, San Diego, CA

Lawrence E. Holder, MD   Clinical Professor, Department of Radiology, University of Florida, Shands-Jacksonville, Jacksonville, FL

James R. Hurley, MD   Associate Professor, Department of Medicine and Radiology, Cornell University Medical College; Associate Director, Division of Nuclear Medicine, The New York Hospital–Weil Cornell Medical Center, New York, NY

Lynne L. Johnson, MD   Director of Nuclear Cardiology, Rhode Island Hospital; Professor of Medicine, Brown University, Providence, RI

John D. Kemp, MD   Professor, Department of Pathology, Microbiology, and Immunology, University of Iowa College of Medicine; Associate Director, Department of Immunopathology Laboratory, University of Iowa Hospitals, Iowa City, IA

Chun Kim, MD   Associate Professor of Radiology, Department of Radiology, Division of Nuclear Medicine, Mount Sinai School of Medicine, New York, NY

E. Edmund Kim, MD, MS   Professor of Radiology & Medicine, Department of Nuclear Medicine and Radiology, University of Texas; Chief, Experimental Nuclear Medicine, Department of Nuclear Medicine, UTMD Anderson Cancer Center, Houston, TX

Lale Kostakogu, MD   Assistant Attending in Nuclear Medicine; Assistant Professor of Radiology, New York Presbyterian Hospital–Weill Cornell Medical College, New York, NY

Eric P. Krenning, MD, PhD   Department of Nuclear Medicine, University Hospital Rotterdam, Rotterdam, The Netherlands

Marvin W. Kronenberg, MD   Professor of Medicine and Radiology, Department of Medicine, Vanderbilt University Medical Center, Nashville, TN

Christopher C. Kuni, MD   Department of Radiology, University of Colorado Health System, University Hospital, Denver, CO

Dik J. Kwekkeboom, MD   Department of Nuclear Medicine, University Hospital of Rotterdam, Rotterdam, The Netherlands

Lamk M. Lamki, MD   Professor of Radiology, Department of Radiology; Chief, Division of Nuclear Medicine, University of Texas Medical School-Houston, Houston, TX

Bengt Långström, MD   Uppsala University PET-Centre, University Hospital, Uppsala, Sweden

Sandra K. Lawrence, MD   Department of Radiology and Radiological Sciences, Vanderbilt University Medical Center, Nashville, TN

Edwin M. Leidholdt, Jr., MD   Clinical Associate Professor of Radiology, University of California, Davis; Regional Radiation Safety Program Manager, Southwestern Service Area VHA National Health Physics Program, US Department of Veterans Affairs, Mare Island, CA

Craig S. Levin, MD   Assistant Professor of Radiology, University of California San Diego School of Medicine; Nuclear Medicine, San Diego VA Medical Center, San Diego, CA

Bruce R. Line, MD   Professor of Diagnostic Radiology; Director, Division of Nuclear Medicine, University of Maryland Medicine, Baltimore, MD

Val J. Lowe, MD   Associate Professor, Department of Radiology; Consultant, Department of Radiology, Mayo Clinic, Rochester, MN

Massoud Majd, MD   Professor, Radiology and Pediatrics, George Washington University School of Medicine; Director of Nuclear Medicine, Children's National Medical Center, Washington, DC

Leon S. Malamud, MD   Temple University Hospital, Philadelphia, PA

William H. Martin, MD   Assistant Professor; Co-Director of Nuclear Cardiology, Department of Radiology and Radiological Sciences, Vanderbilt University Medical Center, Nashville, TN

John G. McAfee, MD   Physician Emeritus, NMD Clinical Center, NIH, Bethesda, MD

John H. Miller, MD   Department of Nuclear Radiology, Children's Hospital, Los Angeles, CA

Gerd Muehllehner, MD   Phillips Medical Systems, Philadelphia, PA

Dieter Munz, MD   Professor and Chairman, Department of Nuclear Medicine, Department of Radiology, Mount Sinai School of Medicine, New York, NY

Patrick B. Murphy, MD   Attending Cardiologist, Mid Central Cardiology, Bloomington, IL

Ronald D. Neumann, MD   Chief, Department of Nuclear Medicine, The National Institutes of Health, Bethesda, MD

Andrew B. Newberg, MD   Division of Nuclear Medicine, University of Pennsylvania Medical Center, Philadelphia, PA

Kjell Oberg, MD   Department of Medical Sciences, University Hospital, Uppsala, Sweden

Robert E. O'Mara, MD   Professor, Department of Radiology, Division of Nuclear Medicine, University of Rochester Medical Center, Strong Memorial Hospital, Rochester, NY

Håkan Örlefors, MD   Department of Medical Sciences, University Hospital, Uppsala, Sweden

C. Leon Partain, MD   Professor, Department of Radiology and Radiological Sciences, Vanderbilt University Medical Center, Nashville, TN

James Patton, PhD   Professor of Radiology and Physics, Department of Radiology and Radiological Sciences, Vanderbilt University Medical Center, Nashville, TN

Michael E. Phelps, PhD   Chairman, Department of Molecular and Medical Pharmacology, UCLA School of Medicine, Los Angeles, CA

Don Poldermans, MD, PhD   Department of Cardiology, Leiden University Medical Center; Department of Cardiology/Epidemiology, Thorax Center, Rotterdam, The Netherlands

Myron Pollycove, MD   US Nuclear Regulatory Commission, Rockville, MD

Steven C. Port, MD, FACC   Clinical Professor of Medicine, University of Wisconsin Medical School, Milwaukee Campus, Aurora Sinai Medical Center, Milwaukee, WI

Thomas A. Powers, MD   Associate Professor; Chief of Emergency Radiology, Department of Radiology, Vanderbilt University Medical Center, Nashville, TN

Robert H. Rubin, MD   Radiology, Nuclear Medicine, Massachusetts General Hospital, Boston, MA

Charles D. Russell, MD, PhD   Professor, Department of Radiology, Division of Nuclear Medicine, University of Alabama at Birmingham, University Hospital and VA Medical Center, Birmingham, AL

Joseph Sam, MD   Fellow in Nuclear Medicine, Department of Radiology, Hospital of the University of Pennsylvania, Philadelphia, PA

Martin P. Sandler, MD   Professor and Chairman, Department of Radiology and Radiological Sciences, Vanderbilt University Medical Center, Nashville, TN

Salil D. Sarkar, MD   Associate Professor of Clinical Nuclear Medicine, Department of Nuclear Medicine, Albert Einstein College of Medicine of Yeshiva University; Chief of Service, Department of Nuclear Medicine, Jacobi Medical Center, Bronx, NY

Sally W. Schwarz, MD   Division of Radiological Sciences, Mallinckrodt Institute of Radiology, St. Louis, MO.

Aldo N. Serafini, MD   Nuclear Medicine Division, University of Miami School of Medicine, Miami, FL

Brahm Shapiro, MD   Professor, Division of Nuclear Medicine, Department of Radiology, University of Michigan; Attending Physician Department of Veterans Affairs Health Systems, Ann Arbor, MI

Barry L. Shulkin, MD   Division of Nuclear Medicine, Department of Radiology, University of Michigan; Department of Veterans Affairs Health Systems, Ann Arbor, MI

Edward B. Silberstein, MD   Professor Emeritus, Departments of Radiology and Medicine; Director Emeritus, Department of Nuclear Medicine, University of Cincinnati Medical Center, Cincinnati, OH

T. P. Singh, MD   Assistant Professor of Pediatrics, Wayne State University School of Medicine; Medical Director, Pediatric Heart Transplant Program; Director, Cardiopulmonary Exercise Physiology Laboratory, Children's Hospital of Michigan, Detroit, MI

James C. Sisson, MD   Division of Nuclear Medicine, Department of Radiology, University of Michigan; Department of Veterans Affairs Health Systems, Ann Arbor, MI

H. Dirk Sostman, MD   Professor and Chair, Radiology Department, Weill Medical College of Cornell University; Radiologist-in-Chief, NY–Weill Cornell Medical Center, New York, NY

Michael G. Stabin, MD, CHP   Department of Radiology and Radiological Sciences, Vanderbilt University, Nashville, TN

Anders Sundin, MD   Department of Radiology, University Hospital, Uppsala, Sweden

Raymond Taillefer, MD   Professor, Department of Radiology, Universite de Montreal; Chief, Department of Nuclear Medicine, Hospital Hotel-Dieu De Montreal, Montreal, Quebec, Canada

Mathew L. Thakur, MD   Department of Radiology, Thomas Jefferson University Hospital, Philadelphia, PA

Mary Tono, BA   Department of Nuclear Medicine, University of California, San Francisco General Hospital, San Francisco, CA

Martin P. Tornai, MD   Departments of Radiology and Biomedical Engineering, Duke University Medical Center, Durham, NC

S. Ted Treves, MD   Professor of Radiology, Harvard Medical School; Chief, Division of Nuclear Medicine, Radiology Department, Children's Hospital, Boston, MA

Timothy G. Turkington, PhD   Associate Research Professor, Departments of Radiology and Biomedical Engineering, Duke University Medical Center, Durham, NC

R. Michael Tuttle, MD   Assistant Professor of Medicine, Cornell School of Medicine, Memorial Sloan Kettering Cancer Center, New York, NY

Jean-Luc C. Urbain, MD   Chairman, Department of Molecular and Functional Imaging, Cleveland Clinic Foundation, Cleveland, OH

Marie-Christiane M. Vekemans, MD   Chen, Hornu, Belgium

Ernst E. van der Wall, MD   Department of Cardiology, Leiden University Medical Center, Department of Cardiology/Epidemiology, Thorax Center, Rotterdam, The Netherlands

João V. Vitola, MD, PhD   Federal University of Parana Medical School, Curitiba, Parana, Brazil

Frans J. Th. Wackers, MD   Professor of Diagnostic Radiology and Medicine; Director, Cardiovascular Nuclear Imaging, Yale University School of Medicine, Department of Diagnostic Radiology and Medicine, New Haven, CT

Richard L. Wahl, MD   Professor of Radiology, Russel H. Morgan Department of Radiology & Radiological Science; Vice Chairman for Technology and Business Development, Director, Division of Nuclear Medicine/PET, Johns Hopkins Medicine, Baltimore, MD

Alan Waxman, MD   Clinical Professor, Department of Radiology, University of Southern California; Co-Director of Imaging; Director of Nuclear Medicine, Cedars-Sinai Medical Center, Los Angeles, CA

Ronald E. Weiner, PhD   Associate Professor, Diagnostic Imaging & Therapeutics, University of Connecticut Health Center, Division of Nuclear Medicine, Farmington, CT

Michael J. Welch, MD, PhD   Professor of Radiology, Division of Radiological Sciences, Mallinckrodt Institute of Radiology, St. Louis, MO

Daniel Worsley, MD   Assistant Professor of Radiology, Department of Radiology, Division of Nuclear Medicine, Vancouver General Hospital, University of British Colombia, Vancouver, BC

Mijin Yun, MD   Instructor, Department of Radiology, Yonsei University and Medical Center, Seoul, Korea

Robert K. Zeman, MD   Professor and Chairman, Department of Radiology, George Washington University School of Medicine; Radiologist-in-Chief, George Washington University Hospital, Washington, DC

Hongming Zhuang, MD   Assistant Professor, Department of Radiology, Division of Nuclear Medicine, University of Pennsylvania, Philadelphia, PA

Harvey A. Ziessman, MD   Professor, Department of Radiology; Director, Division of Nuclear Medicine, Georgetown University Hospital, Washington, DC

Lionel S. Zuckier, MD   Associate Professor and Director of Nuclear Medicine, Department of Radiology, New Jersey Medical School and University Hospital, Newark, NJ

CONTENTS

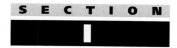

PHYSICS AND INSTRUMENTATION

BASIC PHYSICS OF NUCLEAR MEDICINE

JAMES A. PATTON

Nuclear medicine imaging techniques are performed by means of administering pharmaceuticals that are labeled or tagged with radionuclides so that they are preferentially accumulated in the organs of interest. Images are then obtained with detection systems that are sensitive to the γ-radiation emitted from the administered radiotracers. These images do not possess the spatial resolution of other imaging modalities such as computed tomography and magnetic resonance imaging; however, the information provided to clinicians is generally of a different type, namely functional information. For successful use of these techniques, knowledge of the basic physical principles of nuclear medicine is required. The specific topics include the basic concepts of the atom, the fundamentals of radioactive decay, and the mechanisms by which radiation interacts with matter.

ATOMIC PHYSICS

Early Greek philosophers postulated that all matter was composed of fundamental units arranged in specific patterns to form different types of matter. It is now known that molecules are the smallest subdivisions of matter that retain the original physical and chemical properties of the matter. Molecules can be further broken down into basic fundamental building blocks, called *atoms,* of which all matter is composed. A basic group of substances exist that cannot be broken down into different substances except by the processes of radioactive decay or nuclear reactions. These substances are called *elements,* and each element is composed of a single type of atom. Two or more chemical elements can combine chemically to form compounds by means of bonding of the atoms that compose the individual elements. Thus the atom is the fundamental constituent of matter, and understanding its anatomy is the first step in obtaining knowledge of nuclear medicine physics.

The current simplified concept of the atom was proposed by Bohr in 1913 and is shown in Fig. 1.1. The atom is composed of a positively charged nucleus containing positively charged protons and electrically neutral neutrons, collectively called *nucleons.* Surrounding the nucleus in discrete orbits or shells are enough negatively charged electrons to make the atom electrically neutral. Thus the proton number equals the electron number in the electrically neutral atom. The electron orbits were described as circular by Bohr, but in fact are elliptical. The atomic particles and their fundamental characteristics are shown in Table 1.1. Because the masses of these particles are very small, another scale, based on the atomic mass unit (amu), is often used. One atomic mass unit is defined as 1/12 of the mass of the ^{12}C atom. Recall that 1 g atomic weight (mole) of ^{12}C has a mass of 12 g and contains 6.023×10^{23} atoms (Avogadro's number). One atomic mass unit thus has a mass of 1.66×10^{-24} g. According to this definition, the masses in atomic mass units of the subatomic particles are also shown in Table 1.1. The shells of the atom are denoted by letters of the alphabet, the innermost shell being the *K* shell. The next shell is identified by the letter *L,* the next *M,* and so forth. The shells are also identified by an integer number called the *principal quantum number, n.* For the K shell, $n = 1$; for the L shell $n = 2$, for the M shell $n = 3$, and so forth. In 1925, Pauli presented a modification to the Bohr model of the atom that stated no two electrons can exist in the same energy state. This principle placed a limit on the number of electrons that can exist in each shell. Simply stated, Pauli's principle yields the statement that each

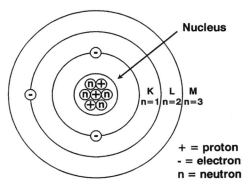

FIGURE 1.1. Current simplified concept of the atom.

J.A. Patton: Department of Radiology and Radiological Sciences, Vanderbilt University Medical Center, Nashville, TN

Table 1.1. *Subatomic particles*

Name	Symbol	Charge	Mass (g)	Mass (amu)	Relative Mass
Electron	e⁻	−1	0.9108×10^{-27}	0.000549	1
Proton	p	+1	1.6724×10^{-24}	1.007277	1,836
Neutron	n	0	1.6747×10^{-24}	1.008665	1,840

shell can contain a maximum of only $2n^2$ electrons and is actually composed of $2n - 1$ subshells, each with slightly different characteristics. These factors are determined by selection rules, a topic beyond the scope of this book.

The electrons are held in their orbits by the Coulomb attractive force between them and the positively charged nucleus and are balanced by centrifugal force as they move around the nucleus. The atom is in its most stable configuration or lowest energy state when the electrons are positioned as closely as possible to the nucleus in the allowed inner orbits. This configuration is called the *ground state.* It is in these positions that the force of attraction on the electrons is greatest, and it is here that the electrons are most tightly bound. The energy required to completely remove an electron from a particular shell within an atom is defined as the *binding energy* of that shell. The binding energy for a particular shell increases with increasing positive charge of the nucleus. For a given atom, binding energy decreases in moving from inner to outer shells. Thus for an electron to move from an inner shell to an outer shell, energy must be supplied to the electron. This process is called *excitation,* and the energy

supplied must be at least equal to the difference in binding energies of the two shells involved in the transition. Conversely, when an electron moves from an outer shell to an inner shell, this same amount of energy must be released in the process. This de-excitation process results in emission of either a characteristic x-ray or an Augér (pronounced *oh-zhay*) electron (Fig. 1.2A). The characteristic x-rays are photons the energies of which are equal to the difference in binding energies of the two shells involved in the transition. They are identified on the basis of the shell in which the original vacancy existed. For example, when an electron drops down from the L shell to fill a vacancy in the K shell, a K x-ray is emitted.

Augér electron emission is an alternative to characteristic x-ray emission. In this process, the energy released by an outer-shell electron filling an inner-shell vacancy is transferred to another orbital electron, usually an outer-shell electron, which is ejected from the atom. The kinetic energy of this electron is equal to the binding energy of the shell being filled minus the sum of the binding energies of the two shells ending up with vacancies after the process is complete. Characteristic x-ray emission or Augér electron emission occurs after each transition. The fluorescent yield is defined for each shell of each element as the probability of characteristic x-ray emission per shell vacancy and increases with increasing positive charge of the nucleus.

The binding energies of electrons in their shells and the energies of characteristic radiation are relatively small. These values are usually stated in terms of the electron volt (eV). This unit is defined as the kinetic energy acquired by a single electron when accelerated through a 1-volt potential difference. Outer

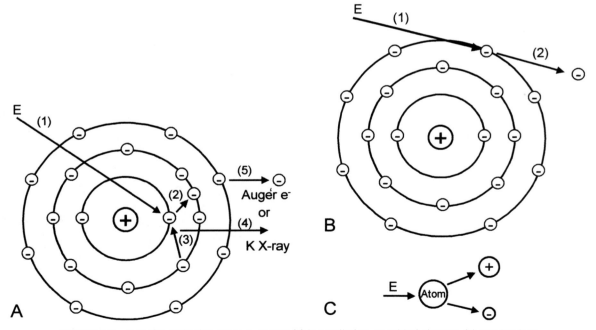

FIGURE 1.2. A: In the excitation process, energy (*E*) is supplied to an orbital electron *(1)*, moving it to an outer shell *(2)*. The atom is de-excited when an electron from the outer shell drops down to fill the vacancy in the inner shell *(3)*. The de-excitation energy is carried off by a characteristic x-ray *(4)* or an Augér electron *(5)*. **B:** In the ionization process, sufficient energy *(1)* is supplied to an orbital electron *(2)* to completely remove it from the atom (*E* > binding energy of electron). **C:** The result of the ionization process is production of a positive and negative ion pair.

shells of light atoms have binding energies of a few electron volts, whereas inner shells of heavy atoms have binding energies that approach 100 keV (1 keV = 1,000 eV). Nuclear processes discussed later involve higher energy values, which are measured in terms of millions of electron volts (1 MeV = 1,000 keV = 1,000,000 eV).

Absorption of sufficient energy by an orbital electron to completely remove it from the atom is called *ionization* (Fig. 1.2B). The electron then has kinetic energy equal to the energy absorbed minus the binding energy of the shell from which it was removed. The result is formation of a positive and negative ion pair (the negative ion is the free electron, and the positive ion is the atom minus the free electron) (Fig.1.2C). If the interaction occurs with an electron in a shell other than the outermost shell, the atom is left in an excited state and it is de-excited by outer-shell electrons dropping down to fill the vacancies, again resulting in characteristic x-ray or Augér electron emission. This process continues until the vacancy moves to the outermost shell, where a free electron is captured to return the atom to its ground state and make it electrically neutral again.

NUCLEAR PHYSICS

The nucleus of an atom is composed of positively charged protons and of neutrons with no charge. Coulomb's law predicts that there would be very strong electrostatic forces of repulsion between the positive charges when brought together. However, within the nucleus, the presence of neutrons in combination with protons provides an environment in which short-range attractive nuclear forces exist that are many times stronger than the repulsive electrostatic forces, and thus a very dense, compact nucleus is formed. In fact, the neutrons may be thought of as glue that helps hold the nucleus together. The relative strengths of these two forces, along with that of the weak force involved in β decay and the gravitational force, are shown in Table 1.2. If the mass of the nucleus is subtracted from the sums of the masses of the individual nucleons, a positive mass difference remains. This difference, called the *mass deficit* or *mass defect,* is explained by the fact that each nucleon gives up a small amount of mass when it is bound within the nucleus. In actuality, this mass is converted to energy and determines the magnitude of the nuclear binding energy that holds the nucleons together. The nuclear binding energy can be calculated with the equation developed by Einstein when he proposed that mass is simply another form of energy. The equation is

$$E = \Delta mc^2$$

Table 1.2. *Forces*

Type	Relative Strength	Comments
Strong or nuclear force	1	Holds nucleus together
Coulomb or electrostatic force	10^{-2}	Results between charged particles; holds atom together
Weak force	10^{-13}	Significant in β decay
Gravitational force	10^{-39}	Result of mass of matter

where E is the binding energy, Δm is the mass defect, and c is the velocity of light. In practice, the mass defect can be calculated with atomic mass units and converted to energy units by use of the energy definition of 1 amu (931.5 MeV). Nuclear binding energy is significantly higher than electron binding energy (on the order of millions of electron volts [MeV]). A relation that is commonly quoted is binding energy per nucleon and is directly related to the stability of the nucleus.

The most fundamental characteristic of an atom is its atomic number (Z), which is the number of protons within the nucleus (also the number of electrons in the electrically neutral atom). Each element has a unique atomic number, and the chemical symbol for the element is synonymous with the atomic number. The number of neutrons within the nucleus is denoted by N. The atomic mass number (A) is the total number of nucleons (neutrons + protons) within the nucleus, thus $A = Z + N$. The atomic mass number is approximately equal to, but not to be mistaken for, the atomic weight, which is the average of the atomic mass numbers of all the naturally occurring atoms of an element weighted according to their natural percentages of abundance.

Any nucleus plus its orbital electrons—that is, any atom—is called a *nuclide*. Nuclides are classified according to nuclear composition and arrangement of nucleons within the nucleus. A nuclear shorthand exists for characterization of nuclides and is of the form, $^A_Z X_N$ where X is the chemical symbol of the element to which the nuclide belongs. Because Z is synonymous with the chemical symbol and $N = A - Z$, the shortened form $^A X$ is generally used, as in ^{131}I ($Z = 53$, $n = 78$) and ^{57}Co ($Z = 27$, $n = 30$). Another form that is acceptable but now less widely used is X-A, as in I-131 and Co-57.

Nuclides that have similar characteristics are often grouped into nuclear families. *Isotopes* are nuclides that have the same atomic number (Z) and thus are nuclides of a particular element. *Isobars* are nuclides with the same atomic mass number (A). *Isotones* are nuclides with the same number of neutrons (N). *Isomers* are nuclides identical in all characteristics except the energy state of the nucleus. An easy way to remember these definitions is as follows: isoto*p*es have the same *p*roton number, isob*a*rs have the same *a*tomic mass number, isoto*n*es have the same *n*eutron number, and isom*e*rs differ only in *e*nergy state. These nuclear families, with examples, are summarized in Table 1.3.

RADIOACTIVE DECAY

It has been observed that most nuclei existing in nature are stable and have high binding energies per nucleon. On the other hand, certain nuclei have lower binding energies per nucleon and are not stable. These nuclei transform themselves randomly and spontaneously to form more stable configurations. These transformations can result in the emission of particles or photons and energy from the nuclei. One important factor in the stability of the nucleus is the neutron to proton ratio. Figure 1.3 shows a plot of neutron number, N, versus proton number (atomic number), Z, for all nuclei. The stable nuclei fall along a narrow band called the *line of stability*. Light nuclei tend to contain the same number of neutrons and protons, and thus the slope is

Table 1.3. *Nuclear families*

Name	A	Z	N	Energy State	Examples
Isotope	Different	Same	Different	Different	^{127}Xe, ^{129}Xe, ^{131}Xe
Isobar	Same	Different	Different	Different	^{131}I, ^{131}Xe, ^{131}Te
Isotone	Different	Different	Same	Different	^{131}I, ^{132}Xe, ^{133}Ce
Isomer	Same	Same	Same	Different	^{99m}Tc, ^{99}Tc

initially approximately unity. As Z increases, the N/Z ratio increases to approximately 1.5. The extra neutrons serve to increase the average distance between protons within the nucleus, thereby reducing the repulsive Coulomb force acting between these particles. If the N/Z ratio deviates to either side of the line of stability because of an excess of protons or neutrons, the nuclides become unstable. Stability is achieved by means of emission of particles from the nucleus. The result is a change in the identity of the nuclide and a more favorable N/Z ratio; that is, unstable nuclei decay toward the line of stability.

Radioactive decay is a random and spontaneous nuclear process in which an unstable parent nucleus transforms into a more stable daughter nucleus through the emission of particles or γ-rays. Energy also is released and carried off by the radioactive emissions. The process is totally unaffected by changes in temperature, pressure, or chemical combinations. The term *radioactive decay* was coined in the early 1900s by investigators who noticed that some elements lost their radioactive properties in a consistent manner that varied from one element to another. It was reasoned that some radioactive atoms were "disintegrating" and producing other atoms. The rate at which the atoms were "decaying" was measured in disintegrations per second. Any unstable or radioactive atom is referred to as a *radionuclide.* The most important factors determining stability are a favorable N/Z ratio, pairing of nucleons, and a high binding energy per nucleon. The greater the variance from these three factors, the greater is the tendency of a nuclide to be unstable.

Radionuclides either occur naturally or are artificially produced. The naturally occurring radionuclides are those that exist in an unstable state in nature. They emit radiation sponta-

neously, and no external influence is necessary to produce radioactive decay. Most of the naturally occurring radionuclides have atomic numbers greater than 82. Two notable exceptions are ^{14}C and ^{40}K. The artificial radionuclides are manufactured, unstable nuclides produced by means of bombarding stable nuclides with high-energy particles in a cyclotron, linear accelerator, or nuclear reactor. All of the radionuclides used in nuclear medicine are in the latter category.

Decay Schemes

All radioactive decay processes can be described with decay schemes that present a detailed analysis of how a radioactive parent is transformed into the ground state of the daughter. Figure 1.4 illustrates the standard format used. An arrow is drawn from the parent to the daughter with the *D-U-I* mnemonic used to indicate that an arrow drawn to the left indicates a decrease in atomic number (positive particle emission), straight down indicates unchanged atomic number (γ-emission), and to the right indicates an increase in atomic number (negative particle emission). Several horizontal lines may be drawn to indicate the various energy states of the daughter. Additional information, usually supplied on the diagram, includes energy and percentage abundance of the transitions and half-lives of the energy states. The decay scheme is actually an energy-level diagram with energy represented by the vertical axis and the lowest-energy state or ground state at the bottom of the diagram.

Radioactive decay processes can also be described with nuclear equations. These are of the general form

$$^{A}_{Z}X \rightarrow ^{A'}_{Z'}Y + W + Q$$

where X represents the parent radionuclide with atomic mass number A and atomic number Z, Y represents the daughter

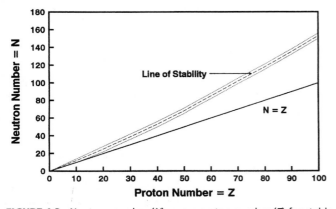

FIGURE 1.3. Neutron number (N) versus proton number (Z) for stable nuclei. The line of stability deviates from the $N = Z$ line (*dashed line*) because of a necessary excess of neutrons. Nuclei to the left and right of the line of stability are radioactive.

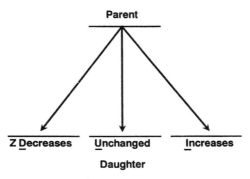

FIGURE 1.4. Standard format used to illustrate decay schemes.

nuclide with atomic mass number A' and atomic number Z', W is the radiation type emitted (may be more than one), and Q is the total energy released in the nuclear transition. These nuclear equations must be balanced as chemical equations so that total charge, total number of nucleons (A), and total energy (remember that mass is one form of energy) are the same on both sides of the equation. Because this equation describes a nuclear decay process, Q is determined by the differences in the mass of the parent nucleus and the sums of the masses of the daughter nucleus and the particles produced in the decay process. This mass difference is converted to energy and released as the daughter products are produced. The magnitude of the energy released in the process can be calculated with Einstein's mass-energy equation.

Decay Processes

There are seven basic nuclear decay processes, which can be grouped into three major categories. These are α transitions, isobaric transitions (including β emission, positron emission, and electron capture), and isomeric transitions (including excited and metastable state transitions and internal conversion). The types of radiation emitted in these processes are summarized in Table 1.4. The transformation of a radioactive parent to the ground state of the daughter may involve one or more of these transitions. Of these seven, only six are important in nuclear medicine imaging. These are β emission, positron emission, electron capture, and the isomeric transitions.

Decay

The α decay process can be described with the equation

$$^{A}_{Z}X \rightarrow {}^{A-4}_{Z-2}Y + {}^{4}_{2}\alpha + Q$$

The α particle is the nucleus of the ^{4}He atom, which consists of two protons and two neutrons and therefore has a charge of $+2$ and a mass of approximately 4 amu. α-Particles usually possess high energy and short range (a few centimeters in air, a fraction of a millimeter in tissue) and are emitted primarily from extremely heavy nuclei (atomic numbers greater than 82). An example of α decay is shown in Fig. 1.5 and is described by the equation

$$^{226}_{88}\text{Ra} \rightarrow {}^{222}_{86}\text{Rn} + {}^{4}_{2}\alpha$$

Because of the large size, high energy, and short range of α particles, they cannot escape body tissues, and therefore they deposit very high radiation doses internally. α-Emitters also typically have very long lifetimes, are members of chains of radioac-

Table 1.4. *Emissions from radioactive decay processes*

Name	Symbol	Charge	Mass (g)
Alpha	α	+2	6.6394×10
Beta	β$^-$	−1	0.9108×10
Positron	β$^+$	+1	0.9108×10
Neutrino	υ	0	0
Gamma	γ	0	0

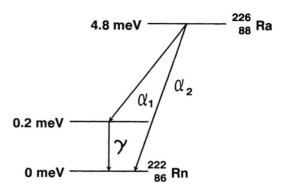

FIGURE 1.5. ^{226}Ra decay scheme illustrating α decay.

tive atoms, and thus have no use in nuclear medicine imaging procedures.

β Decay

Isobaric transitions are decay processes in which the parent and daughter are isobars—members of a nuclear family that have the same atomic mass number (A) but different Z and N. Three isobaric processes are possible—β decay, positron decay, and electron capture. In β-emission the nuclear reaction is of the form

$$^{A}_{Z}X \rightarrow {}^{A}_{Z+1}Y + \beta^- + \upsilon + Q$$

The β particles (β$^-$) are negatively charged electrons that originate in the nucleus and have the same mass and charge as orbital electrons. They have a broad distribution of energy, their velocities approach the speed of light, and they are classified as medium-range particles (several hundred centimeters in air, a few millimeters in tissue). β$^-$ Emission occurs in unstable nuclides that have an unfavorably high N/Z ratio owing to an excess of neutrons. Greater stability is obtained in these nuclides by means of conversion of a neutron to a proton and emission of a β particle. This conversion may be written

$$^{1}_{0}n \rightarrow {}^{1}_{1}p + \beta^- + \upsilon + Q$$

It was originally thought that Q, the energy of the transition, was exactly equal to the energy of the β particle plus that of any associated γ-rays. However, when measurements of β energies were made from a large number of atoms of a particular radionuclide, it was observed that the β particles had a continuous range of energies from zero to a maximum value equal to Q when no γ-rays were involved in the decay process. A typical β spectrum is shown in Fig. 1.6. The average β energy is approximately equal to one-third the maximum energy. To explain the variance in both energies, a new particle was postulated by Pauli in 1931, and its existence was later verified experimentally. This particle, the antineutrino ($\bar{\upsilon}$), has no mass and no charge. It carries off the excess energy in each β decay process ($E_{max} = E_\beta + E_\upsilon$). In some nuclides, after β decay, the nucleus may be left in an excited state, the excess energy carried away by one or more γ-rays as the nucleus moves to the most stable configuration or the ground state.

8 *Physics and Instrumentation*

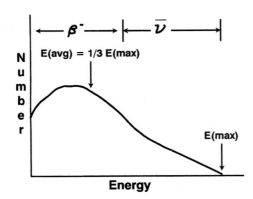

FIGURE 1.6. Typical spectrum of β energies for a particular β decay process. The sum of the energies of the β particle and the neutrino is equal to the total energy given off in the decay process if no γ-rays are involved in the process.

An example of β decay is the transformation of ^{131}I to ^{131}Xe by the nuclear equation

$$^{131}_{53}\text{I} \rightarrow {}^{131}_{54}\text{Xe} + \beta^- + \bar{v}$$

The corresponding decay scheme is shown in Fig. 1.7.

Positron Decay

Positron emission is a second type of isobaric transition. In this decay process, unstable nuclides that have an unfavorably low *N/Z* ratio, because of an excess of protons, are transferred to a more stable configuration according to the nuclear equation

$$^{A}_{Z}X \rightarrow {}^{A}_{Z-1}Y + \beta^+ + v + Q$$

The positron (β$^+$) has the same mass as an orbital electron but is positively charged. The decay process can be described by the conversion of a proton to a neutron with the emission of a positron as indicated by

$$^{1}_{1}p \rightarrow {}^{1}_{0}n + \beta^+ + v + Q$$

Although this reaction appears impossible because the mass of the neutron is greater than the mass of the proton, the equation describes the restructuring of the nucleus. Therefore it is under-

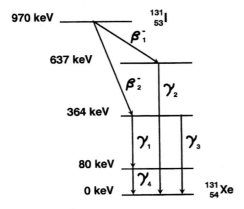

FIGURE 1.7. ^{131}I decay scheme illustrating β decay.

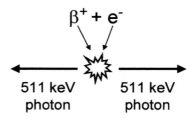

FIGURE 1.8. In the annihilation process, an electron and a positron combine with the masses of the two particles being converted into energy in the form of two 511-keV photons. These annihilation radiations leave their production site at approximately 180 degrees from each other.

stood that part of the energy necessary to form the neutron is supplied by the other nucleons. Positrons decay with a continuous spectrum of energy, as with β decay, and the difference between the expected energy, E$_{max}$, and the observed energy in each decay process is carried off by the neutrino.

A unique characteristic of the positron is that it cannot exist at rest in nature. Once it loses its kinetic energy, the positron immediately combines with a negatively charged electron and undergoes an annihilation reaction in which the masses of the two particles are completely converted into energy in the form of two 0.511-MeV annihilation photons, which leave their production site at 180 degrees from each other (Fig. 1.8). Conservation of energy requires that a minimum energy difference of 1.022 MeV must exist between the parent and the daughter before positron emission can occur. The energy above that value is divided between the positron and the neutrino. As with other processes, the daughter may be left in an excited state, γ-emission being the process by which the daughter moves to the ground state.

An example of positron decay is the decay of ^{15}O to ^{15}N given by the equation

$$^{15}\text{O} \rightarrow {}^{15}\text{N} + \beta^+ + v$$

The corresponding decay scheme is shown in Fig. 1.9.

Electron Capture

The third isobaric transition possibility is electron capture. Like positron emission, electron capture occurs in unstable nuclides that have an unfavorably low *N/Z* ratio. Electron capture is a nuclear decay process in which the nucleus captures one of the inner-shell orbital electrons (most probably from the K shell) of

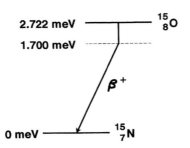

FIGURE 1.9. ^{15}O decay scheme illustrating positron decay.

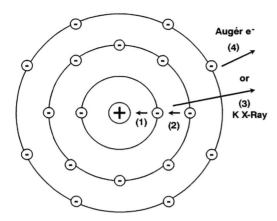

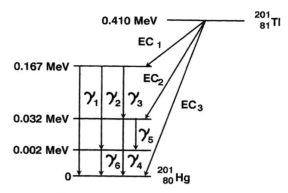

FIGURE 1.11. ^{201}Tl decay scheme illustrating decay by means of electron capture.

FIGURE 1.10. In the electron capture decay process, an inner electron is captured by the nucleus *(1)*. The atom is de-excited when an outer-shell electron drops down to fill the vacancy *(2)*. The de-excitation energy is carried off by a characteristic x-ray *(3)* or an Augér electron *(4)*.

the atom, as illustrated in Fig. 1.10. The general nuclear equation is of the form

$$_Z^A X + e^- \rightarrow _{Z-1}^A Y + \upsilon + Q$$

The daughter produced by means of electron capture is the same as that resulting from positron decay. Positron emission and electron capture are competing decay processes in certain radionuclides. Electron capture can be thought of as reverse β decay in that the electron unites with a proton to form a neutron with excess energy carried off by the neutrino. The equation may be written as

$$_1^1 p + e^- \rightarrow _0^1 n + \upsilon + Q$$

Although the υ carries off some excess energy created in the process, the nucleus can still be left in an excited state, which subsequently leads to γ-emission. After electron capture, the atom also is left in an excited state owing to the vacancy made in the inner-shell of the atom. The atom is de-excited by outer-shell electrons dropping down to fill the vacancies, resulting in characteristic x-ray or Augér electron emission (Fig. 1.10). Detection of the characteristic x-rays is the primary mechanism for identification of electron capture decay processes. An example of electron capture is the decay of ^{201}Tl to ^{201}Hg by the equation

$$_{81}^{201} \text{Tl} + e^- \rightarrow _{80}^{201} \text{Hg} + \upsilon + \gamma$$

The γ-ray is included in this equation because the daughter nucleus is left in an excited state and is immediately de-excited by γ-emission. The corresponding decay scheme is shown in Fig. 1.11.

γ-Emission

Excited-state Transitions

As stated in each of the earlier descriptions of the various decay processes, in many instances the daughter nuclide is left in an excited state. It subsequently is de-excited through the release

of energy in the form of γ-rays. Many times the transition through the excited state is almost instantaneous; that is, the lifetime of the excited state is too short to measure ($<10^{-12}$ seconds). In general, the nuclear equation for excited state transitions can be written as

$$_Z^A X \rightarrow [_Z^{A'} Y]^* + W + Q \rightarrow _Z^{A'} Y + W + Q + \gamma$$

Because the excited state has no measurable lifetime, the middle section of this equation usually is deleted. An example is the decay of ^{123}I to ^{123}Te as illustrated by the equation

$$_{53}^{123} \text{I} + e^- \rightarrow _{53}^{123} \text{Te} + \upsilon + \gamma$$

Thus ^{123}I decays to an excited state of ^{123}Te by means of electron capture. The nucleus immediately goes from the excited state to the ground state by means of emission of a γ-ray. In γ-emission, the de-excitation process can be very simple (only one γ-ray emitted) or very complicated. For example, ^{206}Bi has 74 γ-ray transitions in its decay scheme. γ-Rays may appear on a decay scheme in parallel (side-by-side) to represent alternative modes of decay or in cascade (one after the other) to indicate passage through multiple excited states. The decay scheme for ^{123}I is shown in Fig. 1.12.

Metastable-state Transitions

An excited state of the nucleus that exists for a measurable lifetime ($>10^{-12}$ seconds) is called an *isomeric* or *metastable state*. The metastable state and ground state of the daughter are called

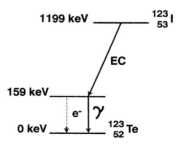

FIGURE 1.12. ^{123}I decay scheme illustrating γ-emission through an excited-state transition.

isomers because they have the same Z and N and differ only in energy state. The general nuclear equations for this decay process may be written as

$$\prescript{A}{Z}{X} \rightarrow \prescript{A^m}{Z}{Y} + W + Q$$
$$\prescript{A^m}{Z}{Y} \rightarrow \prescript{A'}{Z}{Y} + \gamma$$

An m is added to the atomic mass number of the first state of the daughter to indicate a metastable state with a measurable lifetime. The metastable state moves to the ground state through de-excitation by means of γ-emission. The only difference between metastable- and excited-state transitions is the measurable lifetime of the metastable state. An example is the decay of ^{99}Mo to ^{99}Tc through the metastable state, ^{99m}Tc. The decay equations are

$$\prescript{99}{42}{Mo} \rightarrow \prescript{99m}{43}{Tc} + \beta^- + \nu$$
$$\prescript{99m}{43}{Tc} \rightarrow \prescript{99}{43}{Tc} + \gamma$$

The corresponding decay scheme is shown in Fig. 1.13.

Internal Conversion

In many nuclides that undergo de-excitation by means of emitting γ-rays, there is a process that competes with γ-emission. This is the process of internal conversion, and it occurs primarily in metastable-state transitions. In this process, the nucleus, while changing energy states, may occasionally transfer energy from the nucleus to inner-shell orbital electrons, which are subsequently ejected from the atom. We can think of this process as if the γ-ray from the nucleus is internally absorbed by the electron, as illustrated in Fig. 1.14. This conversion electron exits the atom with a kinetic energy equal to the original γ-ray energy minus the binding energy of the electron in its shell. This process leaves the atom in an excited state owing to the vacancy made, and the atom is de-excited by an outer-shell electron dropping down to fill the vacancy and is, therefore, followed by characteristic x-ray or Augér electron emission.

The percentage of internal conversion electrons and γ-rays emitted is given by the internal conversion coefficient, which is defined experimentally for each radionuclide decaying by means

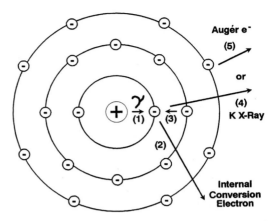

FIGURE 1.14. In the internal conversion process, a γ emitted from the nucleus is captured by an inner-shell electron *(1)*, which is ejected from the atom *(2)*. The atom is de-excited when an outer-shell electron drops down to fill the vacancy *(3)*. The de-excitation energy is carried off by a characteristic x-ray *(4)* or an Augér electron *(5)*.

of the two processes. This coefficient is the ratio of conversion electrons emitted from the atom to γ-rays emitted from the nucleus. It is usually defined for each shell, the highest probability being the K shell coefficient. The decay schemes in Figs. 1.11 through 1.13 illustrate how internal conversion competes with γ-emission.

In selecting a radionuclide for imaging, one must consider, in addition to the half-life, the modes of decay, the energy of the transitions, and the percentage of occurrence of each transition. Table 1.5 details all of the radiation types that result from each of the seven basic processes. Table 1.6 lists the primary radiations from the most common radionuclides used in nuclear medicine imaging.

Decay Equations

Radioactive decay has been considered on a microscopic scale in the past several sections to examine the various types of radioactive decay processes possible. Radioactive decay also can be considered on a macroscopic scale by means of writing decay equations to describe the processes independent of the types of decay.

In a given group of identical atoms of a radionuclide, we cannot predict when a particular atom will decay. However, if there are N radioactive atoms present and ΔN atoms decay in a small increment of time, Δt, we can say that the average rate of decay R, is $\Delta N/\Delta t$. This value also can be called the *activity,*

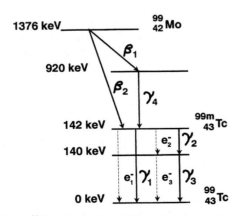

FIGURE 1.13. ^{99}Mo decay scheme illustrating γ-emission through a metastable state transition.

Table 1.5. *Radioactive decay processes*

Process	Possible Radiation Type Emitted
Alpha decay	α
Beta decay	β^-, ν
Positron decay	β^+, ν, 2γ
Electron capture	ν, x-ray, Augér electron
Gamma emission	γ
Internal conversion	IC electron, γ, x-ray, Augér electron

IC, internal conversion.

Table 1.6. *Nuclear decay data for radionuclides used in clinical nuclear medicine imaging*

Nuclide	Half-life	Transition	Energy (keV)	Abundance (%)
^{67}Ga	78 h	EC (9 KeV x-rays)		100
		Gamma 1[a]	93	38
		Gamma 2[a]	185	24
		Gamma 3[a]	300	16
		Gamma 4	394	4
		IC electron 1	93	33
		IC electron 2	185	<1
		IC electron 3	300	<1
^{111}In	68 h	EC (23 KeV x-rays)		100
		Gamma 1[a]	172	90
		Gamma 2[a]	247	94
		IC electron 1	172	10
		IC electron 2	247	6
^{123}I (Fig 1.12)	13 h	EC (27 KeV x-rays)		98
		Gamma[a]	159	84
		IC electron	159	16
^{131}I (Fig 1.7)	8 d	Beta 1	333	7
		Beta 2	606	90
		Gamma 1	284	6
		Gamma 2	637	7
		Gamma 3[a]	364	84
		Gamma 4	80	7
^{99}Mo (Fig 1.13)	66 h	Beta 1	456	18
		Beta 2	1,234	80
		Gamma 4	773	5
^{99m}Tc (Fig 1.13)	6 h	Gamma 1	142	<1
		Gamma 2	2	1
		Gamma 3[a]	140	88
		IC electron 1	142	1
		IC electron 2	2	99
		IC electron 3	140	11
^{201}Tl (Fig 1.11)	73 h	EC (70 KeV x-rays)[a]		
		Gamma 1	167	10
		Gamma 3	135	<3
		IC electron 1	167	15
		IC electron 3	135	8
^{133}Xe	5 d	Beta	346	99
		Gamma[a]	81	37
		IC electron	81	52
^{11}C	20 min	Positron[b]	960	100
^{13}N	10 min	Positron[b]	1,198	100
^{15}O	122 s	Positron[b]	1,732	100
^{68}Ga	68 min	Positron 1[b]	822	1
		Positron 2[b]	1,899	88
		EC (9 KeV x-rays)		11
^{18}F	110 min	Positron[b]	633	97
		EC (0.5 KeV x-rays)		3
^{62}Rb	1.3 min	Positron 1[b]	2,375	12
		Positron 2[b]	3,150	83
		EC (13 KeV x-rays)		5

[a]Transition used for imaging.
[b]511 keV γ-rays result from position annihilation and are used for imaging.
EC, electron capture (characteristic radiation secondary); IC, internal conversion (The energies stated for the internal conversion electrons include those of the resulting characteristic x-rays or Augér electrons.).

A, if appropriate units are used (e.g., curies or becquerels). The decay rate or activity is directly proportional to the number of atoms present and is obtained with the following equation

$$R = A = -\lambda N$$

The proportionality constant, λ, is the decay constant and is the fractional number of atoms decaying per unit of time. The decay constant thus has units of (1/time). The decay constant is a unique value characteristic for each radionuclide. The minus sign in the decay equation indicates that *N* is decreasing with time. *R* is the average decay rate. Measurements of decay rate fluctuate around the average decay rate because radioactive decay is statistical in nature, based on Poisson statistics.

Units of decay rate are disintegrations per second (dps) or

Table 1.7. *Units of decay rate (activity) standard units and system internationale (SI) units*

Standard Unit	Disintegrations per Second	SI Unit	Disintegrations per Second
Curie (Ci)	3.7×10^{10}	Becquerel (Bq)	1
Millicurie (mCi)	3.7×10^{7}	Kilobecquerel (kBq)	10^3
Microcurie (μCi)	3.7×10^{4}	Megabecquerel (MBq)	10^6
Nanocurie (nCi)	3.7×10	Gigabecquerel (GBq)	10^9
Picocurie (pCi)	3.7×10^{-2}		

1 Ci = 37 GBq.
1 Bq = 27.03 pCi.

disintegrations per minute (dpm). Because these values usually are relatively large, activity is generally measured with an alternative scale. The basic conventional unit of activity that has been used in the past is the curie (Ci), which is based on an early observation that 1 g of ^{226}Ra had a decay rate of 3.7×10^{10} dps (only approximately correct). Other units of activity are defined in Table 1.7. Fractional units of activity are specific activity (activity per unit mass) and concentration (activity per unit volume).

A new system of units, the Système Internationale (SI), has been introduced and is now the preferred system. The basic unit of activity in this system is the becquerel (Bq), which corresponds to a decay rate of 1 dps. The units of this system are shown in Table 1.7.

Because the number of atoms (N) remaining to decay at any time (t) is always less than the original number (N_o) present at time $t = 0$, an equation is needed to specify the number of atoms remaining to decay. This equation is

$$N = N_o e^{-\lambda t}$$

This equation says that the number of atoms, N, remaining to decay at any time, t, is equal to the original number, N_o, reduced by the exponential $e^{-\lambda t}$. This exponential is known as the *decay factor*, and e (2.7) is the base of the natural system of logarithms (recall that $e_x = y$ implies that ln $y = x$).

Two other forms of this equation are

$$R = R_o e^{-\lambda t}$$
$$A = A_o e^{-\lambda t}$$

There are several ways to solve problems with these equations. In the past, graphic solutions were performed with semilogarithmic graph paper because plots of exponentials on this type of paper are straight lines. Values of e^x and e^{-x} are tabulated so that mathematic solutions can be easily obtained. Most pocket calculators have natural logarithm calculation capability, making mathematic solutions relatively simple. Decay factors often are tabulated for commonly used radionuclides to simplify activity calculations for technologists.

Physical Half-life

It was previously stated that the decay constant, λ, is uniquely defined for each radionuclide. However, a term related to the lifetimes of radionuclides has a more physical meaning in their routine use. The most commonly used factor is the physical

half-life ($T_{1/2}$). This is the time required for one-half of a group of radioactive atoms to decay or the time for an activity or a decay rate to be reduced to one-half its original value. It can be shown that the half-life and the decay constant are related by

$$\lambda T_{1/2} = 0.693$$

Thus the decay equation may be written as

$$N = N_o e^{-\frac{0.693t}{T_{1/2}}}$$

The decay rate and activity equations can be modified accordingly to yield their most widely used forms, as follows:

$$R = R_o e^{-\frac{0.693t}{T_{1/2}}}$$
$$A = A_o e^{-\frac{0.693t}{T_{1/2}}}$$

Mean Life

Another useful lifetime measurement is the mean life or average life. This is the period of time that it would take for all of the atoms of a radionuclide to decay if the false assumption is made that they decay with the initial decay rate until all of the atoms have decayed. The mean life, $\overline{T}$, is then given by

$$\overline{T} = 1.44 \, T_{1/2}$$

The mean life is a useful relation to use in radiation dose calculations, because the total number of disintegrations occurring in an administered dose is the product of the administered activity and the mean life.

Effective Half-life

In radiation dose calculations based on internally administered radionuclides and in imaging situations, a very important factor to be considered is the rate of disappearance of the radioactivity from the target organ and the body owing to both radioactive decay and biologic excretion. An effective disappearance probability (λ_{eff}) can be defined that is equal to the probability of excretion (λ_b) plus the probability of decay (λ). Thus

$$\lambda_{eff} = \lambda_b + \lambda$$

If the biologic excretion is also exponential in form, then

$$\lambda_b T_{1/2b} = 0.693$$

The effective disappearance is then measured by the effective half-life ($T_{1/2eff}$) which is obtained with

$$T_{1/2eff} = (T_{1/2b} \times T_{1/2})/(T_{1/2b} + T_{1/2})$$

where $T_{1/2b}$ and $T_{1/2}$ are the biologic and physical half-lives, respectively. The mean effective life that can be used in dosimetry calculations (T_{eff}) is then defined as

$$\overline{T}_{eff} = 1.44 \, T_{1/2eff}$$

Radioactive Equilibrium

The decay equations can become more complicated when the radioactive parent decays to a daughter that also is radioactive.

This problem arises because the daughter is decaying at the same time it is being formed by the decay of the parent. A differential equation can be written to characterize this process. The solution yields the Bateman equation, which provides an expression for the activity of the daughter at any time. This equation in its general form is

$$A_d = F\left(\frac{\lambda_d}{\lambda_d - \lambda_p}\right)A_{po}(e^{\lambda_p t} - e^{-\lambda_d t}) + A_{do}(e^{-\lambda_d t})$$

where

A_d = Activity of the daughter at time t
A_{po} = Initial activity of the parent
A_{do} = Initial activity of the daughter
F = Fraction of the parent decaying to the daughter
λ_p = Decay constant of the parent
λ_d = Decay constant of the daughter

There are three special cases that simplify this equation. The first case occurs when the half-life of the daughter is greater than the half-life of the parent ($\lambda_d < \lambda_p$). In this case, the parent decays very rapidly to the daughter, which then decays slowly away. There is never any fixed relation between the parent and the daughter. In the remaining two cases, in which the half-life of the parent is greater than the half-life of the daughter, a constant relation can exist between them that is defined as the condition of radioactive equilibrium.

The second case occurs when the half-life of the parent is many times greater, that is, approaches infinity, than the half-life of the daughter ($\lambda_p << \lambda_d$). In this case, the Bateman equation simplifies to

$$A_d = FA_{po}(1 - e^{-\lambda_d t})$$

If we begin with a pure parent, after several half-lives the daughter activity builds up to the point at which it reaches an equilibrium condition, called *secular equilibrium,* with the parent activity (Fig. 1.15). When equilibrium is reached, the decay rate (activity) of the daughter is equal to the decay rate (activity) of the parent, and the daughter continues to have the same decay rate as the parent as long as no daughter nuclei are removed. An example of secular equilibrium is the decay of ^{226}Ra, which

has a 1,622-year half-life, to ^{222}Rn, which has a 3.8-day half-life.

The third case is of special interest in nuclear medicine. It occurs when the half-life of the parent is greater than the half-life of the daughter ($\lambda_p < \lambda_d$) but does not approach infinity. In this case, the Bateman equation simplifies to

$$A_d = F\left(\frac{\lambda_d}{\lambda_d - \lambda_p}\right)A_{po}(e^{-\lambda_p t} - e^{-\lambda_d t})$$

If we begin with a pure parent, after a few half-lives, the activity of the daughter builds up to a point at which a constant relation exists between parent and daughter. The activity of the daughter can then be calculated from

$$A_d = F(A_p \times T_{1/2p})/(T_{1/2p} - T_{1/2d})$$

The daughter then decays with the half-life of the parent (Fig. 1.16). This condition is defined as *transient equilibrium.* An example is the decay of ^{99}Mo, which has a 66-hour half-life, to ^{99m}Tc, which has a 6-hour half-life. Transient equilibrium forms the basis for the radioisotope generator (Fig. 1.17). In the ^{99}Mo to ^{99m}Tc generator, the activity of ^{99m}Tc builds up to

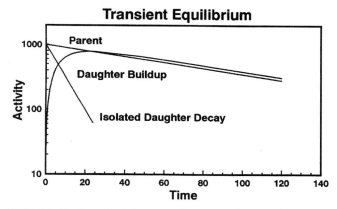

FIGURE 1.16. Plot of activity versus time on semilog scale for a parent and daughter satisfying conditions for transient equilibrium.

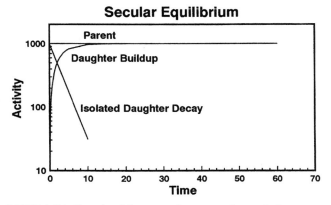

FIGURE 1.15. Plot of activity versus time on semilog scale for a parent and daughter satisfying the conditions for secular equilibrium.

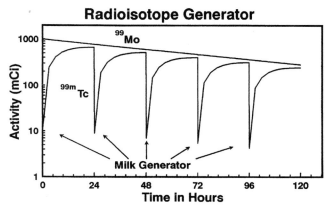

FIGURE 1.17. Plot of activity versus time on semilog scale of ^{99}Mo and ^{99m}Tc in secular equilibrium illustrates the principle of the radioisotope generator.

approximately that of ^{99}Mo in approximately four half-lives. If the ^{99m}Tc is removed (by means of "milking" the generator), the process of buildup immediately begins again. Equilibrium is approached in another four half-lives, at which time the generator can be "milked" again. Thus it is possible to receive a 1-Ci generator calibrated at 8:00 a.m. on Monday, "milk" it once each day, and obtain approximately 3.2 Ci for nuclear medicine procedures during the week.

Statistics

In general, any type of measurement performed has some deviation in the accuracy of the value obtained. If mistakes are excluded from the discussion, there are two basic types of deviations or errors that can contribute to the inaccuracy of a measurement. *Systematic errors* are deviations that appear in every measurement and cause the experimental values obtained to be biased either above or below the actual value by some consistent amount. Repeated measurements yield the same value with the same error. A simple example would be measurement of a specific length with a ruler that is improperly labeled such that 1 inch is actually only $^{15}/_{16}$ inch. Consistent measurements would yield reproducible values, but all values would be shorter than the actual length. The term *accuracy* is used to characterize systematic errors, and measurements that contain systematic errors are said to be *biased*.

Random errors are variations that occur in measurements generally owing to factors over which the observer has no control. These errors can be caused by physical constraints imposed by the methods used to perform the measurements or to actual differences in the variable being measured at the time of each measurement. For example, measurement of a long length with a very short ruler results in random errors due to the limitations of the measurement device. Another example is measurement of the diameter of beans with a micrometer resulting in random errors due to the variability in the diameter of the beans. The terms *precision* and *reproducibility* are used to characterize random errors, and the term *uncertainty* is used as a measure of the random error associated with a measurement.

If a large number of measurements containing random errors are made on a variable and the number of like values versus the measured values is plotted in a frequency distribution, the result is a bell-shaped, or Gaussian, curve (Fig. 1.18). The peak of this curve is the average value or *mean*, and the width of the curve is determined by the magnitude of the random errors associated with the measurements. If a large number of measurements are made and only random errors are associated with the measurements, the actual value should be the mean of the distribution. If N measurements are made and the values obtained are *n1, n2, n3, . . . , nN*, then the mean is

$$\text{Mean} = (n_1 + n2 + n_3 + \ldots + n_N)/N$$

$$mean = \bar{n} = \Sigma \frac{n_i}{N}$$

The Gaussian distribution is characterized with the following equation:

$$P(n) = \frac{1}{\sigma\sqrt{2\pi}} e^{\frac{1}{2}\left(\frac{n - \bar{n}}{\sigma}\right)^2}$$

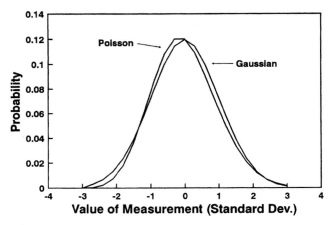

FIGURE 1.18. Plot of Poisson and Gaussian distributions. Measured values are plotted as a function of standard deviations around the mean. The Poisson distribution is defined only for positive values.

where $P(n)$ is the probability of measuring n, and σ is defined as the standard deviation and is a measure of the width of the Gaussian distribution. Because the width of the distribution is determined by the random errors associated with the measurements, the standard deviation is used to characterize the random errors. For the foregoing set of measurements, the standard deviation can be calculated with the following equation:

$$\sigma = \sqrt{\Sigma \frac{(n_i - \bar{n})^2}{n - 1}}$$

For the Gaussian distribution, there is a 68% probability that a measurement will fall within a range around the mean of one standard deviation (mean $\pm$ 1σ). If the ranges are extended to two and three standard deviations (mean $\pm$ 2σ and mean $\pm$ 3σ) the probabilities are increased to 95% and 99%, respectively. These probabilities are referred to as *confidence intervals*.

Radioactive decay is a classic example of random errors associated with a measurement. This is because radioactive decay is completely random. The decay equations defined earlier actually refer to average values of R (decay rate). Multiple measurements of R will yield different values that vary around average or mean values. Radioactive decay is described with Poisson statistics and is represented by the Poisson distribution. Figure 1.18 shows that the Poisson and Gaussian distributions are very similar and essentially overlap when the mean value is large. When a single measurement of n counts is made from a radioactive sample, it is important to know the random error, also known as the *uncertainty*, associated with the measurement. Because the standard deviation (σ) is the best measure of random error, this value can be extracted from the Poisson distribution if the mean value is approximated by n, as follows:

$$\sigma = \sqrt{n}$$

The result of the measurement with its associated error can then be reported as

$$n \pm \sigma = n \pm \sqrt{n}$$

The significance of the confidence intervals can now be described. If there are only random errors associated with the decay process to be considered, then there is a 68% probability that the average value will fall within the measured value $\pm 1\sigma$. Similarly there are a 95% probability and a 99% probability that the average value will fall within the mean $\pm 2\sigma$ and the value $\pm 3\sigma$, respectively. Thus these ranges define the confidence that appropriate measurements are obtained.

It is often more useful to know the percentage error associated with a measurement. In general, the percentage error (percentage uncertainty or percentage standard deviation) is 100 times the error divided by the value in which the error is calculated. For n, this value is

$$\% \ \sigma = \frac{\sigma}{n} \times 100 = \frac{\sqrt{n}}{n} \times 100 = \frac{100}{\sqrt{n}}$$

Measurement of the differences in two decay measurements in a given time period often is needed, for example when a measurement is to be adjusted for background. In general, the error in the sum or the difference of two measurements, A and B, is

$$\sigma_{A+/-B} = \sqrt{(\sigma_A)^2 + (\sigma_B)^2}$$

If two measurements, n_1 and n_2, are obtained, the difference between the two measurements n_n is

$$n_n = n_1 - n_2$$

and the error in the difference is obtained with the following formula:

$$\sigma_{N_n} = \sqrt{n_1 + n_2}$$

The percentage error in the difference is

$$\% \ \sigma_{N_n} = \frac{\sigma_{n_n}}{n_n} = \frac{\sqrt{n_1 + n_2}}{n_1 - n_2} \times 100$$

If n counts are measured in a time interval t, the count rate R from the sample is

$$R = \frac{n}{t}$$

The error in the time measurement usually is extremely small and generally can be ignored. The error in the count rate is then the error in the counts, as follows:

$$\sigma_R = \frac{\sqrt{n}}{t} = \sqrt{\frac{R}{t}}$$

The percentage error (100 times the error divided by the value) in the count rate is then

$$\% \ \sigma_R = \frac{\frac{\sqrt{n}}{t}}{\frac{n}{t}} \times 100 = \frac{100}{\sqrt{n}} = \frac{100}{\sqrt{Rt}}$$

Occasionally, a measurement is made from a sample in one time interval and a measurement of background is made in a longer time interval. In this situation, it is necessary to determine the difference in two count rates and the error associated with this difference. In general, if n_1 counts are measured in t_1 minutes and n_2 counts are measured in t_2 minutes, the net count rate R_n in counts per minute is obtained as follows:

$$R_n = \frac{n_1}{t_1} - \frac{n_2}{t_2} = R_1 - R_2$$

The error in the net count rate is

$$\sigma_{R_n} = \sqrt{(\sigma_{R_1})^2 + (\sigma_{R_2})^2} = \sqrt{\frac{R_1}{t_1} + \frac{R_2}{t_2}}$$

The percentage error in the net count rate is

$$\% \ \sigma_{R_n} = \frac{\sigma_{R_n}}{R_n} = \frac{\sqrt{\frac{R_1}{t_1} + \frac{R_2}{t_2}}}{R_1 - R_2} \times 100$$

INTERACTIONS OF RADIATION WITH MATTER

In general, radiation is an outward flow of energy from an energy source. The radiation can be in the form of particles or electromagnetic radiation propagating through space. The particles can be charged or uncharged and possess kinetic energy ranging from a few electron volts (eV) to billions of electron volts (BeV). Similarly, electromagnetic radiation can possess small amounts of energy per photon (low-energy x-rays and light photons) or relatively large amounts of energy (γ-rays). Radiation interacts with matter through the transfer of energy to its surroundings. Knowledge of these interactions is important because these mechanisms are the means by which radiation dose is delivered to tissues and are the means by which radiation is detected. Radiation can interact with nuclei, electrons, or total atoms, energy being transferred totally or in part to nuclei, electrons, atoms, or even molecules.

Radiation interactions with matter often are classified in terms of specific ionization, linear energy transfer, and range. *Specific ionization* is defined as the number of ion pairs produced along each unit of path length of the trajectory of the particle (ion pairs per millimeter [ip/mm]). *Linear energy transfer* (LET) is a related quantity and is defined as the amount of energy that a particle loses to its surrounding medium for each unit of path length it travels (keV/mm). The *range* of a particle is defined as the distance the particle travels before giving up enough of its kinetic energy so that it no longer interacts with the medium through which it travels. All three of these factors depend on the type of particle (mass and charge), the energy of the particle, and the interacting medium. In general, an average of 34 eV is needed to produce one ion pair.

Charged-particle Interactions

Charged-particle interactions are generally caused by the Coulomb force between charged particles rather than direct physical contact. Charged-particle interactions can result in ionization in which orbital electrons are dislodged from atoms to form positive and negative ions; atomic excitation in which orbital electrons are excited to higher energy levels in the atoms; molecular excitation in which vibrations are produced in molecules; molecular collisions in which atoms or parts of atoms are dislodged from the molecule, resulting in a break in the molecular chain; and bremsstrahlung, which is the production of photons due to deceleration and deflection of particles in the vicinity of other charged particles. Ionized electrons often receive enough energy to produce secondary ionization.

Charged particles can be classified as heavy (protons, deuterons, α particles, and ionized atoms) or light (electrons and positrons). Heavy charged particles generally travel in relatively straight lines and are characterized by high specific ionization, high LET, and short range. In general, a small amount of energy is lost in each interaction, but many interactions occur in a short distance. Heavy-charged-particle interactions have little application in nuclear medicine other than in the production of radioisotopes.

Light-charged-particle interactions are important because interactions of x-rays and γ-rays with matter generally result in the production of free electrons with enough kinetic energy to produce secondary interactions. Electron interactions are similar to those of heavy charged particles. However, because electrons are much smaller, they must travel at high speed to possess the same kinetic energy, and their velocity can approach the speed of light. Also, because of the small mass of electrons, a large amount of energy can be transferred to another particle in a single interaction. Thus the path of an electron can be very tortuous as it travels through a medium owing to the large angles of deflection that can result from some interactions. Electrons generally have a much smaller specific ionization and LET and a longer range than do heavy charged particles.

Photon Characteristics

γ-Rays and x-rays are forms of electromagnetic radiation that transport energy through space as a combination of electric and magnetic fields. Some interactions of these electromagnetic radiations with matter are explained with the theories of wave propagation. Others are explained only with the assumption that the radiation consists of discrete bundles of energy or photons with particle-like characteristics because of their short wavelength and high frequencies. If a photon has at least 15 eV of energy, it is capable of ionizing atoms, and it is referred to as *ionizing radiation*. X-rays, γ-rays, and some ultraviolet rays are types of ionizing radiation.

When a beam of photons is reduced in intensity during its passage through a material, the process is referred to as *attenuation*. Photon attenuation can occur in two ways. Photons can be absorbed or completely removed from the beam and cease to exist, or they can be scattered or deflected from their original line of travel. Photons interact with matter primarily by means of one of five basic processes. These are coherent scattering, photoelectric absorption, Compton scattering, pair production, and photodisintegration. Of these possibilities, only photoelectric absorption and Compton scattering are of consequence in nuclear medicine.

Attenuation Equation

When a photon traverses a medium, a probability of interaction is associated with each of the listed five processes. In general,

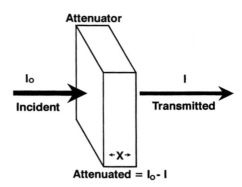

FIGURE 1.19. Attenuation of a beam of photons by an absorber.

this probability is a function of the energy of the photon and the thickness and composition of the material with which the photon interacts. An equation can be written that describes the attenuation of photons by matter. If I_o is the number of photons incident on an absorber of thickness, Δx (Fig. 1.19) and I is the number of transmitted photons, then the number of photons absorbed is as follows:

$$\Delta I_o = I_o - I$$

The fraction of photons absorbed is $\Delta I_o / I_o$ and is directly proportional to the thickness of absorber, Δx. An equation can then be written by inserting a proportionality constant μ as follows:

$$\Delta I_o / I_o = -\mu \Delta x$$

The minus sign indicates that the number of transmitted photons decreases with increasing thickness of the absorber. Applying the techniques of integral calculus, this relation yields the general attenuation equation

$$I = I_o e^{-\mu x}$$

which states that the number of photons transmitted through an absorber, I, is equal to the number of photons incident on the absorber, I_o, reduced by $e^{-\mu x}$, the attenuation factor for the absorber. The quantity μ is the total linear attenuation coefficient and has the units of (1/distance). This factor is defined as the fraction removed from the beam per unit of thickness of the absorber or the probability of interaction in the absorber. The total linear attenuation coefficient, μ, is actually the sum of the linear attenuation coefficients for each of the five possible interactions. Thus

$$\mu = \Omega + \tau + \sigma + \kappa + \pi$$

where Ω, τ, σ, κ, and π are the linear attenuation coefficients for coherent scattering, photoelectric absorption, Compton scattering, pair production, and photodisintegration, respectively. The value of μ depends on the energy of the photon (monochromatic radiation only) and the type of absorbing material and its physical state (solid, liquid, or gas).

To simplify attenuation descriptions, the concept of the half-value layer (HVL) has been defined as the thickness of absorber that reduces the number of transmitted photons in a beam to

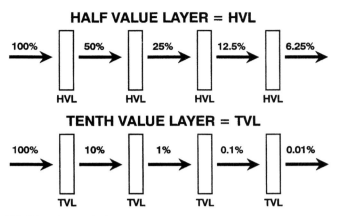

HALF VALUE LAYER = HVL

100% → | → 50% → | → 25% → | → 12.5% → | → 6.25%

HVL   HVL   HVL   HVL

TENTH VALUE LAYER = TVL

100% → | → 10% → | → 1% → | → 0.1% → | → 0.01%

TVL   TVL   TVL   TVL

FIGURE 1.20. A thickness of absorber equal to one half-value layer (HVL) or one tenth-value layer (TVL) reduces the intensity of a photon beam to 50% and 10%, respectively.

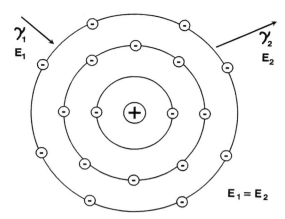

FIGURE 1.21. In coherent scattering (Rayleigh scattering), the incident photon is effectively absorbed by an atom and then re-emitted in a new direction with no loss in energy.

one-half the incident number. The HVL is related to μ as follows:

$$\mu HVL = 0.693$$

and is similar in concept to the half-life in the decay equation. In shielding calculations, the concept of the tenth-value layer (TVL) often is used. The TVL is related to μ as follows:

$$\mu TVL = 2.30$$

The use of the HVL and TVL is shown diagrammatically in Fig. 1.20.

It occasionally is useful to eliminate the physical state of the absorber in attenuation problems. To accomplish this, the concept of the mass attenuation coefficient, μ_m, has been defined by the relation

$$\mu_m = \mu/\rho$$

where ρ is the density of the absorber, and μ_m has the units of cm^2/g. Thus the mass attenuation coefficient of a material for a specific energy is the same whether it is a solid, liquid, or gas.

Coherent Scattering

Coherent or classical scattering (also known as Rayleigh scattering) results from the interaction of a photon with the total atom (Fig. 1.21). In this process, almost no energy is transferred to the atom, and the effect is a change in direction of the photon with no loss in energy. Coherent scattering is a low-energy interaction occurring only at energy below 50 keV. Thus in the diagnostic energy range for imaging (70 to 511 keV) the probability of coherent scattering (Ω) is zero, and therefore is of no importance in nuclear medicine applications.

Photoelectric Absorption

Photoelectric absorption is an extremely important ionization process and is shown diagrammatically in Fig. 1.22. When a

photon undergoes photoelectric absorption, the total energy of the incident photon is transferred to an inner-shell electron. The electron (called the *photoelectron*) is then ejected from the atom with kinetic energy, E_e, equal to the difference between the energy of the incident photon, E_γ, and the binding energy of the electron in its shell, *BE*, as follows:

$$E_e = E_\gamma - BE$$

In general, the most tightly bound inner-shell electrons are involved in the process. However, this is a threshold interaction in that photoelectric absorption cannot occur with an electron unless the energy of the photon is greater than the binding energy of the electron. Thus a photon with energy greater than the binding energy of the K shell most probably will interact with a K-shell electron. It also can interact with electrons in the L and M shells and so on but with decreasing probabilities. However, if the photon has an energy less than the K-shell binding energy

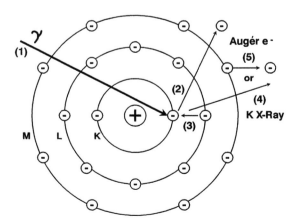

FIGURE 1.22. In the process of photoelectric absorption, a photon is absorbed by an inner-shell electron *(1)*, which is then ejected from the atom *(2)* with an energy equal to the incident proton energy minus the binding energy of the electron. The atom is then de-excited by an outer-shell electron filling the vacancy *(3)*, followed by characteristic x-ray *(4)* or Augér electron emission *(5)*.

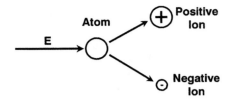

FIGURE 1.23. The end result of photoelectric absorption and Compton scattering is the production of an ion pair (an atom minus 1 electron and the freed electron).

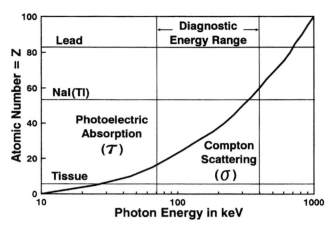

FIGURE 1.25. Plot of atomic number (*Z*) versus photon energy (*E*) illustrating the combinations of *Z* and *E* in which photoelectric absorption (*left of curved line*) and Compton scatter (*right of curved line*) predominate. Three examples are shown (tissue, sodium iodide, and lead). The diagnostic energy range for imaging shown is 70 to 400 keV.

but greater than the L-shell binding energy, it can only interact with L and M shell electrons and so on.

After photoelectric absorption, the rest of the atom is left in an excited state as a positive ion owing to the vacancy made in the inner shell. This vacancy is filled by an outer-shell electron that drops down to take the place of the photoelectron. The resulting de-excitation energy is emitted as a characteristic x-ray or Augér electron, as described earlier. Thus photoelectric absorption produces an ion pair (Fig. 1.23) (the negative ion is the photoelectron, and the positive ion is the atom minus one electron) and characteristic radiation (x-rays or Augér electrons resulting from de-excitation of the positive ion). The photoelectron generally possesses sufficient energy to ionize other atoms.

Photoelectric absorption is a low-energy interaction, and the probability (τ) decreases rapidly with increasing photon energy (proportional to $1/E^3$) (Fig. 1.24). Because photoelectric absorption with a particular shell requires the photon energy to be equal to or greater than the binding energy of the shell, there are discrete changes in the probability at the binding energy of each shell. The probability of photoelectric absorption is strongly dependent on the atomic number (Z) of the absorber (proportional to Z^4) and increases rapidly with increasing Z.

Figure 1.25 combines the two dependencies described and shows the significance of photoelectric absorption in nuclear medicine. For sodium iodide detectors (effective $Z = 53$), the

primary interaction in the diagnostic energy range for imaging (70 to 511 keV) is photoelectric, implying total absorption, which is important for photon detection. For lead collimators ($Z = 82$), the primary interaction also is photoelectric, again implying total absorption. This is important in shielding applications but also yields a source of the characteristic x-rays of lead that must be taken into consideration in patient imaging and sample counting procedures.

Compton Scattering

The other interaction important in nuclear medicine is Compton scattering, shown diagrammatically in Fig. 1.26. Compton

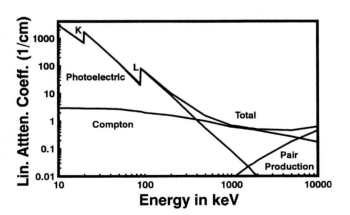

FIGURE 1.24. Plot of linear attenuation coefficients for photoelectric absorption (τ), Compton scattering (σ), and pair production (κ) and the total linear attenuation coefficient ($\mu = \tau + \sigma + \kappa$) versus photon energy.

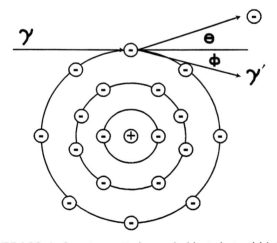

FIGURE 1.26. In Compton scattering, an incident photon (γ) interacts with an outer-shell electron. The electron receives part of the energy of the photon and scatters through an angle (θ). The rest of the energy is carried off by the scatter photon (γ'). The distribution of energy is determined by the angle of scatter (ϕ) of the scattered photon (γ').

Table 1.8. *Energy of scattered photon (γ) and scattered electron (e⁻) versus scattering angle in compton scattering*

Photon Energy[a] (keV)	Scattering Angle (degrees)									
	0		30		45		90		180	
	γ	e⁻	γ	e⁻	γ	e⁻	γ	e⁻	γ	e⁻
70	70	0	69	1	67	3	62	8	55	15
140	140	0	135	5	130	10	110	30	90	50
364	364	0	332	32	301	63	213	151	150	214
511	511	0	451	60	395	116	255	256	170	341

[a]Primary photon energies of ²⁰¹Tl, ⁹⁹ᵐTc, ¹³¹I, and annihilation radiation, respectively.

scattering is the process whereby a photon interacts with a loosely bound outer-shell electron, the electron receiving energy from the photon. The electron recoils at an angle, θ, with respect to the direction of travel of the incident photon. The photon also has its direction of travel altered by an angle, φ. The amount of energy transferred to the electron depends on the angle of scattering of the photon. In Compton scattering interactions, the binding energies of the electrons are small in comparison to the photon energies, and therefore the electrons are considered free. Conservation of energy thus yields the equation

$$E_\gamma = E_{\gamma'} + E_e$$

which states that the energy of the incident photon, E_γ, is equal to the sum of the energies of the scattered photon, $E_{\gamma'}$, and the recoil electron, E_e. Conservation of momentum yields an equation relating the energy of the scattered photon, $E_{\gamma'}$, in keV, to the angle of scatter of the photon, φ:

$$E_{\gamma'} = E_\gamma/[1 + E_\gamma/511)(1 - \cos\phi)]$$

In this equation, 511 is the rest mass of the electron in kiloelectron volts. The scattering angle, φ, of the photon ranges from 0 degrees (no interaction) to 180 degrees (backscatter). Because the electron is assumed to be at rest before interaction, its scattering angle ranges from 0 to 90 degrees. Both θ and φ tend to decrease as the energy of the incident photon increases. The products of Compton scattering are an ion pair (Fig. 1.23; positive ion is the atom minus 1 electron and the electron) and a photon of reduced energy with a new direction of travel. Table 1.8 shows the energies of the scattered photon and electron versus scattering angle of the photon for selected radionuclides used in nuclear medicine.

The probability of Compton scattering (σ) decreases slowly with increasing energy (approximately proportional to $1/E$) and is directly proportional to the electron density (approximately Z/A) of the absorber. The latter phenomenon occurs because the probability that a photon will interact with an atom is determined by the number of electrons in the atom, which is equal to its atomic number.

Figure 1.25 shows that Compton scattering is the dominant interaction for photons within the body ($Z = 8$ for tissue, crossover point is 25 keV; $Z = 20$ for bone, crossover point is 45

keV) throughout most of the diagnostic energy range. Thus if a photon interacts within the body, the interaction most likely is Compton scattering, the original photon being replaced by another photon with decreased energy traveling in a new direction.

Pair Production

Pair production (probability, κ) is a threshold interaction resulting from the primary interaction between a photon and the strong electric field of the nucleus of an atom (Fig. 1.27). In this interaction of the photon, energy is converted to mass in the form of a positive and a negative electron ($e^+ + e^-$). Because the rest mass energy of a single electron is 0.511 MeV, the photon must have at least 1.022 MeV of energy for the interaction to occur. The energy in excess of this value is transferred to the two electrons as kinetic energy. The electrons interact with the medium as previously described until this energy is lost.

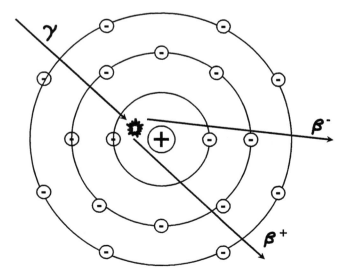

FIGURE 1.27. In a pair-production interaction between a photon with energy greater than 1.022 MeV and the electric field of the nucleus, 1.022 MeV of energy is converted to mass in the form of a positive and a negative electron. The remaining energy is carried off as kinetic energy by the two electrons.

The positive electron then annihilates with a negative electron as previously described (Fig. 1.8). Because pair production is possible only for photons with energy greater than 1.022 MeV, this interaction is of no consequence in nuclear medicine imaging applications.

Photodisintegration

When the photon has very high energy (>7 MeV), it has sufficient energy to produce a photonuclear reaction resulting in the ejection of a nucleon from the nucleus. This process is called *photodisintegration*. The probability (π) of this interaction is very small, and because of the high energy required it is of no consequence in nuclear medicine.

SUGGESTED READING

Bushberg JT, Seibert JA, Leidholdt EM Jr, et al. *The essential physics of medical imaging. Baltimore: Williams and Wilkins, 1994. Chapters 1, 2, 14.*

Chandra R. *Introductory physics of nuclear medicine, 4th ed. Philadelphia: Lea & Febiger, 1992. Chapters 1–3, 6.*

Johns HL, Cunningham JR. *The physics of radiology, 4th ed. Springfield, IL: Charles C Thomas, 1974. Chapters 1, 3–5.*

Sorenson JA, Phelps ME. *Physics in nuclear medicine, 2nd ed. Orlando, FL: Grune & Stratton, 1987. Chapters 1–3, 6, 8, 9.*

Diagnostic Nuclear Medicine, Fourth Edition. Edited by M.P. Sandler, R.E. Coleman, J.A. Patton, F.J.Th. Wackers, A. Gottschalk. Lippincott Williams & Wilkins, Philadelphia 2003.

2

DETECTORS

TIMOTHY G. TURKINGTON
MARTIN P. TORNAI

Radiation detection is fundamental to all diagnostic nuclear medicine procedures. Specific detector devices include survey meters, dose calibrators, well counters, surgical probes, and various imaging devices, such as gamma cameras used for single photon emission computed tomography (SPECT) systems and positron emission tomography (PET) cameras. Because direct detection of charged particles plays a minor role in clinical nuclear medicine and most procedures depend on γ-ray photon detection, the latter phenomenon is the emphasis of this chapter.

Detection of photons depends on the interaction of photons with matter (predominantly through Compton scattering and photoelectric absorption), which causes ionization, which liberates electrons, and excitation of atoms. By means of either direct measurement of the ionization in a detector material or secondary measurement (e.g., with a photomultiplier) of emitted scintillation light, the impinging photons ultimately lead to generation of electrical current. Most devices currently in use in nuclear medicine are gaseous detectors and scintillation detectors.

A distinguishing characteristic of detection techniques used for nuclear medicine imaging is that each detected γ-ray photon is individually evaluated before inclusion in the resulting measurement. This relies on a general principle called *pulse counting* (each detected γ-ray is a pulse) and is the critical feature that in principle allows nuclear medicine techniques to be quantitative. Pulse counting, as used in diagnostic nuclear imaging, is different from other diagnostic imaging techniques (e.g., x-ray imaging), in which detected events are not differentiated but all events are collected indiscriminately over a broad spectral range.

GENERAL RADIATION DETECTION PROPERTIES

Several important properties differentiate the various types of radiation detection devices. A detector type is chosen and optimized for the particular task needed.

T.G. Turkington: Departments of Radiology and Biomedical Engineering, Duke University Medical Center, Durham, NC.
M.P. Tornai: Departments of Radiology and Biomedical Engineering, Duke University Medical Center, Durham, NC.

Efficiency

Radiation detection efficiency is defined as the rate at which a detector is measuring radiation from a source divided by the rate at which radiation is being emitted from the source, as follows:

$$\epsilon = R_d/R_e \qquad [1]$$

where ϵ is the detection efficiency, R_d is the detection rate, and R_e is the emission rate. The efficiency of a detector for detecting radiation from a source is the product of two components—geometric efficiency (how well it surrounds the source geometrically) and intrinsic efficiency (how often the material converts the energy of an impinging particle into a usable electronic signal), as follows:

$$\epsilon = \epsilon_i \cdot \epsilon_g \qquad [2]$$

where ϵ_i is the intrinsic efficiency and ϵ_g is the geometric efficiency. Fig. 2.1 illustrates both effects. Geometric efficiency, ϵ_g, dictates the fraction of radiation that will hit the detector. Intrinsic efficiency, ϵ_i, dictates the fraction of radiation hitting the detector that will stop and generate a signal. Geometric efficiency can be optimized in some cases so that the radioactive source is almost entirely surrounded by detector material. In other cases, the geometric efficiency is small because of limits on detector size and proximity to source. Intrinsic efficiency depends on the detection material, its thickness, and how it is being used, as is discussed later.

Count Rate Capability

When radiation hits a detector, there is some time, a dead time, during which the detector cannot accurately detect another particle. In some cases, this dead time is the result of the time it takes to fully process an event. In other cases, there is dead time simply because a particle interacts with the detector, even if it is not processed, because its effects (e.g., ionization) linger. For many detection systems, both components are present. The smaller the dead time associated with a detector and its associated electronics, the higher is the rate at which radiation can be detected. A detector with shorter dead time and therefore higher count rate capability is generally more desirable. There are many cases in nuclear medicine, however, in which counting rates are

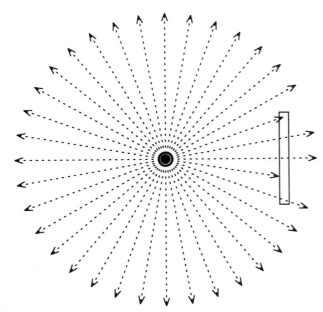

FIGURE 2.1. Radiation detection efficiency. Both geometric and intrinsic efficiency effects are shown. The fraction of radiation directed toward the detector is the geometric efficiency. The fraction impinging on the detector that stops and yields a signal is the intrinsic efficiency.

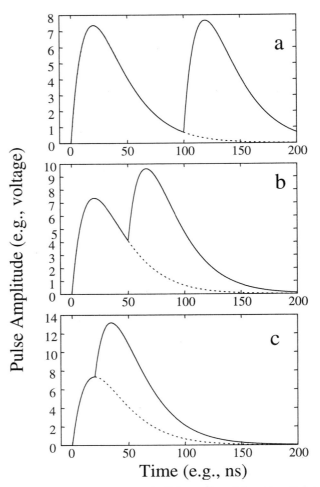

FIGURE 2.2. Pulse pile-up. **A:** Only slight overlap of the pulses. **B:** Substantial overlap, to the degree that both pulses would be corrupted if integrated. **C:** Pulse-detection circuitry may not recognize the presence of two pulses.

low (a few thousand counts per second) such that from a rate perspective, almost any detector would be suitable. High-count-rate needs can be satisfied with a detector with very short dead time or with many independent detectors.

Three examples of signals occurring close together in time are shown in Fig. 2.2. In Fig. 2.2A, the signals arrive far enough apart that both can be differentiated and processed. In Fig. 2.2B, the signals arrive close enough together that neither can be processed without being contaminated by the other. In Fig. 2.2C, the signals are close enough together that they cannot be differentiated as two separate signals, likely resulting in a corrupt measurement. Detector systems that measure pulse magnitude (e.g., energy) would ideally reject both signals in Figs. 2.2B and 2.2C, because neither can be easily measured. It is important, therefore, that such systems recognize the presence of the second pulse, so that both can be rejected. Detection systems that measure simply the presence of signals and not the height, can detect two counts in Fig. 2.2A, one or two counts in Fig. 2.2B, depending on the quality of the signal processing, and one count in Fig. 2.2C.

Detected count rate is plotted against incident radiation rate for three scenarios in Fig. 2.3. The straight line represents a detector system with no dead time, so the detected rate equals the incident rate. The other curves represent a system with a dead time (τ) of 2.5 μs. The upper curve, which approaches a limit of 0.4 MHz ($1/\tau$), would be obtained on a system that always processes the first of two close-together pulses. The lower curve reaches a maximum of $1/(e \cdot \tau)$ and then decreases with increasing incident rate. Such a response occurs when a system actively rejects pulses because of their proximity to other pulses or when any pulse, recorded or not, prevents subsequent pulses

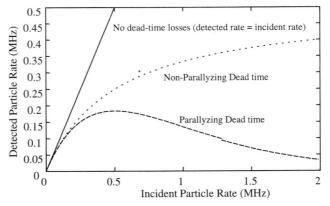

FIGURE 2.3. Count rate losses. Rate responses of three counting systems—ideal (linear, all pulses are counted), nonparalyzing (pulses are missed if they follow too closely after a counted pulse), and paralyzing (pulses are missed if they follow too closely after a another pulse, counted or not.) A dead time (τ) of 2.5 μs is modeled.

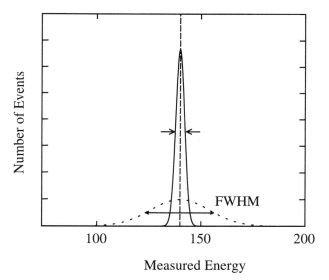

FIGURE 2.4. Energy resolution. Two spectra are shown that represent good (narrow) and poor (wide) energy resolution. The full width at half maximum is indicated for both curves.

from being detected. The latter is called *paralyzing* and the former *nonparalyzing* responses (1,2).

Energy Resolution

The precision with which a detector can measure incident particle energy (or the magnitude of the detected pulse) is called *energy resolution*. The responses of two different detectors to 140-keV radiation are shown in Fig. 2.4. The number of times each energy is registered is shown on the vertical axis. The higher energy resolution curve shows more measurements near the true energy. One frequently used measure of energy resolution is the full width at half maximum (FWHM), depicted on the graph for the two curves. Some detectors do not provide energy information. Others, particularly those needed in nuclear medicine imaging, yield a reasonably precise energy measurement.

SCINTILLATORS

Principles

When a high-energy photon passes through matter, it undergoes Compton scattering, photoelectric absorption, or both (1,2). The energy of the incident photon is transferred to the emitted electrons, a small amount of energy being lost to overcoming the energy binding the electrons to their atoms. The emitted electrons travel through material, ionizing and exciting atoms near their paths. The excited atoms eventually decay to their ground states, giving off electromagnetic radiation. When it is in or near the visible range, this released radiation can be detected and converted into an electronic pulse. This release of light initially stimulated by higher-energy radiation is called *scintillation* (3). This technique for detecting radiation has been used since Rutherford's initial α particle detection experiments.

Scintillator Materials

A key property of scintillating materials is that they are transparent to the light they generate. Many amorphous materials are not, hence scintillators often are grown as highly structured crystals, which can render them more transparent. The following properties differentiate the materials used for scintillation detection:

1. Light output. Each material yields a certain amount of light relative to the energy lost by the incident particle. Higher light output for a given input energy is more desirable. This represents a higher efficiency in conversion from the incident particle energy to light energy. More light energy is equivalent to more light photons, which generally means better energy resolution.

2. Speed or scintillation decay time (λ). The rate at which scintillation light is produced varies greatly from one material to another and ranges from less than 1 ns (10^{-9} s) to hundreds of nanoseconds. A faster scintillator is generally better, because it yields a shorter detector system dead time and thus can count at a higher rate. Figure 2.5 shows pulses from two different scintillators, one fast and one slow, but with the same light output (measured as the area under the curve.) A detector made with a scintillator that yields a high, short curve would have a shorter dead time.

3. Stopping power. The density (ρ) of a material, particularly electron density, and the prevalence of elements with a high atomic number (Z, or effective Z [Z_{eff}]) within it dictate the ability of a material to stop incident radiation. A lower-density, lower-Z material must be thicker than a higher density, higher-Z material to have the same intrinsic detection efficiency for high-energy radiation.

Other important factors that differentiate scintillators include ease of use (ruggedness), expense, and availability. A vast assortment of scintillators are available. Of the materials that make useful scintillators for nuclear medicine, a salt, thallium-activated sodium iodide—NaI(Tl); light output, 38,000 photons/MeV; λ, 230 ns; ρ, 3.67 g/cm³; Z_{eff}, 50.6—is by far the most widespread. The best feature is a high light output. This scintillator has a medium decay time and is moderately dense, but it is not

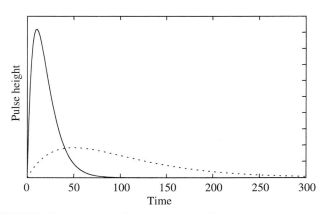

FIGURE 2.5. Long pulse–short pulse. Two pulses with equal area, representing equal energies, but with different time characteristics.

ideal for high-rate counting of high-energy radiation. NaI(Tl) also is highly susceptible to moisture (hygroscopic), which makes it challenging to use and maintain in a hermetically sealed environment.

The next most commonly used scintillator in nuclear medicine, bismuth germanate (BGO), is from a class of crystals called orthosilicates. Orthosilicates tend to have a high density and Z_{eff}, hence excellent stopping powers, and other desirable features, such as fast decay time, useful in high counting rate applications, but none has greater light output than NaI(Tl). BGO has much lower light output than does NaI(Tl) and a slower decay time (light output, 8,000 photons/MeV; λ, 300 ns; ρ, 7.13 g/cm^3; Z_{eff}, 74.2) but is much denser, making it somewhat more suitable for detection of high-energy photons, such as those from positron annihilation. Because of the desirability of density, speed, and energy resolution for the ideal PET scintillator, several good prospects have been evaluated, such as gadolinium oxyorthosilicate (GSO) (4) and lutetium oxyorthosilicate (LSO), and are being put to use (5).

Photomultiplier Tube

Optically connected to the scintillator material is a light detection device. In most cases, this is a photomultiplier tube. As depicted in Fig. 2.6, an incident light photon is stopped in the front thin layer of metal (called the *photocathode*), and an electron is ejected. This electron is accelerated toward an electrode called a *dynode* that has a much higher (positive) voltage than does the photocathode, When the electron hits the dynode, several electrons are ejected. These are accelerated toward a second

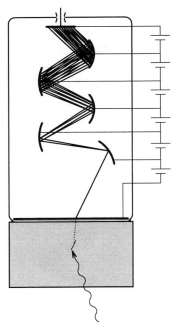

FIGURE 2.6. Photomultiplier with scintillator. Some of the light generated in the scintillator is directed at the photocathode of the photomultiplier tube. A fraction of this light releases photoelectrons when it hits the photocathode. This signal is amplified through the successive dynode stages.

dynode, where the process is repeated. Several more dynodes are held at successively higher voltages, and at each stage, the number of electrons is multiplied. At the final stage (anode) many electrons accumulate and leave the photomultiplier as an electronic pulse. For each scintillation event, many light photons hit the photocathode, some of which are converted to electrons. This electron signal is amplified substantially by the successive dynode stages. The energy resolution is ultimately dependent on the number of electrons ejected at the photocathode, which depends on the number of light photons hitting the photocathode and the conversion efficiency of the photocathode.

Signal Processing

Once the charge signal leaves the photomultiplier, it is processed through several stages of electronics. Although the choice of components depends on the application, it is customary to have a preamplifier stage, which converts the emitted charge signal into a voltage, and additional amplification and pulse shaping. The resulting signal can be fed into a single-channel analyzer (SCA), which determines whether the signal size is within a specified range, or a multichannel analyzer (MCA) which is essentially many SCAs with narrow energy widths that abut one another. An MCA processes a signal and determines which of many possible ranges it was in, much like determining in which bin of a histogram a particular measurement falls into. Similar to an MCA is an analog-to-digital converter (ADC), which assigns a number to the size of the pulse and allows analysis of the spectrum of detected events. An example of energy discrimination signal processing is shown in the pulses of Fig. 2.2. Only the first signal sequence differentiates the independent pulses. The latter two would yield an energy value greater than the magnitude of a single pulse, and thus could be discriminated or rejected with an SCA or MCA unit.

Energy Measurement and Energy Resolution

The energy of a high-energy photon hitting a scintillation detector ideally is proportional to the size of the pulse leaving the photomultiplier tube, because all of the stages (conversion of photon energy into electron kinetic energy, conversion of electron kinetic energy into ionization and excitation of atoms, emission of light from excited atoms, conversion of the light at the photocathode, and amplification of the charge) are linear. In practice, for photons in the range relevant to nuclear medicine, this proportionality is reliable. The important implication is that once a scintillation detector is calibrated (determination of a ratio between incident particle energy and charge emitted from the photomultiplier tube), the calibration factor can be applied to any measured pulse for accurate determination of the energy of the incident particle.

Energy resolution in scintillation detectors is directly related to the number of photoelectrons generated at the photocathode of the photomultiplier tube. The more photoelectrons released, the better is the energy resolution. The number of photoelectrons generated is proportional to the following independent factors:

1. The energy of the incident photon
2. The intrinsic light output and conversion efficiency of the scintillator material
3. The generated light collected at the photocathode
4. The conversion efficiency of the photocathode

Energy resolution is typically expressed as FWHM. The units of this width measure are the same as the units of the energy measurement. For example, a detector may yield 14-keV FWHM energy resolution for 140 keV photons. A commonly used dimensionless or normalized measure of energy resolution comes from dividing the FWHM by the incident photon energy and is expressed as a percentage, as follows:

$$\text{Resolution} = \text{FWHM}/E * 100\% \qquad [3]$$

The 14-keV FWHM measurement for 140 keV photons would therefore be 10% energy resolution. This is a typical value for NaI(Tl) detectors.

Energy Spectrum in Scintillation Detectors

The range of energy values measured in a specific experiment is called the *energy spectrum* (1,2) and can be measured with an MCA or ADC. A perfect radiation detector would always yield the same measurement for the particular incident photon energy. Many factors, however, prevent the actual measured spectrum of a monoenergetic beam of photons from yielding a single value.

There is a limit to the energy resolution of a scintillation detector. Therefore an inherent range of values, centered and peaked at the true value, are measured for a monoenergetic beam of photons. The region in the energy spectrum centered on the true photon energy but blurred by the finite energy resolution is called the *photopeak region*.

Compton Events

In many cases, an incident photon deposits some but not all of its energy in the scintillator. Compton scattering interactions occur between photons and outer-shell electrons. For example, the photon can Compton scatter and leave the detector (Fig. 2.7). Only a fraction of the energy of the incident particle is transferred to the detector. Such Compton events are more prevalent in low-efficiency detectors, those not thick enough to stop the scattered photon. There is a maximum amount of energy a particle can deposit in Compton scattering (when it scatters backward), and there is a corresponding peak in the energy spectrum.

If there is material between the photon source and the detec-

tor, there is a chance that the photon will scatter once or more in that material, entering the detector with less than its initial energy. Such photons add to the energy spectrum everywhere below the photopeak. The energy spectrum of Compton-scattered photons is determined with Eq. 4:

$$E_1 = \frac{E_0}{1 + \frac{E_0}{m_e c^2}(1 - \cos\theta)} \qquad [4]$$

where E_0 is the incident photon energy, E_1 is the scattered photon energy, θ is the scattering angle ($\theta = 0$ means no scattering), m_e is the electron mass, c is the speed of light, and $m_e c^2$ is the energy associated with the electron mass (511 keV). For the maximum scattering angle ($\theta = 180$ degrees, also called *backscattering*) and therefore maximum energy loss, the scattered photon leaves with energy, as determined with Eq. 5:

$$E_1 = \frac{E_0}{1 + \frac{2 \cdot E_0}{m_e c^2}} \qquad [5]$$

For this maximal scattering, the energy imparted to the electron is

$$E_m = \frac{E_0}{1 + \frac{m_e c^2}{2 \cdot E_0}} \qquad [6]$$

The spectrum of energy lost in the scintillation crystal for Compton events in which there is a single scattering and the photon leaves the crystal and therefore has a maximum (the Compton peak) is found with Eq. 6. A peak is observed in the energy spectrum at this maximum value. For photons with an incident energy of 140 keV, the Compton peak is 49.6 keV. For 511-keV photons, the Compton peak is 340 keV.

Backscatter Peak

In some cases, a photon enters the detector after already having scattered. The minimum energy a photon can have after scattering once is found with Eq. 5.

Lead X-rays

Material between the source and the detector—specifically, lead used for collimation—can generate x-rays when hit with the higher-energy emitted radiation. Such x-rays can enter the detector and be counted. These x-rays are recorded at energies unique to the material emitting them. An energy spectrum showing all the aforedescribed effects is shown in Fig. 2.8.

Examples of Scintillation Detectors
Well Counter

In a well counter, a cylinder of thick NaI(Tl) with a hole in the center (Fig. 2.9) has high geometric efficiency for accurate measurement of small amounts (a few microcuries) of radioactivity. An SCA is used to count the events in the photopeak for

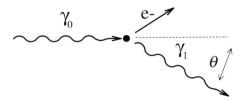

FIGURE 2.7. Compton scattering.

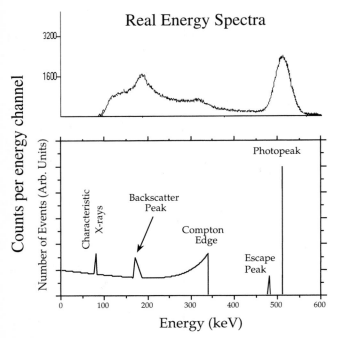

FIGURE 2.8. Real energy spectrum in scintillator. *Top,* measured energy spectrum from 511-keV photons in a 12-mm-thick NaI(Tl) gamma camera. These data were obtained with a low-energy cutoff that precluded detection of lead x-rays. *Bottom,* various components of the spectrum.

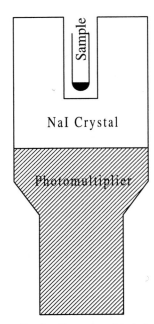

FIGURE 2.9. Schematic of well counter. A hole in the scintillator coupled to the photomultiplier tube is used for sampling.

the sample being measured. The efficiency of the detector can be calibrated for a particular energy so the number of counts can be converted into units of radioactivity. Because the detection efficiency and dead time are both large for this system, severe count-rate losses occur if the sample is more than a few microcuries in strength.

Gamma Camera

A gamma camera, discussed thoroughly in Chapter 3, consists of a large sheet of NaI(Tl) and many photomultipliers that cover the back side. The multiple signals are processed to yield the energy as well as the position at which the photon hit the camera. Some gamma camera designs incorporate quantized or discrete NaI(Tl) or other scintillator or solid-state elements with which to make images.

Positron Emission Tomography

Most conventional PET scanners contain many BGO detectors (6) in a ring to detect the pair of photons emitted from positron annihilation. Some scanners also have sheets of NaI(Tl) (7) or even GSO (4) or LSO (5). Intrinsic efficiency is particularly important in these systems because of the high energy of the radiation and because of the requirement that both emitted photons be detected.

Surgical Probes

Very small scintillators and associated instrumentation are used to make handheld detectors that can be used intraoperatively to allow surgeons to measure regions with a high concentration of radiotracer (8).

GASEOUS DETECTORS

Principles

A simple gas-filled detector is shown in Fig. 2.10. A positively charged wire is located inside a gas-filled cylinder with a conducting wall. When a charged particle passes through the gas, energy is transferred from the particle to ionize atoms by means of Compton scattering with outer-shell electrons. The particle

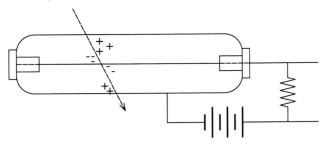

FIGURE 2.10. Simple gas-filled detector. High positive voltage is maintained on the wire in the middle. Liberated electrons (from the passage of radiation) travel toward the wire while the positive ions migrate toward the outer, negative wall of the cylinder.

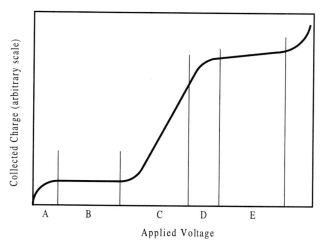

FIGURE 2.11. Gas voltage response. The charge collected in a gas detector as a function of applied voltage. Scales are relative.

of amplification increases linearly with the applied voltage. Above this region, the proportionality breaks down because an increasingly large fraction of the gas atoms are already ionized.

Geiger-Mueller Region (Region E)

At high enough voltage, complete breakdown of the gas is caused by any amount of primary ionization. A system that operates in this region gives a sizable pulse for any ionizing particle that interacts in it. This breakdown must be quenched for the system to be ready to detect another particle. This quenching is accomplished either actively, by means of lowering the applied voltage after a detected pulse, or passively with specific gases.

Spontaneous Breakdown Region (Region >E)

At even higher voltages, gases break down and spontaneously ionize. This region is not useful for particle detection because there would be no additional signal from the interaction of a particle.

Although the actual voltage associated with each region depends on the geometric configuration of the detector, hundreds of volts typically are applied for operations in any of these regions. Because ionization occurs with any gas, air is used in many systems between the electrodes. Gas-filled detectors are less expensive and more portable than scintillator-based detectors. The efficiency for detecting individual photons is not as good as with scintillator-based detectors, and energy is typically not measured per interaction because few photons loose all their energy in the gas.

Examples of Gas-Filled Detectors

Dose Calibrator

A dose calibrator is used to measure radioactive doses. The high voltage is applied to the gas between two concentric cylinders (Fig. 2.12). When a radioactive source is placed in the middle

therefore leaves a track of electrons and ions. If the electric field across the gas is strong enough, the free electrons move toward the positive pole, and the positive ions move toward the negative pole. The result is a collection of charge at the electrodes.

Depending on the amount of voltage applied to the gas and the geometric configuration of the electrodes (wire inside tube, parallel plates, concentric cylinders), a variety of effects may be observed. In general, the size of the collected charge increases with increasing voltage. The levels of response are depicted in Fig. 2.11. In some regions, the charge increases quickly with increasing applied voltage. In other regions, there is little or no increase in collected charge with increasing applied voltage. The regions are described in order of increasing voltage.

Recombination Region (Region A)

At low enough voltages, some of the liberated electrons recombine with ions and therefore do not collect at the positive anode. The number of collected electrons is less than the number of atoms originally ionized. This region is not useful for efficient particle detection.

Ion Chamber Region (Region B)

In this voltage range, recombination is minimal, and most freed electrons are collected at the anode. The collected charge does not vary much with the applied voltage in this region, implying good stability. The output current per incident particle is lower than in the higher-voltage regions.

Proportionality Region (Region C)

At higher voltages, amplification occurs as the electrons are accelerated to high enough energy to produce new ion pairs in collisions with gas molecules, and a limited cascade forms. At the higher voltages in this region, the collected number of electrons can be a thousand times the number of electrons freed by the primary radiation. This region is so named because the amount

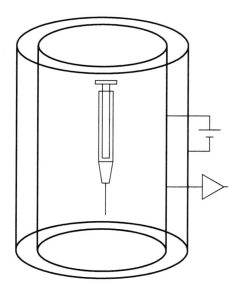

FIGURE 2.12. Diagram of dose calibrator.

of the calibrator, most of the emitted radiation passes through the region between the cylinders, and the gas is ionized. The charge is collected and digitized to yield a measure of the ionization in the gas. This measurement indicates the amount of radiation in the source.

Conversion between radioactivity level and the amount of the ionization depends on the particular radionuclide. For example, a nuclide with multiple emissions per decay has more ionization per decay than does a nuclide with a single emission. The level of ionization also depends on the emitted energy. Therefore it is necessary to have different calibration factors for each radionuclide.

Dose calibrators are used to measure a wide range of radioactivity, from a few microcuries to several hundred millicuries. An example of a calibrator is shown in Fig. 2.13. The device has two rows of buttons. The lower row includes a button for each of the commonly used radionuclides in nuclear medicine. Pushing the appropriate button establishes the calibration between collected current and radioactivity level for that sample. For radionuclides with no preset calibration, manual calibration can be performed with the knob at the left. The upper row of buttons is used to select the order of magnitude (range) of the radioactive source strength.

The geometric efficiency of dose calibrators is high but variable, depending on the location of the source. It is important that sources be located at a position of maximal sensitivity. In

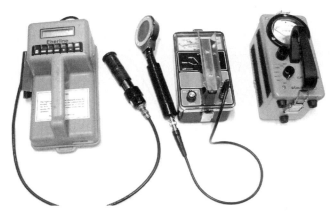

FIGURE 2.14. Three types of portable survey meters.

addition to geometric effects, the volume of the source, if it is in solution, affects the dose measurement because of self-attenuation effects.

Survey Meters

Three handheld surveying devices are shown in Fig. 2.14. At right is an ionization chamber used to measure the current from ionizing particles. Such devices are useful for assessing radioactive dose levels. At the left and in the center are Geiger-Mueller devices. These devices are used to detect individual particles. The rate of detection is shown on a meter and pulses are indicated with an audible response. Geiger-Mueller devices are good for finding spilled material in contaminated regions.

Personal Dosimeters

Small gas-filled tubes containing a charged capacitor can be used to roughly measure personal exposure. When radiation traverses the tube, ionized gas particles discharge the capacitor in proportion to the source strength.

SOLID-STATE DETECTORS

As in gas-filled detectors, in solid-state detectors, radiation ionizes the molecules in a solid, semiconducting material across which there is a voltage. Solid-state detectors have very good energy resolution and have much better stopping power than do gas-filled detectors. High-purity germanium detectors have been used in nuclear medicine, but in very specialized circumstances, because they must be operated at very low temperatures. Solid-state detectors, such as the cadmium telluride (CdTe) are used in some intraoperative surgical probes (8,9).

REFERENCES

1. Knoll GF. *Radiation detection and measurement.* New York: John Wiley & Sons, 1979.

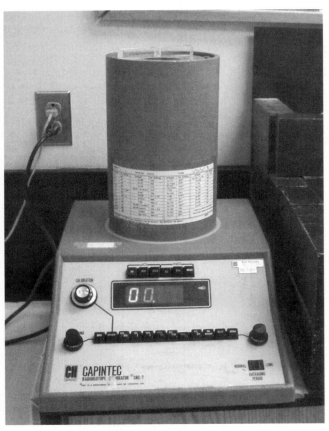

FIGURE 2.13. Dose calibrator.

2. Leo WR. *Techniques for nuclear and particle physics experiments (a how-to approach),* 2nd ed. Berlin: Springer-Verlag, 1994.

3. Birks JB. *Theory and practice of scintillation counting.* Oxford, UK: Pergamon Press, 1964.

4. Takagi K, Fukazawa T. Cerium-activated Gd2SiO5 single crystal scintillator. *Appl Phys Lett* 1983;42:43–45.

5. Melcher CL, Schweitzer JS. A promising new scintillator: cerium-doped lutetium oxyorthsilicate. *Nucl Instrum Methods Phys Med A* 1992;314:212–214.

6. Casey ME, Nutt R. A multicrystal two dimensional BGO detector system for positron emission tomography. *IEEE Trans Nucl Sci* 1986;33:460–463.

7. Karp JS, Muehllehner G. Performance of a position-sensitive scintillation detector. *Phys Med Biol.* 1985;30:643–655.

8. Hoffman EJ, Tornai MP, Janecek M, et al. Intraoperative probes and imaging probes. *Eur J Nucl Med* 1999;26:913–935.

9. Knoll GF. Semiconductor detectors and their applications in medical imaging. *Phys Med* 1993;9:33–39.

SUGGESTED READING

Attix FH. *Introduction to radiological physics and radiation dosimetry.* New York: John Wiley & Sons, 1986.

Sorenson JA, Phelps ME. *Physics in nuclear medicine,* 2nd ed. Orlando, FL: Grune & Stratton, 1987.

ANGER SCINTILLATION CAMERA

L. STEPHEN GRAHAM
CRAIG S. LEVIN
GERD MUEHLLEHNER

The Anger scintillation camera is the standard instrument of choice for imaging both static and dynamic radionuclide distributions in vivo. Since its commercial introduction in 1964 (1), the Anger camera has improved dramatically in all basic performance parameters—field-of-view, uniformity, spatial resolution, energy resolution, and ability to handle high incident count rates. The evolution of this device was shaped by the need for faithful imaging of the 140-keV γ-rays emitted by ^{99m}Tc. The combination of this generator-produced radionuclide and the Anger camera has provided nuclear medicine physicians with a powerful tool that has contributed to the continued growth of the field of nuclear medicine.

Although other approaches to imaging low-energy γ-rays have been explored (e.g., image intensifiers, solid-state detectors, or position-sensitive proportional chambers), changes in the Anger camera have kept this device the instrument of choice for a wide variety of clinical studies. One of the major milestones occurred in 1977, when the prototype of today's single photon emission computed tomography (SPECT) cameras was introduced by Jaszczak et al. (2) on the basis of principles described in 1963 by Kuhl and Edwards (3). Apart from continued improvement in detector performance and stability, recent developments have focused on increases in sensitivity (multiple detectors and the use of magnifying collimators), the addition of features that enhance image quality, such as the ability to perform noncircular orbits, and the use of extremely powerful computers for reconstruction, analysis, and display of images. In all state-of-the-art systems, operation of the camera is fully integrated into the computer. This chapter describes the principles of operation of the modern Anger scintillation camera, describes its fundamental performance parameters, and summarizes recent improvements.

PRINCIPLES OF OPERATION

Figure 3.1 is a block diagram of an Anger camera. A projected image of the radionuclide distribution is formed by means of

L.S. Graham: VA Greater Los Angeles Healthcare System and Biological Imaging, UCLA School of Medicine, Los Angeles, CA.

C.S. Levin: Radiology, UC San Diego School of Medicine and Nuclear Medicine, San Diego VA Medical Center, San Diego, CA.

G. Muehllehner: Philips Medical Systems, Philadelphia, PA.

interactions in a thin thallium-activated sodium iodide [NaI(Tl)] scintillation crystal from γ-ray photons that pass through the collimator holes. Visible and ultraviolet light produced in the crystal at the site of interaction travels outward in all directions and is detected with an array of photomultipliers that convert the light distribution into a set of electronic signals. The position logic circuit converts these voltage pulses into x and y position signals and calculates the centroid of the light distribution. The position signals are then divided by the energy signal so that image size is independent of the incident γ-ray energy. This subset of the electronics is called the *ratio circuit*. Only events that fall within a specific energy range corresponding to the photon energy of the administered radionuclide are used for further processing. The position and energy signals are then corrected with digital processors that compensate for imperfections in the crystal-photomultiplier assembly and in the position logic circuit. Most manufacturers correct the energy signal first as a function of its uncorrected position. The event position is corrected as a function of its corrected energy. Finally, the pro-

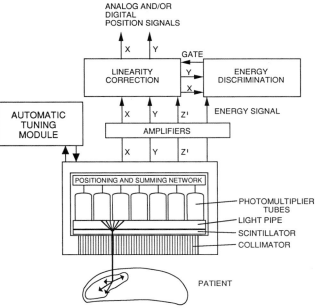

FIGURE 3.1. Anger scintillation camera.

cessed *x* and *y* position information is used to form an image of the radionuclide distribution one event at a time either on an analog display system, such as a high-resolution cathode ray tube (CRT), or in digital memory. A number of vendors include special circuits that automatically balance the photomultiplier tubes. This operation minimizes the effect of drift and aging of electronic components.

Collimation

A collimator projects an image of the radionuclide distribution onto the scintillation crystal by absorbing γ-rays that do not travel in the desired direction. Although collimation was covered in detail in the previous edition, only a brief overview is presented here. The first cameras were fitted with pinhole collimators (4). An inverted, mirror image was formed on the detector, the image size determined by the position of the object relative to the aperture. Because of the pinhole's low sensitivity owing to the small aperture size (3 to 10 mm), pinhole collimators are now commonly used only for imaging small objects, such as the thyroid or lachrymal glands. In these cases, high-resolution images can be obtained because of magnification.

Markedly higher sensitivity for larger objects is obtained with parallel-hole collimators, the most commonly used type (1). The radionuclide distribution is projected onto the scintillation detector without magnification. These collimators can be modified to the appropriate spatial resolution and sensitivity for a variety of clinical needs and to properly handle photons from many different radionuclides. A variant of this design is the slant-hole collimator used for gated blood-pool imaging. If the holes are set at an angle of 30 degrees to the normal configuration, the face of the collimator can be positioned closer to the patient in the left anterior oblique view.

Diverging collimators are used when the object is larger than the field of view of parallel-hole collimators. Because the holes are aligned so they focus to a point behind the detector, the image is minified. These collimators were developed primarily to accommodate large organs, such as the liver, spleen, or both lungs, with a camera having a small field of view (5). The increased field of view must, however, be traded for decreased resolution or lower sensitivity. With the advent of large-field-of-view circular and rectangular detectors, the need for these collimators has largely been eliminated. However, single-axis di-

verging collimators are still used on a few systems for whole-body imaging.

Converging collimators are similar to diverging collimators except that the holes are focused to a point in front of the detector. As such, a converging collimator magnifies the object, usually to a lesser degree than do pinhole collimators, and provides better resolution and sensitivity than does a comparable parallel-hole collimator (6). Because the magnification changes as a function of distance from the surface of the collimator, the projected image looks different from the image obtained with a parallel-hole collimator (7). Objects farther from the face collimator are more highly magnified.

γ-Ray Detection

After passing through the collimator holes, the γ-rays may interact with the NaI(Tl) scintillation crystal. At low energy (< 100 keV) the primary mode of interaction is photoelectric, and the stopping power approaches 100% (Table 3.1). As photon energy increases, the probability of Compton scatter in the crystal increases, and the stopping power decreases rapidly. A γ-ray scattered in the crystal can escape from the crystal, interact by means of a photoelectric event or undergo multiple scattering, and be totally absorbed within the crystal. If all the energy is deposited in the crystal by means of one or more events, the energy signal falls within the photopeak, and the photon is used in image formation.

Table 3.1 shows the probability of a photoelectric interaction and the probability that the total energy will fall within the photopeak as a function of crystal thickness and γ-ray energy (8). If the first interaction in the crystal is a single photoelectric event, all the light is emitted from a region less than 1 mm in diameter. If, however, the γ-ray first interacts by means of one or more Compton scatter interactions and finally deposits all of its energy in the crystal, the position logic circuit calculates a set of *x, y* coordinates that does not correspond to the point of entry into the crystal. This scenario produces a loss of spatial resolution that is even worse at high energy (8,9). At lower energy (<140 keV), loss of spatial resolution is primarily caused by the limited amount of light emitted by the crystal, as discussed later. Thus there are two competing effects. As the energy of the γ-ray increases, more energy can be deposited in the crystal

Table 3.1. *Probabilities of photopeak and photoelectric interactions in sodium iodide for various crystal thicknesses*

Gamma Ray Energy (keV)	Photopeak			Photoelectric		
	6.25 mm	9.52 mm[a]	12.5 mm	6.25 mm	9.52 mm[a]	12.5 mm
100	0.965	0.97	0.990	0.863	0.87	0.882
150	0.707	0.85	0.909	0.568	0.66	0.707
200	0.452	0.60	0.715	0.332	0.43	0.487
280	0.236	0.34	0.444	0.148	0.20	0.245
360	0.143	0.22	0.298	0.078	0.11	0.136
511	0.071	0.12	0.169	0.034	0.045	0.056

[a]Values determined by nonlinear interpolation of data from Anger and Davis (8).
Data from Anger HO, Davis DH. Gamma-ray detection efficiency and image resolution in sodium iodide. *Rev Sci Instrum* 1964;35:693–697.

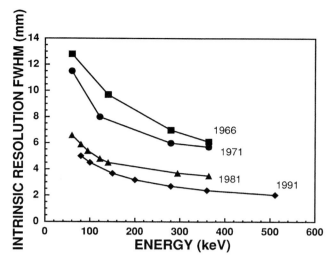

FIGURE 3.2. Intrinsic spatial resolution of Anger camera. Resolution of the Anger camera as a function of energy. **A:** From 1966, a 25-cm field-of-view camera with a 12.5-mm-thick crystal. **B:** From 1971, a 25-cm field-of-view camera with a 12.5-mm-thick crystal. **C:** From 1981, a 38-cm field-of-view camera with 9.5-mm-thick crystal. **D:** From 1991, a 38-cm field-of-view camera with 9.5-mm-thick crystal.

and more light is emitted. Because the amount of light is approximately proportional to the energy of the γ-ray (10), and the brighter the light flashes, the less relative fluctuation there is in the electronic pulses used for positioning, this effect should improve spatial resolution. As the energy of the γ-ray increases, however, a larger fraction of the total photopeak interactions are of the Compton photoelectric type, which produces inaccurate positioning information. Thus the most important improvement in spatial resolution over the years has been at lower energies, as can be seen from the data presented in Fig. 3.2. There have only been slight improvements in intrinsic spatial resolution since 1991. Most state-of-the-art cameras fall in the range of 3.0- to 3.5-mm full width at half maximum (FWHM) at 140 keV.

Light Distribution and Event Localization

The light released from thallium in a NaI(Tl) crystal spreads in all directions. Because it is hygroscopic, NaI is enclosed in a container that has an aluminum entrance window for incoming γ-ray photons and a glass exit window for outgoing scintillation light. To minimize the loss of light at interfaces, a silicon compound or special bonding material is used to optically couple the glass exit window of the detector "can" to the "light pipe" or photomultiplier tubes (many newer cameras no longer have light pipes). When light reaches the photomultiplier tube, many photons interact with its photocathode, which releases electrons known as *photoelectrons*. This signal is then amplified by a series of electrodes called *dynodes* set at increasingly higher voltages. In the photocathode plane, the light intensity has a bell-shaped distribution with its center directly above the point of scintillation. The photomultipliers sample this distribution at discrete intervals. When the photomultipliers are moved closer to the crystal, the bell-shaped distribution becomes narrower, but at

the same time, fewer tubes provide useful signals. Because the limiting factor in spatial resolution—at least for a γ-ray energy of 140 keV—is the statistical accuracy of each photomultiplier tube signal, bringing the photomultipliers closer to the crystal produces larger, more accurate signals. Because the light distribution is narrower in this design, the photomultiplier diameter can be reduced and the number of photomultiplier tubes increased to provide finer sampling of the "light" and cover the same area. State-of-the-art cameras have as many as 107 photomultiplier tubes. The result of positioning the photomultipliers closer to the crystal is an improvement in spatial resolution but at the cost of positional distortion and lack of flood-field uniformity because of incorrect centroid determination.

Two different approaches are currently used to determine the position of x-ray and γ-ray interactions. The basic analog Anger positioning circuit finds the centroid of the light samples taken by the photomultipliers for each event. It has two inherent shortcomings. First, the centroid of the samples obtained with the photomultipliers does not necessarily correspond to the centroid of the light distribution. The result is mispositioning of the event and compression of the positioned events toward the centers of the photomultipliers (11). Second, each signal is treated as if it carried equal position information, thus summing the contributions from the photomultipliers in a less than optimum manner.

Light that reaches the photomultipliers after an x-ray or γ-ray interacts with the NaI is converted into weak electronic signals in the photocathode that are subsequently amplified, first by internal multiplication in the photomultiplier tube itself and then by external electronic preamplifiers. These signals are combined in a position logic circuit that gives each photomultiplier signal different weights to derive the position information. In many newer systems, the event position is calculated from the digitized output of the preamplifiers (described later).

Changes in crystal configuration and light pipe design affect light distribution and thereby the relative signals received by the photomultipliers. When opaque masks are placed between the crystal and light pipe, light can be redirected, and the shape of the light response function can be altered to achieve uniform spatial resolution across the image and improve flood-field uniformity (12). These masks are not commonly used on today's cameras because they limit intrinsic spatial and energy resolution.

An alternative is to amplify the signals from the photomultipliers in a nonlinear preamplifier (13,14) to change the contributions of the photomultiplier signals to the position signals (Fig. 3.3A). This nonlinear amplifier functions in two ways: (a) small signals that are statistically poor in information are eliminated with threshold preamplifiers (13) and (b) large signals are reduced in amplitude (14). Figure 3.3B illustrates the photomultiplier tube output in a camera with a Pyrex heat-resistant glass light pipe. If the scintillation occurs directly under the center of the photomultiplier, that tube receives the largest signal. Small displacements around the center cause only relatively small changes in signal amplitude. Correction for this problem is somewhat complicated by the fact that the shape of the nonlinear response changes with interaction depth in the crystal, which varies with incident photon energy. On average, low-energy photons interact nearer the crystal entrance surface than do high-energy photons. This interaction depth effect, however, does

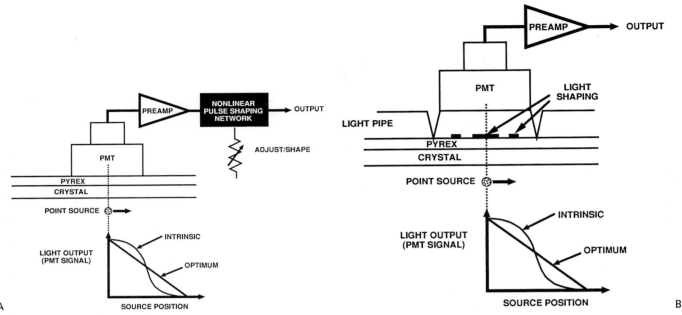

FIGURE 3.3. Light collection from an Anger camera without and with a light pipe. **A:** When a light pipe is not present, a sigmoidal response is obtained. A nonlinear pulse-shaping network can be used to "linearize" the intrinsic response. **B:** The optimum response is a linear decrease in signal intensity as a source is moved away from the central axis of the photomultiplier tube. Without a light pipe, a sigmoidal response is obtained. Use of a light pipe and masks for producing light shaping gives a nearly linear response. (Courtesy of Eric Woronowicz, Ph.D., 1989.)

not significantly change the light distribution because of reflections from the magnesium oxide (MgO) that coats the aluminum entrance window. However, it can affect the total amount of light collected.

Genna et al. (15) in 1981 proposed a digital technique that essentially corresponded to nonlinear amplification with optimum weights in which the photomultiplier signals are digitized and, depending on their amplitude, are transformed into weighted signals that sharply reduce the contribution of the photomultiplier directly above the scintillation. Several vendors now use this general approach. The signal from each photomultiplier tube is digitized with a high-speed analog-to-digital converter (ADC). Event position is calculated with algorithms that can incorporate thresholding and nonlinear response as a function of energy. This approach also provides the opportunity to use sophisticated algorithms for optimizing the final determination of the interaction site.

Energy Discrimination and Correction

After a scintillation event is detected, the energy pulse is examined to assure that only events falling in the photopeak are accepted. As suggested by Svedberg (16), two different approaches can be used to generate the energy pulse (Z' and energy signals in Fig. 3.1). One approach is to use the same signal used for position pulse normalization (Z'). This pulse is optimized to provide the best overall linearity. A second approach is to generate an energy signal that is optimized for uniform signal amplitude over the entire detector area, especially near the edge of the crystal. Even when the latter is used, local variations in light

output or light collection efficiency necessitate use of a digital correction method, as described later.

Good energy discrimination is essential to reduce the amount of radiation that undergoes Compton scattering in a patient and reaches the detector with reduced energy. Because the energy resolution at 140 keV has improved from approximately 16% in 1975 to 8% to 10% today (Fig. 3.2), the energy window must be reduced by an equivalent amount (from 20% to 12%) to take full advantage of the improvement. On an angle-by-angle basis, low-energy photons lose less energy when they are scattered than do high-energy photons. This means it is more likely that scatter events will appear in the photopeak for low-energy photons, and therefore, scattered radiation is more of a problem for low-energy photons than for high-energy photons.

When a collimated point source is moved across the detector face, there may be a variation in point-source sensitivity (counts per unit of time) largely caused by shifts in the photopeak relative to the energy acceptance window. These variations can be caused by changes in the crystal or electronic components and can be reduced by means of proper gain setting and correct tuning of the photomultiplier tubes. The fluctuations also can be caused by an optical design in which the efficiency of light collection varies as a function of position.

Using a simple spatially invariant energy window has the following disadvantages: (a) the energy resolution is worse than it should be because all regions of the camera are treated in common, (b) the point-source sensitivity varies from region to region as the photopeak shifts in relation to the window, and (c) the detector design must be compromised to minimize energy variation at a sacrifice in spatial resolution.

Because shifts in the position of the photopeak are functions of position, it is possible to measure and record the location of the photopeak corresponding to each pixel of a 128 × 128 or finer matrix and to use this information to correct for variations in photopeak position. An event-by-event processor uses the *x, y* coordinates to find the photopeak information for that position and then either moves the energy window (17) or adjusts the energy signal amplitude to compensate for spatial variations in photopeak amplitude (Fig. 3.4). It has been shown (17) that this correction is valid over a wide range of energy-window widths, γ-ray energy, incident count rates, and scatter conditions. A further refinement of this technique involves changing the width of the energy window to compensate for positional variations in energy resolution (18), but this method is not used on current cameras.

Correction for Spatial Nonlinearity

Spatial nonlinearity is systematic error in the positioning of scintillation events. Such distortion is caused by nonlinear changes in the light distributions in the scintillator as a function of location. Because the linear Anger camera arithmetic scheme is not adequate to compensate for these effects, events are not recorded in their true location. The errors are smaller than the positioning error resulting from statistical uncertainty in the number of photons received by each photomultiplier for each event. However, these small distortions cause visible changes in intensity because the displacements are applied to all events in a particular nonlinear region.

Lack of uniformity resulting from spatial distortion is caused by local count compression or expansion (19). To be visually noticeable in an image of line- or orthogonal hole-pattern phantoms, such distortions must exceed several millimeters in spatial displacement. To be seen in clinical images, the distortions must be even more severe. However, nonlinearity can cause unacceptable flood-field variation even when the displacement is less than 1 mm. For example, if a circular area of 20 mm is compressed 0.4 mm toward its center from all directions (as would be the case under the center of a photomultiplier), the effective area is reduced from $100\pi mm^2$ to $92\pi mm^2$. This causes an 8% increase in count density in the perimeter of that area. Thus spatial distortion causes noticeable lack of flood-field uniformity well

before displacement is visually apparent in line-pattern images. Nonlinearity is the primary cause of lack of flood-field uniformity, although local shifts of the photopeak contribute to this problem as well (20).

Distortion can be corrected through event-by-event processing during data collection. First the displacements must be accurately measured by means of acquisition of a high statistics slit or orthogonal hole test pattern image with a fine image matrix (at least 128 × 128 or as high as 512 × 512). Because the true location is known and the actual (distorted) location in the image is measured, a displacement correction can be calculated for all source locations in the field of view. As data are collected, the raw *x* and *y* digital coordinates of each event are corrected in real time by the displacement factors and repositioned. With both energy and nonlinearity corrections applied, the result is uniformity. In some cameras, however, this operation is not totally energy independent. When nuclides other than ^{99m}Tc are used, renormalization maps are needed in most cameras. These are usually based on high-count intrinsic flood images acquired with the radionuclide of interest.

If a scintillation camera is designed for good spatial resolution, large areas of distortion are present. Figure 3.5 (top row) shows an example of a line-pattern image acquired with a large-field-of-view camera both before and after energy and linearity corrections were made. Figure 3.5 (bottom row) shows the energy-corrected flood-field image both before and after linearity correction. This figure clearly shows that distortion can be the most important factor in lack of flood-field uniformity. Because they are inherent in the design, these distortions generally are independent of width of the energy window, incident count rate, and scatter conditions (11).

Through the introduction of digital techniques for spatially

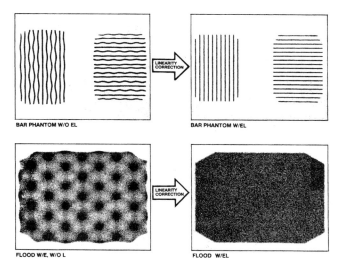

FIGURE 3.5. Lack of linearity without and with energy and linearity correction. **A:** *Top left,* intrinsic slit-pattern image with energy and linearity correction turned off. *Top right,* intrinsic slit pattern image with energy and linearity correction turned on. **B:** *Bottom left,* intrinsic flood with energy correction on and linearity correction off. *Bottom right,* intrinsic flood with energy and linearity correction turned on. (From *Technicare introduces sentinel electronics.* Solon, OH: Technicare Corporation, 1984, with permission.)

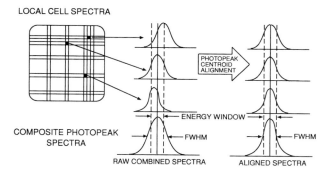

FIGURE 3.4. Energy correction. The energy deposited in the NaI(Tl) crystal by individual events is corrected for spatial variations in amplitude of the energy signal according to measured variations as a function of position (energy map). Alignment of the spectra greatly improves the overall energy resolution of the camera.

varying energy discrimination and removal of spatial distortion, a major constraint has been removed from scintillation camera design. Figure 3.5 shows, as an intermediate step, highly distorted but high-resolution images measured with the analog processor before and after the digital processor corrects for lack of linearity. This increased design freedom can lead to improved spatial resolution compared with that of an analog processor. By means of replacement of the analog positioning circuitry with ADCs and software techniques, even more complex position determination can be done, as can compensation for changes in photon energy.

AUTOMATIC TUNING

For the energy and linearity correction circuits to work properly, it is imperative that the photomultiplier tubes be properly balanced, as they must be when the correction factors are generated, and that all electronic circuits be stable with respect to time. Temporal changes in the gain of the photomultiplier tubes and drifts of electronic components can partially or completely invalidate the corrections and produce significant lack of uniformity (21). Environmental influences on the detector, such as changing magnetic fields and temperature, can also produce a loss of uniformity. To minimize this problem, a number of camera manufacturers have added circuits to monitor photomultiplier tube gain and automatically "tune" the detector. Different techniques are used, but they can be divided into two general categories—on-demand and continuous.

On-demand Tuning

The Epic series of cameras marketed by ADAC Laboratories (Milpitas, CA) includes a system that automatically tunes the detector on demand. In the factory, the photomultiplier tube high voltage in new detectors is set at a nominal voltage (approximately 800 volts). A fully automated microprocessor-controlled system tunes the photomultiplier tubes during flood irradiation with an intense flux of ^{99m}Tc photons. Initially this process involves setting the coarse preamplifier gain so that the analog signal from the individual photomultiplier tubes falls in the dynamic range of the ADCs. This step is followed by automatic adjustment of the fine preamplifier gain on individual tubes so that the global energy resolution is optimized. In the field, the same microprocessor-controlled algorithm is used to "tune" the detector when needed. The microprocessor corrects for large variations in the photomultiplier tube output, but a shift of less than 0.5% in the photopeak centroid for an individual photomultiplier tube does not activate adjustment of the preamplifier. A history of the settings for each photomultiplier tube is maintained in the camera, and any tube that falls outside the satisfactory operational range is flagged. In this situation, service personnel then know that the photomultiplier tube must be replaced (22).

In the current series of cameras manufactured by Marconi (now Philips Medical Systems, formerly Picker International), balance of the photomultiplier tubes is analyzed during daily quality-control uniformity tests. With the aid of split energy windows, tubes that have drifted are identified and the amount of gain shift is quantified (23). These tubes are subsequently recalibrated to restore their output to reference values. A chronologic record of the adjustments is maintained in an on-board database. Any tube that requires frequent adjustments triggers the microprocessor to signal service. These systems also can be accessed by means of modem to monitor (or even adjust) the gain of the photomultiplier tube and to remotely evaluate other service problems. This enables service personnel to identify components that may need replacement before leaving for the job site. The Marconi single head system entails a technique similar to the continuous-tuning method used in cameras manufactured by GE Medical Systems.

A totally different approach is used to tune Elscint cameras. A multistage calibration procedure is implemented, that involves weekly and daily procedures. Once a week, the camera is tuned with a radioactive source. Small software windows are opened in front of each photomultiplier, and the photomultiplier is tuned. After this step, the crystal is illuminated by a light-emitting-diode (LED) optical system, and the response of the photomultiplier tubes is recorded for reference. Thus activation of the optical system to compare the radiation source–measured photomultiplier response with the LED reference data quickly returns the camera to the tuned state (24).

The optical system consists of a single LED placed in the detector housing. Optical fibers are used to transfer light to the crystal that is sensed with the photomultiplier tubes. The signals of each tube are compared with the reference values previously measured with the radioactive source. If a significant shift has occurred, the gain on the tube is adjusted. One cycle requires approximately 20 seconds to complete. The vendor recommends that this be done at least once a day (25).

Continuous Tuning

LEDs are used to tune GE cameras. Technically speaking, the tuning is not continuous, but from a practical standpoint, it is. Each photomultiplier contains an LED mounted in the neck of the tube. At a high frequency (1 to 5 μs every 1 ms), the LED is pulsed, and light travels down the glass walls of the photomultiplier tube to illuminate the photocathode. Some light also enters the crystal and is received by surrounding tubes. The signals from the photomultiplier tubes are fed to individual capacitors (one for each tube) with a time constant of approximately 1 second. The voltages on the capacitors are compared with a reference voltage, and the gain of the tube is adjusted if necessary (26).

A similar approach is used by Toshiba Medical Systems (27). An LED is incorporated in each tube and is pulsed for 0.2 μs, one tube at a time in sequence. One cycle is completed every 200 μs. This process is repeated 255 more times, and the output of each tube is averaged. After 256 cycles, the average output for each tube is compared with reference values, and the preamplifier gain adjusted if necessary. If radiation from the patient strikes the crystal at the same time the LED is pulsed, the γ-ray event takes precedence because of a difference in pulse height. Once the tuning sequence is complete, the data are erased, and the process is repeated. This function is turned off at high count rates.

In the Digitrac and e.cam series, manufactured by Siemens Medical Systems, radiation emitted by the patient is used to tune the camera. The camera can also be calibrated automatically with a point source of ^{99m}Tc (28). During clinical studies, counts are acquired in two narrow tuning windows set on the high side of the photopeak to minimize the acceptance of scatter events. Each tube has two registers (buffers), one for each window, which record the total number of counts. Tuning is initiated when a statistically adequate number of counts are collected in the tuning windows of several tubes. Adjustment of gain for the photomultiplier tube is based on the ratio of the counts in the tuning windows of each tube. A ratio of 1 means the gain is the same as it was when the energy and linearity correction maps were prepared. Each radionuclide requires specific sizes and positions of the tuning windows. These data are stored in lookup tables that are automatically loaded when automatic peaking is initiated.

In a simpler approach used by Summit Nuclear (Hitachi), a microprocessor is used to continuously monitor the high voltage input to the photomultiplier tube (29). The circuit includes a temperature sensor in the detector housing. As needed, the voltage is adjusted back to a set of reference values stored at the time the correction maps were prepared. Additional details concerning some of the methods used for automatic tuning can be found in a review by Graham (21).

Image Formation

Images of radionuclide distributions are formed by means of recording the location of each scintillation event by event. A persistence CRT displays each event in its appropriate x and y location, but the brightness fades slowly. Thus an image can be viewed in real time as the patient is positioned under the camera. However, the image has relatively poor contrast and detail, and persistence CRTs are used only for patient positioning.

Permanent images are formed on film by means of recording the events displayed on a high-resolution CRT either for a predetermined number of counts or for a fixed exposure time. An alternative is to record each event in digital memory by means of adding each count at the appropriate x and y location in a two-dimensional matrix that is displayed as a gray-scale or color image.

SYSTEM PERFORMANCE

The Anger scintillation camera has progressively improved over the 30 years since it became available commercially and has now reached a state of development in which uniformity is very good and system spatial resolution is largely determined by the characteristics of the collimator. This section describes the most important performance parameters with an emphasis on recent improvements.

Resolution and Sensitivity

Intrinsic Spatial Resolution

Intrinsic detector resolution has improved to the point at which it makes a relatively minor contribution to system resolution except when an ultrahigh resolution collimator or close-proximity imaging is used. The following factors have contributed to the improvement: (a) increase in the number of photomultipliers, (b) use of thinner scintillation crystals, (c) improved design freedom through spatial variation of energy windows and removal of spatial distortion for uniformity correction, and (d) direct digitization of photomultiplier tube signals. Manufacturers of scintillation cameras use various combinations of these improvements. The result is that the best intrinsic resolution of present-day large-field-of-view cameras is 2.9 to 4.5 mm as measured with the FWHM.

Since 1974, the Anger scintillation camera has evolved from a device with 19 photomultipliers and a 10-inch (25 cm) field of view to an instrument with either high intrinsic spatial resolution (3 to 4 mm FWHM) with a 10-inch field-of-view camera and 37 photomultipliers (2-inch [5 cm] diameter) or a medium-resolution (5 to 6 mm FWHM), 15-inch (37.5 cm) field-of-view camera with 37 photomultiplier tubes (3-inch [7.5 cm] diameter). Although there were a number of variants, intrinsic spatial resolution (FWHM) slowly improved (Fig. 3.2). As alternative methods for resolution improvements were implemented, a new family of cameras with a large circular or rectangular field of view with 55, 61, 75, 91, or 107 photomultipliers has been developed. This brute-force technique and other refinements improved resolution approximately 1 to 2 mm so that these large-field-of-view cameras now have approximately the same intrinsic resolution as 10-inch-diameter cameras. Most manufacturers of scintillation cameras currently use rectangular crystals.

With the widespread use of ^{99m}Tc radiopharmaceuticals and ^{201}Tl, the performance of scintillation cameras at low energy has become increasingly important. Reducing the thickness of the scintillation crystal from 12.5 mm ($\frac{1}{2}$ inch) to either 9.6 mm ($\frac{3}{8}$ inch) or 6.3 mm ($\frac{1}{4}$ inch) improves intrinsic spatial resolution approximately 1 mm FWHM for energies of 140 keV and less with only a 15% or less reduction in sensitivity (30–33).

Improved intrinsic spatial resolution with a thinner crystal is due to a narrower light spread distribution and improved light collection measured with the photomultiplier tubes. A reduction in the thickness of the Pyrex light pipe alone, however, does not achieve the desired result.

One of the prime requirements of the analog Anger positioning electronics is the "proper" shape of the light-response function. The light-response function is the light intensity measured with a photomultiplier as a function of distance from the center of the photomultiplier (Fig. 3.3). Much effort has been spent on analytic approaches to this problem (34,35) to achieve the proper response by means of manipulation of the light distribution (12), on the use of nonlinear preamplifiers (13), and on delay-line methods (36). In each case, the designer tries to optimize spatial resolution with the constraint of uniform (or nearly uniform) light collection for good energy resolution and of good linearity for acceptable flood-field uniformity.

Collimator and System Resolution

Better collimator spatial resolution can be achieved only at a sacrifice in sensitivity. High-sensitivity collimators typically are used only for fast dynamic studies in which short imaging times preclude collection of an adequate number of counts with higher-resolution and therefore lower-sensitivity collimators.

Overall system resolution (R_s) is determined with both collimator (R_c) and intrinsic spatial resolution (R_i). It can be represented by the formula

$$R_s = \sqrt{R_c^2 + (MR_i)^2}$$

where M is the magnification factor when converging or diverging collimators are used ($M = 1$ for parallel-hole collimators). This relation implies that close to the surface of the collimator, where R_c is low (small FWHM value), system resolution is dominated by the intrinsic resolution, whereas at large distances from the collimator, for example, 15 cm, system resolution is largely determined by collimator performance, particularly for low values (large FWHM) of intrinsic resolution. With standard collimators and imaging situations, system resolution cannot be improved significantly by means of reducing the intrinsic resolution to less than 3 mm. For close-proximity imaging with ultrahigh-resolution collimators, intrinsic resolution less than 3 mm can improve overall system resolution.

Uniformity

If the scintillation camera is exposed to a uniform flux of γ-radiation, the resulting image should have uniform intensity. Because any deviation from this condition can interfere with accurate interpretation of patient images, it is extremely important to verify camera uniformity by acquiring daily flood-field images. This can be done either with a point source of activity if the collimator is removed or with a "sheet" source (a large, uniform source) if the collimator is in place. Many of the digital

correction methods (energy and linearity corrections) were developed to improve uniformity. The result is that most modern scintillation cameras have only negligible uniformity variations for most planar imaging situations. State-of-the-art cameras have integral uniformity values ranging from 2% to 4.5% when measured according to the National Electrical Manufacturers Association protocol (37). Cameras with the best uniformity (2%) include a separate renormalization step that is not used by other vendors.

Unfortunately, photomultipliers (and sometimes associated analog electronic components) tend to become unstable with time. If one or several photomultipliers "drift," hot or cold spots may appear in the flood image. Furthermore, photomultiplier gain can be affected by magnetic fields, such as the earth's magnetic field (38) or a nearby nuclear magnetic resonance unit, which can cause the uniformity to change as a function of detector orientation. This is particularly detrimental in emission computed tomography because of the continual change in orientation of the detector relative to the earth's magnetic field as data are acquired. For this reason, almost all companies now incorporate self-tuning circuitry (see earlier) that adjusts the photomultiplier gain periodically when a change in amplification is detected. Great care must be used in the design of the gain adjustment processor to avoid shifts of the energy spectrum under varying scatter conditions, such as those encountered in emission computed tomography.

Energy Resolution

With improved photomultiplier tubes and the use of energy correction circuits, global energy resolution of state-of-the-art Anger scintillation cameras now falls in the range of 8% to 11%. This means that better elimination of scatter radiation can be achieved by the use of narrower (12% to 15%) pulse height analyzer windows without the loss of a large percentage of photopeak events. A decrease in scatter fraction with improved en-

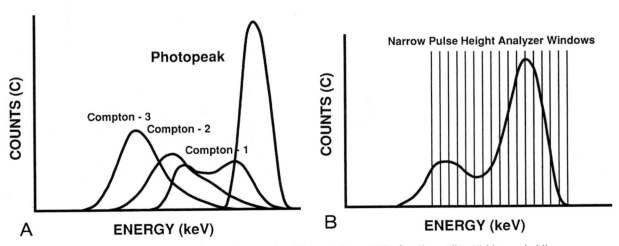

FIGURE 3.6. Elimination of scatter by use of multiple windows. **A:** The first three Kline-Nishina probability coefficients for Compton scattering (single, double, and triple scatter) and the photoelectric peak in a NaI(Tl) crystal. **B:** ^{99m}Tc spectrum in scatter media shows the positioning of 16 narrow pulse height analyzer windows to measure the spectrum on a pixel-by-pixel basis. For ^{99m}Tc the windows cover the energy range from 95 to 161 keV.

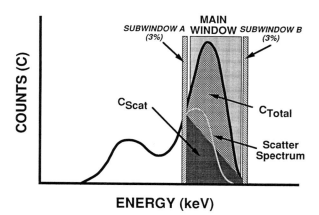

FIGURE 3.7. Triple-energy-window method for scatter removal. Narrow subwindows are positioned just above and below the main window to "measure" the amount of scatter present in the photopeak on a pixel-by-pixel basis. These counts are subtracted from the total counts to "eliminate" scatter and improve contrast. (Modified from Ichihara T, Ogawa K, Motomura N, et al. Compton scatter compensation using the triple-energy window method for single- and dual-isotope SPECT. *J Nucl Med* 1993;34:2216–2221, with permission.)

ergy resolution is well documented (39). The work of Kojima et al. (39) revealed, however, that proper selection of the optimum window depended strongly on the relation between the scatter fraction and the number of primary counts in the image.

In integrated camera-computer systems, several vendors now offer elaborate techniques for "elimination" of scatter radiation. Elscint (now a part of GE Medical Systems) uses a method based on the Klein-Nishina formula for Compton scattering (40,41). Up to 32 images are collected with narrow pulse height analyzer windows (42). For ^{99m}Tc SPECT, 16 images are often acquired for each projection. From this set of images, spectra are generated for each pixel. Data for each pixel are weighted with data from the surrounding pixels to improve the statistics. Figure 3.6A shows the photopeak and single, double, and triple scatter components for ^{99m}Tc. Figure 3.6B presents the multiple, narrow analyzer windows that are used to produce the spectrum for each pixel in the image. Each spectrum is decomposed into the contribution of the photopeak and the summed contribution of several orders of Compton scattering. By separating scatter events from photopeak events, this method makes it possible to remove scatter in different patients and even from different locations within the same patient. The resulting images have markedly improved contrast, but there is an increase in noise. Increased amounts of computer storage are required, however, and high-speed processing is needed to remove the scatter in each projection of a SPECT study.

A computationally simpler method is available for the removal of scatter (43). A conventional pulse height analyzer window is surrounded by two narrow 3% subwindows—one positioned just above and one just below the main window. A trapezoid, defined by the baseline and the number of counts in each of the subwindows, is used as an estimate of the scatter superimposed on the photopeak. A diagram is shown in Fig. 3.7. The number of counts within the trapezoid is subtracted from the counts in the main window on a pixel-by-pixel basis.

Contrast in clinical studies is improved, but image noise increases.

Count Rate Capability

The ability to handle high count rates is often a limiting performance parameter in first-pass cardiac studies. For example, if 4 mCi (148 mBq) of ^{99m}Tc is injected as a bolus with a general-purpose collimator on the camera, a maximum of 10,000 counts/second (cps) are recorded, if there is 50% attenuation. If it is assumed that no counts are lost at such a relatively low count rate, it is easy to calculate that a 20-mCi (740 MBq) injection with a high-sensitivity collimator on the camera, a typical first-pass situation, should yield 100,000 cps. Most state-of-the-art cameras can handle this rate without a significant loss of counts, but many older Anger cameras show a significant loss of counts at this rate.

The count rate capability of the Anger scintillation camera is potentially limited by the decay time of NaI(Tl), by event pulse pileup because all photomultiplier tubes pick up at least some light from every event in a large, continuous crystal, and by the processing and display electronics. Examples of situations in which high count rate capability is needed in an Anger camera are positron coincidence imaging, radionuclide therapy dosimetry imaging, and cardiac first-pass imaging.

After a γ-ray interacts in NaI(Tl), the resulting light is emitted with a decay time of 240 nsec; 1,000 nsec is needed to collect 98% of the light. If it is assumed that the γ-rays arrive at regular time intervals, and if every detected event falls in the energy acceptance window, then 1 million events per second can be handled. However, in clinical studies, one half to two thirds of the incident counts are caused by scattered radiation and are discarded. Nevertheless, every event must be analyzed, and this increases the total dead time. In reality, the incident radiation arrives at random times, and the maximum data rate is further reduced owing to pulse pileup. Typical maximum count rates in older cameras were approximately 100,000 cps with a source in air and less than 30,000 cps in clinical situations.

All modern cameras have four to five stages of derandomizer buffers to improve count rate performance. If two or more events arrive before the camera completes processing a first event, sample-and-hold circuits preserve the events until they can be processed.

Other techniques are used to significantly increase the count rate capability of Anger cameras. One method involves shortening the time during which the electrical signals from the photomultiplier tubes are integrated, but this means that only a fraction of the light emitted by the crystal is collected and used. This previously described technique (44–46) has been applied to Anger cameras (46,47). Because only a fraction of the light is used, there is some loss of energy and spatial resolution. Table 3.2 summarizes calculated count rate capability and loss of spatial resolution as a function of integration time. It is assumed that the pulse is shortened to correspond to the listed integration time. With an integration time as short as 240 nsec, 63% of the light is still collected. When a variable integration time is used (47,48), loss of resolution can be limited. At low count rates, the full integration time is used; at high count rates, shorter

Table 3.2. *Effect of pulse shortening on camera performance*

Output Count rate, 20% Data Loss (cps)	Integration Time (ns)	Percentage Light Emitted	Resolution FWHM (mm)
89,000	1,000	98	4.0
223,000	400	81	4.4
372,000	240	63	5.0
890,000	100	34	6.9

FWHM, full width at half maximum.

integration times are used. Thus for a system with an optimal intrinsic resolution of 4 mm FWHM at 140 keV and an optimal long integration time, high count rate capability can be achieved by means of reducing integration times with only slight degradation in intrinsic spatial resolution (5 mm FWHM). Pulse shortening with variable integration time is one useful option by which the count rate capability of Anger cameras can be improved significantly with only a small loss of intrinsic resolution.

Dead-time Correction

A serious problem remains. It must be determined whether the event of interest is preceded or followed by an event that occurs too close in time to prevent accurate position and energy determination. This loss of accuracy occurs because one pulse stands on the tail of another. A number of techniques have been developed to deal with this problem and fall under the general category of *pulse pileup rejection.* An example of pulse pileup is shown in Fig. 3.8.A.If one of the piled-up events is a photopeak event, then the composite pulse is likely to be eliminated because it will not fall in the energy selection window. This is called *coincidence loss.* More seriously, if two scattered events are summed, they may combine to fall into the energy window, and will be recorded as a single event that will be localized somewhere *between* the two actual events. This is called a *misplaced event.* Thus image quality is degraded without pileup rejection (49, 50) because not only are more good events lost, but also more bad events are accepted.

Pileup rejection circuits generally operate in one of two ways. One approach is to process only the first part of the pulse, as described earlier. This strategy diminishes the effects on the pulses that follow but degrades energy and spatial resolution because the signals are smaller (46). Pulse pileup is not eliminated, but higher counting rates are required before it is prominent (51). A second approach is to measure the length of the output pulse. If it does not return to a value close to the baseline level by a preset time, the pulse is discarded (52). Under this condition, more events are discarded as the count rate increases. Although cameras with this type of pileup rejection have better image quality at high count rates, they also have apparently longer dead times because they do not count these mispositioned events. It has been shown (50,53) that some cameras with apparently high count rate capability achieve this "good" performance by including misplaced events caused by pileup.

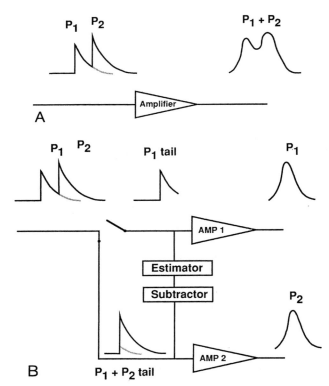

FIGURE 3.8. Pulse pileup. **A:** Effect of pulse pileup when a second pulse (*P₂*) arrives before the first pulse (*P₁*) has been completely processed. The height of the composite pulse (*P₁* + *P₂*) is larger than that of *P₁* alone. **B:** Tail extrapolation circuit that removes the effect of pulse pileup. (Modified from Lewellen TK, Pollard KR, Bice AN, et al. A new clinical scintillation camera with pulse tail extrapolation electronics. *IEEE Trans Nucl Sci* 1990;37:702–706, with permission.)

Use of high-speed electronics has led to the development of a better solution to the problem of pulse pileup (51,54). The incoming pulse to the amplifier is monitored, and the decay of the pulse tail is followed with a circuit called an *estimator* (Fig. 3.8B). If a second pulse arrives before the first pulse has returned to the baseline, the input to the amplifier is immediately switched to a second channel. The estimator extrapolates the first pulse to complete the tail. The extrapolated tail is also routed to the second channel and subtracted from the second pulse. This operation removes the pedestal on which the second pulse is sitting. The cameras that currently use this technique may have multiple levels of extrapolation. Tail extrapolation is particularly attractive because it significantly reduces the number of misplaced events (51) and reduces dead time.

SUMMARY

For planar imaging of radionuclide distributions in humans, the Anger scintillation camera remains the instrument of choice. Although its principal components have not changed substantially, this camera has been perfected and enhanced to the point at which its system resolution is now largely limited by the collimator and uniformity is excellent. Count rate capability has improved in many cameras, but this performance parameter is extremely variable from vendor to vendor.

The limitations imposed by the collimator are severe. Compared with those obtained with other modalities, nuclear medicine images have poor resolution and are limited in image quality because of poor statistics on the number of γ-rays detected. However, the availability of multiple detector systems and magnifying collimators has markedly improved image quality. This improvement is due in part to better statistics and in part to the ability to use collimators with higher resolution (55). In some clinical studies, the improved sensitivity can be used to increase throughput; in others, it may be used to improve image quality. Major performance improvements for radionuclide imaging are possible with SPECT performed with both dedicated imaging instruments and multiple-detector rotating scintillation cameras. Specialized compact devices dedicated to close imaging of specific organs also can greatly improve the performance of scintillation cameras.

REFERENCES

1. Anger HO. Scintillation camera with multichannel collimators. *J Nucl Med* 1964;5:515–531.
2. Jaszczak RJ, Murphy PH, Huard D, et al. Radionuclide emission computed tomography of the head with Tc-99m and a scintillation camera. *J Nucl Med* 1977;18:373–380.
3. Kuhl DE, Edwards RQ. Image separation radioisotope scanning. *Radiology* 1963;80:653–662.
4. Anger HO, Rosenthall DJ. Scintillation camera and positron camera. In: *Medical radioisotope scanning.* Vienna, Austria: International Atomic Energy Agency, 1959:59.
5. Muehllehner G. A diverging collimator for γ-ray imaging cameras. *J Nucl Med* 1969;10:197–201.
6. Moyer, RA. A low-energy multihole converging collimator compared with a pinhole collimator. *J Nucl Med* 1974;15:59–64.
7. Bonte FJ, Graham KD, Dowdey JE. Image aberrations produced by multichannel collimators for a scintillation camera. *Radiology* 1971;98:329–334.
8. Anger HO, Davis DH. Gamma-ray detection efficiency and image resolution in sodium iodide. *Rev Sci Instrum* 1964;35:693–697.
9. Svedberg JB. Computed intrinsic efficiencies and modulation transfer functions for gamma camera. *Phys Med Biol* 1973;18:658–664.
10. Birks JB. *The theory and practice of scintillation counting.* New York: MacMillan, 1964:432.
11. Muehllehner G, Colsher JG, Stoub EW. Correction for nonuniformity in scintillation cameras through removal of spatial distortion. *J Nucl Med* 1980;21:771–776.
12. Martone RJ, Goldman SC, Heaton CC, inventors. Scintillation camera with light diffusion system. US patent 3,784,819. 1974.
13. Kulberg GH, Van Dijk N, Muehllehner G. Improved resolution of the Anger scintillation camera through use of threshold preamplifiers. *J Nucl Med* 1972;13:169–171.
14. Stout KJ, inventor. Radiation sensing device. US patent 3,911,278. 1975.
15. Genna S, Pang S, Smith A. Digital scintigraphy: principles, design and performance. *J Nucl Med* 1981;22:365–371.
16. Svedberg JB. On the intrinsic resolution of a gamma-camera system. *Phys Med Biol* 1972;17:514–524.
17. Steidley JW, Kearns DS, Hoffer PB. Uniformity correction with the Micro-Z processor. *J Nucl Med* 1978;19:712.
18. Knoll GF, Bennet MC, Koral KF, et al. Removal of gamma-camera nonlinearity and nonuniformities through realtime signal processing. In: Di Paola R, Kahn E, eds. *Information processing in medical imaging.* Paris: INSERM, 1980:187–200.
19. Cradduck TD, Fedoruk SO, Reid WB. A new method of assessing the performance of scintillation cameras and scanners. *Phys Med Biol* 1966;11:423–435.
20. Wicks R, Blau M. Effect of spatial distortion on Anger camera field-uniformity correction: concise communication. *J Nucl Med* 1979;20:252–254.
21. Graham LS. Automatic tuning of scintillation cameras: a review. *J Nucl Med Technol* 1986;14:105–110.
22. Hines H, Nelleman P. ADAC Laboratories, Milpitas, CA. Personal communication, 2001.
23. Valentino F. Picker International, Cleveland, OH. Personal communication, 1994.
24. Wainer N. Boston, MA: Elscint. Personal communication, 1994.
25. Bernstein T. Image quality by automatic corrections and calibrations. Boston, MA: Elscint, undated.
26. XR Detector Theory. Rev 0 46-291042G2. GE Medical Systems, Milwaukes, WI., undated.
27. Ichihara T. Internal report. Toshiba Medical Systems, Tustin, CA., undated.
28. ZLC with Digitrac. Siemens Medical Systems no. 917-00000014A-b, 1/84.
29. Enos G. Personal communication, 1994.
30. Sano RM, Tinkel JB, La Vallee CA, et al. Consequences of crystal thickness reduction on gamma-camera resolution and sensitivity. *J Nucl Med* 1978;19:712–713.
31. Chapman D, Newcomer K, Berman D, et al. Half-inch vs quarter-inch Anger camera technology: resolution and sensitivity differences at low photopeak energies. *J Nucl Med* 1979;20:610–611.
32. Royal HD, Brown PH, Claunch BC. Effects of a reduction in crystal thickness on Anger camera performance. *J Nucl Med* 1979;20:977–980.
33. Muehllehner G. Effect of crystal thickness on scintillation camera performance. *J Nucl Med* 1979;20:992–993.
34. Baker RG, Scringer JW. An investigation of the parameters in scintillation camera design. *Phys Med Biol* 1967;12:51–63.
35. Svedberg JB. Image quality of a gamma-camera system. *Phys Med Biol* 1968;13:597–610.
36. Hiramoto T, Tanaka E, Nohara N. A scintillation camera based on delay-line time conversion. *J Nucl Med* 1971;12:160–165.
37. Performance measurements of scintillation cameras. Standards publication NU 1-1994. Washington, DC: National Electrical Manufacturers Association, 1994.
38. Bieszk J. Performance changes of an Anger camera in magnetic fields up to 10 G. *J Nucl Med* 1986;27:1902–1907.
39. Kojima A, Matsumoto M, Takahashi M, et al. Effect of energy resolution on scatter fraction in scintigraphic imaging: Monte Carlo study. *Med Phys* 1993;20:1107–1113.
40. Maor D, Berlad G, Chrem S, et al. Klein-Nishina based energy factors for Compton free imaging (CFI). *J Nucl Med* 1991;32[Suppl]:1000.
41. Berlad G, Maor D, Natanzon A, et al. Compton free imaging (CFI): validation of a new scatter correction method. *J Nucl Med* 1994;35[Suppl]:143P.
42. Elscint Helix procedure manual. Boston, MA: Elscint, undated.
43. Ichihara T, Ogawa K, Motomura N, et al. Compton scatter compensation using the triple-energy window method for single- and dual-isotope SPECT. *J Nucl Med* 1993;34:2216–2221.
44. Asmsel G, Bosshard R, Zajde C. Shortening of detector signals with passive filters for pile-up reduction. *Nucl Instrum Methods* 1969;71:1–12.
45. Brasshard C. Fast counting with NaI spectrometers. *Nucl Instrum Methods* 1971;94:301–306.
46. Muehllehner G, Buchin MP, Dudek JH. Performance parameters of a positron imaging camera. *IEEE Trans Nucl Sci* 1976;23:528–537.
47. Tanaka E, Nohara N, Murayama H. Variable sampling-time technique for improving count rate performance of scintillation detectors. *Nucl Instrum Methods* 1979;158:459–466.
48. Kastner M. A high speed stabilized gated integrator. *IEEE Trans Nucl Sci* 1984;31:447–450.
49. Strand S, Larsson I. Image artifacts at high photon fluence rates in single-crystal NaI(Tl) scintillation cameras. *J Nucl Med* 1978;19:407–413.

50. Lewellen TK, Murano R. A comparison of count rate parameters in gamma-cameras. *J Nucl Med* 1981;22:161–168.
51. Lewellen TK, Pollard KR, Bice AN, et al. A new clinical scintillation camera with pulse tail extrapolation electronics. *IEEE Trans Nucl Sci* 1990;37:702–706.
52. Nicholson PW. *Nuclear electronics.* London: John Wiley & Sons, 1974.
53. Johnston AS, Gergans GA, Kim I, et al. Deadtime of computers coupled with Anger cameras: counting losses and false counts. In: Sorenson IAJA, ed. *Single photon emission computer tomography and other selected topics.* New York: Society of Nuclear Medicine, 1980:219–237.
54. Lewellen TK, Bice AN, Pollard KR, et al. Evaluation of a clinical scintillation camera with pulse tail extrapolation electronics. *J Nucl Med* 1989;29:1554–1558.
55. Muehllehner G. Effect of resolution improvement on required count density in ECT imaging: a computer simulation. *Phys Med Biol* 1985; 30:163–173.

Diagnostic Nuclear Medicine, Fourth Edition. Edited by M.P. Sandler, R.E. Coleman, J.A. Patton, F.J.Th. Wackers, A. Gottschalk. Lippincott Williams & Wilkins, Philadelphia 2003.

4

SINGLE PHOTON EMISSION COMPUTED TOMOGRAPHY

JAMES A. PATTON
THOMAS F. BUDINGER

Nuclear medicine images of radionuclide distributions obtained by means of conventional planar imaging techniques are generally low in contrast because of the presence of overlying and underlying activity that interferes with imaging of the region of interest. This is caused by the superposition of depth information into single data points collected from perpendicular or angled lines of travel of photons from the distribution being studied into holes of the collimator fitted to the scintillation camera (Fig. 4.1A). The resulting planar image shown in Fig. 4.1B is low in contrast (S/B_1) because of the effect of superposition of depth information. This effect can be reduced by means of collecting images from multiple positions around the distribution (Fig. 4.1C) and producing an image of a transverse slice through the distribution (Fig. 4.1D). The resulting tomographic image is of higher contrast (S/B_2) than is the planar image because of the elimination of contributions of activity above and below the region of interest. This is the goal of the techniques provided by single photon emission computed tomography (SPECT); that is, to provide images of slices of radionuclide distributions with image contrast that is higher than that obtained with conventional techniques.

DATA ACQUISITION

Instrumentation

SPECT had its beginning in the early 1960s with the work of Kuhl and Edwards (1). Initial work was conducted with a dual-head scanner with a translation-rotation motion to acquire projection data from transverse planes through the body. Acquired data were projected back into the reconstructed image by means of optical superposition methods and a cathode ray tube and photographic film for display. This system was later updated to a four-detector brain imaging system with an orthogonal geometric configuration while the translation-rotation mode of data collection was maintained (2). The introduction of digital computers in the early 1970s provided important tools for the development of the SPECT technique (3).

The development of the scintillation camera in the 1960s and its ultimate evolution into the imaging system of choice for routine nuclear medicine imaging applications resulted in expenditure of a great deal of effort in extension of the scintillation camera as a tomographic imaging device. The result of these efforts along with the integration of computer systems was the development of the modern day SPECT system as a scintillation camera–computer system with one, two, or three heads and tomographic capability. The scintillation camera collects tomographic data by means of rotating around the region of interest and acquiring multiple planar or projection images during its rotation (Fig. 4.2). It is imperative that the region of interest be included in every projection image. If this is not the case, the resulting truncation of the images will produce artifacts in the final reconstructed images. The camera may move in a continuous motion during acquisition but typically remains stationary during the acquisition of each projection image in a "step and shoot" mode of operation. Complete 360-degree rotation of a

J.A. Patton: Department of Radiology and Radiological Sciences, Vanderbilt University Medical Center, Nashville, TN.

T.F. Budinger: Lawrence Berkeley Laboratory, University of California at Berkeley, Berkeley, CA.

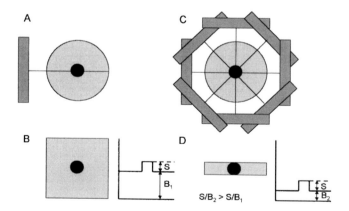

FIGURE 4.1. Routine planar imaging techniques **(A)** provide low-contrast images **(B)** because of the superposition of depth information along the lines of travel of photons from the radionuclide distribution into the holes of the collimator fitted to the scintillation camera. Contrast can be improved by means of collecting images from multiple angles around the distribution **(C)** and producing images of slices through the distribution **(D)**.

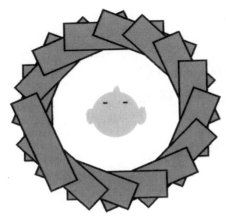

FIGURE 4.2. A scintillation camera collects SPECT data by means of rotating around the region of interest and acquiring multiple planar images from different angular projections.

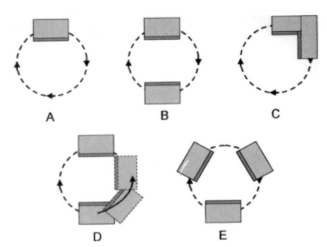

FIGURE 4.4. Options for acquiring SPECT images include single-head (**A**), fixed dual-head, 180-degree (**B**), fixed dual-head, 90-degree (**C**), dual-head, variable-angle (**D**), and triple-head (**E**) geometric configurations of scintillation cameras.

scintillation camera with a rectangular field of view completely samples a cylindrical region of interest. Original camera systems were capable of only circular orbits; however, modern systems have elliptical orbit capability. The collimators are equipped with sensors that detect the presence of the patient and maintain the camera heads close to the patient as the orbit is completed. The preference for elliptical orbits is shown in Fig. 4.3. Because the spatial resolution of collimators used with the scintillation camera degrades with distance from the collimator face, the optimum resolution is obtained in each projection image when the camera is as close to the patient as possible.

Initial SPECT applications were performed with a single-head scintillation camera that acquired data in a 360-degree orbit (Fig. 4.4A). When interest in imaging the myocardium became prominent, experimental work showed that acceptable images could be obtained with a 180-degree orbit (right anterior oblique to left posterior oblique). Although sampling of the region of interest is incomplete, the region of interest lies in the near field of view of the camera throughout the partial orbit where the spatial resolution is optimum, and images of acceptable quality are obtained. Early in the evolution of SPECT, it became evident

that optimum counting statistics for many applications could not be obtained in a reasonable time that could be tolerated by patients. This situation was remedied by the development of multihead scintillation cameras. The first system to evolve was a dual-head camera in a fixed 180-degree geometric configuration that allowed 360-degree acquisition with only a 180-degree rotation of the gantry (Fig. 4.4B). This development provided a twofold increase in the sensitivity of SPECT applications. This increase in sensitivity, however, was not available for cardiac applications with 180-degree acquisition. To address this problem, special purpose, dual-head cameras were developed with the camera heads fixed in a 90-degree configuration (Fig. 4.4C). This made the twofold increase in sensitivity available for cardiac imaging and the acquisition of projections through 180 degrees could be acquired with 90-degree rotation of the dual-head gantry. Because many scintillation cameras must serve multiple purposes in nuclear medicine departments, the next step was development of dual-head, variable-angle scintillation cameras (Fig. 4.4D). These cameras can acquire images with the heads in a 180-degree configuration for routine 360-degree applications, and one head can be moved into a 90-degree configuration with the other head for 180-degree cardiac applications. Even with two detector heads, many SPECT applications are still statistically limited. Because of this limitation, triple-head cameras (Fig. 4.4E) were developed soon after dual-head cameras were introduced. These cameras increase the sensitivity threefold over single-head cameras for 360-degree acquisitions but have only a slight advantage over single-head cameras for cardiac applications because the arc of rotation for acquisitions is 120 degrees per head. Examples of commercially available cameras with these options are shown in Fig. 4.5.

Acquisition Parameters

Collimation

Early SPECT applications with a single-head camera were generally limited to the use of general purpose, parallel-hole collima-

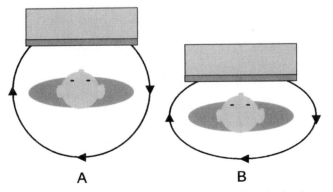

FIGURE 4.3. The optimum spatial resolution in each projection image is obtained when the scintillation camera is as close as possible to the region of interest. Because of this, elliptical orbits are preferred to circular orbits.

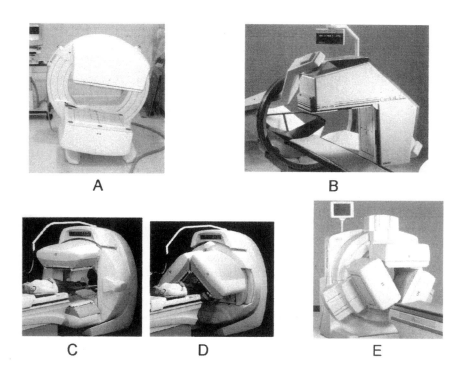

FIGURE 4.5. Commercially available scintillation cameras for SPECT applications include fixed dual-head 180-degree **(A)** and 90-degree **(B)** geometric configurations, dual-head variable-angle **(C–D)** configurations, **(E)** and triple-head configurations.

tors for imaging low-energy radionuclides owing to the sensitivity limitations previously described. The resulting images typically had poor spatial resolution. The emergence of multiple-head cameras and the resulting increase in sensitivity made it possible to improve spatial resolution by the use of high-resolution collimators. These collimators are now the choice for most imaging applications. Medium- and high-energy parallel-hole collimators are used to image medium- and high-energy radionuclides. To increase spatial resolution and improve sensitivity, a special-purpose collimator was developed. As shown in Fig. 4.6, this fan-beam collimator has holes that converge in the transaxial direction while maintaining the conventional parallel-hole configuration in the axial direction. Improved spatial resolution and sensitivity in brain imaging are obtained because of the magnification properties of this collimator.

Matrix Size

There are typically two choices for acquisition matrix sizes for acquiring planar projection images—64 × 64 and 128 × 128.

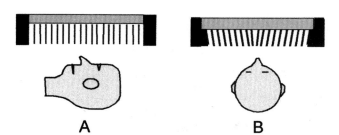

FIGURE 4.6. Fan-beam collimators were designed primarily for brain imaging. The collimator has holes that converge in the transaxial direction **(B)** and maintain the conventional parallel-hole geometry in the axial direction **(A)**.

The decision is based on the size of the smallest object to be imaged in the distribution being studied. Sampling theory states that to resolve frequencies (objects) up to a maximum frequency (smallest object), at least two measurements must be made across one cycle. This maximum frequency is referred to as the *Nyquist frequency*. Because the reconstructed spatial resolution in a SPECT image is typically on the order of 1 to 2 cm, the sampling matrix contains data cells of 5 to 10 mm.

With current large-field-of-view cameras, most imaging applications can be adequately managed with a 64 × 64 pixel array. However, when the smallest object size approaches 1 cm, a 128 × 128 pixel array becomes more appropriate. Acquisition times and count rates from the radionuclide distribution must be considered in this decision, because doubling the matrix size results in reduction by a factor of 4 in counts recorded in each data cell, if imaging times are equal.

Arc of Rotation

Most SPECT acquisitions are accomplished with a 360-degree arc of rotation to completely sample the radionuclide distribution under study. The one exception is cardiac imaging, in which 180-degree acquisition is acceptable (right anterior oblique position to left posterior oblique position) with the myocardium in the near field of the detector. Photons traveling in a posterior direction from the myocardium must travel considerable distances through tissue. Therefore spatial resolution and sensitivity (owing to attenuation) are degraded in the posterior and right posterior oblique views.

Projections per Arc of Rotation

The same sampling theory previously described also applies to the determination of the number of projection views that should be acquired throughout an arc of rotation. With current instrumentation, 120 views are typically obtained with a 360-degree acquisition and 60 views with a 180-degree acquisition. Acquisition times and count rates from the radionuclide distribution must be considered in this decision.

Time per Projection

In general, SPECT techniques necessitate acquisition of as many photon events as possible to produce high-quality images. However, the limiting factor typically is the time a patient can remain motionless during acquisition. This time is typically 20 to 30 minutes and results in imaging times of 20 to 30 seconds for each projection when 120 projections are acquired in a 360-degree rotation with a dual-head camera. Comparable times are used with dual-head cameras in 180-degree acquisitions from the myocardium.

SPECT IMAGE FORMATION

Data Acquisition

SPECT data are acquired as multiple projection images as the heads of the scintillation camera rotate around the region of interest (Fig. 4.7). Each acquired image is actually a set of count profiles measured from different views with the number of count profiles determined by the number of rows of pixels in the acquisition matrix (e.g., 128 for a 128 × 128 matrix size). With parallel-hole collimators, each pixel is the sum of measured photon events traveling along a perpendicular ray and interacting at a point in the detector crystal represented by the pixel location (Fig. 4.8). For 360-degree acquisition with 120 acquired projection arrays, 120 count profiles are acquired at 3-degree increments around the region of interest for each transaxial slice through the radionuclide distribution. An example of two orthogonal count profiles measured from a spherical source is

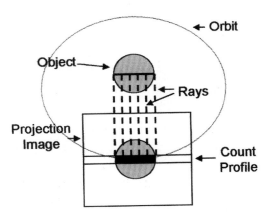

FIGURE 4.8. Single count profile acquired in a single projection image.

shown in Fig. 4.9A. For illustrative purposes, a 10 × 10 array of data cells is superimposed over the image field of view, and numbers are added to represent photons originating from each of the data cells. The count profile acquired at 0 degrees is the sum of measured photons from rows across the distribution. The count profile acquired at 90 degrees is the sum of measured photons from columns through the distribution.

Image Reconstruction

An image of the transaxial slice through the distribution is generated by sequentially projecting the data in each count profile back along the rays from which the data were collected and adding the data to previously backprojected rays. The mathematical term for this process is *linear superposition of backprojections.* Because there is no a priori knowledge of the origin of photons along each ray, the value of each pixel in the count profile is placed in each data cell of the reconstructed image along the ray. This process is shown diagrammatically in Fig. 4.9B for the profile acquired at 0 degrees and in Fig. 4.9C for

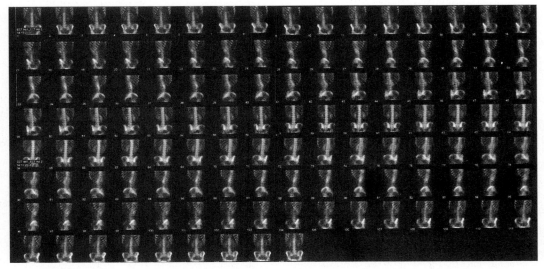

FIGURE 4.7. A data set of 120 planar projection bone images acquired at 3-degree angular increments over 360 degrees.

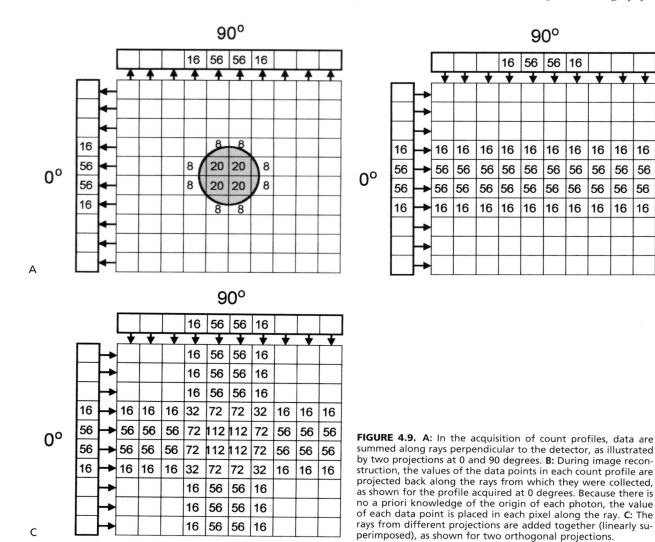

FIGURE 4.9. **A:** In the acquisition of count profiles, data are summed along rays perpendicular to the detector, as illustrated by two projections at 0 and 90 degrees. **B:** During image reconstruction, the values of the data points in each count profile are projected back along the rays from which they were collected, as shown for the profile acquired at 0 degrees. Because there is no a priori knowledge of the origin of each photon, the value of each data point is placed in each pixel along the ray. **C:** The rays from different projections are added together (linearly superimposed), as shown for two orthogonal projections.

the addition of the data from the profile acquired at 90 degrees. Representations of the images resulting from this process are shown in Fig. 4.10B through 4.10C. Uniform projections are used in Fig. 4.10 to illustrate the backprojection principle. In fact, the rays at the periphery of the sphere are of less intensity than at the middle. The classic star-effect blur pattern inherent in backprojection images is evident in these images—each ray of the star corresponds to one projection view. The importance of collecting the appropriate projections is evident from Fig. 4.10, because increasing the number of projections enhances the image contrast and reduces the risk of artifacts from the star effect. This can be seen in Fig. 4.10D, in which two additional sets of projection data at 45 degrees and 135 degrees are projected back into the image.

It is apparent from the data in Figs. 4.9 and 4.10 that the blur pattern inherent in backprojection results in a background that reduces image contrast. To reduce these effects, and to reduce the statistical effects of noise in the images, the mathematical technique of filtering is applied to the count profiles in the projection data before backprojection is performed. A filter is a

mathematical function defined to perform specific enhancements of the profile data. In general, filters enhance edges (sharpen images) and reduce background. The effects of a simple edge-enhancement filter (−1, 2, −1) are shown in Fig. 4.11. In the application of this filter, each data point in the profile is replaced by two times its value and added to the negative of each adjacent data point. The result is that negative numbers are added to the count profiles. Figure 4.11A shows the backprojection of the filtered count profile at 0 degrees. Figure 4.11B shows the effect of adding the filtered backprojected count profile at 90 degrees. It can be observed that the negative data at the edges of one profile cancel unwanted data from other profiles. This effect is shown in Fig. 4.12B through 4.12C. As the number of projections increases, this effect becomes more pronounced (Fig. 4.12D) where the filtered backprojections at 45 degrees and 135 degrees are added to the image. The final step is to set to 0 each pixel in the reconstructed image that has a negative value (Fig. 4.12E). The scanned object is now visible in the image, but many nonzero pixels remain in the image. Addition of multiple projections removes these artifacts and en-

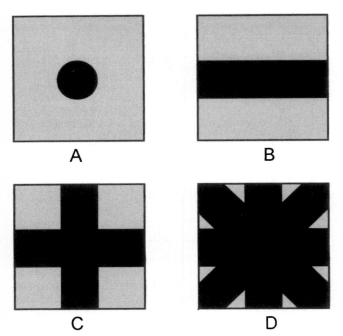

FIGURE 4.10. Backprojection and linear superposition of rays acquired from a uniform sphere (A) at 0 degrees (B), 0 + 90 degrees (C), and 0 + 45 + 90 + 135 degrees (D). Although the rays represent different values, for illustrative purposes all rays are shown with equal intensity.

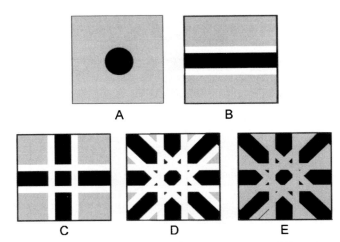

FIGURE 4.12. Backprojection and linear superposition of filtered rays acquired from a uniform sphere (A) at 0 degrees (B), 0 + 90 degrees (C), and 0 + 45 + 90 + 135 degrees (D). Positive values are shown as *black* rays and negative numbers are shown as *white* rays. In D the spherical shape of the object is evident owing to the negative numbers in the image. E: All negative numbers are set to 0.

hances the image of the actual measured distribution. This technique of linear superposition of filtered backprojections has been the image reconstruction algorithm of choice throughout most of the history of SPECT. Figure 4.12 also demonstrates the need to select an appropriate filter for each imaging application. If too many negative numbers are added to the image (over-filtering), valuable image data are removed. If not enough negative numbers are added to the image (under-filtering), unwanted data remain in the image and cause artifacts. Selection of the appro-

priate filter is probably the most important factor in high-quality image reconstruction. The effects of over-filtering and under-filtering are shown in the transverse slices from three patient studies in Fig. 4.13.

The techniques previously discussed are illustrated with data for a single transverse slice. In practice, it is possible to reconstruct as many transverse slices as there are rows in the acquisition matrix. For example, a 64 × 64 matrix provides 64 rows of data that can be used to reconstruct 64 slices. However, because the slice thickness of a single slice often exceeds the spatial resolution of the camera and the data in a single slice often are statistically limited, it is common practice to add two or more adjacent slices to reconstruct thicker slices with improved statistics. The final result of the reconstruction process is a set of transverse

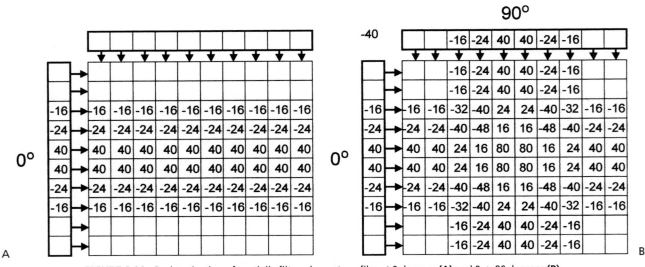

FIGURE 4.11. Backprojection of spatially filtered count profiles at 0 degrees (A) and 0 + 90 degrees (B). The negative values from one projection tend to cancel unwanted positive values from the orthogonal projection.

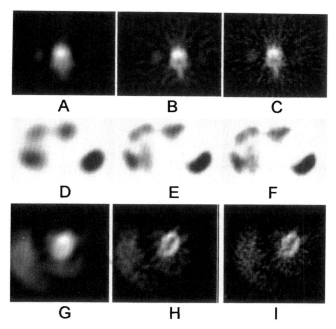

FIGURE 4.13. Transverse images representing three slices from SPECT of a patient with severe metastatic liver disease (**A–C**), bone SPECT of a normal vertebra (**D–F**), and a cardiac perfusion scan (**G–I**) show the effects of over-filtering (**A, D, G**), under-filtering (**C, F, I**), and appropriate filtering (**B, E, H**).

slices. Images of sagittal and coronal slices can easily be generated from this data set by means of reformatting the data (Fig. 4.14). Examples of transverse, sagittal, and coronal slices from a bone SPECT scan are shown in Fig. 4.15.

Filters

Conventional methods for characterizing images and data sets are related to the number of counts in a pixel. Data are defined as being in the *spatial domain,* and the simple filter used to illustrate the effects of filtering on image reconstruction is a *spatial filter.* In practice, filtering of projection data in the spatial domain often is cumbersome and time consuming. This problem is overcome by working in the *frequency domain,* in which the projection data are expressed as a series of sine waves, and a frequency filter is used to modify the data. Conversion of the projection data into the frequency domain is accomplished by means of application of a Fourier transform. The result is that the projection data are represented as a frequency spectrum in which the amplitude of each frequency in the data is plotted (Fig. 4.16A). In SPECT, this frequency spectrum has three distinct components. Background, including the data from the star effect, typically has a very low frequency and therefore dominates the low frequencies of the spectrum. Statistical fluctuations in the data (noise) generally have a high frequency and therefore dominate the high frequencies of the spectrum. True source data lie somewhere in the middle but overlap the background and noise components of the spectrum. The challenge in filtering SPECT data is clearly demonstrated in Fig. 4.16A. The goal is to eliminate as much background and noise from the data while

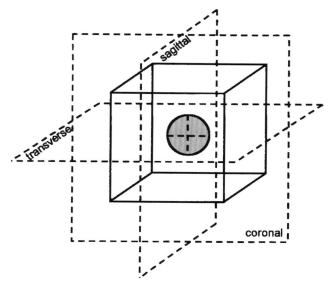

FIGURE 4.14. The result of SPECT reconstruction is a series of transverse images representing slices through the radionuclide distribution. Images of sagittal and coronal slices can be constructed simply by means of reformatting the data.

preserving as many of the source data as possible. The frequency data in the figure are plotted as a function of cycles per pixel. In the earlier discussion of matrix size, the concept of Nyquist frequency was introduced. In the frequency domain, the highest frequency in a data set occurs when one complete cycle covers two pixels. Frequencies higher than this value cannot be imaged. This fact translates into a frequency of 0.5 cycles/pixel as the frequency limit and is defined as the Nyquist frequency. This is why the plot in Fig. 4.16A terminates at 0.5 cycles/pixel. The pixel size used in a particular application can be introduced into this definition so that the Nyquist frequency for the application can be determined. For example, with a pixel size of 0.3 cm, the Nyquist frequency would be 1.67 cycles/cm. Similarly a pixel size of 0.5 cm would define a Nyquist frequency of 1.0 cycles/cm. The smallest object size that could possibly be resolved in an image would be 1 cm.

The first step in filtering the data is to design a filter to remove or reduce the background. This typically is a ramp filter (Fig. 4.16B) and is defined as a high-pass filter because only the amplitude of low-frequency data is reduced while there is no effect on the midrange and high-frequency data that contain the detail in the source (and the noise). The second step is to define a filter to remove or reduce the noise while preserving the detail in the source data. This is accomplished with a low-pass filter (Fig. 4.16C), which provides a window in the spectrum for the acceptance of selected frequencies up to a certain value. A number of low pass filters are available for processing SPECT data. Some have fixed characteristics and others have flexibility in cutoff frequency and the slope of the filter. Some filters are optimized for image data with excellent counting statistics, and others provide the capability for filtering data with poor statistics. The amount of detail in an image and the object size to be resolved (spatial resolution) are important factors to be considered in the selection of a filter. In practice, a low-pass filter can

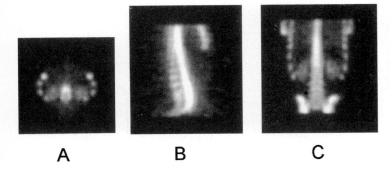

A   B   C

FIGURE 4.15. Images of single transverse (**A**), sagittal (**B**), and coronal (**C**) slices reconstructed from the set of planar projection bone images shown in Figure 4.7.

be applied first to reduce the effects of noise. The ramp filter then is applied to reduce background. The two filters can be combined (Fig. 4.16D). The effect of the two filters on the projection data in this example is shown in Fig. 4.16E. Fig. 4.16E shows that appropriate selection of the cutoff frequency eliminates much of the noise and that selecting an appropriate filter shape preserves most of the source data. Fig. 4.16E also shows that when a cutoff frequency is chosen that is too low, some of the source data are excluded from the final image (over-filtering). When too high a cutoff frequency is chosen, excessive noise is included in the final image (under-filtering). In clinical applications, most imaging systems provide the capability for trying different filters and filter parameters on a single slice of image data to select the appropriate processing algorithm for a specific patient study. Technologists and physicians in the clini-

cal setting often prefer this method of trial and error. Filtering techniques and image reconstruction are described in Prowsner and Prowsner (4).

Iterative Reconstruction

An alternative approach to filtered backprojection that is gaining acceptance in SPECT image reconstruction is the method of iterative reconstruction. Filtered backprojection amplifies statistical noise, which adversely affects image quality. Shepp and Vardi (5) introduced an iterative reconstruction technique in 1982 that was based on the theory of expectation maximization (EM), which has a proven theoretic convergence to an estimate of the actual image distribution that has a maximum likelihood of having projections most similar to the acquired projections.

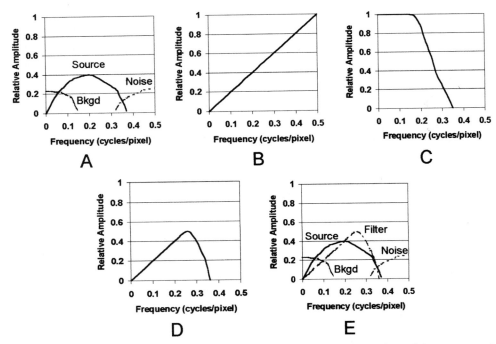

FIGURE 4.16. In the frequency domain, image data can be represented as a series of sine waves, and the data can be plotted as a frequency spectrum that shows the amplitude of each frequency. **A:** Image data have three major components—background, source information, and noise. **B:** A ramp filter is used to eliminate or reduce the contribution of background to the reconstructed image. **C:** A low-pass filter reduces the contribution of noise to the image. Combining the two filters (**D**) produces a window that accepts frequencies primarily from the source distribution (**E**).

Use of these algorithms was very time consuming; several iterations were required to reach a solution, and extensive computer power was needed. Since that time, much effort has been expended in improving and testing algorithms based on this concept. Significant improvements in speed, signal-to-noise ratio, and reconstruction accuracy have resulted from these efforts.

In 1994, Hudson and Larkin (6) developed the technique of ordered sets expectation maximization (OS-EM) for image reconstruction from two-dimensional projection data. This algorithm was based on the concept of dividing the projection data into small subsets (e.g., paired opposite projections in SPECT data) and using the EM algorithm on each subset. The solution of each subset was used as the starting point for the next subset and subsequent subsets were selected to provide the maximum information (e.g., choose the second subset of data to be orthogonal to the first subset). The advantage of this technique is that at the end of the first pass, the entire data set has been processed one time, but n successive approximations to the final solution have been made, where n is the number of subsets. Thus OS-EM is n times faster than the original EM algorithm. Typically only two to three passes through the data set (iterations) are needed for the reconstructed image to converge to a final value that is essentially unchanged by further iterations.

In practice, OS-EM is implemented in SPECT reconstruction (Fig. 4.17). An initial estimate of the final distribution is constructed. This can be accomplished with filtered backprojection, or a simple uniform cylindrical distribution may be used. From this initial estimate, a set of count profiles are generated as an initial estimate of the projection data. This estimated data set is then compared with the initial subset of actual projection data and the error data set (calculated from differences in estimated and actual projection data), and this error data set is used to modify the initial estimate of image data. A second set of estimated projections is generated, and the process is completed. This cycle is repeated until all subsets of actual projections have been used to update the reconstructed image. This process can be repeated a second time, after which the estimate of the final image typically converges to a final solution. As shown in Fig. 4.17, correction for scatter and attenuation effects (see later) can be performed on the acquired projection data during the reconstruction process. The advantage of this technique is that the star effect inherent in filtered backprojection is almost eliminated because the acquired data are distributed within the body contour. Because of this result, the signal-to-noise ratio is gener-

ally improved. Filtering of the data also can be performed to further enhance the reconstructed images.

FACTORS AFFECTING IMAGE QUALITY
Methods for Attenuation Correction

If photons did not interact in materials, then the images of tomographic slices of uniform distributions would be uniform across the slice. However, photons can interact in tissues by means of Compton scattering and to a lesser extent by means of photoelectric absorption. The result is attenuation effects that manifest as a falloff that is depth dependent. This phenomenon is demonstrated by calculated intensities as a function of depth across a uniform cylinder (Fig. 4.18). The ideal constant distribution, with no attenuation, is shown at the top. Examples of the distortion caused by attenuation of the photons of different energies are on the bottom. The two lower plots correspond to the attenuation effects for 140-keV ($\mu = 0.15$) and 511-keV ($\mu = 0.09$) photons in a uniform cylinder of 20 cm diameter. The reconstruction activity in the center of the slice across the cylinder is erroneously low by a factor of approximately 3.5 at 140 keV and 2.5 at 511 keV.

In emission tomography, the goal is to measure and reproduce the position and strength of a radionuclide distribution; therefore the mathematic algorithm must include a method to account for attenuation between the unknown sources and the detectors. This task is far more difficult than that in x-ray tomography, in which the source position and strength are known at all times and only the attenuation coefficients have to be determined. The reconstruction algorithms are similar to those for x-ray computed tomography (CT) with the exception of the need to compensate for attenuation. Attenuation effects have until recently been ignored in commercial SPECT systems. To some extent, clinical results were acceptable because the resulting reconstruction, although not quantitative, shows relative concentrations if the activity distribution is concentrated in the central portion of the section. The usual strategy for gamma-camera techniques is to organize the data into a series of slice projections, each corresponding to a section 10 to 20 mm thick. Each section

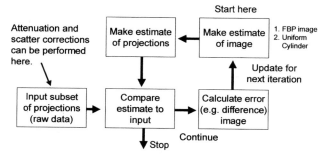

FIGURE 4.17. Steps in iterative reconstruction of SPECT data.

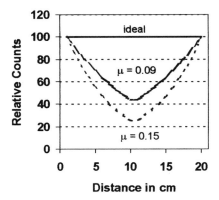

FIGURE 4.18. Plot of attenuated photons versus depth in a 20-cm-diameter uniform phantom for 140-keV photons ($\mu = 0.15$) and 511-keV photons ($\mu = 0.09$). The ideal situation with no attenuation is shown for comparison purposes.

is computed separately. Before reconstruction, compensation for field uniformity must be made (7,8); then one of several methods for attenuation compensation is used. The mathematics are discussed comprehensively by Budinger et al. (9), and Huesman et al. (10) list the computer programs with examples.

Although the methods of correcting for attenuation error are conveniently implemented in positron emission tomography (PET), the techniques are more cumbersome for SPECT. Nevertheless, over the past few years, convenient methods have evolved with iterative approaches (11,12) and direct convolution techniques (13–15). Thus for situations of constant attenuation, the mathematic intractability has been overcome. Three methods are described.

Modification of the Geometric Mean (Method I)

The results of reconstructing projection data that have been modified by means of forming the geometric mean (square root of the product of opposite detected rays) are better than the data obtained when no such maneuver is used; however, serious data distortion still occurs. Application of a correction factor that takes into account the thickness and average activity distribution makes it possible to improve these results. First, the geometric mean of planar projection data is formed by means of multiplying opposing projection rays by one another and calculating the square root. To this modified projection value, a hyperbolic sine correction (sinh) is applied, and then the convolution reconstruction method is used. The sinh correction factor is

$$\frac{e^{\mu}fx}{\sinh(x)} \qquad [1]$$

where μ is the attenuation coefficient, x is one-half the thickness, and f is set from 0.5 to 0.75, depending on the relative amount of activity along the projection line being modified (16). The method of finding the thickness of the object for each projection line involves estimation of the edges of the object from an initial reconstruction before applying the sinh correction. This method works well for sources distributed near the center of the object; however, if the data are statistically poor, as in ^{201}Tl imaging of the heart, the data projections through the posterior thorax contain only a small percentage of the actual photons from the heart. Multiplication of these posterior projections with the less noisy anterior projections can lead to worse results than to use only 180 degrees of anterior projection alone.

Iterative Modification of Pixels (Method II)

If SPECT is performed without consideration of attenuation, the value of each pixel is low because the projected values have been modified by an attenuation effect in accord with the distance between the pixel and the object edge along each ray that passes through that pixel. This modulation is $e^{-\mu di}$, where di is the distance along a particular ray denoted by i (Fig. 4.19).

The overall modification of the source in a particular pixel is merely the sum of these separate modifications divided by the number of projections M:

$$\frac{1}{M}\sum_i e^{-\mu di} \qquad [2]$$

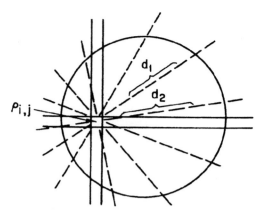

FIGURE 4.19. Iterative method of attenuation correction. Activity in a pixel (*i,j*) is detected as different event rates depending on the distance between the activity location and the edge of the attenuating medium. From analysis of the average attenuation for all views, compensation for distortion can be made by means of the iterative technique.

The method of correction suggested by Chang (12,17) involves first performing a reconstruction to give the distribution $\rho_{i,j}$ modified by

$$\rho_{\text{new }i,j} = \rho_{\text{old }i,j}\frac{1}{\left(\dfrac{1}{M}\sum_i e^{-\mu di}\right)} \qquad [3]$$

The modified data are reprojected, and the differences between the reprojected bin values and the measured projection data are determined. These *difference projections* are used to reconstruct an error image that added to the modified image gives a good result for constant μ. These techniques work well for structures, such as the head, that have more or less constant attenuation coefficients with the exception of 1.5 cm of bone in the skull.

Modification of Projection Data Values before Convolution (Method III)

This procedure was originally developed by Bellini et al. (18) and subsequently evaluated for SPECT (15). First, data for each projection are multiplied by a factor $e^{\mu dk}$, where μ is the attenuation coefficient and dk is defined (Fig. 4.20) as the distance from a centerline to the edge of the object. If we imagine a line through the axis of rotation and parallel to the projection array, the value of dk is the distance between that line and the edge of the object. After modification of each data cell of each projection angle, the projection data are filtered by means of application of a filter the shape of which depends on the attenuation coefficient and the desired spatial resolution. The modified projection values are then backprojected into the image array after multiplication of each value by a factor related to the pixel distance from the centerline. This procedure is rapid, and the filter can be varied to accommodate different noise environments.

Variable Attenuation Distribution

For variable attenuation coefficient situations, two methods have been used with iterative reconstruction techniques. The iterative

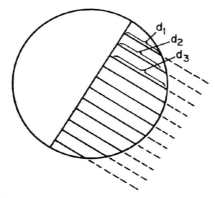

FIGURE 4.20. Attenuation correction with the convolution method. The first stage of the method is to modify each projection before application of a special filter in implementing convolution-type SPECT. To compensate for attenuation involves modification of the projection data by $e^{-\mu di}$.

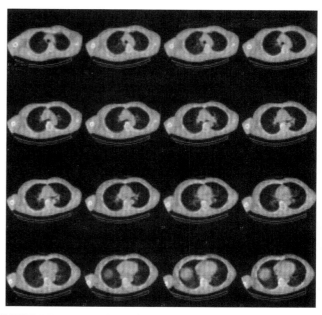

FIGURE 4.21. A partial set of attenuation maps collected with a low-resolution CT scanner mounted on the slipping gantry of a commercial SPECT system. Each map represents attenuation coefficients in a 1-cm transaxial slice through the chest.

reconstruction algorithms involve iterative solutions to the classic inverse problem

$$P = FA \qquad [4]$$

where P is the projection matrix, A is the matrix of true data being sought, and F is the projection operation. The inverse is

$$A = F^{-1}P \qquad [5]$$

which is computed by means of iterative estimation of the data A' and modification of the estimate by means of comparison of the calculated projection set P' to the true observed projections P. The iterative least squares method (16) and maximum likelihood methods (5) are the two approaches to estimating the true data. Both allow incorporation of the attenuation coefficients as weighting factors in the reconstructions. The expectation-maximization algorithm solves the inverse problem by updating each pixel value a_i in accord with

$$a_i^{k+1} = \sum_j p_j \frac{a_i^k f_{ij}}{\sum_i a_i^k f_{ij}} \qquad [6]$$

where P is the measured projection, f_{ij} is the probability that a source at pixel i will be detected in the projection detector j, and k is the iteration. Although first described in 1974 (11) and 1982 (5), these methods have only recently attracted interest, probably because the computational task has only recently been simplified with computer technology. This technique can be incorporated into the OS-EM reconstruction algorithm illustrated in Fig. 4.17.

In practice, the attenuation coefficients are determined from a transmission scan. This is performed on commercial systems with a scanning line source such as ^{153}Gd in conjunction with the scintillation camera to measure sets of transmission projections that can be used to calculate distributions of attenuation coefficients as accomplished in CT. One manufacturer (GE Medical Systems, Milwaukee, WI) uses a low-resolution CT scanner mounted on the slipping gantry of the camera system to measure the attenuation coefficients. The attenuation coefficients are then scaled to the appropriate energy values before

the image reconstruction is performed (19). A set of attenuation maps obtained with this CT scanner approach is shown in Fig. 4.21. Use of these attenuation maps in the OS-EM algorithm allows correction of diaphragmatic attenuation of the inferior wall of the left ventricle in myocardial perfusion studies (Fig. 4.22).

In a second approach, a map of attenuation coefficients is used that is estimated from the outline of the soft tissues and lungs obtained from the first emission reconstruction and assumed values of the attenuation coefficients. This method has undergone evaluation for practical clinical applications in cardiac nuclear medicine.

Variable Spatial Resolution

An important aspect of SPECT is the lack of uniformity of resolution with depth for parallel-hole collimation. This charac-

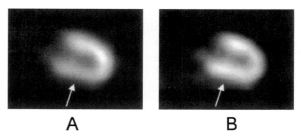

FIGURE 4.22. **A:** Single vertical long axis view of the left ventricle image with ^{99m}Tc sestamibi shows attenuation of the inferior wall. **B:** Same view of the myocardium after attenuation correction with the maps in Fig. 4.21 shows the improvement in image quality that can be obtained with this technique.

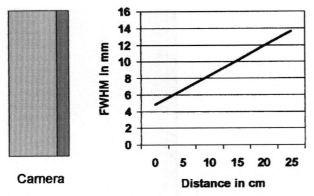

FIGURE 4.23. Plot of spatial resolution (full width at half maximum of a line source of ^{99m}Tc) versus distance from a scintillation camera with a low-energy, high-resolution collimator.

teristic is illustrated in Fig. 4.23 with a plot of spatial resolution versus distance from a scintillation camera with a low-energy, high-resolution collimator. This problem can be solved partially by means of forming the geometric mean (square root of the product of opposing rays) and treating the data as parallel projections for an angular range of 180 degrees. This method, however, is inferior to other techniques that require projections over 360 degrees (12,15).

Other methods to solve the resolution uniformity problem include use of collimators that give a uniform resolution over the range of the object (8), use of moveable focused collimators, as in the Cleon scanner that once was commercially available (20), and incorporation of the spread function data in the reconstruction algorithm (21). Use of measured or theoretic spread function data in an iterative algorithm by means of modifying the weighting factors, as done initially for the effect of attenuation (11), is a promising method for dealing with the collimator problem. The computational approach with an iterative least-squares or maximum likelihood approach may become available on clinical systems in the near future.

Scattered Radiation

Photons emitted by sources within the body that are attenuated by body tissues are either absorbed through the photoelectric process or scattered by the electrons surrounding atoms of the tissue (Compton scattering). These processes lead to the serious attenuation problems discussed earlier. Scattered photons from deep in the body that enter the detection system from erroneous directions have less energy per photon than does unscattered radiation; however, detector systems do not have sufficient energy resolution to eliminate all these photons. Thus scattered photons can contribute as much as 50% of the total collected events in SPECT as well as in PET. This means that a true void deep in a phantom or subject will have an observed false activity that is 20% to 40% of the activity in contiguous regions of the object (22). Unless the scatter contribution is removed before the attenuation correction is applied, amplification of this unwanted background would occur and result in over-correction for attenuation effects. These scattered photons contribute to inaccuracy

in quantitating the amount of radioactivity and degrade the reconstructed images by blurring fine detail and lowering image contrast. The extent and magnitude of scatter increase with the amount of scattering material between the source and the detector. Hence the fraction of detected photons in a projection is a function of the source depth and distance from the edges of the scattering medium.

Scatter Compensation Methods

Simple methods of merely subtracting an estimated background are not applicable generally because Compton scattering depends on the shape of the scattering material (the distribution of attenuation coefficients) and on the distribution of the radionuclide. Scatter contribution also is highly dependent on the collimator and the energy window. For example, the contribution of scatter from sources deep in the subject may be five times greater than the scatter from the sources at the surface near the collimator.

Scatter compensation techniques fall into four general categories—multiple energy window subtraction, energy-weighted compensation, convolution-subtraction technique, and patient-specific scatter modeling.

The method of Compton window subtraction is based on use of a second "scatter" energy window placed below the photopeak window during data acquisition to acquire projection images of the scatter distribution (23). It is assumed that the data obtained from this energy window are estimates of the scatter component in the photopeak window. The scatter compensation consists of subtracting an empirically determined fraction of the scatter data from the photopeak projection images before attenuation correction and image reconstruction. A variant on this energy window method is the dual photopeak window method (24). In this method, two abutting energy windows are used to span the photopeak of the energy spectrum. These methods have provided some image improvement and improved quantitation (25). The use of multiple energy windows below, or even straddling the photopeak window, has resulted in image improvement. These methods, however, suffer from the fact that the scattered photons arriving at a particular energy window depend on the geometric features of the patient, source distribution, and the type of collimator used (26).

The energy-weighted compensation methods are used to estimate scatter correction by means of analyzing the energy spectrum detected at each pixel (27). These spectra are weighted with an energy-weighted function designed to minimize the scatter contribution. This method has been implemented in one commercial system (Siemens, Hoffman Estates, IL).

A third class of methods is used to estimate scatter by means of blurring the projection data, usually by means of convolution of the measured projections with a smoothing kernel (28,29). Some fraction of this blurred projection profile is subtracted from original measured projections. This method requires estimation of the scatter fraction multiplier to be applied to the smoothing data before subtraction.

The scatter modeling methods are patient-specific and therefore able to take into account the fact that the scatter response function varies as a function of both depth inside the scatter medium and distance from the edge of the scatter medium.

Exact scatter response derived from Monte Carlo simulation (22, 30) has been used in both subtraction and iterative reconstruction methods for accurate compensation for scatter. However, the extensive computations and large memory required for Monte Carlo simulation or other exact methods of scatter modeling (26) for every patient make this method impractical at present.

Quantitative Capability

Statistical Precision

The statistical precision of SPECT depends on the number of detected events and the volume of interest. In conventional planar imaging, the signal-to-noise ratio is estimated as the square root of the number of detected events per pixel. However, the act of reconstruction results in propagation of noise that decreases the expected signal-to-noise ratio by factors of eight or more, depending on the resolution sought and the size of the object. The reason for this increase in statistical uncertainty due to reconstruction is illustrated in Fig. 4.24. The variance of a value detected in one projection data cell is equal to the number of events detected and the signal-to-noise ratio therefore is $S/\sqrt{S}$ because the square root of the variance is the expected noise, and S (the detected number of events) is the signal. During the reconstruction, each pixel receives a contribution from all pixels along the particular projection ray (because the ray sum value for all the pixels is placed back into each pixel during backprojection). Under the condition that there are n pixels across the image, the noise in any particular pixel is proportional to the sum of the values of the n pixels. Thus instead of a signal-to-noise ratio of $S/\Sigma\sqrt{S}$, we have $1/\sqrt{S}$, or a decrease in signal-to-noise ratio by the square root of the average number of pixels or resolution elements in projection rays. The formula that deals with the general case is

$$\% \text{ uncertainty} = \frac{1.2 \times 100 \text{ (no. resolution cells)}^{3/4}}{\text{(total no. events)}^{1/2}} \quad [7]$$

The factor 1.2 is based on the convolution kernel (rms, root

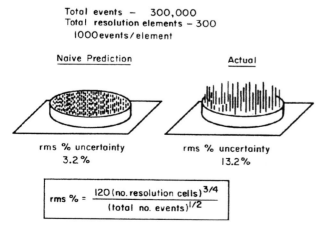

FIGURE 4.24. Magnitude of the decrease in statistical reliability expected from projection images and that after computation of a transverse section. *rms,* root mean square.

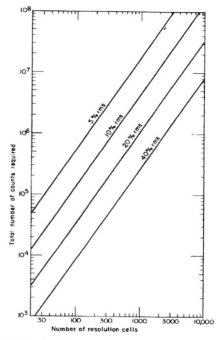

FIGURE 4.25. Relation between the number of detected events and the number of resolution elements in the image for various degrees of statistical certainty.

mean square). Figure 4.25 shows the relation between the total number of events and the number of resolution cells in an image for four levels of uncertainty. Figure 4.24 shows the relation between detected events and the volume of interest. If 300,000 events are collected for a section with 300 pixels (1,000 events/pixel), the root mean square uncertainty is 13.2%. A naive prediction based on $1/\sqrt{S} \times 100$ would give only 3.2% uncertainty. In the foregoing discussion, a uniform distribution is assumed. If the activity is concentrated in a small region of the image, the tomographic uncertainty decreases, as in the case of a single object in a uniform field (31):

$$\% \text{ uncertainty} = \frac{1.2 \times 100 \text{ (total no. events)}^{1/4}}{\text{(average no. events per resolution cell in the target)}^{3/4}} \quad [8]$$

The importance of this modification can be appreciated with evaluation of the uncertainty for cardiac imaging wherein the effective number of resolution elements is almost ten times less than the total number of pixels in a transverse section. Thus for an image of the thorax with 500,000 detected events, the expected uncertainty for heart distribution occupying approximately 135 resolution elements is 7%, but that calculated for the entire thorax of approximately 2,500 resolution elements would be erroneously estimated at 50%. The heart-seeking agents used with ^{99m}Tc allow SPECT of the heart to give more reliable data than ^{201}Tl SPECT from a statistical standpoint because as much as five times more activity is injected.

The arguments presented favor the importance of the effective number of resolution elements in imaging of the heart but indicate the difficulty of imaging the distribution of radionuclides in organs such as the lungs, which occupy most of the resolution elements. Thus the effective number of elements is close to the actual number of image picture elements.

If the resolution cell size decreases by two, the required number of events for constant uncertainty increases by eight. Thus an important goal for instrument design is to increase sensitivity, and an important goal of reconstruction algorithms is to optimize resolution recovery and suppress noise artifacts.

Another aspect of noise propagation peculiar to SPECT and PET is the influence of errors in the attenuation coefficients used to correct the attenuation of projection data. If variable attenuation coefficients are present in the region to be imaged, a transmission study is needed to provide the attenuation. If the transmission data used to correct for variable attenuation have poor statistics, the statistical uncertainty in the resulting SPECT image will be adversely affected.

Quantitative Concentration Recovery (Accuracy)

The quantitative accuracy in a transverse section reconstruction with attenuation compensation depends on the size of the object relative to the resolution. The accuracy or bias related to correct sampling of data is quite different from the precision of a measurement that is dependent on statistics, as discussed earlier. This important concept can be seen from the simulations shown in Fig. 4.26. As the sampling resolution decreases from 10 mm to 2 mm, the reconstruction data have more statistical fluctuation (less precision), but in a region of interest corresponding to the region of the source, the mean value becomes closer to the actual value (more accuracy). For SPECT, collimation is necessary to increase the in-plane resolution, and this results in a decrease in the solid angle and a loss in sensitivity by a larger factor than is the case for PET, as discussed later. Commercially available instruments have resolution of 7 to 10 mm. Thus objects smaller than 15 mm are not quantitatively imaged. This problem is particularly important for tracers that localize in the

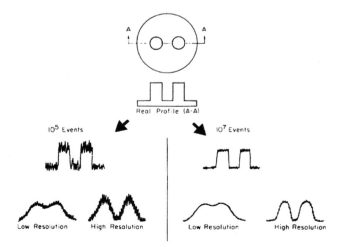

FIGURE 4.26. The quantitative accuracy of the images is controlled by the sampling resolution. A system with good resolution channels the events into the regions of interest from which they originate. However, a system with poor resolution spreads the data outside the anatomic region of interest because of blurring in the poor-resolution system. Statistical uncertainty is a separate consideration.

cerebral gray matter, where activity in the 3.5-mm-wide cerebral cortical ribbon cannot be quantitatively compared with activity in the much larger central gray regions (e.g., caudate nucleus and putamen).

Sensitivity

Quantitative precision requires an adequate number of detected events. Thus for clinically useful SPECT, instrument sensitivity is extremely important and is the major design feature for most instrument development efforts. Sensitivity is the number of events detected for a given source of radiation, and depends mainly on the solid angle of detection. The solid angle is defined as the ratio of area of detector available to a source anywhere in the imaging volume to the area of a sphere with radius R from the center of the volume to the imaging detectors. For example, if 1 cm $\times$ 1 cm is the area of detection for a single gamma camera for an object with a radius of 15 cm from the detector, the single photon solid angle factor is

$$\frac{1 \text{ cm}^2}{4\pi R^2 \text{ cm}^2} = \frac{1}{2835} \qquad [9]$$

Because the positron device can have a ring of detector area, for example, 1 cm thick around the entire circumference, the solid angle factor is

$$\frac{1 \times 2\pi R}{4\pi R^2} = \frac{1}{30} \qquad [10]$$

or almost 100 times better than that of the single photon system for 1-cm resolution. It was on the basis of this incomplete argument that many concluded that SPECT would never compete with PET. However, many other factors must be taken into account.. First, if four arrays of detectors are placed around the object, this advantage is reduced to 25. Second, for PET, the probability of positron detection is the product of the probability of detection by each opposing crystal; thus a crystal efficiency of 80% leads to a PET efficiency of 0.8^2, which is only 64%. The attenuation losses are associated with the total path length through the object in PET and are greater in PET than in SPECT. In addition to the efficiency and attenuation differences, PET requires a larger diameter (e.g., 60 cm for PET and 30 cm for SPECT for the head). Instead of a sensitivity ratio of 100, the expected sensitivity ratio for 1-cm resolution in an instrument for head imaging is

$$\frac{S(\text{PET})}{S(\text{SPECT})} = \frac{15}{a} \qquad [11]$$

where S is sensitivity and a (cm) is the resolution in three dimensions. Having 15 times less sensitivity is not a serious deterrent to SPECT of the brain, but the relative sensitivity for a resolution of 5 mm is 30 and this difference makes SPECT less practical at high resolution. Figure 4.27 shows the relative sensitivity for head and whole-body instruments. An instrument for imaging the thorax or abdomen has much less sensitivity than does the head instrument because of the R^2 influence (Fig. 4.27, *right*).

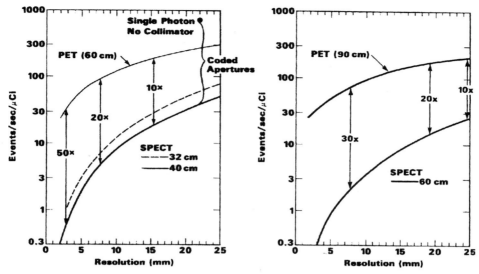

FIGURE 4.27. The calculated sensitivity for SPECT versus that of PET for an instrument designed to image the head (*left*) and one to image the entire body (*right*).

Statistical Parametric Mapping

Quantitative analysis of SPECT studies in brain imaging applications often involves use of regions of interest to measure relative radionuclide activity in specific regions of the brain. Manual techniques are time-consuming and suffer from operator error and difficulty in reproducing the sizes and shapes of regions of interest. The use of standard templates reduces the time required and the reproducibility errors but there are still inherent difficulties in quantitation owing to different sizes and shapes of lesions and brain anatomy. To address these limitations, automated methods with the technique of statistical parametric mapping (32) are currently under study. The software package currently available, SPM'99, was originally designed for the analysis of magnetic resonance and PET images but also has applications in SPECT (33,34). The software provides the capability for transforming images into a standard grid space and has tools for smoothing, coregistration, and performance of statistical analysis of the transformed data by means of general linear modeling techniques. This automated method improves the reliability of quantitative measurements and provides a consistency in multiple study analysis that is not available with other methods.

SINGLE PHOTON EMISSION COMPUTED TOMOGRAPHY WITH POSITRON EMITTERS

The potential of SPECT systems for detection of the 511-keV photons from ^{18}F in fluorodeoxyglucose (FDG) studies of organ metabolism. Applications to lesion detection can be evaluated by means of examination of the equations relative to sensitivity and the physical principles of collimation. As shown in Eq. 11, the sensitivity relative to PET for a resolution of 10 mm is decreased by 15, but this equation is derived for collimator conditions of low-energy photons associated with ^{201}Tl, ^{99m}Tc, and ^{123}I. The lead septa of the collimator for 10-mm resolution for

511-keV photons occupies at least 50% of the area, and the efficiency of ⅜-inch-diameter scintillation camera crystals is 2 to 4 times less than that for the single photon emitters commonly used, further reducing the relative sensitivity. In summary, instead of a sensitivity difference of 15 between three- or four-sided SPECT and PET, we can expect a sensitivity penalty of 45 for 10-mm resolution and approximately 100 for 5-mm resolution. These predictions were verified in studies performed with high-energy SPECT, and the findings indicated that this technique has little application in clinical nuclear medicine (35,36). The single exception is in the evaluation of cardiac FDG intake versus perfusion mismatches. The high signal-to-background ratio, the acceptability of 10-mm spatial resolution, the absence of washout, and the 1.8-hour half-life of ^{18}F allow collection of adequate statistics in a reasonable time for cardiac imaging with this positron emitter. Clinical evaluations with a dual isotope, simultaneous acquisition SPECT protocol and high-energy collimators with ^{18}FDG and ^{99m}Tc sestamibi for the identification of hibernating myocardium have shown that results similar to those from PET can be achieved with this technique (37).

QUALITY ASSURANCE

In addition to the routine quality assurance procedures performed on scintillation cameras, there are two procedures that must be added for cameras with SPECT capability. The first technique is high-quality uniformity correction. Small statistical fluctuations in field uniformity can be tolerated in routine imaging with the scintillation camera. However, the demands for uniformity are much more strict in SPECT. The reason is that lack of field uniformity will appear in each planar projection and be included in the reconstructed data from each projection, resulting in circular artifacts in the final image. To prevent this occurrence, it is necessary to acquire a high-quality flood (30 to 100 million counts) and to use this flood to perform uniformity correction on each planar projection data set before image reconstruction is performed.

The second procedure is center-of-rotation evaluation and correction if necessary. It is imperative that during data acquisition the electronic center of the field of view of the scintillation camera correspond precisely with the mechanical center of rotation of the detector gantry throughout the rotational orbit. Small errors in this correspondence degrade spatial resolution in the reconstructed images and introduce ring artifacts around the mechanical center of rotation. The accuracy of the center of rotation can be evaluated by means of 360-degree acquisition of a point source placed slightly off-center in the imaging field. The x and y positions of the center of the source are then plotted as a function of the angular position of the scintillation camera where x and y are the transaxial and axial positions, respectively. The plot of the axial positions should be a straight line, and the plot of the transaxial positions should be a sine wave. Deviations from these expected values of more than 0.5 pixels are indications of errors that should be corrected by service personnel. In the meantime, these values can be stored and used to correct the positions of planar projection images before image reconstruction (38).

CLINICAL APPLICATIONS

Applications of SPECT to clinical studies preceded x-ray CT, and results of the first quantitative physiologic studies with SPECT were reported in 1975 (39,40). At present, the main interest in SPECT is for heart perfusion imaging with ^{201}Tl and ^{99m}Tc sestamibi and brain imaging with ^{99m}Tc and ^{123}I flow agents and some neuroreceptor ligands. SPECT agents in common use for cerebral blood flow are N-isopropyl-p-(^{123}I)iodoamphetamine (IMP) (41–43) and ^{99m}Tc-labeled hexamethylpropyleneamine oxime (HMPAO). The diffusible gas ^{133}Xe also is being used (44,45). The possibility of revival in brain imaging with SPECT appears to be great because the new compounds concentrate in the brain in proportion to flow (46,47), and images can be obtained over short periods (5 minutes) with a resolution of 7 mm full width at half maximum with appropriate instrumentation. Use of SPECT can provide clinical information similar to perfusion, permeability, and blood volume information obtained with PET but with somewhat less resolution, as discussed earlier.

With the advent of new compounds that concentrate in the heart (48,49), there is renewed interest in SPECT of the heart. A machine designed for dynamic SPECT of the heart is not yet commercially available; however, rotating three-headed gamma-camera systems have demonstrated clinical potential for perfusion imaging with ^{99m}Tc-labeled agents (50–52).

Examination of the liver and kidneys with SPECT has been shown more specific and sensitive in the detection of lesions than is conventional projection imaging (53–55). However, the studies require a data acquisition time of approximately 30 minutes for available devices to obtain adequate statistics to allow reconstruction with distributed sources. Appreciation of the problem is gained if one considers that because of attenuation, only two of 100 photons directed toward the collimator from a source on one side of an abdomen 40 cm in diameter are detected. Yet for quantitative reconstruction, all sources must be detected from all positions with good statistics.

SUMMARY

In SPECT, collimated scintillation camera systems are used to detect γ photons from radionuclides by means of acquisition of multiple-projection images around a patient and use of these data to reconstruct images of slices of the distribution in the patient. These transverse section tomograms yield results similar to those of PET and share with PET the physical problems of attenuation, angular sampling requirements, lack of uniformity of resolution, scatter, and statistical limitations. The severity of these problems is greater for SPECT than for PET; however, they can be compensated for through instrument design and mathematic treatment of the data. Whereas the sensitivity of SPECT in terms of detected events for a given amount of radionuclide in the patient is one-tenth that of PET, the availability of new SPECT radiopharmaceuticals, particularly for imaging of the brain and head, and the practical and economic aspects of SPECT instrumentation make this mode of emission tomography attractive for clinical studies of the heart and brain.

REFERENCES

1. Kuhl DE, Edwards RQ. Image separation radioisotope scanning. *Radiology* 1963;80:653.
2. Kuhl DE, Edwards RQ, Ricci AB, et al. The Mark IV system for radionuclide computed tomography of the brain. *Radiology* 1976;121: 405–413.
3. Kuhl DE, Edwards RQ, Ricci AB, et al. Quantitative section scanning using orthogonal tangent correction. *J Nucl Med* 1973;14:196–200.
4. Prowsner RA, Prowsner ER. Single photon emission computed tomography (SPECT). In: *Essentials of nuclear medicine physics.* Malden, MA: Blackwell Science, 1998:106–135.
5. Shepp LA, Vardi Y, Maximum likelihood reconstruction for emission tomography. *IEEE Trans Med Imaging* 1982;MI-1:113–122.
6. Hudson HM, Larkin RS. Accelerated image reconstruction using ordered subsets of projection data. *J Nucl Med* 1994;13:601–609.
7. Jaszczak RJ, Chang LT, Stein NA. Whole-body single-photon emission computed tomography using dual, large-field-of-view scintillation cameras. *Phys Med Biol* 1979;24:1123.
8. Jaszczak RJ, Coleman RE, Lim CB, et al. Physical factors affecting quantitative measurements using camera-based single photon emission computed tomography (SPECT). *IEEE Trans Nucl Sci* 1981;28:69.
9. Budinger TF, Derenzo SE, Gullberg GT, et al. Trends and prospects for circular ring positron cameras. *IEEE Trans Nucl Sci* 1979;26:2742.
10. Huesman RH, Gullberg GT, Greenberg WL, et al. Users manual: Donner algorithms for reconstruction tomography. Publication 214. Berkeley, CA: Lawrence Berkeley Laboratories, 1977.
11. Budinger TF, Gullberg GT. Three-dimensional reconstruction in nuclear medicine emission imaging. *IEEE Trans Nucl Sci* 1974;21:2–20.
12. Chang L. A method for attenuation correction in radionuclide computed tomography. *IEEE Trans Nucl Sci* 1978;25:638.
13. Derenzo SE, Zaklad H, Budinger T. Analytical study of a high-resolution positron ring detector system for transaxial reconstruction tomography. *J Nucl Med* 1975;16:1166–1173.
14. Gullberg G. The attenuated radon transform: theory and application in medicine and biology [dissertation]. Berkeley, CA: University of California, Berkeley, Lawrence Berkeley Laboratory, 1979.
15. Gullberg GT, Budinger TF. The use of filtering methods to compensate

for constant attenuation in single-photon emission computed tomography. *IEEE Trans Biomed Eng* 1981;28:142.

16. Budinger TF, Derenzo SE, Gullberg GT, et al. Emission computer assisted tomography with single-photon and positron annihilation photon emitters. *J Comput Assist Tomogr* 1977;1:131.

17. Chang L. Attenuation correction and incomplete projection in single photon emission computed tomography. *IEEE Trans Nucl Sci* 1979; 26:2780.

18. Bellini S, Piacentini M, Cafforio C, et al. Compensation of tissue absorbtion in emission tomography. *IEEE Trans Acoust* 1979;27: 213–218.

19. Hasegawa BH, Gingold EL, Reilly SM, et al. Description of a simultaneous emission-transmission CT system. *Proc SPIE* 1990; 1231: 50–60.

20. Stoddard HF, Stoddart HA. A new development in single gamma transaxial tomography: Union Carbide focused collimator scanner. *IEEE Trans Nucl Sci* 1979;26:2742.

21. Formiconi AR, Pupi A, Passeri A. Compensation of spatial system response in SPECT with conjugate gradient reconstruction technique. *Phys Med Biol* 1989;34:69–84.

22. Beck JW, Jaszczak RJ, Coleman RE, et al. Analysis of SPECT including scatter and attenuation using sophisticated Monte Carlo modeling methods. *IEEE Trans Nucl Sci* 1982;29:506.

23. Jaszczak RJ, Floyd CE, Coleman RE. Scatter compensation techniques for SPECT. *IEEE Trans Nucl Sci* 1985;32:786.

24. King MA, Hademenos GJ, Glick SJ. A dual-photopeak window method for scatter correction. *J Nucl Med* 1992;33:605–612.

25. Gilardi MC, Bettinardi V, Todd-Pokropek A, et al. Assessment and comparison of three-scatter correction techniques in single photon emission computed tomography. *J Nucl Med* 1988;29:1971–1979.

26. Frey EC, Tsui BMW. A comparison of scatter compensation methods in SPECT: subtraction-based techniques versus iterative reconstruction with an accurate scatter model. Conference record of the IEEE Nuclear Science Symposium and the Medical Imaging Conference, 25–31 October 1992, Orlando, FL. Piscataway, NJ: IEEE Press, 1992: 1035–1037.

27. DeVito RP, Hamill JJ. Determination of weighting functions for energy-weighted acquisition. *J Nucl Med* 1991;32:343–349.

28. Ljungberg M, Strand SE. Scatter and attenuation correction in SPECT using density maps and Monte Carlo simulated scatter functions. *J Nucl Med* 1990;31:1560.

29. Maski P, Axelsson B, Larson S. Some practical factors influence the accuracy of convolution scatter correction in SPECT. *Phys Med Biol* 1989;34:283.

30. Axelsson B, Msaki P, Israelsson A. Subtraction of Compton-scattered photons in single-photon emission computerized tomography. *J Nucl Med* 1984;25:490–494.

31. Budinger TF, Greenberg WL, Derenzo SE, et al. Quantitative potentials of dynamic emission computed tomography. *J Nucl Med* 1978; 19:309.

32. Friston KJ. Statistical parametric imaging. In: Thatcher RW, Hallet, M, Zeffiro T, et al., eds. *Functional neuroimaging.* New York: Academic Press, 1994:79–93.

33. Johnson LS, Tikofsky RS, Furman V, et al. Reduced cerebral blood flow to white matter of Lyme disease patients demonstrated by statistical parametric mapping of brain SPECT. *J Nucl Med* 1999;40;1197.

34. Tikofsky RS, Jonas SP, Singh D, et al. Statistical parametric mapping (SPM) in the evaluation of dementia: a pilot study. *J Nucl Med* 1999: 40;1205.

35. Martin WH, Delbeke D, Patton JA, et al. FDG-SPECT: correlation with FDG-PET. *J Nucl Med* 1995;36:989–995.

36. Martin WH, Delbeke D, Patton JA, et al. FDG SPECT vs FDG PET for the detection of malignancies. *Radiology* 1996;198:225–241.

37. Sandler MP, Videlefsky S, Delbeke D, et al. Evaluation of myocardial ischemia using a rest metabolism/stress perfusion protocol with 18FDG/99mTc-MIBI and dual isotope simultaneous acquisition SPECT. *J Am Coll Cardiol* 1995;26:870–878.

38. Prowsner RA, Prowsner ER. Quality control. In: *Essentials of nuclear medicine physics.* Malden MA: Blackwell Science, 1998:148–163.

39. Kuhl DE, Alavi A, Hoffman EJ, et al. Local cerebral blood volume in head-injured patients: determination by emission computed tomography of 99m-Tc-labeled cells. *J Neurosurg* 1980;52:309.

40. Kuhl DE, Reivich M, Alavi A, et al. Local cerebral blood volume determined by three-dimensional reconstruction of radionuclide scan data. *Circ Res* 1975;36:610.

41. Hill TC, Holman BL, Lovett R, et al. Initial experience with SPECT (single photon computerized tomography) of the brain using n-isopropyl I-123-p-iodoamphetamine. *J Nucl Med* 1982;23:191.

42. Kuhl DE, Barrio JR, Huang SC, et al. Quantifying local cerebral blood flow by N-isopropyl-p-(^{123}I)iodoamphetamine (IMP) tomography. *J Nucl Med* 1982;23:196–203.

43. Podreka I, Baumgartner C, Suess E, et al. Quantification of regional cerebral blood flow with IMP-SPECT: reproducibility and clinical relevance of flow values. *Stroke* 1989;20:183–191.

44. Devous MDS, Payne JK, Lowe JL. Dual-isotope brain SPECT imaging with technetium-99m and iodine-123: clinical validation using xenon-133 SPECT. *J Nucl Med* 1992;33:1919–1924.

45. Hellman RS, Collier BD, Tikofsky RS, et al. Comparison of single-photon emission computed tomography with (^{123}I)iodoamphetamine and xenon-enhanced computed tomography for assessing regional cerebral blood flow. *J Cereb Blood Flow Metab* 1986;6:747–755.

46. Mayberg HS, Lewis PJ, Regenold W, et al. Paralimbic hypoperfusion in unipolar depression. *J Nucl Med* 1994;35:929–934.

47. Wilhelm KR, Schroder J, Henningsen H, et al. Preliminary results of ^{99m}Tc-HMPAO-SPECT studies in endogenous psychoses. *J Nucl Med* 1989;28:88–91.

48. Maddahi J, Merz R, Van Train KF, et al. Tc-99m MIBI (RP-30) and Tl-201 myocardial perfusion scintigraphy in patients with coronary disease: quantitative comparison of planar and tomographic techniques for perfusion defect intensity and defect reversibility. *J Nucl Med* 1987; 28:654.

49. Watson DD, Smith WH, Teates CD, et al. Quantitative myocardial imaging with Tc-99m MIBI: comparison with Tl-201. *J Nucl Med* 1987;28:653.

50. Budinger T, Araujo L, Ranger N, et al. Dynamic SPECT feasibility studies. *J Nucl Med* 1991;32:955(abst).

51. Sasaki M, Ichiya Y, Kuwabara Y, et al. Rapid myocardial perfusion imaging with ^{99m}Tc-teboroxime and a three-headed SPECT system: a comparative study with ^{201}Tl. *Nucl Med Commun* 1992;13:790–794.

52. Smith AM, Gullberg GT, Christian PE, et al. Kinetic modeling of teboroxime using dynamic SPECT imaging of a canine model. *J Nucl Med* 1994;35:484–495.

53. Biersack HF, Koischwitz D, Lackner K, et al. Single-photon emission computed tomography (SPECT) of the liver with a rotating gamma camera system. *Nuklearmedizin* 1981;10:205–213.

54. Jaszczak RJ, Coleman RE, Lim CB, et al. Lesion detection with single photon emission computed tomography (SPECT) and conventional imaging. *J Nucl Med* 1982;23:97.

55. Raynaud C, Syrota A, Soussaline F, et al. Single photon emission computed tomography in diagnosis of liver metastasis. *J Nucl Med* 1981; 22:P31(abst).

5

POSITRON EMISSION TOMOGRAPHY: METHODS AND INSTRUMENTATION

SIMON R. CHERRY
MICHAEL E. PHELPS

POSITRON EMISSION TOMOGRAPHY

Positron emission tomography (PET) is a unique imaging tool that can be used to visualize and measure many biologic processes in living subjects (1). Modern clinical PET systems now have the ability to simultaneously image the whole brain or heart with 4 to 6 mm spatial resolution and a temporal resolution of seconds. The use of cardiac gating can improve effective temporal resolution to tens of milliseconds. Methods have been developed to image the entire body in a single imaging session. PET has become an important clinical tool, particularly in oncology and the management of neurologic disorders and cardiovascular disease. PET also continues to be a powerful research tool, from clinical research in humans to basic science studies with mice. This chapter provides an overview of (a) the methods and instrumentation used in PET, including the fundamentals of PET imaging, (b) the production and characteristics of commonly used positron emitters, (c) the design of the modern PET scanner, (d) the process of image reconstruction, (e) the correction factors necessary to achieve quantitative PET images, and (f) the use of tracer kinetic models to turn PET images into quantitative biologic assays.

Molecular Imaging with Positron Emission Tomography

The biologic ubiquity of the elements available as positron emitters (compared with elements with suitable energy single γ-ray emitting isotopes) gives PET an unprecedented power to image the distribution and kinetics of natural and analog biologic tracers. Because of the exquisite sensitivity of detection systems to γ-ray emission, these biologic probes can be introduced in trace amounts (nanomolar or even picomolar concentrations) such that they do not disturb the biologic process under investigation. The combination of a tracer that is selective for a specific molecular target or biochemical pathway, an accurate tracer ki-

netic model, and a dynamic sequence of quantitative images from the PET scanner makes it possible to estimate the properties of these targets and the absolute rates of biologic processes in these pathways. Examples of biologic parameters successfully measured with PET include regional blood flow, rates of substrate use (e.g., glucose and oxygen), rates of protein synthesis, neurotransmitter synthesis, receptor binding and density, enzyme activity, and levels of gene expression (1,2). PET imaging systems have an advantage over other in vivo nuclear imaging technologies in that they simultaneously provide high spatial resolution and high sensitivity (the fraction of radioactive decays that lead to a detectable event). This advantage exists largely because no physical collimation is needed, as is discussed later. PET therefore generally provides higher-quality images than either planar nuclear imaging or SPECT, and has greater flexibility in generating natural labeled probes for imaging.

There is also a growing realization of the power of combining PET with pharmacology and drug development (3–5). The synergism results from the common requirements in the development of a drug and a molecular imaging probe. Each is designed to interact with a target molecule or biologic process, the drug to modify the target or process and the imaging probe to measure the properties of the target or the process. Each is designed to be administered systemically, with minimal breakdown by enzyme systems or sequestering by the immune system, and to cross membranes and reach the target with little interaction other than with the target. Because of this commonality, many of the new molecular imaging probes will be labeled drugs originating out of the merger of modern biology, biotechnology, and drug development. These new generations of drugs and molecular imaging probes will focus on the fundamental processes that regulate biologic systems, such as signal transduction, second messengers, and transcription and translation of messenger RNA. With PET, not only can the modifying effects of drugs on a particular biologic process be monitored, but also the drugs themselves can be labeled and introduced in trace amounts, allowing safe determination of the pharmacokinetics in the living human body. PET is a molecular imaging technique that brings together in vivo molecular diagnostics and molecular therapeutics from the fundamental level of genetically engineered and cell transplant models of human disease in mice to the evolving application of these principles in patients.

S.R. Cherry: Department of Biomedical Engineering, UC Davis, Davis, CA.

M.E. Phelps: Department of Molecular and Medical Pharmacology, UCLA School of Medicine, Los Angeles, CA.

Role of Positron Emission Technology in Radiologic Imaging

PET, like SPECT, plays a complementary, but quite distinct role from other commonly used medical imaging modalities, such as magnetic resonance (MR) imaging or x-ray computed tomography (CT). These methods mainly provide anatomic information and are chosen when disruption of normal anatomy by disease is to be expected. There are many situations, however, in which anatomic changes may be completely absent or in which biochemical changes precede anatomic changes. Examples in the brain include neurodegenerative disease, such as Alzheimer's (6), Parkinson's, and Huntington's diseases (7), neurodevelopmental disorders (8), epilepsy (9), psychiatric disorders (10), and drug abuse (11,12). In the care of patients with coronary artery disease and cardiomyopathy, PET helps differentiate ischemic (but viable) and infarcted myocardium (13,14). In cancer throughout the body, PET helps in detecting early disease, grading the degree of malignancy, staging, and differentiating residual tumor or recurrence from necrosis, surgical scarring, and edema (15,16). PET is effective in monitoring patient response to cancer therapy. Gambhir et al. (17) reviewed and analyzed the clinical literature involving more than 20,000 patients with cancer, cardiovascular disease, epilepsy, or Alzheimer's disease. For 20 types of cancer examined, PET was found to be between 8% to 43% more accurate than conventional imaging in diagnosis, staging, detection of recurrence, and assessment of therapeutic response. PET results led to changes in the treatment of 15% to 50% of patients, depending on the clinical situation. The diagnosis of Alzheimer's disease was shown to have 93% accuracy 3 years before the clinical diagnosis of probable Alzheimer's disease could be established. This finding demonstrates that PET provides unique information not available with other modalities and that it has applications in a wide range of diseases.

Looking toward the future, the sequencing of genomes, and determination of the structure and function of proteins is driving biology and medicine to identify the molecular errors of disease and to develop molecular corrections of these errors. This is placing great emphasis on molecular diagnostics, and PET is the leading technology at this time to provide a molecular diagnosis through noninvasive imaging.

FUNDAMENTALS OF POSITRON EMISSION TOMOGRAPHY

The nucleus of an atom contains both neutrons and protons (collectively known as *nucleons*). The number of protons and neutrons in a stable nucleus is such that the repulsive electrostatic force between the positively charged protons is balanced by the attractive strong nuclear forces that act on all nucleons. With cyclotrons, it is possible to produce isotopes that have an excess of protons and are, therefore, unstable. These proton-rich isotopes can decay by two modes—electron capture and positron emission. The result of either decay mode is to convert one of the protons into a neutron, decreasing the atomic number of the atom by one. The result is a better balance between the forces acting on the nucleus.

Electron Capture

In electron capture, the nucleus captures one of the atomic electrons from the inner shells and combines this with a proton to form a neutron. In terms of the nucleus, this can be written as

$$_Z^A N \rightarrow {}_{Z-1}^A N + \nu \tag{1}$$

where Z is the atomic number, A is the mass number, and ν is a neutrino. Energy is released in the decay process because the final daughter state has a lower total energy than the parent state, and this energy is carried off by the neutrino. The likelihood of electron capture increases with atomic number, because the inner-shell electrons tend to be closer to the nucleus and thus are easier to capture. Because this mode of decay does not generally lead to penetrating radiation, it is of limited use for imaging purposes.

Positron Emission

An alternative decay mode is positron emission, whereby a proton in the nucleus is transformed into a neutron and a positron. The positron (e^+) has the same mass as the electron but has a positive charge of exactly the same magnitude as the negative charge of the electron. The nuclear equation for positron emission can be written as

$$_Z^A N \rightarrow {}_{Z-1}^A N + e^+ + \nu \tag{2}$$

For positron emission to be energetically feasible, the difference in total energy between the parent and daughter states has to be at least 1.022 MeV (equal to the energy equivalent of a positron and an electron). It turns out that positron emission, unlike electron capture, is favored in low Z elements. In some higher Z elements, positron emission actually is energetically forbidden because of the 1.022 MeV requirement, and decay can proceed only by means of electron capture. In many intermediate Z, proton-rich nuclei, the two decay modes are competing processes. An example of this, decay of ^{18}F into ^{18}O, is shown in Fig. 5.1. The energy difference between the parent and daughter states (1.65 − 1.022 MeV) is shared between the positron and

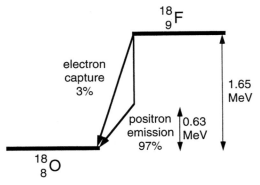

FIGURE 5.1. Decay scheme and energy levels for ^{18}F show competition between positron emission (97%) and electron capture (3%). The total energy of the transition is 1.66 MeV, of which 0.64 MeV is available for positron emission.

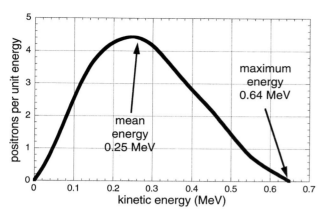

FIGURE 5.2. Typical energy distribution of positrons after emission. The mean energy is approximately one-third the maximum energy. The higher the positron energy, the farther it is likely to travel before annihilation. Thus limits are set on the spatial resolution attainable with PET.

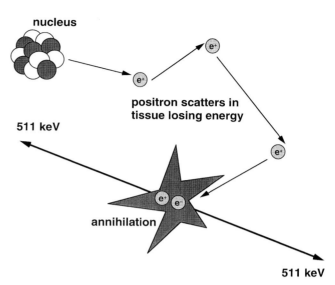

FIGURE 5.3. Proton-rich isotopes can decay by means of positron emission. The positron rapidly loses kinetic energy, scattering off atomic electrons. It slows sufficiently to combine with an electron, and the two particles are annihilated. Their mass is converted into energy in the form of two 511-keV γ-rays, which are emitted back to back.

the neutrino. Emitted positrons therefore have a spectrum of energies (Fig. 5.2). The maximum energy, E_{max}, is equal to

$$E_{max} = E(_Z^A N) - E(_{Z-1}^A N) - 1.022 MeV \qquad [3]$$

Positron Annihilation

The positron has a short lifetime in solids and liquids. It rapidly loses kinetic energy in scattering interactions with atomic electrons. When it reaches thermal energy, essentially at rest, it combines with an electron, and the two particles undergo annihilation. Their mass converts into energy in the form of γ-rays. The energy released in annihilation is 1.022 MeV. To simultaneously conserve both momentum and energy, annihilation must produce two γ-rays with 511 keV of energy that are emitted 180 degrees to each other (Fig. 5.3). The detection of the two 511-keV γ-rays forms the basis for imaging with PET.

Coincidence Detection and Electronic Collimation

There is a relatively high probability that both 511-keV γ-rays will escape from the body without scattering. If both γ-rays can subsequently be detected, we can define the line along which annihilation must have occurred. Because the distance the positron travels before annihilation is generally small, this is a good approximation to the line along which the emitting atom must be located. By having a ring of detectors surrounding the patient, it is possible to build a map of the distribution of the positron-emitting isotope in the body.

One advantage of PET is that it employs electronic collimation. By use of coincidence detection (simultaneous or coincident detection of two γ-rays on opposite sides of the body), the direction from which the γ-rays came is defined. In conventional nuclear medicine techniques, in which only one γ-ray is available, this can be achieved only by use of a lead collimator, drilled with small holes, that mechanically collimates the arriving γ-rays by transmitting γ-rays from only one particular direction

and absorbing all others. The absorption of most of the γ-rays in the lead (only 1 in 10^3 or 10^4 photons typically passes through the holes in the lead collimator) leads to a large reduction in sensitivity compared with that of PET. Another advantage is that all positron-emitting radionuclides produce 511-keV γ-rays, so the PET scanner can be optimized for detection at this one energy. In other nuclear medicine techniques, the γ-ray energy varies with radionuclide, and the camera must be able to image over a range of energy.

Physical Limits of Spatial Resolution in Positron Emission Tomography

Two factors ultimately limit the spatial resolution attainable with PET (18). First, the positron travels a short distance between the site of emission and the site of annihilation. This distance is called the *positron range* and can vary from fractions of a millimeter to several millimeters, depending on the energy spectrum of the emitted positrons and the tissue in which the emission occurs. This effect leads to a blurring of the data that is characterized by an exponential function. A measure of the blurring due to positron range for some commonly used positron-emitting isotopes is shown in Table 5.1.

The other factor that can limit spatial resolution is caused by the residual kinetic energy and momentum of the positron and electron at the moment they annihilate. This leads to the angle between the two γ-rays deviating slightly from 180°. The blurring effect caused by this component depends on the diameter of the PET scanner. For a typical clinical system with a ring diameter of approximately 80 cm, the resolution degradation due to this effect is approximately 1.8 mm. By convolving the noncolinearity and positron range effects, it becomes apparent that the absolute resolution limit in whole-body clinical PET

Table 5.1. *Characteristics of common positron-emitting isotopes*

Isotope	Half-life	β^+ fraction	β^+ E_{max} (MeV)	FWHM (mm)
^{11}C	20.4 min	0.99	0.96	0.28
^{13}N	9.96 min	1.00	1.19	0.45
^{15}O	2.07 min	1.00	1.72	1.04
^{18}F	1.83 h	0.97	0.64	0.22
^{62}Cu	9.74 min	0.98	2.94	2.29
^{68}Ga	68.3 min	0.88	1.90	1.35
^{82}Ru	1.25 min	0.96	3.35	2.6

Values are approximate full width at half maximum (FWHM) of exponential positron range distributions. Because distribution is not gaussian, resolution limits in positron emission tomography due to positron range are not well characterized with this single number. Care should be taken in making any extrapolation to reconstructed image resolution.
E_{max}, maximum energy.

scanners is approximately 2 mm with ^{11}C- or ^{18}F-labeled radiopharmaceuticals. As discussed later, current clinical systems are capable of 4- to 5-mm spatial resolution. In smaller-diameter PET systems (systems dedicated to brain imaging, breast imaging, or animal imaging), a resolution of 1 to 1.5 mm can be achieved because of the smaller contribution from noncolinearity of the γ-rays.

Random and Scattered Coincidence Events

In addition to detection of the true coincidence events, PET imaging with coincidence detection can result in two types of events that are undesirable. A scattered coincidence occurs when one or both of the γ-rays undergo a Compton scatter interaction inside the body. This changes the direction of and reduces the energy of the γ-ray. The change in direction results in misidentification of the γ-ray origin (Fig. 5.4). The fraction of γ-rays scattered depends on the scattering medium and the path length through the body. Therefore the contribution from scattered events is more evident in abdominal imaging than in brain imaging. Although the energy of scattered γ-rays is reduced to less than 511 keV, the most likely scatter angles are small, leading to relatively small losses in energy. The energy resolution of most PET systems is insufficient to reject many of these events, and energy windowing is not an effective means of scatter rejection. Thus many of the scattered events are accepted and subsequently

produce malpositioned data. Correction for these events is discussed later.

Although each annihilation produces two γ-rays, it is common for only one of the two to be detected (the opposing γ-ray may not intersect the detection system or may be scattered out of the system). Random (or accidental) coincidence events (19) occur when two unrelated, single 511-keV γ-rays (not from the same annihilation) strike opposing detectors within the coincidence resolving time of the system (Fig. 5.4). This is accepted as a valid event because it is indistinguishable from a true coincidence event. The random coincidence rate is roughly proportional to the square of the activity in the field of view and is therefore a particular problem for high-count-rate studies. Fortunately, the correction for these events is relatively straightforward.

POSITRON-EMITTING TRACERS AND THEIR PRODUCTION

Positron-Emitting Isotopes

A unique attribute of PET is the availability of isotopes of elements that are the building blocks of all organic molecules. The most important of these are ^{11}C, ^{13}N, and ^{15}O. ^{18}F also is an important and useful radionuclide. Its chemical properties are similar to those of hydrogen and the OH group, allowing it to substitute for hydrogen or OH to produce positron-labeled analog tracers of natural compounds. Fluorine is a widely used element in drug design because of its small size and the strength of the C–F bond. The properties of these positron-emitting isotopes are shown in Table 5.1. With these isotopes, it is possible in theory to label almost any compound of biologic interest. Thousands of positron-emitting compounds have been synthesized (20). These include substances that are present naturally in the body, such as sugars, proteins, amino acids, fatty acids, nucleic acids, hormones, and neurotransmitters, or close analogs of these, which isolate specific pathways of biochemical interest. Drugs can be labeled, and because of the exquisite sensitivity of PET, the pharmacokinetics can be imaged with nanomolar or picomolar concentrations, which are well below the concentrations at which pharmacologic effects become important. It becomes possible, therefore, to examine potentially toxic compounds in the living human body.

There are many other positron-emitting isotopes (e.g., ^{62}Cu,

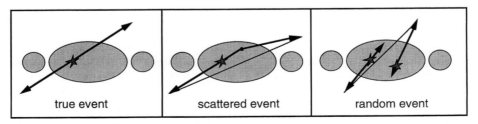

FIGURE 5.4. Three types of events are detected with a PET scanner—true, scattered and random coincidence events. Only true events are part of the desired signal. Random and scattered coincidence is malpositioned and adds a low spatial frequency background to the image. Corrections for random and scattered coincidence must be applied to maximize quantitative accuracy.

^{64}Cu, ^{68}Ga, and ^{124}I), but like many of the single photon isotopes used in conventional nuclear medicine (e.g., ^{99m}Tc, ^{123}I, and ^{67}Ga), they are not isotopes of elements that are ubiquitous in the human body. Therefore they are of most utility for labeling larger biomolecules (e.g., antibodies and peptides), when the label is unlikely to interfere with biologic action.

Production of Positron-Emitting Isotopes

Positron emitters are produced in a cyclotron (21,22). Here stable nuclei are bombarded with protons or deuterons (hydrogen with an added neutron) to produce the proton-rich state necessary for positron emission. Some positron emitters that have parent states that also decay, but with a longer half-life, can be produced in the form of an ion-exchange generator. In this case, the parent is produced by a cyclotron and slowly decays into the daughter positron emitter in the generator. Doses of the positron emitter can be eluted from the generator at regular intervals for use at a PET center. Examples of generator-produced positron emitting isotopes are ^{62}Cu, ^{68}Ga, and ^{82}Rb (23). The ^{68}Ge-^{68}Ga parent-daughter combination is used as a calibration source, and in the sources used for attenuation correction. The slow decay of ^{68}Ge (half-life, 273 days) provides a steady supply of positron-emitting ^{68}Ga, allowing these sources to be used continually over a period of many months before replacement is needed.

Cyclotron Production of Short-lived Positron-Emitting Isotopes

The most useful positron emitters, however, come from stable parent isotopes and therefore cannot be produced as ion-exchange generators. Because of the relatively short half-lives of these isotopes, it is necessary that they be produced close to the PET scanner. Therefore, most PET facilities have their own cyclotrons or receive labeled compounds from regional distribution centers. The technology for medical cyclotrons has advanced dramatically in the last decade (21,22). What started out as large, complicated research machines for nuclear physics groups requiring experienced staff and a large, well-shielded vault, have now become compact, automated, self-shielding, and reliable biomedical devices that can be operated by one technician.

The radioisotope delivery system made by Siemens is typical of a modern PET cyclotron. It accelerates negative hydrogen ions (1 proton, 2 electrons) to 11 MeV. Once the beam of hydrogen ions has reached the desired energy, it is extracted from the cyclotron by passing it through a thin carbon foil that strips off the two electrons. The resulting proton feels the magnetic field of the cyclotron acting in the opposite direction, and the proton leaves the cyclotron and strikes the target (Fig. 5.5). The advantages of this system are that it is possible to have multiple ports on the cyclotron each set up to produce a different isotope and that the beam can be extracted simultaneously into two ports, allowing two isotopes to be produced simultaneously. Other advantages of negative-ion cyclotron designs include easy control, simplified beam shaping, little beam loss (giving rise to less prompt radiation and induced activity, thus reducing shield-

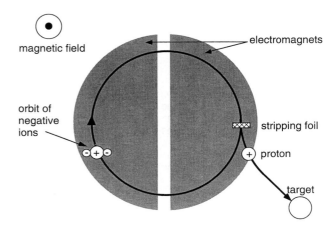

FIGURE 5.5. Schematic shows operation of a negative-ion cyclotron. The H$^-$ ions are accelerated by an alternating electric field to an energy of approximately 10 MeV. At this energy, they are passed through thin carbon foil that strips off the two electrons. The resulting proton is extracted from the beam (because it has positive charge and therefore bends in the opposite direction in the magnetic field) and strikes the target to produce the positron-emitting isotope.

ing requirements), and uniform distribution of beam intensity. The radioisotope delivery system can deliver a 50 μA proton beam through a 1-cm collimator at the target entrance to yield 2 to 3 Ci of ^{18}F, ^{11}C, or ^{15}O and 0.6 Ci of ^{13}N. The entire system can be operated by one technician sitting at a personal computer.

Positron Emission Tomography Tracer Synthesis

There are a number of important considerations in tracer design for PET (24). The availability of isotopes that do not alter the biochemical behavior of the compound of interest is an enormous advantage. However, the half-life of these isotopes is relatively short; therefore synthesis of the labeled product must be rapid. In practice, complex tracers are best labeled with either ^{18}F, ^{11}C, or ^{13}N, because ^{15}O has only a 2-minute half-life and use of this isotope is therefore limited to simple tracers such as H_2O, CO, O_2, and CO_2. Another issue is whether to produce a natural substrate (direct substitution of a positron-emitting atom for a stable atom) or an analog (modification of natural substrate at one or several key locations). The advantage of the analogs is that they can be targeted and limited to interactions in a small section of complex biochemical reaction sequences. This can facilitate subsequent analysis and interpretation of the PET data. The position at which the positron-emitting label is placed (there often is a choice) also is critical. The best labeling position is generally dictated by the biochemical result desired and minimizes the number and amount of labeled metabolites appearing. Often, this requires detailed knowledge of the biochemical reaction sequence for the tracer under consideration.

Taking the positron-emitting isotope from the cyclotron target and synthesizing the labeled tracer of interest can be a labor- and dose-intensive task. A great deal of innovative work centers on the design of automated synthesis devices (21) that take a positron-emitting precursor and turn it into a labeled compound ready for injection into the patient. Such devices, which draw heavily on technology developed for automated gene sequencing and peptide synthesis, are available for producing a range of PET tracers, including ^{18}F-fluorodeoxyglucose (a glucose analog) and L-6-[^{18}F]fluorodopa (a precursor to dopamine). These devices have been integrated with the cyclotron to yield automated systems that produce sterile, pyrogen-free, positron-labeled imaging probes ready for administration to patients. This concept of "electronic generators" has become the base technology for commercial PET radiopharmacies that distribute PET imaging probes to a number of sites, eliminating the need for the many PET centers that are focused on clinical service to run and operate their own cyclotrons.

POSITRON EMISSION TOMOGRAPHY INSTRUMENTATION: DESIGN PRINCIPLES

To image the distribution of positron-emitting isotope in the body, it is necessary to detect both of the 511-keV γ-rays emitted from the positron annihilation in coincidence. To achieve high-quality images, it is important that the detectors used in a PET scanner have high intrinsic spatial resolution, high detection efficiency, and high count-rate capability (minimizing dead-time losses). The ultimate sensitivity of the device (the number of events detected for a given concentration of positron emitter) is strongly related to the product of the detector efficiency and the solid angle coverage of the scanner. Therefore PET scanners typically consist of multiple rings of detectors surrounding the subject. The detector of choice in almost all commercially available PET scanners is a scintillating material coupled to a photomultiplier tube. The 511-keV γ-ray interacts through the photoelectric effect or Compton scattering in the scintillator and deposits all or part of its energy. The scintillator converts this energy into a flash of visible light, which is detected by the photomultiplier tube and converted into a current pulse. If the subsequent coincidence circuitry determines that two γ-rays were detected simultaneously from opposite sides of the body, then an event is registered and stored. These events are subsequently reconstructed with a computer into a series of contiguous tomographic (cross-sectional) images of the body. This image volume can be displayed in transverse, sagittal, or coronal orientation or by means of reslicing the image volume, in any arbitrary orientation.

Intrinsic Spatial Resolution

The intrinsic spatial resolution of a PET system is largely determined by the spatial resolution of the detectors, although for

very-high-resolution systems, there may be a contribution from either the positron range or noncolinearity effects described earlier. Consider passing a point source of radioactivity along a line centered between two detectors of width D. The resulting coincidence point spread function is triangular, with a full width at half maximum of D/2 (Fig. 5.6). In practice, the resolution in the reconstructed images may not be as good as this owing to effects related to data sampling, statistical noise, and the reconstruction algorithm. The reconstructed image resolution is discussed later. However, it is readily apparent that building a high-resolution PET scanner necessitates use of very small individual detector elements or a larger position-sensing detector with very good position resolution.

Detector Efficiency

The efficiency of a detector depends on the stopping power of the scintillator (strongly related to the effective atomic number and density of the material) and the thickness of the scintillator used in the detector. Table 5.2 lists the properties of some commonly available scintillators. Bismuth germanate (BGO) is used in most PET systems because of its unrivaled stopping power for 511-keV γ-rays. Even with BGO, a 3-cm thickness of material is needed to cause 90% of the incoming 511-keV γ-rays to interact. Because both γ-rays must be detected, the overall efficiency for a pair of 3-cm thick detectors is 0.9^2, or 0.81. Despite its good stopping power, BGO has disadvantages relative to other scintillators in that its decay time (the amount of time after the γ-ray interacts over which scintillation light is produced) is quite long, causing count-rate limitations, and its light output (amount of scintillation light generated when a 511-keV γ-ray interacts) is low. A new high-density scintillator, lutetium oxyorthosilicate (LSO) has been introduced and has the advantage of producing large amounts of light with a shorter decay time than that of BGO. LSO has been used in specialized research PET scanners and has been introduced into clinical PET systems.

Energy Resolution and Scattered Events

Events that undergo Compton scattering in the body are misplaced (Fig.5.4). Fortunately, the γ-ray loses energy when scattering occurs, potentially allowing scatter to be rejected by the use of energy discrimination. This is possible because the amount of scintillation light produced is directly proportional to the energy deposited in the scintillator. There are, however, a number of factors that conspire to make the rejection of scatter by means of energy discrimination a difficult problem in PET. First, the amount of scintillation light produced by BGO is not very high, thus the energy resolution, which is inversely proportional

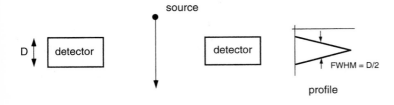

FIGURE 5.6. Line spread function resulting from two detectors in coincidence. The profile is triangular with a full width at half maximum of one-half the detector size. It shows that the resolution in PET is directly influenced by the size of the detectors used.

Table 5.2. *Characteristics of scintillating materials for positron emission tomography*

Scintillator	Effective Z	Decay (µs)	Index of Refraction	Relative Light Yield	Peak Wavelength (nm)
Sodium iodide	50	0.23	1.85	100	410
Bismuth germanate	59	0.30	2.15	13	480
Lutetium oxyorthosilicate	66	0.04	1.82	65	420
Gadolinium oxyorthosilicate	74	0.06	1.85	20	430
Barium fluoride	52	0.62	1.49	13	310
		0.0006		3	220

Z, atomic number.

to the square root of the number of scintillation photons produced, is typically only 20% to 30%. Second, γ-rays, when they scatter in the body, tend to lose only a small amount of energy. Thus the energy of the scattered photons is not much less than 511 keV, and with only 20% energy resolution, these cannot be differentiated from unscattered photons. Third, some unscattered γ-rays interact in the detector through the Compton interaction and deposit only part of their energy. Therefore they have the signature of a scattered event but are true unscattered events. Setting an energy threshold too high results in the loss of true events. In a typical BGO PET system, the energy threshold is set at approximately 350 keV, which is effective in removing some of the scattered events. Still, approximately 30% to 40% of the events detected in a three-dimensional brain study have been scattered. The effect is to add a low spatial frequency background to the PET images, and the result is a slight loss of contrast.

Coincidence Timing and Random Events

To register a valid event, the PET scanner must detect two γ-rays on opposite sides of the body simultaneously. The condition of simultaneity must, in practice, be relaxed somewhat to account for differences in arrival times of the two γ-rays, the finite time to produce scintillation light in the detector, and difference in time delays caused by the processing electronics. The coincidence window for each event usually is set to 12 nanoseconds, requiring that both events occur within ± 12 nanoseconds of each other for an event to be registered. The finite width of the coincidence window, however, allows detection of random (or accidental) events when the two detected γ-rays come from unrelated annihilations. The rate of random coincidence, R, is found as follows:

$$R = 2 \times \tau \times S_1 \times S_2 \qquad [4]$$

where τ is the coincidence time window and S is the rate of single γ-ray events on two detectors. The optimal width of the coincidence time window can be determined experimentally with a plot of the true and random events as a function of τ. If τ is too small, many true events will be discarded; if τ is too large, many random events are accepted. Random events, if not corrected for, add a low-frequency background much as do scattered events, leading to a loss of image contrast, and they can cause image artifacts (19). The fraction of random events in-

creases as the activity in the field of view increases. Doubling the activity doubles the number of true coincidence counts, but because the rate of random events is proportional to the square of the singles event rate, which is roughly proportional to activity, quadrupling of the random-events rate occurs.

Sensitivity

To achieve high sensitivity, the detectors must subtend a large solid angle to the subject. This is why in conventional two-dimensional PET imaging, a ring of detectors is used to capture all the γ-ray pairs emitted from a given slice of the body. To make even better use of the injected dose, modern PET systems consist of multiple rings of detectors that allow multiple slices of the body to be imaged simultaneously (Fig. 5.7). Thin metal shields, called *septa,* are placed between the rings of detectors to help reduce the number of scattered and random coincidences. A modern PET system typically produces 47 to 63 slices from an axial field of view of 10 to 15 cm. These slices can be stacked to provide volumetric image data from the entire heart or brain.

The sensitivity of a single slice of such a system is given by the product of the square of the detector efficiency ε and the solid angle. For a ring of detectors of diameter *d*, each detector measuring *D* cm in width in the axial direction, the sensitivity (in the absence of any scattering or attenuation of γ-rays in the body) at the center of scanner can be approximated as follows:

$$Sensitivity \ (\%) \approx 100 \ \varepsilon^2 \left(\frac{D}{d}\right) \qquad [5]$$

if $D \ll d$. For a typical whole-body PET system with a *d* of

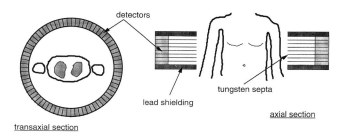

FIGURE 5.7. Transaxial and axial cross-sections through a multiring PET scanner show the interplane septa and lead shielding that help to reduce the single-event rate, improve count-rate performance, and decrease the fraction of random events detected.

80 cm, a D of 4 mm, and $\varepsilon = 0.9$, this results in an absolute sensitivity of only 0.4%. Thus even with complete rings of detectors, slice-based imaging makes poor use of the injected dose.

System Dead-Time and Count-Rate Capability

It takes a finite amount of time to process an event after a 511-keV γ-ray strikes a detector. The rate-determining process usually is collection of the scintillation light by the photomultiplier tubes. The integration time usually is 2 to 3 times the decay time of the scintillator. For BGO, an integration time of 1 microsecond allows collection of more than 90% of the scintillation light. Electronic multiplexing of signals and the coincidence circuitry can, however, also have nonnegligible dead-time components. While an event is being processed, the detector is essentially inactive and cannot perceive another incoming event as a separate event. This event is therefore lost, and the effective sensitivity of the scanner is reduced (25). A simplistic model for dead time in a PET scanner is

$$S = S_0 \exp(-\sigma S_0) \qquad [6]$$

where S_0 is the actual singles rate on the detector, σ is the dead time, and S is the detected singles event rate. With this model, σ is approximately 1 to 3 microseconds for most PET systems. Dead time is not a problem when the PET system consists of a very large number of individual detectors and electronics channels. However, in most PET systems, the detectors entail some form of multiplexing to reduce the complexity of the electronics. This effectively increases the detector area that becomes inactive in the scanner when an event is detected and processed. In some studies in which high doses of short-lived isotopes are used, dead time can become a limiting factor. Dead time leads to a reduction in the number of counts recorded per unit injected dose and can be seen as effectively lowering the sensitivity of the system at high count rates. The count-rate performance of a particular PET system is easily determined by means of monitoring the count rate as a function of the amount of activity within the object of interest.

Noise Equivalent Count Rate

A useful concept in determining the count-rate performance of a PET scanner is the noise equivalent count (NEC) rate. This is the number of counts detected as a function of the activity concentration after correction for the effects of random and scattered events and taking into account dead-time losses. The NEC rate has been shown to be directly proportional to the signal-to-noise ratio in final reconstructed PET images and is thus a good guide to scanner performance (26). It is defined as follows:

$$NEC = \frac{T^2}{T + S + 2kR} \qquad [7]$$

where T is the true count rate, R is the random count rate, and S is the rate of scattered coincidence events. S is defined to include only scattered events that fall within the field of view of the object being imaged. The factor k takes into account that random events are spread rather broadly across the field of view, and only those in the field of view of the object contribute to noise in the image. The factor 2 arises from the use of the delayed coincidence method of correcting for randoms events, which is discussed later. A plot of NEC against activity for a standard 20-cm uniform cylinder often is the easiest way to compare performance among scanners and to predict the signal-to-noise ratio that will be achieved in the final images. It is important that the objects used to obtain the NEC rate be identical if comparisons are to be made, because the NEC rate is highly sensitive to the size and shape of the object in the field of view.

DETECTORS AND SYSTEMS FOR POSITRON EMISSION TOMOGRAPHY

Block Detector

One way to achieve high spatial resolution is to use very small detector elements. Many commercial PET systems today are made with block detectors, which consist of a segmented block of BGO, coupled to four photomultiplier tubes (27,28). Typically, the BGO is 3 cm deep and is segmented into an 8 × 8 array of elements, each approximately 4 mm × 4 mm (Fig. 5.8A). The element in which a γ-ray interacts is determined by looking at the relative light output from the four photomultiplier tubes. Anger-type logic is used to obtain an X position and a Y position from the four photomultiplier tube outputs (P_i) as follows:

$$X = \frac{(P_1 + P_2) - (P_3 + P_4)}{P_1 + P_2 + P_3 + P_4} \qquad [8a]$$

$$Y = \frac{(P_1 + P_3) - (P_2 + P_4)}{P_1 + P_2 + P_3 + P_4} \qquad [8b]$$

The sharing of the scintillation light between the photomulti-

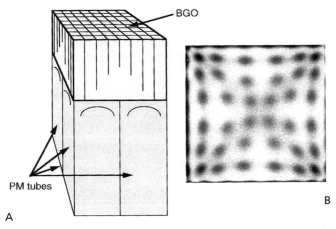

FIGURE 5.8.   A: Schematic shows the BGO block detector commonly used in commercial PET systems. The element in which the γ-ray interacts is determined by looking at the relative outputs of the four photomultiplier tubes. **B:** Image of X and Y (determined from the four photomultiplier tube outputs as shown in Eq. 8) after flood illumination of an 8 × 8 block detector. The individual block elements are clearly resolved. The edge rows and columns that have no light sharing are more difficult to see because they are pushed against the edge of the image.

plier tubes is controlled by the depth of the cuts in the BGO or by the use of a light guide. The aim is to make X and Y close to a linear function of the source position, so that each of the elements in the block can be resolved. Figure 5.8B shows the result of irradiating such a block detector with a flood source of 511-keV γ-rays. The individual elements of the 8 × 8 array are visualized, although there is some lack of linearity toward the edges of the block, which makes the outer elements more difficult to separate.

The great advantage of use of a block detector over use of a simple single-crystal–photomultiplier tube combinations used in the earliest PET systems is that the crystal size is no longer limited by the size of the smallest photomultiplier tube available, and the 16:1 multiplexing of detector elements to photomultiplier tubes results in a much lower cost per detector element. Thus use of a block detector allows dramatic improvement in spatial resolution in a cost-effective way with a very high packing fraction of detectors. A further advantage is that when the output is reduced from 64 crystals into only four photomultiplier tube signals, the electronic requirements are automatically multiplexed to a more manageable scale.

There are limitations to the block detector design. Perhaps the most important is the increase in effective area of the detector unit, which leads to an increase in dead time. Each block has one set of processing electronics. Two events that strike different elements in the block within the integration time set to collect the scintillation light cannot be differentiated. In this situation, only one event is detected (despite the interaction of two γ-rays), and the position of the event is an average (weighted according to the amount of energy deposited by each γ-ray) of the locations of the two γ-rays. This effect, known as *pileup,* leads both to a loss of events and to mispositioning of events (29) at high count rates.

BGO block detectors also do not reach the spatial resolution predicted with the simple point spread function of Fig. 5.6. This is because the position is determined by the relative distribution of light among the four photomultiplier tubes. Because the scintillation light output of BGO is quite low (it is estimated that each 511-keV interaction leads to the production of approximately 150 electrons at the photocathode of the photomultiplier tube), the photomultiplier tube outputs are subject to statistical fluctuation. This appears as fluctuations in the position estimations X and Y and leads to degradation of spatial resolution. The effect is to add approximately 2 mm in quadrature to the predicted full width at half maximum spatial resolution (30). Block detectors also are being developed with LSO scintillator. The faster decay time reduces concerns about dead time, and the higher light output should lead to spatial resolution that is closer to the $D/2$ prediction because of smaller statistical fluctuations in the photomultiplier tube signals.

Another recent modification of the modular block approach is the quadrant sharing detector (31). When the segmented scintillator block is placed across the corners of four larger photomultiplier tubes, the number of photomultiplier tubes needed can be reduced by almost another factor of four (Fig. 5.9). The only disadvantages in comparison to the standard block design are related to count-rate performance (each photomultiplier tube now views four scintillator blocks) and to tube replacement.

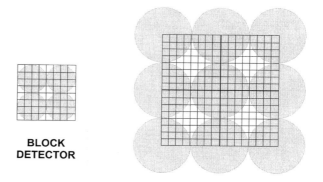

FIGURE 5.9. Comparison of the way photomultiplier tubes (*circles*) are coupled in a standard block detector (*left*) and in a detector in which the scintillator array is shared across the corners of four photomultiplier tubes (*right*). The arrangement on the *right* allows use of larger photomultiplier tubes. The result is almost a factor of four reduction in the number of tubes when the approach is extended to a large panel configuration.

Because the design is interlocking rather than modular, replacement of photomultiplier tubes is somewhat more difficult. These detectors are most easily constructed as large planar panels (rather than segments of a ring), and there are significant gaps (one-half a photomultiplier tube width at each end) between adjacent panels. However, the large cost savings realized with this approach make it attractive for use in whole-body PET scanners.

NaI(Tl) PET Detectors

The other style of detector widely used in clinical PET systems is based on the NaI(Tl) gamma camera. Much like conventional gamma cameras, this detector consists of a plate of NaI(Tl) scintillator coupled to an array of photomultiplier tubes. When the detector is used specifically for PET, however, the thickness of the crystal is increased to approximately 2.5 cm to achieve sufficient stopping power at 511 keV. At this thickness, spatial resolution of approximately 4 to 6 mm can be achieved (32). The other difference is in the pulse-processing electronics. Because the count rates on a detector head are much higher than in single-photon imaging because of the lack of a collimator, a number of tricks, such as local triggering (33) and pulse clipping (32), are used to reduce detector dead time and improve count-rate performance. Rectangular NaI(Tl) detector panels can be configured in a hexagonal geometry to form a PET scanner (34). Recent NaI(Tl) PET detectors are made with curved plates of NaI(Tl) that allow a ring configuration. In one case, a brain scanner has even been made from a single annulus of NaI(Tl) (35).

Other Positron Emission Tomography Detectors

Avalanche photodiode detectors are compact semiconductor photon detectors that may be possible replacements for photo-

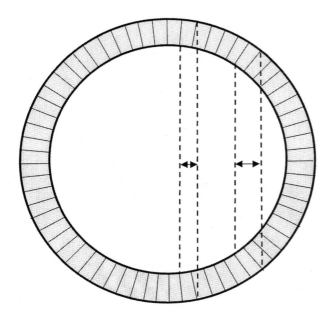

FIGURE 5.10. In a ring geometry scanner, the finite depth of the detector crystals and the fact that the depth of the interaction within the crystal is not known cause an increase in the width of the "strip" viewed with a pair of detectors as a function of radial position. This is known as the *depth of interaction effect* and causes degradation in spatial resolution as the distance from the center of the scanner increases.

multiplier tubes. These devices have relatively high gain (10^3 to 10^4) and high quantum efficiency and are available as individual elements or in arrays. Several groups are exploring detectors based on avalanche photodiode detectors, and prototype PET scanners have already been constructed with these devices (36, 37).

PET detectors generally have to be 2 to 3 cm thick to provide high efficiency. The depth at which the γ-ray interacts inside the scintillator is unknown. This leads to an uncertainty in the position of an event. For a ring scanner geometry, uncertainty increases with radial distance from the center of the scanner (Fig. 5.10). This effect is know as the *depth of interaction effect* and leads to worsening spatial resolution with radial distance. A number of groups have been working on designing depth-encoding detectors, either by using multiple layers of crystals in the detector with different decay times (38) or, by using a thin solid-state photodetector at the far end of the scintillator array and using the ratio of the signals in the photodetectors to determine depth of interaction (39). These approaches are starting to find their way into prototype PET systems and will result in more uniform resolution across the field of view.

The concept of time-of-flight PET is attractive. The basis for this method is to use a very fast scintillator and time the difference in arrival of the two 511-keV photons at the detectors to find the position of the annihilation (40). There are many inherent difficulties in this approach. The fast scintillators, such as barium fluoride (Table 5.2), have much lower stopping power than does BGO, thus the sensitivity of such a machine is lower. Furthermore, the best timing resolution achieved to date is sufficient only to locate the annihilation to within approximately 10 cm. There is a small signal-to-noise gain in using time of flight

but this is negated by the lower efficiency of the fast scintillators and the complex electronics required for such accurate timing. At this time, no time-of-flight PET machines are being produced commercially.

Other novel detector technologies, such as multiwire proportional chamber–based systems (41,42) are being investigated for PET. Although they can obtain high spatial resolution, the sensitivity is generally an order of magnitude lower than that of BGO-based PET systems.

Clinical Positron Emission Tomography Scanners

Clinical whole-body PET scanners fall into two broad categories—those that utilize block detectors consisting of small scintillator elements made from BGO or LSO, and those that use continuous plates of high light-output scintillators such as NaI(Tl).

The ECAT EXACT (CTI/Siemens, Knoxville, TN) (43) and the GE Advance (44) system (GE Medical Systems, Milwaukee, WI) are examples of block-based systems. They consist of multiple rings of BGO block detectors that simultaneously achieve high sensitivity and high resolution and are suitable for a wide range of clinical applications (Fig. 5.11). The ECAT EXACT scanner has 9,216 BGO elements and 576 photomultiplier tubes configured as 24 rings of 348 detectors per ring. Translated into block units, this is 3 rings of 48 blocks. Each block has 8×8 BGO elements of $6.35 \times 6.35 \times 20$ mm. The ring diameter is 82.5 cm, and the axial field of view is 16.2 cm. This system produces 47 image slices, spaced 3.125 mm apart. The GE Advance scanner has 12,096 BGO elements and 672 dual-cathode photomultiplier tubes configured as 18 rings of 672 detectors per ring. This corresponds to 3 rings of 112 blocks. Each block contains 6×6 BGO elements with dimensions of 4 mm (in-plane) $\times 8.1$ mm (axial) $\times 30$ mm (thick). The ring diameter is 92.7 cm, and the axial field of view is 15.2 cm. This system

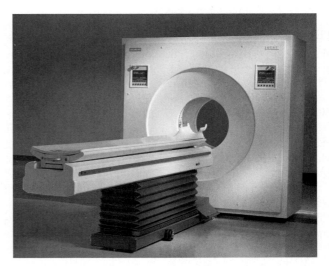

FIGURE 5.11. Photograph shows the CTI/Siemens ECAT EXACT PET system, a typical modern clinical PET scanner. (Courtesy of CTI PET Systems, Inc., Knoxville, TN).

produces 35 image slices spaced 4.25 mm apart. The septa on both these scanners can be retracted under computer control, allowing three-dimensional data acquisition as well as standard two-dimensional acquisition. A timing window of 12 nanoseconds and an energy window of 350 to 650 keV are typical. Reconstructed image planes can be stacked into a volume and resliced into coronal or sagittal sections or sections of any arbitrary orientation relative to the scanner axis. [68]Ge-filled rod sources are used for attenuation and calibration. Extraction of these sources from their shielding and rotation around the field of view also are computer controlled. The EXACT scanner has become available with LSO detector blocks to improve count-rate performance (a limiting factor in three-dimensional data acquisition) for whole-body studies.

The C-PET tomograph (Philips Medical Systems, Best, The Netherlands) is an example of a NaI(Tl)-based system (45). It consists of six curved plates of NaI(Tl) scintillator, each measuring approximately 48 cm (transaxial direction) × 30 cm (axial direction) × 2.5 cm thick. Each plate is viewed with a total of 48 photomultiplier tubes. This is a continuously sampling system and can therefore produce any number of image slices within the 25.6-cm axial field of view (not all the area of the plates are useable owing to edge effects). The higher light output of NaI(Tl) relative to BGO allows use of this system with a tighter energy window, typically 440 to 660 keV.

All three of these scanners are capable of producing high-quality diagnostic images for a range of situations. Figure 5.12. is a representative whole-body image from an [18F]fluorodeoxyglucose (FDG) study of a cancer patient. Images were acquired with an ECAT EXACT scanner.

A trend in recent years has been the use of multiheaded gamma cameras for PET (46). When the collimators are removed from conventional gamma cameras and coincidence circuitry is installed, dual- and triple-headed gamma cameras can be used for PET. The performance is generally inferior to that of the dedicated PET systems described earlier. Performance continues to improve, however, as changes are made in the electronics to deal with the higher count rates, and thicker crystals are used to increase efficiency at 511 keV.

The latest innovation in PET imaging has been combined PET and CT systems that can be used to provide precisely registered anatomic and biologic information in the same imaging session (47). This is particularly powerful in oncology, in which improved diagnostic accuracy results from accurate anatomic localization of the biologic signal from PET and in which these systems can be used for CT-guided biopsy, radiation therapy, and surgical planning. CT also provides information for rapid and high-statistical-quality correction of attenuation for PET data. An initial prototype system was developed by the University of Pittsburgh in collaboration with CTI PET Systems, Inc. (Knoxville, TN) (48). A number of companies now offer dual-modality systems based on integration of existing PET and CT products.

Special Purpose Positron Emission Tomography Systems

Considerable attention has been paid to development of dedicated PET cameras that are optimized for specific tasks. This

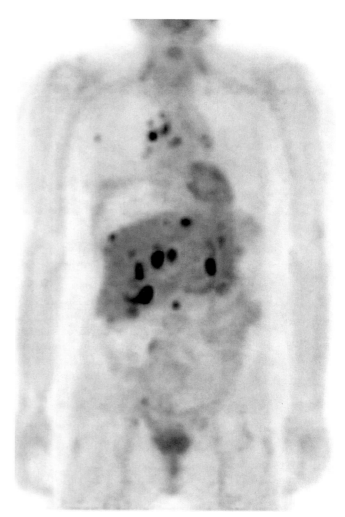

FIGURE 5.12. Whole-body [18F]fluorodeoxyglucose PET study of a patient with ovarian cancer shows a large number of metastatic lesions, particularly in the liver. (Courtesy of CTI PET Systems, Inc., Knoxville, TN).

includes high-resolution systems for brain imaging (35,38) and breast imaging (49–51). There is also much interest in using PET in the study of laboratory animals, because the noninvasive nature of the technique and the flexibility of the chemistry allow measurement of many biologic processes. Several dedicated PET scanners with spatial resolution as high as 1 to 2 mm have been developed for imaging of mice and rats (36,37,42,52–54). Some of these are now becoming commercially available. An image of glucose metabolism in the rat obtained with a microPET P4 animal PET scanner (Concorde Microsystems, Inc., Knoxville, TN) is shown in Fig. 5.13.

DATA ACQUISITION IN POSITRON EMISSION TOMOGRAPHY

Many modern PET scanners can be used to acquire data in two different modes—two-dimensional acquisition with the septa in

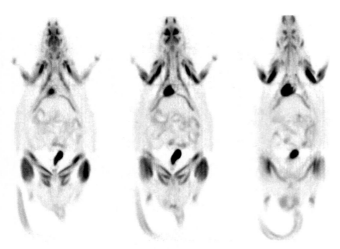

FIGURE 5.13. Whole-body ^{18}[F]fluorodeoxyglucose images of a rat. Images were obtained with a microPET scanner.

place and three-dimensional acquisition with the septa removed. In addition, total-body imaging acquisition protocols that extend the axial scan length by moving the patient sequentially through the scanner have become important. This section describes data acquisition strategies and discusses how raw data are stored in the form of projection matrices known as *sinograms*.

Storing Raw Positron Emission Tomography Data as Sinograms

Each detector pair records the sum of activity along a given line through the body. The data for all possible combinations of detector pairs in a given ring are stored in a sinogram. This is more efficient than storing each recorded event separately, because each detector pair usually records multiple events in a PET study. A typical sinogram from an FDG study of a human brain is shown in Fig. 5.14. Each point in the sinogram represents the sum of all events detected with a particular pair of detectors. The sinogram matrix is organized such that each row represents

the projected activity of parallel detector pairs at a given angle relative to the detector ring. The sinogram itself provides little information on the activity distribution. The data in the sinograms must be reconstructed to convert the projection data into an interpretable image.

Two-dimensional (Slice) Data Acquisition in Positron Emission Tomography

The basic principle of two-dimensional imaging is to take coincidences within a given ring of detectors and form a sinogram from these data. The sinogram is reconstructed to form an image for that detector ring. In this way, we would expect a system with n detector rings to produce n image planes. In practice, to improve sensitivity and axial sampling, coincidences between nearby detector rings also are acquired and averaged together. These are assigned to the slice corresponding to their average axial position. For example, if coincidences between ring 8 and ring 6 are combined, they are assumed to originate from a slice centered on ring 7. Coincidences between immediately adjacent detector rings (e.g., rings 4 and 5) produce image slices that fall halfway between detector rings. In this way, we actually obtain $2n - 1$ image planes, spaced by one-half the detector width, from an n-ring PET scanner.

In modern PET systems, which have small detector elements, several sinograms are combined into a summed sinogram for each image plane to improve sensitivity. This approach is limited to sinograms with small ring differences, because as the ring difference increases, eventually the interplane septa get in the way and prevent detection of events. The averaging process also blurs the data in the axial direction, especially toward the edge of the field of view, where the averaged coincidence lines diverge significantly (Fig. 5.15). This effect becomes intolerable for large ring differences. After considering the trade-off between sensitivity and resolution loss, developers of most modern systems allow a maximum ring difference of ± 5 in forming the two-dimensional data set. Two-dimensional data acquisition leads to $2n - 1$ sinograms, each of which is reconstructed independently to form $2n - 1$ transaxial images, which can be stacked on top of each other to form a three-dimensional image volume.

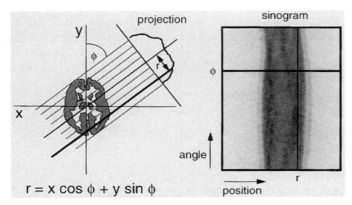

$$r = x \cos \phi + y \sin \phi$$

FIGURE 5.14. PET projection data are conventionally stored in the form of sinograms. Each element in the sinogram represents the activity recorded by a pair of detectors (the projection or sum of all the activity along the line joining the two detectors). The relation between the projection line and its position in the sinogram is shown.

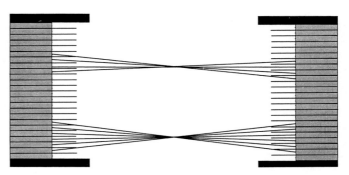

FIGURE 5.15. Axial cross-section through a 24-ring PET scanner shows the standard two-dimensional acquisition mode in which ring differences up to ± 5 are used. Using some of the oblique lines of response helps improve sensitivity but leads to degradation of axial resolution, because all the data contributing to a given slice are assumed to come from within the plane.

Two-dimensional Total Body Acquisition in Positron Emission Tomography

In the management, of patients with cancer, it is vital to assess whether the disease has metastasized, because this is the critical factor in the choice of therapy and in prognosis. Most PET scanners however, cover only a small fraction of the body, typically 15 cm, at one time. The development of total-body PET (55,56) overcomes this limitation because the bed is moved under computer control, and data are acquired at a number of adjacent bed positions to achieve coverage of the entire body. A typical total-body data set obtained with ^{18}F-FDG as the tracer is shown in Fig. 5.12. Total-body imaging has become important in the treatment of patients with cancer and is the most important clinical use of PET. However, challenges remain in reducing the overall scan time, dealing with wide variations in counting rates over different parts of the body, and ultimately providing quantitatively accurate images.

Three-dimensional (Volume) Data Acquisition in Positron Emission Tomography

Even with the addition of neighboring ring coincidences, the sensitivity of PET systems operating in two-dimensional mode is usually less than 1%. A different mode of PET imaging, called *three-dimensional PET acquisition,* can be used to improve sensitivity dramatically removing the interplane septa and allowing coincidences between all detector rings (Fig. 5.16). This leads to a fivefold increase in true sensitivity for a dedicated multiring PET scanner but also results in a higher fraction of scattered coincidence events (57,58). The count rates obtained with the detectors are also much higher, leading under some circumstances to substantial dead time or high rates of random coincidences. A further complication of three-dimensional imaging is that the sinogram data cannot be averaged together in the manner described for two-dimensional imaging. The large ring differences acquired in three-dimensional data sets would result in a severe blurring in the axial direction. It is now necessary to use a fully three-dimensional image reconstruction technique in which the data are reconstructed volumetrically to account for the precise direction of each projection line (59). Although this

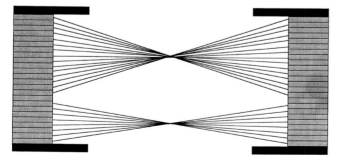

FIGURE 5.16. Axial cross-section of a PET scanner shows three-dimensional data acquisition. All possible lines of response are recorded and reconstructed volumetrically. The exact direction of the line of response is taken into account in the reconstruction.

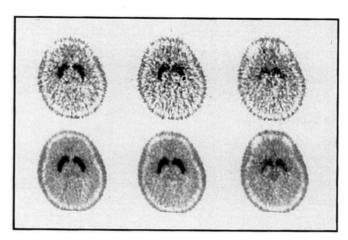

FIGURE 5.17. Comparison of two-dimensional (*top row*) and three-dimensional (*bottom row*) acquisitions for a normal subject after the injection of 6 mCi of [^{18}F]fluorodopa. The acquisition time was 20 minutes in each study. The dramatically improved signal-to-noise ratio is evident in the three-dimensional data set owing to the higher sensitivity.

method is computationally intensive, it does result in all the data being reconstructed in the correct location. The longer reconstruction times and the larger size of the three-dimensional raw projection data sets (n^2 sinograms rather than the $2n - 1$ sinograms in two-dimensional imaging) have limited the use of three-dimensional PET. However, the evolution of faster workstations with rapid data transfer capability onto extremely large disks and multiprocessor boards for reconstruction is turning three-dimensional PET into a viable proposition. A number of scatter correction schemes have been proposed to reduce the scatter to acceptable levels. Three-dimensional acquisition and reconstruction are available on most commercial scanners.

The gain in sensitivity afforded by three-dimensional acquisition is particularly beneficial in low-count-rate studies (e.g., neuroreceptor studies), in which the full sensitivity gain can be realized irrespective of dead-time considerations. Figure 5.17 shows a comparison between 20-minute two-dimensional and three-dimensional acquisitions of data for a normal subject 2 hours after administration of 6 mCi of [^{18}F]fluorodopa. This tracer is concentrated in the caudate and putamen in normal subjects, and these structures are easily identified on the images. The noise level in the three-dimensional data set is clearly much lower than in the two-dimensional study. Three-dimensional data acquisition can lead to signal-to-noise gains of a factor of 2 to 3 for low-count-rate studies or can be used to reduce the imaging time, (improving patient throughput in the clinical environment) or the injected dose (useful for pediatric studies) while maintaining image statistics equivalent to those of the two-dimensional study.

IMAGE RECONSTRUCTION

This section qualitatively describes how to get from the raw PET data in the form of sinograms to a reconstructed image. The standard approach of filtered backprojection is used to reconstruct a single sinogram that represents a single two-dimensional image plane. Reconstruction of a three-dimensional PET data set is more complicated, but many of the principles are the same. Defrise et al. (59) discuss the details of three-dimensional PET reconstruction.

Backprojection

Figure 5.18 shows the sinogram that would be obtained from imaging two cylinders, one twice the diameter of the other but both containing the same activity concentration. Each element in the sinogram represents the sum of activity along a line (the line of response) joining two detectors. Each row in the sinogram forms a one-dimensional projection representing a view of the object from a particular angle (Fig. 5.14). An intuitive approach to image reconstruction is to take each sinogram element and backproject it along the line from which the detected events came (Fig. 5.19). In other words, the events detected for a given detector pair are spread uniformly along a line joining the detector pair. Figure 5.18 shows the outcome of this process after all angles have been backprojected. The resulting image is a crude approximation of the actual object. However, the backprojection process is clearly incorrect, because activity is placed outside the object.

Filtered Backprojection

To obtain the correct image, it can be shown mathematically that each projection has to be filtered before backprojection (60). The filter is a convolution filter, so it is most conveniently applied in frequency (Fourier) space, and the convolution becomes simple multiplication. In broad terms, the filtered backprojection reconstruction process is as follows:

1. Take projection for angle 1 (row 1 in the sinogram).
2. Calculate the Fourier transform of this projection.

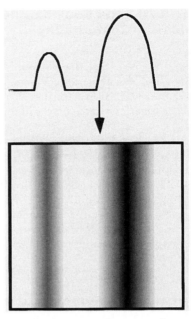

FIGURE 5.19. Backprojection involves spreading each projection across the image matrix at the appropriate angle.

3. Multiply by the reconstruction filter.
4. Calculate the inverse Fourier transform of the filtered projection.
5. Backproject the data for angle 1.
6. Repeat for all other angles in the sinogram.

Figure 5.18 shows a single projection before and after filtering. The negative numbers introduced in the filtering process remove activity placed outside the object in backprojection. The result of backprojecting all the filtered projections (Fig. 5.18) is a faithful representation of the original object.

Reconstruction Filter

The functional form of the reconstruction filter can be derived intuitively from the following argument. In the projection data in Fig. 5.18, the larger cylinder contributes more counts to the projection data, because the path length through the object is larger. Using simple backprojection of the data apparently leads to higher activity in the larger cylinder, even though it has the same activity concentration as the small cylinder. The process of simple backprojection amplifies the activity in large structures relative to smaller structures. In terms of spatial frequency, high frequencies (corresponding to small structures) are underrepresented relative to low frequencies (corresponding to large structures). To correct for the effects of backprojection, it is necessary to weight the lower frequencies less than the higher frequencies. The correct mathematically derived filter (Fig. 5.20) turns out to be a ramp in frequency space (hence the term *ramp filter*). The form of the filter is in agreement with our intuitive argument that higher frequencies should be weighted more than are lower frequencies.

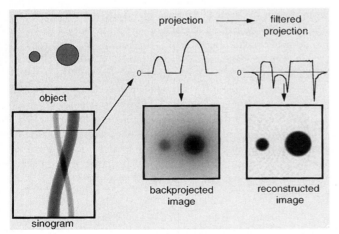

FIGURE 5.18. Principles of image reconstruction: The sinogram is obtained from imaging two cylinders of equal activity. The profile of a single projection line is shown. Simple backprojection of all the projection data leads to a blurred representation of the object. To obtain a faithful representation, the projection must be filtered before backprojection.

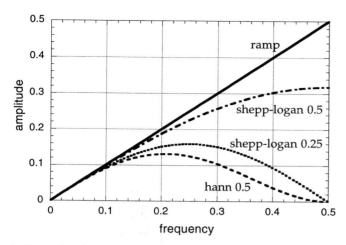

FIGURE 5.20. Common reconstruction filters in frequency space. The ramp filter can be derived mathematically as the appropriate filter to apply. However, it amplifies high-frequency noise components; therefore in practice, the ramp usually is multiplied by a window function whereby the magnitude of the filter is attenuated at high frequencies to produce a compromise between image resolution and noise.

Reconstruction Filter and Image Noise

An unfortunate side effect of the ramp filter is that it also amplifies noise, because statistical fluctuations from one sinogram element to the next contribute roughly equally at all spatial frequencies, whereas true signal tends to have decreasing amplitude with increasing spatial frequency. To counteract this effect, it often is desirable, unless the statistical quality of the data is very good, to attenuate the reconstruction filter at high frequencies. This can be achieved by use of a number of different window functions, such as the Shepp-Logan or the Hann window, which modify the basic ramp-filter shape at higher frequencies. Several different filter forms are shown in Fig. 5.20. A filter factor further characterizes these functions by indicating the point at which the curve turns over or reaches zero. Although these window functions help to control image noise, they also reduce spatial resolution, because reducing the high frequencies is equivalent to smoothing the data. Figure 5.21 shows an FDG brain image reconstructed with the filters shown in Fig. 5.20. The trade-off

between increasing signal-to-noise ratio but decreasing resolution is evident as the filter function changes. The choice of reconstruction filter ultimately depends on the number of counts in the study and the personal preferences of the investigator or physician in trading off image noise and spatial resolution. In clinical PET, the resolution achievable in the reconstructed image almost always is limited by the number of counts contributing to the data set and the need to use a reconstruction that filters the image to an acceptable signal-to-noise level. Typical image resolution achieved in the brain is 5 to 8 mm and in the rest of the body 8 to 15 mm, even though most clinical PET scanners have detectors capable of 4- to 6-mm resolution.

Image Artifacts

It is quite easy to introduce artifacts into the reconstruction if sufficient care is not taken. The most important factor in avoiding reconstruction artifacts is to ensure that the data are sufficiently sampled (61). Sampling theory states that if the highest resolution recorded in the data is R mm, then the data must be sampled at least every $R/2$ mm. Thus for a PET system with detectors with spatial resolution of 6 mm, the sampling (the distance between adjacent elements in the sinogram) should be less than 3 mm. Sufficient angular sampling also is required. Artifacts are readily found when only a subset of the available angular data is used.

Iterative Reconstruction Methods

An alternative reconstruction strategy to filtered backprojection is iterative reconstruction methods (62). These methods start with an initial guess of the image (often a uniform image). This image is then forward-projected to compute the sinogram data that would have been measured for that image. Forward-projection is the inverse process of backprojection and involves summing all the activity along the line joining two detectors. The computed sinogram is compared with the measured sinogram, and the image is updated to account for the differences. If the appropriate cost function (the way in which the difference between the computed and the measured sinogram is calculated) and update equations (the manner in which the image is updated

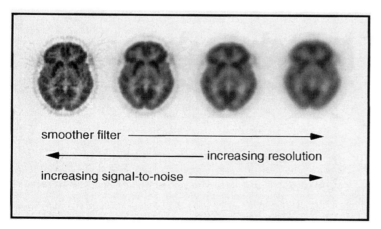

FIGURE 5.21. Effects of reconstruction filters on a [^{18}F]fluorodeoxyglucose study of the brain. The trade-off is evident between spatial resolution and signal-to-noise ratio as smoother filters (increasing attenuation at higher frequencies) are used.

on each iteration) are used, then after several iterations of this process, the computed sinograms start to resemble the measured ones. The goal is to find the image that produces a computed sinogram that is the most consistent with the measured data. The advantage of iterative algorithms is that it is possible to model many aspects of the PET scanner in the forward-projection step. For example, it can take into account that each detector pair does not simply record the activity along a line joining the center of the two detectors but measures the integrated activity along a volume between the two detectors. These algorithms also can give different weight to different sinogram elements, depending on the statistical quality of the data in each element. This can lead to improvements in signal-to-noise ratio and resolution in the reconstructed images. The limitation of iterative techniques, however, is that they are much more computationally intensive (roughly the equivalent of one filtered backprojection reconstruction for each iteration). There is still considerable debate about which "flavor" of algorithm yields the best reconstructed images.

QUANTITATIVE POSITRON EMISSION TOMOGRAPHIC IMAGING

A unique feature of PET is the potential to achieve accurate, quantitative images that directly express the concentration of positron emitter in units of $\mu Ci/cm^3$. Once this is achieved, the data can be processed through a mathematic model that represents the process studied to convert the image into biologic units (nanomoles/min per gram). To achieve absolute quantification, or even relative quantification, a number of important corrections must be made to the raw PET data. Errors still result, however, particularly in structures that have dimensions comparable with or smaller than the image resolution. Cross-registration to high-resolution anatomic images such as MR images can help to quantify these partial volume errors and provide a convenient means for defining anatomically based regions of interest for application to the PET data.

Detector Normalization

A modern PET scanner consists of many thousands of individual detector elements. Because of differences in the exact dimensions of the detectors, the optical coupling to the photomultiplier tube and a whole host of other factors, there can be considerable variation in efficiency among different detectors. In practice, this means that different detector pairs register different count rates when viewing the same activity. To remove these efficiency variations, it is necessary to apply detector normalization factors. These normalization factors are measured by irradiating each detector pair with the same amount of activity. This can be achieved with a thin plane source rotated to different angles in the field of view or by use of a rotating rod source of activity that orbits at the edge of the field of view (63). Adequate counts must be acquired so the normalization is not statistics-limited; that is, the normalization should contain many more counts per detector pair than is actually registered during a clinical scan. Otherwise, noise from the normalization scan is propagated into

the reconstructed image. It is possible to compute normalization factors from a scan of a uniform cylinder that is precisely centered in the scanner in a component-based approach (64). This method has the advantage of generating the normalization factors from a shorter scan, but it gives an estimate rather than a direct measurement of the normalization factors. Normalization files typically are acquired weekly to account for possible changes in photomultiplier tube gain over time.

Attenuation Correction

Attenuation correction is the largest correction factor applied in PET. As the two 511-keV γ-rays pass through the body, there is a high likelihood that one or both of the γ-rays will be absorbed or will be scattered away from the two detectors they would have hit. Attenuation is an exponential process and depends on both the attenuation coefficient of the material and the amount of tissue the γ-rays must pass through. Typical attenuation coefficients at 511 keV are 0.095 cm^{-1} for soft tissue, 0.03 cm^{-1} for lungs, and 0.15 cm^{-1} for bone. The magnitude of the error caused by attenuation can be appreciated with the realization that typically only 1 in every 5 γ-ray pairs escapes from the brain and only 1 in 30 or 40 escapes from the torso without interaction. The attenuation correction factors are therefore very large and must be estimated accurately to recover the original isotope concentration.

The unique nature of annihilation radiation makes it possible to measure the attenuation correction factors directly. Consider the attenuation in a cylinder of cross-section D with attenuation coefficient μ (Fig. 5.22). If the positron-emitter is concentrated at position x, and the number of γ-ray pairs emitted is N_0, the number of γ-ray pairs, N, that escape without being attenuated is as follows:

$$N = N_0 e^{-\mu x} e^{-\mu(D-x)} = N_0 e^{-\mu D} \qquad [9]$$

This expression is the probability of escape for each of the two γ-rays. It is important to notice that attenuation is independent of the source position x. This remains true when the attenuation coefficient is variable within the cross-section under study. Thus wherever the source is along the line joining two detectors, the attenuation is the same. Even if the activity is outside the patient, the attenuation still is the same. It therefore is possible to use an external positron-emitting source (usually a ring source

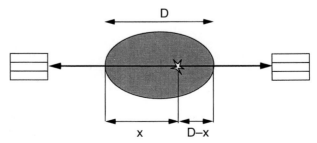

FIGURE 5.22. Attenuation for a given line of response is independent of the source position along the line, because both γ-rays must escape the body (Eq. 9). The combined path length through the body thus is always equal to the width of the body for that projection line.

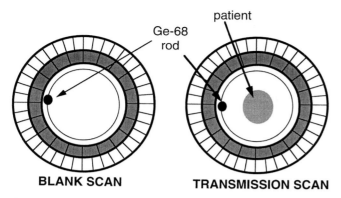

patient

Ge-68
rod

BLANK SCAN   **TRANSMISSION SCAN**

FIGURE 5.23. Blank scan (*left*) and transmission scan (*right*) used for measuring attenuation correction in PET. The source is either a ring or a rotating rod of ^{68}Ge. Blank and transmission scans are generally acquired before activity is injected into the patient.

or a rod source orbiting just inside the field of view) to measure the attenuation correction factors in the following manner.

Blank scan. Acquire data with the external source but nothing else in the field of view. This measurement represents the unattenuated flux N_0 (Fig. 5.23, left).

Transmission scan. Position the patient in the scanner (the patient has not been given an injection of positron emitter at this stage) and acquire another scan with activity from the external source. This represents the attenuated flux N (Fig. 5.23, right).

Attenuation correction factors are calculated for each detector pair by means of calculating the ratio of the blank and the transmission sinograms. High statistics are preferable (but not always practical) in transmission images because the noise associated with statistical fluctuation in the blank and transmission images can propagate through to the final image and introduce bias (65). For this reason, blank and transmission scans often are smoothed before the ratio is calculated.

The transmission scan increases the duration of a study and thus the time during which the patient must lie still. In areas of the body where the attenuation coefficient is reasonably homogeneous (e.g., the brain and parts of the abdomen), it is possible to calculate the attenuation correction according to on the body outline (66). This method has the advantage of accelerating the study and not propagating noise into the reconstructed image. It is, however, less accurate than measured attenuation correction because of the assumptions that have to be made and is therefore of most use when scans are being used in a qualitative or semiquantitative way.

It is possible to acquire a transmission scan after the injection has been administered (67). With a strong rod or point source for the transmission source and knowing the location of that source, the sinogram data can be windowed to accept events from the transmission source alone with minimal contamination from the activity in the patient. It is even possible to perform simultaneous emission-transmission imaging (68), although contamination between the two sets of sinograms can easily cause image artifacts.

Dead-time Correction

It takes a finite time to collect and process the scintillation light from each γ-ray interaction in the detector. During this period, the detector is effectively dead and cannot process another event. If another event does arrive, it is combined with the first event, resulting in a loss of data (two events turn into one) and mispositioning (most PET detectors calculate the position of the event based on the centroid of all the scintillation light received) (29). If the combined energy of the two events is high enough, the event falls outside the energy window of the scanner, and both events are lost. The loss of data is called *dead-time loss*. In most systems, the fraction of time the detector is "dead" is measured on-line and used to correct the data. This correction is an adjustment for the events lost while the system was busy. It cannot reposition the events that were misplaced. In practice, other components of the PET system, such as the coincidence processor, also have dead time, so overall dead-time correction is a complex function of several factors (25). Although dead-time correction becomes a large factor (>1.5) only in high-count-rate studies such as ^{15}O water studies and in three-dimensional studies, it still is important to ensure the correction is accurate over the range of count rates encountered in practical imaging situations.

Randoms Correction

Random or accidental coincidences that occur when two unrelated γ-rays are detected within the coincidence time window can be corrected in one of two ways (19). The most common correction method entails two coincidence circuits. The first of these is used to measure the true coincidences plus the randoms (collectively called *prompt coincidences*) in the standard way. The second circuit has a delay (several hundred nanoseconds) inserted, so all true coincidences are thrown out of coincidence and are not registered. The singles rate on each detector is, however, still the same, thus the randoms rate (Eq. 4) remains, apart from statistical fluctuations, unaltered. To correct for randoms, the counts from the delayed circuit are simply subtracted, usually on-line, from those obtained from the prompt circuit. The random events detected in the prompt coincidence circuit are not the same as those detected in the delayed circuit. Because of this, subtraction of random events increases the statistical noise. Consider a sinogram element that registers T true counts and R random counts. The corrected number of counts, N, is

$$N = Prompts - Delayed = (T + R) - R \quad [10]$$

If Poisson statistics are assumed, the noise, ΔN, is

$$\Delta N = \sqrt{T + 2R} \quad [11]$$

The second correction method involves measuring the singles rate for each detector and calculating the random rate with Eq. 4. Because the singles rate is generally a high statistics measurement, this correction adds little noise but requires accurate knowledge of the coincidence timing window. This is not trivial; small differences in transit time through the electronics cause variations in the effective width of the timing window. The random rates in any given study depend on the rate at which single events are detected. The fraction of random events typically is kept to less than 20% of the total coincidence rate, although in some studies randoms can become a limiting factor and dominate the observed count rate. An example is three-dimensional total body scans passing over the bladder, in which a substantial fraction of the injected dose has accumulated.

Scatter Correction

Scatter has been one of the most intractable problems in PET. Some degree of scatter rejection can be accomplished by applying an energy window to the collected data. Of the residual scatter, the contribution to the reconstructed image in two-dimensional PET imaging is quite small and in many cases is neglected. In three-dimensional PET imaging, there are often as many scattered events as there are unscattered events, and scatter correction often is essential. The most popular correction method is to calculate an estimate of the scatter from an initial reconstruction of the emission scan (approximating the activity distribution) and transmission scan (approximating the distribution of scattering media) (69,70). Although the method does not take into account scatter from outside the field of view, this scatter can be approximately accounted for with a scaling factor. Other approaches to scatter correction include simple background subtraction approaches, deconvolution approaches, and Monte Carlo calculation of the scatter distribution (71–74). These approaches, although often complex and time consuming, are quite successful at removing the scatter and dramatically improving the quantitative accuracy of reconstructed PET images.

Calibration

To reconstruct images in absolute units of μCi/cm^3, it is necessary to calibrate the PET scanner against a standard source. This is commonly done by means of imaging a uniform cylinder. An aliquot from the same cylinder is placed in a vial and well counted against a source of known activity to obtain the absolute activity concentration, which is then related to the counts in the reconstructed PET images (after all corrections have been applied) to obtain the appropriate calibration factor.

Accuracy Limits in Positron Emission Tomography

In addition to the corrections described earlier, corrections for decay of the radionuclide usually are applied during image reconstruction. The accuracy of the quantitative pixel values in the final reconstructed PET images depends critically on how well all the corrections are applied. In the best case, it is estimated that the absolute activity in a region in a PET scan can be measured to approximately 5% (75). Relative accuracy within an image can be as good as 1% to 2%. If any of the corrections are neglected or inappropriately applied, however, the errors can be much larger.

Partial Volume Effects

It is possible to produce highly quantitative PET images provided all correction factors are appropriately applied. This ap-

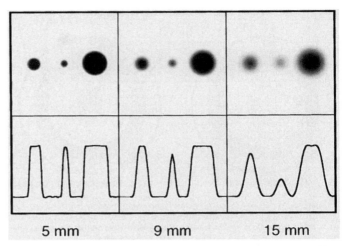

FIGURE 5.24. Partial volume effect. Reconstructed images and profiles through cylinders of diameter 1 cm, 2 cm, and 4 cm, each containing equal activity. As the resolution of the scanner degrades, the recovery of activity in the smaller structures becomes incomplete, and activity is underestimated.

proach works well for all structures that have dimensions greater than twice the spatial resolution of the PET scanner. As the dimension of a structure becomes smaller than this, the activity concentration is progressively overestimated or underestimated, depending on the activity distribution (76). This is illustrated in Fig. 5.24, which shows a profile through structures of different sizes, all containing the same activity concentration relative to a cold background. As the size of the structure decreases, the apparent activity concentration also decreases, and this effect, known as the *partial volume effect,* is caused solely by the limited spatial resolution of the PET scanner. The correction factor needed to obtain the correct value is known as the *recovery coefficient.* Because many structures of interest have dimensions less than twice the image resolution of current clinical systems (e.g., 8 to 10 mm), this is a serious problem and one that is not easy to remedy. For simple geometric shapes, it is possible to calculate the recovery coefficients if the activity distribution is known. This has been applied with some success in cardiac studies, in which the myocardial wall is modeled as a uniform bar (77). High-resolution anatomic images, such as MR images, also can be used to estimate recovery coefficients, if anatomic and functional boundaries in the images coincide (78,79). In many applications, it is not possible to calculate recovery coefficients. In these cases, interpretation of the images must account for the underestimation of activity in small structures that contain high activity levels relative to the background and for the overestimation of activity in small structures that contain little activity relative to the background.

TRACER KINETIC MODELING

The distribution of a labeled tracer in the body after intravenous injection is a dynamic process. When a dynamic sequence of quantitative PET images is obtained starting from the time of injection, it is possible to observe the transport and metabolism of the tracer by organ systems. Figure 5.25 shows a time series

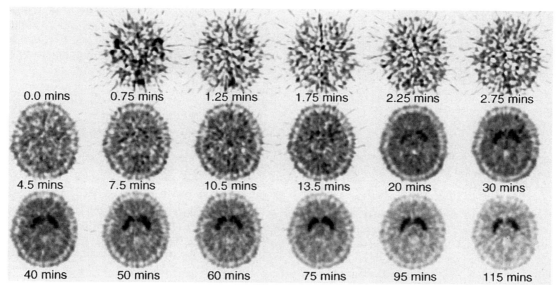

FIGURE 5.25. Time sequence of PET scans after injection of [^{18}F]fluorodopa. The early images progressively reflect blood volume, blood flow, and transport throughout tissues of the brain. Later images reflect the metabolism of [^{18}F]fluorodopa into [^{18}F]fluorodopamine and its storage in vesicles in dopaminergic terminals, which are found predominantly in the caudate nucleus and the putamen.

of PET scans in a single transaxial slice of the brain after injection of [^{18}F]fluorodopa. The distribution evolves from a nonspecific distribution reflecting blood volume and blood flow throughout the brain at early times to one representing the specific location of dopamine synthesizing neurons in the caudate nucleus and putamen. Figure 5.26 shows time versus activity curves for two brain regions—striatum and cerebellum. The aim of tracer kinetic modeling is the mathematic modeling of the fate of the tracer after injection so that the parameters of the model correspond to biologically relevant information. Measurable quantities include total tissue tracer concentration as a function of

time (from the PET data) and blood or plasma concentration as a function of time (from blood sampling). Known information can be used to constrain the model. Tracer kinetic models have been used widely with great success in the biologic sciences and in pharmacology. PET, for the first time, allows performance of quantitative biologic assays in vivo.

Compartmental Models

Most kinetic models used to date are linear compartmental models, in which compartments are used to represent different

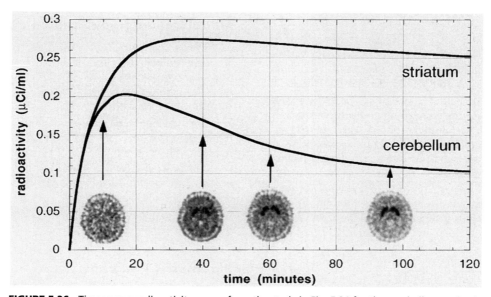

FIGURE 5.26. Time versus radioactivity curves from the study in Fig. 5.24 for the cerebellum and striatum. This information is used with a mathematical model to determine the regional rates of facilitated transport of [^{18}F]fluorodopa into the brain and its metabolism to [^{18}F]fluorodopamine.

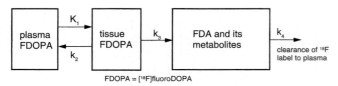

FIGURE 5.27. Simplified compartmental model for transport and metabolism of [^{18}F]fluorodopa.

spatial locations of the tracer (blood, interstitial space, intracellular compartment) as well as different products involving the initial tracer (80). An example is shown in Fig. 5.27, again for [^{18}F]fluorodopa. The arrows between compartments represent the rate at which tracer in one compartment is transported or metabolically transformed into a second compartment. These rate constants usually are represented by k_i, where i identifies the particular rate constant for exchange from one compartment to another. A number of assumptions are made about the compartments. Mixing within the compartment is assumed to be complete and the concentration homogeneous. The rate at which tracer leaves a compartment is assumed proportional to the amount of tracer in the compartment. This leads to first-order differential equations that govern the exchange of the positron-emitting label from one compartment to another as a function of time. Even with fairly simple tracers, extensive knowledge of the transport and metabolism of tracers is required to help formulate the model. With this understanding, it is possible to relate the rate constants to biologically meaningful parameters. In the example in Fig. 5.25, k_3 is the rate constant for converting [^{18}F]fluorodopa into its metabolic product [^{18}F]fluorodopamine, and K_1 is related to the product of blood flow and first-pass extraction of fluorodopa from blood to tissue. To estimate these rate constants, the time versus activity curve is extracted from a time series of data (Fig. 5.25) for tissues of interest (Fig. 5.26), and the compartment model is fitted for the individual rate constants (Fig. 5.27).

Input Function

One compartment to which there is external access is the vascular compartment. This can be seen as the input stage to the model as the tracer is delivered to the tissues through the blood. The time versus activity curve for blood therefore is known as the *input function.* Analysis of arterial blood samples over time gives a good approximation of the time course of tracer delivery to a tissue of interest. This method is not exact because of delay and dispersion effects between the point at which arterial blood is sampled (usually the radial artery) and the arterial blood actually supplying the tissue of interest. The input function is important because it can be considered to drive the model. Both the magnitude and the time course of the input function can have a dramatic effect on the time activity curves for a given tissue of interest.

To avoid the relatively invasive procedure of obtaining arterial blood, it is possible in some circumstances to substitute venous blood samples. These are often obtained from the back of the hand, the hand being heated to open arteriovenous shunts so that

the blood is more "arterial" in nature. Venous blood samples are a good approximation when the extraction of the tracer on any one pass through a capillary bed is low. In certain circumstances, in which a large volume of blood is inside the PET field of view (e.g., cardiac studies or studies including the aorta), it is possible to obtain the input function from rapid dynamic PET imaging and eliminate the need for blood sampling. However, temporal sampling of the PET data can be a limitation, as are partial volume effects from adjacent tissues.

Operational Equation

For any linear compartmental model, one can describe the activity recorded with the PET scanner as the convolution of the input function with a set of exponential functions describing tracer exchange between compartments. Because PET data have limited temporal resolution, and because of the half-life of available positron emitters, we are limited to measuring changes that happen on the time scale of seconds to several hours. Furthermore, because PET picks up the sum of activity in multiple compartments and produces relatively noisy data, it is not possible to unambiguously calculate rate constants from a large number of compartments. The practical limit in PET is three compartments and measurement of up to four separate rate constants. Models often can be simplified by use of analog tracers rather than the natural substrate. These analog tracers are carefully designed such that they follow only a limited segment of a complicated biochemical pathway. FDG, which is an analog of glucose, is a good example of this. It has analogous transport and phosphorylation to glucose but is not further metabolized after entering the cell and becomes effectively trapped. The uptake is proportional to the metabolic rate for glucose of the tissue. For tracers such as FDG, labeled amino acids, and ligands or drugs that react in nearly irreversible ways, even simplified integral equation models based on accumulation of tracer in proportion to the process measured can be used (81).

Model Development and Validation

Any model applied to PET data must be carefully developed and validated with prior knowledge of the transport and metabolism of the tracer of interest (80). In some cases, it is possible to measure directly the biologic parameter of interest in animal studies and compare this with the values obtained through tracer kinetic modeling. Some measure of confidence in how well the model describes the data can be obtained by looking at the residuals. These are the difference between the predicted tissue time versus activity curves obtained with the rate constants estimated from the PET data and the PET data itself. If bias is detected in the residuals, that is, they do not appear random over the time course examined, the model is clearly insufficient to explain the data.

Parametric Imaging

Over recent years, efforts have been made to integrate the image reconstruction process and the biologic model process into a

Table 5.3. *Dosimetry for tracers commonly used in positron emission tomography*

Tracer	Typical Dose (mCi)	Critical Organ	Critical Organ Dose (rad/mCi)	Whole Body Dose (rad/mCi)
[^{18}F] fluorodeoxyglucose	10	Bladder wall	0.241[a]	0.041
[^{18}F]fluorodopa	10	Bladder wall	0.380[b]	0.033
[^{15}O]water	120–300[c]	Lungs	0.002	0.002
[^{13}N]ammonia	20	Bladder wall	0.03	0.006

[a]Voiding schedule required.
[b]With carbidopa.
[c]Total dose injected over multiple runs.
Data from references 82–84.

single operation for well-established models. The result is an image of the rate of the process being measured (metabolic rate for glucose, blood flow, and receptor binding). These parametric images directly display biologic information in quantitative units for the entire imaging field of view, eliminating the need to define regions of interest and apply the model to these one at a time.

DOSIMETRY

Most of the dose in a PET study comes from the deposition of energy by the positron, rather than from the 511-keV γ-rays. The doses therefore are isotope-dependent, and for dosimetry, the dose from the transmission scan can be safely ignored. Table 5.3 shows dose estimates for a range of common PET studies per millicurie of injected tracer (82–84). In general, approximately 10 to 20 mCi of ^{18}F-labeled tracers, 20 to 40 mCi of ^{11}C or ^{13}N-labeled tracers, and up to 180 mCi of ^{15}O-labeled tracers can be injected while still staying within recommended dose limits.

SUMMARY

The more than 500 PET centers worldwide perform a wide range of studies. Modern PET tomographs are capable of producing high-resolution, high-quality images, which are used as diagnostic or prognostic tools and in clinical and basic science research. In patient care, PET often is used semiquantitatively with high signal-to-noise images of biologic processes that form the basis for diagnosis. In clinical research, in which the goal often is to obtain fundamental information on the rate of biologic processes in the body, full quantitative analysis with kinetic modeling and blood sampling is justified. Ultimately, however, the quantitative accuracy of the results is limited primarily by partial volume effects related to the resolution limits of PET and the signal-to-noise ratio in the data, which is related to the sensitivity of the PET scanner. PET is finding a role in the basic

biologic and preclinical sciences with the availability of dedicated small-animal imaging systems that provide molecular imaging assays from metabolism to gene expression.

The challenge in PET instrumentation is to find techniques to improve both spatial resolution and system sensitivity without pushing the cost of the instrument dramatically higher. Research continues into developing more compact accelerator devices for producing positron-emitting isotopes, combined with self-contained automated synthesizer units that produce the labeled imaging probes ready for injection into the patient. The goal is to reach the point at which a wide selection of diagnostic PET imaging probes can be made automatically and inexpensively, either at in-house radiopharmaceutical facilities or at commercial radiopharmacies that supply clinical sites that do not have their own cyclotrons. Another active area of research is reconstruction algorithms. The filtered backprojection methods described earlier, although fast, are far from ideal. Iterative algorithms that accurately model the imaging system and the statistical nature of the data have been shown to improve the signal-to-noise ratio in the images. The relative complexity and long reconstruction times compared with those of filtered backprojection, however, remain obstacles to routine implementation. The challenges in tracer kinetic modeling, apart from development of models for new tracers, are to find ways to handle image noise optimally and to further refine models. Image registration techniques that allow correction of patient movement in long dynamic studies and registration to MR images or CT scans for definition of region of interest are also an important area of development (85).

The last few years have seen PET dramatically extend its reach into routine clinical use. At the other end of the spectrum, PET has expanded into the basic biologic and pharmaceutical sciences. As the technology and methods are further refined, there can only be an increasing role for PET in modern medicine and biology, particularly in the area of molecular diagnostics and the integration of molecular diagnostics with molecular therapeutics.

REFERENCES

1. Phelps ME. PET: the merging of biology and imaging into molecular imaging. *J Nucl Med* 2000;41: 661–681.
2. Phelps ME. PET: a biological imaging technique. *Neurochem Res* 1991; 16:929–940.
3. Burns HD, Hamill TG, Eng W, et al. Positron emission tomography neuroreceptor imaging as a tool in drug discovery, research and development. *Curr Opin Chem Biol* 1999;3:388–394.
4. Tilsley DWO, Harte RJA, Jones T, et al. New techniques in the pharmacokinetic analysis of cancer drugs, IV: positron emission tomography. *Cancer Surv* 1993;17:425–442.
5. Sadzot B, Franck G. Noninvasive methods to study drug deposition: positron emission tomography. *Eur J Drug Metab Pharmacokinet* 1990; 15:135–142.
6. Silverman DHS, Small GW, Phelps ME. Clinical value of neuroimaging in the diagnosis of dementia: sensitivity and specificity of regional cerebral metabolic and other parameters for early identification of Alzheimer's disease. *Clin Positron Imaging* 1999;2:119–130.
7. Playford ED. Positron emission tomography: applications to the investigation of movement disorders. *Eur J Clin Invest* 1994;24:433–440.
8. Mohan KK, Chugani DC, Chugani HT. Positron emission tomography in pediatric neurology. *Semin Pediatr Neurol* 1999;6:111–119.

9. Duncan JS. Positron emission tomography receptor studies. *Adv Neurol* 1999;79:893–899.

10. Baxter LR. Positron emission tomography studies of cerebral glucose metabolism in obsessive compulsive disorder. *J Clin Psychiatry* 1994; 55[Suppl]:54–59.

11. Fowler JS, Volkow ND, Ding YS, et al. Positron emission tomography studies of dopamine-enhancing drugs. *J Clin Pharmacol* 1999; 39[Suppl]:13S–16S.

12. London ED. Positron emission tomography in studies of drug abuse. *NIDA Res Monogr* 1994;138:15–24.

13. Bergman SR. Cardiac positron emission tomography. *Semin Nucl Med* 1998;28:320–340.

14. Schelbert HR. The usefulness of positron emission tomography. *Curr Probl Cardiol* 1998;23:69–120.

15. Silverman DH, Hoh CK, Seltzer MA, et al. Evaluating tumor biology and oncological disease with positron-emission tomography. *Semin Radiat Oncol* 1998;8:183–196.

16. Leskinen S, Lapela M, Lindholm P, et al. Metabolic imaging by positron emission tomography in oncology. *Ann Med* 1997;29:271–274.

17. Gambhir SS, Czernin J, Schwimmer J, et al. A tabulated summary of the FDG PET literature. *J Nucl Med* 2001;42[Suppl]:1S–93S.

18. Levin CS, Hoffman EJ. Calculation of positron range and its effect on the fundamental limit of positron emission tomography system spatial resolution. *Phys Med Biol* 1999;44:781–799.

19. Hoffman EJ, Huang SC, Phelps ME, et al. Quantitation in positron emission tomography, 4: effect of accidental coincidences. *J Comput Assist Tomogr* 1981;5:391–400.

20. Tewson TJ, Krohn KA. PET radiopharmaceuticals: state-of-the-art and future prospects. *Semin Nucl Med* 1998;28:221–234.

21. Satyamurthy N, Phelps ME, Barrio JR. Electronic generators for the production of positron-emitter labeled radiopharmaceuticals: where would PET be without them? *Clin Positron Imaging* 1999;2:233–253.

22. McCarthy TJ, Welch MJ. The state of positron emitting radionuclide production in 1997. *Semin Nucl Med* 1998;28:235–246.

23. Knapp FF, Mirzadeh S. The continuing important role of radionuclide generator systems for nuclear medicine. *Eur J Nucl Med* 1994;21: 1151–1165.

24. Barrio JR. Biochemical principles in radiopharmaceutical design and utilization. In: Phelps ME, Mazziotta JC, Schelbert HR, eds. *Positron emission tomography and autoradiography.* New York: Raven Press, 1986:451–492.

25. Eriksson L, Wienhard K, Dahlbom M. A simple data loss model for positron camera systems. *IEEE Trans Nucl Sci* 1993;40:1548–1552.

26. Strother SC, Casey ME, Hoffman EJ. Measuring PET scanner sensitivity: relating countrates to image signal-to-noise ratios using noise equivalent counts. *IEEE Trans Nucl Sci* 1990;37:783–788.

27. Casey ME, Nutt R. A multicrystal two-dimensional BGO detector system for positron emission tomography. *IEEE Trans Nucl Sci* 1986; 33:460–463.

28. Cherry SR, Tornai MP, Levin CS, et al. A comparison of PET detector modules employing rectangular and round photomultiplier tubes. *IEEE Trans Nucl Sci* 1995;42:1064–1068.

29. Germano G, Hoffman EJ. A study of data loss and mispositioning due to pileup in 2-D detectors in PET. *IEEE Trans Nucl Sci* 1990;37: 671–675.

30. Moses WW, Derenzo SE. Empirical observation of resolution degradation in positron emission tomographs utilizing block detectors. *J Nucl Med* 1993;34:P101(abst).

31. Wong WH, Uribe J, Hicks K, et al. An analog decoding BGO block detector using circular photomultipliers. *IEEE Trans Nucl Sci* 1995; 42:1095–1101.

32. Karp JS, Muehllehner G. Performance of a position-sensitive scintillation detector. *Phys Med Biol* 1985;30:643–655.

33. Mankoff DA, Muehllehner G, Miles GE. A local coincidence triggering system for PET tomographs composed of large-area position-sensitive detectors. *IEEE Trans Nucl Sci* 1990;37:730–736.

34. Karp JS, Muehllehner G, Mankoff DA, et al. Continuous-slice PENN-PET: a positron tomograph with volume imaging capability. *J Nucl Med* 1990;31:617–627.

35. Freifelder R, Karp JS, Geagan M, et al. Design and performance of the HEAD PENN-PET scanner. *IEEE Trans Nucl Sci* 1994;41: 1436–1440.

36. Lecomte R, Cadorette J, Rodrigue S, et al. Initial results from the Sherbrooke avalanche photodiode positron tomograph. *IEEE Trans Nucl Sci* 1996;43:1952–1957.

37. Ziegler SI, Pichler BJ, Boening G, et al. A prototype high-resolution animal positron tomograph with avalanche photodiode arrays and LSO crystals. *Eur J Nucl Med* 2001;28:136–143.

38. Schmand M, Eriksson L, Casey ME, et al. Performance results of a new DOI detector block for a high resolution PET-LSO research tomograph HRRT. *IEEE Trans Nucl Sci* 1998;45:3000–3006.

39. Huber JS, Moses WW, Derenzo SE, et al. Characterization of a 64 channel PET detector using photodiodes for crystal identification. *IEEE Trans Nucl Sci* 1997;44:1197–1201.

40. Ter-Pogossian MM, Mullani NA, Ficke DC, et al. Photon time-of-flight-assisted positron emission tomography. *J Comput Assist Tomogr* 1981;5:227–229.

41. Duxbury DM, Ott RJ, Flower MA, et al. Preliminary results from the new large-area PETRRA positron camera. *IEEE Trans Nucl Sci* 1999; 46:1050–1054.

42. Jeavons AP, Chandler RA, Dettmar CAR. A 3D HIDAC-PET camera with sub-millimetre resolution for imaging small animals. *IEEE Trans Nucl Sci* 1999;46:468–473.

43. Wienhard K, Erikkson L, Grootoonk S, et al. Performance evaluation of the positron scanner ECAT EXACT. *J Comput Assist Tomogr* 1992; 16:804–813.

44. DeGrado TR, Turkington TG, Williams JJ, et al. Performance characteristics of a whole-body PET scanner. *J Nucl Med* 1994;35: 1398–1406.

45. Smith RJ, Adam LE, Karp JS. Methods to optimize whole body surveys with the C-PET camera. Conference Record of the 1999 Nuclear Science Symposium and Medical Imaging Conference, 24–30 October 1999, Seattle, WA. Piscataway, NJ: IEEE Press, 1999:1197–1201.

46. Phelps ME, Cherry SR. The changing design of positron imaging systems. *Clin Positron Imaging* 1998;1:31–45.

47. Townsend DW, Cherry SR. Combining anatomy and function: the path to true image fusion. *Eur Radiol* 2001;11:1968–1974.

48. Beyer T, Townsend DW, Brun T, et al. A combined PET/CT scanner for clinical oncology. *J Nucl Med* 2000;41:1369–1379.

49. Thompson CJ, Murthy K, Picard Y, et al. Positron emission mammography (PEM): a promising technique for detecting breast cancer. *IEEE Trans Nucl Sci* 1995;42:1012–1017.

50. Freifelder R, Karp J. Dedicated PET scanners for breast imaging. *Phys Med Biol* 1997;42:2463–2480.

51. Doshi NK, Silverman RW, Shao Y, et al. MaxPET: a dedicated mammary and axillary region PET imaging system for breast cancer. *IEEE Trans Nucl Sci* 2001;48:811–815.

52. Cherry SR, Shao Y, Silverman RW, et al. MicroPET: a high resolution PET scanner for imaging small animals. *IEEE Trans Nucl Sci* 1997; 44:1161–1166.

53. Del Guerra A, Di Domenico G, Scandola M, et al. High spatial resolution small animal YAP–PET. *Nucl Instrum Methods Phys Res A* 1998; 409:508–510.

54. Weber S, Herzog H, Cremer M, et al. Evaluation of the TierPET system. *IEEE Trans Nucl Sci* 1997;46:1177–1183.

55. Dahlbom M, Schiepers C, Hoffman EJ, et al. Evaluation of PET for whole body imaging. *J Nucl Med* 1990;31:749.

56. Guerrero T, Hoffman EJ, Dahlbom M, et al. Characterization of a whole-body imaging technique for PET. *IEEE Trans Nucl Sci* 1990; 37:676–680.

57. Cherry SR, Dahlbom M, Hoffman EJ. Three-dimensional positron emission tomography using a conventional multislice tomograph without septa. *J Comput Assist Tomogr* 1991;15:655–668.

58. Townsend DW, Geissbuhler A, DeFrise M, et al. Fully three-dimensional reconstruction for a PET camera with retractable septa. *IEEE Trans Med Imaging* 1991;10:505–512.

59. Defrise M, Townsend DW, Geissbuhler A. Implementation of three-dimensional image reconstruction for multi-ring tomographs. *Phys Med Biol* 1990;35:1361–1372.

60. Brooks RA, Di Chiro G. Principles of computer assisted tomography

(CAT) in radiographic and radioisotopic imaging. *Phys Med Biol* 1976; 21:689–732.

61. Huang SC, Hoffman EJ, Phelps ME, et al. Quantitation in positron computed tomography, 3: effect of sampling. *J Comput Assist Tomogr* 1980;4:819–826.
62. Hutton BF, Hudson HM, Beekman FJ. A clinical perspective of accelerated statistical reconstruction. *Eur J Nucl Med* 1997;24:797–808.
63. Hoffman EJ, Guerrero TM, Germano G, et al. PET system calibration and corrections for quantitative and spatially accurate images. *IEEE Trans Nucl Sci* 1989;36:1108–1112.
64. Badawi RD, Lodge MA, Marsden PK. Algorithms for calculating detector normalization coefficients for true coincidences in 3D PET. *Phys Med Biol* 1998;43:189–205.
65. Meikle S, Dahlbom M, Cherry SR. Attenuation correction using count-limited transmission data in positron emission tomography. *J Nucl Med* 1993;34:143–150.
66. Siegel S, Dahlbom M. Implementation and validation of a calculated attenuation correction for PET. *IEEE Trans Nucl Sci* 1992;39:1117–1121.
67. Carson RE, Daube-Witherspoon M, Green MV. A method for postinjection PET transmission measurements with a rotating source. *J Nucl Med* 1988;29:1558–1567.
68. Thompson CJ, Ranger N, Evans AC, et al. Validation of simultaneous PET emission and transmission scans. *J Nucl Med* 1991;32:154–160.
69. Watson CC, Newport D, Casey ME, et al. Evaluation of simulation-based scatter correction for 3-D PET cardiac imaging. *IEEE Trans Nucl Sci* 1997;44:90–97.
70. Ollinger JM, Johns GC. Model-based scatter correction for fully 3D PET. *IEEE Trans Nucl Sci* 1993;40:1264–1268.
71. Grootoonk S, Spinks TJ, Jones T, et al. Correction for scatter using a dual energy window technique with a tomograph operated without septa. *IEEE Trans Nucl Sci* 1991;38:1569–1573.
72. Bergström M, Eriksson L, Bohm C, et al. Correction for scattered radiation in a ring detector positron camera by integral transformation of the projections. *J Comput Assist Tomogr* 1983;7:42–50.
73. Bailey DL, Meikle SR. A convolution-subtraction scatter correction method for 3D PET. *Phys Med Biol* 1994;39:411–424.
74. Holdsworth CH, Levin CS, Farquhar TH, et al. Investigation of accelerated Monte Carlo techniques for PET simulation and 3D PET scanner correction. *IEEE Trans Nucl Sci* 2001:48;74–81.
75. Hoffman EJ, Cutler PD, Guerrero TM, et al. Assessment of accuracy of PET utilizing a 3-D phantom to simulate the activity distribution of 18-F FDG uptake in the human brain. *J Cereb Blood Flow Metab* 1991;11:A17–A25.
76. Hoffman EJ, Huang SC, Phelps ME. Quantitation in positron emission tomography, 1: effect of object size. *J Comput Assist Tomogr* 1979;3:299–308.
77. Gambhir SS, Huang SC, Digby WM, et al. A new method for partial volume and spillover correction in cardiac PET scans. *J Nucl Med* 1989;30:824–825.
78. Meltzer CC, Zubieta JK, Links JM, et al. MR-based correction of brain PET measurements for heterogeneous gray matter radioactivity distribution. *J Cereb Blood Flow Metab* 1996;16:650–658.
79. Rousset OG, Ma Y, Evans AC. Correction for partial volume effects in PET: principle and validation. *J Nucl Med* 1998;39:904–911.
80. Huang SC, Phelps ME. Principles of tracer kinetic modeling in positron emission tomography and autoradiography. In: Phelps ME, Mazziotta JC, Schelbert HR, eds. *Positron emission tomography and autoradiography.* New York: Raven Press, 1986:287–346.
81. Patlak CS, Blasberg RG. Graphical evaluation of blood-to-brain transfer constants from multiple-time uptake data. *J Cereb Blood Flow Metab* 1985;5:584–590.
82. Kearfott KJ. Absorbed dose estimates for positron emission tomography (PET): C15O, 11CO, and CO15O. *J Nucl Med* 1982;23:1031–1037.
83. International Commission on Radiological Protection. *Radiation dose to patients from radiopharmaceuticals.* ICRP publication 53. New York: Pergamon Press, 1988.
84. Brown WD, Oakes TR, Nickles RJ. Revised dosimetry for fluoro-dopa with carbidopa pretreatment. *J Nucl Med* 1993;34:157P(abst).
85. Woods RP, Grafton ST, Holmes CJ, et al. Automated image registration, I: general methods and intrasubject validation. *J Comput Assist Tomogr* 1998;22:139–152.

Diagnostic Nuclear Medicine, Fourth Edition. Edited by M.P. Sandler, R.E. Coleman, J.A. Patton, F.J.Th. Wackers, A. Gottschalk. Lippincott Williams & Wilkins, Philadelphia 2003.

6

NEW TECHNOLOGIES IN NUCLEAR MEDICINE

TIMOTHY G. TURKINGTON
JAMES E. BOWSHER

Nuclear medicine practitioners regularly gain new software and hardware tools for expanding or improving their capabilities. Such tools can range from software updates to entirely new scanners. This chapter describes three innovations that have recently become widespread or are currently becoming widespread—positron emission tomography (PET) with rotating gamma cameras (hybrid PET), x-ray computed tomography (CT) with PET and single positron emission CT (SPECT) systems, and iterative image reconstruction.

POSITRON EMISSION TOMOGRAPHY WITH ROTATING GAMMA CAMERAS

The expanding role of PET, particularly in oncology, has triggered a desire for a range of scanning instruments. At the end of high expense and high performance are multicrystal full-ring systems, which have evolved over years of use in research and clinical practice (1,2). Less expensive dedicated PET scanners also have been developed (3,4). At the modest end are rotating gamma cameras that have been modified for PET in addition to their more customary use for SPECT and planar single photon imaging (5,6). A popular product is a two-head, large-field-of-view rotating system in which the cameras can be positioned at approximately 90 or 180 degrees, allowing whole-body planar scans with simultaneous anterior and posterior views and SPECT scans (90 degrees for cardiac, 180 degrees for other types of imaging.) The capabilities of these systems have been further expanded to allow PET. Although the concept of using gamma cameras in coincidence to image positron emitters is not at all new (7,8), the recent trend toward investigation (9) and commercial availability (10) of these cameras has been possible because of the desirability of imaging with fluorodeoxyglucose (FDG) and because of changes in gamma camera electronics and performance over the last 25 years.

Principles

The positron that is emitted from a PET radiotracer travels a short (~1 mm) distance in the body and then annihilates with an electron. The product of this annihilation is two 511-keV photons, which leave the annihilation site in opposite directions. PET relies on the detection of these photon pairs. Since the photons are emitted in opposite directions, the annihilation point for each pair is assumed to be somewhere on the line connecting these points.

For imaging in coincidence mode, the conventional collimation used for single-photon imaging (parallel hole, converging, diverging, fan beam, cone beam, or pinhole) is removed to allow detected of radiation regardless of its incidence angle on the camera. Events are recorded when 511-keV photons are detected simultaneously in both cameras. As shown in Fig. 6.1, the gantry must rotate during the scan to allow detection of radiation along all the angles at which it can be emitted. The spatial resolution is related to the intrinsic resolution cameras and can be comparable to the spatial resolution of high-end dedicated PET systems (~5 mm).

Limitations

The primary limit of PET on gamma cameras is the rate at which coincidence events are detected. This limit stems from the combination of low detection efficiency for emitted radiation and the limited rate at which the large cameras can count individual photons.

Detection Efficiency

PET detection efficiency depends on the geometric efficiency and the intrinsic detector efficiency. The geometric efficiency is not as good as a that of a full-ring PET system if only a single plane is being imaged but improves with three-dimensional effects (see later). The larger problem is the intrinsic efficiency of the detector for 511-keV photons. Because gamma cameras are optimized (and must remain so) for low-energy single-photon imaging, they have relatively thin (⅜-inch) NaI detectors. This thickness is still enough to stop most 140-keV photons. Thin

T.G. Turkington: Departments of Radiology and Biomedical Engineering, Duke University, Durham, NC.
J.E. Bowsher: Department of Radiology, Duke University, Durham, NC.

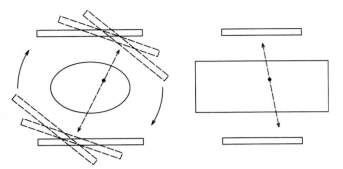

FIGURE 6.1. Simple schematic of PET with rotating gamma cameras.

crystals are efficient for stopping photons from ^{201}Tl and ^{99m}Tc and give good spatial resolution (11). For higher energies, thin crystals are not efficient. Although only 28% of 511-keV photons interact in such a detector, an even smaller fraction (~12%) deposit all their energy there (12).

Singles Count-rate Limits

With the exception of the first-pass cardiac studies, the count-rate capabilities of gamma cameras rarely are pushed beyond a few thousand counts per second (kcps). Much higher rates are required for coincidence imaging. When a photon is detected in one head, the probability that its partner will be detected in the other head is very low (<1%). This low probability is due to photon attenuation and scatter, which cause problems for all PET, and the low detection efficiency is particularly bad for gamma cameras. Even with the huge improvements that have been made to gamma cameras to allow single photon rates greater than 1 Mcps, the detected coincidence rates are typically a few thousand counts per second. Dedicated PET systems with hundreds of independent detector units are capable of much higher singles detection rates, and are therefore able to yield much higher coincidence rates.

One of the confusing factors in discussing detection rates is that the singles rate usually refers to all photon energy detected in the head and the coincidence rate refers only to events in which both photons are at usable energy (photopeak or Compton). The performance of a camera is limited not by the photopeak even rate but by the rate of all scintillation events, because a pulse can cause pileup problems with any previous or successive pulse, regardless of the size of either.

Improvements

Several measures have been taken by camera manufacturers to improve the quality of PET imaging on gamma cameras, including increasing crystal thickness, segmenting the detectors into multiple regions, and using septa to control camera count rates.

Crystal Thickness

The low detection efficiency of $\frac{3}{8}$-inch NaI detectors for 511-keV radiation is a major limitation of gamma camera PET. This thickness is suitable for the lower-energy photons typical of single-photon imaging, especially those from ^{99m}Tc, at 140 keV (11). At this energy and thickness, it is possible to achieve intrinsic spatial resolution of 3.5 mm full width at half maximum or better, and detection efficiency is better than 90%. For higher-energy photons, the detection efficiency decreases, and thicker crystals are desirable. However, when thicker crystals are used, the intrinsic spatial resolution decreases. Therefore any increase in crystal thickness to improve 511-keV detection efficiency degrades lower-energy spatial resolution. Most gamma cameras sold with PET capability have $\frac{5}{8}$-inch- or $\frac{6}{8}$-inch-thick crystals.

The loss of spatial resolution with increasing crystal thickness is caused by the spread of light from the scintillation. Ideally, the light from a scintillation event illuminates a small cluster of photomultiplier tubes, such as a photomultiplier tube and its six neighbors in a hexagonal pattern. Any light spread beyond these central photomultiplier tubes means that generated light is not used for the position calculation. One solution to controlling light spread is to cut grooves on the back of the crystal. Such grooves channel light produced at the front of the crystal and control spread of the light. Such crystals have been implemented in a 1-inch (25 mm) thickness and demonstrate better spatial resolution than untreated $\frac{5}{8}$-inch systems (13).

Singles Count Rates

The singles counting capability of gamma cameras has been improved drastically to achieve PET imaging capability. The improvements have come through several separate measures. The first is shortened integration times. The scintillation light leaving NaI(Tl) has a 230-ns decay constant and therefore requires approximately a microsecond to be fully measured. Full capture of all the light is necessary to achieve the highest possible energy resolution. However, a large fraction of the light is obtained in a much shorter integration. The most sophisticated schemes entail a variable integration time and use of the exponential nature of the light output decay to predict the unmeasured tail.

In a conventional gamma camera, the x, y, and E signals come from a global collection of signals from all photomultiplier tubes. Thus a scintillation event would be corrupted by successive scintillation anywhere in the camera. With digitized information from the photomultiplier tubes, it is possible to reduce the camera area consumed by a single event. Schemes sometimes called *segmentation* or *local zoning* operate the camera in a way that independent scintillations can be recognized simultaneously in different regions of the camera. If a coincidence is detected with a subsequent pileup event in one of the heads, a scheme such as this allows the coincidence event to be used if the pileup photon is far enough away (determined with the segmentation scheme) that it does not affect the energy or position measurement of the original photon (Fig. 6.2).

The use of spatial information to detect and process overlapping events can allow high rates of flux on the detector head. Such schemes can allow better rejection of pileup or processing of events that would otherwise have been rejected or a combination of the two.

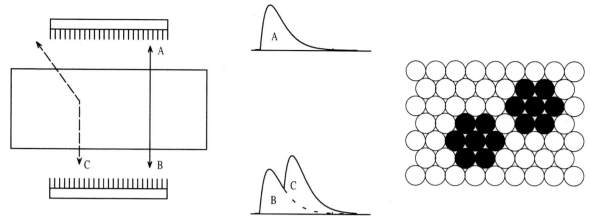

FIGURE 6.2. With newer camera front-end processing schemes, a coincidence event leading to detection of photons *a* and *b* can be processed cleanly even if there is another hit in one of the cameras (*c*), as long as the undesired hit is far enough away from the one in coincidence not to corrupt it. In a conventional gamma camera, only timing is used to differentiate events.

Collimation

As in two-dimensional PET, photons can be prevented from impinging on the detector with lead or tungsten septa (Fig. 6.3). The septa stop several types of events. In *a,* a single photon from outside the field of view is rejected. Although this single-photon event would not cause a coincidence trigger, it would contribute to dead-time losses, which in turn lead to coincidence count-rate limits. In *b,* a scattered event is rejected. If one of the photons is scattered with a significant component in the axial direction, at least one of the photons is rejected by the septa. In *c,* an event with a large axial angle is rejected. Such an event can provide useful information if three-dimensional image reconstruction is used but is lost because of the septa. Events at very large axial angles are possible only when the source is near the middle of the axial field of view. Rejecting such events makes the scanner sensitivity more uniform. In *d,* an event is lost simply because it hit the edge of a septum. Such an event would have provided good information. In *e,* an event in a transaxial plane is shown as accepted. In *f,* an event is shown that is accepted even though it is slightly out of the transaxial plane. Such an event is considered exactly transaxial in two-dimensional reconstruction approximations (14) or can be treated exactly in three-dimensional reconstructions.

If high sensitivity is the primary goal for the PET system, then septa should not be used. This would be the case, for example, if the dose is limited. If the dose is not limited but camera counting rates are limited, use of septa can improve the quality of the events acquired (15).

Images obtained with a large phantom that includes radioactivity out of the field of view are shown in (Fig. 6.4). This phantom includes background radioactivity and small spheres at 8 times the radioactivity concentration of the background. The images are not too different, although much more radioactivity was used in the imaging with septa, demonstrating the higher efficiency of the nonseptal configuration. This central slice is the best case for imaging without septa owing to the high geometric efficiency for detecting radiation at the middle of the

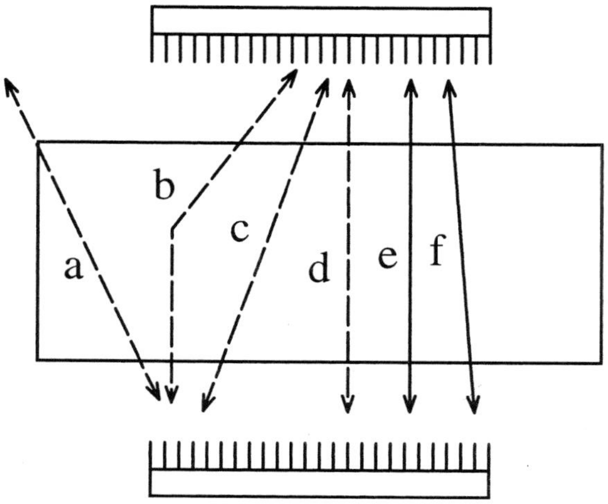

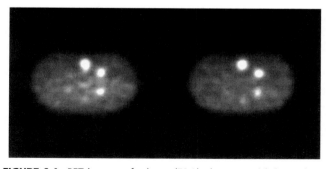

FIGURE 6.4. PET images of a large (50 L) phantom with hot spheres (8× background concentration obtained on a hybrid scanner with 1-inch NaI detectors). The image on the *left* was acquired with no septa with 28 MBq (0.75 mCi) in the phantom. The image on the *right* was acquired with septa, a 12-degree axial acceptance angle, and 130 MBq (3.5 mCi) in the phantom. Both images were reconstructed with a fully three-dimensional iterative image reconstruction algorithm.

FIGURE 6.3. Septa on the gamma camera allow less radiation to hit the detectors, eliminating most radiation from outside the field of view, many scattered events, and radiation with a large axial angle.

scanner, whereas all slices are comparable when imaging is performed with septa.

POSITRON EMISSION TOMOGRAPHIC AND SINGLE PHOTON EMISSION COMPUTED TOMOGRAPHIC SCANNERS WITH X-RAY COMPUTED TOMOGRAPHY

The use of x-ray CT in combination with emission tomography (PET or SPECT) was investigated first with SPECT (16) and then with PET (17). It addresses two distinct issues fundamental to PET and SPECT imaging—attenuation correction and lesion localization.

Attenuation

Attenuation of photons in SPECT and PET leads to loss of quantitative accuracy, lack of image uniformity, and distortions (18–21). Although some software methods exist for correcting regions of uniform attenuation based on determination of the outer body contour (22), proper correction in nonuniform regions requires that the attenuation properties be measured with a transmission scan (23). Conventional techniques make use of the radiation detectors already in place and a sealed radiation source outside the body. In PET, ^{68}Ge, a positron emitter, and ^{137}Cs, a single photon emitter with energy of 662 keV (24,25), are used routinely on commercial systems. In SPECT, several sources have been used, most commonly ^{153}Gd (energy ~ 100 keV) (26).

Several challenging issues are related to radionuclide-based transmission scanning. One is that transmission scanning must be performed after the radiotracer is injected for the protocol to be clinically feasible. Differences in energy between transmission and emission photons can be used to differentiate the origin of the photons in SPECT applications (27) and in some PET applications with ^{137}Cs (24,28). High-intensity transmission sources that overwhelm the emission activity, electronic masks that preclude detection of radiation not in line with the source, and corrections in which data from the emission scan are used to correct the contamination in the transmission scan have been used to address this problem (29).

Another issue is the noise added in transmission-based attenuation correction (30). Transmission scan noise is limited by the duration of the scan, the strength of the radioactive source (often limited by the count-rate capability of the system), and the efficiency of the system for detecting the emissions from the source. It would be desirable to have long transmission scans to reduce the noise added to the emission data in the attenuation correction. However, a transmission scan comparable with or longer than the emission scan is unattractive from a clinical perspective, because the purpose of the transmission scan is simply to correct attenuation effects in the emission data.

Localization of Lesions

PET and SPECT images show functional information. In many cases, the studies are interpreted with the help of anatomic information in x-ray CT and magnetic resonance (MR) images. Images obtained with other modalities typically differ in field of view, pixel size, and slice orientation. For imaging other than of the brain, the morphologic features of the body are different between scans, because the body and its internal features are not rigid. Interpretation of PET or SPECT images is aided by well-registered MR and CT images.

Adding X-ray Computed Tomography to Single Photon Emission Computed Tomography and Positron Emission Tomography

Using x-ray CT in conjunction with a PET or SPECT scanner provides a means of attenuation correction and a way to obtain anatomic images that match the PET or SPECT images as well as possible, because they are acquired close together in time on the same table. Because both image sets are acquired with the patient on the same table, and the relative orientation of the two scanners is known, superior spatial matching of images can be obtained.

The first attempt to merge SPECT and x-ray CT was made by Lang et al. (16), who added a commercial CT system to a commercial SPECT camera. Beyer et al. (17) first added x-ray CT to a PET camera, using rotating, partial-ring PET as the basis. Commercially available nuclear medicine scanners with attached x-ray CT include SPECT cameras with PET imaging capability (31) and dedicated PET systems (32).

Use of the attenuation image provided by x-ray CT for attenuation correction is shown in Fig. 6.5. The attenuation image is shown with a superimposed course grid, signifying the difference between emission CT and CT pixel sizes. The attenuation factor for the line shown is calculated by projecting through the attenu-

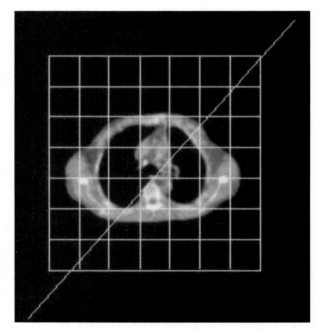

FIGURE 6.5. To determine attenuation along a PET or SPECT radiation path, the CT pixels along that path are traced through and summed.

ation image and summing the attenuation contribution for each pixel on the line. In PET, the resulting factor can be used directly to correct the emission data before reconstruction. In SPECT, the process is more complicated, and accurate correction must be done in the context of an iterative algorithm, but the attenuation factors are still measured by means of tracing through the attenuation image.

Technical Issues

Several technical challenges are associated with dual-modality scanners. These are related both to x-ray attenuation and anatomic localization.

Adjustment of Attenuation Coefficients

Because attenuation of radiation in the body depends on the energy of the radiation, the attenuation factors derived directly from an x-ray CT scan cannot be used directly for correction of higher-energy emission photons. If all image regions were air, water, or a combination of air and water, the attenuation measurement would be essentially a density measurement, and the proportionality factor could be used to scale between values derived from x-rays and those needed for higher-energy photon correction, as follows:

$$\mu_{511}(i) = a \cdot \mu_{x\text{-}ray}(i) \qquad [1]$$

where $\mu_{x\text{-}ray}(i)$ is the attenuation coefficient measured for pixel i by means of x-ray CT, $\mu_{511}(i)$ is the value adjusted to be appropriate for 511 keV (for example) and a is the ratio of attenuation coefficients in water. However, the presence of a higher atomic number (Z) in some materials leads to a different ratio of attenuation coefficients, so a single scaling factor, a, is not valid. For example, the attenuation of x-rays increases more for dense bone (compared with water) than does the attenuation of higher-energy photons, so attenuation correction based on Eq. 1 would over-correct 511-keV photons in the vicinity of bone. These effects have been evaluated and an algorithm has been proposed (33) that entails scaling of Eq. 1 for all pixels at the density of water or lower but contains scaling appropriate for bone for higher-pixel values. In reality, dense bone constitutes a small fraction of the body volume, so the simplistic scaling represented in Eq. 1 is quite good for most situations.

Differences in Body Shape

It is typical to perform fast diagnostic CT with a breath hold. This is not feasible for longer SPECT and PET studies. Therefore if the CT is performed conventionally, the mismatch between images results in inaccuracies in attenuation correction in the vicinity of the diaphragm and the chest wall (34). Systems with low-current x-ray tubes (31) require longer scans. X-ray CT image quality is lost, but there is a better match to the SPECT or PET images.

Use of Contrast Agents

The use of contrast agents to improve the usefulness of x-ray CT images introduces two potential problems related to attenuation

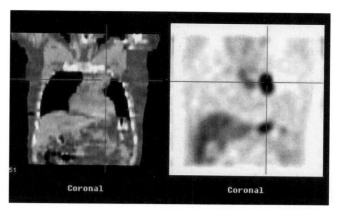

FIGURE 6.6. A ^{67}Ga citrate lymphoma study performed with a gamma camera equipped with x-ray CT. *Left,* x–ray CT images. *Right,* SPECT images. Both have been resliced to produce coronal images. In this display, crosshairs are used to correlate features between the image sets.

correction (35). The first is similar to the bone effect in that contrast medium interferes with the validity of scaling of the attenuation coefficient. That is, tissue that contains contrast material can be opaque to x-rays while hardly different from tissue that does not contain contrast material for 511-keV or even 140 keV photons. In addition, however, the potential for contrast medium to redistribute between transmission and emission scans must be considered.

Example Studies

Two studies from a gamma camera with x-ray CT are shown in Figs. 6.6 and 6.7. The first is a ^{67}Ga citrate SPECT study, the second an FDG PET study.

ITERATIVE IMAGE RECONSTRUCTION

The process of obtaining cross-sectional images of radiotracer distribution from raw projection or sinogram data in PET and SPECT is called *image reconstruction.* Until recently, most clinical images were reconstructed with the filtered backprojection (FBP) algorithm. Currently, however, other algorithms, specifically iterative, statistically based algorithms, are being offered. These more recently available algorithms produce images considerably different from those obtained with the more conventional FBP. The benefits of these algorithms have been explored for many years, but only recently has the computing power of commercial scanners been enough to make their routine use feasible.

In Fig. 6.8, a simple cross-section of the body is superimposed on a grid. The image value at each pixel represents the amount of radioactivity in that region at the time of the scan. For each pixel j, there is a probability that radiation from that pixel will be detected in line of response i for PET or in camera pixel i for SPECT (called bin i for PET and SPECT). The index i is used to describe any of the possible measurements, for example, any pair of PET detectors, or any gamma camera pixel at any

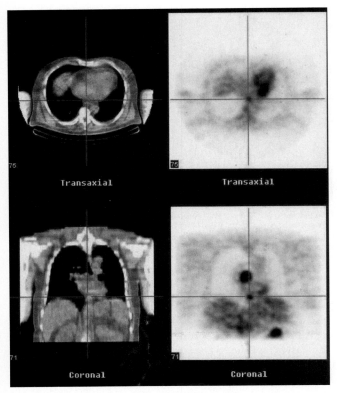

FIGURE 6.7. An [^{18}F]Fluorodeoxyglucose lymphoma study performed with a gamma camera equipped with x-ray CT.

gantry angle. The data acquisition process can be described mathematically as follows:

$$m_i = b_i + \sum_{j=1}^{npix} p_{ij} \lambda_j \qquad [2]$$

where λ_j is the number of photons emitted from pixel j (proportional to the amount of radiotracer in the pixel), m_i is the expected number of photons in bin i, p_{ij} is the probability that an emission from pixel j will be detected in bin i, and b_i is the expected number of background photons detected in bin i. Without considering scatter, p_{ij} is zero for all but a very few combinations of i and j. For example, when a point source is held in front of a gamma camera with a collimator, very few pixels in the camera are illuminated.

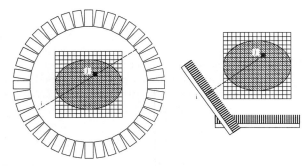

FIGURE 6.8. Detection process for SPECT and PET. Radiation emitted from pixel j has some probability of being detected in bin i.

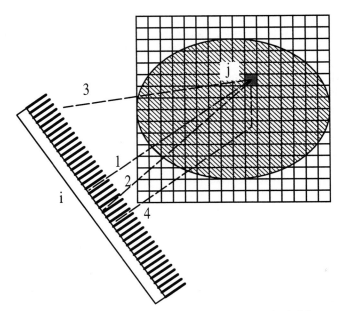

FIGURE 6.9. SPECT detection process with degrading physical factors, including collimator blurring (*2*) and scatter (*4*). Photon (*3*) is rejected by the collimator.

Figure 6.9 shows the acquisition scheme for SPECT when several real physical factors are taken into account. Ray 1 shows the collection of an ideal event. Ray 2 shows the collection of an emitted photon the direction of which is slightly nonperpendicular to the camera face but that still makes it through the collimator. Such events account for the blurring in images obtained with collimated gamma cameras. Ray 3 depicts an emission at an angle too large to be accepted by the camera. For this combination of pixel and detector bin, p_{ij} is zero. Ray 4 shows a scattered photon, emitted from pixel j, scattered, and then detected in a bin far from the ideal one. In equation 2, scatter can be described by p or by b.

The effect of attenuation, which describes the loss of photons otherwise emitted and directed toward a particular bin, can also be included in p, so that a photon trajectory through more tissue would lead to a lower p.

At each detector bin i, the number of photons y_i measured during the SPECT or PET scan is randomly distributed around the expected value m_i according to the Poisson distribution. The image reconstruction task is to estimate all the image pixel values λ_j from the measured projection values y_i. For example, an inversion of Eq. 2 can be written

$$\lambda_j = \sum_{i=1}^{nbin} p_{ji}^{-1} \left(y_i - b_i \right) \qquad [3]$$

where p_{ji}^{-1} represents an inversion of all the probabilities p_{ij}. Mathematically, p_{ij} is a matrix element and p_{ji}^{-1} is an element in the inverse matrix. However, the dimensions of the matrix are so large (the number of image pixels times the number of measurement bins) that direct inversion of the matrix is not feasible as p_{ij} becomes increasingly realistic, modeling the effects of attenuation, scatter, and blur.

In addition to the degrading factors represented in Fig. 6.9, statistical noise further degrades SPECT and PET images. Each measurement y_i typically is only a few counts, and the statistical variations on such low count levels are high. Although no algorithm can "correct" for noise, improvement can be gained by means of statistical weighting of each measurement y_i according to its precision.

Filtered Backprojection (FBP)

FBP follows the form of Eq. 3 to obtain p^{-1}. However, it does so only with a sufficiently simple model of the acquisition. FBP also does not account for the statistical quality of the data.

Maximum Likelihood Expectation Maximization and Ordered Subsets Expectation Maximization

Iterative reconstruction techniques do not require inversion of the detection probabilities p. Instead, estimates of the image are updated to achieve successively better matches between the measured projections y_i and the projections m_i calculated from the image pixel estimates λ_j by means of Eq. 2.

The most thoroughly investigated iterative reconstruction algorithm for PET and SPECT is the maximum likelihood expectation maximization (ML-EM) algorithm (36,37). Mathematically, the algorithm is

$$\lambda_j^{(n+1)} = \frac{1}{\sum\limits_{i=1}^{nbin} p_{ij}} \sum_{i=1}^{nbin} \frac{p_{ij}\lambda_j^{(n)}}{b_i + \sum\limits_{k=1}^{npix} P_{ik}\lambda_k^{(n)}} y_i \qquad [4]$$

Here, $\lambda_j^{(n)}$ is the estimate of the radioactivity at pixel j after iteration n of the algorithm. Each iteration of the algorithm takes the current image estimate, represented by all of the $\lambda_j^{(n)}$, and produces new estimates for each pixel, $\lambda_j^{(n+1)}$. Each iteration of the algorithm essentially takes the current image estimate, calculates what the projections would be if this image were the true radioactivity distribution (in the denominator of the rightmost fraction), and then ultimately updates the image based on

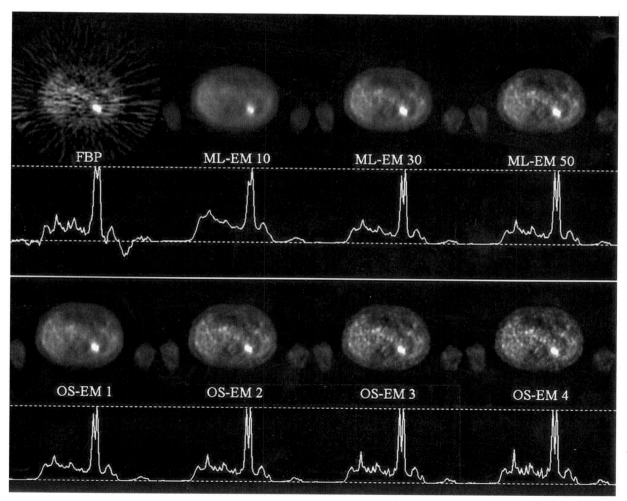

FIGURE 6.10. FDG PET study reconstructed with FBP, ML-EM (10, 30, and 50 iterations), and OS-EM with 28 subsets (1, 2, 3, and 4 iterations). Profiles indicate how well the two bright kidney ducts are resolved as well as the levels of image noise.

the ratio of the measurements y_i to the projection estimate based on the current image estimate.

There are several important properties of the images produced with ML-EM algorithm. Figure 6.10 is an image of a single slice through the liver from an FDG PET study. Several features of this image allow comparison of images, including the presence of two kidney ducts with high uptake, and the liver, the uptake of which is likely uniform. First, the images improve only gradually with each iteration. It can take as many as 50 iterations through the entire data set to produce a good image, with each iteration requiring more computer processing than an FBP reconstruction. Another property is that pixel values cannot be negative. This property can be deduced from the algorithm in Eq. 4. This is different from FBP, in which noise and some artifacts can lead to negative pixels, as demonstrated in the profile in Fig. 6.10. Another property is that resolution and noise both increase with increasing iterations. An important property is the nature of the noise. In general, noise is low in low-activity areas and high in high-activity areas. Although this makes much cleaner-looking images, the interpreter cannot use noise in the background to help differentiate bright spots in the high-uptake areas. With FBP, the noise is relatively constant throughout the image. Some of the important properties of images produced with ML-EM are discussed by Barrett et al. (38) and Wilson et al. (39).

The ML-EM algorithm converges toward the maximum likelihood solution with unlimited iterations (36,37), although in practice the iterations are stopped once sufficient resolution is obtained to control computation times and image noise.

A substantial improvement in speed is made with the ordered subsets expectation maximization algorithm (OS-EM) (40). Similar to ML-EM, this algorithm differs in that it updates the image estimate after processing only a subset of the projections. If the projections are divided into 10 subsets, for example, the images obtained after a single pass through the entire data set (10 image updates) are comparable with images obtained after 10 full iterations through the data in ML-EM. Images produced with OS-EM (28 subsets) are shown in Fig. 6.10.

The iterative reconstruction framework has been used extensively by investigators who have included the degrading physical factors such as attenuation, scatter, and blurring in the acquisition model (41–46).

Other Iterative Algorithms

Whereas the noise in ML-EM and OS-EM typically is controlled by means of limiting the number of iterations and by means of smoothing, other algorithms are designed to converge within a few iterations to a low-noise image. These methods are generally called *maximum a posteriori* or *maximum penalized likelihood* algorithms. These algorithms include penalty functions or prior probability models that encourage less noise in the estimated image (47–50). Models have also been developed to include sophisticated anatomic information, such as that obtained with other imaging modalities (51,52).

REFERENCES

1. DeGrado TR, Turkington TG, Williams JJ, et al. Performance characteristics of a whole-body PET scanner. *J Nucl Med* 1994;35:1398–1406.
2. Brix G, Zaers J, Adam LE, et al. Performance evaluation of a whole-body PET scanner using the NEMA protocol. *J Nucl Med* 1997;38:1614–1623.
3. Karp JS, Muehllehner G, Mankoff DA, et al. Continuous-slice PENN-PET: a positron tomograph with volume imaging capability. *J Nucl Med* 1990;31:617–627.
4. Townsend DW, Wensveen M, Byars LG, et al. A rotating PET scanner using BGO block detectors: design, performance and applications. *J Nucl Med* 1993;34:1367–1376.
5. Patton JA. Instrumentation for coincidence imaging with multihead scintillation cameras. *Semin Nucl Med* 2000;30:239–254.
6. Patton JA, Turkington TG. Coincidence imaging with a dual-head scintillation camera. *J Nucl Med* 1999;40:432–441.
7. Anger HO. Radioisotope cameras. In: Hine GJ, ed. *Instrumentation in nuclear medicine.* Vol. 1. New York: Academic Press, 1967.
8. Muehllehner G, Buchin MP, Dudek JH. Performance parameters of a positron imaging camera. *IEEE Trans Nucl Sci* 1976;23:528–537.
9. Miyaoka RS, Costa WLS, Lewellen TK, et al. Coincidence mode imaging using a standard dual-headed gamma camera. *J Nucl Med* 1996;37:223P.
10. Glass EC, Nelleman P, Hines H, et al. Initial coincidence imaging experience with a SPECT/PET dual head camera. *J Nucl Med* 1996;37:53P.
11. Muehllehner G. Effect of crystal thickness on scintillation camera performance. *J Nucl Med* 1979;20:992–993.
12. Anger HO, Davis DH. Gamma-ray detection efficiency and image resolution in sodium iodide. *Rev Sci Instrum* 1964;35:693–697.
13. Turkington TG, Sampson WH, Coleman RE. Characteristics of a rotating gamma camera with 1-inch sodium iodide detectors for SPECT and PET. *J Nucl Med* 2001;42:98P.
14. Daube-Witherspoon ME, Muehllehner G. Treatment of axial data in three-dimensional PET. *J Nucl Med* 1987;28:1717–1724.
15. Turkington TG. Optimizing rotating gamma camera PET for brain imaging. *IEEE Trans Nucl Sci* 2001;47:1196–1201.
16. Lang TF, Hasegawa BH, Liew SC, et al. Description of a prototype emission-transmission computed-tomography imaging-system. *J Nucl Med* 1992;33:1881–1887.
17. Beyer T, Townsend DW, Brun T, et al. A combined PET/CT scanner for clinical oncology. *J Nucl Med* 2000;41:1369–1379.
18. Huang SC, Hoffman EJ, Phelps ME, et al. Quantitation in positron emission computed-tomography, 2: effects of inaccurate attenuation correction. *J Comput Assist Tomogr* 1979;3:804–814.
19. Zasadny KR, Kison PV, Quint LE, et al. Untreated lung cancer: quantification of systematic distortion of tumor size and shape on non-attenuation-corrected 2-[fluorine-18]fluoro-2-deoxy-D-glucose PET scans. *Radiology* 1996;201:873–876.
20. Wahl RL. To AC or not to AC: that is the question. *J Nucl Med* 1999;40:2025–2028.
21. Farquhar TH, Llacer J, Hoh CK, et al. ROC and localization ROC analyses of lesion detection in whole-body FDG PET: effects of acquisition mode, attenuation correction and reconstruction algorithm. *J Nucl Med* 1999;40:2043–2052.
22. Huang SC, Carson RE, Phelps ME, et al. A boundary method for attenuation correction in positron computed-tomography. *J Nucl Med* 1981;22:627–637.
23. Bailey DL. Transmission scanning in emission tomography. *Eur J Nucl Med* 1998;25:774–787.
24. Karp JS, Muehllehner G, Qu H, et al. Singles transmission in volume-imaging PET with a 137Cs source. *Phys Med Biol* 1995;40:929–944.
25. Shao L, Nellemann P, Muehllehner G. Singles-transmission attenuation correction for dual head coincidence imaging. *J Nucl Med* 1998;39:37P.
26. Bailey DL, Hutton BF, Walker PJ. Improved SPECT using simultaneous emission and transmission tomography. *J Nucl Med* 1987;28:844–851.

27. Gilland DR, Jaszczak RJ, Greer KL, et al. Transmission imaging for nonuniform attenuation correction using a three-headed SPECT camera. *J Nucl Med* 1998;39:1105–1110.

28. Laymon CM, Turkington TG, Gilland DR, et al. Transmission scanning system for a gamma-camera coincidence scanner. *J Nucl Med* 2000;41:692–699.

29. Daube-Witherspoon ME, Carson RE, et al. Post-injection transmission attenuation measurements for PET. *IEEE Trans Nucl Sci* 1988;35:757–761.

30. Dahlbom M, Hoffman EJ. Problems in signal-to-noise ratio for attenuation correction in high-resolution PET. *IEEE Trans Nucl Sci* 1987;34:288–293.

31. Patton JA, Delbeke D, Sandler MP. Image fusion using an integrated, dual-head coincidence camera with x-ray tube–based attenuation maps. *J Nucl Med* 2000;41:1364–1368.

32. Bar-Shalom R, Keidar Z, Engel A, et al. A new combined dedicated PET/CT system in the evaluation of cancer patients. *J Nucl Med* 2001;42:127.

33. Kinahan PE, Townsend DW, Beyer T, et al. Attenuation correction for a combined 3D PET/CT scanner. *Med Phys* 1998;25:2046–2053.

34. Goerres GW, Heidelberg TH, Schwitter MR, et al. Respiratory movement and accuracy of PET-CT-fusion in the thorax. *J Nucl Med* 2001;42:12P.

35. Beyer T, Townsend DW. Dual-modality PET/CT imaging: CT-based attenuation correction in the presence of CT contrast agents. *J Nucl Med* 2001;42:210.

36. Shepp LA, Vardi Y. Maximum likelihood reconstruction for emission tomography. *IEEE Trans Med Imaging* 1982;1:113–121.

37. Lange K, Carson R. EM reconstruction algorithms for emission and transmission tomography. *J Comput Assist Tomogr* 1984;8:306–316.

38. Barrett HH, Wilson DW, Tsui BMW. Noise properties of the EM algorithm, 1: theory. *Phys Med Biol* 1994;39:833–846.

39. Wilson DW, Tsui BMW, Barrett HH. Noise properties of the EM algorithm, 2: Monte-Carlo simulations. *Phys Med Biol* 1994;39:847–871.

40. Hudson HM, Larkin RS . Accelerated image reconstruction using ordered subsets of projection data. *IEEE Trans Med Imaging* 1994;13:601–609.

41. Kadrmas DJ, Frey EC, Karimi SS, et al. Fast implementations of reconstruction-based scatter compensation in fully 3D SPECT image reconstruction. *Phys Med Biol* 1998;43:857–873.

42. Beekman FJ, Kamphuis C, King MA, et al. Improvement of image resolution and quantitative accuracy in clinical single photon emission computed tomography. *Comput Med Imaging Graph* 2001;25:135–146.

43. Tsui BMW, Frey EC, Zhao X, et al. The importance and implementation of accurate 3D compensation methods for quantitative SPECT. *Phys Med Biol* 1994;39:509–530.

44. Gilland DR, Jaszczak RJ, Wang H, et al. A 3D Model of nonuniform attenuation and detector response for efficient iterative reconstruction in SPECT. *Phys Med Biol* 1994;39:547–561.

45. Liang Z, Turkington TG, Gilland DR, et al. Simultaneous compensation for attenuation, scatter and detector response for SPECT reconstruction in 3 dimensions. *Phys Med Biol* 1992;37:587–603.

46. Zeng GL, Gullberg GT, Tsui BMW, et al. 3-Dimensional iterative reconstruction algorithms with attenuation and geometric point response correction. *IEEE Trans Nucl Sci* 1991;38:693–702.

47. Zheng J, Saquib S, Sauer K, et al. Parallelizable bayesian tomography algorithms with rapid, guaranteed convergence. *IEEE Trans Image Process* 2000;9:1745–1759.

48. Mumcuoglu E, Leahy R, Cherry S. Bayesian reconstruction of PET images: methodology and performance analysis. *Phys Med Biol* 1996;41:1777–1807.

49. Fessler JA, Hero AO. Penalized maximum-likelihood image-reconstruction using space-alternating generalized EM algorithms. *IEEE Trans Image Process* 1995;4:1417–1429.

50. Leahy R, Byrne C. Recent developments in iterative image reconstruction for PET and SPECT. *IEEE Trans Med Imaging* 2000;19:257–260.

51. Bowsher JE, Johnson VE, Turkington TG, et al. Bayesian reconstruction and use of anatomical a priori information for emission tomography. *IEEE Trans Med Imaging* 1996;15:673–686.

52. Leahy R, Yan X. Incorporation of anatomical MR data for improved functional imaging with PET. In: Colchester ACF, Hawkes DJ, eds. *Information processing in medical imaging.* New York: Springer–Verlag, 1991:105–120.

Diagnostic Nuclear Medicine, Fourth Edition. Edited by M.P. Sandler, R.E. Coleman, J.A. Patton, F.J.Th. Wackers, A. Gottschalk. Lippincott Williams & Wilkins, Philadelphia 2003.

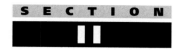

RADIOPHARMACEUTICALS, RADIATION PROTECTION, AND DOSIMETRY

7

RADIOPHARMACEUTICALS

RONALD E. WEINER
MATHEW L. THAKUR

1. INTRODUCTION

A radiopharmaceutical is a combination of radioactive atom (radio), which allows external imaging, and a nonradioactive compound (pharmaceutical), which directs the radioactive tracer to the desired target. The radioactive tracer gives the ability to determine the anatomic location of the tissue in which the tracer has localized. The patient's pathophysiology determines this localization, which leads to the diagnosis, and in some cases the treatment, of the disease. Some pharmaceuticals with suitable functional groups bind the radioactive atoms directly. Others require modification, e.g., chemically attaching a chelating agent, which allows binding of a radionuclide. The compound and radioactive atom should remain intact *in vivo* so that it can provide the appropriate diagnostic information. Therefore, it is important that the radioactive atom binds to the compound with high affinity and that the resultant compound has a high thermodynamic and kinetic stability. The radionuclides used for this purpose are available from three sources: generators, cyclotrons, and nuclear reactors. The source of radionuclide determines its availability, cost, and how the radionuclide use is regulated. Only reactor-produced nuclides are regulated by the Federal Nuclear Regulatory Commission. Generators are portable and are easily transported. Both cyclotron and reactor nuclides are produced and processed in a central commercial facility. The $T_{1/2}$ of some of these nuclides is long enough for shipping to users, radiopharmacies or hospitals, throughout the country without excessive radioactivity decay. Examples are ^{201}Tl, ^{67}Ga, ^{123}I, ^{131}I, and ^{111}In. Their availability is facilitated by the advent of centralized radiopharmacies. Also, many of the radiopharmaceuticals are compounded at the local nuclear medicine laboratories. Thus, these laboratories take on the burden of pharmaceutical manufacturers and are required to perform quality control (QC) analysis of the radiopharmaceuticals produced. These aspects are discussed in the following sections.

2.0 BASIC CHEMISTRY

2.1 Electronic Structure

An atom consists of a positive nucleus with electrons orbiting around the nucleus. For discussion in this chapter, the main

interest is in the outer valence electrons, because these are primarily involved in the interaction that forms bonds between the radionuclide and a pharmaceutical. Quantum numbers (QNs) govern how electrons are placed around the nucleus. The QN define the orbital electron binding energy. The first QN is n, which identifies the principal electron shell and can have values n = 1, 2, 3, etc. These shells are also designated as K (n = 1), L, M, N, etc. The second QN, l or azimuthal QN, can have values l = n − 1, n − 2, . . . , 0. QN, l, defines the ellipticity or shape of electron's orbit. The third QN, m_l (magnetic) can have values m_l = 0, ± 1, ± 2, . . . , ± l. This QN defines the orientation of the orbital in an external magnetic field. The fourth QN is m_s (spin), and m_s can have only two values, − ½ (↓), and ½ (↑). The m_s value can physically be thought of as the angular momentum of an electron. Table 7.1 shows QN for the placement of electrons in the first three shells, n = 1, 2, and 3. The second and third shells are divided into subshells. These subshells are designated s (l = 0), p (l = 2), and d (l = 3) according to the l values for each subshell. These subshells are further subdivided according to the m_l of the subshell. For example, when n = 2, m_l has three values, 1, 0, − 1 and three subshells $2p_x$, $2p_y$, and $2p_z$. Thus, there are four energy levels that can hold eight electrons in the n = 2 shell (Table 7.1). Similarly, in the n = 3 shell, there are nine energy levels with 18 electrons possible.

How are the electrons added to build up the different atoms? Electrons are placed in the lowest energy orbital first. There can be only one electron for each four QNs (Pauli exclusion principle). If two electrons have the same n, l, and m_l, then m_s must be different. Two electrons in the same subshell have opposite spins, ↑↓. When adding electrons to an orbital, the maximum spin multiplicity must be preserved (Hund's rule). Electrons are not paired until each orbital in a degenerate set has been half filled. For example, if three electrons were added to the 2p subshell, each one would be added to each 2p subshell first, i.e., the $2p_x(\uparrow)$, $2p_y(\uparrow)$, and $2p_z(\uparrow)$. A fourth electron would be added to the $2p_x(\uparrow\downarrow)$ level. This concept is important because it partially explains the multiple oxidation states of ^{99m}Tc (see later).

When two atoms combine and form bonds there is a simplistic approach that helps one understand why they combined and why this particular combination is stable. Stability is achieved by the "octet" rule. This rule postulates that atoms attain stability by achieving a noble gas complement of electrons in their

R.E. Weiner: Diagnostic Imaging and Therapeutics, University of Connecticut Health Center, Farmington, CT.
M.L. Thakur: Department of Radiology, Thomas Jefferson University Hospital, Philadelphia, PA.

Table 7.1. *Possible quantum numbers and electron orbitals*

Quantum Numbers			General	
n	1	m_1	Symbol	Explicit
1	0	0	1s	1s
2	0	0	2s	2s
2	1	0	}	$2p_x$
2	1	1	} 2p	$2p_y$
2	1	−1	}	$2p_z$
3	0	0	3s	3s
3	1	0	}	$3p_x$
3	1	1	} 3p	$3p_y$
3	1	−1	}	$3p_z$
3	2	0	}	$3d_{z2}$
3	2	1	}	$3d_{xz}$
3	2	−1	} 3d	$3d_{yz}$
3	2	2	}	$3d_{x2-y2}$
3	2	−2	}	$3d_{xy}$

outer shell (eight electrons in the outer shell). Atoms try to lose or add electrons to complete the octet. For example, fluorine has seven electrons in its outer valence shell. To complete its outer shell this atom tries to add an electron by forming fluoride, $F^- = [Ne]$. An electron can be removed from Na which has a single electron in its valence shell to give $Na^+ = [Ne]$. This electron can be transferred to F. Thus, NaF is very stable because both atoms can achieve a stable octet.

Elements are organized into groups and periods because they share the same valence configuration. Valence is the tendency to lose or gain electrons to form a stable octet. Generally this means that these elements share a variety of chemical properties. This chapter examines only those groups that contain nuclides that are used in nuclear medicine.

Group IA elements have one electron more than the preceding inert gas. Because atoms try to attain a stable octet, it is most likely these atoms would give up their electron to another atom that needs only one electron to complete its shell. If group IA atoms give up an electron they become positively charged and form cations, e.g., Na^+. ^{82}Rubidium (Rb^+), a positron emitter, is used to determine cardiac viability because of its similarities to K^+ (Table 7.2). Group IIA elements, have two electrons in their outer shell. To attain a stable octet, it is most likely these atoms would give up their electrons. Thus for alkaline earths to form compounds, they form doubly charged cations, e.g., Ca^{2+} = [Ar]. Table 7.2 shows the similarities of Sr^{2+} with Ca^{2+} and suggests why ^{89}Sr can be used as an agent that can be incorporated into bone for pain palliation. Group III elements have three electrons in their outer shell and generally attain a stable octet by losing three electrons to another atom. This electron loss gives rise to M^{3+} in aqueous environment, e.g., Y^{3+} = [Kr], Ga^{3+} = $[Ar]3d^{10}$, or In^{3+} = $[Kr]4d^{10}$ (Table 7.2). The octet theory does not quite hold for In and Ga. In these cases, the d shell is stabilized by pairing of all the electrons. In the d shell, there are five levels (Table 7.1), and in the cases of Ga and In, each of the d levels contains two paired electrons (↑↓). Thus it is hard to remove these electrons, so only the s and p electrons in the outer shells are easily removed. Similarly for Tl, the Tl^{1+} state is stabilized by inert pair ($6s^2$). Both thallous (Tl^{1+}) and thallic (Tl^{3+}) are stable oxidation states.

Group IVA elements have four electrons in their outer shell. With this structure it is difficult to lose or gain all four electrons to form a stable octet. It is most likely these atoms would share their electrons with other atoms and form covalent bonds. In a covalent bond, each atom donates an electron to the bond. However, the heavier atoms in this group have more metallic character. Table 7.2 shows that tin, an important atom for preparing ^{99m}Tc compounds, can form two valence states Sn^{2+} and Sn^{4+}. Sn^{3+} is unlikely and Sn^{4+} is more stable state than Sn^{2+}, so that Sn^{2+} can easily lose two electrons (oxidize) to form Sn^{4+}. This is why it is used as a reducing agent. (See Section 2.2.) Similar to Group IVA, Group VA elements have too many electrons, five, to lose or gain all, and therefore these atoms form mostly covalent bonds. Both phosphorous and nitrogen also form coordinate covalent bonds. In this bond both electrons from the donor atom are shared with the recipient atom. These bonds are important in chelate binding. (See Section 2.3.)

Group VI elements have six electrons in their outer shell and might be expected to gain two electrons to form a stable octet. For the lighter elements (group VIA), O^{2-} and S^{2-} are common forms. Oxygen and sulfur form both covalent and coordinate covalent bonds. For the heavier atoms (group VIB), the different electronic structure yields M^{3+} and M^{6+} as stable oxidation states (Table 7.2). All of the electrons in the d shell are unpaired and therefore can be removed rather easily. Examples of these oxidation states in the group are Cr^{3+}, $Cr^{+6}O_4^{2-}$, and $Mo^{+6}O_4^{2-}$. Group VII elements have seven electrons in their outer electron shell. The group VIIA atoms readily gain a single electron to form a stable octet. These halides form simple compounds with metal cations, e.g., $FeCl_3$.

Table 7.2. *Electronic characteristics of useful nuclides*

Element	Group	Electronic Configuration	Ionic Radius, pm	E° V^a
K	IA^b	[Ar]4s	144	−2.90
Rb	IA	[Kr]5s	158	−2.99
Ca	IIA	$[Ar]4s^2$	106	−2.87
Sr	IIA	$[Kr]5s^2$	127	−2.89
Y	IIIB	$[Kr]4d^15s^2$	88	—
Ga	IIIA	$[Ar]3d^{10}4s^24p$	62	−0.35
In	IIIA	$[Kr]4d^{10}5s^25p$	81	−0.34
Tl	IIIA	$[Xe]4f^{14}5d^{10}6s^26p$	95	+0.72 (Tl^{3+})
Sn	IVA	$[Kr]4d^{10}5s^25p^2$	—	—
N	VA	$[He]2s^22p^3$	—	—
P	VA	$[Ne]3s^23p^3$	212 (P^{3-})	—
Cr	VIB	$[Ar]3d^54s^1$	—	−0.74 (Cr^{3+})
Mo	VIB	$[Kr]4d^55s^1$	—	—
O	VIA	$[He]2s^22p^4$	—	—
S	VIA	$[Ne]3s^23p^4$	170 (S^{2-})	—
Tc	VIIB	$[Kr]4d^55s^2$	—	—
Re	VIIB	$[Xe]5d^56s^2$	—	—
F	VIIA	$[He]2s^22p^5$	119 (F^-)	—
I	VIIA	$[Kr]4d^{10}5s^25p^5$	206	—
Co	VIII	$[Ar]3d^74s^2$	—	—
Kr	VIIIA	[Kr]	—	—
Xe	VIIIA	[Xe]	—	—
Sm	Lanthanide	$[Xe]4f^66s^2$	110	−2.30

^{a}for M^{n+} + ne = M(s).
^{b}Chemical abstract service version.
Source: Complied from 6, 72.

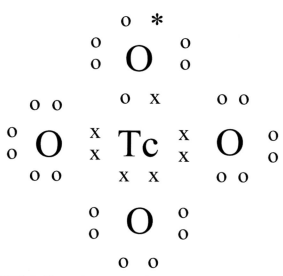

FIGURE 7.1. Electronic structure of TcO_4^- showing the valence electrons of Tc (x), oxygen (o), and an electron contributed by a water proton (*).

Group VIIB elements have a several oxidation states from +1 to +7. This is due to a partially filled d shell (Table 7.2). None of the d shell electrons are paired. Each of the 5 d, along with the 2 s electrons, can be easily removed. Technetium, the most important nuclide in nuclear medicine and a group member, forms a compound pertechnetate ($Tc^{7+}O_4^-$). This represents the most stable oxidation state for Tc (Fig. 7.1). Lastly, the lanthanides have oxidation states of +2, +3, and +4, with the +3 state particularly stable. Filled (14) or half-filled (7) f shells cannot explain these different states, particularly the +3 for Sm.

2.2 Oxidation-Reduction Reactions

In an oxidation-reduction (redox) reaction, one compound is oxidized and the other is reduced. Why are we interested in these reactions? ^{99m}Tc, ^{131}I, and ^{123}I, which are used widely in nuclear medicine, need to undergo redox reactions to label useful compounds. Oxidation of an atom is the loss of electrons and reduction is gain of electrons. Let us examine the reduction of pertechnetate to technetate, TcO_2, using the stannous ion (Sn^{2+}) (Eq. 2.2.1 to 2.2.6). In this case, the oxidation state of Tc is reduced from +7 to +4 (gaining electrons, less positive), and that of Sn is increased from +2 to +4. Tc gains three electrons and Sn loses two electrons. Three atoms of tin and two of Tc are needed so that the gain in electrons to Tc is equal to the loss from Sn (Eq. 2.2.3). Lastly charges (Eq. 2.2.4) and mass (Eq. 2.2.5) also need to be balanced to give the final expression (Eq. 2.2.6).

$$Tc^{7+}O_4^- + Sn^{2+} + H^+$$
$$\rightarrow Tc^{4+}O_2 + Sn^{4+} + H_2O \quad [2.2.1]$$
$$TcO_4^- + 3e \rightarrow TcO_2 \text{ and } Sn^{2+} \rightarrow Sn^{4+} + 2e \quad [2.2.2]$$
$$2\,TcO_4^- + 3\,Sn^{2+} + H^+$$
$$\rightarrow 2\,TcO_2 + 3\,Sn^{4+} + H_2O \quad [2.2.3]$$

$$2(-1) + 3(+2) + 8(+1) \rightarrow 3(+4) \quad [2.2.4]$$
$$8\,(O) + 8\,(H) \rightarrow 4\,(O) + 8\,(H) + 4\,(O) \quad [2.2.5]$$
$$2\,TcO_4^- + 3\,Sn^{2+} + 8\,H^+$$
$$\rightarrow 2\,TcO_2 + 3\,Sn^{4+} + 4\,H_2O \quad [2.2.6]$$

How does one find out which atoms will be reduced and which will be oxidized in a reaction? The ability of a compound to donate or accept electrons is measured and compared to a standard. Hydrogen's ability is used as a standard, and the energy (potential volts) required to remove its electrons is set to 0. Table 7.3 shows the potential volts for a number of redox reactions. For the reactions that are higher in the series (more positive), the atoms on the left are stronger oxidizing agents, and the atoms on the right are weaker reducing agents. For example, F_2 easily accepts its electrons and F^- gives up its electrons grudgingly. What atom could stannous ion reduce from Table 7.3? The energy difference must be positive thus the substance must have a higher E value than stannous ion (−0.14 V). For example, the reduction of ferric to ferrous iron, has a higher E value, + 0.771 V, and the difference (0.911 V) is positive. This suggests that electrons in an acid environment could be transferred from Sn^{2+} to Fe^{3+}. Similarly other compounds can act as electron acceptors for Sn^{2+}, e.g., O_2. Thus both iron and oxygen can interfere with ^{99m}Tc binding reactions by deactivating the stannous ion.

2.3 Coordination Chemistry

Why are we interested in coordination chemistry? What is it? The chemistry of chelate-metal ions interactions is important because metal ions such as ^{99m}Tc, ^{67}Ga, and ^{111}In are used widely in nuclear medicine and form chelate-metal ion complexes. Some examples of ^{99m}Tc chelates presently used are diethylenetetraaminepentaacetic acid (DTPA), 2,3 dimercaptosuccinic acid (DMSA), methylene diphosphonate (MDP), methoxyisobutyl isonitrile (Cardiolite), Ceretec, and mercaptoacetyltriglycine (MAG3). In addition, chelates are coupled to monoclonal antibodies (ProstaScint, OncoScint) and peptides (OctreoScan), allowing the binding of ^{111}In.

What is a chelate? The name comes from the Greek word for "crab's claw." The most familiar chelates are ethylenedi-

Table 7.3. *The electrochemical series*

Reaction	Potential Volts	
$F_2 + 2e \rightarrow 2F^-$	+2.87	easy to accept
$Tl^{3+} + 2e \rightarrow Tl^+$	+1.28	
$O_2 + 4H^+ + 4e \rightarrow + 2H_2O$	+1.23	
$Fe^{3+} + e \rightarrow Fe^{2+}$	+0.771	
$O_2 + 2H^+ + 2e \rightarrow + 2H_2O_2$	+0.69	
$I_2 + 2e \rightarrow 2I^-$	+0.54	
$I_3^- + 2e \rightarrow 3I^-$	+0.54	
$H_2 + e \rightarrow 2H^+$	+0.00	
$Sn^{2+} \rightarrow Sn^{4+} + 2e$ (in 1 N HCl)	−0.14	
$Sn^{2+} + 2e \rightarrow Sn$	−0.14	
$Fe^{2+} + 2e \rightarrow Fe$	−0.44	
$Li^+ + e \rightarrow Li$	−3.03	hard to accept (easy to donate)

aminetetraacetic acid (EDTA) and DTPA (Fig. 7.2**A**). Chelates are molecules that bind to metal ions in a noncovalent manner. Coordinate covalent, ionic, and other bonds hold the chelate tightly to the positively charged metal ion. Noncovalent is an important characteristic for chelates because that means compounding, i.e., radiopharmaceutical, preparation is relatively simple. The number of liganding atoms bound to a metal ion can vary from one to eight and is called coordination number (CN). The most common and important CN are 4, 5, and 6. When CN = 6, the configuration is called octahedral because of its solid geometry. An example is shown in Fig. 7.3.

There are a wide variety of ligand types. If the ligand has only one liganding atom that donates electrons to the metal ion, these ligands are called monodentate (one-toothed) ligands, e.g., NH_3, F^-, CN^-, and H_2O. Ligands that have two liganding atoms each that donate electrons to the metal ion are called bidentate ligands and so on. Presently monodentate ligands; Cardiolite, bidentate ligands; oxine (used to label blood cells with ^{111}In), and tridentate ligands; and Choletec and Hepatolite (hepatobiliary agents, Fig. 7.3) are used. Newer ^{99m}Tc ligands are multidentate, e.g., MAG3. These are more stable because the ^{99m}Tc completely surrounded by liganding groups with less chance for the complex to break down.

The tightness the metal chelate binding is defined by a parameter, stability constant (K). K is determined by the equation, [M-chelate]/[M][chelate] where [M-chelate] is the equilibrium concentration of the metal chelate complex, and [M] and [chelate] are the concentrations of unbound metal and chelate, respectively. A useful function of these constants is to compare the binding of different metal ions to the same chelate or different chelates to the same metal ion. For example, Fe^{3+}-EDTA has a very high stability (K = 25.1) whereas Ca^{2+}-EDTA has a relatively low stability (K = 10.7) (1). Although the binding

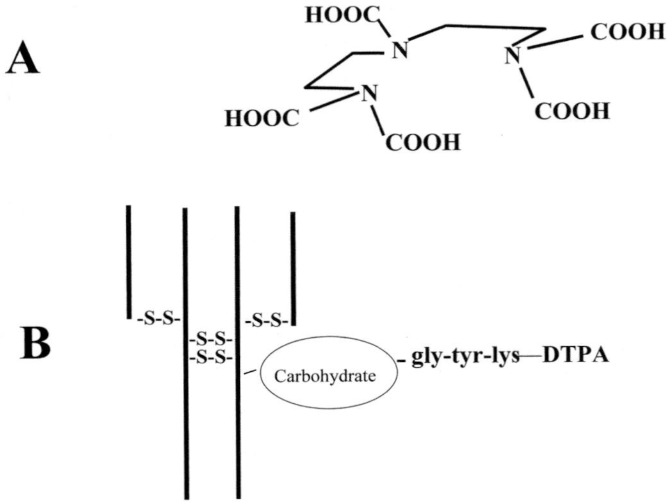

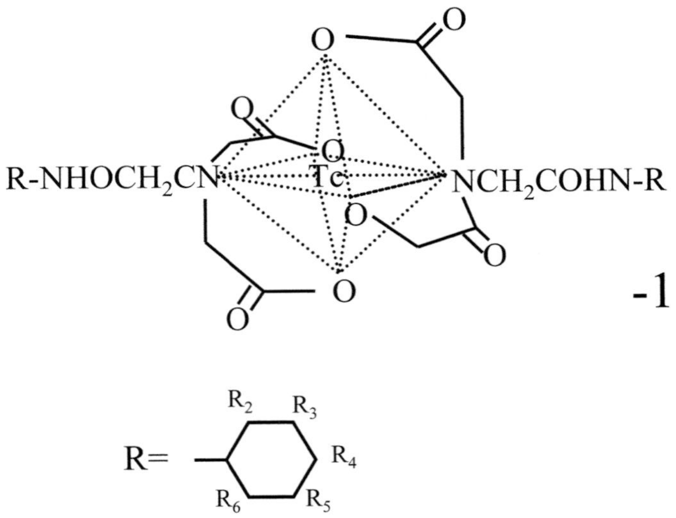

FIGURE 7.3. Proposed general octahedral dimeric structure of ^{99m}Tc iminodiacetate compounds. For Choletec, the R_2, R_4, and R_6 = CH_3 and R_5 = Br. For Hepatolite, R_2 and R_6 = $CH(CH_3)_2$ (33).

stability of the complex is important, equally important is the kinetic stability. A high K does not provide information on how fast the binding or dissociation of the metal ion occurs. Even though a complex has a low affinity constant it may be slow to form or dissociate. Nuclear medicine practitioners are interested in complexes that have high kinetic and metabolic stability. Two to 4 hours of *in vivo* stability is usually sufficient for most nuclear medicine studies. However, [90]Y- or ^{111}In-labeled monoclonal antibodies, which may take days to localize in tumors, require chelates with greater kinetic and metabolic stability.

3.0 RADIONUCLEIDE PRODUCTION METHODS

Radionuclides are produced by three methods: generators, cyclotrons, and nuclear reactors. A generator is a portable system and can easily be transported from the production site to nuclear medicine laboratories for radionuclides use. Cyclotrons and reactors are used to produce nuclides, and then the nuclides are transported across the country.

3.1 Generators

Generators have three basic characteristics. These are (a) a long-lived parent and a short-lived daughter, (b) a daughter with clinically useful nuclear characteristics, and (c) a daughter and parent that are chemically different to facilitate the separation of parent and daughter.

[99m]Tc is a unique element that finds its greatest use as the principle isotope for routine studies in nuclear medicine. It is unique in several respects:

FIGURE 7.2. Structure of **(A)** diethylenetetraaminepentaacetic acid (DTPA) with methylene groups omitted for clarity and **(B)** general structure for coupling a DTPA to antibodies, ProstaScint or OncoScint via the carbohydrate and spacer moiety (47.50).

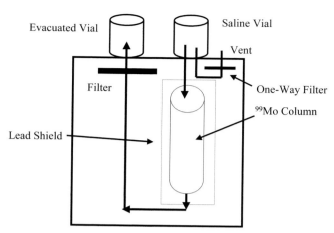

Evacuated Vial   Saline Vial

Vent

Filter

One-Way Filter

^{99}Mo Column

Lead Shield

FIGURE 7.4. Schematic illustration of a typical dry ^{99}Mo/^{99m}Tc generator.

1. It has $T_{1/2}$ of 6 hours, which minimizes the patient's absorbed radiation dose.
2. It emits a single gamma photon of 140 keV, an energy efficiently detected by state-of-the-art gamma cameras.
3. Its transition metal chemistry allows this nuclide to be incorporated into a wide variety of compounds.
4. It is the radioactive decay product (daughter) of a much longer lived radioisotope, ^{99}Mo (67 hours). It therefore can be obtained on a daily basis for up to a week.

The ^{99m}Tc generator system is simple (Fig. 7.4). It consists of a small column of powered alumina (Al_2O_3), which adsorbs the ^{99}Mo as the molybdate anion, ^{99}MoO$_4^{2-}$. The column is placed in a lead shield and is fitted with tubing to allow sterile saline to pass through the column to elute ^{99m}TcO$_4^-$. In the dry-column method, a new vial of saline is place at one end of the column and an evacuated vial at the other end each time the generator is eluted.

3.2 Cyclotron

In a cyclotron, positively charged ions are accelerated by a negatively charged alternating field in two D's (hollow metal structure in the shape of a D) and are used to bombard a target nucleus changing some of the atoms in the target to a new nuclide. Then the new nuclide is purified from the target. Basic elements of a cyclotron beside the D are a high vacuum source, usually a few 10^{-6} mtorr ($\sim 2 \times 10^{-11}$ psi); an ion source in the center; a magnetic field perpendicular to the plane of the D's; a device to measure the beam current; a quadrapole magnet to focus the beam at the target; a shutter to stop the beam; and a bending magnet to direct the beam to target.

To start, the electric field in the gap between the two D's (placed back to back) is set up to accelerate the positively charged ion, p+. The p+ then enters the D. The ion follows the curvature of the D because of the perpendicular magnetic field. The p+ emerges from the D and at a later time the field switches polarity. The charged particle is again accelerated in the gap. This process continues, accelerating the p+ every time it passes

through the gap. The frequency alternates just in time to catch the ion as it enters the gap of the Ds. The time of transit of the particle in the D is independent of the radius. This is important because it is difficult to change the frequency of the electric field if the time of transit did indeed change.

Linear accelerators are also used to produce radionuclides. This instrument operates similarly to a cyclotron. It consists of a long tube containing a number of cylindrical metal tubes (similar to the Ds) with increasing length and under a high vacuum. Ions start at one end and the target is at the other. The potential on the metal tube alternates so that the p+ is accelerated in the gap between these tubes and just drifts or stays at its initial velocity inside the tube. These so-called drift tubes must be successively longer to accommodate the increase in velocity while the frequency is fixed. The advantage of a linear accelerator is that it is simpler to operate. It does not require a magnet. The size of a linear accelerator is one of the constraints.

In the bombardment reaction, there are a number of options including the bombarding particle (protons, deuterons, or alpha particles) and the target material (Table 7.4). To determine which is best, a number of factors are considered. One is the efficiency of the reaction. The accelerated particles are positive and the nucleus is positive and the energy needed to overcome this barrier is the Q-value. There is a probability function that determines the ability of a particle of a particular energy to interact with the nucleus. If the probability is higher, then there is a greater chance that the particle will interact the nucleus. This parameter is called cross section, σ, and the units are in barns (barns = 10^{-24} cm^2). The more interaction there is with a larger σ, the easier it is to smash the atoms. Next is the cost of the target. A target that has low natural abundance usually must be enriched, adding to the cost of the product radionuclide. The contaminants that are produced are also important. These can increase the absorbed dose resulting from the radionuclide and may degrade the image if they emit high-energy photons. Table 7.4 shows different production methods for ^{123}I and the containments and their characteristics for each process.

3.3 Reactors

In a reactor, atoms undergo fission (splitting), and neutrons and heat are produced. Fuel rods contain fissile or fissionable materials, ^{235}U or ^{239}Pu. These materials spontaneously fission and break up into two fragments of about equal size. The basic fission (n, f) reaction is:

$$^{235}U \rightarrow X + Y + \text{2-3 n}_f (1.5 \text{ MeV}) + 200 \text{ MeV (heat)}$$

These high-energy neutrons, n_f, do not have a high probability to cause further fission. Less energetic neutrons do have a high probability of interaction and heavy water (D_2O), graphite, or beryllium are used as moderators to slow down these neutrons. This process gives rise to thermal neutrons = n_t (0.025 eV).

The n_t have a high probability ($\sigma = 580$ barns) of interacting with the uranium and other atoms to produce useful nuclear medicine radionuclides. There are two types of reactions with n_t that produce useful nuclides in reactors. In the fission (n, f) reaction, heavy elements with atomic number greater than 92

Table 7.4. *Bombardment reaction parameters for common nuclides*

Target % Natural Abundance	Reaction	Beam Energy (MeV)	Contaminants
0.2	$^{18}O(p,n)^{18}F$	10–17	
19	$^{68}Zn(p,2n)^{67}Ga$	20	$^{66}Ga < 0.02\%$, $^{65}Zn < 0.2\%$
24	$^{112}Cd(p,2n)^{111}In$	12–22	^{114m}In & $^{65}Zn < 0.08\%$
29.5	$^{203}Tl(p,3n)^{201}Pb \rightarrow {}^{201}Tl$ EC.9.4 h	35–45	$^{200}Tl < 1\%$, $^{202}Tl < 1\%$, $^{203}Pb < 2.5\%$
4.6[a]	$^{124}Te(p,2n)^{123}I$		$^{124}I < 5\%$, $^{24}Na < 0.5\%$
100	$^{127}I(p,5n)^{123}Xe \rightarrow {}^{123}I$ β^+, 2.1 h	40 70	$^{125}I < 2.9\%$, $^{121}Te < 0.1\%$
0.096	$^{124}Xe(p,2n)^{123}Cs \rightarrow {}^{123}Xe\uparrow$ β^+, 8 m	20	

Note: ^{124}I ($T_{1/2}$ = 4.2 d) γ = 511 (50%), 605 (67%); ^{24}Na (15 h) γ = 1,400 (100%), 2,700 (100%); ^{125}I (60 d) γ = 35 (7%); ^{66}Ga (9 h) γ = 511 (114%), 1,039 (57%); ^{65}Zn (245 d) γ = 1,115 (49%), ^{200}Tl (26 h) γ = 368 (88%), 1,210 (35%); ^{202}Tl (12 d) γ = 439 (95%); ^{203}Pb (52 h) γ = 279 (81%); ^{114m}In (50 d) γ = 192 (17%), γ energies in keV and abundance in the parenthesis.
[a]95% enrichment.
Source: Complied from 14, 25, 43, 73, and 74.

are irradiated and yield a number of different radionuclides. For example

$$_{92}U^{235} + n_t \rightarrow {}_{92}U^{236} \rightarrow {}_{53}I^{131} + {}_{39}Y^{102} + 3\,{}_0n^1$$
$$\rightarrow {}_{42}Mo^{99} + {}_{50}Sn^{135} + 2\,{}_0n^1$$

Because many radionuclides are produced at once, isolation of the required radionuclide becomes difficult. The nuclides are produced in a carrier-free or no carrier added (NCA) state, so high specific activity radionuclides are obtained. The ^{235}U that does not undergo fission is recoverable and reusable (reprocessing).

For neutron capture (n, γ), the target nucleus is placed inside the reactor so that the n_t flux irradiates the target. The target captures a neutron and gives off a γ. This means that an element is changed to a different isotope. An example is $^{98}Mo(n, \gamma) \rightarrow {}^{99}Mo$ (67 hours). Other examples are ^{50}Cr (n, γ) $\rightarrow {}^{51}Cr$ (28 days), $^{152}Sm(n, \gamma) \rightarrow {}^{153}Sm$ (1.9 days), $^{124}Xe(n, \gamma) \rightarrow {}^{125}Xe$ (17 hours) $\rightarrow {}^{125}I$ (60 days), $^{88}Sr(n, \gamma) \rightarrow {}^{89}Sr$ (50 days), $^{130}Te(n, \gamma) \rightarrow {}^{131}Te$ (25 minutes) $\rightarrow {}^{131}I$ (8 days).

4.0 TECHNETIUM CHEMISTRY

Two Tc isotopes are used in nuclear medicine, ^{99m}Tc, $T_{1/2}$ = 6 hours, (γ = 140 keV (85%) and ^{99}Tc, $T_{1/2}$ = 2.12 × 10^5 years, β^-_{max} = 292 keV. All the isotopes of Tc are radioactive. Technetium means "artificial" in Greek and it does not exist in the Earth's crust. The aqueous chemistry of Tc is dominated by the oxidizing power of stable, soluble pertechnetate, $Tc^{+7}O_4^-$. To bind a chelate, the Tc in TcO_4^- must be reduced from $Tc^{7+} \rightarrow Tc^{(1-6)+}$. The most commonly used reducing agent in commercial kits is Sn^{2+}. Specific oxidation states can be achieved by adjusting conditions, e.g., concentration of Sn^{2+} or pH, which can increase or decrease the reducing power of the Sn^{2+} ion. However, working with tin presents a number of problems. Sn^{2+} is very unstable because of hydrolysis, which

allows the formation Sn colloids or polymeric species. Other electron acceptors such as dissolved O_2 or other metal ions, Fe^{3+} or Cu^{2+}, in solution can essentially deactivate the Sn^{2+} (Sec 2.2). These problems are solved by freeze-drying the kit solutions. The solutions are freshly prepared then immediately frozen. Also the kits are packed under N_2 to exclude O_2.

The generator eluent contains a significant quantity of ^{99}Tc, the daughter of both ^{99}Mo and ^{99m}Tc, which is an additional labeling problem (Sec 3.1). The percentage of ^{99}Tc increases as a function of time so that at 6 hours postelution it constitutes approximately 40% of the total technetium. The ^{99}Tc competes with the ^{99m}Tc for binding to chelate sites. To overcome this problem, either the chelate concentration is increased or a fresh generator eluent is used to minimize the presence of ^{99}Tc.

Table 7.5 lists the proposed structures and oxidation states of a wide variety of Tc complexes used in nuclear medicine. The chelated, reduced Tc has a wide range of CNs, oxidation states, and geometries. Tc(V) is very common and is stabilized by Tc = O, as an axial ligand. Even if the Tc is chelated, the Tc can be reoxidized to TcO_4^- or reduced further to TcO_2 (hydrolyzed reduced Tc). Newer chelates have been designed with sulfur and

Table 7.5. *Technetium complexes*

Complex	Coordination Number	Oxidation State
Tc(Cardiolite)$^+$	6	I
TcCl$_2$((EtOH)$_2$PPh)$_2$	6	II
Tc(Choletec)$_2^-$	6	III
Tc(Myoview)$^+$	6	V
Tc(Neurolite)^0	5	V
Tc(Ceretec)^0	5	V
Tc(MAG$_3$)$^-$	5	V
[Tc(MDP)$^-$(OH)]$_n$	6	?
TcO$_4^-$	4	VII

Note: Et, C_2H_5; Ph, C_6H_5; MDP, methylene diphosphonate; MAG3, mercaptoacetyltriglycine.
Source: Complied from 2, 3, 4, 17, 24, 33, and 75.

Table 7.6. *Iodine substitution methods*

Methods	Advantages	Disadvantages
Iodine monochloride	High but variable (50%–80%) yield	Low specific activity and very harsh conditions
Chloramine T	High efficiency >90%, high SA Can be easily controlled	Highly reactive
Iodogen	High yield 70%–80%, high SA Can be easily controlled	Slow
Peroxidases	Mildest, good yield, high SA	Poor for 10–100 mCi

Source: 25.

phosphorous ligands, and these may be more stable to reoxidation or reduction than the commonly used nitrogen-based or oxygen-based chelates (Choletec and MDP). The brain agent, Neurolite [Tc(V)-oxo-N,N′-1,2-ethylenediylbis-l-cysteine, diethyl ester], and the renal agent, MAG3 are sulfur-based chelates (23). Myoview [Tc(V)O$_2$\{1,2-bis(bis(ethoxyethyl)phosphino)ethane\}$_2$]$^+$ is a phosphorus-based chelate (4).

5.0 CHEMISTRY OF IODINE

Iodine has three useful radionuclides ^{131}I, ^{123}I, and ^{125}I. These radionuclides are dispensed as the iodide and this form can be oxidized in solution to give I$_2$, which is volatile. The volatility of this form can be minimized by using alkaline pH solutions or adding reducing agents. Iodine chemistry is well understood and has been extensively applied to label several compounds of biologic interest. To label compounds with iodine, two general procedures are used: substitution and exchange reactions. Iodine can be substituted for hydrogen in an aromatic ring of a molecule of interest because the C-H bond is weaker than the C-I bond. To proceed with the reaction, radioactive iodine must be oxidized to I$^+$ to give an electrophilic reactive species. There are a variety of oxidizing agents, which are detailed with their strengths and weaknesses in Table 7.6. In exchange reactions, compounds are initially labeled with nonradioactive iodine and then exchanged with radioactive iodine atoms. This is an equilibrium reaction, which may be slow and require energy to achieve it. This procedure yields low specific activity compounds.

6.0 CHEMISTRY OF OTHER COMMONLY USED NUCLIDES

^{67}Ga, ^{111}In, ^{90}Y, ^{201}Tl, ^{18}F, ^{153}Sm, and ^{32}P are used in a variety of diagnostic and therapeutic applications. ^{67}Ga, ^{111}In, ^{153}Sm, and ^{90}Y are stable in aqueous environment in the +3 oxidation state (5,6). However, each of these nuclides has a tendency to hydrolyze at a wide pH range. These therefore require weak chelates to prevent precipitation and to promote transchelation to higher affinity chelates. For example, ^{67}Ga is available as the weak citrate chelate but ^{67}Ga binds almost immediately to the iron-binding site on transferrin *in vivo* (7). ^{111}In, ^{153}Sm, and ^{90}Y are available as the chloride or acetate salts. These radionuclides are then complexed with high-affinity multidentate chelates (e.g., DTPA) that in some cases are conjugated to antibodies or peptides (Table 7.7) (5,8). ^{111}In complexed with 8-hydroxyquinoline (oxine) is also used to label blood cells. Thallium is stable in both the +1 and +3 oxidation, and the +1 state is soluble at physiologic pH. ^{201}Tl is used as the chloride salt and is incorporated into the myocardium as a K$^+$ mimic. (See Section 8.1.) Fluorine is a very chemically reactive atom (6). It can replace hydrogen in organic compounds and its small size introduces less conformational changes than other halogens. This is why ^{18}F introduced into glucose as 2-deoxy-2-^{18}F-fluoro-D-glucose (FDG) is handled similarly by the glucose carrier system GLUT-1 (9). The most common physiologic form of phosphorus is phosphate. The sodium and potassium phosphates are soluble but most transition metal phosphate complexes are not. The ^{32}P radiopharmaceuticals take advantage of both of these properties.

Table 7.7. *Quality control procedure for non-^{99m}Tc radiopharmaceuticals*

Radiopharmaceutical	Media	Solvent System	R$_f$ Complex	Impurities
^{111}In-ProstaScint	ITLC-SG	0.9% saline	0.0	1.0
^{111}In-OncoScint	ITLC-SG	0.9% saline	0.0	1.0
^{111}In-MyoScint	ITLC-SG	0.5 M citrate buffer, pH 5	0.0	1.0
^{111}In-OcteoScan	Sep-pak −(CH$_2$)$_{18}$	Water [free-^{111}In], methanol [OctreoScan]		
^{90}Y-Zevalin	ITLC-SG	0.9% saline	0.0	1.0
^{131}I-NP-59	TLC-silica gel	Chloroform/acetone (95/5)	0.4	0.0
^{18}F-FDG	TLC-SG 60	Methanol/NH$_4$OH (9:1)	0.83	0.38
	HPLC column	Acetonitrile/water (95/5)	4.1 mL (elution volume)	

Source: 8, 22, 47, 50, 52, 66, 73, and 76.

7.0 QUALITY CONTROL

Purity testing of all commercially available compounds is performed by the manufacturers. However, radiopharmaceuticals manufactured in nuclear medicine laboratories are subject to QC analysis at each local site.

7.1 Chromatography Techniques for Determination of Chemical and Radiochemical Purity

Three types of chromatographic procedures are commonly used: thin layer chromatography (TLC), paper chromatography, and high pressure liquid chromatography (HPLC). Generally a chromatography system consists of a stationery solid matrix and mobile phase solvent that either ascends or descends through the matrix. The sample to be analyzed partitions between the solid and mobile phase. Both solvents and matrices are varied to change the partition (movement) of the sample (Table 7.8). For TLC, adsorbents are layered on a plate made of plastic, Mylar, or glass and dried. For HPLC, adsorbents are packed in either a glass or stainless steel tube called a column. Adsorbents can be ion exchange, normal phase, reverse phase, or surface adsorbents (silica, aluminum oxide, or charcoal). The most common media for chromatographic analysis of radiopharmaceuticals is instant thin layer chromatograph-silica gel (ITLC-SG). Here a glass fiber mesh is impregnated with silica gel and is available in sheets (Table 7.8). In normal phase HPLC, the adsorbent matrix is polar and the solvent pumped through is nonpolar. In such a system, the polar components (contaminants) of the sample are retained on the column and the sample in the nonpolar solvent passes through the column. A more polar solvent (usually water-based) pumped through later, elutes the polar contaminants. For

reverse phase, the matrix is opposite, nonpolar, e.g., $-(CH_2)_{18}$ and $-(CH_2)_9$. Here, the starting solvent is polar and the hydrophobic contaminants are retained on the column. These would then be eluted with a nonpolar solvent miscible with water, e.g., acetonitrile. HPLC is now used routinely for both the purification and purity determination of radiopharmaceuticals.

7.2 Quality Control of ^{99m}Tc Compounds

Most of the ^{99m}Tc radiopharmaceutical solutions should be clear and colorless. However ^{99m}Tc-Ceretec should be blue and the two particulate solutions, ^{99m}Tc-sulfur colloid and ^{99m}Tc-macroaggreagated albumin (MAA), should be cloudy. A common contaminant in ^{99m}Tc solutions is ^{99}Mo, which may have been eluted from the generator. The presence of ^{99}Mo is determined by placing the vial of ^{99m}Tc eluent in a 6-mm thick lead container and then measuring this container in a dose calibrator. Then the ^{99m}Tc activity is measured without the lead container. The ^{99}Mo activity must be less than 0.15 μCi ^{99}Mo/mCi ^{99m}Tc to be administered to a patient. This ratio can be determined because the low energy, 140 keV ^{99m}Tc photon is reduced a million-fold by the lead whereas the higher energy ^{99}Mo photons, 366, 740, and 778 keV, are reduced only by approximately ten-fold.

For radiochemical purity of the common clinical ^{99m}Tc compounds, a variety of TLC procedures are used (Table 7.8). ITLC is preferred because it requires a short (minutes) time for completion. In contrast, Whatman no 1 paper takes approximately 1 hour. In general, approximately 5 μL of the radiopharmaceutical is spotted on a TLC strip and allowed to dry, and the strip is placed in a chromatographic chamber containing the developing solvent. The solvent is allowed to flow to just below the upper end of the strip. The radioactivity is measured as a function of

Table 7.8. *Quality control procedure for ^{99m}Tc radiopharmaceuticals*

Radiopharmaceutical	Media	Solvent System	R$_f$ Complex	Impurities
DTPA, MDP, GH	ITLC-SG	Acetone	0.0	1.0
	ITLC-SG	Water, 0.9% saline	1.0	0.0
IDA analogues	ITLC-SA	20% saline	0.0	1.0
	ITLC-SG	Water	1.0	0.0
Ceretec	ITLC-SG	Methyl ethyl ketone	1.0	0.0
	ITLC-SG	0.9% saline	0.0	1.0
	Whatman No 1	H$_2$O:acetonitrile (1:1)	1.0	0.0
AcuTect	ITLC-SG	Saturated saline	0.0	1.0
	ITLC-SG	Water	1.0	0.0
NeoTect	ITLC-SG	Saturated saline	<0.75	>0.75
	ITLC-SG	Methanol:1 M NH$_4$ (1:1)	<0.4	>0.4
CEA-Scan	ITLC-SG	Acetone	0.0	1.0
Cardiolite	Al Oxide	>95% ethanol	1.0	0.0
Neurolite	Silica gel IB-F	Ethyl acetate	1.0	0.0
Myoview	ITLC-SG	Acetone:dichloromethane (35:65)	0.3–0.75	1.0 and 0.0
MAG3	Sep-pak $-(CH_2)_{18}$ column	0.001 N HCl [^{99m}TcO$_4^-$], ethanol:saline (1:1) [MAG3], column [^{99m}TcO$_2$]		
DMSA	ITLC-SA	Acetone	0.0	1.0

Note: ITLC-SG, Instant thin layer chromatography-silica gel; MAG3, mercaptoacetyl triglycine; SA, silicic acid.
Source: 3, 25, 30, and 55.

the distance it has migrated from the point of application. The R_f, defined the ratio of the radioactivity migration distance to solvent distance, is a compound characteristic. The major impurities, $^{99m}TcO_2$ and $^{99m}TcO_4^-$, usually have R_f values of 0.0 and 1.0, respectively, in the different solvent systems and media (Table 7.8). The percentage of radiopharmaceutical purity is determined by subtracting the percentages of each impurity from 100%.

The presence of Al^{3+} in the $^{99m}TcO_4^-$ eluent, which comes from the alumina absorbent, is also determined. Aluminum interferes with the preparation of sulfur colloid by forming a gelatinous precipitate. Its presence is tested by comparing a drop of a standard Al^{3+} solution, 10 μg/mL, on a paper impregnated with a dye, alizarin. The dye turns pink when complexed with Al^{3+}. A drop of $^{99m}TcO_4^-$ eluent is tested similarly. The color of the drop is compared to this standard to estimate the Al^{3+} concentration.

7.3 Quality Control of Iodine and Other Compounds

There are very few non-^{99m}Tc radiopharmaceuticals that are manufactured in the local radiopharmacy or in a nuclear medicine department. Most of these radiopharmaceuticals are radionuclide salts that are not compounded. Examples are $Na^{123}I$, $^{201}TlCl$, ^{67}Gacitrate, $Na^{32}P$, or $Na^{131}I$. ^{131}I meta-iodobenzylguanidine (MIBG), ^{131}I-Bexxar, ^{32}P-chromic phosphate colloid, and ^{90}Y colloids are prepared at a central facility and shipped throughout the country. There is one ^{131}I-labeled compound, ^{131}I-6β iodomethyl-19-norcholesterol (NP-59), that is not Food and Drug Administration (FDA)-approved and requires QC for its use (Table 7.7). ^{111}In-labeled radiopharmaceuticals are commonly compounded and the QC procedures are shown in Table 7.7. For ^{111}In-WBC or ^{111}In-platelets, the nonbound ^{111}In is removed so that it is unnecessary to test for how much is labeled. However, ^{111}In-WBC viability is determined by the trypan blue exclusion test. Dead white blood cells (WBCs) appear blue under the microscope. Platelet viability is measured by chemically stimulating platelets to aggregate, which is a normal function. Y-90 Zevalin is compounded locally and is subjected to QC analysis (Table 7.7). ^{18}Fl is cyclotron produced (Table 7.4), and the synthesis of FDG is automated because of the isotope's short $T_{1/2}$ (Table 7.7). The presence of impurities is determined by TLC and HPLC analysis (Table 7.8).

8.0 SPECIFIC RADIOPHARMACEUTICALS

8.1 Cardiac Agents

There are four agents that are used to assess myocardial perfusion: $^{201}TlCl$, ^{82}Rb, ^{99m}Tc-sesta 2-methoxyisobutyl isonitrile (MIBI) (^{99m}Tc-Cardiolite), and ^{99m}Tc-Myoview. A fifth one, MyoScint, may be used to diagnose and evaluate acute myocarditis (10) or cardiomyopathies (11). The four radiopharmaceuticals are widely used in nuclear medicine laboratories in the management and diagnosis of coronary artery disease (12).

After injection of $^{201}TlCl$, the radioactivity is rapidly taken up by the normal heart and other muscle tissue, achieving a heart concentration of 4% to 5% of the total injected dose (ID) in 10 to 30 minutes (13). The dose range is 37 to 148 MBq. In the heart, ^{201}Tl has a slow washout ($T_{1/2}$ = 4 to 7 hours), and this provides a long imaging window (~2 hours). In a resting study, 90% of the radioactivity in the blood disappears within 20 minutes, and after exercise only 1.5 minutes is required. Imaging can usually begin at 10- to 15-minutes postinjection (PI). The nuclide also concentrates in the kidney (3%) (14). Thallium uptake into cells is mediated, in part, by the Na^+-K^+-ATPase. Thallous ion has a similar crystal radius (Table 7.2) and hydrated radii to K^+. Intracellular K^+ levels are maintained in myocardial and other cells by this energy requiring membrane bound enzyme. Under identical conditions, in a Na^+-K^+-ATPase model system, thallium uptake was inhibited only 10% to 13% by ouabain, which blocked 50% to 75% of K^+ influx (15).

^{82}Rb, a generator-produced positron emitter [parent, ^{82}Sr ($T_{1/2}$ = 25 d)], can be used similarly to ^{201}Tl (16). This generator is commercially available. The usual dose is 2.22 GBq. Because of its short $T_{1/2}$, it is infused directly into the patient from the generator (Table 7.4). The blood $T_{1/2}$ is also very short, 2.2 minutes, whereas the myocardial $T_{1/2}$ is 6 hours. The heart incorporates 2% to 3% ID, which is intermediate between ^{201}Tl- and ^{99m}Tc-based agents. It is incorporated as a K^+ analogue (Table 7.2).

^{99m}Tc-Cardiolite is a cationic complex (Table 7.5) (17). Both the methyl and butyl groups impart a significant hydrophobic character to the molecule (see mechanism described later). It is prepared from $Cu(1+)(MIBI)_4BF_4$ complex by ligand exchange. ^{99m}Tc is added to the vial, boiled for 10 minutes, and cooled for 15 minutes. The maximum added activity is 5.55 GBq. The preparation is stable for 6 hours after reconstitution. In the QC procedure, one drop of ethanol is spotted with two drops of Cardiolite (Table 7.8). The dose range is 370 to 925 MBq. The blood $T_{1/2}$ is short (~4.3 min) (18). At 5 minutes PI, the myocardium contains 1.2% of ID with a $T_{1/2}$ = 6 hours (3 hours effective). In the rest study, the liver takes up 20% of ID (5 minutes) but has a short $T_{1/2}$ = 30 minutes (rest). Heart activity is comparable to liver at 1 hour and greater at 2 hour PI. In the exercise study, much more Cardiolite is diverted to the heart than the liver. The major excretory pathways are gastrointestinal (GI) tract and urinary tract. Radioactivity in the transverse colon can interfere with images of the apex of the heart.

Myoview has the similar cationic, 1+, characteristic as Cardiolite and the terminal ethoxy groups that also impart hydrophobic character (4). ^{99m}Tc (8.88 GBq maximum) is added to the kit and incubated for 15 minutes at room temperature (RT). The preparation remains within acceptable QC for 8 hours. The dose range is identical to Cardiolite. In normal humans at rest, 1.8% of ID is in heart and 7.5% in liver (5-minutes PI) (19). The liver activity decreases to 0.9% and heart to 1% at 120 minutes. Similar to Cardiolite, there is faster washout through the liver with exercise; heart activity is greater than the liver at 1-hour PI. More activity is excreted through the bladder (40%) than through the GI tract (26%).

The localization mechanism has been studied mainly with Cardiolite, but the structural similarity with Myoview suggests a similar mechanism. Myocardial cells have a high concentration of intracellular K^+ yielding a -90 mV resting potential (20). Compounds that collapse or depolarize these membranes cause lower Cardiolite uptake and enhance washout in model systems (21). Conversely, compounds that hyperpolarize the membrane enhance uptake. This suggests that Cardiolite is drawn to the myocardium by ionic attraction, intercalates in the membrane, and is transported into the cell. Thus the ^{99m}Tc-based agents are able to measure cardiac viability because maintaining the negative membrane potential is an energy-requiring process and dependent on cell viability.

MyoScint is an antimyosin, Fab-fragment antibody with an attached DTPA chelate, which permits labeling with ^{111}In (22). Myosin is the major intracellular muscle protein and is only exposed when the cell is damaged. This protein is soluble in high salt concentration and is not found in the blood after cell rupture. ^{111}In-MyoScint is prepared by adding the contents of vial 1 with 0.5 mg of antibody to vial 2 containing 0.2 M citrate buffer pH 5 and mixing. Then 92.5 MBq of ^{111}InCl$_3$ is added to vial 2 and incubated for at least 10 minutes at RT, and QC analysis is performed (Table 7.7). The citrate buffer rapidly forms a weak ^{111}In complex and allows transchelation to the DTPA-antibody conjugate. Just before injection, the solution is passed through a 0.22 μm filter for sterilization.

8.2 Agents Used for Brain Imaging

Brain perfusion agents have been shown to be clinically effective in the diagnosis of acute ischemic stroke. These agents can detect epilepsy foci during seizures and can establish the diagnosis of Alzheimer's disease (23). ^{111}In-DTPA is use to determine the distribution of cerebrospinal fluid (CSF) and more specifically whether there is a leak of CSF in the central nervous system (5).

There are two agents that are approved for brain perfusion imaging, ^{99m}Tc-Neurolite and ^{99m}Tc-(V)-oxo-d,l-hexamethyl-propyleneamineoxime (HMPAO or exametazime) (^{99m}Tc-Cere-tec). Neurolite is supplied in two vials (2). Vial 1 contains Neurolite, which is stored under acid conditions (~pH 3) to prevent deterioration, and vial 2 contains a neutral pH buffer. The compound is prepared by adding ^{99m}Tc (3.7 GBq maximum) to vial 2. Three ml of saline is injected into vial 1 and mixed, and immediately (less than 30 seconds) 1 mL is withdrawn and added to vial 2. The solution in vial 2 is incubated for 30 minutes at RT, and QC is performed (Table 7.8). The remaining material in vial 1 is discarded. The compound is stable for 6 hours after preparation. The usual dose is 1.1 GBq. Neurolite has high brain uptake, 4.8% to 6.4% ID, at 5 minutes. Blood clearance is rapid with only 5% ID present at 1-hour PI. Excretion is also rapid with 50% ID in urine at 2 hours and 74% at 24 hours. Only 12% of the radioactivity is excreted in feces at 48 hours.

^{99m}Tc-Ceretec has a new formulation that increases its stability in the vial (24). The kit now contains a three-vial system. First, 0.5 mL is removed from vial 1 (methylene blue) and injected in vial 2, which contains phosphate buffer at pH of approximately 7 (must be used within 30 minutes). Next ^{99m}Tc is added to the Ceretec-containing vial 3, followed by the contents of vial 2. The preparation is usable up to 4 hours after reconstitution. The formulation has a relatively low concentra-

tion of tin (8 μg) and therefore fresh generator eluent (within 2 hours) should be used to minimize the presence of oxidants and ^{99}Tc (Table 7.8). Concentration of ^{99m}Tc in the preparation is limited to 2.0 MBq in 5 mL, because autoradiolysis accelerates decomposition. If free ^{99m}Tc in the preparation is greater than 15%, then parotid and choroid plexus uptake will be very high. The usual dose is 1.1 GBq. Brain uptake is 3.5% to 7% ID, which peaks at 1 minute; approximately 15% of brain activity is lost within 2 minutes. There is a slow washout from the brain with $T_{1/2} = 30$ to 71 hours. The liver and kidney uptake is high. Radioactivity is excreted mainly through the GI tract (30% to 50% ID at 48 hours) and kidneys (40% ID at 48 hours).

These compounds pass through the blood–brain barrier via the endothelial cell membrane because of their high lipophilicity (25). Once in the extracellular space, these compounds are converted to hydrophilic species that are incapable of rapid back diffusion. Neurolite is converted to this species by a variety of esterases. These enzymes catabolize the diethyl ester to the ethylendiylbis-cysteine mono ethyl ester (ECM) or the ethylenediylbis-cysteine diacid (EC). Data from cell culture show that uptake is dependent on the brain cell types (26). Brain cells with membrane-bound esterase activity had reduced cell uptake. Without this esterase activity, cells incorporated Neurolite and mostly retained it. This may explain the variation in tumor uptake. A similar esterase enzyme is present in the blood and causes the conversion of the parent compound to ECM or EC so that the ^{99m}Tc is rapidly excreted in the urine.

In contrast to Neurolite, Ceretec is converted to the hydrophilic species by either reduction or oxidation of the ^{99m}Tc. Oxidation of the ^{99m}Tc-Ceretec complex is accelerated by PO$_4$, excess Sn^{2+}, and autoradiolysis (27). Phosphate is presumably the factor that stimulates oxidation in the blood. Similar to Neurolite, Ceretec can be converted by redox activity both extracellularly and intracellularly (28). Because redox function may vary locally, the brain tumor uptake can increase or decrease.

The QC for ^{111}In-DTPA is performed by the manufacturer and the dose is 55.5 MBq. After intrathecal injection, the ^{111}In-DTPA moves with the flow of CSF up the spinal canal to the head (5). The radiopharmaceutical migrates to the basal cisterns, over the top of the cerebral cortex to the parasagittal space, and finally to the arachnoid villi where it exits. The ^{111}In-DTPA does not normally enter the ventricle space. The complex then appears in the blood and is rapidly excreted by the kidneys (65% ID in the first 24 hours).

8.3 Venous Clot Detection

For more than 25 years, the development of radiopharmaceuticals for the detection of thrombi and emboli by hot-spot imaging has been an elusive goal of radiopharmaceutical chemists (29). Recent research efforts to develop a clot-binding agent have targeted the GPIIb/IIIa receptor expressed on activated platelets. Fibrinogen present in the blood adheres to this receptor and forms a bridge between platelets. Fibrinogen binds via two Arg-Gly-Asp (RGD) sequences on the α and γ chains. There are 40,000 to 80,000 GPIIb/IIIa molecules at the platelet's surface and activation brings additional molecules to the surface. Recently AcuTect, a peptide dimer that contains a RGD mimetic sequence [S-aminopropyl-L-cysteine (apc)-GD], has been approved for deep vein thrombus (DVT) detection (30). The apc-GD sequence contains a cyclize methionine group, which confers rigidity to the conformation and a D-amino acid, which makes the apc-RG sequence more resistant to proteolysis. To label AcuTect with ^{99m}Tc, radioactivity (less than 1.85 GBq and less than 1.85 GBq/mL) is added to the kit and heated at 100°C for 15 minutes. After cooling (10 to 15 minutes), the AcuTect is ready for injection and QC (Table 7.8). The usual radiopharmaceutical dose is 740 to 925 MBq containing 75 to 100 μg of peptide. Whole body images demonstrated rapid renal and GI excretion (31). After a day, 80% ID is excreted in the kidneys and only 10% via the GI tract (30). The blood $T_{1/2}$ is short, 2 hours, and soft tissue uptake was minimal. At 4-hours PI, 40% of the radioactivity in blood and 45% of radioactivity in urine is still bound to AcuTect. AcuTect has a high RGD specificity and affinity. The concentration of AcuTect to achieve a 50% inhibition of fibrinogen (IC_{50}) binding to platelets was 6.8 nM. In contrast, the IC_{50} was 12,900 nM for vitronectin binding to platelets.

8.4 Lung Imaging

The most frequent lung imaging procedure in nuclear medicine is the ventilation/perfusion (V/Q) study for the detection of pulmonary embolism (32). The V/Q study consists of comparing the lung ventilation image and perfusion image. The objective is to determine a mismatch between these two images that indicates a perfusion deficit in a fully ventilated lung segment. ^{99m}Tc-MAA is used to determine regional lung perfusion (16). The aggregates with the average size, 10 to 40 μm (range 15 to 90 μm), lodge in the lung capillary bed (capillary diameter, 8.2 ± 1.5 μm). A dose of 74 to 185 MBq are injected into the antecubital vein, which flows from the heart directly into the pulmonary circulation. On the first pass 90% of the MAA is extracted, and it provides an image of regional blood flow. The

wide range of particle size means that larger vessels may be blocked. However, the number of vessels actually compromised is a small fraction (1%) of the total. If 1×10^6 particles are injected, there is a 125-fold safety factor. Administration of 125×10^6 particles would raise pulmonary arterial pressure about 10% to 20%.

MAA is prepared by adding ^{99m}TcO$_4$ and incubating for various times depending on the kit manufacturer (16). MAA is usually stored at 4°C before and after addition of ^{99m}Tc. The particles will settle with time so it is important to mix the vial at all stages. A large gauge (18 to 21 G) needle is recommended for injection to prevent clumping of the particles in the needle hub. The minimum particle number to give good uniformity of the image is 60,000 with a maximum of 1,200,000. MAA is removed from lung following fragmentation into smaller particles by mechanical movement within the arterioles. These particles are incorporated into the liver and are proteolytically digested. Finally the ^{99m}TcO$_4^-$ is released into blood and excreted through the kidney (30% to 75% ID) and the GI tract. The T_B (biologic $T_{1/2}$) in the lung is approximately 5.6 hours.

^{133}Xe, ^{81m}Kr, and ^{99m}Tc-DTPA aerosol are used for the ventilation portion of this study (25). Probably the most commonly used is reactor-produced ^{133}Xe that has a long $T_{1/2}$ and can easily be kept on hand (Table 7.9). However, it has a low energy and low abundance γ photon, which degrades image quality. The patient is asked to inhale ^{133}Xe gas (370 to 555 MBq) mixed with air in a closed system, to hold the breath to establish an equilibrium, and finally to exhale into a collecting bag. Images are taken during this sequence. Because ^{81m}Kr is also a noble gas, the ventilation study is performed similarly to the ^{133}Xe procedure. However, because of the short $T_{1/2}$ only the initial wash in phase can be performed but it allows repeat images (Table 7.9). This isotope also has better γ photons with higher abundance. The disadvantage is that the generator for ^{81m}Kr is only useful for 1 day because the parent, ^{81}Rb, has a short $T_{1/2} = 4.6$ hours.

Table 7.9. *Nuclear characteristics of non-^{99m}Tc radionuclides*

Nuclide	$T_{1/2}$	Principle Radiations (γ = keV, β = MeV, Augér = keV)
^{14}C	5730 y	$\beta_{max} = 0.156$, $\beta_{mean} = 0.045$
^{18}F	110 m	$\gamma = 511$ (194%)^a
^{32}P	14 d	$\beta_{max} = 1.7$, $\beta_{mean} = 0.695$
^{51}Cr	27.7 d	$\gamma = 320$ (9%)
^{57}Co	270 d	$\gamma = 14$ (9%), 122 (86%), 136 (11%)
^{67}Ga	3.25 d	$\gamma = 93$ (38%), 184 (24%), 300 (22%)
^{81m}Kr	13 s	$\gamma = 190$ (67%)
^{82}Rb	75 s	$\gamma = 511$ (190%)
^{89}Sr	50 d	$\beta_{max} = 1.46$, $\beta_{mean} = 0.58$
^{90}Y	2.7 d	$\beta_{max} = 2.3$, $\beta_{mean} = 0.94$
^{111}In	2.8 d	$\gamma = 171$ (91%), 245 (94%), Augér = 0.6, 2.4, 19.2, 25.4, & 22.3
^{123}I	13.3 hr	$\gamma = 159$ (83%)
^{125}I	60 d	$\gamma = 35$ (7%)
^{131}I	8 d	$\gamma = 364$ (82%), 637 (7%), 723 (2%); $\beta_{max} = 0.606$, $\beta_{mean} = 0.19$
^{133}Xe	5.3 d	$\gamma = 81$ (37%)
^{153}Sm	1.9 d	$\gamma = 103$ (28%), $\beta_{max} = 0.81$, $\beta_{mean} = 0.24$
^{201}Tl	3.08 d	$\gamma = 69$, 80 (95%), 135 (2.5%), 167 (10%)

^{a}Number in the parentheses is gamma photon abundance, the number of photons emitted per disintegration.
Source: Complied from 25, 77.

Alternatively ^{99m}Tc-DTPA is made into an aerosol by a nebulizer (25). About 1.1 to 1.48 GBq ^{99m}Tc-DTPA is injected into the nebulizer and air or oxygen is forced through it to produce the aerosol droplets (0.5 to 3 μm). A small aliquot of ethanol may be added to the nebulizer, which will enhance droplet formation. The patient inhales the aerosol using a closed system. The aerosol is exhaled into a filter to trap the activity and minimize external contamination. About 10% of the activity is deposited in the lungs, which allows imaging. Lung deposition is dependent on the particle size with the small particles being deposited peripherally and larger ones more centrally. Imaging is performed similarly to the two other agents.

8.5 Hepatobiliary Agents

These agents are mainly used to diagnose bile duct obstructions and alterations in liver function. These agents are extracted by the liver and excreted unmodified through the common bile duct, gallbladder, and finally into the small intestine. The iminodiacetate (HIDA) derivatives were developed in the 1970s (16). These have a dimeric octahedral structure (Fig. 7.3). For preparation, ^{99m}Tc activity is added to the kit vial and incubated for a period of time at RT as directed by the manufacturer. The usual dose is 74 to 111 MBq, which is increased to 185 to 259 MBq in patients with high bilirubin values. The blood clearance is normally rapid, with only 17% ID remaining at 10-minutes PI. This clearance is slowed in jaundiced patients, to 34% or more at 10 minutes. The liver is visualized at 5-minutes PI with maximum uptake at 11 minutes. Gallbladder is visualized at 10- to 15-minutes PI, and intestinal activity appears at 30- to 60-minutes PI. Urinary excretion is low, 1% of ID at 3-hours PI in patients with normal bilirubin, but excretion is increased by three-fold in jaundiced patients.

The various HIDA derivatives consist of modifications at different positions on the benzyl ring (Fig. 7.3). These profoundly influenced the biodistribution and hepatic throughput. These molecules are actively taken up by an anionic binding carrier protein on the hepatocyte membrane (33). A variety of organic anions, e.g., bilirubin, are taken up by this carrier. Excretion into bile canaliculi is rate limiting. HIDA has a low affinity for albumin but changes at benzyl positions 3, 4, or 5 can enhance binding (Fig. 7.3). Binding to albumin reduces renal excretion but also limits liver uptake. This binding is particularly related to the length of the added -(CH$_2$)$_n$ chain and suggests that HIDA derivatives bind to albumin in a manner similar to fatty acids. In diabetics, in whom fatty acid concentration is increased, HIDA binding to albumin could be reduced and renal excretion increased. In hemolytic jaundice, the bilirubin is albumin bound. In obstructive jaundice, the bilirubin is conjugated with glucuronic acid to make it more soluble and nonprotein bound. It is readily excreted in the urine and can compete with HIDA compounds for liver entry.

8.6 Renal Agents

Table 7.10 shows the available agents and their general uses. Among them, ^{99m}Tc-DTPA is very easy to prepare (16). It requires only the addition of ^{99m}TcO$_4^-$ to the DTPA vial and a short incubation (Table 7.10). QC is standard (Table 7.8), and the dose is 259 to 555 MBq. Although the exact structure of the ^{99m}Tc-DTPA is unknown, it is likely to be similar to In-DTPA (34). Thus ^{99m}Tc is bound tightly to this small chelate so that the total size is approximately 400 Da, and the complex is uncharged. This allows ^{99m}Tc-DTPA to pass easily through the glomerular pores whose average diameter is 8 nm (Albumin = 68,000 Da, 6-nm size). There is little or no protein or red blood cell (RBC) binding of ^{99m}Tc-DTPA that would slow or prevent filtration and invalidate glomerular filtration rate (GFR) measurements (Table 7.11). ^{99m}Tc-DTPA has the slowest blood clearance because of low extraction ratio. Because of this low extraction ratio, imaging is difficult in patients with poor renal function.

The agent ^{99m}Tc-MAG3 requires heating after the addition of pertechnetate to the kit vial (Table 7.10). The QC uses a reverse phase C$_{18}$ minicolumn (Table 7.8), and the dose injected is 185 to 370 MBq (3). In contrast to DTPA, ^{99m}Tc-MAG3 has a much shorter blood T$_{1/2}$ and a high extraction ratio (Table 7.11). This radiopharmaceutical is actively transported into the tubules by a mechanism that is specific for organic acids, e.g., probenecid or para-aminohippurate. Fig. 7.5 shows the structure

Table 7.10. *Characteristics of the different renal radiopharmaceuticals*

Radiopharmaceutical	Mechanism	Uses	Preparation
DTPA	Glomerular filtration	Renal perfusion Collecting system GFR	1–2 min + ^{99m}Tc Good for 6–12 hr
MAG3	Low GF (20%) Active tubular secretion Inferior for anatomy	Renal function Tubular dysfunction	10 min at 100°C Good for 6 hr
DMSA	Low GF	Renal parenchyma only	10–15 min + ^{99m}Tc
	Tubular secretion	Cortical binding	Good for 4 hr
GH	Glomerular filtration Cortical binding Tubular secretion	Renal perfusion (L) Collecting system (E) ATN	15 min + ^{99m}Tc store at 2–8°C Good for 6 hr

Note: ATN, Acute tubular necrosis; E, early; GF, glomerular filtration; GFR, glomerular filtration rate; L, late.
Source: 3, 25, 35, 78, and 79.

Table 7.11. *Biological properties of renal agents*

Property	DTPA	GH	DMSA	Hippuran	MAG3
Blood T$_{1/2}$ (min)	70	27	54	30	3,17
Plasma clearance (mL/min)	100–120	—	—	600–700	340
Protein binding (%)	4–15	50–75	75–90	50–70	80–90
RBC (%)	~0	—	—	15	~5
ID renal uptake (%)					
1 hr	4	9	24	87	53
6 hr	2	12	41	—	—
Urinary excretion (%)					
2 hr	50	50	16	70	70
6 hr	73	64	26	—	90
24 hr	96	71	37	—	—
Extraction ratio (%)	20	—	4–5	88	80

Note: DMSA, 2,3-dimercaptosuccinic acid; DTPA, diethylenetetraaminepentaacetic acid; GH, ^{99m}Tc glucoheptonate; Hippuran, iodohippuranic acid; MAG3, mercaptoacetyltriglycine.
Source: 3, 16, 25, and 80.

of MAG3. In the peritubular capillaries, these compounds pass through the basement membrane, are actively transported into the tubular cells, and then secreted into the tubule lumen. MAG3 is not reabsorbed because the pK$_a$ of its carboxylic acid (3.4) is much lower than the pH of urine. Urine pH is usually 5.0 but could be as low as 4.

The third agent, ^{99m}Tc-DMSA, is prepared by the simple addition of radioactivity to the kit vial (35). The ID ranges from 74 to 185 MBq. QC is performed using ITLC-SG (Table 7.8). However there are activity (less than 1480 MBq) and volume (1 to 4 mL) restrictions to minimize autoradiolysis. The precise localization mechanism of DMSA is unknown and the structure has not been well characterized. It is known that probenecid does not reduce uptake (16). There is high protein binding that reduces urinary excretion (Table 7.11). Uptake in the renal parenchyma is high only after 1 hour and continues to increase. Animals studies suggest that more than 96% of this activity is cortex-bound.

^{99m}Te-glucoheptonate (GH) is also easily prepared and needs only a short incubation with ^{99m}Tc (Table 7.10). Although GH has the advantage of rapid blood disappearance, it is an intermediate agent to assess either parenchymal binding or tubule function. It has less cortical uptake compared to DMSA and less

urinary excretion than MAG3 (Table 7.11). Thus it is only used when the other agents are unavailable.

8.7 Bone-Seeking Agents

Bone-imaging radiopharmaceuticals provide useful diagnostic information for a wide variety of neoplastic and nonneoplastic osseous disorders (36). Bone imaging in the ^{99m}Tc era was initiated with ^{99m}Tc-labeled polyphosphate, in which each phosphate group is connected by an ester (oxygen) bond (16). This eventually led to the development of diphosphonates in which the oxygen (ester) is replaced by carbon (phosphonate). This change reduced diphosphonate hydrolyses by blood esterases. Presently, MDP is the most commonly used bone radiopharmaceutical. The preparation is simple with the addition of ^{99m}Tc to the kit vial and short 10- to 15-minute incubation. The preparation is usable for 6 hours after ^{99m}Tc addition, and QC is done using ITLC-SG (Table 7.8). The usual ID is 740 to 925 MBq. Biodistribution is rapid with radioactivity deposited in the bone (45% to 55%), urine (56% to 59%), and blood (3% to 5%) at 3-hours PI. The ^{99m}Tc-MDP is loosely protein bound, with little RBC binding, which allows rapid renal excretion. Imaging is usually performed at 2-hours PI. Because renal function is important for ^{99m}Tc-MDP clearance, factors that impair renal function, such as chemotherapeutic drugs, degrade image quality (37).

Bone-seeking agents are taken up at the sites of active bone formation (38). Increased vascularity in bone lesions alone does not account for this increased uptake. To form bone, Ca^{2+} and PO$_4^-$ ions are actively transported into osteoblast-produced vesicles. Amorphous (noncrystalline) calcium phosphate (ACP) forms first in the vesicle, and then there is a transition to hydroxyapatite (HA). Eventually the vesicles rupture and the formed ACP or HA migrates to the bone organic matrix. It is likely that the ^{99m}Tc-MDP is actively transported into these vesicles as the intact complex similar to the phosphate compounds. Diphosphonates are thought to bind to Ca^{2+} in the bone crystal via one set of oxygens of the phosphonate groups.

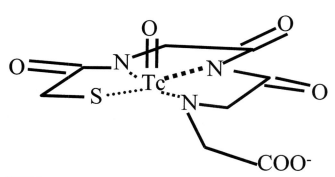

FIGURE 7.5. Proposed structure of MAG3 (3).

The ^{99m}Tc is bound to the other set of oxygens. As the ACP is formed, the ^{99m}Tc-MDP would be bound to the growing crystalline material. In addition, ^{99m}Tc-diphosphonates bind preferentially to ACP compared to HA, and there is more ACP in growing bone compared to mature bone.

8.8 Thyroid Treatment Agents

^{131}NaI is the preferred agent for the treatment of hyperthyroidism and thyroid cancer (25). ^{131}I is concentrated in the thyroid and a few other tissues. It also has a high energy β particle that is effective in destroying thyroid tissue (Table 7.9). Patients are treated with a specific amount of ^{131}I activity, based on MBq/g of tissue, the 24-hour uptake value [which is determined after an oral diagnostic dose (185 kBq)], and the mass of the gland. The mass of the thyroid is estimated by palpation and thyroid imaging with ^{99m}TcO$_4$$^-$. It is assumed that the biologic $T_{1/2}$ is constant for all patients. Each 37 kBq deposited gives 5.2 cGy to the thyroid (39). For example, a 60-g thyroid and 2.96 MBq/g with 75% uptake would give 18,720 cGy to the thyroid.

In addition to the thyroid, iodine is absorbed in salivary glands, gastric mucosa, and GI tract and then taken up by thyroid. The major pathways for excretion are kidney (90%), salivary glands, exhaled air, and sweat (25). As a result when a patient is going home after a high-dose therapy, a variety of common household items, e.g., silverware, cups, towels, bathtub, and soap, get contaminated with ^{131}I. ^{131}I passes through the placenta and is concentrated in the fetal thyroid. Fetal thyroid uptake starts at tenth week of gestation. ^{131}I is also concentrated in breast and excreted in the breast milk. The concentration in milk can be as high as 33-fold greater than the plasma value.

8.9 Inflammation and Infection Detection Agents

For many years ^{67}Ga citrate was used for the detection of both acute and chronic abscesses and inflammatory processes. However, with the development of ^{111}In-oxine or ^{99m}Tc-HMPAO labeled white blood cells (^{111}In- or ^{99m}Tc-WBC), ^{67}Ga is now used mostly to identify chronic inflammatory processes (40). Since its introduction in 1977, ^{111}In-WBC has been successfully used to identify sites of acute inflammation and infection (41). In more recent years, ^{99m}Tc-WBC has replaced ^{111}In-WBC as the inflammation detection agent of choice (42).

^{67}Ga is a cyclotron-produced radionuclide and is used as described in Section 6.0. The preparation contains a high concentration of citrate, 0.12 M (43). The adult dose for imaging chronic infections is 148 to 222 MBq. The radioactivity is excreted very slowly (13). In humans, the radioactivity is initially distributed in the liver (5% ID), spleen (1%), kidney (2%), and skeleton (24%). This remains constant as a function of time. However during this time, a large amount of activity appears in the bowel, which tends to obscure lesions. ^{67}Ga is delivered to the inflammation site by transferrin, where it is translocated to abscess-related proteins (44).

^{111}In-WBC and ^{99m}Tc-WBC are both prepared similarly. Briefly approximately 50 mL of the patients' blood is removed,

the white cell fraction is isolated from the plasma, and this fraction is incubated for approximately 15 minutes with ^{111}In-oxine or ^{99m}Tc-Ceretec at RT (5,24). The plasma is added back to cells, and the cells centrifuged to remove nonbound activity. The cells are resuspended in plasma and finally injected into the patient. ^{99m}Tc-Ceretec is prepared as described in Section 8.2 except the methylene blue is not added to the preparation (24). The dose is 555 to 740 MBq. ^{111}In-oxine is prepared by adding oxine in ethanol to 37 to 185 MBq of ^{111}In in acetate buffer, and the resultant ^{111}In-oxine is extracted in a nonmiscible organic solvent (5). The organic layer is removed, solvent is evaporated, and the resultant complex dissolved in ethanol and added to the cells. The hydrophobic ^{111}In-oxine complex can intercalate into the cell's membrane and eventually pass into the cytoplasm. Then the ^{111}In is translocated to cytosolic proteins with higher ^{111}In affinity. The patient dose is limited to 18.5 MBq because of the high-absorbed dose to the spleen (0.8 cGy/MBq). The blood cells should be injected within 4 hours of removal from the patient; otherwise the ability of the WBC to migrate to inflammatory foci may be compromised. Labeled cells are actively incorporated into an inflammatory or infection site as a normal part of the infection fighting process (44).

8.10 Oncologic Agents

During the past 10 years or so there has been an explosive growth of agents for diagnosis and treatment of cancer. These agents include monoclonal antibodies; ProstaScint, OncoScint, and CEA-Scan peptides; OctreoScan and NeoTect and small molecules; Miraluma, FDG, MetaStron, and Quadramet.

8.10.1 Diagnostic Agents

^{67}Ga citrate still remains useful for imaging of a number of soft tissue tumors (45) such as Hodgkin's disease, non-Hodgkin's lymphoma, lung cancer, hepatoma, and melanoma. The usual dose is 296 to 370 MBq. The biodistribution has been described (Sec 8.9). The mechanism of ^{67}Ga tumor localization has been studied extensively (7). Data suggest that ^{67}Ga binds to transferrin and is incorporated in tumors by the upregulation of transferrin receptors (TFRs) on cancer cells. It is thought that iron requirements for DNA synthesis, in rapidly growing tumors, necessitate TFR upregulation.

^{111}In-ProstaScint can be used to determine the extent of prostate cancer once the initial diagnosis is made and can be used to detect the extent of recurrence in the face of rising PSA after a radical prostatectomy (46). ProstaScint is a whole IgG$_1$, murine monoclonal antibody that was generated from human prostatic cell line. It is directed against the cytosolic portion of prostate specific membrane antigen. Presently, it is believed that only broken or leaky cells incorporate ProstaScint. The antibody, containing a DTPA chelate, is coupled specifically via a spacer molecule to the carbohydrate portion of the IgG (Fig. 7.2**B**). DTPA binding to the carbohydrate moiety prevents the DTPA from coupling to amino acids required for antigen binding and preserves the antibody's affinity. Furthermore, the spacer molecule positions the DTPA away from the antibody minimizing any steric hindrance by the antibody that could reduce the ^{111}In-

DTPA affinity. For preparation, 185 to 222 MBq of ^{111}InCl$_3$ is added to vial 1 containing 0.5 M acetate buffer (47). The acetate buffer raises the solution pH ($\sim$4 to 6) and forms a weak ^{111}In complex that prevents hydrolysis and possible precipitation at this pH. The contents of vial 1 is added to vial 2 containing 0.5 mg of antibody and then incubated for 30 minutes at ambient temperature. In this process, the ^{111}In is transchelated to the DTPA-antibody conjugate. Adding the ^{111}InCl$_3$ directly to the protein without the acetate buffer could hydrolyze the ^{111}In and the HCl could denature the antibody. The antibody solution is filtered (0.22 μm) before injection to remove any aggregates formed. The dose is 167 to 204 MBq, and the preparation is stable for 8 hours after reconstitution. For QC analysis, the sample is mixed with DTPA, incubated for a few minutes, spotted, and chromatographed (Table 7.7). The prevalence of adverse reactions is minimal (4% to 5%), and the incidence of human anti-mouse antibody (HAMA) is low (8%). For the second infusion, however, 19% of patients were documented to have had an elevated HAMA titer. ^{111}In-Prostascint has a T$_{1/2}$ = 67 hours in the blood and is excreted very slowly. Only 10% of the ID appears in the urine after 72-hours PI. Ninety-six hours PI or longer is usually required for the background to be sufficiently reduced for imaging. The ^{111}In is taken up by the liver, spleen, bone marrow, and kidneys.

^{111}In-OncoScint is used to image recurrence for colorectal and ovarian cancer (48,49). The monoclonal antibody is directed against a tumor-associated antigen, TAG-72 (50). TAG-72, a high molecular weight, mucin-like glycoprotein is expressed on 94% of colorectal adenocarcinomas and 100% of ovarian cancers tested. The ^{111}In-binding site is a DTPA covalently coupled to the antibody in a manner similar to ProstaScint (Fig. 7.2**B**). ^{111}In-OncoScint is prepared in a manner identical to ProstaScint, using the two-vial system. Injections and QC procedures are also performed similarly (Table 7.7). ^{111}In-OncoScint has a long blood T$_{1/2}$ and slow urinary excretion. Radioactivity accumulates mainly in the liver, spleen, and bone marrow. Liver radioactivity can obscure liver metastases. Lesser but definite activity is seen in the kidney, bowel, bladder, male genitalia, and breast nipples. OncoScint is now approved for repeat use. Patients should be tested for HAMA before a second injection. A HAMA of less than 50 ng/mL would not interfere with the study. Adverse reactions were 2% to 4%, and only 0.7% of the patients experienced serious (anaphylaxis) reactions.

^{99m}Tc-CEA-Scan is used to determine both extent and location of colorectal cancer in initial staging or recurrence (51). This agent, a Fab$'$, is specific for carcinoembryonic antigen (CEA). CEA is expressed extracellularly on a variety of cancer cells, including GI tract cancer. CEA-Scan can bind circulating (shed) CEA (greater than 250 ng/mL). ^{99m}Tc binds to sulfhydryl groups present on the antibody. ^{99m}TcO$_4^-$ (740 to 1,110 MBq) is added to the vial containing CEA-Scan and incubated for 30 minutes at RT. The solution is filtered (0.22 μm) and is injected within 4 hours of preparation. Both HAMA and adverse reactions were reported to have a low (less than 1%) frequency. ^{99m}Tc-CEA-Scan has a rapid blood clearance (T$_{1/2}$ = 1 hour). The urinary excretion is 28% of the ID within 24 hours. The radioactivity is incorporated in the kidneys, liver, spleen, and

bone marrow. The liver activity recedes as a function of time and allows the detection of important liver metastases.

OctreoScan is a somatostatin analog, octreotide, modified by adding DTPA (Fig. 7.2**A**) to Phe^1 for ^{111}In binding (52). Somatostatin is an endogenous growth hormone inhibitor and acts by binding to somatostatin receptors (SSTRs) expressed on a variety of cell types. ^{111}In-OctreoScan is used to localize a wide variety of neuroendocrine tumors because of SSTR upregulation on these cancer cells (53,54). It is prepared by adding 111 MBq of ^{111}InCl$_3$ (contains 3.5 μg FeCl$_3$ to minimize nonspecific indium binding) to a vial containing 10 μg of pentetreotide and incubating 30 minutes at RT (52). A Sep-pak C$_{18}$, minicolumn is used to perform QC (Table 7.7). The adult diagnostic dose is 185 to 222 MBq and is usable for 6 hours after preparation. ^{111}In-OctreoScan is rapidly cleared from the blood and excreted into the urine, 25% of the ID after 3 hours and 50% after 6 hours. Hepatobiliary excretion is minor, less than 2% appears in the feces after 72 hours.

Because ^{111}In-OctreoScan detects both small cell lung cancer (SCLC) and non-small cell lung cancer (nSCLC) with high sensitivity (53), a ^{99m}Tc-based somatostatin analogue, NeoTect, was developed to provide an noninvasive method to differentiate malignant versus benign pulmonary masses detected by computed tomography (CT) or chest x-ray film. ^{99m}Tc-NeoTect is easy to prepare (55). It has short blood clearance (t$_\alpha$ = 4 minutes) and imaging is performed at 2- to 4-hours PI. The agent localizes in the kidneys, spleen, bladder, thyroid, and bone. At 4-hours PI, 70% to 80% of the circulating radioactivity in blood and 61% of excreted radioactivity in urine is still bound to NeoTect. Protein binding is 10% to 20%. NeoTect has high affinity (K$_D$ $\sim$2 nM) for SSTR subtypes 2, 3, and 5. Even though the presence of SSTR has not yet been demonstrated on nSCLC cells, it is argued that the high sensitivity in this disease is due to lymphocyte cells or other SSTR-containing cells at the tumor site (56). A small (4% to 5%) fraction of patients experienced adverse reactions to NeoTect.

^{99m}Te-Miraluma (Cardiolite) is used to detect malignant breast lesions as an adjunct to mammography and to avoid repeated biopsies (57). Little activity, approximately 1% ID, is taken up by the lesions but the uptake in normal breast tissue is even lower.

FDG is approved for detection of tumors in lung, colorectal, and head and neck cancer and melanoma and lymphoma (58). Despite the very short T$_{1/2}$ of ^{18}F (Table 7.9) and the fact that it is cyclotron-produced, this compound is available throughout the USA. The usual dose is 370 MBq. There is rapid decline of FDG in blood (59). At 10-minutes PI, only approximately 15% of the initial value remains in the blood with a T$_{1/2}$ = 0.2 to 0.3 minute. FDG is distributed in the in heart (3% to 4%) and brain (2% to 3%). Radioactivity is excreted in the urine and appears in the bladder. Imaging is performed 40 to 60 minutes after injection. FDG is incorporated in tumors by GLUT-1 upregulation in actively growing cancers (9). FDG is partially metabolized by phosphorylation and trapped inside the cell. Radioactivity does not appear in either the liver or kidney because of the presence of phosphatases. These enzymes dephosphorylate FDG and allow its diffusion out of the cell.

8.10.2 Therapeutic Agents

Studies are in progress to determine if ^{111}In-OctreoScan or ^{90}Y-labeled OctreoScan derivatives can be used as therapeutic agents for the treatment of neuroendocrine tumors (60). Patients were treated with ^{111}In-OctreoScan doses ranging from 6 to 11 GBq with a slow infusion every few weeks for multiple times. The cumulative dose for patients ranged from 20 to 74 GBq. A similar procedure was used for the ^{90}Y-labeled OctreoScan derivatives. For both agents, the kidney was the dose-limiting organ, and the main toxicity appeared to be hemopoietic. The therapeutic effectiveness of high-dose ^{111}In-OctreoScan is dependent on the nuclear localization of ^{111}In-OctreoScan and short penetration range (0.02 to 10 μm) in tissue (cell diameter $\approx$ 10 μm) of the Auger electrons (Table 7.9). In contrast, ^{90}Y, a pure high-energy β emitter, has an 11-mm range in tissue and an intermediate $T_{1/2}$ (Table 7.9). This long range allows ^{90}Y-labeled peptide-bound cells, and cells in the vicinity, to be irradiated.

MetaStron ([89]SrCl) is used for the relief of intractable pain from widespread metastatic bone lesions secondary to prostate cancer, breast cancer, and other malignancies (61). [89]Sr is a pure β emitter with a maximum range of 8 mm in tissue, which provides minimal radiation of soft tissue distant from the lesions in which it concentrates (Table 7.9). The absence of a γ photon does not permit verification of bone lesion uptake. However, the lesions are continually irradiated for an extended period because of its long $T_{1/2}$. MetaStron that is not incorporated in bone is rapidly cleared from the blood into the urine (62). Urinary output is greatest in the first 2 days after injection. The skeleton takes up to 50% of the ID. The recommended dose is 148 MBq. The main limitation to ^{89}Sr and other bone-seeking therapeutic agents is bone marrow toxicity. MetaStron causes a 15% to 30% decrease in platelets and leukocytes levels from the preinjection value. However, 12 weeks are required for full recovery. Ionic strontium is incorporated into bone in a similar manner to calcium (Table 7.2) (38).

Quadramet, an ethylene diamine tetramethylene phosphonic acid (EDTMP) complex of [153]Sm^{3+}, would be used similarly as MetaStron (63). This nuclide has a shorter $T_{1/2}$, shorter (3 mm) range in tissue, and has a γ photon that allows imaging of the bone localization (Table 7.9). It is transported and stored frozen ($-20°C$) to minimize autoradiolysis. The dose is 37 MBq/kg. [153]Sm-EDTMP rapidly clears from the blood (99% in 5 hours), and an average of 35% of the dose is excreted in the urine during the first 6-hours PI. Skeletal uptake depends on the number of bony metastases but ranges from approximately 56% to 77% of the administered dose. This radiopharmaceutical, similar to MetaStron, causes myelosuppresion resulting in a platelet and WBC concentration decline of 40% to 50% of the preinjection value. Only 6% to 8% of patients experienced grade 3 and 4 toxicity for either platelet or WBC values. These counts returned to pretreatment levels by 6 to 8 weeks in all patients. This radiopharmaceutical localizes in bone by a mechanism identical to ^{99m}Tc-MDP (38).

There are two labeled antibodies, ^{131}I-Bexxar (64) and ^{90}Y-Zevalin (8), which are in clinical trials for treatment of patients with B-cell lymphoma. Zevalin was recently (Feb. 2002) approved by the FDA. The clinical trial results have been promising, with a response in 70% to 80% of the patients. Both anti-

bodies are whole murine IgG and target CD-20, a B-cell antigen that is over expressed in lymphoma. ^{90}Y-Zevalin has a DTPA-based chelate bound to antibody. The structure is similar to ProstaScint and OncoScint except the spacer and point of attachment are different (Fig. 7.2**B**). [90]Y is produced from a long-lived ($T_{1/2}$ = 28 years) ^{90}Sr generator (65). The long tissue range (see previous discussion) of ^{90}Y means that ^{90}Y-Zevalin can also irradiate nearby cells when it binds to the target cell. For the therapy, first a test dose of ^{111}In-Zevalin is given to determine if the antibody has a normal distribution (8). Normally the antibody is distributed in the liver, spleen, and bone marrow. Before ^{111}In-Zevalin is administered, Rituxan (400 to 500 mg), a nonradioactive anti-CD-20 antibody is infused. This saturates the circulating CD-20 sites in the blood and any nonspecific sites in the liver and other tissues. A week later, ^{90}Y-Zevalin is injected, which is again preceded by Rituxan infusion. The dose is 15 MBq/kg. Myelotoxicity is the main side effect. Platelets are reduced to a mean of 50,000/μL in 6 to 14 days, and absolute neutrophil count (ANC) is reduced to 1,000/μL in 8 to 14 days.

Bexxar, the ^{131}I-labeled antibody, is used similarly to Zevalin (64). [131]I is thought to irradiate normal tissues less than ^{90}Y because of the lower maximum range in tissue (2.4 mm). Myelotoxicity was similar but took longer to achieve (Table 7.9). It is labeled using the iodogen method. A test diagnostic dose (185 MBq) is used to determine the therapeutic dose. For therapeutic procedure, 450 to 475 mg of the nonradioactive antibody is infused first, and then the therapeutic dose is injected to achieve a 65 to 75 cGy total body absorbed dose. Thyroid uptake must be blocked with approximately 100 mg of I^- [Lugol's or saturated solution of KI (SSKI)]. Myelotoxicity is dose limiting. Platelets are reduced to a mean of 60,000/μL in 35 days, ANC to 1,000/μL in 46 days, and hemoglobin to 11.1 g/dL in 46 days.

8.11 Imaging Adrenal Disorders

There are two agents for adrenal imaging, [131]I-6β-iodomethyl-19-norcholesterol (NP-59) and ^{131}I-meta-iodo-benzylguanidine (MIBG) (66). NP-59 is used to image disorders of the adrenal cortex, which produces the corticosteroids. These disorders are Cushing's disease, aldosteronism, and hyperandrogenism. It is also used in primary aldosteronism to distinguish bilateral hyperplasia and adrenal adenoma and to characterize an adrenal mass as a complement to CT. Even though NP-59 has been used for over 20 years, the FDA has not yet approved it. To use this compound, the filing of an investigational new drug application to the FDA is required, and patients must sign informed consent forms approved by the institutional review board. It is prepared by first synthesizing the nonradioactive iodinated compound, and then it is labeled with ^{131}I by exchange techniques. QC is required before use (Table 7.7). The preparation is formulated using 1.6% tween-80 and 6.6% ethanol, which keep the NP-59 in solution. Occasional mild reactions have been observed mainly due to either the tween-80 or ethanol. It is stored frozen ($-20°C$) to minimize autoradiolysis. After injection, radioactivity accumulates in the liver, gallbladder, and GI tract. Liver uptake gives rise to deiodination and free I^- in the blood. The thyroid can incorporate the free I^-. Lugol's or SSKI is given at least 2 hours before NP-59 administration and blocks 90% of thyroid uptake. Imaging is started at 3- to 5-days PI because of slow blood clearance. The dose is limited to 37 MBq because of the high (~4 cGy/MBq) radiation dose to the adrenal. NP-59 is incorporated in the cortex as a cholesterol analogue. All steroid hormones are made by converting cholesterol to pregnenolone in the mitochondria. The ^{131}I is at position C-6 of the cholesterol backbone. Cortical enzymes do not modify the cholesterol backbone at this position to produce pregnenolone (67). However, the C-6 position is modified for the conversion of pregnenolone to progesterone and other corticosteroids. Thus it is likely that NP-59 is partially converted to a corticosteroid and thus enzymatically trapped in the adrenal cortex.

MIBG is used to image disorders of the adrenal medulla (66). Medulla synthesizes and secretes catecholamines—epinephrine and norepinephrine. The medulla is like a group of sympathetic nerve cells without axons. This agent is used to diagnose pheochromocytomas, neuroblastoma, and neurofibromatosis. The manufacturer uses exchange labeling to attach ^{131}I to MIBG and it requires no QC locally. It is stored frozen ($-20°C$) to minimize autoradiolysis. Imaging is started at 1- to 3-days PI because the blood $T_{1/2}$ in patients with normal renal function is 5 days. Urinary excretion is 50% of ID at 24-hours PI and only 10% of ID is metabolized into ^{131}I, iodohippuric acid, or iodobenzoic acid. The tiny (1 cm × 6 mm) normal medulla is not imaged. At 1- to 2-days PI, most radioactivity is in the bladder and liver. Heart activity (adrenergic innervation) is seen only on initial (2- to 4-hours PI) images. Liver uptake gives rise to deiodination and free I^- in the blood. The I^- could subsequently be incorporated into the thyroid. Lugol's or SSKI given before MIBG administration blocks thyroid uptake. The dose is limited to 18.5 MBq because of the high adrenal absorbed dose, 0.94 cGy/MBq. A wide variety of drugs, e.g., antihypersensives, amitriptyline and derivatives, imipramine and derivatives, sympathetic amines and cocaine, taken by patients give rise to false-negative images. Data from animal and *in vitro* experiments show that there are two mechanisms for MIBG localization. Uptake-2 is a high-capacity, low-affinity uptake with a fast ($T_{1/2}$ ~1 hour) washout. In the high-affinity, low-capacity uptake-1, MIBG follows the reuptake of norepinephrine. After transmitting the signal to next neuron, norepinephrine is actively transported back (reuptake) into the original neuron and placed back into storage vesicles.

8.12 Miscellaneous *In Vitro* and *In Vivo* Procedures

A few nonimaging procedures that are occasionally performed are described in this section. To measure RBC mass, 1 MBq of ^{51}Cr-labeled RBC (^{51}Cr-RBC) is used, and a 370-kBq dose of ^{125}I human serum albumin (HSA) is used to measure plasma volume (25). Plasma volume is usually performed to confirm the red cell mass value. In these procedures, ^{51}Cr-RBC and ^{125}I-HSA are injected, and blood samples are withdrawn at specific times PI. The RBC mass is determined from the hematocrit values, the radioactivity injected, and the radioactivity concentration in the blood. This value is compared to standard values determined from the height and weight of the patient. ^{125}I-HSA is available commercially. To label the RBCs, the blood is mixed

with acid citrate dextrose in a vial, $Na_2^{51}CrO_4$ is added and incubated 30 minutes at RT. During this time CrO_4^{2-} diffuses into RBCs and then ascorbate is added. Ascorbate reduces the CrO_4^{2-} to Cr^{3+} and locks the ^{51}Cr inside the RBCs. RBC survival measurements also use ^{51}Cr-RBC (1.85 to 3.7 MBq) (25). This procedure is an accurate indicator of low-grade RBC destruction in patients suspected of hemolytic anemia. The blood is labeled, reinjected, and withdrawn three times a week for 2 weeks, and the blood $T_{1/2}$ is compared to normal values.

The Schilling's test is used to identify patients with pernicious anemia (25). This is caused by inadequate absorption of B_{12} in the ileum. In this procedure, an 18.5 kBq capsule of ^{57}Co vitamin B_{12} is given orally, and after 1 hour, stable vitamin B_{12} is administered intramuscularly. The large excess of vitamin B_{12} exchanges with any ^{57}Co vitamin B_{12} present on transcobalamin, the blood B_{12} transport protein. Most of the radioactive ^{57}Co that has been absorbed in the small intestine is excreted into the urine. One complete 24-hour urine is collected. The percentage excretion is compared to a standard. If it is abnormal (less than 5%), the test is repeated and the capsule is given with intrinsic factor. This additional test determines if there is a deficiency of intrinsic factor, a component in the stomach that aids transintestinal tract B_{12} transport.

^{14}C-urea breath test is used to determine if the stomach has been colonized by *Helicobacter pylori* (*H. pylori*) (68). *H Pylori* is implicated in the formation of ulcers. *H. pylori* has a unique enzyme, urease, that cleaves ^{14}C-urea (37 kBq) given orally, to form ammonia and carbon dioxide. ^{14}Carbon dioxide would appear in the breath. The patient exhales into a weak alkaline solution that traps the ^{14}carbon dioxide. A suitable scintillator is added to the solution, and the mixture is measured for radioactivity.

^{111}In-labeled platelets (1.85 to 5.55 MBq) are used to determine platelet survival (69). This is used in patients with thrombocytopenia to differentiate production versus destruction disorders. Platelets are separated from the patient's blood and labeled with ^{111}In-oxine (5). The labeled platelets are injected, blood is withdrawn at various times PI, and the radioactivity measured and plotted as a function of time (69). This blood $T_{1/2}$ value is compared to normal value of 7 days. For QC, aggregation and recovery [number of platelets circulating immediately after injection (normal 50% to 60%)] are performed. Recovery indicates the percentage of damaged platelets lost immediately.

^{32}P and ^{90}Y colloids are used to perform a synovectomy during the course of rheumatoid arthritis or hemophilia, are instilled into the peritoneal cavity to treat ovarian cancer, or are infused directly into tumors to deliver high β radiation doses (Table 7.9) (70). ^{32}P-chromic phosphate colloidal ($CrPO_4$) is prepared by a precipitation technique or a reduction method. ^{32}P in the form of phosphoric acid is treated with chromic nitrate to precipitate the chromic phosphate that is heated to greater than 400°C. This material is machined to break down the particles to correct size, but the variability of the particle size is high. Alternatively, chromium is reduced in the presence of radioactive phosphoric acid and gelatin to form the colloid. Unreacted material is removed by dialysis. To prepare ^{90}Y colloid, a ^{90}YCl solution is treated with sodium silicate in water to obtain uniform suspension of ^{90}Y silicate. To prepare ^{90}Y resin particles (a cross-linked styrene divinylbezene copolymer), ionic ^{90}Y is adsorbed to a cation exchange resin with a 29 to 35 μm particle size.

^{32}P sodium phosphate is principally used in the therapy of polycythemia vera when phlebotomy alone is unable to control erythrocytosis or thrombocytosis (71). QC is performed by the manufacturer. For polycythemia vera, the dose is 1.9 to 3.7 MBq/kg of body surface (dose should not exceed 185 MBq) and the ^{32}P is given intravenously. If remission does not occur within 3 months, the dose may be increased up to 25% for retreatment. The ^{32}P is incorporated into bone and irradiates the hemopoietic tissue with the high energy β particle (Table 7.9).

REFERENCES

1. Fisher RB, Peters, DG. *Quantitative chemical analysis,* 3rd ed. Philadelphia: WB Saunders, 1968:404–448.
2. *Neurolite.* Package insert. Arlington Heights, IL: Amersham Healthcare, 1994.
3. *TechneScan MAG3.* Package insert. St. Louis: Mallinckrodt Medical, 1995.
4. *Myoview.* Package insert. Arlington Heights, IL: Amersham Healthcare, 1996.
5. Weiner RE, Thakur ML. Chemistry of Gallium and Indium radiopharmaceuticals. In: Welch M, ed. *Textbook of radiopharmaceuticals.* September 2002. West Sussex, UK: JohnWiley (*In press*).
6. Cotton FA, Wilkinson G. *Advanced inorganic chemistry,* 5th ed. New York: Interscience, 1988:123–979.
7. Weiner RE. The mechanism of ^{67}Ga localization in malignant disease. *Nucl Med Biol* 1996;23:745–751.
8. Wiseman GA, White CA, Stabin M et al. Phase I/II 90Y-Zevalin (yttrium-90 ibritumomab tiuxetan, IDEC-Y2B8) radioimmunotherapy dosimetry results in relapsed or refractory non-Hodgkin's lymphoma. *Eur J Nucl Med* 2000;27:766–777.
9. Chung J-K, Lee YJ, Kim C, et al. Mechanisms related to [^{18}F]fluorodeoxyglucose uptake of human colon cancers transplanted in nude mice. *J Nucl Med* 1999;40:339–346.
10. Narula J, Malhotra A, Yasuda T, et al. Usefulness of antimyosin antibody imaging for the detection of active rheumatic myocarditis. *Am J Cardiol* 1999;84:946–950.
11. Nanas JN, Margari ZJ, Lekakis JP, et al. Indium-111 monoclonal antimyosin cardiac scintigraphy in men with idiopathic dilated cardiomyopathy. *Am J Cardiol* 2000;85:214–220.
12. Sodee DB, Port SC, O'Donnell JK, et al. Cardiovascular system. In: Early PJ, Sodee DB, eds. *Principles and practice of nuclear medicine.* St. Louis: Mosby, 1995:370–442.
13. Weiner RE, Thakur ML. Metallic radionuclides: applications in diagnostic and therapeutic nuclear medicine, *Radiochim Acta* 1995;70/71: 273–287.
14. *Thallous chloride ^{201}Tl.* Package insert. St. Louis: Mallinckrodt, 1990.
15. Sands H, Delano ML, Camin LL, et al. Comparison of the transport of $^{42}K^+$, $^{22}Na^+$, $^{201}Tl^+$, and $[^{99m}Tc(dmpe)_2 \cdot Cl_2]^+$ using human erythrocytes. *Biochim Biophys Acta* 1985;812:665–670.
16. Kowalsky RJ, Perry JR. *Radiopharmaceuticals in nuclear medicine practice.* Norwalk, CT: Appleton & Lange, 1987:211–378.
17. *Cardiolite.* Package insert. Billerica, MA: DuPont Pharmaceuticals Co, 1998.
18. Leppo JA, DePuey EG, Johnson LL. A review of cardiac imaging with sestamibi and teboroxime. *J Nucl Med* 1991;32:2012–2022.
19. Jain D, Wackers FJT, Mattera J, et al. Biokinetics of technetium-99m-tetrofosmin: myocardial perfusion imaging agent: implications for a one-day imaging protocol. *J Nucl Med* 1993;34:1254–1259.
20. Guyton AC. *Textbook of medical physiology,* 8th ed. Philadelphia: WB Saunders, 1991:98–110.
21. Carvalho PA, Chiu ML, Kronauge JF, et al. Subcellular distribution and analysis of technetium-99m-MIBI in isolated perfused rat hearts. *J Nucl Med* 1992;33:1516–1521.
22. *MyoScint.* Package insert. Malvern, PA: Centocor, 1996.
23. Therapeutics and Technology Assessment Subcommittee of the American Academy of Neurology. Assessment of brain SPECT. *Neurology* 1996;46:278–285.
24. *Ceretec.* Package insert. Arlington Heights, IL: Amersham Healthcare, 1996.
25. Saha GP. *Fundamentals of nuclear pharmacy,* 4th ed. New York: Springer-Verlag, 1998:47–327.
26. Jacquier-Sarlin MR, Polla BS, Slosman DO. Cellular basis of ECD brain retention. *J Nucl Med* 1996;37:1694–1697.
27. Hung JC, Corlija M, Volkert WA, et al. Kinetic analysis of technetium-99m d,1-HM-PAO decomposition in aqueous media. *J Nucl Med* 1988;29:1568–1576.
28. Jacquier-Sarlin MR, Polla BS, Slosman DO. Oxido-reductive state: the major determinant for cellular retention of technetium-99m-HMPAO. *J Nucl Med* 1996;37:1413–1416.
29. Weiner RE, Thakur ML. New developments in radiolabeled blood cells. In: Sampson CS, ed. *Textbook of radiopharmacy,* 3rd ed. Reading, UK: Harwood Academic Publishers, 1999:105–123.
30. *AcuTect.* Package insert. Londonderry, NH: Diatide, 1998.
31. Taillefer R, Thérasse E, Turpin S, et al. Comparison of early and delayed scintigraphy with ^{99m}Tc-Apcitide and correlation with contrast-enhanced venography in detection of acute deep vein thrombosis. *J Nucl Med* 1999;40:2029–2035.
32. Sostman HD, Neumann RD, Gottshalk A. Evaluation of patients with suspected thromboembolism. In: Sandler MP, Coleman RE, Wackers FJT et al., eds. *Diagnostic nuclear medicine,* 3rd ed. Baltimore: Williams & Wilkins, 1995:584–611.
33. Loberg MD, Porter DW, Ryan JW. Review and current status of hepatobiliary imaging agents. In: *Radiopharmaceuticals II: Proceedings of the 2nd International Symposium on Radiopharmaceuticals.* New York: Society of Nuclear Medicine, 1979:519–543.
34. Mäcke HR, Riesen A, Ritter W. The molecular structure of indium-DTPA. *J Nucl Med* 1989;30:1235–1239.
35. *DMSA.* Package insert. Arlington Heights, IL: Amersham Healthcare, 1993.
36. Charron M, Brown ML. Primary and metastatic bone disease. In: Sandler MP, Coleman RE, Wackers FJT, et al., eds. *Diagnostic nuclear medicine,* 3rd ed. Baltimore: Williams & Wilkins, 1995:649–668.
37. Hladik WB III, Nigg LL, Rhodes BA. Drug-induced changes in the biologic distribution of radiopharmaceuticals. *Sem Nucl Med* 1982;12:184–194.
38. Spencer RP, Weiner RE, Hosain F: Bone imaging radiopharmaceuticals. In: Henkin RE, Boles MA, Dillehay GL, et al., eds. *Nuclear medicine,* 2nd ed. St. Louis: Mosby Yearbook, 1996:1125–1140.
39. Becker DV, Hurely JR. Radioiodine treatment of hyperthyroidism. In: Sandler MP, Coleman RE, Wackers FJT, et al., eds. *Diagnostic nuclear medicine,* 3rd ed. Baltimore: Williams & Wilkins, 1995:943–958.
40. Neumann RD, McAfee JG. Gallium-67 imaging in infection. In: Sandler MP, Coleman RE, Wackers FJT, et al., eds. *Diagnostic nuclear medicine,* 3rd ed. Baltimore: Williams & Wilkins, 1995:1493–1507.
41. Preston DF. Indium-111 label in inflammation and neoplasm imaging. In: Early PJ, Sodee DB, eds. *Principles and practice of nuclear medicine.* St. Louis: Mosby, 1995:714–724.
42. Coleman M, Datz ML. Detection of inflammatory disease using radiolabeled cells. In: Sandler MP, Coleman RE, Wackers FJT, et al., eds. *Diagnostic nuclear medicine,* 1995:1509–1524.
43. *Gallium citrate.* Package insert. ^{67}Ga injection. St. Louis: Mallinckrodt, 1992.
44. Weiner RE, Thakur ML. Imaging infection/inflammations: pathophysiologic basis and radiopharmaceuticals. *Qtr J Nucl Med* 1999;43:2–8.
45. Neumann RD, Kemp JD, Weiner RE. Gallium-67 imaging for detection of malignant disease. In: Sandler MP, Coleman RE, Wackers FJT, et al., eds. *Diagnostic nuclear medicine,* 3rd ed. Baltimore: Williams & Wilkins, 1995:1243–1260.
46. Blend MJ, Sodee DB. ProstaScint: an update. In: Freeman LM, ed.

Nuclear medicine annual 2001. Philadelphia: Lippincott Williams & Wilkins, 2001:109–137.

47. *ProstaScint.* Package insert. Princeton, NJ: Cytogen, 1996.
48. Blend MJ, Bhadkamkar VA. Impact of radioimmunoscintigraphy on the management of colorectal and ovarian cancer patients: a retrospective study. *Cancer Invest* 1998;16:431–441.
49. Pinkas L, Robins PD, Forstrom LA, et al. Clinical experience with radiolabelled monoclonal antibodies in the detection of colorectal and ovarian carcinoma recurrence and review of the literature. *Nucl Med Commun* 1999;20:689–696.
50. *OncoScint.* Package insert. Princeton, NJ: Cytogen, 1992.
51. *CEA-Scan.* Package insert. Morris Plains, NJ: Immunomedics, 1996.
52. *OctreoScan.* Package insert. St. Louis: Mallinckrodt, 1994.
53. Krenning EP, Kwekkeboom DJ, Bakker WH, et al. Somatostatin receptor scintigraphy with [^{111}In-DTPA-D-Phe^1] and [^{123}I-Tyr^3]-octreotide: the Rotterdam experience with more than 1000 patients. *Eur J Nucl Med* 1993;20:716–731.
54. Gibril F, Reynolds JC, Chen CC, et al. Specificity of somatostatin receptor scintigraphy: a prospective study and effects of false-positive localizations on management in patients with gastrinomas. *J Nucl Med* 1999;40:539–553.
55. *NeoTect.* Package insert. Londonderry, NH: Diatide, 1999.
56. Blum JE, Handmaker H, Rinne NA. The utility of a somatostatin-type receptor binding peptide radiopharmaceutical (P829) in the evaluation of solitary pulmonary nodules. *Chest* 1999;115:224–232.
57. Buscombe JR, Cwikla JB, Holloway B, et al. Prediction of the usefulness of combined mammography and scintimammography in suspected primary breast cancer using ROC curves. *J Nucl Med* 2001;42:3–8.
58. Gambhir SS, Czernin J, Schwimmer J, et al. A tabulated summary of the FDG PET literature. *J Nucl Med* 2001;42:1S–93S.
59. Phelps ME, Hoffman EJ, Selin C, et al. Investigation of [^{18}F]2-fluoro-2-deoxyglucose for the measure of myocardial glucose metabolism. *J Nucl Med* 1978;19:1311–1319.
60. Weiner RE, Thakur ML. Radiolabeled peptides in diagnosis and therapy. *Sem Nucl Med* 2001;31:296–311.
61. Robinson RG, Preston DF, Spicer JA, et al. Radionuclide therapy of intractable bone pain: emphasis on strontium-89. *Sem Nucl Med* 1992;22:28–32.
62. *Metastron.* Package insert. Arlington Heights, IL: Amersham Healthcare, 1993.
63. *Quadramet.* Package insert. North Billerica, MA: Dupont Pharma, 1997.
64. Kaminski MS, Estes J, Zasadny KR, et al. Radioimmunotherapy with iodine (131)I tositumomab for relapsed or refractory B-cell non-Hodgkin lymphoma: updated results and long-term follow-up of the University of Michigan experience. *Blood* 2000;96:1259–1266.
65. Hsieh BT, Ting G, Hsieh HT, Shen LH. Study on the preparation of carrier-free ^{90}Y for medical research. *Radioact & Radiochem* 1992;3:26–30.
66. Gross MD, Shulkin BL, Shapiro B, et al. Adrenal scintigraphy and therapy of neuroendocrine tumors with radioiodinated metaiodobenzylguanidine. In: Sandler MP, Coleman RE, Wackers FJT, et al., eds. *Diagnostic nuclear medicine,* 3rd ed. Baltimore: Williams & Wilkins, 1995:1023–1045.
67. McGilvery RW. *Biochemistry a functional approach,* 3rd ed. Philadelphia: WB Saunders, 1983:726–732.
68. Desroches JJ, Lahaie RG, Picard M, et al. Methodological validation and clinical usefulness of carbon-14-urea breath test for documentation of presence and eradication of *Helicobacter pylori* infection. *J Nucl Med* 1997;38:1141–1145.
69. Rodriques M, Sinzinger H, Thakur M, et al. Labelling of platelets with indium-111 oxine and technetium-99m hexamethylpropylene amine oxine: suggested methods. International Society of Radiolabelled Blood Elements (ISORBE). *Eur J Nucl Med* 1999;26:1614–1616.
70. Weiner RE, Spencer RP. Therapeutic use of particulate radiopharmaceuticals. In: Arshady R, ed. *Radioactive and magnetic microparticles for medical applications.* London: Citus Books, 2001:321–360.
71. Murray T, Hilditch TE. Therapeutic applications of radiopharmaceuticals. In: Sampson CS, ed. *Textbook of radiopharmacy,* 3rd ed. Reading, UK: Harwood Academic Publishers, 1999:369–385.
72. Cotton FA, Wilkinson G, Gaus PL. *Basic inorganic chemistry,* 2nd ed. New York: John Wiley and Sons, 1987:545–554.
73. Hichwa, RD. Production of PET radioisotopes and principles of PET imaging. In: Henkin RE, Boles MA, Dillehay GL, et al.., eds. *Nuclear medicine,* 2nd ed. St. Louis: Mosby Yearbook, 1996:279–291.
74. *Indium chloride.* Package insert. Sterile solution. St. Louis: Mallinckrodt, 1995.
75. Deutsch E. Inorganic radiopharmaceuticals. In: *Radiopharmaceuticals II: Proceedings of the 2nd International Symposium on Radiopharmaceuticals.* New York: Society of Nuclear Medicine, 1979:129–146.
76. Chaly T, Dahl JR. Thin layer chromatographic detection of kryptofix 2.2.2 in the routine synthesis of [^{18}F]2-fluoro-2-deoxy-D-glucose. *Nucl Med Biol* 1989;16:385–387.
77. Lederer CM, Shirley VS, eds. *Table of isotopes,* 7th ed. New York: John Wiley and Sons, 1978:207–536.
78. *DTPA.* Package insert. Kirkland, Canada: Draximage Inc., 1998.
79. *Glucoceptate.* Package insert. St. Louis: Mallinckrodt, 1991.
80. Eshima D, Taylor A Jr. Technetium-99m (^{99m}Tc) Mercaptoacetyltriglycine: update on the new ^{99m}Tc renal tubular function agent. *Sem Nuc Med* 1992;22:61–73.

Diagnostic Nuclear Medicine, Fourth Edition. Edited by M.P. Sandler, R.E. Coleman, J.A. Patton, F.J.Th. Wackers, A. Gottschalk. Lippincott Williams & Wilkins, Philadelphia 2003.

8

ACCELERATORS AND POSITRON EMISSION TOMOGRAPHY (PET) RADIOPHARMACEUTICALS

SALLY W. SCHWARZ
GREG G. GAEHLE
MICHAEL J. WELCH

Although several hundred positron emission tomography (PET) radiopharmaceuticals have been administered to humans, the number of compounds that are routinely used is relatively small. The only PET radiopharmaceutical currently approved by the United States Food and Drug Administration (FDA) is ^{82}Rb-labeled rubidium chloride, which is produced from a strontium-rubidium (^{82}Sr/^{82}Rb) generator. However, by far the most widely used PET radiopharmaceutical is ^{18}F-fluorodeoxyglucose (FDG). The FDA has awarded a new drug application (NDA) for FDG to one location, St. Joseph's Hospital, Peoria, Illinois. The most widely used PET radiopharmaceuticals, other than FDG, are labeled with the short half-life nuclides ^{18}F, ^{11}C, ^{13}N, and ^{15}O (Table 8.1). Although several generators have been described for the production of positron emitting nuclides, a limited number of generator compounds are currently used in humans.

PARTICLE ACCELERATORS

PET radioisotopes are generally produced by charged particle accelerators. In a cyclotron, charged particles such as protons, deuterons, ^{3}H particles, and α particles are accelerated inside flat evacuated metallic cylinders called dees. The simplest cyclotron configuration has two dees. The circular path of the particle is maintained by placing the dees between the poles of an electromagnetic field. The positively charged particles or negative ions are produced in an ion source located in the center of the cyclotron.

As the charged particle is attracted into the cyclotron and

moves along the circular path under the magnetic field it gradually increases its energy because of a high-voltage alternating electric field. The electric field is alternated rapidly at approximately 10^{12} times per second in a typical case, causing the particle to be accelerated as it reaches the gap between the dees. When the particle reaches the periphery of the dees it has attained high energy. It exits the cyclotron and is deflected onto a target where the nuclear reaction occurs (Table 8.2).

The majority of cyclotrons built before 1980 accelerated positively charged particles, primarily protons ($^1_1$H) or deuterons($^2_1$H$^+$). Medical cyclotrons marketed today accelerate negative ions. The first negative-ion cyclotron designed specifically for PET was built by Computer Technology and Imaging, Inc. (CTI), and the most popular cyclotron produced by CTI is the RDS 111. The ion source is located at the center of the RDS 111 cyclotron as shown in Fig. 8.1. Today negative-ion cyclotrons are produced by a number of companies. Table 8.3 lists various manufacturers and the parameters of the machines. The General Electric (GE) PETtrace, Ebco TR 13/8, IBA Cyclone 10/5, and CGR-Sumitomo negative-ion cyclotrons accelerate both hydrogen ions and deuterium ions.

This negative-ion design allows for a simple deflection system, in which the beam is extracted from the machine by interaction with a very thin carbon foil, avoiding the need for conventional positive-ion extraction apparatus required for positive-ion cyclotrons. The carbon foil strips electrons from the H$^-$ ion resulting in the formation of the positively charged proton spe-

S.W. Schwarz: Division of Radiological Sciences, Mallinckrodt Institute of Radiology, St. Louis, MO.

G.G. Gaehle: Division of Radiological Sciences, Mallinckrodt Institute of Radiology, St. Louis, MO.

M.J. Welch: Division of Radiological Sciences, Mallinckrodt Institute of Radiology, St. Louis, MO.

Table 8.1. *Properties of Some Common PET Radioisotopes*

Radioisotope	Half-Life (Minutes)	Maximum β⁺ Energy (keV)	Comment
^{18}Fluorine	109.7	635	Can ship short distances
^{68}Gallium	68.3	1880	Generator daughter
^{11}Carbon	20.4	970	On-site generator
^{13}Nitrogen	9.96	1190	On-site generator
^{15}Oxygen	2.07	1700	On site generator
^{82}Rubidium	1.25	3350	Generator daughter

Table 8.2. *Common PET Radioisotopes and Their Production Methods in Cyclotrons Using Protons and Deuterons*

Nuclide	Half-Life	Production Method	Target Material	Comment
^{18}F	109.7 min	^{18}O(p,n)^{18}F	^{18}O-water	Enriched isotope
		^{20}Ne(d,α)^{18}F	Ne gas	Yields F$_2$
^{11}C	20.4 min	^{14}N(p,α)^{11}C	N$_2$ gas	Used in cyclotrons
		^{10}B(d,n)^{11}C	Boric oxide	Not common
		^{11}B(d,2n)^{11}C	Boric oxide	Not common
		^{14}N(d,αn)^{11}C	N$_2$ gas	Not common
^{13}N	9.96 min	^{16}O(p,α)^{13}N	Water	Used in cyclotrons
		^{13}C(d,n)^{13}N	CO$_2$ gas	Requires deuterons
^{15}O	2.07 min	^{14}N(d,n)^{15}O	N$_2$ gas	Requires deuterons
		^{15}N(p,n)^{15}O	[^{15}N]N$_2$ gas	Enriched gas
		^{16}O(p,pn)^{15}O	O$_2$ gas	Not common

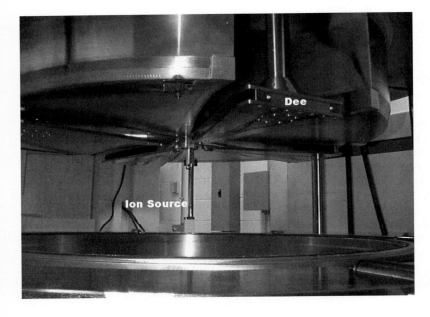

FIGURE 8.1. Interior of the CTI RDS 111 cyclotron shows the ion source located in the center of the dees.

cies that then changes direction without a deflector because of the change in the particles charge that reverse the effects of magnetic containment. The proton bombards the target material in a manner similar to that in a positive-ion cyclotron. With the negative-ion machines it is possible to place the carbon foil so that it only partially intersects the accelerated particle beam.

Table 8.3. *Beam Characteristics of Several Negative-Ion Commercial Cyclotrons for PET*

Company & Model	Proton Energy (MeV)	Deuteron Energy (MeV)	Beam Current (μA)
CTI RDS 111	11	None	80
Ebco TR 13/8	13	8	50
Ebco TR 19	13-19	9	75(p), 75(d)
GE Minitrace	10	5	50
GE PETtrace	16	8	75 (p), 60 (d)
IBA Cyclone 30	15-30	9-15	350
IBA Cyclone 10/5	10	5	50
IBA Cyclone 18/9	18	9	40

This allows a second carbon foil to be placed in the vacuum chamber further down the perimeter to extract the negative-ion beam at a second point in the machine. This design allows for simultaneous production of two radioisotopes.

Although the companies listed previously produce negative-ion cyclotrons, most cyclotrons installed over the last 5 years have been CTI or GE cyclotrons. CTI currently markets two cyclotrons, an RDS 111 and an RDS Eclipse (Fig. 8.2).

The Eclipse, introduced in 2001, is likely to become the preferred CTI cyclotron. It is an 11-MeV ion cyclotron that uses two target ports with rotating carousels, each of which can hold up to four targets. The Eclipse operates with beam currents as high as 65 μamp. Multiple runs at 60 μamp and 2-hour saturation have been carried out. With two ^{18}F targets irradiated, yields as high as 6 Ci have been obtained.

GE markets the PETtrace (Fig. 8.3). This GE cyclotron is a dual-particle machine (proton and deuteron) with energies of 16 and 10 MeV, respectively. The PETtrace cyclotron has dual-bombardment capabilities specifically designed to be user friendly with a full range of optional synthesis modules.

Over the past 20 years several low-cost accelerators have been

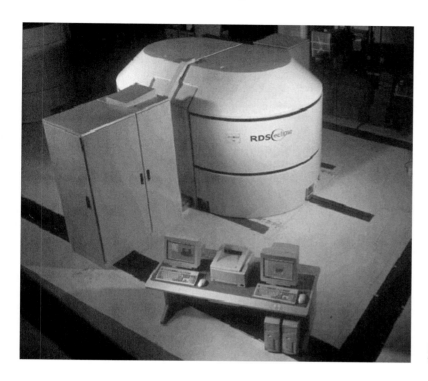

FIGURE 8.2. RDS Eclipse, 11-MeV negative-ion cyclotron that has 65 μamp beam current potential.

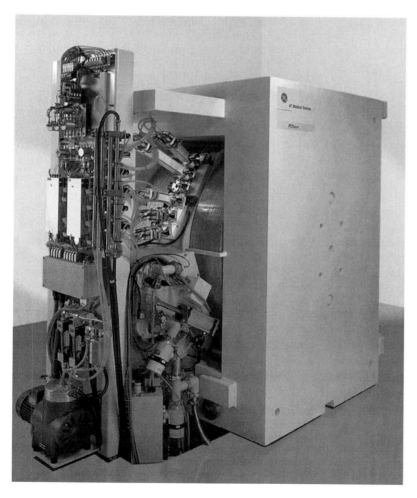

FIGURE 8.3. The GE negative-ion PETtrace allows acceleration of either hydrogen or deuterium ions.

proposed, some to produce the full range of PET radionuclides and some specifically for the shorter lived nuclides. These accelerators were described in a recent review article (1) but have had little impact on the market. Although ^{18}F-FDG is widely used, it still seems that there is a need for a dedicated machine capable of producing ^{15}O-labeled radiopharmaceuticals and possibly ^{13}N-ammonia, but only a few dedicated low-energy accelerators are currently used.

Compounding Process and Procedure Verification

All PET radiopharmaceutical formulation should follow the United States Pharmacopeia (USP) XXV guidelines for PET compounding. These guidelines require written procedures that include the definition that all starting materials of a specified grade will be used (2). Standards for identity testing should be written for acceptance of each raw material. For critical components, a certificate of analysis should be obtained from the supplier and at least one identity test should be performed as part of standard material acceptance testing. Components, containers, closures, and supplies used in the radiosynthesis of PET radiopharmaceuticals should be stored in a controlled access area according to written procedures. These raw materials must be logged in and assigned lot numbers and expiration dates based on the manufacturer's expiration date or assigned an expiration date based on the physical and chemical properties of the component, material, or supply. Chemical reactions with the radiopharmaceutical storage container should also be investigated because the container can be a potential source of impurities. Validation of the final product container must be provided indicating that no material is leached from the container or closure system into the final PET radiopharmaceutical.

Batch production records and quality control (QC) records are essential. Written procedures for each PET radiopharmaceutical intended for intravenous administration require sterile membrane filtration (0.22 μm), and particulate filtration (0.45 μm) is required for PET radiopharmaceuticals intended for inhalation. The information contained on the radiopharmaceutical label should include the name of the radiopharmaceutical, the lot number, the total radioactivity and radioactive concentration at the time and date of calibration, the expiration time and date, and the name and quantity of any added preservative or stabilizer. The label should also state "Caution: Radioactive Material."

Quality Control

Radiopharmaceuticals administered for PET procedures usually incorporate radionuclides that possess very short physical half-lives (e.g., $T_{1/2}$ of ^{18}F = 109.7 minutes, ^{11}C = 20.4 minutes, ^{13}N = 9.96 minutes, and ^{15}O = 2.07 minutes). The radionuclides are then synthetically incorporated into the final PET radiopharmaceutical, which must be analyzed, meet quality assurance specifications, and be fully documented before administration to humans (3). The USP requires various types of QC information such as radionuclidic identity; radionuclidic, radio-

ochemical, and chemical purity; and sterility and pyrogen testing. It is important that each analytical test be validated and the limits for each test be specified.

Cyclotron targets and the target materials used to produce these PET radionuclides must be of high quality and monitored by the PET center because, together with the nuclear reactions, these materials determine the radionuclidic, radiochemical, and chemical purity of the radionuclide. For example, ^{18}F is produced in the CTI machine using a silver body target and ^{18}O enriched water. Other radionuclides that could be formed during the bombardment are due to proton irradiation of the foil material (havar metal), producing radiometal contaminants. For example, irradiation of a silver target body can cause production of ^{109}Cd. The critical nuclear parameters include the beam current, particle energy, threshold energy (Fig. 8.4), and the purity of the target substance.

Radionuclide production can be analyzed for radionuclidic impurities through multichannel analysis (MCA), or pulse height γ-ray spectroscopy. The radionuclidic purity determination can be made three to four half-lives after the end of bombardment (EOB) with little interference from the main 511-keV photopeak of the positron emitters.

Radionuclide identity can be accomplished before release of the radiopharmaceutical by decay analysis using a dose calibrator computer program to calculate $T_{1/2}$. The QC method for determining radiochemical purity is usually based on a chromatographic method with simultaneous radioactivity detection. Various types of chromatographic methods such as thin layer chromatography (TLC) or high-performance liquid chromatography (HPLC) can be used. HPLC allows in-line measurement of chemical and radiochemical purity. These chromatographic methods are performed using standards for comparing R_f value or retention time or for generating standard curves.

Chemical impurities separated by HPLC are generally easy to detect if they are ultraviolet (UV) absorbing. Compounds that

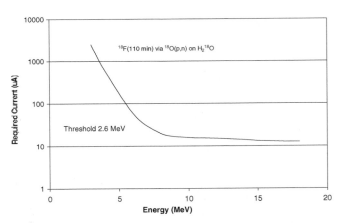

Beam Current Required to Produce 1 Ci of F-18 with a 2 Hour Bombardment at Various Energies MeV

FIGURE 8.4. Beam current required for proton and deuteron reactions.

are poorly absorbing can be detected by pulsed amperometric detectors (PADs). The mass quantities of radioactive active ingredients contained in a PET radiopharmaceutical can vary from nanogram to milligram quantities. The chemical purity requirement is to verify the chemical identity of the drug product, including stereoisomeric purity. Gas chromatography methods can be used for the measurement of the residual solvents such as ethanol, acetonitrile, and ethanol. Chemical purity analysis also requires verification of the absence of any chemical impurities or solvent residues in the final preparation. The analyses also require an injection of a known standard each time QC is performed. In this way the accuracy of the system is determined each time. For PET radiopharmaceuticals labeled with a radionuclide with a $T_{1/2}$ less than 20 minutes, the USP allows QC procedures to be performed on an initial QC subbatch before the patient batch.

Tests should be done to ensure sterility, apyrogenicity, isotonicity, and suitable acidity (pH) before administration to humans. The injectable drug product should be formulated as an isotonic solution and sterilized by filtration through a 0.22 μm filter as a final step in the radiosynthetic procedure. The pH and isotonicity can be adjusted to physiologic values before the final filtration by the addition of sterile buffers or a sodium chloride solution. Verification of apyrogenicity should be made using the USP bacterial endotoxin test (BET) on each batch of nongaseous radiopharmaceutical prepared for intravenous human administration. The USP limit for endotoxins is 175 endotoxin units (EU) per volume (V), which is the maximum administered total dose in milliliters. If the $T_{1/2}$ is equal to or greater than 20 minutes, a 20-minute endotoxin "limit test" must be performed prerelease. A standard 60-minute test must also be performed on each batch. Sterility should be determined after release on each batch of parenteral radiopharmaceutical intended for human use. USP methods require inoculation of the radiopharmaceutical into both tryptic soy broth and fluid thioglycolate media within 24 hours after the end of synthesis (EOS). Because an entire lot of a PET radiopharmaceutical may be administered to one or several subjects, depending on the radioactivity remaining in the container at the time of administration, administration of the entire quantity of the lot to a single patient should be anticipated for each lot prepared. Each PET radiopharmaceutical intended for inhalation should incorporate a particulate filter (0.45 μm) as a component of the administration procedure.

The radionuclidic purity should be determined by γ-ray spectrum using multichannel pulse height analysis or a germanium detector.

With every major change or initial production of a new radiopharmaceutical, three independent production runs should be performed to verify the drug product quality, strength, and purity.

Although PET radiopharmaceuticals have a limited life because of the physical half-life of the radionuclide, stability studies must be performed for the time period from the EOS to administration. The stability of the active ingredients should also be determined for a known container under set storage conditions.

FDA APPROVED PET RADIOPHARMACEUTICALS

^{82}Rb-Rubidium Chloride

^{82}Rb is currently the only FDA-approved PET radiopharmaceutical. The approved indication is for PET myocardial perfusion imaging. It is used in the diagnosis of infarction to distinguish normal from abnormal regions of myocardial perfusion in patients with suspected myocardial infarction. Studies have been performed to evaluate myocardial blood flow (MBF) using ^{82}Rb. Several studies comparing ^{82}Rb PET and ^{201}Tl single photon emission computed tomography (SPECT) have demonstrated the diagnostic accuracy of using ^{82}Rb for the detection of coronary artery disease (CAD). A study from the Cleveland Clinic (4) demonstrated increased sensitivity with ^{82}Rb PET over ^{201}Tl SPECT (95% vs. 75%) using angiography as the gold standard. A study at the University of Michigan (5) demonstrated increased specificity with ^{82}Rb PET over ^{201}Tl SPECT (85% vs. 53 %). To quantify MBF, mathematical modeling has been used to isolate the tracer delivery mechanism from the tracer retention mechanism (6,7).

^{82}Rb is a generator-produced isotope from the decay of ^{82}Sr ($T_{1/2} = 25.3$ days). ^{82}Sr is produced in high-energy accelerators by irradiation of ^{98}Mo by 700- to 800-MeV protons. ^{82}Rb decays with a $T_{1/2}$ of 75 seconds. It decays 95% by positron emission and 5% by electron capture. In addition to the annihilation photon from β^+ annihilation, it emits a 776 keV gamma (15% abundance) and a 1,395 keV gamma (0.5% abundance). ^{85}Sr is produced during production of ^{82}Sr in approximately equal amounts at EOB and has a $T_{1/2}$ of 64.8 days.

Rubidium is an alkali metal and forms ionic solids. In solution rubidium forms a +1 cation. It is distributed *in vivo* similar to potassium ions, and it accumulates in the cells of the myocardium as a function of blood flow and/or viability.

The ^{82}Rb infusion system is marketed by Bracco Diagnostics and consists of the ^{82}Rb generator and the mobile infusion cart. The infusion cart contains two shields, one for the generator and one for the waste bottle; an in-line dosimeter for measurement of the ^{82}Rb; and an electronic infusion control system. The generator is a mixture of ^{82}Sr/^{85}Sr adsorbed on the surface of a stannic oxide column. During elution of the ^{82}Rb some strontium is also eluted, which is referred to as breakthrough. This breakthrough is a radionuclidic impurity, and daily QC must be performed to determine the amount of ^{82}Sr and ^{85}Sr that is present. The allowable limits for ^{82}Sr is 0.02 μCi/mCi ^{82}Rb, and for ^{85}Sr the limit is 0.2 μCi/mCi ^{82}Rb. After the first elution of the day, the ^{82}Rb is allowed to decay, and the total amount of strontium is assayed. Using ratios provided by the manufacturer, the amount of ^{82}Sr and ^{85}Sr can be calculated. The ^{82}Rb generator can be reeluted after 12.5 minutes (10 half-lives) and is typically replaced every 30 days.

United States Pharmacopeia (USP) PET Radiopharmaceuticals

^{18}F-Fluorodeoxyglucose (FDG) Injection

FDG is currently dispensed and distributed according to the USP monograph requirements for FDG, because the FDA has not finalized the regulatory status of PET radiopharmaceuticals. The approved indications for FDG are lung, esophageal, colorectal, head and neck, and esophageal cancer; lymphoma; melanoma; refractory seizures; and myocardial viability. The indication for breast cancer is under consideration.

FDG is used widely in many aspects of PET diagnostic nuclear medicine including diagnosis of cancer and diseases of the brain and heart. The mechanism of FDG trapping follows the glucose biochemical pathway. FDG is transported into the cell and metabolized by phosphorylation with hexokinase to FDG-6 phosphate (Fig. 8.5). However, unlike glucose, FDG-6-phosphate is then trapped in the cell because of the stereochemical and structural demands of the enzyme responsible for further catabolism.

The direct measurement of glucose metabolism with FDG also yields valuable information about tumor localization and quantitation, and several extensive review articles are available on the clinical aspects of FDG in oncology applications (8) and in neurooncology (9). For tumor staging and assessment of treatment response, FDG and PET often distinguish viable tumor from nontumor masses (10), because of increased glucose utilization in malignant tumors. This transformation is often associated with downregulation of glucose-6-phosphate and the upregulation of glucose transporters (especially GLUT-1) and hexokinase (11). FDG and PET have demonstrated the potential for noninvasive tumor staging because of their ability to detect lymph node metastases from breast and lung cancers, melanoma, and head and neck carcinomas (12,13). The amount of FDG uptake strongly correlates with response to therapy; a decrease in FDG uptake after therapy indicates a positive response. Several recent review articles include various types of carcinoma such as breast, glioma, colorectal, and lung (14,15). It is important to note that all cells metabolize glucose, and, therefore, FDG is not tumor specific; this can present a significant problem particularly after therapy when macrophages, which exhibit high uptake of FDG,

replace tumor cells. Cellular uptake can also be affected by high blood sugar levels. FDG transport competes with glucose for membrane-bound transporters (16). This can be controlled by requiring the patient to fast 4 to 6 hours before FDG injection (17).

^{18}F decays 97% by positron emission and 3% by electron capture, with a β max of 0.635 MeV. ^{18}F fluoride was first produced for ^{18}F-FDG production by the $^{20}Ne(d, \alpha)^{18}F$ nuclear reaction. The use of a neon gas target passivated with F_2, and filled with 0.1% F_2 in neon, provides labeled fluorine gas, $^{18}F^{19}F$. This production of ^{18}F involving F_2 gas is inherently carrier added and therefore has limits on the specific activity that can be obtained. The effect of target purity on the chemical form of ^{18}F during ^{18}F-F_2 production has been described (18). Currently the proton irradiation of ^{18}O-labeled water by the nuclear reaction $^{18}O(p, n)^{18}F$ is the preferred method of producing ^{18}F, with yields of greater than one Ci at EOB. The target is constructed of metals such as silver, titanium, nickel, or stainless steel. The target has small cavities for the target water, which range in volume from 0.1 to 4 mL; the small cavities are covered by thin metal foils such as havar metal, which is an alloy containing chromium, cobalt, iron, manganese, molybdenum, nickel, and vanadium. The major problem in producing ^{18}F using ^{18}O enriched water is the limited availability and high cost of the isotopically enriched target material. To aid in the conservation of the ^{18}O-labeled water, unused target material can be recovered by ion exchange chromatography (19).

The nucleophilic fluorination method developed by Hamacher et al. (20) for production of FDG, using the nucleophilic displacement reaction with 1,3,4,6-tetra-O-acetyl-2-trifluoromethansulfonyl-β-D-mannopyranose (mannose triflate) (Fig. 8.6), is the most commonly used method today for the routine production of ^{18}F-FDG. After displacement, acid hydrolysis of the acetylated intermediate 2-^{18}F-fluro-1,3,4,6-tetra-O-acetyl-^{d}-glucose (TA-^{18}F-FDG) gives 2-^{18}F-FDG (Fig. 8.7) in good

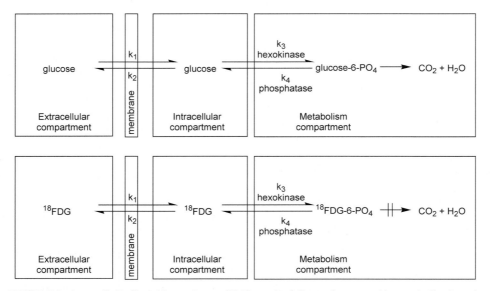

FIGURE 8.5. Intracellular fluorodeoxyglucose (FDG) uptake follows glucose and is metabolized to glucose-6-PO_4. Further metabolism is blocked, trapping FDG in the cell.

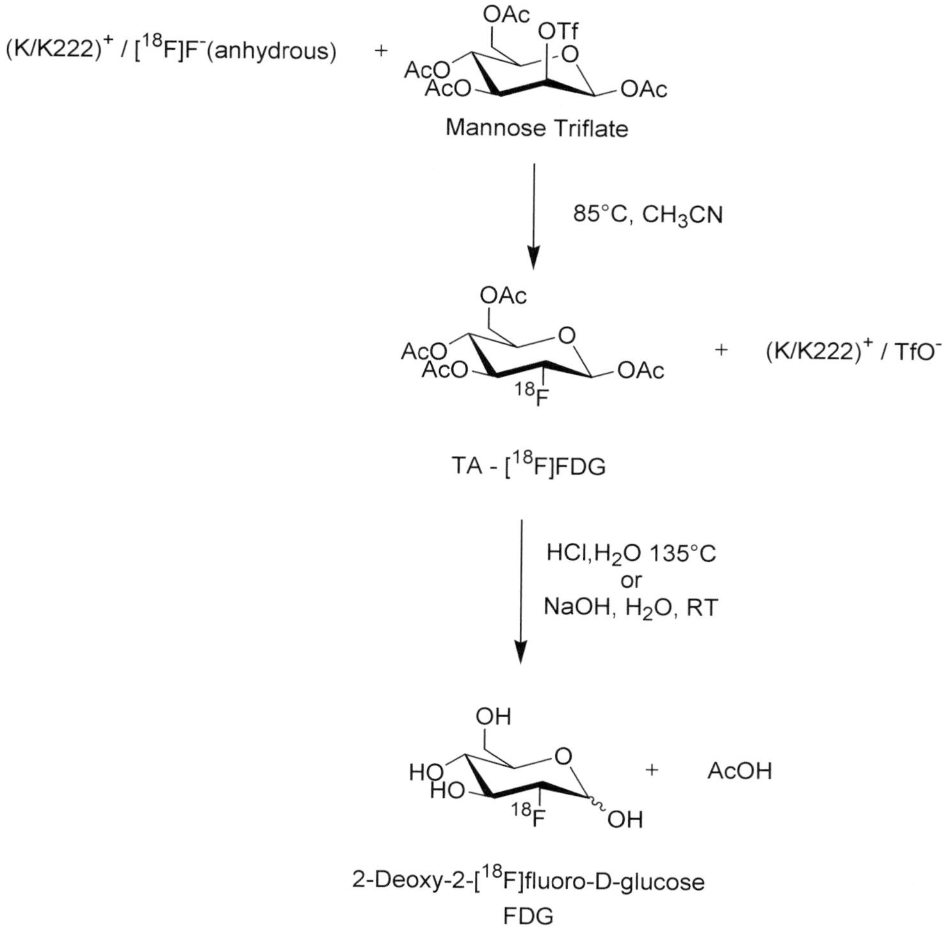

(K/K222)+ / [18F]F-(anhydrous)
+
OAc
OTf
O
AcO
AcO
OAc
Mannose Triflate
85°C, CH3CN
OAc
O
AcO
AcO
18F
OAc
+
(K/K222)+ / TfO-
TA - [18F]FDG
HCl,H2O 135°C
or
NaOH, H2O, RT
OH
O
HO
HO
18F
OH
+
AcOH
2-Deoxy-2-[18F]fluoro-D-glucose
FDG

FIGURE 8.6. Fluorodeoxyglucose synthetic scheme using Kryptofix chemistry with acid or base hydrolysis.

FDG18
SYNTHESIZER

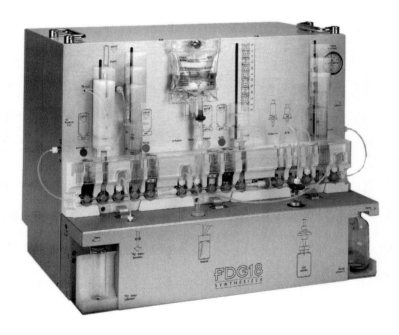

FIGURE 8.7. Fluorodeoxyglucose synthesizer produced by Coincidence Technologies and recently acquired by GE Medical Systems.

yield. The Hamacher synthesis uses Kyrptofix 2.2.2 as a phase transfer catalyst to increase the reactivity of the fluoride ions. Because Kryptofix is a toxic substance, any radiosynthesis using Kryptofix 2.2.2 must include a QC method to determine the concentration in the final product. USP requires that the concentration must be less than 50 μg/mL. The USP approved method to test for the presence of Kryptofix, developed by Chaly and Dahl (21), involves a rapid, simple, TLC QC procedure using a silica gel thin-layer chromatographic plate developed in a mixture of methanol/ammonium hydroxide (9:1). The developed plate is dried, and iodine vapor is used for visualization. A yellow spot (R_f = 0.4) indicates the presence of Kryptofix 2.2.2. The USP test takes about 30 minutes to complete. Mock et al. (22) have also developed a color spot test for FDG that can determine the presence of Kryptofix to as low as 2.0 μg/mL in about 5 minutes. The test uses pretreated strips of plastic-backed silica gel TLC (Eastman Kodak) that is saturated with iodoplatinate reagent and overspotted with drops of ^{18}F-FDG and Kryptofix standard solutions.

Füchtner et al. (23) reported a method of base hydrolysis of the FDG acetylated intermediate, which can be used with either electrophilic or nucleophilic procedures. Overall the base hydrolysis reportedly can increase yield, reduce the overall time of the reaction, and avoid formation of the chemical impurity 2-deoxy-2-chloro-D-glucose formed during acid hydrolysis. The alkaline hydrolysis can cause epimerization of the FDG to 2-^{18}F-flurodeoxy-D-mannose (FDM). Meyer et al. (24) has reported that controlling base concentrations, reaction times, and temperatures limits the FDM formation to 0.5%.

FDG synthesis modules available on the market employ several chemistry methods to prepare the ^{18}F-FDG. The Coincidence Technologies FDG synthesizer (Fig. 8.7) uses the nucleophilic substitution method (20). The resulting tetra acetyl-^{18}F-glucose is trapped on a standard reverse phase extraction cartridge, and the acetyl groups are removed using base hydrolysis. The CTI Quadrax synthesizer employs Kryptofix nucleophilic

radiofluorination with base hydrolysis. The original CTI FDG synthesizer uses Kryptofix chemistry with acid hydrolysis. Ebco and Nuclear Interface (Fig. 8.8) modules use a nucleophilic reaction with either Kryptofix or tetrabutylammonium (25) hydrogen carbonate then hydrolysis with HCl.

One of the original FDG synthesis modules was developed by GE using direct nucleophilic exchange on a quaternary 4-aminopyridinium resin (26). The overall FDG yields of this module were about 30% to 40% decay corrected, so it is not currently marketed. GE has recently purchased the Coincidence Technologies FDG synthesis module that uses Kryptofix nucleophilic radiofluorination with base hydrolysis. The yield of this synthesis module is routinely 60% to 75%.

The radiochemical purity of FDG can be determined by using silica gel 60 TLC plates developed in acetonitrile/water (95:5). This system allows separation of FDG (R_f = 0.4); ^{18}F-fluoride (R_f = 0.1) and TA-^{18}F-FDG, the nonhydrolyzed intermediate (R_f = 0.6).

The radionuclide identity test is performed prerelease by decay analysis to determine the half-life of the radionuclide, which for FDG is 109.7 ±3% minutes (USP). Radionuclidic purity should be determined on a defined interval by γ-ray spectrum using multichannel pulse height analysis or a germanium detector.

Other potential FDG impurities include 2-chloro-2deoxyglucose and 2-fluoro-2-deoxymannose. Ion chromatography (IC) with PAD (10 to 100 pmol) has been used to analyze for the presence of 2-chloro-2-deoxyglucose (27). HPLC analysis with a Dionex PA 1 column eluted with 0.1 M NaOH (24) can be used to analyze for the presence of 2-fluoro-2-deoxymannose. The mass is detected using UV absorption at 206, with an in-line radioactive detector to analyze for the presence of FDM.

Additional prerelease QC requirements are set for pH (range must be between 4.5 and 7.5) and BET (<175 EU/V). To

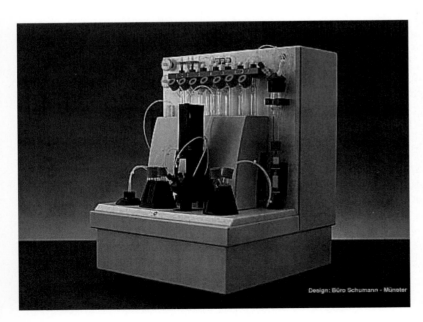

FIGURE 8.8. Nuclear Interface FDG synthesis module.

insure sterility, the final product is filtered through a 0.22 μm filter before injection. Residual solvent concentrations such as acetonitrile (0.04% w/v), ethanol, and ether (0.5% w/v) must be tested before release of ^{18}F-FDG. Gas chromatographic methods have been developed for the measurement of residual solvents, which allow precision and linearity over the range of concentration levels required by the FDA (3). To ensure the sterile process, the final filter must be tested for integrity after filtration. Sterility testing release is performed after release, but inoculation of the media is required within 24 hours after EOS. USP specification for specific activity is no carrier added.

^{13}N-Ammonia Injection

^{13}N-ammonia is labeled with the positron emitting radionuclide, ^{13}N ($T_{1/2}$ = 9.96 minutes). It decays 100% by β^+ emission with a maximum β^+ energy of 1.2 MeV. ^{13}N-ammonia injection was added to the USP in 1990.

^{13}N-ammonia injection has attracted interest as an imaging agent to study brain (28), liver (29,30), and myocardial perfusion (31,32). Perfusion studies have been performed with subjects both at rest and during exercise (33,34). Recently, myocardial blood flow (MBF) was quantified using ^{13}N-ammonia and a two-tissue compartmental model. The results were compared with the argon inert gas technique, and good quantitative correlation was found between the two techniques (35).

The myocardial uptake of ^{13}N-ammonia has been demonstrated to be proportional to the coronary blood flow (36). The advantages of ^{13}N-ammonia over ^{201}Tl imaging includes better resolution, the ability to quantitate flow, and the ability to perform multiple serial studies within a brief period under varied conditions (37). Also ^{13}N-ammonia has been evaluated for predicting contractile recovery after acute myocardial infarction (38). Quantitative flow measurements have been assessed for detection and localization of CAD (32).

When ^{13}N-ammonia is injected intravenously, it rapidly clears from the circulation, 85% leaving the blood in the first minute (39) and only 0.4% remaining in the circulation after 200 seconds (28). The ^{13}N-ammonia is taken up mainly by the myocardium, the brain, the liver, and the kidneys (40,41). Cardiac imaging is based on myocardial tissue uptake of ^{13}N-ammonia, which is related to regional MBF. Localization in myocardial cells is due to diffusion of ^{13}N-ammonia across the capillary, retention by metabolism to ^{13}N-glutamine by glutamine synthetase (28,42), and subsequent trapping within the tissues by incorporation into the cellular pool of amino acids.

Previously ^{13}N-ammonia was produced by chemical reduction of ^{13}NO$_x$ species with Devarda's alloy or other reducing reagent, and the ^{13}N-ammonia was distilled before use (43). The synthetic methods reported by Wieland et al. (44) and Channing (45) use an in-target high-yield production of ^{13}N-ammonia by proton irradiation of a pressurized aqueous mixture of ethanol (5mM). The addition of ethanol as a hydroxy radical scavenger greatly enhances the yield of ^{13}N-ammonia (46). ^{13}N-ammonia is produced by the nuclear reaction ^{15}O(p, α)^{13}N, employing protons on dilute aqueous ethanol. The ethyl alcohol is 95% diluted in sterile water for injection. The target chamber can be constructed of titanium or silver. When ^{13}N-ammonia is transferred from the target through a strong anion-exchange membrane, all anionic impurities are removed. The aqueous ethanol mixture is convenient because it is suitable for human intravenous injection after sterilization by final filtration through the 0.22 μm vented filter into a sterile vial or syringe. Before production the target and product delivery lines are flushed with the sterile water/ethanol mixture to help insure aseptic process.

Because ^{13}N-ammonia has a $T_{1/2}$ less than 20.0 minutes, the USP allows preparation of a subbatch for QC testing before preparation of the patient batch. Each QC subbatch should be tested for radionuclide identity, pH between 4.5 to 7.5, chemical and radiochemical purity equal to or greater than 95% BET (<175 EU/mL) at EOS. Final product should be filtered through a 0.22 μm filter to ensure sterility. Every batch should be inoculated for sterility within 24-hours EOS. The USP specification for specific activity is no carrier added.

Because the primary aqueous anionic ^{13}N species after irradiation are nitrite and nitrate, radiochemical purity testing can alternately be performed using a strong anion exchange ion chromatography (IC) with a Wescan Anion/Ranion column, 100 × 4.6 mm (available through Alltech Associates, Deerfield, Illinois) or equivalent, eluted with 4 mM p-hydroxybenzoic acid, pH 8.5, at a flow rate of 2.0 mL/minute. The effluent can be monitored for conductivity and radioactivity. Strong cation exchange IC can be performed on a cation column (Waters cation M/D, 150 × 3.9 mm) using 3 mM nitric acid in 0.1 M ethylenediaminetetraacetic acid (EDTA) as the eluent at a flow of 1.0 mL/minute. Retention time for ^{13}N-ammonia is approximately 5 minutes. Radiochemical purity can be determined using an inline, flow-through NaI detector.

Because ^{13}N-ammonia can be synthesized by different methods, chemical purity must be assessed for potential impurities. If Devarda's alloy is used to reduce the ^{13}N-nitrate/nitrite; the presence of aluminum must be determined to be equal to or less than 10 μg/mL. The USP details a spectrophotometric assay to test for the presence of aluminum. A colorimetric test for formaldehyde, which can be formed during synthesis, is available commercially (Fast Formalert; Baxter Healthcare, McGaw Park, Illinois). A detection limit of 2 ppm has been reported (45).

Radionuclide identity must be performed to assure the $T_{1/2}$ = 9.96 minutes ±3%. The radionuclidic purity is analyzed by either multichannel pulse height analysis and/or multichannel scaling. Most radionuclidic impurities formed are usually removed by the anion exchange resin treatment after removal from the target. The primary radionuclidic impurity remaining is ^{15}O, most likely present as ^{15}O-water, produced by the ^{16}O(p, n)^{15}O nuclear reaction.

^{11}C-Sodium Acetate Injection

^{11}C-labeled acetate PET has been used to assess oxidative myocardial metabolism since the mid 1980s (47–51). Endogenous acetate differs from ^{11}C-acetate only at the carboxylic carbon where a stable carbon atom is replaced by a ^{11}C atom. ^{11}C-acetate is converted to acetyl coenzyme A by the enzyme acetyl CoA synthetase after myocardial uptake. Acetyl coenzyme A enters the tricarboxylic acid cycle (TCA or Krebs cycle) and is predominately metabolized to the end product ^{11}C-CO$_2$, which is then cleared from the myocardium. Because the TCA cycle is closely linked to oxidative phosphorylation, ^{11}C-acetate metabolism can provide an index of oxidative metabolism.

Myocardial oxidative metabolism relative to MBF can be used to evaluate the location, extent, and severity of myocardial cardiotoxicity. ^{15}O-water can be used to measure MBF under normal and pathologic states, and ^{11}C-acetate can be used to assess oxidative metabolism. Alternatively, ^{11}C-acetate can be used exclusively to evaluate regional oxidative metabolism and regional MBF (52,53). Miller et al. (54) developed a method to construct quantitatively accurate three-dimensional (3D) images of myocardial oxidative consumption from serial images of myocardial washout of ^{11}C-acetate. The 3D functional display permits assessment of the inferoposterior wall and also permits viewing of the myocardium from all angles. Hicks et al. (55) obtained results that showed that right ventricular ^{11}C-acetate clearance rate constants, obtained by PET imaging, provided a noninvasive evaluation of right ventricular oxidative metabolism. Porenta et al. (56) used gated cardiac PET imaging with ^{11}C-acetate as a noninvasive method for near simultaneous assessment of MBF oxygen requirements and contractile function.

Synthetic methods have been developed by Pike et al. (57) and Norenberg et al. (58) to produce ^{11}C-acetate. The syntheses incorporates ^{11}C-CO$_2$ produced in a cyclotron by the nuclear reaction ^{14}N(p, α)^{11}C, that is trapped in liquid nitrogen. The ^{11}C-CO$_2$ is released into freshly prepared methyl magnesium bromide in diethyl ether at room temperature. Hydrochloric acid is added to the reaction vessel, the phases are allowed to separate, and the aqueous layer is withdrawn from the reaction vessel. Sodium bicarbonate in water for injection is added to the reaction vessel, heated at 60°C for 5 minutes, and finally filtered through a 0.22 μm filter.

Each batch of ^{11}C-acetate should be adjusted for isotonicity. USP prerelease QC specifications include radionuclidic identity, pH between 4.5 to 8.5, radiochemical purity equal to or greater than 95%, and BET (<175 EU/mL) at EOS. An in-process 20-minute endotoxin limit test can be performed prerelease of the ^{11}C-acetate, followed by the 60-minute test completed after release. Final product should be filtered through a 0.22 μm filter to assure sterility. Every batch should be inoculated for sterility testing within 24 hours EOS. Specific activity must be greater than 100 mCi (3.7 GBq)/μmole.

Several radiochemical purity methods have been used for ^{11}C-acetate. One HPLC method (58) uses a reverse-phase C-8 column (Alltech, 10 μm, 4/6 × 250 mm) eluted with 7 mN H$_3$PO$_4$ at a flow rate of 2 mL/minute. A radioactive detector can be placed in-line with the HPLC following the UV detector. The acetate mass is detected using a UV detector at 210 nm, and the results are compared with a standard compound injection. Another method used a BioRad fast organic acid column (100 × 7.8 mm) eluted with 10% acetonitrile 10% in 0.007 N sulfuric acid at a flow rate of 1.0 mL/minute. Mass is detected using UV light at 210 nm, and radioactivity is detected with an in-line flow through NaI detector. The retention time for ^{11}C-acetate is approximately 3 minutes.

Chemical purity concerns for ^{11}C-acetate include trace amounts of magnesium and bromide ions, which could present a toxicologic concern. Magnesium is analyzed using IC with a Waters cation M/D (150 × 3.9 mm) eluted with 3 mM nitric acid in 0.1 M EDTA at a flow of 1.0 mL/minute. Retention time for Mg^{+2} is approximately 12 minutes. Bromide is also analyzed using IC with a Dionex anion column (250 × 4 mm) eluted with 2.0 mM Na$_2$CO$_3$/1.0 mM NaHCO$_3$ at a flow rate of 1.2 mL/minute with suppressed conductivity. Bromide elutes with a retention time of approximately 7 minutes. Gas chromatographic methods have been developed that can be used to determine the concentration of diethyl ether or other solvents that may be present in the preparation (3).

^{18}F Sodium Fluoride Injection

^{18}F sodium fluoride injection was first used for bone imaging in 1962 (59) and was added as a PET radiopharmaceutical to the USP in 1991. Tracer kinetics indicate optimal imaging time is approximately 60- to 90-minutes postinjection. A recent study has evaluated renal and whole blood kinetics by comparing ^{18}F-fluoride and ^{99m}Tc-MDP. Several studies have used ^{18}F-fluoride in combination with FDG to qualitatively and quantitatively evaluate benign skeletal lesions and malignant skeletal metastases (60).

USP prerelease QC specifications for ^{18}F-fluoride include radionuclidic identity, pH between 4.5 to 8.0, radiochemical purity equal to or greater than 95%, BET (<175 EU/mL) at EOS. Every batch should be filtered through a 0.22 μm filter to assure sterility and inoculated for sterility testing within 24-hours EOS. Specific activity is no carrier added.

^{18}F sodium fluoride can be prepared by trapping the ^{18}F-fluoride on an anion exchange resin (AG1-X9) in the carbonate form prepared according to the method of Schlyer et al. (19). The ^{18}F-fluoride is eluted with 0.02 M potassium carbonate solution. An aliquot of the ^{18}F-fluoride is added to 0.9% NaCl through a sterile 0.22 μm filter. Radiochemical purity must be greater than 95%, which can be assessed using ion chromatography.

Radiochemical purity can be analyzed using IC with a Dionex anion column (250 × 4 mm) eluted with 2 mM Na$_2$CO$_3$/1 mM NaHCO$_3$ at a flow rate of 1.2 mL/minute with suppressed conductivity. Fluoride elutes with a retention time of approximately 3.5 minutes.

^{18}F Fluorodopa Injection

The positron-emitting fluorinated L-DOPA analog 6-^{18}F-fluoro-L-3,4-dihydroxyphenylalanine (FDOPA) (Fig. 8.9) has been used as an imaging agent for brain dopamine neurons (61–63). The chemical structure of FDOPA differs from L-DOPA only at the 6 position of the catechol moiety where a fluorine atom replaces a hydrogen atom. ^{18}F FDOPA injection was added to the USP in 1991. The cell bodies of the central dopaminergic neurons are located in the pars compacta of the substantia nigra and ventral tegmental area (64). FDOPA is converted to 6-^{18}F-flurodopamine by decarboxylation (Fig. 8.9) and is actively stored in sympathetic synaptic vesicles; it can be released by sympathetic nerve stimulation (63). In certain brain disorders L-DOPA is deficient. In the rhesus monkey, after pe-

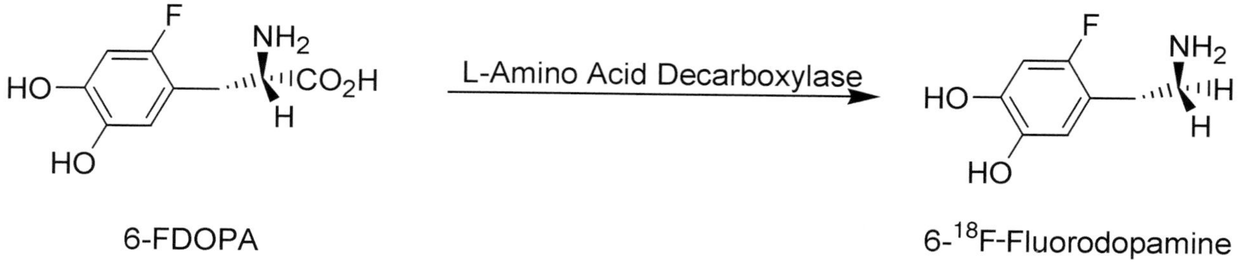

FIGURE 8.9. Fluorodopa decarboxylation to fluorodopamine.

ripheral intravenous administration of FDOPA, fluorodopamine was synthesized and retained in the striatum, the part of the brain with the highest density of dopaminergic nerve fibers (65). Baboon studies using FDOPA were also performed to test the validity of FDOPA as an analog of L-DOPA. It was determined that FDOPA was converted to ^{18}F-fluorodopamine, acting as false neurotransmitter. These studies showed that the radioactivity released by reserpine was most probably resulting from ^{18}F-fluorodopamine release (66). This suggested that FDOPA was decarboxylated and stored in vesicles as ^{18}F-fluorodopamine (63). Dopamine receptor binding studies have confirmed that both 5- and 6-fluorodopamine have high affinities and properties similar to dopamine at D_2 sites (67). In an attempt to understand the role of the dopaminergic system in Parkinson's disease (PD) and other neurologic disorders, studies of presynaptic dopaminergic function of FDOPA have been conducted in animals and in humans (62,68,69). In hemiparkinsonian patients, a reduced accumulation of ^{18}F activity has been found in the contralateral striatum (70). Because dopamine cannot cross the blood–brain barrier, its precursor, FDOPA, the analog of L-DOPA that crosses the blood–brain barrier, is administered. Often carbidopa, a drug routinely used in combination with L-DOPA in the treatment of PD, is given by oral administration. Carbidopa does not cross the blood–brain barrier but acts only peripherally. It inhibits peripheral decarboxylation of L-DOPA (as well as FDOPA) by aromatic amino acid decarboxylase. By preventing the peripheral breakdown of FDOPA, a greater amount of radiotracer reached the brain. The only labeled compounds present in plasma of subjects pretreated with carbidopa (as long as 120 minutes after FDOPA injection) are FDOPA and 3-O-methyl-6-6-[^{18}F]fluorodopa (71). A recent study investigated the improved FDOPA availability induced by catechol-O-methyltransferase (COMT) inhibitor entacapone used in the treatment of advanced PD. In the presence of a decarboxylase inhibitor such as L-DOPA, COMT becomes the major metabolizing enzyme for L-DOPA (72). It was concluded that prolonged FDOPA availability induced by COMT inhibition required prolonged PET imaging.

PET scanning with FDOPA has proven valuable in characterizing aberrations of dopaminergic function in PD (73–75) and other movement disorders such as dystonia (76) and Huntington's disease (77).

The first commonly used synthetic method was developed by Adam et al. (78). ^{18}F-fluorine gas was produced by the nuclear reaction ^{20}Ni(d, α)^{18}F. This synthetic method produced FDOPA in nearly equivalent amounts with the 2-^{18}F-fluorodopa isomer. FDOP had to be separated from the starting material and the 2-^{18}F-fluorodopa isomer using an extensive high pressure liquid chromatography purification procedure.

In 1990, Luxen et al. (79) developed a regioselective radiofluorodemercuration procedure. The use of a mercury intermediate proved to give higher yields, whereas increasing the pressure in the neon target increased the recovery of ^{18}F and the specific activity (80). The fluorine exchange for the mercury is highly selective and eliminates the need for a chromatographic purification step. Luxen et al. (81) have reviewed methods for the radiosynthesis of FDOPA by nonradioselective electrophilic fluorination, radioselective fluorodemetallation, and nucleophilic substitution, as well as reviewing metabolic FDOPA studies to emphasize the importance of the biochemical component in the development of FDOPA for PET.

The recent FDOPA synthesis of Namavari et al. (82) has been adapted by deVries as a one-post synthesis. The reaction is a fluorodestannylation followed by acidic removal of the protecting groups. Overall, yield of the reaction was approximately 30%. A Nuclear Interface synthesis module was modified to perform the FDOPA synthesis. The Nuclear Interface DOPA fluorodestannylation reaction is carried out in fluorotrichloromethane. The protecting groups are removed by hydrolysis with HBr.

USP prerelease QC procedures required are radionuclide identity, pH (4.0 to 5.0), radiochemical (>95%) and chemical purity, and BET (<175 EU/mL). The final preparation must be isotonic and sterilized by final filtration through a 0.22 μm filter. Each batch must be inoculated for sterility testing within 24-hours EOS. Radionuclidic purity must be analyzed on a defined schedule. The USP value for the specific activity specification is greater than 100 mCi/mmol (83).

Radiochemical purity can be assessed with HPLC analysis using a Nucleosil column ([18]C, 5 μ, 100 Å) eluted with 0.07 M KH_2PO_4 equipped with an in-line NaI detector. FDOPA elutes with a retention of approximately 8 minutes. Mass is determined using UV absorbance at 280 nm (84). Enantiomeric purity can be determined by HPLC injection equipped with a chiral ligand exchange HPLC column (85). As specified in the USP the radioactivity of the L-isomer must be greater than 95% of the total.

Chemical purity must be defined based on the synthetic methods employed. If mercury-containing starting materials are used, a test must be performed to show that the level of mercury is less than 0.5 μg/mL. To analyze for the presence of mercury-containing starting materials or reagents, an HPLC QC can be used with a C-18 column eluted with 50 mM tetrabutylammonium iodide (TBAI) in 60% acetonitrile:40% water with UV detection at 270 nm (79). This method is rapid, and the retention time is 6.6 minutes (86). The distribution of impurities is dependent on the synthetic method used. Pike et al. (87) recommend an upper acceptable limit of 50 μg for this compound, a potent neurotoxin when it is converted to the L-6-hydroxydopamine *in vivo* (88).

If the FDOPA is synthesized using a fluorodestannylation reaction, the stannous content of the radiopharmaceutical must be determined. USP defines a heavy metals test to determine that the content of metallic impurities does not exceed the specified heavy metal, although the current USP monograph for FDOPA does not state a limit for tin in FDOPA.

^{15}Oxygen Radiopharmaceuticals

^{15}O radiopharmaceuticals were among the first positron emitting tracers to be used in living animals (89). These investigators used ^{15}O-oxygen administered by inhalation to study "oxygen metabolism" in tumors. In the early 1960s ^{15}O was used by the group at Hammersmith Hospital (90–92) to study lung function. The most common compounds that are prepared are ^{15}O-oxygen, ^{15}O-water, and ^{15}O-CO. Several procedures have been described for the production of these compounds, the most common procedure to produce ^{15}O-oxygen, ^{15}O-carbon monoxide, and ^{15}O-carbon dioxide is

$$N_2/O_2 \text{ (0.5–2\%)} \Longrightarrow O^{15}O \xrightarrow[\substack{\text{charcoal} \\ 450°}]{\substack{\text{charcoal} \\ 950°}} \begin{array}{c} CO^{15}O \\ \\ C^{15}O \end{array}$$

O-15 labeled water can be prepared by several methods. These are:

1. $CO^{15}O + H_2 \rightleftharpoons H_2CO_2{}^{15}O \rightleftharpoons CO_2 + H_2{}^{15}O$
2. $N_2/H_2 \text{ (0.1–1\%)} \rightarrow H_2{}^{15}O$
3. $O^{15}O + H_2 \xrightarrow{\text{Pd catalyst}} H_2{}^{15}O$

In the first technique the oxygen of $CO^{15}O$ is exchanged with water, in the second $H_2{}^{15}O$ is produced directly in the target, and in the third the conversion takes place in a shielded device located near the PET scanner. Using the CTI RDS series of cyclotrons enriched ^{15}N-enriched nitrogen target gas is used. Interestingly, in Japan full reimbursement by health insurance is approved only for ^{15}O gas inhalation studies for patients with cerebral vascular disease. Studies of this type are being carried out in Japan and elsewhere (93–96).

Because of the short half-life of ^{15}O, a limited number of complex molecules have been prepared. ^{15}O-butanol has been synthesized; it is a more accurate tracer than ^{15}O-water for quantifying brain blood flow. ^{15}O-hydrogen peroxide has also been prepared (97,98).

Other PET Radiopharmaceuticals

Besides the compounds discussed previously many compounds have been labeled with ^{13}N, ^{11}C, and ^{18}F. These compounds have been labeled to study brain function and cardiac function, as well as various parameters of tumors. At present it is difficult to predict which of these compounds will be introduced into clinical practice over the next 5 years. Reviews of the compounds under investigation are discussed in a forthcoming radiopharmaceutical textbook [Welch MJ, Redvanly CS, eds. *Handbook of radiopharmaceuticals. Radiochemistry and Applications.* 2002 (*in press*).] Two agents that are likely to be applied clinically in the next few years are 3′-deoxy-3′-fluorothymidine and ^{18}F-fluorocholine (99). 3′-deoxy-3′-fluorothymidine is a thymidine analog that has been shown to be resistant to degradation and is retained in proliferating tissue by the action of thymidine kinase 1. This agent is likely to be useful for monitoring treatment response of tumors. Fluorocholine is a choline analog that has been shown to be useful in imaging of prostate cancer.

Radiopharmaceuticals with Medium Half-Life Radionuclides

A series of radiopharmaceuticals currently under evaluation are agents to image tissue hypoxia. These agents have potential application in studying hypoxia in the brain and heart, as well as in tumors. Misonidazole analogs have been labeled with ^{123}I and ^{99m}Tc for SPECT, as well as ^{18}F for PET studies (100). ^{18}F fluoromisonidazole (FMISO) has been evaluated for several years. It has been shown to be retained in hypoxic tissue in the brain, heart, and tumors, and studies have shown imageable differences between normal and hypoxic tissues. This and other nitroimidazole-based agents show low cellular uptake and slow clearance from normal tissues (101,102). Copper-(11)-diacetyl-bis(N^4-methylthiosemicarbazone) (Cu-ATSM) is one of a class of bis-thiosemicarbazones that have been shown to display uptake that is either flow dependent or hypoxia selective (103–105). Cu-ATSM can be labeled with a series of copper radionuclides with half-lives ranging from 10 minutes to 12 hours. These nuclides can be readily prepared from a generator (^{62}Cu) (106) or produced using a biomedical cyclotron (107, 108).

Another series of compounds being investigated are agents to measure the efficacy of gene therapy. In this category compounds have been labeled with either ^{18}F or the longer half-live PET isotopes, ^{124}I or ^{76}Br. These agents have been developed as reporter probes for imaging HSV1-TK expression. These are uracil analogs labeled with ^{124}I (109) and acycloguanosine analogs labeled with ^{18}F (110–112). Both of these classes of substrates are phosphorylated by HSV1-TK to their monophosphates and are metabolically trapped in cells.

REFERENCES

1. McCarthy TJ, Welch MJ. The state of positron emitting radionuclide production in 1997. *Sem Nucl Med* 1998;28:235–246.
2. United States Pharmacopeia (USP). 1999:91–93.
3. Channing MA, Huang BX, Eckelman WC. Analysis of residual solvents in 2-[18F]FDG by GC. *Nucl Med Biol* 2001;28:469–471.

4. Go RT, Marwick TH, MacIntyre WJ et al. A prospective comparison of rubidium-82 PET and thallium-201 SPECT myocardial perfusion imaging utilizing a single dipyridamole stress in the diagnosis of coronary artery disease. *J Nucl Med* 1990;31:1899–1905.

5. Stewart RE, Schwaiger M, Molina E et al. Comparison of rubidium-82 positron emission tomography and thallium-201 SPECT imaging for detection of coronary artery disease. *Am J Cardiol* 1991;67:1303–1310.

6. Herrero P, Markham J, Shelton ME et al. Noninvasive quantification of regional myocardial perfusion with rubidium-82 and positron emission tomography. *Circulation* 1990;82:1377–1386.

7. Herrero P, Markham J, Shelton ME et al. Implementation and evaluation of a two-compartment model for quantification of myocardial perfusion with rubidium-82 and positron emission tomography. *Circ Res* 1992;70:496–507.

8. Ak I, Stokkel MPM, Pauwels EKJ. Positron emission tomography with 2-[18F]fluoro-2-deoxy-D-glucose in oncology. *J Cancer Res Clin Oncol* 2000;126:560–574.

9. Roelcke U, Leenders KL. PET in neuro-oncology. *J Cancer Res Clin Oncol* 2001;127:2–8.

10. Smith TA. FDG Uptake, tumour characteristics and response to therapy: a review. *Nucl Med Commun* 1998;19:97–105.

11. Pauwels EKJ, Sturm EJC, Bombardieri E. Positron-emission tomography with [18F]fluorodeoxyglucose. Part I. Biochemical uptake mechanism and its implication for clinical studies. *J Cancer Res Oncol* 2000;126:549–559.

12. Nieweg OE, Kim EE, Wong W-H et al. Positron emission tomography with fluorine-18-deoxyglucose in the detection and staging of breast cancer. *Cancer* 1993;71:3920–3925.

13. Wahl RL, Cody RL, Hutchins GD et al. Primary and metastatic breast carcinoma: initial clinical evaluation with PET and the radiolabeled glucose analog 2-[F-18]-fluoro-deoxy-2-D-glucose (FDG). *Radiology* 1991;179:3920–3925.

14. van der Hiel B, Pauwels EKJ, Stokkel MPM. Positron emission tomography with 2-[18F]-fluoro-2-deoxy-D-glucose in oncology. Part IIIa: Therapy response monitoring in breast cancer, lymphoma and gliomas. *J Cancer Res Clin Oncol* 2001;127:269–277.

15. Stokkel MPM, Draisma A, Pauwels EKJ. Positron emission tomography with 2-[18F]-fluoro-2-deoxy-D-glucose in oncology. Part IIIb: Therapy response monitoring in colorectal and lung tumors, head and neck cancer, hepatocellular carcinoma and sarcoma. *J Cancer Res Clin Oncol* 2001;127:278–285.

16. Lindholm P, Minn H, Leskinen-Kallio S et al. Influence of the blood glucose concentration on FDG uptake in cancer—a PET study. *J Nucl Med* 1993;34:1–6.

17. Rigo P, Paulus P, Kaschten BJ et al. Oncological applications of positron emission tomography with fluorine-18 fluorodeoxyglucose. *Eur J Nucl Med* 1996;23:1641–1674.

18. Bida GT, Ehrenkaufer RL, Wolf AP et al. The effect of target-gas purity on the chemical form of F-18 during 18F-F2 production using the neon/fluorine target. *J Nucl Med* 1980;21:758–762.

19. Schlyer DJ, Bastos MA, Alexoff D et al. Separation of [18F]fluoride from [180]water using anion exchange resin. *Int J Radiat Applic Instrum A Appl Radiat Isotopes*1990;41:531–533.

20. Hamacher K, Coenen HH, Stocklin G. Efficient stereospecific synthesis of NCA 2-[18F]fluoro-2-deoxy-D-glucose using aminopolyether supported nucleophilic substitution. *J Nucl Med* 1986;27:235–238.

21. Chaly T, Dahl JR. Thin layer chromatographic detection of Kryptofix 2.2.2. in the routine synthesis of [18F]-2-fluoro-deoxyglucose. *Nucl Med Biol* 1989;16:385–387.

22. Mock BH, Winkle W, Vavrek MT. A color spot test for the detection of Kryptofix 2.2.2 in [18F]FDG preparations. *Nucl Med Biol* 1997;24:193–195.

23. Füchtner F, Steinbach J, Mading P et al. Basic hydrolysis of 2-[18F]fluoro-1,3,4,6-tetra-O-Acetyl-D-glucose in the preparation of 2-[18F]fluoro-2-deoxy-D-glucose. *Appl Radiat Isotopes* 1996;47:61–66.

24. Meyer G-J, Matzke KH, Hamacher K et al. The stability of 2-[18F]fluoro-deoxy-D-glucose towards epimerisation under alkaline conditions. *Appl Radiat Isotopes* 1999;51:34–41.

25. Brodak JW, Dence CS, Kilbourn MR et al. Robotic production of

26. Toorongian SA, Mulholland GK, Jewett DM et al. Routine production of 2-deoxy-2-[18F]fluoro-D-glucose by direct nucleophilic exchange on a quaternary 4-aminopyridinium resin. *Nucl Med Biol* 1990;17:273–279.

27. Alexoff DL, Casati R, Fowler JS et al. Ion chromatographic analysis of high specific activity 18FDG preparations and detection of the chemical impurity 2-deoxy-2-chloro-D-glucose. *Int J Radiat Applic Instrum A Appl Radiat Isotopes* 1992;43:1313–1322.

28. Phelps ME, Hoffman EJ, Coleman RE et al. Tomographic images of blood pool and perfusion in brain and heart. *J Nucl Med* 1976;17:603–612.

29. Chen BC, Huang SC, Germano G et al. Noninvasive quantification of hepatic arterial blood flow with nitrogen-13-ammonia and dynamic positron emission tomography. *J Nucl Med* 1991;32:2199–2206.

30. Hayashi N, Tamaki N, Yonekura Y et al. Imaging of the hepatocellular carcinoma using dynamic positron emission tomography with nitrogen-13 ammonia. *J Nucl Med* 1985;26:254–257.

31. Hutchins GD, Schwaiger M, Rosenspire KC et al. Noninvasive quantification of regional blood flow in the human heart using N-13 ammonia and dynamic positron emission tomographic imaging. *J Am Coll Cardiol* 1990;15:1032–1042.

32. Muzik O, Duvernoy C, Beanlands RS et al. Assessment of diagnostic performance of quantitative flow measurements in normal subjects and patients with angiographically documented coronary artery disease by means of nitrogen-13 ammonia and positron emission tomography. *J Am Coll Cardiol* 1998;31:534–540.

33. Krivokapich J, Smith GT, Huang SC et al. 13N ammonia myocardial imaging at rest and with exercise in normal volunteers. Quantification of absolute myocardial perfusion with dynamic positron emission tomography. *Circulation* 1989;80:1328–1337.

34. Tamaki N, Yonekura Y, Yamashita K et al. Value of rest-stress myocardial positron tomography using nitrogen-13 ammonia for the preoperative prediction of reversible asynergy. *J Nucl Med* 1989;30:1302–1310.

35. Kotzerke J, Glatting G, van den Hoff J et al. Validation of myocardial blood flow estimation with nitrogen-13 ammonia PET by the argon inert gas technique in humans. *Eur J Nucl Med* 2001;28:340–345.

36. Walsh W, Harper PV, Resnekov L et al. Noninvasive evaluations of regional myocardial perfusion in 112 patients using a mobile scintillation camera and intravenous nitrogen-13-labeled ammonia. *Circulation* 1976;54:266–275.

37. Niemeyer MG, Kuijper AF, Gerhards LJ et al. Nitrogen-13 ammonia perfusion Imaging: relation to metabolic imaging. *Am Heart J* 1993;125:848–854.

38. Lancellotti P, Melon PG, de Landsheere CM et al. The role of early measurement of nitrogen-13 ammonia uptake for predicting contractile recovery after acute myocardial infarction. *Int J Cardiac Imaging* 1998;14:261–267.

39. Harper PV, Lathrop KA, Krizek H et al. Clinical feasibility of myocardial imaging with 13NH3. *J Nucl Med* 1972;13:278–280.

40. Schelbert HR, Phelps ME, Huang SC et al. N-13 ammonia as an indicator of myocardial blood flow. *Circulation* 1981;63:1259–1272.

41. Monahan WG, Tilbury RS, Laughlin JS. Uptake of 13N-labeled ammonia. *J Nucl Med* 1972;13:274–277.

42. Harper PV, Schwartz J, Beck RN et al. Clinical myocardial imaging with nitrogen-13 ammonia. *Radiology* 1973;108:613–617.

43. Tilbury RS, Dahl JR, Monahan WG et al. The production of 13N-labeled ammonia for medical use. *Radiochem Radionel Lett* 1977;8:317–323.

44. Wieland B, Bida G, Padgett H et al. In-target production of [13N]ammonia via proton irradiation of dilute aqueous ethanol and acetic acid mixtures. *Int J Radiat Applic Instrum A Appl Radiat Isotopes* 1991;42:1095–1098.

45. Channing MA, Dunn BB, Kiesewetter DO et al. The quality of [13N]ammonia produced by using ethanol as a scavenger. *J Labeled Cpds Radioph* 1994;35:334–336.

46. Ferrieri R, MacDonald K, Schlyer DJ et al. Proton irradiation of dilute aqueous ethanol for in-target production of [13N]ammonia:

studies on the fate of ethanol. *J Labelled Comp Radiopharm* 1993;32: 461–463.

47. Brown M, Marshall DR, Sobel BE et al. Delineation of myocardial oxygen utilization with carbon-11-labeled acetate. *Circulation* 1987; 76:687–396.

48. Brown MA, Myears DW, Bergmann SR. Validity of estimates of myocardial oxidative metabolism with carbon-11 acetate and positron emission tomography despite altered patterns of substrate utilization. *J Nucl Med* 1989;30:187–193.

49. Brown MA, Myears DW, Bergmann SR. Noninvasive assessment of canine myocardial oxidative metabolism with carbon-11 acetate and positron emission tomography. *J Am Coll Cardiol* 1988;12: 1054–1063.

50. Buxton DB, Schwaiger M, Nguyen A et al. Radiolabeled acetate as a tracer of myocardial tricarboxylic acid cycle flux. *Circ Res* 1988;63: 628–634.

51. Henes CG, Bergmann SR, Walsh MN et al. Assessment of myocardial oxidative metabolic reserve with positron emission tomography and carbon-11 acetate. *J Nucl Med* 1989;30:1489–1499.

52. Gropler RJ, Siegel BA, Geltman EM. Myocardial uptake of carbon-11-acetate as an indirect estimate of regional myocardial blood flow. *J Nucl Med* 1991;32:245–251.

53. Sun KT, Yeatman LA, Buxton DB et al. Simultaneous measurement of myocardial oxygen consumption and blood flow using [1-carbon-11]acetate. *J Nucl Med* 1998;39:272–280.

54. Miller TR, Wallis JW, Geltman EM et al. Three-dimensional functional images of myocardial oxygen consumption from positron tomography. *J Nucl Med* 1990;31:2064–2068.

55. Hicks RJ, Kalff V, Savas V et al. Assessment of right ventricular oxidative metabolism by positron emission tomography with C-11 acetate in aortic valve disease. *Am J Cardiol* 1991;67:753–757.

56. Porenta G, Cherry S, Czernin J et al. Noninvasive determination of myocardial blood flow, oxygen consumption and efficiency in normal humans by carbon-11 acetate positron emission tomography imaging. *Eur J Nucl Med* 1999;26:1465–1474.

57. Pike VW, Eakins MN, Allan RM et al. Preparation of [1-11C]acetate—an agent for the study of myocardial metabolism by positron emission tomography. *Int J Appl Radiat Isotopes* 1982;33:505–512.

58. Norenberg JP, Simpson NR, Dunn BB et al. Remote synthesis of [11C]acetate. *Appl Radiat Isotopes* 1992;43:943–945.

59. Blau M, Nagler W, Bender MA. Fluorine-18: a new isotope for bone scanning. *J Nucl Med* 1962;3:332–334.

60. Cook GJ, Fogelman I. Detection of bone metastases in cancer patients by 18F-fluoride and 18F-fluorodeoxyglucose positron emission tomography. *Q J Nucl Med* 2001;45:47–52.

61. Firnau G, Garnett ES, Sourkes TL et al. [18F] fluoro-dopa: a unique gamma emitting substrate for dopa decarboxylase. *Experientia* 1975; 31:1254–1255.

62. Garnett ES, Firnau G, Nahmias C. Dopamine visualized in the basal ganglia of living man. *Nature* 1983;305:137–138.

63. Chiueh CC, Zukowska-Grojec Z, Kirk KL et al. 6-Fluorocatecholamines as false adrenergic neurotransmitters. *J Pharmacol Exp Ther* 1983;225:529–533.

64. Anden NE, Carlsson A, Dahlstrom A et al. Demonstration and mapping out of nigro-neostriatal dopamine neurons. *Life Sci* 1964;3: 523–530.

65. Firnau G, Sood S, Chirakal R et al. Cerebral metabolism of 6-[18]fluoro-L-3,4-dihydroxyphenylalanine in the primate. *J Neurochem* 1987; 48:1077–1082.

66. Firnau G, Garnett ES, Chan PK et al. Intracerebral dopamine metabolism studied by a novel radioisotope technique. *J Pharm Pharmacol* 1976;28:584–585.

67. Firnau G, Garnett S, Marshall AM et al. Effects of fluoro-dopamines on dopamine receptors (D1, D2, D3, sites). *Biochem Pharmacol* 1981; 30:2927–2930.

68. Garnett S, Firnau G, Nahmias C et al. Striatal dopamine metabolism in living monkeys examined by positron emission tomography. *Brain Res* 1983;280:169–171.

69. Martin WR, Palmer MR, Patlak CS et al. Nigrostriatal function in humans studied with positron emission tomography. *Ann Neurol* 1989;26:535–542.

70. Martin WRW, Adam MJ, Bergstom M et al. *In vivo study of dopa metabolism in Parkinson's disease.* New York: Raven Press, 1986: 97–102.

71. Boyes BE, Cumming P, Martin WR et al. Determination of plasma [18F]-6-fluorodopa during positron emission tomography: elimination and metabolism in carbidopa treated subjects. *Life Sci* 1986;39: 2243–2252.

72. Ruottinen HM, Niinivirta M, Bergman J et al. Detection of response to COMT inhibition in FDOPA PET in advanced Parkinson's disease requires prolonged imaging. *Synapse* 2001;40:19–26.

73. Martin WR, Stoessl AJ, Adam MJ. Positron emission tomography in Parkinson's disease: glucose and dopa metabolism. In: Yahr MD, Bergmann KJ, eds. *Advances in neurology: Parkinson's disease.* New York: Raven Press, 1986:45:95–98.

74. Leenders KL. Parkinson's disease and PET tracer studies. *J Neural Transm* 1988;27:219–225.

75. Leenders K, Palmer A, Turton D. DOPA uptake and dopamine receptor binding visualized in the human brain in vivo. In: Fahn S, Marsden CD, Jenner P, Teychenne P, eds. *Recent developments in Parkinson's disease.* New York: Raven Press, 1986:103–114.

76. Lang AE, Garnett ES, Firnau G et al. Positron tomography in dystonia. *Adv Neurol* 1988;50:249–253.

77. Leenders KL, Frackowiak RS, Quinn N et al. Brain energy metabolism and dopaminergic function in Huntington's disease measured in vivo using positron emission tomography. *Mov Disord* 1986;1:69–77.

78. Adam MJ, Ruth TJ, Grierson JR et al. Routine synthesis of L-[18F]6-fluorodopa with fluorine-18 acetyl hypofluorite. *J Nucl Med* 1986; 27:1462–1466.

79. Luxen A, Perlmutter M, Bida G. Remote, semiautomated production of 6-[18F]fluoro-L-dopa for human studies with PET. *Appl Radiat Isotopes* 1990;41:275–281.

80. Casella V, Ido T, Wolf AP et al. Anhydrous F-18 labeled elemental fluorine for radiopharmaceutical preparation. *J Nucl Med* 1980;21: 750–757.

81. Luxen A, Guillaume M, Melega WP et al. Production of 6-[18F]fluoro-L-dopa and its metabolism in vivo—a critical review. *Int J Radiat Applic Instrum B Nucl Med Biol* 1992;19:149–158.

82. Namavari M, Bishop A, Satyamurthy N et al. Regioselective radiofluorodestannylation with [18F]F2 and [18F]CH3 COOF: a high yield synthesis of 6-[18F]fluoro-L-dopa. *Appl Radiat Isotopes* 1992;43: 989–996.

83. United States Pharmacopeia (USP). 25.2001:2068-2071.

84. Chen J, Huang S, Finn R. Quality control procedure for 6-[18F]fluoro-L-dopa: a presynaptic PET imaging ligand for brain dopamine neurons. *J Nucl Med* 1989;30:1249–1256.

85. Gunther K, Martens J, Schickedanz M. Resolution of optical isomers by thin layer chromatography (TLC). Enantiomeric purity of L-dopa. *Anal Chem* 1985;322:513–514.

86. Dunn B, Channing M, Adams H et al. A single column, rapid quality control procedure for 6-[18F]fluoro-L-dopa and [18F]fluorodopamine PET imaging agents. *Nucl Med Biol* 1991;18:209–213.

87. Pike VW, Kensett MJ, Turton DR et al. Labelled agents for PET studies of the dopaminergic system—some quality assurance methods, experience and issues. *Int J Radiat Applic Instrum A Appl Radiat Isotopes* 1990;41:483–492.

88. Sachs C, Jonsson G. Selective 6-hydroxy-DOPA induced degeneration of central and peripheral noradrenaline neurons. *Brain Res* 1972; 40:563–568.

89. Ter-Pogossian M, Powers W. The use of radioactive oxygen-15 in the determination of oxygen content in malignant neoplasms. *Radioisotopes Sci Res* 1958;3:1–11.

90. Dyson NA, Sinclair JD, West JB. A comparison of the uptakes of oxygen-15 and oxygen-16 in the lung. *J Physiol* 1960;152:325–336.

91. Dollery CT, West JB. Metabolism of oxygen-15. *Nature* 1960;189: 1121.

92. West JB, Dollery CT. Absorption of inhaled radioactive water vapour. *Nature* 1961;189:588.

93. Iwama T, Akiyama Y, Morimoto M et al. Comparison of positron emission tomography study results of cerebral hemodynamics in patients with bleeding- and ischemic-type Moyamoya disease. *Neurosurg Focus* 1998;5:1–7

94. Yamauchi H, Fukuyama H, Hagahama Y et al. Long-term changes of hemodynamics and metabolism after carotid artery occlusion. *Neurology* 2000;54:2095–2102.

95. Yamauchi H, Fukuyama H, Nagahama Y et al. Evidence of misery perfusion and risk for recurrent stroke in major cerebral arterial occlusive disease from PET. *J Neurol Neurosurg Psychiatry* 1996;61:18–25.

96. Grubb RL Jr, Derdeyn CP, Fritsch SM et al. The importance of hemodynamic factors in the prognosis of symptomatic carotid occlusion. *JAMA* 1998;280:1055–1060.

97. Kabalka GW, Lambrecht RM, Sajjad M et al. Synthesis of [15O]labeled butanol via organoborane chemistry. *Int J Appl Radiat Isotopes* 1985;36:853–855.

98. Takahashi K, Murakami M, Hagami E et al. Radiosynthesis of ^{15}O-labelled hydrogen peroxide. *J Labelled Comp Radiopharm* 1989;27:1167–1175.

99. Shields AF, Grierson JR, Dohmen BM et al. Imaging proliferation *in vivo* with [F-18]FLT and positron emission tomography. *Nature Med* 1998;4:1334–1336.

100. Nunn A, Linder K, Strauss HW. Nitroimidazoles and imaging hypoxia. *Eur J Nucl Med* 1995;22:265–280.

101. Shelton ME, Dence CS, Hwang DR et al. Myocardial kinetics of fluorine-18 misonidazole: a marker of hypoxic myocardium. *J Nucl Med* 1989;30:351–358.

102. Martin GV, Caldwell JH, Graham MM et al. Noninvasive detection of hypoxic myocardium using fluorine-18-fluoromisonidazole and positron emission tomography. *J Nucl Med* 1992;33:2202–2208.

103. Dearling JL, Lewis JS, Mullen GE et al. Design of hypoxia-targeting radiopharmaceuticals: selective uptake of copper-64 complexes in hypoxic cells in vitro. *Eur J Nucl Med* 1998;25:788–792.

104. Lewis JS, McCarthy DW, McCarthy TJ et al. Evaluation of 64Cu-ATSM in vitro and in vivo in a hypoxic tumor model. *J Nucl Med* 1999;40:177–183.

105. Lewis JS, Sharp TL, Laforest R et al. Tumor uptake of copper-diacetyl-bis(*N*4-methylthiosemicarbazone): effect of changes in tissue oxygenation. *J Nucl Med* 2001;42:655–661.

106. Haynes NG, Lacy JL, Nayak N et al. Performance of a 62Zn/62Cu generator in clinical trials of PET perfusion agent 62Cu-PTSM. *J Nucl Med* 2000;41:309–314.

107. McCarthy DW, Shefer RE, Klinkowstein RE et al. Efficient production of high specific activity 64Cu using a biomedical cyclotron. *Nucl Med Biol* 1997;24:35–43.

108. McCarthy DW, Bass LA, Cutler PD et al. High purity production and potential applications of copper-60 and copper-61. *Nucl Med Biol* 1999;26:351–358.

109. Tjuvajev JG, Finn R, Watanabe K et al. Noninvasive imaging of herpes virus thymidine kinase gene transfer and expression: a potential method for monitoring clinical gene therapy. *Cancer Res* 1996;56:4087–4095.

110. Alauddin MM, Conti PS, Mazza SM et al. Synthesis of 9-[(3-[18F]fluoro-1-hydroxy-2-propoxy)methyl]guanine ([18F]FHPG): a potential imaging agent of viral infection and gene therapy using PET. *Nucl Med Biol* 1996;23:787–792.

111. Barrio JR, Namavari M, Srinivasan A et al. Carbon-8 radiofluorination of purines: a general approach to probe design for gene therapy in humans. *J Labelled Comp Radiopharm* 1997;40:348.

112. Shiue C-Y, Hustinx R, Zhuang H et al. 9-[(3-[18F]fluoro-1-hydroxy-2-propoxy)methyl]guanine ([18F]FHPG): a promising agent for monitoring HSV1-tk gene transfer to tumors. *J Labelled Comp Radiopharm* 1999;42:S13–15.

9

RADIATION PROTECTION

JERROLD T. BUSHBERG
EDWIN M. LEIDHOLDT, JR.

The use of ionizing radiation in nuclear medicine carries with it a responsibility to both patient and staff to maximize the diagnostic and therapeutic benefit while minimizing the potential for adverse health effects. Shortly after the discovery of the x-ray by Roentgen in 1895, the potential for acute health hazards of ionizing radiation became apparent. However, the risks of delayed effects from ionizing radiation were not known, and many early users did not believe that anyone could be hurt by something that could not be detected by any of the human senses. Many experiments on the biologic effects of ionizing radiation began in the early 1900s, and the first radiation protection standards were proposed by the British Roentgen Society in 1915. We now realize that these pioneers had a very limited knowledge of the hazards of ionizing radiation and of the principles of radiation protection.

Some uncertainties remain regarding the risks to humans of certain health effects from ionizing radiation, particularly cancer and genetic effects from low-dose and low-dose rate radiation. Despite this, however, more scientific data are available today on the health effects of ionizing radiation than on any other physical agent or chemical. The use of most forms of ionizing radiation is heavily regulated at both the national and state levels.

QUANTITIES AND UNITS IN RADIATION DOSIMETRY

Absorbed Dose

The amount and rate of energy deposition in tissue are major determinants of biologic effects. The *absorbed dose* is defined as the amount of energy imparted to matter by ionizing radiation per unit mass (1–4). The Système Internationale (SI) unit of absorbed dose is the gray (Gy). A gray is defined as one joule (J) of energy deposited per kilogram (kg) of matter. The traditional unit of absorbed dose is the rad, originally an acronym for *r*adiation *a*bsorbed *d*ose. A rad is defined as 0.01 J/kg; thus,

one rad is equal to 0.01 gray. Absorbed dose is defined for all types of ionizing radiation and matter. Absorbed dose to soft tissue is most relevant in radiation protection.

A disadvantage to the quantity absorbed dose is that it is difficult to measure directly, especially in radiation protection applications. Instead, it is usually inferred from measurements of other quantities, such as ionization per mass of air.

The x-rays and γ-rays used in nuclear medicine deposit their energy in matter by photoelectric absorption and Compton scattering. The absorbed dose can be calculated from the mass energy absorption coefficient of a material, if the fluence (number of photons per unit area) and the energies of the photons are known. The absorbed dose to an organ or tissue from a radiopharmaceutical includes energy deposition from both particulate radiations and photons.

Although one gray (100 rad) is a very large radiation dose to man, it represents an extremely small energy deposition per mass of matter. The energy in a gray, if deposited as heat, would raise the temperature of water by approximately 2.4×10^{-4}°C.

Exposure

The intensity of x radiation or γ radiation at a particular location can be expressed as the radiation's ability to ionize air at that location. *Exposure* is defined as the total amount of ionization (electrical charge) produced per mass of air, when all the electrons produced in that mass of air are completely stopped in air (1,2). The SI unit of exposure is the coulomb per kilogram (C/kg). The traditional unit of radiation exposure is the roentgen (R). A roentgen is defined as the amount of x-radiation or γ radiation that produces 2.58×10^{-4} coulomb of charge per kilogram of air.

Exposure is a useful quantity for several reasons. It is a direct measure of ionization; ionization is the initiating event in most biologic damage. Exposure can be easily measured by portable air-filled ionization chambers. Furthermore, the atomic numbers of the elements constituting air are close to those of the elements comprising soft tissue and so exposure is nearly proportional to the absorbed dose to soft tissue over a considerable range of photon energies.

It is important to appreciate the limitations inherent in the use of exposure:

J.T. Bushberg: Department of Radiology, and Environmental Health & Safety, UC Davis Medical Center, Sacramento, CA.

E.M. Leidholdt: Radiology, University of California, Davis, and Southwestern Service Area VHA National Health Physics Program, US Department of Veterans Affairs, Mare Island, CA.

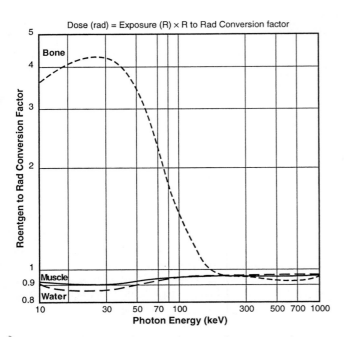

FIGURE 9.1. The roentgen-to-rad conversion factor versus photon energy for water, muscle, and bone. (From Bushberg JT, Seibert JA, Leidholdt EM, et al. *The essential physics of medical imaging*, 2nd edition Philadelphia: Lippincott Williams & Wilkins, 2002, with permission.)

1. It is defined only for x-rays and γ-rays (i.e., not energetic charged particles).
2. It is difficult to measure for photons with energies greater than a few MeV.
3. It is defined for ionization in air only.
4. An ambient air ionization chamber is affected by atmospheric pressure and temperature, which determine the mass of air in the fixed volume of the chamber. Corrections for variations in atmospheric pressure and temperature are usually modest.

The ratio of absorbed dose per unit of radiation exposure (i.e., rad/roentgen) is called the *f-factor* and has been determined for various tissues. Thus, if the exposure and the energy of the x-rays or γ-rays are known, the absorbed dose can be determined. The f-factors for water, muscle, and bone are shown in Fig. 9.1. Notice that the exposure in roentgens is within approximately 10% of the absorbed dose to soft tissue in centigray (rad) over the range of photon energies encountered in nuclear medicine.

Kerma and Air Kerma

Ionizing electromagnetic radiations, such as x-rays and γ-rays, deposit energy in matter by a two-stage process. First, they interact with atoms by the photoelectric process; Compton effect; and, for very high energy photons, pair production, releasing or creating energetic electrons. Second, the energetic electrons deposit energy in matter by ionization and excitation.

The amount of kinetic energy per mass of matter given to these energetic electrons in the first stage is called *kerma* (1,2), originally an acronym for *kinetic energy released in matter*. The SI unit of kerma is the gray, defined earlier in this chapter.

When matter is irradiated by low-energy photons, the released electrons also have low energies and travel only short distances. In this case, the kerma and absorbed dose at a particular location are nearly equal. On the other hand, high-energy photons generate high-energy electrons that may travel considerable distances in matter. In this case, the kerma and absorbed dose at a particular location may differ significantly.

Air-filled ionization chamber instruments may be calibrated to indicate air kerma rate instead of exposure rate. Air kerma and exposure are nearly proportional over a wide range of photon energies. An exposure of one roentgen is equivalent to an air kerma of 8.76 mGy.

Equivalent Dose and Dose Equivalent

The absorbed dose and dose rate are not the only determinants of biologic damage. An additional factor is the microscopic energy deposition pattern. In interacting with an absorber, all forms of ionizing radiation liberate charged particles that, for the purpose of predicting their microscopic energy deposition patterns, can be described by mass, charge, and kinetic energy. The average number of ion pairs formed by a particular radiation per unit path-length is referred to as its *specific ionization* and is expressed in units of ion pairs per micrometer. A related quantity is the *linear energy transfer* (LET), which is the average energy deposited locally per unit path-length. LET is commonly expressed in keV/μm.

Those forms of radiation that produce dense ionization patterns (i.e., high LET radiations) have been shown to produce greater amounts of irreparable damage in both cellular and complex biologic systems per unit dose than low LET radiations. Radiobiologists describe this difference in biologic response by comparing a particular "test" radiation to a standard radiation (often 250 kVp x-rays). A biologic end point is selected for observation (e.g., 37% cell survival in irradiated cell cultures), and the doses necessary to produce this end point for the test and standard radiations are determined experimentally. The ratio of the dose required for the standard radiation to the dose required for the test radiation is referred to as the *relative biologic effectiveness* (RBE) of the test radiation. The RBEs of various radiations typically range from 1 to about 80 for both mammalian systems and cells in culture (5).

This information has been used to establish modifying *radiation weighting factors* (w_R) to the absorbed dose that express the relative biologic hazards of specified forms of radiation. These weighting factors have been established for both particulate and electromagnetic radiations of various energies and are listed in Table 9.1.

The absorbed dose (in gray or rad) can be modified to represent the biologic hazard of the radiation by multiplying the absorbed dose by the radiation weighting factor for that type of radiation. This product is referred to as the *equivalent dose* (4). If an individual is exposed to more than one type of radiation, the equivalent dose is the sum of the products of the absorbed doses from each type of radiation and the weighting factors.

$$H_T = \sum_R w_R \cdot D_{T.R} \qquad [1]$$

where $D_{T.R}$ is the average absorbed dose to an organ or tissue

Table 9.1. *Radiation Weighting Factors*

Type and Energy of Radiation	Radiation Weighting Factor (w_T)
Photons (x- and γ-rays), all energies	1
Electrons and muons, all energies	1
Neutrons, energy <10 keV	5
10 keV to 100 keV	10
>100 keV to 2 MeV	20
>2 MeV to 20 MeV	10
>20 MeV	5
Protons, other than recoil protons, energy >2 MeV	5
alpha particles, fission fragments, heavy nuclei	20

Source: Adapted from 4.

T from radiation of type R (3,4). The SI unit of equivalent dose is the sievert (Sv); thus, one gray of a radiation with a radiation weighting factor of one will yield an equivalent dose of one Sv. The traditional unit of equivalent dose is the rem (originally an acronym for *roentgen-equivalent-m*an); one rem is equal to 0.01 Sv.

For example, if a person were to accidentally ingest a mixture of radioactive materials from which the dose to the gastrointestinal tract is 50 mGy (5 rad) from α-particles, 30 mGy (3 rad) from β-particles, and 20 mGy (2 rad) from γ-rays, the absorbed dose would be

$$D = 50 \text{ mGy} + 30 \text{ mGy} + 20 \text{ mGy} =$$
$$100 \text{ mGy} = 10 \text{ rad}$$

However, the equivalent dose to the gastrointestinal tract would be

$$H = (50 \ mGy)(20) + (30 \ mGy)(1) + (20 \ mGy)(1p6$$
$$= 1.05 \ Sv = 105 rem.$$

The quantity equivalent dose coexists with an older but similar quantity, *dose equivalent* (1,2,3). The dose equivalent, similar to the equivalent dose, is intended to reflect the biologic harm from absorbed doses of different types of radiation. It is calculated as the sum of the products of the absorbed doses from each type of radiation and quality factors (Q), similar to the radiation weighting factors w_R, which reflect the relative harm from different types of radiation.

$$H = \sum_R Q_R \cdot D_R \qquad [2]$$

where D_R is the absorbed dose from radiation R at a point and Q_R is the quality factor for that type of radiation (1–3). The quality factors are listed as a function of LET in Table 9.2.

Table 9.2. *Quality Factors as a Function of the Linear Energy Transfer of the Radiation*

Quality Factor	Linear Energy Transfer L (keV/μm)
1	L $\leq$ 10
0.32 L $-$ 2.2	10 < L < 100
$300/\sqrt{L}$	L $\geq$ 100

Note: The quality factor is one for photons and electrons, because the linear energy transfer of electrons is less than 10 keV per μm.
Source: Adapted from 3.

The units of dose equivalent are the sievert (Sv) and the rem (traditional). The major distinction between the two quantities is that dose equivalent is computed from the absorbed dose at a point, whereas the equivalent dose is calculated from the average dose to a tissue or organ. The quantity dose equivalent is used in the current U.S. Nuclear Regulatory Commission (NRC) regulations.

Effective Dose

A common problem in personnel dosimetry occurs when the body is exposed to ionizing radiation in a nonuniform manner, either from external sources (e.g., the fluoroscopist who wears a lead apron) or internal sources (e.g., a person who inhales ^{131}I). In 1977, in an attempt to compare detriment from nonuniform exposure of the body with detriment from uniform exposure of the body, the International Commission on Radiological Protection (ICRP) proposed a new scheme for dose limitation (6). The scheme defined a weighted average of the dose equivalents to the various tissues and organs of the body.

$$E = \sum_T w_T \cdot H_T \qquad [3]$$

where the H_T are the average dose equivalents to the various tissues or organs of the body and the tissue weighting factors w_T, listed in Column 2 of Table 9.3, reflect the relative risk of detrimental effects. The sum of the tissue weighting factors w_T is one.

$$\sum_T w_T = 1.0 \qquad [4]$$

The weighted equivalent dose E became known as the *effective dose equivalent* (ede). In 1990, the ICRP revised the scheme, with new tissue weighting factors (Table 9.3, Column 3) (4). The weighted equivalent dose was then given the name *effective*

Table 9.3. *Tissue Weighting Factors(w_T)*

Tissue	Tissue Weighting Factors (ICRP Publication 26, 1977)	Tissue Weighting Factors (ICRP Publication 60, 1990)
Gonads	0.25	0.20
Red bone marrow	0.12	0.12
Colon		0.12
Lung	0.12	0.12
Stomach		0.12
Bladder		0.05
Breast	0.15	0.05
Liver		0.05
Esophagus		0.05
Thyroid	0.03	0.05
Skin		0.01
Bone surfaces	0.03	0.01
Remainder	0.30	0.05
Sum	1.00	1.00

Note: The U.S. Nuclear Regulatory Commission's system of dose limitation (contained in Title 10 Part 20, of the Code of Federal Regulations) incorporates the ICRP 26 tissue weighting factors. ICRP Publications 26 and 60 describe how the remainder terms are to be applied to organs not assigned weighting factors.

dose to distinguish it from the ede, which was based on the older tissue weighting factors. However, the system of dose limitation mandated by the NRC uses the older 1977 weighting factors. The quantities effective dose equivalent and effective dose are specified in the same units as equivalent dose, i.e., sievert (Sv) or rem (traditional).

To illustrate the concept of effective dose, one can compare the risk from 50 μSv (5 mrem) equivalent dose to the gonads with a similar exposure to the whole body. The effective dose from the gonadal exposure is

$$E = \left(\text{equivalent dose to the gonads}\right)$$
$$\cdot \left(\text{tissue weighting factor for the gonads}\right)$$
$$= 50 \ \mu Sv \times 0.20 = 10 \ \mu Sv.$$

In other words, the detriment from a gonadal dose of 50 μSv is similar to that from a uniform exposure of 10 μSv (1 mrem) to the entire body.

The effective dose concept permits the risk of stochastic effects from nonuniform exposures of the body to be estimated. The ICRP estimates the risk of fatal cancer, for working adults, to be 4×10^{-2} deaths per Sv (4×10^{-4} per rem) (4). The ICRP estimates the risk to be two or three times higher for infants and children and substantially lower for adults older than 50 years (7).

A possible disadvantage to the quantity effective dose is that it fails to account for nonuniform irradiation of individual tissues and organs. The dose distribution within a particular organ or tissue from incorporated radioactivity can be very nonuniform, particularly when the distribution of radioactivity is not uniform and when the radionuclide emits charged particles of short range.

Committed Equivalent Dose and Committed Effective Dose

Another facet of radiation dosimetry is the situation in which radioactive material is injected into the body, inhaled, ingested, or absorbed through the skin. The exposure from incorporated radioactivity continues until the activity is eliminated from the body by biologic excretion and radioactive decay. If a radionuclide has a sufficiently long half-life and the biologic excretion is sufficiently slow, the activity irradiates the individual over the remainder of his or her life. The *committed equivalent dose* is the equivalent dose to a particular tissue or organ over a specified length of time.

$$H_{c,T}(\tau) = \int_0^{\tau} \dot{H}_T(t)dt \qquad [5]$$

where $\dot{H}_T(t)$ is the equivalent dose rate to the organ or tissue T from radioactivity throughout the body at time t and τ is the specified time interval (4). The *committed effective dose* is the sum of committed equivalent doses to the various organs and tissues of the body, each weighted by the appropriate tissue weighting factor w_T.

$$E_c(\tau) = \sum_T w_T \cdot H_{c,T}(\tau) \qquad [6]$$

The units of committed equivalent and effective dose are the

sievert (Sv) and rem (traditional). If the length of time τ is not specified, it is assumed to be 50 years for adults and from intake to age 70 years for children (4).

Dosimetric Quantities for Populations

For a comparison of the possible effects of various sources of radiation on a population, the *collective effective dose* is defined as the sum of the effective doses of each person in the population (4). The SI unit of collective effective dose is the man-sievert. For example, if 100 people were each exposed to one mSv (100 mrem), the collective effective dose would be 0.1 man-sievert (10 man-rem). This concept necessarily implies (a) linearity between radiation dose and detrimental effect and (b) that there is no threshold level for the detriment. The reliability of these assumptions are difficult to prove; however, most scientists believe that calculations made in this manner lead to a conservative estimate of detriment.

The *genetically significant dose* is a measure of genetic detriment to a population. It is defined as the dose that, if given to every member of the population, would produce the same genetic detriment as the actual doses received by the various individuals.

SOURCES OF EXPOSURE

Natural Sources of Radiation Exposure

Natural sources of radiation include cosmic rays and cosmogenic and primordial radionuclides. Cosmic rays are an external source of exposure, cosmogenic radionuclides are primarily an internal source, whereas primordial radionuclides, primarily radon, contribute to both the external and internal exposure, as well as exposure to the bronchial epithelium from airborne activity. The exposures from radionuclides in the soil and cosmic rays vary significantly throughout the world (8,9,10). The average annual effective dose equivalent to the populations of the United States and Canada from all natural sources is estimated to be approximately 3 mSv (300 mrem) per year. Medical exposures from diagnostic x-ray and nuclear medicine sources add approximately 0.54 mSv (54 mrem) (11) per year to this value. These estimates of medical exposure are based on surveys performed circa 1980 and may not reflect current values. Adding the exposures from common products, such as tobacco (12,13,14), raises the average annual effective dose equivalent to 3.6 mSv (360 mrem) from natural and technology based sources of radiation. The components of the average annual effective dose equivalent to the population of the United States are listed in Table 9.4.

REGULATIONS PERTAINING TO THE USE OF RADIATION

Advisory Bodies

A number of advisory groups publish information and recommendations relevant to protection against ionizing radiation. Although the recommendations of these groups do not carry the force of law, they often become "standards of practice" and may

Table 9.4. *Contributions to the Annual Effective Dose Equivalent of the Population of the United States Circa 1980–1982*

Source	Number of People Exposed (thousands)	Average Annual Effective Dose Equivalent in the Exposed Population (mSv)	Average Annual Effective Dose Equivalent in the U.S. Population (mSv)	% of Total Average Annual Effective Dose Equivalent in the U.S. Population
Natural sources				
Radon	230,000	2.0	2.0	55
Cosmic radiation	230,000	0.27	0.27	8
Cosmogenic radionuclides	230,000	0.01	0.01	<1
External terrestrial	230,000	0.28	0.28	8
Internal radionuclides	230,000	0.39	0.39	11
Occupational	930	2.3	0.009	<<1
Nuclear fuel cycle	—	—	0.0005	<<1
Consumer products				
Tobacco	50,000	—	—	
Other	120,000	0.05–0.3	0.05–0.13	3
Miscellaneous	25,000	0.006	0.0006	<<1
Environmental				
Sources				
Medical				
Diagnostic x-rays	—[a]	—	0.39	11
Nuclear medicine	—[a]	—	0.14	4
Rounded total	230,000		3.6	100

[a]The number of examinations is known, but not the number of exposed persons.
Source: Adapted from 13.

be incorporated into regulations by regulatory agencies. The ICRP, founded in 1928, is the most eminent of these bodies. It is composed of internationally recognized experts in many fields relevant to radiation protection. It was founded to provide guidance relevant to the use of x-rays and radium in medicine but has since broadened its interests to encompass other sources and uses of radiation and radioactive material. However, it retains a special relationship with the profession of radiology.

The National Council on Radiation Protection and Measurements (NCRP) is a prestigious nonprofit corporation chartered by Congress in 1964. Its members consist of experts in ionizing and nonionizing radiation and related disciplines. It has a role similar to that of the ICRP but provides recommendations with a national rather than international perspective. The ICRP and NCRP have issued well over 200 monographs relevant to radiation protection.

Regulatory Agencies

The NRC is a Federal agency charged with regulating the production and use of radioactive material created by nuclear reactors, called *byproduct material,* or that can be used to fuel nuclear reactors. It was established by the Energy Reorganization Act of 1974, which abolished the U.S. Atomic Energy Commission and transferred its licensing and regulatory functions to the NRC. The NRC has no jurisdiction over radioactive materials produced by particle accelerators and naturally occurring radioactive materials other than uranium and thorium.

The NRC's regulations are contained in Title 10 of the Code of Federal Regulations (CFR). Portions of these regulations relevant to the medical use of byproduct material include Part 19 (10 CFR 19), which requires the training of workers in radiation safety precautions and notification of workers of their radiation

exposures; Part 20 (10 CFR 20), entitled *Standards for Protection Against Radiation,* which establishes a system for the limitation of radiation doses to workers and members of the public and contains regulations on many other topics, including the disposal of radioactive waste; and Part 35 (10 CFR 35), entitled *Medical Use of Byproduct Material,* which contains regulations regarding to the use of radioactive material in nuclear medicine and radiation oncology (15–17). In addition to promulgating regulations, the NRC issues advisory documents containing suggested methods for complying with the regulations (18–27).

At the time of writing, the NRC has published an extensive revision of Part 35 as a final regulation. The stated goal of the revision is to "focus NRC's regulations on those medical procedures that pose the highest risk to workers, patients, and the public, and to structure its regulations to be risk-informed and more performance based . . ." (28). The new Part 35 is less prescriptive than the previous Part 35, particularly regarding the use of radiopharmaceuticals for routine diagnostic procedures. For example, the previous Part 35 requires the use of syringe radiation shields when administering radiopharmaceuticals by injection, except when the use of a shield is contraindicated in the case of a specific patient, whereas the use of syringe shields, although still regarded as good practice, is not specifically required by the new Part 35.

The NRC has an inspection and enforcement program to ensure compliance with their regulations. The NRC periodically inspects facilities it has licensed. Should violations be discovered, the NRC can levy fines, place additional restrictions on the use of byproduct material, and even withdraw permission to use byproduct material. In extreme circumstances, the NRC can seek criminal penalties against individuals.

The NRC is permitted to transfer its responsibilities for regulating byproduct material to state governments, provided that the states establish and enforce regulations similar to those of the NRC. States granted these powers are called *agreement states.* Thirty-two states are currently agreement states.

The shipping of radioactive material is regulated by the U.S. Department of Transportation (DOT). The regulations of the DOT are contained in Title 49 of the Code of Federal Regulations. The production of radiopharmaceuticals, the testing in humans of radiopharmaceuticals under development, and the administration of radioactive substances to humans for basic research are regulated by the U.S. Food and Drug Administration (FDA), whose regulations are contained in Title 21 of the Code of Federal Regulations.

Standards for Protection against Radiation

As mentioned in the preceding section, the NRC has promulgated *Standards for Protection Against Radiation* (10 CFR 20) to protect persons who are occupationally exposed to radiation and members of the public. These regulations incorporate, with modifications, the system for dose limitation published in ICRP Publications 26 and 30 (6,29). This system was intended to prevent deterministic effects (effects not occurring for doses below a threshold and whose severities increase with increasing dose beyond the threshold; these effects include cataracts, reduction in fertility, and hematologic consequences of bone marrow depletion) and limit the probability of stochastic effects (effects whose probabilities increase with increasing dose but whose severities are unaffected by dose, such as cancer and hereditary defects).

The system of dose limitation imposes two requirements: (a) all exposures must be maintained as low as reasonably achievable (ALARA), social and economic factors being taken into account, and (b) the exposures to individuals must not exceed the limits provided in the regulations. These NRC regulations adopt, with modifications, the system proposed in ICRP Publications 26 and 30 for summing doses from radionuclides incorporated into the body and doses from sources external to the body and provide a set of limits for the sums.

Summing Internal and External Doses

Doses to an individual from sources external to the body are usually determined by a dosimeter worn on the part of the body, other than the extremities, likely to receive the greatest dose. The body dosimeter indicates the deep dose equivalent and the shallow dose equivalent from external sources. The *deep dose equivalent* is the dose equivalent at a depth of 1 cm of tissue and the *shallow dose equivalent* is the dose equivalent at a depth of 0.007 cm of tissue. The NRC's main modifications to the ICRP Publication 26 system are

1. The NRC requires the deep dose equivalent to be determined for the part of the body, other than the extremities, receiving the highest exposure.
2. Under the NRC scheme, all organs and tissues of the body (except the skin and the lenses of the eyes) are assumed to receive the deep dose equivalent from external sources.

The committed dose equivalent and committed effective dose equivalent are due only to exposure from radionuclides incorporated into the body. The *committed dose equivalent* ($H_{T,50}$) is the dose equivalent to a tissue or organ T over the 50 years following the ingestion or inhalation of radioactivity. The *committed effective dose equivalent* ($H_{E,50}$) is the weighted average of the committed dose equivalents to the various organs and tissues of the body

$$H_{E,50} = \sum_T w_T \cdot H_{T,50} \qquad [7]$$

where the tissue weighting factors w_T are those from ICRP Publication 26 (Table 9.3, Column 2). The *total effective dose equivalent* is the sum of the deep dose equivalent and the committed effective dose equivalent.

Dose Limits

The dose limits for persons who are occupationally exposed are

1. Total effective dose equivalent: 0.05 Sv (5 rem) per year
2. The sum of the deep dose equivalent and the committed dose equivalent to any individual organ or tissue: 0.5 Sv (50 rem) per year
3. Shallow dose equivalent to the skin or any extremity: 0.5 Sv (50 rem) per year
4. Eye dose equivalent (dose equivalent to the lens of the eye): 0.15 Sv (15 rem) per year

Occupational exposures to minors (persons younger than 18 years) may be no more than 10% of the previously mentioned limits. The dose to an embryo or fetus, from the occupational exposure of a declared pregnant woman, may not exceed 0.005 Sv (0.5 rem) over the duration of the pregnancy. (A declared pregnant woman is a woman who has voluntarily chosen to declare her pregnancy in writing to her employer.) Efforts must be made to avoid substantial variation above a uniform monthly exposure rate.

The total effective dose equivalent to "individual members of the public" shall not exceed one mSv (100 mrem) per year. The dose of radiation in an unrestricted area may not exceed 0.02 mSv (2 mrem) in any 1 hour. Individual members of the public include employees who are not occupationally exposed. For example, a dietitian whose office is adjacent to the radiopharmacy in nuclear medicine would be considered an individual member of the public.

Based on the estimated risk of cancer per unit of effective dose and in an attempt to maintain the risk to radiation workers comparable to those of workers in industries deemed to be safe, both the ICRP and the NCRP recommend occupational dose limits more stringent than those currently set by the NRC (Table 9.5).

Annual Limits on Intake and Derived Air Concentrations

In practice, the committed dose equivalent and committed effective dose equivalent are rarely used for demonstrating compliance with the dose limits. Instead, compliance is usually demonstrated by one of two methods. In the first method, an individu-

Table 9.5. *Comparison of Current U.S. Nuclear Regulatory Commission Dose Limits*

	Recommendations		Regulations
	ICRP Publication 60 (1990)	**NCRP Report No. 116 (1993)**	**U.S. NRC 10 CFR 20**
Occupational limits			
Effective dose	50 mSv *and* 100 mSv in 5 years	50 mSv *and* 10 mSv × age (y)	50 mSv (effective dose equivalent[a])
Lens of eye	150 mSv	150 mSv	150 mSv
Skin, hands, feet	500 mSv	500 mSv	500 mSv
Any organ or tissue	—	—	500 mSv
Embryo or fetus	2 mSv external dose to abdomen and limit intakes to 1/20 of an ALI for remainder of pregnancy[b]	Equivalent dose to fetus 0.5 mSv per month[b]	Dose to fetus 5 mSv during entire pregnancy
Public dose limits			
Effective dose	1 mSv *and, if needed,* higher values provided 5 mSv not exceeded over 5 years	1 mSv for continuous exposures *and* 5 mSv for infrequent exposures	1 mSv (effective dose equivalent[c])

Note: Largely based upon recommendations of the ICRP published in 1977 and 1979, with the current recommendations of the ICRP and NCRP. All limits are annual limits, unless otherwise specified.
[a]The effective dose equivalent is similar to the effective dose, but based upon tissue weighing factors published by the ICRP in 1977.
[b]After pregnancy is known.
[c]Exclusive of the dose contribution from patients administered radioactive material.

al's intake of radioactive material is estimated and compared to an *annual limit on intake* (ALI). The ALI is the activity of a radionuclide that, if inhaled or ingested, would produce a committed dose equivalent of 0.5 Sv (50 rem) in any individual organ or tissue or a committed effective dose equivalent of 0.05 Sv (5 rem). ALIs for inhalation of airborne radioactive materials of interest in nuclear medicine are listed in Table 9.6. ALIs are not listed for noble gases because very little of the inhaled activity is retained in the body; most of the dose from them is due to external exposure from the cloud of gas surrounding the exposed individual. When the ALI is determined by the limit on the committed dose equivalent to an organ (0.5 Sv), as is the case for ^{131}I, the name of the organ is listed after the ALI, followed in parentheses by the activity that would cause a committed effective dose equivalent of 0.05 Sv.

Alternatively, the air concentration of a radionuclide may be measured and compared to its *derived air concentration* (DAC).

Table 9.6. *Annual Limits on Intake (ALIs) and Derived Air Concentrations (DACs) Established by the NRC for Radionuclides Likely to Become Airborne in the Nuclear Medicine Department*

Radiochemical	ALI for Inhalation (μCi)	DAC (μCi/ml)	Airborne Effluent Concentration (μCi/ml)
^{99m}Tc aerosol	20,000	1 × 10^{-4}	3 × 10^{-7}
^{131}I (any form)	50 (thyroid) 200[a]	2 × 10^{-8}	2 × 10^{-10}
^{133}Xe	not defined[b]	1 × 10^{-4}	5 × 10^{-7}

Note: ALIs and DACs pertain to restricted areas, whereas airborne effluent concentrations apply to effluents released to unrestricted areas.
[a]Whenever the concentration of a particular radionuclide is limited by the dose to a specific organ, the critical organ is listed after the ALI, followed by the activity that would cause an effective dose equivalent of 0.05 mSv (5 rem).
[b]ALI is not listed, because the vast majority of the dose is from photons emitted from the cloud of gas surrounding the worker and very little is from gas inhaled by the worker.

The DAC is the concentration of a radionuclide in air that, if breathed under conditions of light activity for 2,000 hours, would result in the inhalation of the ALI. Table 9.6 also lists the DACs of airborne radioactive materials likely to be encountered in nuclear medicine.

If an individual is exposed to a single airborne radionuclide and his or her exposure from external sources is less than one tenth of the dose limit (0.5 rem for a nonpregnant adult worker), it is sufficient to demonstrate that his or her intake is less than an ALI. However, if these conditions are not met, it must be demonstrated that the dose to each organ does not exceed 50 rem, and the total effective dose equivalent does not exceed 5 rem.

Example Assume that a worker could receive a deep dose equivalent up to 2.5 rem in a year from external sources. What is the maximal activity of ^{131}I that could be inhaled by this worker without causing the worker to exceed the limits?

Solution To ensure that the dose equivalent to the worker's thyroid does not exceed 50 rem

$$\frac{2.5\,rem}{50\,rem} + \frac{intake}{50\,\mu Ci} \leq 1$$
$$intake \leq 47.5\,\mu Ci$$

To ensure that the worker's total effective dose equivalent does not exceed 5 rem

$$\frac{2.5\,rem}{5\,rem} + \frac{intake}{200\,\mu Ci} \leq 1$$
$$intake \leq 100\,\mu Ci$$

The maximal permissible intake of ^{131}I is therefore the smaller of the two, or 47.5 μCi.

PERSONNEL DOSIMETRY

Personnel dosimetry is the determination of the exposures of people to ionizing radiation. Personnel dosimeters are devices worn to measure doses to persons from external sources of radiation. There are many devices available today that may serve as personnel dosimeters. One way to assess currently available devices is to compare them to an ideal dosimeter. An ideal dosimeter would have the following characteristics:

1. The response of the dosimeter would be independent of radiation energy (linear energy response).
2. The response of the dosimeter would be independent of its orientation relative to the direction of the incident radiation. This is called geometry independence.
3. The dosimeter would be sensitive enough to record exposure slightly over background [~20 μGy/week (2 mrad/week)] and have a range large enough to record serious overexposures [e.g., ~5 Gy (500 rad)].
4. The dosimeter would respond only to ionizing radiation, would not be affected by other environmental conditions (e.g., heat and humidity), and would not lose stored information with time.
5. The dosimeter would indicate separately the doses from α, β, γ, and neutron radiations of various energy ranges.
6. The radiation dose would be readable immediately but also permanently recorded for future analysis.
7. The dosimeter would be tissue equivalent so that the results can be expressed directly as absorbed dose to tissue.
8. The dosimeter would be small, lightweight, rugged, easy to use, and inexpensive.

No dosimeter available today meets all of the ideal characteristics. In fact, some of the ideal characteristics are not satisfied by any currently available dosimeters.

The NRC requires all persons whose doses from external sources are likely to exceed 10% of the occupational limits listed above to wear dosimeters (16). The NRC requires dosimeters used to measure the dose to the body to indicate the deep, eye, and shallow dose equivalents and extremity dosimeters (wrist or finger dosimeters) to indicate shallow dose equivalents. The deep dose equivalent is the dose equivalent at a tissue depth of 1 cm, the eye dose equivalent is the dose equivalent at a tissue depth of 0.3 cm, and the shallow dose equivalent is the dose equivalent at a tissue depth of 0.007 cm. The NRC also requires personnel dosimeters other than pocket ion chambers and electronic dosimeters to be processed by a dosimetry processor accredited by the National Voluntary Laboratory Accreditation Program (NVLAP) of the U.S. National Institute of Standards and Technologies.

Film Badge Dosimeters

The film badge, despite its limitations, is still a widely used personnel dosimeter. All film badges are constructed in a manner similar to that in Fig. 9.2. A piece of film, coated with a radiation-sensitive photographic emulsion and contained in a light-tight and moisture-resistant envelope, is sandwiched between a series of plastic and metal filters in a plastic holder. The holder also has an "open window" section in which there is no plastic or metal filter in front of the film. This open window permits a portion of the film to detect all radiation with the exception of α and weak β particles. The metal filters provide different attenuation factors for photons, and thus the relative darkening behind these filters, called the filter pattern, helps to identify the energy of the x-rays and γ-rays. In addition, the metal filters help to compensate for the overresponse of the film to low-

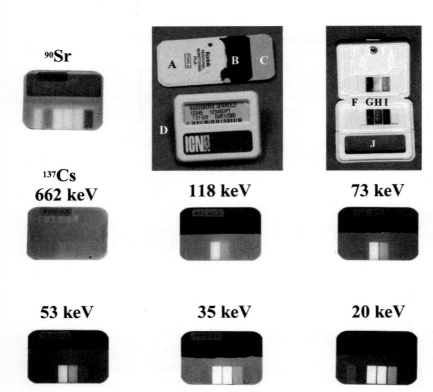

FIGURE 9.2. A film pack (*A*) consists of a black (light opaque) envelope (*B*) containing the film (*C*). The film pack is placed in the plastic film badge (*D*) sandwiched between two sets of Teflon (*F*), lead (*G*), copper (*H*), and aluminum (*I*) filters. Film badges typically have an area where the film pack is not covered by a filter or the plastic of the badge and thus is directly exposed to the radiation. This "open window" area (*J*) is used to detect medium and high-energy β radiation that would otherwise be attenuated. The relative darkening on the developed film (filter patterns) provides a crude but useful assessment of the energy of the radiation exposure. The diagram shows typical filter patterns from exposure to a high-energy β emitter (90Sr), a high-energy γ emitter (137Cs), and x-rays with effective energies from 20 to 118 keV. Film badge and filter patterns courtesy of ICN Worldwide Dosimetry Service, Irvine, CA. (From Bushberg JT, Seibert JA, Leidholdt EM, et al. *The essential physics of medical imaging,* 2nd ed. Philadelphia: Lippincott Williams & Wilkins, 2002, with permission.)

energy photons resulting from the high photoelectric cross section of the silver halide (AgBr) crystals in the film.

These films are typically used for 1-month periods and returned to the vendor, where they are developed and read. The optical density of each area of the film is measured by a densitometer. The radiation dose is determined by comparing the optical densities to predetermined standards.

Advantages of Film Badges

1. Film has a broad dose range: 0.1 mGy to 15 Gy (0.01 to 1,500 rad) for x-rays and γ-rays and 0.5 mGy to 10 Gy (0.05 to 1,000 rad) for high-energy β⁻-particles.
2. Plastic and metal filters in the film badge permit it to distinguish between penetrating radiation (i.e., photons) and nonpenetrating radiation (β⁻-particles and low-energy x-rays). The energy of the photons can be grossly evaluated as high, medium, or low energy.
3. The developed film provides a permanent record of the exposure that can be reanalyzed at a future date.
4. Film badges are small, lightweight, easy to use, and inexpensive.

Disadvantages of Film Badges

1. Film is sensitive to environmental effects such as heat and humidity. For example, a film badge left on the dash of a car on a hot summer day may be rendered unreadable by the heat.
2. Film must be processed by the film badge supplier, and thus the evaluation of an exposure cannot be made immediately. In the event of a suspected serious overexposure, the film can be sent to the vendor and processed within approximately 48 hours.
3. The film packets cannot be used for periods much more than a month.

Thermoluminescent and Optically Stimulated Luminescent Dosimeters

Thermoluminescent dosimeters (TLDs) and optically stimulated luminescent (OSL) dosimeters have a wide range of applications in radiation dosimetry. Both use storage phosphors. Storage phosphors are inorganic crystalline materials in which excited electrons become trapped in metastable states. When ionizing radiation interacts with the material, the energy deposition raises electrons from the valence band into the higher energy conduction band, where some settle into metastable electron traps. The electron vacancies left in the valence band by the removal of the electrons are called *holes*. Larger radiation doses to the phosphor cause more valence electrons to inhabit these electron traps. The trapped electrons can be released by heating or exposure to light. The released electrons fall to the valence band, filling the holes, with the emission of visible or ultraviolet (UV) light photons. The amount of emitted light can be measured with a photomultiplier tube (PMT), permitting determination of the dose to the phosphor. These visible or UV photons interact with the PMT,

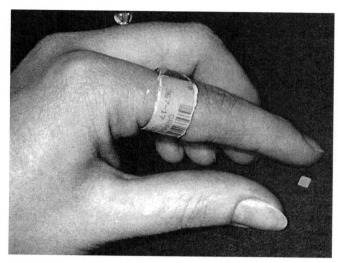

FIGURE 9.3. A small chip of LiF (*shown above*) is sealed in a ring (underneath the identification label) which is worn on the palmar surface so that the chip would face a radiation source held in the hand. (From Bushberg JT, Seibert JA, Leidholdt EM, et al. *The essential physics of medical imaging,* 2nd ed. Philadelphia: Lippincott Williams & Wilkins, 2002, with permission.)

producing an electrical current in it. The PMT amplifies this current through a process of electron multiplication. The current from the PMT is integrated (accumulated) to produce a signal whose amplitude is proportional to the absorbed dose to the dosimeter.

In most radiation detectors designed to detect energetic x-rays and γ-rays, high atomic number materials are preferred, to maximize the sensitivity of the detector. However, for personnel dosimetry, it is often desirable that the detector material have an effective atomic number similar to that of soft tissue, so that the dose to the dosimeter material is nearly proportional to that of soft tissue over a wide range of x-ray and γ-ray energies.

A TLD is "read" by heating it, typically to 300°C to 400°C, in a light-tight enclosure in front of a PMT. Lithium fluoride (LiF) is the TLD material most commonly used for personnel dosimetry. Because its effective atomic number is similar to that of soft tissue, the absorbed dose to LiF is similar to that of soft tissue over a wide range of x-ray and γ-ray energies. Its electron traps are sufficiently "deep" so that there is relatively little loss of trapped electrons at normal ambient temperatures, even over several months. Body dosimeters using LiF usually have two or more chips; single chips are used in finger rings to monitor extremity exposures (Fig. 9.3). The lower limit of detection of LiF is about 0.1 mGy (10 mrad). Other TLD materials, such as aluminum oxide activated with carbon, can be used if smaller doses must be assessed. However, measures must be taken to compensate for their nonlinear energy responses relative to soft tissue.

Advantages of TLDs

1. LiF TLDs have a very wide dose-response range: 0.1 mGy to 1000 Gy (0.01 to 100,000 rad).
2. LiF TLDs are tissue equivalent (Z ≈ 7), which means that

the quantity of light emitted by a TLD is nearly proportional to dose to soft tissue over a wide range of x-ray and γ-ray energies.

3. They can be reused following heating at high temperature for several hours. This process is referred to as *annealing*.
4. They are very small and so can be used on finger rings.
5. They are lightweight and as easy to use as film.

Disadvantages Of TLDs

1. TLDs cannot be read without a TLD reader, which is expensive and requires periodic calibration. Most TLDs are returned to the vendor to be processed (read).
2. Once the TLD is processed, the radiation exposure information is lost from the TLD crystal; it cannot be reprocessed at a later date.
3. TLDs are also susceptible to environmental effects (heat and humidity), and the information stored on the TLD will eventually fade or degrade with time.

OSL dosimeters are increasingly being used instead of film and TLDs. After exposure to ionizing radiation, the material is read by stimulating it with light from a laser and measuring the intensity of the emitted light with a PMT. The light emitted by the phosphor can be distinguished from the stimulating light either by stimulating with a light frequency (color) different from that of the stimulated emissions or by using a pulsed laser and measuring the decaying stimulated emissions after the laser pulse has ended.

The material most commonly used in OSL personnel dosimeters is aluminum oxide, activated with a trace amount of carbon (Al_2O_3:C). It has a reasonably low effective atomic number and it provides about a tenfold greater sensitivity than LiF TLDs. It can be read several times, permitting verification of measurements. It can be reused after erasure with intense light, to release most trapped electrons. A disadvantage of aluminum oxide, compared to LiF, is that its effective atomic number is not as close to that of soft tissue.

Pocket Ion Chambers

The pocket ion chamber is a simple electroscope. It consists of an air-filled cylinder containing a central insulated electrode that can be charged with respect to the outside case. A quartz fiber located on the end of the central electrode is deflected in proportion to the charge. This fiber can be viewed through a simple optical system in which it appears as a hairline cursor on a superimposed exposure scale. The dosimeter is charged before use so that the quartz fiber is deflected to indicate a reading of zero exposure. Radiation causes ionization of the air in the chamber. These ions partially neutralize the stored charge, causing the quartz fiber to experience less repulsion and therefore to move closer to its uncharged position. This movement is seen as a uprange deflection of the hairline on the exposure scale (Fig. 9.4).

Advantages of Pocket Ion Chambers

1. The most significant advantage of this instrument is that it can be read immediately by the user without a loss of information.

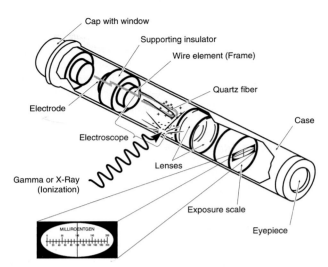

FIGURE 9.4. Cross section of an analog pocket ion chamber. (From Bushberg JT, Seibert JA, Leidholdt EM, et al. *The essential physics of medical imaging*, 2nd ed. Philadelphia: Lippincott Williams & Wilkins, 2002, with permission.)

2. Pocket ion chambers are manufactured with several range scales (e.g., 0 to 200 mR, 0 to 5 R, or 0 to 500 R).
3. They are reusable, lightweight, and small.

Disadvantages of Pocket Ion Chambers

1. Many models are unable to detect low-energy photons or any particulate radiation because of the thick chamber wall. However, special low energy models are available.
2. The dosimeter may spontaneously discharge if dropped on a hard surface, resulting in a spurious high exposure reading.
3. They are fragile and may break if dropped.
4. When they are recharged for reuse, the prior exposure information is lost; therefore, they provide no permanent record.

Electronic Personnel Dosimeters

Electronic personnel dosimeters may use Geiger-Mueller (G-M) tubes or silicon solid-state diodes as detectors. Their major advantage is that, like pocket ion chambers, they provide the user a visible display of his or her current exposure. Older models were generally unreliable, fragile, bulky, and insensitive to low energy x-rays and γ-rays. Recent models have overcome many of these limitations and will no doubt become more commonly used in the future (Fig. 9.5). The better models use solid-state diodes.

Advantages of Electronic Personnel Dosimeters

1. They can be read immediately by the user without any loss of information.
2. They are reusable.
3. Some models can be programmed to sound an alarm at a preset dose-rate.
4. The best models have very high sensitivity, accurately mea-

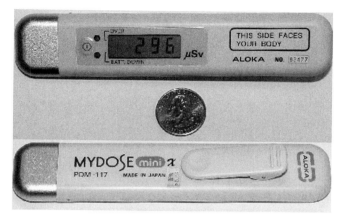

FIGURE 9.5. Electronic personal dosimeter. (Courtesy of Saint-Gobain Crystals and Detectors, Solon OH.)

sure doses over a wide range [1 μGy to 1 Gy (0.1 mrad to 100 rad)], and have a linear energy response to photons over a wide energy range (±20% from 20 keV to 6 MeV).

Disadvantages of Electronic Personnel Dosimeters

1. They are more expensive than film and TLD badges.
2. They are bulky compared to film and TLD badges.
3. Less expensive models may be unable to detect low-energy photons or any particulate radiation and may have a nonlinear energy response.
4. They require periodic replacement of electrical batteries.

Common problems encountered with all personnel dosimeters include erroneous high exposures resulting from the dosimeter having been inadvertently left in a radiation field or having been contaminated with radioactive material and false-low exposures from not being worn.

Bioassays

A bioassay is a measurement to assess the amount of radioactive material incorporated in the body. Bioassays for radionuclides emitting penetrating radiations can be performed by sensitive detectors external to the body, whereas those for other radionuclides usually rely on assays of excreta, most often urine. The most common bioassay in nuclear medicine is the measurement of the activities of ^{125}I or ^{131}I in the thyroid glands of staff handling large activities of these isotopes. This assay is usually performed using a thyroid uptake probe equipped with a sodium iodide (NaI) scintillation detector. In all bioassays, the detector efficiency must be known. The efficiency of the thyroid probe is determined by counting a known activity of the isotope of interest in a thyroid phantom, such as the American National Standards Institute (ANSI) thyroid phantom, which simulates the attenuation of the average adult neck. For any bioassay procedure, the *minimum detectable activity* must be determined to ensure that the procedure is capable of detecting a sufficiently small activity (30). The minimum detectable activity is reduced (the bioassay becomes more sensitive) as the detection efficiency

and counting time are increased and as the background count-rate is reduced. Methods have been developed that permit the effective dose to the person to be estimated from the activity measured during the bioassay (18,31–33).

RADIATION SURVEY INSTRUMENTS AND SURVEY PROCEDURES

Radiation surveys are performed in the nuclear medicine laboratory to evaluate external radiation fields from a variety of sources and to detect and measure contamination of facilities and personnel. These surveys are an important part of keeping occupational radiation exposures ALARA. External radiation fields can be measured with a portable ionization chamber (ion chamber) or, under the appropriate conditions, a G-M survey instrument.

Portable Ionization Chamber Survey Meters

Theory of Operation

An ion chamber survey meter for measuring exposure-rate or air kerma consists of an air-filled chamber containing two electrodes, a battery to provide a voltage between the electrodes, and a sensitive electrometer to measure the current flowing between the electrodes (Fig. 9.6). The walls of the chamber must be made of a material whose effective atomic number is similar to that of air. Exposure to radiation causes partial ionization of the air in the chamber. Ionization of the air from x-rays and γ-rays results primarily from electrons released following photoelectric or Compton interactions in the chamber walls. The ions are attracted to the electrodes, producing an ionization current that is measured by the electrometer. The ion chamber can thus

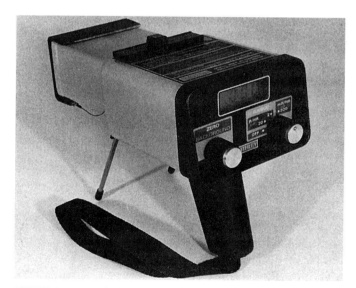

FIGURE 9.6. Portable air-filled ionization chamber survey meter. This particular instrument measures exposure-rates ranging from about 0.1 mR/hour to 20 R/hour. (Photograph courtesy Inovision Radiation Measurements.) (From Bushberg JT, Seibert JA, Leidholdt EM, et al. *The essential physics of medical imaging*, 2nd ed. Philadelphia: Lippincott Williams & Wilkins, 2002, with permission.)

be considered a current generator whose output current is proportional to the rate of internal air ionization. When the radiation source is x-rays or γ-rays, the current is proportional to the exposure-rate (e.g., mR/hour). Most ion chambers have plastic or metal caps that must be placed over the thin entrance windows of the chambers for measurements of higher energy photons. The cap can also be used to determine if the indicated exposure-rate is partially caused by β-radiation.

Advantages of The Ion Chamber

1. The exposure-rate can be accurately measured over a wide range of photon energies. The measured exposure is typically within ±10% of the actual exposure between 40 keV and several MeV.
2. Ion chamber survey meters have a wide exposure range, typically 0.001 to 500 R/hour.
3. Ion chamber survey meters will not saturate in moderately high radiation fields and express minimal dose-rate effects (typically less than 10% error between 10 mR/hour and 10 R/hour).
4. Changes in atmospheric temperature and pressure do affect measurements from ambient air ion chambers; however, correction factors are typically minor.

Disadvantages of Ion Chambers

1. The response times of these instruments are moderately slow and thus careful observation is required to make accurate measurements.
2. The very small electrical charge produced by each interaction causes ion chambers to be relatively insensitive. An ion chamber would not be the instrument of choice to locate minor contamination or a low-activity source. A more suitable instrument for these applications would be a G-M survey meter.

Geiger-Mueller Survey Instruments

Theory of Operation

The most common and versatile portable radiation survey instrument in the nuclear medicine laboratory is the G-M survey meter. These instruments are available from many vendors in a variety of designs. The typical instrument consists of a handheld probe housing the G-M tube, connected by a cable to a separate case containing the detector circuitry and display (Fig. 9.7).

A G-M detector consists of a thin, cylindrical metal shell with a wire mounted at the center of the cylinder. The detector is typically filled with a noble gas (e.g., helium or argon) and a small amount (~5%) of a halogen such as chlorine or an organic compound such as ethyl alcohol (quenching gas). A potential difference (voltage) of approximately 900 volts is applied between the shell and the central wire, which is the positive electrode (anode). As in the ion chamber, radiation produces ion pairs in the sensitive volume. However, in the case of the G-M counter, the large potential difference across the tube accelerates the electrons toward the anode, supplying them with sufficient kinetic energy to produce additional ionization. This avalanche

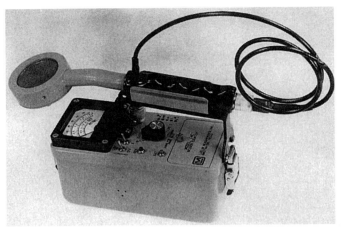

FIGURE 9.7. Portable G-M survey meter with thin-window "pancake" probe. (Photograph courtesy Ludlum Measurements, Inc.) (From Bushberg JT, Seibert JA, Leidholdt EM et al. *The essential physics of medical imaging,* 2nd ed. Philadelphia: Lippincott Williams & Wilkins, 2002, with permission.)

continues as secondary ionizations trigger additional gas ionization, eventually resulting in a large number of electrons being collected on the anode. This cascade effect, resulting in approximately 10^9 electrons being collected per ionization event, produces (in a typical G-M instrument) a signal of about 1 volt, which is used to activate a counting circuit. The counting circuit registers each avalanche as a count. The number of counts per minute (cpm) is proportional to the amount of radiation incident on the G-M tube.

Most G-M tubes contain quenching gases to prevent the positive ions, which slowly drift to the cathode, from triggering additional avalanches. The time between the initial avalanche and the neutralization is typically about 100 milliseconds. During this time interval, referred to as the *deadtime* of the detector, the detector is insensitive to additional interactions.

The magnitude of the multiplication effect, and thus the voltage pulse, is independent of the type or energy of the initial ionizing radiation. Therefore, the magnitudes of the pulses from a G-M counter cannot be used to determine the energies of incident charged particles and photons. However, discrimination between electrons (β-particles and conversion electrons) and photons is possible by sliding a metal or plastic sleeve over a portion of the G-M tube to absorb the electrons. The thickness of the wall of the G-M tube determines the minimum electron energy detectable.

A G-M detector is extremely sensitive to charged particles of sufficient energy to penetrate the wall of the tube; almost every charged particle reaching the interior of the tube is registered as a count. Flat large-area thin-window probes, called pancake probes, are especially useful for surveys for radioactive contamination (Fig. 9.7). The high sensitivity of these detectors to charged particles allows them to detect small amounts of activity.

G-M detectors are relatively insensitive to x-rays and γ-rays, relative to other detectors such as NaI scintillators. Most x-rays and γ-rays pass through the gas without interaction. Most photons that are detected interact with the wall of the tube, with the resultant electrons entering the gas.

G-M survey meters may be calibrated to indicate either exposure-rate (mR/hour) or count-rate (cpm). Those calibrated to indicate exposure-rate (mR/hour) usually exhibit a nonlinear energy response relative to an air-filled ion chamber. If calibrated with a high-energy γ-ray source (typically ^{137}Cs, 662 keV γ-rays), they overrespond by as much as a factor of five for photons in the range of 40 to 100 keV. An energy response curve supplied by the manufacturer can be used to correct the indicated exposure-rate, if the energy of the incident photons is known. Some manufacturers offer energy compensated G-M probes in which the G-M tube is covered by a sleeve of higher atomic number metal; the increased photoelectric absorption of lower energy photons by the sleeve gives the detector a flat energy response, permitting accurate measurement of exposure-rate over a wide range of photon energies. However, the energy-compensated probe is not very useful for contamination surveys, because the metal sleeve attenuates most charged particles, and it is much less sensitive to low energy photons than an uncompensated probe.

Advantages of G-M Detectors

1. G-M detectors are extremely sensitive to charged particles of sufficient energy to penetrate the walls of the tubes. G-M instruments equipped with thin window pancake probes are very useful for locating radioactive contamination.
2. G-M survey meters are useful for locating areas of high exposure-rate, although for most meters, the indicated exposure-rate may be substantially in error.
3. G-M detectors are relatively inexpensive, portable, lightweight, and rugged and thus are the instrument of choice for most surveys in the nuclear medicine laboratory.

Disadvantages and Limitations of G-M Detectors

1. Most probes exhibit considerable energy dependence, causing significant errors when exposure-rates are measured for photons of energies other than that for which the detector was calibrated. Energy compensated G-M probes have a response relatively independent of photon energy, but at the cost of reduced sensitivity to low energy photons and insensitivity to charged particles.
2. Deadtime count losses cause the G-M detector to indicate a falsely low interaction rate at high interaction rates. In extremely high radiation fields, the interaction rate may be so high that the long deadtime inherent in G-M detectors results in complete saturation of the detector system. Depending on the design of the instrument, this will result in either a continuous full scale or a zero reading on the meter. The latter is obviously a serious and potentially dangerous limitation of the G-M detector; therefore, ion chambers should always be used to evaluate high-radiation fields. The count-rate of a G-M detector is typically limited to about 300,000 cpm. This permits a typical G-M tube to measure exposure rates up to about 200 mR/hour, although smaller tubes can measure higher exposure rates.
3. G-M detectors, even with very thin windows, are relatively insensitive to contamination from certain radionuclides, such

as ^{125}I and ^{51}Cr. The weak Augér electrons from these radionuclides are unable to penetrate the entrance window and most of their x-rays or γ-rays pass through the gas without interaction. Other types of instruments, such as portable scintillation survey meters, are preferable for these radionuclides.

Use of Portable Survey Instruments

Portable survey instruments should be calibrated at least annually. Following calibration, a small check source (typically one μCi of ^{137}Cs for G-M instruments and 10 μCi of ^{137}Cs for ion chamber survey meters) is placed against the detector and the indicated reading recorded on the instrument. On each day of use of a meter, the same check source is placed against the meter at the same location; if the reading is not within ± 20% of the reading when last calibrated, the instrument should be recalibrated. The instrument's battery should also be checked each day that the instrument is used.

Surveys with a G-M detector for radioactive contamination are usually performed with the instrument set to its most sensitive scale while the probe is moved slowly approximately 1 cm above the surface to be surveyed. Most G-M survey instruments have speakers that provide an audible indication of the count rate, enabling the operator to locate sites of contamination or excessive exposure without looking at the meter.

Wipe Tests for Removable Contamination

Depending on the survey technique, portable radiation survey instruments may fail to detect surface contamination less than approximately 4 kBq (~0.1 μCi) of ^{99m}Tc per 100 cm^2. Although this amount of activity does not constitute a serious personnel hazard, it is good practice to detect and eliminate all unnecessary sites of contamination.

Contamination is simply the presence of noncontained radioactive material in an amount and/or location that is undesirable. Contamination can be either fixed or removable (transportable). This distinction is important with regard to the potential for spread of the contamination to other facilities or personnel. Removable contamination is detected and measured by wipe tests. A piece of filter paper or similar material is wiped over a surface area of approximately 100 cm^2 (~4 × 4 inches) and counted in an appropriate detector.

The activity on a wipe sample can be assayed using a G-M survey instrument, a proportional counter, a liquid scintillation counter, or a NaI(Tl) well counter or probe system. The selection of one particular instrument over another will be a function of the radionuclide in question, availability of instrumentation, desired minimum detectable activity, accuracy of result, and speed of analysis. In most nuclear medicine laboratories, a NaI(Tl) well detector is the instrument of choice for assaying wipe test samples because of its high detection efficiency for x-ray and γ-ray emitting radionuclides. If the NaI(Tl) well detector is connected to a multichannel analyzer, the energy spectrum of an unknown radionuclide can be readily displayed and the radionuclide identified by matching its energy spectrum with previously collected spectra from radionuclides used in the laboratory. This information can be extremely useful in tracing a source of contamination.

Regulatory agencies in the United States commonly require contamination levels to be recorded in units of disintegrations per minute (dpm)/100 cm². The measured count-rate must be corrected for the background count-rate of the detector and the detection efficiency for the specific radionuclide. For most NaI(Tl) well counters, a conservative estimate of the detection efficiency for common radionuclides used in nuclear medicine is 50%. Thus, when the detector efficiency has not been determined, multiplying the observed counts per minute by two, after subtracting background, should provide a reasonable estimate of the disintegrations per minute.

Location, Frequency, and Action Levels for Radiation Surveys

As mentioned earlier in this chapter, at the time of writing, the NRC has promulgated revisions to their medical use regulations (10 CFR Part 35) as final regulations (28). The previous NRC regulations required areas where radiopharmaceuticals were routinely prepared or administered to be surveyed at the end of each day of use and all areas where radiopharmaceuticals or radioactive waste were stored to be surveyed weekly with a portable radiation survey meter (18). The previous regulations also required surveys for removable contamination (wipe tests) to be performed weekly of all areas where radiopharmaceuticals were routinely prepared, administered, or stored (18).

The revised NRC medical use regulations specifically require surveys at the end of each day of use with a portable radiation survey meter only of areas where radiopharmaceuticals requiring a written directive, i.e., iodine-131 sodium iodide and therapeutic radiopharmaceuticals, are prepared or administered. Tests for removable contamination are not specifically required by the revised regulations.

Nonetheless, even if not required by regulation, it is prudent to perform surveys with a portable radiation survey meter, at the end of each day of use, for contamination and exposure rate, of all areas of the nuclear medicine department where any radiopharmaceuticals are routinely prepared or administered. The instrument used should be able to detect exposure rates as low as 0.1 mR/h. A Geiger-Mueller survey meter equipped with a large area thin-window detector is recommended for these surveys. Action levels should be established for the surveys; if the measurements exceed the action levels, the individual performing the survey most notify the Radiation Safety Officer.

It is common practice to remove any contamination found by either survey meter or wipe test. If proper precautions are taken, most contamination occurs on disposable plastic-backed paper that can be discarded into the radioactive waste. Typically, contaminated surfaces not protected by disposable coverings are cleaned until the removable contamination is less than 3 Bq (~200 dpm) per 100 cm². In the infrequent case in which contamination by a short-lived radionuclide in a controlled area cannot be completely removed, it is common practice to remove the majority of the contamination, cover the area with an impermeable material to prevent the spread of contamination, cover with a sheet of lead to reduce the exposure rate to staff,

label with a warning sign and the date, and allow the contamination to decay in place.

The NRC also requires surveys to be performed of radiation levels in restricted and unrestricted areas and of radioactive material in effluents to demonstrate compliance with the dose limit for individual members of the public [one mSv (100 mrem) per year] (16). Very sensitive dosimeters, such as those using aluminum oxide TLDs, may be placed in unrestricted areas to demonstrate compliance with respect to external sources of radiation.

PRINCIPLES AND APPLICATIONS OF RADIATION PROTECTION

Sources of Exposure in Nuclear Medicine

The average body dose of a nuclear medicine technologist in a busy 500-bed hospital is approximately 2 mSv (200 mrem) per year. Technologists who routinely elute generators or primarily perform positron emission tomography (PET) imaging may receive substantially higher doses. The exposure received by the individual technologist is determined by factors such as

1. The activities and photon energies of the radionuclides used.
2. The radiopharmaceuticals' biodistribution and biologic half-life in the patients.
3. Lengths of the imaging procedures. Critically ill and uncooperative patients typically require more positioning time and may require retakes because of patient motion.
4. The distance from the patient to the technologist during imaging. The computer and camera console should be as far from the patient as is practical in an imaging room.

Although the nuclear medicine technologists' hands are exposed to large dose-rates for short periods during radiopharmaceutical preparation and injection, the majority of the effective dose to the technologists is from activity in the patient during imaging (34). Over the last 25 years, the replacement of older radiopharmaceuticals with ones labeled with short-lived non-β-particle emitting radionuclides has permitted the administration of much larger activities to patients. These large activities, although necessary for good image quality, produce much higher exposure-rates in the vicinity of the patient. Typical exposures to imaging personnel from various nuclear medicine procedures are listed in Table 9.7.

Protection against External Exposure

Three techniques can be used to reduce radiation exposure from sources external to the body: decreasing time, increasing distance, and using shielding. These radiation protection principles are ubiquitous in all aspects of health physics and have special applications in nuclear medicine.

Time

Limiting radiation exposure from high-radiation fields occasionally encountered in nuclear medicine can be accomplished in

Table 9.7. *Typical Exposure Rate at 1 Meter from Adult Nuclear Medicine Patient after Radiopharmaceutical Administration*

Study	Radiopharmaceutical	Activity (mCi)[a]	Exposure Rate at 1 m (mR/hr)
Thyroid cancer therapy	^{131}I (NaI)	200	~35
Tumor imaging	^{18}F (FDG)	10	~5.0
Cardiac gated imaging	^{99m}Tc RBC	20	~0.9
Bone scan	^{99m}Tc MDP	25	~1.2
Tumor imaging	^{67}Ga citrate	3	~0.4
Liver-spleen scan	^{99m}Tc sulfur colloid	4	~0.2
Myocardial perfusion imaging	^{201}Tl chloride	3	~0.1

Note: FDG, ^{18}F-fluorodeoxyglucose; MDP, methylene diphosphonate; RBC, red blood cell.
[a]Multiply by 37 to obtain MBq.
Source: 45.

many cases by simply reducing the time spent working with or near the source. Typically, the highest radiation fields encountered in the nuclear medicine laboratory are associated with the preparation of the radiopharmaceuticals. The amount of time spent preparing vials and syringes of radiopharmaceuticals in the radiopharmacy is usually directly proportional to one's experience in these tasks. Training technologists initially with nonradioactive solutions is a good way to provide the needed experience while preventing unnecessary radiation exposure.

Distance

Perhaps the most effective and commonly used radiation protection precaution employed in nuclear medicine is the use of distance to reduce exposure. With some exceptions, the dimensions of most radiation sources are small compared to the distances between the sources and personnel. Under these conditions, the radiation field intensity can be assumed to decrease inversely with the square of the distance. The effect of this inverse square law can be seen in the example in Table 9.8 demonstrating the effectiveness of remote handling devices in reducing radiation exposure from unshielded radionuclides. Long tongs or forceps

Table 9.8. *Effect of Distance on Exposure with Common Radionuclides Used in Nuclear Medicine*

Radionuclide 370 MBq (10 mCi)	[a]Exposure Rate (mR/hr) at 1 cm	[a]Exposure Rate (mR/hr) at 10 cm (~4 inches)
^{67}Ga	7,500	75
^{99m}Tc	6,200	62
^{123}I	16,300	163
^{131}I	21,800	218
^{133}Xe	5,300	53
^{201}Tl	4,500	45

[a]Calculated from the Γ_{20}.
Source: 45.

should always be used, when handling unshielded sources or vials containing large activities, to reduce the radiation dose to the hands.

It is important to keep in mind that the patient is a radiation source. Facilities should be designed so that, following patient positioning, staff can adequately monitor both the patient and acquisition of the image while maintaining a large distance between themselves and the patient. In particular, imaging rooms should be as large as is reasonable and computer consoles in the imaging rooms should be placed as far as possible from the location of the patient being imaged.

The exposure rate at a particular distance from an unshielded radioactive source is a function of its decay scheme and is expressed as the *exposure rate constant* (Γ). Γ is the exposure rate from x-rays and γ-rays above a specified minimum energy (e.g., (Γ_{20} is the exposure rate constant for all photons with energies above 20 keV) per unit activity and at a unit distance. Γ is commonly expressed as roentgens per hour from 1 mCi at 1 cm, which has the units: R • cm^2/mCi • hour. The exposure-rate from any activity and at any distance may be calculated as

$$\dot{X} = \Gamma A/r^2 \qquad [8]$$

where Γ is the exposure rate constant, A is the activity of the source, and r is the distance from the source. The exposure rate constants of radionuclides commonly used in nuclear medicine are listed in Table 9.9. The dramatic effect of distance on lowering the exposure rate is shown in Table 9.8 for radionuclides commonly used in nuclear medicine.

Table 9.9. *Exposure Rate Constants(Γ_{20} and Γ_{30})[a] and Half Value Layers (HVL) of Lead for Radionuclides of Interest to Nuclear Medicine*

Radionuclide	Γ_{20} (Rcm^2/mCihr)[b]	Γ_{30} (Rcm^2/mCihr)[b]	Half Value Layer in Pb (cm)[c,d]
^{57}Co	0.56	0.56	0.02
^{60}Co	12.87	12.87	1.2
^{51}Cr	0.18	0.18	0.17
^{137}Cs	3.25	3.25	0.55
^{18}F	5.66	5.66	0.39
^{11}C, ^{13}N	5.85	5.85	0.39
^{67}Ga	0.75	0.75	0.1$^-$
^{123}I	1.63	0.86	0.04
^{125}I	1.47	0.26	0.002
^{131}I	2.18	2.15	0.3
^{111}In	3.24	2.0	0.1
^{192}Ir	4.61	4.61	0.60
^{99}Mo[e]	1.47	1.43	0.7
^{99m}Tc	0.62	0.60	0.03
^{201}Tl	0.45	0.45	0.02
^{133}Xe	0.53	0.53	0.02

[a]Γ_{20} and Γ_{30} calculated from the absorption coefficients of Hubbell and Seltzer (46) and the decay data table of Kocher (47).
[b]Multiply by 27.03 to obtain uGycm^2/GBqhr at 1 meter.
[c]The first HVL will be significantly smaller than subsequent HVLs for those radionuclides with multiple photon emissions at significantly different energies (e.g., Ga-67) because the lower energy photons will be preferentially attenuated in the first HVL.
[d]Some values were adapted from (48). Other values were calculated by the authors.
[e]with Tc-99m in equilibrium
Source: 45.

Shielding

In addition to time and distance, shielding of the radiation source is commonly used to reduce the exposure rate to personnel. The choice of shielding material is a function of the type of radiation and its energy. β^--radiation is best shielded with low atomic number (Z) materials, such as plastic or water, to minimize the production of bremsstrahlung x-rays, which are much more penetrating than the β^--particles. When large activities of high-energy β^--emitters are to be shielded, lead shielding outside the plastic shield will help attenuate the bremsstrahlung that is produced.

External radiation fields from radionuclides used in nuclear medicine consist primarily of x-rays and γ-rays. High-atomic number materials such as lead are very effective in attenuating these forms of radiation.

The half-value layer (HVL) is the thickness of a specified shielding material that reduces the intensity of the incident radiation by one half. When shielding is placed in a narrow beam of monoenergetic x-rays or γ-rays, the attenuation of the beam is exponential.

$$\dot{X} = \dot{X}_o e^{-\mu x} \qquad [9]$$

where $\dot{X}$ is the exposure-rate with the shielding in the beam, $\dot{X}_o$ is the exposure-rate at the same point without the shielding, x is the thickness of the shielding, and μ, called the linear attenuation coefficient, is a constant that varies with the atomic number and density of the shielding material and the energy of the incident photons. For such narrow monoenergetic beams of γ-rays, one HVL reduces the intensity of the beam by half, two HVLs reduce the intensity by one fourth, three HVLs reduce it by one eighth, and so on. The general formula for the reduction factor is $1/2^n$ where n is equal to the number of HVLs. The HVL is a function of the radionuclide being shielded and the shielding material.

For polyenergetic photon beams, such as those from radionuclides emitting photons of widely different energies, or x-rays from an x-ray tube, attenuation is not exponential. The lower energy photons are more readily attenuated and, in this case, the first HVL is less than the second HVL.

Nearly all actual shielding situations involve wide beams of x-rays or γ-rays. In this case, even if the incident photons are monoenergetic, attenuation is not exponential. The buildup of scattered photons in the beam causes the attenuation to be less than predicted by Equation 9. Nonetheless, for the photon-emitting radionuclides commonly used in nuclear medicine and high atomic number shielding materials such as lead, narrow beam HVLs can be used for approximate shielding calculations. The HVLs of lead for several radionuclides common to nuclear medicine are listed in Table 9.9.

Lead aprons (0.5 mm lead equivalent), which are commonly worn in diagnostic x-ray departments to shield personnel from low-energy scattered radiation, are not usually recommended for use in nuclear medicine departments because they do not provide very effective attenuation for the higher energy photons from radiopharmaceuticals (~65% attenuation for 140 keV γ-rays).

The 511 keV annihilation photons from ^{18}F and other positron-emitting radiopharmaceuticals require much thicker shielding than most other radionuclides used in nuclear medicine. Most facilities routinely performing PET establish a separate and more heavily shielded dose preparation station for PET radiopharmaceuticals. Much thicker vial and syringe shields are used for PET radiopharmaceuticals.

Considerations in Shield Construction

When erecting or relocating a shield, the following points should be considered:

1. All six sides adjacent to the shield should be considered in terms of affording adequate protection for both radiation workers and others. In particular, the bottoms of bench-top work areas should be sufficiently shielded to protect the lower part of the body.
2. The working surface must be able to support the weight of the shielding.
3. Consideration must be given to the radiation exposure to the head of a person manipulating objects behind the shield. Leaded glass is commonly used for this purpose. Mirrors located over or in storage areas often permit sources to be manipulated without direct radiation exposure to the head.
4. After construction, the shield should be evaluated by placing a source behind the shield and measuring the exposure rates in surrounding areas.

Radiopharmaceutical Preparation Areas

Table-top lead shields with leaded glass windows are used to protect the heads and bodies of persons preparing doses of radiopharmaceuticals (Fig. 9.8). Most commercial table-top shields

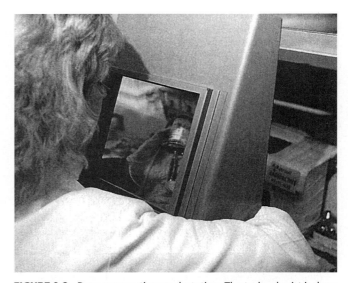

FIGURE 9.8. Dose preparation work station. The technologist is drawing the radiopharmaceutical from a vial shielded by a "lead pig" into a syringe contained in a syringe shield. Further protection from radiation exposure is afforded by working behind the lead L-shield with a leaded glass window. The technologist is wearing a lab coat and disposable gloves to prevent contamination. A film badge is worn on the lab coat to record whole body exposure and a thermoluminescent dosimeter finger ring is worn inside the glove to record the extremity exposure. (From Bushberg JT, Seibert JA, Leidholdt EM, et al. *The essential physics of medical imaging,* 2nd ed. Philadelphia: Lippincott Williams & Wilkins, 2002, with permission.)

do not have lead in their bases; a separate sheet of lead should be placed on the table top beneath the table-top shield. Shielding is commonly placed against the wall behind the dose preparation area to protect personnel in the adjacent room.

Syringe and Vial Shields

All stock solutions of radioactive material should be stored in vial shields. Virtually all radionuclides shipped to nuclear medicine departments arrive in lead vial shields that are adequate for the purpose of radiation safety. Commercial vial shields with leaded glass windows are helpful because they permit the fluid level in the vial to be seen while withdrawing an aliquot with a syringe.

Syringe shields made from lead or tungsten with lead-glass windows are commonly used to reduce exposures during radio-pharmaceutical preparation and administration (Fig. 9.9). Syringe shields can reduce exposure to the technologists' hands by 50% during radiopharmaceutical preparation and as much as 80% during injection (34).

Shielding during Imaging

Techniques that minimize the exposure to technologists during imaging procedures will substantially reduce their annual effective doses. To that end, fixed or mobile leaded glass or acrylic shields between the computer terminal and the location of the patient being imaged can be used to protect the technologist. This is particularly important in situations in which the computer terminal and imaging equipment are in close proximity.

Personnel Contamination Protection and Incorporation of Radioactivity into the Body

Small amounts of radioactivity on the skin or in the body can produce large radiation doses. For example, the intake of 37

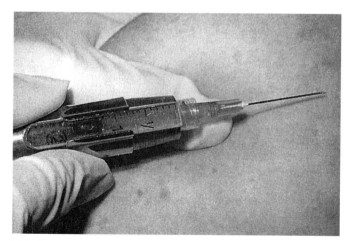

FIGURE 9.9. Syringe shield for a 3-cc syringe. The barrel is made from high Z material (e.g., lead or tungsten) in which a leaded glass window is inserted so that the syringe graduations and the dose can be seen. (From Bushberg JT, Seibert JA, Leidholdt EM et al. *The essential physics of medical imaging*, 2nd ed. Philadelphia: Lippincott Williams & Wilkins, 2002, with permission.)

kBq (1 μCi) of ^{131}I NaI will produce a dose to the thyroid of approximately 0.01 Gy (1 rad). In addition, it is often difficult or impossible to significantly hasten the elimination of radioactivity once it has been incorporated into the body. Incorporation of radioactivity into the body can occur by inhalation, ingestion, or absorption through the skin or through wounds. For these reasons, it is important to handle unsealed radioactive material in such a manner as to prevent it from coming into contact with the skin and to minimize the release of radioactivity into the air.

The degrees of hazard of radioactive materials as potential internal contaminants vary widely and are determined by the following factors: (a) the types and energies of the particles and photons emitted, (b) the physical half-lives of the radionuclides, (c) the kinetics of the materials in the body, and (d) the potentials of the materials to become airborne or to be absorbed through the skin. Radionuclides emitting α-particles are, in general, more hazardous than those emitting electrons, and those emitting energetic electrons tend to be more hazardous that those mainly emitting photons. Radioactive materials of longer physical half-life tend to be more hazardous than those of shorter half-life. The kinetics of the radioactive material in the body are important; materials retained by the body tend to be more hazardous than those which are rapidly eliminated. Also, those which concentrate in or near radiosensitive tissues (e.g., the bone marrow) are, in general, more hazardous than those which are more uniformly distributed in the body or concentrate in less radiation sensitive tissues. The most hazardous radionuclides commonly used in nuclear medicine are ^{131}I, ^{125}I, ^{89}Sr, and ^{32}P.

Radiation Protection–Practical Considerations

Provided that the radioactive material is not likely to become airborne, the main precautions when handling unsealed radioactivity resemble the universal precautions used to protect staff from blood-borne pathogens. The following is a list of basic rules that should be observed when working with radioactive material:

1. Unsealed radioactive material should be handled in designated work areas posted with radioactive material warning signs. The work surfaces should be covered with plastic-backed absorbent paper or other suitable material that will absorb spills and prevent the spread of contamination. The paper should be replaced regularly.
2. Lab coats or other protective clothing must be worn when in rooms where unsealed radioactivity is used. Lab coats should be buttoned while handling radioactivity. This protective clothing should be changed if contaminated and should not be worn outside the work area.
3. Disposable impermeable gloves should be worn when handling unsealed radioactive material and replaced frequently.
4. Hands should be washed after removing the disposable gloves and surveyed with a suitable survey instrument. The hands should also be washed and the hands and clothing surveyed before eating, drinking, or smoking, and at the end of the workday.
5. Body dosimeters should be worn in the department and

finger dosimeters should be worn whenever eluting generators, handling radioactivity, or positioning patients.

6. All radioactive material should be kept in adequately shielded containers when not in use. Mirrors should be placed behind open storage areas to reduce exposure to the head.

7. All potentially volatile or gaseous radioactive materials (e.g., ^{131}I and ^{133}Xe) should be stored and used in a fume hood with adequate air flow (i.e., average face velocity between 100 and 150 ft/minute).

8. No eating, drinking, or smoking should be allowed in rooms in which radionuclides are stored or used nor should storage of food or beverages be permitted.

9. All containers of radioactive material should be clearly labeled with radionuclide name, chemical form, activity, and date and time of assay.

10. Pipetting should never be done by mouth. Instead, remote or mechanical pipetting devices should be used.

11. Work areas should be kept as clear and clutter free as possible.

12. All spills should be contained and cleaned up immediately to minimize the spread of contamination. Spills should be cleaned from the areas of low contamination toward the area of highest contamination.

13. Office, study, and reading areas should be located as far away from radionuclide storage areas as practical.

14. Syringe and vial shields should always be used for preparing and administering doses of radiopharmaceuticals to patients.

15. Long tongs or forceps should be used to reduce the radiation dose to the hands when handling unshielded vials and other sources.

16. All preparations of radiopharmaceutical stock solutions and patient doses should be performed behind a leaded glass drawing station.

17. G-M meter surveys of the laboratory area should be conducted at the end of the work day to evaluate and document exposure-rates and contamination.

18. The recapping of needles should be discouraged to reduce the hazards of blood-borne pathogens. However, when recapping a needle is necessary, the cap must not be held with the hands.

Radioactive Aerosols and Gases

A number of radioactive noble gases (e.g., ^{133}Xe and ^{81m}Kr) and ^{99m}Tc-DTPA aerosol are used in nuclear medicine for lung ventilation studies. In addition, radioiodine in the form of NaI can evolve a radioactive gas. The risk to workers from airborne radioactivity depends on the radionuclide, its chemical form, its concentration in the air, and the duration of time that persons are exposed to it. The dose from radioactive noble gases is mostly due to external exposure from the cloud of gas, because little of the gas is absorbed from the lungs. For most other airborne radioactive material, there is significant uptake and retention of radioactivity by the body. The methods for protecting personnel from airborne radioactivity are to minimize the activity that is released, use dilution to minimize the concentration of radioac-

tivity in the air, and limit the time that people are exposed to airborne radioactivity.

The primary method of protecting workers and the public from airborne radioactivity is to minimize the release of activity to the atmosphere. For example, vials of radioactive iodine should be kept tightly capped. Solutions of radioiodine in the form of NaI should be maintained at a basic pH, because the volatility is enhanced at low pH.

Filters or traps are commonly used to minimize the release of activity to the atmosphere. In nuclear medicine, disposable filters are used to collect the ^{99m}Tc aerosol and charcoal traps are commonly used to collect ^{133}Xe exhaled by patients during pulmonary-ventilation studies. Many traps are equipped with monitors that continuously measure the concentration of xenon in the exhaust from the traps. The charcoal cartridges should be replaced when indicated by the exhaust monitors. When a trap is not equipped with an exhaust monitor, the exhaust gas should be collected periodically and counted to ensure that the trap is functioning acceptably.

Significant activities of volatile or gaseous radioactive materials should be stored and manipulated in fume hoods. The average air velocity at the face of the fume hood should be between 100 and 150 ft/minute with the sash of the hood at a reasonable working height (typically about 45 cm). The fume hood should be free of clutter that might create areas of reduced air flow. The average face velocity should be measured at least annually, and the hood marked with the date of the inspection, the average face velocity, and the maximal acceptable sash height. The fan for the hood should be located at the exhaust (roof) end of the ducting and the ducting should terminate in a stack far from building air intakes.

Rooms in which ventilation studies are performed should be at a negative pressure with respect to surrounding rooms, so that the air flow at doorways is into rather than out of the ventilation study rooms, thereby limiting the loss of radioactive gas or aerosol into surrounding rooms (inflow exceeds exhaust flow). The room exhaust should be entirely released to the exterior of the building away from intake vents; it should not be recirculated. In addition, the exhaust flow must be sufficient to keep the average airborne concentration in the room substantially less than the DAC specified by the NRC for that radionuclide. (DACs for certain radionuclides of interest to nuclear medicine are listed in Table 9.6.) The average air activity concentration in the room is calculated from the following equation.

$$C = \frac{A/T}{Q} \qquad [10]$$

where C is the average air concentration, A is the average activity released in a specified time period (typically a month), T is the time period, and Q is the room's exhaust flow (typically in cubic feet per minute). The ventilation rates in rooms in which radioactive gases are used should be periodically measured to verify that the air exhaust rate substantially exceeds the supply rate and that the average air concentration of the radioactive gas is ALARA.

For example, assume that a room used for ^{133}Xe lung ventilation studies has an exhaust air flow of 400 cubic feet per minute, that an average of 10 ventilation studies are performed per month, and that an average activity of 10 mCi is used per study. If it assumed that 25% of the ^{133}Xe is lost to the room, the average air concentration is

$$C = \frac{(0.25)(10pts)(10mCi/pt)/(1 month)}{400 cu.ft./min}$$

Converting millicuries to microcuries and cubic feet to milliliters and recognizing that there are approximately 10,000 working minutes in a month, the average air concentration is

$$C = 2.2 \times 10^{-7} \ \mu Ci/mL$$

which is much less than the DAC for ^{133}Xe listed in Table 9.6.

More detailed information on radiation protection principles can be found in several publications (35–37).

PROTECTION OF THE NUCLEAR MEDICINE PATIENT

Ensuring Intended Radiopharmaceutical Administration

Among the most important aspects to protecting the nuclear medicine patient is to ensure that appropriate studies are performed correctly on the intended patients and that female patients who may be pregnant or are nursing children by breast are identified before the administration of radiopharmaceuticals. Each nuclear medicine department should have written procedures regarding the administration of radiopharmaceuticals to patients; staff members must be trained in these procedures on employment and regularly thereafter. The following procedures are recommended for routine diagnostic studies:

1. All requests for patient studies must be reviewed by a nuclear medicine staff physician for appropriateness. The request for a study should then be sent to the technologists in writing. It is the responsibility of the physician to ensure that the desired procedure is clearly described.
2. Each vial of a radiopharmaceutical must be labeled to identify the radiopharmaceutical. When a vial of a radiopharmaceutical is placed in a vial radiation shield, the shield must be conspicuously labeled with the name of the radiopharmaceutical.
3. The activity of each dose of a photon-emitting radiopharmaceutical should be assayed using a dose calibrator before administration, even if it is a precalibrated unit dose prepared by a commercial radiopharmacy.
4. The radiopharmaceutical and prescribed activity or activity range for each procedure should be posted near the dose calibrator and/or contained within the department's policy and procedure manual. Alternatively, the nuclear medicine physician may specify the radiopharmaceutical and activity to be administered in writing for each patient.
5. Each syringe containing a radiopharmaceutical must be labeled to identify the radiopharmaceutical. Whenever a syringe of a radiopharmaceutical is placed in a syringe radiation shield obscuring the label on the syringe, the shield must be conspicuously labeled to identify the radiopharmaceutical,

even if the syringe is to be immediately administered to a patient.
6. The patient must be identified by two independent means (e.g., requesting the patient to recite his or her name and social security number) at the time of radiopharmaceutical administration. The information received from the patient, the approved request for the procedure, and the label on the syringe shield must be compared. If more than one dose is to be administered to a patient, the patient must be properly identified at the time of each administration.
7. All female patients of childbearing potential must be asked if they might be pregnant or are breast-feeding a child before the administration of a radiopharmaceutical. It should not be assumed that adolescent female patients are sexually inactive.

Written Directives

The NRC requires each of its medical licensees administering specified higher risk radiopharmaceuticals to develop and implement written procedures to ensure that the radiopharmaceuticals are administered to patients as directed by the nuclear medicine physician (17,28). A written directive, specifying the patient, radiopharmaceutical, activity, and route of administration, must be prepared and signed by the physician before the administration of an activity of ^{131}I NaI exceeding 1.11 MBq (30 μCi) or any administration of a radiopharmaceutical for therapeutic purposes. Before each administration, the patient's identity must be carefully verified as the individual named in the written directive, and the administration must be in accordance with the directive. The licensee must maintain all written directives and records of the administrations for 3 years. It is recommended that a standard form be used for written directives. Fig. 9.10 shows such a form.

Patients Who May Be Pregnant or Are Nursing Children

If a pregnant woman is administered a photon-emitting radiopharmaceutical, x-rays or γ-rays from the radioactivity in maternal tissues will irradiate the embryo or fetus. Moreover, many radiopharmaceuticals or their radioactive products cross the placenta and directly irradiate the fetus. In particular, unbound radioiodine crosses the placenta and the fetal thyroid begins to concentrate iodine at about the end of the first trimester (38). Many radiopharmaceuticals or their radioactive products are excreted in breast milk. Furthermore, some radiopharmaceuticals excreted by the breast can impart large doses to the breasts of the lactating mother.

Before diagnostic administrations, female patients of childbearing age, including adolescent girls, should be asked if they might be pregnant or are nursing infants by breast. Also, patient waiting and reception areas should be posted with prominent signs requesting such patients to notify the staff. Patients who might be pregnant or are breast-feeding must be referred to a nuclear medicine staff physician who will determine whether the study should be performed and, if the study is to be performed, any modifications to the procedure and precautions to be followed by the patient. A pregnancy test can be performed

CHECKLIST FOR RADIOPHARMACEUTICAL THERAPY OR ADMINISTRATION OF ^{131}-I AS SODIUM IODIDE

Radiopharmaceutical Prescription
(completed by Nuclear Medicine Attending Physician)

Patient_____

Social Security Number_____Date of Birth_____

Procedure_____
_____

Radiopharmaceutical Prescribed_____ in the Chemical Form of_____

Route of Administration_____Activity Prescribed_____millicuries

Signature of Nuclear Medicine Attending Physician_____Date_____

Radiopharmaceutical Administration
(Two Nuclear Medicine staff members shall verify that the patient's identity,
radionuclide, chemical form, activity, and route of administration match the above prescription.)

Patient identification: The patient's identity has been verified immediately prior to administration of the radiopharmaceutical and compared to the prescription above by at least two of the following methods:

_____1. Asking the patient to state and spell his/her full name and compare with the prescription above.
_____2. Comparing stated social security number with prescription above.
_____3. Comparing stated date of birth with prescription above.
_____4. Comparing stated address with patient's record and prescription above.
_____5. Comparing photographic identification (e.g., driver's license) with prescription above and patient's appearance.
_____6. Comparing in-patient identification wrist band with patient record and prescription above.
_____7. Relative or friend attests to patient's identify:
Name of attestor_____Relationship to patient_____

Pregnant or breast-feeding: If patient is female and between 12 and 50 years of age, pregnancy test was performed and negative AND patient was asked if she is breast-feeding a child._____

Radiopharmaceutical dosage verification: (completed by person administering radiopharmaceutical)

Radiopharmaceutical being administered_____ in the chemical form of_____
Radiopharmaceutical lot number_____
Measured activity_____millicuries at_____
Route of administration_____
Date and time of administration_____

Signature of person administering dose_____

Signature of person verifying patient's identity, radiopharmaceutical, activity, and route of administration_____

FIGURE 9.10. Checklist for radiopharmaceutical therapy or administration of ^{131}I as sodium iodide.

if it is uncertain whether the patient is pregnant. If the radiopharmaceutical is [131]I NaI or if the radiopharmaceutical is intended for therapeutic purposes, the possibility of pregnancy should be eliminated by a human chorionic gonadotropin (hCG) test, unless the patient is a premenarchal child, is in a certain postmenopausal state, or has had a documented hysterectomy or tubal ligation.

When the patient is pregnant, the physician should consider other diagnostic modalities and radiopharmaceuticals that might reduce or even avoid the irradiation of the fetus. The physician may wish to ask a medical physicist to estimate the radiation dose to the fetus from the intended procedure. Estimations of fetal dose are relatively simple when the radiopharmaceutical does not cross the placenta. Reducing the administered activity will reduce the fetal dose; however, it must first be ascertained whether the patient is capable of remaining immobile for the increased duration of the study. Because of the proximity of the bladder to the uterus, the patient should be advised to drink fluids and void frequently to reduce the fetal dose from radiopharmaceuticals eliminated via the kidneys. The physician should discuss the potential risks, alternatives, and precautions with the patient. It is prudent to have the patient sign a statement acknowledging the discussion and consenting to the study.

Patients who are nursing children by breast must be counseled by the nuclear medicine physician to cease breast-feeding until the radionuclide in the milk has reached a sufficiently low concentration. For ^{99m}Tc-labeled radiopharmaceuticals, this is typically 24 hours or less. As in the case of the pregnant patient, the physician should consider whether the study is necessary, alternate diagnostic modalities, and other radiopharmaceuticals that might reduce the length of time that cessation of nursing is required. Table 9.10 contains recommendations for the cessa-

tion of breast-feeding following the administration of common radiopharmaceuticals. The patient should be instructed to manually express and discard her breast milk during this period to avoid discomfort and maintain lactation. The physician should discuss the potential risks, alternatives, and precautions with the patient; provide written instructions that include a description of the possible consequences of failing to follow the instructions; and ask the patient to sign a statement acknowledging the discussion and consenting to the study. NRC regulations regarding patients who are nursing infants are discussed later in the section about release of patients after radiopharmaceutical administration.

Radiolabeled Blood Products

Certain procedures, such as ^{111}In-labeled and ^{99m}Tc-labeled leukocyte scans, studies using ^{99m}Tc-labeled erythrocytes prepared *in vitro,* and ^{51}Cr erythrocyte studies, require the *in vitro* labeling and reinjection of blood elements into the patient. Tragic consequences can occur if blood or blood components from a patient with blood-borne pathogens are mistakenly reinjected into another patient. Each nuclear medicine department should have stringent procedures requiring the labeling of blood samples and identification of the patient at the time the blood is drawn and again before reinjection to avoid such accidents. All staff must be trained in such procedures on employment and regularly thereafter.

Determination of Activities of Radiopharmaceutical Doses

Before administration to patients, the activities of photon-emitting radiopharmaceuticals are commonly measured using instru-

Table 9.10. *Recommendations for Cessation of Breast Feeding after Administration of Radiopharmaceutical to Mothers*

Radiopharmaceutical	Administered Activity[a]	Imaging Procedure	Safe Breast Milk Concentration (μCl/ml)	Cessation of Breast Feeding until Breast Milk Is Safe
[99m]Tc sodium pertechnetate	10 mCi	Thyroid scan and Meckel's scan	8.2×10^{-2}	24 hrs
[99m]Tc kits (general rule)	5–25 mCi	All	8.2×10^{-2}	24 hrs
[99m]Tc DTPA	10–15 mCi	Renal scan	1.2×10^{-1}	17 hrs
[99m]Tc MAA	3–5 mCi	Lung perfusion scan	1.2×10^{-1}	10 hrs
[99m]Tc sulfur colloid	5 mCi	Liver spleen scan	1.6×10^{-1}	15 hrs
[99m]Tc MDP	15–25 mCi	Bone scan	2.1×10^{-1}	17 hrs
[67]Ga citrate	6–10 mCi	Infection and tumor scans	2.1×10^{-3}	4 wks
[201]Tl chloride	3 mCi	Myocardial perfusion	2.4×10^{-3}	3 wks
Sodium [123]I	30 μCi	Thyroid uptake	1.2×10^{-4}	3 days
	50–400 μCi	Thyroid scan	1.2×10^{-4}	5 days
Sodium [131]I	5 μCi	Thyroid uptake	4.1×10^{-7}	68 days
Sodium [131]I	10 mCi	Thyroid cancer Scan or Graves Therapy	4.1×10^{-7}	Discontinue[b]
Sodium [131]I	29.9 mCi	Outpatient therapy for hyperfunctioning nodule	4.1×10^{-7}	Discontinue[b]
Sodium [131]I	100 mCi or more	Thyroid cancer treatment (ablation)	4.1×10^{-7}	Discontinue[b]

[a]Multiply by 37 to obtain MBq.
[b]Discontinuance is based not only on the excessive time recommended for cessation of breast feeding but also on the high dose the breasts themselves would receive during the radiopharmaceutical breast transit.
Source: 49.

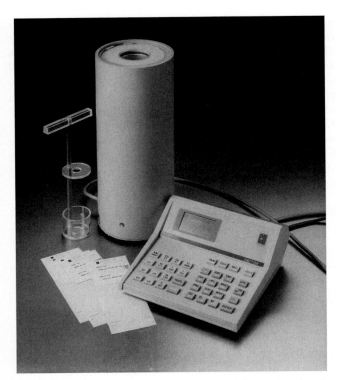

FIGURE 9.11. Dose calibrator. Detector is a well-type ion chamber filled with pressurized argon. The plastic vial and syringe holder (shown to left of ionization chamber) is used to place radioactive material into the detector. This reduces exposure to the hands and permits the activity to be measured in a reproducible geometry. (Photograph courtesy Capintec, Inc.) (From Bushberg JT, Seibert JA, Leidholdt EM et al. *The essential physics of medical imaging,* 2nd ed. Philadelphia: Lippincott Williams & Wilkins, 2002, with permission.)

ments called *dose calibrators.* In the typical dose calibrator, the detector is a cylindrical ion chamber surrounding a well for the syringe or vial being assayed (Fig. 9.11). Most of these ion chambers are filled with a high atomic number gas, such as argon, and are pressurized to permit the assay of activities of a few microcuries. Because the ion chamber is sealed, pressure and temperature corrections are not necessary. The electrical current from the ion chamber is measured and multiplied by a user-selected calibration factor for the radionuclide being assayed, and the activity is displayed. In the case of radionuclides with significant low-energy photon emissions, such as ^{123}I, ^{125}I, and ^{133}Xe, the attenuation by the syringe or vial containing the radionuclide can significantly affect the measurement.

Radiopharmaceuticals, such as ^{32}P and ^{89}Sr, that do not emit x-rays or γ-rays, are usually obtained as unit doses from commercial radiopharmacies. The stated activity, corrected for radioactive decay, is usually relied on. If adjustment of the activity is needed, it is usually performed using volumetric measurements. However, it is prudent to use the dose calibrator for an approximate measurement of the activity.

MEDICAL EVENTS (MISADMINISTRATIONS)

The medical use regulations of the NRC define certain serious errors in the administration of radiopharmaceuticals to patients as *medical events* (28). The former regulations called these *misadministrations* (17). The medical use regulations define a medical event as

A. The administration of byproduct material that results in one of the following conditions (1 or 2) unless its occurrence was the direct result of patient intervention (e.g., ^{131}I therapy patient takes only one half of the prescribed dosage and refuses to take the remainder):

1. A dose that differs from the prescribed dose by more than 0.05 Sv (5 rem) effective dose equivalent, 0.5 Sv (50 rem) to an organ or tissue, or 0.5 Sv (50 rem) shallow dose equivalent to the skin; and one of the following conditions (i or ii) has also occurred:

   (i) The total dose delivered differs from the prescribed dose by 20% or more.

   (ii) The total dosage (i.e., administered activity) delivered differs from the prescribed dosage by 20% or more or falls outside the prescribed dosage range. Falling outside the prescribed dosage range means the administration of activity that is greater or less than a predetermined range of activity for a given procedure that has been established by the licensee.

2. A dose that exceeds 0.05 Sv (5 rem) effective dose equivalent, 0.5 Sv (50 rem) to an organ or tissue, or 0.5 Sv (50 rem) shallow dose equivalent to the skin from any of the following:

   (i) An administration of a wrong radioactive drug containing byproduct material

   (ii) An administration of a radioactive drug containing byproduct material by the wrong route of administration

   (iii) An administration of a dose or dosage to the wrong individual

   (iv) An administration of a dose or dosage delivered by the wrong mode of treatment

B. Any event resulting from intervention of a patient or human research subject in which the administration of byproduct material or radiation from byproduct material results or will result in unintended permanent functional damage to an organ or a physiological system, as determined by a physician. Patient intervention means actions by the patient or human research subject, whether intentional or unintentional, that affect the radiopharmaceutical administration.

When a medical event is discovered, whenever possible, immediate action should be taken to protect the patient. Methods include the use of emetics or gastric lavage to remove orally administered radiopharmaceuticals and the use of blocking agents such as potassium iodide for ^{131}I NaI. Delay in the implementation of such measures drastically reduces their effectiveness. NCRP Report No. 65 provides useful guidance (39).

NRC regulations require the licensee to notify the NRC no later than the next calendar day after discovery of the event and the referring physician within 24 hours, followed by a written report to the NRC within 15 days (17,28). The patient, or patient's responsible relative or guardian, must also be notified within 24 hours, unless the referring physician informs the licensee either that he or she will inform the patient or that, based on medical judgment, notifying the patient would be harmful. The licensee is not required to notify the patient or the patient's responsible relative or guardian without first consulting the referring physician. If a verbal notification is made, the patient or patient's responsible relative or guardian must be informed that a written description of the event can be obtained from the licensee on request. The written report to the NRC must state whether the licensee informed the patient or the patient's relative or guardian or, if not, why not. The report to the NRC must *not* include the patient's name or other identifying information. Whenever a medical event is suspected, the current NRC regulations should be consulted to ensure that all legal requirements are met.

The NRC's medical use regulations also require that the NRC be notified, within the next calendar day after discovery, of either of the following (28):

1. Any dose to an embryo or fetus exceeding 50 mSv (5 rem) dose equivalent from an administration of a radiopharmaceutical to a pregnant woman unless the dose to the embryo or fetus was specifically approved in advance by the nuclear medicine physician.
2. Any dose to a nursing child, resulting from an administration of a radiopharmaceutical to a breast-feeding patient, that exceeds 50 mSv (5 rem) total effective dose equivalent or that causes unintended permanent functional damage to an organ or physiological system.

The proposed regulations require notification of the pregnant woman or mother, notification of the referring physician, and a written report, as described previously for a medical event.

Reduction of Patient's Radiation Dose

The radiopharmaceutical chosen for a procedure significantly affects the radiation dose to the patient. In particular, ^{123}I NaI should be used instead of ^{131}I NaI for routine thyroid uptake measurements and imaging. Also, ^{123}I-labeled radiopharmaceuticals should be used, whenever possible, instead of diagnostic radiopharmaceuticals labeled with ^{131}I. Whenever ^{131}I-labeled radiopharmaceuticals, other than NaI, are used (e.g., ^{131}I hippuran), the patient's thyroid should be first blocked with nonradioactive iodine to limit the thyroidal uptake of unbound radioiodine.

The radiation doses to patients from radiopharmaceuticals that are excreted in the urine can be reduced significantly by encouraging the patients to drink fluids and void frequently. It is important, of course, to first screen for patients for whom this recommendation is contraindicated, such as patients suffering from congestive heart failure.

Release of Patients after Administration of Radiopharmaceuticals

Until May 29, 1997, a medical facility licensed by the NRC was not permitted to release a patient following the administration of a radiopharmaceutical unless the measured dose rate from the patient was less than 5 mrem/hour at a distance of 1 meter, or the activity in the patient was less than 30 millicuries. On and after that date, a medical facility licensed by the NRC is permitted to release from its control any patient administered a radiopharmaceutical, provided that the total effective dose equivalent to any other individual from the patient is not likely to exceed 5 mSv (500 mrem) (17,28). If the total effective dose equivalent

to another individual is likely to exceed 1 mSv (100 mrem), the licensee must provide the released patient with written instructions on actions to maintain doses to others ALARA. If the dose to a nursing child could exceed 1 mSv (100 mrem) if there were no interruption of breast-feeding, the instructions must include guidance on the interruption or discontinuance of breast-feeding and information on the consequences of failure to follow the guidance. NRC Regulatory Guide 8.39 provides guidance on compliance with these regulatory requirements (24). The NRC requires that records regarding the basis for the release of patients and provision of instructions to patients nursing infants by breast be retained in certain situations.

Patients administered radiopharmaceuticals for diagnostic nuclear medicine procedures can be immediately released; the doses to others from these patients are not likely to exceed 5 mSv (24). In fact, the only common nuclear medicine diagnostic procedure in which the dose to others is likely to exceed 1 mSv is the ^{131}I NaI whole-body thyroid cancer survey.

RADIOPHARMACEUTICAL THERAPIES

Radiopharmaceuticals are used for therapy in a number of diseases. The most common are the use of activities of 110 MBq to 1 GBq (~3 to 30 mCi) of ^{131}I NaI for the treatment of hyperthyroidism and 2 to 7.5 GBq (~50 to 200 mCi) of ^{131}I NaI for the treatment of thyroid carcinoma. Activities up to 555 MBq (15 mCi) of ^{32}P as sodium phosphate are used for the treatment of diseases of the bone marrow such as polycythemia vera, thrombocythemia, and certain leukemias and for palliation of pain in patients with multiple skeletal metastases from cancer. Activities of approximately 150 MBq (4 mCi) of ^{89}Sr chloride or 260 GBq (70 mCi) of ^{153}Sm-EDTMP are administered for palliation of pain in patients with multiple skeletal metastases from cancer. A variety of monoclonal and polyclonal antibodies, the majority of which are labeled with ^{131}I, are under investigation for radioimmunotherapy of cancer. The properties of these radionuclides are summarized in Table 9.11.

All radionuclides used for therapy emit a significant fraction of their decay energy as charged particles. The properties that make these radionuclides useful in therapy also render them relatively hazardous to medical staff, the patients' families, and the public. The primary precaution for radionuclides, such as ^{32}P and ^{89}Sr, emitting only charged particles is to control contamination from the patients. External exposure from x-rays

Table 9.11. *Physical Properties of Radionuclides Commonly used for Therapy*

Nuclide	Half-Life Energy (days)	Maximum β^- Energy (keV)	Average β^- Emissions (keV)	x- and γ- Ray (keV)
^{131}I	8.04	807	182	364 (81%) others <723
^{32}P	14.3	1710	695	none
^{153}Sm	1.93	810	233	103 (29%)
^{89}Sr	50.6	1491	583	rare

(bremsstrahlung) is negligible. In the case of therapeutic radionuclides with significant photon emissions, such as ^{131}I, precautions must be taken against both contamination and external exposure.

The dose usually arrives precalibrated for the correct activity at the time of administration. The activity should be measured using a dose calibrator, preferably twice, before it is administered to the patient. Before administration of the dose, a written directive must be prepared by the nuclear medicine staff physician naming the patient and specifying the radionuclide, chemical form, activity to be administered, and route of administration. The identity of the patient must be carefully verified, preferably by at least two independent means. (See the section on written directives earlier in this chapter.) If the patient is female and of childbearing age, the precautions described previously in the section on pregnant and nursing patients should be taken. The administration must be in accordance with the directive. Although a technologist may administer therapeutic quantities of radioactive material, it is recommended that the nuclear medicine staff physician directly supervise the administration of the dose.

Release of Therapy Patients

As mentioned previously, medical facilities licensed by the NRC are permitted to administer radiopharmaceuticals for therapeutic purposes to outpatients, provided that the total effective dose equivalent to any other individual from the patient is not likely to exceed 5 mSv (500 mrem) (17,28). Therefore, a decision must be made whether to immediately release the patient after treatment or to hospitalize the patient for radiation protection purposes. When a decision is made to hospitalize the patient for radiation protection purposes, it must be further decided when the hospitalized patient should be released. Usually, the hospitalized patient is released when the remaining activity decreases to a predetermined amount. NRC Regulatory Guide 8.39 provides calculational methods for estimating doses to individuals from the released patient (24). Patients being treated with ^{32}P, ^{89}Sr, and ^{153}Sm; most patients being treated for hyperthyroidism with ^{131}I; and many patients being treated with ^{131}I for thyroid cancer may be treated without being hospitalized, except when hospitalization is required for medical reasons. However, each patient should be interviewed regarding his or her home and work situation before administration of the radiopharmaceutical and instructed in radiation safety precautions to be followed after treatment. It may occasionally be necessary to hospitalize patients for radiation safety reasons, who otherwise could be immediately released, for example, if the patient lives with a pregnant woman or small children in a small apartment, or if it is believed that the patient is unlikely to follow radiation safety precautions.

Radiation safety precautions should be given, both verbally and in writing, to released therapy patients. The following is an example of such precautions for ^{131}I:

Safety Precautions Following Administration of Radioactive ^{131}I: greater than 370 MBq (10 mCi) The dose of radioactive iodine that you have received is beneficial to you, but it is desirable that other persons not be unnecessarily exposed to radiation. The

following precautions will help minimize the radiation exposure to other persons.

A. During the first 5 days
   Much of the radioactivity in your body will be eliminated in your urine. Also, some radioactivity will be found in your saliva and perspiration. To minimize the spread of radioactivity:
   1. Wash cups, plates, and eating utensils immediately after use or use disposables.
   2. Do not kiss anyone.
   3. Do not share towels and washcloths with others.
   4. Sleep in a separate bed.
   5. Wash any clothing you have worn (including pajamas, underwear, towels, and bed linens) separately from those used by other members of your family.
   6. Do not touch or hold infants or pregnant women.
   7. Stay at least 3 feet away from other people, except for very brief contact.
   8. Flush the toilet twice after using it. If you spill any urine on the toilet or elsewhere, wash the area three times using toilet paper and flush it down the toilet.
   9. Wash your hands frequently, especially before touching another person.
B. During the next 5 days
   Your thyroid gland will contain significant radioactivity. To minimize the radiation exposure to others:
   1. Sleep in a separate bed.
   2. Avoid sitting close to others (within 2 feet) for hours at a time (for example, at a movie theater).
   3. Do not hold infants or young children, except for short periods.
C. If you are breast-feeding an infant, you must discontinue breast-feeding. If you feed your child by breast after you have received the radioactive iodine, your child will receive some of the radioactive iodine. This would likely damage your child's thyroid gland and may increase the chance of your child developing cancer. The extent of the damage to the child's thyroid and the probability of developing cancer will depend on the actual radiation dose that the child received.

The precautions described in Items A and C listed above are sufficient for patients administered ^{32}P or ^{89}Sr for therapeutic purposes or activities of ^{131}I NaI between 37 to 370 MBq (1 to 10 mCi).

Precautions Regarding the Hospitalized Therapy Patient

The following radiation safety precautions are recommended for hospitalized ^{131}I therapy patients:

1. Room selection: The patient must be confined to a private room selected to minimize the exposure to staff and other patients. Corner rooms with two exterior walls are often used. Adjacent rooms, other than infrequently occupied rooms such as storage rooms, usually must be placed off limits, unless shielding is used. The patient's room must have a private toilet.
2. Training of staff: The nursing staff on the ward and the ward team (medical students, residents, fellows, and staff physicians) must be trained in radiation safety precautions. Written instructions to nursing staff should be placed in the patient's chart, and a warning label indicating that the

patient contains radioactive material should be placed on the cover of the patient's chart. Housekeeping personnel must be instructed not to enter the room and not to remove anything from the room. Dietetics personnel must be instructed to provide disposable table service and not to enter the room when delivering meals. Personnel on all shifts must receive training.

3. Room preparation: The majority of the ^{131}I will be excreted in the urine in the first 24 hours; however, ^{131}I will also be found in perspiration and saliva. Surfaces likely to become contaminated should be covered with plastic or plastic-backed absorbent paper to aid in decontamination. These include the floor of the room and bathroom, the mattress, the pillows, toilet seat, rim of the toilet bowl, tops of all tables and night stands, and anything the patient is likely to touch (e.g., the phone, light switches, TV and bed controls).

4. The patient's door should be posted with a "Caution–Radioactive Materials" warning sign and instructions that the room not be released for general use without the approval of the RSO and that visitors and ancillary personnel contact the nursing station or Radiation Safety Office before entering the room.

5. Radiation safety instructions for the patient: The patient should be instructed in radiation safety precautions. These include not leaving the room, keeping distance from and not touching visitors, flushing the toilet twice after use, and frequent hand washing. Male patients should be asked to sit when urinating into the toilet. Patients for whom it is not contraindicated for medical reasons should be encouraged to drink fluids and urinate frequently while confined.

6. Personnel dosimetry: Nursing staff providing care for the patient should be issued dosimeters.

7. Administration of the dose: The therapy dose should be transported to the patient's room on a cart and should be shielded to reduce the exposure rate at 1 meter to less than 2 mR/hour.

8. Survey of dose-rates in adjacent areas: Promptly after administration of the dose, the dose rates should be measured in all adjacent occupied areas, including rooms above and below (unless demonstrated not to be required by previous measurements), to verify that the dose rates in unrestricted areas (including hallways) do not exceed 20 μSv/hour (2 mrem/hour) and that no member of the public (which includes nearby patients, visitors, and office workers) will receive more than 1 mSv (100 mrem) in a year. Access must be restricted to any areas in which the dose rate exceeds 20 μSv/hour (2 mrem/hour).

9. Care of these patients is similar to the treatment of isolation patients. All food should be served with disposable plates and utensils that will be discarded after use into a designated radioactive waste container. Used linens must not be sent to the laundry without being released by the radiation safety staff. Nursing staff must promptly notify nuclear medicine or radiation safety of spills of excreta in the room, medical emergencies, or the patient's death. Nurses and ward team members should wear their assigned radiation dosimeters and disposable shoe covers and gloves when entering the room. This protective clothing should be removed and placed in radioactive waste containers when personnel leave the room. If the nurses' duties are likely to cause their clothing to become contaminated, they should wear aprons or isolation gowns. Used aprons or gowns should be placed in the contaminated linen container in the patient's room at the end of each shift. If the patient is medically stable, discontinuing the routine monitoring of the patient's vital signs can significantly reduce the exposure to nursing staff. If this monitoring is discontinued, the nursing staff should check on the patient as frequently as necessary from the doorway of the patient's room. If monitoring of vital signs is necessary, a sphygmomanometer should be left in the patient's room. The head of the stethoscope should be placed in a disposable glove before being placed against the patient.

10. Visitors should be informed of the contamination and exposure hazard and be instructed to remain outside the patient's room or wear protective clothing and remain at or beyond a safe distance (as determined by radiation safety) from the patient during the visit. No direct patient contact should be permitted. Pregnant women and children younger than 18 years should be discouraged from visiting the patient in the hospital.

11. Release of the patient: The NRC and most state regulatory agencies require that patients not be discharged from the hospital until the total effective dose equivalent to any other individual from the patient is unlikely to exceed 5 mSv (500 mrem). The methods described in NRC Regulatory Guide 8.39 can be used to calculate an amount of activity remaining in the patient, below which the patient may be released from hospitalization (24). The activity remaining in the patient can be easily estimated from the exposure-rate at a fixed distance from the patient. The exposure-rate is initially measured with an ionization chamber at a fixed distance (typically 1 to 3 meters) from the patient's abdomen approximately 15 minutes after the dose has been administered. The exposure rate at the same distance, when the activity in the patient has fallen to A mCi, will be approximately

$$\dot{X} = \frac{A}{A_o}\dot{X}_o \qquad [11]$$

where $\dot{X}_o$ is the initial exposure rate (mR/hour) and A_o is the administered activity (mCi). For example, if a decision has been made to release a patient when the remaining activity is 30 mCi and the exposure rate at 1 meter from a patient shortly after the administration of a 100-mCi dose is 20 mR/hour, the patient may be discharged when the exposure rate is

$$\dot{X}_{30mCi} = \frac{30mCi}{100mCi}\left(20mR/h\right) = 6mR/h$$

Patients are usually discharged between 24 and 48 hours after administration of the radioiodine.

12. Discharge instructions to patients: The patient should be interviewed regarding his or her situation at home and at work. The patient should be given, both verbally and in writing, radiation safety precautions to be followed after discharge from the hospital. (The earlier section on safety

precautions following administration of radioactive [131]I: 370 MBq to 1.11 GBq (10 to 30 mCi) is recommended.)

13. Decontamination of the patient's room: Once the patient is discharged, all protective coverings and trash should be removed and treated as radioactive trash. Linens may be stored for decay or treated as radioactive trash. The room must be decontaminated and surveyed before it is released for routine use. The room is surveyed with a sensitive survey instrument, such as a G-M survey meter with a thin window pancake probe and with wipe tests. Current NRC regulations do not permit the room to be reassigned until the removable contamination on each wipe sample is less than 200 dpm/100 cm^2 wiped (17). The proposed NRC medical use regulations do not specify a limit for removable contamination (28).

The recent introduction of radioimmunotherapy with ^{131}I-labeled monoclonal antibodies directed toward various tumors has increased the number of therapies with high activities of radioiodine. These patients are typically in much poorer health than thyroid cancer patients and often require longer hospitalization. This fact, together with an increased likelihood of acute medical intervention and life support, greatly enhances the possibility of radioiodine contamination of healthcare personnel and facilities. Special efforts should be made to adequately train these individuals in appropriate radiation safety practices. Pathology personnel should also be trained and prepared to deal with this complication. Health physics assistance may be necessary to evaluate and monitor radiation fields and to help with contamination control if patients require surgery or autopsy within a few days following the radiotherapy dose.

The precautions for hospitalized patients treated with ^{32}P, ^{89}Sr, or ^{90}Y are identical to those listed above for therapy with ^{131}I, except that there is little external exposure from these patients. Dose rates need not be measured in adjacent rooms following administration, adjacent rooms are not placed off limits, and nursing staff need not be issued dosimeters. Additional recommendations and precautions for managing patients who have received therapeutic amounts of radionuclides may be found in NCRP Report No. 37 (40). A revision of this document is being prepared by the NCRP.

MISCELLANEOUS ASPECTS OF RADIATION SAFETY IN NUCLEAR MEDICINE

Receiving Radiopharmaceutical Packages

The NRC (16) and agreement states require procedures to be established for the receipt of packages of radioactive material to minimize the potential for contamination and personnel exposure. If packages are received in a mailroom or warehouse rather than directly by the nuclear medicine department, the mailroom or warehouse staff must be instructed in radiation safety precautions, including the requirement to immediately report packages that are damaged or appear to be leaking.

The packages should first be inspected visually to confirm their integrity. The external surfaces of most radioactive packages must be surveyed by wipe tests for removable contamination.

In addition, the radiation levels emitted by packages containing especially large activities must be measured. All packages known to contain radioactive materials and showing evidence of damage or leakage must also be surveyed for contamination and radiation levels. The NRC requires these surveys to be performed within 3 hours of receipt or, if received outside of normal working hours, within 3 hours of the beginning of the next working day. Most institutions monitor all radioactive packages for removable contamination and radiation levels to avoid accidentally failing to perform one of these tests of a package for which it is required. If removable contamination is found, personnel should take precautions to prevent its spread. If the removable contamination on the external surface, as determined by wiping an area of 300 cm^2, exceeds 110 Bq (6,600 dpm), or if the radiation levels from the package exceed specified limits, the final delivery carrier and the NRC or the state radiologic health organization must be immediately notified. These limits are 2 mSv/hour (200 mrem/hour) at the surface of the package and 0.1 mSv/hour (10 mrem/hour) at 1 meter, unless the package was delivered using an exclusive use vehicle, as defined in NRC regulations. Although not required by regulations, some departments perform wipe tests of the innermost containers (the vials and syringes), using swabs or forceps to minimize exposure to the hands, to ensure that the inner containers are not leaking or badly contaminated. When the receipt of this material is properly recorded, it should be stored in a manner that minimizes radiation exposure to personnel. If the shipping package is not reusable, it is usually surveyed for contamination in a low-background area, using a thin-window G-M survey meter, all radioactive warning labels are rendered unrecognizable, and it is discarded as nonradioactive waste.

Radioactive Waste

There are a number of methods for disposal of radioactive waste. These include (a) decay in storage, followed by disposal as nonradioactive waste; (b) disposal into the sanitary sewer system; (c) shipment to a recipient licensed to receive the waste; (d) incineration; and (e) shipment to a licensed radioactive waste burial site. The NRC and agreement states permit patient excreta to be discarded into the sanitary sewer without regard for its radioactivity (16).

Because of significant increases in the cost of radioactive waste disposal and the loss of some disposal options, minimization of radioactive waste is important. Items that are not radioactive should not be discarded into the radioactive waste. In particular, disposable shipping cartons from radioactive material shipments should be surveyed in a low-background area with a portable G-M survey meter and, if they are not contaminated, discarded into the normal trash once their warning labels have been removed or rendered unrecognizable.

Decay in storage is an attractive option for the nuclear medicine department, because of the short half-lives of most radionuclides used. The NRC permits its licensees to discard as ordinary trash radioactive waste containing radionuclides with half-lives less than 120 days, provided that any radiation warning labels are obliterated, and the material is surveyed with a sensitive survey meter in a low-background area to determine that its radioactivity cannot be distinguished from background. It is recommended that the radioactive waste be segregated by half-life into the categories of (a) ^{18}F and any other short-lived positron emitters, (b) ^{99m}Tc, (c) radionuclides with half-lives less than 6 days (i.e., ^{67}Ga, ^{111}In, ^{123}I, ^{133}Xe, ^{153}Sm, and ^{201}Tl), and (d) others (e.g., ^{131}I and ^{89}Sr), to minimize the volume of waste in storage.

Many commercial radiopharmacies will accept the return of used syringes and vials. However, this constitutes the shipping of radioactive materials and is subject to either NRC or agreement state regulations and also DOT regulations. Many departments prefer to decay this material in storage to avoid the shipping requirements.

Radioactive materials may also be shipped to a licensed radioactive waste burial site. There are only three such sites in the United States that are currently accepting low-level radioactive waste. Because of an organization of the states into regional compacts under the federal Low-Level Radioactive Waste Policy Act of 1980, not all states have access to all of these radioactive waste burial sites. Even when available, this disposal option is very expensive and subject to complicated regulatory requirements.

The NRC (16) and agreement states permit the sewer disposal of radioactive material, provided that it is soluble or readily dispersible biologic material. The disposals must not exceed limits on the activity that may be released annually and monthly limits on the average concentration of activity in the sewage. However, some local agencies have established regulations regarding the sewer disposal of radioactive waste that are more restrictive than state and federal regulations.

An institution may request permission from the NRC or agreement state agency to permit the incineration of radioactive waste. The application must demonstrate that releases of airborne radioactivity from the stack will be within permissible limits. The ash must be monitored and, if it contains significant amounts of radioactivity, must be treated as radioactive waste.

Shipping Radioactive Materials

The transportation of radioactive materials, including radioactive waste, is regulated by the DOT. DOT regulations (Title 49 of the Code of Federal Regulations) contain requirements for shipping papers, packaging, and package labeling. The DOT also requires training of workers who ship radioactive materials. Returning used syringes, used vials, and unused doses to a radiopharmacy constitutes shipping of radioactive materials and is subject to DOT regulations. DOT regulations largely conform to the standards of the International Atomic Energy Agency.

Most radiopharmaceuticals and ^{99}Mo/^{99m}Tc generators are shipped to nuclear medicine departments in Type A packages. Type A packages must prevent the loss of contents and must maintain their radiation shielding properties during normal transportation, including rough handling. The shipper of a Type A package must maintain documentation showing that the package design has been tested and was capable of withstanding DOT-specified water spray, free drop, stacking, and penetration tests. A Type A package must be labeled on two opposite sides with DOT-approved Radioactive I, II, or III labels; the proper

label is determined by the maximal radiation levels at the surface and at 1 meter from the package. A Type A package must be equipped with a security seal that would indicate that the package had been opened. A Type A package must be accompanied by shipping papers, which describe the contents; written emergency response information; and an emergency response telephone number that is monitored 24 hours a day while the shipment is being transported.

Limited quantities of radioactive material, as defined in DOT regulations, may be shipped as excepted packages, thereby avoiding most of complicated regulatory requirements regarding Type A packages. Used syringes, used vials, and unused doses are commonly returned to commercial radiopharmacies as *excepted packages, limited quantity.* Used ^{99}Mo/^{99m}Tc generators are typically returned to the vendor as either excepted packages, limited quantity, or as empty radioactive packages. These are shipped in strong tight packages that will not leak radioactive materials under conditions normally incident to transportation. Testing and certification of the package design and shipping papers are not required. The radiation levels at the surface of an excepted package may not exceed 5 μSv/hour (0.5 mrem/hour), and the removable contamination on the surface of the package must be within limits specified by DOT regulations. Commercial radiopharmacies and vendors of generators typically provide detailed instructions for preparing return shipments.

RADIATION ACCIDENTS

A radiation accident may be defined as a substantial inadvertent exposure to ionizing radiation or unintentional contamination with a radionuclide. Several texts and reviews of the preparation for and response to radiation accidents are available (41–44). Although clinically significant radiation accidents are rare, it is prudent for each hospital to have a written procedure to cope with such accidents. Emergency room and employee health staff should also have regular training in such accidents. The radiation accident victims most likely to be treated are hospital staff members who have contaminated their skin, splashed radioactivity into their eyes, or punctured themselves with contaminated sharps.

Radiation accidents may be classified into those caused by irradiation by external sources and those involving contamination of the victims by radioactive material. It should be noted that more than one type of accident may occur in a given circumstance. For example, an individual may be exposed and contaminated in the same accident.

Irradiation by External Sources

Exposure to a source of radiation causes an individual to be *irradiated.* Under most circumstances, the exposure ends once the radiation source is turned off, removed, or shielded or the individual is removed from the area. Unless the exposure is massive, the clinical effects of the radiation injury are not immediately apparent. The actual symptoms and ultimate injury depend on the absorbed dose, tissues exposed, and penetrating capabilities of the radiation. Unless there has been a massive exposure to neutrons, the individual does not become radioactive and may be handled without special precautions. Medical management in such cases is initially symptomatic, with particular care being taken to assess the absorbed dose by using biologic criteria such as nausea, vomiting, diarrhea, skin erythema, lymphocyte count, and chromosomal aberration frequency.

Contamination

The second major type of radiation accident is *contamination* with a radionuclide. The contamination may be on the surface of the skin (external contamination), may be within the body (internal contamination), or may be in the form of an embedded object. Contamination usually refers to unsealed radionuclides rather than sealed sources.

External contamination rarely reaches levels that cause acute medical effects. There are a few instances in which there may be absorption of the radionuclide through the skin, such as contamination with tritium or radioiodine. α-Emitting radionuclides do not pose a hazard if the skin is intact because the particles are unable to penetrate to the viable layer of the dermis. Energetic β-particles can cause skin erythema and in some cases skin necrosis. As a practical matter, these effects are seen only in circumstances in which there is very high specific activity (such as fresh fallout from nuclear weapons). Skin contamination with γ-emitting radionuclides usually poses more hazard to the sensitive internal organs than to the skin itself. The major hazard associated with external contamination is that it may become internal, through inhalation, through transdermal absorption, by absorption through wounds, or, more likely, through ingestion. The medical management of external contamination consists of removal of the contamination. Simply removing the outer clothing often removes 70% to 90% of external contamination, with the remainder usually being on the hands, face, and hair. After the clothing is removed, washing with soap and water usually removes 90% to 95% of surface contamination.

In instances in which there is a physical injury associated with external contamination, the transportation of such a patient into the emergency room area must be carefully controlled to prevent spread of the contamination to personnel, facilities, and equipment. Overall, emergency room management is a matter of having some form of protective clothing available (such as shoe covers, water-repellent gowns or coveralls, surgical masks, and gloves). If time permits, the floor should be covered and the area roped-off. Medical stabilization of the patient always takes priority. After the patient is stabilized, removal of external contamination can be performed.

Management of internal contamination is a much more difficult problem. Early diagnosis and treatment are necessary to have much effect in most cases. As an example, a substantial fraction of soluble transuranic radionuclides activity administered intravenously or absorbed through wounds will concentrate in bone. The vast majority of this activity is localized in the osseous tissues within 2 hours. The best early treatment is specific to the radionuclide and its chemical form. Unfortunately, this type of information is often difficult to obtain within the first 2 hours after an accident. Most early treatment of internal contamination is based on preplanning and educated guesses.

NCRP Report No. 65 provides guidance for the management of internal contamination (39).

The major treatment methods for internal contamination use one or more of the following principles:

1. Blocking or isotopic dilution (e.g., oral administration of nonradioactive potassium iodide to prevent thyroidal uptake of radioactive iodine). Suspected or known exposure to radioactive iodine can be conveniently treated by having the patient drink a glass of water containing 5 drops of saturated solution of potassium iodide (SSKI) (39).
2. Limiting the uptake (e.g., administration of aluminum-containing antacids to reduce uptake from the gastrointestinal tract).
3. Increasing the transit through the body (treatment with fluids in the case of tritium contamination or administration of cathartics in the case of ingestion).
4. Local removal (e.g., debridement of a contaminated wound).
5. Decorporation (e.g., administration of chelating agents such as calcium- or zinc-DTPA for treatment of transuranic internal contamination).

The amount of internal contamination from inhalation can be assessed if the concentrations in the atmosphere and the occupancy time are known. Lacking these, other facts about the accident are also useful. Accidents in which there was a grinding procedure suggest large particles, which are usually deposited in the anterior nose and pharynx. An accident involving a fire would suggest much smaller particles that may well be deposited much further down in the bronchial tree or in alveoli. To assess the possibility of internal contamination, nasal swabs may be useful; such samples should be obtained as early as possible following a contamination accident because the nose and nasopharynx clear relatively quickly. Swab samples should be obtained from each nostril to ensure that there is, in fact, inhalation rather than contamination of a nares by a finger.

Whole body counters are very sensitive devices that are used at many nuclear power plants to assess internal contamination. Unfortunately, they are cumbersome and their extreme sensitivities often render them useless when clinically significant amounts of radionuclides are present. In cases in which a whole body counter cannot be used, a γ-camera may provide useful information. A relatively crude photopeak analysis can be performed and localization of radionuclide within the body by imaging methods is often possible. There should always be follow-up of patients suspected of having internal contamination with analysis of serial urine and/or fecal samples. Follow-up thyroid counting is useful in those patients who have internal contamination with radioiodine.

RADIATION SAFETY PROGRAMS AT MEDICAL INSTITUTIONS
Radioactive Materials License

Any individual or institution wishing to perform nuclear medicine or to use radioactive materials for research or radiation oncology must first apply to the NRC or pertinent agreement state agency for a license. A license application must be prepared describing the facilities where the radioactive material is to be used, the persons who are to supervise the use of the material and their qualifications, the uses of the material (i.e., uptake, dilution, and excretion studies; imaging studies; or therapies), and the possession limits for certain categories of material. Under current NRC licensing procedures, the license application must also contain proposed procedures for such matters as receiving and opening packages of radioactive material, testing dose calibrators, handling radioactive material safely, dealing with spills of radioactive material, and surveying of use areas for exposure and contamination, as well as proposed procedures for personnel dosimetry, radiopharmaceutical therapies, and disposal of radioactive waste. At the time of writing, the NRC has proposed a simplification of the licensing process to accompany the proposed revision of 10 CFR Part 35 discussed previously in the section on regulatory agencies. Under this simplified process, instead of submitting proposed procedures in the application, the applicant must merely submit statements committing to developing and implementing the written procedures regarding these issues (27). The NRC (25,27) and agreement state agencies provide suggested procedures. When the license is issued, all commitments made by the applicant in the license application become legally binding. A common cause of violations found during inspections by the NRC and agreement state agencies is unawareness of provisions of the license.

Radiation Safety Officer

Each facility performing nuclear medicine must designate a RSO. In small departments, the RSO is usually the nuclear medicine physician. Hospitals with large nuclear medicine programs may have a full-time RSO. This person will usually hold a doctorate or masters degree in an appropriate discipline and may be certified by the American Board of Radiology, the American Board of Medical Physics, the American Board of Science in Nuclear Medicine, or the American Board of Health Physics. In very large programs, such as those at research and teaching hospitals, the RSO may be assisted by other health physicists, technicians, and clerical personnel. The duties of the RSO include investigating incidents, writing procedures, performing periodic radiation surveys, training personnel, monitoring personnel dosimetry, directing action during emergencies such as spills and personnel contamination, performing periodic audits of users of radioactive material, and preparing license applications and amendment requests.

Radiation Safety Committee

The former NRC medical use regulations required each medical institution licensed to use radioactive materials to have a radiation safety committee (17). The NRC's revised medical use regulations removed the requirement for a radiation safety committee for less complex medical use programs (28). Under the revised regulations, only medical use programs wih two or more of the following types of use – (a) radiopharmaceuticals requiring written directives, (b) manual brachytherapy, (c) photon-emitting remote-afterloading brachytherapy devices, (d) teletherapy devices with radioactive sources (e.g., ^{60}Co machines), and (e)

gamma stereotactic radiosurgery devices – are required to establish a radiation safety committee. Agreement state regulations may differ from those of the NRC.

The regulations require that the committee oversee all uses of byproduct material permitted by the NRC license. The NRC requires the committee to include an authorized user for each type of use permitted by the license (e.g., if nuclear medicine is performed, a nuclear medicine physician must be a member of the committee), the radiation safety officer, a representative of nursing, and a representative of management who is neither an authorized user nor the radiation safety officer (28).

Typically, such committees meet at least quarterly. The committees review the qualifications of proposed authorized users and a proposed radiation safety officer prior to submitting license applications or license amendment requests to the NRC or an agreement state agency, review the doses to workers, review incidents and corrective action taken, and perform an annual review of the radiation safety program.

Some medical institutions, typically large research and teaching hospitals, are issued *licenses of broad scope*. The NRC's regulations regarding broad scope licenses, in most cases, require the establishment of a radiation safety committee. In a broad scope license, the radiation safety committee is delegated the authority to approve authorized users for clinical and research uses of radioactive material, to approve extensive changes to facilities, and to approve new uses of radioactive materials, without obtaining amendments to the license.

Training Program

One of the most important aspects of a radiation safety program is the training of workers who enter restricted areas. These workers must be trained before assuming their duties and regularly thereafter, and their training must be commensurate with the complexity of their duties and the magnitude of the risk. Workers who must be trained include nuclear medicine physicians and technologists, nurses who provide care for radiopharmaceutical therapy patients, and other staff who may routinely enter restricted areas. Housekeepers who clean the nuclear medicine department or who work on wards where radiopharmaceutical therapy patients are confined, maintenance personnel who enter restricted areas, and hospital security personnel also should receive limited training commensurate with the risks encountered. In addition, all nursing staff should receive some general training because they encounter patients who have been administered radiopharmaceuticals for diagnostic purposes. NRC regulations require this training to describe the sources of radiation, the health risks associated with ionizing radiation, precautions to minimize exposure, applicable portions of regulations and license conditions, the requirement to report to the appropriate supervisor anything that might cause a violation of regulations or license conditions or unnecessary exposure of persons to radiation, and the workers' right to obtain their radiation exposure reports (15). Women must be notified of their right, should they become pregnant, to declare their pregnancies, thereby causing their embryos or fetuses to be subject to a more restrictive dose limit. (See the section on standards for protection against radiation earlier in this chapter.)

REFERENCES

1. International Commission on Radiation Units and Measurements. *Radiation quantities and units*. Bethesda, MD: International Commission on Radiation Units and Measurements, 1980; ICRU report no 33.

2. National Council on Radiation Protection and Measurements. *SI Units in radiation protection and measurements*. Bethesda, MD: National Council on Radiation Protection and Measurements, 1985; NCRP report no 82.

3. International Commission on Radiation Units and Measurements. *Quantities and units in radiation protection dosimetry*. Bethesda, MD: 1993; ICRU report no 51.

4. International Commission on Radiological Protection. 1990 Recommendations of the International Commission on Radiological Protection. ICRP publication 60. *Ann ICRP* 1991;21(1-3).

5. National Council on Radiation Protection and Measurements. *The relative biological effectiveness of radiations of different quality*. Bethesda, MD: National Council on Radiation Protection and Measurements, 1990; NCRP report no 104.

6. International Commission on Radiological Protection. Recommendations of the International Commission on Radiological Protection. ICRP publication 26. *Ann ICRP* 1977;1(3).

7. International Commission on Radiological Protection. *Summary of the current ICRP principles for protection of the patient in nuclear medicine*. Oxford: Pergamon Press, 1993.

8. United Nations Scientific Committee on the Effects of Atomic Radiation. *Sources and effects of ionizing radiation, 1993*. Report to the General Assembly. United Nations, New York: United Nations Scientific Committee on the Effects of Atomic Radiation, 1993.

9. National Technical Information Service. *A citizen's guide to radon, what it is and what to do about it*. OPA-86-004. Springfield, VA: National Technical Information Service, 1986.

10. National Council on Radiation Protection and Measurements. *Limitation of exposure to ionizing radiation*. Bethesda, MD: National Council on Radiation Protection and Measurements, 1993; NCRP report no 116.

11. National Council on Radiation Protection and Measurements. *Exposure of the U.S. population from diagnostic medical radiation*. Bethesda, MD: National Council on Radiation Protection and Measurements, 1989; NCRP report no 100.

12. National Council on Radiation Protection and Measurements. *Radiation exposure of the U.S. population from consumer products and miscellaneous sources*. Bethesda, MD: National Council on Radiation Protection and Measurements, 1987; NCRP report no 95.

13. National Council on Radiation Protection and Measurements. *Ionizing radiation exposure of the population of the United States*. Bethesda, MD: National Council on Radiation Protection and Measurements, 1987; NCRP report no 93.

14. National Council on Radiation Protection and Measurements. *Exposure of the U.S. population from occupational radiation*. Bethesda, MD: National Council on Radiation Protection and Measurements, 1989; NCRP report no 101.

15. US Nuclear Regulatory Commission. *Notices, instructions, and reports to workers: inspection and investigations*. Title 10 of the Code of Federal Regulations, Part 19. Washington, DC: US Government Printing Office, January 1, 2001.

16. US Nuclear Regulatory Commission. *Standards for protection against radiation*. Title 10 of the Code of Federal Regulations, Part 20. Washington, DC: US Government Printing Office, January 1, 2001.

17. US Nuclear Regulatory Commission. *Medical use of byproduct material*. Title 10 of the Code of Federal Regulations, Part 35. Washington, DC: US Government Printing Office, January 1, 2001.

18. US Nuclear Regulatory Commission. *Regulatory guide 8.9: acceptable concepts, models, equations, and assumptions for a bioassay program*. Revision 1. Washington, DC: US Government Printing Office, July, 1993.

19. US Nuclear Regulatory Commission. *Regulatory guide 8.10: operating philosophy for maintaining occupational radiation exposure as low as is reasonably achievable*. Washington, DC: US Government Printing Office, September, 1975.

20. US Nuclear Regulatory Commission. *Regulatory guide 8.13: instruction concerning prenatal radiation exposure*. Revision 3. Washington, DC: US Government Printing Office, June, 1999.

21. US Nuclear Regulatory Commission. *Regulatory guide 8.18: information relevant to ensuring that occupational radiation exposure at medical institutions will be as low as reasonably achievable*. Revision 1. Washington, DC: US Government Printing Office, October, 1982.

22. US Nuclear Regulatory Commission. *Regulatory guide 8.23: radiation safety surveys at medical institutions*. Washington DC: US Government Printing Office, January, 1981.

23. US Nuclear Regulatory Commission. *Regulatory guide 8.33: quality management program*. Washington, DC: US Government Printing Office, October, 1991.

24. US Nuclear Regulatory Commission. *Regulatory guide 8.39: Release of patients administered radioactive materials*. Washington, DC: US Government Printing Office, April, 1997.

25. US Nuclear Regulatory Commission. *Regulatory guide 10.8: guide for the preparation of applications for medical programs*. Revision 2. Washington, DC: US Government Printing Office, August, 1987.

26. US Nuclear Regulatory Commission. *Appendix X to regulatory guide 10.8: guidance on complying with new part 20 requirements*. Washington DC: US Government Printing Office, 1992.

27. US Nuclear Regulatory Commission. *NUREG-1556: Consolidated guidance about materials licenses, vol 9, Program-specific guidance about medical use licenses, draft report for comment*. Washington, DC: US Government Printing Office, August, 1998.

28. 10 CFR Parts 20, 32, and 35-Medical Use of Byproduct Material; Final Rule, *Federal register*. Washington, DC: US Government Printing Office, April 24, 2002:20250–20397.

29. International Commission on Radiological Protection. Limits for intakes of radionuclides by workers. ICRP publication 30 (four parts, including supplements). *Annals of the ICRP*. Elmsford, NY: Pergamon Press, 1979–1988.

30. National Council on Radiation Protection and Measurements. *A handbook of radioactivity measurements procedures*, 2nd ed. Bethesda, MD: National Council on Radiation Protection and Measurements, 1985; NCRP report no 58.

31. International Commission on Radiological Protection. *Individual monitoring for intake of radionuclides by workers: design and interpretation*. ICRP publication 54. Elmsford, NY: Pergamon Press, 1988.

32. Lessard ET, Yihua X, Skrable KW et al. *Interpretation of bioassay measurements*. US Nuclear Regulatory Commission. NUREG/CR-4884. Washington DC: US Government Printing Office, July, 1987.

33. Eckerman KF, Wolbarst AB, Richardson AC. *Limiting values of radionuclide intake and air concentration and dose conversion factors for inhalation, submersion, and ingestion*. Federal guidance report No. 11. Washington DC: US Government Printing Office, September, 1988; EPA-520/1-88-20.

34. Barrall RC, Smith SI. Personal radiation exposure and protection from Tc-99m radiation. In: Kereiakes JG, Corey KR, eds. *Biophysical aspects of the medical use of technetium-99m*. AAPM monograph no 1. Cincinnati, OH: University of Cincinnati, 1976.

35. International Commission on Radiological Protection. *The handling, storage, use and disposal of unsealed radionuclides in hospitals and medical research establishments*. ICRP publication 25. Elmsford, NY: Pergamon Press, 1977.

36. US Department of Health, Education and Welfare (USDHEW). *Radiation safety in nuclear medicine: a practical guide*. Washington, DC: US Government Printing Office, 1981; USDHEW Publ FDA-82 8180.

37. National Council on Radiation Protection and Measurement (NCRP). *Radiation protection for medical and allied health personnel*. Washington, DC: National Council on Radiation Protection and Measurements, 1989; NCRP report no 105.

38. Mettler FA, Upton AC. *Medical effects of ionizing radiation*, 2nd ed. Philadelphia: WB Saunders, 1995:330.

39. National Council on Radiation Protection and Measurements (NCRP). *Management of persons accidentally contaminated with radionuclides*. Washington, DC: National Council on Radiation Protection and Measurements, 1980; NCRP report no 65.

40. National Council on Radiation Protection and Measurements (NCRP). *Precautions in the management of patients who have received therapeutic amounts of radionuclides.* Washington, DC: National Council on Radiation Protection and Measurements, 1970; NCRP report no 37.

41. Hubner KF, Fry SA, eds. The medical basis for radiation accident preparedness. In: *Proceedings of a conference, Oak Ridge, TN.* New York: Elsevier, 1980.

42. Shleien B. *Preparedness and response in radiation accidents.* US Department of Health & Human Services. Washington, DC: US Government Printing Office, 1984; FDA-83 8211.

43. Leonard RB, Ricks RC. Emergency department radiation accident protocol. *Ann Emerg Med* 1980;9:9.

44. Gusev IA, Guskova AK, Mettler FA, eds. *Medical management of radiation accidents.* 2nd ed. Boca Raton, FL: CRC Press, 2001.

45. Bushberg JT, Seibert JA, Leidholdt EM, et al. *The essential physics of medical imaging,* 2nd edition Philadelphia: Lippincott Williams & Wilkins, 2002.

46. Hubbell, JH, Seltzer SM. *Tables of x-ray mass attenuation coefficients and mass energy-absorption coefficients 1 keV to 20 MeV for elements Z = 1 to 92 and 48 additional substances of dosimetric interest.* National Institute of Standards and Technology, 1995, NISTIR 5632.

47. Kocher DC. Radioactive decay data tables. Technical Information Center, US Department of Energy, 1981, DOE/TIC-11026.

48. Goodwin PN. Radiation safety for patients and personnel. In: *Freeman and Johnson's clinical radionuclide imaging,* 3rd ed. WB Saunders, 1984: 370.

49. Conte AC, Bushberg JT. Essential science of nuclear medicine. In: Brant WE, Helms CA, eds. *Fundamentals of diagnostic radiology.* Baltimore: Williams & Wilkins, 1994.

Diagnostic Nuclear Medicine, Fourth Edition. Edited by M.P. Sandler, R.E. Coleman, J.A. Patton, F.J.Th. Wackers, A. Gottschalk. Lippincott Williams & Wilkins, Philadelphia 2003.

10

RADIOPHARMACEUTICAL DOSIMETRY

JERROLD T. BUSHBERG
MICHAEL G. STABIN

The objective of internal radiation dosimetry calculations is to determine the absorbed energy per unit mass (i.e., dose) to various organs delivered from internally deposited radionuclides (radiopharmaceuticals). The first systematized formulation for determining the radiation absorbed dose from internally deposited radionuclides was developed by Marinelli et al. (1), in 1948. This work was extended and standardized by Loevinger et al. (2) in 1956 and later developed by Loevinger and Berman (3) into a generalized formalism for internal dose calculations applicable to all radionuclides. In 1968, this system was adopted by the Society of Nuclear Medicine's Medical Internal Radiation Dose Committee (MIRD). The MIRD schema (4), with subsequent revisions and additions, is currently the most widely accepted method for estimating the internal radiation dose from radionuclides of general interest in nuclear medicine.

As a practical matter, physicians engaged in the clinical practice of nuclear medicine are rarely called on to perform dosimetry calculations. The organ doses for approved diagnostic radionuclides are determined by the radiopharmaceutical supplier and provided as part of the package insert. There are, however, circumstances in which dose calculations must be performed. Examples include requests for use of new diagnostic agents, requests for use of an old agent by a new route of administration, certain therapeutic administrations, or other situations not covered by the standard dose estimates provided in the package insert (e.g., dose to a pregnant woman). In addition, the original dosimetry provided by the manufacturer is rarely updated as new (often more accurate) information becomes available. It is also important that the clinician have at least some understanding of the most common method by which radiation doses are calculated. Unfortunately it is impossible to present such material without the presentation of some algebraic formulas and symbols not always familiar to the reader. The level of presentation of material in this section is a compromise, allowing the reader actually

to perform model calculations by the MIRD method while avoiding more complex dosimetry analyses.

PARAMETERS AND UNITS

One way to think about calculating organ doses from internally administered radiopharmaceuticals is to organize and define those parameters or variables that are the necessary determinants of the absorbed dose in tissue. This process begins by identifying three major categories of parameters to be considered:

1. Radionuclide parameters: These are parameters related only to the physical and immutable properties of the radionuclide.
2. Biologic parameters: These are parameters related only to the biologic system and the pharmacokinetics of the radiopharmaceutical.
3. Combined parameters: These are parameters that are a function of both the radionuclide and the biologic system.

Radionuclide Parameters

The term used to indicate the total average energy available from a given radionuclide per nuclear transformation is the mean energy per disintegration (Δ), which is expressed in the unit gram-rad per microcurie-hour (g-rad/μCi-hr). Nuclear transformation is usually referred to as disintegration (dis). The unit of radiation quantity, or activity, is expressed in μCi, which is equal to 3.7×10^4 disintegrations/second or 1.33×10^8 disintegrations/hour. The unit for radiation dose is the rad, which is defined in terms of absorbed energy per gram of material (energy/g). If we choose the unit of time to be hours (i.e., dis/hour), the equivalent units of Δ are energy/dis, as shown below.

$$\Delta_t = \frac{g-rad}{\mu Ci - hr} = \frac{g \cdot \left(\frac{energy}{g}\right)}{\left(\frac{dis}{hr}\right) \cdot hr} = \frac{energy}{dis} \qquad [1]$$

The expression Δ_i is used to denote the energy per disintegration for a particular radiation emission. The i is used to denote the general equation as it applies to any value of i (i.e., $\Delta_1, \Delta_2, \Delta_3,$

J.T. Bushberg: Environmental Health & Safety, and Department of Radiology, UC Davis Medical Center, Sacramento, CA.

M.G. Stabin: Department of Radiology and Radiological Sciences, Vanderbilt University, Nashville, TN.

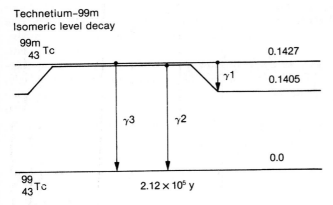

Technetium–99m
Isomeric level decay

FIGURE 10.1. Decay scheme and radiation emission information for ^{99m}Tc. **Top:** Decay scheme. **Bottom:** Radiation emission information. *K, L, M, X, Y,* orbital shells; *Int Con Elect,* internal conversion electron; *Augér Elect,* Augér electron.

scheme and spectrum of emissions is considerably more complex, consisting of three isomeric transitions (γ_1, γ_2, γ_3) and a number of particulate radiations, as well as low-energy characteristic x-rays. The Δ_i for each type of radiation is calculated from the relationship

$$1 = 2\ 3\ 4$$
$$\Delta_i = 2.13\ n_i\ E_i$$

Code	Symbol	Explanation
1.	Δ_i	Mean energy per disintegration for the *i*th emission.
2.	2.13	A conversion constant to convert MeV/disintegration to g-rad/μCi-hr.
3.	n_i	Mean number (average number) of *i*th-type radiation emitted per disintegration.
4.	E_i	Mean energy of the *i*th particle or photon emitted (in MeV).

Two other important parameters of the radionuclide are the quantity of radioactivity initially administered (A_o), expressed in μCi, and the characteristic physical half-life (T_p), expressed in hours. The physical half-life is an immutable property of the radionuclide and is defined as the time necessary to decrease a quantity of radioactivity from a specified radionuclide by one half (e.g., T_p for ^{99m}Tc = approximately 6 hours).

A summary of these radiation-specific variables, their relationship, and units is shown in Table 10.1.

etc.). When the value *i* appears in any equation, it denotes the general form applicable to any discrete entity. Values of δ_i have been calculated for the principal particulate and electromagnetic (photon) emissions resulting from the nuclear transformation process. The photons include γ- and x-rays, and the particulate radiations include α and β^- particles, positrons (β^+), internal conversion electrons (ICEs), and Augér electrons (AEs). One can appreciate the contribution of these various radiations to the overall energy emitted by considering, for example, the decay scheme and radiations from ^{99ms}Tc (Fig. 10.1).

Although we usually think of ^{99m}Tc as a relatively simple monoenergetic 140-keV photon emitter, the actual decay

Table 10.1. *Variables That Identify or Quantify Some Aspects of the Radiation Source (Radionuclide)*

Symbol	Quantity	Describes	Equivalent	Units
i		ith type of radiation photon or particle (i.e., γ, x-ray, ICE, AE)		
n_i		Mean number of the ith type of radiation emitted per disintegration		
E_i		Mean energy of radiation i		MeV/particle or photon
Δ_i	Mean energy per disintegration for radiation i	Total average energy emitted as radiation i per disintegration		g-rad/μCi-hr
A_o	Activity	Quantity of radioactivity present at time = 0 expressed as the number of disintegrations per second (dps)	2.13 $n_i\overline{E}$	μCi
T_p	Physical half-life	Time required to decrease a quantity of radioactivity by one-half	3.7×10^4 dps	hours (hr)

Table 10.2. *Variables That Identify or are a Function of the Biologic System*

Symbol	Quantity	Describes	Units
r	Region	A specific tissue or organ system	
r_k	Target	Identity of the target tissue for which the dose is being calculated	
r_h	Source	Identity of the source tissue in which some fraction of the activity is distributed	
f_h	Fractional uptake	The fraction of the administered activity taken up by the source tissue (r_b)	
m_k	Mass	Mass of the target tissue	grams (g)
T_b	Biologic half-life	The time required by the source tissue (r_b) to biologically eliminate one-half of the deposited radiopharmaceutical from the source organ	hours (hr)

Biologic Parameters

Biologic parameters identify the target organs for which the dose is being calculated (r_k), the various source organs in which the radiopharmaceutical is distributed (r_h), the fraction of the injected activity localized in each source organ (f_h), the mass of the target organ (m_k) in grams, and the biologic half-life of the radiopharmaceutical in a specified source organ (T_b). The biologic half-life expressed in hours is defined as the time necessary for the egress of one half of the initially deposited radiopharmaceutical from a specified source organ. This will, of course, depend only on the pharmacokinetics of the radiopharmaceutical in an individual patient and not on any of the decay characteristics of the radionuclide. For the majority of radiopharmaceuticals, or in the absence of more accurate kinetics data, the biologic elimination rate is assumed to follow a single exponential function (i.e., e^{-x}). These factors are summarized in Table 10.2.

Combined Parameters (Physically and Biologically Dependent)

The final category of parameters includes quantities that are functions of both the physical characteristics of the radionuclide and the biologic system in which it is located. As we have seen, the quantity referred to as *half-life* is a generic term that represents the time required for activity to decrease by one half of its original value. The effective half-life (T_e) represents the time required for the activity initially present in a specified source organ to decrease by one half. The effective half-life is a function of the combined effects of physical decay and biologic elimination of the radiopharmaceutical from the source organ. The quantitative relationship between T_p, T_b, and T_e is

$$T_e = \frac{T_p \cdot T_b}{T_p + T_b}$$

If T_b is infinite (i.e., the material is not excreted) or very long compared with T_p (e.g., ^{99m}Tc sulfur colloid in the liver), T_p becomes controlling and the T_e is effectively equal to T_p. This can be proved by inserting a larger number for T_b relative to T_p in Eq. 3.

The fraction of each *i*th type of radiation emitted from a radionuclide in a source organ (r_h) that is absorbed in a specified target organ (r_k) is symbolized as $\phi_i(r_k \leftarrow r_h)$ and referred to as the absorbed fraction (i.e., energy emitted by r_h and absorbed by r_k for each Δ_i). The value of the absorbed fraction (ϕ_i) depends on (a) the type and energy of the radiation emitted and (b) the geometric relationships, elemental composition, and attenuation characteristics of the source, target, and interposing tissues.

The radiation emission data are known with a high degree of accuracy for most radionuclides; however, the complex interactions and energy deposition patterns represented in the absorbed fraction $\phi_i(r_k \leftarrow r_h)$ for a particular combination of radionuclide, source, and target are best estimated by computer algorithms that employ the Monte Carlo technique (5,6). The Monte Carlo technique determines the energy deposited in tissue by tracing the randomly generated, but probabilistically determined, pathways and interactions of emissions from a large number of disintegrations and by averaging the results.

The anatomic model used for many years in these calculations was that of a 70-kg "standard" or "reference" hermaphrodite person. Various simplifications regarding elemental composition, organ size, position, contents, and geometry were made. Figs. 10.2 and 10.3 show the dimensions of the reference hermaphrodite phantom and the geometric simplifications and relationships of the principal organs. Calculations of absorbed dose using this phantom are thus really estimates of doses to the organs of this phantom and, hopefully, are somewhat representative of an average of the adult population. Significant improve-

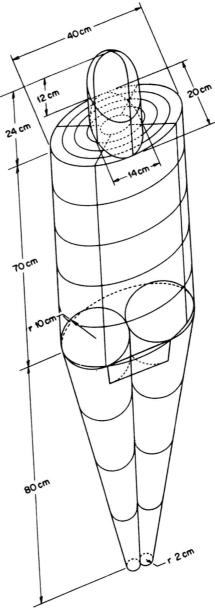

FIGURE 10.2. Exterior of the adult human phantom. Dimensions and coordinate system of adult human phantom. (From Snyder WJ, Ford MR, Warner GG. Estimates of absorbed fraction for photon sources uniformly distributed in various organs of the heterogeneous phantom. *nm/MIRD Pamphlet #5* (Revised). New York: Society of Nuclear Medicine, 1978, with permission.)

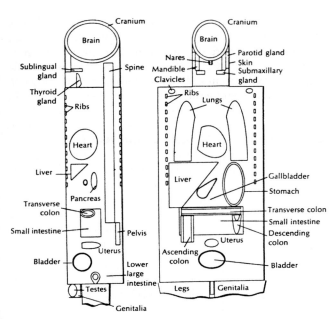

FIGURE 10.3. Computer plots of phantom sections. Computer plots of sections through adult hermaphrodite phantom illustrating the shape of the internal organs and their relative position. (From Smith EM, Warner GG. Estimates of radiation dose to the embryo from nuclear medicine procedures. *J Nucl Med* 1976;17:836–839, with permission.)

$$\overset{①}{\overline{(D)(r_k)}} = \frac{\overset{②}{\underset{h}{\Sigma}} \overset{③}{A_o} \bullet \overset{④}{f} \bullet \overset{⑤}{1.44T_e} \overset{⑦}{\underset{i}{\Sigma}} \overset{}{\Delta_i} \overset{⑨}{\Phi_i} \overset{}{(r_k \leftarrow r_h)}}{\underset{⑥}{m_k}} \qquad [4]$$

Code	Symbol	Quantity	Describes	Equivalence	Units
1.	$D(r_k)$	absorbed dose	Energy-deposited per unit mass of the target organ (r_k)	$\dfrac{100 \text{ erg}}{\text{g}}$	rad
2.	Σ_h		The sum of all the determinations from emissions originating within both the target organ and all other organs		
3.	A_o	activity	Activity at time 0	3.7×10^4 dps	µCi
4.	f	fractional	Fraction of the administered activity in a source organ		
5.	$1.44T_e$		The "average" life of the radioactivity in a source organ	$\dfrac{1.44 T_p \cdot T_b}{T_p + T_b}$	hr
6.	m_k	mass	Mass of the target organ		g
7.	Σ_i		Sum of all the emissions		
8.	Δ_i	mean energy per disintegration for radiation i	Total average energy emitted as radiation i per disintegration	$2.13 n_i E_i$	g-rad/µCi-hr
9.	ϕ_i $(r_k \leftarrow r_h)$	absorbed fraction	The fraction of the energy emitted by the radionuclide in the source organ (r_h) that is deposited in the target organ (r_k)		

ments to this model have been made over the years. First in the category of improvements was the addition of certain improved organ systems, including the heart (7), brain (8), peritoneal cavity (9), prostate gland (10), esophagus (11), and subregions of the brain (12). A significant improvement in the ability to extend dose calculations to more individuals was realized in the pediatric phantom series of Cristy and Eckerman (13) and the pregnant woman phantom series of Stabin et al. (14). The pediatric phantom series consisted of six phantoms, representing individuals of age 0 (newborn), 1 year, 5 years, 10 years, 15 years, and 18 years (adult). The Cristy and Eckerman adult phantom is slightly different than the original adult phantom described in MIRD Pamphlet No. 5, Revised (15).

The basic MIRD expression of mean absorbed dose in a particular target organ $\bar{D}(r_k)$ from all source organs is shown in Eq. 4. This equation takes into account all of the physical and biologic variables discussed thus far.

Note that the summation sign $[\Sigma_i, \Delta_i, \phi_i(r_k \leftarrow r_h)]$ *indicates that one must sum the individual products of the amount of energy released by radiation (Δ_i) per disintegration (Δ_i) and the fraction of that energy absorbed by the designated target $[\phi_i(r_k \leftarrow r_h)]$.* The symbol ($\Sigma_h$) reflects the need to calculate the target organ dose by adding together not only the individual doses from activity located within the target organ itself (i.e., $r_k = r_h$—the

Table 10.3. *Conventional and SI radiologic Units and Conversion Factors*

Quantity	Conventional units		Multiply by the conventional units to obtain SI units	SI units	
	Name	Symbol		Name	Symbol
Activity	Curie	Ci	3.7×10^{10}	Becquerel[a]	Bq
Exposure	Roentgen	R	2.58×10^{-4}	Coulomb per kilogram	C/kg
Absorbed dose	Radiation absorbed dose	rad	10^{-2}	Gray[b]	Gy
Dose equivalent	Roentgen-equivalent man	rem	10^{-2}	Sievert	Sv

[a]Bq, 1 disintegration/sec (dis sec^{-1}).
[b]Gray, 1 Joule/kg.

self-irradiating dose) but also the dose resulting from other source tissues irradiating the target tissue.

Simplified Dose Calculation Technique

The cumulated activity ($\bar{A}_h$) represents the total number of disintegrations from the specified amount of activity in the source organ. This can be seen by a simple analysis of units [i.e., $\bar{A}_h$ = A_o (dis/time) • T_e (time) = dis].

The cumulated activity in the source organ, expressed in μCi-hr, can be represented by a single term ($\bar{A}_h$) incorporating the biodistribution and kinetics information as shown in Eq. 5.

$$\bar{A}_h = A_o \cdot f_h \cdot 1.44\, T_e \qquad [5]$$

The MIRD Committee has further simplified the dose calculation procedure by combining the appropriate values of Δ_i, ϕ_i ($r_k \leftarrow r_h$), and m_k for each combination of source, target, and radionuclide into a so-called *S* factor as shown in Eq. 6.

$$S(r_k \leftarrow r_h) = \frac{\sum \Delta_i \phi_i (r_k \leftarrow r_h)}{m_k} \qquad [6]$$

The *S* factor thus represents the mean absorbed dose in the target organ per unit cumulated activity in a designated source organ in rad/μCi-hr. Thus, the equation for calculating the absorbed dose to r_k reduces to

$$\overset{①}{\overline{D(r_k)}} = \overset{②}{\underset{\Sigma_h}{|}}\overset{③}{\underset{\bar{A}_h}{|}}\overset{④}{\underset{S(r_k \leftarrow r_h)}{|}} \qquad [7]$$

Code	Symbol	Quantity	Equivalence	Units
1.	$\overline{D(r_k)}$	target organ dose	$\Sigma_h A_h S$ $(r_k \leftarrow r_h)$	rad
2.	Σh	sum of the determinations from emissions originating within both the target organ and all other organs		
3.	$\bar{A}_h$	cumulated activity	$A_o \cdot f \cdot$ $1.44 T_e$	μCi-hr
4.	$S(r_k \leftarrow r_h)$	S factor	$\Sigma_i \Delta_i \phi_i$ $(r_k \leftarrow r_h)$	rad/μCi-hr

The MIRD Committee has compiled *S* factors for more than 110 radionuclides and 20 source/target combinations (16).

A WORD ABOUT UNITS

The traditional radiologic units of Ci, R, rad, and rem are maintained throughout this section rather than switching to the equivalent Système Internationale (SI) units (Bq, C/kg, Gy, and Sv, respectively) because the former are still the most commonly used units in nuclear medicine in the United States. The relationship between these two systems is given in Table 10.3. Other units are chosen for their utility in a given example or because of common usage. Although any variety of units may be employed in a radiation dose calculation, care must be taken to

ensure unit consistency throughout (i.e., not mixing seconds with hours or μCi with Ci), and some effort should be made to choose units that are best suited to a particular problem or that follow some logical and/or established convention. One could express velocity in furlongs per fortnight, but this would hardly be a very useful term!

EXAMPLES OF DOSE CALCULATIONS

The simplest example of a MIRD calculation would be a situation in which the radiopharmaceutical instantaneously localized in a single organ and remained there with an infinite biologic half-life.

For the purpose of demonstrating the basic MIRD technique, a hypothetical situation is presented below in Example 1.

EXAMPLE 1
A patient is injected with 3 mCi (111 MBq) of ^{99m}Tc sulfur colloid. Estimate the radiation absorbed dose to the
(a) liver
(b) testes
(c) red bone marrow
(d) total body

Assumptions

1. All of the injected activity is uniformly distributed in the liver.
2. The uptake of ^{99m}Tc sulfur colloid in the liver from the blood is essentially instantaneous.
3. There is no biologic removal of ^{99m}Tc sulfur colloid from the liver.

In this case the average dose $\bar{D}$ to any target organ (r_k) can be estimated by applying the simplified MIRD formulation in Eq. 7.

$$\bar{D}(r_k) = \sum_h \bar{A}_h\, S(r_k \leftarrow r_h) \qquad [7]$$

Step 1. Calculate the cumulated activity ($\bar{A}_h$) in the source organ (i.e., liver). By inserting the appropriate values into Eq. 5 we have

$$\bar{A}_h = \left(3000\ \mu Ci\right)\left(1\right)\left(1.44\right)\left(6\ hr\right) = 2.60 \times 10^4\ \mu Ci-hr$$

Note that because $T_b = \infty$, $T_e = T_p$.

Step 2. Find the appropriate S factors for each target/source combination and the radionuclide of interest (i.e., ^{99m}Tc). A reproduction of the appropriate MIRD table for this calculation is shown in Table 10.4. The appropriate *S* factors are found at the intersection of the source organ (i.e., liver) column and the individual target organs (i.e., liver, testes, red marrow, or total body) row. [A complete listing of *S* factors is contained in MIRD Pamphlet #11 (16).]

Target (r_k)	Source (r_h)	S Factor
Liver	Liver	4.6×10^{-5}
Testes	Liver	6.2×10^{-8}
Red bone marrow	Liver	1.6×10^{-6}
Total body	Liver	2.2×10^{-6}

Table 10.4. *Absorbed Dose Per Unit Cumulated Activity (rad/μCi-hr)* [99m]*Technetium (Half-Life 6.02 Hours)*[a]

Target organs (r$_k$)	| Source organs (r$_b$)									
	Adrenals	Bladder contents	Stomach contents	SI contents	ULI contents	LLI contents	Kidneys	Liver	Lungs	Other tissue (muscle)
Adrenals	3.1E−03	1.5E−07	2.7E−06	1.0E−06	9.1E−07	3.6E−07	1.1E−05	4.5E−06	2.7E−06	1.4E−06
Bladder wall	1.3E−07	1.6E−04	2.7E−07	2.6E−06	2.2E−06	6.9E−06	2.8E−07	1.6E−07	3.6E−08	1.8E−06
Bone (total)	2.0E−06	9.2E−07	9.0E−07	1.3E−06	1.1E−06	1.6E−06	1.4E−06	1.1E−06	1.5E−06	9.8E−07
GI (stom wall)	2.9E−06	2.7E−07	1.3E−04	3.7E−06	3.8E−06	1.8E−06	3.6E−06	1.9E−06	1.8E−06	1.3E−06
GI (SI)	8.3E−07	3.0E−06	2.7E−06	7.8E−05	1.7E−05	9.4E−06	2.9E−06	1.6E−06	1.9E−07	1.5E−06
GI (ULI wall)	9.3E−07	2.2E−06	3.5E−06	2.4E−05	1.3E−04	4.2E−06	2.9E−06	2.5E−06	2.2E−07	1.6E−06
GI (LLI wall)	2.2E−07	7.4E−06	1.2E−06	7.3E−06	3.2E−06	1.9E−04	7.2E−07	2.3E−07	7.1E−08	1.7E−06
Kidneys	1.1E−05	2.6E−07	3.5E−06	3.2E−06	2.8E−06	8.6E−07	1.9E−04	3.9E−06	8.4E−07	1.3E−06
Liver	4.9E−06	1.7E−07	2.0E−06	1.8E−06	2.6E−06	2.5E−07	3.9E−06	4.6E−05	2.5E−06	1.1E−06
Lungs	2.4E−06	2.4E−08	1.7E−06	2.2E−07	2.6E−07	7.9E−08	8.5E−07	2.5E−06	5.2E−05	1.3E−06
Marrow (red)	3.6E−06	2.2E−06	1.6E−06	4.3E−06	3.7E−06	5.1E−06	3.8E−06	1.6E−06	1.9E−06	2.0E−06
Oth tiss (musc)	1.4E−06	1.8E−06	1.4E−06	1.5E−06	1.5E−06	1.7E−06	1.3E−06	1.1E−06	1.3E−06	2.7E−06
Ovaries	6.1E−07	7.3E−06	5.0E−07	1.1E−05	1.2E−05	1.8E−05	1.1E−06	4.5E−07	9.4E−08	2.0E−06
Pancreas	9.0E−06	2.3E−07	1.8E−05	2.1E−06	2.3E−06	7.4E−07	6.6E−06	4.2E−06	2.6E−06	1.8E−06
Skin	5.1E−07	5.5E−07	4.4E−07	4.1E−07	4.1E−07	4.8E−07	5.3E−07	4.9E−07	5.3E−07	7.2E−07
Spleen	6.3E−06	6.6E−07	1.0E−05	1.5E−06	1.4E−06	8.0E−07	8.6E−06	9.2E−07	2.3E−06	1.4E−06
Testes	3.2E−08	4.7E−06	5.1E−08	3.1E−07	2.7E−07	1.8E−06	8.8E−06	6.2E−08	7.9E−09	1.1E−06
Thyroid	1.3E−07	2.1E−09	8.7E−08	1.5E−08	1.6E−08	5.4E−09	4.8E−08	1.5E−07	9.2E−07	1.3E−06
Uterus (nongrvd)	1.1E−06	1.6E−05	7.7E−07	9.6E−06	5.4E−06	7.1E−06	9.4E−07	3.9E−07	8.2E−08	2.3E−06
Total body	2.2E−06	1.9E−06	1.9E−06	2.4E−06	2.2E−06	2.3E−06	2.2E−06	2.2E−06	2.0E−06	1.9E−06

Target organs (r$_b$)	| Source organs (r$_b$)									
	Ovaries	Pancreas	R marrow	Cort bone	Tra bone	Skin	Spleen	Testes	Thyroid	Total body
Adrenals	3.3E−07	9.1E−06	2.3E−06	1.1E−06	1.1E−06	6.8E−07	6.3E−06	3.2E−08	1.3E−07	2.3E−06
Bladder wall	7.2E−06	1.4E−07	9.9E−07	5.1E−07	5.1E−07	4.9E−07	1.2E−07	4.8E−06	2.1E−09	2.3E−06
Bone (total)	1.5E−06	1.5E−06	4.0E−06	1.2E−05	1.0E−05	9.9E−07	1.1E−06	9.2E−07	1.0E−06	2.5E−06
GI (stom wall)	8.1E−07	1.8E−05	9.5E−07	5.5E−07	5.5E−07	5.4E−07	1.0E−05	3.2E−08	4.5E−08	2.2E−06
GI (SI)	1.2E−05	1.8E−06	2.6E−06	7.3E−07	7.3E−07	4.5E−07	1.4E−06	3.6E−07	9.3E−09	2.5E−06
GI (ULI wall)	1.1E−05	2.1E−06	2.1E−06	6.9E−07	6.9E−07	4.6E−07	1.4E−06	3.1E−07	1.1E−08	2.4E−06
GI (LLI wall)	1.5E−06	5.7E−07	2.9E−06	1.0E−06	1.0E−06	4.8E−07	6.1E−07	2.7E−06	4.3E−09	2.3E−06
Kidneys	9.2E−07	6.6E−06	2.2E−06	8.2E−07	8.2E−07	5.7E−07	9.1E−06	4.0E−08	3.4E−08	2.2E−06
Liver	5.4E−07	4.4E−06	9.2E−07	6.6E−07	6.6E−07	5.3E−07	9.8E−07	3.1E−08	9.3E−08	2.2E−06
Lungs	6.0E−08	2.5E−06	1.2E−06	9.4E−07	9.4E−07	5.8E−07	2.3E−06	6.6E−09	9.4E−07	2.0E−06
Marrow (red)	5.5E−06	2.8E−06	3.1E−05	4.1E−06	9.1E−06	9.5E−07	1.7E−06	7.3E−07	1.1E−06	2.9E−06
Oth tiss (musc)	2.0E−06	1.8E−06	1.2E−06	9.8E−07	9.8E−07	7.2E−07	1.4E−06	1.1E−06	1.3E−06	1.9E−06
Ovaries	4.2E−03	4.1E−07	3.2E−06	7.1E−07	7.1E−07	3.8E−07	4.0E−07	0.0	4.9E−09	2.4E−06
Pancreas	5.0E−07	5.8E−04	1.7E−06	8.5E−07	8.5E−07	4.4E−07	1.9E−05	5.5E−08	7.2E−08	2.4E−06
Skin	4.1E−07	4.0E−07	5.9E−07	6.5E−07	6.5E−07	1.6E−05	4.7E−07	1.4E−06	7.3E−07	1.3E−06
Spleen	4.9E−07	1.9E−05	9.2E−07	5.8E−07	5.8E−07	5.4E−07	3.3E−04	1.7E−08	1.1E−07	2.2E−06
Testes	0.0	5.5E−08	4.5E−07	6.4E−07	6.4E−07	9.1E−07	4.8E−08	1.4E−03	5.0E−10	1.7E−06
Thyroid	4.9E−09	1.2E−07	6.8E−07	7.9E−07	7.9E−07	6.9E−07	8.7E−08	5.0E−10	2.3E−03	1.5E−06
Uterus (nongrvd)	2.1E−05	5.3E−07	2.2E−06	5.7E−07	5.7E−07	4.0E−07	4.0E−07	0.0	4.6E−09	2.6E−06
Total body	2.6E−06	2.6E−06	2.2E−06	2.0E−06	2.0E−06	1.3E−06	2.2E−06	1.9E−06	1.8E−06	2.0E−06

ULI, upper large intestine; LLI, lower large intestine; SI, small intestine.
[a]From Snyder WS, Ford MR, Warner GG, Watson SB: *Absorbed Dose Per Unit Accumulated Activity for Selected Radionuclides and Organs* (MIRD Pamphlet No. 11). New York: Society of Nuclear Medicine, 1975.

Step 3. Organize the assembled information in a table of organ doses.

Target organ (r$_k$)	$\bar{A}_b$(μCi-hr)	$S(r_k \leftarrow r_b)$ (rad/μCi-hr)	$\bar{D}(r_k)$ (rad)
1. Liver	$2.60 \times 10_4 \times 4.6 \times 10^{-5}$	=	1.2
2. Testes	$2.60 \times 10_4 \times 6.2 \times 10^{-8}$	=	0.002
3. Red bone marrow	$2.60 \times 10_4 \times 1.6 \times 10^{-6}$	=	0.042
4. Total body	$2.60 \times 10_4 \times 2.2 \times 10^{-6}$	=	0.057

Note that the relatively small dose to target organs other than the liver is mostly due to (a) only a small fraction of the isotropically emitted penetrating radiation (i.e., γ-rays) being intercepted by the other organ systems (e.g., testes and red bone marrow) *or* (b) the relatively large mass over which the radiation is distributed (e.g., total body).

The first example is simplified by the fact that there was only one source organ (liver) and no biologic elimination of the radiopharmaceutical. The second example is a more complex but realistic dosimetry problem.

EXAMPLE 2

A patient receives 20 mCi of ^{99m}Tc methylene diphosphonate for a bone scan. Estimate the radiation absorbed dose to the

(a) Red bone marrow
(b) Bladder wall

Assumptions

1. Thirty-five percent of the activity is uniformly distributed in the bone where T_b = 18.6 days. (Note: 18.6 days × 24 hours/day = 446.4 hours.)
2. Sixty percent of the activity is in the bladder where T_b = 0.67 hours.
3. Five percent of the activity is uniformly distributed in the whole body where T_b = 0.43 hours.
4. The uptake in all of the source organs was essentially instantaneous.

We will still use the formalism in Eq. 7.

Step 1. Calculate $\tilde{A}_b$ for each source organ, remembering

$$\tilde{A}_b = A_o \cdot f_h \cdot 1.44\, T_e \text{ and } T_e = \frac{T_p \cdot T_b}{T_p + T_b}$$

Source Organ	A_o (μCi)	f_b	1.44	T_e (hr)	$\tilde{A}_b$ (μCi-hr)
Bone	20,000 × 0.35 × 1.44 × 5.94				= 5.99×10^4
Bladder contents	20,000 × 0.60 × 1.44 × 0.603				= 1.04×10^4
Total body	20,000 × 0.05 × 1.44 × 0.40				= 5.78×10^2

Step 2. Find the appropriate S factors for each target/source combination.

Note that because the injected activity is localized in multiple source organs, for every target organ (i.e., red bone marrow and bladder wall) there are three sources of radiation (i.e., bone, bladder contents, and total body). An additional complication is that S factors in Table 10.4 have been calculated separately for cortical (cort) and trabecular (tra) bone. Thus, one must assume that the cumulated activity ($\tilde{A}_b$) in the bone is equally divided between the two bone tissues and therefore consider each as an individual source organ. The permutations of target/source combinations and associated S factors are as follows.

Target (r_k)	Source (r_b)	S factor (rad/μCi-hr)
Red bone marrow	Cort bone	4.1×10^{-6}
Red bone marrow	Tra bone	9.1×10^{-6}
Red bone marrow	Bladder contents	2.2×10^{-6}
Red bone marrow	Total body	2.9×10^{-6}
Bladder wall	Cort bone	5.1×10^{-7}
Bladder wall	Tra bone	5.1×10^{-7}
Bladder wall	Bladder contents	1.6×10^{-4}
Bladder wall	Total body	2.3×10^{-6}

It is interesting to note that the dose per unit activity (S factor) for the trabecular bone irradiating the bone marrow (9.1×10^{-6}) is more than twice as large as the S factor for the cortical bone irradiating the bone marrow (4.1×10^{-6}), even though the activity is evenly distributed between the two bone tissues. This occurs because in the dosimetric model, marrow is only associated with trabecular bone, so that nonpenetrating

radiations (i.e., ICEs and AEs) from the trabecular bone interact with the marrow and dose from cortical bone is due only to penetrating radiations (i.e., x-rays and the 140-keV gamma ray).

Yet another complication arises in that we have calculated an ($\tilde{A}$) for the *remainder of the body* (in this problem total body minus bone and bladder contents), whereas we have available S values for the *total body*. Cloutier et al. (17) showed how to correct either the ($\tilde{A}$) values or the S values for this problem. Although the ($\tilde{A}$) correction is technically easier (18), correction of the S values is a more intuitive process. The S value correction is performed as follows.

$$S(r_k \leftarrow RB) = S(r_k \leftarrow TB)\left(\frac{m_{TB}}{m_{RB}}\right) - \sum_b S(r_k \leftarrow r_b)\left(\frac{m_b}{m_{RB}}\right)$$

where

$S(r_k \leftarrow RB)$ is the S-value for "remainder of the body" irradiating target region r_k

$S(r_k \leftarrow TB)$ is the S-value for the total body iradiating target region r_k

$S(r_k \leftarrow r_b)$ is the S-value for source region h irradiating target region r_k

m_{TB} is the mass of the total body

m_{RB} is the mass of the remainder of the body, i.e., the total body minus all other source organs used in this problem, and

m_h is the mass of source region h.

For this problem the S values for remainder of body irradiating the red marrow and the bladder wall are 2.7×10^{-6} and 1.9×10^{-6} rad/μCi-hr, respectively, instead of 2.9×10^{-6} and 2.3×10^{-6} rad/μCi-hr.

Step 3. Organize the assembled information into a table of organ doses for each target from each source.

Target (r_k) = Red bone marrow (RM)

Source organ	$\tilde{A}_b$ (mCi-hr)	S(rad/μCi-hr)		D_{rk} (rad)
Cort bone (CB)	½ (5.99×10^4) × 4.1×10^{-6}		=	0.123
Tra bone (TrB)	½ (5.99×10^4) × 9.1×10^{-6}		=	0.272
Bladder contents (BC)	1.04×10^4 × 2.2×10^{-6}		=	0.023
Total body (TB)	5.78×10^2 × 2.7×10^{-6}		=	0.002

The total dose to red bone marrow is the sum of the dose from each source: $\bar{D}(r_kLT\$sd>k) = \sum \bar{D}(r_k \leftarrow r_h) = \sum \bar{D}(RM \leftarrow CB) + \bar{D}(RM \leftarrow TrB) + \bar{D}(RM \leftarrow BC) + \bar{D}(RM \leftarrow TB)$ (i.e., $\bar{D}(r_k) = 0.123 + 0.272 + 0.023 + 0.002 = 0.42$ rad (420 mrad, 4.2 mGy).

Target (r_k) = Bladder wall (BW)

Source organ	$\tilde{A}_b$ (μCi-hr)	S($r_k \leftarrow r_h$) (rad/μCi-hr)		D_{rk} (rad)
Cort bone (CB)	½ (5.99×10^4) × 5.1×10^{-7}		=	0.015
Tra bone (TrB)	½ (5.99×10^4) × 5.1×10^{-7}		=	0.015
Bladder contents (BC)	1.04×10^4 × 1.6×10^{-4}		=	1.700
Total body (TB)	5.78×10^2 × 1.9×10^{-6}		=	0.001

As before, $\bar{D}(r_k) = \sum_b \tilde{A}_b\, S(r_k \leftarrow r_h) = 0.015 + 0.015 + 1.700 + 0.001 = 1.7$ rad (1,700 mrad or 17 mGy). Note that the dose to the bladder wall is almost entirely (98.2%) due to activity in the bladder. From these calculations one can appreciate how the effective half-life (T_e) of activity in an organ affects

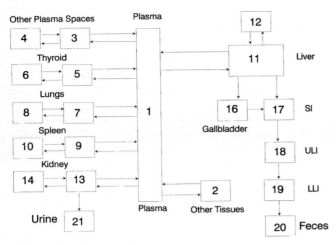

FIGURE 10.4. Compartmental model for ^{99m}Tc compound of example 3.

the dose to a target. In this situation, a recommendation to have the patient void 1 to 2 hours after the administration of the activity not only improves the scintigram but can reduce the dose to the bladder wall by as much as 75% (19). Minimization of bladder radiation dose through optimization of bladder voiding schedules for many radiopharmaceuticals was given in MIRD Dose Estimate Report No. 14, revised (20).

EXAMPLE 3

This example employs a model with several source organs, in which the kinetics of an agent have been determined in a population of adult volunteers but for which dose estimates are desired for children of all ages, as well as adults. Very few investigators have the time or resources to study the kinetics of radiopharmaceuticals in children and adults, so it is typical to use a single set of $(\bar{A})$ values with S values determined for several different age groups. A diagram of the model is shown in Fig. 10.4. The $(\bar{A})$'s determined from the experimental studies with this ^{99m}Tc-labeled compound are

Thyroid	35 µCi-hr
Lungs	200 µCi-hr
Liver	550 µCi-hr
Gallbladder	120 µCi-hr
Small Intestine	630 µCi-hr
Upper Large Intestine	850 µCi-hr
Lower Large Intestine	400 µCi-hr
Kidneys	520 µCi-hr
Spleen	210 µCi-hr
Urinary Bladder	2000 µCi-hr
Remainder of Body	450 µCi-hr

The dose estimates for this problem would be calculated exactly the same as for Example 2, except that there are a lot more calculations to do. The easiest way to perform the calculation may be in a matrix format. If the set of dose estimates we want is a 1 × 14 matrix (dose estimates for 14 target organs—thyroid, lungs, liver, gallbladder, small intestine, upper large intestine, lower large intestine, kidneys, urinary bladder, spleen, ovaries, testes, red marrow, and total body), this can be found by multiplication of a 1 × 11 matrix of residence times (for the 11 source organs listed previously) and a 11 × 14 matrix of S-values.

Table 10.5. *Radiation Dose Estimates for the Compound of Example 3*

	Estimated Radiation Dose (mGy/mBq)					
Organ	Newborn	1-yr-old	5-yr-old	10-yr-old	15-yr-old	Adult
Adrenals	3.6E−02	1.9E−02	1.1E−02	7.4E−03	4.8E−03	3.7E−03
Brain	3.3E−03	1.4E−03	7.8E−04	4.8E−04	3.0E−04	2.5E−04
Breasts	9.6E−03	4.3E−03	2.4E−03	1.4E−03	7.7E−04	6.2E−04
Gallbladder wall	3.6E−01	1.7E−01	5.7E−02	3.4E−02	2.5E−02	2.2E−02
LLI wall	3.7E−01	1.5E−01	8.2E−02	5.2E−02	3.2E−02	2.5E−02
Small intestine	2.3E−01	1.0E−01	5.7E−02	3.6E−02	2.2E−02	1.8E−02
Stomach	3.7E−02	1.8E−02	1.1E−02	7.1E−03	4.5E−03	3.5E−03
ULI wall	4.8E−01	2.1E−01	1.1E−01	7.0E−02	4.2E−02	3.3E−02
Heart wall	1.7E−02	8.3E−03	4.7E−03	3.1E−03	2.0E−03	1.5E−03
Kidneys	2.9E−01	1.2E−01	6.9E−02	4.8E−02	3.4E−02	2.8E−02
Liver	9.0E−02	4.3E−02	2.4E−02	1.7E−02	1.1E−02	8.7E−03
Lungs	5.4E−02	2.2E−02	1.1E−02	7.5E−03	5.3E−03	3.6E−03
Muscle	2.3E−02	1.2E−02	6.7E−03	4.4E−03	3.0E−03	2.5E−03
Ovaries	8.9E−02	4.7E−02	2.9E−02	2.0E−02	1.4E−02	1.1E−02
Pancreas	4.5E−02	2.2E−02	1.3E−02	8.9E−03	5.5E−03	4.4E−03
Red marrow	1.4E−02	7.8E−03	5.7E−03	4.5E−03	3.2E−03	2.6E−03
Bone surfaces	3.1E−02	1.5E−02	8.1E−03	5.5E−03	3.8E−03	3.0E−03
Skin	1.1E−02	4.9E−03	2.6E−03	1.7E−03	1.1E−03	8.8E−04
Spleen	2.9E−01	1.2E−01	6.5E−02	4.3E−02	2.8E−02	2.0E−02
Testes	4.5E−02	2.4E−02	1.3E−02	8.2E−03	4.7E−03	3.3E−03
Thymus	8.4E−03	3.9E−03	2.2E−03	1.4E−03	9.1E−04	7.1E−04
Thyroid	2.8E−01	2.1E−01	1.1E−01	5.0E−02	3.3E−02	2.0E−02
Urinary bladder wall	1.0E+00	4.4E−01	2.3E−01	1.6E−01	1.2E−01	9.7E−02
Uterus	1.1E−01	6.0E−02	3.7E−02	2.5E−02	1.6E−02	1.3E−02
Effective dose equivalent (mSv/mBq)	1.9E−01	8.8E−02	4.7E−02	3.1E−02	2.1E−02	1.7E−02

LLI, lower large intestine; ULI, upper large intestine.

$$[\bar{D}] = [\bar{A}] \times [S]$$

In addition, we can repeat this calculation six times to obtain dose estimates for each member of the Cristy-Eckerman phantom series, thus simulating a set of dose estimates for children of various ages and adults. Table 10.5 gives dose estimates for these six ages for the cumulated activities shown previously.

Note how the dose estimates increase with decreasing age, because the organs get smaller and closer together. The overall increase for any organ going from an adult to a newborn is typically about a factor of 10 for ^{99m}Tc. An adjustment that might reasonably be made to this set of dose estimates is to decrease cumulated activities for the urinary bladder and gastrointestinal tract organs to reflect more rapid clearance in young children. Note also the calculation of a new quantity, the effective dose equivalent (EDE), instead of the total body dose (the total energy absorbed in the body divided by the mass of the total body). The EDE is calculated by multiplying the dose estimates (after conversion to dose equivalent) for individual organs by a risk-related weighting factor (Table 10.6)(21) and adding up the individual weighted dose equivalents to a single value. For "Remainder of Body," choose the five organs with the highest doses that do not have a specifically assigned weighting factor and assign each a weighting factor of 0.06. For example, for the adult

Organ	Dose Equivalent (mSv/mBq)	Weighting Factor	Weighted Dose Equivalent (mSv/mBq)
Ovaries	0.011	0.25	0.0028
Breasts	0.00062	0.15	0.000093
Lungs	0.0036	0.12	0.00043
Red marrow	0.0026	0.12	0.00031
Thyroid	0.020	0.03	0.00060
Bone surfaces	0.0030	0.03	0.000090
Urinary bladder	0.097	0.06	0.0058
ULI wall	0.033	0.06	0.0020
Kidneys	0.028	0.06	0.0017
LLI wall	0.025	0.06	0.0015
Gallbladder wall	0.022	0.06	0.0013
TOTAL (EDE)			0.017 mSv/mBq

Table 10.6. *Organ Weighting Factors Assigned in ICRP 30 for the Effective Dose Equivalent and in ICRP 60 for the Effective Dose*

Organ	Weighting factors	
	ICRP 30	ICRP 60
Gonads	0.25	0.20
Red marrow	0.12	0.12
Colon		0.12
Lungs	0.12	0.12
Stomach		0.12
Bladder		0.05
Breasts	0.15	0.05
Liver		0.05
Esophagus		0.05
Thyroid	0.03	0.05
Skin		0.01
Bone surfaces	0.03	0.01
Remainder	0.30	0.05

ICRP, International Commission on Radiological Protection.

Similarly, the effective dose would be calculated as shown later. The weighting factor for the remainder is divided equally among ten organs not explicitly mentioned in this list but which were assigned by the International Commission on Radiation Protection (ICRP) [adrenals, brain, upper large intestine (ULI), small intestine, kidneys, muscle, pancreas, spleen, thymus, and uterus]. Esophagus and skin are not routinely treated, because they generally receive a low dose or are not given in the standard phantoms and because their weighting factors are relatively low.

	Dose Equivalent (mSv/MBq)	Weighting Factor	Weighted Dosed Equivalent (mSv/MBq)
Ovaries	1.1E-02	0.2	2.2E-03
Red Marrow	2.6E-03	0.12	3.1E-04
LLI Wall	2.5E-02	0.12	3.0E-03
Lungs	3.6E-03	0.12	4.3E-04
Stomach	3.5E-03	0.12	4.2E-04
Urin Bladder Wall	9.7E-02	0.05	4.9E-03
Breasts	6.2E-04	0.05	3.1E-05
Liver	8.7E-03	0.05	4.4E-04
Thyroid	2.0E-02	0.05	1.0E-03
Bone Surfaces	3.0E-03	0.01	3.0E-05
Adrenals	3.7E-03	0.005	1.9E-05
Brain	2.5E-04	0.005	1.3E-06
ULI Wall	3.3E-02	0.005	1.7E-04
Small Intestine	1.8E-02	0.005	9.0E-05
Kidneys	2.8E-02	0.005	1.4E-04
Muscle	2.5E-03	0.005	1.3E-05
Pancreas	4.4E-03	0.005	2.2E-05
Spleen	2.0E-02	0.005	1.0E-04
Thymus	7.1E-04	0.005	3.6E-06
Uterus	1.3E-02	0.005	6.5E-05
TOTAL (ED)			1.3E-02

Although originally derived for an adult working population (21), the ICRP has proposed the quantity as useful in nuclear medicine and applicable to all age groups (22). This quantity is thought by many to be better than total body dose in comparing radiopharmaceuticals, procedures, and so forth. It is important, however, not to attach too much significance to the number, because it is a derived quantity based on many assumptions, subject to change. Indeed, a new set of weighting factors has already been published by the ICRP (23); the new quantity associated with these new weighting factors is called effective dose (ED). Toohey and Stabin (24) studied the difference between EDE, ED, and total body dose for a large number of radiopharmaceuticals and found that the ratio of ED/EDE was typically around 0.8 in adults but that both quantities are higher than total body dose, sometimes by factors of more than 10. The MIRD Committee has advised caution in the use of this quantity in nuclear medicine (25), pointing out that the quantity is especially not to be applied to therapy situations or to evaluate the risk to an individual.

LIMITATIONS OF THE MIRD METHOD

The MIRD formulation is a significant improvement over other previously used methods, specifically the widely used formulation recommended by the ICRP in 1959 (26). However, the MIRD method as traditionally applied usually includes several assumptions, limitations, and simplifications, which include

1. Activity is assumed to be uniformly distributed in the source organs.
2. Energy deposition is averaged over the entire mass of the target organ (i.e., no microdosimetric models are considered).
3. Simple geometric shapes and interorgan relationships are used to approximate human anatomy.
4. The phantoms used for a reference adult (i.e., 154 lb and 5 ft 8 in.), adolescent, and child are only an approximation of the physical dimensions of any particular individual.
5. Each organ is assumed to be of homogeneous density and composition.
6. Minor dose contributions from bremsstrahlung radiation and Coster-Kronig transitions are ignored.
7. With a few exceptions, low-energy photons and all particulate radiation are assumed to be absorbed locally (i.e., nonpenetrating).

The general MIRD dose equation (Eq. 4) does not, however, contain these assumptions. It is a generally applicable absorbed dose equation whose application is only limited by the assumptions inherent in the specific values for the parameters entered. If the absorbed fractions, for instance, are derived for tissue or cellular level geometries (instead of whole organ geometries), the absorbed doses will be accurate for this domain. Some approaches exist for overcoming some of these limitations. Although it is beyond the scope of this chapter to discuss them all in detail and evaluate their impact on the accuracy of dose calculations, we will give a brief overview of some of these developing areas, to provide some understanding of how the field of internal dose assessment is developing currently.

PATIENT-SPECIFIC DOSE CALCULATIONS

Some have attempted to overcome the limitations of the use of standardized hermaphrodite phantoms to approximate the geometry of the human body. Fusion of anatomic and physiologic image information has been accomplished in several centers (27–29), providing the ability to develop three-dimensional (3D) distributions of dose based on actual patient images. Registration of anatomic [computed tomography (CT) and magnetic resonance imaging (MRI)] and physiologic [positron emission tomography (PET) and single photon emission computed tomography (SPECT)] images is needed for transporting particles from the different anatomically defined source regions to the target regions. Patient positioning on different devices is often difficult to maintain, and the patient's body habitus may be different (e.g., postprandial vs. preprandial). For this reason, various techniques using deformable mappings have been developed and used (30). The images to be fused include CT, whole body planar, PET, and SPECT scans.

Voxel Source Kernel Methods

As a step in the direction of providing precalculated dose conversion factors for use with 3D voxel data, voxel source kernels were developed by Williams et al. (31) and the MIRD Committee (32). These dose conversion factors in principle allow calculation of 3D-dose information from patient-specific data, but only in limited spatial areas in which there are no changes in material composition or density. (These kernels were developed only for a soft tissue medium and thus do not work in lung or bone or where soft tissue/bone or lung interfaces occur.)

Patient-Specific Computer Codes

Two groups have attempted to permit the introduction of tumor-like regions in the standard phantoms, to estimate tumor dose contributions to other organs (33,34). The idea of providing patient-specific dose distributions based on voxel information of patient-specific image data has been studied by several authors, including the 3D-ID code at Memorial Sloan-Kettering Cancer Center (27), the SIMIND code from the University of Lund (28), and the RTDS code at the City of Hope Medical Center (29). Stabin and Yoriyaz (35) have shown that the MCNP computer code may be used with patient image data to perform voxel-based radiation transport of electrons and photons in a heterogeneous tissue medium.

SMALL SCALE AND MICRODOSIMETRY

When there is significant uptake of the radiopharmaceutical in a target organ of interest, the averaging of the dose over the entire organ system is an oversimplification of the actual energy deposition pattern. If dose estimation formulas are to be successfully used to provide a quantitative variable in a dose-response risk projection model, then the appropriate dose(s) to be considered may be not only the average organ system dose but also the detailed energy deposition pattern over short (i.e., macromolecular or cellular) ranges. This is especially important for nonpenetrating radiations (e.g., low-energy photons, ICE, AE, β^-, β^+) in radiobiologically critical targets.

For example, the work of Rao et al. (36) with mouse testes demonstrated that intratesticular administration of thallous chloride resulted in a significant concentration of the thallium cation in the basal layer (≥ 10 μm) of the seminiferous epithelium. This region is generally populated with spermatogonia, which are the stem cells for sperm. The authors demonstrated that ^{201}Tl, which emits predominantly low-energy mercury x-rays, AEs, and ICEs, was two to four times more effective in reducing testis weight and sperm number than ^{204}Tl (an energetic β-emitter) per unit activity administered. However, this result is contrary to what one would expect by considering only the total testicular dose (rad) per microcurie of ^{201}Tl and ^{204}Tl in the organ as calculated by conventional dosimetry, or 8.3 and 54.0 rad, respectively. Thus, it appears that the abundance of low-energy electrons emitted during ^{201}Tl decay, which deliver the majority of their energy over a very short range, have a more significant influence over the measured biologic effect than the average total energy deposited per gram would have predicted. Although it is likely that the intravenous route of administration of ^{201}Tl in the clinical setting and blood-testis barrier prevent the inorganic thallous ion from being in intimate contact with the germinal layer of the seminiferous tubules, it is important to note that the estimate of average dose to the testes would not have represented this biologically significant dose distribution pattern.

On the other hand, if one were to consider ^{111}In platelet scintigraphy, the situation may be reversed. A 5-rad organ dose to the spleen is predicted during radioplatelet imaging with modest amounts (<200 μCi) of injected activity. It is important to remember, however, that the 5-rad splenic dose calculation was made by dividing the energy from radiation absorbed in the spleen during decay by the organ's entire mass. This simplification ignores the fact that a significant fraction of the particulate radiation emitted by ^{111}In is in the form of low-energy (0.6 to 25.4 keV) AEs, which undoubtedly deposit some of their energy within the platelet itself or in adjacent platelets that have formed small platelet aggregates. Thus, in this case, the estimated average dose may overestimate the actual energy deposition pattern realized by sensitive sites within cells of the spleen.

Calculational Techniques

Calculating absorbed dose as a function of distance from point or extended photon or electron-emitting sources has been facilitated for many years by the formulas of Loevinger et al. (37) and the point kernels of Berger (38). Through the use of the formulas of Loevinger et al. or the point kernels of Berger, dose as a function of distance may be estimated for most source geometries. Development of the actual techniques and examples is beyond the scope of this chapter. More recently, similar efforts have been attempted by Cross et al. (39), Werner et al. (40), and Howell et al. (41). Certain radiation transport codes are also available that can simulate the transport and absorption of photon and electron energy. Current examples include the EGS code series (42) and the MCNP code (43). The point kernels of Berger and Cross et al. were generated by similar codes. Most of these authors have produced very similar results, differing only slightly at short distances or at high energies. Useful applications of these results have been published by a number of authors, including Howell et al. (41), Faraggi et al. (44), Hui et al. (45), and Werner et al. (29), usually for activity in and around tumors of various sizes.

The problems discussed (dose to the testes from thallium isotopes and dose to the spleen from ^{111}In platelets), however, can be addressed through use of these methods, to evaluate where the energy is actually deposited. One of the barriers encountered in this analysis is knowledge of the microscopic distributions of the radionuclides. This information is not accessible by current external imaging techniques, although some information may be gleaned from autoradiography studies.

Intracellular Dosimetry

Since the introduction of [111]In 8-hydroxyquinoline (In-Oxine) as a cellular radiolabel by McAfee and Thakur (46) in 1976, the use of this lipid-soluble chelate and its chemical analogs (e.g., tropolone) for cell labeling has rapidly expanded. The diagnostic

Table 10.7. *Doses and Dose Rates for Cellular Radiolabels*

Cells	Nuclide	Dose Rate[a] (rad-hr)	T_c (hr)	Dose (rad)[a]
Neutrophils	[99m]Tc	91	3	390
	[111]In	187	5.5	1,480
	[51]Cr	115	6	990
Platelets	[99m]Tc	125	5.7	1,030
	[111]In	213	42	12,900
	[51]Cr	193	93	25,900

[a]Assumes 1 mCl uniformly distributed in 1.3×10^8 neutrophils or 7.5×10^9 platelets typically contained in 30 ml of whole blood. Modified from Bassano and McAfee (56).

utility of ^{111}In-labeled formed blood elements (specifically platelets and granulocytes) has been demonstrated by numerous investigators (47–55). Of more recent concern has been the intracellular dose to these circulating blood cells and its potential radiobiologic significance.

Bassono and McAfee (56) have calculated cellular radiation doses to neutrophils and platelets for a number of radionuclides of clinical interest. Table 10.7 shows the dose and dose rate estimates for ^{111}In based on this work, together with those of ^{99m}Tc and ^{51}Cr for comparison. Note that although the dose and dose rates shown here are considerably higher than those seen from commonly used radiopharmaceuticals and organ system dosimetry, this is mainly a result of the relatively small mass represented by these cells. Studies of structure, function, survival, and margination of these cells have not demonstrated any significant abnormalities (57,58). Although the fact that platelets are enucleated and both platelets and neutrophils are postmitotic may help explain their relative radioresistivity, such is not the case for lymphocytes, which have large nuclei, long mitotic futures, and variable mitotic rates. It has been known for some time that lymphocytes are among the most radiosensitive targets in the body, and several investigators have evaluated the effect of intracellular ^{111}In in lymphocytes (59,60).

Microdosimetry

Dosimetry at the cellular level or DNA level is yet another level of dosimetry, called microdosimetry by some, and is distinguished from small-scale dosimetry by its stochastic nature. Much of the work in this field, useful in radiation detection as well as tissue dosimetry, has been developed by Harold Rossi. A summary of some of the concepts of microdosimetry is given in an article by Rossi and Zaider (61). Some applications of these concepts have been attempted by Makrigiorgos et al. (62, 63), Gardin et al. (64), and Leichner (65). Although these calculations are possible, the interpretation of the results is uncertain at present, and more development is needed.

ACCURACY OF DOSE CALCULATIONS

The time integrated activity ($\bar{A}_b$) used for each initial organ dose estimate generated during the investigational new drug (IND) phase of radiopharmaceutical development is usually based on laboratory animal data, which may or may not be representative of human biodistribution and kinetics. The animal model assumption and biodistribution kinetics will always be associated with some error in attempting to predict the human dosimetry. In an analysis of data sets for several radiopharmaceuticals first using animal data and then using human data gathered in clinical trials, the animal data typically predicted correctly the organ that received the highest absorbed dose and determined most estimates for most organs within a factor of two (66). Sparks and Aydogan (67) studied a large number of data sets in which both animal and human kinetics were used to calculate human dose estimates and found that the choice of extrapolation method could have a significant impact on the dose estimates and that the variability in the predicted values of human doses could be considerable.

Another consideration is the applicability of human dosimetry data when they are available. If the data are based primarily on normal healthy adult volunteers, it is clear that biodistribution and kinetics for this group will be different from a patient population of dissimilar ages and in whom the normal metabolic process may be compromised by the presence of various pathophysiologic conditions. In addition, our estimate of the impact on human health from a particular dose-response model may be off by an order of magnitude in either direction. Some MIRD Dose Estimate Reports (e.g., 68) attempt to address the issue of the impact of disease states on the radiation dose estimates, but in general this area is not well studied.

Considering this, one may ask, why bother to do these calculations at all if they are fraught with so many assumptions and potential errors? The answer is that this system and other dose estimate models give us a yardstick for comparison from which we can make some decisions regarding the safety or potential hazards of future radiopharmaceuticals. In addition, the calculated dose estimates also serve as a guide to the safe and selective use of currently used radiopharmaceuticals in various patient populations. As more detailed information regarding the dose-response relationship becomes available the utility of our cumulative knowledge base of radiopharmaceutical dosimetry will have even greater significance. In addition, as more success is achieved with the use of patient-specific data for internal dose calculations, particularly in situations involving therapy, more confidence will be gained in the reported numbers.

MIRD PUBLICATIONS AND DOSE ESTIMATES

Since the publication of the first MIRD schema in 1968 (4), the committee has published a number of pamphlets containing additional information, refinements, and simplifications of the technique. In addition, various task groups of the committee periodically publish dose estimate reports in the *Journal of Nuclear Medicine* that use the MIRD formalisms and the best available human and animal data to estimate organ doses in humans from radiopharmaceuticals, either in routine clinical use or under current clinical evaluation. Information on MIRD documents is available through the Society of Nuclear Medicine.

For the most commonly used diagnostic and therapeutic radiopharmaceuticals, Appendix 1 summarizes typically administered adult dose, the organ receiving the highest radiation dose and its dose, gonadal dose, and the adult ED. For most of these same radiopharmaceuticals, Appendix 2 provides a table of effective doses per unit activity administered in 15-, 10-, 5-, and 1-year-old patients, and Appendix 3 provides a table of absorbed doses to the embryo/fetus per unit activity administered to the mother at early gestation and 3-, 6-, and 9-months gestation.

REFERENCES

1. Marinelli LD, Quimby EH, Hine GJ. Dosage determination with radioactive isotopes; practical considerations in therapy and protection. *Am J Roent Radium Ther* 1948;59:260.
2. Loevinger R, Holt JG, Hine GJ. Internally administered radioisotopes. In: Hine GJ, Brownell GL, eds. *Radiation dosimetry.* New York: Academic Press, 1956.
3. Loevinger R, Berman M. A formalism for calculation of absorbed dose from radionuclides. *Phys Med Biol* 1968;13:205.
4. Loevinger R, Berman M. A schema for absorbed dose calculations for biologically distributed radionuclides. *J Nucl Med* 1968;(Suppl 1, Pamphlet 1).
5. Ellett WH, Callahan AB, Brownell GL. Gamma-ray dosimetry of internal emitters. I. Monte Carlo calculations of absorbed dose from point sources. *Br J Radiol* 1964;37:45.
6. Ellett WH, Callahan AB, Brownell GL. Gamma-ray dosimetry of internal emitters. II. Monte Carlo calculations of absorbed dose from uniform sources. *Br J Radiol* 1965;38:541.
7. Coffey J, Cristy M, Warner G. MIRD Pamphlet No 13: specific absorbed fractions for photon sources uniformly distributed in the heart chambers and heart wall of a heterogeneous phantom. *J Nucl Med* 1981;22:65–71.
8. Eckerman KF, Cristy M, Warner GG. Dosimetric evaluation of brain scanning agents. In: Watson EE, Schlafke-Stelson AT, Coffey JL et al., eds. *Third international radiopharmaceutical dosimetry symposium.* HHS Publication FDA 81-8166. Rockville, MD: US Dept. of Health and Human Services, Food and Drug Administration, 1981:527–540.
9. Watson EE, Stabin MG. A model of the peritoneal cavity for use in internal dosimetry. *J Nucl Med* 1986;27:979(abst).
10. Stabin MG. A model of the prostate gland for use in internal dosimetry. *J Nucl Med* 1994;35:516.
11. Eckerman KF, Ryman JC. *External exposure to radionuclides in air, water, and soil.* Federal Guidance Report No. 12, EPA Report No. EPA 402-R-93-081. Washington, DC: US Government Printing Office, 1993.
12. Crady DL, Bolch WE, Weber DA et al. Specific absorbed fractions for photon sources in a revised dosimetric model of the brain. *Health Physics* 1993;64(Suppl):S17.
13. Cristy M, Eckerman K. *Specific absorbed fractions of energy at various ages from internal photon sources.* ORNL/TM-8381 V1-V7. Oak Ridge, TN: Oak Ridge National Laboratory, 1987.
14. Stabin MG, Watson EE, Cristy M et al. *Mathematical models and specific absorbed fractions of photon energy in the adult female at various stages of pregnancy.* ORNL/TM-12907, 1995.
15. Snyder W, Ford M, Warner G. *Estimates of specific absorbed fractions for photon sources uniformly distributed in various organs of a heterogeneous phantom.* MIRD Pamphlet No. 5 (revised). New York: Society of Nuclear Medicine, 1978.
16. Snyder WS, Ford MR, Warner GG et al. *"S" absorbed dose per unit cumulated activity for selected radionuclides and organs.* nm/MIRD Pamphlet #11. New York: Society of Nuclear Medicine, 1975.
17. Cloutier R, Watson E, Rohrer R et al. Calculating the radiation dose to an organ. *J Nucl Med* 1973;14:53–55.

18. Coffey J, Watson E. Calculating dose from remaining body activity: a comparison of two methods. *Med Phys* 1979;6:307–308.

19. Smith EM, Warner GG. Practical methods of dose reduction to the bladder wall. In: Cloutier RJ, Coffey JL, Snyder WS et al., eds. *Radiopharmaceutical dosimetry, proceedings of a symposium at Oak Ridge, April 1976.* Bureau of Radiological Health Publication (EDS)76-8044. Washington, DC: US Government Printing Office, 1976.

20. Thomas SR, Stabin MG, Chen CT et al. MIRD Pamphlet No. 14, Revised: a dynamic urinary bladder model for radiation dose calculations. *J Nucl Med* 1999;40:102S–123S.

21. International Commission on Radiological Protection. *Limits for intakes of radionuclides by workers.* ICRP Publication 30. New York: Pergamon Press, 1979.

22. International Commission on Radiological Protection. *Protection of the patient in nuclear medicine.* ICRP Publication 52. New York: Pergamon Press, 1987.

23. International Commission on Radiological Protection. *1990 recommendations of the International Commission on Radiological Protection*. ICRP Publication 60. New York: Pergamon Press, 1991.

24. Toohey RE, Stabin MG. Comparative analysis of dosimetry parameters for nuclear medicine. In Stelson A, Stabin M, Sparks R, eds. *Proceedings of the Sixth International Radiopharmaceutical Dosimetry Symposium, May 7–10, 1996.* Gatlinburg, TN: Oak Ridge Associated Universities, 1999:532–551.

25. Poston J. Application of the effective dose equivalent to nuclear medicine patients. *J Nucl Med* 1993;34:714–716.

26. International Committee on Radiological Protection. Report of ICRP Committee II on permissible dose for internal radiation. *Health Phys* 1959;3:1.

27. Sgouros G. Treatment planning for internal emitter therapy: methods, applications, and clinical implications. In Stelson A, Stabin M, Sparks R, eds. *Proceedings of the Sixth International Radiopharmaceutical Dosimetry Symposium, May 7–10, 1996.* Gatlinburg, TN: Oak Ridge Associated Universities, 1999:13–25. .

28. Tagesson M, Ljungberg M, Strand S-E. The SIMDOS Monte Carlo code for conversion of activity distributions to absorbed dose and dose-rate distributions. In Stelson A, Stabin M, Sparks R, eds. *Proceedings of the Sixth International Radiopharmaceutical Dosimetry Symposium, May 7–10, 1996.* Gatlinburg, TN: Oak Ridge Associated Universities, 1999:425–440.

29. Liu A, Williams L, Lopatin G et al. A radionuclide therapy treatment planning and dose estimation system. *J Nucl Med* 1999;40:1151–1153.

30. Zijdenbos AP, Dawant BM, Margolin R. Morphometric analysis of white matter lesions in MR images: method and validation. *IEEE Trans Med Imaging* 1994;13:716–724.

31. Williams LE, Liu A, Raubitschek AA et al. A method for patient-specific absorbed dose estimation for internal beta emitters. *Clin Cancer Res* 1999;Oct 5(10 Suppl):3015s–3019s

32. Bolch W, Bouchet L, Robertson J et al. MIRD Pamphlet No. 17: the dosimetry of nonuniform activity distributions—radionuclide S values at the voxel level. *J Nucl Med* 1999;40:11S–36S.

33. Johnson T, McClure D, McCourt S. MABDOSE I: Characterization of a general purpose dose estimation code. *Med Phys* 1999;26:1389–1395.

34. Clairand I, Ricard M, Gouriou J et al. DOSE3D: EGS4 Monte Carlo code-based software for internal radionuclide dosimetry. *J Nucl Med* 1999;40:1517–1523.

35. M. Stabin and H. Yoriyaz. Photon specific absorbed fractions calculated in the trunk of an adult male phantom. *Health Phys* 2002;80:21–44.

36. Rao DV, Govelitz DF, Sastry KSR. Radiotoxicity of thallium-201 in mouse testes: inadequacy of conventional dosimetry. *J Nucl Med* 1983;24:145.

37. Loevinger R, Japha E, Brownell G. Discrete radioisotope processes. In: Hine G, Brownell G, eds. *Radiation dosimetry.* New York: Academic Press, 1956:694–802.

38. Berger, M. MIRD Pamphlet No 7. Distribution of absorbed dose around point sources of electrons and beta particles in water and other media. *J Nucl Med* 1971;12(Suppl 5):5.

39. Cross W, Freedman N, Wong P. *Tables of beta-ray dose distributions in water.* AECL-10521. Chalk River, Ontario, Canada: Chalk River Nuclear Laboratories, 1992.

40. Werner B, Rahman M, Salk W. Dose distributions in regions containing beta sources: uniform spherical source regions in homogeneous media. *Med Phys* 1991;18:1181–1191.

41. Howell R, Rao D, Sastry K. Macroscopic dosimetry for radioimmunotherapy: nonuniform activity distributions in solid tumors. *Med Phys* 1989;16:66–74.

42. Bielajew A, Rogers D. PRESTA: the parameter reduced electron-step transport algorithm for electron Monte Carlo transport. *Nucl Instrum Methods* 1987;B18:165–181.

43. Briesmeister, JF. *MCNP—a general Monte Carlo N-particle transport code.* LA-12625-M. Los Alamos, NM: Los Alamos National Laboratory, 1993.

44. Farragi M, Gardin I, Labriolle-Vaylet C et al. The influence of tracer localization on the electron dose rate delivered to the cell nucleus. *J Nucl Med* 1994;35:113–119.

45. Hui T, Fisher D, Press O et al. Localized beta dosimetry of ^{131}I-labeled antibodies in follicular lymphoma. *Med Phys* 1992;19:97–104.

46. McAfee JG, Thakur ML. Survey of radioactive agents for in vitro labeling of phagocytic leukocytes. I. Soluble agents. *J Nucl Med* 1976;17:480.

47. Goodwin DA, Bushberg JT, Doherty PW et al. In-111 labeled autologous platelets for location of vascular thrombi in humans. *J Nucl Med* 1978;19:626.

48. Davis HH, Siegel BA, Joist JH et al. Scintigraphic detection of atherosclerotic lesions and venous thrombi in man by indium-111-labeled autologous platelets. *Lancet* 1978;1:1185.

49. Smith N, Chandler S, Hawker RJ et al. Indium-labeled autologous platelets as diagnostic aid after renal transplantation. *Lancet* 1979;1:1241.

50. Thakur ML, Lavender JP, Arnot RN et al. Indium-111 labeled autologous leukocytes in man. *J Nucl Med* 1977;18:1014.

51. Doherty PW, Bushberg JT, Lipton MJ et al. The use of indium-111-labeled leukocytes for abscess detection. *Clin Nucl Med* 1978;3:108.

52. Ezekowitz MD, Burow RD, Heath PW et al. The diagnostic accuracy of indium-111 platelet scintigraphy in the diagnosis of left ventricular thrombi. *Am J Cardiol* 1983;51:1563–1564.

53. Goss TP, Monahan JJ. Indium-111 white blood cell scan. *Orthop Rev* 1981;10:91.

54. Ezekowitz MD, Wilson DA, Smith EO et al. The comparison of indium-111 platelet scintigraphy and two-dimensional echocardiography in the diagnosis of left ventricular thrombi. *N Engl J Med* 1982;306:1509–1513.

55. Thakur ML, Gottschalk AG, eds. *In-111 labeled neutrophils, platelets and lymphocytes.* New York: Trivirum Publishing Co, 1980.

56. Bassano DA, McAfee JG. Cellular doses of labeled neutrophils and platelets. *J Nucl Med* 1979;20:255.

57. Zakhireh B, Thakur ML, Malech HL et al. Indium-111 labeled human polymorphonuclear leukocytes: viability, random migration, chemotaxis, bacterial capacity and ultrastructure. *J Nucl Med* 1979;20:741.

58. Welch MJ, Mathias CJ. Platelet viability following In-111 oxine labeling in electrolyte solutions. In: Thakur ML, Gottschalk AG, eds. *In-111 labeled neutrophils, platelets and lymphocytes.* New York: Trivirum Publishing Co, 1980:93–102.

59. Rannie GH, Thakur ML, Ford WL. Indium-111 labeled lymphocytes: preparation, evaluation and comparison with Cr-51 lymphocytes in rats. *Clin Exp Immunol* 1977;29:509.

60. Chisholm PM, Danpure HJ, Healey G et al. Cell damage resulting from the labeling of rat lymphocytes and HeLa S3 cells with In-111 oxine. *J Nucl Med* 1979;20:1308.

61. Rossi H, Zaider M. Elements of microdosimetry. *Med Phys* 1991;18:1085–1092.

62. Makrigiorgos G, Ito S, Baranowska-Kortylewicz J et al. Inhomogeneous deposition of radiopharmaceuticals at the cellular level: experimental evidence and dosimetry implications. *J Nucl Med* 1990;31:1358–1363.

63. Makrigiorgos G, Adelstein S, Kassis A. Limitations of conventional internal dosimetry at the cellular level. *J Nucl Med* 1989;30:1856–1864.

64. Gardin I, Linhart N, Petiet A et al. Dosimetry at the cellular level of

Kupffer cells after technetium-99m-sulphur colloid injection. *J Nucl Med* 1992;33:380–384.

65. Leichner P. *Macrodosimetry and microdosimetry in radioimmunotherapy.* DOE/ER/61195. Omaha: University of Nebraska Medical Center, 1991.

66. Stabin M. *Radiation dosimetry and the predictive value of preclinical models.* Presentation, Washington, DC: Drug Information Association, July 13, 1989.

67. Sparks RB, Aydogan B. Comparison of effectiveness of some common animal data scaling techniques in estimating human radiation dose. In: Stelson A, Stabin M, Sparks R, eds. *Proceedings of the Sixth International Radiopharmaceutical Dosimetry Symposium, May 7–10, 1996.* Gatlinburg, TN: Oak Ridge Associated Universities, 1999:705–716.

68. Atkins H et al. MIRD Dose Estimate Report No. 3—Summary of current radiation dose estimates to humans with various liver conditions from 99mTc sulfur colloid. *J Nucl Med* 1975;16:108A–108B.

Appendix 10.1. *Summary of Typically Administered Adult Dose; Organ Receiving the Highest Radiation Dose and its Dose; Gonadal Dose and the Adult Effective Dose for Some Commonly Used Diagnostic and Therapeutic Radiopharmaceuticals*

Radiopharmaceutical	Typical Activity Administration (Adult) MBq	mCi	Highest Organ Dose[d] mGy	Organ	rad	Gonadal Dose[d,f] mSv (ov/ts)	rem (ov/ts)	Effective Dose or Effective Dose Equivalent[d,e] mSv	rem	Reference
^{14}C Urea Normal	0.037	0.001	4.44E−03	Bladder wall	4.44E−04	ov 8.88E−04 ts 8.88E−04	ov 8.88E−05 ts 8.88E−05	1.15E−03	1.15E−04	1
^{14}C Urea Heliobacter positive	0.037	0.001	1.33E+00	Bone surfaces	1.33E−01	ov 4.44E−02 ts 2.81E−03	ov 4.44E−03 ts 2.81E−04	1.48E−01	1.48E−02	1
^{57}Co Cyanocobalamin IV no carrier	0.037	0.001	1.89E+00	Liver	1.89E−01	ov 6.29E−02 ts 3.59E−02	ov 6.29E−03 ts 3.59E−03	2.15E−01	2.15E−02	2
^{57}Co Cyanocobalamin IV with carrier	0.037	0.001	5.92E−02	Liver	5.92E−03	ov 3.03E−03 ts 5.92E−03	ov 3.03E−04 ts 5.92E−04	9.62E−03	9.62E−04	2
^{57}Co Cyanocobalamin Oral no flushing	0.037	0.001	5.92E−03	Liver	5.92E−04	ov 5.55E−04 ts 2.55E−02	ov 5.55E−05 ts 2.55E−03	7.03E−04	7.03E−05	2
^{57}Co Cyanocobalamin Oral with flushing	0.037	0.001	2.33E−02	Liver	2.33E−03	ov 3.03E−03 ts 1.70E−02	ov 3.03E−04 ts 1.70E−03	3.70E−03	3.70E−04	2
^{51}Cr Sodium chromate RBC's	5.6	0.151	8.96E+00	Spleen	8.96E−01	ov 4.59E−01 ts 3.53E−01	ov 4.59E−02 ts 3.53E−02	1.46E+00	1.46E−01	2
^{18}F Fluoro-deoxyglucose	370	10.000	5.92E+01	Bladder	5.92E+00	ov 5.55E+00 ts 4.44E+00	ov 5.55E−01 ts 4.44E−01	7.03E+00	7.03E−01	1
^{67}Ga Citrate	185	5.000	1.17E+02	Bone surfaces	1.17E+01	ov 1.52E+01 ts 1.04E+02	ov 1.52E+00 ts 1.04E+01	1.85E+01	1.85E+00	1
^{123}I Hippuran	14.8	0.400	2.81E+01	Bladder wall	2.81E+00	ov 1.02E−01 ts 7.10E−03	ov 1.02E−02 ts 7.10E−04	1.78E−01	1.78E−02	1
^{123}I MIBG	14.8	0.400	9.92E−01	Liver	9.92E−02	ov 1.21E−01 ts 8.44E−02	ov 1.21E−02 ts 8.44E−03	1.92E−01	1.92E−02	1
^{123}I Sodium iodide (0% uptake)	14.8	0.400	1.33E+00	Bladder wall	1.33E−01	ov 1.45E−01 ts 1.02E−01	ov 1.45E−02 ts 1.02E−02	1.92E−01	1.92E−02	2
^{123}I Sodium iodide (5% uptake)	14.8	0.400	9.32E+00	Thyroid	9.32E−01	ov 1.78E−01 ts 8.14E−02	ov 1.78E−02 ts 8.14E−03	5.62E−01	5.62E−02	2
^{123}I Sodium iodide (15% uptake)	14.8	0.400	2.81E+01	Thyroid	2.81E+00	ov 1.78E−01 ts 7.84E−02	ov 1.78E−02 ts 7.84E−03	1.11E+00	1.11E−01	2
^{123}I Sodium iodide (25% uptake)	14.8	0.400	4.74E+01	Thyroid	4.74E+00	ov 1.63E−01 ts 7.70E−02	ov 1.63E−02 ts 7.70E−03	1.63E+00	1.63E−01	2
^{123}I Sodium iodide (35% uptake)	14.8	0.400	6.66E+01	Thyroid	6.66E+00	ov 1.63E−01 ts 7.40E−02	ov 1.63E−02 ts 7.40E−03	2.22E+00	2.22E−01	2
^{123}I Sodium iodide (45% uptake)	14.8	0.400	8.44E+01	Thyroid	8.44E+00	ov 1.63E−01 ts 7.10E−02	ov 1.63E−02 ts 7.10E−03	2.81E+00	2.81E−01	2
^{123}I Sodium iodide (55% uptake)	14.8	0.400	1.04E+02	Thyroid	1.04E+01	ov 1.63E−01 ts 6.81E−02	ov 1.63E−02 ts 6.81E−03	3.40E+00	3.40E−01	2

(continued)

Appendix 10.1. *(continued)*

Radiopharmaceutical	MBq	mCi	Highest Organ Dose mGy	Organ	Highest Organ Dose rad	Gonadal Dose mSv	Gonadal Dose rem	(ov/ts)	Effective Dose or Effective Dose Equivalent mSv	Effective Dose or Effective Dose Equivalent rem	Reference
125I Albumin	0.74	0.020	5.11E-01	Heart	5.11E-02	1.48E-01	1.48E-02	ov	2.52E-01	2.52E-02	2
						1.18E-01	1.18E-02	ts			
131I Hippuran	0.74	0.020	6.81E-01	Bladder wall	6.81E-02	1.18E-02	1.18E-03	ov	3.85E-02	3.85E-03	1
						8.88E-03	8.88E-04	ts			
131I MIBG	0.74	0.020	6.14E-01	Liver	6.14E-02	4.88E-02	4.88E-03	ov	1.48E-01	1.48E-02	2
						4.37E-02	4.37E-03	ts			
131I Sodium iodide (0% uptake)	37.00	100	2.26E+03	Bladder wall	2.26E+02	1.55E+02	1.55E+01	ov	N/A	N/A	2
						1.37E+02	1.37E+01	ts			
131I Sodium iodide (5% uptake)	37.00	100	2.66E+05	Thyroid	2.66E+04	1.63E+02	1.63E+01	ov	N/A	N/A	2
						1.07E+02	1.07E+01	ts			
131I Sodium iodide (15% uptake)	37.00	100	7.77E+05	Thyroid	7.77E+04	1.59E+02	1.59E+01	ov	N/A	N/A	2
						1.04E+02	1.04E+01	ts			
131I Sodium iodide (25% uptake)	37.00	100	1.33E+06	Thyroid	1.33E+05	1.59E+02	1.59E+01	ov	N/A	N/A	2
						9.99E+01	9.99E+00	ts			
131I Sodium iodide (35% uptake)	37.00	100	1.85E+06	Thyroid	1.85E+05	1.55E+02	1.55E+01	ov	N/A	N/A	2
						9.62E+01	9.62E+00	ts			
131I Sodium iodide (45% uptake)	37.00	100	2.37E+06	Thyroid	2.37E+05	1.55E+02	1.55E+01	ov	N/A	N/A	2
						9.62E+01	9.62E+00	ts			
131I Sodium iodide (55% uptake)	37.00	100	2.92E+06	Thyroid	2.92E+05	1.52E+02	1.52E+01	ov	N/A	N/A	2
						9.62E+01	9.62E+00	ts			
111In Pentetreotide also known as Octreoscan	222	6.0	1.27E+02	Spleen	1.27E+01	5.99E+00	5.99E-01	ov	1.20E+01	1.20E+00	1
						3.77E+00	3.77E-01	ts			
111In White blood cells	18.5	0.5	1.09E+02	Spleen	1.09E+01	2.42E+00	2.42E-01	ov	1.18E+01	1.18E+00	4
						5.55E-01	5.55E-02	ts			
81mKr Krypton gas	370	10	1.70E-03	Breast	1.70E-04	6.29E-05	6.29E-06	ov	9.99E-03	9.99E-04	2
						6.29E-06	6.29E-07	ts			
15O Water	370	10	7.03E-01	Heart	7.03E-02	3.15E-01	3.15E-02	ov	3.44E-01	3.44E-02	1
						2.74E-01	2.74E-02	ts			
32P Phosphate	148	4.0	1.63E+03	Red marrow	1.63E+02	1.10E+02	1.10E+01	ov	3.26E+02	3.26E+01	2
						1.10E+02	1.10E+01	ts			
153Sm Lexidronam also know as Quadramet	2590	70	1.08E+04	Bone surfaces	1.08E+03	2.25E+01	2.25E+00	ov	N/A	N/A	4
						1.40E+01	1.40E+00	ts			
89Sr Chloride also known as Metastron	148	4.0	2.52E+03	Bone surfaces	2.52E+02	1.15E+02	1.15E+01	ov	N/A	N/A	2
99mTc Apcitide also known as AcuTect	740	20	4.44E+01	Bladder wall	4.44E+00	4.66E+00	4.66E-01	ov	6.88E+00	6.88E-01	4,5
						3.92E+00	3.92E-01	ts			

Radiopharmaceutical	MBq	mCi		Critical organ			ov/ts				
99mTc Depreotide also known as NeoTect	740	20	6.66E+01	Kidneys	6.66E+00	3.11E+00	ov	3.11E-01	1.70E+01	1.70E+00	4.5
						2.29E+01	ts	2.29E+00			
99mTc Disofenin also know as HIDA (iminodiacetic acid)	185	5.0	2.04E+01	Gallbladder	2.04E+00	3.52E+00	ov	3.52E-01	3.15E+00	3.15E-01	1
	1.15E+02	ts	1.15E+01			2.78E-01	ts	2.78E-02			
99mTc DMSA (dimercaptosuccinic acid) also known as Succimer	185	5.0	3.33E+01	Kidneys	3.33E+00	6.48E-01	ov	6.48E-02	1.63E+00	1.63E-01	1
						3.33E-01	ts	3.33E-02			
99mTc Exametazime also known as Ceretec and HMPAO	740	20	2.52E+01	Kidneys	2.52E+00	4.88E+00	ov	4.88E-01	6.88E+00	6.88E-01	1
						1.78E+00	ts	1.78E-01			
99mTc Macro aggregated albumin (MAA)	148	4.0	9.77E+00	Lungs	9.77E-01	2.66E-01	ov	2.66E-02	1.63E+00	1.63E-01	
						1.63E-01	ts	1.63E-02			
99mTc Medronate also know as Tc-99m Methyenedi-phosphonate (MDP)	740	20	4.66E+01	Bone surfaces	4.66E+00	2.66E+00	ov	2.66E-01	4.22E+00	4.22E-01	1
						1.78E+00	ts	1.78E-01			
99mTc Mertiatide also know as MAG3 Normal renal function	370	10	4.07E+01	Bladder wall	8.14E+00	2.00E+00	ov	4.00E-01	2.59E+00	5.18E-01	1
						1.37E+00	ts	2.74E-01			
99mTc Mertiatide also know as MAG3 Abnormal renal function	370	10	3.07E+01	Bladder wall	6.14E+00	1.81E+00	ov	3.63E-01	2.26E+00	4.51E-01	1
						1.26E+00	ts	2.52E-01			
99mTc Mertiatide also know as MAG3 Acute unilateral renal blockage	370	10	7.40E+01	Kidneys	1.48E+01	1.41E+00	ov	2.81E-01	3.70E+00	7.40E-01	1
						7.40E-01	ts	1.48E-01			
99mTc Neurolite also known as ECD and Bicisate	740	20	5.40E+01	Bladder wall	5.40E+00	5.77E+00	ov	5.77E-01	8.14E+00	8.14E-01	
						2.59E+00	ts	2.59E-01			
99mTc Pentetate also know as Tc-99m DTPA	370	10	2.29E+01	Bladder wall	2.29E+00	1.55E+00	ov	1.55E-01	1.81E+00	1.81E-01	3
						1.07E+00	ts	1.07E-01			
99mTc Pyrophosphate	555	15	3.50E+01	Bone surfaces	3.50E+00	2.00E+00	ov	2.00E-01	3.16E+00	3.16E-01	1
						1.33E+00	ts	1.33E-01			
99mTc Red blood cells	740	20	1.33E+01	Kidneys	1.33E+00	2.74E+00	ov	2.74E-01	5.18E+00	5.18E-01	1
						1.70E+00	ts	1.70E-01			
99mTc Sestamibi also know as Cardiolite	740	20	2.89E+01	Gallbladder	2.89E+00	6.73E+00	ov	6.73E-01	6.66E+00	6.66E-01	1

(continued)

Appendix 10.1. *Summary of Typically Administered Adult Dose; Organ Receiving the Highest Radiation Dose and its Dose; Gonadal Dose and the Adult Effective Dose for Some Commonly Used Diagnostic and Therapeutic Radiopharmaceuticals*

Radiopharmaceutical	Typical Activity Administration (Adult)		Highest Organ Dose[d]			Gonadal Dose[d,f]				Effective Dose or Effective Dose Equivalent[d,e]		Reference
	MBq	mCi	mGy	Organ	rad	mSv	rad	rem	ov/ts	mSv	rem	
Rest						2.81E+00	2.81E-01	2.81E-01	ts			
^{99m}Tc Sestamibi also know as Cardiolite	740	20	2.44E+01	Gallbladder	2.44E+00	5.99E+00	5.99E-01	5.99E-01	ov	5.85E+00	5.85E-01	1
Stress						2.74E+00	2.74E-01	2.74E-01	ts			
^{99m}Tc Sodium pertechnetate	370	10	2.11E+01	ULI wall	2.11E+00	3.70E+00	3.70E-01	3.70E-01	ov	4.81E+00	4.81E-01	1
						1.04E+00	1.04E-01	1.04E-01	ts			
^{99m}Tc Sulfur colloid	296	8.0	2.22E+01	Spleen	2.22E+00	6.51E-01	6.51E-02	6.51E-02	ov	2.78E+00	2.78E-01	1
						1.66E-01	1.66E-02	1.66E-02	ts			
^{99m}Tc Technegas	740	20	8.14E+01	Lungs	8.14E+00	3.03E-01	3.03E-02	3.03E-02	ov	1.11E+01	1.11E+00	1
						4.51E-02	4.51E-03	4.51E-03	ts			
^{99m}Tc Tetrofosmin also know as Myoview Rest	740	20	2.66E+01	Gallbladder	2.66E+00	6.22E+00	6.22E-01	6.22E-01	ov	5.62E+00	5.62E-01	1
						1.78E+00	1.78E-01	1.78E-01	ts			
^{99m}Tc Tetrofosmin also know as Myoview Stress	740	20	2.00E+01	Gallbladder	2.00E+00	5.62E+00	5.62E-01	5.62E-01	ov	5.18E+00	5.18E-01	1
						2.15E+00	2.15E-01	2.15E-01	ts			
^{201}Tl Thallous chloride (with contaminants)	74	2.0	4.59E+01	Thyroid	4.59E+00	7.40E+00	7.40E-01	7.40E-01	ov	1.18E+01	1.18E+00	3
						1.48E+01	1.48E+00	1.48E+00	ts			
^{133}Xe Xenon gas (rebreathing for 5 minutes)	555	15	6.11E-01	Lungs	6.11E-02	4.05E-01	4.05E-02	4.05E-02	ov	4.44E-01	4.44E-02	2
						3.83E-01	3.83E-02	3.83E-02	ts			

References:

1, Annals of the International Commission on Radiological Protection Publication 80. Radiation dose to patients from radiopharmaceuticals. Tarrytown, NY: Elsevier Science, 1999. Note: Consult this reference for dosimetry information on other radiopharmaceuticals.

2, The International Commission on Radiological Protection Publication 53. Radiation dose to patients from radiopharmaceuticals. Elmsford, NY: Pergamon Press, 1988. Note: Consult this reference for dosimetry information on other radiopharmaceuticals.

3, Stabin MG, Stubbs JB, Toohey RE. Radiation dose estimates for radiopharmaceuticals, NUREG/CR-6345. Washington DC: Department of Energy and the Department of Health and Human Services, 1996.

4, Courtesy of Richard B. Sparks PhD. CDE Inc, Knoxville, TN.

5, Information supplied by the manufacturer.

Notes:

[a] Modified and reproduced with permission from Bushberg J et al. The essential physics of medical imaging, 2nd ed. Baltimore: Lippincott Williams & Wilkins, 2001.

[b] If reference is 1, then effective dose is given. If reference is 2, 3, or 4, then effective dose equivalent is given.

[c] N/A, not applicable. The effective dose is not a relevant quantity for therapeutic doses of radionuclides because it provides an estimate of effective stochastic risk (e.g., cancer and genetic detriment) and is not relevant to deterministic (i.e., nonstochastic) risks (e.g., acute radiation syndrome).

[d] Radiation dose per typical activity administered to an adult.

[e] Although the effective dose (and effective dose equivalent) was developed for (and thus incorporates assumptions relevant to) a healthy occupationally exposed population (as compared with an ill elderly population characteristic of medical imaging) its application in medicine has been recommended by the ICRP and, at the very least, offers a relative basis upon which doses may be compared between various diagnostic examinations (nuclear medicine, diagnostic x-rays) using ionizing radiation.

Appendix 10.2. *Effective Dose Per Unit Activity Administered to 15-, 10-, 5-, and 1-year-old Patients for Some Commonly Used Diagnostic Radiopharmaceuticals[c]*

Radiopharmaceutical	15 Years Old		10 Years Old		5 Years Old		1 Year Old		Reference
	mSv/MBq	rem/mCi	mSv/MBq	rem/mCi	mSv/MBq	rem/mCi	mSv/MBq	rem/mCi	
[18]F Fluoro-deoxyglucose	0.025	0.093	0.036	0.133	0.050	0.185	0.095	0.352	1
[67]Ga Citrate	0.130	0.481	0.200	0.740	0.330	1.221	0.640	2.368	1
[123]I Sodium iodide (0% uptake)	0.016	0.059	0.024	0.089	0.037	0.137	0.037	0.137	2
[123]I Sodium iodide (5% uptake)	0.053	0.196	0.080	0.296	0.150	0.555	0.290	1.073	2
[123]I Sodium iodide (15% uptake)	0.110	0.407	0.170	0.629	0.350	1.295	0.650	2.405	2
[123]I Sodium iodide (25% uptake)	0.170	0.629	0.260	0.962	0.540	1.998	1.000	3.700	2
[123]I Sodium iodide (35% uptake)	0.230	0.851	0.350	1.295	0.740	2.738	1.400	5.180	2
[123]I Sodium iodide (45% uptake)	0.290	1.073	0.440	1.628	0.940	3.478	1.800	6.660	2
[123]I Sodium iodide (55% uptake)	0.350	1.295	0.530	1.961	1.100	4.070	2.100	7.770	2
[111]In Pentatreotide also known as Octreoscan	0.071	0.263	0.100	0.370	0.160	0.592	0.280	1.036	1
[111]In White blood cells	0.836	3.093	1.240	4.588	1.910	7.067	3.380	12.506	2
[99m]Tc Disofenin also know as HIDA (iminodiacetic acid)	0.021	0.078	0.029	0.107	0.045	0.167	0.100	0.370	1
[99m]Tc DMSA (dimercaptosuccinic acid) also known as Succimer	0.011	0.041	0.015	0.056	0.021	0.078	0.037	0.137	1
[99m]Tc Exametazime also known as Ceretec and HMPAO	0.011	0.041	0.017	0.063	0.027	0.100	0.049	0.181	1
[99m]Tc Macro aggregated albumin (MAA)	0.016	0.059	0.023	0.085	0.034	0.126	0.063	0.233	1
[99m]Tc Medronate also know as [99m]Tc Methyenedi-phosphonate (MDP)	0.007	0.026	0.011	0.041	0.014	0.052	0.027	0.100	1
[99m]Tc Mertiatide also know as MAG3	0.009	0.033	0.012	0.044	0.012	0.044	0.022	0.081	1
[99m]Tc Bicisate also known as ECD and Neurolite	0.014	0.052	0.021	0.078	0.032	0.118	0.060	0.222	2
[99m]Tc Pentetate also know as ^{99m}Tc DTPA	0.006	0.023	0.008	0.030	0.009	0.033	0.016	0.059	1
[99m]Tc Pyrophosphate	0.007	0.026	0.011	0.041	0.014	0.052	0.027	0.100	1
[99m]Tc Red blood cells	0.009	0.033	0.014	0.052	0.021	0.078	0.039	0.144	1
[99m]Tc Sestamibi also know as Cardiolite (Rest)	0.012	0.044	0.018	0.067	0.028	0.104	0.053	0.196	1
[99m]Tc Sestamibi also know as Cardiolite (Stress)	0.010	0.037	0.016	0.059	0.023	0.085	0.045	0.167	1
[99m]Tc Sodium pertechnetate	0.017	0.063	0.026	0.096	0.042	0.155	0.079	0.292	1
[99m]Tc Sulfur colloid	0.012	0.044	0.018	0.067	0.028	0.104	0.050	0.185	1
[99m]Tc Tetrofosmin also know as Myoview (Rest)	0.010	0.036	0.013	0.048	0.022	0.081	0.043	0.159	1
[99m]Tc Tetrofosmin also know as Myoview (Stress)	0.008	0.030	0.012	0.044	0.018	0.067	0.035	0.130	1
[201]Tl Thallous chloride	0.293	1.084	1.160	4.292	1.500	5.550	2.280	8.436	3

References:
1, Annals of the International Commission on Radiological Protection Publication 80. Radiation dose to patients from radiopharmaceuticals. Tarrytown, NY: Elsevier Science, 1999.
2, Courtesy of Richard B. Sparks PhD. CDE Inc, Knoxville, TN.
3, Radiation Internal Dose Information Center, Oak Ridge, TN, 2001.
Notes:
[a]Modified and reproduced with permission from Bushberg J et al. The essential physics of medical imaging, 2nd ed. Baltimore: Lippincott Williams & Wilkins, 2001.
[b]If reference is 1, then effective dose is given. If reference is 2 or 3, then effective dose equivalent is given.
[c]Although the effective dose (and effective dose equivalent) was developed for (and thus incorporates assumptions relevant to) a healthy occupationally exposed population (as compared with an ill elderly population characteristic of medical imaging) its application in medicine has been recommended by the ICRP and, at the very least, offers a relative basis upon which doses may be compared between various diagnostic examinations (nuclear medicine, diagnostic x-rays) using ionizing radiation.

Appendix 10.3. *Summary of Absorbed Dose Estimates to the Embryo/fetus Per Unit Activity Administered to the Mother for Some Commonly Used Radiopharmaceuticals*

Radiopharmaceutical	Dose at different stages of gestation								Source
	Early		3 Months		6 Months		9 Months		
	mGy/MBq	rad/mCi	mGy/MBq	rad/mCi	mGy/MBq	rad/mCi	mGy/MBq	rad/mCi	
[57]Co Cyanocobalamin (normals, no flushing dose)	1.5000	5.5500	1.0000	3.7000	1.2000	4.4400	1.3000	4.8100	1
[18]F Fluoro-deoxyglucose	0.0270	0.0999	0.0170	0.0629	0.0094	0.0348	0.0081	0.0300	1
[67]Ga Citrate	0.0930	0.3441	0.2000	0.7400	0.1800	0.6660	0.1300	0.4810	1
[123]I Sodium iodide (25% uptake)	0.0200	0.0740	0.0140	0.0518	0.0110	0.0407	0.0098	0.0363	1
[125]I Albumin	0.2500	0.9250	0.0780	0.2886	0.0380	0.1406	0.0260	0.0962	1
[131]I Sodium iodide (25% uptake)	0.0720	0.2664	0.0680	0.2516	0.2300	0.8510	0.2700	0.9990	1
[111]In Pentetreotide also known as Octreoscan	0.0820	0.3034	0.0600	0.2220	0.0350	0.1295	0.0310	0.1147	1
[111]In White blood cells	0.1300	0.4810	0.0960	0.3552	0.0960	0.3552	0.0940	0.3478	1
[99m]Tc Disofenin also know as HIDA (iminodiacetic acid)	0.0170	0.0629	0.0150	0.0555	0.0120	0.0444	0.0067	0.0248	1
[99m]Tc DMSA (dimercaptosuccinic acid) also known as Succimer	0.0051	0.0189	0.0047	0.0174	0.0040	0.0148	0.0034	0.0126	1
[99m]Tc Exametazime also known as Cerete and HMPAO	0.0087	0.0322	0.0067	0.0248	0.0048	0.0178	0.0036	0.0133	1
[99m]Tc Macro aggregated albumin (MAA)	0.0028	0.0104	0.0040	0.0148	0.0050	0.0185	0.0040	0.0148	1
[99m]Tc Med-ronate also know as Tc-99m Methyenediphosphonate (MDP)	0.0061	0.0226	0.0054	0.0200	0.0027	0.0100	0.0024	0.0089	1
[99m]Tc Mertiatide also know as MAG3	0.0180	0.0666	0.0140	0.0518	0.0055	0.0204	0.0052	0.0192	1
[99m]Tc Bicisate also known as ECD and Neurolite	0.013	0.0481	0.01	0.0370	0.0055	0.0204	0.0044	0.0163	2
[99m]Tc Pentetate also know as Tc-99m DTPA	0.0120	0.0444	0.0087	0.0322	0.0041	0.0152	0.0047	0.0174	1
[99m]Tc Pyrophosphate	0.0060	0.0222	0.0066	0.0244	0.0036	0.0133	0.0029	0.0107	1
[99m]Tc Red blood cells	0.0064	0.0237	0.0043	0.0159	0.0033	0.0122	0.0027	0.0100	1
[99]Tc Sestamibi also know as Cardiolite (Rest)	0.0150	0.0555	0.0120	0.0444	0.0084	0.0311	0.0054	0.0200	1
[99]Tc Sestamibi also know as Cardiolite (Stress)	0.0120	0.0444	0.0095	0.0352	0.0069	0.0255	0.0044	0.0163	1
[99m]Tc Sodium pertechnetate	0.0110	0.0407	0.0220	0.0814	0.0140	0.0518	0.0093	0.0344	1
[99m]Tc Sulfur colloid	0.0018	0.0067	0.0021	0.0078	0.0032	0.0118	0.0037	0.0137	1
[99m]Tc Teboroxime also know as Cardiotec	0.0089	0.0329	0.0071	0.0263	0.0058	0.0215	0.0037	0.0137	1
[201]Tl Thallous chloride	0.0970	0.3589	0.0580	0.2146	0.0470	0.1739	0.0270	0.0999	1
[133]Xe Xenon gas (rebreathing for 5 minutes)	0.00041	0.00152	0.000048	0.00018	0.000035	0.00013	0.000026	0.00010	1

References
1, Stabin MG. Fetal dose calculation workbook (ORISE 97-0961). Oak Ridge, TN: Radiation Internal Dose Information Center, Oak Ridge Institute for Science and
2, Courtesy of Richard B. Sparks PhD, CDE Inc, Knoxville, TN.
Notes:
[a]Modified and reproduced with permission from Bushberg JT et al. The Essential Physics of Medical Imaging 2nd ed. Baltimore: Lippincott Williams & Wilkins, 2001.

11

RADIOBIOLOGY

S. JULIAN GIBBS

It has been recognized for almost a century that ionizing radiation, in sufficient doses, produces damage in living systems (1). However, despite decades of intensive research worldwide, it has not been established conclusively that small doses, such as those encountered by staff and patients in diagnostic procedures in the healing arts, are harmful. Neither has it been demonstrated that such doses are safe, i.e., devoid of injurious effects. This dilemma led the scientific community, on grounds of prudence, to establish the no-threshold model, which states that any dose of radiation, however small, *may* carry a small probability of biologic damage. Estimates of risk in this chapter are based on this model. It must be emphasized at the outset that there is a large uncertainty in these risk estimates, not only in their magnitudes, but also in whether these risks exist at all. There are no confirmed data demonstrating that any patient has ever been harmed by current techniques of the diagnostic use of ionizing radiation in the healing arts.

The public, the media, and even some scientists have confused the no-threshold model with established fact. The model fits available data, but not to the exclusion of other models. Some data support the concept of beneficial effects of small doses of radiation, called radiation hormesis (2). It seems clear that the facts lie somewhere between the two extremes, but their precise location in this space is unknown. We must proceed, however, with the information we have to estimate risks to patients and staff from diagnostic radiation in the healing arts and to determine that those risks are within the range that society considers acceptable (Table 11.1). To do otherwise could ignore a radiation dose that might be avoided or could prevent a patient from receiving a clinically indicated procedure.

It is first necessary to provide basic information dealing with radiation effects at the cellular level to create rational understanding of effects in intact organisms, especially humans.

CELLULAR RADIOBIOLOGY

Radiation effects result from the chemical events that follow ionization within a cell. Ion pairs are created randomly, either in biologically important molecules (direct action) or through damage to these molecules as a result of free radicals formed by radiolysis of water (indirect action). Overwhelming experimental evidence points to DNA as the target molecule. Numerous alterations in DNA have been described, including alteration or deletion of bases; strand breaks, or disruption of the sugar-phosphate backbone, of either one (single-strand break) or both (double-strand break) of the double helix; and cross-linking, or production of covalent bonds, between the two chains.

Transformation and Mutation

Relatively modest DNA damage involving only one or a few molecules per cell, which results from small radiation doses, is thought to be associated with subtle changes in cell chemistry. These apparently minor chemical changes, however, can lead to serious alterations in cell function. *In vitro* transformation has been demonstrated in mammalian cells exposed to doses as small as 10 mGy. Frequency of transformation is relatively low, of the order of 10^{-2} per Gy. Transformed cells are characterized by loss of contact inhibition in culture, and the generation of malignant tumors when injected in sufficient numbers into susceptible animals (5). In other cases, rather severe damage, such as deletion of large numbers of base pairs, may result in cells that are not perceptibly altered (6). Some relatively large regions of DNA contain no genetic information essential for cell survival or func-

Table 11.1. *One in a Million Risks*

Risk	Quantity
Existence, male, age 60	20 min
Living in New York	2 days
Living in Denver	2 months
Living in stone building	2 months
Drinking Miami water	1 year
Living near PVC plant	10 years
Travel by canoe	6 min
Travel by bicycle	10 miles
Travel by automobile	300 miles
Travel by commercial air	1,000 miles
Working in coal mine	1 hour
Typical factory work	10 days
Smoking	1.4 cigarettes
Drinking wine	500 cc

Source: 3, 4.

S.J. Gibbs: Radiology and Radiological Sciences, Vanderbilt University, Nashville, TN.

tion. Specific locus mutations *in vitro* have been studied by a number of investigators. Frequency is much lower than that of transformation, typically of the order of 10^{-4} to 10^{-6} per Gy (7).

Cell Death

More severe DNA damage, especially strand breaks, has been associated with cell death. Three modes of radiation-induced cell death have been described. *Reproductive cell death,* or loss of clonogenicity, has been extensively studied in cultured mammalian cells. Classically, cell survival curves have been generated using the target theory model (8) shown in Fig. 11.1**A**. With high linear energy transfer (LET) radiation (e.g., heavy charged particles), the survival curve is exponential.

$$S = e^{-D/D_0}$$

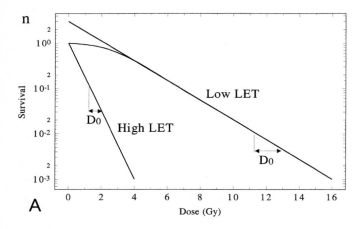

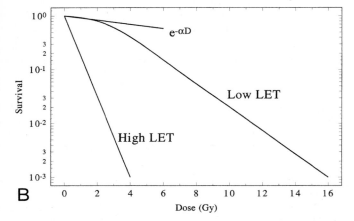

FIGURE 11.1. Cell survival curves, hypothetical. **A:** Target theory. The curve following exposure to neutrons or charged particles *(high LET)* is exponential, characterized by D_0, the reciprocal of the slope. From exposure to x-rays, γ-rays, or electrons *(low LET)*, there is a shoulder resulting from repair of sublethal damage at low doses. The curve is characterized by D_0 and n, the intercept of the linear portion of the curve extrapolated to zero dose. **B:** Theory of dual radiation action. The curve following exposure to high-LET radiation is exponential, characterized by α the reciprocal of D_0. The initial slope in the curve from low-LET radiation, characterized by $e^{-\alpha D}$, estimates effects from small doses. Downward concavity comes from the βD^2 term.

where S is the surviving fraction, D is radiation dose, and D_0 is a parameter, the reciprocal of the slope. This is known as the single-target model. With low-LET radiation (e.g., x-ray) the curve is exponential with a shoulder.

$$S = 1 - (1 - e^{-D/D_0})n$$

where n is the extrapolation number, the intercept on the ordinate of the extrapolation of the linear portion of the curve. This is the multihit or multitarget model. A cell survival curve can be characterized using this model by specifying D_0 and, with low-LET radiation, n. In general, D_0 is smaller, i.e., the curve is steeper, with high LET radiation.

An alternative to target theory is the theory of dual radiation action, which models survival curves as

$$S = e^{-(\alpha D + \beta D2)}$$

where α and β are parameters, as shown in Fig. 11.1**B** (9). In general, α is more than β. Thus, with low LET radiation at low doses or low dose rates, the $(\beta D^2$ term is negligible. At higher doses, the curve remains concave downward. At high LET β ≈ 0. The model is broadly applicable to a number of radiation effects, including carcinogenesis.

For most mammalian cells in culture exposed to low-LET radiation, D_0 is about 1 to 2 Gy, and n is 2 to 3. Several investigators have shown by ingenious techniques that most mammalian cells *in vivo* exhibit similar radiosensitivity. The major exceptions are lymphocytes and bone marrow colony forming cells, for which the D_0 is about 0.7 Gy (10).

Programmed cell death, or apoptosis, is a mode of cell death in which the first visible sign is chromatin condensation. The dying cell then disintegrates to form a cluster of apoptotic bodies that are membrane bound and that are soon phagocytosed. Because membranes remain intact until phagocytosis, no cellular contents are released, and no inflammatory response occurs. In irradiated radioresponsive tumors, brief waves of apoptotic bodies are seen (Fig. 11.2), peaking about 4-hours postexposure, with a D_0 of about 4 Gy (11). Apoptosis is an active, genetically programmed process. Presence of p53 tumor suppressor gene is required for radiation-induced apoptosis in mouse thymocytes (12). It plays a role in a number of physiologic processes, e.g., embryonic development (10). Its overall importance in radiobiology is not yet fully understood or appreciated.

Interphase cell death, not genetically programmed, requires very large doses that disrupt cellular membranes and organization or, in extreme cases, molecules, such as denaturation of proteins. This is the classically described mode of death of nondividing cell populations. It is of limited importance in radiobiology. The doses required to produce it occur only in such things as nuclear explosions and then only when the exposed individuals are close enough to the detonation to be killed by blast or heat.

Modifying Factors

A number of factors and conditions may either increase or decrease the magnitude of the effect of a given dose. In general, these factors must be present at the time of exposure.

Physical factors generally interact at the level of ionization.

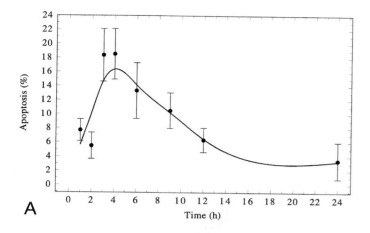

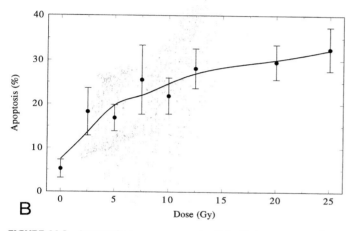

FIGURE 11.2. Apoptosis, or programmed cell death, in mouse ovarian tumors irradiated *in vivo*. **A:** Time course. A brief wave of apoptosis occurs after single exposure of 2.5 Gy, peaking at 4- to 6-hours postexposure and returns to control levels at 24 hours. **B:** Dose-response curve at 4 hours after single exposure. The response appears to saturate at about 10 Gy, with little further increase at doses above 12.5 Gy. Error bars in both plots represent standard deviations. (From Stephens LC, Hunter NR, Ang KK et al. Development of apoptosis in irradiated murine tumors as a function of time and dose. *Radiat Res* 1993;135:75–80, with permission.)

LET, or the spatial density of ion pairs produced along the track of an ionizing particle, affects not only the shape but also the slope of the cell survival curve (Fig. 11.1). Densely ionizing particles, such as neutrons or heavy charged particles, will deposit a lethal dose in any cell they traverse. Conversely, sparsely ionizing particles, such as photons, may deposit only a single interaction in a cell, resulting in sublethal damage. Only when a second particle deposits an independent second event in the same cell will the cell be killed—the origin of the D^2 term in the theory of dual radiation action (13). *Dose rate* directly affects damage. If a dose is protracted over time by either low dose rate or fractionation, injury is less than that caused by the same dose delivered in a single brief exposure (13). *Heat* sensitizes cells to lethal effects of low LET radiation (10).

Chemical factors generally interact at the level of the initial physical chemical event, promptly after the physical event of ionization. *Oxygen* sensitizes cells to lethal effects of radiation.

Cells exposed in total absence of oxygen are much more resistant. The oxygen enhancement ratio measured as change in D_0 is usually about two to three. The mechanism is thought to be interaction of molecular oxygen with radicals produced by radiolysis of water, yielding more reactive hydroperoxyl radicals (10, 13). *Radioprotectors,* generally chemicals containing sulfhydryl groups, protect cells and organisms from lethal radiation effects, presumably acting as free radical scavengers (14). *Radiosensitizers* have the opposite effect, especially on hypoxic cells (10). These factors are effective only with low LET radiation.

Biologic factors are intrinsic to the cell population at the time of exposure. *Repair* of sublethal damage occurs between dose fractions or during exposure at low dose rate (15). Radiation injury may be regarded as equilibrium between damage and repair—at high dose rates, the equilibrium shifts toward damage, whereas at lower dose rates it may shift toward survival. *Cell cycle* stage is a major player. Cells in M and G_2 are the most sensitive, whereas those in late S are most resistant, with early S and G_1 intermediate (10). The difference in sensitivity, measured as D_0, between the most sensitive and most resistant phases is generally a factor of two to three. Nondividing cells—those not in the cell division cycle—are among the most resistant.

MAMMALIAN RADIOBIOLOGY

Biologic effects of radiation in mammals fall into two categories. *Stochastic* effects are those in which the probability of occurrence is a function of dose, the effect being all or nothing. They are the result of subtle alterations in cell chemistry, such as transformation or mutation. *Deterministic* effects are those in which the severity is a function of dose. They are generally the result of cell killing—the more cells killed, the more severe the effect.

Stochastic Effects

Available data are consistent with the widely held hypothesis of the absence of a threshold dose for these effects, the major examples of which are cancer and genetic effects. As the dose approaches zero, the probability of occurrence approaches zero—but is not zero for the smallest doses for which conclusive data are available, about 50 to 100 mSv. Thus, if a threshold dose exists, it is quite small.

The problem with extending the database to smaller doses is that radiation mimics nature. Radiation-induced cancer or mutation cannot be distinguished by any known method from spontaneous cancer or mutation. The only observable event in an irradiated population is increased incidence of the stochastic effect. A tiny increment on a substantial spontaneous incidence is undetectable unless the study population is quite large. For example, Land (16) estimated that a prospective study to examine the risk of screening mammography in asymptomatic women would require enrolling 60 million subjects at age 35, half of whom get screening mammography, with all followed for life. Even this large study population would yield a statistical power of only 0.5.

Data from studies of stochastic effects in a number of exposed populations have been extensively reviewed by the Committee on the Biological Effects of Ionizing Radiation (BEIR) of the U.S. National Research Council (17) and the United Nations Scientific Committee on the Effects of Atomic Radiation (UN-SCEAR) (18). Two alternative models are used to estimate risk. The additive model results in absolute risk, for example cancer deaths per million person years per sievert. The multiplicative model produces relative risk, essentially the incidence of the effect in the exposed population divided by incidence in controls. It is sometimes expressed as excess relative risk, or relative risk minus one. That is, a relative risk of 1.5 and excess relative risk of 0.5 both project a 50% increase in the event in the exposed population. The multiplicative model is generally more conservative and fits most data better; it is, therefore, used for risk estimation in this chapter.

Cancer

Radiation-induced cancer was observed as early as 1904 (19). However, despite the accumulation of anecdotal evidence, can-

cer was not widely recognized as a risk of low-dose radiation until excess leukemia appeared in the Japanese atomic bomb survivors (Fig. 11.3) beginning shortly after World War II (20).

Japanese Atomic Bomb Survivors

The Hiroshima and Nagasaki populations of more than 75,000 survivors have been intensively studied. Although deaths from solid tumors greatly outnumber those from leukemia, the relative risk of leukemia has been greater than that of solid tumors. Relative risk is normalized to spontaneous incidence, which for leukemia is quite low in the Japanese population. The temporal increase in deaths from solid tumors (Fig. 11.3**A**) reflects both the increase in spontaneous cancer in the aging population and the long latent period for radiation-induced solid tumors, now thought to be the remainder of the lifespan of exposed subjects. However, it appears that virtually all excess leukemia deaths occurred within 25 years of exposure (Fig. 11.3**B**). Although

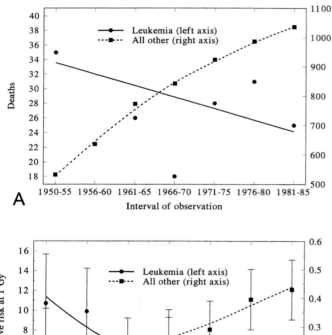

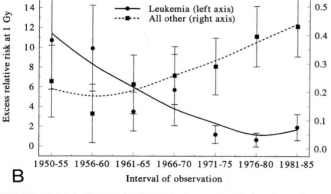

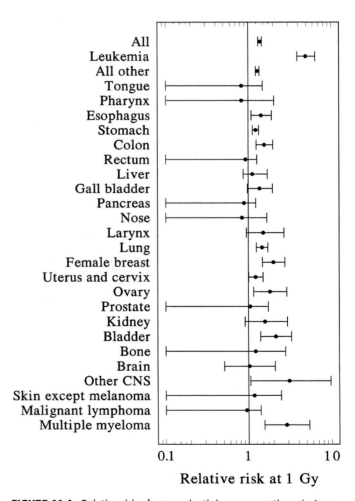

FIGURE 11.3. **A:** Cancer deaths in Japanese atomic bomb survivors, 1950–1985. Deaths from leukemia generally decreased from a maximum in the early years, whereas deaths from all other cancers increased as the population aged. **B:** Excess relative risk per gray for leukemia also peaked in early years and has declined, whereas risk of other tumors has increased. Error bars represent standard errors. (From Shimizu Y, Kato H, Schull WJ. Life span study report 11. Part 2. Cancer mortality in the years 1950–85 based on the recently revised doses (DS86). Hiroshima, Japan: Radiation Effects Research Foundation, 1988, technical report RERF TR 5-88, with permission.)

FIGURE 11.4. Relative risk of cancer death by organ or tissue in Japanese atomic bomb survivors. Excess (relative risk > 1) has been found in nearly all organs, but in many cases is not statistically significant because of the small numbers involved. Error bars represent 90% confidence limits. (From Shimizu Y, Kato H, Schull WJ. Life span study report 11. Part 2. Cancer mortality in the years 1950–85 based on the recently revised doses DS86. Hiroshima, Japan: Radiation Effects Research Foundation, 1988, technical report RERF TR 5-88, with permission.)

there has been an increase in cancer death rate in most organs and tissues in the Japanese atomic bomb survivors, only leukemia; cancers of the esophagus, stomach, colon, lung, female breast, ovary, and bladder; and multiple myeloma are clearly statistically significant (Fig. 11.4). Lack of significance for many organs relates to small numbers of cases (e.g., 52 deaths in the study population from prostate cancer).

Most earlier studies of cancer risk in the Japanese survivors have used death as the end point. Death is sharply defined, and cause of death can be determined retrospectively from death certificates. However, recent studies have used cancer incidence as the end point, so nonfatal cancer can be included in the calculation of detriment (21–23). As shown in Table 11.2, risk of cancer incidence is generally greater than that for cancer death, reflecting either curative treatment or intercurrent death from other causes.

The dose response (Fig. 11.5) for radiation-induced cancer in carefully controlled animal experiments can be fit by a curve from the theory of dual radiation action.

$$I = (\alpha D + (\beta D^2)e^{-(\alpha D + (\beta D2)}$$

where I is incidence and D is dose. The initial $\alpha D + \beta D^2$ expression defines the carcinogenic process, with the βD^2 term accounting for the upward concavity. The exponential term includes cell killing at higher doses. However, for solid tumors in the Japanese atomic bomb survivors, there are no significant

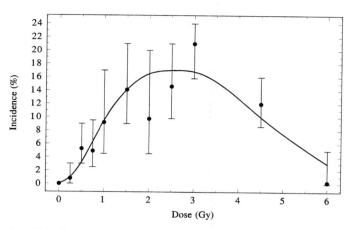

FIGURE 11.5. Dose response curve for radiation-induced myeloid leukemia in mice. In carefully controlled animal experiments, the curve typically extrapolates to spontaneous incidence at zero dose, is initially concave upward, reaches a maximum, and then declines at high doses. Transformed cells are killed by large doses, accounting for the reduced effectiveness. (From Mole RH, Papworth DG, Corp MJ. The dose response for x-ray induction of myeloid leukemia in male CBA.H mice. *Br J Cancer* 1983;47:285–291, with permission.)

Table 11.2. *Cancer in Japanese Atomic Bomb Survivors*

Organ or Tissue	Incidence 1958–87[a]			Mortality 1950–85[b]		
	ERR[c] at 1 Sv	EAR[d] per 10^4 PY Sv	AR[e] %	ERR[c] at 1 Sv	EAR[d] per 10^4 PY Sv	AR[e] %
Digestive system	0.38	10.4	7.8	0.24	3.39	6.6
Esophagus	0.28	0.30	6.5	0.43	0.34	12.7
Stomach	0.32	4.8	6.5	0.23	2.07	6.3
Colon	0.72	1.8	14.2	0.56	0.56	15.1
Liver	0.49	1.6	10.9	0.12	0.05	3.9
Gallbladder	0.12	0.18	2.2	0.37	0.22	8.2
Respiratory system	0.80	4.4	16.3	0.40	1.29	10.1
Lung	0.95	4.4	18.9	0.46	1.25	11.4
Female breast	1.6	6.7	31.9	1.00	1.02	22.1
Uterus	−0.15	−1.1	−3.3	0.22	0.60	5.3
Ovary	0.99	1.1	17.7	0.81	0.45	18.7
Prostate	0.29	0.61	7.0	0.05	0.03	1.9
Urinary tract	1.2	2.1	22.3	1.02	0.55	22.7
Thyroid	1.2	1.6	25.9			
Total solid tumors	0.63	29.7	11.6	0.29	7.41	7.9
Lymphoma	0.62	0.56	14	−0.05	−0.02	−1.8
Multiple myeloma	0.25	0.08		1.86	0.21	32.5
Leukemia	3.9	2.7	50	3.92	2.29	55.4
ALL	9.1	0.62	70			
AML	3.3	1.1	46			
CML	6.2	0.9	62			
Other	3.6	0.21	51			

Note: ALL, Acute lymphocytic leukemia; AML, acute myelogenous leukemia; CML, chronic myelogenous leukemia.
[a]Except lymphoma, myeloma, and leukemia. 1950–1987. Data from 21, 22.
[b]Data from 20.
[c]Excess relative risk.
[d]Excess absolute risk.
[e]Attributable risk.

deviations from linearity at doses below 2 Sv. Exclusion of cases with doses greater than 2 Sv eliminates only 55 cases from a total of 8,613 cases in a study population of 79,972 (21). For leukemia in this population, the data were consistent with linear nonthreshold models except for acute myelogenous leukemia, which showed statistically significant upward concavity (22). Radiation can interact with other factors in the carcinogenic process. Risk of cancer in the Japanese survivors depended not only on dose, but also on age at exposure, interval since exposure, and sex.

Other Irradiated Populations

Studies of the Japanese atomic bomb survivors have provided the most extensive, quantitative data dealing with radiation carcinogenesis. However, excess cancer has been identified in a large number of other populations. Most have followed exposure from medical sources; a few instances of nonmedical exposure are important.

Excess leukemia was identified in several studies, including patients receiving therapeutic radiation for ankylosing spondylitis (25) and for carcinoma of the uterine cervix (26,27). Statistically significant association between diagnostic x-ray exposure and adult-onset leukemia was detected in some (28,29), but not all (30), case-control studies.

Excess breast cancer was first seen in women who had undergone repeated fluoroscopy to the chest (31). Numerous other populations with excess breast cancer were subsequently identified, including, in Canada (32) and Massachusetts (33), women who had been treated for tuberculosis by repeated pneumothorax under fluoroscopic control and women who had been treated with small therapeutic doses of radiation for acute postpartum mastitis (34). The BEIR V committee concluded from these and other data that breast cancer risk was greater in women irradiated before age 20 than in those irradiated later in life, that breast cancer risk is influenced by hormonal status, and that there was little effect of dose protraction (17).

Lung cancer was extensively studied in uranium miners (Fig. 11.6) who worked in an atmosphere contaminated with radon and its radioactive progeny (35). The interaction of radiation with smoking appears to be multiplicative rather than additive. Excess lung cancer has also been detected in the ankylosing spondylitis patients (26).

Elevated stomach cancer was detected in patients treated with therapeutic irradiation for peptic ulcer between 1937 and 1955, with a relative risk of 3.7 from the fractionated dose of 16 to 17 Gy (36).

Radiogenic thyroid cancer was studied in a number of populations, of which the most extensive were young people who were epilated for tinea capitis on arrival in the new state of Israel (37) and infants who were irradiated for thymic enlargement (38). Effects of internally deposited ^{131}I are difficult to interpret because of problems of dosimetry. Older studies suggested that the relative effectiveness per unit dose of internal emitters was less than one-half that of external radiation (39). Patients treated with ^{131}I for thyrotoxicosis were studied. Doses were generally very large (50 to 100 Gy), resulting in extensive death of cells that might have been transformed. Further, the incidence of thyroid cancer among thyrotoxicosis patients is quite high, mak-

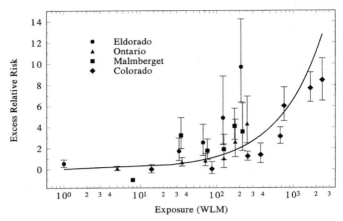

FIGURE 11.6. Lung cancer in four cohorts of uranium miners as a function of occupational exposure in working level months (WLM). The four groups were miners at Eldorado and Ontario in Canada, Malmberget in Sweden, and the Colorado Plateau in the United States. One WLM represents 1 typical month (22 working days) in an atmosphere containing radioactive particulates (radon and its progeny) in a concentration equivalent to a "working level," which has a complicated definition depending on ventilation and so forth. Curve represents fitted power function. Risk, expressed as excess relative risk, is increased at higher exposures. There is considerable discordance in the data amongst the four cohorts, probably the result of cofactors such as smoking. Conversion of exposure in WLM to dose equivalent to bronchial epithelium requires a number of assumptions, leading to considerable uncertainty in the results. Current data suggest a range of 60 to 200 mSv/WLM. (From Committee on the Biological Effects of Ionizing Radiation. *Health risks of radon and other internally deposited alpha-emitters (BEIR IV).* Washington, DC: National Academy Press, 1988, with permission.)

ing control groups difficult to identify (40). Relative risks varied from 1.01 to 9.1, depending on control group selected (17). Follow-up of more than 10,000 subjects who had undergone diagnostic procedures using ^{131}I in Sweden (average thyroid dose 0.5 Gy) yielded a relative risk of thyroid cancer of 1.27 (95% confidence interval 0.94 to 1.67). However, many of these studies were ordered because of suspected thyroid tumors and many subsequent tumors were either medullary or poorly differentiated, and one was a sarcoma—none of which have been seen in excess numbers in other irradiated populations (41). Thyroid cancer was extensively investigated in Marshall Islanders exposed from nuclear weapons testing in 1954 to external γ radiation from fallout and to ingested radioiodides (Table 11.3) (42).

Tab e 11.3. *Thyroid Tumors in Marshall Islanders Exposed to Radioactive Fallout*

Atoll	Age at Exposure (v)	Dose (Gy)	Nodules (%)	Cancer (%)
Rongelap	1	≥15	66.7	0
	2–9	8–15	81.2	6.2
	≤10	3.4–8	13.3	6.7
Alingnae	<10	2.8–4.5	28.6	0
	≤10	1.4–1.9	33.3	0
Utirik	<10	0.6–1.0	7.8	1.6
	≤10	0.3–0.6	12.0	2.0
Controls	<10		2.6	0.9
	≤10		7.8	0.8

Source: 42.

Children living in portions of Nevada and Utah were exposed to radioactive fallout from weapons testing in 1952 to 1955, resulting in thyroid doses up to 1 Gy. The relative risk of thyroid cancer was found to be 1.9, which was not statistically significant (43). Finally, a large and detailed animal study found essentially no difference in the effectiveness per unit dose of external versus internal radiation in thyroid carcinogenesis (44). The BEIR V committee estimated the effectiveness ratio for ^{131}I compared with x-rays as 0.66, but with a 95% confidence interval of 0.14 to 3.15. It now seems clear that the juvenile thyroid is more sensitive than the adult, females are more sensitive than males to both spontaneous and radiogenic thyroid cancer by a factor of about three, and radiogenic thyroid cancer is commonly accompanied or preceded by benign nodules and its histology is usually low-grade papillary. Tumor growth is promoted by hormonal stimulation (17).

Excess cancer of the esophagus has been observed in the ankylosing spondylitics. In fact, esophageal cancer is the major tumor seen to continue in excess more than 25-years postexposure (25).

Colon cancer in excess incidence has been unequivocally identified in the Japanese atomic bomb survivors. Other studies, however, are not so convincing. Statistically significant associations between colon cancer and therapeutic radiation for benign gynecologic conditions were established in some (45,46), but not all (47,48), studies. No excess colon cancer deaths were seen in a 30-year follow-up of a large series of patients irradiated for carcinoma of the uterine cervix (27). Excess colon cancer was detected in the ankylosing spondylitics (25). However, these results have been excluded from risk estimations because of the well-known associations between ankylosing spondylitis and ulcerative colitis and between ulcerative colitis and colon cancer (17). Radiogenic cancer of the small intestine has been detected in experimental animals but not in humans.

In the liver, excess cancer has been seen mainly in human and animal populations with intrahepatic concentrations of radionuclides. Thorotrast, containing 25% colloidal ^{232}ThO$_2$, was used extensively as a radiologic contrast agent until about 1955. Three major epidemiologic studies of its association with liver cancer were summarized by the BEIR IV committee, showing, for example, 413 excess liver cancers in a population of 2,334 in the largest study (34). No excess liver cancers were detected in the ankylosing spondylitics (25) or in patients irradiated for carcinoma of the uterine cervix (27).

The recognition in the mid-1920s of "radium jaw" in watch-dial painters (49), the result of ingestion of minute quantities of ^{226}Ra, and sometimes ^{228}Ra, from "tipping" their artists' brushes on their tongues, led to abandonment of the technique and to the first standards for occupational radiation protection (50). Osteogenic sarcoma is the common result of the high-LET radiation of radium (35). In addition, low-LET radiation is associated with bone cancer in the ankylosing spondylitis patients (25) and in the long-term follow-up for occurrence of second cancers following radiotherapy (27), but low-LET occupational exposure in British radiologists (51) was not associated with bone cancer.

Radiation was noted to increase the incidence of tumors of the nervous system in several populations, including the previously mentioned Israeli tinea capitis subjects (52) and the anky-

losing spondylitics (25). Mortality from brain cancer was about three times greater in early American radiologists than in other medical specialists (53), suggesting an effect of occupational exposure. Associations between intracranial meningiomas and diagnostic exposure were reported (54–56). Although the dose-response curve remains unknown, available data clearly indicate that the brain is relatively sensitive to radiation carcinogenesis.

Organs of the genital system, except the ovary, appear relatively insensitive to radiogenic cancer (17). The urinary tract, especially the bladder, is somewhat sensitive, as seen in the ankylosing spondylitics (25) and in women therapeutically irradiated for benign uterine bleeding (46).

Both animal and human studies have detected excess parathyroid disease, including hyperparathyroidism, hyperplasia, adenomas, and, occasionally, cancer (17). The paranasal sinuses were found sensitive to the carcinogenic influence of high-LET radiation in the radium-dial painters and Thorotrast subjects (35). No associations with low-LET exposure were identified (17).

Death from radiogenic skin cancer, occurring in an area of radiodermatitis, was observed as early as 1904 (19). In the Israeli tinea capitis studies, excess basal cell carcinoma was noticed on the skin of the head, face, and neck in white, but not nonwhite, subjects (57), suggesting an interaction of ionizing radiation with ultraviolet exposure.

Excess multiple myeloma was seen in 12 of 17 irradiated populations, with the greatest risk occurring in those exposed to internal emitters (58). No excess Hodgkin's disease was identified in irradiated populations; non-Hodgkin's lymphomas were shown to be elevated in some populations, but not in others (17).

Radiogenic cancers of the pharynx and larynx were observed as a late complication of high-dose therapeutic radiation (17). Salivary gland tumors were noted in excess incidence in patients treated with external radiation (52) and ^{131}I (59) and associated with diagnostic exposure (60). Data on pancreatic cancer following radiation exposure are sparse and inconsistent, perhaps related to the well-known difficulty of detection of the disease (17).

Prenatal Exposure

A great deal of attention has been devoted to study of the relationship of prenatal diagnostic radiation exposure to childhood cancer since the first report by Stewart and associates (61) in 1956. Numerous studies soon followed, with conflicting results. A prospective study, which is less sensitive but more specific than retrospective case-control studies, found a significant association between prenatal exposure and childhood leukemia, but not other cancers, in white children—but no such association in blacks. Furthermore, there was a similar level of association with childhood accidental death (62). If one accepts the results of this study as showing that prenatal radiation is carcinogenic, then one must also accept its role in the etiology of accident proneness. In all of these studies, it is presumed that the prenatal diagnostic exposure was rational—that is, the attending physician had a valid reason for prescribing the exposure. One large scale study investigated the effects of routine pelvimetry at term, finding no significant association with childhood cancer (63). Early reports in the Japanese survivors exposed *in utero* showed no increase in childhood cancer; however, as this population has reached middle age, excess cancer has been detected (64).

Risk of Radiation-Induced Cancer

The BEIR V committee estimated that the risk of radiogenic cancer, averaged over both sexes and all ages, following acute whole-body exposure to low-LET radiation at high dose rate, is 8% per sievert (17). They further estimated that this risk estimate should be reduced by a factor of two or more for small doses or low dose rate. The UNSCEAR committee concluded that this dose and dose-rate effectiveness factor (DDREF) is close to 1 for solid tumors and 2 for leukemia, or about 1.7 overall, with a 90% confidence interval of 1.1 to 3.1 (18).

Genetic Effects

There are obvious uncertainties in estimation of risk of radiogenic cancer because of inconsistencies in the human data. However, there are no directly confirmed data dealing with human genetic effects of radiation. Thus, genetic risk estimation depends on a general knowledge of human genetics and extrapolation from animal studies.

In 1955, Macht and Lawrence (65) reported increased likelihood of congenital anomalies in offspring of radiologists as compared with children of other physicians. In 1990, Gardner et al., (66) reported the increased incidence of leukemia and lymphoma among children in and around the Sellafield nuclear plant in the United Kingdom, associated with occupational exposure of the fathers. However, extensive analysis of eight indicators of genetic effect in offspring of the Japanese atomic bomb survivors (stillbirths, congenital anomalies, childhood death, childhood cancer, chromosomal rearrangements, protein electrophoretic behavior and enzyme activity, sex ratio, and childhood physical development) failed to demonstrate any statistically significant genetic effect (67). The average dose to the parents was 0.4 Sv, in the range of the doubling dose estimated from early animal experiments.

Animal data, on the other hand, have been so convincing as to make certain the existence of a genetic effect of radiation. Data from Muller's (68) studies in the 1920s using the geneticist's favorite organism, *Drosophila*, were used for decades for the estimation of genetic risk. The "megamouse studies" at Oak Ridge National Laboratory in the 1950s and early 1960s (Fig. 11.7), named for the size of the study population, examined specific-locus recessive mutations in mice (69). They were major contributors to early BEIR and UNSCEAR estimates of the doubling dose, in the range of 0.5 to 2.5 Sv. The doubling dose is the dose required to double the spontaneous mutation rate. Usual early calculations used the human spontaneous mutation rate and the radiation response of mice, generally half the radiation response of the male mouse at low dose rates, because the female was much less sensitive. Thus, the doubling dose was for a mythical creature with the spontaneous mutation rate of humans and half the radiation response of a male mouse. The direct method of risk estimation avoided these complications by examining the frequency of dominant mutants in first generation offspring. For example, if the frequency of skeletal defects in mice was 4×10^{-4} per Gy per gamete and in humans about

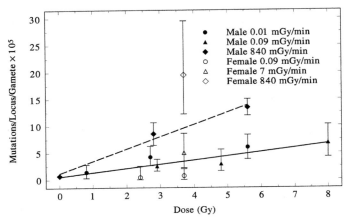

FIGURE 11.7. The "megamouse studies": specific locus mutations in mice exposed to x-rays, showing effects of sex and dose rate. Error bars represent 90% confidence intervals. *Solid line* is linear regression of low dose rate data for males (0.01 and 0.09 mGy/min combined) and *dashed line* is linear regression for high dose rate (840 mGy/minute) data for males. No regression is possible for females because the spontaneous mutation rate was so low as to be statistically unacceptable, even in a population of hundreds of thousands. The dose rate effect is as expected in both sexes; damage is proportional to dose and dose rate. At low dose rates, the mutation rate in females given up to 4 Gy was no greater than the spontaneous rate in males, but at high dose rates females were more sensitive than males. (From Russell WL. The nature of the dose-rate effect of radiation on mutation in mice. *Jpn J Genet* 1964;40(Suppl):128–140, with permission.)

20% of serious dominant disorders involve the skeleton, then the frequency of serious first-generation dominant disorders in humans should be about 2,000 per million live births per sievert (70).

Genetic Risk

The BEIR V Committee concluded that the human doubling dose is not likely to be less than the value of approximately 1 Sv from animal studies (17). Indeed, reappraisal of data from the first-generation offspring of Japanese atomic bomb survivors indicated that this value probably overestimated the risk (71). The UNSCEAR 1993 report concluded that the doubling dose is not likely to be less than 2 Sv. Their best estimate of the doubling dose for low dose rate exposure was 4 Sv (18).

The National Council on Radiation Protection and Measurements has estimated that the genetically significant dose to the average U.S. citizen is approximately 1.3 mSv per year. About 1 mSv comes from natural sources in the environment, and about 0.3 mSv is from manmade radiation, including medical, consumer products (tobacco, luminous watch dials, smoke detectors, etc.), occupational, and miscellaneous sources (72). Thus, the total genetic radiation burden of the population is approximately 40 mSv per generation. The estimated increased incidence of genetic disease is so small as to be nearly impossible to detect in a study population of finite size, as shown in Table 11.4, especially because about 75% is from unavoidable natural sources that have been with humans since the beginning of time.

Deterministic Effects

Deterministic effects occur in all exposed individuals, provided doses exceed thresholds. Thus, the statistical problems obvious

Table 11.4. *Estimated Incidence of Genetic Disease from Environmental Exposure (40 mSv per Generation)*

	Incidence (per Million Live Births)		Effects of 40 mSv per Generation (per Million Live Births)			
			UNSCEAR[a]		BEIR[b]	
Genetic Disease	UNSCEAR[a]	BEIR[b]	First Generation	Equilibrium	First Generation	Equilibrium
Autosomal dominant	10,000		60	400		
Clinically severe		2500				
Clinically mild		7500			20–80	100
X-linked		400			4–60	300
Autosomal recessive	2500	2500	0.2	60	<4	<20
Chromosomal anomalies						Very slow ↑
Structural	400	600	10	16	<20	Very little ↑
Numeric	3400	3800	Very small	Very small	<4	<4
Congenital anomalies	60,000	20,000–30,000	Not estimated		40	40–400
Multifactorial diseases	600,000		Not estimated			
Heart disease		600,000			Not estimated	
Cancer		300,000			Not estimated	
Other		300,000			Not estimated	
Total			70	480		

[a]Data from 18.
[b]Data from 17.

in estimation of risk of stochastic effect do not exist for deterministic effects. These effects are a concern in radiation oncology and some interventional radiologic procedures, but are never encountered in patients from the doses employed in diagnostic medicine.

Acute Radiation Syndromes

The best known deterministic effects are the acute radiation syndromes. They are a serious concern in the event of radiation accidents or nuclear war but are not a consideration in the analysis of risks of diagnostic or occupational exposure. The dose levels given in relation to these effects are for acute whole-body exposures. The acute radiation syndromes were recently reviewed by Hall (73).

The *hematopoietic* or *bone marrow syndrome* is the result of killing of proliferating cells of the hematopoietic series in the bone marrow, resulting in depression of circulating leukocytes and platelets and the possibility of death within 60 days. The threshold dose is about 250 mSv for detectable suppression of white count, 1 Sv for symptoms, and 3 Sv for death within 60 days. Individuals receiving doses in this range go first into prodromal phase, characterized by nausea and vomiting within hours of exposure. Recovery usually follows within about 24 hours, and there may be several symptom-free days. White cells in circulation at the time of exposure are relatively unaffected and continue to function through their normal lifespan. However, they are not replaced by the failing bone marrow. Symptoms of the hematopoietic syndrome begin as white and platelet counts fall and consist of chills, fever, fatigue, petechial hemorrhages in the skin, ulceration of the oral mucosa, and epilation. The LD$_{50/60}$ (the dose that kills half the population within 60 days) has been estimated as about 3 to 4 Sv. However, several Chernobyl workers survived doses up to about 8 Sv with only supportive care. The LD$_{50/60}$ with treatment may be as great as 7 Sv. Bone marrow transplantation was used for 13 Chernobyl victims; only two survived, one of whom showed signs of autologous marrow repopulation. Apparently only one transplant was successful. The dose window for effective marrow transplantation is quite narrow. Below 8 Sv it should be unnecessary and above 10 Sv it is ineffective because of the results of the gastrointestinal syndrome.

At doses above 10 Sv, the *gastrointestinal syndrome* results in death within about 10 days from denudation of the epithelial lining of the small intestine, the result of killing of proliferating cells in the crypts of Lieberkuhn. Characteristic symptoms are nausea, vomiting, and extended diarrhea. Several Chernobyl victims, in whom bone marrow transplants failed, died of this syndrome 7 to 10 days postexposure.

The *cerebrovascular* or *central nervous system (CNS) syndrome* occurs following doses above about 100 Gy. All systems are severely damaged at this dose. However, the CNS syndrome evolves so rapidly that death occurs within 48 hours, before the other syndromes have a chance to develop. Symptoms usually begin in minutes and consist of severe nausea and vomiting followed by disorientation, loss of muscular coordination, respiratory distress, seizures, coma, and death. The precise cause of death is not fully known. The most widely held view is a direct effect on the microvasculature, resulting in massive intracranial edema. However, animal studies showed that the dose required to produce this syndrome is greater if the head alone is irradiated, rather than the whole body.

Cataract

A great deal of attention in the medical literature has been devoted to risk of radiogenic cataract from small radiation doses, such as diagnostic or occupational exposure. Most early studies of patient dosimetry from diagnostic procedures included determination of dose to the optic lens. However, human data from a number of exposed populations indicate a clear threshold (Fig.

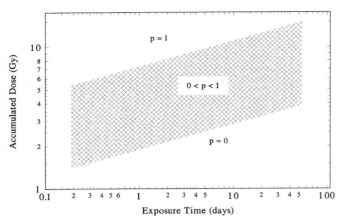

FIGURE 11.8. Time-dose isoeffect plot for radiogenic cataract. Any point (combination of time over which radiation is administered and total accumulated dose) falling below the shaded area is virtually certain to be below the threshold for clinically significant cataract. Any point above the shaded area is virtually certain to produce such a cataract. Any point within the shaded area falls in the range of biologic variation, and may or may not produce a progressive cataract in a given individual. (From Merriam GR, Szechter A, Focht EF. The effects of ionizing radiation on the eye. *Front Radiat Ther Oncol* 1972;6:346–385, with permission.)

11.8)—0.6 to 1.5 Gy in Japanese atomic bomb survivors and about 2 Gy in patients receiving fractionated radiotherapy (74, 75). The International Commission on Radiological Protection has concluded that the threshold for progressive, vision-impairing cataract in the general population from highly protracted exposure is not likely to be less than 8 Sv. This is well beyond the levels encountered by virtually all individuals from environmental, occupational, or medical diagnostic sources.

Sterility

The germinal cells of testes and ovaries, especially at certain stages of their production and maturation, are highly radiosensitive. Threshold doses for temporary sterility are rather small (Table 11.5). Permanent sterilization, however, requires large doses or protracted doses delivered at rather high dose rates (74).

Other Organs and Tissues

Threshold doses for production of deterministic effects in adults are much greater than those employed in diagnostic medicine.

Table 11.5. *Threshold Doses for Sterility*

Tissue/Effect	Acute Dose (Sv)	Protracted Dose (Sv)	Protracted Dose Rate (Sv/y)
Testes			
Temporary sterility	0.15	Not applicable[a]	0.4
Permanent sterility	3.5	Not applicable	2
Ovaries			
Sterility	2.5–6	6	>0.2

[a]Threshold depends on dose rate rather than total dose.
Source: 74.

Table 11.6 lists the doses required to produce such effects in 5% (ED$_5$, an effective threshold) and 50% (ED$_{50}$, the median effective dose) of exposed subjects in 5 years. In growing children, the required doses are much smaller, but still beyond diagnostic levels (Table 11.7). The data in Tables 11.6 and 11.7 are for conventionally fractionated therapeutic doses. For smaller fields, the required doses are somewhat greater; conversely, for larger fields, they are smaller. Acute doses to produce the effect will be smaller. Growth retardation, measured as decreased adult height, was seen in Japanese atomic bomb survivors who were younger than 5 years old at exposure and whose dose equivalent was greater than 1 Sv (18).

Effects on Embryo and Fetus

Just as the growing child is more sensitive than the adult, the embryo is even more sensitive to deterministic effects. Gestational age at exposure determines the nature of the effect, as shown in Fig. 11.9 (77,78). The only effect observed from preimplantation exposure in mice is early prenatal death. A large portion of medical exposure of the unrecognized pregnancy occurs during this period. If the mouse data could be extrapolated directly to humans, then the continuing pregnancy could be taken as evidence that there was no effect from that exposure. There were no survivors in the Hiroshima and Nagasaki populations who were exposed during the first 2 weeks of gestation. Thus, human and animal data are consistent but do not provide

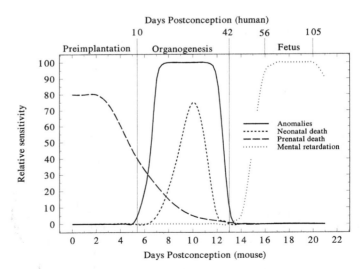

FIGURE 11.9. Influence of gestational age on deterministic effects in mice and mental retardation in humans. Prenatal death is the overwhelming probability from preimplantation exposure, whereas congenital anomalies and neonatal death are most likely from exposure during major organogenesis in mice. In the Japanese atomic bomb survivors, maximum sensitivity to mental retardation occurred from exposure between eighth and fifteenth weeks of gestation. Note that human development does not map linearly to mouse development. In humans, the fetal period occupies most of pregnancy; in mice it is a minor component. (From Russell LB, Russell WL. An analysis of the changing radiation response of the developing mouse embryo. *J Cell Physiol* 1954;43(Suppl 1):103–149; Otake M, Schull WJ. In utero exposure to A-bomb radiation and mental retardation: a reassessment. *Br J Radiol* 1984;57:409–414, with permission.)

Table 11.6. *Estimated Total Accumulated Dose for Deterministic Effects in Adults 5 Years After Fractionated Radiotherapy*

Organ	Treated Field	Injury	ED$_5$ (Gy)	ED$_{50}$ (Gy)
Bone marrow	Whole	Hypoplasia	2	5
Ovary	Whole	Permanent sterility	2–3	6–12
Testis	Whole	Permanent sterility	5–15	20
Lens	Whole	Cataract	5	12
Kidney	Whole	Nephrosclerosis	23	28
Liver	Whole	Liver failure	35	45
Lung	Lobe	Fibrosis	40	60
Heart	Whole	Pericarditis	40	>100
Thyroid	Whole	Hypothyroidism	45	150
Pituitary	Whole	Hypopituitarism	45	200–300
Brain	Whole	Necrosis	50	>60
Spinal cord	5 cm²	Necrosis	50	>60
Breast	Whole	Atrophy, necrosis	>50	>100
Skin	100 cm²	Ulcer, fibrosis	55	70
Eye	Whole	Panophthalmitis	55	100
Esophagus	75 cm²	Ulcer, stricture	60	75
Bladder	Whole	Ulcer, contracture	60	80
Bone	10 cm²	Necrosis, fracture	60	150
Ureter	5–10 cm	Stricture	75	100
Muscle	Whole	Atrophy	>100	

Source: 74, 76.

conclusive proof that conclusions drawn from the mouse studies may be applied directly to humans.

Exposure of the pregnant mouse during the period of major organogenesis leads to congenital anomalies and neonatal death. The sensitive period for induction of a specific anomaly is brief; exposure must occur at a critical stage of development or differentiation of the involved tissues. An exception is the CNS, which is rapidly developing throughout organogenesis. Thus, the spectrum of anomalies in irradiated populations is weighted toward CNS anomalies, which was also seen in pregnant patients treated in the early days of radiotherapy (79).

The major effects seen in Japanese survivors irradiated *in utero* were growth retardation, especially microcephaly (80) and mental retardation (78). Survivors exposed within 3,000 m of the hypocenter were shorter, lighter in weight, and smaller in head circumference than those exposed at distances greater than 3,000 m (81). Microcephaly (head smaller than two standard deviations below the mean for age) was seen after exposures in the first 25 weeks of pregnancy, with maximum sensitivity in the first 16 weeks (Fig. 11.10). Mental retardation was not seen from exposure before 8 weeks or after 25 weeks. Maximum sensitivity occurred at 8 to 15 weeks; at 16 to 25 weeks, sensitiv-

ity was about half of the maximum (Fig. 11.11). These effects were reflected in IQ scores and school performance.

Most data, both from human studies and animal experiments, are consistent with a threshold of approximately 100 mSv for early prenatal death and for teratogenic effects (82). The National Council on Radiation Protection and Measurements (NCRP) has concluded that statistically significant increase in these effects is not likely below about 150 mSv (83). However, a few studies have shown effects, including human microcephaly down to about 50 mSv (81). Although there is agreement that these effects are deterministic, the magnitude of the threshold dose remains uncertain. The International Committee on Radio-

Table 11.7. *Estimated Total Accumulated Dose for Deterministic Effects in Growing Children 5 Years After Fractionated Radiotherapy*

Organ	Field	Injury	ED$_5$ (Gy)	ED$_{50}$ (Gy)
Breast	5 cm²	No development	10	15
Cartilage	5 cm²	Arrested growth	10	30
Bone	10 cm²	Arrested growth	20	30
Muscle	10 cm²	Hypoplasia	20–30	40–50

Source: 18, 74, and 76.

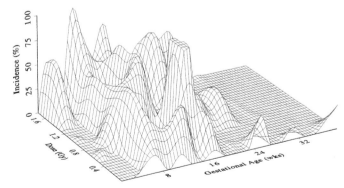

FIGURE 11.10. Influence of gestational age and dose on incidence of microcephaly in Hiroshima atomic bomb survivors irradiated *in utero*. There was a general dependence on dose. There were a total of 8 cases in the 115 individuals exposed to doses less than 100 mGy. These followed exposure at all gestational ages. Virtually all cases that were exposed to more than 100 mGy followed exposure in the first 25 weeks of pregnancy. (From Miller RW, Mulvihill JJ. Small head size after atomic irradiation. In: Sever JL, Brent RL, eds. *Teratogen update: environmentally induced birth defect risks.* New York: Alan R. Liss, 1986:141–143, with permission.)

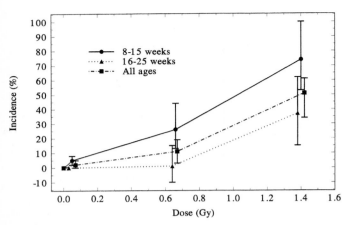

FIGURE 11.11. Dose response for mental retardation in Japanese atomic bomb survivors exposed *in utero*. No cases were seen from exposure before 8 weeks gestational age. Maximum sensitivity occurred from exposure 8 to 15 weeks gestational age. Sensitivity at 16 to 25 weeks was about half that at 8 to 15 weeks. (From Otake M, Schull WJ. In utero exposure to A-bomb radiation and mental retardation: a reassessment. *Br J Radiol* 1984;57:409–414, with permission.)

logical Protection (ICRP) has concluded that the threshold for radiation protection purposes should be taken as 100 mSv (84). Early mouse studies indicated that the incidence of prenatal death was well above 50% and that incidence of congenital anomalies approached 100% at 2 Sv delivered at the times of peak sensitivities (77). The shape of the dose response curve between 0.1 and 2 Sv remains unclear.

Assessment of risk of human mental retardation from exposure *in utero* is a bit clearer. Maximum likelihood analysis of data from the Japanese indicated an incidence of severe retardation of 43% at 1 Sv and a threshold of 200 to 400 mSv, with a lower 95% confidence limit of about 100 mSv, delivered during the period of maximum sensitivity, gestational age 8 to 15 weeks (85). IQ scores declined by about 30 per Sv from exposure during this interval (86). Response was significantly less (about half) at 16 to 25 weeks and near zero at other times.

RISK ASSESSMENT

A number of indicators of risk, e.g., whole-body and critical organ doses, have been used in older publications. More recently, the effective dose has become the standard. The effective dose provides an estimate of the uniform whole-body dose that would carry the same risk of stochastic effect as the dose actually administered nonuniformly over the body, or over only part of the body, as in medical or occupational exposure. The concept was introduced by Jacobi (87) in 1975. He defined detriment, the probability of stochastic effect weighted by severity of that effect

$$G = \sum s_i \, \alpha_i \, d_i.$$

where s is the severity, α the probability of the effect per unit dose, and d is the average dose to the ith organ. If the dose is uniform to the total body (D_{TB}), then

$$G = \sum s_i \, \alpha_i \, D_{TB} = D_{TB} \sum s_i \, \alpha_i$$

The effective dose, for the total body, is then

$$D_E = D_{TB} = \frac{\sum s_i \, \alpha_i \, d_i}{\sum s_i \, \alpha_2}.$$

Defining a weight factor for each organ as the fraction of total body stochastic effect attributable to that organ

$$w_i = \frac{s_i \, \alpha_i}{\sum s_i \, \alpha_i}.$$

then simplifies the effective dose to

$$D_E = \sum w_i \, d_i.$$

The ICRP (88) adopted a simplified version of the Jacobi effective dose, which they called effective dose equivalent in 1977. They eliminated the severity factors and used only lethal cancer or genetic effect expressed in the first two postirradiation generations as end points. Laws and Rosenstein (89) adapted the effective dose to apply to somatic effects only. In 1990, the ICRP (84) returned to the effective dose concept, defining the product $s_i \, \alpha_i$ as detriment. They concluded that detriment, which is a weighted probability of stochastic effect, is 5.6% per Sv for the adult working population and 7.3% per Sv for the entire population (Table 11.8). Risk is greater in the entire population because of inclusion of children, whose radiosensitivity is greater. Inclusion of older retired adults, whose genetic risk is zero and whose cancer risk substantially lower, in the entire population mitigates but does not completely counteract the effect of the children.

The ICRP has provided organ weight factors for calculation of effective dose, shown in Fig. 11.12 (84). The same set of factors is used for either the working or the entire population. Differences are beyond the precision of the method. The effective dose, calculated for a given set of exposure circumstances,

Table 11.8. *Detriment (Percent per Sv)*

Tissue or Organ	Adult Workers	Entire Population
Bladder	0.24	0.29
Bone marrow	0.83	1.04
Bone surface	0.06	0.07
Breast	0.29	0.36
Colon	0.82	1.03
Esophagus	0.19	0.24
Liver	0.13	0.16
Lung	0.64	0.80
Ovary (cancer)	0.12	0.15
Gonads (genetic)	0.80	1.33
Skin	0.03	0.04
Stomach	0.80	1.00
Thyroid	0.12	0.15
Remainder	0.47	0.59
Subtotals (rounded)		
Fatal cancer	4.0	5.0
Nonfatal cancer	0.8	1.0
Severe hereditary effects	0.8	1.3
Total (rounded)	5.6	7.3

Source: 84.

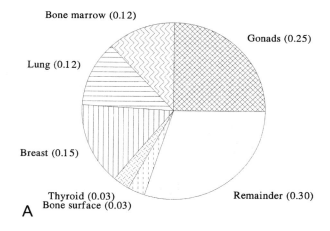

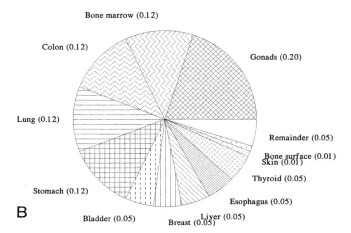

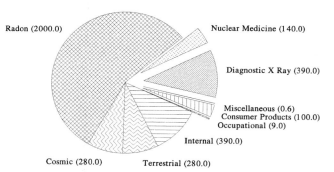

FIGURE 11.13. Annual radiation dose, average, 3,600 μSv/year to U.S. population, from all sources. Natural sources (radon and progeny, cosmic, terrestrial, and internal) account for 3,000 μSv/year, whereas manmade sources (diagnostic x-ray, nuclear medicine, consumer products, occupational, and miscellaneous) contribute only 600 μSv/year. The healing arts account for the majority of manmade radiation exposure. (From National Council on Radiation Protection and Measurements. Ionizing radiation exposure of the population of the United States. Bethesda, MD: National Council on Radiation Protection and Measurements, 1987, NCRP report no 93, with permission.)

FIGURE 11.12. Organ weight factors for calculation of ICRP 1977 effective dose equivalent **(A)** and 1990 effective dose **(B)**. The effective dose equivalent or effective dose is calculated from organ doses. It is an estimate of the uniform whole-body dose carrying the same risk of stochastic effect as the dose administered nonuniformly. In general, the 1990 effective dose is less than the 1977 effective dose equivalent, calculated from the same organ dose data. [From International Commission on Radiological Protection. 1990 Recommendations of the International Commission on Radiological Protection. ICRP publication 60. *Ann ICRP* 1991;21(1-3); International Commission on Radiological Protection. Recommendations of the International Commission on Radiological Protection. ICRP publication 26. *Ann ICRP* 1977; 1 (3), with permission.]

e.g., occupational or a given diagnostic procedure or set of procedures, can then be compared with environmental exposure (Fig. 11.13). The NCRP has calculated this average exposure to the American population, from all sources, as effective dose equivalent (72). That is, they used the 1977 ICRP method (88). In general, 1990 effective doses are less than 1977 effective dose equivalents. The ratio ranges from about 0.6 for ^{99m}Tc gluconate to very nearly 1.0 for ^{99m}Tc-MAA (18). The major factor in this difference was the large weight for remainder in the 1977 method (Fig. 11.12**A**), which was required by the paucity of data on specific organ risks at the time. The commission recommended that the remainder be estimated by the five organs (excluding those with specific weights), each assigned a weight of 0.06, which overestimated the influence of the remainder on

effective dose equivalent in many cases (92). For thyroid studies the effective dose is greater than effective dose equivalent by a factor of up to 1.6 for radioiodide uptake. The weight factor for the thyroid was reduced for the 1990 effective dose, in accord with new data. Thus, the 1990 effective dose and 1977 effective dose equivalent may be used interchangeably only for crude first-order approximations.

Effective dose equivalents in children and adults are presented for most radiopharmaceuticals in Table 11.9. Similar data for exposure *in utero* are presented in Tables 11.10 and 11.11 and for exposure during lactation in Table 11.12. These data have replaced specific organ doses, critical organ doses, and so forth, as indices of patient dose in most recent publications. The data in Tables 11.9 through 11.12 apply to healthy individuals. Isotope distribution may vary with disease states, possibly producing differences in radiation dose distribution and effective dose equivalent or effective dose. ICRP Publication 53 and its supplement (90,91) provide some examples of alteration of effective dose equivalent in certain diseases. They also provide doses to specific organs used in calculation of effective dose equivalent.

The major advantage of effective dose equivalent or effective dose calculated for a diagnostic procedure is that it can be compared with environmental radiation as an estimate of the radiation burden to the patient. For example, the effective dose equivalent of a typical study using 500 mBq (about 15 mCi) of ^{99m}Tc pertechnetate with blocking is about 2.8 mSv (Table 11.9), the equivalent of about 11 months of natural background (Fig. 11.13). It may be tempting to calculate detriment from the patient effective dose equivalent, but this tacitly assumes that the linear nonthreshold model is established fact. Such is definitely not the case. Results of the calculation could be worse than worthless—they could be misleading.

RECOMMENDATIONS

Diagnostic nuclear medicine procedures deliver small radiation doses to the patient. The effective dose equivalent or effective

Table 11.9. *Effective Dose Equivalents from Diagnostic Nuclear Medicine Procedures*

Isotope	Pharmaceutical	Conditions of Administration[a]	Effective Dose Equivalent (mSv/mBq)[b]				
			Adult	Age 15	Age 10	Age 5	Age 1
^{3}H	Water		1.6×10^{-2}	1.6×10^{-2}	1.8×10^{-2}	2.4×10^{-2}	4.5×10^{-2}
	Inulin		1.2×10^{-3}	1.5×10^{-3}	2.4×10^{-3}	3.8×10^{-3}	7.5×10^{-3}
	Neutral fat and free fatty acids		2.2×10^{-1}				
^{11}C	Erythrocytes		6.9×10^{-3}	8.4×10^{-3}	1.4×10^{-2}	2.2×10^{-2}	4.2×10^{-2}
	Spiperone		5.9×10^{-3}	7.8×10^{-3}	1.2×10^{-2}	1.8×10^{-2}	3.4×10^{-2}
^{14}C	CO	20 s inhalation	6.6×10^{-3}	8.0×10^{-3}	1.3×10^{-2}	2.1×10^{-2}	4.0×10^{-2}
		1 h continuous	4.3×10^{-3}	5.3×10^{-3}	5.3×10^{-3}	1.4×10^{-2}	2.6×10^{-2}
	CO_2	20 s inhalation	1.7×10^{-3}	2.0×10^{-3}	3.1×10^{-3}	4.9×10^{-3}	9.4×10^{-3}
		1 h continuous	1.1×10^{-3}	1.3×10^{-3}	2.0×10^{-3}	3.1×10^{-3}	6.0×10^{-3}
	Inulin		1.1×10^{-2}	1.3×10^{-2}	2.1×10^{-2}	3.3×10^{-2}	6.5×10^{-2}
	Neutral fat and free fatty acids		2.1				
^{13}N	N_2 gas	20 s inhalation	3.7×10^{-4}	5.8×10^{-4}	8.4×10^{-4}	1.3×10^{-3}	2.5×10^{-3}
		1 h continuous	4.2×10^{-4}	6.5×10^{-4}	9.4×10^{-4}	1.4×10^{-3}	2.9×10^{-3}
	N_2 solution		4.0×10^{-4}	6.2×10^{-4}	8.9×10^{-4}	1.4×10^{-3}	2.7×10^{-3}
	NH_3		2.7×10^{-3}	3.2×10^{-3}	4.9×10^{-3}	7.7×10^{-3}	1.5×10^{-2}
	L-Glutamate		1.3×10^{-2}	1.7×10^{-2}	2.9×10^{-2}	3.9×10^{-2}	7.7×10^{-2}
^{15}O	CO	20 s inhalation	1.1×10^{-3}	1.5×10^{-3}	2.4×10^{-3}	3.9×10^{-3}	7.6×10^{-3}
		1 h continuous	7.6×10^{-4}	1.0×10^{-3}	1.6×10^{-3}	2.6×10^{-3}	5.1×10^{-3}
	CO_2	20 s inhalation	5.4×10^{-4}	6.8×10^{-4}	1.1×10^{-3}	1.7×10^{-3}	3.3×10^{-3}
		1 h continuous	4.0×10^{-4}	5.0×10^{-4}	7.8×10^{-4}	1.2×10^{-3}	2.4×10^{-3}
	O_2 gas	20 s inhalation	3.9×10^{-4}	5.7×10^{-4}	8.5×10^{-4}	1.3×10^{-3}	2.7×10^{-3}
		1 h continuous	4.3×10^{-4}	6.4×10^{-4}	9.5×10^{-4}	1.5×10^{-3}	3.0×10^{-3}
^{18}F	F^-		2.7×10^{-2}	3.4×10^{-2}	5.2×10^{-2}	8.6×10^{-2}	1.7×10^{-1}
	FDG		2.7×10^{-2}	3.2×10^{-2}	4.7×10^{-2}	7.3×10^{-2}	1.3×10^{-1}
^{22}Na	Na^+		2.8	3.3	4.9	8.0	1.5×10^1
^{24}Na	Na^+		3.4×10^{-1}	3.9×10^{-1}	6.1×10^{-1}	1.0	1.9
^{28}Mg	Mg^{2+}		8.3×10^{-1}	9.8×10^{-1}	1.6	3.0	6.4
^{32}P	PO_4^{3-}		2.2	3.0	5.1	1.0×10^1	2.2×10^1
^{33}P	PO_4^{3-}		3.3×10^{-1}	4.4×10^{-1}	7.5×10^{-1}	1.5	3.2
^{35}S	SO_4^{2-}		9.8×10^{-2}	1.2×10^{-1}	2.0×10^{-1}	3.4×10^{-1}	6.8×10^{-1}
^{34m}Cl	Cl^-		8.6×10^{-3}	1.8×10^{-2}	2.9×10^{-2}	4.6×10^{-2}	9.0×10^{-2}
^{36}Cl	Cl^-		8.0×10^{-1}	9.6×10^{-1}	1.6	2.8	5.6
^{38}Cl	Cl^-		1.6×10^{-2}	1.8×10^{-2}	3.0×10^{-2}	4.9×10^{-2}	9.7×10^{-2}
^{38}K	K^+		2.7×10^{-2}	3.6×10^{-2}	5.5×10^{-2}	9.4×10^{-2}	1.7×10^{-1}
^{42}K	K^+		1.9×10^{-1}	2.3×10^{-1}	3.8×10^{-1}	6.4×10^{-1}	1.3
^{43}K	K^+		1.7×10^{-1}	2.0×10^{-1}	3.0×10^{-1}	4.8×10^{-1}	9.0×10^{-1}
^{45}Ca	Ca^{2+}		2.1	2.8	4.8	8.9	1.9×10^1
^{47}Ca	Ca^{2+}		1.4	1.8	2.9	5.0	1.1×10^1
^{48}Sc	Nonabsorbable marker	Oral fluid	1.4	1.8	2.8	4.4	7.8
		Oral solid	1.5	1.8	2.9	4.4	8.0
^{47}Sc	Nonabsorbable marker	Oral fluid	5.6×10^{-1}	7.3×10^{-1}	1.3	2.1	4.2
		Oral solid	5.7×10^{-1}	7.4×10^{-1}	1.3	2.2	4.3
^{51}Cr	$CrCl_3$		1.1×10^{-1}	1.4×10^{-1}	2.1×10^{-1}	3.1×10^{-1}	5.5×10^{-1}
	EDTA		2.3×10^{-3}	3.1×10^{-3}	4.6×10^{-3}	7.0×10^{-3}	1.3×10^{-2}
	Platelets		2.4×10^{-1}	3.5×10^{-1}	5.3×10^{-1}	8.2×10^{-1}	1.5
	Erythrocytes		2.6×10^{-1}	3.3×10^{-1}	5.2×10^{-1}	8.0×10^{-1}	1.5
		Denatured	4.0×10^{-1}	5.4×10^{-1}	8.3×10^{-1}	1.3	2.3
	Leukocytes		1.9×10^{-1}	2.8×10^{-1}	4.3×10^{-1}	6.7×10^{-1}	1.3
	Nonabsorbable marker	Oral fluid	3.4×10^{-2}	4.7×10^{-2}	7.7×10^{-2}	1.2×10^{-1}	2.3×10^{-1}
		Oral solid	3.4×10^{-2}	4.8×10^{-2}	7.8×10^{-2}	1.2×10^{-1}	2.3×10^{-1}
^{52}Fe	$Fe^{2+, 3+}$	Oral	1.0	1.1	1.9	3.4	7.0
^{55}Fe	$Fe^{2+, 3+}$	Parenteral	5.9	8.0	1.3×10^1	2.3×10^1	4.6×10^1
		Oral	5.9×10^{-1}	8.1×10^{-1}	1.3	2.3	4.6
^{59}Fe	$Fe^{2+, 3+}$	Parenteral	1.3×10^1	1.5×10^1	2.4×10^1	3.7×10^1	6.8×10^1
		Oral	2.0	2.5	4.0	6.2	1.1×10^1
^{57}Co	Bleomycin		5.6×10^{-2}	7.1×10^{-2}	1.0×10^{-1}	1.6×10^{-1}	2.8×10^{-1}
	Vitamin B_{12}	IV, Carrier free	5.8	7.3	1.1×10^1	1.6×10^1	2.8×10^1
		IV, Carrier	5.8×10^{-1}	7.3×10^{-1}	1.1	1.6	2.9
^{58}Co	Vitamin B_{12}	IV, Carrier free	1.1×10^1	1.3×10^1	2.0×10^1	2.9×10^1	4.9×10^1
		IV, Carrier	1.1	1.3	2.0	2.9	5.0
^{64}Cu	$Cu^{+, 2+}$		5.3×10^{-2}	6.6×10^{-2}	1.0×10^{-1}	1.5×10^{-1}	2.8×10^{-1}
^{67}Cu	$Cu^{+, 2+}$		2.2×10^{-1}	2.7×10^{-1}	4.1×10^{-1}	6.1×10^{-1}	1.2
^{62}Zn	Zn^{2+}		4.9×10^{-1}	6.6×10^{-1}	1.0	1.6	3.1

(continued)

Table 11.9. *(continued)*

Isotope	Pharmaceutical	Conditions of Administration[a]	Effective Dose Equivalent (mSv/mBq)[b]				
			Adult	Age 15	Age 10	Age 5	Age 1
^{65}Zn	Zn^{2+}		1.1×10^1	1.3×10^1	1.9×10^1	2.8×10^1	4.8×10^1
^{69m}Zn	Zn^{2+}		2.1×10^{-1}	2.5×10^{-1}	3.9×10^{-1}	6.1×10^{-1}	1.2
^{66}Ga	Citrate		3.4×10^{-1}	4.3×10^{-1}	7.0×10^{-1}	1.2	2.3
^{67}Ga	Citrate		1.2×10^{-1}	1.6×10^{-1}	2.5×10^{-1}	4.0×10^{-1}	7.9×10^{-1}
^{68}Ga	Citrate		2.7×10^{-2}	3.4×10^{-2}	5.6×10^{-2}	9.5×10^{-2}	1.9×10^{-1}
	EDTA		4.0×10^{-2}	5.2×10^{-2}	7.5×10^{-2}	9.5×10^{-2}	1.8×10^{-1}
^{72}Ga	Citrate		3.5×10^{-1}	4.4×10^{-1}	7.0×10^{-1}	1.1	2.1
^{72}As	AsO_3^{3-}, AsO_4^{3-}		4.8×10^{-1}	5.9×10^{-1}	9.2×10^{-1}	1.4	2.7
^{74}As	AsO_3^{3-}, AsO_4^{3-}		6.3×10^{-1}	7.6×10^{-1}	1.2	1.8	3.4
^{76}As	AsO_3^{3-}, AsO_4^{3-}		3.9×10^{-1}	4.8×10^{-1}	7.6×10^{-1}	1.2	2.4
^{75}Se	SeO_3^{2-}		3.5	4.4	6.8	9.6	1.6×10^1
	Methionine		3.0	3.8	6.5	9.2	1.5×10^1
	Methylcholesterol		1.7	2.1	3.1	4.5	7.7
	Bile acid		1.1	1.3	1.8	2.9	6.2
^{76}Br	Br^-		3.0×10^{-1}	3.5×10^{-1}	5.5×10^{-1}	8.6×10^{-1}	1.6
^{77}Br	Br^-		7.8×10^{-2}	9.1×10^{-2}	1.3×10^{-1}	2.0×10^{-1}	3.5×10^{-1}
	Spiperone		8.7×10^{-2}	1.1×10^{-1}	1.6×10^{-1}	2.4×10^{-1}	4.2×10^{-1}
^{82}Br	Br^-		4.3×10^{-1}	4.9×10^{-1}	7.3×10^{-1}	1.1	1.9
^{81m}Kr	Kr		2.7×10^{-5}	4.0×10^{-5}	5.7×10^{-5}	8.8×10^{-5}	1.7×10^{-4}
^{82}Rb	Rb^+		4.8×10^{-3}	6.7×10^{-3}	1.0×10^{-2}	1.8×10^{-2}	3.3×10^{-2}
^{81}Rb	Rb^+		3.1×10^{-2}	3.7×10^{-2}	5.7×10^{-2}	1.1×10^{-1}	2.2×10^{-1}
	Erythrocytes	Denatured	2.7×10^{-1}	3.8×10^{-1}	5.8×10^{-1}	9.1×10^{-1}	1.7
^{64}Rb	Rb^+		3.6	4.4	6.6	1.1×10^1	2.0×10^1
^{86}Rb	Rb^+		3.9	4.8	7.7	1.4×10^1	2.9×10^1
^{85}Sr	Sr^{2+}		8.5×10^{-1}	1.0	1.5	2.3	4.3
^{87m}Sr	Sr^{2+}		6.7×10^{-3}	8.1×10^{-3}	1.3×10^{-2}	2.1×10^{-2}	4.1×10^{-2}
^{89}Sr	Sr^{2+}		2.9	3.8	6.5	1.2×10^1	2.5×10^1
^{99m}Tc	Albumin	IV	7.9×10^{-3}	9.7×10^{-3}	1.5×10^{-2}	2.3×10^{-2}	4.2×10^{-2}
		Intrathecal lumbar	1.1×10^{-2}				
		Intrathecal cisternal	6.8×10^{-3}				
	Citrate		8.3×10^{-3}	1.0×10^{-2}	1.5×10^{-2}	2.2×10^{-2}	3.9×10^{-2}
	Colloid, large		1.4×10^{-2}	1.8×10^{-2}	2.8×10^{-2}	4.1×10^{-2}	7.3×10^{-2}
	Colloid, small		1.4×10^{-2}	1.9×10^{-2}	2.9×10^{-2}	4.3×10^{-2}	7.6×10^{-2}
	DMSA		1.6×10^{-2}	1.9×10^{-2}	2.7×10^{-2}	4.0×10^{-2}	6.9×10^{-2}
	DTPA	IV	6.3×10^{-3}	7.8×10^{-3}	1.1×10^{-2}	1.7×10^{-2}	3.0×10^{-2}
		Intrathecal lumbar	1.1×10^{-2}				
		Intrathecal cisternal	6.6×10^{-3}				
	HM-PAO		9.3×10^{-3}	1.1×10^{-2}	1.7×10^{-2}	2.6×10^{-2}	4.8×10^{-2}
	MAG3		7.3×10^{-3}	9.3×10^{-3}	1.2×10^{-2}	1.2×10^{-2}	2.2×10^{-2}
	MIBI	Resting	8.5×10^{-3}	1.1×10^{-2}	1.7×10^{-2}	2.6×10^{-2}	5.0×10^{-2}
		Exercise	8.5×10^{-3}	9.7×10^{-3}	1.5×10^{-2}	2.2×10^{-2}	4.3×10^{-2}
	Plasmin		1.1×10^{-2}	1.5×10^{-2}	2.2×10^{-2}	3.4×10^{-2}	6.0×10^{-2}
	Gluconate, glucoheptonate		9.0×10^{-3}	1.1×10^{-2}	1.6×10^{-2}	2.4×10^{-2}	4.2×10^{-2}
	Penicillamine		1.3×10^{-2}	1.6×10^{-2}	2.3×10^{-2}	3.4×10^{-2}	5.9×10^{-2}
	Pertechnetate	IV, no blocking	1.3×10^{-2}	1.6×10^{-2}	2.5×10^{-2}	4.0×10^{-2}	7.3×10^{-2}
		IV, blocking	5.5×10^{-3}	6.6×10^{-3}	9.8×10^{-3}	1.5×10^{-2}	2.6×10^{-2}
		Oral, no blocking	1.5×10^{-2}	1.9×10^{-2}	2.9×10^{-2}	4.6×10^{-2}	8.4×10^{-2}
	IDA derivatives		2.4×10^{-2}	2.9×10^{-2}	4.4×10^{-2}	7.0×10^{-2}	1.5×10^{-1}
	Fibrinogen		8.1×10^{-3}	9.9×10^{-3}	1.5×10^{-2}	2.4×10^{-2}	4.3×10^{-2}
	Erythrocytes		8.5×10^{-3}	1.1×10^{-2}	1.6×10^{-2}	2.5×10^{-2}	4.6×10^{-2}
	Denatured erythrocytes		4.1×10^{-2}	5.6×10^{-2}	8.4×10^{-2}	1.3×10^{-1}	2.2×10^{-1}
	Phosphates, phosphonates		8.0×10^{-3}	1.0×10^{-2}	1.5×10^{-2}	2.5×10^{-2}	5.0×10^{-2}
	Aerosols	Fast clearance	7.0×10^{-3}	9.1×10^{-3}	1.3×10^{-2}	2.0×10^{-2}	3.6×10^{-2}
		Slow clearance	1.5×10^{-2}	2.2×10^{-2}	3.1×10^{-2}	4.6×10^{-2}	8.5×10^{-2}
	Heparin		7.3×10^{-3}	9.3×10^{-3}	1.4×10^{-2}	2.1×10^{-2}	3.8×10^{-2}
	Macroaggregated albumin		1.2×10^{-2}	1.8×10^{-2}	2.5×10^{-2}	3.8×10^{-2}	6.9×10^{-2}
	Nonabsorbable markers	Oral fluids	2.4×10^{-2}	2.9×10^{-2}	4.7×10^{-2}	7.3×10^{-2}	1.3×10^{-1}
		Oral solids	2.4×10^{-2}	2.9×10^{-2}	4.6×10^{-2}	7.1×10^{-2}	1.3×10^{-1}
	Albumin microspheres		1.1×10^{-2}	1.6×10^{-2}	2.2×10^{-2}	3.3×10^{-2}	6.2×10^{-2}
	Platelets		2.2×10^{-2}	2.9×10^{-2}	4.4×10^{-2}	6.7×10^{-2}	1.2×10^{-1}
	Leukocytes		1.7×10^{-2}	2.3×10^{-2}	3.5×10^{-2}	5.4×10^{-2}	9.8×10^{-2}

(continued)

Table 11.9. *(continued)*

Isotope	Pharmaceutical	Conditions of Administration[a]	Effective Dose Equivalent (mSv/mBq)[b]				
			Adult	Age 15	Age 10	Age 5	Age 1
^{111}In	In^{3+}		2.6×10^{-1}	3.3×10^{-1}	4.9×10^{-1}	7.5×10^{-1}	1.4
	DTPA	IV	2.5×10^{-2}	3.1×10^{-2}	4.5×10^{-2}	6.7×10^{-2}	1.2×10^{-1}
		Intrathecal lumbar	1.4×10^{-1}				
		Intrathecal cisternal	1.2×10^{-1}				
	Aerosols	Fast clearance	2.8×10^{-2}	3.6×10^{-2}	5.3×10^{-2}	7.9×10^{-2}	1.4×10^{-1}
		Slow clearance	2.9×10^{-1}	3.9×10^{-1}	5.6×10^{-1}	8.4×10^{-1}	1.5
	Nonabsorbable markers	Oral fluids	3.0×10^{-1}	3.7×10^{-1}	6.0×10^{-1}	9.3×10^{-1}	1.7
		Oral solids	3.1×10^{-1}	3.8×10^{-1}	6.1×10^{-1}	9.4×10^{-1}	1.7
	Platelets		7.0×10^{-1}	9.3×10^{-1}	1.4	2.1	3.7
	Leukocytes		5.9×10^{-1}	7.9×10^{-1}	1.2	1.8	3.2
	Bleomycin		1.6×10^{-1}	2.0×10^{-1}	2.9×10^{-1}	4.4×10^{-1}	7.7×10^{-1}
^{113m}In	In^{3+}		1.3×10^{-2}	1.7×10^{-2}	2.8×10^{-2}	4.6×10^{-2}	9.2×10^{-2}
	Hydroxide, colloidal		1.7×10^{-2}	2.3×10^{-2}	3.6×10^{-2}	5.7×10^{-2}	1.1×10^{-1}
	DTPA		1.4×10^{-2}	1.8×10^{-2}	2.7×10^{-2}	4.2×10^{-2}	7.9×10^{-2}
	Aerosols	Fast clearance	1.8×10^{-2}	2.5×10^{-2}	3.6×10^{-2}	5.6×10^{-2}	1.1×10^{-1}
		Slow clearance	2.6×10^{-2}	3.8×10^{-2}	5.5×10^{-2}	8.5×10^{-2}	1.7×10^{-1}
	Nonabsorbable markers	Oral fluids	2.7×10^{-2}	3.3×10^{-2}	5.6×10^{-2}	9.1×10^{-2}	1.8×10^{-1}
		Oral solids	2.8×10^{-2}	3.4×10^{-2}	5.5×10^{-2}	9.1×10^{-2}	1.8×10^{-1}
^{123}I	I$^-$	Thyroid uptake 0%	1.3×10^{-2}	1.6×10^{-2}	2.4×10^{-2}	3.7×10^{-2}	$6.7 \times 10^{-}$
		Uptake 25%	1.1×10^{-1}	1.7×10^{-1}	2.6×10^{-1}	5.4×10^{-1}	1.0
	Amphetamine		3.2×10^{-2}	4.3×10^{-2}	6.2×10^{-2}	9.4×10^{-2}	$1.7 \times 10^{-}$
	Fibrinogen		2.7×10^{-2}	3.3×10^{-2}	5.3×10^{-2}	8.3×10^{-2}	$1.6 \times 10^{-}$
	Albumin	IV	2.6×10^{-2}	3.2×10^{-2}	5.0×10^{-2}	8.0×10^{-2}	$1.5 \times 10^{-}$
		Intrathecal lumbar	3.9×10^{-2}				
		Intrathecal cisternal	2.8×10^{-2}				
	Microaggregated albumin		2.4×10^{-2}	3.1×10^{-2}	4.7×10^{-2}	7.2×10^{-2}	$1.3 \times 10^{-}$
	Hippuran		1.5×10^{-2}	1.9×10^{-2}	2.8×10^{-2}	4.3×10^{-2}	7.8×10^{-2}
	MIBG		1.8×10^{-2}	2.3×10^{-2}	3.4×10^{-2}	5.0×10^{-2}	9.0×10^{-2}
	Rose bengal		7.6×10^{-2}	9.4×10^{-2}	1.5×10^{-1}	2.4×10^{-1}	4.7×10^{-1}
^{124}I	I$^-$	Thyroid uptake 0%	1.1×10^{-1}	1.3×10^{-1}	2.0×10^{-1}	3.1×10^{-1}	5.6×10^{-1}
		Uptake 25%	6.5	1.0×10^{1}	1.5×10^{1}	3.3×10^{1}	6.1×10^{1}
^{125}I	I$^-$	Thyroid uptake 0%	1.2×10^{-2}	1.5×10^{-2}	2.3×10^{-2}	3.7×10^{-2}	7.3×10^{-2}
		Uptake 25%	7.1	1.0×10^{1}	1.3×10^{1}	2.5×10^{1}	4.0×10^{1}
	Fibrinogen		1.2×10^{-1}	1.5×10^{-1}	2.4×10^{-1}	3.9×10^{-1}	7.7×10^{-1}
	Albumin		3.4×10^{-1}	4.1×10^{-1}	6.8×10^{-1}	1.1	2.2
	Nonabsorbable markers	Oral fluids	1.5×10^{-1}	1.9×10^{-1}	3.3×10^{-1}	5.4×10^{-1}	1.0
		Oral solids	1.6×10^{-1}	2.0×10^{-1}	3.4×10^{-1}	5.6×10^{-1}	1.1
	Hippuran		1.0×10^{-2}	1.3×10^{-2}	2.0×10^{-2}	3.1×10^{-2}	6.0×10^{-2}
	Antipyrene		1.3×10^{-2}	1.6×10^{-2}	2.6×10^{-2}	4.1×10^{-2}	8.0×10^{-2}
	Thalamate		9.7×10^{-3}	1.2×10^{-2}	1.9×10^{-2}	3.0×10^{-2}	5.7×10^{-2}
	PVP		1.2	1.5	2.3	3.5	6.6
	T4		1.2×10^{-1}	1.4×10^{-1}	2.3×10^{-1}	3.8×10^{-1}	7.6×10^{-1}
	T3		4.9×10^{-2}	6.1×10^{-2}	1.0×10^{-1}	1.7×10^{-1}	3.3×10^{-1}
	rT3		3.6×10^{-2}	4.6×10^{-2}	7.7×10^{-2}	1.2×10^{-1}	2.4×10^{-1}
	Diiodothyronine		3.6×10^{-2}	4.5×10^{-2}	7.6×10^{-2}	1.2×10^{-1}	2.4×10^{-1}
^{131}I	I$^-$	Thyroid uptake 0%	7.2×10^{-2}	8.8×10^{-2}	1.4×10^{-1}	2.1×10^{-1}	4.0×10^{-1}
		Uptake 25%	1.1×10^{1}	1.7×10^{1}	2.5×10^{1}	5.6×10^{1}	1.0×10^{2}
	Fibrinogen		5.6×10^{-1}	6.9×10^{-1}	1.1	1.8	3.6
	Albumin	IV	8.6×10^{-1}	1.1	1.7	2.8	5.4
		Intrathecal lumbar	9.0×10^{-1}				
		Intrathecal cisternal	8.4×10^{-1}				
	Macroaggregated albumin		5.0×10^{-1}	7.0×10^{-1}	1.0	1.6	3.1
	Nonabsorbable markers	Oral fluids	9.3×10^{-1}	1.1	2.0	3.2	6.3
		Oral solids	9.5×10^{-1}	1.2	2.0	3.3	6.5
	Microaggregated albumin		2.4×10^{-2}	3.1×10^{-2}	4.7×10^{-2}	7.2×10^{-2}	1.3×10^{-1}
	Hippuran		6.6×10^{-2}	8.3×10^{-1}	1.3×10^{-1}	1.9×10^{-1}	3.7×10^{-1}
	Antipyrine		7.8×10^{-2}	9.5×10^{-2}	1.5×10^{-1}	2.3×10^{-1}	4.4×10^{-1}

(continued)

Table 11.9. *(continued)*

Isotope	Pharmaceutical	Conditions of Administration[a]	Effective Dose Equivalent (mSv/mBq)[b]				
			Adult	**Age 15**	**Age 10**	**Age 5**	**Age 1**
^{131}I	Norcholesterol		1.5	2.2	3.4	6.8	1.3×10^1
	PVP		9.7×10^{-1}	1.2	1.8	2.7	5.1
	T4		4.4×10^{-1}	5.2×10^{-1}	8.5×10^{-1}	1.4	2.6
	T3		2.7×10^{-1}	3.3×10^{-1}	5.4×10^{-1}	8.7×10^{-1}	1.7
	rT3		2.2×10^{-1}	2.7×10^{-1}	4.5×10^{-1}	7.3×10^{-1}	1.4
	Diiodothyronine		2.2×10^{-1}	2.7×10^{-1}	4.4×10^{-1}	7.2×10^{-1}	1.4
	MIBG		2.0×10^{-1}	2.6×10^{-1}	4.0×10^{-1}	6.1×10^{-1}	1.1
	Rose bengal		9.1×10^{-1}	1.1	1.9	3.2	6.3
^{127}Xe	Gas	30 s inhalation	1.4×10^{-4}	1.8×10^{-4}	2.7×10^{-4}	4.1×10^{-4}	7.5×10^{-4}
		10 m rebreathe	1.2×10^{-3}	1.5×10^{-3}	2.2×10^{-3}	3.5×10^{-3}	6.3×10^{-3}
^{133}Xe	Gas	30 s inhalation	1.9×10^{-4}	2.6×10^{-4}	4.0×10^{-4}	6.4×10^{-4}	1.3×10^{-3}
		10 m rebreathe	1.3×10^{-3}	1.5×10^{-3}	2.5×10^{-3}	4.1×10^{-3}	8.3×10^{-3}
^{129}Cs	Cs$^+$		4.7×10^{-2}	5.4×10^{-2}	8.1×10^{-2}	1.2×10^{-1}	2.2×10^{-1}
^{130}Cs	Cs$^+$		2.4×10^{-3}	2.6×10^{-3}	3.9×10^{-3}	5.9×10^{-3}	1.1×10^{-2}
^{131}Cs	Cs$^+$		4.9×10^{-2}	5.4×10^{-2}	7.8×10^{-2}	1.2×10^{-1}	2.1×10^{-1}
^{134m}Cs	Cs$^+$		5.1×10^{-3}	4.9×10^{-3}	6.6×10^{-3}	8.7×10^{-3}	1.5×10^{-2}
^{131}Ba	Ba^{2+}		5.0×10^{-1}	7.0×10^{-1}	1.1	1.8	3.4
	Nonabsorbable markers	Oral fluids	4.5×10^{-1}	6.6×10^{-1}	1.1	1.7	3.1
		Oral solids	4.6×10^{-1}	6.7×10^{-1}	1.1	1.7	3.2
^{133m}Ba	Ba^{2+}		4.1×10^{-1}	6.4×10^{-1}	1.1	1.9	3.8
^{135m}Ba	Ba^{2+}		3.1×10^{-1}	3.8×10^{-1}	6.7×10^{-1}	1.1	2.3
^{140}La	DTPA		1.9×10^{-1}	2.3×10^{-1}	3.5×10^{-1}	5.3×10^{-1}	9.9×10^{-1}
^{169}Yb	DTPA	IV	4.6×10^{-2}	5.8×10^{-2}	8.9×10^{-2}	1.4×10^{-1}	2.5×10^{-1}
		Intrathecal lumbar	2.3×10^{-1}				
		Intrathecal cisternal	2.2×10^{-1}				
^{198}Au	Colloid		1.5	2.1	3.3	5.3	1.0×10^{-1}
^{197}Hg	HgCl$_2$		3.2×10^{-1}	4.0×10^{-1}	5.8×10^{-1}	8.7×10^{-1}	8.8×10^{-1}
	BMHP		3.9×10^{-1}	5.0×10^{-1}	7.5×10^{-1}	1.1	1.4
	Chlormerodrin		1.8×10^{-1}	2.3×10^{-1}	3.4×10^{-1}	5.2×10^{-1}	9.8×10^{-1}
^{203}Hg	Chlormerodrin		1.7	2.2	3.3	4.9	8.8
^{201}Tl	Tl$^{+, 3+}$		2.3×10^{-1}	3.6×10^{-1}	1.5	2.0	3.0

[a]IV unless otherwise specified.
[b]Multiply numbers in table by 3.7 to convert to rem/mCl.
Source: 90, 91.

Table 11.10. *Estimated Dose to Embryo from Maternal Diagnostic Nuclear Medicine Procedures*

Isotope	Pharmaceutical	Embryo Dose (mGy/mBq to Mother)
^{99m}Tc	Albumin	4.9×10^{-3}
	Lung aggregate	9.5×10^{-3}
	Polyphosphate	9.7×10^{-3}
	Pertechnetate	1.0×10^{-2}
	Stannous glucoheptonate	1.1×10^{-2}
	Sulfur colloid	8.6×10^{-3}
^{123}I	NaI (15% uptake)	8.6×10^{-3}
	Rose bengal	3.5×10^{-2}
^{131}I	NaI (15% uptake)	2.7×10^{-2}
	Rose bengal	1.8×10^{-1}

Source: 93.

Table 11.11. *Estimated Fetal Thyroid Dose from Maternal Radioiodine*

Gestation Period	Fetal/Maternal Ratio (Thyroid Gland)	Dose to Fetal Thyroid (mGy/mBq)
10–12 weeks	—	2.7×10^{-7} (precursors)
12–13 weeks	1.2	1.9×10^{-4}
Second trimester	1.8	1.6×10^{-3}
Third trimester	7.5	—
Term	—	2.2×10^{-3}

Source: 93

Table 11.12. *Estimated Dose to Mother and Breast-Feeding Child from Diagnostic Nuclear Medicine Procedures During Lactation*

Radiopharmaceutical	Effective Dose Equivalent (mSv/mBq)	
	Mother	**Child**
^{99m}Tc pertechnetate	1.1×10^{-2}	3.0×10^{-2}
^{131}I iodohippurate	5.0×10^{-2}	7.0
^{51}Cr EDTA	2.5×10^{-3}	1.5×10^{-3}
^{125}I fibrinogen	1.1×10^{-1}	3.2

Source: 18.

dose is the best estimate of the radiation burden to the patient from that dose. The linear nonthreshold model suggests that these doses carry small risks of stochastic effects. It is not certain, however, that this model is really the best fit to available data in this dose range. Therefore, all recognized authorities recommend that medical needs of the patient take precedence over potential radiation risk. That is, radiation exposure for a procedure that is clinically justified should not be an overriding concern. All effort should obviously be made to optimize the procedure so as to minimize exposure to both patients and staff. On the other hand, procedures whose purposes are nonmedical, such as mass screening, occupational, medicolegal, insurance, or research, should be carefully weighed as to what benefit is received by whom versus the radiation burden to the subject.

The most frequent source of radiation exposure problems in diagnostic medicine is the unwitting exposure of an early, unrecognized pregnancy. The question is at what dose level should consideration be given to termination of the pregnancy on grounds of radiation effect to the embryo. Although there are no clear data, there is reason to believe that the embryo and fetus are more sensitive to stochastic effects, in particular cancer, than the adult or even the child. However, the problem of the applicability of the linear nonthreshold model again enters. In any event, even by the most conservative models, the probability of a stochastic effect from such an exposure is very small and therefore difficult to deal with. However, thresholds for deterministic effects in the early embryo are in the range of 50 to 150 mGy. It is possible to deliver doses in this range in diagnostic medicine, especially from a complicated workup. In years past, several authors recommended specific dose levels for recommending therapeutic abortion (94,95). Now it seems more reasonable to consider an action range rather than an action level. Doses to the embryo below about 50 mGy should carry little or no risk of deterministic effect. Doses in the range of 50 to 150 mGy may be associated with small, perhaps statistically insignificant, risk, and the patient should be so counseled. Above 150 mGy, however, the risk is likely to be statistically significant, and pregnancy termination should be considered.

These recommendations are not intended for blind application to any specific case. They should be tempered with judgment. The patient still comes first.

REFERENCES

1. Rollins WH. *Notes on x-light.* Boston: Privately published, 1904.
2. Sagan LS, ed. Radiation hormesis. Proceedings of a conference held at Oakland CA, Aug. 14–16, 1985. *Health Phys* 1987;52:519–680.
3. Pochin EE. *Why be quantitative about radiation risk estimates?* L.S. Taylor lecture series, no. 2. Washington, DC: NCRP Publications, 1978.
4. Wilson R. Risks caused by low levels of pollution. *Yale J Biol Med* 1978;51:37–51.
5. Borek C. In vitro cell transformation by low doses of x-irradiation and neutrons. In: Yuhas JW, Tennant RW, Regan JD, eds. *Biology of radiation carcinogenesis.* New York: Raven Press, 1976:309–326.
6. Rinchik EM, Stoye JP, Frankel WN et al. Molecular analysis of viable spontaneous and radiation-induced albino (c)-locus mutations in the mouse. *Mutat Res* 1993;286:199–207.
7. Thacker J. Radiation-induced mutation in mammalian cells at low doses and dose rates. In: Nygaard OF, Sinclair WK, Lett JT, eds. *Effects of low dose and low dose rate radiation.* New York: Academic Press, 1992:77–124.
8. Lea DE. *Actions of radiations on living cells,* 2nd ed. Cambridge, UK: Cambridge University Press, 1955.
9. Kellerer AM, Rossi HH. A generalized formulation of the theory of dual radiation action. *Radiat Res* 1978;75:471–488.
10. Hall EJ. *Radiobiology for the radiologist,* 4th ed. Philadelphia: JB Lippincott, 1994.
11. Stephens LC, Hunter NR, Ang KK et al. Development of apoptosis in irradiated murine tumors as a function of time and dose. *Radiat Res* 1993;135:75–80.
12. Lowe SW, Schmitt EM, Smith SW et al. p53 is required for radiation-induced apoptosis in mouse thymocytes. *Nature* 1993;362:847–849.
13. Kollmorgen GM, Bedford JS. Cellular radiation biology. In: Darymple GV, Gaulden ME, Kollmorgen GM et al., eds. *Medical radiation biology.* Philadelphia: WB Saunders, 1973:100–127.
14. Bacq ZM, Alexander P. *Fundamentals of radiobiology.* New York: MacMillan, 1961.
15. Elkind MM, Sutton H. Radiation response of mammalian cells grown in culture. I. Repair of x-ray damage in surviving Chinese hamster cells. *Radiat Res* 1960;13:556–593.
16. Land CE. Estimating cancer risks from low doses of ionizing radiation. *Science* 1980;209:1197–1203.
17. Committee on the Biological Effects of Ionizing Radiation. *Health effects of exposure to low levels of ionizing radiation (BEIR V).* Washington, DC: National Academy Press, 1990.
18. United Nations Scientific Committee on the Effects of Atomic Radiation. *Sources and effects of ionizing radiation.* New York: United Nations, 1993.
19. Upton AC. Cancer research 1964: thoughts on the contributions of radiation biology. *Cancer Res* 1964;24:1861–1868.
20. Shimizu Y, Kato H, Schull WJ. *Life span study report 11. Part 2. Cancer mortality in the years 1950–85 based on the recently revised doses (DS86).* Hiroshima, Japan: Radiation Effects Research Foundation, 1988, technical report RERF TR 5-88.
21. Thompson DE, Mabuchi K, Ron E et al. Cancer incidence in atomic bomb survivors. Part II: Solid tumors, 1958–1987. *Radiat Res* 1994; 137(Suppl):S17–S67.
22. Preston DL, Kusumi S, Tomonaga M et al. Cancer incidence in atomic bomb survivors. Part III: Leukemia, lymphoma and multiple myeloma, 1950–1987. *Radiat Res* 1994;137(Suppl):S68–S97.
23. Ron E, Preston DL, Mabuchi K et al. Cancer incidence in atomic bomb survivors. Part IV. Comparison of cancer incidence and mortality. *Radiat Res* 1994;137(Suppl):S98–S112.
24. Mole RH, Papworth DG, Corp MJ. The dose response for x-ray induction of myeloid leukemia in male CBA.H mice. *Br J Cancer* 1983;47: 285–291.
25. Darby SC, Doll R, Gill SK et al. Long-term mortality after a single treatment course with x-rays in patients treated for ankylosing spondylitis. *Br J Cancer* 1987;55:179–190.
26. Boice JD Jr, Blettner M, Kleinerman RA et al. Radiation dose and leukemia risk in patients treated for cancer of the cervix. *J US Natl Cancer Inst* 1987;79:1295–1311.
27. Boice JD Jr, Enghohm G, Kleinerman RA et al. Radiation dose and second cancer risk in patients treated for cancer of the cervix. *Radiat Res* 1988;116:3–55.
28. Stewart A, Pennypacker W, Barber R. Adult leukemia and diagnostic x-rays. *Br Med J* 1962;3:882–890.
29. Gibson R, Graham S, Lilienfeld A et al. Irradiation in the epidemiology of leukemia among adults. *J US Natl Cancer Inst* 1972;48:301–311.
30. Linos A, Gray J, Orvis A. Low dose radiation and leukemia. *N Engl J Med* 1980;302:1101.
31. MacKenzie I. Breast cancer following multiple fluoroscopies. *Br J Cancer* 1965;19:1–9.
32. Miller AB, Howe GR, Sherman GJ et al. Breast cancer mortality following irradiation in a cohort of Canadian tuberculosis patients. *N Engl J Med* 1989;321:1285–1289.
33. Hrubec Z, Boice J, Monson R et al. Breast cancer after multiple chest fluoroscopies: second follow-up of Massachusetts women with tuberculosis. *Cancer Res* 1989;49:229–234.

34. Shore R, Hildreth N, Woodward E et al. Breast cancer among women given x-ray therapy for acute postpartum mastitis. *J US Natl Cancer Inst* 1986;77:689–696.

35. Committee on the Biological Effects of Ionizing Radiation. *Health risks of radon and other internally deposited alpha-emitters (BEIR IV).* Washington, DC: National Academy Press, 1988.

36. Griem ML, Justman J, Weiss L. The neoplastic potential of gastric irradiation. *Am J Clin Oncol* 1984;7:675–677.

37. Ron E, Modan B. Thyroid and other neoplasms following childhood scalp irradiation. In: Boice JD Jr, Fraumeni JF Jr, eds. *Radiation carcinogenesis: epidemiology and biological significance.* New York: Raven Press, 1984:139–151.

38. Shore RE, Woodward ED, Hempelmann LH. Radiation-induced thyroid cancer. In: Boice JD Jr, Fraumeni JF Jr, eds. *Radiation carcinogenesis: epidemiology and biological significance.* New York: Raven Press, 1984:131–138.

39. National Council on Radiation Protection and Measurement. *Induction of thyroid cancer by ionizing radiation.* Bethesda, MD: National Council on Radiation Protection and Measurement, 1985, NCRP report no 80.

40. Hoffman DA. Late effects of I-131 therapy in the United States. In: Boice JD Jr, Fraumeni JF Jr, eds. *Radiation carcinogenesis: epidemiology and biological significance.* New York: Raven Press, 1984:273–280.

41. Holm L-E, Wicklund KE, Lundell GE et al. Thyroid cancer after diagnostic doses of iodine-131: a retrospective study. *J US Natl Cancer Inst* 1988;80:1132–1136.

42. Conard RA. Late radiation effects in Marshall Islanders exposed to fallout 28 years ago. In: Boice JD Jr, Fraumeni JF Jr, eds. *Radiation carcinogenesis: epidemiology and biological significance.* New York: Raven Press, 1984:57–71.

43. Rothman RJ. Significance of studies of low-dose radiation fallout in the western United States. In: Boice JD Jr, Fraumeni JF Jr, eds. *Radiation carcinogenesis: epidemiology and biological significance.* New York: Raven Press, 1984:73–82.

44. Lee WR, Chiacchierini RP, Shlein B et al. Thyroid tumors following I-131 or localized x-irradiation to the thyroid and the pituitary glands in rats. *Radiat Res* 1982;92:307–319.

45. Brinkley D, Haybittle JL. The late effects of artificial menopause by x-radiation. *Br J Radiol* 1969;42:519–521.

46. Smith PG, Doll R. Late effects of x-irradiation in patients treated for metropathia haemorrhagica. *Br J Radiol* 1976;49:224–232.

47. Dickson RJ. The late results of radium treatment for benign uterine hemorrhage. *Br J Radiol* 1969;42:582–594.

48. Wagoner JK. Leukemia and other malignancies following radiation therapy for gynecological disorders. In: Boice JD Jr, Fraumeni JF Jr, eds. *Radiation carcinogenesis: epidemiology and biological significance.* New York: Raven Press, 1984:153–159.

49. Blum T. Osteomyelitis of the mandible and maxilla. *J Am Dent Assoc* 1924;11:802–805.

50. Taylor LS. *Radiation protection standards.* Cleveland, OH: CRC Press, 1971.

51. Smith PG, Doll R. Mortality from cancer and all causes among British radiologists. *Br J Radiol* 1981;54:187–194.

52. Shore RE, Albert RE, Pasternack BS. Follow-up study of patients treated by x-ray epilation for tinea capitis: resurvey of posttreatment illness and mortality experience. *Arch Environ Health* 1976;31:17–24.

53. Matanoski GM. The current mortality rates of radiologists and other physician specialists: specific causes of death. *Am J Epidemiol* 1975;101:199–210.

54. Preston-Martin S, Paganini-Hill A, Henderson BE et al. Case control study of intracranial meningiomas in women in Los Angeles County, California. *J US Natl Cancer Inst* 1980;65:67–73.

55. Soffer D, Pittalura S, Feiner M et al. Intracranial meningiomas following low-dose irradiation to the head. *J Neurosurg* 1983;59:1048–1053.

56. Rubinstein AB, Shalit MN, Cohen ML et al. Radiation-induced cerebral meningioma: a recognizable entity. *J Neurosurg* 1984;61:966–971.

57. Harley N, Kolber AB, Shore RE et al. The skin dose and response for the head and neck in patients irradiated with x ray for tinea capitis: implications for environmental radioactivity. In: *Proceedings of the 16th Midyear Topical Meeting of the Health Physics Society.* Springfield, VA: National Technical Information Service, 1983:125–142.

58. Cuzick J. Radiation-induced myelomatosis. *N Engl J Med* 1981;304:204–210.

59. Land CE. Carcinogenic effects of radiation on the human digestive tract and other organs. In: Upton AC, Albert RE, Burns FJ et al., eds. *Radiation carcinogenesis.* New York: Elsevier, 1986:347–378.

60. Preston-Martin S, Thomas DC, White SC et al. Prior exposure to medical and dental x-rays related to tumors of the parotid gland. *J US Natl Cancer Inst* 1988;80:943–949.

61. Stewart A, Webb J, Giles D et al. Malignant disease in childhood and diagnostic irradiation in utero. *Lancet* 1956;1:447.

62. Diamond EL, Schmerler H, Lilienfeld AM. The relationship of intra-uterine radiation to subsequent mortality and development of leukemia in children. *Am J Epidemiol* 1973;97:283–313.

63. Oppenheim BE, Griem ML, Meier P. Effects of low-dose prenatal irradiation in humans: analysis of Chicago Lying-In data and comparison with other studies. *Radiat Res* 1974;57:508–544.

64. Yoshimoto Y, Kato H, Schull WJ. *Risk of cancer among in utero children exposed to A-bomb radiation: 1950–84.* Hiroshima, Japan: Radiation Effects Research Foundation, 1988, RERF technical report 4-88.

65. Macht SH, Lawrence PS. National survey of congenital malformation, resulting from exposure to roentgen radiation. *Am J Roentgenol* 1955;73:442–466.

66. Gardner MJ, Snee MP, Hall AJ et al. Results of case-control study of leukaemia and lymphoma among young people near Sella-field nuclear plant in West Cumbria. *Br Med J* 1990;300:423–428.

67. Neel JV. Update on the genetic effects of ionizing radiation. *JAMA* 1991;66:698–701.

68. Muller HJ. Artificial transmutation of the gene. *Science* 1927;66:84–87.

69. Russell WL. The nature of the dose-rate effect of radiation on mutation in mice. *Japan J Genet* 1964;40(Suppl):128–140.

70. Selby PB, Selby PR. Gamma-ray-induced dominant mutations that cause skeletal abnormalities in mice. I. Plan, summary of results and discussion. *Mutat Res* 1977;43:357–375.

71. Schull WJ, Otake M, Neel JV. Genetic effects of the atomic bombs: a reappraisal. *Science* 1981;213:1220–1227.

72. National Council on Radiation Protection and Measurements. *Ionizing radiation exposure of the population of the United States.* Bethesda, MD: National Council on Radiation Protection and Measurements, 1987, NCRP report no 93.

73. Hall EJ. *Radiobiology for the radiologist,* 4th ed. Philadelphia: JB Lippincott, 1994.

74. International Commission on Radiological Protection. Nonstochastic effects of ionizing radiation. ICRP publication 41. *Ann ICRP* 1984;14(3).

75. Merriam GR, Szechter A, Focht EF. The effects of ionizing radiation on the eye. *Front Radiat Ther Oncol* 1972;6:346–385.

76. Rubin P, Casarett GW. A direction for clinical radiation pathology. The tolerance dose. *Front Radiat Ther Oncol* 1972;6:1–16.

77. Russell LB, Russell WL. An analysis of the changing radiation response of the developing mouse embryo. *J Cell Physiol* 1954;43(Suppl 1):103–149.

78. Otake M, Schull WJ. In utero exposure to A-bomb radiation and mental retardation: a reassessment. *Br J Radiol* 1984;57:409–414.

79. Goldstein L, Murphy DP. Microcephalic idiocy following radium therapy for uterine cancer during pregnancy. *Am J Obstet Gynecol* 1929;18:1890–195.

80. Miller RW, Mulvihill JJ. Small head size after atomic irradiation. In: Sever JL, Brent RL, eds. *Teratogen update: environmentally induced birth defect risks.* New York: Alan R. Liss, 1986:141–143.

81. Committee on the Biological Effects of Ionizing Radiations. *The effects on populations of exposure to low levels of ionizing radiation (BEIR III).* Washington, DC: National Academy of Sciences, 1980.

82. Brent RL, Gorson RO. Radiation exposure in pregnancy. *Curr Probl Radiol* 1972;2:1–48.

83. National Council on Radiation Protection and Measurements. *Medical exposure of pregnant and potentially pregnant women.* Bethesda, MD:

National Council on Radiation Protection and Measurement, 1977, NCRP report no. 54.

84. International Commission on Radiological Protection. 1990 Recommendations of the International Commission on Radiological Protection. ICRP publication 60. *Ann ICRP* 1991;21(1-3).

85. Otake M, Yashimaru H, Schull WJ. *Severe mental retardation among the prenatally exposed survivors of the atomic bombing of Hiroshima and Nagasaki: a comparison of the old and new dosimetry systems.* Hiroshima, Japan: Radiation Effects Research Foundation, 1987, RERF technical report 16-87.

86. Schull WJ, Otake M. *Effects on intelligence of prenatal exposure to ionizing radiation.* Hiroshima, Japan: Radiation Effects Research Foundation, 1986, RERF technical report 7-86.

87. Jacobi W. The concept of effective dose—a proposal for the combination of organ doses. *Radiat Environ Biophys* 1975;12:101–109.

88. International Commission on Radiological Protection. Recommendations of the International Commission on Radiological Protection. ICRP publication 26. *Ann ICRP* 1977;1(3).

89. Laws PW, Rosenstein M. A somatic dose index for diagnostic radiology. *Health Phys* 1978;35:629–642.

90. International Commission on Radiological Protection. Radiation dose to patients from radiopharmaceuticals. ICRP publication 53. *Ann ICRP* 1987;18(1–4).

91. International Commission on Radiological Protection. Addendum 1 to radiation dose to patients from radiopharmaceuticals. *Ann ICRP* 1991;22(3):1–28.

92. Gibbs SJ. Influence of organs in the ICRP's remainder on effective dose equivalent computed for diagnostic radiation exposures. *Health Phys* 1989;56:515–520.

93. Kereiakes JG, Rosenstein M. *Handbook of radiation doses in nuclear medicine and diagnostic radiology.* Boca Raton, FL: CRC Press, 1980.

94. Hammer-Jacobsen E. Therapeutic abortion on account of x-ray examination during pregnancy. *Dan Med Bull* 1959;6:113–121.

95. Dekaban AS. Abnormalities in children exposed to x-radiation during various stages of gestation: tentative timetable of radiation to the human fetus. *J Nucl Med* 1968;9:471–477.

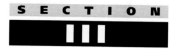

CARDIOVASCULAR

12

DIGITAL TECHNIQUES FOR THE ACQUISITION, PROCESSING, AND ANALYSIS OF NUCLEAR CARDIOLOGY IMAGES

GUIDO GERMANO
DANIEL S. BERMAN

Unlike many other imaging modalities, nuclear medicine has been associated with computers and digital images since its inception. Computers not only control the acquisition of nuclear data, but also images are retained in digital form for routine processing, display, quantification, and storage. This chapter provides a review of the use of computers in nuclear cardiology today. In its first section, various types of nuclear cardiology images are reviewed with respect to their dimensionality and mode of acquisition. A second section examines the processing necessary to pass from the acquired (raw) data to the final images, on which visual or quantitative analysis is performed. A third section describes methods of quantitative analysis of cardiac images aimed at extracting global and regional information on myocardial perfusion and function. Finally, future applications of computers in nuclear cardiology are briefly discussed.

The reader should be familiar with the basic principles of computer operation covered in Section I, Physics and Instrumentation, of this book, as well as with the principles of single photon emission computed tomography (SPECT), outlined in Chapter 4. Today SPECT imaging represents the vast majority of all cardiac nuclear procedures performed in the United States, and consequently it is given special prominence in our review.

IMAGE ACQUISITION

There are a large number of acquisition protocols and techniques used in nuclear cardiology today, most of them based on the Anger scintillation camera or a variation of this camera (see

G. Germano: Medicine and Radiological Sciences, UCLA School of Medicine, and Artificial Intelligence Program, Department of Medicine, Cedars-Sinai Medical Center, Nuclear Medicine, Los Angeles, CA.
D.S. Berman: Department of Imaging, Cedars-Sinai Medical Center, and Department of Medicine, UCLA School of Medicine, Los Angeles, CA.

Chapter 3). In our discussion, we shall classify nuclear cardiology datasets based on their dimension, as summarized in Table 12.1.

Planar

A static planar study by definition requires a two-dimensional (2-D) acquisition, because counts are collected in two dimensions (X and Y in the image). In planar imaging the camera is fixed relative to the patient, so the 2-D image obtained reflects the projection of the three-dimensional (3-D) distribution of radioactivity in the patient's myocardium. This is why planar images are also called projection images or projections. Because planar images cannot differentiate between overlapping structures, image contrast suffers, and it is necessary to acquire more than one projection image to localize abnormalities. The planar projections most commonly used for myocardial perfusion imaging are the anterior, the 45-degree left anterior oblique (LAO), and a left lateral view.

Gated Planar

Electrocardiogram (ECG)-gated planar studies require the acquisition of a planar image for each phase or interval of the cardiac cycle, resulting in a 3-D dataset spanning X, Y, and time. Because the cardiac cycle is divided in as many as 8 to 64 intervals, data from many different cycles (up to several hundreds) must be averaged to ensure adequate count statistics. Figure 12.1

Table 12.1. *Nuclear Cardiology Datasets*

Study	Dimensionality	Variables	# Images
Standard planar	2	X, Y	1–4
Gated planar	3	X, Y, time	8–64
First pass	3	X, Y, time	500–5000
Standard SPECT	3	X, Y, Z	30–120
Gated SPECT	4	X, Y, Z, time	240–1920
Dynamic SPECT	4	X, Y, Z, time	180–3000

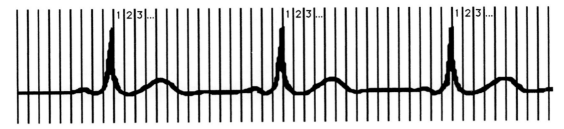

FIGURE 12.1. Electrocardiographic gating. Each cardiac cycle (defined by two successive R-wave peaks) is divided into a number of fixed-length temporal intervals or frames. Data collected during homologous frames in different cycles are summed together, because they refer to the same phase of the cardiac cycle.

explains the way in which counts are accumulated in gated planar acquisition: Counts collected during the *n*th interval from the occurrence of each R-wave trigger are accumulated in the same projection image (frame *n*). Acquisition stops when a preset number of counts has been collected or when a predetermined period has elapsed. Figure 12.1 is based on the most common gating approach, referred to as fixed temporal resolution with forward-gating; in this approach, all gating intervals have the same length (generally, between 10 and 100 milliseconds), based on the average duration of the cardiac cycle. Other gating approaches include (a) fixed temporal resolution with backward-gating, in which the gating intervals are synchronized from the R-wave backward, and applied to the latest heartbeat's data stored in a memory buffer; (b) a combination of forward and backward gating; and (c) the variable temporal resolution method, in which the R-R duration is dynamically adjusted to match the average length of the latest few heart cycles, and the length of the gating intervals (which remain constant in number) changes accordingly (1). ECG-gated planar studies are performed for the purpose of assessing myocardial function and may employ equilibrium blood pool agents such as ^{99m}Tc-labeled red blood cells or myocardial perfusion agents.

First Pass

The first-pass acquisition technique uses very fine temporal sampling (20 to 100 frames/second) to look at the initial transit of a radionuclide bolus through the central circulation. As with gated planar imaging, a succession of planar images is acquired, resulting in a 3-D dataset spanning X, Y, and time; however, the overall duration of the study is much shorter. Key to the successful application of the first-pass technique is the administration of a compact bolus, which ideally should result in a full-width–half-maximum of less than 2 seconds in the superior vena cava. Acquisition is completed in less than 1 minute and can be performed in any desired view, because distinct temporal relationships in the arrival and disappearance of radioactivity from the various cardiac chambers allows their separation with first-pass studies.

Of note, first-pass studies typically average data over multiple heart cycles (generally 4 to 10), and can therefore also benefit from ECG gating. The first-pass technique is used principally for the assessment of left ventricular (LV) and right ventricular (RV) function.

SPECT

In SPECT imaging, the camera's detector(s) rotate around the patient, collecting a planar image every few degrees. Then, the 3-D distribution of radioactivity is reconstructed from this set of 2-D projection images, resulting in a 3-D dataset spanning X, Y, and Z. The tomographic reconstruction process was first described by Bracewell (2) for astronomical applications and subsequently applied to medical tomography by Shepp and Logan (3). The most popular form of tomographic reconstruction from projections in nuclear medicine is backprojection. Figure 12.2 shows a graphical explanation of backprojection, with

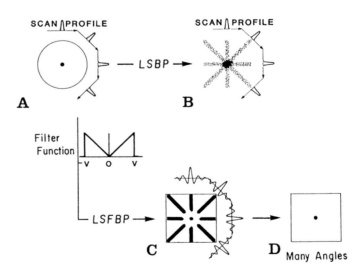

FIGURE 12.2. Reconstruction of tomographic images via backprojection. The counts in scan profiles collected at different angles around a point source **(A)** can be uniformly backprojected onto an image matrix [linear superimposition of back projections (LSBP)]. The original point source distribution is recreated, but at the cost of blurring and loss of contrast; moreover, the characteristic star artifact is produced **(B)**. Alternatively, the profile counts can be first processed by a filter function shaped like a ramp in the Fourier domain and an oscillating damped curve in the space domain, and then backprojected onto the image matrix [linear superimposition of filtered back projections (LSFBP)] **(C)**. The curve sections below zero cancel the star artifact, the cancellation being closer to perfect the more profiles are used for reconstruction **(D)**. In modern tomography, LSFBP is universally preferred to LSBP. (From Phelps ME, Hoffman EJ, Gado M, et al: Computerized transaxial reconstruction. In DeBlanc H, Sorenson J, eds. *Non invasive brain imaging, computerized tomography and radionuclides.* Society of Nuclear Medicine, Reston, VA: 1975:111–145, with permission.)

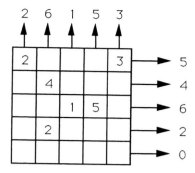

FIGURE 12.3. Algebraic reconstruction technique (ART) of tomographic images. Each point in the profiles of Fig. 12.2 is the sum of a row, a column, or a diagonal distribution of image matrix pixels. A system of equations can then be constructed and solved for those pixels. The concept is exemplified in this figure by showing the numeric components of two representative profiles, along the horizontal and the vertical direction. For other angles, the sum of fractional pixels must be considered.

the 2-D projection images (perpendicular to the plane of the page) simplified into one-dimensional (1-D) profiles, and the 3-D radioactivity distribution simplified into a 2-D point source. Each profile represents the integrated sum of the activity distribution along that particular angle. In standard backprojection [linear superimposition of back projections (LSBP)], the counts in each profile are uniformly "smeared" back onto the tomographic image matrix, with consequent loss of resolution and contrast and creation of the characteristic star artifact. In filtered backprojection [linear superimposition of filtered back projections (LSFBP)], each profile is filtered with a damped oscillating function before backprojection, so as to eliminate the star artifact and recover image contrast and resolution. The canonic filter function used corresponds to a ramp in the frequency or Fourier domain; as we shall see, filters are usually described in terms of their shape in this domain.

Filtered backprojection is not the only reconstruction method used in nuclear cardiology, although it is by far the most widely used. Increasing attention is being focused on iterative or algebraic reconstruction techniques (ARTs) that also use the projection images as input but aim at finding the exact mathematical solution to the problem of activity distribution in the field of view (FOV) by considering the value in each pixel of the reconstructed image as an unknown and each point in a profile (projection image) as an equation. The basic concept of ART is shown in Fig. 12.3, again applied to a simple 2-D activity distribution and two representative profiles.

For cardiac applications, standard SPECT studies are principally performed for the purpose of assessing myocardial perfusion and therefore use myocardial perfusion agents.

Gated SPECT

Gated SPECT studies are to SPECT imaging what gated planar studies are to planar imaging. In essence, a number (usually 8 or 16) of projection images is acquired at each projection angle, with each image corresponding to a specific portion of the cardiac cycle; each set of projections corresponding to a given phase

(interval) of the cardiac cycle is then reconstructed into a 3-D SPECT dataset, resulting in a four-dimensional (4-D) dataset spanning X, Y, Z, and time. Of note, summing all projections at each angle before reconstruction yields what is generally referred to as the ungated or summed gated SPECT dataset, essentially equivalent to a static SPECT study (Fig. 12.4). Gated SPECT may be used either with perfusion agents (gated perfusion SPECT) or less commonly with equilibrium blood pool agents (gated blood pool SPECT). In the former, a gated SPECT acquisition will produce a static SPECT dataset (summed gated SPECT), from which perfusion is assessed and a larger gated SPECT dataset, from which function is evaluated. The strong appeal and recent extraordinary diffusion of the gated SPECT technique is a direct consequence of the ease and modest expense with which perfusion assessment can be upgraded to perfusion/function assessment.

The normal fluctuation of the cardiac cycle during gated acquisitions has led to the building of tolerances in the count collection process. The beat length acceptance window aims at eliminating data from cardiac cycles that are too short or too long, while still accepting a sensible range of data, and it can be seen as analogous to the energy acceptance window that is positioned on the radioisotope's photopeak before acquisition (4). Let us assume that the expected cardiac cycle duration is 1 second (heart rate = 60 beats/minute): A beat length acceptance window of 20% allows accumulation of data from cardiac cycles having a duration within ± 10% of the expected duration (in our case, within a 900- to 1,100-millisecond range). An acceptance window of 100%, somewhat counterintuitively, allows accumulation of data from cycles having duration within ± 50% of the expected (in our case, within a 500- to 1,500-millisecond range). This is *not* equivalent to accepting 100% of the cycles, which is instead consistent with having a window of infinite width. Although choosing a narrow acceptance window would ensure the integrity of the gated SPECT dataset by eliminating counts from arrhythmic cycles, the window is often set to a wider value to preserve the integrity of the perfusion SPECT data. In fact, because the latter is derived by summing the various intervals of the gated study, if too many counts are rejected because of

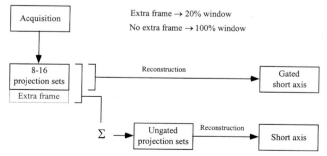

FIGURE 12.4. A gated single photon emission computed tomography (SPECT) acquisition produces a static SPECT dataset from which perfusion is assessed and a larger gated SPECT dataset from which function is evaluated (short axis = reoriented SPECT images). The cardiac beat length acceptance window ought to be set so as not to compromise perfusion assessment. [From Germano G, Berman DS. Gated SPECT. In: *Nuclear cardiac imaging: principles and applications*, 3rd ed. New York: Oxford University Press, 2002 *(in press)*, with permission.]

gating problems not only would the gated information be unreliable, but artifacts also might appear in the summed SPECT data. This entire problem can be overcome if all rejected counts are automatically accumulated in an extra frame (a ninth frame in eight-frame gated SPECT imaging) and added back during generation of the summed perfusion SPECT study. With this approach, summed perfusion SPECT data will be exactly the same as if it had been acquired without gating, whereas only data from cycles with acceptable beat length will contribute to the gated SPECT dataset. Although the extra frame feature is not currently standard on camera equipment, its diffusion is expected to increase in the future. Our advice is to use as wide an acceptance window as possible if no extra frame is available to "save" rejected counts or a 20% to 30% acceptance window if that feature is available (Fig. 12.4).

Dynamic SPECT

Dynamic SPECT studies can be thought of as a succession of consecutive static SPECT acquisitions acquired to follow a dynamic process, such as the change in myocardial radionuclide distribution with time. A 4-D dataset is produced spanning X, Y, Z, and time, but there is no gating involved. Dynamic planar or dynamic SPECT acquisitions ranging from 15 seconds to 1 to 2 minutes have been effectively employed with multidetector cameras to image ^{99m}Tc-teboroxime, a myocardial perfusion agent with rapid uptake and washout (5,6).

List Mode

When a projection image is produced as the result of a standard acquisition, one knows the number of counts associated with every pixel in the image. However, one does not know *at what time* each individual count was accumulated in that pixel, nor does one know *what energy* that particular count had (one only knows that its energy was within a range specified by the energy acquisition window). List mode acquisition aims at overcoming these limitations by collecting extra information about each count and delaying generation of the projection image until the acquisition is complete.

In temporal list mode acquisition, each individual count is stored in a memory bin, which contains information on the count's location in the XY detector plane and the exact time of its arrival (as determined by the camera's internal clock). This approach may be useful in achieving more accurate binning of gated data but requires substantially more memory and more postacquisition processing than standard acquisition. For instance, 200,000 counts accumulated in a projection image would occupy $(64)2 = 4,096$ memory locations if a 64×64 pixel^2 matrix is used, as opposed to 200,000 memory locations in temporal list mode. Moreover, the individual memory location in list mode would have to be larger, because it must contain the additional timing information.

In energy list mode, the exact energy associated with each individual count is digitized and stored in a memory bin together with the count's XY location (7). Commitment to a specific energy window at the acquisition stage is no longer necessary: One can collect all the counts in the energy spectrum and process them at a later time to remove undesired counts. This approach may be useful to identify and remove scattered radiation, because it has been suggested that optimal scatter correction would require knowledge of the full spectral distribution of Compton photons (8). As a particularly interesting case, the problem of correcting for isotope crosstalk in simultaneous dual isotope myocardial perfusion SPECT may be best approached using this form of acquisition.

IMAGE PROCESSING AND DISPLAY

Image Restoration

Even in a well-functioning gamma camera system, there are known inaccuracies of the hardware acquisition chain that need to be compensated in software before the data is analyzed. For instance, the nonlinearity of the X and Y positioning signals across the face of the detector would typically result in "pincushion" or "barrel" distortion of the image, easily detectable with the use of straight-line test patterns (9). The common approach to correcting these and other image nonuniformities is that of acquiring a very high-count image of a uniform radiation field or flood. For multidetector cameras, an image per detector is acquired. Each pixel in this test image would have the same value (within statistical precision) if uniformity were perfect. Therefore, the differences in counts between pixels in the image can be used to generate a correction matrix to be applied to all subsequent clinical studies. Correction will generally occur "on the fly" during acquisition, so that any projection data available for processing will have been already corrected for nonuniformities.

Another image restoration technique important for SPECT acquisitions is the center of rotation (COR) correction, which ensures perfect alignment of the mechanical axis of rotation of the camera detector(s) with the electronic axis of rotation of the image reconstruction matrix. Without this correction, "tuning fork" artifacts and general image degradation may appear in the reconstructed images. The usual way to perform the COR correction is to acquire a 360-degree SPECT study of a point source, then plot the (x,y) position of the point source's centroid on the projection images as a function of the projection angle. If alignment were perfect, the Y (axial) coordinate of the point source would be constant, while the X (transaxial) coordinate would describe a sinusoidal curve of amplitude proportional to the source's distance from the physical axis of rotation. Deviations from this ideal behavior are used to compute correction matrices to be stored in the computer hard disk and applied to all subsequent studies. On multidetector cameras, COR correction also allows to check the registration of the different detectors. COR correction can be performed less often than nonuniformity correction (weekly vs. daily). Motion correction algorithms, which realign the projection data before reconstruction, have recently been developed and validated (10).

Image Enhancement

Image enhancement is the process of altering the acquired image or set of images so as to make them ready for visual or quantitative analysis. Enhancing an image may consist in changing its temporal or spatial resolution, contrast, and uniformity. Because these parameters are interrelated, maximizing one can be done only at the expense of others. A trade-off depending on the particular study or type of analysis desired is usually sought. Most types of image enhancement involve the use of filters. Images are generally thought of and represented in the conventional 2-D or 3-D space, i.e., in the space domain. However, filters are just as often defined in the frequency or Fourier domain. We shall now attempt to briefly explain the relationship between these two concepts.

Space and Frequency Domain

The often misunderstood concept of frequency domain is easier to appreciate if one thinks of it as of a different way to express size and distance relationship between physical objects in an image. In the simplified case in Fig. 12.5, rectangular objects of different sizes regularly repeat themselves along the horizontal direction, spaced by a distance equal to their horizontal dimension. In spatial domain terms, one would say that the first object repeats itself every 20 pixels, the second every 10 pixels, and the third every 2 pixels. In frequency domain terms, one could equivalently say that the frequency of occurrence of the objects is 0.05 times per pixel (or, in common parlance, 0.05 cycles/pixel), 0.1 cycles/pixel, and 0.5 cycles/pixel, respectively. This reasoning can be extended to a 2-D or 3-D situation, the basic concept remaining the following: Distance or size in the spatial domain corresponds (with inverse relationship) to frequency in the frequency domain. Consequently, small structures in an image are said to have high frequency, and image resolution is often expressed as a percentage of the Nyquist frequency (Ny), i.e., the highest frequency that can be displayed in the image matrix (9). The Nyquist frequency is by definition equal to 0.5 cycles/pixel, and it obviously depends on the pixel size of the image matrix, which in turn depends on the matrix size and the acquisition/reconstruction zoom factor. To be accurate, what we refer to as frequency should be more correctly termed *spatial frequency*, because an analogous relationship to the one between space and spatial frequency exists between time and temporal frequency. An example of the latter relationship is the phase analysis technique, which is chiefly used in first-pass and blood pool imaging.

The mathematical operator that allows us to pass from the space to the frequency domain is the Fourier transform. The reason why the Fourier transform and the frequency or Fourier domain are so extensively used in image processing is because the relatively complex operation of convolution of two functions in the physical space is equivalent to the simple multiplication of their Fourier transforms in the frequency domain. Of particular relevance to nuclear cardiology, filtering a count profile can be accomplished by multiplying the Fourier transforms of the filter and the profile.

Filters

In the frequency domain, high frequencies correspond to small structures or areas of sharp changes in image intensity [i.e., bone edges in an x-ray film of the hand, brain gyri in a SPECT, positron emission tomography (PET) or magnetic resonance (MR) study of the head, small tumors in whole body planar or SPECT studies, or a small defect in a SPECT or PET myocardial perfusion study], whereas low frequencies correspond to relatively large and uniform image areas. If one wants to increase the resolution of an image, one can amplify its high frequencies or attenuate its low frequencies; if one wants to blur the image, one must do the opposite. The filters most used in nuclear medicine are passive filters, of which a low-pass and a high-pass representative example are shown in Fig. 12.6. By displaying filters in the frequency domain, one gains an intuitive appreciation of their operation: Low-pass filters let low frequencies pass, while progressively attenuating higher frequencies. Because image noise has high frequency, low-pass or smoothing filters are applied to projection images before reconstruction and serve the purpose of reducing statistical noise early in the processing chain.

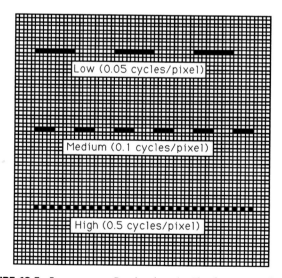

FIGURE 12.5. Frequency or Fourier domain. The frequency of occurrence of the long, medium, or short objects can be expressed as the inverse of the number of pixels between two consecutive objects. The frequency of 0.5 cycles/pixels (Nyquist frequency) is the highest achievable, because the unit of image resolution is 1 pixel. As a general rule, high frequencies are associated with small objects and low frequencies with large, uniform objects.

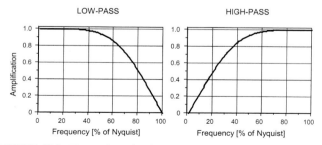

FIGURE 12.6. Curves (transfer functions) describing a representative low-pass **(left)** and high-pass filter **(right)** in the frequency domain. A low-pass filter progressively attenuates (amplification <1) higher frequencies, whereas a high-pass filter increasingly attenuates lower frequencies. [From Germano G. The physics of myocardial SPECT imaging. *J Nucl Med* 2001 *(in press)*, with permission.]

(Preamplifiers are used in hi-fi stereo equipment for essentially the same reason.) The price to pay, of course, is a loss of contrast and edge definition in the image. High-pass filters, on the other hand, reduce the influence of large, uniform structures: Their use is essentially limited to the ramp filter used during filtered backprojection reconstruction to minimize the star artifact, as seen in Fig. 12.2.

The most popular low-pass filters used in nuclear cardiology belong to the Hanning and the Butterworth families. Hanning filters had been traditionally employed to process ^{201}Tl images; Butterworth filters were initially preferred for ^{99m}Tc images, but their flexibility and ease of design have made them the filters of choice in most nuclear medicine procedures today.

A Butterworth filter in the frequency (f) domain is shaped like a curve described by the equation

$$B(f) = \frac{1}{1 + \left(\frac{f}{f_c}\right)^{2n}} \qquad [1]$$

where f_c is the critical or cutoff frequency, and n the order of the filter. From simple mathematical considerations it is apparent that any Butterworth filter has amplitude 1 when f is small (low frequencies), amplitude 0 when f is large (high frequencies), and amplitude 0.5 at $f = f_c$. However, the mode of transition from one to zero can be profoundly altered by acting on the filter's parameters n and f_c. Essentially, the order of a Butterworth filter controls the slope of the transition, while its critical frequency f_c controls the location of the slope's middle point (Fig. 12.7). *NOTE:* It is important to be aware of the fact that there is some confusion as to the units of measurement for the critical frequency of a Butterworth filter. Although some prefer to express it as a 0 to 1 numeric range, 1 being the highest attainable frequency or 100% of the Nyquist frequency; others point out that the Nyquist frequency is by definition equivalent to 0.5 cycles/pixel and adopt a 0 to 0.5 range instead. In other words, the *same* cutoff or critical frequency can be reported as 0.3 or 0.6 on two different camera systems. Whether a critical frequency is expressed in cycles/pixel or as a fraction of the Nyquist frequency, it should be clear that any measurement expressed in frequency terms must always be accompanied by knowledge of the pixel size value.

Generally speaking, the smaller the area encompassed by the response curve of a filter in the frequency domain, the fewer the spatial frequencies that are not attenuated and the smoother the resulting image. Fig. 12.8 shows that application of Butterworth filters of increasingly lower critical frequency results in reconstructed images that are increasingly smoother. Varying the order of a Butterworth filter has a more subtle effect on the final image, with higher order generally corresponding to slightly smoother images.

In addition to passive filters, active filters such as the Metz and Wiener adaptive filter (11) have gained some degree of popularity in nuclear cardiology. Their appeal lies in the ability to provide both amplification and attenuation of frequencies in selected ranges (so as to, ideally, reduce noise without unduly penalizing resolution) (Fig. 12.9); however, limited clinical validation makes it difficult at this time to assess their comparative value vis-á-vis passive filters.

Image Reorientation (SPECT)

SPECT images that are the direct product of tomographic reconstruction are termed *transaxial,* because they represent planes (slices) perpendicular to the long axis of the patient but usually not perpendicular to the long axis of the left ventricle. Moreover, the angle of intersection between the transaxial images and the left ventricle is not standardized, because the heart's orientation in a patient's chest varies amongst different individuals. To avoid artifactual inhomogeneities in the regional count densities caused by this variable angle and more effectively compare images from different patients, most visual and quantitative analysis is performed on the short-axis images, which are perpendicular to the left ventricle's long axis.

The transformation of transaxial into short-axis images is realized via the reorientation process. Reorientation typically consists of two operator-guided steps. First, a midventricular transaxial image is selected, and the left ventricle's long axis is manually drawn on that image (Fig. 12.10, **left**). The image volume is then reformatted along planes perpendicular to the transaxial plane and parallel to the left ventricle's long axis. The operator selects a sagittal image and draws the left ventricle's long axis in that plane (Fig. 12.10, **center**). The orientation of the long axis in the transaxial and the sagittal plane uniquely defines its orientation in the 3-D space, and the image volume is finally reformatted along planes perpendicular to that direction, generating a set of short-axis images (Fig. 12.10, **right**). It has been demonstrated that incorrectly performed reorientation can result in serious artifacts (12) and that the subjective operator-guided process is prone to interobserver and intraobserver variability.

Several algorithms have been proposed to automate the reorientation process. In one approach, an isosurface representing the left ventricle is generated using the marching cubes algorithm, and a nonlinear estimate of the left ventricle's long axis is determined from the normals to the polygons forming the isosurface (13). Other algorithms exploit the fact that the left ventricle has roughly ellipsoidal shape; therefore, its midsurface or "skeleton" can be fitted to a quadratic function in the 3-D space, with the major axis of the ellipsoid coinciding with that of the left ventricle's long axis (14,15). By virtue of being auto-

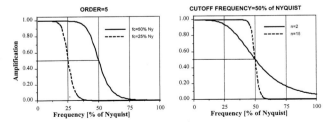

FIGURE 12.7. (Left) Butterworth filters of the same order ($n = 5$) but different critical frequency f_c (50% and 25% of Nyquist), and **(right)** Butterworth filters with the same critical frequency (50% of Nyquist) but different order ($n = 2$ and $n = 15$). These graphs show that the order of a Butterworth filter controls the slope of its transfer function, while its critical frequency f_c controls the location of the slope's middle point.

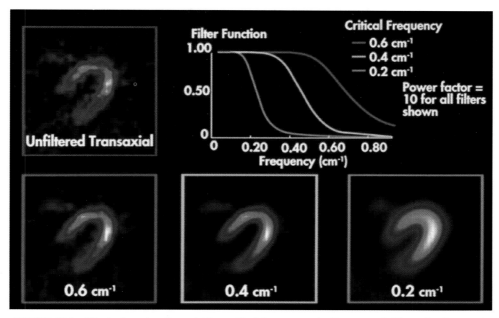

FIGURE 12.8. Effect of varying the cutoff or critical frequency of a Butterworth filter of order *n* = 5. Filtration is usually applied to the projection images before reconstruction, but its effect is shown on the reconstructed transaxial images. Because Butterworth filters are low-pass filters, application of any of them results in smoother images compared with no filtering. Lower critical frequencies correspond to increased smoothing, with the optimal value depending on the specific radioisotope and protocol used. Note that the power factor of a filter equals (by definition) twice its order and that all frequencies are expressed in cycles/cm rather than in cycles/pixel. (From Dupont Pharmaceutical Company, Billerica, MA, with permission.)

matic, these computer-based approaches eliminate the subjectivity in axis alignment, an important source of error in perfusion SPECT studies.

Scatter Correction

At the present, scatter correction is not routinely used with either planar or SPECT myocardial imaging. Both in planar and in

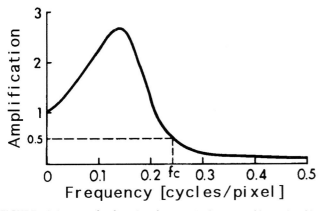

FIGURE 12.9. Transfer function for a typical Wiener filter. This filter amplifies mid-frequencies and attenuates higher ones. Note that the top frequency value of 0.5 cycles/pixel is equivalent to the 100% of Nyquist value in Fig. 12.6. (From Miller TR, Rollins, ES. A practical method of image enhancement by interactive digital filtering. *J Nucl Med* 1985;26:1075–1080, with permission.)

SPECT imaging, the great majority of the radiation emitted from the heart is scattered by the surrounding tissue through Compton-type interactions (see Chapter 1). Scattered γ-rays typically carry incorrect positional information and, if imaged, result in reduced lesion contrast (much as background activity in planar images). Most scattered radiation can be prevented from reaching the camera's detector by using a collimator; however, some scatter is always present because collimators must be efficient enough to yield images of good counting statistics. Rejection of scattered radiation that reaches the detector is routinely performed at the time of data acquisition by using an energy discrimination window centered on the isotope's photopeak; but once again, the window cannot be too tight for statistical reasons, i.e., excessive counts would be rejected. Consequently, scatter correction methods have been introduced that can be applied to the projection data at the image enhancement step. Most scatter correction methods rely on modern cameras' ability to acquire data in multiple energy windows. One popular approach uses a standard window centered on the isotope's photopeak and another at lower energy in the Compton region of the spectrum. The scatter image is scaled and subtracted from the photopeak image (16), yielding in first approximation, a scatter-purged image. Because scatter in the photopeak region is different from scatter at lower energies, alternative approaches have used two windows adjacent to each other and positioned on the photopeak so as to split it (17), a window centered on the photopeak and two small subwindows on both sides of the main window (18), or as many as 5 to 30 separate windows variously distributed on the spectrum (19).

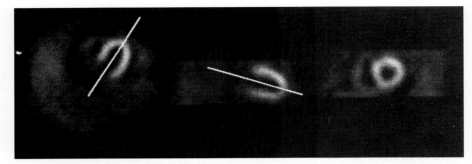

FIGURE 12.10. Reorientation of transaxial into short-axis images. The left ventricle long axis is determined in a transaxial image (**left**) and a vertical long axis image (**center**). Then, the image volume is resliced perpendicular to the left ventricle, resulting in doughnut-like short axis images (**right**).

Even a cursory review of the literature on scatter correction algorithms will reveal that no one algorithm is universally accepted. This is, at least in part, a consequence of the lack of comparative data on their relative efficacy, especially in clinical images. This limitation could be overcome through the acquisition of data in energy list mode and their successive sorting and processing as required by the various algorithms.

Attenuation Correction

Photon attenuation is a concept that applies to SPECT or planar imaging (its correction, however, is for practical purposes limited to SPECT), and is perhaps the single most serious impediment to absolute quantitation in myocardial SPECT. Photon attenuation refers to the partial absorption of radioactivity arising in the patient by the tissue structure of the body. In cardiac imaging, attenuation affects different areas of the heart differently, thus preventing an accurate measurement of relative amount of radioactivity in a given myocardial region. A recently developed approach to attenuation correction that has quickly become commercially applied in nuclear cardiology is the simultaneous emission/transmission technique. Transmission images can be acquired using a modified x-ray tube, a flood source, or a line source positioned opposite the detector. Their goal is that of providing pixel-specific tissue attenuation information from which spatially varying correction coefficients can be derived and used to modify the related emission images (20). Line sources are the most widely employed means of generating transmission images. In one approach, a tightly collimated line source (containing the same or a different isotope as was injected in the patient) is moved across the detector and electronically synchronized with a scanning window designed to acquire transmission information (transmitted through the patient), while the remainder of the detector acquires the emission data (emitted by the patient). In another approach, a stationary line source is positioned between two of a triple-detector camera's detectors, and transmission data is collected by the third detector, equipped with a fan-beam collimator (20). Whatever the method, it is generally accepted that attenuation correction ought to be performed in conjunction with scatter correction, downscatter correction (if the isotope used to generate transmission information has higher energy than the injected isotope), and compensation for resolution nonuniformities (20). It is hoped that these correc-

tions will eliminate or minimize differences between images of normal male and female patients, as well as nonuniformities in a given patient study caused by nonuniform tissue attenuation. To date, however, the implementation of attenuation correction with SPECT has not become widespread. Because the ability to perform attenuation correction based on simultaneously acquired transmission/emission data requires considerable expense to purchase the transmission hardware, its success will ultimately depend on full clinical validation of its incremental diagnostic and prognostic value and clear demonstration of its cost effectiveness compared with alternative approaches and techniques.

Background Subtraction in Planar Images

SPECT does not require background subtraction, because it maps the 3-D distribution of a radioisotope onto a 3-D image volume. On the other hand, planar imaging compresses that same 3-D distribution into a 2-D image, which will contain contributions from structures underlying and overlying the heart. These spurious contributions, cumulatively termed background, reduce the visibility of perfusion defects in the myocardium. A processing approach that minimizes background contributions is the bilinear interpolative background subtraction technique developed by Goris et al. (21), and later modified by Watson et al. (22). In this approach, a human operator defines the heart's location by sizing and positioning a rectangular boundary region tightly around the heart in the planar image. The region serves as a mask in that all pixels outside it are zeroed. The value of each pixel P(x,y) inside the mask is modified by subtracting from it an estimated, spatially variant background value based on the shortest distance of P(x,y) from the four sides of the mask and the pixel values at the mask's boundary. In different implementations of interpolative background subtraction, the boundary region is irregular, polygonal, or elliptical, no one method being clearly superior to the others.

Image Display

Image display is specific to the particular type of images being displayed. For example, a complete set of projection images is usually viewed by endless loop cine display of the image sequence, so as to give the impression of rotation around the patient and allow the viewer to identify patient or organ motion that occurred during acquisition. Static SPECT studies are displayed not as 3-D volumes, but as a series of 2-D images presented side by side, for immediate visualization of perfusion in the entire myocardium. Specifically, at Cedars-Sinai the images are arranged in four rows of 8 (16 short-axis, 8 vertical, and 8 horizontal long-axis): Left to right, the short-axis images progress from apex to base, the vertical long-axis images from the septal to the lateral wall, and the horizontal long-axis from the inferior to the anterior wall of the left ventricle. When two studies (i.e., rest and stress perfusion) are displayed together, their rows are interlaced to permit easier comparison of homologous images. By convention, the myocardial apex will point upward in the horizontal long-axis images and rightward in the vertical long-axis images (Fig. 12.11).

As for gated SPECT studies, because each image is now displayed over the 8 to 16 frames of the cardiac cycle, showing all 2-D myocardial slices simultaneously would result in too much information to easily interpret. We therefore recommend a 5-slice display in which three representative short-axis slices (apical, midventricular, and basal), as well as one vertical long axis and one horizontal long axis midventricular tomogram, are viewed in a cine format. Nuclear cardiology images are displayed in a gray or monochrome scale or a multicolor format. A ten-step color scale is often used to visually assess myocardial thickening or gauge the relative activity of different organs or structures in the image.

Three-dimensional displays are implemented through surface or volume rendering techniques. Surface rendering is essentially equivalent to threshold-based segmentation plus surface extraction. The extracted surface is approximated by a wire mesh tiled with a mosaic of polygons or by the outward faces of the voxels (cuberilles) belonging to the surface itself; in either case, the main depth cue is derived from simulated illumination of the

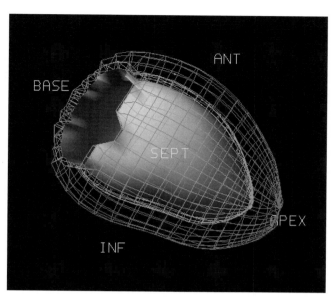

FIGURE 12.12. Three-dimensional display of a gated perfusion single photon emission computed tomography study. The shaded surface, inner grid, and outer grid represent the endocardium, endocardium at end-diastole, and epicardium, respectively, and cineing through the acquisition frames will give the illusion of a pulsating heart.

surface (Fig. 12.12). Surface rendering is the least computationally demanding form of rendering, because it discards all nonsurface information about the rendered object. That notwithstanding, interactive manipulation of surface-rendered images requires real-time redrawing of all the polygons in the wire mesh and may prove computationally onerous.

Volume rendering visualizes data from the entire image volume, as opposed to from just a surface. This is accomplished by tracing rays from each pixel in the rendered image plane to the sampled image volume (backward mapping) or by directly mapping the sampled image volume onto the rendered image plane (forward mapping). The advantages of volume rendering are that the final image retains more information and does not suffer from artifacts consequent to incorrect surface determination (23); however, every voxel in the image volume must be processed, and the algorithm is more computationally expensive.

IMAGE ANALYSIS AND QUANTIFICATION

The goal of a nuclear cardiac study is to gain information on the state of the heart, and various types of computerized image analysis allow us to extract that information from processed cardiac images. Region of interest (ROI) analysis measures the average number of counts in a group of contiguous image pixels; in case of a dynamic acquisition, time-activity curves can be generated and then fitted to a variety of mathematical functions. Parametric imaging aims at extracting distinctive information from an image or set of images, presenting it in a succinct and visually effective manner. Forms of image analysis essential to quantification include "segmentation" to isolate the heart from neighboring structures, as well as the application of edge detection or

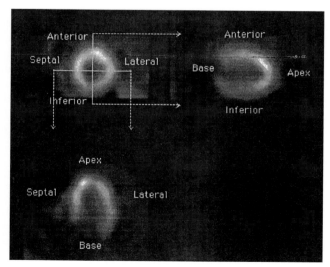

FIGURE 12.11. Standardized display of myocardial perfusion images. A midventricular short-axis image **(top left)**, vertical long-axis image **(top right)**, and horizontal long-axis image **(bottom)** are shown. The solid lines depict the locations of the displayed vertical and horizontal long-axis views.

pattern recognition algorithms to precisely outline the boundaries of the LV cavity or the myocardium.

ROIs and Time-Activity Curves

A ROI is a 2-D or 3-D curve encompassing a number of contiguous pixels or voxels, and is used to measure the average activity (average number of counts) in various regions of planar or SPECT images. As a general rule, ROIs should be large enough to average out statistical noise but small enough to minimize the count loss from the partial volume effect. Partial volume penalizes objects of dimensions smaller than twice the image resolution, making the apparent concentration of activity in those objects lower than the true concentration (Fig. 12.13) (24). Thus, an ROI centered on the maximal-count pixel of a large object will yield measurements fairly independent of the ROI's size, whereas an ROI centered on the maximal-count pixel of a small object will yield measurements of value inversely proportional to the ROI's size. Based on the reconstructed resolution [10- to 20-mm full width at half maximum (FWHM)] of current camera systems, the LV cavity can be considered a large object, but the myocardial wall cannot. This requires that extreme caution be used when collecting data from myocardial ROIs. On the other hand, the partial volume effect is very helpful in the assessment of systolic myocardial thickening from gated SPECT imaging, because it can be assumed that myocardial "brightness" (in the image) and actual myocardial thickness are linearly proportional, making the apparent myocardial brightening between diastole and systole a good proxy for myocardial thickening.

All dynamic acquisition protocols produce image datasets from which time-activity curves can be derived. A time-activity curve is a discrete function displaying the average count activity in a fixed ROI as a function of the temporal frame at which imaging takes place. In planar first-pass imaging, a ROI can be positioned on the LV cavity so that the initial transit of a bolus of radioactivity through the left ventricle can be followed. Because frames in first-pass studies are very tightly spaced (each lasting on the order of 10 milliseconds), the temporal resolution of the related time-activity curve is excellent, allowing the extraction of information such as time of arrival, the rise time, and the time to maximum. In dynamic myocardial SPECT imaging, it is possible to place an ROI on a myocardial wall and derive a time-activity curve showing a radioisotope's uptake and washout from the myocardium (5). A time-activity curve is a discrete sequence of data points, but it can be approximated by or fitted to a continuous mathematical function of time. Fitting consists in (a) selecting a type of function whose general shape matches that of the time-activity curve and then (b) iteratively varying the function's parameters to improve the match. In the least-squares fitting method, the optimal match is obtained by minimizing the squared distances of the data points from the fitting function. The fitting process reduces the statistical variability intrinsic to the data, thus representing a form of smoothing.

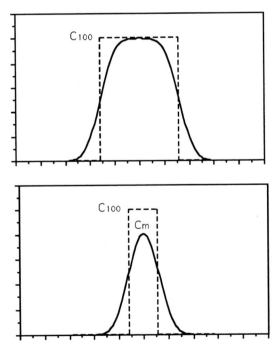

FIGURE 12.13. Partial volume effect. When an object containing a uniform concentration of radioactivity (*dashed line, top*) is larger than twice the resolution of the nuclear camera system; the imaged distribution (*solid line, top*) is somewhat blurred but its maximum value coincides with the original concentration C100. If, however, the object is smaller (*dashed line, bottom*), the maximum value of the imaged distribution Cm is lower than C100 (*solid line, bottom*). In other words, the recovery coefficient of the activity distribution in the bottom graph is <1. (From Hoffman EJ, Huang SC, Phelps ME. Quantitation in positron emission computed tomography: 1. Effect of object size. *J Comput Assist Tomogr* 1979;3:299–308, with permission.)

Phase Analysis and Parametric Images

An interesting generalization of the ROI concept is to consider each pixel in the image as an ROI; in other words, time-activity curves can be generated for every pixel in the image. The main application of this technique is phase analysis of gated planar first-pass or blood pool studies, although the same analysis can be performed for each voxel in gated SPECT blood pool studies. Phase analysis is based on the principle that every function can be expressed as the sum of a series of sine and/or cosine functions of different frequencies and amplitudes. Because time-activity curves for a gated blood pool study are periodic functions without major discontinuities, in their case the series can be truncated to its first harmonic component. In other words, every time-activity curve can be expressed by the equation

$$f(t) = A_0 + A_1 \cos(\phi_t + \phi_1)$$

where A_0, A_1, and ϕ_1 are different for each (x,y) pixel in the LV blood pool. A phase image is then the collection of all the phases $\phi_1(x,y)$ of the pixel-specific time-activity curves; if the left ventricle contracts synchronously or in phase, all $\phi_1(x,y)$ will be similar in value, and the phase image representation of the left ventricle will have uniform brightness or color. Similarly, two amplitude images can be built by collecting all the $A_0(x,y)$ and $A_1(x,y)$ values. An example of phase and amplitude images

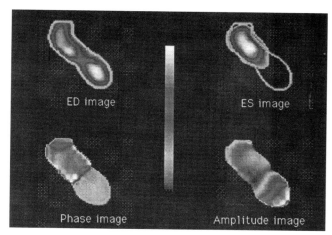

FIGURE 12.14. ⁹⁹ᵐTechnetium-sestamibi first-pass study of a normal patient. **(Top)** End-diastolic (ED) and end-systolic (ES) images with superimposed end-diastolic contour, and **(bottom)** phase and amplitude images. Note the uniformity of color in the left ventricular (LV) portion of the phase image, indicating uniform contraction of the LV myocardium. The amplitude image has a wider range of colors in the same area, reflecting the fact that different parts of the myocardium move by different amounts, albeit in phase.

for a gated planar first-pass study performed on a normal patient is shown in Fig. 12.14.

The phase and amplitude images in Fig. 12.14 are parametric images, because they focus on a particular piece of information or parameter in the original image set and present it in a condensed, more readily interpretable format. Specifically, they are "true" parametric images, because, all together, they contain full information on the study from which they originate. To the extent that the first harmonic approximation of time-activity curves is valid, the entire gated planar first-pass or blood pool study can be reconstituted from the knowledge of the three parameters $A_0(x,y)$, $A_1(x,y)$, and $\phi_1(x,y)$.

Most parametric images do not contain enough information to allow mathematical reconstruction of the original image data; however, they are important because of their synthetic power and immediate ability to convey physiologic meaning. Fig. 12.12 is a parametric image because only the endocardial and epicardial LV surfaces are shown and not the entire 3-D myocardium. Other examples of parametric images are the perfusion polar maps (Fig. 12.15), which contain one maximal count circumferential profile from each short-axis image in the stress or the rest dataset and display the profiles as concentric annuli or rings having either the same thickness (distance-weighted polar maps) or thicknesses representative of the volume of the myocardium in the individual slices (volume-weighted polar maps) (25). Parametric images are also useful to visualize cardiac function, including ejection fraction (EF), stroke volume, myocardial motion, and myocardial thickening.

Image Segmentation and Edge Detection

Every type of cardiac quantification must start with the isolation (segmentation) of the structure to be quantified. The simplest form of image segmentation is thresholding. If the heart is the

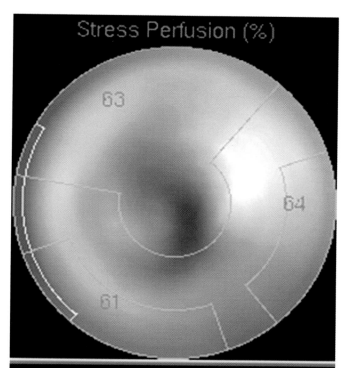
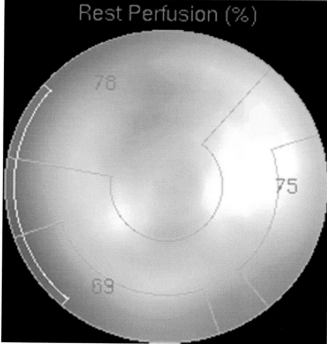

FIGURE 12.15. Distance-weighted two-dimensional polar maps for a stress **(top)** and a rest **(bottom)** perfusion single photon emission computed tomography study of the same patient. The standard coronary artery territories are superimposed on the images and demonstrate a stress perfusion abnormality in the left anterior descending coronary territory.

"hottest" structure in an image, setting to zero all the pixels below a certain fraction of the image's maximal pixel count will reduce or eliminate extracardiac activity. Unfortunately, in myocardial perfusion studies, hepatic activity may be well above that of the heart (26) and pulmonary, splenic, and intestinal uptake is often of concern. In addition, the relatively poor image resolution causes spillover of activity (24), so that organs containing radioactivity and in close proximity of one another may appear connected (e.g., the left and right ventricle in gated blood pool SPECT studies). In planar studies, it is especially problematic to separate the ventricles from the atria.

More sophisticated approaches to segmentation have been devised that use adaptive thresholding or knowledge of the expected location, size, and shape of the heart. An example of segmentation of the left ventricle in a planar ^{99m}Tc-sestamibi image with prominent intestinal uptake is shown in Fig. 12.16. In this case, the heuristic criteria used are that the left ventricle ought to be in the upper right area of the image, have size within the physiologic range, and have a doughnut-like shape. In gated studies, isolation of the LV cavity or myocardium can also be effected by identifying and clustering pixels whose count value changes the most during the cardiac cycle, based on the assumption that count variations are a consequence of motion of activity-containing structures.

Once segmentation has identified and isolated the heart in the image volume, heart edges, or boundaries are generally determined using some form of edge detection. Edge detection may involve thresholding (27), Gaussian fitting of count profiles across the myocardium (28), or moment analysis (29) or gradient analysis of the count distribution in the myocardium (30) or the LV cavity (31). Gradient analysis typically identifies the LV epicardial and/or endocardial surfaces as the collections of the local minima and maxima of the count distributions across the left ventricle, although this approach is quite sensitive to noise and may require the combined use of smoothing techniques. Another approach, applicable to perfusion SPECT imaging, starts by extracting the maximal count or midmyocardial surface and then estimates the location of the endocardium and epicardium by assuming a fixed myocardial thickness (32). Regardless of the methodology used, edge detection should ideally succeed even in the presence of discontinuities in the image data (Fig. 12.17). This is often feasible, if the discontinuities are "filled in" using appropriate constraints based on the geometry and smoothness of the immediately adjacent areas.

Quantitation of SPECT Perfusion

Quantitation of SPECT myocardial perfusion is based on the measurement of myocardial counts in a number of regions or samples covering the entire myocardium, followed by their comparison to the normal count distribution for a similar patient. Perfusion is not measured in absolute terms (mL/minute/g) but is generally normalized to the myocardial region with the highest uptake. Given the large amount of perfusion data contained in a SPECT image, a parametric approach is used in which either the maximal or the average count value in a region is taken to

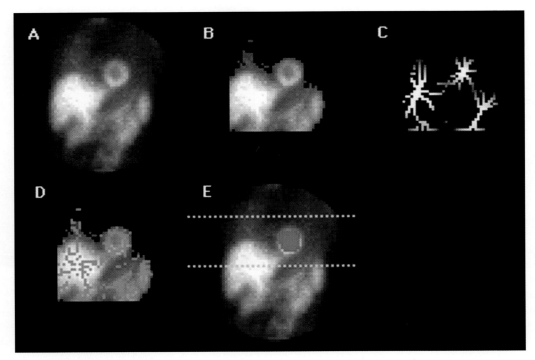

FIGURE 12.16. Automatic segmentation of the left ventricular (LV) myocardium in a projection image. The image **(A)** is masked **(B)**, then iteratively convolved with a two-dimensional Gaussian function **(C)**. A second convolution process is followed by local maxima extraction (dots in **D**). A ring encompassing the best star in **C** is sought in **D**. This ring bounds the LV myocardium (red patch in **E**). (From Germano G, Kavanagh PB, Chen J, et al. Operator-less processing of myocardial perfusion SPECT studies. *J Nucl Med* 1995;36:2127–2132, with permission.)

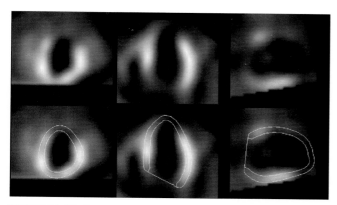

FIGURE 12.17. Representative short axis and horizontal and vertical long axis ^{99m}Tc-sestamibi images **(left to right)** of a patient with a severe apical perfusion defect. Use of an appropriate edge detection algorithm will result in the generation of accurate contours **(bottom)**.

be representative of the entire region. The number of samples depends on the sampling scheme. Traditional sampling involves the extraction of a maximal count circumferential profile from each short-axis image in the stress and the rest data sets, according to a hybrid sampling scheme that models the LV myocardium as having cylindrical shape in its most basal two thirds and spherical shape at the apex (32) (Fig. 12.18). The circumferential

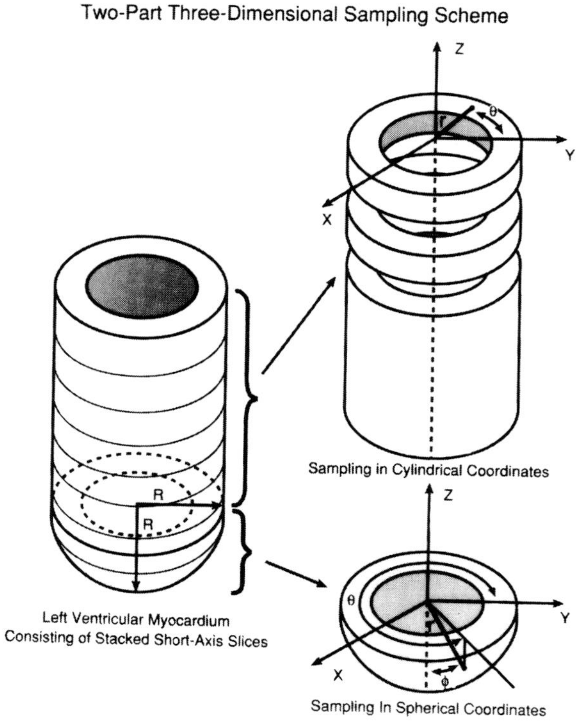

Two-Part Three-Dimensional Sampling Scheme

Sampling in Cylindrical Coordinates

Left Ventricular Myocardium Consisting of Stacked Short-Axis Slices

Sampling In Spherical Coordinates

FIGURE 12.18. Traditional sampling for maximal count circumferential profiles extraction from stacked perfusion single photon emission computed tomography images (short axis). (From Garcia EV, Bateman TM, Berman DS, et al. Computer techniques for optimal radionuclide assessment of the heart. In: Gottschalk A, Hoffer PB, Potchen EJ, eds. *Diagnostic nuclear medicine,* vol 1, 2nd ed. Baltimore: Williams & Wilkins, 1988:259–290, with permission.)

profiles (each comprising 36 to 60 equally spaced maximal count samples) are combined in 2-D polar maps. Thus, polar maps contain a variable number of circumferential profiles (proportional to the number of short-axis slices, i.e., to the size of the myocardium), which are displayed as concentric annuli or rings having either the same thickness (distance-weighted polar maps) or thicknesses representative of the volume of the myocardium in the individual slices (volume-weighted polar maps) (25). More recent sampling schemes are independent of the size of the myocardium and use a fixed number of sample points (33) (e.g., 24 latitudinally, 32 longitudinally). The sampling grid may follow an ellipsoidal template that is fitted to the midmyocardial surface, thus maximizing the perpendicularity of the sampling profiles to the myocardium (34), and the resulting polar maps contain a standard number of data points, unrelated to myocardial size.

Quantitative assessment of SPECT perfusion abnormalities usually requires a number of steps. The first is the determination of the normal perfusion distribution of the radioisotope, defined as the mean and variance of the homologous pixel count values from the polar maps of at least 20 to 30 patients with a low likelihood of coronary artery disease studied with that radioisotope (the distribution is gender-specific and, to a lesser extent, protocol-specific). Then, the optimal criteria for detection of perfusion abnormalities are developed in a pilot population consisting of at least 60 normal and abnormal patients, with perfusion defects of different size, severity, and location adequately represented. The ideal goal is that of determining, for each pixel, the fractional number of standard deviations below normal at which perfusion in that pixel is deemed abnormal, although for practical purposes that determination is made for clusters of pixels or segments (typically, the myocardium is divided into 17 or 20 segments). Finally, the normal limits and criteria for abnormality are validated in a prospective population of characteristics similar to the pilot one, with coronary angiography as the gold standard for abnormalities. Myocardial pixels with abnormal perfusion can be "blacked out" in the 2-D polar map, so as to give an immediate impression of the extent of abnormality; moreover, the percentage of abnormal pixels can be expressed as a numeric value for each segment, vascular territory, myocardial wall, or for the entire myocardium (34,35). Recently developed software algorithms are also capable of automatically generating semiquantitative segmental perfusion scores analogous to those used in visual assessment of perfusion (32–34) (Fig. 12.19).

Quantitation of Gated SPECT Function

Global and regional parameters of LV function quantitated from gated perfusion SPECT images include ejection fraction, end-diastolic volume (EDV), end-systolic volume (ESV), and regional myocardial wall motion and thickening. Diastolic function assessment is generally not performed with gated SPECT (because it would require too large a number of gating intervals), nor is RV assessment, although the latter is feasible with gated blood pool SPECT (36). Quantitation of gated SPECT function is mostly based on 3-D geometry and not counts: For example, the LV cavity volume is the product of an individual voxel's

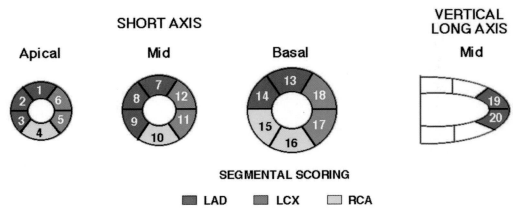

FIGURE 12.19. Diagrammatic representation of segmental division of the single photon emission computed tomography slices and the assignment of individual segments to individual coronary arteries using the 20-segment model. Each segment is scored using a 0 to 4 scale (0, normal; 1/2/3, slightly/moderately/ severely reduced; 4, absent perfusion). LAD, left anterior descending coronary artery; LCX, left circumflex coronary artery; RCA, right coronary artery. (From Berman DS, Germano G. An approach to the interpretation and reporting of gated myocardial perfusion SPECT. In Germano G, Berman DS, eds. *Clinical gated cardiac SPECT.* Armonk, NY: Futura Publishing, 1999:147–182, with permission.)

volume and the number of voxels bound by the LV endocardium and valve plane. The left ventricular ejection fraction (LVEF) value is given by the simple ratio

$$LVEF = (EDV - ESV)/EDV$$

Detection of the 3-D surfaces necessary for function quantitation is generally accomplished using one of the edge detection techniques described earlier, and 3-D sampling is conducted in the same way as for perfusion, leading to perfect registration of perfusion and function data in gated perfusion SPECT.

The published literature on gated SPECT quantitation indicates that measurements of LVEF and ES or ED volumes are overall quite accurate, as determined for a variety of radiopharmaceuticals and validated against a large number of "gold standards" (37). The reproducibility of these measurements is by definition perfect if the algorithm used to derive them is completely automatic, but is generally very good even if some degree of manual operation is required. The repeatability (agreement of the quantitative measurements from separate gated SPECT studies of the same patient) is also excellent, making gated SPECT an ideal technique for serial assessment of patients undergoing medical or surgical therapy.

There are some limitations to quantitation of global function from gated SPECT. For example, it has been shown that the relatively low resolution of nuclear cardiology images can lead to an underestimation of the LV cavity size in patients with small ventricles, particularly at end-systole, the end result being an overestimation of the LVEF (38). This phenomenon can be alleviated by magnifying the left ventricle either in acquisition (by employing a larger acquisition zoom) and/or in reconstruction (by employing zoomed centered or zoomed off-axis reconstruction). Conversely, gated SPECT imaging is usually performed with 8-frame gating, which leads to mild underestimation of the LVEF (as a result of the smoothing of the time-volume curve) compared with 16-frame gating. However, the degree of underestimation has been shown to be small

(three to four LVEF percentage points) and remarkably uniform over a wide range of EFs (28).

Quantitative measurements of regional function from gated perfusion SPECT can be obtained by measuring the excursion of the endocardium from end diastole (ED) to end systole (ES) [wall motion, (30,39,40)], by measuring the apparent brightening of the myocardium from ED to ES resulting from the partial volume effect [wall thickening, (32,41,42)], or by a combination of the two (39). Although published validation studies for gated SPECT-derived measurements of myocardial wall motion and thickening are not as numerous as for volumes and LVEF, this is likely to change in the future. As with SPECT perfusion, quantitative measurements of abnormal regional function, as well as semiquantitative segmental scores for myocardial wall motion and thickening, can be automatically generated by software. Gated blood pool SPECT is unable to measure epicardial surfaces or myocardial thickening but is superior to perfusion SPECT for combined LV and RV function assessment.

There are a number of additional quantitative parameters, indirectly related to perfusion or function, that can be measured from a typical cardiac SPECT study as routinely performed at most institutions (Fig. 12.20). Among them, the lung/heart ratio (43), the transient ischemic dilation (TID) ratio (ratio of the LV cavity volumes poststress and at rest) (44), and the LV mass (volume bound by the LV epicardium, endocardium, and valve plane) (45).

FUTURE DIRECTIONS

A complete discussion of future applications of computers to nuclear cardiology is beyond the scope of this chapter; however, it is useful to highlight some select issues beyond image processing and analysis. An important area of software development will involve improving the portability and ease of exchange of image files. Most nuclear medicine companies have agreed to

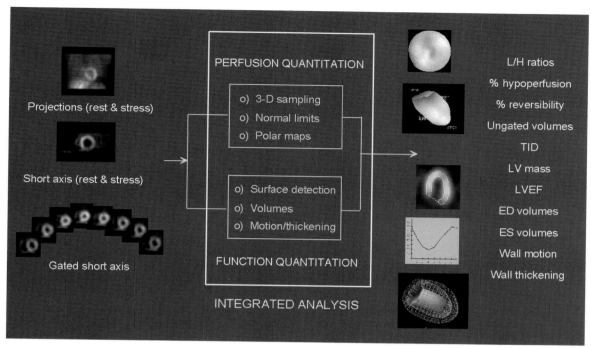

FIGURE 12.20. Quantitative parameters that can be measured from a rest/stress gated perfusion single photon emission computed tomography protocol. (From Germano G, Berman DS. Quantitative gated perfusion SPECT. In Germano G, Berman DS, eds. *Clinical gated cardiac SPECT.* Armonk, NY: Futura Publishing, 1999:115–146, with permission.)

support the Digital Imaging and Communications in Medicine (DICOM) Standard, which specifies a nonproprietary data interchange protocol, digital image format, and file structure for biomedical images and image-related information. Ideally, DICOM compliance would allow data to be acquired on one vendor's computer; transferred across a local- or wide-area network; and processed, quantified, and/or displayed on another vendor's (or a low-cost, nonproprietary) workstation. In reality, different vendors' DICOM implementations are not always perfectly compatible, but practical progress to achieve this goal is expected in the near future. Also, because DICOM interfaces to other information systems provide for shared management of patient, procedure, and results information related to images, it is hoped that the nuclear cardiology images will soon be integrated with those pertaining to other imaging modalities. This opportunity is responsible for the increasing activity in the development of image correlation and registration techniques, an obvious example of which relates to the merging of anatomic modalities, such as magnetic resonance imaging (MRI) or computed tomography (CT), with functional modalities like SPECT. Integration of image and nonimage data is proceeding in concert with the diffusion of radiology information systems (RIS) and hospital-wide information systems (HIS), and advances in the compression and transmission of large image datasets will occur in the context of telemedicine and local- or wide-area networks. Additional areas of technical development will include the development and validation of criteria for abnormality of regional wall motion and thickening, approaches for quantitatively assessing diastolic function, and methods incorporating the degree of reversibility of defects into criteria for abnormality in perfusion

SPECT studies, as well as, potentially, methods for artifact recognition.

A drive to standardize the format and content of nuclear cardiology reports is under way (46) and will likely lead to much greater uniformity in how perfusion and function information is related to the referring physician. Automatic generation of standardized reports will require algorithms to translate quantitative parameter values into natural language, including statements on patient prognosis as derived from a continually growing number of single- and multicenter patient databases. The role of outcomes research and data mining is sure to increase in the future and will be key to improving patient care while reducing costs.

REFERENCES

1. Bacharach SL, Bonow RO, Green MV. Comparison of fixed and variable temporal resolution methods for creating gated cardiac blood-pool image sequences. *J Nucl Med* 1990;31:38–42.
2. Bracewell R, Riddle A. Inversion of fan-beam scans in radioastronomy. *Astrophys J* 1967;150:427–434.
3. Shepp LA, Logan BF. The Fourier reconstruction of a head section. *IEEE Trans Nucl Sci* 1974;-21(3):21–43.
4. Germano G, Berman D. Acquisition and processing for gated perfusion SPECT: technical aspects. In: G Germano and D Berman, eds. *Clinical gated cardiac SPECT.* Armonk, NY: Futura Publishing, 1999:93–113.
5. Chua T, Kiat H, Germano G et al. Technetium-99m teboroxime regional myocardial washout in subjects with and without coronary artery disease. *Am J Cardiol* 1993;72:728–734.
6. Smith AM, Gullberg GT, Christian PE. Experimental verification of technetium 99m-labeled teboroxime kinetic parameters in the myocardium with dynamic single-photon emission computed tomography:

reproducibility, correlation to flow, and susceptibility to extravascular contamination. *J Nucl Cardiol* 1996;3:130–142.

7. Lewellen TK, Miyaoka RS, Kohlmyer SG et al. An XYE acquisition interface for General Electric Starcam Anger cameras. *Proc IEEE Med Imag Conf* 1991;vol 3:1861–1865.

8. Pollard KR, Lewellen TK, Kaplan MS et al. Energy-based scatter corrections for scintillation camera images of iodine-131. *J Nucl Med* 1996; 37:2030–2037.

9. Sorenson JA, Phelps ME. *Physics in nuclear medicine,* 2nd ed. Orlando, FL: Grune & Stratton, 1987.

10. Matsumoto N, Berman D, Kavanagh P et al. Quantitative validation of a new patient motion correction program for myocardial perfusion SPECT. *J Nucl Med* 2000;41(5):45P–46P (abst).

11. King MA, Schwinger RB, Doherty PW et al. Two-dimensional filtering of SPECT images using the Metz and Wiener filters. *J Nucl Med* 1984; 25:1234–1240.

12. DePuey EG, Garcia EV. Optimal specificity of thallium-201 SPECT through recognition of imaging artifacts [see comments]. *J Nucl Med* 1989;30:441–449.

13. Mullick R, Ezquerra NF. Automatic determination of LV orientation from SPECT data. *IEEE Trans Med Imaging* 1995;14:88–99.

14. Cauvin JC, Boire JY, Maublant JC et al. Automatic detection of the left ventricular myocardium long axis and center in thallium-201 single photon emission computed tomography. *Eur J Nucl Med* 1992;19: 1032–1037.

15. Germano G, Kavanagh PB, Su HT et al. Automatic reorientation of three-dimensional, transaxial myocardial perfusion SPECT images [see comments]. *J Nucl Med* 1995;36:1107–1114.

16. Jaszczak RJ, Greer KL, Floyd CE Jr et al. Improved SPECT quantification using compensation for scattered photons. *J Nucl Med* 1984;25: 893–900.

17. King MA, Hademenos GJ, Glick SJ. A dual-photopeak window method for scatter correction. *J Nucl Med* 1992;33:605–612.

18. Ogawa K, Harata Y, Ichihara T et al. A practical method for position-dependent Compton-scatter correction in single photon emission CT. *IEEE Trans Med Imaging* 1991;10:408–412.

19. Hannequin PP, Mas JF. Photon energy recovery: a method to improve the effective energy resolution of gamma cameras. *J Nucl Med* 1998; 39:555–562.

20. Cullom S, Case J, Bateman T. Attenuation correction in myocardial perfusion SPECT. In: DePuey EG, Garcia EV, Berman DS, eds. *Cardiac SPECT imaging,* 2nd ed. New York: Lippincott Williams & Wilkins, 2001:89–102.

21. Goris ML, Daspit SG, McLaughlin P et al. Interpolative background subtraction. *J Nucl Med* 1976;17:744–747.

22. Watson DD, Campbell NP, Read EK et al. Spatial and temporal quantitation of plane thallium myocardial images. *J Nucl Med* 1981;22: 577–584.

23. Wallis JW, Miller TR. Volume rendering in three-dimensional display of SPECT images [see comments]. *J Nucl Med* 1990;31:1421–1428.

24. Hoffman EJ, Huang SC, Phelps ME. Quantitation in positron emission computed tomography: 1. Effect of object size. *J Comput Assist Tomogr* 1979;3:299–308.

25. Germano G, Van Train K, Kiat H et al. Digital techniques for the acquisition, processing, and analysis of nuclear cardiology images. In: Sandler MP, ed. *Diagnostic nuclear medicine.* Baltimore: Williams & Wilkins, 1995:347–386.

26. Chua T, Kiat H, Germano G et al. Rapid back to back adenosine stress/rest technetium-99m teboroxime myocardial perfusion SPECT using a triple-detector camera. *J Nucl Med* 1993;34:1485–1493.

27. Nichols K, DePuey EG, Rozanski A. Automation of gated tomographic left ventricular ejection fraction. *J Nucl Cardiol* 1996;3(6 Pt 1): 475–482.

28. Germano G, Kiat H, Kavanagh PB et al. Automatic quantification of ejection fraction from gated myocardial perfusion SPECT. *J Nucl Med* 1995;36:2138–2147.

29. Goris ML, Thompson C, Malone LJ et al. Modelling the integration of myocardial regional perfusion and function. *Nucl Med Commun* 1994;15(1):9–20.

30. Faber TL, Stokely EM, Peshock RM et al. A model-based four-dimensional left ventricular surface detector. *IEEE Trans Med Imaging* 1991; 10:321–329.

31. Faber TL, Stokely EM, Templeton GH et al. Quantification of three-dimensional left ventricular segmental wall motion and volumes from gated tomographic radionuclide ventriculograms. *J Nucl Med* 1989; 30:638–649.

32. Faber TL, Cooke CD, Folks RD et al. Left ventricular function and perfusion from gated SPECT perfusion images: an integrated method. *J Nucl Med* 1999;40:650–659.

33. Ficaro E, Kritzman J, Corbett J. Development and clinical validation of normal Tc-99m sestamibi database: comparison of 3D-MSPECT to CEqual. *J Nucl Med* 1999;40(5):125P (abst).

34. Germano G, Kavanagh PB, Waechter P et al. A new algorithm for the quantitation of myocardial perfusion SPECT. I: technical principles and reproducibility. *J Nucl Med* 2000;41:712–719.

35. Sharir T, Germano G, Waechter PB et al. A new algorithm for the quantitation of myocardial perfusion SPECT. II: validation and diagnostic yield. *J Nucl Med* 2000;41:720–727.

36. Germano G, Van Kriekinge S, Berman D. Quantitative gated blood pool SPECT. In: Germano G, Berman D, eds. *Clinical gated cardiac SPECT.* Armonk, NY: Futura Publishing, 1999:339–347.

37. Germano G, Berman D. Quantitative gated perfusion SPECT. In: Germano G, Berman D, eds. *Clinical gated cardiac SPECT.* Armonk, NY: Futura Publishing, 1999:115–146.

38. Nakajima K, Taki J, Higuchi T et al. Gated SPECT quantification of small hearts: mathematical simulation and clinical application. *Eur J Nucl Med* 2000;27:1372–1379.

39. Germano G, Erel J, Lewin H et al. Automatic quantitation of regional myocardial wall motion and thickening from gated technetium-99m sestamibi myocardial perfusion single-photon emission computed tomography. *J Am Coll Cardiol* 1997;30:1360–1367.

40. Yang KT, Chen HD. Evaluation of global and regional left ventricular function using technetium-99m sestamibi ECG-gated single-photon emission tomography. *Eur J Nucl Med* 1998;25:515–521.

41. Stollfuss JC, Haas F, Matsunari I et al. Regional myocardial wall thickening and global ejection fraction in patients with low angiographic left ventricular ejection fraction assessed by visual and quantitative resting ECG-gated 99mTc-tetrofosmin single-photon emission tomography and magnetic resonance imaging. *Eur J Nucl Med* 1998;25:522–530.

42. Fukuchi K, Uehara T, Morozumi T et al. Quantification of systolic count increase in technetium-99m-MIBI gated myocardial SPECT. *J Nucl Med* 1997;38:1067–1073.

43. Bacher-Stier C, Sharir T, Kavanagh PB et al. Postexercise lung uptake of 99mTc-sestamibi determined by a new automatic technique: validation and application in detection of severe and extensive coronary artery disease and reduced left ventricular function. *J Nucl Med* 2000;41: 1190–1197.

44. Mazzanti M, Germano G, Kiat H et al. Identification of severe and extensive coronary artery disease by automatic measurement of transient ischemic dilation of the left ventricle in dual-isotope myocardial perfusion SPECT. *J Am Coll Cardiol* 1996;27:1612–1620.

45. Maruyama K, Hasegawa S, Mu X et al. Assessment of left ventricular mass index by quantitative gated myocardial SPECT: comparison with echocardiography. *J Nucl Med* 2000;41(5):153P (abst).

46. Wackers F. Intersocietal Commission for the Accreditation of Nuclear Medicine Laboratories (ICANL) position statement on standardization and optimization of nuclear cardiology reports. *J Nucl Cardiol* 2000; 7:397–400.

Diagnostic Nuclear Medicine, Fourth Edition. Edited by M.P. Sandler, R.E. Coleman, J.A. Patton, F.J.Th. Wackers, A. Gottschalk. Lippincott Williams & Wilkins, Philadelphia 2003.

13

GENERAL CONCEPTS OF VENTRICULAR FUNCTION, MYOCARDIAL PERFUSION AND EXERCISE PHYSIOLOGY RELEVANT TO NUCLEAR CARDIOLOGY

MARVIN W. KRONENBERG
LEWIS C. BECKER

Knowledge of ventricular mechanics, the physiology of the coronary circulation, and exercise physiology is necessary for the accurate interpretation of radionuclide ventriculographic and myocardial perfusion images. This chapter outlines these important basic concepts. For further elaboration, and for subcellular and cellular mechanisms, the reader is referred to the texts in the list of suggested readings.

VENTRICULAR FUNCTION

Basic Concepts

Ventricular function is controlled by four major factors: preload, afterload, heart rate and rhythm, and contractility (Fig. 13.1). *Left ventricular performance* can be measured in several ways, some of which include stroke volume (volume ejected per beat), cardiac output (blood flow per minute), cardiac index (cardiac output per M^2 body surface area), and the ejection fraction (percent of end-diastolic volume ejected per beat). *Preload* is defined as the myocardial tension at end-diastole. It is estimated by myocardial segment length in the isolated muscle and by end-diastolic volume in the intact heart. *Afterload* is defined as the resistance to myocardial fiber shortening or the impedance to chamber contraction. Afterload may be estimated by the systolic load in papillary muscle experiments and by the systolic blood pressure or calculated wall stress in the intact heart. *Contractility* is defined as the intensity or quality of myocardial contraction. Each of these factors has multiple determinants. In addition to the properties of the veins and the arteries, neural and humoral factors greatly influence cardiac performance by affecting preload, afterload, heart rate, and contractility. Also, the contiguous adjacent structures—the lungs, pericardium, and pleura—affect cardiac function by influencing the filling and emptying of the heart. In conditions of heart failure, hypertrophy and dilatation are important modifying, compensatory mechanisms.

The *cardiac cycle* illustrates a sequence of electrical events that trigger mechanical events, producing pressure and flow. Figure 13.2 demonstrates these events for the left heart. In response to atrial depolarization, the atria contract, increasing the atrial pressure and left ventricular diastolic pressure (a wave). In response to ventricular electrical depolarization, the left ventricle contracts. Isovolumic contraction is analogous to isometric contraction, in which the myocardial force or pressure increases, but no external work is performed. When the intraventricular pressure rises to a level sufficient to open the aortic valve, forward flow begins. The greatest flow occurs in early systole. The aortic pressure rises and then falls as ejection subsides. At the end of ventricular ejection, ventricular pressure falls to a level just below the aortic diastolic pressure, and the aortic valve closes. The aortic pressure tracing shows a dicrotic notch resulting from the elastic recoil pressure of the aorta. Left ventricular pressure then falls (isovolumic relaxation) to a level low enough to allow the mitral valve to reopen, and the process of rapid ventricular filling ensues. The heart sounds correspond to atrial contraction (S_4), mitral valve closure (S_1), aortic valve closure (S_2), and rapid ventricular filling (S_3), respectively.

M.W. Kronenberg: Department of Medicine, Vanderbilt University Medical Center, Nashville, TN.

L.C. Becker: Department of Medicine, Johns Hopkins Medical Institutions, Baltimore, MD.

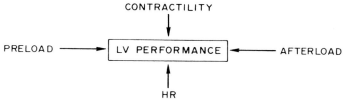

FIGURE 13.1. Determinants of left ventricular performance. HR, heart rate; LV, left ventricular.

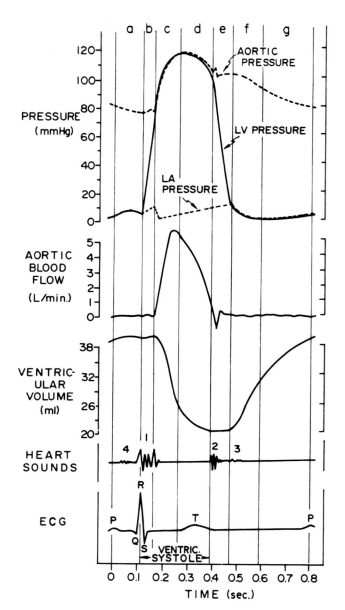

FIGURE 13.2. The cardiac cycle. Electrical events, followed by left heart flow and pressure, are illustrated. *a,* atrial contraction; *b,* isovolumic ventricular contraction; *c,* rapid ventricular ejection; *d,* slow ventricular ejection; *e,* isovolumic ventricular relaxation; *f,* rapid ventricular filling; *g,* slow ventricular filling. ECG, electrocardiogram; LA, left atrial; LV, left ventricular. (From Berne RM, Levy M. *Cardiovascular physiology,* 6th ed. St. Louis: Mosby, 1992, with permission.)

The ventricular volume increases during atrial contraction and then decreases during the rapid ejection of blood (stroke volume) after aortic valve opening. These events are followed by rapid ventricular filling in early diastole, then a period of slow ventricular filling. The same electrical and mechanical events and the same pressure-volume relations apply to the right ventricle. Rapid heart rates reduce the ejection time somewhat and reduce the slow ventricular filling period markedly.

A useful method for depicting ventricular function is the relationship between pressure and volume. Figure 13.3 shows

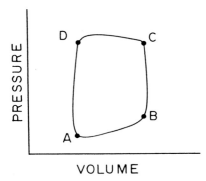

FIGURE 13.3. The ventricular pressure-volume relationships. See text for details.

such a *pressure-volume loop.* In the isolated papillary muscle, this can be portrayed as a force-length relationship. Because left ventricular pressure and volume are more easily measured in the intact heart than myocardial force and segment length, these are the more common modes for expression. The curve AB depicts the diastolic filling of the left ventricle. The curve BC demonstrates isometric contraction before reaching the level of pressure sufficient to open the aortic valve at point C. The curve CD represents isotonic contraction (ejection at relatively constant pressure after the aortic valve has opened). At the end of ejection, when ventricular pressure falls below the aortic diastolic pressure, the aortic valve closes. The curve DA represents isometric or isovolumic relaxation, an active process of relaxation of the left ventricular muscle, allowing pressure to diminish to levels sufficient to open the mitral valve and restart ventricular filling at point A. The diastolic pressure-volume relationship AB represents ventricular *compliance (dV/dP),* which is a measure of ventricular distensibility. The systolic pressure-volume relationship measured by BCD is a measure of ventricular systolic function, stiffening or *elastance,* as stored power is turned into kinetic energy.

There are several ejection-phase indices of cardiac performance. The stroke volume (mL/beat) is represented by the distance on the volume axis between C and D. The ejection fraction is calculated as (EDV − ESV)/EDV, where EDV is the end-diastolic volume (B), and ESV is the end-systolic volume (D). Normal values for the left ventricle range from 0.50 to 0.70, and this index of global left ventricular performance is often calculated in the practice of nuclear cardiology from the estimated left ventricular cavity volume using myocardial perfusion images and from red blood cell labeled images (radionuclide ventriculograms). An isovolumic index of contractility is the rate of rise of pressure *(dP/dt).*

Preload

The early studies of Frank, Starling, and Wiggers demonstrated that increasing myocardial stretch (length) produced stronger contractions (force). Studies in the frog ventricle by Frank in the late 1800s led to studies in the intact dog on right heart bypass (to control left ventricular filling characteristics) and also to elegant studies in the papillary muscle. Each of these emphasized the relationship between preload (ventricular stretch or volume) and a measure of cardiac performance (e.g., stroke volume, stroke work, cardiac output). As noted in Fig. 13.4, the normal relationship between the end-diastolic volume (or pressure) and performance is curvilinear. Thus, as the ventricle is filled (stretched), ventricular performance (as measured by an ejection-phase index) increases, but asymptotically, so that beyond certain limits further stretch does not increase stroke volume, but merely raises the level of end-diastolic ventricular pressure and volume. Under steady state conditions, this relationship is a reflection of myocardial contractility. Conditions or agents that enhance contractility are termed *positive inotropic stimuli.* Under these conditions, stroke volume can be increased for any given level of pressure or volume, such that the ventricle contracts to a greater degree for the same end-diastolic volume. Conversely, ventricular function can be depressed by so-called *negative inotropic factors,* with a lower stroke volume for the same level of diastolic volume.

The "operating point" for the intact heart is a more narrow range of diastolic pressure and volume. In practice, the description of ventricular function as normal, enhanced, or depressed is often based on single observations of ventricular contraction, stroke volume, or cardiac output. However, the care of patients with congestive cardiac failure is based on optimizing cardiac output while avoiding the excessively high end-diastolic pressures and volumes that produce pulmonary and systemic venous pressure elevation and congestion. Conversely, inadequate ventricular filling leads to low cardiac output syndromes, which may be reversed by appropriate volume loading. Clinical examples associated with increased ventricular preload include valvular regurgitant lesions, intracardiac shunts (congenital or acquired), and pulmonary or systemic arteriovenous fistulas. Such alterations in preload can produce abnormalities of diastolic pressure and volume, even when myocardial contractility is still normal. Conversely, decompensated myocardial failure (as in dilated cardiomyopathies) is a common cause of excessive preload.

Ventricular filling is determined by the degree of active (energy requiring) relaxation of the myocardium (active calcium removal from the cytoplasm surrounding actin and myosin),

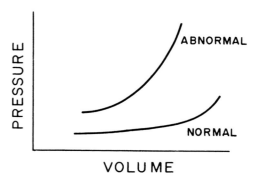

FIGURE 13.5. Ventricular compliance. Normal and abnormal curves are shown. In the normal state, there is a large change in volume for a small change in pressure (*dV/dP*), thus compliance is high.

venous return of blood, atrial contraction, the duration of diastole, and importantly, ventricular compliance (1) and perhaps diastolic "suction" (2). The term *compliance* (*dV/dP*) defines the relationship between diastolic pressure and volume (Fig. 13.5). The normal curve is nonlinear and demonstrates a large change in volume with a minimal increase in diastolic pressure, which remains low. The abnormal curve shows that small changes in volume are accompanied by large increases in diastolic pressure, and the diastolic pressures are higher at similar volumes. Chamber compliance itself is multifactorial. The ventricular size, its wall thickness, the completeness of active myocardial relaxation, the material properties of the ventricular wall (fibrous tissue versus normal), external compressive forces, and internal restriction to filling (such as endocardial fibroelastosis) all determine compliance. The pericardium itself has a pressure-volume relationship. Normally, the pericardium is a thin, compliant structure, and progressive increments of fluid added to the pericardial space cause minimal increases in pressure until a threshold level at which further increments in volume cause marked increases in the intrapericardial pressure. This condition of decompensated pericardial tamponade limits ventricular preload, and cardiac output can be subnormal in spite of a normal myocardium. Such would be the case with acute hemopericardium. Similarly, a thickened pericardium can limit ventricular filling and cause the syndrome of chronic constrictive pericarditis. Removal of pericardial fluid or the pericardium itself produces a more normal ventricular diastolic pressure-volume relationship. Chronic disorders of the myocardium, such as hypertrophy, fibrosis after infarction, and infiltrative disorders such as amyloidosis, reduce compliance. Transient myocardial ischemia causes stiffening and reduced compliance also (discussed later). Finally, right ventricular dilatation affects left ventricular filling (see the section on ventricular interaction).

Afterload

Afterload is the resistance to fiber shortening or ventricular systolic emptying. A combination of inertial forces, aortic impedance, and arteriolar tone (systemic vascular resistance) constitutes the ventricular afterload. Valvular aortic stenosis is an example of excess afterload resulting from high outflow *impedance,* whereas

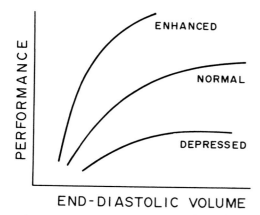

FIGURE 13.4. The Frank-Starling mechanism. Greater end-diastolic volume produces greater ventricular performance. Curves for normal, enhanced, and depressed contractility are shown.

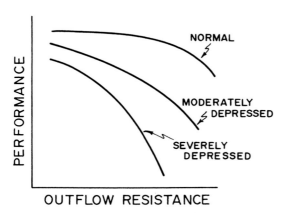

FIGURE 13.6. Concept of afterload regulation of ventricular performance. Ventricular performance (e.g., stroke volume) decreases as outflow resistance increases. The role of afterload is greatest when ventricular function is severely depressed. (From Cohn JN, Franciosa JA. Vasodilator therapy of cardiac failure. *N Engl J Med* 1977;297:27, with permission.)

systemic hypertension can cause increased vascular *resistance.* The systolic arterial pressure and left ventricular wall stress (discussed later) are related to ventricular afterload. Figure 13.6 demonstrates the concept of the inverse, curvilinear relationship between ventricular performance and afterload (outflow resistance). Curves from ventricles with normal, moderately depressed, and severely depressed contractility are shown. For each curve, performance diminishes as the afterload increases. Conversely, reducing afterload increases performance. At low levels of afterload, the performance of each ventricle is roughly similar, but at greater levels of afterload, ventricles with reduced contractility, which operate on depressed curves and have lower stroke volume (3,4).

Contractility

Contractility is a broad term that describes the quality or intensity of myocardial contraction or fiber shortening. It may be influenced by diverse stimuli, such as ischemia, hypoxia, acidosis, drugs (both positive and negative inotropic agents), and intrinsic disorders of the myocardium.

The cellular mechanisms underlying contractility have been studied extensively, but estimation of contractility in the intact state has been difficult because cardiac performance (as an estimate of contractility) is also influenced by preload, afterload, and heart rate (Fig. 13.1). Such ejection phase indices as cardiac output, ejection fraction, stroke volume, stroke work, and V_{cf} (the velocity of circumferential fiber shortening) are each interdependent and dependent on loading conditions and heart rate. Thus, they reflect the contractile state only if changes in loading conditions and heart rate are excluded. Other nonejection phase indices, such as isovolumic dP/dt (the rate of rise of pressure during isovolumic systole), estimate contractility better because they are less influenced by loading conditions, but maximal dP/dt is affected by loading conditions and thus is generally inadequate when loading conditions change (5).

To circumvent the problem of loading conditions, there has

been extensive study of the contractile state in the isolated supported heart, in intact animal models, and in human subjects (6–13). The end-systolic pressure-volume relationship (ESPVR) and modifications have received much attention as indices of contractility that are relatively independent of loading conditions. The ESPVR incorporates pressure afterload into the estimate of contractility, whereas other estimates of contractility, such as the ejection fraction and dP/dt at maximal pressure, do not account for systolic afterload. Figure 13.7 demonstrates the concept of the generally linear relationship of end-systolic pressure and volume in the isolated supported heart. Several manipulations of ventricular pressure and volume are shown. Using the ESPVR concept, the myocardium is considered to have systolic behavior somewhat analogous to a spring. In a spring, there is a linear relationship between force and length such that greater stretch produces greater tension, and, similarly, in the heart there is a linear relationship between the afterload (as end-systolic pressure) and the end-systolic volume. Figure 13.7A demonstrates that preload may vary widely (*solid lines*), and when the ventricle is allowed to eject after reaching the same systolic pressure, in each case the ventricle ejects to the same end-systolic volume. Thus, under such conditions, regardless of preload, the end-systolic volume is determined by the level of end-systolic pressure. The pressure-volume loops (*dashed lines*) show that

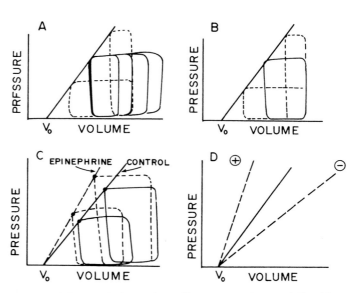

FIGURE 13.7. Ventricular end-systolic pressure-volume relationship (ESPVR) in the isolated, supported heart. **A:** Solid lines represent cardiac cycles at four levels of end-diastolic volume and demonstrate that the ventricle contracts to similar end-systolic volume, dependent on the systolic pressure and relatively independent of the end-diastolic pressure or volume. Dashed lines represent cardiac cycles at two other levels of end-diastolic pressure. The curve connecting the end-systolic pressure-volume points is linear. V_o represents ventricular volume when P = 0. **B:** Pressure-volume loops from similar end-diastolic volumes. The end-systolic pressure determines the end-systolic volume. **C:** The ESPVR is shifted leftward by the positive inotropic drug epinephrine. **D:** Positive inotropic drugs shift the ESPVR leftward, and negative inotropic drugs shift the ESPVR rightward. V_o is relatively constant in the isolated heart, in spite of changes in contractility. (From Suga H, Sagawa K, Shoukas AA. Load independence of the instantaneous pressure-volume ratio of the canine left ventricle and effects of epinephrine and heart rate on the ratio. *Circ Res* 1974;32:314, with permission.)

end-systolic volume may become larger or smaller depending on the systolic pressure afterload against which the ventricle ejects. When the end-systolic pressure-volume points are connected, the relationship is linear. Figure 13.7**B** illustrates that the ESPVR is relatively independent of end-diastolic volume. Here, with end-diastolic volume set constant, the ventricle is allowed to eject at low, medium, and high levels of systolic pressure. Under such conditions the end-systolic pressure determines the level of end-systolic volume, and the linearity is apparent. Thus, under constant contractile conditions, the ESPVR is an index of contractility, which is expressed in terms of ventricular elastance (E) and described by the equation $E_{es} = P_{es}/(V_{es}-V_o)$, where P and V are end-systolic (es) pressure and volume, and V_o represents the volume when $P = 0$. In Fig. 13.7**C**, the pressure-volume relationship, which was defined under control conditions in one contractile state, is shifted leftward when an infusion of epinephrine produces a new steady state of increased contractility. In Fig. 13.7**D,** to summarize, the pressure-volume relationship shifts leftward under positive inotropic states and shifts rightward with negative inotropic conditions.

There are some modifiers to the general concept. First, in acute experiments performed in the isolated heart, V_o is relatively constant. In the intact animal and in humans, V_o is more variable, partly as a result of acute changes in contractility and partly because of chronic adaptation by ventricular dilatation to conditions such as congestive cardiac failure. Second, in contrast to the engineering model of the spring, myocardial elastance increases with time during the cardiac cycle and is maximal at end-systole. This is termed *time-varying elastance* and is probably a result of the interaction of calcium and the contractile apparatus, fiber properties, chamber geometry, and the sequence of activation. Third, further careful work has shown that the ESPVR is somewhat curvilinear (9), especially at high contractile states, and that all indices of contractility may have this property because of the time-varying enhancement of contractility during systole. Further enhancements to the measurement of contractility have included the linearity of preload recruitable stroke work (10) and preload adjusted maximal power (12), a measurement of the maximum rate of ventricular work (instantaneous ventricular pressure × rate of volume change) adjusted for end-diastolic volume. This latter index holds promise for future noninvasive study because the rate of rise of the arterial pressure and the decrease in ventricular volume may be estimated noninvasively (13). However, further study is necessary before clinical application.

The ESPVR concept has been applied in clinical studies, with volume or dimension estimates by contrast ventriculography, echocardiography, or radionuclide ventriculography. Pressure afterload may be estimated by direct intraarterial recording or by indirect sphygmomanometer measurements, sometimes extrapolated to end-systolic pressure by using the so-called calibrated carotid pulse tracing (13,14). Ventricular wall stress is an important measure of afterload (Fig. 13.8). Within the ventricle, tension, or force per unit area, is compensated by wall thickness and yields the term *stress.* Stress-shortening relations (stress-V_{cf}) usefully incorporate compensatory mechanisms such as hypertrophy into the afterload estimate (15,16). This index of contractility also allows easier comparison between ventricles of different

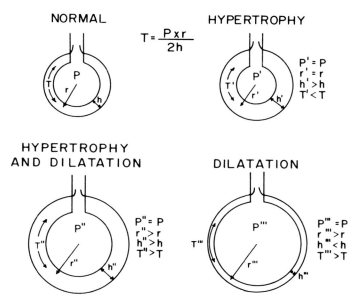

FIGURE 13.8. Compensatory mechanisms. As a consequence of heart failure, the left ventricle may dilate to produce an adequate stroke volume. Hypertrophy may accompany dilation or may occur alone as a response to systemic hypertension. The Laplace equation demonstrates the effects of hypertrophy, dilation, and the combination on wall tension (*T*). Increasing wall thickness (*h*) reduces tension and myocardial oxygen demand. However, increasing systolic pressure (*P*) or the ventricular end-diastolic radius (*r*) increases wall tension above normal and increases myocardial oxygen consumption. (From Shepard JT, Vanhoutte PM. *The human cardiovascular system.* New York: Raven Press, 1979:73, with permission.)

sizes. However, the assumptions in all such calculations may be compromised in the frequent case of regional ventricular dyssynergy following myocardial infarction.

Rhythm and Conduction Abnormalities

Cardiac conduction normally proceeds from the sinoatrial node through the atrioventricular node and His bundle to ramify into the left and right bundle branch systems and Purkinje fibers. This rapid electrical depolarization produces an orderly sequence of atrial contraction followed by ventricular contraction. Well-timed atrial systole may increase the stroke volume by 10% to 20%. Conversely, atrial arrhythmias such as atrial fibrillation reduce the end-diastolic volume and stroke volume, other factors remaining equal. The contributions of sinus rhythm and the atrial systolic transport mechanism to end-diastolic volume may be especially important in low cardiac output syndromes (i.e., reduced systolic performance) or in hearts with poor compliance.

Given a normal sequence of atrial and ventricular activation (normal sinus rhythm), the heart rate has obvious importance in generating the cardiac output (stroke volume × heart rate). Thus, bradycardia must reduce cardiac output, if stroke volume remains constant. Also, there are rate-dependent changes in contractility. Faster rates increase the strength of contraction through calcium mechanisms. This effect is most pronounced at rates in the 60 to 100 beats/minute range.

Ventricular premature contractions have several deleterious

effects. Early in diastole, the ventricular volume may be small. By itself, this would reduce stroke volume. Also there is reduced contraction based on a lower than normal amount of calcium available for transport to the active sites on actin and myosin. Postpremature beats tend to be more forceful contractions, probably as a result of greater calcium available to the contractile apparatus and a larger end-diastolic volume. Frequent premature ventricular contractions and salvos of such beats may severely reduce the cardiac output.

Conduction disorders, such as right or left bundle branch block, disrupt the normal sequence of ventricular depolarization and contraction. This out-of-phase contraction sequence produces unusual motion of the interventricular septum, which can be observed on echocardiography and radionuclide ventriculography. This sequence also reduces septal perfusion. The combination of dyssynchrony and hypoperfusion reduces contractility (17). As many as 20% to 25% of patients with congestive heart failure have QRS prolongation. In some this is due to bundle branch block, but in most others this is due to a nonspecific intraventricular conduction abnormality. Recently, experiments with simultaneous ventricular depolarization using pacing leads in the right ventricular apex and in veins on the lateral wall of the left ventricle have shown acute improvements in ventricular mechanics (18), ventricular synchrony, and ejection fraction (19). Further, blinded clinical trials have also shown improved exercise capacity over 6 months of "resynchronization" therapy (20).

Myocardial Efficiency

Cardiac energetics can be categorized into the amount of energy used for external mechanical work, the amount still available as potential energy following contraction, and the amount dissipated as heat during systole. For a meticulous analysis of this topic the reader is referred to the monograph of Sagawa and associates. Cardiac mechanical efficiency may be expressed as the ratio of external mechanical work divided by total oxygen consumption. Considerable interest has centered on methods for judging cardiac mechanical efficiency in patients. External work may be estimated by formulas that account for stroke work per minute (developed pressure × stroke volume × heart rate per minute). Oxygen consumption may be measured in catheterization laboratories by measuring the arterial/coronary sinus oxygen difference and estimating myocardial blood flow. Recent work has emphasized the noninvasive estimation of mechanical efficiency using the work-metabolic index. For the numerator of the equation, echocardiography is used to estimate stroke volume, which is multiplied by the peak systolic pressure to estimate external work. For the denominator, the ^{11}C acetate decay rate has been validated as an estimate of myocardial oxygen consumption, (21,22). Using these methods, the β-adrenergic blocking drug, metoprolol, was recently shown to produce an improvement in mechanical efficiency in patients with congestive heart failure (23).

Regional Left Ventricular Performance

All of the foregoing discussion relates to measurements of global (overall) ventricular performance. Such concepts are applicable to the normal heart or to the heart that is affected uniformly by generalized disorders of contractility. Coronary artery disease produces regional functional abnormalities that are acute or chronic. For example, a myocardial infarction in the distribution of the left anterior descending coronary artery may cause septal, anterior, and apical akinesis. Such regional disorders modify regional function. Their effect on global left ventricular performance depends on the extent of the regional abnormality and secondary compensatory events, such as increased contraction and hypertrophy of the remaining normal myocardium.

Compensatory Adjustments

Left Ventricular Factors

The left ventricle responds to a chronic, pathologic increase in afterload or preload by myocardial hypertrophy, dilatation, or both. This process is termed *ventricular remodeling*. The Laplace equation describes the relationship between wall tension, pressure, radius, and wall thickness (Fig. 13.8). Wall tension increases with dilation. It is reduced when there is adequate compensatory hypertrophy. When pressure and volume increase beyond the ability of hypertrophy to compensate, tension (or wall stress) rises to inappropriately high levels. Eventually left ventricular dysfunction occurs. This results in inadequate ventricular performance and is characterized by reduced forward output, unusually high filling pressures with their congestive consequences, or both. If the adjustment is inadequate, further dilatation may occur. Such dilatation further stretches the myofibrils and the actin and myosin subunits. Theoretically, when dilatation is extreme, cardiac output may decline (descending limb of Frank-Starling relationship). Secondary pulmonary hypertension and right ventricular dysfunction may occur. Systemic hypertension and myocardial infarction are the two commonest causes of ventricular dilatation and hypertrophy. After myocardial infarction, remodeling involves both the infarct regions (expansion) and the noninfarcted regions, which also dilate and hypertrophy (24). The right ventricle is anatomically thinner and less well-suited for compensating for this pressure and volume stress. Thus, right ventricular dilatation occurs and leads to right atrial hypertension, volume overload, or both plus annular dilatation and possible tricuspid valvular regurgitation as well. The right ventricle is quite sensitive to pressure or volume overload and its contractility declines under such stress (25).

Neurohormonal Factors and Cytokines

The systemic arterial blood pressure is determined by the blood volume, the characteristics of the arteries and veins, and the characteristics of the heart as a pump. In the presence of inadequate pump performance, high-pressure and low-pressure mechanoreceptors (baroreceptors) form the afferent limb for central sympathetic and vagal compensatory activity. Consequently, the heart rate increases. Norepinephrine is released from adrenergic fibers in the heart in an attempt to increase contractility and in the arterioles for regional vasoconstriction. Such vasoconstriction occurs in the skin, the splanchnic circulation, and the renal afferent arterioles. The systemic capacitance vessels constrict to increase right heart venous return, which increases preload in an attempt to increase cardiac performance. Hormonal adjustments are proportional to the degree of left ventricular dysfunction (26) and include elevated levels of circulating norepinephrine, renin, angiotensin II, aldosterone, and arginine vasopressin, the latter two being related to increasing the circulating blood volume. In addition, the circulating concentration of endothelin is elevated in heart failure, and recent work has shown progressively increased levels of tumor necrosis factor-α related to the severity of congestive heart failure (27).

Arteriolar vasoconstriction helps normalize the blood pressure, but at a higher level of peripheral resistance. Volume adjustments increase preload but commonly at the cost of pulmonary or peripheral edema. The chronically elevated levels of circulating catecholamines and the excess sympathetic activation are associated with downregulation of β-adrenergic receptors (28). This leads to less myocardial responsiveness to these positive inotropic factors plus chronotropic downregulation such that the heart rate is relatively lower than normal for the amount of circulating norepinephrine. Such chronotropic downregulation of the sinoatrial node is especially pronounced during exercise. Inadequate cardiac output also leads to changes in oxyhemoglobin dissociation, which favors oxygen unloading.

Gradually, the heart, arteries, and veins come to a new operating point based on these circulatory adjustments. These adjustments may be sufficient to produce a normal cardiac output without circulatory congestion (asymptomatic left ventricular dysfunction) or may be inadequate to compensate for progressive myocardial dysfunction and lead to symptomatic dysfunction (congestive heart failure).

Ventricular Interaction

The right ventricle responds to the same mechanisms for altering performance as the left. Right and left ventricular interaction can be important. When examined in series, left heart failure can cause right heart failure. However, when examined in parallel, they interact through the interventricular septum, through common muscle fibers, and through the pericardium, which surrounds both chambers. For example, pulmonary hypertension can produce right ventricular hypertrophy and dilatation, eventually bowing the interventricular septum toward the left ventricle and adversely changing both the systolic and diastolic left ventricular pressure-volume relations.

Cardiopulmonary Interaction

Cardiopulmonary interactions have been incompletely characterized. However, several obvious models of interaction have been described. For instance, marked decreases in the intrapleural pressure on inspiration can reduce left ventricular performance by sequestering blood in the pulmonary circuit, thereby reducing left ventricular filling. Also, positive end-expiratory ventilatory pressure can reduce venous return to the right heart and limit cardiac output. Hypoxia has complex effects, with a primary depressant effect on the myocardium and a secondary stimulatory effect produced by adrenergic norepinephrine release. Local pulmonary reflexes may alter the heart rate.

Hemodynamic Effects of Pharmacologic Therapy in Heart Failure

Using the conceptual models outlined previously, one can see that *positive inotropic agents* increase the stroke volume for the same level of preload (Fig. 13.4) and reduce the end-systolic volume for the same level of afterload. (Fig. 13.7**C** and **D**). They increase the cardiac output and arterial blood pressure, thereby reducing the secondary vascular volume shifts and neurohormonal compensations for hypotension, hypovolemia, and reduced perfusion. *Negative inotropic agents* produce the opposite effects. *Afterload-reducing drugs* act by reducing vascular resistance and the arterial blood pressure. Such vasodilation improves stroke volume (Fig. 13.6).

Of all these potential effects, angiotensin-converting enzyme inhibitors and β-adrenergic blocking drugs have made the greatest clinical impact in treating heart failure. In addition to their hemodynamic effects (emphasized here), each class of drugs has important, beneficial effects on myocardial cells and vessels. Angiotensin-converting enzyme inhibitors reduce afterload, but importantly have also lessened ventricular remodeling (29) and have reduced the morbidity and mortality of heart failure (30, 31). A large body of work has now accumulated showing that β-adrenergic receptor blockade, while initially a negative inotropic influence, can, over a period of weeks to months, improve the responsiveness to circulating neurohormones, improve exercise capacity and the left ventricular ejection fraction (32), and increase survival (33) in many patients with systolic dysfunction and heart failure.

Positive inotropic drugs have been studied extensively. Dobutamine stimulates β1-, β2-, and α-adrenergic receptors, and milrinone is a phosphodiesterase inhibitor, which potentiates the effects of cyclic AMP and is also a vasodilator. Both have been clinically useful as acute intravenous infusions for treating decompensated congestive heart failure (34). The use of positive inotropic drugs as oral agents for treating heart failure has been generally unsuccessful. The β-adrenergic agonists caused receptor downregulation with no benefit, and the phosphodiesterase inhibitors showed excess mortality compared with placebo. Calcium sensitizing drugs, such as vesnarinone, were also associated with excess mortality. Of the positive inotropic drugs, only digitalis has shown a positive effect, consisting of reduced morbidity from heart failure among patients with severe left ventricular dysfunction.

Diagnostic Usefulness of Drugs in Ventricular Dysfunction

Positive inotropic drugs (e.g., dobutamine) and vasodilators (e.g., dipyridamole and adenosine) have been employed for pharmacologic stress testing and for the evaluation of myocardial viability (35). Dobutamine's effect on ventricular function has been studied using echocardiography during its infusion. At low doses, the drug may increase the contractility of viable, "hibernating" or "stunned" myocardium. At higher doses, its net effect may be to produce ischemia. This biphasic response of viable myocardium presages functional improvement after myocardial revascularization (36).

Dipyridamole prevents the reuptake of adenosine, potentiates its effects on its receptors, and produces both coronary (37) and systemic vasodilation. Because of systemic vasodilation, ventricular afterload is reduced. In normal subjects, the left ventricular ejection fraction increases and wall motion remains normal or is enhanced. However, in patients with significant coronary atherosclerosis the drug may induce myocardial ischemia and the ejection fraction fails to increase or may decrease, and there may be new wall motion abnormalities. This is the basis for the dipyridamole echo test (38) and for prior studies of dipyridamole radionuclide ventriculography (39). Infusion of adenosine would be expected to produce similar effects. The effects of dipyridamole and adenosine on myocardial blood flow and perfusion are discussed in a later section (see the section on pharmacologic alteration of myocardial perfusion).

MYOCARDIAL PERFUSION

Normal Regulation of Coronary Blood Flow

Anatomic Factors

The left and right coronary arteries provide the major conduits for blood flow to the left and right ventricles and atria. A much smaller contribution, more important for the atria and right ventricle than the left ventricle, is provided by channels originating directly from the heart's cavities and running into the inner layers of the wall. Although the epicardial arteries usually provide only a minor portion of the total coronary vascular resistance, their contribution may be considerable under circumstances of atherosclerotic narrowing or spasm.

The major site of coronary vascular resistance normally resides in small intramural arteries and arterioles 10 to 40 μm in diameter, which exhibit important degrees of vasomotive constriction and dilation in response to various metabolic, humoral, and/or neural stimuli. Many of these small intramural arteries arise as perforating vessels from the epicardial arteries and course directly through the ventricular wall to the subendocardium, where they branch profusely to form a subendocardial vascular plexus or network. This network provides the major source of intercoronary collateral flow in the event of a coronary artery occlusion, although large epicardial artery-to-epicardial artery connections also play an important role.

As in other organs, the myocardial capillaries serve as semipermeable membranes for delivery of oxygen and nutrients and removal of metabolic waste products. The transport of molecules occurs between the capillary lumen and interstitial space via passive diffusion, pinocytosis, or passage through interendothelial pores. Capillary density is normally high (2 to 5 × 10^5 capillaries per mm², with one capillary per muscle fiber), although the density can be reduced by disease processes, such as left ventricular hypertrophy. Whether a given capillary bed is perfused at any given moment is controlled by arteriolar precapillary sphincters. During hypoxia the sphincters relax, resulting in an increase in effective capillary density and in a reduction in effective intercapillary distance.

Perfusion Pressure

Coronary blood flow is determined by the interaction between perfusion pressure and coronary vascular resistance (flow = perfusion pressure divided by resistance). Because the major portion of coronary blood flow occurs in diastole, perfusion pressure is often assumed to be equal to aortic diastolic pressure. However, in the presence of atherosclerotic stenoses of the coronary arteries, very significant pressure drops may occur along the course of the major epicardial arteries, reducing effective perfusion pressure markedly. Depending on the distribution of coronary stenoses, perfusion pressure may be significantly lower in one coronary bed than an adjacent one, encouraging the growth and development of intercoronary collaterals from the high- to the low-pressure bed.

The concept of perfusion pressure must also take into account the presence of backpressure, that is, pressure at the level of the myocardial capillaries. The effective coronary driving pressure is actually equal to the perfusion pressure minus the backpressure. In most cases, the backpressure is equal to tissue pressure and is determined by the level of the left ventricular diastolic pressure. This is especially true for the subendocardial layer of the left ventricle, which is directly compressed when left ventricular cavity pressure rises. However, coronary sinus pressure may determine backpressure if it exceeds left ventricular diastolic pressure, as in some patients with right ventricular infarction or severe pulmonary hypertension.

Coronary Resistance

Extrinsic Compressive Forces

One of the most remarkable things about the heart is that during systolic contraction the intramural coronary vessels are compressed and coronary blood flow is effectively throttled. Blood is squeezed into the coronary veins and also backward into the epicardial arteries, which store the blood until the next beat (capacitive function). Systolic compressive forces are believed normally to be higher in the inner than the outer portion of the left ventricular wall, causing a greater reduction in systolic flow in the deeper layers. This deficit in myocardial perfusion must be made up for in diastole, and, in fact, about 85% of total coronary flow is diastolic under normal conditions. Because of greater inhibition of subendocardial perfusion in systole, diastolic perfusion of this region is higher to keep flow uniform across the wall. This compensation is mediated by greater dilatation of resistance vessels in the subendocardium, leading to some loss of total subendocardial vascular reserve. These concepts explain the critical dependence of subendocardial perfusion on diastolic hemodynamics. Subendocardial blood flow is affected out of proportion to subepicardial flow by decreases in effective diastolic perfusion pressure. Reduced diastolic pressure, in turn, could be due to a generalized drop in arterial pressure, a localized coronary artery stenosis, a rise in left ventricular filling pressure, or a shortening of diastolic time per beat as a result of an increase in heart rate. Because the subendocardium must normally use some of its vasodilatory reserve to maintain baseline perfusion, the subendocardium is especially vulnerable to ischemia and to ischemic damage during stress. The adequacy of subendocardial flow has been assessed experimentally using the diastolic pressure-time index (DPTI) divided by the systolic pressure-time index (SPTI), essentially an estimate of the supply/demand balance of the subendocardium (40).

The potential exists for imaging reduced subendocardial perfusion in patients with coronary artery disease using techniques with high spatial resolution. Contrast agents that track regional myocardial perfusion may be injected intravenously and imaged during the first pass through the coronary circulation (microbubbles for echocardiography, gadolinium-DTPA for magnetic resonance, and iodinated contrast agents for ultrafast computed tomography). Positron emission tomography (PET) and single photon emission computed tomography (SPECT) have too low a spatial resolution for imaging flow differences between layers of the left ventricular wall.

Metabolic Regulation

The most potent factor regulating coronary blood flow is the tight coupling that exists between coronary blood flow and myocardial oxygen demand, necessitated by the almost complete dependence of the myocardium on aerobic metabolism. In theory, myocardial oxygen delivery could be increased by either an increase in coronary blood flow or an increase in oxygen extraction, although the latter mechanism is limited by the high degree of extraction that exists under normal conditions. In practice, however, myocardial blood flow increases and decreases *pari passu* with changes in oxygen requirements, whereas increased extraction is generally found only when vasodilator reserve is exhausted. The close coupling between myocardial oxygen consumption and flow is adjusted on a second-by-second basis and represents the dominant mechanism for regulation of coronary blood flow.

The major determinants of myocardial oxygen consumption are heart rate, myocardial contractility, and wall stress (Fig. 13.8). Maximal exercise, associated with increases in all three major determinants of myocardial oxygen consumption, may cause as much as a fourfold increase in coronary blood flow with an opposite reduction in coronary vascular resistance. This increase is impressive, but it does not represent the full maximal vasodilating capacity of the coronary bed, which can be elicited by administration of potent arteriolar vasodilating agents, such as adenosine or dipyridamole. Under these conditions, as much as a sixfold increase in flow may occur.

Tight coupling of myocardial oxygen demands and flow results in the phenomenon of coronary autoregulation. Over a wide range of perfusion pressure, from about 50 to 150 mm Hg, coronary flow stays relatively constant as coronary vascular resistance adjusts to balance the change in pressure. Below 50 mm Hg, however, the vasodilating capacity of at least a portion of the ventricular wall is exceeded, further autoregulation is no longer possible, and coronary flow falls abruptly. Above 150 mm Hg, the coronary vessels cannot or do not constrict further, and coronary flow increases rapidly. The concept of coronary autoregulation explains why relatively large changes in hemodynamics, above and below the normal level, may have little effect on the level of coronary blood flow.

A related phenomenon is *coronary reactive hyperemia* (Fig. 13.9). Following release of a brief coronary occlusion, flow increases above the previous baseline value (hyperemia) and the excess flow delivered to the myocardium ("repayment") equals or exceeds the amount of flow "debt" incurred during the occlusion. The amount and duration of hyperemia depend on the

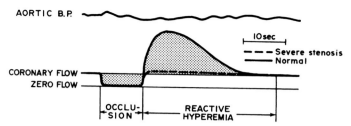

FIGURE 13.9. Reactive hyperemia. A flow meter implanted around a coronary artery is used to measure flow during and following a 10-second total occlusion of the artery. Flow drops to zero during occlusion and the dotted area between normal and zero flow represents the "flow deficit." On release of occlusion, flow increases to four to five times baseline (reactive hyperemia) and the dotted area under this portion of the curve represents "flow repayment," which can be seen to exceed the "flow debt." In the presence of a severe upstream stenosis, the reactive hyperemic response is markedly blunted or eliminated (*dashed line*). B.P., blood pressure. (From Olsson RA. Myocardial reactive hyperemia. *Circ Res* 1975;37:263, with permission.)

duration of occlusion, but the peak flow response is maximal after 15 to 30 seconds of occlusion. Reactive hyperemia has been measured in patients undergoing cardiac surgery using a Doppler flow meter placed over an epicardial coronary artery (41). It has also been identified in patients undergoing angioplasty following balloon deflation, using an intracoronary Doppler flow velocity catheter (42), and after reversal of transient coronary spasm using thallium perfusion imaging (43).

Despite its importance, the precise mechanism responsible for the metabolic regulation of coronary flow is uncertain. A number of chemical mediators have been proposed, including oxygen, potassium, and calcium, but the most likely mediators are one or more of these: adenosine, other nucleotides, prostaglandins, carbon dioxide, and/or hydrogen ion. These substances are all produced rapidly during ischemia and can cause relaxation of arterial smooth muscle. For example, adenosine is produced during metabolism of high-energy adenine nucleotides, diffuses across the myocardial cell membrane into the interstitial space, and is thought to interact with adenosine receptors to relax arteriolar smooth muscle and cause a decrease in coronary vascular resistance. ATP-sensitive potassium channels also contribute to reactive hyperemia by opening during ischemia, resulting in hyperpolarization and relaxation of vascular smooth muscle. Blockade of these channels by glibenclamide reduces reactive hyperemia by nearly 50% (44). It is likely that no single mediator exists, but rather that the tight coupling of metabolic needs and flow is a complex process that can be modulated by a number of compounds.

Neural and Humoral Regulation

The large and small coronary vessels and myocardial conduction tissue receive an abundant supply of autonomic nerves. Cardiac sympathetic nerves arise from the sympathetic ganglia, including the stellate ganglion, and densely innervate the epicardial coronary arteries and veins, as well as the intramural arteries, venules, and capillaries. Efferent parasympathetic cholinergic innervation arrives via the vagal nerves and supplies the coronary vessels and conduction system.

Sympathetic stimulation causes an increase in heart rate and myocardial contractility, resulting in an increase in myocardial metabolism and a compensatory rise in coronary blood flow via metabolic autoregulation. Vagal stimulation, in contrast, causes a striking bradycardia, modest decrease in myocardial contractility and a resultant decrease in myocardial metabolism. The coronary arteries constrict in response to these effects on the myocardium, although the direct effect of vagal stimulation is to produce mild coronary dilation.

Infusions of adrenergic or cholinergic agonist drugs produce a much greater effect than can be elicited by more physiologic neural stimulation. For example, infusion of phenylephrine or methoxamine, both α-adrenergic agonists, can produce a two-fold coronary constrictor response, compared with a 10% to 25% increase produced by selective sympathetic stimulation. Dobutamine, a synthetic sympathomimetic amine that stimulates β-adrenergic receptors, produces an increase in myocardial contractility and a secondary increase in myocardial blood flow. It is used in conjunction with echocardiography or perfusion imaging to diagnose coronary artery disease in patients who are unable to exercise (45). During dobutamine infusion, the presence of a coronary stenosis limits the flow increase that can occur through that vessel, leading to a maldistribution of perfusion and/or the appearance of a left ventricular wall motion abnormality (resulting from an imbalance between myocardial oxygen supply and demand).

A number of endogenous and exogenous humoral substances can produce significant coronary vasoconstriction. Among these are angiotensin, vasopressin, serotonin, and the prostaglandins thromboxane A_2 and leukotriene D. Humoral coronary vasodilators include adenosine, acetylcholine, histamine, and the prostaglandins (PG) PGE_1 and prostacyclin (PGI_2). Infusion of these humoral agents can produce several-fold changes in coronary vascular resistance.

Pharmacologic Alteration

Potent coronary vasoactive substances have been developed for experimental, as well as therapeutic, manipulation of the coronary circulation. The most familiar of these are the nitrate preparations, including nitroglycerin and the longer acting isosorbide dinitrate. Nitrates cause a relaxation of arterial smooth muscle, particularly in the large epicardial coronary arteries, resulting in an increase in vessel caliber and a reversal of coronary spasm. Nitric oxide (NO) is believed to represent the direct mediator of these effects by increasing cellular levels of cyclic guanosine monophosphate (cGMP), which in turn inhibits calcium release from internal stores and calcium influx through membrane channels. NO is derived from organic nitrates following their conversion to inorganic nitrite in the presence of intracellular thiols such as cysteine. Nitroprusside, another nitrovasodilator, releases NO directly.

Administration of nitroglycerin sublingually causes a transient increase in coronary blood flow lasting 1 to 2 minutes, related to a dilation of arteriolar resistance vessels, combined with a longer lasting (up to 30 minutes) increase in epicardial vessel diameter, which is not associated with altered flow unless a significant coronary stenosis is present. Prolonged intravenous infusion of nitroglycerin similarly results in coronary dilation, usually without an increase in coronary blood flow, unless ath-

erosclerotic narrowings are present and cause the epicardial arteries to become an important site of vascular resistance. If nitroglycerin is given within a few minutes of radionuclide tracer injection during an exercise perfusion study, perfusion defects are often obliterated because of an increase in flow to the ischemic region at a time when significant amounts of tracer are still circulating in the blood.

Nonnitrate vasodilators, such as adenosine and dipyridamole, exert potent dilatory effects on resistance arterioles, resulting in large increases in coronary blood flow. In contrast to nitrates, the effects on epicardial conductance arteries are minimal. Dipyridamole has been used in conjunction with radionuclide perfusion imaging to increase coronary blood flow and uncover occult coronary stenoses, as with exercise (37,46). This drug works by blocking the cellular uptake and metabolism of adenosine, thereby increasing its concentration at vascular smooth muscle receptors. Its effects can be reversed by aminophylline. In contrast to exercise, there is generally little change in heart rate or blood pressure following dipyridamole and therefore little change in myocardial oxygen demands. Radionuclide tracers, such as ^{201}Tl- or ^{99m}Tc-based tracers like sestamibi or tetrofosmin, are injected following a 4-minute intravenous infusion of the drug, and imaging is performed several minutes later. A perfusion defect signifies the presence of a flow limiting coronary artery stenosis (usually reducing arterial diameter by ($\geq$50%). Whereas flow increases several fold in response to dipyridamole in myocardium perfused by nonstenotic coronary arteries, the flow increase is blunted in areas fed by stenotic vessels; this is the basis of the maldistribution of tracer uptake that occurs in patients with coronary artery disease. There is also evidence that collateral-dependent regions of myocardium may experience an actual decrease in flow below baseline (coronary steal) because of a decrease in collateral driving pressure (discussed later). Adenosine itself has also been used to increase myocardial blood flow in conjunction with radionuclide perfusion imaging (47). Because of its very short half-life, adenosine must be continued for several minutes after the tracer is injected to ensure that its uptake is completed while flow is increased. Calcium-blocking drugs, such as nifedipine, verapamil, and diltiazem, are also coronary vasodilators. These drugs inhibit the transsarcolemmal passage of calcium through voltage-gated calcium channels and have potent effects on both arteriolar resistance vessels and epicardial conductance arteries. They represent an important class of agents for reversal of coronary spasm and treatment of myocardial ischemia.

Coronary constrictor agents, such as ergonovine, are occasionally used clinically to provoke coronary artery spasm (48). In certain patients with rest angina, spontaneous coronary spasm may be responsible for attacks of episodic ischemia. Ergonovine is believed to induce spasm only in those susceptible individuals in whom spontaneous spasm is already occurring. Often spasm occurs at the site of an atherosclerotic plaque, but sometimes the coronary arteries appear normal. Ergonovine has been used in conjunction with thallium imaging to noninvasively detect spasm-induced perfusion defects, but because of the risk of inducing complete heart block, ventricular fibrillation, or difficult-to-reverse coronary spasm, ergonovine testing should be done only in the cardiac catheterization laboratory. Emergency intracoronary administration of vasodilators can then be performed if necessary.

Endothelium-Dependent Vasomotion

Normal regulation of vasomotor tone *in vivo* is critically dependent on a normally functioning vascular endothelium. The endothelium participates in the metabolism of circulating vasoactive compounds such as angiotensin, bradykinin, and serotonin, and synthesizes vasodilator substances such as prostacyclin and NO, as well as constrictor substances such as endothelin. Many vasodilating substances (e.g., acetylcholine and bradykinin) produce their effect *in vivo* by stimulating specific endothelial cell receptors, leading to production of NO from L-arginine by the enzyme NO synthase. NO is then released from the endothelium and diffuses to overlying smooth muscle, where it produces relaxation through an increase in cGMP (49). The dilatation of an epicardial coronary artery that occurs during an increase in flow (i.e., during exercise or during an infusion of adenosine) is endothelium dependent (50). Coronary atherosclerosis, as well as the presence of coronary risk factors such as hypertension and hypercholesterolemia, are associated with endothelial dysfunction and impaired endothelium-dependent vasodilation (51). Nitroglycerin and nitroprusside release NO directly and are considered *endothelium-independent* vasodilators (see earlier discussion). Endothelial dysfunction occurs in epicardial coronary arteries, as well as in the microcirculation, impeding both large coronary artery dilatation and coronary blood flow regulated at the level of small resistance vessels. Tonic release of vasodilator prostanoids and NO contributes to resting conduit and resistance vessel tone, peak functional hyperemia, and metabolic vasodilatation in humans (52).

Myocardial Ischemia

Coronary Stenoses

Obstruction to coronary blood flow is usually caused by atherosclerotic narrowing in the epicardial coronary arteries, most often proximally at sites of turbulence, bending, or vessel bifurcations. Much less commonly, coronary obstruction may be related to embolization, vasculitis, dissection, or myocardial muscle bridging.

When hemodynamically significant, a coronary stenosis produces a pressure gradient within the artery, with downstream pressure falling below upstream pressure. The severity of stenosis is most related to the minimum luminal area available for passage of blood, but it is also affected by the length and the shape of the narrowing. Eccentric stenoses may cause greater turbulence and loss of kinetic energy, resulting in larger pressure gradients. Stenosis severity is most often assessed by coronary angiography and is usually expressed as a percentage diameter stenosis relative to the diameter of an adjacent normal arterial segment. Experimentally, it has been determined that at least 50% diameter narrowing is required to reduce the maximal coronary flow response and that a stenosis must exceed 90% before resting flow is reduced. These general concepts have been confirmed in patients with coronary artery disease using a Doppler flow velocity catheter at the time of coronary angiography or by using noninvasive quantitative PET perfusion imaging (53,54).

The severity of coronary artery disease in a patient is often described in terms of the most severe diameter stenosis in the three major arteries: anterior descending, circumflex, and right. Although convenient, this approach ignores the length of narrowings, the presence of lesions in series, and the diffuseness of arterial involvement. The narrowings are often estimated visually without actual measurements, resulting in reports that appear more quantitative than they really are. Furthermore, measurements of percentage diameter narrowing assume that the adjacent comparison segments are truly normal and are not themselves narrowed by disease, which is only infrequently the case. Studies by Marcus and associates (41), comparing coronary angiographic data with physiologic measurements of coronary flow obstruction, showed that the angiographic estimates of severity correlate poorly with true obstruction except when the stenosis is judged very severe (>90%) or very slight (<10%).

An additional problem in relating anatomic narrowings to physiologic effects is that the degree of stenosis is probably not fixed in most cases but rather is dynamic and changing in response to a wide variety of factors. Decreases in distending pressure appear to increase stenosis severity by partial collapse of the stenotic segment. The opposite occurs with increases in distending pressure. Increased flow through a stenotic segment results in increased turbulence and energy loss, a fall in downstream pressure, and a possible increase in stenosis severity as a result of collapse of the distal end of the stenosis. Various humoral and neural stimuli could also have important effects on stenosis severity by constriction of arterial smooth muscle in the stenotic segment.

As a stenosis increases in severity, compensatory arteriolar dilatation must occur to maintain normal flow, using in the process a portion of the vasodilator reserve of the involved myocardium. Clinically, this loss of reserve is detected by a reduction in ratio of flow during maximal coronary vasodilation (usually induced by adenosine or a similar drug) to the baseline blood flow. This is most often assessed with an intracoronary flow velocity catheter. The normal flow ratio of four to six is reduced to two to four with moderate coronary stenoses and to one to two with severe stenoses. Reduced flow reserve in patients with coronary artery disease has also been reported using quantitative PET perfusion imaging (55).

Increasing stenosis severity also leads to a progressive reduction in distal coronary pressure and increasing vulnerability to subendocardial ischemia, because perfusion of the endocardial layers of the left ventricle is critically dependent on distal coronary pressure. Paradoxically, even though exercise increases epicardial coronary *flow* through a severe stenosis, subendocardial *perfusion* may actually decrease, because ischemia can increase the left ventricular filling pressure and increase the subendocardial diastolic compressive forces.

Coronary Collaterals

Coronary collateral vessels are vascular channels that connect large coronary arteries to one another. Native coronary collaterals are small, thin-walled structures with an endothelial lining and a sparse smooth muscle layer. Ischemia, however, can induce these primitive collaterals to develop into a major vascular network that can substantially modify the effects of coronary artery occlusion. Thus, following the onset of occlusion or the development of a severe stenosis (>80% diameter), a pressure gradient develops between occluded and nonoccluded vascular beds that stretches the collaterals, leading to rupture of the internal elastic lamina and migration of monocytes into the vessel wall. Over the next 1 to 2 weeks vascular growth occurs by mitotic division of endothelial cells, smooth muscle cells, and fibroblasts, resulting in larger, relatively thin-walled channels. A series of angiogenic factors produced in the myocardium, including vascular endothelial growth factor (VEGF) and fibroblast growth factor (FGF), contribute importantly to this growth of new blood vessels. Subsequently, over a period of months, the vessel wall becomes thicker and more organized by continued cellular proliferation and synthesis of elastin and collagen, so that the collateral vessel ultimately resembles a normal coronary artery. Experimentally, the functional capacity of collateral channels is near maximal by 4 weeks after coronary occlusion. Although effective resistance through immature native collaterals may be 60 to 80 times greater than minimal resistance through normal coronary vessels, the resistance falls to only two to three times normal in well-developed mature collaterals. Myocardium totally dependent on collaterals may have completely normal flow under resting conditions and may also possess substantial vascular reserve, with maximal flow as much as 50% of normal. Exercise perfusion imaging in patients may fail to detect a total coronary artery occlusion if collateralization of the occluded region is extensive, particularly if exercise heart rate is less than maximal (56).

Flow through collaterals is primarily dependent on the pressure gradient existing between the myocardial region perfused by the occluded or stenosed artery and the adjacent myocardial regions. Native immature collaterals may exhibit some vasomotion to neural, humoral, or pharmacologic stimuli, but the response is minimal because of the sparse numbers of smooth muscle cells present. Fully developed collaterals, however, have thick muscle coats and substantial neural connections are therefore capable of significant vasomotor activity.

Coronary steal is a vasodilator-induced decrease in collateral flow to a collateral-dependent region (57). This response is seen with small vessel arteriolar-type dilators, such as dipyridamole or adenosine, and is most likely to occur in the setting of multivessel disease, where the arteries supplying collateral flow are themselves narrowed by coronary stenoses. An increase in flow through these stenosed arteries leads to a decrease in downstream pressure (see earlier discussion), which reduces the pressure head across the collaterals and causes a decrease in collateral perfusion. This mechanism is believed to account for the high prevalence of myocardial ischemia (chest pain or electrocardiographic changes) seen in patients with severe coronary artery disease given dipyridamole during radionuclide perfusion imaging.

Relation Between Perfusion, Function, and Other Manifestations of Ischemia

A decrease in blood flow to a region of myocardium is associated with metabolic, functional, and electrocardiographic abnormalities, usually accompanied by the symptom of angina pectoris. Decreased oxygen delivery results in a cessation of aerobic metabolism, switch over to anaerobic glycolysis, buildup of lactic acid with tissue acidosis, and depletion of tissue high-energy phosphates. There is an almost immediate decrease in regional mechanical function, apparently related to an inability to cycle calcium normally to the myofilaments. Alterations in membrane function cause cell depolarization and relative inexcitability of the ischemic tissue, resulting in electrocardiographic ST segment abnormalities and QRS changes. All of these alterations are completely reversible if flow is restored within 15 to 20 minutes, although mechanical dysfunction may persist for hours to days before returning to normal (stunned myocardium) (Fig. 13.10) (58). Stunning is caused in part by oxygen-free radicals generated during reperfusion (41), and the dysfunction associated with stunning can be transiently reversed by catecholamines or calcium. Longer ischemic durations result in progressive cellular necrosis, beginning with the most vulnerable subendocardial layers and proceeding in wave-like fashion toward the epicardium (60).

Of the various clinical manifestations of ischemia, regional mechanical dysfunction appears first, followed by electrocardiographic abnormalities, and finally by the symptom of chest pain. When monitoring patients with unstable angina in the coronary care unit, it is common to see electrocardiographic changes without chest pain as a manifestation of early ischemia. Chest pain may occur seconds to minutes later or not at all (silent ischemia). Rest thallium imaging under these circumstances may demonstrate perfusion defects, despite the absence of chest pain or electrocardiographic abnormalities, which redistribute over sev-

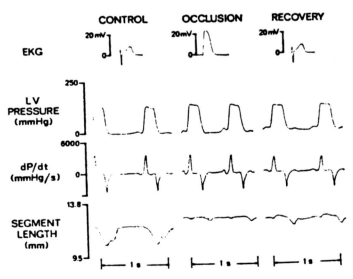

FIGURE 13.10. "Stunned myocardium." Myocardium remains dysfunctional after a brief (5-minute) occlusion of the coronary artery, despite normalization of the surface electrocardiogram. Residual dysfunction is denoted by increased myocardial segment length and markedly depressed shortening in the previously ischemic zone 5 minutes after release of the occlusion, and dysfunction may persist for up to 2 hours after such a brief occlusion. dP/dt, rate of rise of ventricular pressure; LV, left ventricle. (From Heyndrickx GR, Millard RW, McRitchie RJ et al. Regional myocardial function and electrophysiologic alterations after brief coronary occlusions in conscious dogs. *J Clin Invest* 1975;56:978, with permission.)

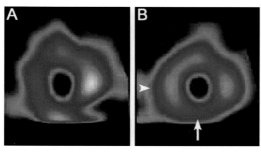

FIGURE 13.11. Single photon emission computed tomography short-axis views following injection of ^{201}Tl at rest. **A:** Rest injection in the absence of chest pain demonstrates an extensive anterior, septal, and inferior defect. **B:** Delayed imaging 6 hours later shows normalization of the anterior and septal walls (*arrowhead*), with a persistent defect in the inferior wall (*arrow*). These findings demonstrate asymptomatic resting ischemia of the anterior and septal regions and infarction in the inferior wall.

eral hours (Fig. 13.11). Reduced blood flow can be associated with a proportional down-regulation of contractility and oxygen demands, resulting in myocardial dysfunction without the usual signs of ischemia (i.e., no chest pain or electrocardiographic or metabolic abnormalities). This phenomenon is known as hibernating myocardium (61). Function can be promptly restored to normal by increasing blood flow, commonly by means of percutaneous transluminal coronary angioplasty or bypass surgery. Hibernating myocardium can be detected by a rest-injected thallium study that demonstrates an initial perfusion defect filling in over 3 to 4 hours (indicative of regional myocardial viability). PET may also be used to detect hibernating myocardium. A perfusion defect accompanied by evidence of metabolic activity in a region with reduced contractile function (perfusion-metabolism mismatch) identifies myocardium that is viable but ischemic at rest and, therefore, hibernating.

EXERCISE PHYSIOLOGY

Normal Mechanisms and Types of Cardiac Stress

Ventricular function can be examined more effectively and minor dysfunction may be exposed more easily if a stress is applied to the heart. Electrical pacing or handgrip (isometric exercise) may be used, but rhythmic (isotonic, dynamic) exercise is most often employed.

Three major adjustments occur during *rhythmic exercise.* First, in response to the metabolic demands of the exercising muscles, those arterioles dilate, and the muscular blood flow increases. Second, to prevent systemic hypotension, the central nervous system produces arteriolar constriction in the nonexercising beds, such as the renal and splanchnic circulations. Also, the splanchnic venous capacitance vessels constrict. These changes help maintain the arterial pressure, in spite of vasodilation in the exercising muscular beds, and they increase the venous return to the right heart. The mechanical pumping effects of exercising muscles help return blood to the right heart as well. The splanchnic and renal circulations are capable of withstanding such vaso-

constriction, because their resting flow is considerably greater than their metabolic demands.

The third compensation is thermal. The excess heat produced by the exercising muscles is dissipated by cutaneous vasodilation, mediated by temperature-sensitive cells in the hypothalamus. The greater the degree of muscular and skin vasodilation, the greater the splanchnic and renal vasoconstriction. These homeostatic mechanisms help preserve cardiac and cerebral perfusion.

The heart and lungs are the limiting factors in maintaining adequate tissue perfusion and oxygenation. The heart rate, stroke volume, blood pressure, and the inotropic state of the myocardium increase during exercise. An increase in heart rate is the primary means for increasing the cardiac output. Although the stroke volume increases slightly during the initial phases of rhythmic exercise, it may decrease slightly during prolonged exercise, apparently as a result of dilation of the cutaneous veins with a reduction in venous return and end-diastolic volume. However, with increased sympathetic stimulation of the myocardium, contractility is enhanced and the end-systolic volume decreases. Through these mechanisms the stroke volume increases by 10% to 20% during supine exercise. The stroke volume decreases when standing, but it increases during upright exercise to levels equal to supine resting stroke volume. By the combination of slightly improved stroke volume and tachycardia, the cardiac output rises threefold to sixfold during moderately severe rhythmic exercise. The arterial systolic blood pressure increases usually by 50%, based on the level of resting vasoconstriction, the character of the arterial walls, and the cardiac performance. The increased contractile state is also evident by tachycardia, shorter systolic ejection time, smaller end-systolic volume, increased *dP/dt*, and an increase in the ratio of peak systolic pressure to end-systolic volume.

All of these mechanisms cause an increase in myocardial oxygen consumption. However, in the face of such increased demand, the increase in the heart rate reduces the coronary diastolic filling time, and coronary atherosclerosis may limit coronary blood flow, causing myocardial ischemia in the susceptible heart. The rate-pressure product, heart rate multiplied by the systolic arterial blood pressure, correlates roughly with myocardial oxygen consumption and is an index of the severity of the exercise stress.

Isometric exercise has been employed in some instances for the evaluation of ischemic heart disease. The major effects of static exercise are an increase in the arterial blood pressure and moderate increase in heart rate. Under extreme conditions, the arterial blood pressure may increase more than during rhythmic exercise, but conventional rhythmic exercise testing produces greater heart rate responses and greater oxygen demands. It is difficult to maintain and quantitate the effects of isometric exercise, and this limits its usefulness for testing cardiac reserve, whether by conventional electrocardiography or by imaging methods.

Atrial pacing has been used to increase myocardial oxygen demands and coronary blood flow, particularly in patients who are unable to perform rhythmic exercise. However, pacing causes little increase in contractility or coronary flow compared with dynamic exercise.

Cold pressor testing has been used in the clinical laboratory as a type of stress in conjunction with blood pool or perfusion imaging. The cold pressor response is obtained by immersing one hand in ice water for 1 to 2 minutes. Systolic blood pressure usually increases 10%, but heart rate is unchanged. Coronary artery diameter decreases and focal coronary spasm may be elicited in patients with variant angina or coronary atherosclerosis. This response is probably mediated by α-adrenergic receptors in the coronary arteries stimulated through neural reflexes. Endothelial dysfunction enhances catecholamine-mediated coronary vasoconstriction (62). Sufficient coronary constriction or spasm may be associated with radionuclide perfusion defects, but this test is much less efficient than dynamic exercise for uncovering occult coronary artery disease.

Effects of Ischemia on Ventricular Performance

Myocardial ischemia is usually a localized phenomenon, resulting from excess myocardial oxygen demands compared with supply (e.g., myocardial blood flow). Transient myocardial ischemia may be produced by primary reduction in supply, such as by coronary ligation in the experimental animal or by coronary spasm in humans. More commonly, coronary stenoses limit supply, and demand is increased by physical activity, excess endogenous circulating catecholamines, or positive inotropic agents.

Regional ischemia, as noted earlier, reduces contraction (Fig. 13.10). Ischemia also hampers the active process of diastolic relaxation. The remaining, normally perfused myocardium attempts to compensate for ischemic regional dysfunction by enhanced contraction, probably the result of ventricular dilation and the Frank-Starling mechanism.

These important local effects may be accompanied by global hemodynamic derangements, if the area of ischemia is sufficiently large. The inadequate regional contraction may cause an increase in end-systolic volume. The end-diastolic volume may increase subsequent to the increase in end-systolic volume. The myocardium stiffens as a consequence of ischemia, and compliance thus becomes abnormal (Fig. 13.5). Incomplete relaxation can cause further elevation of the diastolic ventricular pressures, both early and late in diastole. These global changes in systole and in diastole can resolve after ischemia is relieved or may become chronic, as after infarction when fibrous scar replaces the normally compliant myocardium.

Both contrast and radionuclide ventriculography can detect and quantitate these abnormalities in systolic performance. Compliance abnormalities can be measured only by a combination of pressure and volume, but abnormal left ventricular filling rates resulting from reduced compliance may be seen using radionuclide ventriculography in some patients.

Coronary Blood Flow During Dynamic Exercise

Because of the tight coupling of myocardial blood flow and myocardial oxygen demands, coronary flow increases during exercise. Total myocardial oxygen consumption per beat increases about 60%. Myocardial oxygen demands are often approximated by the rate-pressure product but are also influenced by the inotropic state of the heart, left ventricular volume, and left ventricular wall thickness.

Left ventricular function during exercise is ordinarily not limited by coronary blood flow except in the presence of coronary artery disease. An exception may be during vigorous sprint exercise without a gradual warm-up, when systolic blood pressure increases rapidly, possibly leading to a transient subendocardial supply/demand imbalance.

In the presence of coronary stenoses, the normal increase in coronary flow during exercise is prevented. It is believed that flow increases in myocardium perfused by narrowed arteries but not to the extent necessary to keep up with increased oxygen demands. However, some evidence suggests that flow may actually fall below baseline levels in ischemic regions during stress. Maseri and associates (63) have shown that the washout of ^{133}Xe gas from an ischemic region slows markedly during pacing-induced ischemia after the region has been preloaded with the radioactive xenon. Similarly, Selwyn and coworkers (64) have demonstrated that the uptake of ^{82}Rb, a very short half-life cationic flow tracer, is reduced below baseline during ischemic episodes.

An absolute reduction in regional myocardial perfusion could occur during exercise if distal coronary pressure were to fall sufficiently, left ventricular diastolic pressure were to rise to inhibit subendocardial perfusion, or both were to occur together, which may often be the case. In addition, exercise-induced coronary vasoconstriction may often occur, particularly in the presence of endothelial dysfunction. At the far end of the spectrum, coronary spasm may occur during exercise, recognizable by the appearance of ST segment elevation during or following exercise.

The appearance of a perfusion defect during exercise signifies only that the perfusion of the area with the defect is less than that of the surrounding myocardium. Flow to the ischemic region could be increased or decreased in an absolute sense and the images would look the same. Similarly, flow to the apparently normal area may actually be normal or abnormal: One can only determine that the normal areas have the highest flow within the left ventricle.

REFERENCES

1. Gaasch WH, Levine HJ, Quinones MA et al. Left ventricular compliance: mechanisms and clinical implications. *Am J Cardiol* 1976;38: 645–653.
2. Udelson JE, Bacharach SL, Cannon RO III et al. Minimum left ventricular pressure during β-adrenergic stimulation in human subjects. Evidence for elastic recoil and diastolic "suction" in the normal heart. *Circulation* 1990;82:1174–1182.
3. Weber KT, Janicki JS, Hefner LL et al. Determinants of stroke volume in the isolated canine heart. *J Appl Physiol* 1974;37:742–747.
4. Cohn JN, Franciosa JA. Vasodilator therapy of heart failure. *N Engl J Med* 1977;297:27–31.
5. Wallace AG, Skinner NS Jr, Mitchell JH. Hemodynamic determinants of the maximal rate of rise of left ventricular pressure. *Am J Physiol* 1963;205:30–36.
6. Suga H, Sagwa K. Instantaneous pressure-volume relationships and their ratio in the excised, supported canine left ventricle. *Circ Res* 1974; 35:117–126.
7. Grossman W, Braunwald E, Mann T et al. Contractile state of the left ventricle in man as evaluated from end-systolic pressure-volume relations. *Circulation* 1977;56:845–852.

8. Carabello BA, Spann JF. The uses and limitations of end-systolic indices of left ventricular function. *Circulation* 1984;69:1058–1064.

9. Burkhoff D, Sugiura S, Yue DT et al. Contractility-dependent curvilinearity of end-systolic pressure-volume relations. *Am J Physiol* 1987; 252(Heart Circ Physiol 21):H1218–H1227.

10. Glower DD, Spratt JA, Snow ND et al. Linearity of the Frank-Starling relationship in the intact heart: the concept of preload recruitable stroke work. *Circulation* 1985;71:994–1009.

11. Little WC, Cheng C-P, Mumma M et al. Comparison of measures of left ventricular contractile performance derived from pressure-volume loops in conscious dogs. *Circulation* 1989;80:1378–1387.

12. Kass DA, Beyar R. Evaluation of contractile state by maximal ventricular power divided by the square of end-diastolic volume. *Circulation* 1991;84:1698–1708.

13. Marmor A, Sharir T, Shlomo IB et al. Radionuclide ventriculography and central aorta pressure change in noninvasive assessment of myocardial performance. *J Nucl Med* 1989;30:1657–1665.

14. Borow KM, Green LH, Grossman W et al. Left ventricular end-systolic stress-shortening and stress-length relations in humans. *Am J Cardiol* 1982;50:1301–1308.

15. Colan SD, Borow KM, Neumann A. Left ventricular end-systolic wall-stress velocity of fiber shortening relation: a load independent index of myocardial contractility. *J Am Coll Cardiol* 1984;4:715–724.

16. Ross J Jr. Cardiac function and myocardial contractility: a perspective. *J Am Coll Cardiol* 1983;1:52–62.

17. Park RC, Little WC, O'Rourke RA. Effect of alteration of left ventricular activation sequence on the left ventricular end-systolic pressure-volume relation in closed-chest dogs. *Circ Res* 1985;57:706–717.

18. Kass DA, Chen CH, Curry C et al. Improved left ventricular mechanics from acute VDD pacing in patients with dilated cardiomyopathy and ventricular conduction delay. *Circulation* 1999;99:1567–1573.

19. Kerwin WF, Botvinick EH, O'Connell JW et al. Ventricular contraction abnormalities in dilated cardiomyopathy: effect of biventricular pacing to correct interventricular dyssynchrony. *J Am Coll Cardiol* 2000;35:1221–1227.

20. Cazeau S, Leclercq C, Lavergne T et al. Effects of multisite biventricular pacing in patients with heart failure and intraventricular conduction delay. *N Engl J Med* 2001;344:873–880.

21. Brown MA, Myears DW, Bergmann SR. Noninvasive assessment of canine myocardial oxidative metabolism with carbon-11 acetate and positron emission tomography. *J Am Coll Cardiol* 1988;12:1054–1063.

22. Beanlands RSB, Bach DS, Raylman R et al. Acute effects of dobutamine on myocardial oxygen consumption and cardiac efficiency measured using carbon-11 acetate kinetics in patients with dilated cardiomyopathy. *J Am Coll Cardiol* 1993;22:1389–1398.

23. Beanlands RSB, Nahmias C, Gordon E et al. The effects of β_1-blockade on oxidative metabolism and the metabolic cost of ventricular work in patients with left ventricular dysfunction. A double-blind, placebo-controlled, positron-emission tomography study. *Circulation* 2000; 102:2070–2075.

24. McKay RG, Pfeffer MA, Pasternak RC et al. Left ventricular remodeling after myocardial infarction: a corollary to infarct expansion. *Circulation* 1986;74:693–702.

25. Konstam MA, Cohen SR, Salem DN et al. Comparison of left and right ventricular end-systolic pressure-volume relations in congestive heart failure. *J Am Coll Cardiol* 1985;6:1326–1334.

26. Francis GS, Benedict C, Johnstone DE et al. Comparison of neuroendocrine activation in patients with left ventricular dysfunction with and without congestive heart failure. A substudy of the Studies of Left Ventricular Dysfunction (SOLVD). *Circulation* 1990;82:1724–1729.

27. Torre-Amione G, Kapadia S, Lee J et al. Tumor necrosis factor α and tumor necrosis factor receptors in the failing human heart. *Circulation* 1996;93:704–711.

28. Colucci WS, Ribiero JP, Rocco MB et al. Impaired chronotropic response to exercise in patients with congestive heart failure. Role of postsynaptic β-adrenergic desensitization. *Circulation* 1989;80:314–323.

29. Konstam MA, Rousseau MF, Kronenberg MW et al. Effects of the angiotensin converting enzyme inhibitor enalapril on the long-term progression of left ventricular dysfunction in patients with heart failure. *Circulation* 1992;86:431–438.

30. The SOLVD Investigators. Effect of enalapril on survival in patients with reduced left ventricular ejection fractions and congestive heart failure. *N Engl J Med* 1991;325:293–302.

31. Pfeffer MA, Braunwald E, Moye LA et al. On behalf of the SAVE Investigators. Effect of captopril on mortality and morbidity in patients with left ventricular dysfunction after myocardial infarction: results of the survival and ventricular enlargement trial. *N Engl J Med* 1992;327:669–677.

32. Packer M, Bristow MR, Cohn JN et al. for the US Carvedilol Heart Failure Study Group. Effect of carvedilol on morbidity and mortality in chronic heart failure. *N Engl J Med* 1996;334:1349–1355.

33. Hjalmarson A, Goldstein S, Fagerberg B et al. Effects of controlled-release metoprolol on total mortality, hospitalizations, and well-being in patients with heart failure: the metoprolol CR/XL randomized intervention trial in congestive heart failure (MERIT-HF). MERIT-HF Study Group. *JAMA* 2000;283:1295–1302.

34. Biddle TL, Benotti JR, Creager MA et al. Comparison of intravenous milrinone and dobutamine for congestive heart failure secondary to either ischemic or dilated cardiomyopathy. *Am J Cardiol* 1987;59:1345–1350.

35. Dilsizian V, Bonow RO. Current diagnostic techniques of assessing myocardial viability in patients with hibernating and stunned myocardium. *Circulation* 1993;87:1–20.

36. Qureshi U, Nagueh SF, Afridi I et al. Dobutamine echocardiography and quantitative rest-redistribution 201Tl tomography in myocardial hibernation. Relation of contractile reserve to 201Tl uptake and comparative prediction of recovery of function. *Circulation* 1997;95:626–635.

37. Gould KL. Noninvasive assessment of coronary stenoses by myocardial perfusion imaging during pharmacologic coronary vasodilatation. I. Physiologic basis and experimental validation. *Am J Cardiol* 1978;41:267–278.

38. Picano E, Lattanzi F. Dipyridamole echocardiography. A new diagnostic window on coronary artery disease. *Circulation* 1991;83(Suppl III):III-19–III-26.

39. Cates CU, Kronenberg MW, Collins HW et al. Dipyridamole radionuclide ventriculography: a test with high specificity for severe coronary artery disease. *J Am Coll Cardiol* 1989;13:841–851.

40. Buckberg GB, Fixler DE, Archie JP et al. Experimental subendocardial ischemia in dogs with normal coronary arteries. *Circ Res* 1972;30:67–81.

41. White CW, Wright CB, Doty DB et al. Does visual interpretation of the coronary arteriogram predict the physiologic importance of a coronary stenosis? *N Engl J Med* 1984;310:819–824.

42. Doucette JW, Corl PD, Payne HM et al. Validation of a Doppler guidewire for intravascular measurement of coronary artery flow velocity. *Circulation* 1992;85:1899–1911.

43. Kronenberg MW, Roberton RM, Born ML et al. Thallium-201 uptake in variant angina: probable demonstration of myocardial reactive hyperemia in man. *Circulation* 1982;66:1332–1338.

44. Aversano T, Ouyang P, Silverman H. Blockade of the ATP-sensitive potassium channel modulates reactive hyperemia in the canine coronary circulation. *Circ Res* 1991;69:618–622.

45. Pennell DJ, Underwood SR, Swanton RH et al. Dobutamine thallium myocardial perfusion tomography. *J Am Coll Cardiol* 1991;18:1471–1479.

46. Albro PC, Gould KL, Westcott RJ et al. Noninvasive assessment of coronary stenoses by myocardial imaging during pharmacologic coronary vasodilation. III. Clinical trial. *Am J Cardiol* 1978;42:751–760.

47. Verani MS, Mahmarian JJ, Hixson JB et al. Diagnosis of coronary artery disease by controlled coronary vasodilation with adenosine and thallium-201 scintigraphy in patients unable to exercise. *Circulation* 1990;82:80–87.

48. Schroeder JS, Bolen JL, Quint RA et al. Provocation of coronary spasm with ergonovine maleate. New test with results in 57 patients undergoing coronary arteriography. *Am J Cardiol* 1977;40:487–491.

49. Griffith TM, Lewis MJ, Newby AC et al. Endothelium-derived relaxing factor. *J Am Coll Cardiol* 1988;12:797–806.

50. Inoue T, Tomoike H, Hisano K et al. Endothelium determines flow-dependent dilation of the epicardial coronary artery in dogs. *J Am Coll Cardiol* 1988;11:187–191.

51. Reddy KG, Nair RN, Sheehan HM et al. Evidence that selective endothelial dysfunction may occur in the absence of angiographic or ultrasound atherosclerosis in patients with risk factors for atherosclerosis. *J Am Coll Cardiol* 1994;23:833–843.

52. Duffy SJ, Castle SF, Harper RW et al. Contribution of vasodilator prostanoids and nitric oxide to resting flow, metabolic vasodilation, and flow-mediated dilation in human coronary circulation. *Circulation* 1999;100:1951–1957.

53. Miller DD, Donohue TJ, Younis LT et al. Correlation of pharmacological ^{99m}Tc-sestamibi myocardial perfusion imaging with poststenotic coronary flow reserve in patients with angiographically intermediate coronary stenosis. *Circulation* 1994;89:2150–2160.

54. Goldstein RA, Kirkeeide RL, Demer LL et al. Relation between geometric dimensions of coronary artery stenoses and myocardial perfusion reserve in man. *J Clin Invest* 1987;79:1473–1478.

55. Dayanikli F, Grambow D, Muzik O et al. Early detection of abnormal coronary flow reserve in asymptomatic men at high risk for coronary artery disease using positron emission tomography. *Circulation* 1994;90:808–817.

56. Rigo P, Becker LC, Griffith LSC et al. The influence of coronary collaterals on the results of thallium-201 myocardial stress imaging. *Am J Cardiol* 1979;44:452–458.

57. Becker LC. Conditions for vasodilator-induced coronary steal in experimental myocardial ischemia. *Circulation* 1978;57:1103–1110.

58. Heyndrickx GR, Millard RW, McRitchie RJ et al. Regional myocardial functional and electrophysiological alterations after brief coronary occlusion in conscious dogs. *J Clin Invest* 1975;56:978–985.

59. Bolli R, Jeroudi MO, Patel BS et al. Marked reduction of free radical generation and contractile dysfunction by antioxidant therapy begun at the time of reperfusion. Evidence that myocardial "stunning" is a manifestation of reperfusion injury. *Circ Res* 1989;65:607–622.

60. Reimer KA, Lowe JE, Rasmussen MM et al. The wavefront phenomenon of ischemic cell death. I. Myocardial infarct size vs. duration of coronary occlusion in dogs. *Circulation* 1977;56:786–794.

61. Rahimtoola SH. Coronary bypass surgery for chronic angina—1981: a perspective. *Circulation* 1982;65:225–241.

62. Baumgart D, Haude M, Görge G, Liu F et al. Augmented α-adrenergic constriction of atherosclerotic human coronary arteries. *Circulation* 1999;99:2090–2097.

63. Maseri A, L'Abbate A, Pesola A et al. Regional myocardial perfusion in patients with atherosclerotic coronary artery disease at rest and during angina pectoris induced by tachycardia. *Circulation* 1977;55:423–433.

64. Selwyn AP, Forse G, Fox K et al. Patterns of disturbed myocardial perfusion in patients with coronary artery disease. Regional myocardial perfusion in angina pectoris. *Circulation* 1981;64:83–90.

SUGGESTED READING

Becker LC. Increasing coronary blood flow. In: Wagner GS, ed. *Myocardial infarction: measurement and intervention.* The Hague: Martinus Nijhoff Publishers, 1982:415–456.

Berne RM, Rubio R. Coronary circulation. In: Berne RM, ed. *Handbook of physiology.* Section 2: The cardiovascular system. Volume I. The heart. Bethesda, MD: American Physiological Society, 1979:873–952.

Braunwald E, Sonnenblick EH, Ross J Jr. *Mechanisms of contraction of the normal and failing heart,* 2nd ed. Boston: Little, Brown and Company, 1976.

Colucci WS, Braunwald E. Pathophysiology of heart failure. In: Braunwald E, Zipes DP, Libby P, eds. *Heart disease.* 6th ed. Philadelphia: WB Saunders, 2001:503–533.

Eichhorn EJ, Bristow MR. Medical therapy can improve the biological properties of the chronically failing heart. A new era in the treatment of heart failure. *Circulation* 1996;94:2285–2296.

Hoffman JIE. Key references: coronary blood flow. *Circulation* 1980;62:187–198.

LeWinter MM, Osol G. Normal physiology of the cardiovascular system. In: Fuster V, Alexander RW, O'Rourke RA, eds. *Hurst's the heart,* 10th ed. New York: McGraw-Hill, 2001:63–94.

Little WC. Assessment of normal and abnormal cardiac function. In: Braunwald E, Zipes DP, Libby P, eds. *Heart disease,* 6th ed. Philadelphia: WB Saunders, 2001:479–502.

Marcus ML. *The coronary circulation in health and disease.* New York: McGraw-Hill, 1983.

Olsson RA, Bunger R, Spann JAE. Coronary circulation. In: Fozzard HA, Haber E, Jennings RB et al., eds. *The heart and cardiovascular system. Scientific foundations,* 2nd ed. New York: Raven Press, 1986:1390–1425.

Opie LH. Mechanisms of cardiac contraction and relaxation. In: Braunwald E, Zipes DP, Libby P, eds. *Heart disease,* 6th ed. Philadelphia: WB Saunders, 2001:443–478.

Sagawa K, Maughan L, Suga H et al. *Cardiac contraction and the pressure-volume relationship.* New York: Oxford University Press, 1988.

Schaper W, Bernotat-Danielowski S, Nienaber C et al. Collateral circulation. In: Fozzard HA, Haber E, Jennings RB et al., eds. *The heart and cardiovascular system. Scientific foundations,* 2nd ed. New York: Raven Press, 1991:1427–1464.

Shepherd JT, Vanhoutte PM. *The human cardiovascular system: Facts and concepts.* New York: Raven Press, 1979.

Diagnostic Nuclear Medicine, Fourth Edition. Edited by M.P. Sandler, R.E. Coleman, J.A. Patton, F.J.Th. Wackers, A. Gottschalk. Lippincott Williams & Wilkins, Philadelphia 2003.

14

RADIONUCLIDE EVALUATION OF LEFT VENTRICULAR FUNCTION

PATRICK B. MURPHY
STEVEN C. PORT

There are many techniques available to the clinician for the assessment of ventricular function. All the commonly used clinical imaging modalities, including conventional x-ray, computed tomography (CT) x-ray, magnetic resonance imaging (MRI), ultrasound, and γ-ray, provide useful information about ventricular function. Because of its excellent spatial resolution and freedom from contamination by surrounding structures, contrast angiography has been the standard to which all of those have been compared. Of the noninvasive methods, the radionuclide techniques are unique because the radioactivity that is injected for the purpose of imaging the heart temporarily remains in the cardiac chambers in a concentration that is directly proportional to the volume of blood in those chambers, making the technique inherently quantitative. All the other noninvasive and invasive techniques require mathematical assumptions about the geometry of a ventricle to quantitate ventricular function. Such assumptions work well some of the time, but when the shape of a ventricle is distorted by localized infarction, severe hypertrophy, or marked dilatation, the accuracy of geometric approaches is questionable. One could argue that the radionuclide methods should be the standard to which others, including contrast angiography, are compared.

Although many different names have been used for the radionuclide methods of evaluating ventricular function, the term *radionuclide angiography* (RNA) is used here. It is a generic term, which is appropriate because it acknowledges that it is not only the ventricles that are imaged but the great vessels, the atria, and other blood-filled organs as well. RNA is performed in two distinctly different ways, the gated equilibrium radionuclide angiography (ERNA) and the first-pass radionuclide angiography (FPRNA). Each technique has its own particular strengths and weaknesses and the student or practitioner of radionuclide cardiac imaging should be thoroughly familiar with the unique attributes and technical requirements of each technique. In this chapter, the two techniques are described separately and then compared.

EQUILIBRIUM RADIONUCLIDE ANGIOGRAPHY

Equilibrium radionuclide imaging is known by other names: gated blood pool imaging (GBP), radionuclide ventriculography (RNV), or simply MUGA (multigated acquisition). Since Strauss and Zaret (1,2) showed its use for measuring left ventricular ejection fraction (LVEF) and detecting regional ventricular dysfunction, there have been major enhancements in the hardware and software necessary for data acquisition and processing. Blood pools in the body consist mainly of the cardiac chambers, great vessels, and spleen. Those organs contain large amounts of free blood as opposed to blood intermixed with tissue such as in the liver or kidney. Spatial resolution of the photons can be maximized so that anatomically correct representations of the cardiac chambers and great vessels may be produced. With the use of a physiologic trigger, such as an electrocardiogram (ECG) gate that links the acquisition to the cardiac cycle, elegant cinematic displays of the change in radioactivity within the cardiac chambers and great vessels can be generated. If the radionuclide has long enough biologic and physical half-lives, then images may be acquired in multiple views or during multiple physiologic conditions such as the sequential stages of an exercise test.

Imaging Agents

The only radionuclide that has been used clinically for ERNA is ^{99m}Tc. Initially, ^{99m}Tc-human serum albumin was used to create an intravascular tag. However, image quality was, by present standards, relatively poor and acquisition times were prolonged because the large amount of albumin sequestered in the pulmonary arterial tree caused a low signal-to-background ratio (3). The use of labeled albumin was virtually replaced in the late 1970s by the more efficient method of labeling red blood cells (RBCs) *in vivo* (4,5). The RBC tag had a much more favorable target-to-background ratio compared with labeled albumin.

P.B. Murphy: Attending Cardiologist, Mid Central Cardiology, Bloomington, IL.

S.C. Port: Clinical Professor Of Medicine, University Of Wisconsin Medical School, Milwaukee Clinical Campus, Aurora Sinai Medical Center, Milwaukee, WI.

RBC Labeling Techniques

Technetium labeling of RBCs requires that the technetium be reduced so that it will bind with intracellular protein. The reduced form of technetium binds to the globin chain of the hemoglobin molecule. The initial reducing agent used was the iron ion found in iron ascorbate. Although that was effective, separation by column chromatography was necessary and labeling efficiency was not high. A higher binding efficiency was found with the use of the stannous ion (6). Standardized kit formulations using stannous pyrophosphate were subsequently developed and have greatly facilitated the clinical application of this type of RBC labeling. The optimal dose of tin will maximize the percentage of technetium bound inside the RBC and minimize the extravascular and circulating free technetium. An inadequate amount of stannous ion will result in free technetium remaining outside the RBC, thus increasing background contamination of the images. An excess amount of stannous ion results in the reduction of technetium before its entrance into the cell, thereby preventing its binding to intracellular protein and again increasing background activity. There are currently three RBC labeling protocols in use: *in vivo, in vitro,* and *modified in vivo* (in "vivtro") techniques.

In Vivo Technique

The *in vivo* labeling technique, as the name describes, takes place within the bloodstream. Pretreatment of the RBC is performed with an intravenous injection of 10 to 20 μg per kg of stannous pyrophosphate (7,8). The stannous ion is allowed to circulate for 30 minutes, which results in maximum uptake by the RBCs. A dose of 15 to 30 mCi (550 to 1100 MBq) of ^{99m}Tc pertechnetate is then injected intravenously. The RBCs will be labeled over the succeeding 5 to 10 minutes. Some of the free circulating pertechnetate will be taken up by the thyroid, the kidneys, and the gastric mucosa. A large percentage of the unbound pertechnetate will be excreted by the kidneys. The labeling efficiency of this method ranges from 85% to 95%. The *in vivo* technique is considered the easiest to perform because it is the least labor intensive and it results in the lowest radiation exposure to personnel. It also has the benefit of the injection of a small bolus of ^{99m}Tc pertechnetate that facilitates adjunctive first-pass imaging.

In Vitro Technique

In contrast, the *in vitro* method is the most technically complex and time-consuming approach. A small amount (10 to 20 cc) of the patient' blood is withdrawn into a syringe. Stannous citrate is then added to provide approximately 1.5 μg of stannous ion and additionally to help prevent coagulation of the blood. After 5 minutes of gentle agitation, the syringe is centrifuged. The supernatant that contains any excess stannous ions is then discarded. The resultant packed RBCs are then mixed with 15 to 30 mCi (550 to 1110 MBq) of ^{99m}Tc pertechnetate. After another 5 minutes of gentle agitation, the mixture is considered properly incubated and is reinjected into the patient. After 5 to 10 minutes, the tagged RBCs are considered to be in equilibrium throughout the blood volume. The labeling efficiency of the *in vitro* technique is routinely above 95% (9). However, the increased time, blood handling, and radiation exposure for the technologists and the need for a centrifuge have precluded clinical acceptance of the *in vitro* technique.

Modified In Vivo Technique

The *modified in vivo* or in vivtro technique represents a compromise between the two previous methods. Increased labeling efficiency, compared with the *in vivo* technique, is achieved by tagging the RBCs with ^{99m}Tc pertechnetate outside the body, whereas less labor and exposure for the technologist is achieved by *in vivo* RBC preparation with stannous ion. In this technique, stannous pyrophosphate is injected intravenously. After 30 minutes, 5 mL of blood are withdrawn into a shielded syringe containing 15 to 30 mCi (550 to 1110 MBq) of ^{99m}Tc pertechnetate and 1 mL of acid-citrate-dextrose (ACD) solution. After 10 minutes of incubation, the RBCs are reinjected. Five to 10 minutes are then adequate for equilibrium throughout the total blood volume.

Compared with the *in vitro* method, this technique is less time consuming, but the tagging efficiency of 90% to 93% is lower (10). In general, image quality will be better than that achieved with the *in vivo* technique. As a result, the in vivtro technique has become the method of choice in many clinical facilities (Fig. 14.1).

Factors that May Modify RBC Labeling

There are several drugs, intravenous solutions, and clinical conditions that may theoretically interfere with RBC labeling (11, 12). Heparin, because of its clinical ubiquity, is probably of most concern. Heparin may reduce the labeling efficiency by oxidizing the stannous ion and complexing with the pertechnetate. One cannot avoid studying patients receiving heparin, but direct injection of the tin or the pertechnetate into intravenous lines that contain heparin should be avoided. Solutions of dextrose, mannitol, and sorbitol, and the presence of antibodies to the

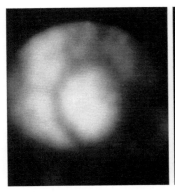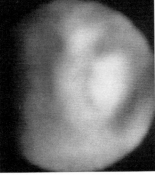

FIGURE 14.1. Red blood cell (RBC) labeling. On the left is an example of a good quality RBC tag performed using the modified *in vivo* technique. The cardiac chambers are clearly delineated and the background activity is low. On the right is an example of a poor quality tag that was performed using the *in vivo* technique. Note the poor target-to-background ratio.

RBCs, as can occur in certain autoimmune diseases or after treatment with methyldopa or quinidine, may also reduce labeling efficiency.

Instrumentation

Camera

The goal of ERNA is to obtain images of the cardiac chambers and great vessels with as high a spatial resolution as possible. The small field-of-view (SFOV) cameras provide higher resolution images than do the large field-of-view (LFOV) systems. SFOV cameras are most adaptable to ERNA because they can be more easily manipulated into the appropriate positions and can typically touch the chest during the acquisition of all views. The LFOV systems can certainly provide diagnostic quality images and are used frequently. Multicrystal gamma-cameras have been used but are not recommended because of their lower spatial resolution.

Collimation

The collimator should be selected to meet the demands of the particular type of study to be acquired. For most resting ERNA studies where the clinical question is the evaluation of ventricular function, a standard parallel hole, low energy, all-purpose collimator is adequate. With LFOV detectors, a slant hole collimator may be useful because it requires less angulation of the large head making oblique views easier and more comfortable to acquire. High-resolution collimators do improve image quality, but the gain in resolution is achieved by prolonging imaging time. For most resting studies, however, time is not usually important so high-resolution collimators should be used if available.

For exercise studies, there is a premium on the count rate because time is limited. Some laboratories have used high-sensitivity collimators during exercise, but the degradation in resolution may not be worth the higher count flux. In general, the all-purpose collimator is most often used for exercise acquisitions.

Computer/Software

All commercially available computers designed for nuclear imaging systems are capable of acquiring ERNA data. Where systems differ is in the software. Ideally, the software should allow a variety of frame rates and pixel matrixes for both acquisition and processing. The system should permit both 64×64 and 128×128 acquisitions at frame rates of 8 to at least 32 frames per cycle. Arrhythmia detection and editing are essential. It is particularly helpful to be able to perform a time correction of the data as it is being acquired. Standard temporal and spatial filters, as well as Fourier filtering, are necessary and available on most, if not all, systems. Both frame mode and list mode acquisition protocols should be available. The software for data processing should allow manual, automatic, and semiautomatic approaches. It is incumbent on the operator to perform a validation study of the particular processing protocol chosen.

Data Acquisition

Imaging Angles

Most facilities employ three standard views for routine diagnostic work. The ability to view a study cinematically as it is progressing allows the technologist to reposition a patient or the detector to achieve an optimal image.

The primary view for quantitative analysis in ERNA is the so-called best septal view. This view is typically obtained with the detector in a 40-degree to 50-degree left anterior oblique (LAO) position. A slight caudal tilt enhances separation of the left atrium and the left ventricle. Ideally, the best septal view provides a true short axis view in which the left ventricle appears spherical and there is clear separation of the two ventricles. Because this is the view that will be used for almost all the quantitative analyses applied to the study, several angles should be tested until the best possible angle is identified. Furthermore, this is the only view that can isolate that part of the left ventricle perfused by the circumflex coronary artery. Either too shallow or too steep an angle will compromise that ability (Fig. 14.2).

Two additional views are obtained to visualize the remaining walls of the left ventricle and other cardiac structures. An anterior view is obtained by simply positioning the detector parallel to the chest or by rotating the detector approximately 45 degrees anteriorly from the best septal view. The third view is the left lateral view that can be acquired by placing the patient in a right decubitus position with the detector parallel to the left chest or by rotating the detector 45 degrees more laterally than the best septal view.

Most important is that the technologist understands the anatomy of the cardiac chambers so that the appropriate anatomic views are acquired even if the angles do not conform to what one would predict.

Gating

Gating is the technique that links the acquisition of the image data to the cardiac cycle. Most ERNA studies are acquired in the so-called frame mode. In a frame mode acquisition, the car-

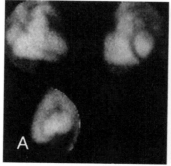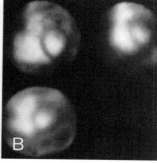

FIGURE 14.2. **A:** Examples of correctly positioned anterior, best septal, and lateral views of a resting equilibrium radionuclide angiogram (EqRNA) examination. **B:** Three examples of septal views. The upper left image shows a true best septal view. The image at the upper right is an example of too shallow a septal view and the lower image is that of too steep a view. Note that the left ventricle and right ventricle can be separated in all three examples but only the upper left image is the correct one.

diac cycle is arbitrarily divided up into a fixed number of frames and the data from each cycle are divided up and stored as individual frame memory bins. Individual beat information is lost once that beat has been added to the data. Theoretically, any physiologic event that varies with the cardiac cycle could be used to gate an acquisition. The ECG is the most convenient and is universally used for ERNA. The accuracy of the gate depends on the QRS recognition scheme used by the computer and the quality of the ECG signal. There is usually a small time lag between the onset of electrical depolarization and the onset of systolic contraction, so the peak (R wave) or the nadir (S wave) of the QRS complex actually corresponds fairly closely to end-diastole. However, the lag between the QRS and the onset of contraction varies from subject to subject and can be prolonged if there is a conduction delay such as left bundle branch block so that end-diastole may actually occur in frame 2 or 3 of the study.

There are a number of gating schemes for ERNA. The standard method is the forward gating technique. In this case, the ECG signal is used to identify the beginning of frame 1 of the acquisition. Frame time is calculated as the average RR interval divided by the number of assigned frames. In the example of a 16-frame study, the events recorded during the first sixteenth of the RR cycle will be stored in frame 1, the information from the second sixteenth time interval of the cardiac cycle in the second frame, and so on until the last frame is acquired. The accuracy of this approach depends heavily on the constancy of the RR interval during the acquisition. If a beat is longer than the previous beats, then the last frame acquired will not correspond to the end of the cycle. If a beat is shorter than the previous beats, then the last frame acquired will contain data from the beginning of the beat following the short beat. Variable beat length most significantly affects the diastolic portion of the cardiac cycle so that the end of the left ventricular (LV) time-activity curve may appear quite distorted (Fig. 14.3). One approach to avoiding beat variability is to use an RR interval screening method (window) whereby the computer analyzes the beat length of each cycle and accepts or rejects the beat based on

predetermined criteria. Fortunately, the systolic portion of the cardiac cycle is insignificantly affected by most minor variations in cycle length. With appropriate attention to RR window selection, accurate representations of both the systolic and diastolic portions of the LV time-activity curve could routinely be obtained (13).

Reverse Gating

Instead of assigning frame number 1 to the R wave, in reverse gating, the last frame is assigned to end on the R wave. As a result, the end-diastolic (ED) portion of the time-activity curve is protected and any distortions tend to occur in early systole. A compromise is the use of a combined forward-reverse gating technique. The first two thirds of the cycle are gated in a forward direction and the end of the cycle in a reverse direction, and the two portions of the curve are joined. The forward gating improves the accuracy of the information obtained early in systole, whereas the backward gating portion preserves the ED data (14).

Alternate R Wave Gating

Another approach is alternate R wave gating (15). With this technique, frame 1 of the study is identified by every other R wave. Once a cycle is initiated, it is continued through the next R wave and ends with third R wave. The resultant time-activity curve encompasses two complete cardiac cycles and the diastolic portion of the first of the two cycles contains less distortion than would be seen in standard forward gating. Application of the alternate R wave gate is appropriate when evaluation of diastolic function is the clinical question at hand.

R-R Window and Arrhythmia Rejection

All commercially available systems have beat length acceptance criteria as part of the standard ERNA acquisition protocol. The appropriate RR window for a given study depends on the subject's rhythm, the type of study, and the desired level of physiologic accuracy. Obviously, the narrower the RR window, the more homogeneous the beat lengths and the more physiologic the resultant time-activity curve. The tradeoff is always accuracy versus time because the narrower the window the longer the acquisition. For most routine clinical applications, a 10% to 15% window is appropriate. Virtually all premature beats will fall outside such a window. However, a number of sinus beats will also be rejected if there is any significant sinus arrhythmia, which is common. Increasing the window will decrease acquisition time but at the expense of the diastolic portion of the time-activity curve. During an exercise study, the time available for imaging is very brief but the heart rate during exercise is usually so regular that the RR window is usually not important.

List Mode

List mode acquisition is the most memory intensive method. The scintigraphic data are stored continuously without any pre-

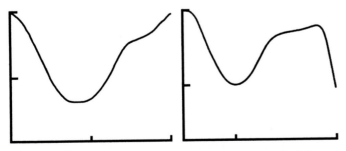

FIGURE 14.3. The left ventricular time-activity curve on the left was acquired in frame mode with software that allowed analysis and time correction of each accepted beat before storing the beat in memory. As a result there is preservation of the integrity of the diastolic portion of the curie. Studies acquired in such a fashion will always have the last frame return to end-diastole. On the right is an example of a similar curve acquired with a standard frame mode acquisition. Minor changes in heart rate within the beat acceptance window result in the last frame occurring at different times in the diastolic portion of the cardiac cycle. The shape of the curve is typical of this common problem.

set framing criteria. Time markers and the ECG signal are also stored. After the acquisition is terminated, the operator has the ability to screen all the cycles stored during the acquisition. The data can then be reformatted into a cycle that contains as many beats of whatever length is desired. With this approach the operator can set a very narrow RR window and then screen the resultant cycle to see if there are enough beats in the window to provide accurate statistics. If not, the window can be adjusted to accept more beats until the optimal combination of window length and statistics is produced. List mode allows formatting of multiple beat lengths for the study of the effects of cycle length or arrhythmia on ventricular function. Time-activity curves with very high temporal resolution can be generated with this technique because the timing markers are usually stored at 10-millisecond intervals. As a result, the list mode acquisition is particularly appropriate for studies of diastolic function.

Frame Rate and Frame Counts

Selection of the number of frames for an ERNA study depends on the clinical question being asked, the software capabilities, and the time available for acquisition. The greater the number of frames obtained during the cardiac cycle, the better the temporal resolution of the ventricular time-activity curve and, therefore, the more representative of the true cyclic variations in chamber volume. The influence of the frame rate on the measurements of systolic and diastolic function has been examined. It has been shown that the systolic phase of the cycle could be adequately assessed with as few as 16 frames per cycle, whereas the diastolic variables were best measured using 32 to 48 frames per cycle (14). Practically, it is advisable to acquire all LAO views at 32 frames per cycle so that both systole and diastole can be adequately evaluated in all clinical studies. The other views of the acquisition can be acquired at 24 or even 16 frames per cycle. For exercise studies, in which the scanning time is at a premium and in which the interest is usually in systolic function, a frame rate of 16 frames per cycle is a good compromise between temporal resolution and statistics per frame.

To maintain image quality and statistical reliability for quantitation, a minimum number of counts must be contained in each frame. Most authorities believe that the absolute minimum number of counts per frame is 125,000, but would also agree that a more typically acceptable number would be 250,000 counts per frame (16). Whichever minimum number is selected, an increase in the number of frames will proportionally increase the scanning time to maintain the same count rate per frame.

Stress Protocols

Exercise

The evaluation of ventricular function during exercise is helpful diagnostically and, in particular, prognostically. ERNA can be applied to bicycle exercise in both the upright and supine positions. Treadmill exercise is unsuitable for equilibrium studies because of chest motion. Several commercially available exercise tables equipped with cycle ergometers have been specifically designed for simultaneous radionuclide imaging. Supine bicycle

exercise places maximum strain on the legs and many patients will stop exercising with leg fatigue before achieving an adequate cardiovascular stress. That is especially true in older or deconditioned subjects. Semisupine or upright exercise is better tolerated. Supine cycling is accompanied by higher LV ED pressure but lower peak heart rates than is upright cycling, but the overall stress on the heart is fairly similar at any given workload (17).

There is no absolutely correct imaging sequence for acquisition of an exercise ERNA. The resting LAO study should be performed in the same position as the exercise study so that the change in volumes and/or function will reflect the cardiac status rather than any change in position. Graded exercise using 3-minute stages works reasonably well because the heart rate usually reaches a plateau in about 1 minute, and 2 minutes remain for acquisition. Because it is difficult to predict when a subject will stop exercising, it is wise to acquire each stage of the study although it is not necessary to process all stages. The peak exercise stage should be extended as long as the patient can safely continue to insure image quality. However, the workload should never be lowered during the acquisition to prolong the exercise. Decreases in workload of as little as 25% are accompanied by immediate improvement in regional and global ventricular function that could result in underestimation of the magnitude of ischemia (18).

The primary view for an exercise study is, of course, the best septal view that allows generation of the quantitative data to be analyzed and reported. Wall motion abnormalities may be assessed in the septal, inferior, lateral, or posterior walls in the best septal view. If there is a specific clinical question regarding the anterolateral wall or apex or if one wants to obtain maximum sensitivity for left anterior descending coronary artery disease (CAD), it may be useful to quickly rotate the detector to the anterior view once the septal view has enough statistics. Although not necessary in most cases, an immediate postexercise image may be of value in predicting recovery of function after revascularization in ventricular segments with severe motion abnormalities at rest (19,20).

Alternatives to Exercise: Pacing, Cold Pressor, and Pharmacologic Stress

Several options are available to challenge the coronary circulation and ventricular function in subjects who are unable to exercise. They include atrial pacing, cold pressor testing, catecholamine infusions, and coronary vasodilators. Before the widespread application of pharmacologic testing, atrial pacing was proposed as a mechanism of increasing myocardial oxygen demand, thereby provoking ischemia (21). Cold pressor testing stresses the heart by peripheral vasoconstriction induced during immersion of an extremity in ice water. That results in elevation of systolic and diastolic blood pressure, as well as changes in the distribution of coronary blood flow. In patients with significant CAD, regional ventricular ischemia can be produced (22).

Catecholamine infusion is another approach to increasing myocardial oxygen demand in an effort to induce ischemia. Isoproterenol, dopamine, and dobutamine have all been tested, but only intravenous dobutamine has received significant clinical acceptance. Dobutamine is usually started at 5 μg/kg/minute, and the infusion rate is progressively increased every 5 minutes to 10, 20, 30, 40, and up to 50 µg/kg/minute or until a target heart rate is reached or symptoms preclude continuation of the test (23). As with an exercise test, each stage of the infusion should be imaged. Ischemic or arrhythmic effects can be reversed by either discontinuing the infusion or by intravenous administration of a rapidly acting beta blocker. Dobutamine produces a fairly consistent increase in heart rate and typically a modest elevation in blood pressure. Occasionally, the blood pressure and heart rate may suddenly drop during the infusion.

Standard Data Processing

There are as many approaches to processing of ERNA data as there are vendors of gamma-cameras and software. It is beyond the scope of this chapter to review every nuance of data processing. However, the basic routines necessary to the processing of all studies are discussed. The operator is advised to view a cinematic display of the best septal view before beginning processing. That will provide a good visual sense of the spatial relationships between the two ventricles and between the ventricles and the atria, which becomes important during the creation of the regions-of-interest for the ventricular time-activity curve.

Left Ventricular Time-Activity Curve: Creating the Regions-of-Interest

Because all the quantitative data that will be used to describe the function of the left ventricle are derived from the LV time-activity curve, every effort should be made to generate a curve that, as accurately as possible, reflects the changes in volume throughout the cardiac cycle. Most important to that process, of course, is the information density or counts within each frame and the sharpness of separation between the ventricle and surrounding chambers throughout the cardiac cycle, both of which are determined before processing begins. Despite all the temporal and spatial filters available to the operator, technically inadequate raw data cannot be resurrected during processing. Given whatever raw data is available, the subsequent accuracy of the time-activity curve is highly dependent on the accuracy of the regions-of-interest (ROI). There are three ways to generate the ROI; manual, semiautomatic, and automatic.

As its name implies, the manual method requires the operator to draw all the ROI to be used for the time-activity curve (Fig. 14.4). Because this is a labor intensive approach, it is usually restricted to drawing only the ED and end-systolic (ES) ROI. The ED ROI is usually drawn on frame 1 of the study. That ROI can then be used to generate a preliminary curve whose nadir identifies the ES frame. The operator can then draw the ES ROI. Two curves now exist, one from the ED ROI and the other from the ES ROI. The two curves can be interpolated to create the final LV time-activity curve.

The semiautomatic method requires the operator to identify the left ventricle by manually drawing an initial ROI at ED. The program will then use an automated edge-detection algorithm to identify the LV perimeter in every frame of the study including the ED frame. All the computer-generated ROI should be visually inspected in a large enough format to be easily checked

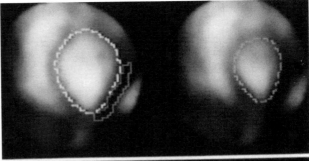
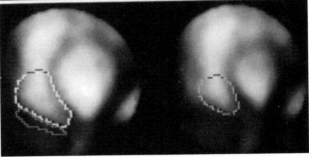

FIGURE 14.4. To calculate the left (*top*) or right (*bottom*) ventricular ejection fraction manually, regions-of-interest (ROIs) are hand drawn around the chamber at end-diastole (*left*) and at end-systole (*right*) taking care to avoid nonventricular activity. A crescent-shaped background ROI is placed near the lateral border of the ventricle at end-diastole. For left ventricular processing, the background ROI avoids the activity from the adjacent spleen.

for accuracy. In the semiautomated or interactive approach, the operator can then reject and recreate any ROI that either excludes ventricular activity or includes nonventricular activity.

In the fully automated method, the operator does not get the opportunity to review and adjust the computer-determined ROI (Fig. 14.5). Operators should not be lulled into accepting automated ROI without visual inspection of each ROI. No algorithm is infallible. The automated approaches are not supplied for their accuracy, but rather for their speed and consistency. In direct comparisons of results obtained with manual and automated ROI, the manual method actually had the smallest intraobserver and interobserver variabilities (24). As a routine quality control technique, it is advisable to process each clinical study using both a manual and either an automated or semiautomated method.

Background Correction

For accurate quantitative analysis of ERNA data, the time-activity curve must be corrected for the contribution of adjacent, noncardiac activity. When viewed in the LAO position, the left ventricle is adjacent to the lung and descending aorta. Occasionally, splenic or gastric activity is superimposed on the LV chamber. There will be some activity contained in the pulmonary vasculature, especially in patients with high pulmonary pressures, and some activity in the myocardium itself. There is also a variable contribution from the left atrium that is difficult, if not impossible, to quantify. Background activity is estimated by drawing a ROI lateral to the left ventricle in the best septal view.

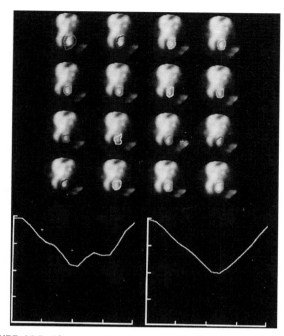

FIGURE 14.5. The computer can automatically generate regions-of-interest (ROIs) on each frame of the study once an initial, manual ROI is drawn to orient the computer to the borders of the chamber (*top, left*). As the time-activity curve on the left illustrates, the computer-generated ROIs not infrequently include noncardiac activity. A semiautomatic program allows the operator to selectively override the computer to correct any errant ROIs, which then corrects the time-activity curve (*right*).

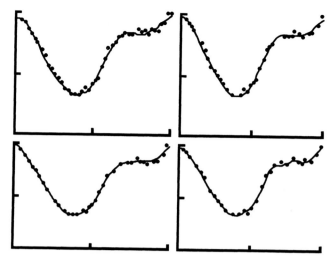

FIGURE 14.6. Applying a Fourier transform to the raw data eliminates noise. The figure shows the effects of increasing the number of harmonics used in the filtering process. With three harmonics (*top left*), the fitted curve appears to inadequately represent the true physiologic details of the actual data curve whereas six harmonics (*lower right*) appear to introduce variability that was not present in the raw data. Four (*top right*) or five (*bottom left*) harmonics appear to be adequate at average resting heart rates.

Typically, a 2 to 3 pixel-wide crescent-shaped ROI, placed 1 to 3 pixels away from the LV ROI, is used to quantify the background (Fig. 14.4). The average count per pixel in that ROI is assumed to be representative of the entire background and is subtracted from each pixel count within the LV ROI. Care must be taken that "hot" noncardiac sites are not incorporated into the background ROI, e.g., liver or spleen. If that occurs, an artificially high ejection fraction (EF) would be calculated.

Temporal and Fourier Filtering

Once the background correction has been applied, the time-activity curve should be reviewed using a display of each data point. The operator should identify any points that do not appear to belong to the curve of that subjects data and then reexamine the ROI that produced those values. If necessary, the ROI should be redrawn. Even after the ROI are reviewed, the unfiltered time-activity curve may show fluctuations in counts that are not physiologic but due, instead, to the randomness of γ-photon emissions and unavoidable admixture of nonventricular activity in a ROI. To eliminate such random noise in the data, the time-activity curve is typically subjected to a temporal filter that in its simplest form might be a 1-2-1 frame smoothing. There are multiple mathematical models for generating a "best fit" curve. Fourier filtering is somewhat more complex. It analyzes the data in the frequency domain and fits a curve that

contains one or more frequencies (harmonics). Figure 14.6 shows the effects of applying Fourier filtering using progressively more harmonics in the filter. The optimal number of harmonics depends, to some degree, on the segment of the time-activity curve that is of interest but four or five harmonics seems to be quite sufficient (25).

Left Ventricular Ejection Fraction

Once the data processing is completed, the LVEF can be calculated as

$$\frac{\left\lceil \text{ED counts-Bkgd counts}\right\rceil - \left\lceil \text{ES counts-Bkgd counts}\right\rceil}{\text{ED counts-Bkgd counts}}$$

Because background counts cancel out of the numerator, the term simplifies to

$$\frac{\text{ED counts-ES counts}}{\text{ED counts-Bkgd counts}}$$

Consequently, LVEF varies directly with the background activity. An inappropriately high background would spuriously increase LVEF and insufficient background would lower the LVEF. The normal range for the LVEF at rest is approximately 0.50 to 0.80.

Another index of the systolic performance of the left ventricle is the systolic ejection rate, expressed as the peak or the mean (26,27). It is calculated using the first derivative of the time-activity curve. There has been no clinical demonstration that application of the ejection rate is diagnostically or prognostically more useful than LVEF.

Right Ventricular Ejection Fraction

A right ventricular (RV) time-activity curve may also be generated from ERNA data. Again, the best septal view must be used to ensure separation of the left and right ventricles (28). In that projection, however, there is incomplete separation of the right atrium from the right ventricle. The inclusion of atrial counts into the RV ES ROI may result in a spuriously low right ventricular ejection fraction (RVEF). Correct identification of the pulmonary valve may also be problematic in an ERNA study. Phase images, which are useful in localizing valve planes, may be particularly helpful during RV processing. The range of normal values for the RVEF as measured from standard ERNA data is 0.46 to 0.70 (29). When the RVEF is the main clinical question, then standard ERNA is not the procedure of choice. Alternative methods such as the gated first-pass technique or traditional first-pass RNA may be used in that setting.

Left Ventricular Diastolic Filling

Several indices of diastolic filling of the left ventricle can be calculated from the LV time-activity curve. Because of the complexity of the diastolic portion of the LV time-activity curve, it is important to acquire the data with sufficient temporal resolution. A minimum of 32 frames per cardiac cycle is necessary and, as indicated earlier, a 4th- or 5th-order Fourier filter or other polynomial filter should be applied to the data before calculating any filling parameters. The most often cited indexes of diastolic function are the peak filling rate (PFR) and the time from end-systole to the time at which the peak filling rate occurs (tPFR). The PFR is calculated by taking the first derivative of the time-activity curve (Fig. 14.7).

The first major positive peak in the first derivative curve corresponds to the point in the time-activity curve at which counts are increasing at their fastest rate. The PFR is typically measured in counts/second and normalized to ED counts to yield end-diastolic volumes/second (EDV/second). The tPFR should be expressed in milliseconds.

The second major positive peak in the first derivative curve corresponds to the most rapidly increasing count rate during atrial systole and has been referred to as the atrial filling rate (AFR), a somewhat misleading term because it is the ventricle that is filling. Calculation of the ratio of the PFR to the AFR or vice versa is useful as a quantitative descriptor of the relative contributions of early rapid filling and late (atrial) filling of the left ventricle. The PFR and the AFR have been shown to correspond to the E and A waves of the Doppler echocardiographic mitral velocity waveform (30).

Normal values for the PFR and tPFR have been reported from many laboratories (31). As a general rule, at rest, the normal PFR should exceed 2.5 EDV/second, and the tPFR should be less than 180 milliseconds. The AFR is typically 1.0 EDV/second and the PFR/AFR ratio is usually greater than 2.5.

Measurement of Left Ventricular Volume

LV volume has been measured with ERNA using either geometric or count proportional approaches. The geometric method

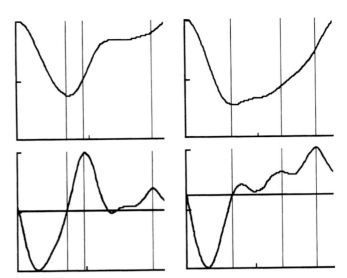

FIGURE 14.7. Normal (*left*) and abnormal (*right*) time-activity curves (*upper*) and their respective first-derivative curves (*lower*). Note the timing of the first major positive peak in the first-derivative that identifies the point at which counts are increasing in the ventricle at their most rapid rate, i.e., the peak filling rate (PFR). The time from end-systole (the nadir of the time-activity curve) to the PFR is the tPFR. The second positive peak in the first-derivative curve reflects the peak atrial contribution to left ventricular filling (AFR). Note the relative heights of the early and late filling peaks of the first-derivative curve on the left compared with that on the right where the atrial contribution to filling is abnormally large and the early peak filling rate is both delayed and reduced.

uses the same mathematical assumptions that are applied to contrast angiographic data (32). The geometric approach to ERNA data suffers from its reliance on spatial resolution that cannot compare to contrast angiographic or other high-resolution imaging modalities.

Count Proportional Methods with Blood Sampling

By definition, at equilibrium, the counts recorded from any chamber are directly proportional to the volume of that chamber. The relationship between counts and volume for any subject can be determined by withdrawing a known sample of blood and recording its activity. That relationship can then be used to calculate the volume of any chamber whose count rate can be measured. In practice, a small amount of labeled blood is withdrawn and counted *in vitro* using the gamma-camera. Then, the background corrected, ED counts from the LV ROI are used to generate an approximate LV EDV as

$$\frac{\text{ED counts corrected for the time per frame}}{\text{counts/ml of the reference blood sample}}$$

The EDV calculated in that manner is not, however, the actual EDV because the counts recorded from the left ventricle are subject to attenuation and to the accuracy of the ROI, neither of which influences the counts recorded *in vitro* from the reference blood sample. In lieu of measuring the attenuation, a regression equation can be used to calculate the absolute LV EDV from the attenuated radionuclide EDV (33). Other investigators have used chest wall markers to measure the distance from the detector to the center of the LV chamber. That distance and an assumed coefficient of attenuation are then used to correct the ED counts for attenuation (34). Still others have actually measured attenuation directly by counting a sealed source in air and then again *in vivo* (35,36). Standard errors of the estimate for EDV and ESV using blood sampling methods have been ± 36 mL and ±33 mL, respectively.

Count-Proportional Methods without Blood Sampling

An alternative count-proportional method for calculating chamber volume is based on the idea of defining a reference volume within the image itself. One group suggested calculating the geometric volume of a cylindrically shaped segment of the aorta and then determining the counts in the same cylinder to establish the relationship of counts to volume for a given subject (37). Another approach assumes the reference volume to be a rectangular solid whose dimensions are the diameter of the left ventricle and the sides of a pixel. Ventricular volume can then be expressed in terms of the counts in the hottest pixel, the size of the pixel matrix, and the total counts recorded from the left ventricle (38–40). The advantages of this approach are its applicability to any system, its freedom from blood sampling, and its suitability to automation. Standard errors of the estimate for ED and ES volumes of the LV range from 23 to 34 mL and 10 to 36 mL, respectively, when using these methods.

Phase and Amplitude Images

Phase images derive their name from the fact that they are graphic representations of the timing of events in the cardiac cycle. The change in counts in each pixel in the image is analyzed in the frequency domain and a single harmonic Fourier filter, i.e., a cosine curve is fit to the data. Each pixel's cosine curve can be characterized by its amplitude and its relationship to the time of onset of the cardiac cycle, i.e., the R wave of the ECG signal. The beginning of the first frame is typically assigned a phase angle of 0 degrees that results in a value of 180 degrees for end-systole and 360 degrees for the end of diastole (the next R wave). In the normal situation, most, if not all, pixels in the two ventricles are filling and emptying at virtually the same time and atrial pixels are all filling and emptying together, but are 180 degrees out of phase with the ventricular pixels. By assigning colors to each phase angle, a color coded, graphic display of the timing of events can be generated (Fig. 14.8). Phase images may be particularly helpful in identifying ventricular asynchrony as occurs in disturbances of conduction, in preexcitation syndromes, and in arrhythmias (41). They are routinely used in automated processing algorithms for identification of ROI borders.

Amplitude images derive their name from their relationship to the height of the fitted cosine curve described earlier. They represent the maximum change in counts between the peak and nadir of the fitted cosine curve. They are analogous to a stroke volume image. In the stroke volume image, ES counts are subtracted from ED counts, and the resultant difference is color

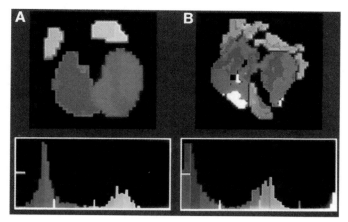

FIGURE 14.8. Normal **(A)** and abnormal **(B)** phase images (*upper*) and their respective phase angle histograms (*lower*). In the normal example, the pixels in both ventricles are of a fairly uniform color, and the histogram shows a narrow distribution of phase angles consistent with synchronous contraction throughout both chambers. The phase angles of the atrial pixels are 180 degrees out of phase with the ventricular pixels as one would expect because the atria fill while the ventricles empty. In the abnormal case, the pixels within the ventricles show several different phase angles. The septal and apical pixels in the left ventricle have phase angles that are similar to those of the atrial pixels indicating that this part of the left ventricle is 180 degrees out of phase with the rest of the chamber, which is typical of a dyskinetic segment. There is a band of black pixels in the left ventricle indicating that there is no change in counts throughout the cardiac cycle in this area, which is typical of an akinetic segment.

coded. If ES counts exceed ED counts, as occurs routinely in the atria and the aorta or in a dyskinetic ventricular segment, the negative value is set to zero so that such pixels drop out of the image. Hence, the atria, the aorta, and dyskinetic segments would not appear on a stroke volume image, but do appear in the amplitude image that does not recognize positive and negative values. Usually, the pixel with the largest change in counts during the cycle is assigned the brightest color, and all other pixels are scaled appropriately. It is then relatively straightforward to identify groups of pixels whose colors indicate smaller amplitudes and, therefore, reduced systolic function (Fig. 14.9).

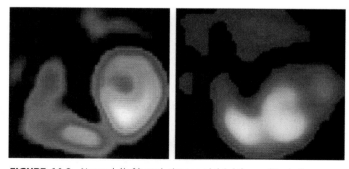

FIGURE 14.9. Normal (*left*) and abnormal (*right*) amplitude images. Pixels are color coded in direct relationship to the change in counts from end-diastole to end-systole. In these figures, the bright colors represent higher stroke counts. In the normal example, there is a shell of bright pixels around the periphery of the left ventricle, which is where most of the change in counts during systole occurs. Near the aortic valve, the darker color occurs because end-systolic volume is located there, which results in a smaller change in counts. On the right is an example of a patient with posterolateral dysfunction.

Such images may be helpful in identifying regional ventricular dysfunction.

Data Analysis and Interpretation

When reviewing ERNA data, care should be taken to review each study in a systematic manner so that errors of omission do not occur. When looking at the views provided, they should be assessed for the spatial relationships, temporal relationships, and size and function of the cardiac chambers. To do that, the images should be reviewed in cinematic display, preferably simultaneously. Once the interpreting physician has assessed the data qualitatively, the clinical impression should be compared with the quantitative results. Discordance between qualitative and quantitative results should be resolved by either reprocessing or reevaluation of the cinematic displays.

Chamber Orientation

In the anterior view, the right ventricle is seen in the foreground with the left ventricle slightly posterior and to the right (Fig. 14.10). Although there is overlap between the right ventricle and the inferior wall of the left ventricle in this view, the higher count density of the left ventricle typically allows clear visualization of the inferior wall. The other segments of the left ventricle that are well seen in this view are the anterolateral wall and the apex. The body, apex, and outflow tract of the right ventricle are typically seen in this projection. The right atrium is usually easily identified and occasionally the superior and inferior vena cavae are seen. The left atrium is usually hidden behind the great vessels and the left ventricle. The pulmonary artery extends from the RV outflow tract upwards and toward the left lung crossing the ascending aorta. Part of the ascending aorta is almost always visible. The separation between the liver and the right ventricle should be noted in the anterior view.

In the best septal view, the two most prominent features are the two ventricles separated by a very well-delineated interventricular septum. It is probably the best view for assessing LV and RV chamber enlargement and is the best view to assess septal hypertrophy. The septum, lateral, and inferoapical walls of the LV are seen in this view. The more horizontal the heart, the more inferior wall is seen; the more vertical the heart, the more the apex is seen.

Above the left ventricle, the left atrium, especially the left atrial appendage is usually well-delineated and left atrial enlargement is usually obvious in this projection. The right atrium is largely obscured by the right ventricle in the best septal view, but may be seen at RV end-systole and may include both vena cavae. Both the pulmonary artery and aorta are also seen.

The lateral view offers the only totally unobstructed view of the inferior wall of the left ventricle and is, therefore, an important view to acquire. It may be the only view in which an inferior wall motion abnormality is detected. There is considerable overlap between the LV apex and the right ventricle in this view, and it is occasionally impossible to assess apical wall motion. The anteroseptal wall of the left ventricle is well seen. The left atrium and mitral valve plane are usually well seen in the lateral view. The right atrium is not visible.

Chamber Size

The evaluation of chamber or great vessel size is largely subjective and relative. With enough clinical experience on a given gamma-camera-computer system, the interpreter can fairly accurately identify varying degrees of chamber enlargement. Surrounding structures or other chambers in the same view are often the best references for assessing chamber size and are independent of the zoom factor used for acquisition or the distance of the chambers from the detector. For the left ventricle, calculation of an absolute volume and comparison to normal limits for a given laboratory is the ideal way of defining LV chamber enlargement. The right ventricle is typically smaller in its anteroposterior (AP) dimension than is the left ventricle in the LAO view. When the AP dimension of the right ventricle exceeds that of the left ventricle, the right ventricle may be enlarged, but when the LV chamber is small because of hypertrophy, the right ventricle may appear relatively large even though it is normal in size. Moreover, the size of the RV inflow tract is quite variable, and mild increases in RV size are difficult to distinguish from normal variants. The atria are the most difficult to evaluate. Depending on the imaging angle and cardiac orientation, the right atrium has a variable profile, appearing considerably larger in some normal subjects than in others. The left atrial appendage is visible in the best septal view, and if it is clearly identifiable throughout the cardiac cycle, it usually signifies left atrial enlargement. Usually the left atrial appendage becomes very small or frankly invisible during atrial systole.

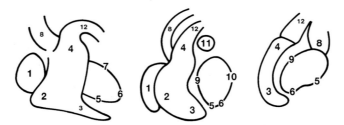

FIGURE 14.10. The commonly visualized chambers, vessels, and ventricular segments in the anterior (*left*), best septal (*middle*), and lateral (*right*) views of a standard equilibrium radionuclide angiogram (EqRNA). 1, right atrium; 2, right ventricular (RV) inflow; 3, RV apex; 4, RV outflow; 5, left ventricular (LV) inferior wall; 6, LV apex; 7, LV anterolateral wall; 8, Ascending aorta; 9, LV septum; 10, LV lateral or true posterior wall; 11, left atrium, 12, pulmonary artery.

Pulmonary Artery

The pulmonary artery is best assessed in the anterior and the best septal views. The pulmonary artery is usually comparable in size to the ascending aorta. When enlarged, there may be increased pulmonary artery pressure. Associated signs that need to be evaluated when looking at the size of a pulmonary artery include the size and function of the right ventricle and the activity in both lung fields. When there is significant pulmonary artery hypertension leading to a large pulmonary artery, the right ventricle is often dilated and hypocontractile. When pulmonary activity is increased it may signify left-sided failure as the cause of pulmonary hypertension. A rare cause of a large pulmonary artery would be a pulmonary embolus.

Aorta

Both the ascending and proximal descending aorta and occasionally the entire descending thoracic aorta may be evaluated qualitatively for size and tortuosity. In the best septal view, the ascending aorta may be seen and evaluated for significant dilatation. Mild dilatation is often missed on ERNA studies, and this is certainly not the study of choice for that diagnosis. Tortuosity and aneurysmal dilatation of the descending aorta may be seen on this view as well. The ERNA does not have the resolution necessary to identify a dissection of the aorta.

Pericardial Space

Surrounding the ventricular blood pools are the myocardium, the pericardial fat, and any pericardial fluid. The tracer-free space surrounding the ventricular cavities is enlarged when a pericardial effusion is present. However, because the thicknesses of the myocardium and pericardial fat vary, small pericardial effusions may be quite difficult to detect with certainty. When a pericardial effusion is large, there will be a proportionately large "halo" or darkened area around the heart (Fig. 14.11). In the anterior view, the space between the liver and the RV blood pool should be routinely examined. Enhanced separation of those two structures usually signifies the presence of a pericardial effusion. If the silhouette surrounding the LV blood pool appears enlarged in the LAO view but there is normal separation between the

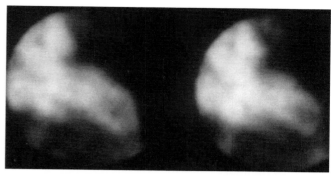

FIGURE 14.12. Patients with anterior and especially apical infarcts may have mural thrombi at the site of akinetic or dyskinetic myocardium. In this case, the anterior view shows a large space-occupying mass in an anteroapical left ventricular aneurysm at end-diastole (*left*) and end-systole (*right*). Given the appearance of this mass and its location within an aneurysmal segment, the overwhelming likelihood is that it represents a thrombus.

right ventricle and the liver, then the increased silhouette is typically not as a result of a pericardial effusion.

Left Ventricular and Left Atrial Thrombi

Ventricular thrombi can be directly visualized in gated equilibrium studies (Fig. 14.12). They are typically found in association with ventricular segments that are akinetic, dyskinetic, or aneurysmal. The clots have been visualized and described as either an irregularity along the myocardium or as a space-occupying lesion and, thus, an area of decreased count activity in the left ventricle.

Left atrial thrombi are not typically visualized directly but the absence of the left atrial appendage in the best septal or steep LAO views is consistent with a left atrial thrombus (41).

Assessment of Rhythm and Conduction

Normal Sinus Rhythm

The anterior view, in which both the right atrium and the two ventricles are seen, is the best view for assessment of rhythm and conduction abnormalities. In normal sinus rhythm, the right atrium may be seen to contract at the end of ventricular filling just before contraction of the ventricles. Atrial contraction must be distinguished from the change in atrial size resulting from filling that can occur during any rhythm. Unequivocal contraction of the atria occurs virtually exclusively in sinus rhythm. Only the very rare patient with a slow atrial or atrioventricular (AV) nodal tachycardia will show organized atrial contraction and a one-to-one relationship to the ventricles.

Atrial Flutter-Fibrillation

Atrial fibrillation results in a loss of organized atrial activity, and the atria do not appear to contract. The atria are usually dilated unless the fibrillation is of recent origin. The same is true of atrial flutter, although on occasion, in a well-organized and not too rapid flutter, a two-to-one or larger atrial to ventricular contraction ratio can be observed in the cine display. An extremely

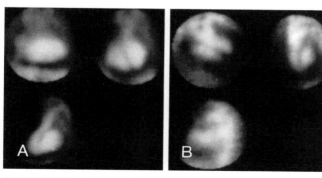

FIGURE 14.11. A pericardial effusion is characterized by an increase in the silhouette surrounding the cardiac chambers, in particular the ventricles. In the anterior view, the space between the liver and the right ventricular chamber is typically wider. Panel A shows a study from a subject with a moderate sized effusion, and Panel B shows a large effusion.

rare and typically transient cause of the atria failing to contract is atrial standstill from an atrial infarction.

Pacemaker Rhythm

There are two basic types of pacing, atrial or AV sequential pacing, which reproduce the normal hemodynamics of synchronized atrial and ventricular systole that are present in sinus rhythm and ventricular pacing, in which case, ventricular and atrial contractions may be completely asynchronous. Scintigraphically, atrial pacing cannot be distinguished from sinus rhythm. With AV sequential pacing, the timing of atrial and ventricular contractions appears normal but the ventricle is stimulated from the apex, which creates an apical to basal wave of contraction through the ventricle that is easily distinguished from the normal pattern of ventricular depolarization. With ventricular pacing, both AV synchrony and the normal ventricular contraction pattern are lost.

Bundle Branch Block

In right bundle branch block, the septum is activated via the left Purkinje system, as is normally the case, and the ventricular contraction pattern appears normal. A phase image, however, may disclose the delayed onset of contraction in the right ventricle (42). Left bundle branch block results in paradoxical septal motion that may be well seen in the best septal view. The phase image may be helpful in identifying or confirming the presence of left bundle branch block (Fig. 14.13). Paradoxical motion of the septum toward the right ventricle during LV systole may be distinguished from septal dyskinesia resulting from infarction by the absence of the early motion of the septum toward the LV cavity in the setting of septal infarction.

Assessment of Systolic Function

The evaluation of regional and global ventricular systolic function is probably the most important clinical role for ERNA. The

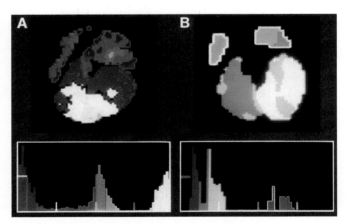

FIGURE 14.13. Phase images are particularly helpful in recognizing conduction abnormalities. **A:** Systolic contraction begins at the apex of the right ventricle and left ventricle and spreads upward toward the base of the heart. A sequence that is distinctly different from normal (see Fig. 14.8A) and that is typical of pacemaker rhythm. **B:** The left ventricle contracts considerably later than the right ventricle. (Note the distinctly separate ventricular peaks on the phase histogram.) This pattern is typical of left bundle branch block where depolarization and hence contraction are delayed in the left ventricular myocardium.

ventricular segments in the three typical views of an ERNA study are indicated in Fig. 14.11. An assessment should be recorded and reported for each of the segments. Regional dysfunction of the right ventricle is distinctly less common than global dysfunction and typically results from RV infarction in association with inferior infarction of the left ventricle (43). Regional dysfunction may also be seen in RV dysplasia, although even here the most common finding is a dilated and diffusely abnormal right ventricle (44). Many different types of parametric images are available to help the physician assess regional LV function including, stroke volume, regional LVEF, amplitude, and phase images. However, one should never be lulled into trusting such images without an independent evaluation of the cinematic display. Parametric images are arithmetic constructs whose validity depend on the statistical strength of the raw data and the confounding influence of adjacent or overlying structures.

Regional LV Function

Regional systolic contraction or regional wall motion can be described in terms of synergy and synchrony. Synergy refers to the force of contraction and synchrony to the timing of contraction. The conventional terms for describing the severity of abnormal synergy (asynergy) are hypokinesia, akinesia, and dyskinesia. Abnormal synchrony is referred to as asynchrony. Although the degrees of asynchrony have no special designations, the phase angle generated from a phase image can be used to quantify the degree of asynchrony. The extent of a regional wall motion abnormality is defined by the amount of the ventricular perimeter involved and should also be assessed and recorded routinely.

Normal

Normal wall motion is relatively simple to identify when all ventricular segments appear to contract at the same time, at the same rate, and to the same extent. Differentiating normal contraction from a synchronously contracting chamber, whose segments move somewhat less vigorously than normal, can be a very subjective decision and one that can only be made confidently with a lot of experience. In such a situation, quantitative information such as the regional LVEF or regional shortening statistics may be helpful. Altering the speed of the cinematic display can alter the subjective appreciation of the vigor of contraction and, therefore, the display speed should be kept within a narrow range for the sake of consistency.

Hypokinesia

The term signifies a reduction in the extent of contraction. Contraction is still present. Regional hypokinesia is best detected by comparison to other, more vigorously contracting segments in the same ventricle. As indicated earlier, when normally contracting segments are not present in the same ventricle, it may be difficult to recognize mild degrees of diffuse hypokinesia. The terms mild, moderate, and severe are used to characterize the spectrum of reduced wall motion between normal and akinesia. Contrast angiographers have used chord shortening to quantify regional systolic motion, and a similar approach has been applied to radionuclide data even though the resolution of the typical RNA is not ideally suited to such an approach (45).

Akinesia

Akinesia signifies the absence of detectable contraction. In general, akinetic segments are fibrotic and devoid of viable myocardium (46). However, both stunned and hibernating myocardium may appear akinetic and, by inference, nonviable, yet may recover function with time or after revascularization.

Dyskinesia

A dyskinetic wall segment is one that passively bulges outward while the surrounding ventricular segments contract inward toward the center of the chamber. The pathologic substrate for dyskinetic myocardium is typically a thinned, fibrotic tissue devoid of any viable myocardial cells (46). Dyskinesia is typical of an aneurysm although some aneurysms appear akinetic rather than dyskinetic. As mentioned for akinesia, even dyskinesia may occasionally be seen in viable but stunned or hibernating myocardium.

Paradoxical Movement

The term paradoxical is used to characterize the motion of the ventricular septum that occurs in the presence of left bundle branch block or in certain RV overload states. The septum appears to move toward the LV cavity early in systole and then bulge toward the RV chamber as the rest of the left ventricle contracts. Although out of phase with the rest of the left ventricle, the paradoxically moving segment does contract. This is in contrast to a dyskinetic segment that does not contract at all. Dyskinesia can occur anywhere in the ventricle, whereas paradoxical movement is restricted to the septum.

Aneurysm

An aneurysm of the ventricle is typically formed by a thin wall of fibrous tissue. Angiographically, an aneurysm appears as a noncontractile part of the ventricle whose margins are clearly separable from the surrounding myocardium typically by a neck or waist formed by the contraction of the surrounding muscle (Fig. 14.14). An aneurysm may be dyskinetic or akinetic. The most common locations for an aneurysm are the apex and anterior wall. Inferior and posterior aneurysms occur less often. Identification of an aneurysm may be important in a patient's clinical course. They are associated with an increased incidence of ventricular arrhythmias, congestive heart failure (CHF), and ventricular thrombi, the latter with the potential for systemic embolization.

Regional Ejection Fraction

The term *regional ejection fraction* has been applied to represent the EF of a varying number of subdivisions of the ventricle ranging in size from 1 pixel to one third of the chamber. It may be of assistance in helping the interpreting physician detect regional dysfunction (47). Advantages of the regional EF over standard wall motion analysis include the facts that it is objective and that it represents three-dimensional data rather than two-dimensional data. Because of the latter, it should be clear that regional wall motion and regional EF are not equivalent. Com-

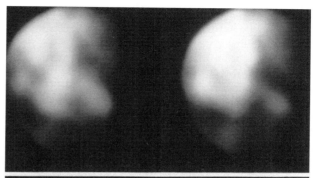
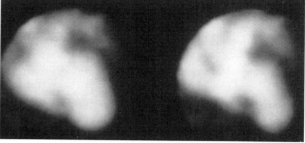

FIGURE 14.14. A small apical aneurysm is shown in the top panel with end-diastole on the left and end-systole on the right. The normal contraction of the base of the left ventricle makes the apical aneurysm appear very discrete and creates the narrow neck at end-systole. *Below,* the aneurysm is large and not as discrete because the myocardium outside the aneurysm does not contract normally.

parisons of regional EFs from one study to the next, or from one patient to another, presupposes that the alignment of the ventricles is identical and that the center of the ventricle remains in the same place, assumptions that are not always true.

Quantitative Regional Wall Motion

As in contrast angiography, regional wall motion may be quantified by calculating regional shortening fractions of a number of radii drawn from the center of the ventricle to the perimeter of the chamber at both ED and ES (48). Rotation of the chamber during systole challenges the assumption that the center of the chamber remains constant, but the technique is fairly reproducible and is certainly valid for comparisons between interventions in the same individual. It is the latter application that is most suited to the use of this type of analysis (45). Quantification of regional wall motion is desirable because the qualitative analysis of wall motion is very subjective and interobserver variability is substantial. However, any geometric analysis of standard blood pool data is dependent on the variable resolution of the images.

Global Systolic Function: Left Ventricular Ejection Fraction

The performance of the entire ventricular chamber can be called global systolic function. The EF is used to quantify global ventricular function and typically ranges from 0.50 to 0.80 at rest and approximately 0.56 to 0.86 during exercise. Those values will vary somewhat among laboratories. Reductions in LVEF at rest are usually characterized as mild (0.40 to 0.49), moderate (0.30 to 0.40), and severe (<0.30).

The three major determinants of LV function are preload, afterload, and the intrinsic contractility of the left ventricle itself. Preload refers to the amount of initial loading of the ventricle just before its contraction, i.e., the degree to which the muscle fibers are stretched from their resting state. Afterload refers to those forces that resist the ejection of blood from the left ventricle, i.e., peripheral resistance. The systolic blood pressure is a relative measure of peripheral vascular resistance. In general, increasing afterload results in less complete emptying of the ventricle. Myocardial contractility refers to the intrinsic inotropic state of the muscle and clinically can be thought of as the contractile performance of the ventricle at any given preload and afterload. An increase in contractility as might occur with an increase in catecholamines will result in the ventricle contracting to a smaller ES volume, thus increasing the EF. A decrease in contractility will result in a decrease in EF. Because of that direct relationship, the EF is used clinically as a surrogate for contractility and works quite well as long as the loading conditions on the ventricle are within a physiologic range. The power of the EF as a clinical predictor of outcome in various cardiac diseases is testimony to its relationship to the intrinsic state of the myocardium. However, when loading conditions are changed, as occurs with the increased afterload of sudden hypertension or severe aortic stenosis or the decreased afterload of mitral insufficiency, EF may not reflect the contractility of the myocardium. EF, unlike contractility, varies with loading conditions. As a result, investigators have looked for measurements other than EF that might more accurately reflect myocardial contractility regardless of loading conditions (49,50).

Diastolic Left Ventricular Function

The interpretation of the diastolic filling portion of the LV time-activity curve depends on both qualitative and quantitative assessment of the data. The qualitative assessment may be the more valuable of the two because there are certain characteristic patterns of abnormal filling that recur frequently in clinical practice and because quantitation varies so much from laboratory to laboratory (15). Figure 14.15 shows several LV time-activity curves that are representative of the common patterns of abnormal diastolic filling. Prolongation of isovolumic relaxation, delayed and/or decreased early rapid filling, and exaggeration of the atrial contribution to filling are the typical disturbances of the normal filling pattern. They may occur alone or in combination. An exaggeration of the atrial contribution to filling associated with a variable decrease in the early PFR is typical of both normal aging (51) and hypertension (52). Prolongation of isovolumic relaxation is typical of hypertrophic myopathy (53) and delayed and decreased rapid filling is typical of CAD (54).

The isovolumic relaxation period may be measured, but is typically short and may occupy only the time between two frames of a standard ERNA acquisition. Delayed early rapid filling may be quantified by prolongation of the tPFR. Decreased early rapid filling can be measured as a reduced PFR. The contribution of the atrium may be expressed as the absolute AFR or the ratio of the atrial to early rapid filling rates (AFR/PFR) or

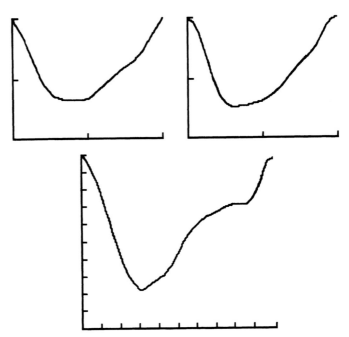

FIGURE 14.15. Typical clinical examples of abnormal diastolic filling patterns. In the curve on the upper left, the time at which peak filling occurs (tPFR) is prolonged due largely to a prolongation of the isovolumic relaxation phase. The atrial contribution to filling is increased. At the top right, the tPFR is prolonged largely because of decreased early rapid filling resulting in a reduced peak filling rate. In the lower curve, the only abnormality is as exaggerated atrial contribution to filling.

its inverse PFR/AFR. Normal values for PFR, tPFR, and AFR vary substantially depending on the type of acquisition, frame rate, and, in the case of the ERNA, the gating technique (15, 55).

It must be understood that the analysis of filling patterns and the timing of filling events represent the changes in volume during diastole, but obviously do not reflect the changes in intraventricular pressure. It is possible, therefore, to encounter normal filling times and a normal appearing filling pattern and still have abnormal diastolic pressure.

Regurgitant Fraction and Left-to-Right Shunts

In an intact cardiac system, blood flows from one chamber to the next in one direction only, and so the amount of blood pumped per beat from one ventricle must equal that pumped from the other ventricle. Therefore, the stroke counts of the two ventricles must be equal. Any abnormality of structure or valve function that results in blood flow deviating from that unidirectional pattern will alter that fundamental relationship of stroke counts between the two ventricles.

In the case of mitral insufficiency or aortic insufficiency, LV stroke counts will be higher than RV stroke counts because each stroke of the left ventricle contains the counts destined to go forward in the circulation, as well as the counts that will travel backward across the insufficient valve. The RV stroke counts represent only those counts going forward in the circulation. Hence, the ratio of LV to RV stroke counts will exceed one by a fraction related to the magnitude of the insufficiency (56). The same concept applies to left-to-right shunts at the ventricular level, although, in that case, RV stroke counts are also increased above normal because the right ventricle participates in the shunt (57). In contrast, RV stroke counts will exceed LV stroke counts in the presence of tricuspid or pulmonary insufficiency or with a left-to-right shunt at the atrial level.

Stroke count ratios derived from ERNA have been found to be similar to the flow ratios measured at cardiac catheterization. Some authors believe that the RV/LV ratio may be compared directly to the Qp/Qs ratio derived from oximetry. But because these numbers are derived during an equilibrium study, the exact location of a shunt or regurgitant lesion cannot be ascertained. Furthermore, the radionuclide data are highly dependent on the accuracy of the ventricular ROI, which are particularly problematic for the right ventricle because of right atrial overlap and difficulty identifying the pulmonary valve. The right atrial overlap becomes even more of a problem when the right atrium is enlarged. As a result, reported LV to RV stroke count ratios usually exceed one in normal individuals. Other noninvasive techniques, such as Doppler echocardiography or first-pass RNA, are probably more accurate in detecting and quantifying both left-to-right shunts and valvular insufficiency.

Tomographic (Single Photon Emission Computed Tomography) ERNA

ERNA may be acquired using a tomographic technique. When initially described, only the ED and ES frames were stored for reconstruction (58–60), but with the expanded memory and increased speed of newer computers, all frames may be reconstructed. After routine RBC labeling, the subject may be imaged with standard tomographic equipment using a step and shoot protocol for 16 to 32 stops. At each stop, the acquisition is gated as is done in routine ERNA, except that the number of frames per cardiac cycle is usually limited to approximately 8 to 12 because of time and memory constraints. Each stop is imaged for approximately 1 minute so that the entire acquisition takes no longer than an average three-view planar ERNA study. The raw data then consist of 16 or 32 separate 8- to 12-frame ERNA acquisitions. Tomographic reconstruction of each of the 8 frames of the study can then be performed to create axial and standard short axis and vertical and horizontal long axis images. Regional wall motion may then be interrogated tomographically. The advantages of tomographic ERNA include the ability to examine regional wall motion throughout the entire depth of the ventricles, the freedom of the reconstructed data from background activity, and the fact that the acquisition does not require the technologist to identify specific imaging angles. At this time, however, it is not clear what real clinical benefit is achieved by acquiring an ERNA study tomographically. In very specific situations, such as a large LV aneurysm in which it may be difficult to accurately assess the margins of the aneurysm and the contraction pattern of the myocardium that may be hidden from view in a planar study, a tomographic acquisition would be helpful (59). The tomographic study may also be useful for

measurement of chamber volume by calculation of the total number of three-dimensional pixels, i.e., voxels in the chamber of interest (60).

FIRST-PASS IMAGING

First-pass RNA is distinguished from ERNA in two fundamental ways. First, no labeling of RBCs is performed, and second, all usable data are acquired during the initial transit of a radionuclide bolus through the central circulation. The first-pass study relies on the temporal separation of chambers to generate chamber specific data as opposed to the requisite spatial separation in an ERNA study. Inherent in the first-pass study is the ability to track the transit of the radionuclide through the heart and great vessels, which makes it possible to detect abnormalities of tracer transit as is found in congenital heart disease, shunts, and valvular insufficiency. Although the concept of first-pass RNA was first employed in 1927 (61) to measure the circulation time in man, it was not until 1969 that a ^{99m}Tc injection was used to sequentially visualize the heart and great vessels in patients (62). At that time, the technology was considered to be an improvement over contrast angiography because it was less invasive and less hazardous to the patient and did not disturb the circulatory function.

Imaging Agents

The requirements of a radionuclide for first-pass imaging are basically twofold: First, it must remain intravascular for the duration of the initial transit through the central circulation. Second, it must be safe for injection in a sufficiently large dose to generate the count rates necessary for this type of imaging.

^{99m}Tc Agents

Because of its high specific activity, ^{99m}Tc has been used for many years in nuclear medicine procedures. As we have seen previously, ^{99m}Tc pertechnetate is presently used in ERNA studies. This agent may also be given as a bolus and is a very adequate agent for first-pass RNA. This agent may be used solely for a first-pass study or in conjunction with RBC labeling for an ERNA study. An alternate technetium agent, diethylenetriamine penta-acetic acid (DTPA) is more commonly used because it is more rapidly cleared from the circulation by the kidneys. Of the technetium-based myocardial perfusion imaging agents, sestamibi has been satisfactorily used for first-pass RNA (63,64), as have teboroxime (65,66) and tetrofosmin (67).

Ultra-Short-Lived Radionuclides

Although the 6-hour half-life of ^{99m}Tc is relatively short, the agents to which it is complexed have varying biologic clearance times. Therefore, radiation exposure limits the number of first-pass acquisitions that can be performed at a given time. Agents with extremely short half-lives reduce the radiation exposure and allow more studies to be performed in a short period.

^{195m}Au has a half-life of 30.5 seconds. It is easily produced from a portable mercury generator. The correlation between first-pass EFs using ^{195m}Au and those using ^{99m}Tc products exceeded 0.9 (68). The short half-life allows numerous studies to be performed on the same patient without extreme radiation exposure and with extremely low background radiation from previous injections (69).

^{191m}Ir has an extremely short half-life of 4.9 seconds, requiring the subject be connected to the portable generator. Studies have shown its clinical utility for evaluating LV function and for quantitation of left-to-right shunts (70). The 4.9-second half-life makes ^{191m}Ir particularly attractive for pediatric imaging.

^{178m}Ta was initially used to evaluate global LV function. The half-life of this agent is 9.3 minutes, which makes it easier to use than ^{191m}Ir. However, its primary photopeak of 55 to 65 keV make it suboptimal for standard gamma-cameras. With the clinical validation of a new type of gamma-camera, the multiwire proportional detector, and the development of an efficient portable ^{178m}Ta generator, satisfactory first-pass RNA has been performed with this radionuclide (71).

Instrumentation

At rest, there are, on average, 6 to 10 beats, and at peak exercise 4 to 6 beats, during a typical first-pass study. As such, first-pass studies must have very high count rates to ensure the necessary count density for both image quality and statistical reliability of EFs and volumes. Although first-pass EFs may be generated with lower count rates, at least 150,000 counts/second and preferably ≥200,000 counts/second are necessary for adequate image quality, especially at end-systole.

Multicrystal Gamma-Camera

Historically, multicrystal gamma-camera systems were the first and only devices that could reliably record the count rates necessary for first-pass imaging. The initial multicrystal systems were able to record counts in excess of 250,000 to 300,000 counts/second while maintaining enough spatial resolution for regional wall motion analysis. The latest generation of multicrystal gamma-cameras continues to deliver count rates in the same range but with enhanced energy and spatial resolution. To deliver such high count rates, the early multicrystal systems did sacrifice spatial resolution to the point that they were not particularly useful for other types of imaging. That may not be true of the newer generation of multicrystal cameras. Early systems were very large, very heavy, and not portable. Newer systems are substantially smaller and portable (Fig. 14.16).

Single-Crystal Gamma-Cameras

Conventional single-crystal gamma-cameras could count fairly linearly up to 60,000 counts/second, but at higher rates there was substantial data loss and peak count rates with a clinical dose of technetium rarely exceeded 100,000 counts/second with a collimator. As such, single-crystal cameras could not be used for high count rate first-pass RNA. More recent developments in camera-computer systems, specifically, all-digital front-end technology, allow single-crystal systems to achieve count rates up to 200,000 counts/second. Clinically accurate, high count rate first-pass RNA has been performed with these newer single-crystal systems (72,73).

Collimation

To achieve adequate count rates, high-sensitivity and ultra-high sensitivity collimators are appropriate for first-pass studies. Some tradeoff between sensitivity and resolution is necessary and will depend on the system in use. Collimators whose holes are aligned with the acquisition matrix offer the best combination of sensitivity and resolution.

Computer/Software

All current generation computer systems have enough speed and storage capacity for acquisition and processing of first-pass data. However, appropriate software is not universally available. First-pass acquisitions may be performed with either 64 × 64 or

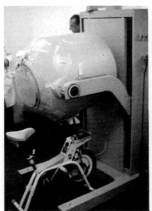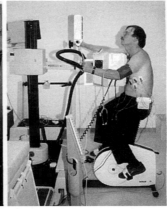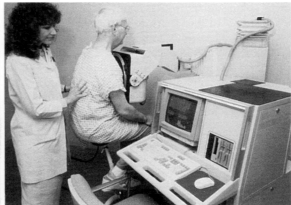

FIGURE 14.16. The evolution of cameras dedicated to first-pass imaging: (*left*) Baird Atomic System 77; (*middle*) Scinticor SIM400; (*right*) proportional-wire camera. (Courtesy of Dr. Jeffrey Lacy.)

smaller matrixes. The 32 × 32 matrix has been used for some single-crystal systems (72), whereas the multicrystal systems now use a 20 × 20 matrix. The smaller matrixes increase the counts/pixel and are especially helpful in maintaining the integrity of the ES image in which the count density often becomes very marginal with a 64 × 64 matrix.

Data Acquisition

Injection Techniques

Unlike the equilibrium study, the first-pass study requires bolus injection of a small volume with a high, specific activity. The quality of the first-pass study is very dependent on the discreteness of the bolus. Consequently, the radionuclide must be injected into as large a bore vein as close to the central circulation as possible. In practice, there are only two sites that work well for that purpose, the medial antecubital and the external jugular veins. Lateral antecubital veins are reasonable alternatives. No other peripheral veins are acceptable. For the arm veins, an 18-gauge cannula is preferred whereas a 20-gauge cannula is adequate for the external jugular vein (Fig. 14.17). When the RVEF is of primary interest, it is helpful to prolong the radionuclide injection so that more RV beats are available for data processing.

Radionuclide Dose

The appropriate radionuclide dose depends on the sensitivity of the gamma-camera, the number of injections to be made, the size of the individual, and the specific radionuclide being used. With a multicrystal camera, doses as low as 8 to 10 mCi (296 to 370 MBq) may be used, although 20 to 25 mCi (740 to 925 MBq) are recommended because lower doses may yield suboptimal statistics in large individuals or in cases in which there are few beats available for processing. For single-crystal gamma-cameras, the dose should not be lower than 15 mCi (555 MBq) and should preferably be ±25 mCi (925 MBq) in

the average adult. For the ultra-short-lived radionuclides, the doses can be substantially higher and doses of 50 mCi (1850 MBq) have been reported.

Imaging Angles

Because of the temporal separation of cardiac chambers, first-pass radionuclide studies can theoretically be acquired in any view. Typically, however, studies are acquired in either a shallow right anterior oblique (RAO) view or a straight anterior projection. The shallow RAO view works well because it helps separate the atria from the ventricles and projects the left ventricle away from the descending aorta. It is also a convenient view for direct comparison to contrast angiography. When the right ventricle is the chamber of primary concern, the 30-degree RAO view enhances right atrial-RV separation. The anterior view works best for exercise studies because it is much easier to stabilize the chest against the detector. When the circumflex coronary artery is in question, an LAO view is useful. It should be noted that the count density in the left atrium is larger in first-pass studies than in equilibrium studies because of the activity in the bolus. As a result, a standard LAO view results in considerable left atrial-LV overlap and an underestimation of LVEF. For shunt studies, as much of the lung fields as possible, particularly the right lung field, should be in the field of view, even to the exclusion of part or all of the left ventricle if necessary.

ECG Recording

For high count rate first-pass acquisitions using a multicrystal camera, no ECG signal is necessary. The counts within the time-activity curve from a ventricular ROI are sufficient for the manual or automated identification of ED and ES frames. When count rates may be lower, as frequently occurs with single-crystal camera acquisitions, it is helpful to store an ECG signal that can then be used to facilitate data processing. Whether or not an ECG signal is stored, it is helpful to verify the cardiac rhythm before injection. Occasionally, the rhythm may be so irregular as to preclude a good quality first-pass study.

Frame Rates

The optimal frame rate depends on the heart rate—the higher the heart rate, the faster the frame rate. At resting heart rates of 50 to 100 beats/minute, 20 frames/second (50 milliseconds/frame) is adequate. At heart rates of 150 to 200, frame rates of 40 to 100 frames/second are necessary (74). Rather than constantly adjusting the frame rate, most laboratories compromise on 40 to 50 frames/second for both rest and exercise studies. Data are usually acquired for 30 seconds from the time of injection to ensure that the entire transit is acquired.

Patient Positioning

First-pass studies cannot usually be repeated if an error in positioning is made. Therefore, it is important to verify that the chambers of interest will be in the field of view before study

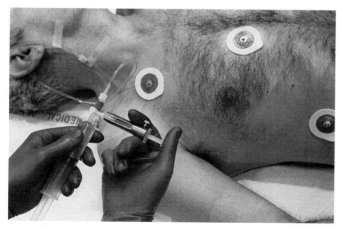

FIGURE 14.17. A typical setup for an external jugular vein approach to first-pass studies. The technique is well-tolerated, carries no additional risk compared with the antecubital approach, and leaves the patient's arms free for holding on to a handrail and for blood pressure recordings.

acquisition. Placing a uniform flood source or an exposed dose syringe behind the patient provides an image of the chest that allows identification of the lungs and mediastinum. Alternatively, a 1 mCi test dose can be injected for positioning. When more than one study is performed, the background activity from a preceding injection can be used for positioning.

Stress Protocols

Bicycle Exercise Studies

First-pass RNA is particularly well suited to the evaluation of ventricular function during exercise. The only caveat in acquiring such studies is that the chest must be relatively motionless with regard to the detector. Historically, that led to the use of bicycle ergometry as the method of choice for exercise first-pass studies. Although initial studies used supine bicycle exercise for correlation with data obtained in the cardiac catheterization laboratory, upright bicycle ergometry proved better for stabilizing the chest and was better tolerated (75,76) (Fig. 14.18). Any graded exercise protocol is acceptable and because the acquisition time at peak exercise is so short, no time is required for stabilization of the heart rate. However, care should be taken to stabilize the patient's chest against the detector to minimize motion. Exercise should be continued until the bolus is seen to clear the left ventricle. If technetium is used, a maximum of two injections may be made during the exercise study unless a resting study is not performed on the same day. For most clinical studies, rest and peak exercise acquisitions are sufficient.

Treadmill Exercise

During treadmill exercise, there is considerably more motion of the chest than during bicycle exercise. In fact, there is often so much motion that, until recently, first-pass RNA was never performed during treadmill exercise. With the introduction of a motion-detection scheme that uses an external radioactive source attached to the chest, the image distortion resulting from chest motion has been considerably reduced. Clinically satisfactory first-pass RNA can now be routinely performed during treadmill exercise (64,65,77,78). The external marker affixed to the chest is used to track chest wall and presumably cardiac motion. It must have a principal photopeak that lies outside the spectrum of the ^{99m}Tc so that both the marker photopeak and the technetium photopeak may be acquired simultaneously. Both ^{241}Am and ^{125}I have been used for that purpose. (Fig. 14.18)

Standard Data Processing

Analysis of Ventricular Function

First-pass data processing can be divided into four major steps. The first step is the creation of the time-activity curve from a ROI surrounding the ventricle of interest. Second is the selection of the beats to be included in the final analysis. Third is background subtraction, and fourth is the creation of the final representative cycle from which all quantitative data are obtained. For details of data processing, the reader is referred to previously published articles describing those routines (75–81). Some of the more important aspects of processing are discussed here.

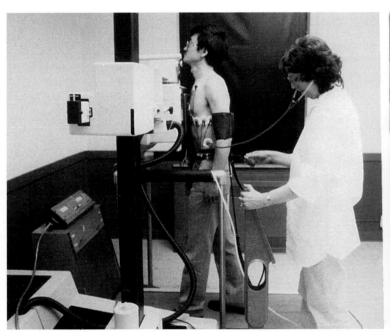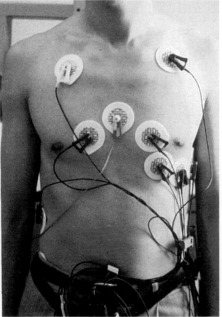

FIGURE 14.18. First-pass radionuclide angiography can be performed during treadmill exercise (*left*); however, a scheme for motion detection and correction is mandatory. In this case, an external sealed source containing ^{241}Am is affixed to the chest (what appears to be an electrode right over the middle of the sternum) so that a dual energy acquisition (using the 140 keV peak of ^{99m}Tc and the 50 keV of the americium) can be performed.

Region-of-Interest Selection

An initial ventricular ROI is usually drawn manually on images generated by adding 20 to 40 frames of raw data together. That ROI is used to generate a time-activity curve from which an initial representative cycle is created. For both the left and right ventricles, the improved ventricular images from that initial representative cycle should then be used to draw separate ED and ES ROI (Fig. 14.19). Various parametric images such as stroke volume and phase images may be helpful in drawing the ROI. As in the processing of equilibrium data, the LV and RV ROI may be manually, semiautomatically, or automatically drawn.

Beat Selection

Once the final LV ROI has been identified, the operator has the opportunity to select those beats from the ventricular time-activity curve to be included in the final analysis. For routine processing, ventricular premature beats, and, whenever possible, postextrasystolic beats should be excluded (Fig. 14.20). In ventricular bigeminy, when there are frequent premature ventricular contractions (PVCs), or when there is extremely irregular atrial fibrillation, data processing becomes extremely difficult and often impossible. When such rhythms are present, the study should be postponed or an ERNA acquisition performed.

Background Correction—Left Ventricle

There are several different approaches to background correction in first-pass studies. However, the most accurate appears to be the so-called lung frame method (81). In this method, the distribution of counts in an image taken from the late pulmonary phase, just before appearance of the radionuclide in the left ven-

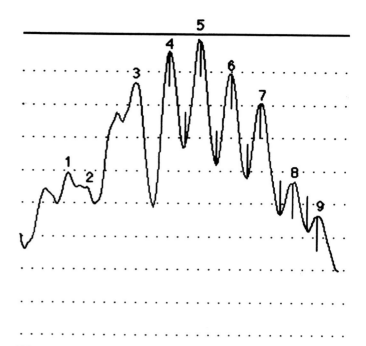

FIGURE 14.20. Beat selection is important during first-pass processing. In this example, beats numbered 3, 4, 5, and 6 are sinus beats; beat number 2 is a premature ventricular contraction (PVC); and beat number 3 is a post-PVC beat. The inclusion of PVC beats and post-PVC beats would spuriously lower or raise the ejection fraction, respectively.

tricle, is used to correct the LV phase. An adjustment for pulmonary washout is made. Background correction is crucial in the calculation of LVEF and, unlike the background correction in ERNA, changes in the background frame can cause large changes in the calculated LVEF. Occasionally, studies are encountered that cannot be appropriately corrected using the lung frame method because of persistent RV activity throughout the pulmonary phase. In such situations, application of a regression equation to the uncorrected data may be the only way to generate an accurate LVEF.

Representative Cycle

After final beat selection and background correction, the individual beats are added together, frame by frame, to create the final representative cycle, which may be displayed in a cine loop for analysis of regional wall motion. As in ERNA, a host of parametric images may be created from the representative cycle. The most commonly used parametric images are the regional EF and stroke volume images (Fig. 14.21). However, all parametric images are very count dependent for accuracy and very high count rate first-pass data are necessary for their routine clinical application.

The ED and ES counts of the representative cycle are used to calculate the LVEF using the same formula as that described previously for ERNA. LVEFs calculated by this measurement technique have correlated closely with EFs measured during cardiac catheterization (80,82,83). Systolic ejection rates and diastolic filling parameters are also calculated from the representative cycle.

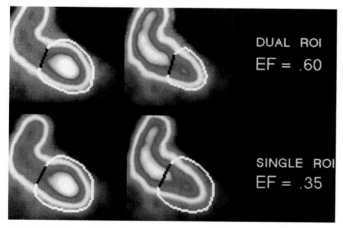

FIGURE 14.19. Although first-pass processing may be performed with a single region-of-interest (ROI) around the left ventricle at end-diastole (*bottom left*), movement of the aortic valve toward the apex and filling of the left atrium during left ventricular systole bring a variable, but sometimes significant, amount of nonventricular activity into the single ROI at end-systole (*bottom right*). Using a separate end-systolic ROI (*top right*) avoids that problem. In this case, because of a dilated left atrium, the dual ROI left ventricular ejection fraction (LVEF) is much higher than the single ROI LVEF. In general, dual ROI ejection fractions are 5 to 10 ejection fraction units higher than their single ROI counterparts.

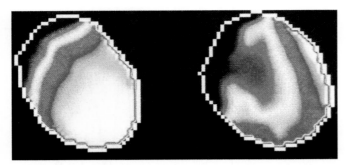

FIGURE 14.21. Parametric images may be helpful in defining localized abnormalities of contraction as indicated previously (see Fig. 14.9). One of the most commonly used images is the regional ejection fraction image generated by color coding the ejection fraction of each pixel in the ILV image. A normal, homogeneous pattern is shown on the left and an example with clear regional dysfunction is shown on the right.

The accuracy of the first-pass LVEF is directly related to the statistical content of the data. The error in the measurement increases as the ED counts in the representative cycle decreases (84).

Although most exercise studies performed using bicycle exercise are free of major cardiac motion, mild degrees of motion occur frequently. A motion-correction scheme can be applied to the representative cycle that uses a center of mass algorithm to identify the location of the ventricle throughout the LV phase and that then corrects each frame of the representative cycle accordingly.

Right Ventricular Function

The first-pass technique is the method of choice for measurement of RVEF because of the ability to acquire the study in the RAO view, which maximizes right atrial-RV separation. Although the bolus does provide temporal separation of chambers, there is still a large quantity of activity in the right atrium during the majority of the RV phase. To exclude right atrial activity from the RVEF calculation, both ED and ES ROI are necessary (85) (Fig 14.22).

Measurement of Left Ventricular Volume

Geometric Method

As in ERNA, LV volume may be calculated by measuring the area of the left ventricle and the length of the major axis in pixels. The pixel measurements can be converted to centimeters and the modified Sandler-Dodge equation (discussed earlier) can then be used to calculate LV volume. This approach has been validated (86). It is very dependent, however, on the criteria used for definition of the LV borders and on the accuracy of the LV ROI.

Count-Proportional Methods

The reference volume approach described for ERNA data has been successfully applied to first-pass data as well. The variables that must be measured include the total counts in the left ventricle (T) and the counts in the hottest pixel in the LV (Nmax). With the size of a pixel (m) as a given, the volume of the LV is calculated as

$$\frac{1}{3} \frac{(T)^{3/2}}{(Nmax - 3.5)} m^3$$

The correlation coefficient between EDV measured with that approach and the EDV measured at cardiac catheterization exceeded 0.93 for both multicrystal and single-crystal systems (87). The standard error of the estimate for EDV is ±35 mL. The stroke volume may then be calculated as the product of EDV and EF and cardiac output as the product of the stroke volume and the heart rate.

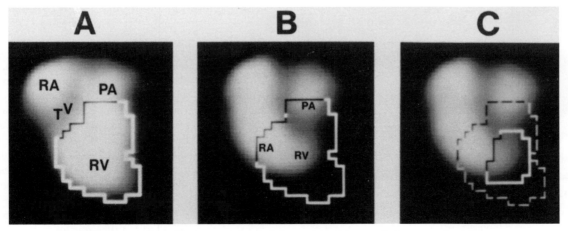

FIGURE 14.22. As indicated in Fig. 14.19 for the left ventricle, right ventricular processing is best accomplished by using separate end-diastolic and end-systolic region-of-interest (ROI). **Panel A:** A ROI is drawn around the right ventricle at end-diastole. **Panel B:** The end-systolic frame is shown with the ROI from **Panel A.** Note the inclusion of right atrial (*RA*) and pulmonary arterial (*PA*) activity within the ROI. Inclusion of that much nonventricular activity in a single end-diastolic ROI would underestimate the true right ventricular ejection fraction. **Panel C:** A separate end-systolic ROI is drawn that excludes the atrial and pulmonary atrial activity.

Measurement of Pulmonary Transit Time and Pulmonary Blood Volume

The transit time between any two chambers may be calculated by generating a time-activity curve from the chambers of interest and measuring the time between the peaks of the curves (88). The mean transit time through the pulmonary circulation is calculated as the difference between the mean transit times of the pulmonary artery and the left atrium.

The product of the pulmonary mean transit time and the cardiac output is the pulmonary blood volume. An increase in pulmonary blood volume from rest to exercise may be used as a criterion for the diagnosis of CAD (89). In one study, an increase of more than 1.06 in the ratio of pulmonary blood volumes from exercise to rest had a sensitivity of 79% and a specificity of 100% in the detection of CAD involving the left ventricle (90). Other studies, though, have failed to confirm that clinical correlation.

Data Analysis and Interpretation

Normal Anatomy and Tracer Transit

The analysis of tracer transit through the central circulation is unique to first-pass RNA. The expected sequential appearance of the radionuclide in the superior vena cava, right atrium, right ventricle, pulmonary circulation, left side of the heart, and then the aorta should be confirmed in every study. Deviations from that sequence may indicate a congenital abnormality (Fig. 14.23). In the absence of a prolonged injection, prolongation of tracer transit through the right heart suggests pulmonary hypertension, tricuspid or pulmonary valve insufficiency, or a left-to-right intracardiac shunt. With a good bolus injection and normal tracer transit through the right heart and lungs, prolonged tracer transit through the left heart suggests mitral or aortic insufficiency or a left-to-right shunt. Left side valvular

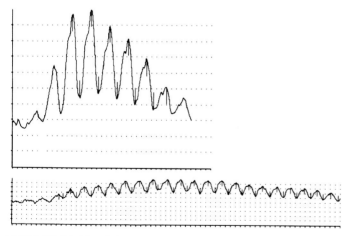

FIGURE 14.23. Visualizing tracer transit is helpful in detecting valvular insufficiency. Normal tracer transit through the left ventricle is shown *above* and markedly prolonged left ventricular tracer transit because of left sided valvular insufficiency is shown *below*. Correlation with the images may permit the interpreter to distinguish between mitral and aortic insufficiency based on an enlarged left atrium or ascending aorta, respectively.

insufficiency can be quantified from first-pass data using a stroke count approach or a curve analysis technique.

Left Ventricular Systolic Function

The evaluation of both systolic and diastolic ventricular function begins with the inspection of the time-activity curve of the LV ROI. Review of the beat selection, the background frame selection, and, in the case of the exercise study, the presence of cardiac motion is important for the quality control of each study. Otherwise, the definitions and principles presented for the analysis of systolic function using ERNA apply to first-pass data as well. In the anterior first-pass left ventriculogram, the anterolateral, apical, and inferoseptal walls are visible. In an RAO first-pass left ventriculogram, the anterior, apical, and inferior walls are visible. The correlation between regional wall motion in the RAO first-pass study and wall motion in contrast ventriculography has been shown to be clinically acceptable (72). The weakest correlation occurred in the inferior wall probably as a result of background oversubtraction. Because the first-pass study is acquired in only one projection and resolution is somewhat limited, it may be difficult to separate regional wall motion abnormalities in contiguous or overlapping segments. One typical example of that shortcoming is the appearance of anterior hypokinesia on a study acquired in the anterior view in a subject whose pathology actually involves the circumflex coronary artery. In that case, the three-dimensional effect of the posterior wall motion is interpreted in two-dimensional analysis as a problem with the anterior wall.

Parametric Images

As described earlier for ERNA, a variety of parametric images can be generated to assist in the analysis of regional ventricular function. Phase and amplitude, stroke volume, regional EF, and mean transit time images may be helpful in certain clinical situations. They have the advantage of being more representative of the three-dimensional changes in counts throughout the ventricle than the cinematic display of the representative cycle. However, parametric images require very high count rates for accuracy. The potential diagnostic benefits of high count density parametric images have been thoroughly described (91).

Left Ventricular Diastolic Function

The same approach used for evaluating diastolic function in ERNA studies may be applied to first-pass data as well. First-pass studies are usually acquired at frame rates fast enough for the evaluation of diastole. A frame time of 25 milliseconds is roughly equivalent to a 32 frames/cycle gated acquisition at a heart rate of 60 beats/minute (frame time 31 milliseconds). The PFR, tPFR, and filling fractions may all be calculated (92,93). Because of the potential sensitivity of those measurements to the changing concentration of the radionuclide during the LV phase, it is considered important to select beats from both the ascending and descending limbs of the LV time-activity curve.

Assessment of Valvular Insufficiency

As indicated earlier, prolongation of tracer transit through the left heart is typical of mitral or aortic insufficiency. Using the pulmonary time-activity curve as a monoexponential input function, the LV time-activity curve may be deconvoluted so that the primary LV curve and the contribution from the regurgitation may be quantified. The degree of insufficiency calculated in that fashion has been correlated with standard invasive data (94). Others have taken a similar approach to that used in ERNA and compared the total stroke count outputs of the left and right ventricles. The correlation between regurgitant fractions measured in that way and those measured at catheterization was 0.86 (95). Others have attempted to quantify tricuspid insufficiency (96).

Left-to-Right Shunts

The application of radionuclides to the detection and quantitation of intracardiac and extracardiac shunts is an extension of indicator dilution theory. Any measurable, nondiffusible indicator injected into the central circulation has a finite circulation time and a typical monoexponential appearance and disappearance when sampled downstream from the injection site. In the case of an intracardiac left-to-right shunt as occurs with atrial and ventricular septal defects, injection of an indicator proximal to the shunt with sampling distal to the shunt yields a curve that is not monoexponential because of the early reappearance of the indicator that is shunted through the defect. The FPRNA can be used to create such a curve after injection of the indicator, in this case a radionuclide, into a peripheral vein with sampling downstream represented by the externally recorded appearance and clearance of the tracer in the lungs. Standard curve analysis techniques, such as the exponential and γ variate mathematical fits, can then be performed on a pulmonary time-activity curve to separate that curve into a primary component and a shunt component. The areas of those two components are proportional to systemic and shunt flows and allow calculation of the ratio of pulmonary to systemic flow, or Qp/Qs, which is an index of the severity of the shunt (Figs. 14.24). With that type of analysis, shunts with a Qp/Qs as small as 1.2/1 have been accurately detected. The early reports using this technique showed excellent correlations with invasive oximetry readings (97,98).

Accurate detection and quantitation of left-to-right shunts is completely dependent on the integrity of the bolus entering the lung. If the bolus is delayed by virtue of a poor injection or by prolonged transit through the right heart as might occur with significant tricuspid or pulmonary insufficiency, then the pulmonary curve will deviate from a true monoexponential even without a shunt. In such a situation, it may be impossible to quantify a left-to-right shunt. However, it is almost always possible to visually confirm the presence of a left-to-right shunt. The sequential appearance of the radionuclide bolus in the right atrium, right ventricle, pulmonary circulation, and left ventricle is obvious on a normal study, and the LV phase is typically free of any RV activity. In the case of an intracardiac left-to-right shunt, activity appears in the right and left ventricles simultaneously so that a clear LV phase cannot be identified (Fig. 14.25).

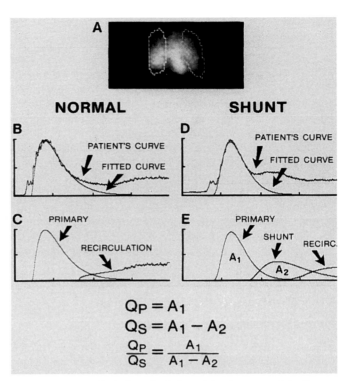

$$Q_P = A_1$$
$$Q_S = A_1 - A_2$$
$$\frac{Q_P}{Q_S} = \frac{A_1}{A_1 - A_2}$$

FIGURE 14.24. Calculation of a left-to-right shunt. **Panel A:** Shows a frame of the first-pass study selected because of the clear definition of the pulmonary activity. Manually drawn region-of-interest (ROI) are placed around each lung. The time-activity curve from the pulmonary ROI is indicated in panels **B** and **D** as the patient's curve. The superimposed mathematical fit is also shown. Panels **C** and **E** show the fitted curves alone. The areas *A1* and *A2* are used to calculate the Qp/Qs.

Therefore, the presence of a clearly identifiable LV image during the first-pass virtually excludes a significant intracardiac left-to-right shunt. A patent ductus arteriosus, however, does not involve the right ventricle and cannot be excluded by that visual method.

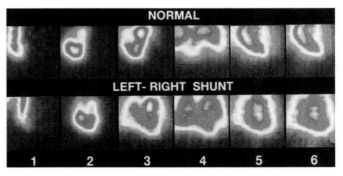

FIGURE 14.25. Serial images of a normal patient and a patient with a left-to-right intracardiac shunt are shown. Images 1 to 4 show the tracer appearing in the superior vena cava, right atrium, right ventricle, and lungs in both patients. In images 5 and 6, the normal patient shows a clearly identifiable left ventricular (LV) chamber, whereas the patient with the shunt shows activity in both ventricles because the tracer crosses from left to right at the same time it appears in the left ventricle. No clear LV chamber can be identified. When the serial images show an LV phase as clearly as it is shown in the normal example here, a significant left-to-right intracardiac shunt is excluded.

First-pass RNA has also been used to detect right-to-left shunts. By placing a ROI over a systemic artery that is uncontaminated by pulmonary activity, early appearance of a radionuclide bolus in the systemic circulation following intravenous injection is consistent with a right-to-left shunt (99). Right-to-left shunts are most often seen in congenital heart disease in children, and the preferred radionuclide method for detection and quantitation remains the intravenous injection of macroaggregated albumin. A ratio is generated from the activity that bypasses the lung through the shunt to arrive in organs such as the brain and kidney and the activity in the lung (100).

Clinical Applications of Ventricular Function Imaging

Diagnosis of Coronary Artery Disease

When coronary blood flow is lower than the demand for flow, the ischemic cascade is initiated. Regional metabolic dysfunction ensues that leads to regional mechanical dysfunction, which may then, if enough myocardium is involved, lead to global ventricular dysfunction. Electrocardiographic changes and symptoms tend to occur last. Because RNA is an excellent test for the detection of regional and global ventricular dysfunction, it has been applied to the diagnosis of CAD. The typical ischemic response includes a new or worsened regional wall motion abnormality, an increase in ES volume, a decrease in EF, a variable increase in EDV, and alterations of diastolic filling. However, all or none of those responses may occur depending on the amount of myocardium rendered ischemic.

Left Ventricular Ejection Fraction Response to Exercise

Early experience with exercise RNA suggested that normal subjects increase their LVEF by at least 0.05 during dynamic exercise. Failure to increase the LVEF by at least 0.05 became a criterion for the diagnosis of CAD, and reports appeared suggesting that use of that criterion had an extremely high sensitivity for the diagnosis of coronary disease (101–104). However, as indicated earlier, localized ischemia may occur without any change in EF if the overwhelming majority of the ventricle is not ischemic. Furthermore, after much more experience with exercise RNA, it is clear that there are many reasons for the EF failing to increase by at least 0.05 during exercise. Men and women appear to respond differently to exercise with men relying more on a decrease in ES volume and a concomitant increase in EF, and women relying more on an increase in EDV and less on increasing EF (105,106). Healthy older volunteers appear to have blunted EF responses to exercise (107). Isometric exercise results in an acute drop in EF (108), and the type of exercise protocol may have a dramatic effect on the EF response to exercise (109). In addition, the resting EF appears to influence the EF response to exercise (110). The EF response may be altered by severe hypertension or by valvular heart disease. An inadequate exercise effort, defined as a rate-pressure product less than 25,000, may also decrease the sensitivity for coronary disease (111). As a result of the numerous factors that can affect the LVEF other than CAD, the use of EF criteria for the diagnosis of CAD has poor specificity (89,112). In the largest study on the subject, the specificity for diagnosis of CAD of a failure to increase the LVEF during exercise by at least 0.05 had a specificity of 79%. Sensitivity was fairly high at 89% (112).

Although EF criteria do not perform well for the diagnosis of any coronary involvement, exercise RNA has been used successfully to distinguish severe coronary disease from mild or no disease. In general, exercise LVEF varies inversely with the extent and severity of the coronary disease (112,113). As a result, exercise LVEF can be used to identify patients with a large ischemic burden, those most likely to have multivessel or left main disease (114–115), and those most likely to benefit from revascularization procedures (116).

Regional Wall Motion

In contrast to abnormalities of the global EF during exercise, the detection of a regional abnormality of ventricular function either at rest or during exercise is highly specific for CAD. Regional dysfunction may be seen in certain cardiomyopathies but that is exceptionally rare. The specificity of a new or worsened regional wall motion abnormality during exercise has been reported to be as high as 93% (112). Unfortunately, the sensitivity of an exercise-induced wall motion abnormality is quite low in part because of the fact that exercise RNA is usually performed in only one view and in part because of the limited spatial resolution of the exercise RNA. As indicated previously, various parametric images may be used to assist in detecting regional ventricular dysfunction. However, no large prospective studies have been performed to rigorously test their performance in the diagnosis of CAD.

Although not typically applied as diagnostic criteria, abnormalities of diastolic function are common in patients with CAD because of the impairment in ventricular relaxation seen with ischemia. Reduced and delayed PFRs, as well as decreased first-third filling fractions, have been described in patients with coronary disease, including those with normal systolic function (55, 117,118). When blood flow is normalized, diastolic function may improve (119).

Pharmacologic Interventions

A large body of evidence exists that supports the diagnostic sensitivity and specificity of myocardial perfusion imaging in conjunction with the use of the coronary vasodilators dipyridamole (120) and adenosine (121). There is also evidence to suggest that catecholamine administration coupled with myocardial perfusion imaging is useful for detecting coronary disease (122). There is considerably less evidence that radionuclide ventricular function imaging during pharmacologic stimulation is useful diagnostically. ERNA has been found to be modestly sensitive but quite specific for the diagnosis of coronary disease when performed after a dipyridamole infusion (123) and has been performed with some success during dobutamine infusion (124).

Combined Function-Perfusion Imaging

Early attempts at combined function-perfusion imaging used the simultaneous injection of ultra-short-lived radionuclides, such as ^{195m}Au (125) and ^{191}Ir (126), along with ^{201}Tl. With that approach, a first-pass study could be acquired during the injection and a perfusion image could be acquired soon thereafter when the gold or iridium had decayed to background levels. Difficulties with the generators for gold and iridium prevented widespread application of those techniques.

The advent of the technetium perfusion imaging agents makes it possible to perform combined ventricular function and myocardial perfusion imaging with a single radionuclide injection. At the time of injection of the radionuclide, a first-pass study can be acquired and perfusion imaging can be performed subsequently (63–67). The combined study can provide all the regional and global functional information and quantitative SPECT perfusion data both at rest and during exercise. The functional impact of any given perfusion abnormality can be directly and quantitatively assessed. Preliminary evidence suggests that diagnostic sensitivity is enhanced using the combined approach (64). Routine addition of function to perfusion imaging appears to improve the detection of multivessel disease compared with the perfusion data alone (127). In addition, diagnostic confidence is enhanced with the availability of both function and perfusion data. Perhaps most importantly, the addition of functional data adds the rest and/or exercise LVEF, two prognostically powerful variables in patients with coronary disease.

Assessment of Prognosis in Chronic Stable Coronary Artery Disease

It has long been appreciated that the prognosis of patients with stable CAD is directly related to the contractile state of the left ventricle. Large series of both medically and surgically treated patients have been followed for several years, and the data from different investigators confirm that the resting LVEF measured either invasively or noninvasively is a powerful predictor of subsequent outcome (128,129). After the introduction of rest and exercise RNA, a large series of patients with stable CAD was followed during medical management after baseline catheterization and rest and exercise RNA were obtained. As noted in previous studies, the resting radionuclide LVEF was a powerful predictor of subsequent outcome. However, the peak exercise LVEF proved to be even more powerful in predicting subsequent mortality (130,131). The change in EF from rest to exercise was of no prognostic significance when a multivariable analysis was performed. Furthermore, when the radionuclide data were compared with the clinical and catheterization-derived variables, it was shown that the combination of the exercise EF and the clinical data contained almost all the prognostic information available from a catheterization. Figure 14.26 shows mortality plotted against the exercise EF. Patients with an exercise LVEF greater than 0.50 have an excellent long-term outlook. Mortality begins to increase sharply once LVEF drops below 0.35. In a much smaller patient group, and using ERNA, the resting LVEF proved to be a more important predictor of outcome than the exercise LVEF (132).

Other investigators have suggested that the change in the EF from rest to exercise is prognostically important. In a study of patients with three-vessel CAD who were mildly symptomatic, those subjects whose LVEF fell during exercise had more subsequent events than those subjects whose LVEF did not fall during exercise (133). In that study, all patients who died showed a decrease in LVEF and at least 1 mm of ST segment depression during exercise. Although there is some controversy about which of the three variables, resting LVEF, exercise LVEF, and the exercise-rest LVEF is most important in differing patient populations, there is certainly universal agreement that the LVEF can be used to stratify patients into high, low, and intermediate probabilities for subsequent cardiac events.

As yet, no prospective study has been performed that used the results of exercise RNA to assign patients to medical or revascularization treatment strategies. In a nonprospective, nonrandomized study of subjects with normal resting LV function, it was shown that those subjects with the greatest fall in LVEF during exercise preoperatively showed the most benefit in terms of pain relief and longevity following bypass surgery (116). That type of data suggests that the exercise RNA can be used for segregating patients into those who should be treated medically and those who should receive some interventional strategy.

Assessment of Acute Myocardial Infarction

Diagnosis

RNA performed in patients who have sustained an acute myocardial infarction (MI) can be used to localize and size the infarct, diagnose coexistent complications such as RV infarction or a ruptured interventricular septum, and predict both the short-term, in-hospital event rate and subsequent posthospital event rate. For a resting study during an acute MI, an ERNA is preferred because it allows one to assess all the segments of both ventricles. During inferior wall infarction, it is advisable to acquire a first-pass study during the injection of the labeled red cells or the technetium pertechnetate (in the case of *in vivo* labeling). The first-pass portion of the study provides the best measurement of RVEF, and the gated portion of the study provides the high-resolution wall motion assessment of the right and left ventricles and the LVEF. Having the first-pass study available also allows detection and quantitation of any shunt resulting from a ruptured septum.

Right Ventricular Infarction

It has been shown that more than 30% of inferior wall infarctions are accompanied by RV infarction (134). Scintigraphic

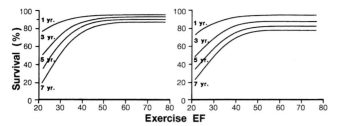

FIGURE 14.26. Overall survival (*left*) and infarct-free survival (*right*) are shown plotted against the exercise first-pass left ventricular ejection fraction (LVEF). Survival rates decrease rapidly once the exercise LVEF drops below 0.35. (Courtesy of Dr. Robert Jones.)

methods for the detection of RV infarction include RV uptake of technetium pyrophosphate and regional and global RV dysfunction on RNA. The advantage of the RNA is that it not only identifies the RV infarct but defines its extent and severity. It has been shown repeatedly that RV dysfunction associated with an acute inferior infarction often improves over time even without revascularization. Even severe RV dysfunction may improve in a matter of days (135) (Fig. 14.27).

Ruptured Septum and Acute Mitral Regurgitation

A ruptured interventricular septum is an uncommon but catastrophic complication of acute infarction, more often inferior infarction. The diagnosis may be established at the bedside by detecting an oxygen step-up in the right ventricle or pulmonary artery, by demonstration of flow across the septum using Doppler echocardiography, or by detection of a left-to-right shunt using RNA. Because of its widespread availability and increasing clinical experience, echocardiography is probably the test of choice in this setting. The same is true for mitral regurgitation resulting from papillary muscle dysfunction or frank rupture.

Assessment of Prognosis

The resting radionuclide LVEF acquired at bedside early in the course of acute MI has been used to risk stratify patients into groups with varying probabilities of death or ventricular fibrillation during their hospitalization (136). The identification of coexisting RV infarction recently was shown to carry a worse short- and long-term prognosis compared with those patients without RV infarction (137). For those patients that survive their infarcts, RNA has been used to predict subsequent outcome. As

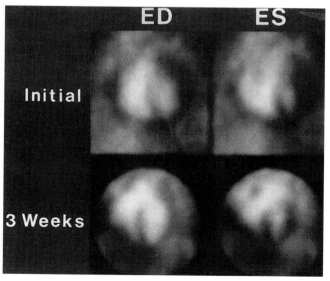

FIGURE 14.27. The equilibrium radionuclide angiogram (EqRNA) at the *top* was acquired soon after the patient presented with what appeared to be an inferior wall myocardial infarction (MI). The study suggested that the MI was primarily right ventricular (RV) in location. In this case, in which a thrombolytic was not administered, there is spontaneous improvement in RV function 3 weeks after the initial event.

in patients with stable CAD, both the resting (138) and the exercise LVEF (139,140) have been shown to be highly predictive of subsequent event rates. Predischarge stress RNA has also been used to discriminate between subjects with low and high risk for future events and performs better than stress ECG in that capacity (141,142). There is, however, little data that addresses the role of stress RNA after infarction in the interventional era. Considerably more focus has been given to the use of perfusion imaging for assessment of residual myocardial viability in the infarct area and detection of ischemia in segments remote from the infarct very soon after successful thrombolysis so that rapid decisions can be made regarding the need for catheterization and possible revascularization.

Assessment of Myocardial Viability

The assessment of myocardial viability plays an important role in patients with CAD. In either stunned or hibernating myocardium, severe ventricular dysfunction may be present even though the myocardium is still viable. Identification of such tissue has become increasingly important because contractile function may be improved by restoration of blood flow. Despite, the profoundly depressed baseline function of stunned or hibernating myocardium, the viability of such muscle can be confirmed by demonstrating transiently improved function following acute afterload reduction, ventricular extrasystoles, inotropic stimulation, and immediately following cessation of exercise.

Systolic function of severely hypokinetic segments may improve after administration of nitroglycerin. Originally described during contrast ventriculography, the technique has been has also been performed using RNA (143,144). Improved function following nitroglycerin administration is a marker for improvement after revascularization. Catecholamines were also initially used in the catheterization lab to demonstrate inotropic reserve in severely depressed myocardial segments. More recently, low-dose dobutamine infusions have been performed during echocardiographic examination to detect viable muscle. RNA could be used in place of echocardiography, although some would argue that the ability to visualize wall thickening is an important part of the assessment of the catecholamine response (145). Immediately following cessation of exercise, there is an increase in EF and an improvement in the systolic function of myocardial segments that were severely abnormal at rest and which remained so during exercise (18,19,109). Furthermore, identification of that response proved to be a marker for improvement in resting function following revascularization (20). The radionuclide assessment of myocardial viability using ventricular function analysis has been largely replaced by perfusion imaging protocols using either single photon or positron techniques. Whether perfusion and function should both be evaluated or whether one assessment should follow the other if the result is not conclusive has never been tested.

Evaluation of the Patient with Dyspnea or Congestive Heart Failure

There are many causes of dyspnea, both cardiac and noncardiac, but when a cardiac cause of dyspnea is being considered and the physical examination does not suggest any significant valvular heart disease, then a resting and, if necessary, an exercise RNA can often provide a diagnosis. If resting LV and RV function are normal in a patient being evaluated for dyspnea, especially dyspnea on exertion, then an exercise study should be performed. It may be useful to combine RNA, spirometry, and respiratory gas exchange measurements as a so-called cardiopulmonary stress test so that both cardiac and pulmonary causes, as well as the relative contribution of each, may be assessed (146).

In recent years, increasing attention has been paid to diastolic LV function as a cause of shortness of breath or CHF. It has been estimated that isolated diastolic dysfunction may be the cause of 30% of cases diagnosed with CHF (147,148). RNA is particularly well suited for distinguishing systolic from diastolic causes of CHF (Fig. 14.28). As indicated previously, diastolic dysfunction may be recognized visually by inspection of the LV volume curve and may be quantified by measurement of the PFR, tPFR, and the AFR.

Cardiomyopathy

Idiopathic Dilated

As its name implies, the sine qua non of the idiopathic dilated cardiomyopathy is the finding of a dilated and diffusely hypocontractile left ventricle. RNA is an ideal method for establishing the diagnosis. The etiology of diffuse LV dysfunction may not be apparent from a radionuclide, or for that matter, any type of ventriculogram. Findings that may be helpful in distinguishing idiopathic from so-called ischemic cardiomyopathies include the status of the right ventricle and the presence of akinetic or dyskinetic segments. There tends to be more involvement of the right ventricle in idiopathic dilated myopathies than in ischemic myopathies. In fact, the ratio of LV to RV EDV has been used to discriminate ischemic from nonischemic myopathies (149). However, one should recognize that RV dysfunction is a frequent finding with any long-standing LV dysfunction regardless of the etiology. The presence of akinetic or dyskinetic LV segments is very suggestive of an ischemic rather than an idiopathic cardiomyopathy. Occasionally, infiltrative myopathies, such as ventricular dysplasia, or inflammatory myocardial disease, such as sarcoid, may cause localized akinesia or dyskinesia. Associated findings in dilated cardiomyopathies are dilatation of the left and right atria and enlargement of the pulmonary artery, the latter a sign of pulmonary hypertension and atrial fibrillation.

The exercise response may be helpful in distinguishing ischemic from nonischemic causes of diffuse LV dysfunction. When resulting from coronary disease, the diffusely hypokinetic ventricle typically results from three-vessel disease. During exercise, such ventricles fail to increase the EF and typically show a drop in LVEF. In contrast, it is quite typical for patients with idiopathic dilated myopathies to show substantial increases in LVEF during exercise (150).

Hypertrophic Cardiomyopathy

Subjects with either concentric or asymmetric hypertrophic cardiomyopathy typically have small EDVs because of the thick-

ened myocardium and their EFs are, therefore, typically quite high. Consequently, their left ventricles appear to be hyperdynamic but there is no evidence that such ventricles have any intrinsically greater contractility than normal. In the LAO view, septal hypertrophy may be recognized on an ERNA. On the basis of radionuclide data, it has been demonstrated that diastolic dysfunction is present in the majority of patients with hypertrophic cardiomyopathy. In fact, it is the diastolic dysfunction that accounts for most of the clinical symptomatology in these patients. RNA has been used to demonstrate improvement in diastolic function when patients with hypotrophic myopathy are treated with drugs such as calcium blockers that appear to have a direct effect on diastolic filling (151).

Restrictive Cardiomyopathy

In restrictive cardiomyopathy, the primary pathologic disturbance is the impairment of LV diastolic filling. As such, RNA may be used to assist in the diagnosis. A recent study suggested that RNA could be helpful in distinguishing restrictive cardiomyopathy from constrictive pericardial disease (152). In restrictive disease, early diastolic filling is typically delayed and/or reduced whereas in constrictive disease, early diastolic filling tends to be more rapid than normal.

Doxorubicin (Adriamycin) Cardiotoxicity

In patients undergoing chemotherapy with doxorubicin, there is a significant risk of developing cardiotoxicity, which is characterized by a decrease in LV systolic function. The cardiotoxicity is dose-related and is infrequently seen at cumulative doses of under 400 mg/m². If the dose exceeds 500 mg/m², the probability of cardiotoxicity increases dramatically (153). RNA has become the procedure of choice for serial evaluation of patients during doxorubicin therapy (154–156). The primary measurement is the LVEF at rest. A study should be performed before any therapy so that baseline LV function is known. Thereafter, studies may be repeated at the discretion of the oncologist, but once the cumulative dose exceeds 250 mg/m², more frequent follow-up is recommended. Once the dose reaches 450 to 500 mg/m², LVEF should be checked before each dose. A decrease in LVEF 10 to 15 EF units or a decrease to below 0.45 is considered significant. If a significant decrease in LVEF is documented and the clinical decision is to proceed with further therapy, then the LVEF should be measured before each dose. When the radionuclide data are equivocal or when the cumulative dose exceeds 500 mg/m² without radionuclide evidence of toxicity, myocardial biopsy may be useful (157).

Valvular Heart Disease

The primary role of RNA in valvular heart disease is the serial evaluation of LV size and LVEF. As indicated previously, both FPRNA and ERNA have been used to quantify valvular insufficiency using stroke count and curve analysis techniques, but in practice the simplicity and accuracy of Doppler echocardiography make it the test of choice for that purpose. In stenotic valvular lesions, the only established role of RNA is to evaluate LV and RV function.

Aortic and Mitral Insufficiency

Patients with aortic insufficiency should be followed with serial measurements of LVEF and LV volumes. There is sufficient evidence to indicate that when the resting LVEF drops below 0.50, the prognosis for recovery of LV function after valve replacement decreases. Furthermore, once the LVEF drops below 0.50, there is a significantly greater risk of patients becoming symptomatic or even developing heart failure (158) and once the LVEF drops below 0.40, there is a higher long-term mortality even after valve replacement (159). Echocardiographic measurements of the EDV and ES volume are also predictive of subsequent outcome. Radionuclide volumes have not yet been used for that purpose. It has been shown that the LVEF may decrease during exercise in asymptomatic patients with aortic insufficiency (160,161), but there is no convincing evidence that the exercise LVEF is of any prognostic significance.

In patients with mitral insufficiency, the LVEF has also been shown to be of prognostic value. The clinical outcome and postoperative mortality of patients undergoing mitral valve replacement for mitral insufficiency were related to the preoperative LVEF. As in aortic insufficiency, when the LVEF dropped below 0.50, the clinical outcome was poorer (162). Because mitral insufficiency causes ventricular unloading compared with aortic insufficiency, the measured LVEF may be less reflective of actual ventricular contractility. Following mitral valve replacement, it is common to see the LVEF fall because the ventricle must now contract solely against systemic resistance (163). As a result, a method of evaluating LV contractile function that is independent of the loading conditions would be useful in patients with mitral insufficiency.

Assessment of Patients with Chronic Obstructive Pulmonary Disease

The major determinant of RV function is its afterload, the pulmonary artery pressure or resistance. Elevated pulmonary artery pressures, either transient or chronic, will result in a decrease in RV systolic function.

RV systolic function tends to be reduced in patients with pulmonary hypertension. The relationship is not, however, linear, because many subjects with pulmonary hypertension may maintain normal RV systolic function for some time. In the setting of chronic obstructive pulmonary disease (COPD), RVEF does tend to be lower than normal and is inversely related to the pulmonary hypertension (164). An abnormal resting RVEF in a patient with COPD may be predictive of subsequent cor pulmonale (165). Patients with COPD and normal RV function at rest may show abnormal responses of the RVEF to exercise (166).

Congenital Heart Disease

Congenital heart disease may be detected and characterized with FPRNA in children (167,168) and in adults (169). However, given the spatial resolution of echocardiography, MRI, and fast-CT, there is little, if any, primary role for radionuclide studies in the anatomic description of congenital heart lesions. However, FPRNA may still play a significant role in the detection and quantitation of left-to-right shunts. Left-to-right shunts are reliably detected on a FPRNA study. As indicated previously, any significant intracardiac left-to-right shunt can be detected visually by the absence of a clear LV phase (Fig. 14.25). Quantitatively, shunts with a Qp/Qs of less than 1.2/1 cannot be reliably distinguished from normal.

Serial Evaluation of LV Function: Reproducibility of Radionuclide LVEF

As indicated earlier, the serial measurement of EF may be important for the longitudinal evaluation of disease progression or regression, the response to specific therapy, or the toxicity of agents like doxorubicin. Because it is noninvasive, accurate, and quantitative, RNA is the technique of choice for this purpose. Variability data are available for both first-pass RNA and ERNA (170–172). At rest, the first-pass LVEF showed a mean difference of 0.04 ± 0.04 between measurements in the same subjects on different days. For ERNA, the mean differences for same-day studies and separate-day studies were 0.03 ± 0.03 and 0.04 ± 0.03 respectively (160). Of note is the finding that the variability was greater in subjects with normal ventricles (0.05 ± 0.04) than in those with reduced LV function (0.02 ± 0.02). Intraobserver and interobserver variability for processing the same data are inconsequential.

FPRNA VERSUS ERNA

Historically, the choice of performing a first-pass or a gated study depended on the type of gamma-camera and the particular software available. Currently, both FPRNA and ERNA can be adequately performed with several different gamma-cameras, and most current computers are fast enough and have sufficient storage capacity to handle either type of data. Virtually all clinical applications have been performed with both techniques. The selection of a procedure should be dictated by the clinical question at hand. Laboratories should have both modalities available and should be familiar with the acquisition of both types of studies. In general, ERNA offers a higher spatial resolution but a relatively prolonged acquisition time and can only provide quantitative data in the best septal view. The FPRNA trades spatial resolution for speed.

For most studies of LV function at rest, the equilibrium method is preferred. At rest, time is not a significant factor, so the acquisition can be prolonged as much as necessary to achieve high count rates and maximum spatial resolution. Multiple views of the heart may be obtained. For the evaluation of RV function at rest, a combined FPRNA and ERNA is recommended. The first-pass method remains the procedure of choice for measurement of RVEF whereas the ERNA data offer better resolution of regional wall motion and multiple views.

During exercise, the speed of the first-pass study is a major

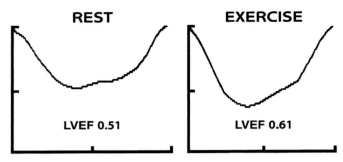

REST   **EXERCISE**

LVEF 0.51   **LVEF 0.61**

FIGURE 14.28. These curves were obtained in a man complaining of dyspnea on exertion. Regional wall motion and left ventricular ejection fractions were normal at rest and during exercise, but diastolic dysfunction was obvious on both studies. When pulmonary causes of dyspnea are not apparent, rest and exercise ventricular function studies may be particularly helpful in identifying the cause. They may be combined with spirometry and blood gas measurements as a so-called cardiopulmonary stress test to quantify the relative contributions of the heart and lungs to the patient's dyspnea.

advantage and FPRNA is, therefore, the procedure of choice for evaluation of LV function during exercise. When there is a specific question about ischemia in the circumflex distribution, an exercise ERNA may be more appropriate than an exercise FPRNA because of the difficulty with left atrial-LV overlap in LAO first-pass studies. The presence of arrhythmia such as very irregular atrial fibrillation, frequent premature beats or bigeminy is problematic for both techniques. FPRNA, however, is more susceptible to compromise by arrhythmia because of the paucity of beats available for analysis.

For the evaluation of diastolic LV function at rest, the ERNA is preferred because of the ability to accumulate a large number of counts per frame throughout the cycle that decreases the percent error in the calculation of diastolic filling parameters (Figs. 14.28 and 14.29). FPRNA is certainly the preferred method of detecting and quantifying left-to-right shunts.

Nonimaging Probes

As yet, nonimaging probes have not assumed a significant role in clinical practice. They have been used successfully for research to evaluate changes in LV function in ambulatory subjects or to assess serial changes in LV function during spontaneous ischemic episodes in unstable patients. They have the benefit of displaying real-time variations in LV function and have excellent temporal resolution. There are portable, freestanding units to assess the stationary patient, and there are miniaturized detectors that can be strapped to the patients chest for ambulatory monitoring. Measurement of LVEF with the stationary probe correlates fairly well with values obtained with a standard gamma-camera. Discordance is more common when there are regional wall motion abnormalities.

The miniaturized probes may be secured to the chest with a vest-like garment. The LVEF measured with this type of probe has correlated well with the LVEF from a standard gamma-camera (173,174). With the aid of a patient recorder diary, changes in LV function may be correlated with normal activities in much the same manner as is done with an ambulatory ECG recordings. Silent ischemia may be readily detected with these particular probes (175) (Fig. 14.30).

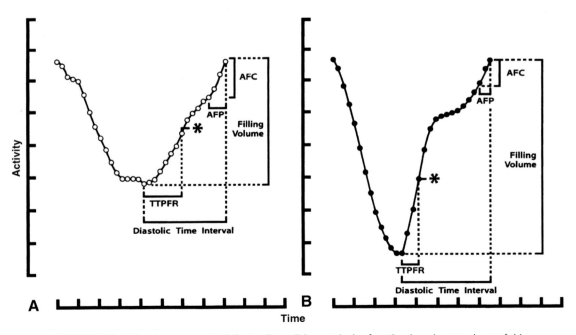

FIGURE 14.29. It has been suggested that radionuclide ventricular function imaging may be useful in distinguishing constrictive from restrictive heart disease. In restriction **(Panel A),** early filling tends to be delayed thus prolonging the time at which peak filling occurs (tPFR). In constriction **(Panel B),** early filling is more rapid than usual thus shortening the tPFR. (From Aroney CN, Ruddy TD, Dighero H et al. Differentiation of restrictive cardiomyopathy from pericardial constriction: assessment of diastolic function by radionuclide angiography. *J Am Coll Cardiol* 1989;13:1007–1014, with permission.)

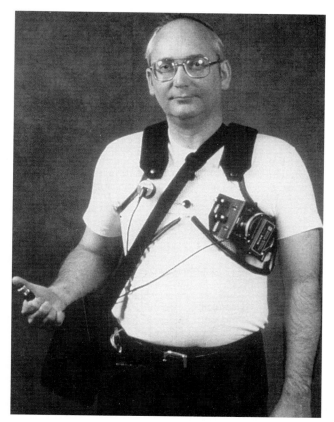

FIGURE 14.30. The "vest" is a miniaturized on-imaging probe that has been used to evaluate changes in LVEF during routine daily activities and mental stress. (Courtesy of Capintec, Inc.)

REFERENCES

1. Strauss HW, Zaret BL, Hurley PJ et al. A scintigraphic method for measuring left ventricular ejection fraction in man without cardiac catheterization. *Am J Cardiol* 1971;28:575–580.
2. Zaret BL, Strauss HW, Hurley PJ et al. A noninvasive scintiphotographic method of detecting regional ventricular dysfunction in man. *N Engl J Med* 1971;284:1174–1180.
3. Strauss HW, McKusick KA, Boucher CA et al. Of linens and laces—the eighth anniversary of the gated blood pool scan. *Sem Nucl Med* 1979;9:296–308.
4. Pavel DG, Zimmer AM, Patterson VN et al. *In vivo* labeling of red blood cells with Tc-99m: a new approach to blood pool visualization. *J Nucl Med* 1979;18:308.
5. Thrall SH, Freitas JE, Swanson D et al. Clinical comparison of cardiac blood pool visualization with technetium-99m red blood cells labeled *in vivo* and with technetium-99m human serum albumin. *J Nucl Med* 1978;19:796–803.
6. Lin M, Winchell HS, Shipley BA. Use of FE (II) or SN (II) alone for technetium labeling of albumin. *J Nucl Med* 1971;12:204–211.
7. Hamilton RG, Alderson PO. A comparative evaluation of techniques for rapid and efficient *in vivo* labeling of red blood cells with Tc-99m pertechnetate. *J Nucl Med* 1971;18:1010.
8. Kato M. *In vivo* labeling of red blood cells with Tc-99m with stannous pyridoxylideneamines. *J Nucl Med* 1979;20:1071.
9. Hegge FN, Hamiton GW, Larson SM et al. Cardiac chamber imaging: a comparison of red blood cells labeled with Tc-99m *in vitro* and *in vivo*. *J Nucl Med* 1978;19:129–134.
10. Callahan RG, Froelich JW, McKusick KA et al. A modified method for the *in vivo* labeling of red blood cells with Tc-99m: concise communication. *J Nucl Med* 1982;23:315–318.
11. Parker DA, Karvelis KC, Thral JH et al. Radionuclide ventriculography: methods. In: Gerson MC, ed. *Cardiac nuclear medicine*. New York: McGraw-Hill, 1991:84.
12. Hladik WB III, Nigg KK, Rhodes BA. Drug-induced changes in the biologic distribution of radiopharmaceuticals. *Sem Nucl Med* 1982; 12:184–211.
13. Juni JR, Chen CC. Effects of gating modes on the analysis of left ventricular function in the presence of heart rate variation. *J Nucl Med* 1988;29:1272–1278.
14. Bacharach SL, Green MV, Borer JS. Instrumentation in data processing in cardiovascular medicine: evaluation of ventricular function. *Sem Nucl Med* 1979;9:257–272.
15. Clements IP, Sinak LJ, Gibbons RG et al. Determination of diastolic function by radionuclide ventriculography. *Mayo Clin Proc* 1990;65: 1007–1019.
16. Parker DA, Karvelis KC, Thral JH et al. Radionuclide ventriculography: methods. In: Gerson MC, ed. *Cardiac nuclear medicine*. New York: McGraw-Hill, 1991:88–89.
17. Freeman MR, Berman DS, Staniloff H et al. Comparison of upright supine bicycle exercise in the detection and evaluation of extent coronary artery disease by equilibrium radionuclide ventriculography. *Am Heart J* 1981;102:182–189.
18. Seaworth JF, Higginbotham MB, Coleman RE et al. Effect of partial decreases in exercise work load on radionuclide indexes of ischemia. *J Am Coll Cardiol* 1983;2:522–529.
19. Rozanski A, Elkayam U, Berman DS et al. Improvement of resting myocardial asynergy with cessation of upright bicycle exercise. *Circulation* 1983;67:529–535.
20. Rozanski A, Berman D, Gray R et al. Preoperative prediction of reversible myocardial asynergy by postexercise radionuclide ventriculography. *N Engl J Med* 1982;307:212–216.
21. Stratman HG, Kennedy HL. Evaluation of coronary artery disease in the patient unable to exercise: alternatives to exercise stress testing. *Am Heart J* 1989;117:1344–1365.
22. Stratton JR, Halter JB, Hallstrom AP et al. Comparative plasma catecholamine and hemodynamic responses to hand grasp, cold pressor, and supine bicycle exercise testing in normal subjects. *J Am Coll Cardiol* 1983;2:93–104.
23. Iskandrian AS, Verani MS, Heo J. Pharmacologic stress testing: mechanism of action, hemodynamic responses, and results in detection of coronary artery disease. *J Nucl Cardiol* 1994;1:94–111.
24. Jensen FT, Lund O, Erlandsen M. Reliability of three computer methods in the analysis of ECG gated radionuclide left ventriculography: interrecording, interobserver, and intraobserver variability. *Angiology* 1991;42:866–877.
25. Bacharach SL, Green MV, Vitale D et al. Optimum Fourier filtering of cardiac data: a minimum-error method: concise communication. *J Nucl Med* 1983;24:1176–1183.
26. Johnson LL, Marshall M, Johnson YE et al. Radionuclide angiographic evaluation of left ventricular function by resting ejection rate during the first third of systole in patients with chronic aortic regurgitation. *Am Heart J* 1982;104:92–100.
27. Bacharach SL, Green MV, Borer JS et al. Left ventricular peak ejection rate, filling rate, and ejection fraction - frame rate requirements at rest and exercise: concise communication. *J Nucl Med* 1979;20:189–193.
28. Maddahi J, Berman DS, Matsuoka DT et al. A new technique for assessing right ventricular ejection fraction using rapid multiple-gated equilibrium blood pool scintigraphy: description, validation and findings in chronic coronary artery disease. *Circulation* 1979;60:581–589.
29. Winzelberg GG, Boucher CA, Prohous GM et al. Right ventricular function in the aortic and mitral disease. *Chest* 1981;79:520.
30. Spirito P, Maron BJ, Bonow RO. Noninvasive assessment of left ventricular diastolic function: comparative analysis of Doppler echocardiographic and radionuclide angiographic techniques. *J Am Coll Cardiol* 1986;7:518–526.
31. Bonow RO, Bacharach SL, Green MV et al. Impaired left ventricular diastolic filling in patients with coronary artery disease: assessment with radionuclide angiography. *Circulation* 1981;64:315–322.
32. Sandler H, Dodge HT. The use of single plane angiocardiograms for

the calculation of left ventricular volume in man. *Am Heart J* 1968; 75:325–334.

33. Dehmer GJ, Lewis SE, Hillis LD et al. Nongeometric determination of left ventricular volumes from equilibrium blood pool scans. *Am J Cardiol* 1980;45:293–300.

34. Links JM, Becker LC, Shindledecker JG et al. Measurement of absolute left ventricular volume from gated blood pool studies. *Circulation* 1982;65:82–91.

35. Mauer AH, Siegel JA, Denenberg BS et al. Absolute left ventricular volume from gated blood pool imaging with use of esophageal transmission measurement. *Am J Cardiol* 1983;51:853–858.

36. Fearnow EC, Jaszczak RJ, Harris CC et al. Esophageal source measurement of Tc-99m attenuation coefficients for use in left ventricular volume determinations. *Radiology* 1985;157:517–520.

37. Bourguignon MH, Douglas KH, Links JM et al. Fully automated data acquisition processing and display in equilibrium radioventriculography. *Eur J Nucl Med* 1981;6:343.

38. Nickel O, Schad N, Andrews EJ et al. Scintigraphic measurement of left ventricular volumes from the count-density distribution. *J Nucl Med* 1982;23:404–410.

39. Massardo T, Gal RA, Grenier RP et al. Left ventricular volume calculations using a count based ratio method applied to multigated radionuclide angiography. *J Nucl Med* 1990;31:450–456.

40. Levy WC, Cerqueira MD, Matsuoka DT et al. Four radionuclide methods for left ventricular volume determination: comparison of a manual and an automated technique. *J Nucl Med* 1992;33:763–770.

41. Gerwitz H, Wilner A, Garriepy S. Diagnosis of left-ventricular mural thrombus by means of radionuclide ventriculography. *J Nucl Med* 1981;22:610–612.

42. Frais MA, Botvinick EH, Shosa DW et al. Phase image characterization of ventricular contraction in left and right bundle branch block. *Am J Cardiol* 1982;50:95.

43. Starling MR, Dell'Italia LJ, Chaudhuri TK et al. First transit and equilibrium radionuclide angiography in patients with inferior transmural myocardial infarction. Criteria for the diagnosis of associated hemodynamically significant right ventricular infarction. *J Am Coll Cardiol* 1984;4:923.

44. Hrooka Y, Urabe Y, Imaizumi T et al. The usefulness of equilibrium radionuclide ventriculography in the diagnosis of arrhythmogenic right ventricular dysplasia and a report of cases of a familial occurrence. *Jpn Circ J* 1988;52:511–517.

45. Zaret BL, Wackers FJ. Radionuclide methods for evaluating the results of thrombolytic therapy. *Circulation* 1987;76(II):8–17.

46. Hackel DB, Wagner G, Ratliff NB et al. Anatomic studies of the cardiac conducting system in acute myocardial infarction. *Am Heart J* 1972;83:77–81.

47. Bodenheimer MM, Banka VS, Fooshee CM et al. Comparative sensitivity of the exercise electrocardiogram, thallium imaging and stress radionuclide angiography to detect the presence and severity of coronary heart disease. *Circulation* 1979;60:1270.

48. Sheehan FH, Dodge HT, Mathey DG et al. Application of the centerline method: analysis of change in regional left ventricular wall motion in serial studies. In: *Computers in cardiology.* Long Beach, CA: IEEE Computer Society, 1982:9–12.

49. Ramanathan KB, Erwin SW, Sullivan JM. Relationship of peak systolic pressure/end systolic volume ratio to standard ejection phase indices and ventricular function curves in coronary disease. *Am J Med Sciences* 1984;288:162–168.

50. Watkins J, Slutsky R, Tubau J et al. A scintigraphic study of the relationship between left ventricular peak-systolic pressure and endsystolic volume in normal subjects and patients with coronary artery disease. *Br Heart J* 1982;48:39.

51. Bonow RO, Vitale DF, Bachararch SL et al. Effects of aging on asynchronous left ventricular regional function and global ventricular filling in normal human subjects. *J Am Coll Cardiol* 1988;11:50–58.

52. Inouye I, Massie B, Loge D et al. Abnormal left ventricular filling: an early finding in mild to moderate systemic hypertension. *Am J Cardiol* 1984;53:120–126.

53. Betocchi S, Bonow RO, Bacharach SL et al. Isovolumic relaxation period in hypertrophic myopathy: assessment by radionuclide angiography. *J Am Coll Cardiol* 1986;7:74–81.

54. Bonow RO, Bacharach SL, Green MV et al. Impaired left ventricular diastolic filling in patients with coronary artery disease: assessment with radionuclide angiography. *Circulation* 1981;64:315–323.

55. Bonow RO. Radionuclide angiographic evaluation of left ventricular diastolic function. *Circulation* 1991;84(Suppl I):208–215.

56. Rigo P, Alderson DO, Robertson RM et al. Measurement of aortic and mitral regurgitation by gated cardiac blood pool scans. *Circulation* 1979;60:306.

57. Rigo P, Chevigne M. Measurement of left to right shunts by gated radionuclide angiography: concise communication. *J Nucl Med* 1982;23:1070.

58. Maublant J, Bailly P, Mestas D et al. Feasibility of gated single-photon emission transaxial tomography of the cardiac blood pool. *Radiology* 1983;146:837–839.

59. Tamaki N, Mukai T, Ishii Y et al. Multiaxial tomography of heart chambers by gated blood-pool emission computed tomography using a rotating gamma-camera. *Radiology* 1983;547–554.

60. Underwood SR, Walton S, Laming PJ et al. Left ventricular volume and ejection fraction determined by gated blood pool emission tomography. *Br Heart J* 1985;53:216–222.

61. Blumgart HL, Weiss S. Studies on the velocity of blood flow. VII. The pulmonary circulation time in normal resting individuals. *J Clin Invest* 1927;4:399–425.

62. Mason DT, Ashburn WL, Harbert JC et al. Rapid sequential visualization of the heart and great vessels in man using the wide-field anger scintillation camera. *Circulation* 1969;39:19–28.

63. Jones RH, Borges-Neto S, Potts JM. Simultaneous measurement of myocardial perfusion and ventricular function during exercise from a single injection of technetium-99m sestamibi in coronary artery disease. *Am J Cardiol* 1990;66:68E–71E.

64. Borges-Neto S, Coleman RE, Potts JM et al. Combined exercise radionuclide angiocardiography and single photon emission computed tomography perfusion studies for assessment of coronary disease. *Sem Nucl Med* 1991;21:223.

65. Johnson LL, Rodney RA, Vaccarino RA et al. Left ventricular perfusion and performance from a single radiopharmaceutical and one camera. *J Nucl Med* 1992;33:1411–1416.

66. Williams KA, Taillon LA, Draho JM et al. First-pass radionuclide angiographic studies of left ventricular function with technetium-99m-teboroxime, technetium-99m sestamibi and technetium-99m-DTPA. *J Nucl Med* 1993;34:394–399.

67. Takahashi N, Tamaki N, Tadamura E et al. Combined assessment of regional perfusion and wall motion in patients with coronary artery disease with technetium-99m-tetrofosmin. *J Nucl Cardiol* 1994;1:29–38.

68. Mena I, Narahara KA, de Jong R et al. Gold-195m, an ultra-short-lived generator-produced radionuclide: clinical application in sequential first pass ventriculography. *J Nucl Med* 1983;24:139–144.

69. Dymond DS, Elliott AT, Flatman W et al. The clinical validation of gold-195m: a new short half-life radiopharmaceutical for rapid, sequential, first pass angiocardiography in patients. *J Am Coll Cardiol* 1983;2:85–92.

70. Treves S, Cheng C, Samuel A et al. Iridium-191 angiocardiography for the detection and quantitation of left-to-right shunting. *J Nucl Med* 1980;21:1151–1157.

71. Verani MS, Lacy JL, Guidry GW et al. Quantification of left ventricular performance during transient coronary occlusion at various anatomic sites in humans: a study using tantalum-178 and a multiwire gamma-camera. *J Am Coll Cardiol* 1992;19:297–306.

72. Gal R, Grenier RP, Carpenter J et al. High count rate first-pass radionuclide angiography using a digital gamma-camera. *J Nucl Med* 1986;27:198–206.

73. Nichols K, DePuey EG, Gooneratne N et al. First-pass ventricular ejection fraction using a single-crystal nuclear camera. *J Nucl Med* 1994;35:1292–1300.

74. Bowyer KW, Konstantinow G, Rerych SK et al. Optimum counting intervals in radionuclide cardiac studies: In: *Nuclear cardiology: selected computer aspects.* New York: Society of Nuclear Medicine, 1978:85.

75. Rerych SK, Scholz PM, Newman GE et al. Cardiac function at rest and during exercise in normals and in patients with coronary heart disease. Evaluation by radionuclide angiocardiography. *Ann Surg* 1978;187:449.

76. Berger HI, Reduto LA, Johnstone DE et al. Global and regional left ventricular response to bicycle exercise in coronary artery disease. *Am J Med* 1979;66:13–21.

77. Potts JM, Borges-Neto S, Smith LR et al. Comparison of bicycle and treadmill radionuclide angiocardiography. *J Nucl Med* 1991;32: 1918–1922.

78. Friedman JD, Berman DS, Kiat H et al. Rest and treadmill exercise first-pass radionuclide ventriculography: validation of left ventricular ejection fraction measurements. *J Nucl Cardiol* 1994;4:382–388.

79. Jengo MA, Mena I, Blaufuss A et al. Evaluation of left ventricular function (ejection fraction and segmental wall motion) by single pass radioisotope angiography. *Circulation* 1978;57:326.

80. Marshall RC, Berger HJ, Costin JC et al. Assessment of cardiac performance with quantitative radionuclide angiocardiography. *Circulation* 1977;56:820–829.

81. Gal R, Grenier RP, Schmidt DH et al. Background correction in first-pass radionuclide angiography: comparison of several approaches. *J Nucl Med* 1986;27:1480–1486.

82. Scholz PM, Rerych SK, Moran JF et al. Quantitative radionuclide angiocardiography. *Cathet Cardiovasc Diagn* 1980;6:265–283.

83. Bodenheimer MM, Banka VS, Fooshee CM et al. Quantitative radionuclide angiography in the right anterior oblique view: comparison with contrast ventriculography. *Am J Cardiol* 1978;41:718–725.

84. Wackers FJT. First-pass radionuclide angiocardiography. In: Gerson MC, ed. *Cardiac nuclear medicine*. New York: McGraw-Hill, 1991: 67–80.

85. Morrison DA, Turgeon J, Ouitt T. Right ventricular ejection fraction measurements: contrast ventriculography versus gated blood pool and gated first-pass method. *Am J Cardiol* 1984;54:651–653.

86. Anderson PAW, Rerych SK, Moore TE et al. Accuracy of left ventricular end-diastolic dimension determinations obtained by radionuclide angiocardiography. *J Nucl Med* 1981;22:500.

87. Gal R, Grenier RP, Port SC et al. Left ventricular volume calculation using a count-based ratio method applied to first-pass radionuclide angiography. *J Nucl Med* 1992;33:2124–2132.

88. Jones RH, Sabiston DC Jr, Bates BB et al. Quantitative radionuclide angiocardiography for determination of chamber to chamber cardiac transit times. *Am J Cardiol* 1972;30:855–864.

89. Osbakken MD, Boucher CA, Okada RD et al. Spectrum of global left ventricular responses to supine exercise: limitation in the use of ejection fraction in identifying patients with coronary artery disease. *Am J Cardiol* 1983;51:28.

90. Hanley PC, Gibbons RJ. Value of radionuclide-determined changes in pulmonary blood volume for the detection of coronary artery disease. *Chest* 1990;97:7–11.

91. Schad N, Andrews ES, Fleming JW. *Colour atlas of first-pass functional imaging of the heart.* Hingham, Boston: MTP Press Ltd., 1985.

92. Reduto LA, Wickemeyer WJ, Young JB et al. Left ventricular diastolic performance at rest and during exercise in patients with coronary artery disease. *Circulation* 1981;63:1228–1237.

93. Polak JF, Kemper AJ, Bianco JA et al. Resting early peak diastolic filling rate: a sensitive index of myocardial dysfunction in patients with coronary artery disease. *J Nucl Med* 1982;23:471–478.

94. Philippe L, Mena I, Darcourt J et al. Evaluation of valvular regurgitation by factor analysis of first-pass angiography. *J Nucl Med* 1988; 29:159–167.

95. Janowitz WR, Fester A. Quantitation of left ventricular regurgitant fraction by first pass radionuclide angiocardiography. *Am J Cardiol* 1982;49:85–92.

96. Kanishi Y, Tatsuta N, Hikasa Y et al. Assessment of tricuspid regurgitation by analog computer analysis of dilution curves recorded by scintillation camera. *Jpn Circ* 1982;J46:1147.

97. Maltz DL, Treves S. Quantitative radionuclide angiocardiography: determination of Qp:Qs in children. *Circulation* 1973;47: 1048–1056.

98. Askenazi J, Ahnberg DS, Korngold E et al. Quantitative radionuclide angiocardiography: detection and quantitation of left-to-right shunts. *Am J Cardiol* 1976;37:382–387.

99. Peter CA, Armstrong BE, Jones RH. Radionuclide quantitation of right-to-left intracardiac shunts in children. *Circulation* 1981;64:572.

100. Dogan AS, Rezai K, Kirchner PT et al. A scintigraphic sign for detection of right-to-left shunts. *J Nucl Med* 1993;34:1607–1611.

101. Rerych SK, Scholz PM, Newman GE et al. Cardiac function at rest and during exercise in normals and patients with coronary artery disease. *Ann Surg* 1978;187:449.

102. Borer JS, Kent KM, Bacharach SL et al. Sensitivity, specificity and predictive accuracy of radionuclide cineangiography during exercise in patients with coronary artery disease. *Circulation* 1979;60:572.

103. Berger H, Reduto L, Johnstone D et al. Global and regional left ventricular response to bicycle exercise in coronary artery disease: assessment by quantitative radionuclide angiocardiography. *Am J Med* 1979;66:13.

104. Jengo JA, Oren V, Conant R et al. Effects of maximal exercise stress on left ventricular function in patients with coronary artery disease using first pass radionuclide angiocardiography. A rapid noninvasive technique for determining ejection fraction and segmented wall motion. *Circulation* 1979;59:60–65.

105. Gibbons RJ, Lee KL, Cobb F et al. Ejection fraction response to exercise in patients with chest pain and normal coronary arteriograms. *Circulation* 1981;64:952–957.

106. Higginbotham MB, Morris KB, Coleman RE et al. Sex-related differences in the normal cardiac response to upright exercise. *Circulation* 1984;70:357.

107. Port SC, Cobb FR, Coleman E et al. Effect of age on the response of the left ventricular ejection fraction to exercise. *N Engl J Med* 1980; 303:1133–1137.

108. Peter CA, Jones RH. Effects of isometric handgrip and dynamic exercise on left ventricular function. *J Nucl Med* 1980;21:1131.

109. Foster C, Dymond DS, Anholm JD et al. Effect of exercise protocol on the left ventricular response to exercise. *Am J Cardiol* 1983;51: 859–864.

110. Port SC, McEwan P, Cobb FR et al. Influence of resting left ventricular function on the left ventricular response to exercise in patients with coronary artery disease. *Circulation* 1981;63:856.

111. Brady TJ, Thrall JH, Lo K et al. The importance of adequate exercise in the detection of coronary heart disease by radionuclide ventriculography. *J Nucl Med* 1980;21:1125.

112. Jones RH, McEwen P, Newman GE et al. Accuracy of diagnosis of coronary artery disease by radionuclide measurement of left ventricular function during rest and exercise. *Circulation* 1981;64:586–601.

113. DePace NL, Iskandrian AS, Hakki A et al. Value of left ventricular ejection fraction during exercise in predicting the extent of coronary artery disease. *J Am Coll Cardiol* 1983;1:1002.

114. Johnson SH, Bigelow C, Lee KL et al. Prediction of death and myocardial infarction by radionuclide angiocardiography in patients with suspected coronary artery disease. *Am J Cardiol* 1991;67:919–926.

115. Gibbons RJ, Fyke FE III, Clements IP et al. Noninvasive identification of severe coronary artery disease using exercise radionuclide angiography. *J Am Coll Cardiol* 1988;11:28–34.

116. Jones RH, Floyd RD, Austin EH et al. The role of radionuclide angiocardiography in the preoperative prediction of pain relief and prolonged survival following coronary artery bypass grafting. *Ann Surg* 1983;197:743.

117. Austin EH, Jones RH. Radionuclide left ventricular volume curves in angiographically proved normal subjects and patients with three-vessel coronary disease. *Am Heart J* 1983;106:1357.

118. Miller TR, Goldman KJ, Sampathkumaran KS et al. Analysis of cardiac diastolic function: application in coronary artery disease. *J Nucl Med* 1983;24:2–7.

119. Bonow RO, Kent KM, Rosing DR et al. Improved left ventricular diastolic filling in patients with coronary artery disease after percutaneous transluminal angioplasty. *Circulation* 1982;66:1159–1167.

120. Leppo JA. Dipyridamole-thallium imaging: the lazy man's stress test. *J Nucl Med* 1989;30:281–287.

121. Verani MS, Mahmarian JJ, Hixson JB et al. Diagnosis of coronary artery disease by controlled coronary vasodilation with adenosine and

122. thallium-201 scintigraphy in patients unable to exercise. *Circulation* 1990;82:80–87.

122. Pennell DJ, Underwood SR, Swanton RH et al. Dobutamine thallium myocardial perfusion tomography. *J Am Coll Cardiol* 1991;18:1471–1479.

123. Cates CU, Kronenberg MW, Collins HW et al. Dipyridamole radionuclide ventriculography: a test with high specificity for severe coronary artery disease. *J Am Coll Cardiol* 1989;13:841–851.

124. Bahl VK, Vasan RS, Malhotra A et al. A comparison of dobutamine infusion and exercise during radionuclide ventriculography in the evaluation of coronary arterial disease. *Int J Cardiol* 1992;35:49–55.

125. Narahara KA, Mena I, Maublaut JC et al. Simultaneous maximum exercise radionuclide angiography and thallium stress perfusion imaging. *Am J Cardiol* 1984;53:812.

126. Verani MS, Lacy JL, Ball ME et al. Simultaneous assessment of regional ventricular function and perfusion utilizing iridium-191m and thallium-201 during a single exercise test. *Am J Cardiol Imaging* 1988;2:206.

127. Palmas W, Friedman JD, Kiat H et al. Improved identification of multiple-vessel coronary artery disease by addition of exercise wall motion analysis to Tc-99m-sestamibi myocardial perfusion SPECT. *J Nucl Med* 1993;34:1308.

128. Harris PJ, Harrell FE Jr, Lee KL et al. Nonfatal myocardial infarct in medically treated patients with coronary artery disease. *Circulation* 1980;62:240–248.

129. CASS Principal Investigators. Coronary artery surgery study (CASS): a randomized trial of coronary bypass surgery. Survival data. *Circulation* 1983;68:989.

130. Pryor DB, Harrel FE, Lee KL et al. Prognostic indicators from radionuclide angiography in medically treated patients with coronary artery disease. *Am J Cardiol* 1984;53:18.

131. Lee KL, Pryor DB, Pieper KS et al. Prognostic value of radionuclide angiography in medically treated patients with coronary artery disease. *Circulation* 1990;82:1705–1717.

132. Talierao CP, Clements IP, Zingmeister AR et al. Prognostic value and limitations of exercise angiography in medically treated coronary artery disease. *Mayo Clin Proc* 1988;63:573–582.

133. Bonow RO, Kent KM, Rosing DR et al. Exercise-induced ischemia in mildly symptomatic patients with coronary artery disease and preserved left ventricular function: identification of subgroups at risk of death during medical therapy. *N Engl J Med* 1984;311:1339.

134. Isner JM, Roberts WC. Right ventricular infarction complicating left ventricular infarction secondary to coronary artery disease. *Am J Cardiol* 1978;42:885.

135. Steele P, Kirch D, Ellis J et al. Prompt return to normal of depressed right ventricular ejection fraction in acute inferior infarction. *Br Heart J* 1977;39:1319.

136. Ony L, Green S, Reiser P et al. Early prediction of mortality in patients with acute myocardial infarction: a prospective study of clinical and radionuclide risk factors. *Am J Cardiol* 1986;57:33.

137. Zehender M, Kasper W, Kauder E et al. Right ventricular infarction as an independent predictor of prognosis after acute inferior myocardial infarction. *N Engl J Med* 1993;328:81–88.

138. The Multicenter Post-Infarction Research Group. Risk stratification and survival after myocardial infarction. *N Engl J Med* 1983;309:331.

139. Morris KG, Palmieri ST, Califf RM et al. Value of radionuclide angiography for predicting specific cardiac events after acute myocardial infarction. *Am J Cardiol* 1985;55:318.

140. Mazzotta G, Camerini A, Scopinaro G et al. Predicting cardiac mortality after uncomplicated myocardial infarction by exercise radionuclide ventriculography and exercise-induced ST-segment elevation. *Eur Heart J* 1992;13:330–337.

141. Corbett JR, Dehmer GJ, Lewis SE et al. The prognostic value of submaximal exercise testing with radionuclide ventriculography before hospital discharge in patients with recent myocardial infarction. *Circulation* 1981;64:535–544.

142. Hung J, Goris ML, Nash E et al. Comparative value of maximal treadmill testing, exercise thallium myocardial perfusion imaging and exercise radionuclide ventriculography for distinguishing high- and low-risk patients soon after acute myocardial infarction. *Am J Cardiol* 1984;53:1221.

143. Helfrant RH, Pine R, Meister SG et al. Nitroglycerin to unmask reversible asynergy. *Circulation* 1974;50:108–113.

144. Salel AF, Berman DS, DeNardo GL et al. Radionuclide assessment of nitroglycerin influence on abnormal left ventricular segmental contraction in patients with coronary heart disease. *Circulation* 1976;53:975–981.

145. Bavilla F, Gheorghiade M, Alam M et al. Low-dose dobutamine in patients with acute myocardial infarction identifies viable but not contractile myocardium and predicts the magnitude of improvement in wall motion abnormalities in response to coronary revascularization. *Am Heart J* 1991;122:1522–1531.

146. Boucher CA, Anderson MD, Schneider MS et al. Left ventricular function before and after reaching the anaerobic threshold. *Chest* 1985;87:145–150.

147. Soufer R, Wohlgelernter D, Vita NA et al. Intact systolic left ventricular function in clinical congestive heart failure. *Am J Cardiol* 1985;55:1032–1036.

148. Cohn JN, Johnson G, VA Cooperative Study Group. Heart failure with normal ejection fraction. *Circulation* 1990;81(Suppl III):4A.

149. Iskandrian AS, Helfeld H, Lemlek J et al. Differentiation between primary dilated cardiomyopathy and ischemic cardiomyopathy based on right ventricular performance. *Am Heart J* 1992;123:768–773.

150. Schoolmeester WL, Simpson AG, Saverbrunn BJ et al. Radionuclide angiographic assessment of left ventricular function during exercise in patients with a severely reduced ejection fraction. *Am J Cardiol* 1981;47:804.

151. Bonow RO, Rosing DR, Bacharach SL et al. Effects of verapamil on left ventricular systolic function and diastolic filling in patients with hypertrophic cardiomyopathy. *Circulation* 1981;64:787–796.

152. Aroney CN, Ruddy TD, Dighero H et al. Differentiation of restrictive cardiomyopathy from pericardial constriction: assessment of diastolic function by radionuclide angiography. *J Am Coll Cardiol* 1989;13:1007–1014.

153. VonHoff DD, Layard MW, Basa P et al. Risk factors for doxorubicin-induced congestive heart failure. *Ann Intern Med* 1979;91:710.

154. Alexander J, Dainiak N, Berger HJ et al. Serial assessment of doxorubicin cardiotoxicity with quantitative radionuclide angiocardiography. *N Engl J Med* 1979;300:278.

155. Gottdiener JS, Mathisen DJ, Borer JS et al. Doxorubicin cardiotoxicity: assessment of late left ventricular dysfunction by radionuclide cineangiography. *Ann Intern Med* 1981;94:430.

156. Choi BW, Berger HJ, Schwartz PE et al. Serial radionuclide assessment of doxorubicin cardiotoxicity in cancer patients with abnormal baseline resting left ventricular performance. *Am Heart J* 1983;106:638.

157. Mason JW, Bristow MR, Billingham ME et al. Invasive and noninvasive methods of assessing adriamycin cardiotoxic effects in man: superiority of histopathologic assessment using endomyocardial biopsy. *Cancer Treat Rep* 1978;62:857.

158. Bonow RO. Radionuclide angiography in the management of asymptomatic aortic regurgitation. *Circulation* 1991;84(Suppl I):296–302.

159. Cohn LH. Timing of surgery in chronic mitral and aortic valve regurgitation. *J Am Coll Cardiol Curr J Rev* 1993; July/August:49–51.

160. Borer JS, Bacharach SL, Green MV et al. Exercise-induced left ventricular dysfunction in symptomatic and asymptomatic patients with aortic regurgitation: assessment with radionuclide cineangiography. *Am J Cardiol* 1978;42:351–357.

161. Huxley RL, Gaffney FA, Corbett JR et al. Early detection of left ventricular dysfunction in chronic aortic regurgitation as assessed by contrast angiography, echocardiography, and rest and exercise scintigraphy. *Am J Cardiol* 1983;51:1542–1550.

162. Crawford MH, Souchek J, Oprian CA. Determinants of survival and left ventricular performance after mitral valve replacement. *Circulation* 1990;81:1173–1181.

163. Levine HJ, Gaasch WH. Ratio of regurgitant volume to end-diastolic volume: a major determinant of ventricular response to surgical correction of chronic volume overload. *Am J Cardiol* 1983;52:406–410.

164. Brent BN, Mahler D, Matthay RA et al. Noninvasive diagnosis of

pulmonary arterial hypertension in chronic obstructive pulmonary disease: right ventricular ejection fraction at rest. *Am J Cardiol* 1984; 53:1349–1353.

165. Berger HJ, Matthay RA, Loke J et al. Assessment of cardiac performance with quantitative radionuclide angiocardiography: right ventricular ejection fraction with reference to findings in chronic obstructive pulmonary disease. *Am J Cardiol* 1978;41:897–905.

166. Matthay RA, Berger HJ, Davies RA et al. Right and left ventricular exercise performance in chronic obstructive pulmonary disease: radionuclide assessment. *Ann Intern Med* 1980;93:234.

167. Hurley PJ, Wesselhoeft H, James AE Jr. Use of nuclear imaging in the evaluation of pediatric cardiac disease. *Sem Nucl Med* 1972;2: 353.

168. Kriss JP, Enright LP, Hayden WG et al. Radioisotopic angiocardiography: findings in congenital heart disease. *J Nucl Med* 1972;13:31.

169. Gal R, Port SC. Radionuclide angiography in congenitally corrected transposition of the great vessels in an adult. *J Nucl Med* 1987;28: 116–118.

170. Marshall RC, Berger HJ, Reduto LA et al. Variability in sequential measures of left ventricular performance assessed with radionuclide angiocardiography. *Am J Cardiol* 1978;41:531.

171. Upton MT, Rerych SK, Newman GE et al. The reproducibility of radionuclide angiographic measurements of LV function in normal subjects at rest and during exercise. *Circulation* 1980;62:126–132.

172. Wackers FJT, Berger HJ, Johnstone DE et al. Multiple gated cardiac blood pool imaging for left ventricular ejection fraction: validation of the technique and assessment of variability. *Am J Cardiol* 1979; 43:1159.

173. Tamaki N, Gill JB, Moore RH et al. Cardiac response to daily activities and exercise in normal subjects assessed by an ambulatory ventricular function monitor. *Am J Cardiol* 1987;59:1164–1169.

174. Broadhurst P, Cashman P, Crawley J et al. Clinical validation of a miniature nuclear probe system for continuous on-line monitoring of cardiac function and ST-segment. *J Nucl Med* 1991;32:37–43.

175. Breisblatt WM, Weiland FL, McLain JR et al. Usefulness of ambulatory radionuclide monitoring of left ventricular function early after acute myocardial infarction for predicting residual myocardial ischemia. *Am J Cardiol* 1988;62:1005–1010.

15

MYOCARDIAL PERFUSION IMAGING

FRANS J. TH. WACKERS

Since the mid-1970s, when ^{201}Tl became commercially available for clinical use, stress and rest radionuclide myocardial perfusion imaging has been widely employed for imaging of the heart and for the assessment of regional myocardial perfusion (1). Myocardial perfusion imaging was initially performed using the planar projection imaging technique. In the early 1980s single photon emission computed tomography (SPECT) was developed and during the subsequent decade SPECT imaging has become the most commonly performed cardiac imaging modality. Because planar myocardial perfusion imaging is only infrequently used for cardiac imaging and no new technical advances have been made, for a detailed discussion on planar cardiac imaging we refer to previous editions of this chapter (2). In our laboratory we use planar imaging only for very obese patients, whose weight can not be supported by the SPECT imaging table or for patients who can not lie still during SPECT image acquisition.

^{99m}Tc-labeled agents with better characteristics for clinical imaging than ^{201}Tl were developed in the late 1980s and were approved for clinical imaging in the early 1990s (3–5). At the time of this writing, approximately 75% of all stress myocardial perfusion studies in the United States are performed using ^{99m}Tc-sestamibi or ^{99m}Tc-tetrofosmin, whereas ^{201}Tl is used as the stress-imaging agent in only 25% of all studies.

Over the years radionuclide myocardial perfusion imaging has become an important diagnostic tool in the routine armamentarium of the clinical cardiologist. As discussed in this chapter, the most important clinical indications for performing radionuclide myocardial perfusion imaging are the detection of coronary artery disease and risk stratification of patients with disease.

SPECT IMAGE ACQUISITION

For SPECT imaging, a continuous series of 32 or more planar projection images is acquired in a 180-degree to 360-degree arc around the patient. Technical details of the acquisition of SPECT myocardial perfusion images are discussed in Chapter

12. Specific aspects of cardiac image acquisition using various radiopharmaceuticals are summarized in Table 15.1. We also refer to the "Updated Imaging Guidelines for Nuclear Cardiology Procedures: Part 1" published by the American Society of Nuclear Cardiology (6).

NORMAL SPECT MYOCARDIAL PERFUSION IMAGES

Reconstructed slices of the heart are displayed as short-axis, horizontal long-axis, and vertical long-axis slices. The display of SPECT myocardial perfusion images is standardized (Fig. 15.1). This is important for exchange, transfer, and interpretation of images acquired in different laboratories. The standardized nomenclature for SPECT images and the designation of coronary territories are shown in Figs. 15.2 to 15.5.

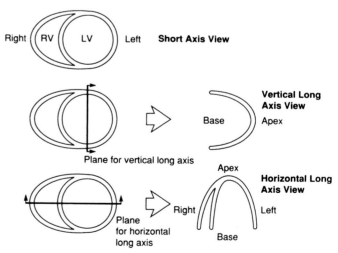

FIGURE 15.1. Standardized display of SPECT myocardial perfusion images. The short axis slices are displayed with the right ventricle left and the left ventricle right. The short axis slices are displayed as a horizontal row of images, starting with the apical slice on the left and the basal slices on the right. The vertical long axis slices are cut from the septum toward the lateral wall, displaying the septal slices on the left and the lateral slices on the right. The horizontal long axis slices are cut from the inferior wall towards the anterior wall, displaying the inferior wall slices on the left and the anterior wall slices on the right.

F.J.Th. Wackers: Cardiovascular Nuclear Imaging, Yale University School of Medicine, Department of Diagnostic Radiology, New Haven, CT.

Table 15.1. *Summary of Typical Acquisition Parameters for SPECT Myocardial Perfusion Imaging with* ^{201}Tl *and* ^{99m}Tc-Labeled Agents

	^{201}Tl	^{99m} Tc-Agents	^{99m} Tc-Agents
Dose	3.5–4 mCi	Low: 10–15 mCi	High: 20–30 mCi
Start imaging after injection:			
During exercise	10–15 min	15–30 min	15–30 min
During pharmacologic	5–10 min	45–60 min	45–60 min
At rest	45 min	45–60 min	45–60 min
Imaging interval:			
Redistribution	3–4 hrs		
Stress-Rest, Rest-Stress		1–4 hrs	1–4 hrs
Imaging position	Supine or prone	Supine or prone	Supine or prone
Collimator	Low-energy, all-purpose	Low-energy, high-resolution	Low-energy, high resolution
Orbit	Circular 180°	Circular, 360° or 180°	Circular, 360° or 180°
Energy peak	70 keV	140 keV	140 keV
	167 keV		
Energy window	20% and 30% symmetric	20% symmetric	20% symmetric
Matrix	64 × 64	64 × 64	64 × 64
Pixel size	6.4 ± 0.2mm	6.4 ± 0.2mm	6.4 ± 0.2mm
Acquisition type	Step-and-shoot	Step-and-shoot	Step-and-shoot
No. of projections	32	64	64
Time/projection	40 s	25 s	20s
Total imaging time	22 min	27 min	22 min

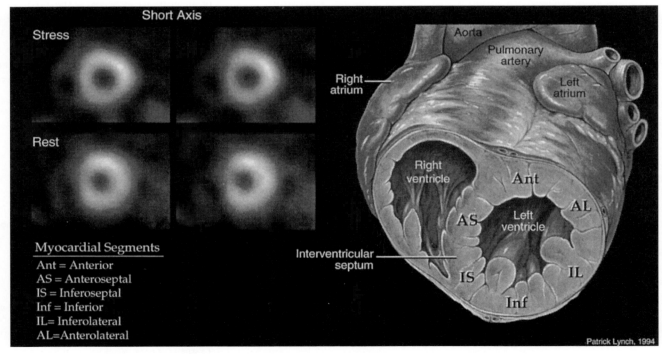

FIGURE 15.2. Anatomy of the left ventricle on short axis SPECT slices. Schematic anatomic drawing of the left ventricle as displayed in reconstructed short axis slices. Stress/rest scintigraphic short axis slices are shown in the left upper corner.

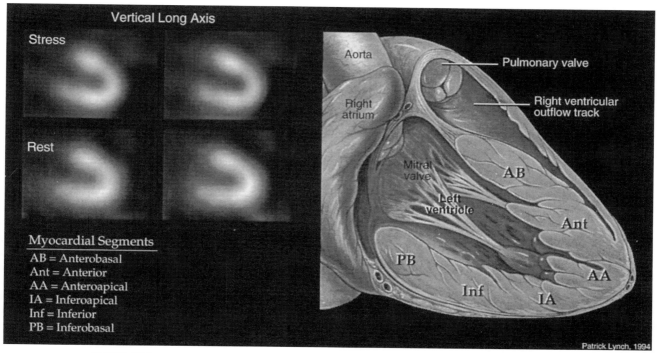

FIGURE 15.3. Anatomy on the left ventricle on vertical long axis SPECT slices. Schematic anatomic drawing of the left ventricle displayed in reconstructed vertical long axis SPECT slice is shown. Stress/rest scintigraphic vertical long axis slices shown in the left upper corner.

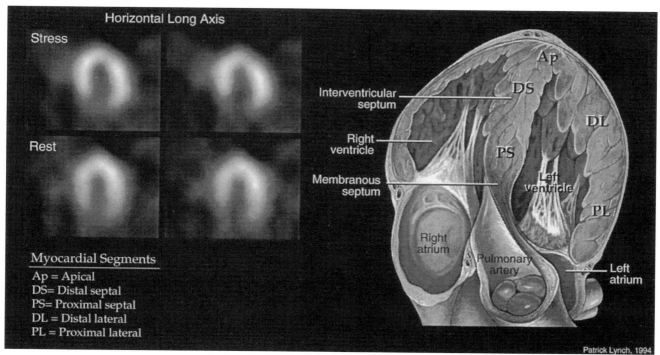

FIGURE 15.4. Anatomy of the left ventricle on horizontal long axis SPECT slices. Schematic anatomic drawing of the left ventricle as displayed in reconstructed horizontal long axis slices. Stress/rest scintigraphic horizontal long axis slices are shown in the upper left corner.

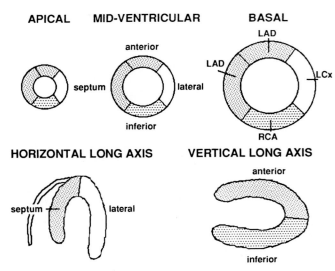

APICAL   MID-VENTRICULAR   BASAL

HORIZONTAL LONG AXIS   VERTICAL LONG AXIS

FIGURE 15.5. Anatomic segments and coronary artery territories on SPECT myocardial perfusion imaging.

Varying Spectrum of Normal SPECT Images

As can be appreciated by quantitative analysis, even on normal SPECT images the relative myocardial uptake of a radiotracer is not perfectly homogeneous. Slight regional variations can be appreciated, although these generally do not exceed 20% of maximal radiotracer uptake.

On apical and midventricular short-axis slices, it is normal to observe slightly less uptake of radiotracer in the septal wall, as compared with the lateral wall (Fig. 15.6). Furthermore, there may be slightly less inferoseptal uptake in male patients in basal slices as a normal variant. Radiotracer distribution in females tends to be more homogeneous in the basal slices. The most apical short-axis slices (without ventricular cavity) often show inhomogeneous radiotracer distribution ("coffee bean" appearance) resulting from partial volume effect and because of the relative eccentric location of the apex relative to the detector orbit (see later). The most basal short-axis slices usually show an apparent septal defect. This is a normal finding that represents the *membranous portion* of the basal septum.

In contrast to planar imaging, in which each view is an independently acquired and unique image, the vertical long-axis slices and the horizontal long-axis slices are reconstructed from the same raw data as the short-axis slices. Thus, no new information is to be expected on these images. The main purpose for analyzing long-axis slices is to inspect the apex and base of the heart. These areas are not well displayed on short-axis slices and may appear erroneously inhomogeneous because of partial volume effect. Only slices that clearly show left ventricular cavity should be analyzed. On the horizontal long-axis slices the septum is usually shorter than the lateral wall, a normal finding caused by the membranous portion of the septum.

Artifacts on SPECT Images

Artifacts occur frequently on reconstructed SPECT slices. However, an experienced and alert interpreter usually can recognize their presence (7).

Diaphragmatic Attenuation

The most frequent and difficult to deal with artifact on SPECT imaging is that caused by diaphragmatic attenuation. SPECT imaging is performed with the patient lying in supine position. We have shown previously that with the patient in supine position the left ventricular inferior wall is attenuated in approximately 25% of patients. False-positive inferior wall defects occur frequently on SPECT images (Fig. 15.7). To recognize this potential SPECT artifact a number of quality assurance measures can be taken. In our laboratory we acquire *two additional planar images* after SPECT image acquisition is completed: one left lateral view with the patient lying supine and another left lateral view with the patient lying on his or her right side. This additional set of images will alert the interpreter to the possibility of inferior wall attenuation on SPECT. Analysis of regional wall motion on electrocardiogram (ECG)-gated SPECT images may also be helpful for recognizing inferior wall attenuation artifacts. Normal wall motion of an apparent fixed defect is suggestive of attenuation artifact. Other investigators recommended different patient positioning during SPECT imaging to recognize attenuation artifacts: either in the prone or the upright position. It is likely that attenuation artifacts will continue to limit the specificity of SPECT imaging, until attenuation correction devices have been thoroughly validated and are routinely used for clinical SPECT imaging.

Breast Artifacts

On SPECT imaging, breast attenuation artifacts are often less extensive and less dense than on planar imaging. Nevertheless, they are at times difficult to distinguish from true myocardial perfusion defects (Fig. 15.8). To detect the potential of breast artifacts on SPECT imaging, inspection of the "rotating projection images" before interpretation is an essential part of quality assurance. On cine display of the projection images (Fig. 15.9), one can observe the "breast shadow" moving over the heart, a sign that should alert to the potential of breast artifacts on reconstructed slices. Again, visual analysis of ECG-gated SPECT images is most helpful for recognizing breast attenuation artifacts. Normal regional wall motion in an area with an apparent fixed defect is highly suggestive of artifact. In the future, attenuation correction software may solve the problem of breast artifacts.

Upward Creep

During SPECT acquisition, the heart may change from a vertical position immediately after exercise to a more horizontal position towards the end of SPECT image acquisition when the patient is rested. This change in position of the heart was observed to occur in particular in subjects who exercised well. The explanation for the observation is that during SPECT acquisition the patient's breathing pattern changes from deep after exercise to more shallow during recovery, with flattening of the diaphragm. This change in position of the heart has been coined "upward creep" and has been shown to cause artifactual inferior wall defects (8). To avoid these artifacts, it has been recommended that image acquisition should not be started immediately after

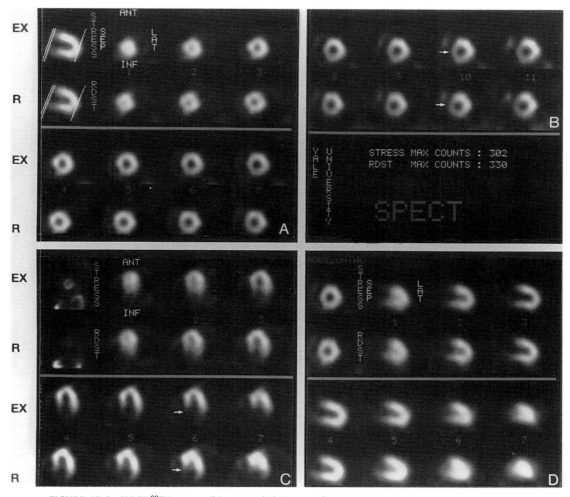

FIGURE 15.6. SPECT ^{99m}Tc-sestamibi myocardial images after exercise and at rest in a normal subject showing normal variation of radiopharmaceutic distribution. On the midventricular short axis slices **A**, the inferior septal areas have slightly less activity than the lateral wall. On the basal slices **B**, an apparent septal defect is present (*arrow*). This is the membranous portion of the septum. This is also seen in the horizontal long axis slices **C** where the septum is shorter (*arrow*) than the lateral wall. Vertical long axis slices are shown in **D**. (Reproduced by permission from Wackers FJTh. Artifacts in planar and SPECT myocardial perfusion imaging. *Am J Cardiac Imaging* 1992;6:42–58.)

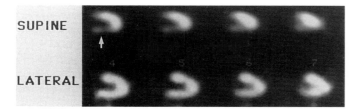

FIGURE 15.7. Vertical long axis ^{201}Tl SPECT images of the patient shown in Figure 25.21. Images acquired with the patient lying on his back (supine) are shown in the *top* panel. An inferior wall myocardial perfusion defect in present (*arrow*). The patient was turned on the right side (lateral) and SPECT imaging was repeated. This time the vertical long axis images are normal. The erroneous inferior wall defect on supine imaging is caused by attenuation by the left hemidiaphragm. Turning the patient onto her right side diminishes diaphragmatic attenuation. (Reproduced by permission from Wackers FJTh. Artifacts in planar and SPECT myocardial perfusion imaging. *Am J Cardiac Imaging* 1992;6:42–58.)

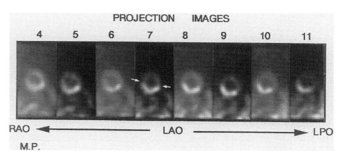

FIGURE 15.8. Serial consecutive planar projection images of the patient in Fig. 15.9 with breast artifact. The breast shadow can be seen to be moving over the heart on frames 5–11 (*arrows*).

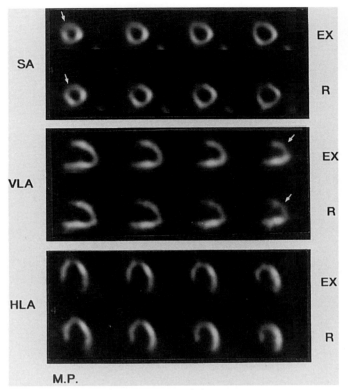

FIGURE 15.9. ²⁰¹Tl SPECT images with breast artifacts. On exercise (*EX*), short axis slices show that an anterior apical myocardial perfusion defect (arrows) is present. On the delayed redistribution (*R*) images, the anterior wall defect appears to be larger. The inconsistency of location of the defects is caused by change in position of the breast during repeat imaging. On the horizontal or vertical long axis slices anterior defects can be appreciated as well. (Reproduced by permission from Wackers FJTh. Artifacts in planar and SPECT myocardial perfusion imaging. *Am J Cardiac Imaging* 1992;6:42–58.)

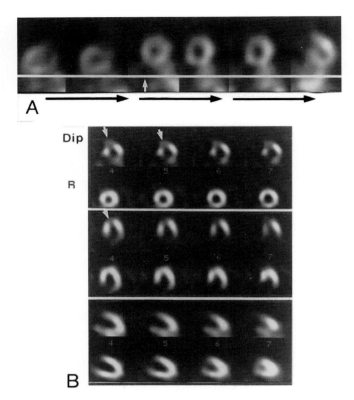

FIGURE 15.10. A. Selected planar projection images from LPO (*left*) to RAO position, before SPECT reconstruction. During acquisition of the LAO planar projection image position the patient moved upwards on the table (*arrow*) The *white bar* is a reference for initial position of the inferior wall. **B.** ²⁰¹Tl SPECT myocardial perfusion images of the same patient as **A**. The initial images after infusion of dipyridamole (*Dip*) demonstrate apparent antero-apical defects (*arrows*). The redistribution (*R*) images are entirely normal. This is an example of marked distortion of image due to patient motion. Inspection of the planar projection images is essential for quality assurance and recognition of motion. (Reproduced by permission from Wackers FJTh. Artifacts in planar and SPECT myocardial perfusion imaging. *Am J Cardiac Imaging* 1992;6: 42–58.)

exercise but should be delayed for approximately 10 minutes to allow the patient to recover from the exercise effort. This delay may be advantageous, because this time allows for acquisition of a planar anterior image for assessment of exercise-induced increased lung uptake before starting SPECT imaging. Upward creep is not a problem using ⁹⁹ᵐTc-labeled agents, because it is standard to start imaging no sooner than 15 minutes after termination of exercise.

Patient Motion

Many patients find it difficult to lie still for 20 to 30 minutes on the imaging table with the arms extended over the head. Motion artifacts may seriously degrade the quality of SPECT images and may cause artifacts on reconstructed slices. This is dependent on the type of motion, the degree of motion, and the number of camera heads. Typical motion artifacts show the heart as if it is "broken up" but also may mimic myocardial perfusion defects (Figs. 15.10 **A** and **B**). Improved table design and different imaging positions could minimize this problem. Several investigators have noted that patients generally tolerate the prone or upright position better than the supine position, and less motion was observed using those unconventional posi-

tions. Patient motion is best detected on the rotating projection images, i.e., cine display of all planar projection images. This is an essential part of quality assurance before interpretation of the reconstructed slices. Presently, most vendors have motion correction software included in the standard software package. However, this software cannot correct for all types of patient motion. Thus, it is better to prevent patient motion than to rely on motion correction software. For some patients it may be impossible to remain motionless on the imaging table. Repeat imaging is often equally unsuccessful. In these patients it is best to repeat imaging by planar technique.

Center of Rotation and Field Uniformity

Other artifacts typical for SPECT imaging, but usually less of a problem with improved technology and strict adherence to periodic equipment quality assurance, are those of the center-of-rotation offset and flood field nonuniformity. Offset of the center-of-rotation can produce typical artifacts. These artifacts are best observed on the horizontal long-axis slices as defects and "smearing" or "hurricane sign" near the apex (Fig. 15.11). Furthermore, center-of-rotation offset can cause a severe degradation of image resolution. Field nonuniformity causes typical ring artifacts. The latter artifacts are related to the mechanics of the SPECT gamma-camera and can be avoided by routine gamma-camera quality control. Center-of-rotation and uniformity are usually not a major source of problems in a well-run nuclear cardiology laboratory in which quality assurance tests are performed on a regularly scheduled basis.

Orbit-Related Artifacts

Another potential artifact is related to the orbit of the SPECT camera. Because the heart is eccentric in the chest, a circular orbit, and in particular a "body contour" orbit, brings the camera head(s) at varying distances from the target organ. With varying distance the resolution of the gamma-camera varies at each stop. Varying resolution may create typical artifacts—180 degrees diametrically opposed defects on the short-axis slices (9) (Fig. 15.12). These artifacts can be avoided by using a 360-degree acquisition orbit or by moving the patient laterally over the imaging table and thus bringing the heart in the center of the orbit. Unfortunately most vendors (and even the ASNC Imaging Guidelines for Nuclear Cardiology Procedures) recommend a 180-degree orbit for routine imaging (6). Depending

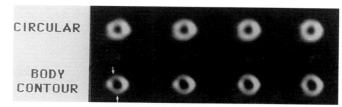

FIGURE 15.12. Effect of gamma-camera orbit. Short axis SPECT slices using a circular orbit (i.e., the heart is in the center of rotation of the camera head) are shown (*top*). The images are normal. Short axis SPECT slices using a body contour orbit are shown in bottom panel. Varying spatial resolution causes a typical artifact of 180° diametrical defects (*arrow*). (Reproduced by permission from Wackers FJTh. Artifacts in planar and SPECT myocardial perfusion imaging. *Am J Cardiac Imaging* 1992;6:42–58.

on the degree of eccentricity of the heart and the patient's body habitus, these artifacts may be disturbing in particular in the first apical short-axis slices. A normal variant, that often is referred to as the "insertion of the right ventricle," is due to image acquisition with a 180-degree circular orbit.

Artifacts Caused by Reconstruction and Display

During processing of a SPECT perfusion study, incorrect assignment of the left ventricular long axis on either the midtransaxial or midventricular long-axis slices, may result in reconstructed slices that are distorted and not comparable. Furthermore, the line-up of stress-rest slices depends on subjective selection of comparable slices by the computer operator. Pseudoreversibility can be created by incorrect alignment of slices (Fig. 15.13). Careful inspection of long-axis selection and the line-up of all reconstructed slices is an important aspect of quality control.

Artifactual Defects Resulting from Intense Hepatic Activity

Intense hepatic or bowel activity adjacent to the heart may occur with ^{99m}Tc-labeled imaging agents. This may create artifactual myocardial perfusion defects after filtered back projection (Fig. 15.14). Germano et al. (10) showed that adjustment of appropriate prereconstruction filters may minimize such artifacts (see also Chapter 12).

Artifacts on Polar Map

Although the concept of creating a polar map or bull's-eye plot is attractive from the point of view of data reduction, it should be realized that this display is not a true image of the heart. Artifacts are extremely difficult to recognize once a polar map image has been created. An excellent discussion of the appearance of artifacts on topographic bull's-eye plot can be found in the publication by DePuey et al. (11).

Artifacts on SPECT imaging may be treacherous. The ability to differentiate artifacts form true perfusion abnormalities distinguishes the expert from the novice interpreter.

Although SPECT imaging with ^{99m}Tc-labeled agents is consistently of better quality than SPECT imaging with ^{201}Tl (Fig.

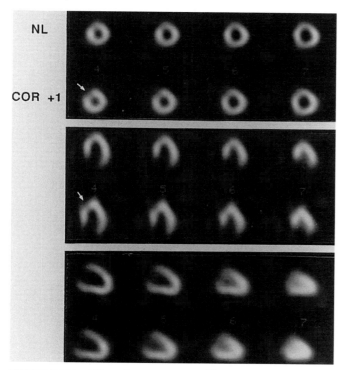

FIGURE 15.11. Offset of center rotation. ^{99m}Tc-sestamibi images of a normal subject. The original SPECT slices are shown on top (*NL*). One pixel center of rotation offset was introduced (*bottom*). Small artifactual defects are present on the short axis slices and long-axis slices (*arrow*). (Reproduced by permission from Wackers FJTh. Artifacts in planar and SPECT myocardial perfusion imaging. *Am J Cardiac Imaging* 1992;6:42–58.)

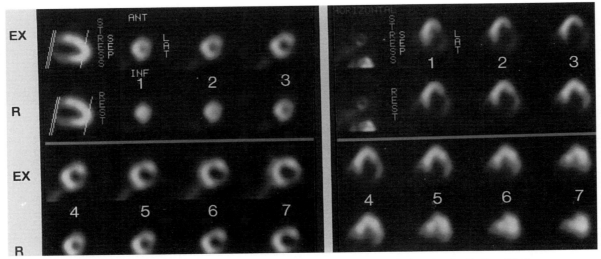

FIGURE 15.13. Pseudoreversibilty caused by misalignment of exercise (*EX*) and redistribution (*R*) slices in a patient with a fixed inferior wall defect. During processing the short-axis and horizontal long axis slices were not lined up correctly. Stress short axis slice no. 1 corresponds to rest slice no. 3. Without paying attention to the selection of slices, one could erroneously interpret these images as showing a reversible inferior wall defect. (Reproduced by permission from Wackers FJTh. Artifacts in planar and SPECT myocardial perfusion imaging. *Am J Cardiac Imaging* 1992:6:42–58.)

15.15), artifacts are a potential problem with all imaging agents. It is important that the interpreter always be alert to the possibility of artifacts.

RELATIVE ACCUMULATION OF RADIOPHARMACEUTICALS

Myocardial perfusion images are analyzed for *relative differences* in radiotracer accumulation. This represents an important limitation for image analysis. In patients suspected of ischemic heart disease, a myocardial segment with relatively less activity is considered to be the abnormal area, representing either exercise-induced myocardial ischemia or infarction, whereas normal-ap-

pearing segments presumably are supplied by arteries without significant disease. However, in patients with triple-vessel coronary artery disease, only the myocardial segment(s) supplied by the most severely stenosed artery(ies) may show myocardial perfusion defect(s), whereas the other segments also supplied by

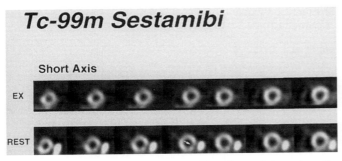

FIGURE 15.14. SPECT reconstruction artifact due to intense hepatic and intestinal activity. Exercise/rest short axis 99mTc-sestamibi SPECT images in patient with intense bowel activity at rest. The exercise (*EX*) image is normal. The septum on the EX image is relatively "hot" due to hypertrophy in this patient with hypertension. The resting images show intense uptake adjacent to the inferior lateral wall. Filtered backprojection using a standard Butterworth filter causes an artifactual defect in the inferior lateral wall (*arrow*). In patients with intense activity adjacent to the heart, the filter should be adjusted.

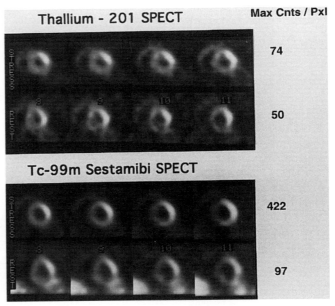

FIGURE 15.15. Comparison of 201Tl SPECT imaging with 99mTc-sestamibi SPECT imaging in the same patient. Interval between the two studies was 5 days. The difference in quality of SPECT imaging using different radiopharmaceutics can be appreciated. Count density per pixel in projection images is substantially higher with 99mTc-sestamibi than with 201Tl. 99mTc-sestamibi SPECT images are of better quality than the 201Tl images. Nevertheless, both images show the presence of a fixed septal defect.

stenosed arteries, but relatively less severe, may appear to be normal. Obviously this may result in an underestimation of the extent of disease. Usually in patients with multivessel coronary artery disease, one or more arteries will be most severely diseased and result in abnormal myocardial perfusion images. However, it is conceivable that in patients who have balanced disease of all major arteries no regional defect can be discerned.

Nevertheless, the overall sensitivity of SPECT myocardial perfusion imaging in patients with multivessel disease is high, greater than 90%. However, only 30% of these patients may have abnormalities in multiple territories suggesting multivessel disease. Recent data suggest that attenuation correction devices may be important for enhancing the accurate detection of multivessel disease (12).

In many patients with hypertension, the septum has been noted to be "hotter" than the lateral wall. This creates an apparent mild lateral wall myocardial perfusion defect. However, the amount of regional myocardial radiotracer uptake not only cor-relates with regional myocardial blood flow but also correlates with regional myocardial mass. In patients with hypertension, septal hypertrophy is a cause for relatively *increased* radiotracer uptake rather than *decreased* uptake in the lateral wall.

Unless accurate absolute quantification of radiotracer uptake is realized, the analysis of relative radiotracer uptake carries the potential for erroneous conclusions.

ECG-GATED MYOCARDIAL PERFUSION IMAGING

State-of-the-art SPECT myocardial perfusion imaging involves the acquisition of SPECT images in ECG-gated mode for simultaneous assessment of myocardial perfusion and function. Technical aspects of ECG-gated image acquisition and processing are discussed in Chapter 12. ECG-gated images should be interpreted from endless loop cine display on computer screen. Re-

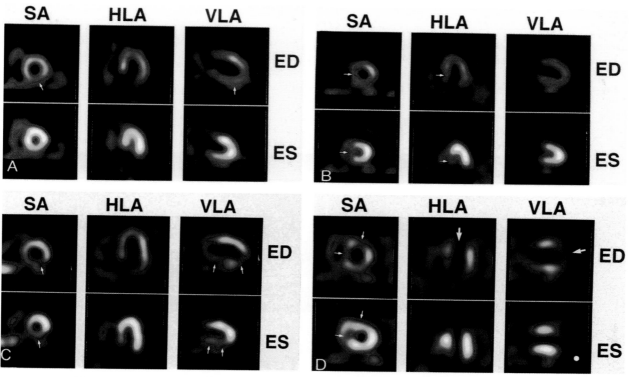

FIGURE 15.16. ECG-gated ^{99m}Tc-sestamibi SPECT images. The end-diastolic (*ED*) and end-systolic (*ES*) frames are shown in short axis (*SA*), horizontal long axis (*HLA*), and vertical long axis (*VLA*) slices. **A.** Normal image: During systole, homogenous thickening of the myocardium can be appreciated. The ED images show somewhat less uptake (*arrow*) in the inferior wall on the SA and VLA images. Because of the normal contraction shown in the ES images, this mild apparent defect is mostly likely caused by subdiaphragmatic attenuation. **B.** Patient with a septal infarct: The ED images show a septal perfusion defect on the SA and HLA slices (*arrows*). During systole, this area does not show contraction, and the presence of akinesis confirms scarred myocardium. **C.** Inferior wall ischemia: The ED images show an inferoseptal myocardial perfusion defect (*arrow*). During ES the intensity of color increases, indicating myocardial thickening. This patient had reversible ischemia of the inferior wall on SPECT slices. **D.** Patient with infarction and ischemia: The ED postexercise images show a large anteroapical and septal myocardial perfusion defect on the horizontal and vertical long axis slices. The anteroapical segment (*long arrow*) does not contract during systole. However, the anterior and septal wall (*small arrow*) show increased color intensity during systole, indicating myocardial viability (*arrows*). (Reproduced by permission from Wackers FJTh, Maniawski P, Sinusas AJ. Evaluation of left ventricular wall function by ECG-gated Tc-99m-sestamibi imaging. In: Beller GA, Zaret BL, eds. *Nuclear cardiology: state of the art and future direction.* St. Louis: Mosby, 1993:85–100.)

gional wall motion is best analyzed from linear gray scale display, whereas regional wall thickening is best analyzed by observing changes in color intensity. The latter phenomenon is caused by partial volume effect and enhanced recovery of counts during myocardial thickening (13).

Good correlation has been reported between visual analysis of regional wall motion on SPECT images and visual analysis of regional wall motion on echocardiography (14). Visual analysis of regional wall motion and wall thickening on gated SPECT images may be helpful for the recognition of artifactual attenuation defects resulting from breast or diaphragm. For instance, if one suspects that an apparent fixed myocardial perfusion defect is actually caused by attenuation, normal regional wall thickening in the same area on gated SPECT substantially increases the likelihood of attenuation (Fig. 15.16**A, B, C,** and **D**). Analysis of *isolated* end-diastolic stress and end-diastolic rest SPECT images has been proposed as a means to enhance the sensitivity of detecting coronary artery disease (15). Assessment of regional wall motion on gated SPECT images is largely performed by visual analysis. Recently, some investigators have published software for quantifying regional wall thickening on gated SPECT images (16,17).

The most widely accepted clinical use of ECG-gated SPECT is for the determination of global left ventricular ejection fraction (LVEF) and volumes (18–20). A number of commercially available and well-validated software packages exist (Fig 15.17). The technical aspects for computing LVEF from gated SPECT are discussed in Chapter 12. Numerous studies have demonstrated excellent to good correlation between LVEFs derived from gated SPECT by various gated SPECT software packages and those derived by other independent methods (i.e., equilibrium or first-pass radionuclide angiography). Gated SPECT provides a simple and relatively accurate means to evaluate global left ventricular function. However, one should be aware of certain limitations. The reliability and accuracy of LVEF depends on the count density of the study, the amount of extracardiac gastrointestinal activity, the size of the left ventricle, and the stability of heart rate during acquisition. The best results for LVEF are obtained from a high-dose SPECT study after exercise (minimal gastrointestinal activity), in an average-sized person who is in regular sinus rhythm (21,22). Gated SPECT LVEF always is a *resting* LVEF, even when calculated from stress images. After an injection of radiotracer during stress, the actual acquisition of SPECT images occurs with the patient resting on the imaging table.

Some investigators have reported that LVEF on poststress images may be significantly lower than that derived from the companion rest image (23). This has been explained as "poststress stunning." In our experience such decreased poststress LVEF (for more detail see Fig. 15.23 and Fig. 15.42) occurs only in a minority (approximately 10 to 15%) of patients and usually in patients with severe multivessel coronary artery disease. As can be anticipated, the prevalence of poststress stun-

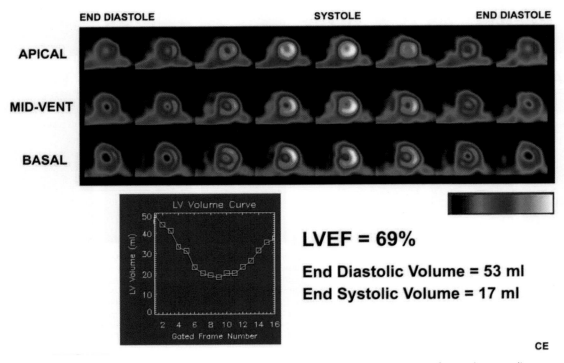

FIGURE 15.17. Computation of left ventricular ejection fraction (LVEF) from a 16-frame electrocardiogram (ECG)-gated single photon emission computed tomography study. *Top:* Display of 16 images (from end diastole through systole to end diastole) of representative apical, midventricular, and basal stress slices. The change in color throughout the cardiac cycle is due to myocardial wall thickening and relatively less partial volume effect (i.e., improved recovery of counts). The color scale ranges from white (maximum) to black (minimum). *Bottom:* Left ventricular volume curve generated from the same ECG-gated slices. Global LVEF, end-diastolic volume, and end-systolic volume are shown.

ning appears to be affected by the time interval after termination of exercise. The shorter the time interval, the higher the likelihood of depressed poststress LVEF.

OPTIMAL SPECT IMAGING

Careful attention to technical details is important for optimal SPECT imaging. Because of the potential of motion during image acquisition, the patient should be immobilized using straps or devices that make it more comfortable for the patient to remain still. The technologist should be attentive to potential patient motion. Motion may involve movement of the patient's body and may also involve a change in position of the heart within the chest (upward creep).

The standard patient position is supine with the arms up over the head. This makes it feasible to bring the camera head(s) as close as possible to the patient's chest. However, it is feasible to acquire adequate SPECT images without artifacts with the patient's arms along the sides of the body. Thus, this is an acceptable alternative position in patients who have problems in folding the arms over the head.

Quality Assurance of SPECT Image Interpretation

The clinical interpretation of SPECT images should follow a systematic approach (7). We propose the following routine:

1. Inspection of cine display of rotating planar projection images (Fig. 15.18). This should always be the first step before interpretation of SPECT images. The rotating images allow assessment of overall study quality: (a) Is the left ventricle well visualized? (b) Is there excessive extracardiac activity? Is there extracardiac activity immediately adjacent to the heart? (c) Is there patient motion or upward creep of the heart? (d) Is there a breast shadow obscuring the heart in certain

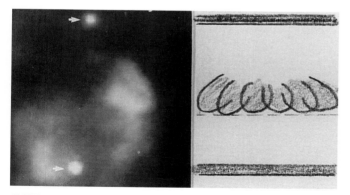

FIGURE 15.18. Cine display of projection images. Inspection of cine display of all 32 images acquired for SPECT reconstruction is an important step in quality control prior to image interpretation. Upward creep and/or body motion can be readily recognized in this display. Two point sources on the patient's chest in the field of view (*arrows*) can also be used as fixed reference marks. They should move on the cine display in a straight line. Presently, we use a white reference bar that can be positioned at the inferior wall (*LV*) (see Figs. 15.8 and 15.10).

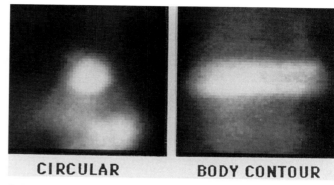

FIGURE 15.19. Inspection of cine display of 32 planar projection images for quality control of SPECT imaging. When the heart is excentric in the camera orbit, as for example, when the gamma-camera follows the *body contour*, the heart will move from the left of the screen to the right of the screen. When the heart is in the center of the orbit, as with a *circular* orbit with the imaging table moved laterally to position the heart in the center, the heart pivots in the center on the rotating image. The more the heart is off-center, the more likely artifacts occur (see Fig. 15.12).

projections? (e) Is the orbit of the detector head around the heart circular (the heart "pivots" in the center of the screen) or elliptical (the heart "runs" across the screen from one side to the other) (Fig. 15.19).
2. Did the patient continue to exercise after injection of the radiotracer for 1 to 2 minutes?
3. Was timing of imaging appropriate after injection of radiotracer?
4. Was an appropriate dose of the radiopharmaceutical administered? What is the count density in the left ventricle? Software used in our laboratory displays automatically the maximal number of counts in the "hottest" pixel in the heart in one of the anterior projection images.
5. Are displayed reconstructed tomographic slices appropriately chosen? Are stress and rest slices paired and aligned correctly (Fig. 15.13)?
6. Are there artifacts that are potentially due to motion (Fig. 15.10**A** and **B**), breast (Figs. 15.8 and 15.9), or diaphragmatic attenuation (Fig. 15.7)? If needed, one should inspect the cine of the rotating planar images again. Inspection of cine display of ECG-gated slices may be helpful.
7. Quantification (polar map or circumferential profiles) is compared with visual analysis.
8. Was ECG-gating optimal? "Blinking" on cine display of the left ventricle indicates that there was a problem resulting from arrhythmia. Is the LVEF volume curve appropriate?

IMAGE INTERPRETATION

SPECT images are interpreted by visual analysis, often aided by computer quantification (Figs. 15.20–15.23). Interpretive reproducibility has been shown to be moderate to excellent and can be significantly improved by quantitative analysis (23a). It is helpful to divide the numerous reconstructed short-axis slices in three groups: apical slices, midventricular slices, and basal slices. After interpretation of all short-axis slices, the apex and base should be reviewed on the long-axis slices. The following defines the various image patterns:

Normal. Homogeneous uptake of the radiopharmaceutical throughout the myocardium. Regional variation of not more than 20% of maximal counts is within normal range. Quantitative analysis allows for comparison of regional myocardial uptake to that of normal image files (Fig. 15.20).

Defect. A localized myocardial area with decreased radiotracer uptake. Defects may vary in intensity, from slightly reduced activity to almost total absence of activity. A visual approach for assessing the presence and severity of myocardial perfusion defects involves segmentation of the heart and subjective scoring. The following is a widely used scoring system: 0, normal; 1, mildly reduced; 2, moderately reduced; 3, severely reduced; and 4, absent uptake. This scoring is applied to either a 17- or 20-segment model (2). From this subjective scoring, summed scores can be derived for stress and rest images. Quantitative computer analysis allows for objective comparison of inhomogeneous uptake to that of normal image files (Fig. 15.21). The severity of myocardial perfusion defects is usually expressed as percent of normal activity (19).

Reversible Defect. A defect that is present on the initial stress images and is no longer present or present to a lesser degree on the resting or delayed images. This pattern usually indicates myocardial ischemia. Visually discernible reversibility corresponds quantitatively to at least 25% improvement of defect. Quantitative analysis allows for objective comparison of relative radiotracer uptake on stress and rest images relative to normal

data files (Fig. 15.21). Defect reversibility may be enhanced by sublingual administration of nitroglycerine immediately before rest injection of radiotracer.

Fixed Defect. A defect that is unchanged and present on both exercise and rest (delayed) images. This pattern generally indicates infarction and scar tissue. However, in some patients with fixed ^{201}Tl defects on 2- to 4-hour delayed imaging, improved uptake can be noted after a new resting injection or on 24-hour redistribution imaging. Quantitative analysis allows for objective comparison of relative radiotracer uptake on stress and rest images relative to normal data files (Fig. 15.22).

Reverse Defect. The initial images are either normal or show a defect, whereas the delayed or rest images show a more severe defect. This pattern is frequently observed in patients who have undergone thrombolytic therapy or percutaneous coronary angioplasty. This phenomenon is thought to be caused by initial excess of tracer uptake in a reperfused area with a mixture of scar tissue and viable myocytes. Initial accumulation is followed by rapid clearance from scar tissue. Although the significance of this finding is controversial, it does not represent evidence of exercise-induced ischemia.

Lung Uptake. Normally no, or very little, radiotracer is noted in the lung fields on postexercise images (Fig. 15.23). Increased lung uptake can be quantified as lung-to-heart ratio (normal <0.5 for ^{201}Tl and <0.4 for ^{99m}Tc-labeled agents). This important abnormal finding indicates exercise-induced ischemic left ventricular dysfunction (24).

Transient Left Ventricular Dilation. Occasionally, the left ventricle appears to be larger following exercise than on the

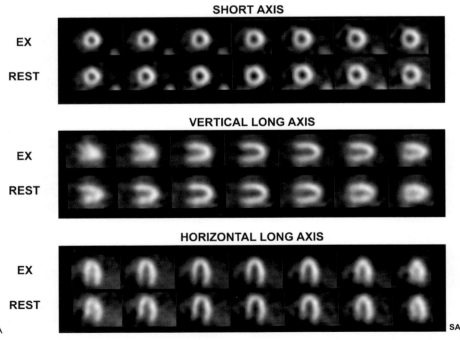

FIGURE 15.20. A: Normal exercise (EX)-rest single photon emission computed tomography (SPECT) ^{99m}Tc-sestamibi myocardial perfusion images. Reconstructed slices are displayed in standard format as shown in Fig. 15.1. Visually the images show homogeneous radiotracer uptake in all displayed slices. *(Figure continues.)*

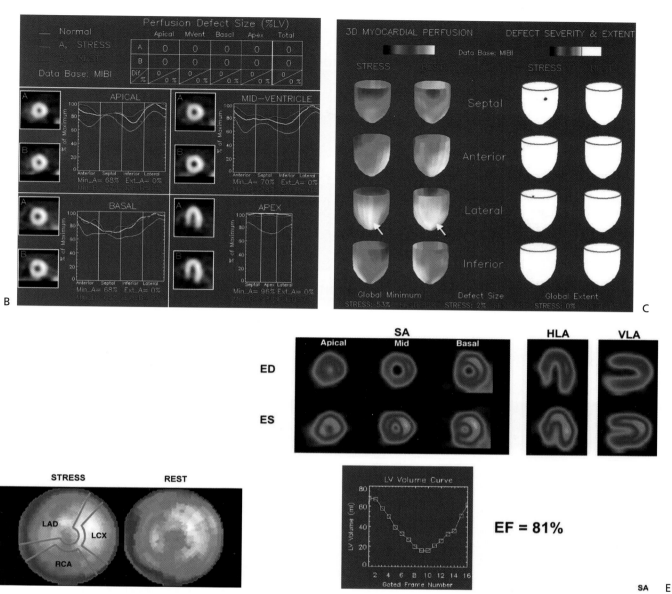

FIGURE 15.20. *Continued.* **B:** Quantification of images in **A** using circumferential profile analysis. Circumferential count distribution profiles of three representative apical, midventricular, and basal slices and of one horizontal long-axis slice are shown. The exercise profiles are shown in *yellow* and the rest profiles in *red*. All profiles are normalized to maximal activity within each individual slice (*local maximum*) and are compared with a normal data file (*white curve*). The profiles are plotted starting in the anterior wall and then counterclockwise towards the septum and inferior and lateral wall. For quantitative analysis 36 interpolated count distribution profiles are generated from apex to base (not shown). Total myocardial perfusion defect size is calculated from these 36 interpolated circumferential profiles in comparison to normal data files. Defect size is expressed as percent of left ventricle and shown in the table (*top*). In this example of a normal subject, all points of the profiles are above the lower limit of normal curve. There is no quantifiable perfusion defect. **C:** *Left:* Three-dimensional display of stress and rest relative radiotracer uptake in the entire left ventricle on the basis of 36 interpolated circumferential count distribution profiles from apex to base. The shape of the left ventricle is normalized to a bullet shape and displayed with the septal, anterior, lateral, and inferior walls facing the observer. Relative radiotracer uptake is normalized to the ventricular area with maximal count density (*global maximum*). On both the stress and rest images, maximal uptake is in the midventricular lateral wall (*arrows*). *Right:* Display of defect extent and severity relative to a normal data file. Because the images are normal, no area is displayed. The color scale is depicted on top; white is maximum and black is minimum. **D:** Polar map or bull's eye display of the same normal SPECT images. Similar to **C**, relative radiotracer uptake is displayed normalized to the global maximum. Relative radiotracer distribution is displayed as concentric rings, with the apex in the center and the base of the left ventricle at the periphery of the map. The color scale is similar to the one in **C**. The coronary artery territories of the left anterior descending coronary artery (LAD), the left circumflex coronary artery (LCX), and the right coronary artery (RCA) are indicated. **E:** 16-frame ECG-gated SPECT images. The end-diastolic (ED) and end-systolic (ES) images are shown for three short-axis slices (SA), one horizontal long-axis slice (HLA), and one vertical long-axis slice (VLA). The change in color from ED to ES is due to normal wall thickening. Global left ventricular ejection fraction (LVEF) is normal at 81%. Regional wall thickening and motion are normal. The color scale is the same as in **C**.

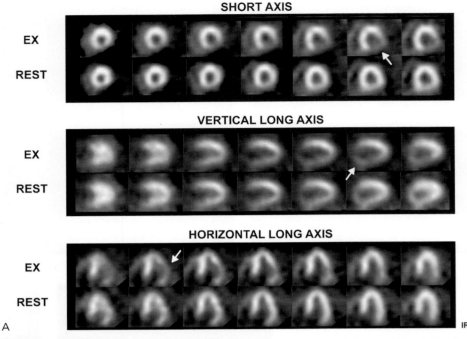

A

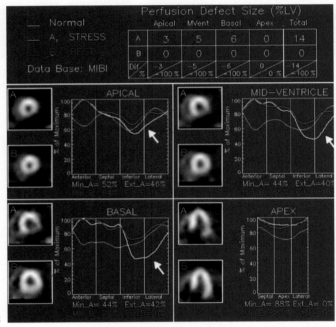

B

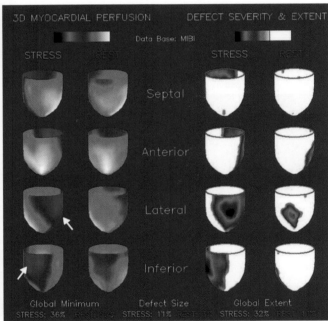

C

FIGURE 15.21. **A:** Abnormal single photon emission computed tomography (SPECT) myocardial perfusion imaging of a patient with extensive stress-induced inferolateral ischemia. The images show an extensive inferolateral myocardial perfusion defect (*arrows*), extending from apex to base. The resting images are normal: a completely reversible myocardial perfusion defect. **B:** Quantification of the images in **A** using circumferential profile analysis. The display is the same as in Fig. 15.20. In the apical, midventricular, and basal slices, the yellow stress profiles are well below the lower limit of normal (*white curve*) in the inferolateral wall (*arrows*). The apex is not involved. The rest (*red*) profiles are almost completely within normal range. Total defect size is calculated from 36 interpolated circumferential profiles (not shown) involving the entire left ventricle from apex to base. As shown in the table, the stress defect is computed to involve 14% of the left ventricle; the rest defect is 0%. This is quantitatively a large reversible defect. **C:** *Left:* Three-dimensional display of stress and rest relative radiotracer uptake. There is a large inferolateral myocardial perfusion defect on the stress images (*arrows*) that has almost completely normalized at rest. *Right:* The extent and severity relative to the lower limit of normal distribution are displayed. The considerable improvement at rest can be appreciated. *(Figure continues.)*

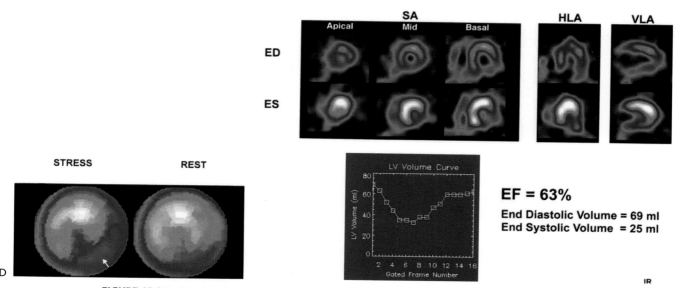

FIGURE 15.21. *Continued.* **D:** The polar map display shows a large inferolateral defect at stress (*arrow*) and almost complete normalization at rest. **E:** 16-frame electrocardiogram-gated SPECT images. The display is the same as in Fig. 15.20. Visual analysis of regional wall motion and thickening on cine display showed mild hypokinesis of the inferolateral wall on the poststress images. Nevertheless, global left ventricular ejection fraction is preserved at 63% because of normal contraction in the remaining walls.

rest or delayed image (Fig. 15.24). This pattern also has been associated with exercise-induced left ventricular dysfunction and greater amount of myocardium at risk (25). Closer observation of this pattern suggests that there is cavity dilation (with thinning of the wall) rather than global left ventricular dilation. Thus, this pattern may well be due to subendocardial ischemia.

Transient Right Ventricular Visualization. The right ventricle is more clearly visualized on the poststress images than on the rest images (Fig. 15.24). This pattern again indicates transient left ventricular dysfunction during stress. (26)

Quantitative Analysis

A number of validated software packages are commercially available for quantification of SPECT myocardial perfusion and function (CPS-QGS, Emory Toolbox, 4D-MSPECT, and Wackers-Liu CQ). The basic principles of SPECT quantification are similar for each of these software packages. Normalized relative radiotracer uptake in reconstructed slices is compared and quantified against normal data files. The relative radiotracer uptake on SPECT images is displayed either as polar plots (bull's eye plots) (27) or as circumferential count distribution profiles (19). In our laboratory, we prefer the circumferential count profile display (see disclosure at the end of chapter). Circumferential count profiles with display of the lower of the normal curve are generated for each of the short-axis slices and displayed with a curve representing the lower limit of normal myocardial count distribution. This provides a readily understandable graphic and quantitative measure of how abnormal the patient's image is compared with a normal database. Figures 15.20, 15.21, 15.22, and 15.24 show representative clinical examples of quantitative SPECT imaging.

Importance of Quantitative Image Analysis

We believe that reliable quantification of myocardial perfusion images (by any method) is extremely important and should be used routinely for the following reasons:

1. Quantification provides *greater confidence* in interpretation. Graphic display of relative count distribution serves as an objective and consistent second observer. The normal database serves as a fixed benchmark against which images are compared.
2. Quantification provides *enhanced intraobserver* and *interobserver interpretive reproducibility* (28).
3. Quantification provides a reproducible means of measuring the *degree of abnormality*. It is well established that the more abnormal a myocardial perfusion image is, the poorer is the patient's outcome.

Quantification of rest LVEF from myocardial perfusion images provides additional important prognostic information.

In our view, quantitative analysis is *complementary* to visual analysis. Interpretation should start with visual inspection of images. First, visual inspection of the unprocessed rotating planar images. Second, visual analysis of reconstructed SPECT slices in three orthogonal cuts. Images should be inspected for overall quality and the presence of possible artifacts. Third, quantitative display then serves to *confirm* the visual impression. Quantitative analysis should not, and cannot, be expected to provide entirely new information. We refer to this process as "quantitative analysis with visual overread."

Table 15.2 provides a comparative categorization of myocardial perfusion abnormalities by commonly used subjective scoring and computer quantification.

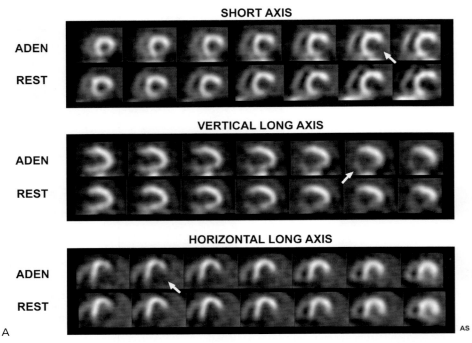

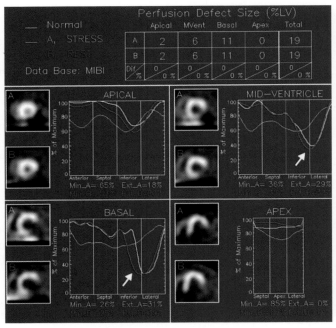

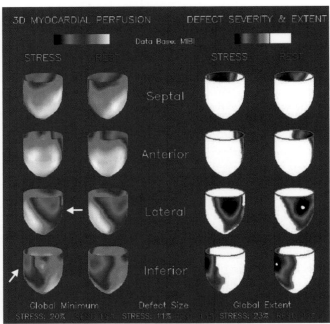

FIGURE 15.22. A: Abnormal single photon emission computed tomography (SPECT) myocardial perfusion imaging of a patient with a large inferolateral infarction without ischemia. The images show an extensive inferolateral myocardial perfusion defect (*arrows*), extending from apex to base. The defect is unchanged at rest. **B:** Quantification of images in **A** using circumferential profile analysis. The display is the same as in Fig. 15.20. In the midventricular and basal slices, the *yellow* stress profiles are well below the lower limit of normal (*white curve*) in the inferolateral wall (*arrows*). In the apical slice, the yellow profile is just below the normal limit. The apex itself is not involved. The rest (*red*) profiles are almost superimposed on the stress profiles. There is no appreciable improvement. The table shows that stress defect is computed to involve 19% of the left ventricle; the rest defect is also 19%. This is quantitatively a large fixed inferolateral defect. **C:** *Left:* Three-dimensional display of stress and rest relative radiotracer uptake. There is a large inferolateral myocardial perfusion defect on the stress images (*arrows*) that is almost identical at rest. *Right:* The extent and severity relative to the lower limit of normal distribution are displayed . No improvement in defect size can be appreciated. (*Figure continues.*)

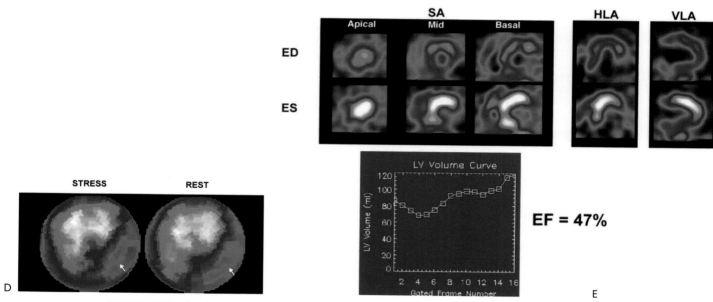

FIGURE 15.22. *Continued.* **D:** The polar map display shows a large fixed inferolateral defect both at stress and at rest (*arrows*). **E:** 16-frame electrocardiogram-gated poststress SPECT images. The display is the same as in Fig. 15.20. Visual analysis of regional wall motion and thickening on cine display showed akinesis of the inferolateral wall. The regional wall motion in the remote anteroseptal walls is normal. The anterolateral wall is severely hypokinetic resulting from tethering of the infarcted area. Global left ventricular ejection fraction is depressed at 47%.

CLINICAL VALUE OF MYOCARDIAL PERFUSION IMAGING

Acute Myocardial Infarction

Acute myocardial infarction is a pathologic condition of severely reduced resting regional myocardial blood flow and regional myocardial cell death. Resting radionuclide myocardial perfusion imaging is a reliable noninvasive means to detect acutely decreased regional myocardial blood flow.

Characteristic Images of Myocardial Infarction

On radionuclide myocardial perfusion images, myocardial infarction is visualized as an area with decreased tracer accumulation. Because the remaining normally perfused myocardium is visualized, the anatomic location and relative extent of myocardial infarction can be determined. Myocardial infarctions at various anatomic locations display characteristic myocardial perfusion images. Examples of SPECT images in patients with acute myocardial infarction are shown in Figs. 15.25 and 15.26.

Location of Myocardial Infarction

Accurate localization and sizing of acute myocardial infarction by noninvasive methods has clinical relevance. The location and size of infarction is of prognostic importance. For instance, patients with anterior wall infarction have a poorer prognosis than patients with inferior wall infarction. Moreover, involvement of the septum in anterior wall infarction indicates a large infarction and is associated with a mortality rate three times higher than in infarction at other locations. Excellent correlation between postmortem location and size of myocardial infarction and location and size on myocardial perfusion imaging has been documented (29).

Importance of Myocardial Infarction Size

The outcome of a patient with acute myocardial infarction is directly related to the total amount of infarcted and necrotic myocardium (30). Because of the early application of radionuclide imaging in patients with acute myocardial infarction, the potential value of myocardial perfusion imaging to assess the extent of myocardial damage (noninvasively and quantitatively) has been recognized.

Because the normal and/or viable myocardium is visualized with a myocardial perfusion imaging agent, a perfusion defect can be expressed as a percentage of the total visualized left ventricle. Moreover, because myocardial perfusion images demonstrate both acute and old infarction, the *total* amount of irreversibly damaged myocardium can be quantified. Early after acute myocardial infarction, LVEF or the extent of abnormal regional wall motion may not be an accurate measurement of the total amount of irreversible damage, because stunned (but viable) dysfunctional myocardium may be present. Thus, myocardial perfusion imaging appears particularly suited for early quantitative assessment of infarct size. Indeed, in patients who had conventional (i.e., noninterventional) treatment of myocardial infarction, the size of myocardial perfusion defects correlated well with postmortem size of infarction (29). In experimental canine models the area at risk for infarction correlated well with the SPECT defect size. Also, in clinical studies in patients with acute infarction, it was feasible to visualize the area at risk, the salvaged

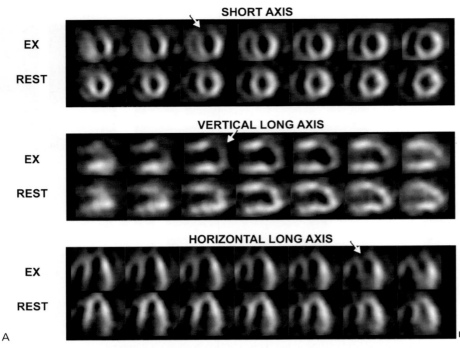

SHORT AXIS

EX

REST

VERTICAL LONG AXIS

EX

REST

HORIZONTAL LONG AXIS

EX

REST

A

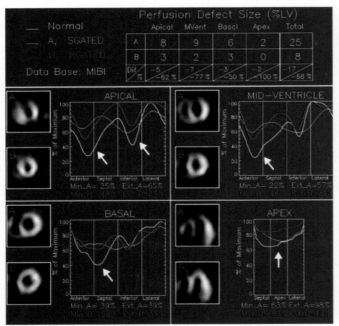

B

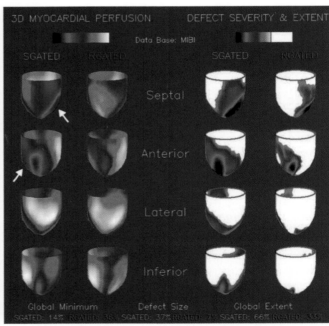

C

FIGURE 15.23. **A:** High-risk stress-rest single photon emission computed tomography (SPECT) myocardial perfusion images. The reconstructed slices show a large anteroapical and septal myocardial perfusion defect (*arrows*) that is almost completely reversible at rest. In addition, there is transient left ventricular cavity dilation (best appreciated in the two last short-axis slices at the right. **B:** Quantification of the images in **A.** The exercise circumferential profile (*yellow*) is below the lower limit of normal in the anteroseptal and inferior walls in the apical slices (*arrows*). The rest circumferential profile (*red*) shows partial improvement in the anterior wall and is completely reversible in the inferior wall. In midventricle and base of the left ventricle, the stress defect in the anteroseptal area is almost completely reversible. The defect in the apex is also reversible. Quantitatively the exercise defect size is large: 25% of left ventricle. The rest defect is moderate (8% of left ventricle) resulting from incomplete reversibility in the anterior wall. The ischemic burden is large: 20% of left ventricle. The size and extent of the defect, and in addition the visual suggestion of transient dilation of the left ventricle, implies that this is a high-risk study. **C:** *Left:* Three-dimensional display of the myocardial perfusion defect shown in **A.** The extensive involvement of the left ventricle is well visualized. *Right:* The partial reversibility of the defect in the anterior wall can be appreciated. *(Figure continues.)*

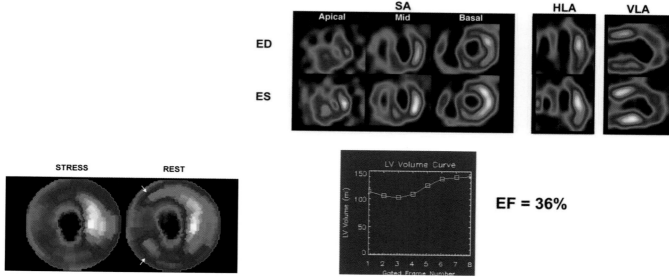

FIGURE 15.23. *Continued.* **D:** The polar map display shows a large anteroseptal and inferoseptal and apical defect at stress (*arrows*). The partial reversibility in anterior and inferior wall can be appreciated at rest (*arrows*). **E:** 16-frame electrocardiogram-gated SPECT images. The display is the same as in Fig. 15.20. Visual analysis of regional wall motion indicates severe akinesis and hypokinesis of a large portion of the anteroapical and anteroseptal wall. Left ventricular ejection fraction is severely depressed at 36%. In view of the substantial reversibility of the defect in areas with left ventricular dysfunction, these gated SPECT images suggest severe postexercise ischemic stunning.

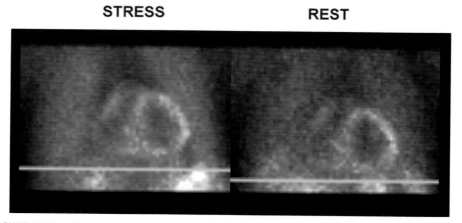

FIGURE 15.24. Abnormal anterior planar projection images. There is increased ^{99m}Tc-tetrofosmin uptake in both lungs after exercise. The patient had severe multivessel coronary artery disease. At rest lung uptake is normal. The heart is enlarged. Left ventricular ejection fraction by gated single photon emission computed tomography was depressed at 43%.

Table 15.2. *Comparative Characterization of Abnormal SPECT results*

Defect size	Small	Medium	Large
Vascular territories	<1/2	1	2 or 3
SSS[a]	4–8	9–13	>13
Polar maps (% of LV)[b]	<10%	10%–20%	>20%
Circumf. profile (%of LV)[c]	<5%	5%–10%	>10%

[a]Summed Stress Score.
[b]Compared with gender-matched normal file and reflects extent only.
[c]Circumferential profiles: based on Wackers-Liu-CQ: Sum of defects in 36 interpolated slices. Compared to normal data files and incorporates both extent and severity.

area, and the ultimate infarction (31,32). In patients with old infarction, an inverse relationship exists between the size of planar or SPECT myocardial perfusion defects and the LVEF (33).

Detection of Acute Myocardial Infarction

Resting myocardial perfusion imaging with either ^{201}Tl or ^{99m}Tc-labeled agents is a very sensitive and reliable means for detecting acute myocardial infarction in the very early hours after onset of acute chest pain. This was first demonstrated with [201]Tl (34) and subsequently confirmed using ^{99m}Tc-labeled agents (31).

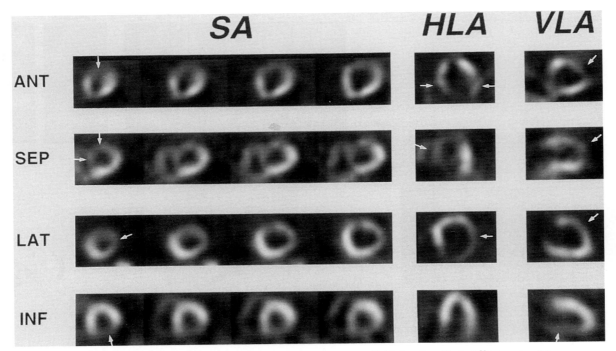

FIGURE 15.25. SPECT ^{99m}Tc-sestamibi images of acute myocardial infarction. Typical ^{99m}Tc-sestamibi SPECT images of acute myocardial infarction, in short axis (*SA*) horizontal long axis (*HLA*), and vertical long axis (*VLA*) slices. From top to bottom: anterior (*ANT*), anteroseptal (*SEP*), lateral (*LAT*), and inferior (*INF*) infarctions. Defects are indicated by *arrows*.

Time of Imaging

A clear relationship exists between diagnostic yield of myocardial perfusion imaging in acute myocardial infarction and the timing of imaging after onset of acute chest pain (Fig. 15.27). Wackers et al. (34) showed that all patients studied within 6 hours of onset of chest pain had abnormal ^{201}Tl images. Of patients studied between 6 and 24 hours after chest pain, 88% had perfusion defects, whereas only 72% of patients studied later than 24 hours after onset of symptoms had myocardial perfusion defects. The overall sensitivity of planar ^{201}Tl myocardial imaging for detection of acute infarction was 82%. Numerous subsequent studies have confirmed the excellent sensitivity (94%) and specificity (92%) for overall detection of myocardial infarction using either planar or SPECT resting myocardial perfusion imaging. For clinical imaging in patients with acute chest pain it is important to realize that images can be abnormal when serum biomarkers for cardiac injury are still within normal range.

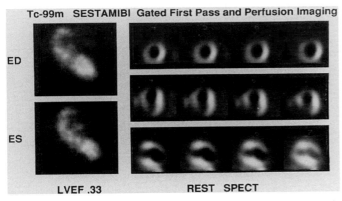

FIGURE 15.26. Simultaneous assessment of myocardial perfusion and function. ^{99m}Tc-sestamibi imaging in acute myocardial infarction allows assessment of both function and perfusion. In this patient with large anteroseptal infarction, the injection of sestamibi was utilized for first-pass radionuclide angiography *(left)*. The end-diastolic and systolic frames are shown. Global left ventricular ejection fraction was severely depressed at 0.33. On the right are resting SPECT images in short axis, and vertical and horizontal long axis slices. A large anteroseptal myocardial perfusion defect is present.

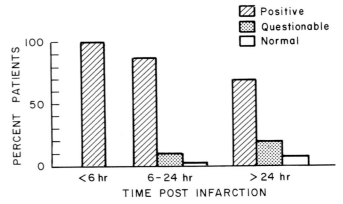

FIGURE 15.27. ^{201}Tl imaging results and time after infarction. Results of ^{201}Tl myocardial imaging in 200 patients with acute myocardial infarction in relation to time interval after onset of chest pain. (Reproduced by permission from Wackers FJTh. Thallium-201 myocardial imaging. In: Wackers FJTh, ed. *Thallium-201 and technetium-99m pyrophosphate myocardial imaging in the coronary care unit.* The Hague: Martinus Nijhoff Publishers, 1980:70–104.)

Myocardial Perfusion Imaging and Reperfusion Therapy for Acute Myocardial Infarction

Early interventions in patients with acute myocardial infarction by percutaneous coronary revascularization or thrombolysis can potentially salvage jeopardized myocardium. Myocardial perfusion imaging has been used as an objective means to document restoration of blood flow to the infarct region, as well as to visualize the extent of salvaged viable myocardium (31,32). The ^{99m}Tc-labeled agents, sestamibi and tetrofosmin, have characteristics that are well suited for application in patients who undergo interventions for acute myocardial infarction. Because of stable binding within myocardial cells and slow clearance, it is feasible to administer these agents immediately before or at the time of an intervention (thrombolysis or primary angioplasty). Imaging can then be performed later at a convenient time. Extensive clinical experience has been accumulated using ^{99m}Tc-sestamibi for this clinical application. When ^{99m}Tc-sestamibi is administered *before* thrombolytic therapy, the perfusion defect visualizes the *myocardium at risk*. When ^{99m}Tc-sestamibi is injected *after* thrombolytic therapy, the hypoperfused area reflects the *ultimate infarction* (Fig. 15.28). This basic concept has been validated in experimental animal models of coronary artery occlusion and reperfusion (35). Thus, if the perfusion defect on the second image is smaller than on the first image, myocardial salvage and patency of the infarct artery is most likely achieved by reperfusion therapy. Wackers et al. (31) and Gibbons et al. (32) published the first reports on the usefulness of ^{99m}Tc-sestamibi in the setting of thrombolytic therapy to assess the efficacy of therapy (Fig. 15.29). Their initial findings using planar and SPECT ^{99m}Tc-sestamibi imaging have been confirmed in numerous subsequent publications and in studies of hundreds of patients.

The experience with ^{99m}Tc-sestamibi in acute myocardial infarction can be summarized as follows. The myocardial area at risk varies greatly in individual patients with acute myocardial infarction. There is no good correlation between the risk area as demonstrated with ^{99m}Tc-sestamibi imaging and the anatomic site of the occlusion of the infarct artery, i.e., distal or proximal. The area at risk in an acute anterior infarction is larger than that in acute inferior infarction. A decrease in size of myocardial perfusion defect (i.e., defect size before thrombolytic therapy compared with that after thrombolytic therapy) is predictive of reperfusion of the infarct artery and subsequent improvement of left ventricular regional wall motion. Serial myocardial perfusion imaging showed that in many patients (approximately 40%) defect size *continues to decrease* days after thrombolytic therapy was administered. The size of a myocardial perfusion defect correlates well with LVEF at hospital discharge (33). Patients with collateral circulation to the infarct artery have smaller ultimate infarct size than patients without collateral circulation.

Serial ^{99m}Tc-sestamibi imaging has been shown to be a potentially useful tool to assess the clinical efficacy of various revascularization strategies in the acute phase of acute myocardial infarction (36). The patient serves as his or her own control and, consequently, smaller numbers of patients need to be recruited for clinical trials.

An interesting and incompletely understood observation is that the improvement of myocardial perfusion observed on serial imaging immediately after the acute intervention continues dur-

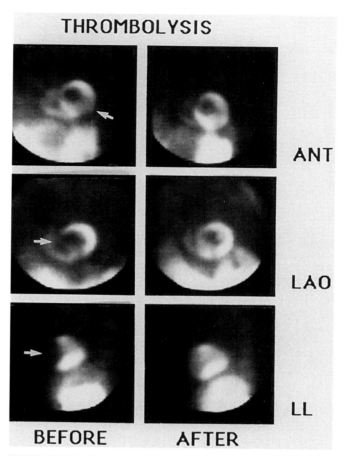

FIGURE 15.28. Planar myocardial perfusion imaging with ^{99m}Tc-sestamibi before and after thrombolytic therapy in a patient with an acute anteroseptal myocardial infarct. ^{99m}Tc-sestamibi was injected immediately before initiation of thrombolytic therapy and imaging was performed 2 hours later. Because of the lack of significant redistribution of ^{99m}Tc-sestamibi, the distribution of myocardial blood flow at the time of injection is "frozen" in time. The images before thrombolytic therapy show an anteroseptal myocardial perfusion defect *arrows* that was quantified as 53%. The patient was reinjected with ^{99m}Tc-sestamibi after thrombolytic therapy was completed. These images show improved perfusion of the anteroseptal segments, indicating successful reperfusion of the infarct artery. The perfusion defect size after thrombolytic therapy was 35%, consequently 18% of myocardium has been salvaged by thrombolytic therapy. (Reproduced by permission from Wackers FJTh, Gibbons RJ, Verani MS, et al. Serial quantitative planar technetium-99m-isonitrile imaging in acute myocardial infarction: efficacy for noninvasive assessment of thrombolytic therapy. *J Am Coll Cardiol* 1989;14:861–873.)

ing the subsequent months. This further improvement of myocardial perfusion is only in part explained by recovery of stunned regional myocardial dysfunction (37).

Myocardial Perfusion Imaging for the Assessment of Prognosis after Acute Myocardial Infarction

Myocardial perfusion imaging during the acute and subacute phase of infarction provides prognostic information in two ways: (a) assessment of the extent of myocardial damage and (b) the detection of residual jeopardized myocardium. Furthermore, using ECG-gated SPECT imaging also resting LVEF can be

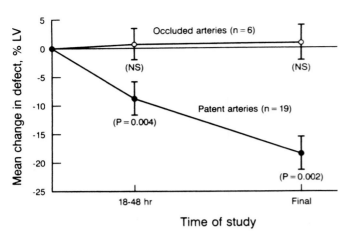

FIGURE 15.29. Serial SPECT myocardial perfusion imaging after thrombolysis for acute myocardial infarction. In patients with occluded coronary arteries and unsuccessful thrombolytic therapy, no change in myocardial defect size occurred. In contrast, patients who had successful thrombolytic therapy with reperfusion of the infarct artery (patent arteries) had a significant decrease in perfusion defect at 18–48 hours after onset of chest pain. Interestingly, there was a further decrease in defect size during subsequent days (Reproduced by permission from Pellikka. PA, Behrenbeck R, Verani MS, Mahmarian JJ, Wackers FJTh, Gibbons RJ. Serial changes in myocardial perfusion using tomographic technetium-99m-hexakis-2-methoxy-2-methyl-propyl-isonitrile imaging following reperfusion therapy of myocardial infarction. *J Nucl Med* 1990;31:1269–1275.)

determined. Cerquiera et al. (38) showed that in patients who had thrombolytic therapy for acute infarction, a relationship existed between SPECT myocardial perfusion defect size and long-term survival (Fig. 15.30).

Nestico et al. (39) noted that prominent visualization of the right ventricle at rest after acute myocardial infarction was a poor prognostic sign. These patients had a lower mean LVEF, larger left ventricular ^{201}Tl defects, and more complex ventricular arrhythmias. It is likely that visualization of the right ventricle in these cases is caused by increased right ventricular afterload.

Risk Evaluation at Hospital Discharge.

Cerquiera et al. (38) showed that in patients who had thrombolytic therapy for acute infarction, a relationship exists between SPECT myocardial perfusion defect size and long-term survival (Fig. 15.30).

At hospital discharge, stress myocardial perfusion imaging has important prognostic value by demonstrating stress-induced myocardial ischemia within the infarct area and/or in the territories of remote coronary arteries. Gibson et al. (40) demonstrated that quantitative analysis of predischarge ^{201}Tl stress images was superior to the stress ECG in identifying patients with multivessel disease and in predicting subsequent cardiac events. Predischarge exercise tests after acute myocardial infarction are usually *submaximal* exercise tests. To improve diagnostic yield of myocardial perfusion imaging in this patient population, alternative modes of stress have been investigated. Brown et al. (41) showed that dipyridamole or adenosine vasodilation myocardial perfusion imaging early (days 3 to 5) after acute infarction can be employed safely and identifies accurately patients at increased

risk for in-hospital and out-of-hospital complications (Fig. 15.31).

Stress Myocardial Perfusion Imaging in Patients after Thrombolytic Therapy

Dakik et al. (42) showed that after thrombolytic therapy for acute myocardial infarction, predischarge stress SPECT myocardial perfusion imaging identified patients at high risk for subsequent events, as well as low-risk patients (Fig. 15.32).

Unstable Angina

An important portion of coronary care unit admissions consists of patients with suspected acute coronary syndrome or unstable angina. This diagnosis is mostly tentative and based on the cardiologist's judgment of history and symptoms. Objective evidence of myocardial ischemia would be extremely helpful in patient management.

Wackers et al. (43) evaluated the value of ^{201}Tl myocardial imaging in patients with unstable angina who were studied *during a pain-free period* (<18 hours) after an anginal episode. A definite relationship was observed between the time of imaging after last anginal attack and the results of imaging (Fig. 15.33). Fifty percent of patients studied within 6 hours after the last anginal attack had abnormal ^{201}Tl images, compared with only 27% of patients studied later. Patients, who had perfusion defects, showed filling-in of the defects on delayed redistribution imaging, indicating viable myocardium. Others have confirmed these observations in patients with unstable angina. These findings suggest that in patients with unstable angina, regional hypoperfusion exists and persists longer than can be judged from the patient's clinical status or electrocardiographic ST segment changes. Transient myocardial perfusion defects on resting ^{201}Tl scans can also be observed in selected patients with severe but stable angina pectoris. In general, patients with coronary artery disease without history of infarction who demonstrate reversible resting defects have more severe coronary artery disease and a poorer prognosis than patients with chest pain syndromes and normal ^{201}Tl images. Bilodeau et al. (44) extended these observations using ^{99m}Tc-sestamibi imaging. When a patient was injected with ^{99m}Tc-sestamibi *during pain,* the presence of a myocardial perfusion defect, particularly if not present in the absence of pain, was highly sensitive and specific for severe coronary artery disease.

Myocardial Imaging for Triage of Patients in the Emergency Department

In daily practice, numerous patients (8 million patients in the United States alone) are seen in emergency departments with acute chest pain and nondiagnostic ECGs. Their clinical diagnosis is uncertain. These patients were often admitted to "rule-out myocardial infarction." After clinical observation and costly hospital admission, more than half of these patients do not have an acute coronary syndrome. Wackers et al. (45) and subsequently many others (46,47) have shown that resting myocardial perfusion imaging can be used to better triage these patients

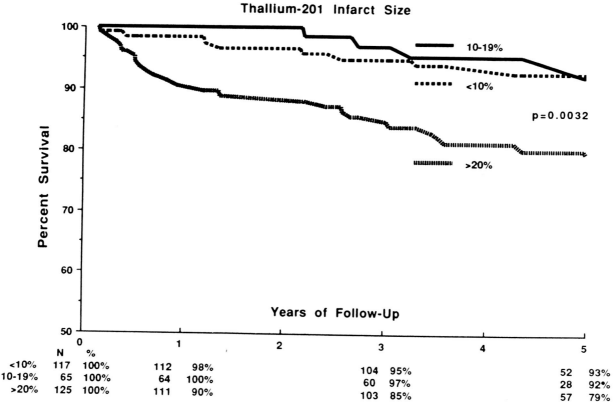

FIGURE 15.30. [201]Tl SPECT infarct size and percent survival during followup after thrombolytic therapy for acute myocardial infarction. Patients with large (≥20%) myocardial perfusion defects after thrombolytic therapy for myocardial infarction, had significantly poorer prognosis then patients with a small or moderate sized myocardial perfusion defects. (Reproduced by permission from Cerqueira MD, Maynard C, Ritchie JL, Davis KB, Kennedy JW. Long-term survival in 618 patients from the western Washington streptokinase in myocardial infarction trials. *J Am Coll Cardiol* 1992;20:1452–1459.)

(Fig. 15.34). Clinical studies in well over 6,000 patients have shown that resting myocardial perfusion imaging is highly sensitive (>90%) for detecting acute myocardial infarction and, most importantly, has a very high negative predictive value (>99%). If a patient with acute chest pain has a normal resting myocardial perfusion image, it is highly unlikely that the patient has an ongoing acute coronary syndrome. Many hospitals have instituted dedicated chest pain centers where patients with acute chest pain are evaluated using a combination of biomarkers of myocardial injury, rest imaging and early stress testing with or without radionuclide myocardial perfusion imaging. Resting imaging is a more effective diagnostic methodology in patients with *ongoing chest pain* than biomarkers. Biomarkers may not yet be positive during the very early hours of acute coronary syndrome, whereas myocardial perfusion images are already abnormal. If resting imaging is negative, early stress testing is safe and appropriate. This allows for management decisions to be made at an earlier point in time. The purpose of chest pain centers is twofold: to rule out acute coronary syndrome and to rule out significant chronic coronary artery disease. Because one third of patients can either not perform adequate physical exercise or have resting ECG changes precluding exercise ECG interpretation, stress myocardial perfusion imaging plays an important role in

the complete evaluation of chest pain center patients (48). With discriminate use of rest and stress radionuclide myocardial perfusion imaging in a chest pain center, less and more appropriate patients with acute chest pain are hospitalized and more patients are sent home (Fig. 15.35).

Chronic Coronary Artery Disease

Pathophysiologic Basis for Stress Myocardial Perfusion Imaging

Patients with chronic stable coronary artery disease usually are asymptomatic at rest. However, during exercise they may develop symptoms of angina pectoris. The pathophysiologic basis of this clinical syndrome is that at rest (even in the presence of a significant coronary stenosis) regional myocardial blood flow is adequate to meet myocardial oxygen demands. However, during exercise, the same coronary artery stenosis limits appropriate augmentation of myocardial blood flow (coronary reserve) to meet increased metabolic demands (Fig. 15.36). Thus, insufficient regional oxygen supply to the myocardium supplied by a diseased coronary artery leads to local myocardial ischemia and clinical angina pectoris. Under these circumstances regional inhomogeneity of myocardial blood flow exists, which can be visu-

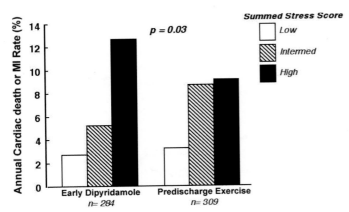

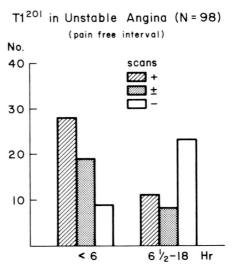

FIGURE 15.31. Risk stratification of patients with acute myocardial infarction by early vasodilation and predischarge stress testing. Annual cardiac death or recurrent myocardial infarction (MI) rate as a function of the summed stress score, categorized as low (0 to 4), intermediate (5 to 8), or high (>8), for dipyridamole and submaximal exercise [99m] Tc-sestamibi single photon emission computed tomography imaging. Event rate increased as scores increased. The ability to predict cardiac events was significantly better for early dipyridamole studies than for predischarge exercise studies for each summed score. (Modified from Brown KA, Heller GV, Landin RS et al. Early dipyridamole Tc-99m-sestamibi single photon emission computed tomographic imaging 2 to 4 days after acute myocardial infarction predicts in-hospital and postdischarge cardiac events: comparison with sub-maximal exercise imaging. *Circulation* 1999;100:2060–2066, with permission.)

FIGURE 15.33. Planar ^{201}Tl imaging results and time after angina. Relationship between results of ^{201}Tl myocardial perfusion imaging in patients with unstable angina and the time of imaging after the last anginal episode. Symbols: + = abnormal ^{201}Tl image, ± = questionable ^{201}Tl images, − = normal ^{201}Tl image. (Reproduced by permission of the American Heart Association from Wackers FJTh, Lie Kl, Liem KL, et al. Thallium-201 scintigraphy in unstable angina pectoris. *Circulation* 1978;57:738.)

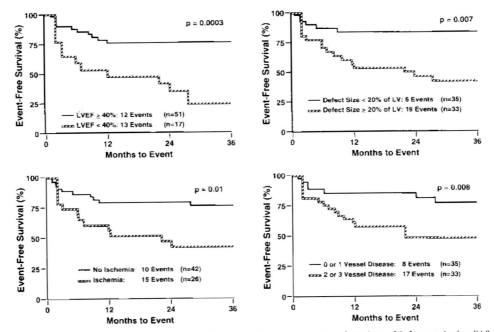

FIGURE 15.32. Kaplan-Meier curves showing event-free survival as a function of left ventricular (LV) ejection fraction (EF) **(A)**, perfusion defect size **(B)**, presence of myocardial ischemia **(C)** and the extent of coronary artery disease **(D)**. Events were defined as cardiac death, myocardial reinfarction, unstable angina, or congestive heart failure. (From Dakik HA, Mahmarian JJ, Kimball KT et al. Prognostic value of exercise 201-T1 tomography in patients treated with thrombolytic therapy during acute myocardial infarction. *Circulation* 1996;94:2735–2742, with permission.)

SHORT AXIS

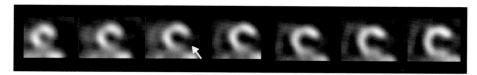

VERTICAL LONG AXIS

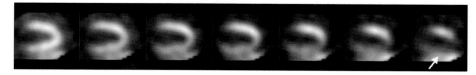

HORIZONTAL LONG AXIS

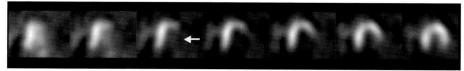

A

WR

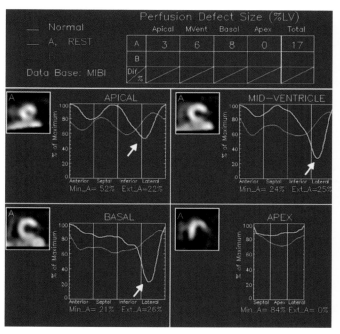

B

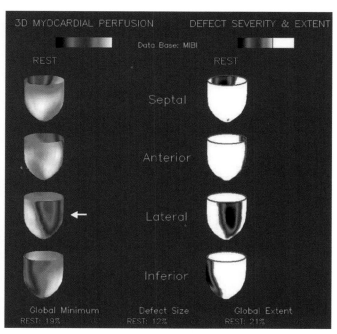

C

FIGURE 15.34. A: Abnormal rest single photon emission computed tomography (SPECT) myocardial perfusion imaging in a 52-year-old man who presented with acute chest pain. The patient was injected with 20 mCi of ^{99m}Tc-sestamibi. The resting SPECT images show a large inferolateral myocardial perfusion defect (*arrows*). B: Quantification of defect in **A** using circumferential profile analysis. The display is the same as in Fig. 15.20. In the apical, midventricular, and basal slices the count distribution profiles are below the lower limit of normal (*white curve*) in the inferolateral wall (*arrows*). The apex is not involved. Quantitatively the rest defect is large and involves 17% of the left ventricle. C: 8-frame electrocardiogram-gated SPECT images. The display is the same as in Fig. 15.20. Visual analysis of cine display indicated hypokinesis of a large portion of the inferolateral wall. *(Figure continues.)*

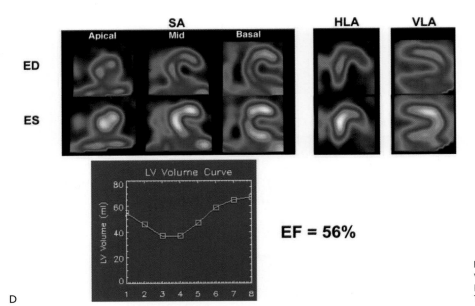

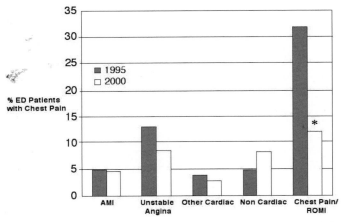

D

EF = 56%

FIGURE 15.34. *Continued.* Global resting left ventricular ejection fraction is, nevertheless, preserved at 56% because of vigorous contraction in the remaining walls.

alized by myocardial perfusion imaging. After intravenous injection of a radiolabeled myocardial perfusion imaging agent (either at exercise or at rest), the radiotracer clears rapidly from the blood (Fig. 15.37) and accumulates within the heart according to regional distribution of blood flow (Figs. 15.38 and 15.39). Although myocardial perfusion imaging agents are extracted relatively rapidly from the blood , an "ischemic steady state" of 1 to 2 minutes after tracer injection is required for sufficient tracer accumulation and visualization of perfusion defects.

FIGURE 15.35. Impact of the selective use of radionuclide myocardial perfusion imaging in a chest pain center on patient admissions. The distribution of admission diagnoses in patients hospitalized directly from the emergency department (ED) are shown. Each diagnosis category is expressed as a percentage of all patients with chest pain presenting to the emergency department. The proportion of patients with chest pain directly admitted to rule-out myocardial infarction (ROMI) decreased significantly during 3 years of chest pain center operation, whereas the proportion of the other diagnoses remained unchanged. AMI, acute myocardial infarction. *$p < 0.0001$. (From Abbott BG, Abdel-Aziz I, Nagula S et al. Selective use of single-photon emission computed tomography myocardial perfusion imaging in a chest pain center. *Am J Cardiol* 2001;87:1351–1355, with permission.)

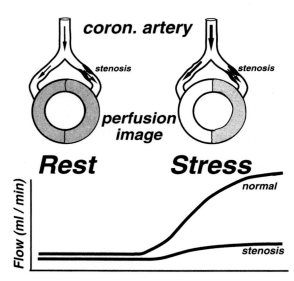

FIGURE 15.36. Schematic representation of the principle of rest/stress myocardial perfusion imaging. *Top:* Two branches of a coronary artery are schematically shown, one is normal (*left*), and one has a significant stenosis (*right*). *Middle:* Myocardial perfusion images of the territories supplied by the two branches. *Bottom:* Schematic representation of coronary blood flow in the branches at rest and during stress. At rest, myocardial blood flow is equal in both coronary artery branches. When a myocardial radiotracer is injected at rest, uptake is homogenous (normal image). During stress, coronary blood flow increases 2.0–2.5 times in the normal branch, but not to the same extent in the stenosed branch, resulting in heterogenous distribution of blood flow. This heterogeneity of blood flow can be visualized with ^{201}Tl or ^{99m}Tc-sestamibi as an area with relatively decreased uptake (abnormal image with a myocardial perfusion defect). (Reproduced by permission from Wackers FJTh. Exercise myocardial perfusion imaging. *J Nucl Med* 1994;35:726–729.)

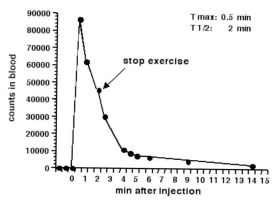

FIGURE 15.37. Blood disappearance curve of ^{99m}Tc-sestamibi after injection at peak exercise in a normal subject. Maximal blood activity is at 0.5 minute. At 2 minutes after injection, blood activity is 50% of maximum. Blood levels are minimal at approximately 6 minutes after injection. This figure illustrates the importance of continuation of exercise for at least 2 minutes after injection at peak exercise.

Exercise Protocol

In most U.S. laboratories, treadmill exercise is the preferred method of stress in conjunction with myocardial perfusion imaging. The speed and grade of the treadmill can easily be adjusted to the physical condition and agility of the patient. In many other countries, the upright bicycle is the preferred exercise modality. In preparation for the exercise test, the patient should be in a fasting state. Diabetic patients should take their regular dose of insulin and have a light breakfast at least 1 hour before the test.

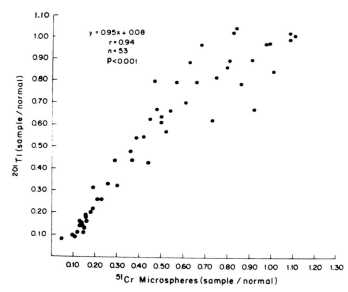

FIGURE 15.38. Transmural myocardial ^{201}Tl uptake and regional myocardial blood flow. Relationship between transmural myocardial ^{201}Tl uptake and relative regional myocardial blood flow as estimated by radioisotope microsphere technique in experimental animals. Activities are expressed as ratios between infarct sample and the mean of normal samples obtained in each individual study. The microsphere estimate of transmural regional myocardial blood flow correlates well with transmural ^{201}Tl uptake. (Reproduced by permission from DiCola VC, Downing SE, Donabedian RK, Zaret BL. Pathophysiological correlates of thallium-201 myocardial uptake in experimental infarction. *Cardiovasc Res* 1977;11:141.)

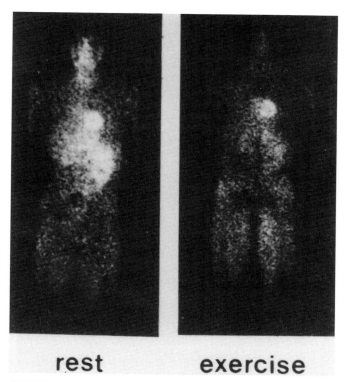

FIGURE 15.39. Whole body distribution of ^{201}Tl at rest and following exercise. At rest, ^{201}Tl accumulates in the heart, liver, spleen, kidneys, and gastrointestinal tract, proportional to the relative distribution of cardiac output. Following exercise, ^{201}Tl activity in the heart is prominent. Most of the remaining ^{201}Tl activity is accumulated in the exercising muscles of the thighs. Note the almost absent activity in the splanchnic region. (Reproduced by permission from Wackers FJTh, Busemann Sokole E, Samson G, van der Schoot JB. Atlas of TI-201 myocardial scintigraphy. *Clin Nucl Med* 1977;2:64.)

Several standardized exercise protocols exist. The most widely used protocol is the one designed by Bruce. According to this protocol the subject starts out at 1.7 mph on a 10% grade (Table 15.3). Subsequently, every 3 minutes the speed and grade of the treadmill are increased until the patient reaches a predefined end point of exercise.

Generally accepted end points for exercise are (a) angina pectoris or reproduction of the patient's symptoms, (b) severe fatigue, (c) hypotension, (d) ventricular arrhythmias, or (e) severe electrocardiographic ST-segment depression (e.g., 3 mm or more) at 0.08 milliseconds after the J-point. The age-predicted target heart rate should be considered a guideline for adequate exercise, but is in itself *not* a good end point, because maximal

Table 15.3. *Bruce Graded Treadmill Exercise Protocol*

Stage	Speed (mph)	Grade (%)	Time (min)	METS[a]
1	1.7	10	3	5
2	2.5	12	3	7
3	3.4	14	3	10
4	4.2	16	3	13
5	5.0	18	3	16

[a]METS, metabolic equivalents.

attainable heart rate may vary importantly among individuals of the same age. A knowledgeable and experienced physician, assisted by a nurse or technician, should supervise each stress test and monitor heart rate, blood pressure, electrocardiographic changes, and symptoms each 2 to 3 minutes. Serious complications as the direct result of stress testing are rare (approximately 1:10,000). The physician who administers the stress test should be trained in advanced cardiac life support.

An intravenous line should be in place in an antecubital vein for injection of radiopharmaceutical. When an end point of exercise is reached, the radiopharmaceutical is rapidly injected in the intravenous line and flushed with a bolus of 10 mL of saline. The patient is then encouraged to exercise for another 1 to 2 minutes at the same level of exercise. This continuation of exercise after the injection of the radionuclide is important because it takes approximately 2 minutes for 50% of the injected radiopharmaceutical to be cleared from the blood (Fig. 15.37). Consequently, it is crucial that during myocardial radiotracer uptake, heart rate and, presumably, myocardial blood flow are maintained at a steady state. If the patient cannot continue to exercise at the same level, speed and grade of the treadmill can be decreased to a lower level.

Pharmacologic Stress Protocol

A considerable number (40% to 50%) of patients referred for stress testing are unable to perform adequate physical exercise on a motor-driven treadmill. This is in particular the case in patients with neurologic or orthopedic problems, patients with claudication because of severe peripheral arterial disease, patients with severe lung disease, or patients on β-blockers medication. In these patients, several alternative methods to evaluate the presence of significant coronary artery disease are available: coronary vasodilatation with dipyridamole or adenosine or β-adrenergic stress with dobutamine.

Pharmacologic Vasodilation

Intravenous infusion of dipyridamole or adenosine is a practical and clinically proven useful alternative to physical exercise for provoking myocardial perfusion abnormalities (49). Adenosine is a direct potent dilator of the coronary resistance vasculature and markedly increases coronary blood flow. Dipyridamole achieves the same result in an indirect way: Dipyridamole inhibits reabsorption of adenosine back into the myocytes, thus, increasing blood and tissue adenosine level (Fig. 15.40) Adenosine is activated at adenosine receptor sites. These receptors can be blocked with aminophylline or xanthine derivatives.

Infusion of dipyridamole or adenosine results in a threefold to fourfold increase of coronary artery blood flow. However, no such increase occurs in zones supplied by coronary arteries with hemodynamically significant stenosis. This produces *inhomogeneity of regional myocardial blood flow* that can be visualized by myocardial perfusion imaging (Fig. 15.36).

Extensive clinical experience exists with dipyridamole and adenosine infusion. Dipyridamole is infused over a 4-minute period (0.568 mg/kg). At approximately 4 minutes after the completion of infusion, maximal coronary dilatory effect is achieved. This usually is associated with a modest (~10 bpm) increase in heart rate and approximately 10 mm Hg decrease in systolic blood pressure. At this time of maximal vasodilatory effect, a myocardial perfusion imaging agent is injected intravenously. In many centers, dipyridamole infusion is combined, if at all feasible, with simultaneous low-level treadmill exercise. Even minimal exercise decreases the incidence of subjective side effects and decreases subdiaphragmatic tracer uptake, which can be a considerable problem with ^{99m}Tc-labeled agents.

Because of the short half-life of adenosine, the infusion protocol can be shorter than that of dipyridamole. Adenosine is infused intravenously with a maximal dose of 140 µg/kg/minute. The radiopharmaceutical is injected at 1.5 to 2 minutes after start of infusion and continued for 2 to 3 minutes. Myocardial perfusion imaging is performed as described earlier. The advantage of direct adenosine infusion is the rapid onset of vasodilatation (<1 minute), and short half-life (30 seconds). This makes it a safe drug in high-risk patients.

In patients with significant coronary artery disease, transient myocardial perfusion defects can be observed after pharmacologic vasodilation (Fig. 15.41). During the infusion of vasodila-

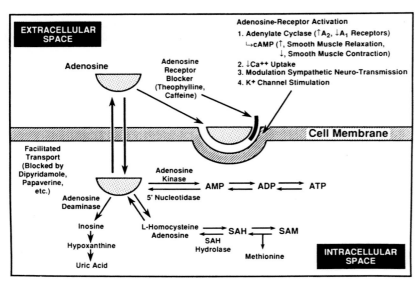

FIGURE 15.40. Mechanism of adenosine pharmacologic vasodilation. Adenosine is synthesized intracellularly from ATP or S-adenosyl homocysteine (SAM). Adenosine leaves the cell to act on surface membrane receptors, and then reenters the cell to be metabolized to ATP, S-adenosyl homocysteine, or uric acid. Theophylline and caffeine are competitive blockers at the receptor sites. *AMP* = Adenosine monophosphate; *SAH* = S-adenosyl-L-homocysteine. (Reproduced by permission from Verani MS. Adenosine thallium-201 myocardial perfusion scintigraphy. *Am Heart J* 1991;122:269–278.)

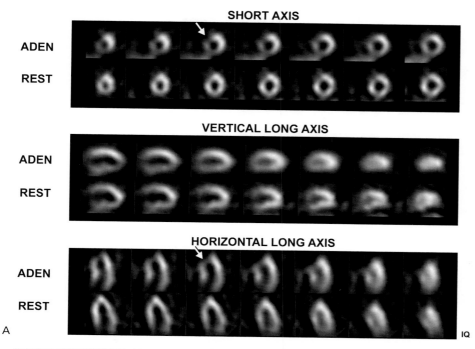

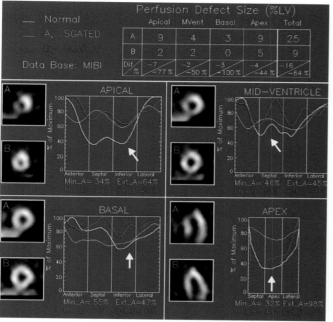

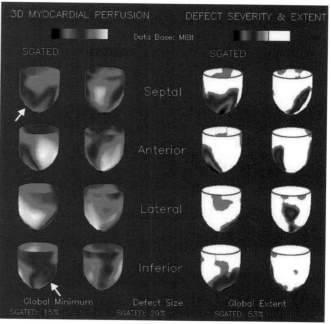

FIGURE 15.41. **A:** Abnormal adenosine-rest single photon emission computed tomography (SPECT) myocardial perfusion images. There is an extensive apical-septal and inferior defect (*arrows*) that shows substantial reversibility at rest. **B:** Quantification of the images in **A.** In the apical slices, the adenosine circumferential profile (*yellow*) is below the lower limit of normal in the inferoseptal segments (*arrow*). There is some extension into the anterior wall. On the resting circumferential profile, (*red*) radiotracer uptake has improved substantially in the same areas. In the midventricular slices the defect is in the septal-inferior area (*arrow*) and is almost completely reversible at rest. In the basal slices, there is a mild inferolateral reversible defect. The apex itself shows a fixed defect. Quantitatively the exercise defect size is large: 25% of left ventricle. The rest defect is moderate (9% of left ventricle) resulting from incomplete reversibility in the apical areas. The ischemic burden is large: 16%. **C:** *Left:* Three-dimensional display of the myocardial perfusion defect shown in **A.** The large inferoseptal defect extends from apex to base (*arrows*). There is minor involvement of the anterior wall as well. There is clearly partial improvement rest. *Right:* By comparison to normal data files, the substantial improvement in the septum and inferoapical walls can be appreciated. (*Figure continues.*)

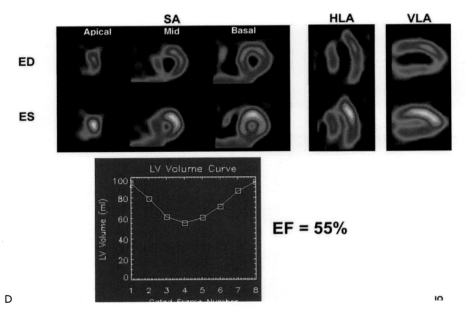

D

FIGURE 15.41. *Continued.* **D:** 8-frame electrocardiogram-gated SPECT images. The display is the same as in Fig. 15.20. Visual analysis of cine-display suggested normal regional wall motion and wall thickening. Left ventricular ejection fraction is preserved at 55%.

tors, most patients with abnormal myocardial perfusion images do have *heterogeneity of blood flow but no true myocardial ischemia.* Only 10% to 25% of patients may clinically manifest ischemia with ECG changes. The underlying pathophysiology of vasodilation-induced ischemia is "coronary steal." In this situation, the markedly increased coronary blood flow in the normal myocardial zones steals blood, via collaterals, away from the vascular bed supplied by a critical stenosis. This undesirable effect of dipyridamole can be reversed relatively quickly by intravenous administration of aminophylline. Because of the short half-life of adenosine, termination of adenosine infusion is usually sufficient to relieve symptoms. Adenosine causes significantly more side effects than dipyridamole. The most worrisome side effect of adenosine is that of high degree atrioventricular (AV) block. The frequency of second- and third-degree AV block is significantly higher in patients with a baseline PR interval of more than 200 milliseconds. However, if this occurs, it will revert quickly by discontinuation of the infusion of adenosine. The half-life of dipyridamole is considerably longer (20 to 45 minutes), and aminophylline is often needed to control side effects.

Dobutamine Pharmacologic Stress

Dobutamine infusion is employed in patients who cannot perform physical exercise and who have contraindications for dipyridamole or adenosine infusion because of bronchospastic pulmonary disease or in patients who are on xanthine derivatives or had caffeine. Dobutamine increases myocardial oxygen demand by increasing myocardial contractility, heart rate, and systolic blood pressure. The increase in coronary blood flow is similar to that during physical exercise (twofold to threefold) and less than that with adenosine or dipyridamole. Because of these selection criteria, it can be inferred that patients who require dobutamine stress already represent a relatively high-risk group.

The dobutamine infusion protocol is as follows: Starting with intravenous infusion of 5 μg/kg/minute, the dose is increased

every 3 minutes, if tolerated, to a maximal dose of 40 μg/kg/minute. The radiopharmaceutical is injected during infusion of the maximal dose, and infusion is continued for 2 to 3 minutes. Myocardial perfusion imaging is performed as described earlier.

Myocardial perfusion imaging after pharmacologic vasodilatation and stress has been reported to yield sensitivities and specificities for the detection of coronary artery disease similar to that of exercise imaging. Nevertheless, compared with exercise, the extent and severity of myocardial perfusion defects may be less with dipyridamole and dobutamine. In contrast, images acquired with adenosine are similar to those acquired after exercise (49).

Imaging Protocols

The timing of imaging after injection at peak stress and at rest varies for different radiopharmaceuticals and protocols. Table 15.1 summarizes the details of imaging.

The image acquisition protocol should be strictly standardized in each laboratory for timing of imaging, sequence of imaging, and duration of imaging. In each laboratory camera-specific detailed acquisition protocols should be prepared to ensure consistency in quality.

[201]Tl

The patient is injected with [201]Tl (3.5 mCi) at peak exercise. Imaging is performed within 5 minutes of termination of exercise and delayed redistribution imaging is performed 3 to 4 hours later. In selected patients (see chapter 16), ^{201}Tl may be reinjected at rest either the same day (1 mCi) or on a different day (3.5 mCi). Rest imaging is started approximately 45 minutes after injection.

[99m]Tc-labeled agents

Two basic protocols are employed for ^{99m}Tc-labeled imaging agents, a two-day protocol or a 1-day "split-dose" protocol.

Using the 2-day protocol, 25 to 30 mCi of ^{99m}Tc-sestamibi or ^{99m}Tc-tetrofosmin is administered on one day at rest and a similar dose is administered on another day at peak stress. After physical exercise, imaging can be started at approximately 15 to 30 minutes after injection. After pharmacologic stress, subdiaphragmatic activity usually is still too intense for good quality images. After pharmacologic stress, it is recommended to start imaging at 45 to 60 minutes after injection. After injection of ^{99m}Tc-sestamibi or ^{99m}Tc-tetrofosmin at rest, imaging is also delayed at least 45 to 60 minutes to allow sufficient clearance of radiotracer from the liver. Using the 1-day protocol, the total dose administered to the patient per day is split in two: a low dose of 10 to 15 mCi is administered first, followed 3 hours later by the high dose of 20 to 25 mCi of ^{99m}Tc-sestamibi. Although there is a preference to perform the rest study first and the exercise study second, this sequence can be reversed without significant effect on the detection of coronary artery disease (50). *The previously outlined time intervals may have to be adjusted in individual patients. If subdiaphragmatic radioactivity is very intense at the scheduled time of imaging, it is recommended to delay imaging until the gastrointestinal activity has cleared. Some investigators recommend drinking of water to enhance movement of radiotracer through the bowel. Drinking milk or eating a fatty meal has, in our experience, no significant effect on clearing of gastrointestinal activity.*

Dual-Isotope Imaging

According to this protocol, rest imaging is performed first with ^{201}Tl (3.5 mCi). As soon as rest ^{201}Tl imaging is completed, the patient is stressed and 25 to 30 mCi of ^{99m}Tc-sestamibi is injected at peak stress. Stress imaging is then performed 15 minutes after completion of exercise. The advantage of this sequential protocol is the relatively short time in which rest and stress imaging can be completed, and it has gained widespread popularity (51). Fig. 15.42 shows an example of dual-isotope images. The interpreter of dual-isotope images should keep in mind that ^{201}Tl and ^{99m}Tc have different physical characteristics and that different injected doses are used. Consequently a different and heavier filter is required for the ^{201}Tl images. This may give the impression that on the ^{201}Tl images the left ventricular cavity is smaller than on the sestamibi images. However, this is not due to transient dilation of the left ventricle but results from the difference in the applied filter. In addition, defect reversibility may appear greater on ^{201}Tl rest images than on sestamibi rest images because of the greater contribution of scattered photons. Recently, *simultaneous acquisition* dual-isotope imaging has been reported to be feasible. Because of potential problems and necessity for correction of cross talk of ^{99m}Tc in the ^{201}Tl window, this alternative acquisition protocol should still be considered experimental.

Detection of Coronary Artery Disease

Since its introduction in the mid-1970s, numerous clinical studies have reported the clinical usefulness of radionuclide stress imaging for detection of coronary artery disease in patients with chest pain syndromes. In 1994, the American Medical Association commissioned a Diagnostic And Therapeutic Technology Assessment (DATTA) review of SPECT myocardial perfusion imaging (52). This extensive review of the literature revealed

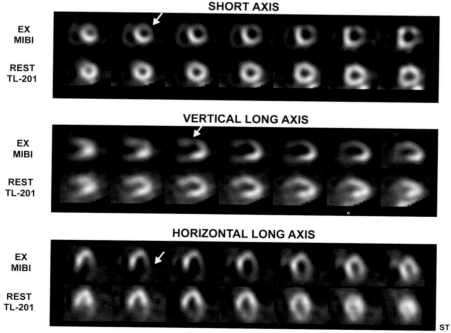

FIGURE 15.42. A: Abnormal dual isotope resting ^{201}Tl-stress ^{99m}Tc-sestamibi single photon emission computed tomography (SPECT) myocardial perfusion images. The reconstructed slices show a large anterolateral myocardial perfusion defect (*arrows*), extending from apex to base, that is almost completely reversible. *(Figure continues.)*

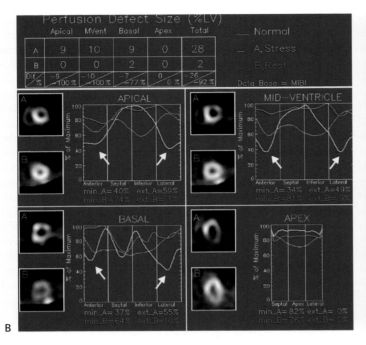

B

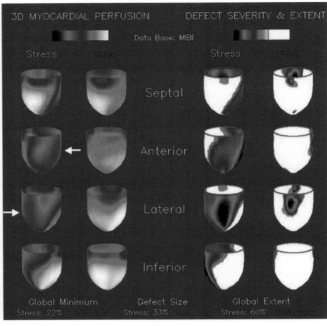

C

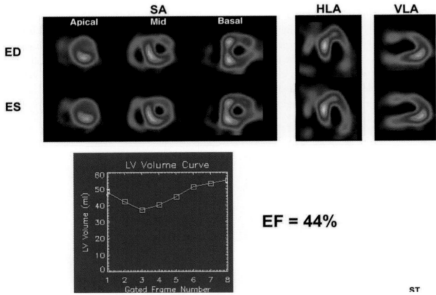

EF = 44%

D

ST

FIGURE 15.42. *Continued.* **B:** Quantification of defect size using circumferential profile analysis. The display is the same as in Fig. 15.20. In the apical, midventricular, and basal slices the yellow stress profiles are below the lower limit of normal (*white curve*) in the anterior and lateral walls (*arrows*). The apex is not involved. The rest (*red*) profiles are almost completely within normal range. By quantitative analysis the stress defect involves 28% of the left ventricle, the rest defect is 2%. This is quantitatively a large reversible defect. **C:** *Left:* Three-dimensional display of the myocardial perfusion defect shown in **A.** The extensive involvement of the left ventricle is well visualized (*arrows*). *Right:* The nearly complete reversibility of the defect in the anterolateral wall can be appreciated. **D:** 8-frame electrocardiogram-gated stress SPECT images. The display is the same as in Fig. 15.20. Visual analysis of cine-display indicated hypokinesis of the inferolateral wall. Left ventricular ejection fraction is depressed at 44%. Because of the substantial reversibility of the defect, this observation suggest poststress ischemic stunning.

sensitivities for planar imaging ranging from 67% to 96% and sensitivities for SPECT imaging ranging from 83% to 98%. The range of specificities for planar imaging varied from 40% to 100% and from 53% to 100% for SPECT imaging (Fig. 15.43). Since the introduction of ^{99m}Tc-labeled myocardial perfusion imaging agents, numerous studies have shown that comparable diagnostic yield was achieved (Table 15.4) (53–58). A relatively recent study in 235 patients showed an overall sensitivity of 95% and specificity of 76% for angiographic (≥50% stenosis) coronary artery disease, with a normalcy rate in low-likelihood patients of 93% (58). Fig. 15.44 shows the diagnostic yield for identifying disease in individual coronary arteries. The relatively low specificity of SPECT imaging suggests that artifacts resulting

Table 15.4. *Sensitivity, Specificity, and Normalcy Rate for Detection of Coronary Artery Disease by SPECT Imaging*

Author	# Pts	Sensitivity (%)	Specificity (%)	Normalcy Rate (%)
Kiat et al., 1989 (53)	36	93	75	100
Iskandrian et al., 1989 (54)	39	82	100	
Kahn et al., 1989 (55)	38	95		
Solot et al., 1993 (56)	128	97	71	
Van Train et al., 1994 (57)	161	89	36	81
Azzarelli et al., 1999 (58)	235	95	77	93
Average	637	92	72	91

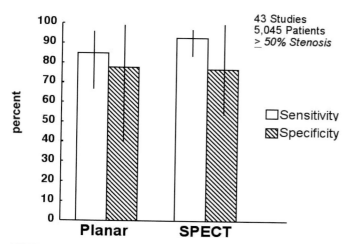

FIGURE 15.43. Sensitivity and specificity of planar and single photon emission computed tomography (SPECT) for detection of angiographic coronary artery disease based a meta-analysis of the literature commissioned by the American Medical Association (52).

from attenuation and motion are not always recognized. Referral bias has been proposed as another potential explanation for the limited specificity of SPECT imaging (59). Referral bias is explained as follows. With the increasing clinical acceptance of stress myocardial perfusion imaging in patients suspected of having coronary artery disease, patients with abnormal myocardial perfusion studies are preferentially referred for cardiac catheterization, whereas patients with normal myocardial perfusion images are generally not referred. This practice limits angiographic confirmation of true-negative patients. Patients with angiographic normal coronary arteries are likely to be referred because of abnormal perfusion (false-positive) images. To circumvent this problem, it is preferred to assess the "normalcy rate" of myocardial perfusion imaging in normal subjects as a surrogate for specificity.

An important advantage of the ^{99m}Tc-labeled agents is that the quality of SPECT images is consistently better than that of ^{201}Tl SPECT imaging (Fig. 15.15).

High-Risk Coronary Artery Disease Myocardial Perfusion Images

The more severe a patient's coronary artery disease, the more extensive are the perfusion abnormalities on stress myocardial perfusion images. Therefore, it is important that myocardial perfusion abnormalities are described in terms that reflect the extent and severity of findings or, preferably, that image quantification is used. Patients with the largest area of ischemia or scar are at the highest risk for future cardiac death or infarction. As mentioned previously, the identification of multivessel coronary artery disease and of left main disease is confounded by the fact that abnormal radionuclide myocardial perfusion images depend on the presence of *relative differences* in radiotracer uptake. When coronary artery disease is diffuse, the detection may become problematic. In clinical practice most patients with left main coronary artery disease have abnormal stress myocardial perfusion images. However, the expected typical left main pattern [i.e., defects in the distribution of the left anterior descending coronary artery and left circumflex coronary artery (anteroseptal and posterolateral myocardial perfusion defects)] is found in only approximately one third of patients. Nevertheless, most patients (approximately 90%) have multiple defects, and often it is this image pattern that indicates high-risk disease.

High-risk patterns on stress myocardial perfusion images (Figs. 15.23 and 15.24) can be characterized as follows:

- Multiple defects in two or more coronary artery territories
- Large stress-induced defects
- Large defect reversibility
- Increased pulmonary radiotracer uptake after stress
- Transient dilatation of the left ventricle after stress
- Transient visualization of the right ventricle after stress
- Depressed resting LVEF

The patterns of transient left ventricular dilation, increased radiotracer lung uptake, and transient increased right ventricular visualization are different manifestations of stress-induced left ventricular dysfunction and herald severe coronary artery disease. These patterns have been shown to be potent predictors of adverse outcome.

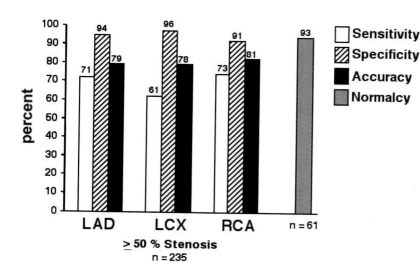

FIGURE 15.44. Sensitivity, specificity, accuracy, and normalcy rate of ^{99m}Tc-tetrofosmin single photon emission computed tomography imaging for detection of disease in individual coronary arteries in 235 consecutive patients. Normalcy rate was assessed in 61 patients with low likelihood of coronary artery disease. LAD, left anterior descending coronary artery; LCX, left circumflex coronary artery; RCA, right coronary artery. (Modified from Azzarelli S, Galassi AR, Foti R et al. Accuracy of 99m-tetrofosmin myocardial tomography in the evaluation of coronary artery disease. *J Nucl Cardiol* 1999;6:183, with permission.)

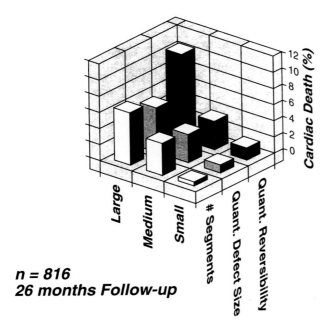

$n = 816$
26 months Follow-up

FIGURE 15.45. Prognostic importance of size and type of myocardial perfusion abnormality. Data are from 816 patients with stable coronary artery disease enrolled in the Multicenter Study on Silent Myocardial Ischemia (MSSMI). The patients had 26 months follow-up. All patients had quantitative planar ^{201}Tl stress imaging. The graph relates the size of exercise defects, defect reversibility, and number of abnormal segments to cardiac death rate during follow-up. The highest cardiac death rate occurred in patients with the most abnormal images. In particular, patients with greatest defect reversibility had the highest cardiac death rate.

High-risk patterns on either planar or SPECT imaging are highly specific (approximately 95%) for multivessel coronary disease; however, the sensitivity is only about 70%. Therefore, the absence of the foregoing scintigraphic characteristics does not rule out the possibility of multivessel disease.

Stress Myocardial Perfusion Imaging and Prognosis

Data on sensitivity and specificity for detection of *angiographic* coronary artery disease by SPECT imaging are relatively dated,

i.e., originating from the early to mid-1990s. However it is doubtful that these data will be updated for present methodology and technology in the foreseeable future. Of far greater clinical significance than angiographic correlation is the *prognostic value* of stress SPECT myocardial perfusion imaging. In the 1980s, the literature on the prognostic value was almost exclusively based on planar ^{201}Tl imaging. However, since the early 1990s an abundance of published data confirmed similar prognostic value of SPECT stress myocardial perfusion imaging.

Brown et al. (60) were the first to demonstrate that the number of reversible planar ^{201}Tl defects was the most important statistically significant predictor of future cardiac events. Similarly, Ladenheim et al. (61) and others demonstrated that the extent and severity of ^{201}Tl defects correlated with the occurrence of cardiac events (Fig. 15.45). Since then, numerous analyses have confirmed that the *extent of myocardial perfusion abnormalities* on planar or SPECT imaging in patients after acute infarction, as well as in patients with chronic coronary artery disease, is a powerful predictor of future hard cardiac events (i.e., cardiac death and nonfatal myocardial infarction (62) (Fig. 15.46). There are some data (63) to suggest that the site of future acute myocardial infarction is better predicted by the location of a SPECT stress-induced perfusion defect than by the most severe stenosed artery on coronary angiography (77% vs. 62%).

On the other hand, the presence of *normal* stress myocardial perfusion images by quantitative analysis, even in patients with known coronary artery disease, was associated with a very favorable prognosis (64–68) (Fig. 15.47 and Table 15.5). The (rare) coronary events occurred predominantly in patients with a high likelihood of, or known, coronary artery disease. Interestingly, cardiac events occurred particularly in patients with a positive exercise ECG and in patients who had undergone prior coronary angioplasty. It was observed that the "warranty" for a favorable prognosis of normal stress myocardial perfusion images appeared to expire approximately 2 years after the index stress test.

These data on abnormal and normal test results indicate that the extent of myocardial perfusion defects, or lack thereof, provides significant functional and prognostic information that sur-

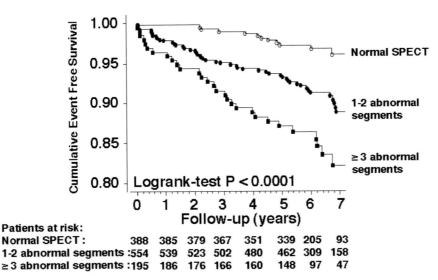

Patients at risk:

	0	1	2	3	4	5	6	7
Normal SPECT :	388	385	379	367	351	339	205	93
1-2 abnormal segments :	554	539	523	502	480	462	309	158
≥ 3 abnormal segments :	195	186	176	166	160	148	97	47

FIGURE 15.46. Kaplan-Meier cardiac survival curves according to the number of abnormal segments on ^{201}Tl single photon emission computed tomography (SPECT). The more abnormal segments on ^{201}Tl SPECT the lower survival. The number of patients examined each year is indicated. ^{201}Tl, ^{201}thallium; SPECT, single photon emission computed tomography; o, normal ^{201}Tl SPECT; °, presence of 1 to 2 abnormal segments; l, presence of ≥3 abnormal segments. (From Vanzetto G, Ormezzano O, Fagret D et al. Long term additive prognostic value of thallium-201 myocardial perfusion imaging over clinical and exercise stress test in low-to-intermediate risk patients. Study in 1,137 patients with 6 year-follow-up. *Circulation* 1999;100:1521, with permission.)

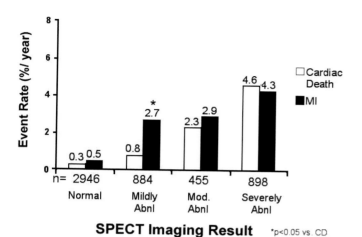

FIGURE 15.47. Cardiac event rate as a function of the degree of stress myocardial perfusion abnormalities. Event rate increases as stress single photon emission computed tomography images are more abnormal. However, patients with mildly abnormal images have low risk for cardiac death but intermediate risk for myocardial infarction. MI, myocardial infarction. (From Hachamovitch R, Berman DS, Shaw LJ et al. Incremental prognostic value of myocardial perfusion single photon emission computed tomography for the prediction of cardiac death. *Circulation* 1998;97:535, with permission.)

passes that of anatomic information derived from coronary angiography. Haronian et al. (69) demonstrated with ^{99m}Tc-sestamibi imaging during percutaneous transluminal coronary angioplasty (PTCA) balloon occlusion that the coronary angiogram is of limited value in predicting the extent of the area at risk for a given coronary artery stenosis. Zeiher et al. (70) showed that apparently false-positive ^{201}Tl myocardial perfusion images in patients with normal epicardial coronary angiograms could be explained by abnormal coronary flow reserve.

Independent and Incremental Prognostic Value of Stress Myocardial Perfusion Imaging

In clinical practice, a diagnostic test is not used in isolation. Other clinical and diagnostic data are usually available. The prognostic value of stress myocardial perfusion imaging, as was

Table 15.5. *Yearly Cardiac Event Rate in Patients with Normal Myocardial Perfusion Images*

	n	Cardiac Death	Nonfatal MI
Wackers et al., 1985 (64)	95	0%	1.0%
Brown et al., 1994 (65)	234	0%	0.5%
Raiker et al., 1993 (66)	208	0%	0.5%
Hachamovitch et al., 1998 (67)	2946	0.3%	0.5%
Soman et al., 1999 (68)	473	0.2%	0.0%

MI, myocardial infarction.

discussed earlier, is extremely important and supports the validity and accuracy of the test. However, if similar information can be derived from other less costly and more readily available tests, it may not be cost effective to perform radionuclide myocardial perfusion imaging. Numerous investigators have demonstrated the incremental prognostic value of successive data (clinical, exercise ECG, stress radionuclide imaging, and coronary angiography) in patients with suspected coronary artery disease. Stress myocardial perfusion imaging variables provided significantly greater prognostic information than the combination of clinical and angiographic data. The extent of the perfusion abnormality on quantitative SPECT was consistently the single most important prognostic predictor (Fig. 15.47).

In a series of seminal and large database analyses, Hachamovitch et al. (71,74–76) categorized patients into low, intermediate, and high risk for cardiac events on the basis of clinical, historical, and exercise information. In each clinical risk category, radionuclide imaging further enhanced risk stratification with respect to the occurrence of future cardiac events (Fig. 15.48). In all clinical subgroups, *normal* perfusion studies were associated with an exceedingly low yearly event rate (<1%). Hachamovitch et al. (76) also demonstrated that incremental value and enhanced risk stratification can be achieved in men and women and in young and older adult patients. Patients with low pretest risk generally have a relatively low cardiac event rate and do not need any testing. Several investigators proposed a strategy of hierarchical testing. Patients with intermediate to high risk for coronary artery disease (and who have normal rest-

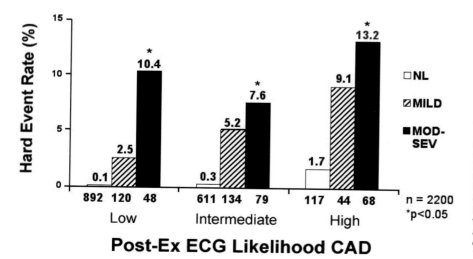

FIGURE 15.48. Incremental prognostic value derived from stress myocardial perfusion imaging over and beyond risk stratification in low-, intermediate-, and high-risk group on the basis of clinical, historical- and exercise information. In each postexercise-electrocardiogram risk category, the results of stress myocardial perfusion imaging [i.e., normal (NL), mild, and moderate-severe (MOD-SEV)] provides enhanced risk stratification for cardiac events (death and myocardial infarction). HE, hard events (i.e. death, myocardial infarction). (From Berman DS, Hachamovitch RH, Kiat H et al. Incremental value of prognostic testing in patients with known or suspected ischemic heart disease: a basis for optimal utilization of single-photon emission computed tomography. *J Am Coll Cardiol* 1993;6:665, with permission.)

ing ECG) should have first exercise ECG. If the result of exercise ECG is normal, the patient is at low risk and perfusion imaging will not provide additional new information. If the exercise ECG is abnormal and/or the posttest risk is intermediate, stress SPECT imaging is appropriate for further evaluation (77,78).

Shaw et al. (79) analyzed the costs of two diagnostic approaches in patients referred for the evaluation of chest pain in a multicenter database study. One group of 5,826 patients underwent first stress SPECT imaging followed by cardiac catheterization if SPECT images were abnormal, whereas the other group of 5,423 patients was directly referred for cardiac catheterization. They found no differences in short-term or long-term outcome. However, the total diagnostic cost and the long-term follow-up cost was 30% to 41% lower when SPECT imaging was performed as the first step of the evaluation (Fig 15.49). Similar cost savings for the noninvasive diagnostic strategy in comparison to the primary invasive diagnostic strategy were reported in the European EMPIRE study.

In an observational study of 5,183 patients, Hachomovitch et al. (76) showed that a significant association existed between the degree of abnormality on stress SPECT imaging and the occurrence of death or myocardial infarction (Fig. 15.47). However, for patients with mildly abnormal SPECT images there was a differential risk. These patients were at low risk for cardiac death (0.8% per year) but at intermediate risk for myocardial infarction (2.7% per year). This suggests that patients with mildly abnormal myocardial perfusion images are best treated with aggressive risk factor modification. In fact, Bateman et al. (80) observed that the outcome in patients with non-high-risk myocardial perfusion imaging who were treated with aggressive medical management had a better outcome than patients treated with coronary interventions. Sharir et al. (81,82) further demonstrated the incremental prognostic importance of LVEF and end-systolic volume derived from gated SPECT images. Poststress LVEF was the best predictor for cardiac death, whereas the amount of ischemia was the best predictor for nonfatal myocar-

dial infarction (Fig. 15.50**A** and **B**). The important message from these studies for the practicing clinician is that nuclear cardiology reports should describe *the degree of abnormal perfusion and function* on stress SPECT images and that prognostic implications should be conveyed to referring physicians.

Monitoring the Effect of Revascularization with Perfusion Imaging

An important purpose for performing stress myocardial perfusion imaging is not only to detect significant coronary artery disease, but also to provide guidance in patient management decisions. Patients with markedly abnormal and high-risk stress myocardial perfusion images usually will be considered candidates for coronary revascularization, either by coronary bypass surgery or percutaneous coronary interventions, such as angioplasty, stenting, and brachytherapy. Stress myocardial perfusion imaging plays a role in monitoring the effect of revascularization.

Surgical Revascularization

Although many patients have stress myocardial perfusion imaging before revascularization, this is not routinely performed after coronary bypass surgery and is, according to guidelines, only indicated when symptoms reoccur. Because many patients have nonspecific ST-T segment changes on the baseline ECG after surgery, myocardial perfusion imaging is preferred over exercise electrocardiography to evaluate these patients. With knowledge of the details of revascularization, tomographic localization of perfusion abnormalities allows determination of whether clinical ischemia is likely to be caused by coronary graft closure or by newly developed disease in other coronary arteries. Alazraki et al. (83) followed 336 patients randomized to coronary bypass graft surgery or coronary angioplasty in the Emory Angioplasty versus Surgery Trial (EAST) study with quantitative ^{201}Tl SPECT imaging. At 1 year after revascularization, stress-induced ischemia occurred more often after angioplasty than after surgery

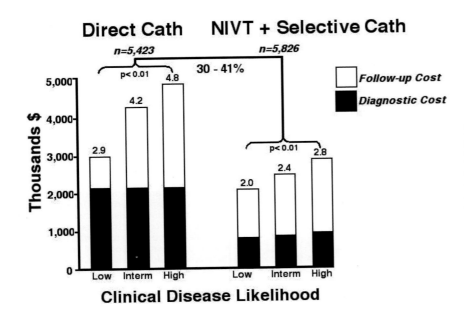

FIGURE 15.49. Cost savings achieved by noninvasive testing (NIVT) and selective catheterization (Cath) in comparison to direct cardiac catheterization of patients suspected of having coronary artery disease. The patients are grouped according to clinical likelihood of having coronary artery disease. The total cost included both initial diagnostic cost and later follow-up cost. The noninvasive testing strategy resulted in 30% to 41% cost savings. (From Shaw LJ, Hachamovitch R, Berman DS et al. The economic consequences of available prognostic strategies for the evaluation of stable angina patients: an observational assessment of the value of precatheterization ischemia. Economics of noninvasive diagnosis (END) multicenter study group. *J Am Coll Cardiol* 1999;33:661, with permission.)

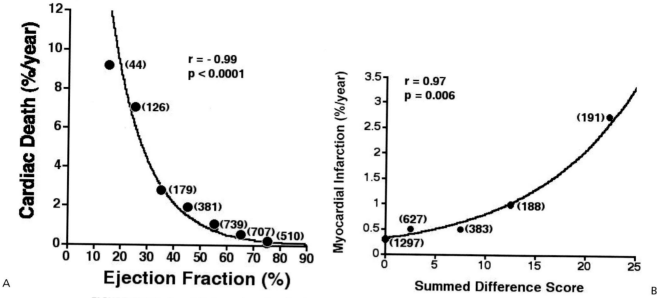

FIGURE 15.50. A and B: Annual cardiac death rate as a function of poststress left ventricular ejection fraction calculated from electrocardiogram-gated ^{99m}Tc-sestamibi single photon emission computed tomography (SPECT) images. **B:** Nonfatal acute myocardial infarction rate as a function of the degree of stress-induced myocardial ischemia on resting ^{201}Tl/stress ^{99m}Tc-sestamibi SPECT imaging. (From Sharir T, Germano G, Kang X et al. Prediction of myocardial infarction versus cardiac death by gated myocardial perfusion SPECT: risk stratification by the amount of stress-induced ischemia and poststress ejection fraction. *J Nucl Med* 2001;42:831–837, with permission.)

(46% vs, 27%, $p < 0.001$). Quantitative ^{201}Tl SPECT imaging effectively stratified patients according to the occurrence of subsequent cardiac events at 3-year follow-up.

Percutaneous Coronary Intervention

Stress myocardial perfusion imaging may be particularly useful after coronary intervention of patients with multivessel coronary artery disease. Often the most severe stenosis in the "culprit" vessel was dilated and stented. However, a question often remains whether the stenoses in other vessels are of significance. During interpretation of SPECT images the interpreter can focus on a particular vascular territory. The optimal timing of imaging after percutaneous coronary intervention remains unclear. Initial investigators reported a high incidence of false-positive myocardial perfusion abnormalities early after percutaneous transluminal coronary angioplasty, presumably because of delayed return of coronary flow reserve within the territory of the dilated artery (84). Because these data were published, substantial progress has been made with interventional techniques and technology, i.e., coronary stenting and brachytherapy. At present, the general experience is that most patients have normal myocardial perfusion images within the first week of successful coronary intervention. At approximately 4 weeks after the intervention, a good correlation has been demonstrated between stress-induced myocardial perfusion abnormalities and the presence or absence of restenosis, independent of clinical symptoms (85).

Garzon and Eisenberg (86) performed a meta-analysis of all studies, between the years 1975 and 2000, examining the diagnostic abilities of exercise treadmill testing, stress nuclear imaging, and stress echocardiography at 6 months after percutaneous coronary interventions for detection of restenosis. The pooled analysis demonstrated that nuclear perfusion imaging has a sensitivity of 87% and specificity of 78% for detection of restenosis. However, these investigators suggested that the value of routine testing after coronary interventions to detect restenosis would decline as the rates of restenosis are substantially reduced with the use of coronary stenting and other adjunctive therapies. Galassi et al. (87) observed that exercise ^{99m}Tc-tetrofosmin SPECT imaging was more accurate for identifying in-stent restenosis than exercise symptoms and exercise electrocardiography. They suggested that repeat coronary angiography should be based primarily on clinical findings that are corroborated by noninvasive testing.

In our own laboratory we often perform electrocardiographic treadmill stress testing shortly after percutaneous coronary interventions to assess functional status and exercise-induced symptoms. Stress myocardial perfusion imaging is performed in patients who develop symptoms suggestive of restenosis or at 6 months in those who are asymptomatic. SPECT imaging allows the determination of whether clinical ischemia is caused by restenosis at the site of angioplasty or by progression of disease in other coronary arteries.

Berman et al. (88) performed a retrospective databank analysis of 421 patients who had serial quantitative SPECT myocardial perfusion imaging with a mean interval of 2.5 years. Patients, particularly those with extensive defects, who underwent coronary revascularization during the interval (either by coronary bypass surgery or percutaneous coronary intervention) had significant improvement of myocardial perfusion abnormalities.

Risk Stratification before Noncardiac Surgery

Vasodilator myocardial perfusion imaging has found a major clinical application in evaluating risk for perioperative cardiac events in patients scheduled for major noncardiac surgery. It is well known that patients with severe peripheral vascular disease often have associated significant coronary artery disease, which may, or may not, be clinically apparent. In these patients, perioperative morbidity and mortality is related to underlying coronary artery disease. In patients who required peripheral vascular surgery, Boucher et al. (89) and many others demonstrated that dipyridamole ^{201}Tl imaging correctly predicted the occurrence of subsequent cardiac events (90,91). However, the predictive value of myocardial perfusion imaging was only 15% to 30%. Eagle et al. (92) demonstrated that clinical variables, such as age, prior myocardial infarction, diabetes mellitus, history of angina, or congestive heart failure, should be taken into consideration and that these variables substantially increase or decrease the surgical risk. However, not every patient scheduled for a surgical procedure requires preoperative testing for the presence of coronary artery disease. The American Heart Association and the American College of Cardiology (AHA/ACC) published extensive guidelines for preoperative cardiac stress testing in patients scheduled for noncardiac surgery in which the type of surgery and clinical risk factors are weighted (93). Table 15.6 provides a simplified version of these guidelines for deciding whether or not a particular patient needs testing (94). If testing is indicated, in most patients pharmacologic vasodilation myocardial perfusion imaging with adenosine or dipyridamole is the most appropriate test. For minor surgery, risk stratification is usually not indicated, whereas for major surgery (e.g., abdominal aortic aneurysm repair), risk stratification is appropriate. As can be anticipated, the incidence of future cardiac events is related to the *extent* of perfusion abnormalities (90,95). Short-term prognosis is determined by the presence of evidence of ischemia, i.e., reversible myocardial perfusion defects, whereas long-term prognosis is determined by the presence of fixed defects (90). In the latter situation, a fixed defect (i.e., scar) can be considered a surrogate for LVEF.

Selection of Patients for Stress Myocardial Perfusion Imaging

Although the sensitivity and specificity of myocardial perfusion imaging is better than that of routine ECG exercise testing, stress

Table 15.6. *Shortcut to Noninvasive testing in Preoperative Patients*

- Intermediate clinical predictors are present, i.e., Canadian class 1 or 2 angina, prior myocardial infarct based on history or pathologic Q waves, compensated or prior CHF, or diametes
- Poor functional capacity, i.e., less than 4 METS
- High-risk surgical procedure, i.e., semi-emergency major operations; aortic repair or peripheral vascular; prolonged surgical procedures with large fluid shifts and/or blood loss

---

If 2 of 3 factors are present, noninvasive testing is appropriate.
(From Leppo JA, Dahlberg ST: The question: to test or not to test in preoperative cardiac risk evaluation. *J Nucl Cardiol* 1998;5:332, with permission.)

myocardial perfusion imaging is not a perfect diagnostic test. Some false-negative results can be expected in patients with angiographic coronary artery disease, and false-positive results may also occur. According to Bayes' theorem, the significance of a test result relates not only to the sensitivity and specificity of the test but also to the prevalence of disease in the population under study. Assuming that myocardial perfusion stress imaging has an approximate sensitivity of 90% and a specificity of 80%, a positive result obtained in a population with a very low prevalence of coronary artery disease (e.g., <3%) will have a low predictive value of only 13%, because, compared with expected true-positive results, a relatively large absolute number of false positives can be anticipated. However, in a patient population with a high prevalence of coronary artery disease (e.g., 90%), a positive result has a predictive value of 99%. In this setting, relative to true-positive results, only a few false positives are obtained. On the other hand, in a population with a high prevalence of disease, a relatively large number of false-negative results are also obtained and the predictive value of a negative test for absence of coronary artery disease is only 51%. Thus, in a population with a low prevalence of coronary artery disease (such as young, asymptomatic subjects), a positive test is of little practical value, whereas in a population with a high prevalence of coronary artery disease (50- to 60-year-old men with typical angina pectoris), a negative test is of little practical diagnostic value. The magnitude of difference between pretest probability of disease (determined by patient's age, symptoms, and a stress ECG) and posttest probability (determined by the results of stress myocardial perfusion imaging) is a measurement for the practical value of the test (Fig. 15.51). Stress myocardial perfusion imaging has optimal discriminative value in the patient population with a pretest probability of coronary artery disease ranging from about 40% to 70%. This population includes patients with atypical chest pain and asymptomatic patients with known major risk factors or with a positive stress ECG.

We, and others, observed that in patients with a low to intermediate pretest likelihood for coronary artery disease and normal rest ECG, radionuclide exercise myocardial does not always yield incremental value (78,79). Patients with normal exercise electrocardiography had normal exercise myocardial perfusion images; myocardial perfusion imaging, thus, provided no additional information. However, of patients with abnormal exercise electrocardiography, one half had normal exercise myocardial perfusion images. Consequently, we proposed a step-wise diagnostic approach in this population of patients: exercise electrocardiography first and exercise myocardial perfusion imaging second, only in patients with abnormal exercise electrocardiography.

Stress Myocardial Perfusion Imaging in Patients with Left Bundle Branch Block

In patients with complete left bundle branch block, the electrical conduction abnormality precludes the use of conventional electrocardiographic criteria for the localization of acute infarction or detection of exercise-induced ischemia. In patients with left bundle branch block, and without history of myocardial infarction, resting myocardial perfusion images generally are normal, although the septum often is thinner than normal. In patients with documented acute or old infarction, resting myo-

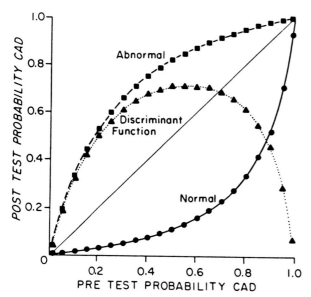

FIGURE 15.51. Probability of coronary artery disease. Pre- and posttest probability of coronary artery disease (*CAD*) for abnormal and normal results of quantitative ^{201}Tl stress imaging (sensitivity 90%, specificity 95%). The curve describes the difference between posttest probability of a normal and an abnormal test result, indicating the range of disease prevalence for which ^{201}Tl stress imaging discriminates most effectively between the presence or absence of disease. [201]Tl stress imaging is most useful when the pretest prevalence of coronary artery disease is 40–70%. Example: In a patient with a pretest probability of coronary artery disease of 60%, a positive ^{201}Tl stress test increases the probability of coronary artery disease to approximately 90%, but a negative test decreases it to about 15%. In contrast, in a very high or a very low pretest probability of disease, no clinically meaningful diagnostic improvement will be gained by either a positive or negative test result. Symbols: ■ = abnormal; ▲ = posttest probability difference; ● = normal. (Reproduced by permission from Hamilton GW, Trobaugh G, Ritchie JC, Gould KL, DeRouen TA, Williams DL. Myocardial imaging with [201]Tl: an analysis of clinical usefulness based on Bayes' theorem. *Semin Nucl Med* 1978;8:358.)

cardial perfusion defects were similar to those seen in infarct patients without conduction abnormalities. Thus, *resting* radionuclide myocardial perfusion imaging is extremely helpful in precisely localizing the site of acute or old infarction in left bundle branch block.

On the other hand false-positive anteroseptal myocardial perfusion defects have been observed frequently after exercise in patients with complete left bundle branch block and normal coronary arteries. In an experimental canine study, Hirzel et al. (96) demonstrated that right ventricular electrical pacing (mimicking left bundle branch block) produced diminished septal blood flow, thus providing a possible explanation for the perfusion defects observed in patients with left bundle branch block. However, the flow heterogeneity measured only 20%, which is generally not sufficient to be detected on planar or SPECT myocardial perfusion imaging. We believe that there is another possible explanation for the apparent defects. Many patients with left bundle branch block may have left ventricular dilatation and left ventricular dysfunction. Using quantitative techniques, we observed a relationship between the presence of myocardial perfusion abnormalities and the degree of left ventricular dilatation (97). Thus, it is conceivable that partial volume effect resulting

from altered geometry and thinning of the dilated left ventricle provides an alternative explanation for the observed defects.

The anatomic location of myocardial perfusion defects in left bundle branch block defects should be considered. Whereas anteroseptal perfusion defects may be not indicative of coronary artery disease, involvement of the apex contiguous with anteroseptal perfusion defects and inferior location are suggestive of coronary artery disease.

False-positive localized anteroseptal defects in left bundle branch block can be avoided by using pharmacologic vasodilation instead of physical exercise (98). The mechanism of improved specificity is unclear. Nevertheless, it is presently considered standard practice to use pharmacologic vasodilation in patients with complete left bundle branch block.

Prognostic Value of Myocardial Perfusion Imaging in Patients with Left Bundle Branch Block

Similar to observations made in patients without left bundle branch block, in patients with left bundle branch block the extent and size of stress myocardial perfusion defects is of prognostic significance (99). The size of myocardial perfusion abnormalities stratified patients in high- and low-risk groups with a threefold difference in hard cardiac events regardless of the presence or absence of coronary artery disease. This is in agreement with the notion that abnormal image patterns in left bundle branch block are not just artifacts resulting from abnormal electrical conduction but that they reflect anatomic left ventricular changes, i.e., dilation and dysfunction.

Dilated Cardiomyopathy

The number of patients with congestive heart failure is increasing steadily. Most patients have ischemic cardiomyopathy, but a substantial number of patients have nonischemic dilated cardiomyopathy. For clinical management decisions it is important to be able to distinguish between these two etiologies. The advent of ECG-gated SPECT myocardial perfusion imaging has made it possible to discern these entities noninvasively with some certitude. It is not uncommon that patients referred for nonspecific complaints are identified for the first time as having a cardiomyopathy because of normal myocardial perfusion images with depressed LVEF. In idiopathic cardiomyopathy, the left ventricle is dilated and shows homogeneous or diffusely inhomogeneous radiotracer uptake. In addition global and regional wall motion is diffusely depressed (Fig. 15.52). Large, localized defects, involving more than 40% of the circumference of the left ventricle, and regional wall motion abnormalities strongly favor ischemic etiology of cardiomyopathy (100) (Fig. 15.53). However, fixed defects have also been reported in patients with idiopathic dilated cardiomyopathy. These are scarred areas often located in the left ventricular apex and inferior wall.

NEW APPROACHES FOR THE DIAGNOSIS OF CORONARY ARTERY DISEASE

In this chapter we discussed the time-honored methods of evaluating stress-induced heterogeneity of myocardial blood flow as

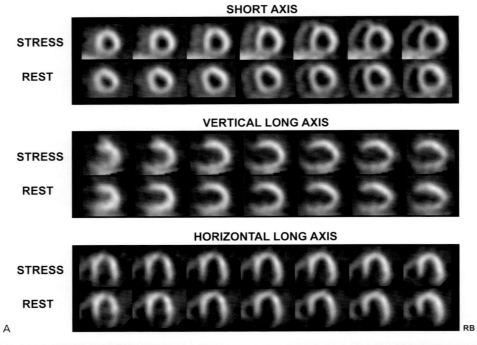

SHORT AXIS

STRESS

REST

VERTICAL LONG AXIS

STRESS

REST

HORIZONTAL LONG AXIS

STRESS

REST

A

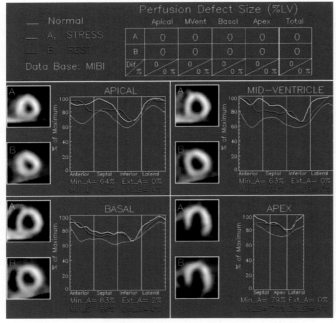

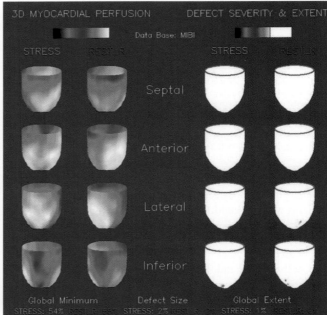

FIGURE 15.52. A: Stress-rest ^{99m}Tc-sestamibi single photon emission computed tomography (SPECT) images of a patient with an idiopathic dilated cardiomyopathy. The left ventricle is markedly enlarged and dilated. There are no distinct myocardial perfusion defects. **B:** Quantification of myocardial perfusion using circumferential profile analysis. The display is the same as in Fig. 15.20. All circumferential profiles are within normal range. No defect is quantified. **C:** *Left:* Three-dimensional display of SPECT images shown in **A.** There is relatively decreased radiotracer uptake in the inferior wall at stress and rest. *Right:* When compared with normal data files this decrease is within normal range, suggesting that it is most likely resulting from attenuation. *(Figure continues.)*

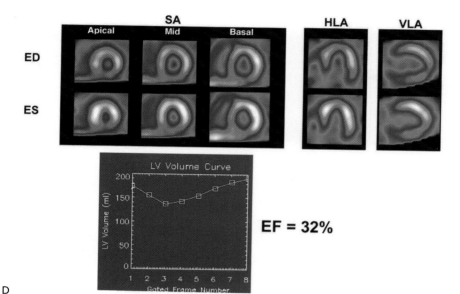

FIGURE 15.52. *Continued.* **D:** 8-frame gated SPECT images. End-diastolic and end-systolic frames of electrocardiogram-gated SPECT images in **A** are shown. Visual analysis of regional wall motion on cine display shows diffuse hypokinesis of all left ventricular wall segments. Global left ventricular ejection fraction is severely depressed at 32%.

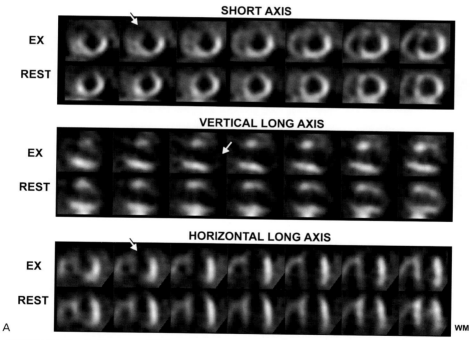

FIGURE 15.53. A: Stress-rest ⁹⁹ᵐTc-sestamibi single photon emission computed tomography (SPECT) images of a patient with an ischemic cardiomyopathy. The patient has severe multivessel coronary artery disease and sustained several previous infarcts. The left ventricle is enlarged and dilated. On the poststress images, there is additional transient left ventricular dilation. There is a large anteroapical and septal myocardial perfusion defect (*arrows*), extending from apex to midventricle. There is some minor reversibility at rest in the midventricular area. *(Figure continues.)*

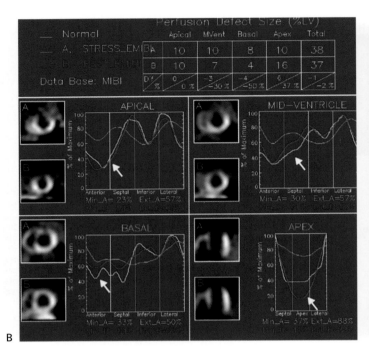

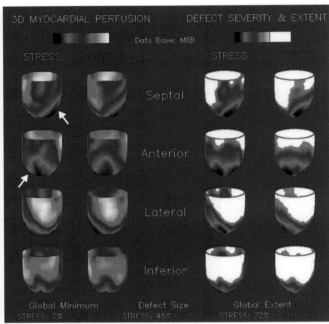

B

C

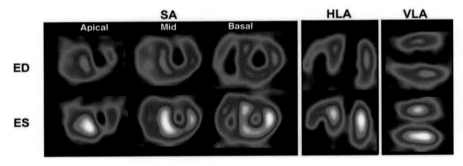

D

EF = 40%

FIGURE 15.53. *Continued.* **B:** Quantification of defect size using circumferential profile analysis. The display is the same as in Fig. 15.20. In the apical, midventricular, and basal slices, the yellow stress profiles are below the lower limit of normal (*white curve*) in the anteroseptal and lateral walls (*arrows*). The apex is also involved. The rest (*red*) profiles show only minor reversibility in the midventricular and basal slices. By quantitative analysis, the defect is very large both at stress (38%) and at rest (37%) **C:** *Left:* Three-dimensional display of the myocardial perfusion defect shown in **A.** The extensive involvement of the left ventricle is well visualized (*arrows*). The is no appreciable change between stress and rest *Right:* In comparison to normal data files, there is no change in defect extent and severity. **D:** End-diastolic and end-systolic frames of the electrocardiogram-gated SPECT images in **A.** Visual analysis of regional wall motion on cine display showed diffuse hypokinesis with akinesis in the anteroapical and septal segments. Global left ventricular ejection fraction is depressed at 40%.

a means of detecting coronary artery disease. For the continued growth of the field it is important that other avenues are explored as well.

It is likely that, depending on the severity of induced myocardial ischemia, metabolic changes occur on a cellular level as a consequence of changes in regional myocardial nutrient blood flow. Indeed Abramson et al. (101), using ^{18}F-fluorodeoxyglucose (FDG) metabolic PET imaging after physical or vasodilator stress, observed regionally increased FDG uptake in selected patients with significant angiographic coronary artery disease. Another approach may be to pursue the direct visualization of myocardial ischemia. Nitroimidazoles are compounds that are specifically retained in severely hypoxic tissue. Weinstein et al. (102) demonstrated focal ^{99}Tc-nitroimidazole uptake in an experimental animal model of acute myocardial ischemia.

These and other novel approaches deserve further exploration.

DISCLOSURE STATEMENT

Through an agreement between Yale University School of Medicine and Eclipse Systems, Inc., Branford, CT, Frans J. Th. Wackers, M.D. receives royalties from sales of the Wackers-Liu CQ software for SPECT quantification shown in this chapter.

REFERENCES

1. Wackers FJTh, van der Schoot JB, Busemann Sokole E et al. Noninvasive visualization of acute myocardial infarction in man with thallium-201. *Br Heart J* 1975:37:741.

2. Wackers FJTh. Myocardial perfusion imaging. In: Sandler MP, Coleman RE, Wackers FJTh et al., eds. *Diagnostic nuclear medicine,* 3rd ed. Baltimore: Williams & Wilkins, 1996:443–516.
3. Wackers FJTh, Berman DS, Maddahi J et al. Technetium-99m hexakis 2-methoxyisobutyl isonitrile: human biodistribution, dosimetry, safety, and preliminary comparison to thallium-201 for myocardial perfusion imaging. *J Nucl Med* 1989;30:301–311.
4. Kiat H, Maddahi J, Roy LT et al. Comparison of technetium-99m-methoxy isobutyl isonitrile and thallium-201 for evaluation of coronary artery disease by planar and tomographic methods. *Am Heart J* 1989:117:1–11.
5. Jain D, Wackers FJTh, Mattera J et al. Biokinetics of ^{99m}Tc-tetrofosmin, a new myocardial perfusion imaging agent: implications for a one-day imaging protocol. *J Nucl Med* 1993;34:1254–1259.
6. DePuey EG, Garcia EV, eds. Updated imaging guidelines for nuclear cardiology procedures, Part 1. *J Nucl Cardiol* 2001;8:G1–G54.
7. Wackers FJTh. Artifacts in planar and SPECT myocardial perfusion imaging. *Am J Cardiac Imaging* 1992;6:42–58.
8. Friedman J, Van Train K, Maddahi J et al. "Upward creep" of the heart: a frequent source of false-positive reversible defects during thallium-201 stress-redistribution SPECT. *J Nucl Med* 1989;30:1718–1722.
9. Maniawski PJ, Morgan HT, Wackers FJTh. Orbit related variation in spatial resolution as a source of artifactual defects in Tl-201 SPECT. *J Nucl Med* 1991;32:871–875.
10. Germano G, Chua T, Kiat H et al. A quantitative phantom analysis of artifacts due to hepatic activity in technetium-99m-myocardial perfusion SPECT studies. *J Nucl Med* 1994;35:356–359.
11. DePuey EG, Garcia EV, Berman DS, eds. *Cardiac SPECT imaging,* 2nd ed. Philadelphia: Lippincott, Williams & Wilkins, 2000.
12. Duvernoy CS, Ficaro EP, Karabajakian MZ et al. Improved detection of left main coronary artery disease with attenuation-corrected SPECT. *J Nucl Cardiol* 2000;7:639–648.
13. Wackers FJTh, Maniawski P, Sinusas AJ. Evaluation of left ventricular wall function by ECG-gated Tc-99m-sestamibi imaging. In: Beller GA, Zaret BL, eds. *Nuclear cardiology: state of the art and future direction.* St. Louis: Mosby, 1993:85–100.
14. Chua T, Yin LC, Thiang TH et al. Accuracy of the automated assessment of left ventricular function with gated perfusion SPECT in the presence of perfusion defects and left ventricular dysfunction: correlation with equilibrium radionuclide ventriculography and echocardiography. *J Nucl Cardiol* 2000;7:301–311.
15. Taillefer R, DePuey EG, Udelson JE et al. Comparison between the end-diastolic images and the summed images of gated Tc-99m-Tc-sestamibi SPECT perfusion study in detection of coronary artery disease in women. *J Nucl Cardiol* 1999;6:169–176.
16. Shen MYH, Liu Y, Sinusas AJ et al. Quantification of regional myocardial wall thickening on ECG-gated SPECT imaging. *J Nucl Cardiol* 1999;6:583–595.
17. Calnon DA, Kastner RJ, Smith WH et al: Validation of a new counts-based gated single photon emission computed tomography method of quantifying left ventricular systolic function: comparison with equilibrium radionuclide angiography. *J Nucl Cardiol* 1997;4:464.
18. Germano G, Kiat H, Kavanagh PB et al. Automated quantification of ejection fraction from gated myocardial perfusion SPECT. *J Nucl Med* 1995;36:2138–2147.
19. Liu YH, Sinusas AJ, Deman P et al. Quantification of SPECT myocardial perfusion images: methodology and validation of the Yale-CQ method. *J Nucl Cardiol* 1999;6:190–203.
20. Faber TL, Cooke CD, Folks RD et al. Left ventricular function and perfusion from gated SPECT perfusion images: an integrated method. *J Nucl Med* 1999;40:650–659.
21. Vallejo E, Dione DP, Sinusas AJ et al. Assessment of left ventricular ejection fraction with quantitative gated SPECT: accuracy and correlation with first-pass radionuclide angiography. *J Nucl Cardiol* 2000;7:461–470.
22. Nichols K, Yao S-S, Kamran M et al. Clinical impact of arrhythmias on gated SPECT cardiac myocardial perfusion and function assessment. *J Nucl Cardiol* 2001;8:19.
23. Johnson LL, Verdesca SA, Aude WY et al. Postischemic stunning can affect left ventricular ejection fraction and regional wall motion on post-stress gated sestamibi tomograms. *J Am Coll Cardiol* 1997;30:1641–1648.
23a. Wackers FJTh, Bodenheimer M, Fleiss JL et al. and the MSSMI Tl-201 Investigators. Factors affecting uniformity in interpretation of planar Tl-201 imaging in a multicenter trial. *J Am Coll Cardiol* 1993;21:1064–1074.
24. Gill JB, Ruddy TD, Newell JB et al. Prognostic importance of thallium uptake by the lungs during exercise in coronary artery disease. *N Engl J Med* 1987;317:1485–1489.
25. Marcassa C, Galli M, Baroffio C et al. Transient left ventricular dilation at quantitative stress-rest sestamibi tomography: clinical, electrocardiographic, and angiographic correlates. *J Nucl Cardiol* 1999;6:397–405.
26. Williams KA, Schneider CM. Increased stress right ventricular activity on dual isotope perfusion SPECT. *J Am Coll Cardiol* 1999;34:420.
27. Klein JL, Garcia EV, DePuey EG et al. Reversibility bull's-eye: a new polar bull's-eye map to quantify reversibility of stress-induced SPECT thallium-201 myocardial perfusion defects. *J Nucl Med* 1990;31:1240–1246.
28. Wackers FJTh, Bodenheimer M, Fleiss JL et al. and the MSSMI Tl-201 Investigators. Factors affecting uniformity in interpretation of planar Tl-201 imaging in a multicenter trial. *J Am Coll Cardiol* 1993;21:1064–1074.
29. Wackers FJTh, Becker AE, Samson G et al. Location and size of acute transmural myocardial infarction estimated from thallium-201 scintiscans. A clinicopathological study. *Circulation* 1977;56:71–78.
30. Page DL, Caulfield JB, Kastor JA et al. Myocardial changes associated with cardiogenic shock. *N Engl J Med* 1971;285:134.
31. Wackers FJTh, Gibbons RJ, Verani MS et al. Serial quantitative planar technetium-99m-isonitrile imaging in acute myocardial infarction: efficacy for noninvasive assessment of thrombolytic therapy. *J Am Coll Cardiol* 1989;14:861–873.
32. Gibbons RJ, Verani MS, Behrenbeck T et al. Feasibility of tomographic ^{99m}Tc-hexakis-2-methoxy-2-methylpropyl-isonitrile imaging for the assessment of myocardia area at risk and the effect of treatment in acute myocardial infarction. *Circulation* 1989;80:1278–1286.
33. Christian TF, Behrenbeck T, Pellikka PA et al. Mismatch of left ventricular function and infarct size demonstrated by technetium-99m isonitrile imaging after reperfusion therapy for acute myocardial infarction: identification of myocardial stunning and hyperkinesia. *J Am Coll Cardiol* 1990;16:1632–1638.
34. Wackers FJTh, Busemann Sokole E, Samson G et al. Value and limitations of thallium-201 scintigraphy in acute phase of myocardial infarction. *N Engl J Med* 1976;295:1.
35. Verani MS, Jeroudi MO, Mahmarian JJ et al. Quantification of myocardial infarction during coronary occlusion and myocardial salvage after reperfusion using cardiac imaging with technetium-99m hexakis 2-methoxyisobutyl isonitrile. *J Am Coll Cardiol* 1988;12:1573–1581.
36. Gibbons RJ, Holmes DR, Reeder GS et al. Immediate angioplasty compared with the administration of a thrombolytic agent followed by conservative treatment for myocardial infarction. *N Engl J Med* 1993;328:685–691.
37. Castro PF, Corbolan R, Baeza R et al. Effect of primary angioplasty on left ventricular function and myocardial perfusion as determined by Tc-99m sestamibi scintigraphy. *Am J Cardiol* 2001;87:1181–1184.
38. Cerqueira MD, Maynard C, Ritchie JL et al. Long-term survival in 618 patients from the western Washington streptokinase in myocardial infarction trials. *J Am Coll Cardiol* 1992;20:1452–1459.
39. Nestico PE, Hakki A, Felsher J et al. Implication of abnormal right ventricular thallium uptake in acute myocardial infarction. *Am J Cardiol* 1986;58:230.
40. Gibson RS, Watson DD, Craddock GB et al. Prediction of cardiac events after uncomplicated myocardial infarction: a prospective study comparing predischarge exercise thallium-201 scintigraphy and coronary angiography. *Circulation* 1983;68:321.
41. Brown KA, Heller GV, Landin RS et al. Early dipyridamole Tc-99m-sestamibi single photon emission computed tomographic imaging 2 to 4 days after acute myocardial infarction predicts in-hospital and

post-discharge cardiac events: comparison with sub-maximal exercise imaging. *Circulation* 1999;100:2060–2066.

42. Dakik HA, Mahmarian JJ, Kimball KT et al. Prognostic value of exercise 201-Tl tomography in patients treated with thrombolytic therapy during acute myocardial infarction. *Circulation* 1996;94: 2735–2742.

43. Wackers FJTh, Lie KI, Liem KL et al. Thallium-201 scintigraphy in unstable angina pectoris. *Circulation* 1978;57:738.

44. Bilodeau L, Theroux P, Gregoire J et al. Technetium-99m sestamibi tomography in patients with spontaneous chest pain: correlations with clinical, electrocardiographic and angiographic findings. *J Am Coll Cardiol* 1991;18:1684–1691.

45. Wackers FJTh, Lie KI, Liem KL et al. Potential value of thallium-201 scintigraphy as a means of selecting patients for the coronary care unit. *Br Heart J* 1979;41:111.

46. Tatum JL, Jesse RL, Kontos MC et al. Comprehensive strategy for the evaluation and triage of the chest pain patient. *Ann Emerg Med* 1997;29:116–125.

47. Heller GV, Stowers SA, Hendel RC et al. Clinical value of acute rest technetium-99m tetrofosmin tomographic myocardial perfusion imaging in patients with acute chest pain and nondiagnostic electrocardiograms. *J Am Coll Cardiol* 1998;31:1011.

48. Abbott BG, Abdel-Aziz I, Nagula S et al. Selective use of single-photon emission computed tomography myocardial perfusion imaging in a chest pain center. *Am J Cardiol* 2001;87:1351–1355.

49. Levine MG, Ahlberg AW, Mann A et al. Comparison of exercise, dipyridamole, adenosine, and dobutamine stress with the use of Tc-99m tetrofosmin tomographic imaging. *J Nucl Cardiol* 1999;6: 389–396.

50. Heo J, Kegel J, Iskandrian AS et al. Comparison of same-day protocols using technetium-99m-sestamibi myocardial imaging. *J Nucl Med* 1992;33:186–191

51. Berman DS, Kiat H, Friedman JD et al. Separate acquisitions rest thallium-201/stress technetium-99m sestamibi dual-isotope myocardial perfusion single-photon emission computed tomography: a clinical validation study. *J Am Coll Cardiol* 1993;22:1455–1464.

52. Henkin RE, Kalousdian S, Kikkawa RM et al. Diagnostic and therapeutic technology assessment (DATTA), myocardial perfusion imaging utilizing single-photon emission-computed tomography (SPECT). *Washington manual of therapeutic technology*. Washington, DC: 1994:2850.

53. Kiat H, Maddahi J, Roy L et al. Comparison of technetium 99m methoxy isobutyl isonitrile and thallium-201 for evaluation of coronary artery disease by planar and tomographic methods. *Am Heart J* 1989;117:111.

54. Iskandrian AS, Heo J, Long B et al. Use of technetium-99m isonitrile (RP-30A) in assessing left ventricular perfusion and function at rest and during exercise in coronary artery disease, and comparison with coronary arteriography and exercise thallium-201 SPECT imaging. *Am J Cardiol* 1989;64:270.

55. Kahn JK, McGhie I, Akers MS et al. Quantitative rotational tomography with ^{201}Tl and ^{99m}Tc 2-methoxly-isobutyl-isonitrile. *Circulation* 1989;79:1282.

56. Solot G, Hermans J, Merlo P et al. Correlation of 99Tcm-sestamibi SPECT with coronary angiography in general hospital practice. *Nucl Med Commun* 1993;14:23.

57. Van Train KF, Garcia EV, Maddahi J et al. Multicenter trial validation for quantitative analysis of same-day rest-stress technetium-99m-sestamibi myocardial tomograms. *J Nucl Med* 1994;35:609.

58. Azzarelli S, Galassi AR, Foti R et al. Accuracy of 99m-tetrofosmin myocardial tomography in the evaluation of coronary artery disease. *J Nucl Cardiol* 1999;6:183.

59. Rozanski A, Diamond GA, Berman D et al. The declining specificity of exercise radionuclide ventriculography. *New Engl J Med* 1983;309: 518–522.

60. Brown KA, Boucher CA, Okada RD et al. Prognostic value of exercise thallium-201 imaging in patients presenting for evaluation of chest pain. *J Am Coll Cardiol* 1983;1:994.

61. Ladenheim ML, Pollock BH, Rozanski A et al. Extent and severity of myocardial hypoperfusion as predictors of prognosis in patients with suspected coronary artery disease. *J Am Coll Cardiol* 1986;7:464.

62. Vanzetto G, Ormezzano O, Fagret D et al. Long term additive prognostic value of thallium-201 myocardial perfusion imaging over clinical and exercise stress test in low-to-intermediate risk patients. Study in 1,137 patients with 6 year-follow-up. *Circulation* 1999;100:1521.

63. Candell-Riera J, Pereztol-Valdez O, Santana-Boado C et al. Relationship between the location of the most severe myocardial perfusion defects, the most severe coronary artery stenosis, and the site of subsequent myocardial infarction. *J Nucl Med* 2001;42: 558–563.

64. Wackers FJTh, Russo DJ, Russo D et al. Prognostic significance of normal quantitative planar thallium-201 stress scintigraphy in patients with chest pain. *J Am Coll Cardiol* 1985;6:27.

65. Brown KA, Altland E, Rowen M. Prognostic value of normal Tc-99m sestamibi cardiac imaging. *J Nucl Med* 1994;35:554–557.

66. Raiker K, Sinusas AJ, Zaret BL et al. One-year prognosis of patients with normal Tc-99m-sestamibi stress imaging. *Circulation* 1993; 88(Suppl):1486.

67. Hachamovitch R, Berman DS, Shaw LJ et al. Incremental prognostic value of myocardial perfusion single photon emission computed tomography for the prediction of cardiac death. *Circulation* 1998;97: 535.

68. Soman P, Parsons A, Lahiri N et al. The prognostic value of a normal Tc-99m-sestamibi SPECT study in suspected coronary artery disease. *J Nucl Cardiol* 1999;6:252–256.

69. Haronian HL, Remetz MS, Sinusas AJ et al. Myocardial risk area defined by technetium-99m sestamibi imaging during percutaneous transluminal coronary angioplasty: comparison with coronary angiography. *J Am Coll Cardiol* 1993;22:1033–1043.

70. Zeiher, AM, Drause T, Schachinger V et al. Impaired endothelium-dependent vasodilation of coronary resistance vessels is associated with exercise-induced myocardial ischemia. *Circulation* 1995;91:2345.

71. Berman DS, Hachamovitch RH, Kiat H et al. Incremental value of prognostic testing in patients with known or suspected ischemic heart disease: a basis for optimal utilization of single-photon emission computed tomography. *J Am Coll Cardiol* 1993;6:665.

72. Palmas W, Friedman JD, Diamond GA et al. Incremental value of simultaneous assessment of myocardial function and perfusion with technetium-99m sestamibi for prediction of extent of coronary artery disease. *J Am Coll Cardiol* 1995;25:1024.

73. Mahmarian JJ, Mahmarian AC, Marks GF et al. Role of adenosine thallium-201 tomography for defining long-term risk in patients after acute myocardial infarction. *J Am Coll Cardiol* 1995;25:1333.

74. Hachamovitch R, Berman DI, Kiat H et al. Effective risk stratification using exercise myocardial perfusion SPECT women: gender-related differences in prognostic nuclear testing. *J Am Coll Cardiol* 1996;28: 34.

75. Hachamovitch R, Berman DS, Kiat H et al. Exercise myocardial perfusion SPECT in patients without known coronary artery disease: incremental prognostic value and impact on subsequent patients management. *Circulation* 1996;93:905.

76. Hachamovitch R, Shaw LJ, Berman DS. The ongoing evolution of risk stratification using myocardial perfusion imaging in patients with known or suspected coronary artery disease. *Acc Curr Rev* 1999;8:66.

77. Christian TF, Miller TD, Bailey KR et al. Exercise tomographic thallium-201 imaging in patients with severe coronary artery disease and normal electrocardiogram. *Ann Intern Med* 1994;121:825.

78. Mattera JA, Arain SA, Sinusas AJ et al. Exercise testing with myocardial perfusion imaging in patients with normal baseline electrocardiograms: cost saving with a stepwise diagnostic strategy. *J Nucl Cardiol* 1998;5:498.

79. Shaw LJ, Hachamovitch R, Berman DS et al. The economic consequences of available prognostic strategies for the evaluation of stable angina patients: an observational assessment of the value of precatheterization ischemia. Economics of noninvasive diagnosis (END) multicenter study group. *J Am Coll Cardiol* 1999;33:661.

80. Bateman TM, O'Keefe JH, Dong VM et al. Coronary angiography rates following stress SPECT scintigraphy. *J Nucl Cardiol* 1995;2: 217.

81. Sharir T, Germano G, Kavanagh PB et al. Incremental prognostic

value of post-stress left ventricular ejection fraction and volume by gated myocardial perfusion single photon emission computed tomography. *Circulation* 1999;100:1035–1042.

82. Sharir T, Germano G, Kang X et al. Prediction of myocardial infarction versus cardiac death by gated myocardial perfusion SPECT: risk stratification by the amount of stress-induced ischemia and poststress ejection fraction. *J Nucl Med* 2001;42:831–837.

83. Alazraki NP, Krawczynska EG, Kosinski AS et al. Prognostic value of thallium-201 single-photon emission computed tomography for patients with multivessel coronary artery disease after revascularization (the Emory Angioplasty versus Surgery Trial [EAST]). *Am J Cardiol* 1999;84:1369–1374.

84. Manyari DE, Knudson M, Kloibar R et al. Sequential thallium-201 myocardial perfusion studies after successful percutaneous transluminal coronary artery angioplasty: delayed resolution of exercise-induced scintigraphic abnormalities. *Circulation* 1988;77:86.

85. Miller DD, Verani MS. Current status of myocardial perfusion imaging after percutaneous transluminal coronary angioplasty. *J Am Coll Cardiol* 1994;24:260.

86. Garzon PP, Eisenberg MJ. Functional testing for the detection of restenosis after percutaneous transluminal coronary angioplasty: a meta-analysis. *Can J Cardiol* 2001;17:41–48.

87. Galassi AR, Foti R, Azzarelli S et al. Usefulness of exercise tomographic myocardial perfusion imaging for detection of restenosis after coronary stent implantation. *Am J Cardiol* 2000;85:1362–1364.

88. Berman DS, Kang X, Schisterman E et al. Serial changes on quantitative perfusion SPECT in patients undergoing revascularization or conservative therapy. *J Nucl Cardiol* 2001;8:428–437.

89. Boucher CA, Brewster DC, Darling RC et al. Determination of cardiac risk by dipyridamole-thallium imaging before peripheral vascular surgery. *N Engl J Med* 1985;312:389.

90. Hendel RC, Whitfield SS, Villegas BJ et al. Prediction of late cardiac events by dipyridamole thallium imaging in patients undergoing elective vascular surgery. *Am J Cardiol* 1992;70:1243–1249.

91. Lette J, Waters D, Bernier H et al. Preoperative and long term risk cardiac assessment. Predictive value of 23 clinical descriptors, 7 multivariants scoring systems and quantitative dipyridamole imaging in 360 patients. *Ann Surg* 1992;216:192.

92. Eagle KA, Singer DE, Brewster DC et al. Dipyridamole-thallium scanning patients undergoing vascular surgery. Optimizing preoperative evaluation of cardiac risk. *JAMA* 1987;257:2385–2189.

93. ACC/AHA Task Force Report. Guidelines for perioperative cardiovascular evaluation for noncardiac surgery. *J Am Coll Cardiol* 1996; 27:910–948.

94. Leppo JA, Dahlberg ST. The question: to test or not to test in preoperative cardiac risk evaluation. *J Nucl Cardiol* 1998;5:332.

95. Brown KA, Rowen M. Extent of jeopardized viable myocardium determined by myocardial perfusion imaging best predicts perioperative cardiac events in patients undergoing noncardiac surgery. *J Am Coll Cardiol* 1993;21:335–340.

96. Hirzel HO, Senn M, Neusch K et al. Thallium-201 scintigraphy in complete left bundle branch block. *Am J Cardiol* 1984;53:764.

97. Hodge J, Mattera J, Fetterman R et al. False-positive Tl-201 defects in left bundle branch block: relationship to left ventricular dilatation. *J Am Coll Cardiol* 1987;9:139A(abst).

98. O'Keefe JH, Bateman TM, Barnhart CS. Adenosine thallium-201 is superior to exercise thallium-201 for detecting coronary artery disease in patients with left bundle branch block. *J Am Coll Cardiol* 1993; 21:1332.

99. Nallamothu N, Bagheri B, Acio ER et al. Prognostic value of stress myocardial perfusion single photon emission computed tomography imaging in patients with left bundle branch block. *J Nucl Cardiol* 1997;4:487.

100. Danias PG, Ahlberg AW, Clark III BA et al. Combined assessment of myocardial perfusion and left ventricular function with exercise technetium-99m sestamibi gated single-photon emission computed tomography can differentiate between ischemic and nonischemic dilated cardiomyopathy. *Am J Cardiol* 1998;82:1253–1258.

101. Abramson BL, Ruddy TD, DeKemp RA et al. Stress perfusion/metabolism imaging: a pilot study for a potential new approach to the diagnosis of coronary artery disease in women. *J Nucl Cardiol* 2000; 7:205–212.

102. Weinstein H, Reinhardt CP, Leppo JA. Direct detection of regional myocardial ischemia with technetium-99m nitroimidazole in rabbits. *J Nucl Med* 1998;39:598–607.

Diagnostic Nuclear Medicine, Fourth Edition. Edited by M.P. Sandler, R.E. Coleman, J.A. Patton, F.J.Th. Wackers, A. Gottschalk. Lippincott Williams & Wilkins, Philadelphia 2003.

16

ASSESSMENT OF MYOCARDIAL VIABILITY

ROBERT O. BONOW

In patients with chronic coronary artery disease, left ventricular function is among the most important determinants of long-term prognosis (1–5). In general, patients with normal or near-normal left ventricular systolic function have an excellent outcome whether treated with medical therapy or with revascularization procedures. In contrast, the large subgroup of patients with moderate to severe left ventricular dysfunction is at considerable risk of death during the course of medical therapy (Fig. 16.1). Patients with impaired ventricular function at particular risk are those with inducible myocardial ischemia, poor exercise tolerance, or evidence of complex ventricular ectopic activity. Hence, exercise testing and arrhythmia monitoring are commonly used in the risk stratification of patients with left ventricular dysfunction.

Testing to evaluate the presence and extent of viable but dysfunctional myocardium in such patients is less well established, but an increasing database indicates the clinical importance of assessing myocardial viability in patients with coronary artery disease and impaired ventricular function (6,7). It has been firmly established that a large subset of patients with left ventricular dysfunction undergoing myocardial revascularization will manifest marked improvement in ventricular function after myocardial revascularization (6–12), including normalization of ventricular function in some patients. The term for this potentially reversible form of left ventricular dysfunction is *myocardial hibernation,* indicating a condition in which myocardial contractility has been reduced in the setting of a sustained reduction in myocardial blood supply (9–12). The concept of hibernation has been challenged in recent years, and an alternative concept has been proposed of persistent left ventricular dysfunction caused by repeated episodes of myocardial ischemia leading to repetitive stunning (13,14). Independent of the mechanism, which is difficult to determine clinically, the important clinical issue is that viable but dysfunctional myocardium in patients with chronic coronary artery disease will improve in function only if identified and revascularized.

Although the percentage of patients who have an important

reversal of left ventricular dysfunction after revascularization varies among reported series (probably related to patient selection factors and revascularization techniques), it is not inconsequential. It has been shown in several surgical series that 25% to 40% of patients (Fig. 16.2) with chronic coronary artery disease and left ventricular dysfunction have the potential for marked improvement in ventricular function (15,16). These findings have several implications. First, given the important relation between left ventricular function and survival (Fig. 16.1), the improvement in ventricular function after revascularization may translate into an improvement in survival. Although definitive data that tie improved function to improved survival are lacking, many recent retrospective studies have begun to establish this point, as discussed later. Second, the decision to proceed with revascularization in patients with moderate to severe left ventricular dysfunction often is difficult. Such patients undergo coronary artery bypass surgery or coronary angioplasty with considerable risk of procedure-related morbidity and mortality. The perioperative mortality associated with surgical revascularization of patients with left ventricular dysfunction is approximately 10%. Hence, accurate methods to detect viable myocardium distal to a coronary stenosis, with the potential for reversal of left ventricular dysfunction, are essential to select in a prospective manner patients for whom these risks are justified.

At present, several clinically reliable physiologic markers of viability can be used for this purpose. These include indexes of regional coronary blood flow, regional wall motion, and regional systolic wall thickening. These are accurate markers of viability when they are normal or nearly normal but have major limitations in the identification of viable myocardium when severely reduced or absent. In the setting of hibernating myocardium, by definition, indexes of regional perfusion and systolic function (regional wall motion and wall thickening) will be severely reduced or absent despite maintenance of tissue viability (9–12). Thus these three indexes are imprecise in differentiating hibernating myocardium from myocardial scar.

Although measures of baseline systolic function are imprecise indicators of viability, contractile reserve is maintained in viable, hibernating myocardium, and this index can be assessed readily with low-dose dobutamine echocardiography (6,17–19). Numerous studies attest to the accuracy of dobutamine echocardiography in unmasking dysfunctional but viable myocardium and

R.O. Bonow: Department of Medicine, Division of Cardiology, Northwestern University Medical School and Northwestern Memorial Hospital, Chicago, IL.

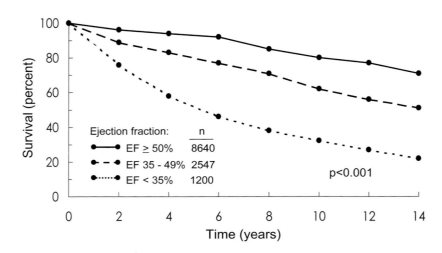

FIGURE 16.1. Influence of resting left ventricular ejection fraction (*EF*) on survival during medical therapy in patients in the Coronary Artery Surgery Study (CASS) Registry. (Modified from Emond M, Mock MB, Davis KB, et al. Long-term survival of medically treated patients in the Coronary Artery Surgery Study (CASS) Registry. *Circulation* 1994;90:2645–2657, with permission of Lippincott Williams & Wilkins.)

in predicting recovery of function after revascularization. This remains an exciting area of current investigation.

During the past decade, numerous studies have demonstrated that nuclear cardiology techniques involving single-photon methods as well as positron emission tomography (PET) also provide critically important information about viability in patients with left ventricular dysfunction. This chapter reviews the strengths, applications, and limitations of nuclear cardiology procedures for the assessment of myocardial viability.

201TL IMAGING TO ASSESS MYOCARDIAL VIABILITY

In the setting of reduced blood flow and oxygen availability, tissue viability can be maintained only if persistent metabolic activity is maintained at a sufficient level to meet the energy demands required to maintain a number of fundamental cellular processes. This includes sufficient energy, among other processes, to prevent irreversible configurational changes of struc-

tural and contractile proteins, to prevent ischemic contracture of myocytes, to prevent disruption of mitochondria, and to maintain sarcolemmal, sarcoplasmic reticulum, and mitochondrial membrane integrity. Maintenance of membrane integrity also implies preservation of electrochemical gradients across the sarcolemma. These processes can persist only if a critical level of blood flow is maintained. Sufficient blood flow is necessary both to deliver the substrates for the metabolic processes and to wash out the byproducts of these processes. For example, the metabolites of the glycolytic pathway include lactate and hydrogen ion (20,21), which have inhibitory effects on glycolytic enzymes. The intracellular accumulation of lactate and hydrogen ion result ultimately in termination of glycolysis, depletion of high-energy phosphates, cell membrane disruption, and cell death. The dependence on a critical level of blood flow as well as preservation of membrane function suggests that in theory imaging agents that reflect regional myocardial blood flow and membrane integrity should provide excellent information regarding tissue viability. Because retention of ^{201}Tl with time is an active process that is a function of cell viability and cell mem-

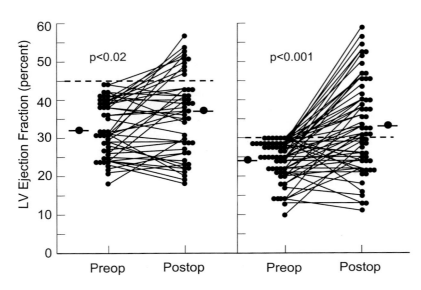

FIGURE 16.2. Left ventricular ejection fraction at rest measured with radionuclide ventriculography before (*Preop*) and after (*Postop*) coronary artery bypass surgery in patients with preoperative left ventricular dysfunction in two surgical series (15,16). Although the operation resulted in only a small increase in mean ejection fraction, substantial increases in ejection fraction were observed in a substantial subset of patients, and ejection fraction normalized in many patients. (From Bonow RO. The hibernating myocardium: implications for management of congestive heart failure. *Am J Cardiol* 1995;75:17A–25A (left panel) and Elefteriades JA, Tolis G Jr., Levi E, et al. Coronary artery bypass grafting in severe left ventricular dysfunction: excellent survival with improved ejection fraction and functional state. *J Am Coll Cardiol* 1993; 22:1411–1417 (right panel), with permission of Elsevier Publishing Company.)

brane activity, ^{201}Tl should perform well as a marker of myocardial viability.

Thallium Redistribution as a Marker of Viability

The single most important index of viability with ^{201}Tl imaging is the demonstration of reversibility of a perfusion defect, that is, net accumulation of ^{201}Tl in a myocardial territory with contractile dysfunction relative to the washout of ^{201}Tl in a normally perfused territory. Myocardial regions that are precariously balanced, with such a marked reduction in flow as to cause contractile dysfunction at rest, are likely to manifest even greater flow inhomogeneity relative to normal regions during either exercise or pharmacologic stress imaging. Hence a large number (if not most) of these regions manifest reversible ^{201}Tl perfusion defects when a standard stress-redistribution imaging protocol is used. The demonstration of stress-induced reversible ischemia in regions with contractile dysfunction is evidence of the viability of these regions and of the potential for substantial improvement in function after revascularization. The positive predictive value of a reversible ^{201}Tl defect regarding improvement in function after coronary artery bypass surgery or angioplasty is excellent.

In contrast, the negative predictive value of an irreversible ^{201}Tl defect is relatively poor. Many regions of severely ischemic or hibernating myocardium do not demonstrate appreciable reversibility of ^{201}Tl defects during conventional exercise-redistribution imaging. Fifty percent or more of regions with apparently "irreversible" ^{201}Tl defects improve in function after successful revascularization (22–26). Hence because of this poor negative predictive accuracy, it is now accepted that standard stress-redistribution ^{201}Tl scintigraphy does not have satisfactory precision in differentiating hibernating myocardium from fibrotic myocardium in patients with coronary artery disease and left ventricular dysfunction. It is well established that modifications in imaging protocols with ^{201}Tl considerably enhance the ability of ^{201}Tl imaging to depict viable myocardium (6,12,27). These include late redistribution imaging and ^{201}Tl reinjection techniques.

Late Thallium Redistribution Imaging

In a considerable number of patients, late imaging, 24 to 72 hours after stress, elicits ^{201}Tl redistribution in many defects that appear to be irreversible 3 to 4 hours after stress, and this late ^{201}Tl redistribution is evidence of viable myocardium (25, 28–30). As many as 54% of defects irreversible 3 to 4 hours after stress show reversibility 24 hours after stress, although this number is as low as 22% in some studies. ^{201}Tl redistribution is a continual process (31), and a truly irreversible defect on early redistribution images will not reverse at a later time. However, it is also true that in a number of viable regions, the magnitude of defect reversal at 3 to 4 hours may be minimal and poorly detected. Hence the defect may not reverse appreciably on qualitative interpretation, and the increase in relative tracer activity also may not exceed the reproducibility limit by quantitative analysis. In such regions, late redistribution imaging may enhance the certainty that the defect has reversed itself.

The positive predictive value of late redistribution is greater than 90% (29) for improvement after revascularization; thus that a defect has reversed itself on late images is an excellent marker of viable myocardium. However, even though imaging 24 hours after stress helps identify a greater number of reversible defects than does imaging 3 to 4 hours after stress, there are important limitations of late-redistribution imaging. The negative predictive accuracy of the presence of an irreversible defect at 24 hours appears little better than that of the presence of an irreversible defect at 3 to 4 hours. It has been shown, for example, that 37% of irreversible defects at 24 hours improve after revascularization (29). Moreover, 39% of irreversible defects at 24 hours show improvement according to results of quantitative analysis when ^{201}Tl is reinjected while the patient is at rest (32). Hence it appears that a considerable number of dysfunctional but viable myocardial segments do not demonstrate redistribution after a stress ^{201}Tl study, no matter how lengthy the redistribution period.

Thallium Reinjection Imaging

Reinjection of ^{201}Tl, either after the standard 3- to 4-hour redistribution image (33–35) or after a late 24-hour redistribution image (32), facilitates late uptake of ^{201}Tl in many viable regions with apparently irreversible defects and can be used to differentiate viable and infarcted myocardium. The available data indicate that the reinjection technique provides greater accuracy for the detection of viable myocardium than either early or late redistribution imaging. As many as 49% of "irreversible" defects on 4-hour redistribution images (33) and 39% of such defects on 24-hour redistribution images (32) show improved or normal uptake after ^{201}Tl reinjection (32,33). A number of studies of patients with left ventricular dysfunction have shown the efficacy of thallium reinjection imaging for prediction of improved wall motion after revascularization (6,26,33,36,37).

An imaging protocol that includes stress and redistribution images with ^{201}Tl reinjection as necessary will provide most of the viability information that can be obtained from ^{201}Tl imaging. Rarely do late redistribution images after reinjection provide important additional information not achieved with the earlier three-image acquisitions (38).

On the other hand, a protocol that includes three sets of ^{201}Tl image acquisitions (stress, redistribution, and reinjection) creates logistical constraints for the laboratory and inconvenience for the patient. Several modifications of the reinjection technique to streamline the imaging protocol are currently in clinical practice. The first of these involves the routine reinjection of ^{201}Tl 3 to 4 hours after stress without acquiring redistribution images. This approach improves efficiency and helps with identification of viable myocardium in most patients in whom the redistribution images would have been misleading by showing persistent defects. This approach has an important limitation, however, because a number of patients with left ventricular dysfunction have reduced regional myocardial perfusion at rest. This is the definition of *myocardial hibernation*. In a subset of these patients, ^{201}Tl redistribution occurs after exercise or pharmacologic stress. However, reinjection of ^{201}Tl at rest increases ^{201}Tl uptake in the normally perfused territories to a greater extent

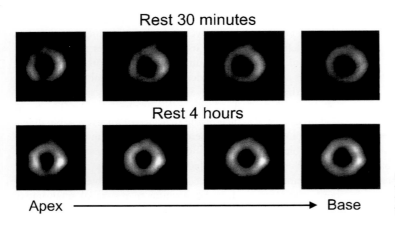

Rest 30 minutes

Rest 4 hours

Apex ──────────────────▶ Base

FIGURE 16.3. Rest-redistribution thallium imaging in a patient with severe heart failure and left ventricular dysfunction (ejection fraction, 29%). Substantial redistribution of thallium is evident in the anterior, septal, and inferior left ventricular myocardium.

than in the hypoperfused territories, resulting in the appearance of relative ^{201}Tl "washout" compared with the redistribution image. This differential uptake of ^{201}Tl results in a defect on stress images that improves or normalizes on the redistribution images but then reappears on the reinjection images (33,39). In such patients, the reinjection images may mirror the stress images, and it is the redistribution image, not the reinjection image, that provides the important information regarding reversibility of a defect and, hence, viability. Although this effect occurs in only a small subset of patients, elimination of the redistribution data creates uncertainties regarding the interpretation of an irreversible defect when a stress-reinjection protocol is used (39).

The second modification of the reinjection protocol is early reinjection of ^{201}Tl immediately after completion of acquisition of the stress images (40–42). Imaging is repeated 3 to 4 hours later. This allows both the reinjected ^{201}Tl dose and the initial stress ^{201}Tl dose to redistribute together for several hours before imaging is performed. Although this method is attractive in concept, the available data indicate mixed results. One study had favorable results with an early reinjection protocol (41). However, two other studies have shown that defects that persist 3 hours after early reinjection show later reversal if either 24-hour

redistribution imaging or ^{201}Tl reinjection is performed (40, 42).

Rest-Redistribution Thallium Imaging

Exercise ^{201}Tl imaging produces the uncertainty of whether a defect on stress images represents ischemic myocardium that must be unmasked with further redistribution or reinjection images. Exercise imaging also imposes questions regarding which of the many possible imaging protocols to unmask viable myocardium is most efficacious and logistically practical. If the sole clinical issue to be addressed is the viability of one or more left ventricular regions with systolic dysfunction, and not whether there is also inducible ischemia, rest-redistribution ^{201}Tl imaging is a practical approach that can yield accurate viability data. A resting protocol to assess viability must include both initial images (indicating regional perfusion) and subsequent redistribution images (Fig. 16.3). Although early experience with resting ^{201}Tl protocols yielded mixed results regarding the predictive accuracy of rest-redistribution imaging (43–45), results of recent studies indicate that quantitative analysis of regional ^{201}Tl activity in rest-redistribution studies can be used to predict recovery

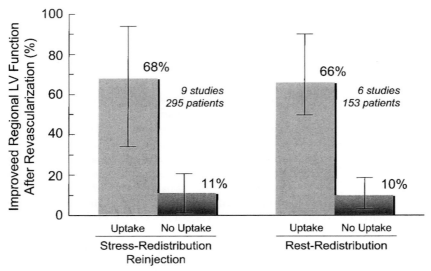

FIGURE 16.4. Likelihood of improvement in regional left ventricular function based on published reports of stress-redistribution-reinjection and rest-redistribution thallium imaging. *Horizontal bars* connected by *vertical lines* indicate the range of reported values in individual studies. (From Bonow RO. Assessment of myocardial viability with thallium-201. In: Zaret BL, Beller GA, eds. *Nuclear cardiology: state of the art and future directions.* St. Louis: Mosby, 1998:503–512, with permission of Mosby.)

of regional left ventricular function (46). The results compare favorably with the results of ^{201}Tl exercise-reinjection imaging and metabolic PET (47).

The data available from comparisons of rest-redistribution imaging and stress-redistribution-reinjection imaging indicate similar positive and negative predictive values for recovery of regional function after revascularization (48). Both techniques have high sensitivity, yielding a negative predictive value greater than 90% (Fig. 16.4). However, specificity is much lower, yielding a positive predictive value less than 70%. A limitation of this analysis is that that thallium data are considered in a binomial manner rather than as a continuum. When data are assessed across the continuum of thallium activity in dysfunctional regions (Fig. 16.5), a nearly linear relation has been observed between regional thallium activity and likelihood of recovery after revascularization (19). This continuous relation between thallium activity and myocardial viability is confirmed with histologic studies of myocardial biopsy specimens obtained at surgery (49). These results show a significant inverse relation between thallium uptake and the degree of myocardial interstitial fibrosis (Fig. 16.6).

There are cogent reasons to consider exercise imaging for most patients with left ventricular dysfunction. The demonstration of exercise-induced ischemia has important prognostic implications that under most conditions identifies the patient as a candidate for revascularization therapy. Although this may be true of all patients with coronary artery disease, it is especially true of patients with left ventricular dysfunction. Evidence of inducible ischemia superimposed on impaired left ventricular function at rest characterizes a subgroup of patients at considerable risk of death during medical therapy.

Another consideration that favors stress imaging is the observation that many persistent defects on rest-redistribution images have only a mild decrease in relative ^{201}Tl activity. Although the ^{201}Tl uptake in such a region indicates it is viable, this does not ensure improvement in function if revascularization is performed. Only slightly more than 60% of mild persistent defects on rest-redistribution studies improve after revascularization

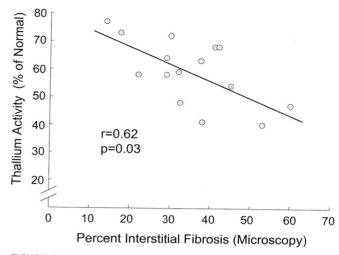

FIGURE 16.6. Regional thallium activity in dysfunctional myocardial regions assessed by means of SPECT and plotted as a function of the percentage of interstitial fibrosis in myocardial biopsy specimens obtained in the same regions. (From Zimmerman R, Mall G, Rauch B, et al. Residual 201Tl activity in irreversible defects as a marker of myocardial viability: clinicopathological study. *Circulation* 1995;91:1016–1021, with permission of Lippincott Williams & Wilkins.)

(46). Defect reversibility is a better predictor of improvement after revascularization than is level of ^{201}Tl activity per se (37). Many persistent defects on thallium rest-redistribution images exhibit greater flow heterogeneity with exercise, indicating the presence of a more severe defect than is present on the rest study (47). The result is an exercise-induced defect with partial reversibility at rest, which is more convincing evidence of viability than is a persistent resting defect. Thus the exercise-redistribution-reinjection ^{201}Tl protocol has the attraction, not present in the rest-redistribution ^{201}Tl protocol, that it provides important information regarding both jeopardized myocardium and viable myocardium. On the other hand, the same ischemia and viability information can be obtained when rest-redistribution ^{201}Tl imaging is performed as part of a dual-isotope stress-rest

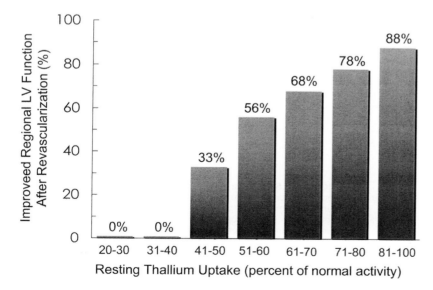

FIGURE 16.5. Nearly linear relation between the percentage of peak thallium activity on rest-redistribution images and the likelihood of segmental improvement after revascularization. Although various cutoff values have been proposed as "thresholds" for viability, this figure indicates the continuous nature of this relation. (From Perrone-Filardi P, Pace L, Prastaro M, et al. Dobutamine echocardiography predicts improvement of hypoperfused dysfunctional myocardium after revascularization in patients with coronary artery disease. *Circulation* 1995;91:2556–2565, with permission of Lippincott Williams & Wilkins.)

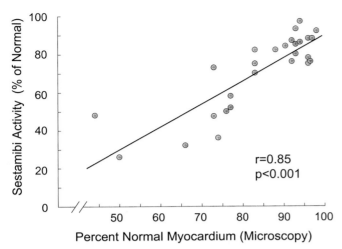

FIGURE 16.7. Regional sestamibi activity assessed on SPECT images in dysfunctional myocardial regions plotted as a function of the percentage of viable myocardium in myocardial biopsy specimens obtained in the same regions. (From Dakik HA, Howell JF, Lawria GM, et al. Assessment of myocardial viability with 99mTc-sestamibi tomography before coronary bypass graft surgery: correlation with histopathology and postoperative improvement in cardiac function. *Circulation* 1997;96: 2892-2898, with permission of Lippincott Williams & Wilkins.)

protocol. The rest-redistribution ^{201}Tl protocol can be incorporated readily into the daily routine of laboratories that have adopted a dual-isotope [99m]Tc-^{201}Tl imaging protocol for stress-rest imaging. Thus a ^{99m}Tc-based perfusion tracer can be used to assess stress perfusion and ^{201}Tl to assess resting perfusion. Resting perfusion defects can then be further evaluated with redistribution imaging before the stress ^{99m}Tc study or 24 hours after the ^{99m}Tc study.

99MTC PERFUSION IMAGING TO ASSESS VIABILITY

[99m]Tc sestamibi, like ^{201}Tl, requires intact sarcolemmal and mitochondrial processes for retention. This agent has been shown to be an excellent marker of cellular viability (50–52). In both experimental and clinical settings in which ^{99m}Tc sestamibi delivery to dysfunctional myocardium is adequate, such as after reperfusion to previously ischemic or damaged myocardium, the uptake and retention of ^{99m}Tc sestamibi tracks with markers of myocardial viability rather than with pure markers of perfusion (51,53–55). However, ^{99m}Tc-sestamibi does not redistribute as avidly as does ^{201}Tl after its initial uptake, either during exercise or at rest. Thus compared with ^{201}Tl, ^{99m}Tc sestamibi would appear to have inherent weaknesses for viability assessment in clinical situations in which blood flow is severely impaired and tracer delivery is reduced (56). This hypothesis was supported by results of initial studies comparing rest-exercise ^{99m}Tc sestamibi imaging to exercise-redistribution-reinjection ^{201}Tl imaging. These results showed that use of ^{99m}Tc sestamibi leads to underestimates of viable myocardium in patients with chronic coronary artery disease and left ventricular dysfunction (57–60).

A number of subsequent studies have provided consistent and convincing evidence indicating the potential of ^{99m}Tc sestamibi for viability assessment in patients with left ventricular dysfunction. First, ^{99m}Tc sestamibi is well established as an excellent perfusion tracer for detecting inducible myocardial ischemia, whether left ventricular function is normal or depressed, and ischemic myocardium is viable myocardium. As is the case with ^{201}Tl imaging, myocardial regions with systolic dysfunction that manifest reversible ischemia during ^{99m}Tc sestamibi imaging have a very high likelihood of recovery of function after revascularization. Moreover, a number of studies have shown that a quantitative analysis of ^{99m}Tc sestamibi activity in regions with perfusion defects at rest provides important insights into the potential for improved function with revascularization (61–66). As with ^{201}Tl imaging, there is a continuous inverse relation between regional ^{99m}Tc sestamibi activity and the extent of interstitial fibrosis measured in myocardial biopsy specimens (63,65) (Fig. 16.7). This observation translates into a continuous relation, similar to that observed during ^{201}Tl imaging, between regional ^{99m}Tc sestamibi activity and the likelihood of improvement in regional function after revascularization (Fig

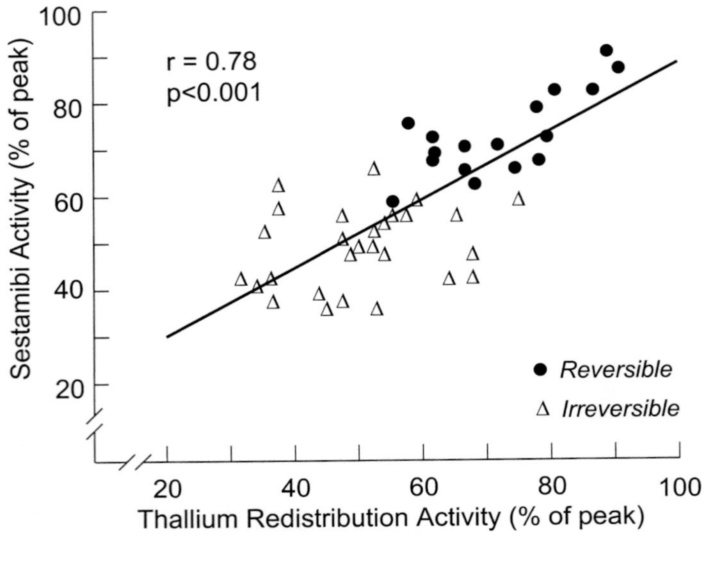

FIGURE 16.8. Comparison of regional sestamibi activity at rest and redistribution thallium activity on rest-redistribution images of dysfunctional myocardium in patients before coronary bypass surgery. Both tracers show a continuous relation relative to the likelihood of functional improvement after revascularization. (From Udelson JE, Coleman PS, Matherall JA, et al. Predicting recovery of severe regional ventricular dysfunction: comparison of resting scintigraphy with thallium-201 and technetium-99m sestamibi. *Circulation* 1994;89:2552-2561, with permission of Lippincott Williams & Wilkins.)

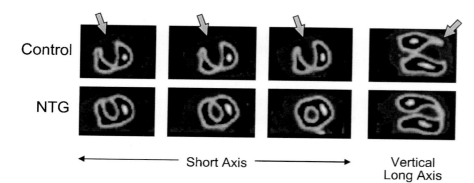

Control

NTG

← ——— Short Axis ——— →   Vertical Long Axis

FIGURE 16.9. Nitrate-enhanced sestamibi image shows enhanced tracer uptake in the anterior wall and apex in areas of diminished sestamibi uptake at rest (*arrows*) after nitrate administration. (From Maurea S, Cuocolo A, Soricelli A, et al. Enhanced detection of viable myocardium by technetium-99m-MIBI imaging after nitrate administration in chronic coronary artery disease. *J Nucl Med* 1995;36:1945-1952, with permission of the Society of Nuclear Medicine.)

16.8). Regional ^{99m}Tc sestamibi activity at rest correlates more strongly with ^{201}Tl imaging redistribution activity than with the initial uptake of ^{201}Tl when resting ^{99m}Tc sestamibi imaging is compared directly with rest-redistribution ^{201}Tl imaging in the same patients (62,67,68). Another approach with which to optimize viability assessment with ^{99m}Tc sestamibi is administration of nitroglycerin (Fig 16.9). Several studies have shown that use of nitrates improves detection of viable myocardium, presumably because of enhancement of collateral blood flow (69–73).

^{99m}Tc sestamibi can be used for viability assessment by means of one or a combination of three approaches—reversibility of stress-induced defects, severity of resting defects, or nitrate-enhanced ^{99m}Tc sestamibi imaging at rest. The combination of all three of these approaches would optimize the use of ^{99m}Tc sestamibi for detecting viable but dysfunctional myocardium.

Investigations with ^{99m}Tc tetrofosmin for assessing myocardial viability are limited. Because both agents require active processes for mitochondrial uptake, ^{99m}Tc tetrofosmin should perform in a similar manner to ^{99m}Tc sestamibi, but this concept has not been firmly established in a large enough number of patients to provide definitive conclusions at this time.

POSITRON EMISSION TOMOGRAPHY

PET is established as an exceptional tool for identifying viable myocardium in patients with impaired left ventricular function (74–77). Several PET methods have been developed for this purpose. The method with the greatest cumulative clinical experience and the most extensive documentation in the literature is imaging with ^{18}F-fluorodeoxyglucose (FDG), a marker of regional exogenous glucose use, to identify preserved metabolic activity in regions of severely underperfused and dysfunctional myocardium (74,77–82). Thus PET imaging can be used to assess directly the persistent metabolic activity necessary to maintain cellular viability.

^{18}F-Fluorodeoxyglucose Imaging for Viability Assessment

A pattern of enhanced uptake of FDG relative to blood flow in regions with reduced perfusion, called *FDG–blood flow mismatch* (Fig. 16.10) indicates viable myocardium in which the metabolic substrate preference has been shifted toward greater glucose use rather than use of fatty acids or lactate (78–82). The finding of FDG–blood flow mismatch in myocardial regions with impaired systolic function was shown in several studies to be an accurate marker for differentiating viable from nonviable myocardium. The cumulative experience from six studies, including a total of 146 patients with left ventricular dysfunction undergoing myocardial revascularization procedures, indicates that the finding of FDG–blood flow mismatch has a positive accuracy of 82% and a negative accuracy of 83% in prediction of recovery of regional function after myocardial revascularization (6,79, 82–86).

Identification of viable tissue with FDG–blood flow mis-

^{13}NH$_3$ ^{18}FDG

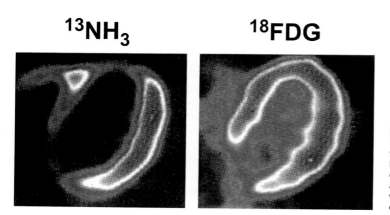

FIGURE 16.10. PET assessment of myocardial viability. Transaxial PET images show FDG–blood flow mismatch in the anterior and septal walls as a marker of underperfused but metabolically active and viable myocardium. (From Maddahi J, Schelbert H, Brunken R, et al. Role of thallium-201 and PET imaging in evaluation of myocardial viability and management of patients with coronary artery disease and left ventricular dysfunction. *J Nucl Med* 1994;35:707-715, with permission of the Society of Nuclear Medicine.)

match has several important, clinically relevant implications. First, augmentation of regional systolic function after revascularization, as predicted with FDG–blood flow mismatch, results in a tangible and predictable increase in ejection fraction. In several studies, global left ventricular function significantly and consistently increased after revascularization in patients with FDG–blood flow mismatch on pre-revascularization PET studies. The average ejection fraction increased from 32% before to 45% after revascularization (74,84,86,87). There is also evidence that the extent and magnitude of FDG–blood flow mismatch in a patient with left ventricular dysfunction can be used to predict the magnitude of recovery in global left ventricular function after revascularization (74,88).

^{18}F-Fluorodeoxyglucose Imaging Compared with Thallium Imaging

In keeping with the limitations of ^{201}Tl redistribution imaging for assessment of myocardial viability, several studies have shown that metabolic PET imaging with FDG is superior to standard exercise-redistribution ^{201}Tl scintigraphy for this assessment, when both techniques are performed on the same patients (89–92). Between 38% and 47% of irreversible ^{201}Tl defects on 3- to 4-hour redistribution images in these studies were determined to be metabolically active on the corresponding PET images. Similarly, 51% of persistent defects on late (24-hour) redistribution images were metabolically active with FDG uptake on PET images (93). These data provide further evidence that early and late redistribution imaging leads to overestimates of the presence and severity of myocardial fibrosis.

A much better concordance between PET and ^{201}Tl imaging is obtained with ^{201}Tl reinjection methods (94–96). Among patients with chronic coronary artery disease and left ventricular dysfunction who underwent both stress-redistribution-reinjection ^{201}Tl imaging and PET imaging with FDG, most segments with ^{201}Tl defects identified as viable with ^{201}Tl reinjection had FDG uptake and hence metabolic evidence of myocardial viability (94–96). Although overall concordance between the ^{201}Tl reinjection and FDG uptake data is excellent, the frequency with which irreversible ^{201}Tl defects (even with reinjection) manifest FDG uptake remains a subject of uncertainty and debate.

^{18}F-Fluorodeoxyglucose Imaging Compared with ^{99m}Tc Sestamibi Imaging

Only two studies have been conducted to compare quantitative regional ^{99m}Tc sestamibi activity with regional FDG activity in the same patients (60,61). Unfortunately, these two investigations reached conflicting conclusions regarding the correlation between regional ^{99m}Tc sestamibi activity as an index of viability compared with FDG activity. These differences may reflect the small numbers of patients studied or differences between the methods used in the two studies. No firm conclusions can be drawn regarding comparisons between ^{99m}Tc sestamibi and PET imaging until more data are available.

Alternative Positron Emission Tomographic Techniques for Identifying Viable Myocardium

Three methods to assess viability with PET without using FDG have been described, but these have not been studied extensively. Identification of preserved oxidative metabolism by means of PET with ^{11}C acetate has been shown to be an accurate marker for viable myocardium in patients with left ventricular dysfunction and for prediction of recovery of regional left ventricular function after revascularization (83). Other PET methods for assessment of myocardial viability include the use of ^{15}O water to determine the amount of perfusable tissue within dysfunctional myocardial segments (97,98) and analysis of ^{82}Rb uptake and washout kinetics in regions with impaired systolic function (99). Each of these three PET applications have thus far been used in examinations of only a small number of patients, and each report has been from only a single institution. Greater clinical experience is needed before these methods can be recommended for routine purposes.

SINGLE PHOTON EMISSION TOMOGRAPHY VERSUS POSITRON EMISSION TOMOGRAPHY FOR VIABILITY ASSESSMENT

Because viability requires both intact membrane function and maintenance of metabolic processes, markers of cell-membrane integrity should be, in theory, equally efficacious for assessing myocardial viability as are indicators of metabolic activity. Thus the relative accuracy of PET or single photon emission tomography (SPECT) methods in identifying viable myocardium are related less to the underlying physiologic processes being measured than to the ability to image these processes with existing SPECT or PET detectors. In this regard, there are several advantages to PET approaches, including improved image resolution, the ability to correct for photon attenuation, and the ability to assess metabolic activity independent of perfusion. Advantages of SPECT imaging include the ability to assess inducible ischemia along with viability as part of a routine comprehensive imaging protocol. Identification of inducible ischemia provides both prognostic information and viability information (ischemic myocardium, by definition, is viable myocardium). Viability also can be assessed with ^{201}Tl or ^{99m}Tc sestamibi imaging for all patients without the standardized and controlled metabolic conditions necessary for FDG PET studies. With these considerations in mind, the principal advantage of PET is the availability of routine attenuation-correction algorithms (75,76). The current SPECT protocols share the limiting feature of photon attenuation of a low-energy radioisotope, in which apparently irreversible ^{201}Tl or ^{99m}Tc sestamibi defects suggesting fibrosis may be merely attenuation artifacts in viable tissue. Thus it is anticipated that imaging with ^{201}Tl or with ^{99m}Tc-based agents will not achieve the accuracy of PET for viability assessment until techniques to correct for photon attenuation are perfected for SPECT. However, effective attenuation-correction algorithms are on the horizon for routine use with multiheaded SPECT systems (100).

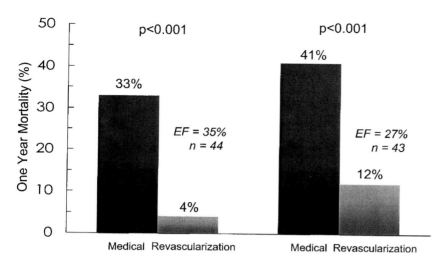

FIGURE 16.11. One-year mortality rates among patients with left ventricular dysfunction and evidence of viable myocardium, determined according to FDG–blood flow mismatch on PET images by Eitzman et al. (101) (*left*) and Di Carli et al. (102) (*right*). In both series, patients treated medically had a higher 1-year mortality rate than did patients undergoing myocardial revascularization.

PROGNOSTIC IMPLICATIONS OF VIABILITY ASSESSMENT

Medical Therapy versus Revascularization in Patients with Viable Myocardium

The demonstration of viable myocardium in patients with coronary artery disease and left ventricular dysfunction appears to indicate a particularly poor prognosis with medical therapy. The available data indicate that these patients have improved survival with revascularization therapy. These observations, initially made with PET, have now been confirmed with SPECT.

Several investigators using PET have reported that myocardial revascularization in patients with underperfused but metabolically active myocardium significantly improves survival compared with the survival results obtained with medical therapy. Two separate studies, summarized in Fig. 16.11, reported outcomes in a total of 87 patients with left ventricular dysfunction (mean ejection fraction, 31%). Eitzman et al. (101) reported a 1-year mortality rate of 33% among patients treated medically. The mortality rate was only 4% among patients undergoing coronary artery bypass surgery or angioplasty. The mortality

rates with medical therapy versus revascularization were 41% and 12%, respectively, in the data reported by Di Carli et al. (102). Many of the patients in the study by Di Carli et al. were referred for PET evaluation from the heart failure program at their institution. In addition to improved survival, patients with myocardial viability by PET who underwent revascularization also had significant relief of symptoms of heart failure (102) and better objective exercise tolerance (103) than did patients treated medically.

Parallel findings have been reported in studies of SPECT with [201]Tl. In studies of patients with evidence of myocardial viability at thallium imaging, Gioia et al. (104) and Cuocolo et al. (105) assessed outcome among those treated medically compared with that among those undergoing myocardial revascularization. Survival rate with and survival rate without myocardial infarction were significantly higher among patients treated with revascularization (Fig 16.12). Thus far no prognostic data have been reported from studies of the use of ^{99m}Tc sestamibi or ^{99m}Tc tetrofosmin.

Data from clinical studies with PET and thallium SPECT provide concordant information suggesting that patients with

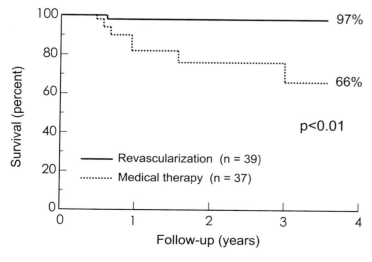

FIGURE 16.12. Survival rate among patients with left ventricular dysfunction and viable myocardium assessed by means of ^{201}Tl SPECT. The survival rate is greater among patients undergoing myocardial revascularization than it is among patients treated medically. (From Cuocolo A, Petretta M, Nicolai E, et al. Successful coronary revascularization improves prognosis in patients with previous myocardial infarction and evidence of viable myocardium at thallium-201 imaging. *Eur J Nucl Med* 1998;25:60-68, with permission of the European Society of Nuclear Medicine.)

coronary artery disease and left ventricular dysfunction, who have evidence of viable myocardium within dysfunctional regions, represent a group at particularly high risk during the course of medical therapy. This risk appears to be reduced significantly by a strategy of myocardial revascularization. There are major limitations of these studies that should be addressed, and because of these limitations, definitive conclusions cannot be reached at this time. These studies all represent retrospective, nonrandomized series involving relatively small numbers of patients. In addition, patient selection biases may have been present, and the factors used to select some patients for revascularization and others for medical therapy are unspecified. It is unclear whether other predictors of outcome, such as severity of angina or inducible myocardial ischemia, were used to guide the selection toward revascularization. Prospectively designed, randomized trials involving large numbers of patients clearly are required to resolve these issues (106). However, the overall concordance of the available results thus far obtained with three independent imaging methods at multiple centers supports the concept that patients with left ventricular dysfunction and evidence of myocardial are a group at high risk with a high rate of cardiac events. This poor prognosis appears to be reduced considerably by means of a strategy of revascularization of the viable but underperfused myocardium. These observations support the concept that methods to detect myocardial viability and ischemia have important clinical relevance to the care of patients who have had myocardial infarction and to that of patients with heart failure.

Selection of Patients for Revascularization

Another important issue regarding the prognostic implications of identifying viable myocardium is the importance of this assessment in the selection of patients with left ventricular dysfunction for myocardial revascularization. This issue addresses whether revascularization should be undertaken primarily for patients with evidence of myocardial viability or whether revascularization should be considered in the treatment of all patients with coronary artery disease and left ventricular dysfunction, with or without evidence of viable myocardium. The latter, aggressive strategy must be balanced by the high operative risk of 10% or greater among patients with severe left ventricular dysfunction and the fact that even with surgery, patients with severe left ventricular dysfunction have a relatively poor long-term outcome.

Several series have provided important data that serve to address this particular question. Pagley et al. (107) reported the outcome among patients with left ventricular dysfunction (mean ejection fraction, 28%) after coronary artery bypass surgery, all of whom underwent preoperative thallium imaging. Patients with evidence of myocardial viability had a significantly lower perioperative and long-term postoperative mortality rate than did patients without myocardial viability (Fig. 16.13). The perioperative mortality rate for the group without viable myocardium was 10%. Similar findings were reported by Haas et al. (108), who used metabolic PET. In that study, 34 patients with left ventricular dysfunction (mean ejection fraction, 28%) underwent preoperative PET and were referred for bypass surgery on the basis of myocardial viability. Another 35 patients (mean ejection fraction, 29%) did not undergo preoperative imaging and were referred for surgery on the basis of clinical and angiographic findings. The group with viable evidence of myocardium on preoperative PET studies had significantly better perioperative and long-term survival than did the group who did not undergo viability assessment (Fig 16.14). The perioperative mortality for the latter group was 11%. There were no early deaths in the group with preoperative viability assessment.

The caveats mentioned earlier apply to interpretation of these data regarding the application of viability measures for selecting patients with left ventricular dysfunction for myocardial revascularization. The available data represent retrospective analyses of clinical databases, and there are important potential patient-selection biases. To date no large-scale, randomized, prospectively designed trials have been conducted to address this issue. In the absence of definitive trial data, however, the current data are remarkably consistent.

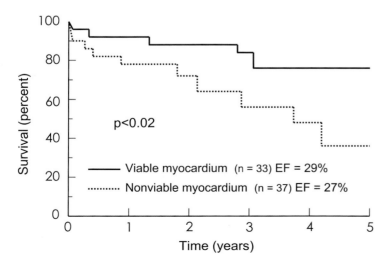

FIGURE 16.13. Survival rate among patients with left ventricular dysfunction undergoing coronary artery bypass surgery, all of whom underwent preoperative perfusion imaging with [201]Tl. Perioperative and long-term postoperative survival rates were significantly greater among patients with evidence of substantial myocardial viability than among patients with less evidence of viable myocardium. (From Pagley PR, Beller GA, Watson DD, et al. Improved outcome after coronary artery bypass surgery in patients with ischemic cardiomyopathy and residual myocardial viability. *Circulation* 1997;95:793–800, with permission of Lippincott Williams & Wilkins.)

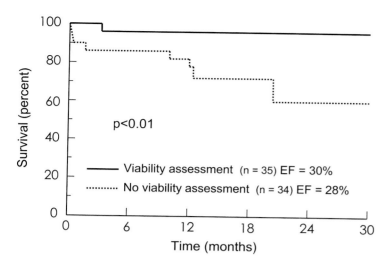

FIGURE 16.14. Survival rate in patients with left ventricular dysfunction undergoing coronary artery bypass surgery. One group of patients underwent preoperative viability assessment with FDG PET. The decision to proceed with surgery was based on evidence of viable myocardium. The second group did not undergo preoperative viability assessment, and the decision for revascularization was based on clinical and angiographic findings. Perioperative and long-term postoperative survival rates were significantly greater among patients whose decision for revascularization was driven by evidence of myocardial viability. (From Haas F, Haehnel CJ, Picker W, et al. Preoperative positron emission tomographic viability assessment and perioperative and postoperative risk in patients with advance ischemic heart disease. *J Am Coll Cardiol* 1997;30:1693–1700, with permission of Elsevier Publishing Company.)

SUMMARY

Identification of myocardial viability in patients with left ventricular dysfunction has several important clinical implications. Recovery of left ventricular function after revascularization appears to translate into an improvement in prognosis and an amelioration of symptoms. Although it is important to interpret the results of the studies reported to date with some degree of caution, because of the caveats mentioned previously, the overall concordance of the results supports the concepts (a) that patients with viable but dysfunctional myocardium are a high risk group with a high cardiac event rate and (b) that this poor prognosis can be reduced considerably with revascularization of the viable but underperfused myocardium.

Nuclear cardiology techniques have the unique potential to help differentiate viable tissue on the basis of perfusion, cell-membrane integrity, and metabolic activity. Thereby greater precision can be achieved than with investigation of regional anatomic features or function. Despite basic and clinical research in this area for more than a decade, a number of issues regarding the clinical applications of these techniques have not been fully resolved. First, the relative efficacy of PET compared with that of ^{201}Tl or ^{99m}Tc sestamibi is a principal issue, and larger-scale studies comparing these two methods in the evaluation of patients undergoing revascularization are essential. Although there may be subgroups of patients for whom PET provides more accurate and reliable results than can be obtained with ^{201}Tl imaging, these subgroups are not fully defined at present. Second, the efficacy of ^{99m}Tc sestamibi imaging relative to that of these other modalities in the assessment of myocardial viability also requires further investigation. The properties of the newer technetium-based perfusion tracers for viability assessment warrant similar study. Third, single-photon approaches to metabolic imaging (such as ^{123}I labeled fatty acids) appear promising (109, 110). Further investigation of these agents compared with ^{201}Tl or FDG in imaging of the same patient populations is needed.

The clinical relevance of viability assessment with these and other imaging modalities requires extensive study. More than 80% of dysfunctional myocardial regions identified as viable with various imaging techniques may improve after revascularization, but the specific patients likely to benefit clinically from this information are not fully delineated. At present, identification of viable myocardium is only one factor that enters the equation to recommend or not recommend revascularization in the care of patients with impaired left ventricular function. As in the care of any other patient with coronary artery disease, this decision should be based on clinical manifestations, coronary anatomic features, left ventricular function, and evidence of inducible ischemia. Increasingly, however, determination of the viability of myocardial territories to be revascularized plays a pivotal role in decision making. Definitive, accurate, and cost-effective methods are essential to make this determination. Nuclear cardiology techniques will be called on with increasing frequency for this purpose.

REFERENCES

1. Hammermeister KE, DeRouen TA, Dodge HT. Variables predictive of survival in patients with coronary disease: selection by univariate and multivariate analysis from the clinical, electrocardiographic, exercise, arteriographic, and quantitative angiographic evaluations. *Circulation* 1979;59:421–430.
2. Harris PJ, Harrel FE, Lee KL, et al. Survival in medically treated coronary artery disease. *Circulation* 1979;60:1259–1269.
3. Mock MB, Ringqvist I, Fisher LD, et al. Survival of medically treated patients in the Coronary Artery Surgery Study (CASS) registry. *Circulation* 1982;66:562–568.
4. Emond M, Mock MB, Davis KB, et al. Long-term survival of medically treated patients in the Coronary Artery Surgery Study (CASS) Registry. *Circulation* 1994;90:2645–2657.
5. Bonow RO, Epstein SE. Indications for coronary artery bypass surgery: implications of the multicenter randomized trials. *Circulation* 1985;72[Suppl V]:23–30.
6. Bonow RO. Identification of viable myocardium. *Circulation* 1996; 94:2674–2680.
7. Beller GA. Comparison of thallium-201 scintigraphy and low-dose dobutamine echocardiography for the noninvasive assessment of myocardial viability. *Circulation* 1996;94:2681–2684.
8. Rahimtoola SH. Coronary bypass surgery for chronic angina—1981: a perspective. *Circulation* 1982:65:225–241.

9. Braunwald E, Rutherford JD. Reversible ischemic left ventricular dysfunction: evidence for "hibernating" myocardium. *J Am Coll Cardiol* 1986;8:1467–1470.

10. Rahimtoola SH. The hibernating myocardium. *Am Heart J* 1989; 117:211–213.

11. Ross J Jr. Myocardial perfusion-contraction matching: implications for coronary artery disease and hibernation. *Circulation* 1991;83: 1076–1083.

12. Dilsizian V, Bonow RO. Current diagnostic techniques of assessing myocardial viability in hibernating and stunned myocardium. *Circulation* 1993;87:1–20.

13. Camici PG, Wijns W, Borgers M, et al. Pathophysiology of chronic reversible left ventricular dysfunction due to coronary artery disease (hibernating myocardium). *Circulation* 1997;96:3205–3214.

14. Wijns W, Vatner SF, Camici PG. Mechanisms of disease: hibernating myocardium. *N Engl J Med* 1998;339:173–181.

15. Elefteriades JA, Tolis G Jr, Levi E, et al. Coronary artery bypass grafting in severe left ventricular dysfunction: excellent survival with improved ejection fraction and functional state. *J Am Coll Cardiol* 1993;22:1411–1417.

16. Bonow RO. The hibernating myocardium: implications for management of congestive heart failure. *Am J Cardiol* 1995;75:17A–25A.

17. Cigarroa CG, deFilippi CR, Brickner E, et al. Dobutamine stress echocardiography identifies hibernating myocardium and predicts recovery of left ventricular function after coronary revascularization. *Circulation* 1993;88:430–436.

18. La Canna G, Alfieri O, Giubbini R, et al. Echocardiography during infusion of dobutamine for identification of reversible dysfunction in patients with chronic coronary artery disease. *J Am Coll Cardiol* 1994; 23:617–626.

19. Perrone-Filardi P, Pace L, Prastaro M, et al. Dobutamine echocardiography predicts improvement of hypoperfused dysfunctional myocardium after revascularization in patients with coronary artery disease. *Circulation* 1995;91:2556–2565.

20. Opie LH. Effects of regional ischemia on metabolism of glucose and fatty acids: relative rates of aerobic and anaerobic energy production during myocardial infarction and comparison with effects of anoxia. *Circ Res* 1976;38[Suppl I]:52–74.

21. Camici P, Ferrannini E, Opie LH. Myocardial metabolism in ischemic heart disease: basic principles and application to imaging by positron emission tomography. *Prog Cardiovasc Dis* 1989;32:217–238.

22. Gibson RS, Watson DD, Taylor GJ, et al. Prospective assessment of regional myocardial perfusion before and after coronary revascularization surgery by quantitative thallium-201 scintigraphy. *J Am Coll Cardiol* 1983;1:804–815.

23. Liu P, Kiess MC, Okada RD, et al. The persistent defect on exercise thallium imaging and its fate after myocardial revascularization: does it represent scar or ischemia? *Am Heart J* 1985;110:996–1001.

24. Manyari DE, Knudtson M, Kloiber R, et al. Sequential thallium-201 myocardial perfusion studies after successful percutaneous transluminal coronary artery angioplasty: delayed resolution of exercise induced scintigraphic abnormalities. *Circulation* 1988;77:86–95.

25. Cloninger KG, DePuey EG, Garcia EV, et al. Incomplete redistribution in delayed thallium-201 single photon emission computed tomographic (SPECT) images: an overestimation of myocardial scarring. *J Am Coll Cardiol* 1988;12:955–963.

26. Ohtani H, Tamaki N, Yonekura Y, et al. Value of thallium-201 reinjection after delayed SPECT imaging for predicting reversible ischemia after coronary artery bypass grafting. *Am J Cardiol* 1990;66: 394–399.

27. Hendel RC. Single-photon perfusion imaging for the assessment of myocardial viability. *J Nucl Med* 1994;35[Suppl]:23S–31S.

28. Gutman J, Berman DS, Freeman M, et al. Time to completed redistribution of thallium-201 in exercise myocardial scintigraphy: relationship to the degree of coronary artery stenosis. *Am Heart J* 1983;106: 989–995.

29. Kiat H, Berman DS, Maddahi J, et al. Late reversibility of tomographic myocardial thallium-201 defects: an accurate marker of myocardial viability. *J Am Coll Cardiol* 1988;12:1456–1463.

30. Yang LD, Berman DS, Kiat H, et al. The frequency of late reversibility in SPECT thallium-201 stress-redistribution studies. *J Am Coll Cardiol* 1990;15:334–340.

31. Watson DD. Methods for detection of myocardial viability and ischemia. In: Zaret BL, Beller GA, eds. *Nuclear cardiology.* St. Louis: Mosby, 1992:65–76.

32. Kayden DS, Sigal S, Soufer R, et al. Thallium-201 for assessment of myocardial viability: quantitative comparison of 24-hour redistribution imaging with imaging after reinjection at rest. *J Am Coll Cardiol* 1991;18:1480–1486.

33. Dilsizian V, Rocco TP, Freedman NMT, et al. Enhanced detection of ischemic but viable myocardium by the reinjection of thallium after stress-redistribution imaging. *N Engl J Med* 1990;323:141–146.

34. Rocco TP, Dilsizian V, McKusick KA, et al. Comparison of thallium redistribution with rest "reinjection" imaging for detection of viable myocardium. *Am J Cardiol* 1990;66:158–163.

35. Tamaki N, Ohtani H, Yonekura Y, et al. Significance of fill-in after thallium-201 reinjection following delayed imaging: comparison with regional wall motion and angiographic findings. *J Nucl Med* 1990; 31:1617–1623.

36. Nienaber CA, de la Roche J, Camarius H, et al. Impact of 201 thallium reinjection imaging to identify myocardial viability after vasodilation-redistribution SPECT. *J Am Coll Cardiol* 1993;21:283A(abst).

37. Kitsou AN, Srinivasan G, Quyyumi AA, et al. Stress-induced reversible and mild-to-moderate irreversible thallium defects: are they equally accurate for predicting recovery of regional left ventricular function after revascularization? *Circulation* 1998;98:501–508.

38. Dilsizian V, Smeltzer WR, Freedman NMT, et al. Thallium reinjection after stress-redistribution imaging: does 24-hour delayed imaging following reinjection enhance detection of viable myocardium? *Circulation* 1991;83:1247–1255.

39. Dilsizian V, Bonow RO. Differential uptake and apparent thallium-201 "washout" after thallium reinjection: options regarding early redistribution imaging before reinjection or late redistribution imaging after reinjection. *Circulation* 1992;85:1032–1038.

40. Kiat H, Friedman JD, Wang FP, et al. Frequency of late reversibility in stress-redistribution thallium-201 SPECT using an early reinjection protocol. *Am Heart J* 1991;122:613–619.

41. van Eck-Smit BLF, van der Wall EE, Kuijper AFM, et al. Immediate thallium-201 reinjection following stress imaging: a time-saving approach for detection of myocardial viability. *J Nucl Med* 1993;34: 737–743.

42. Dilsizian V, Bonow RO, Quyyumi AA, et al. Is early thallium reinjection after postexercise imaging a satisfactory method to detect defect reversibility? *Circulation* 1993;88:1064.

43. Berger BC, Watson DD, Burwell LR, et al. Redistribution of thallium at rest in patients with stable and unstable angina and the effect of coronary artery bypass surgery. *Circulation* 1979;60:1114–1125.

44. Iskandrian AS, Hakki A, Kane SA, et al. Rest and redistribution thallium-201 myocardial scintigraphy to predict improvement in left ventricular function after coronary artery bypass grafting. *Am J Cardiol* 1983;51:1312–1316.

45. Mori T, Minamiji K, Kurogane H, et al. Rest-injected thallium-201 imaging for assessing viability of severe asynergic regions. *J Nucl Med* 1991;32:1718–1724.

46. Ragosta M, Beller GA, Watson DD, et al. Quantitative planar rest-redistribution 201Tl imaging in detection of myocardial viability and prediction of improvement in left ventricular function after coronary bypass surgery in patients with severely depressed left ventricular function. *Circulation* 1993;87:1630–1641.

47. Dilsizian V, Perrone-Filardi P, Arrighi JA, et al. Concordance and discordance between stress-redistribution-reinjection and rest-redistribution thallium imaging for assessing viable myocardium. *Circulation* 1993;88:941–952.

48. Bonow RO. Assessment of myocardial viability with thallium-201. In: Zaret BL, Beller GA, eds. *Nuclear cardiology: state of the art and future directions.* St. Louis: Mosby, 1998:503–512.

49. Zimmerman R, Mall G, Rauch B, et al. Residual 201Tl activity in irreversible defects as a marker of myocardial viability: clinicopathological study. *Circulation* 1995;91:1016–1021.

50. Freeman I, Grunwald AM, Hoory S, et al. Effect of coronary occlusion

and myocardial viability on myocardial activity of technetium-99m-sestamibi. *J Nucl Med* 1991;32:292–298.

51. Sinusas AJ, Watson DD, Cannon JM, et al. Effect of ischemia and postischemic dysfunction on myocardial uptake of technetium-99m-labeled methoxyisobutyl isonitrile and thallium-201. *J Am Coll Cardiol* 1989;14:1785–1793.

52. Beanlands RSB, Dawood F, Wen WH, et al. Are the kinetics of technetium-99m methoxyisobutyl isonitrile affected by cell metabolism and viability? *Circulation* 1990;82:1802–1814.

53. Edwards NC, Ruiz M, Watson DD, et al. Does Tc-99m sestamibi given immediately after coronary reperfusion reflect viability? *Circulation* 1990;82:III-542(abst).

54. Li QS, Matsumura K, Dannals R, et al. Radionuclide markers of viability in reperfused myocardium: comparison between 18F-2-deoxyglucose, 201Tl, and 99mTc-sestamibi. *Circulation* 1990;82:III-542(abst).

55. Christian TF, Behrenbeck T, Pellikka PA, et al. Mismatches of left ventricular function and perfusion with Tc-99m-isonitrile following reperfusion therapy for acute myocardial infarctions: identification of myocardial stunning and hyperkinesia. *J Am Coll Cardiol* 1990;16:1632–1638.

56. Bonow RO, Dilsizian V. Thallium-201 and technetium-99m-sestamibi for assessing viable myocardium. *J Nucl Med* 1992;33:815–818.

57. Cuocolo A, Pace L, Ricciardelli B, et al. Identification of viable myocardium in patients with chronic coronary artery disease: comparison of thallium-201 scintigraphy with reinjection and technetium-99m methoxyisobutyl isonitrile. *J Nucl Med* 1992;33:505–511.

58. Marzullo P, Sambuceti G, Parodi O. The role of sestamibi scintigraphy in the radioisotopic assessment of myocardial viability. *J Nucl Med* 1992;33:1925–1930.

59. Marzullo P, Parodi O, Reisenhofer B, et al. Value of rest thallium-201/technetium-99m sestamibi scans and dobutamine echocardiography for detecting myocardial viability. *Am J Cardiol* 1993;71:166–172.

60. Sawada SG, Allman KC, Muzik O, et al. Positron emission tomography detects evidence of viability in rest technetium-99m sestamibi defects. *J Am Coll Cardiol* 1994;23:92–98.

61. Dilsizian V, Arrighi JA, Diodati JG, et al. Myocardial viability in patients with chronic ischemic left ventricular dysfunction: comparison of 99mTc-sestamibi, 201 thallium, and 18F-fluorodeoxyglucose. *Circulation* 1994;89:578–587.

62. Udelson JE, Coleman PS, Matherall JA, et al. Predicting recovery of severe regional ventricular dysfunction: comparison of resting scintigraphy with thallium-201 and technetium-99m sestamibi. *Circulation* 1994;89:2552–2561.

63. Medrano R, Lowry RW, Young JB, et al. Assessment of myocardial viability with 99mTc sestamibi in patients undergoing cardiac transplantation: a scintigraphic/pathological study. *Circulation* 1996;94:1010–1017.

64. Maes AF, Borgers M, Flameng W, et al. Assessment of myocardial viability in chronic coronary artery disease using technetium-99m sestamibi SPECT: correlation with histologic and positron emission tomographic studies and functional follow-up. *J Am Coll Cardiol* 1997;29:62–68.

65. Dakik HA, Howell JF, Lawria GM, et al. Assessment of myocardial viability with 99mTc-sestamibi tomography before coronary bypass graft surgery: correlation with histopathology and postoperative improvement in cardiac function. *Circulation* 1997;96:2892–2898.

66. Schneider CA, Voth E, Gawlich S, et al. Significance of rest technetium-99m sestamibi imaging for the prediction of improvement of left ventricular dysfunction after Q wave myocardial infarction: importance of infarct location adjusted thresholds. *J Am Coll Cardiol* 1998;32:648–654.

67. Sansoy V, Glover DK, Watson DD, et al. Comparison of thallium-201 resting redistribution with technetium-99m-sestamibi uptake and functional response to dobutamine for assessment of myocardial viability. *Circulation* 1995;92:994–1004.

68. Kauffman GJ, Boyne TS, Watson DD, et al. Comparison of rest thallium-201 imaging and rest technetium-99m sestamibi for assessment of myocardial viability in patients with coronary artery disease

and severe left ventricular dysfunction. *J Am Coll Cardiol* 1996;27:1592–1597.

69. Bisi G, Sciagra R, Santoro GM, et al. Rest technetium-99m sestamibi in combination with short-term administration of nitrates: feasibility and reliability for prediction of postrevascularization outcome of asynergic territories. *J Am Coll Cardiol* 1994;24:1282–1289.

70. Galli M, Marcassa C, Imperato A, et al. Effects of nitroglycerin by technetium-99m sestamibi tomoscintigraphy on resting global myocardial hypoperfusion in stable patients with healed myocardial infarction. *Am J Cardiol* 1994;74:843–848.

71. Maurea S, Cuocolo A, Soricelli A, et al. Enhanced detection of viable myocardium by technetium-99m-MIBI imaging after nitrate administration in chronic coronary artery disease. *J Nucl Med* 1995;36:1945–1952.

72. Bisi G, Sciagra R, Santoro GM, et al. Technetium-99m-sestamibi imaging with nitrate infusion to detect hibernating myocardium and predict postrevascularization recovery. *J Nucl Med* 1995;36:1994–2000.

73. Sciagra R, Bisi G, Santoro GM, et al. Caomparison of baseline-nitrate technetium-99m sestamibi with rest-redistribution thallium-201 tomography in detecting viable hibernating myocardium and predicting post-revascularization recovery. *J Am Coll Cardiol* 1997;30:384–391.

74. Schelbert HR, Buxton D. Insights into coronary artery disease gained from metabolic imaging. *Circulation* 1988;78:496–505.

75. Bonow RO, Berman DS, Gibbons RJ, et al. Cardiac positron emission tomography: a report for health professionals from the Committee on Advanced Cardiac Imaging and Technology of the Council on Clinical Cardiology, American Heart Association. *Circulation* 1991;84:447–454.

76. Schelbert HR, Bonow RO, Geltman E, et al. Clinical use of positron emission tomography: position paper of the Cardiovascular Council of the Society of Nuclear Medicine. *J Nucl Med* 1993;34:1385–1388.

77. Schelbert H. Metabolic imaging to assess myocardial viability. *J Nucl Med* 1994;35[Suppl]:8S–14S.

78. Marshall RC, Tillisch JH, Phelps ME, et al. Identification and differentiation of resting myocardial ischemia and infarction in man with positron computed tomography, 18F-labeled fluorodeoxyglucose and N-13 ammonia. *Circulation* 1983;67:766–778.

79. Tillisch JH, Brunken R, Marshall R, et al. Reversibility of cardiac wall-motion abnormalities predicted by positron tomography. *N Engl J Med* 1986;314:884–888.

80. Brunken R, Tillisch J, Schwaiger M, et al. Regional perfusion, glucose metabolism, and wall motion in patients with chronic electrocardiographic Q wave infarctions: evidence for persistence of viable tissue in some infarct regions by positron emission tomography. *Circulation* 1986;73:951–963.

81. Maddahi J, Schelbert H, Brunken R, et al. Role of thallium-201 and PET imaging in evaluation of myocardial viability and management of patients with coronary artery disease and left ventricular dysfunction. *J Nucl Med* 1994;35:707–715.

82. Tamaki N, Yonekura Y, Yamashita K, et al. Positron emission tomography using fluorine-18 deoxyglucose in evaluation of coronary artery bypass grafting. *Am J Cardiol* 1989;64:860–865.

83. Gropler RJ, Geltman EM, Sampathkumaran K, et al. Functional recovery after coronary revascularization for chronic coronary artery disease is dependent on maintenance of oxidative metabolism. *J Am Coll Cardiol* 1992;20:569–577.

84. Lucignani G, Paolini G, Landoni C, et al. Presurgical identification of hibernating myocardium by combined use of technetium-99m hexakis 2-methoxyisobutylisonitrile single photon emission tomography and fluorine-18 fluoro-2-deoxy-D-glucose positron emission tomography in patients with coronary artery disease. *Eur J Nucl Med* 1992;19:874–881.

85. Carrel T, Jenni R, Haubold-Reuter S, et al. Improvement in severely reduced left ventricular function after surgical revascularization in patients with preoperative myocardial infarction. *Eur J Cardiothorac Surg* 1992;6:479–484.

86. vom Dahl J, Altehoefer C, Sheehan FH, et al. Recovery of myocardial function following coronary revascularization: impact of viability and

long-term vessel patency as assessed by preoperative F-18 FDG PET and serial angiography. *J Nucl Med* 1993;34:23P(abst).

87. Bessozi MC, Brown MD, Hubner KF, et al. Retrospective post-therapy evaluation of cardiac function in 208 coronary artery disease patients evaluated by positron emission tomography. *J Nucl Med* 1992;33:885(abst).

88. Nienaber CA, Brunken RC, Sherman CT, et al. Metabolic and functional recovery of ischemic human myocardium after coronary angioplasty. *J Am Coll Cardiol* 1991;18:966–978.

89. Brunken R, Schwaiger M, Grover-McKay M, et al. Positron emission tomography detects tissue metabolic activity in myocardial segments with persistent thallium perfusion defects. *J Am Coll Cardiol* 1987;10:557–567.

90. Tamaki N, Yonekura Y, Yamashita K, et al. Relation of left ventricular perfusion and wall motion with metabolic activity in persistent defects on thallium-201 tomography in healed myocardial infarction. *Am J Cardiol* 1988;62:202–208.

91. Brunken RC, Kottou S, Nienaber CA, et al. PET detection of viable tissue in myocardial segments with persistent defects at Tl-201 SPECT. *Radiology* 1989;65:65–73.

92. Tamaki N, Yonekura Y, Yamashita K, et al. SPECT thallium-201 tomography and positron tomography using N-13 ammonia and F-18 fluorodeoxyglucose in coronary artery disease. *Am J Card Imaging* 1989;3:3–9.

93. Brunken RC, Mody FV, Hawkins RA, et al. Positron emission tomography detects metabolic activity in myocardium with persistent 24-hour single photon emission computed tomography 201Tl defects. *Circulation* 1992;86:1357–1369.

94. Bonow RO, Dilsizian V, Cuocolo A, et al. Identification of viable myocardium in patients with chronic coronary artery disease and left ventricular dysfunction: comparison of thallium-201 with reinjection and PET imaging with 18F-fluorodeoxyglucose. *Circulation* 1991;83:26–37.

95. Tamaki N, Ohtani H, Yamashita K, et al. Metabolic activity in the areas of new fill-in after thallium-201 reinjection: comparison with positron emission tomography using fluorine-18-deoxyglucose. *J Nucl Med* 1991;32:673–678.

96. Perrone-Filardi P, Bacharach SL, Dilsizian V, et al. Regional left ventricular wall thickening: relation to regional uptake of 18F-fluoro-deoxyglucose and thallium-201 in patients with chronic coronary artery disease and left ventricular dysfunction. *Circulation* 1992;86:1125–1137.

97. Yamamoto Y, de Silva R, Rhodes CG, et al. A new strategy for the assessment of viable myocardium and regional myocardial blood flow using 15O-water and dynamic positron emission tomography. *Circulation* 1992;86:167–178.

98. de Silva R, Yamamoto Y, Rhodes CG, et al. Preoperative prediction of the outcome of coronary revascularization using positron emission tomography. *Circulation* 1992;86:1738–1742.

99. Gould KL, Haynie M, Hess MJ, et al. Myocardial metabolism of fluorodeoxyglucose compared to cell membrane integrity for the potassium analogue Rb-82 for assessing infarct size in man by PET. *J Nucl Med* 1991;32:1–9.

100. Garcia EV. Quantitative myocardial perfusion single-photon emission computed tomographic imaging: quo vadis? (where do we go from here?) *J Nucl Cardiol* 1994;1:83–93.

101. Eitzman D, Al-Aouar Z, Kanter HL, et al. Clinical outcome of patients with advanced coronary artery disease after viability studies with positron emission tomography. *J Am Coll Cardiol* 1992;20:559–565.

102. Di Carli MF, Davidson M, Little R, et al. Value of metabolic imaging with positron emission tomography for evaluating prognosis in patients with coronary artery disease and left ventricular dysfunction. *Am J Cardiol* 1994;73:527–533.

103. Di Carli MF, Asgarzadie F, Schelbert HR, et al. Quantitative relation between myocardial viability and improvement in heart failure symptoms after revascularization in patients with ischemic cardiomyopathy. *Circulation* 1995;92:3436–3444.

104. Gioia G, Powers J, Heo J, et al. Prognostic value of rest-redistribution tomographic thallium-201 imaging in ischemic cardiomyopathy. *Am J Cardiol* 1995;75:759–762.

105. Cuocolo A, Petretta M, Nicolai E, et al. Successful coronary revascularization improves prognosis in patients with previous myocardial infarction and evidence of viable myocardium at thallium-201 imaging. *Eur J Nucl Med* 1998;25:60–68.

106. Bonow RO, Camici PG, DiCarli MF, et al. Imaging in heart failure. *J Nucl Cardiol* 2001;8:296–305.

107. Pagley PR, Beller GA, Watson DD, et al. Improved outcome after coronary artery bypass surgery in patients with ischemic cardiomyopathy and residual myocardial viability. *Circulation* 1997;95:793–800.

108. Haas F, Haehnel CJ, Picker W, et al. Preoperative positron emission tomographic viability assessment and perioperative and postoperative risk in patients with advance ischemic heart disease. *J Am Coll Cardiol* 1997;30:1693–1700.

109. Tamaki N, Kawamoto M, Yonekura Y, et al. Regional metabolic abnormality in relation to perfusion and wall motion in patients with myocardial infarction: assessment with emission tomography using an iodinated branched fatty acid analog. *J Nucl Med* 1992;33:659–667.

110. Murray G, Schad N, Ladd W, et al. Metabolic cardiac imaging in coronary artery disease with severe left ventricular dysfunction: assessment of myocardial viability with 123I-iodophenylpentadecanoic acid imaged by a multicrystal camera and correlation with transmural myocardial biopsy. *J Nucl Med* 1992;33:1269–1277.

17

MYOCARDIAL HOTSPOT IMAGING

LYNNE L. JOHNSON

ADVANTAGES OF HOTSPOT AGENTS IN CARDIAC IMAGING

The development of nuclear imaging agents for the heart has focused primarily on perfusion because the driving clinical use is for diagnosis and prognosis in coronary artery disease. In the new era of molecular cardiology, the biochemical pathways for the biologic and pathologic mechanisms of the cell are being elucidated. This information is used to identify the structure of specific inducible gene products, receptors, phospholipids, and other important cellular molecules and protein structures that can serve as targets. This approach represents a direct way to observe pathobiologic mechanisms and presents a way to widely increase the clinical applications of cardiac imaging. This section discusses tracers that target specific physiologic and pathologic cellular processes in the myocardium. They are commonly called *hotspot imaging agents.*

IMAGING MYOCARDIAL NECROSIS AND APOPTOSIS

The development of more accurate serum markers for necrosis, such as the troponins, and the success of thrombolytic treatment or early angioplasty to salvage myocardium have reduced the role of nuclear imaging in the management of acute myocardial infarction. Antimyosin antibody is no longer available in the United States and is rarely used worldwide. Several new agents, however, show promise in the management of acute coronary syndromes and rejection after cardiac transplantation. These indications are discussed, and a brief historical perspective on infarct imaging is provided.

Assessment of regional left ventricular wall motion or wall thickening with echocardiography, radionuclide angiography, cine magnetic resonance imaging (MRI), or gated single photon emission computed tomography (SPECT) is not an accurate technique for diagnosing or localizing myocardial scarring. Function studies can result in overestimation of scarring or miss

a small scar. Abnormal wall motion is common in the distribution of an occluded or highly stenotic coronary vessel in the absence of scarring and in the presence of normal resting blood flow (1). The observation of this discordance between function and viability led to coining of the term *hibernation* (2–4). Experimental studies have shown that the most likely mechanism for this phenomenon is frequent and recurrent ischemic episodes and postischemic stunning that lead to chronic dysfunction (5). Myocardium that slowly recovers function after acute myocardial infarction also is stunned. With successful and early reperfusion, the amount of residual necrosis usually is very small and is localized to the subendocardium. It is not uncommon to find completely normal regional and global left ventricular function after a small, nontransmural reperfused infarction.

Use of a perfusion tracer alone does not give an accurate estimate of the presence or extent of myocardial necrosis. When injected during coronary occlusion, a perfusion tracer demarcates the risk region that is larger than the ultimate area of necrosis in the presence of successful thrombolysis (6). Even when injected several days after the infarction, use of a perfusion tracer may lead to overestimation of the scar. Systolic thinning alone may make the counts in viable but stunned myocardium appear low because of a partial volume effect (7). Using the size of the perfusion defect leads to overestimation of recent necrosis in the presence of additional scarred areas from remote infarctions. A perfusion tracer is insensitive for detecting non–Q wave infarctions because of the limited resolution of nuclear imaging cameras to detect transmural count differentials. In the thrombolytic era, an increasingly larger percentage of myocardial infarctions are non–Q wave. Contrast-enhanced cine MRI shows promise for visualizing non–Q wave myocardial infarction and for viability assessment (8).

99MTC PYROPHOSPHATE

Uptake of ^{99m}Tc pyrophosphate in the region of the heart was observed on bone scans 20 years ago (9). It turned out that these patients with cardiac uptake of ^{99m}Tc pyrophosphate had recent myocardial infarctions. Because this radiopharmaceutical binds to calcium in bone, it was hypothesized and subsequently found that the mechanism of uptake into necrotic myocardium is bind-

L.L. Johnson: Nuclear Cardiology, Rhode Island Hospital and Department of Medicine, Brown University, Providence, RI.

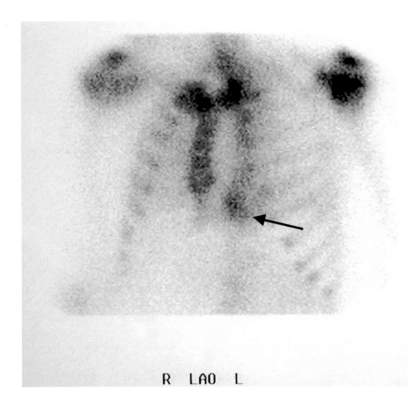

R LAO L

FIGURE 17.1. Forty-five-degree left anterior oblique planar
99mTc pyrophosphate image of 67-year-old man being evaluated for metastatic prostate cancer. *Arrow* points to focal uptake of tracer corresponding to the inferoapical region of the left ventricle. This incidental finding indicates recent myocardial necrosis. (Images provided by Dr. Richard Noto.)

ing to intracellular calcium in the acute infarct (10). During severe ischemia, there is a calcium flux across the sarcolemma. As the intracellular concentration of the electrolyte increases, the cell becomes irreversibly damaged, and calcium is deposited in the mitochondria. Some severely ischemic myocytes that have accumulated intracellular calcium may be capable of recovery, and therefore uptake of pyrophosphate is not specific for irreversible myocyte necrosis. In experimental studies, maximal uptake of pyrophosphate was observed at the infarct border, where flow was only moderately reduced (11). A correlate of these experimental observations, is a "donut" pattern of tracer uptake seen in patients that corresponds to the periphery of large infarcts.

Because it requires time for calcium to accumulate in an infarct, there is a 24- to 48-hour lag between vessel occlusion at the infarct and development of a positive scan result. Pyrophosphate therefore cannot be used in the emergency department to diagnose infarction. Planar imaging usually is sufficient to establish a diagnosis, but SPECT helps separate myocardial from rib activity in equivocal cases. However, even when tomography is used, it may be difficult to resolve small infarcts from blood pool activity.

The diagnostic accuracy of pyrophosphate for myocardial infarction was reported in a study of 52 patients who underwent pyrophosphate imaging and later died and underwent necropsy (12). The sensitivity was 89%, the specificity was 100%, and the predictive value for a positive scan result was 100% and for a negative scan, 72%. The reduced sensitivity is caused by difficulty detecting small regions of myocardial uptake from faint but persistent blood pool activity. The importance of knowing that 99mTc pyrophosphate is taken up into areas of recent myo-

cardial infarction is to be alert to finding and interpreting cardiac uptake on bone scans. Older patients referred for bone scans as part of an evaluation for metastatic cancer frequently have coronary artery disease and may have unrecognized areas of recent infarction (Fig. 17.1).

ANTIMYOSIN ANTIBODY IMAGING

A discussion of antimyosin antibody imaging is useful because this modality represents a known standard for hotspot imaging for acute myocardial necrosis and is used for historical comparison with new agents. Because of the observation that human heavy-chain myosin is the least soluble of the myocardial contractile proteins, Khaw et al. (13) developed a murine antibody to this highly insoluble protein for in situ infarct labeling. In addition to being highly insoluble, the antigen heavy-chain myosin protein composes approximately 10% of the cardiac myocyte. This yields a large number of antibody binding sites, many more than tumor antigenic binding sites. Properties of the antibody include a high specificity for binding to necrotic myocardium (14,15). The antibody can bind to the antigen (heavy-chain myosin) only by passing through holes in the sarcolemmal membrane. The degree of ischemia leading to sarcolemmal disruption signifies irreversible cell injury and subsequent cell death. In comparison with that of pyrophosphate, antimyosin uptake is more specific for myocyte necrosis.

The radiopharmaceutical in clinical comprises Fab fragments of murine monoclonal immunoglobulin G antimyosin antibody labeled with 111In. This is accomplished by means of transchelation labeling of diethylenetriaminepentaacetic acid (DTPA) antibodies with ^{111}In in citrate buffer at pH 5.5. The citrate buffer prevents the indium from forming a colloid and allows the indium to transchelate to the DTPA-coupled antibody at a pH that minimizes damage to the protein. The blood pool clearance for ^{111}In antimyosin is slow with a half-life ($t_{1/2}$) of 6 to 12 hours. By 24 hours after injection, the blood pool has cleared sufficiently in most patients to yield diagnostic infarct imaging. Significant extracardiac sources of ^{111}In activity include the kidneys, which are the target organs, and the liver, which accumulates ^{111}In presumably because of transchelation of the ^{111}In from the chelate antibody complex to transferrin and subsequent uptake into the reticuloendothelial system. To improve specific activity and decrease nonspecific binding, Khaw et al. charge modified antimyosin with polylysine (16). Techniques to label the antibody with ^{99m}Tc also have been developed (17,18).

Uptake of the antibody into infarcts varies with the degree of necrosis and can approach 1% to 3% of the injected doses into large infarcts. Uptake also depends on antibody delivery and infarct location. Experimental studies showed more intense uptake in reperfused than in nonreperfused infarcts, reflecting differences in blood flow (delivery) to the infarct zone (19). The safety and diagnostic accuracy of planar antimyosin imaging were evaluated in a multicenter clinical trial in which 497 patients with chest pain were enrolled in 25 sites in the United States and Europe (20). The investigators used electrocardiographic and enzyme criteria as the standard of reference for myocardial infarction. The overall sensitivity for detecting myocardial necrosis was 89% with a higher sensitivity for detecting Q-wave infarction (94%) than for detection of non–Q-wave infarction (82%). The specificity was 95% as assessed from data on patients admitted to the hospital with chest pain syndromes determined clinically not to be ischemic in origin at hospital discharge. Thirty-seven percent of scans performed on patients with the clinical diagnosis of unstable angina showed uptake of antimyosin in the heart. The pathophysiologic mechanism of unstable angina involves an unstable atherosclerotic plaque that develops transient thrombus with spontaneous lysis. This observation probably represents the scan correlate of an elevated troponin value, which has been reported to identify a worse prognosis among patients with unstable angina (21).

The window for positive results of ^{111}In antimyosin scanning is wide. In a multicenter study to evaluate the duration of scan positivity, the findings were 65% positive at 2 to 4 months, 62% at 4 to 6 months, 51% at 6 to 8 months, 46% at 8 to 10 months, and 29% at 10 to 12 months (22,23). The presumed mechanism of late positive results is antimyosin binding to strands of myosin imbedded in the scar. In the late injection study, it was observed that antimyosin uptake late after infarction is faint and that tracer washes out rapidly from the myocardium.

Simultaneous dual isotope imaging with a perfusion tracer (^{201}Tl) and an infarct avid tracer (^{111}In antimyosin) was reported (24). This approach allowed mapping of perfusion and necrosis on the same image. [111]In and ^{201}Tl can be imaged well together because the major photopeaks are well separated with minimal cross-talk, and the half-lives (and doses) of the two are almost equivalent. Eighty-seven patients underwent dual isotope imaging over a 4-year period. Results for the first 42 were reported

(24). Patients were given an injection of 2 mCi of ^{111}In antimyosin at bedside within 48 hours of the onset of chest pain and underwent imaging 48 hours later. Images with two different tracers were interpreted simultaneously. Corresponding short axis, vertical long axis, and horizontal long axis slices were lined up on a color video display for qualitative interpretation. [201]Tl defects with ^{111}In antimyosin uptake corresponding in size and location were classified as matches. [201]Tl defects without corresponding ^{111}In antimyosin uptake were classified as mismatches, and regions of uptake of both ^{201}Tl and ^{111}In antimyosin in the same segments were classified as overlap. During 6 weeks of follow-up evaluation, 39 patients had additional ischemic events. Thirty-eight of these 39 patients had dual isotope scan patterns interpreted as mismatches or overlap, yielding a high sensitivity (97%). Most of these patients had multiple patterns of uptake of the two tracers in their hearts, such as a matched or unmatched pattern in one vascular territory and an overlap pattern in another vascular territory. Of the 48 patients who were event-free up to 6 weeks, the dual isotope scan patterns were almost evenly divided between matched and unmatched or overlap patterns, yielding a specificity of only 56%. Reasons for this poor specificity include reduced ^{111}In antimyosin tracer delivery into the bed of an infarct with total infarct vessel occlusion and poor collateral vessels or reduced thallium uptake into stunned or hibernating myocardium.

[99m]TC D-GLUCARIC ACID IMAGING

Glucaric acid (glucarate) is a six-carbon acid sugar that is the end product of uridine diphosphoglucose metabolism and therefore is a naturally occurring compound in humans. In the development of a technetium label for antimyosin antibody fragments, glucarate was used as a transchelator and found serendipitously to localize in areas of experimental myocardial infarction (25). Because of its small molecular weight (210 d) and lack of antigenicity, glucarate has unique properties as an imaging agent regarding both blood pool clearance and safety. Studies with swine showed a biexponential blood washout with a first-component $t_{1/2}$ of 5.0 ± 0.9 minutes, a second-component $t_{1/2}$ of 54.3 ± 13.5 minutes, and an overall $t_{1/2}$ of 25.2 minutes. Focal uptake in the risk region could be seen by 41 ± 15 minutes after injection with minimal bone and moderate liver uptake (26). A phase I trial with healthy human volunteers has been completed by Taillefer. The blood pool clearance curve best approximated a triexponential equation. An initial, rapid distribution phase with a $t_{1/2}$ of 9.0 minutes was followed by a redistribution phase with a $t_{1/2}$ of 54.4 minutes and a final elimination phase with a biologic $t_{1/2}$ of 26.5 hours. The main route of excretion is renal, 67% of the injected dose being excreted in 24 hours. The mean administered dose was 859 ± 73 MBq (23.2 ± 2.0 mCi). Estimated radiation doses were highest to the testes (0.035 mGy/MBq) followed by the kidney (0.032 mGy/MBq), thyroid (0.019 mGy/MBq), and wall of the lower large intestine (0.017 mGy/MBq) (Amiscan 101 Study Report).

Glucarate uptake under conditions of ischemia and necrosis have been investigated in a variety of experimental models. In experiments of occlusion-reperfusion conducted with dogs, rats, and rabbits, investigators have found tracer uptake only in tri-phenyl-tetrazolium chloride (TTC)–negative myocardium (necrosis positive) and not in regions that were ischemic-reperfused and TTC positive (necrosis negative) (27–30). When uptake of ^{99m}Tc glucarate was compared with that of ^{111}In antimyosin in rabbits there were positive correlations for both reperfused and nonreperfused areas of infarction, but counts in the infarct were higher for ^{99m}Tc glucarate (30). Better uptake in reperfused infarcts probably occurs because the smaller molecular size of ^{99m}Tc glucarate allows better access to low-flow regions. In a swine model of severe ischemia caused by fixed 80% coronary artery stenosis with pacing, ^{99m}Tc glucarate was taken up in the risk region with minimal necrosis according to TTC staining and early scattered myocyte death at electron microscopic examination (26). That the tracer was injected during pacing and uptake was clearly visualized on in vivo planar scans performed 2 hours later suggests ^{99m}Tc glucarate is taken up by severely ischemic-necrotic myocytes almost immediately as the cells are irreparably damaged. Khaw et al. (25) performed fractional extraction of radioactivity from infarcted tissues into nuclear, mitochondrial, and cytosolic fractions and found greater than 75% of radioactivity in the nuclear fraction. From these results, they proposed the mechanism for ^{99m}Tc glucarate uptake as binding to the highly basic histones in the nuclei of irreparably damaged myocytes.

Mariani et al. (31) in Genoa performed an early clinical trial of ^{99m}Tc glucarate imaging with 28 patients who came to the emergency department with acute ischemic syndromes. The patients were given injections in the emergency department and underwent three-view planar imaging an average of 3 hours after the injection. Eighteen patients received thrombolytic therapy, and a final diagnosis of acute myocardial infarction was confirmed in 23 and angina in 5 cases. In this small sample, the sensitivity of ^{99m}Tc glucarate imaging in the detection of acute myocardial infarction was time dependent. Fourteen patients given injections within 9 hours of the onset of chest pain had positive scan results (Fig. 17.2). The other nine scans with false-negative results were those of patients given injections more than 9 hours after the onset of pain. The time between injection and imaging did not affect the positive results of the scan. Scans that clearly showed focal uptake in the infarct region imaged 3 hours after injection also had clearly positive results as late as 23 hours after injection despite decay of the technetium. The results of this pilot study support the experimental data, which showed ^{99m}Tc glucarate is taken up soon after the onset of necrosis and can be imaged soon after injection and that the time window for positive scan results is early in the course of infarction. These

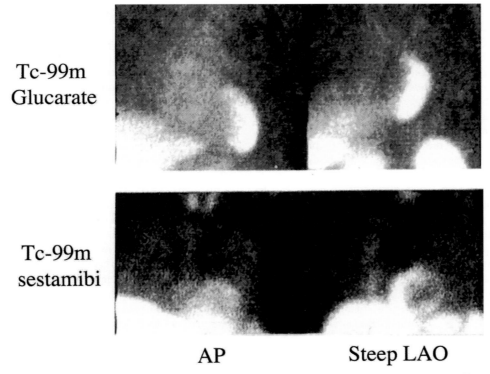

FIGURE 17.2. Anterior (*left*) and steep left anterior oblique (*right*) planar images obtained with ^{99m}Tc glucarate (*top*) and ^{99m}Tc sestamibi (*bottom*). The patient had arrived in the emergency department 3.5 hours after onset of chest pain. Glucarate imaging was performed 3.5 hours after the onset of chest pain, and the sestamibi scan was performed 2 days later. The extensive uptake of ^{99m}Tc glucarate in the anterolateral wall corresponds in extent and location to the perfusion defect. (Images provided by Dr. Giuliano Mariani and adapted from Mariani G, Villa G, Rossettin PF, et al. Detection of acute myocardial infarction by 99mTc-labeled D-glucaric acid imaging in patients with acute chest pain. *J Nucl Med* 1999; 40:1832–1839, with permission.)

properties are different from those of antimyosin and suggest that ^{99m}Tc glucarate may find clinical use for early diagnosis of necrosis in patients with non–ST-segment elevation myocardial infarction. A phase II clinical trial is in progress.

IMAGING APOPTOSIS: ANNEXIN V

As part of the process of embryologic development, regulation of the immune system, necessary cell death in viral illness, and response to hormonal stimulation and withdrawal, the organism must have a mechanism for eliminating cells that have completed their useful function or are detrimental (32). This physiologic process is *apoptosis,* or programmed cell death. Apoptosis is energy dependent and orderly. Cells autodigest their components and enclose noxious chemical substances into lipid-enclosed vesicles that can undergo phagocytosis without provoking an inflammatory response. Apoptosis also plays a role in disease. Loss of normal apoptosis contributes to neoplastic growth. Apoptosis has been observed in several pathologic cardiac conditions, including hypoxia, myocardial ischemia and reperfusion, myocardial infarction, right ventricular dysplasia, rejection of heart transplants, and dilated cardiomyopathy (33–36). Apoptosis of macrophages has been observed in unstable atherosclerotic lesions (37). Triggers to apoptosis in pathologic states identified to date include radiation, myocardial cell stretch, pressure overload, and the presence of oxygen radicals, nitric oxide, or cytokines such as tumor necrosis factor α. Once triggered, the apoptotic process becomes irreversible through activation of a proteolytic cascade of cysteine proteases called *caspases.* Early in the process of apoptosis there is a rearrangement of the phospholipids in the cell membranes. Two enzymes, called *translocase* and *floppase,* maintain a phospholipid called *phosphatidylserine* (PS) on the inner leaflet of the membrane. When apoptosis is triggered, these two enzymes are inactivated, and another enzyme called *scramblase* is activated and flips PS to the outer leaflet of the membrane. In this location, PS is available to bind with a ligand.

Annexin V is an endogenous human protein with a high affinity for PS on the cell membrane. It is an acute-phase reactant, but its precise function in the body is unknown. Annexin has a high affinity for PS, comparable with receptor-ligand affinity, making it an excellent agent for imaging exposed PS and potentially identifying and quantifying apoptosis. The genes coding for human annexin have been identified and cloned, and the protein is produced by means of recombinant technology. Radiolabeling of annexin V with ^{99m}Tc can be accomplished by means of several approaches. The method for products used in clinical trials involves to diaminedisulfide (N2S2) with subsequent reduction of technetium to label the protein (38).

IMAGING TRANSPLANT REJECTION AND MYOCARDIAL INFARCTION

Blankenberg et al. (39) at Stanford University performed proof of concept experiments documenting uptake of radiolabeled annexin V in an animal model of apoptosis. A group of investigators (40,41) at Columbia University have shown that nitric oxide

triggers apoptosis in experimental animals. They went on to demonstrate increased expression of inducible nitric oxide synthase in biopsy specimens of right ventricle from patients with allograft rejection (42). These experimental data show that ^{99m}Tc annexin-V imaging may be a good agent for diagnosing and quantifying allograft rejection in heart transplantation. Proof of concept for uptake in animal models of transplant rejection has been shown (43,44). Clinical trials are in progress. One possible limitation to using this method to quantify cardiac rejection in patients is that apoptotic cell density does not correlate directly with the severity of the rejection at biopsy. Preliminary results have shown positive scan results in some patients with biopsy-proven rejection, but the uptake has been faint, and SPECT is needed. Some patients have diffuse uptake, others have focal uptake. More severe rejection correlates with a greater percentage of positive scan results but not with more intense tracer uptake.

Apoptotic cells have been identified in areas of severe ischemia and infarction in animal models (34,35). There is debate surrounding the importance of this mode of cell death vis-à-vis necrotic cell death in acute myocardial infarction. The methods used to detect apoptosis are based on identifying DNA fragmentation and include the ladder method based on finding 180-base-pair lengths or multiples thereof, and terminal deoxynucleotidyl transferase–mediated deoxyuridine triphosphate–biotin nick end labeling (TUNEL). It is unclear whether these methods are accurate when tissue is intermixed in both apoptotic and necrotic cells. This distinction may not be important for imaging. As enzymes are deregulated in severe ischemia leading to necrotic death, PS is exposed and may be bound by annexin V. More specifically, annexin V is a marker for PS expression regardless of the route by which it is expressed. In a pilot study, Hofstra et al. (45) in the Netherlands documented uptake of ^{99m}Tc annexin V in patients with acute myocardial infarction. They reported the results obtained for 7 patients who arrived for treatment within 6 hours of the onset of chest pain. The patients underwent SPECT early (3.4 hours) and late (20.5 hours) after injection. Scan results were positive in 6 of 7 cases. At early imaging, blood pool activity was still too high to see focal myocardial uptake, but at late imaging, the focal uptake was clearly seen (Fig. 17.3). Additional clinical trials are in progress.

HYPOXIA-AVID IMAGING AGENTS

Tissue hypoxia occurs in tumors and in ischemic myocardium. The classes of agents described in this section have a dual purpose—tumor imaging and myocardial imaging. The location and extent of tumor hypoxia is a major factor in determining the success of cancer therapy. Although myocardial ischemia (hypoxia) due to an imbalance between oxygen supply and demand is a common clinical problem, perfusion imaging is successful in assessing extent and severity. Possible uses of hypoxia-avid hotspot imaging agents are not yet defined.

Tracers developed to image hypoxia have low redox potential. They become reduced by receiving electrons from disturbed mitochondrial electron transport chains in hypoxic cells with disturbed electron flow. The reduced complexes are trapped intra-

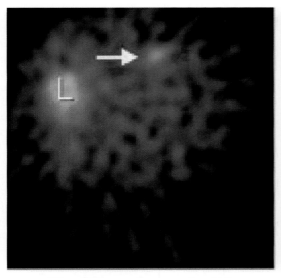 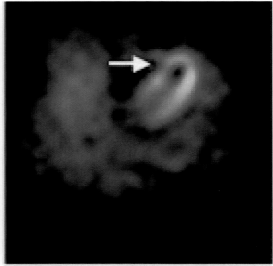

Tc-99m Annexin V   Tc-99m Sestamibi Rest

FIGURE 17.3. *Right,* transverse ^{99m}Tc sestamibi tomographic images of acute anteroseptal infarction (*arrow*) 22 hours after reperfusion by means of primary percutaneous transluminal coronary angioplasty. *Left,* increased uptake of ^{99m}Tc annexin V in the anteroseptal region (*arrow*) 4 hours after injection. *L,* liver. (Images provided by Dr. L. Hofstra and modified from Hofstra L, Liem IH, Dumont EA, et al. Visualization of cell death in vivo in patients with acute myocardial infarction. *Lancet* 2000;356:209–212, with permission.)

cellularly. Two classes of agents have been developed. The *nitroimidazoles* undergo reduction of the nitro functional group. The metal-containing *dithiosemicarbazone* complexes undergo reduction of copper complex exposed to oxygen-depleted cells. Two important questions confront investigators developing hypoxia agents for the heart. The first question is at what tissue oxygen level is the agent retained? The second is how often and in what clinical conditions do these levels of hypoxia occur? The answers to these questions are not readily obtainable because of limitations in measuring probes and experimental models. The unit for reporting oxygen concentration commonly used in medicine is *torr,* approximately equal to millimeters of mercury. Sensing microelectrode probes and chromophores with phosphorescence quenching can be used to measure tissue oxygen. Each technique has limitations for measuring transmural oxygen and requires direct application to the tissue. Retention of a compound can be measured in cell culture under different oxygen levels as well as anoxic conditions. These experiments do not take into account diffusion distances found in tissue. Perfused rat hearts are used to measure uptake and retention of tracers, but there are limitations to both blood and buffer perfused setups. The oxygen-carrying capacity of the buffer-perfused hearts is low and requires high flow rates to achieve normoxia. Even under these conditions, there are transient hypoxic periods during every cardiac cycle. Determining the level of myocardial blood flow necessary for tracer retention experimentally is easier than oxygen measurements, and the results are more readily applicable to humans.

NITROIMIDAZOLES

The nitroimidazoles are compounds used in therapeutic doses as radiation sensitizers and as antibiotics (46,47). The efficacy of these agents is based on retention in tissue with low oxygen levels. Radioactive labeling with ^{99m}Tc has been achieved by means of complexing moieties through a ligand and leaving a reactive site. The mechanism for retention in therapeutic doses probably involves covalent intracellular binding, but when the agent is given in tracer amounts for imaging, the retention mechanism of the reactive products is not known. The oxygen level extrapolated from cell culture required for retention of 50% of maximal value was approximately 0.04 torr. Because of the technical limitations mentioned earlier, this value is probably too low and cannot be extrapolated to in vivo conditions. This remains an area of active investigation.

The first nitroimidazole compound investigated was BMS-181321. Using Langendorff buffer-perfused rat hearts, Ng et al. (48) showed increasing retention curves as oxygen levels decreased. Using an extracorporeal coronary perfusion open chest swine model, Stone et al. (49) investigated the relation between coronary blood flow and tracer retention. Reduced flow to the left anterior descending coronary artery was maintained during tracer injection. Retention began to increase as flow decreased to less than 1.0 mL/g/min and continued to increase as flow decreased to 0.2 mL/g/min. Using an open-chest canine model, Shi et al. (50) found results similar to those found by Stone et al.: increasing retention with progressively reduced coronary blood flow. However, in vivo imaging showed poor target to background ratios and inability to differentiate visually hypoxic from normoxic areas. Target to background uptake depends on washout from normoxic tissue as well as retention in hypoxic tissue. This first compound had relatively slow washout from normoxic tissue. To improve washout from normoxic tissue, chemical modifications to the original compound were made. The 2-nitroimidazole moiety was removed from the parent compound;

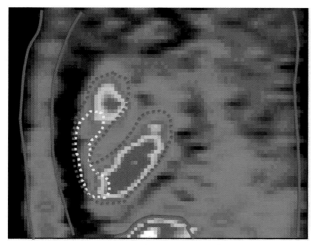 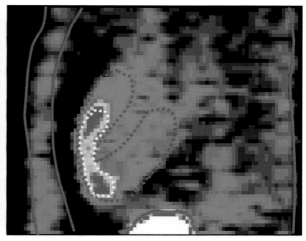

Left Lateral
Tl-201

Left Lateral
Tc-99mBRU 59-21

FIGURE 17.4. Left lateral planar images from an experimental study of left anterior descending coronary artery occlusion in canine model. *Left,* thallium images show an anteroapical perfusion defect. *Right,* [99m]Tc BRU 59-21 images show maximal tracer uptake in borders of anterior infarction. (Images provided by Adrian Nunn, Bracco Diagnostics, Princeton, NJ.)

the result was the compound called ^{99m}Tc-HL91. With an open-chest dog model of prolonged low flow, Okada et al. (51) showed hotspots in the risk region within 60 minutes of tracer injection. These hotspots continued to improve to a target to background ratio of 3.0 over 4 hours. Another modification of the original compound was to move the nitroimidazole moiety to the 6 position on the chelate ring and substitute an oxygen atom for the $-CH_2$ group in the 5 position. This compound, called BRU-59-21, has been studied in several animal models. In a canine infarct model, investigators at Bracco Diagnostics (52,53) in-

jected both ^{201}Tl and ^{99m}Tc BRU-59-21 into animals and found uptake of the radiolabeled nitroimidazole at the infarct border (Fig. 17.4). Uptake was fond in two different closed-chest swine models: fixed coronary stenosis with pacing (demand) and transient coronary occlusion. In the first study, tracer was injected during the third minute of 5 minutes of pacing. Focal hotspots were visualized in the risk region with in vivo imaging by 3 hours after injection. Several of the animals showed focal subendocardial necrosis with TTC staining. The nadir of endocardial blood flow in the risk region was 0.2 mL/g/min. In the second

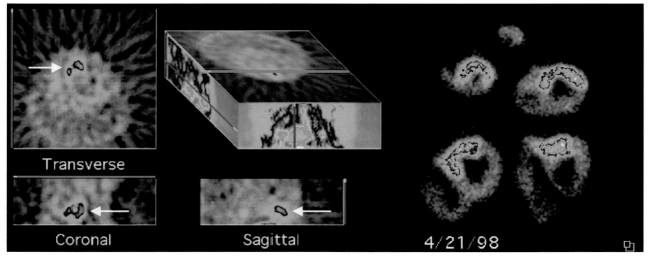

FIGURE 17.5. In vivo SPECT image (*left*) and ex vivo heart slices imaged on the detector from an experiment with domestic swine that entailed 6 minutes of occlusion of the left anterior descending coronary artery. [99m]Tc BRU 50-21 was injected 2 minutes before occlusion. Focal uptake is present in the ischemic risk region. Triphenyl-tetrazolium chloride staining showed no necrosis. (From Johnson LL, Schofield L, Donahay T, et al. Myocardial uptake of a ^{99m}Tc-nitroheterocycle in a swine model of occlusion and reperfusion. *J Nucl Med* 2000;41:1237–1243, with permission.)

study, tracer was injected at varying intervals in relation to a period of transient (6 minutes) coronary occlusion to investigate the timing between injection and positive scan results in transient ischemia. Endocardial blood flow in the risk region decreased to similarly low levels of 0.19 mL/g per minute. Hotspots were seen at in vivo imaging when tracer was injected 5.0 and 2.2 minutes before occlusion but not when it was injected 15 minutes before and 15 minutes after occlusion (Fig. 17.5).

DITHIOSEMICARBAZONES

A group of investigators in Japan developed a generator system that elutes copper nuclides as glycine complexes (54). This generator system is in clinical use in combination with the perfusion agent Cu(II)-pyruvaldehyde-*bis*(N4-methyl-thiosemicarbazone) (Cu-PTSM). Experimental studies showed that Cu-PTSM can be easily reduced by the electron transport system of normal mitochondria—Cu(II) to Cu(I)—and the reduced species retained in cells. It was hypothesized that a derivative of Cu-PTSM with a lower redox potential would be selectively retained in cells with abnormal mitochondria and might function as an effective hypoxia-avid imaging agent. Fuibayashi et al. (55) added a single methyl group on the ligand backbone to produce the copper complex to Cu(II)-diacetyl-*bis*(N4-methylthiosemicarbazone) (Cu-ATSM). The redox potential of Cu-ATSM is 100 mV lower than that of Cu-PTSM and close to that of the reduced form of nicotinamide adenine dinucleotide (NADH). They showed that disturbing the electron transport chain with rotenone increased reduction of the complex. With isolated perfused rat hearts subjected to normoxia, hypoxia, and reoxygenation, the investigators found greater than 80% retention under hypoxia compared with 20% under normoxic conditions. In rats with left anterior descending coronary artery occlusion, there was an inverse relation between relative thallium uptake and Cu-ATSM uptake (55). This same group of investigators compared uptake of ^{64}Cu-ATSM and ^{11}C-acetate (as a flow tracer) in rats given injections and killed within 20 minutes of occlusion before necrosis occurred. The investigators performed autoradiography on the heart slices (56). Areas of reduced ^{11}C-acetate corresponded to areas of increased ^{64}Cu-ATSM uptake. As relative blood flow expressed as normalized acetate values decreased, ^{64}Cu-ATSM uptake increased to 30% to 40% of normal when blood flow decreased and ceased at less than 20%. These results suggest that uptake at low flow is limited by poor delivery of tracer to the ischemic tissue.

In summary, two classes of hypoxia-avid hotspot imaging agents have been developed. A major clinical drive for their development is tumor imaging to help guide therapy. Cardiac uses for these agents have yet to be defined. Demand ischemia is well diagnosed with perfusion tracers. Use in the emergency department to identify acute rest ischemia secondary to transient coronary artery occlusion may be limited by the need to administer the injection at the time of occlusion. Uptake in infarct border zones may be useful in quantifying salvageable myocardium. It is unclear whether patients with chronic ischemic heart disease due to epicardial or microvascular disease have tissue hypoxia of sufficient severity at rest to retain one of these tracers

and if so what it may mean clinically. Hypoxia is a necessary condition for development of tumor angiogenesis and angiogenesis occurring after myocardial infarction. With the advent of angiogenesis therapy, the need to localize regional hypoxia to guide therapy may become important. These are areas of active research.

REFERENCES

1. Vanoverschelde JLJ, Wijns W, Borgers M, et al. Chronic myocardial hibernation in humans: from bench to bedside. *Circulation* 1997;95: 1961–1971.
2. Rahimtoola S. The hibernating myocardium. *Am Heart J* 1989;117: 211–221.
3. Diamond GA, Forrester JS, deLuz L, et al. Post-extrasystolic potentiation of ischemic myocardium by atrial stimulation. *Am Heart J* 1978; 95:204–209.
4. Vanoverschelde JLJ, Wijns W, Depre C, et al. Mechanisms of chronic regional postischemic dysfunction in humans: new insights from the study of noninfarcted collateral-dependent myocardium. *Circulation* 1993;87:1513–1523.
5. Shen YT, Vatner SF. Mechanism of impaired myocardial function during progressive coronary stenosis in conscious pigs: hibernation versus stunning? *Circ Res* 1995;76:479–488.
6. Wackers FJT, Gibbons RJ, Verani MS, et al. Serial quantitative planar technetium-99m isonitrile imaging in acute myocardial infarction: efficacy for noninvasive assessment of thrombolytic therapy. *J Am Coll Cardiol* 1989;4:861–873.
7. Sinusas AJ, Qing XS, Vitols PJ, et al. Impact of regional ventricular function, geometry, and dobutamine stress on quantitative ^{99}mTc-sestamibi defect size. *Circulation* 1993;88:2224–2234.
8. Kim RJ, Wu E, Rafael A, et al. The use of contrast-enhanced magnetic resonance imaging to identify reversible myocardial dysfunction. *N Engl J Med* 2000;343:1445–1453.
9. Parkey RW, Bonte FJ, Meyer SL, et al. A new method for radionuclide imaging of acute myocardial infarction in humans. *Circulation* 1974; 50:540–546.
10. Buja M, Tofe A, Kulkarni PV, et al. Sites and mechanisms of localization of technetium-99m phosphorous radiopharmaceuticals in acute myocardial infarcts and other tissues. *J Clin Invest* 1977;60:724–740.
11. Beller GA, Khaw BA, Haber E, et al. Localization of radiolabeled cardiac myosin-specific antibody in myocardial infarcts comparison with technetium-99m stannous pyrophosphate. *Circulation* 1977;55: 74–78.
12. Poliner LR, Buja LM, Parkey RW, et al. Clinicopathologic findings in 52 patients studied by technetium-99m stannous pyrophosphate myocardial scintigraphy. *Circulation* 1979;59:257–267.
13. Khaw BA, Beller GA, Haber E, et al. Localization of cardiac myosin-specific antibody in myocardial infarction. *J Clin Invest* 1976;58: 439–446.
14. Khaw BA, Fallon JT, Beller GA, et al. Specificity of localization of myosin-specific antibody fragments in experimental myocardial infarction, histologic, histochemical, autoradiographic and scintigraphic studies. *Circulation* 1979;60:1527–1531.
15. Khaw BA, Scott J, Fallon JT, et al. Myocardial injury: quantification by cell sorting initiated with antimyosin fluorescent spheres. *Science* 1982;217:1050–1053.
16. Torchilin VP, Klibanov AL, Nossiff ND, et al. Monoclonal antibody modification with chelate-linked high-molecular-weight polymers: major increases in polyvalent cation binding without loss of antigen binding. *Hybridoma* 1987;6:229–240.
17. Rhodes BA, Zamora PO, Newell KD, et al. Technetium-99m labeling of murine monoclonal antibody fragments. *J Nucl Med* 1986;27: 685–693.
18. Senior R, Bhattacharya S, Manspeaker P, et al. ^{99}mTc-antimyosin antibody imaging for the detection of acute myocardial infarction in human beings. *Am Heart J* 1993;126:536–542.
19. Johnson LL, Lerrick KS, Coromilas J, et al. Measurement of infarct

size and percentage myocardium infarcted in a dog preparation with single photon emission computed tomography, thallium-201 and indium-111 monoclonal antimyosin Fab. *Circulation* 1987;76:181–190.

20. Johnson LL, Seldin DW, Becker LC, et al. Antimyosin imaging in acute transmural myocardial infarctions: results of a multicenter clinical trial. *J Am Coll Cardiol* 1989;13:27–35.

21. Antman EM, Tanasijevic MJ, Thompson, et al. Cardiac-specific troponin I levels to predict the risk of mortality in patients with acute coronary syndromes. *N Engl J Med* 1996;355:1342–1349.

22. Matsumori A, Yamada T, Tamaki N, et al. Persistent uptake of indium-111-antimyosin monoclonal antibody in patients with myocardial infarction. *Am Heart J* 1990;120:1026–1030.

23. Tamaki N, Yamada T, Matsumori A, et al. Indium-111-antimyosin antibody imaging for detecting different stages of myocardial infarction: comparison with technetium-99m-pyrophosphate imaging. *J Nucl Med* 1990;31:136–142.

24. Johnson LL, Seldin DW, Keller AM, et al. Dual isotope thallium and indium antimyosin SPECT imaging to identify acute infarct patients at further ischemic risk. *Circulation* 1990;81:37–45.

25. Khaw BA, Nakazawa A, O'Donnell SM, et al. Avidity of technetium 99m glucarate for the necrotic myocardium: in vivo and in vitro assessment. *J Nucl Cardiol* 1997;4:283–290.

26. Johnson LL, Schofield L, Mastrofrancesco P, et al. Technetium-99m glucarate uptake in a swine model of limited flow increased demand. *J Nucl Cardiol* 2000;7:590–598.

27. Yaoita H, Fischman AJ, Wilkinson R, et al. Distribution of deoxyglucose and technetium-99m-glucarate in the acutely ischemic myocardium. *J Nucl Med* 1993;34:1303–1308.

28. Ohtani H, Callahan RJ, Khaw BA, et al. Comparison of technetium-99m-glucarate and thallium-201 for the identification of acute myocardial infarction in rats. *J Nucl Med* 1992;33:1988–1993.

29. Orlandi C, Crane PD, Edwards DS, et al. Early scintigraphic detection of experimental myocardial infarction in dogs with technetium-99m-glucaric acid. *J Nucl Med* 1991;32:263–268.

30. Narula J, Petrov A, Pak KY, et al. Very early non-invasive detection of acute experimental nonreperfused myocardial infarction with 99mTc-labeled glucarate. *Circulation* 1997;95:1577–1584.

31. Mariani G, Villa G, Rossettin PF, et al. Detection of acute myocardial infarction by 99mTc-labeled D-glucaric acid imaging in patients with acute chest pain. *J Nucl Med* 1999;40:1832–1839.

32. Blankenberg F, Narula J, Strauss HW. In vivo detection of apoptotic cell death: a necessary measurement for evaluation therapy for myocarditis, ischemia and heart failure. *J Nucl Cardiol* 1999;6:531–539.

33. Gottlieb RA, Burleson KO, Kloner RA, et al. Reperfusion injury induces apoptosis in rabbit cardiomyocytes. *J Clin Invest* 1884;94:1621–1628.

34. Kajstura J, Cheng W, Reiss K, et al. Apoptotic and necrotic myocyte cell deaths are independent contributing variables in infarct size in rats. *Lab Invest* 1996;74:86–107.

35. Fliss H, Gattinger D. Apoptosis in ischemic and reperfused rat myocardium. *Circ Res* 1996;79:949–956.

36. vanHeerde WL, Robert-Offerman S, Dumont E, et al. Markers of apoptosis in cardiovascular tissues: focus on annexin-V. *Cardiovasc Res* 2000;45:549–559.

37. Bjorkerud S, Bjorkerud B. Apoptosis is abundant in human atherosclerotic lesions especially in inflammatory cells (macrophages and T cells) and may contribute to accumulation of gruel and plaque instability. *Am J Pathol* 1996;149:367–380.

38. Tait JF, Brown DS, Gibson DF, et al. Development and characterization of annexin V mutants with endogenous chelation sites for (99m) Tc. *Bioconjug Chem* 2000;11;6:918–925.

39. Blankenberg FG, Katsikis PD, Tait JF, et al. In vivo detection and imaging of phosphatidylserine expression during programmed cell death. *Proc Natl Acad Sci U S A* 1998;95:6349–6354.

40. Pinsky DJ, Aji W, Szabolcs M, et al. Nitric oxide triggers programmed cell death (apoptosis) of adult rat ventricular myocytes in culture. *Am J Physiol* 1999;277:H1189–H1199.

41. Yang X, Ma N, Szabolcs M, et al. Upregulation of COX-2 during cardiac allograft rejection. *Circulation* 2000;101:430–438.

42. Szabolcs MJ, Ravalli S, Minanov O, et al. Apoptosis and increased expression of inducible nitric oxide synthase in human allograft rejection. *Transplantation* 1998;65:804–812.

43. Vriens PW, Blankenberg FG, Stoot JH, et al. The use of technetium TC99m annexin V for in vivo imaging of apoptosis during cardiac allograft rejection. *J Thorac Cardiovasc Surg* 1998;116:844–853.

44. Oguro Y, Krams SM, Martinez OM, et al. Radiolabeled annexin V imaging: diagnosis of allograft rejection in an experimental rodent model of liver transplantation. *Radiology* 2000;214:795–800.

45. Hofstra L, Liem IH, Dumont EA, et al. Visualization of cell death in vivo in patients with acute myocardial infarction. *Lancet* 2000;356:209–212.

46. Nunn A. The biology of technetium based hypoxic tissue localising compounds. In: Machulla HJ. *Imaging of hypoxia: tracer developments*. Dordrecht, The Netherlands: Kluwer Academic Publishers, 1999:19–45.

47. Nunn A, Linder K, Strauss HW. Nitroimidazoles and imaging hypoxia. *Eur J Nucl Med* 1995;22:265–280.

48. Ng CK, Sinusas AJ, Zaret BL, et al. Kinetic analysis of technetium-99m-labeled nitroimidazole (BMS-181321) as a tracer of myocardial hypoxia. *Circulation* 1995;92:1261–1268.

49. Stone CK, Mulnix T, Nickles RJ, et al. Myocardial kinetics of a putative hypoxic tissue marker, 99mTc-labeled nitroimidazole (BMS-181321), after regional ischemia and reperfusion. *Circulation* 1995;92:1246–1253.

50. Shi CQX, Sinusas AJ, Dione DP, et al. Technetium-99m-nitroimidazole (BMS181321), a positive imaging agent for detecting myocardial ischemia. *J Nucl Med* 1995;36:1078–1086.

51. Okada RD, Johnson G, Nguyen KN, et al. 99mTc-HL91 "hot spot" detection of ischemic myocardium in vivo by gamma camera imaging. *Circulation* 1998;97:2557–2566.

52. Johnson LL, Schofield L, Donahay T, et al. Myocardial uptake of a 99mTc-nitroheterocycle in a swine model of occlusion and reperfusion. *J Nucl Med* 2000;41:1237–1243.

53. Johnson LL, Schofield L, Mastrofrancesco P, et al. Technetium-99m-nitroimidazole uptake in a swine model of demand ischemia. *J Nucl Med* 1998;39:1468–1475.

54. Mastumoto K, Fujibayashi Y, Yonekura Y. Application of the new zinc-62;copper-62 generator: an effective labeling method for 62 Cu-PTXM. *Nucl Med Biol* 1992;19:36–44.

55. Fujibayashi Y, Taniuchi H, Yonejura Y, et al. Copper-62-ATSM: a new hypoxia imaging agent with high membrane permeability and low redox potential. *J Nucl Med* 1997;38:1155–1160.

56. Fujibayashi Y, Cutler CS, Anderson CJ, et al. Comparative studies of Cu-64-ATSM and C-11-acetate in an acute myocardial infarction model: ex vivo imaging of hypoxia in rats. *Nucl Med Biol* 1999;26;1:117–121.

Diagnostic Nuclear Medicine, Fourth Edition. Edited by M.P. Sandler, R.E. Coleman, J.A. Patton, F.J.Th. Wackers, A. Gottschalk. Lippincott Williams & Wilkins, Philadelphia 2003.

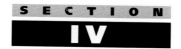

PULMONARY

EVALUATION OF PATIENTS WITH SUSPECTED VENOUS THROMBOEMBOLISM

H. DIRK SOSTMAN
ALEXANDER GOTTSCHALK

Pulmonary embolism (PE) is not itself a disease. Rather, it is a potentially fatal complication of deep vein thrombosis (DVT). Accordingly, these two processes must be considered together. Although effective therapy is available for venous thromboembolism, the therapy itself can produce considerable morbidity. An accurate diagnosis is mandatory. The clinical manifestations and laboratory findings of pulmonary embolism are nonspecific. Additional evaluation with imaging studies is essential. However, accurate imaging tests are invasive, and noninvasive imaging tests are imperfectly accurate.

These simple facts are at the center of diagnostic evaluation and clinical treatment of patients believed to have PE. Despite this underlying simplicity, the attendant details can be problematic. Many of the issues in diagnosis and management of suspected PE revolve around the appropriate performance, interpretation, and utilization of imaging tests, the subjects of this chapter.

PRETEST PROBABILITY

Epidemiology

Subclinical PE may be extremely common if the autopsy data represent the true picture, because pathologic studies have shown PE present at as many as 70% of autopsies when the emboli are sought zealously (1). The occurrence of clinically significant PE probably depends on several factors. These include the degree of vascular occlusion produced by the emboli, the pulmonary vascular reserve, the age of the embolized thrombus, and the presence of associated medical or surgical conditions affecting cardiac function, pulmonary vascular smooth muscle function, and fibrinolytic activity.

There is uncertainty about patient selection and the accuracy of diagnostic tests as used in clinical studies defining the fre-

quency of PE. Therefore interpretation of results is not straight-forward. The prevalence of PE in large series of patients with clinical evidence of PE referred for ventilation-perfusion (V/Q) scans has ranged from 25% to 50%. A reasonable point estimate would be approximately 33%, which was the frequency observed in the Prospective Investigation of Pulmonary Embolism Diagnosis (PIOPED) (2). However, most of the prevalence data in the literature emanate from academic, tertiary care hospitals and associated clinics. The prevalence of PE in other types of inpatient and outpatient settings may be quite different (consider, for example, the possible differences between private suburban family practice offices and inner city public hospitals).

For clinical practice, we want to know the actual pretest probability for an individual patient. If this and the operating characteristics of the diagnostic test (e.g., the likelihood ratios for positive and negative results) are known, a reasonable estimate of the probability that an individual patient has the disease can be derived. The starting point for assessment of pretest probability is the relative risk of venous thrombosis in certain groups to which individual patients may belong.

The clinical groups at high risk of venous thrombosis and PE are well known. Certain discrete types of coagulopathy, such as deficiency of antithrombin III, protein C, or protein S, are associated with high risk of thrombosis. A variety of clinical conditions in which venous stasis or intimal injury is present place the patient at high risk of DVT and PE. Such conditions, which can be transient, include pelvic and lower extremity trauma (including surgery), prolonged general anesthesia, burns, pregnancy and the postpartum state, venous obstruction (previous DVT, extrinsic mass or fibrosis), occupational venous stasis, congestive heart failure, immobility (long automobile and airplane trips are notorious risk factors), obesity, cancer, advanced age, and certain drugs (e.g., estrogens). These risk factors can be additive.

The approximate prevalence of PE in a particular population may or may not be known. It usually is possible, however, for the clinician to have an initial estimate of the relative risk of venous thromboembolism in an individual patient before a detailed clinical and imaging evaluation begins.

H. Dirk Sostman: Radiology Department, Weill Medical College of Cornell University, and NY-Weill Cornell Medical Center, New York, NY.

A. Gottschalk: Department of Radiology, Michigan State University, East Lansing, MI.

Course of Disease

Dalen and Alpert (3) estimated that 11% of patients with PE experience sudden death. They further estimated that the diagnosis of PE is not made in 63% of cases, and no treatment is given. This group has an estimated 30% mortality rate, presumably owing to recurrent emboli. In the other 26% of cases, the diagnosis is made and treatment is given. In this group the mortality rate is thought to decrease to 8%. Thus proper diagnosis and therapy are believed to reduce mortality significantly. However, Dalen and Alpert based their estimates of the consequences of not treating patients on results for series in which the diagnosis of PE was made on clinical grounds alone (4). Because the clinical diagnosis of PE is inaccurate, the 30% death rate ascribed to PE in patients not given anticoagulants is likely also to be inaccurate. We must recognize that we do not know precisely the efficacy of anticoagulant therapy.

Only limited data are available concerning the long-term outcome for patients who survive the initial episode of PE. Owing to the interplay between fibrinolysis and organization, the degree of net residual vascular obstruction is variable. Resolution of acute PE has not been documented to occur in less than 24 hours. The documented rates of resolution vary from 1 or 2 days to several weeks or months. At a 4-month follow-up evaluation, 60% or more of all patients with PE have at least improvement in pulmonary blood flow, and 40% have complete recovery. However, 35% of patients may have incomplete resolution of scintigraphic abnormalities. Older patients, patients with larger emboli, and patients with coexisting congestive heart failure are more likely to have incomplete resolution and residual perfusion defects on V/Q scans. Accordingly, follow-up scans are highly useful in defining the new baseline for the patient for possible future diagnostic encounters (5).

Clinical Assessment

The clinical manifestations among patients with PE are variable and relatively nonspecific (6–8). Although numerous signs and symptoms have been touted as establishing a diagnosis, none has been found truly discriminatory after objective assessment. The "classic" triad of dyspnea, pleurisy, and hemoptysis, for example, was present in only a small number of patients with confirmed PE in the Urokinase Pulmonary Embolism Trial. However, many patients do have characteristic clinical features. Among patients with confirmed PE without preexisting cardiac or pulmonary disease, either dyspnea or tachypnea occurred in 96%. When the clinical diagnosis of DVT also was present, 99% of patients with a diagnosis of PE were included. Unfortunately, dyspnea and tachypnea occur in a wide variety of both serious and trivial clinical disorders, and thus these findings are not specific for PE.

Reliable exclusion or confirmation of acute PE by means of electrocardiography or blood chemical analysis is not currently possible. The Pco_2 and Po_2 lack sensitivity and specificity, although they can serve in assessment of the severity of the acute event. Po_2 cannot be used to exclude an embolus, because as many as 15% of patients with PE may have a Po_2 greater than 80 mm Hg when breathing ambient air. The use of blood mark-ers for coagulation has been studied extensively and some, such as D-dimer levels, may have an adjunctive role in clinical evaluation, possibly in combination with alveolar dead-space measurements (9).

The clinical examination also has been shown to be inaccurate for DVT. The signs and symptoms used to make a clinical diagnosis of DVT—calf pain and tenderness, unilateral lower limb swelling, positive Homan sign—occur with equal frequency among patients with and those without confirmed thrombi. In approximately 50% of patients with clinically suspected DVT, no thrombus is found at further testing. Autopsy studies show the poor sensitivity of clinical examination. In only 11% to 25% of cases of autopsy-proven DVT was the diagnosis suspected before death. However, if the clinical signs and symptoms suggest DVT, there is greater likelihood that a thrombus is present than there is if the results of clinical examination are normal. More recent analysis has suggested that a limited number of clinical findings are relatively accurate predictors of the occurrence of DVT (10), but this remains to be confirmed by independent evaluations.

The low sensitivity of symptoms, signs, and results of clinical laboratory tests implies that a significant number of silent cases of PE and DVT occur. Among patients at high risk, unremarkable results of a clinical examination do not reliably exclude thromboembolic disease. Conversely, the diagnosis must be confirmed, even when the clinical features are classic for DVT or PE, because of the low specificity of clinical and laboratory evaluation.

Overall Assessment of Pretest Probability

Although objective testing is crucial to the diagnosis of venous thromboembolism, the population under a particular physician's care is probably well-defined experientially, and the clinical assessment of the probability that disease exists likely is much more useful than has been suggested. In the PIOPED, the pretest estimate of the likelihood of PE by experienced clinicians was almost as accurate as the V/Q scan categorization (Table 18A.1). These clinical estimates were not made according to set criteria, and thus it is impossible for them to be tested or improved on in other studies. In addition to the overall assessment, results of recent analyses suggest that V/Q scan interpretive criteria can be usefully adjusted according to the patient's history (see later, Diagnostic Criteria: Newer Data and the PIOPED II).

Table 18A.1. *Ventilation-Perfusion (V/Q) Scintigraphy versus Clinical Assessment*

V/Q scintigraphy		Clinical assessment	
Category	PPV (%)	Category (%)	PPV (%)
High	87	80–100	74
Intermediate	29	20–79	31
Low–normal	11	0–19	9

Positive predictive value (PPV) in the PIOPED study for pulmonary embolism of the pretest clinical assessment and the V/Q scan categories of high, intermediate, and low through normal.
Data from The PIOPED Investigators. Value of the ventilation/perfusion scan in acute pulmonary embolism. *JAMA* 1990;263:2753–2759.

APPROACH TO THE IMAGING EVALUATION

The goal of diagnostic imaging is to direct therapy. Because anticoagulation is appropriate for patients who have either PE or DVT, the finding of either a venous thrombus or a pulmonary embolus is sufficient to begin anticoagulant therapy. When considering venous thrombi, some physicians usually treat the patient only for thrombi in the popliteal vein or more proximal deep veins. Others selectively or always treat the patients for calf thrombi or superficial thrombi. Thrombosis of calf veins without proximal extension is unlikely to result in PE.

In examination of the lungs to establish the diagnosis of acute PE, the finding of a single embolus is sufficient. The therapeutic effort rarely is directed at managing the event that has already occurred. It is directed at preventing a subsequent event (11). Demonstrating the presence of the disease process is sufficient, and quantification of the size or number of emboli usually is not necessary. However, when clinical concern relates to possibly recurrent embolism or evaluation of clot burden for possible lytic therapy, quantification of disease may be useful.

VENOUS IMAGING

Role in the Diagnostic Evaluation

There is, of course, a strong correlation between PE and DVT, because PE is a manifestation of the process of venous thromboembolism, which normally begins with DVT. Accordingly, DVT and PE must be considered together in diagnostic evaluation and patient care. A patient with respiratory symptoms initially needs an imaging evaluation for possible PE. The study should be directed at the chest. If the diagnosis remains uncertain, venous imaging can be performed instead of additional noninvasive pulmonary imaging or invasive pulmonary angiography. Noninvasive venous imaging is safe, more pleasant for the patient, and more widely available than is arteriography. However, venous imaging of patients with documented PE often does not show DVT, and further pulmonary imaging may be needed if the findings at venous imaging are normal. This may be due to modality-specific false-negative results of imaging or to embolization of the entire venous thrombus.

Radiologic Venous Imaging Techniques

Contrast venography is the diagnostic standard of reference for DVT. Extensive experience has shown that identification of well-defined filling defects in fully opacified veins is accurate for detection of DVT but that negative findings at conventional venography have been shown to exclude clinically significant DVT (12). However, venography does have limitations, including difficulties in venous cannulation, incomplete filling of the venous system, and other technical problems in as many as 5% of cases (13); discomfort in as many as 8% of patients, even when nonionic contrast material is used; and a variety of local and systemic reactions to contrast material, including induced DVT in as many as 8% of cases, even when nonionic contrast material is used (14,15).

The limitations of conventional venography led to develop-ment of noninvasive tests for DVT. Compression ultrasonography and its refinements have been investigated extensively (16–20). The sensitivity and specificity of ultrasonography for proximal (above-knee) DVT in patients with symptoms is very high, more than 95%. However, ultrasonography also has limitations. It is less accurate in the diagnosis of recurrent DVT, although follow-up studies after acute episodes can improve accuracy in subsequent diagnostic encounters; it is operator dependent, particularly for calf DVT; and accuracy in the diagnosis of pelvic DVT has not been demonstrated. Ultrasonography is significantly less sensitive (~65%) for asymptomatic DVT (20) and therefore is not recommended as a screening procedure for patients at high risk who do not have symptoms.

Venous imaging with magnetic resonance (MR) for detecting DVT is used at a few centers. Published accuracy figures show sensitivity and specificity greater than 95% for all sites of DVT, including those in patients without symptoms. MR imaging is more sensitive than is ultrasonography in areas known to be difficult to image with ultrasound (pelvis, adductor canal, calf), but the specificity of the two techniques is equivalent (21,22). There is some suggestion, based on anecdotal data and personal experience, that MR imaging is a superior method for differentiating acute and chronic DVT. Although advanced MR technology is not required, experience with normal flow-related signal loss in the pelvic veins is necessary to avoid errors, and accuracy can be expected to be institution-specific at this stage of development and dissemination In addition, MR imaging is limited by high expense and lack of scanner availability.

"Direct" computed tomographic (CT) venography has been performed with direct pedal injection of iodinated contrast medium. It is subject to the same complications as is conventional venography. However, several investigators have begun to perform "indirect" CT venography—CT imaging of the lower extremities after CT pulmonary arteriography without administration of additional contrast material. Acceptable image contrast between DVT and blood can be obtained with this approach. The accuracy for detecting DVT is high (sensitivity, 98%; specificity, 96%) compared with that of ultrasonography (23,24), but ultrasonography is an admittedly imperfect standard of reference. Nevertheless, the technique of indirect CT venography combined with CT pulmonary angiography will increase the diagnostic yield of venous thromboembolism among patients who undergo this combined procedure.

PULMONARY IMAGING

Role in the Diagnostic Evaluation

The emphasis placed on venous imaging in the evaluation of patients with suspected venous thromboembolism should not obscure the central role of pulmonary imaging of patients with respiratory or thoracic symptoms. For these patients, the diagnostic investigation should be directed first at the thorax.

Chest Radiograph

Chest radiography is not an accurate method of diagnosing PE (25). Most patients who have PE, and many undergo evaluation for PE with normal results, have abnormal chest radiographic findings (26). The most suggestive signs of PE on chest radiographs are focal oligemia or changes in the size of the proximal pulmonary artery, but these signs can be difficult to interpret unless good comparison images are available. The nonspecific findings commonly associated with PE include consolidation, atelectasis, small pleural effusion, and diaphragmatic elevation. Parenchymal abnormalities from PE usually resolve within 1 to 4 weeks. Pleural fibrosis and linear scars may remain. Although cavitation can occur in bland infarcts, it is uncommon without coexisting infection.

The chest radiograph is used to exclude clinical mimics of PE, including rib fracture and pneumothorax. If V/Q scintigraphy is performed, the chest radiograph is needed for comparison with the V/Q study. High quality posteroanterior and lateral chest radiographs should be obtained at the same time as the V/Q scan. If radiography is performed with portable equipment, the patient's position should be recorded accurately. For a patient with suspected acute PE, the chest radiograph should be obtained as close in time to the V/Q scan as possible, but certainly within 12 hours of the V/Q scan. If the patient has intervening symptoms, another chest radiograph should be obtained before scanning.

Other Noninvasive Pulmonary Imaging Techniques

There has been considerable interest in helical CT for detecting PE. Results of several studies have been quite good (27–32), an overall sensitivity of 80% to 85% and specificity of 90% to 95%. These results have led some authors to advocate wholesale replacement of the V/Q scintigraphy with helical CT. This proposal is being actively debated, but it has already been adopted in clinical practice at some centers. Because the sensitivity of CT is lower than that of perfusion scintigraphy, a critical question concerns clinical outcome among untreated patients with normal CT findings. Data are sparse. Results of one study suggested that PE recurred within 3 months in 3 of 109 (2.8%) untreated patients with intermediate V/Q, negative CT, and negative lower extremity ultrasound findings (33). Those of another study suggested that the risk of subsequent PE after normal findings are obtained at CT angiography is 1%, not significantly different from the 3.1% rate for low-probability results of V/Q scans (34). A review of studies published before June 1999 suggested that the sensitivity of CT was only 68% at a specificity of 91% (35). Recently published studies conducted with improved CT technique suggest better results than this (36,37). It is likely that continued technical improvements, such as multidetector scanners, which allow thin collimation and very high pitch, will further improve the sensitivity of CT for subsegmental emboli. Likewise, increasing observer experience will likely improve results.

The probably lower sensitivity of CT seems to be one of its few major disadvantages compared with scintigraphy. Like CT, MR imaging can depict PE directly as intravascular filling defects on cross-sectional images. Experience with MR imaging in examinations of patients with suspected PE is more limited than that with CT. In addition, MR techniques are still evolving. Studies of contrast-enhanced pulmonary MR angiography by Meaney et al. (38) and Gupta et al. (39) met the criteria for level 1 studies. In the study by Meaney et al., the sensitivity of MR angiography was 100%; the specificity, 95%; the positive predictive value, 87%; and the negative predictive value, 100%. In the study by Gupta et al., among 36 patients, the sensitivity and specificity per embolus (per zone) were 68% and 99.7%, whereas the sensitivity and specificity per patient were 85% and 96%. These important studies must be confirmed at other centers and with other patient populations, particularly because some studies suggest that MR imaging may be less accurate than is CT (40). At many centers, helical CT is a realistic option in the care of patients with suspected PE. Clinical application of MR imaging is limited to highly motivated centers with appropriate expertise in and technology for MR imaging.

The PIOPED II has begun to enroll patients. The purpose of PIOPED II is to determine the extent to which helical CT is an efficacious, minimally invasive test for PE and thereby to reduce the need for pulmonary angiography and V/Q scintigraphy. PIOPED II is a multicenter, prospective study in which imaging will be performed with multidetector scanners with thin collimation and high pitch. When the study is completed, the results should provide the best data currently available to assess the different modalities used to image PE. PIOPED II is described in more detail later.

Ventilation-Perfusion Scintigraphy: Image Acquisition

Normal scintigraphic studies of the lungs show homogenous patterns of evenly matched ventilation (V) and perfusion (Q) that correlate precisely with the aerated lung seen on the chest radiograph. Pathophysiologic states commonly are associated with scintigraphically detectable perturbations of ventilation and perfusion. These perturbations generally result in regional heterogeneity of pulmonary perfusion and ventilation rather than overall changes.

Vascular occlusive processes include PE, extrinsic vascular compression, pulmonary vasculitis, and congenital abnormalities. These processes usually leave alveoli structurally intact, and ventilation usually is preserved in regions of vascular occlusion. Accordingly, V/Q mismatch is the hallmark of this type of pathophysiologic condition. Airspace occlusion may be associated with pneumonia, pulmonary infarction, and other airspace disorders. The degree of ventilation and perfusion loss can vary independently, but both usually are reduced concomitantly. Therefore a V/Q match typically is present and usually is associated with a radiographic opacity. Obstructive physiologic characteristics are present in disorders such as emphysema, bronchitis, bronchiectasis, and asthma, which predominately affect the conducting and exchanging air spaces. Alveolar hypoxia results, and the corresponding pulmonary arteries constrict, thus redistributing blood to better ventilated alveoli and preserving the matching of ventilation and blood flow. Matched V/Q abnormalities are seen with this type of physiologic process as well, but corresponding radiographic opacities are less common. In restrictive lung disease, chronic inflammation and fibrosis may eventually obliterate alveoli and capillaries. However, the airways remain functional, and regional ventilation may be increased relative to perfusion. The configuration and pattern of perfusion abnormalities usually are different from the vascular occlusive state. Mixtures of these pathophysiologic states are extremely common among individual patients.

Perfusion Imaging

Perfusion scintigraphy of the lung is accomplished by inducing microembolization of radiolabeled particles in the pulmonary arterioles. The number of particles that impact in a particular volume of the lung is proportional to the pulmonary arterial blood flow to that region. Perfusion scintigraphy provides a visual representation of the regional distribution of pulmonary blood flow at the time of radiopharmaceutical injection.

Particulate embolization does cause a minor degree of obstruction of pulmonary blood flow, but this effect is almost never physiologically significant. An even distribution of radioactivity in the vascular bed requires injection of 60,000 or more particles. The usual 2 to 4 mCi ^{99m}Tc (140-keV photon) macroaggregated albumin (MAA) patient dose contains approximately 500,000 particles, so injections of a low number of particles and statistically invalid scans are rarely a problem. Freshly prepared MAA should be used, because breakdown products in the preparation, such as ^{99m}Tc pertechnetate, can cause spurious extrapulmonary uptake. The intravenous injection of labeled particles should be performed with the patient supine, and the radiopharmaceutical should be injected slowly over 5 to 10 seconds while the patient takes moderately deep breaths. This method ensures that pulmonary blood flow is evenly distributed, which is important for adequate visualization of the upper lung and other physiologically hypoperfused regions. The syringe containing the radiopharmaceutical should be agitated immediately before the injection to ensure a homogeneous suspension of the labeled particles. One must not allow blood to clot within the syringe, because clots will adsorb the radioactive aggregates and cause an uneven distribution of activity (Fig. 18A.1). If the radiopharmaceutical must be injected through intravenous tubing, the fluid must be flowing rapidly. Even so, a portion of the dose may adhere to the tubing, and injections through tubing are discouraged. Injection into central venous or pulmonary arterial catheters should be avoided, because streaming or selective catheter position may result in uneven distribution of the injected particles.

In the PIOPED II, imaging for perfusion scintigraphy can be performed in the following three ways. In the first, a wide-field-of-view gamma camera equipped with a low-energy, all-purpose collimator is used to obtain eight views of the thorax (anterior, posterior, right and left posterior and anterior oblique, and right and left lateral) in a routine manner (Fig. 18A.2). For each view, 750,000 counts are obtained, except for the lateral views. The lateral view with the best perfusion is imaged for 500,000 counts, the time is recorded, and the second lateral view is acquired for the same length of time. In the second method, a comparably equipped gamma camera is used to obtain the posterior view for 750,000 counts, and all other views are obtained in the same time. In the third method, if a high-resolution, low-energy collimator is used, the counts are reduced to 600,000 and 400,000 if the lateral views are obtained as in the

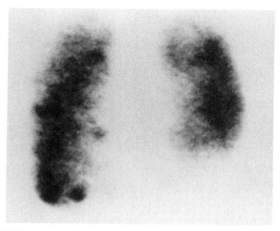

FIGURE 18A.1. Radionuclide absorption by clotted blood within syringe. This is an old case showing "hot clots" due to absorption of ^{99m}Tc macroaggregated albumin to blood that has clotted in the syringe used for injecting the radiopharmaceutical (we are happy to say we do not have any recent examples). The cutoff of the left costophrenic angle on this posterior view is evident because of the use of a small-field-of-view camera. There is marked inhomogeneity of lung activity as a result of the small number of free particles remaining (e.g., the spurious right upper lobe defect). Such a study should not be interpreted. A perfusion examination performed 18 hours later was normal.

first technique. Regardless of the technique used, we suggest that contiguous surfaces of the lung be displayed next to each other on the readout (e.g., left posterior oblique, then posterior, then right posterior oblique, and so on). The lungs should be approximately 1.25 inches (3 cm) long (superior-inferior) on the readout.

Perfusion scintigraphy is sensitive but not specific. As discussed earlier in the description of physiologic patterns, nearly all pulmonary diseases can cause a significant decrease in pulmonary arterial blood flow to affected lung zones (41,42).

Ventilation Imaging

Abnormalities in the perfusion scan that are matched by zones of abnormal ventilation are less likely to represent PE, whereas mismatched abnormalities (reduced perfusion with preserved ventilation, that is, the vascular occlusive state) have a high correspondence with PE, given normal chest radiographic findings in the same lung region (41). Therefore most nuclear physicians consider it essential to obtain both ventilation and perfusion images to ensure accurate categorization when findings on perfusion scans are abnormal.

^{133}Xe (80-keV photon) gas has been used for many years and is still used widely for ventilation studies. Use of this agent requires apparatus for administering the gas and for trapping exhaled gas. This ventilation apparatus includes a tightly sealing face mask or mouthpiece, a spirometer, tubing with intake and exhaust valves, and a shielded charcoal trap. If a wide-field-of-view scintillation camera and an all-purpose collimator are used to perform a ventilation study *before the perfusion imaging is done*, we recommend the following technique. A first-breath image of 100,000 counts or 10 to 15 seconds is obtained after administration of 15 to 20 mCi (550 to 770 MBq) of ^{133}Xe

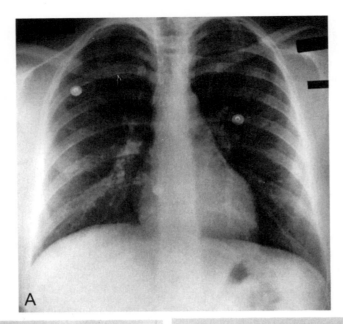

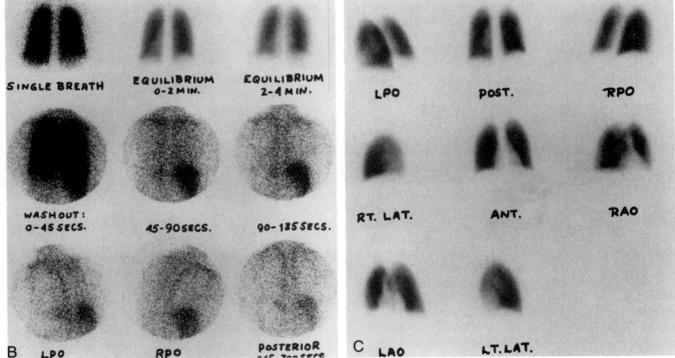

FIGURE 18A.2. Example of a ventilation-perfusion study with normal results. Chest radiograph **(A)**, ¹³³Xe ventilation scan **(B)**, and ^{99m}Tc macroaggregated albumin eight-view perfusion scan **(C)**. On the ventilation study, the camera intensity is purposely increased for the "washout" phase, and posterior oblique views are obtained. An incidental finding in **(B)** is ¹³³Xe uptake in subcutaneous and hepatic fat. *LPO*, left posterior oblique; *PRO*, right posterior oblique, *POST.*, posterior; *LAT.*, lateral; *ANT.*, anterior; *RAO*, right anterior oblique; *LAO*, left anterior oblique.

into the intake port as the patient inspires maximally. Then the patient rebreathes gas in a closed-spirometer system while three 75-second equilibrium images are made in posterior, right posterior oblique, and left posterior oblique projections. The equilibrium phase should last 4 minutes. The intake valves of the system are then readjusted so that the patient breathes ambient air, and

washout images are obtained at 45- to 60-second intervals such that the washout phase lasts at least 5 minutes. The first three washout images are standard posterior views. Next, right and left posterior oblique images and a final posterior image are made. The posterior oblique equilibrium and washout views are obtained to better localize zones of abnormal lung volume and

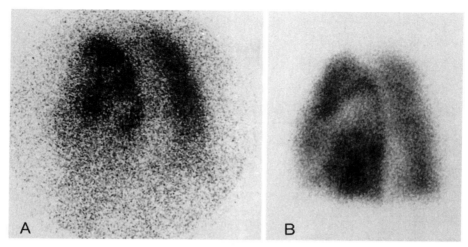

FIGURE 18A.3. Use of posterior oblique washout view to help localize areas of abnormal ventilation on a ^{133}Xe study. The left posterior oblique view of the ^{133}Xe scan **(A)** shows abnormal areas of ^{133}Xe retention that correspond well to perfusion deficits on the left posterior oblique view of the ^{99m}Tc microaggregated albumin scan **(B)**.

xenon retention with respect to their anterior-posterior location (Fig. 18A.3). If a dual-headed camera is used, it is not necessary to obtain oblique views in either the equilibrium or washout phases, but these still should be made for the same time intervals.

The equilibrium image has a radioactivity distribution corresponding to the aerated lung volume. Images made during washout from normal lungs show rapid and symmetric clearance of activity from the lungs (usually within 90 seconds). In contrast to the first-breath image, which indicates ventilatory abnormality as a deficit in radioactivity in the lung, washout images show zones with abnormal ventilation as hotspots as delayed clearance of ^{133}Xe produces areas of focal retained activity on a background of decreasing activity from normal lung regions. To obtain maximum information from the washout images, one first must use a sufficiently long (>3 minutes) rebreathing period to allow the radionuclide to enter abnormal lung zones through collateral air drift.

Obtaining the ventilation study before the perfusion is the most accurate technique to use with ^{133}Xe. It allows optimum images in the washout portion of the ventilation study because no ^{99m}Tc is present in the lungs to produce scatter. This scatter occurs in the same energy window as ^{133}Xe primary photons and can obscure ^{133}Xe retention. Because of current computer capability, postperfusion ^{133}Xe ventilation technique is being used at many centers. It is more efficient, because the ventilation study is not needed if the results of the perfusion study are normal. If this technique is used, the most optimal view to see the perfusion defect usually is selected, and technetium downscatter from MAA is subtracted with a computer before xenon is used.

Radioaerosols are a means for imaging regional ventilation and are available commercially in the form of small and efficient aerosol nebulizers. Radioaerosols are small particles, rather than gases. The usual radioaerosol agent is ^{99m}Tc-labeled diethylene-triaminepentaacetic acid (DTPA) (Fig. 18A.4). Typically, 30 mCi (1,110 MBq) of ^{99m}Tc DTPA is placed in the nebulizer,

and inhalation of the aerosol continues until 1 mCi (37 MBq) is in the lungs. The radioaerosol inhalation study usually is performed before the perfusion scintigram is obtained. To yield uniform apex-to-base deposition, the inhalation study should be performed with the patient in the supine position. In the PIO-PED II, many of the study centers are using aerosols with the following preperfusion technique. A 200,000- to 250,000-count posterior aerosol image is made and the time recorded. All other views are obtained with this time comparable with the perfusion scan. The counts for the all the images can be kept constant, except for the lateral views, which are proportionately reduced. The count rate for the aerosol ventilation study should be no more then 25% of the count rate for the perfusion scan; 20% or less is ideal. If central deposition is found, at least 250,000 counts must be collected. If postperfusion aerosol images are obtained, and the perfusion defects are in the bases, the erect position can be used. It is important to monitor the region of the perfusion deficit on a computer to be sure the count within the deficit at least doubles on the postperfusion aerosol study. The use of ^{99m}Tc pyrophosphate aerosols yields a longer residence time, which is important in examinations of smokers (42).

In Europe and Australia, an ultrafine dry dispersion of ^{99m}Tc-labeled carbon particles (Technegas) has become popular. The benefits are speed and ease of administration, deep peripheral penetration with minimal bronchial deposition, and prolonged pulmonary retention. Comparison with radioactive gases usually has been favorable (43). This agent is not yet generally available in the United States.

It is not obvious that any one of the aforementioned agents is ideal for ventilation studies. Results of comparisons of the various techniques are limited but suggest that there is no major diagnostic difference (44,45). It is common for many institutions to use more than one agent at different times. An institution that uses one of the radioactive gases for routine V/Q scintigraphy might use the convenient aerosols for portable examinations in the intensive care unit. Accordingly, considera-

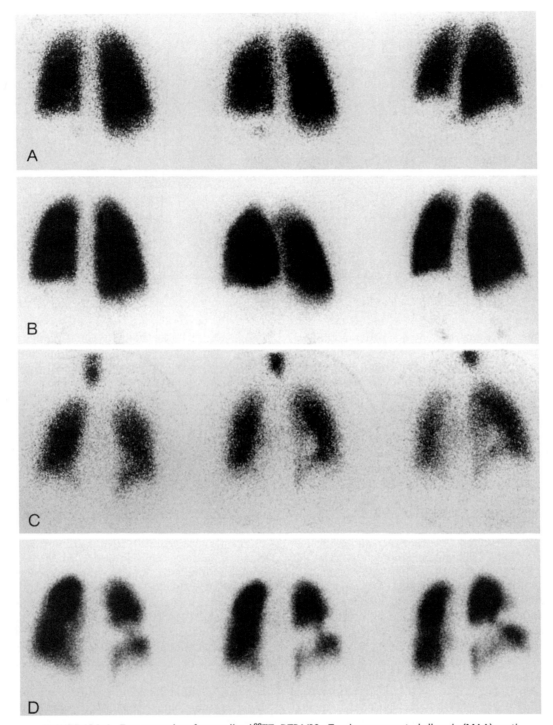

FIGURE 18A.4. Two examples of aerosolized ^{99m}Tc DTPA/99mTc microaggregated albumin (MAA) ventilation-perfusion studies. Normal **(A)** and abnormal **(C)** ventilation scans with corresponding normal **(B)** and abnormal **(D)** perfusion scans. In both examples, posterior and both posterior oblique views are shown in each panel. **A:** Normal ^{99m}Tc-DTPA aerosol ventilation study. **B:** Normal ^{99m}Tc MAA perfusion study. Faint gastric **(A)** and renal **(B)** activity from the ^{99m}Tc DPTA is apparent, as is the precise correspondence of the lung images of ventilation **(A)** and perfusion **(B)**. **C:** Deficit in activity in the right lower lobe on the aerosol ventilation images. Aerosol ventilation imaging, like ^{81m}Kr and the early phases (first breath and equilibrium) of ^{153}Xe studies, shows abnormal ventilation as a deficit in activity. **D:** Corresponding ^{99m}Tc MAA perfusion images. There are perfusion deficits in the right lower lobe (matched by abnormal ventilation) and in the right upper lobe anterior segment (a mismatched deficit). The two studies can be compared simply with multiple-view ventilation images.

tions such as cost, patient logistics, and referral patterns will determine which of these ventilation agents is best suited for a specific institution.

Ventilation-Perfusion Scintigraphy: Image Interpretation

Diagnostic Criteria: Older Data

Truly normal results of a perfusion scan have long been accepted to exclude PE for practical purposes (the morbidity and mortality of missed PE have been thought less than those from pulmonary arteriography or anticoagulant therapy). It is the perfusion portion of the examination that is important in consideration of possible PE—as long as perfusion is normal, findings on the ventilation images or chest radiograph can be abnormal, and the scan is still read as normal in the sense of being negative for PE (Fig. 18A.5). A normal scan result usually stops the evaluation for PE and diverts attention to other possibilities.

Although it is sensitive, perfusion scintigraphy is not specific for PE. Nearly all pulmonary diseases, including neoplasms, infections, and chronic obstructive pulmonary disease, can produce decreased pulmonary blood flow to affected regions (46). To overcome this problem, Wagner et al. (47) and DeNardo et al. (48) suggested combined V/Q lung imaging. McNeil et al. (41), highlighted the findings of numerous investigators by pointing out that abnormalities in the perfusion scan that are matched by abnormal ventilation usually are not caused by PE but that the presence of mismatched abnormalities coexisting with a normal chest radiograph has a high correlation with angiographic demonstration of PE. Alderson et al. (49) later showed that the overall diagnostic accuracy of scintigraphic detection of pulmonary emboli improved significantly when ^{133}Xe ventilation studies were added to the perfusion scan and chest radiograph.

Neumann et al. (50) introduced the concept of segmental equivalents—that two subsegmental perfusion defects can be added to produce the same diagnostic significance as a single segmental defect. Results of a subsequent retrospective study by Kotlyarov and Reba (46) supported the usefulness of this approach.

Extensive work by Biello et al. (51,52) further categorized perfusion defects matched by ventilatory or radiographic abnormalities and provided grounds for reducing the number of "indeterminate" diagnoses. Further evaluation of this work (53) indicated that this diagnostic scheme provides improved interobserver consistency and a 30% reduction in indeterminate readings compared with the results with an older scheme.

Experience has clearly shown that a scintigraphic perfusion study demonstrating multiple large, often bilateral, wedge-shaped, pleura-based perfusion defects with normal ventilation and a clear chest radiograph in the corresponding areas has a high correspondence with PE (Fig. 18A.6). The most important cause of error in this situation is previous, unresolved PE (see later, Pulmonary Embolism Mimics). A scan pattern of this type usually is read as "high probability of PE" and results in a clinical diagnosis of PE, which is followed by appropriate therapy.

Table 18A.2 shows two sets of commonly used diagnostic criteria—the Biello criteria (52) and the revised PIOPED criteria with modifications based on retrospective review of the database of proven cases provided by the PIOPED investigators (54,55). Certain definitions are important to understanding and proper use of these criteria. In all these criteria, *small* is defined as a defect involving less than 25% of the area of an average-sized pulmonary arterial segment; *moderate* is equivalent to 25% to

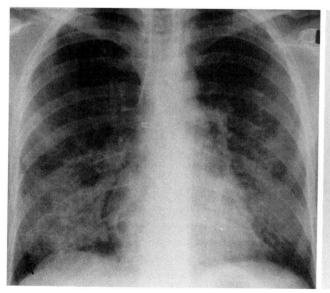

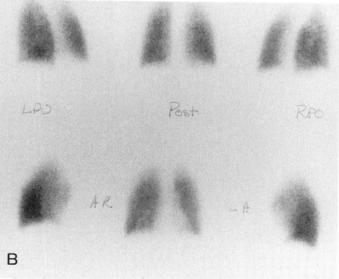

FIGURE 18A.5. The findings on a perfusion scintigram can be normal or nearly normal despite the presence of considerable pulmonary disease. The perfusion scan findings govern categorization of the study as to the likelihood of pulmonary embolism. In the imaging examination of this patient with resolving adult respiratory distress syndrome, the chest radiograph **(A)** shows diffuse opacities, but the perfusion scan **(B)** is essentially normal. The study is therefore correctly interpreted as negative for PE.

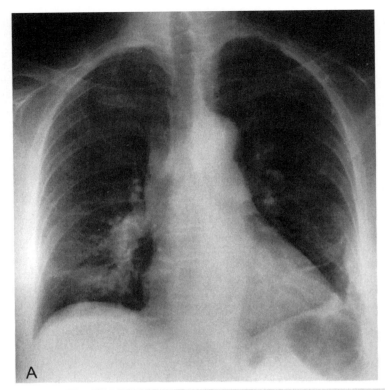

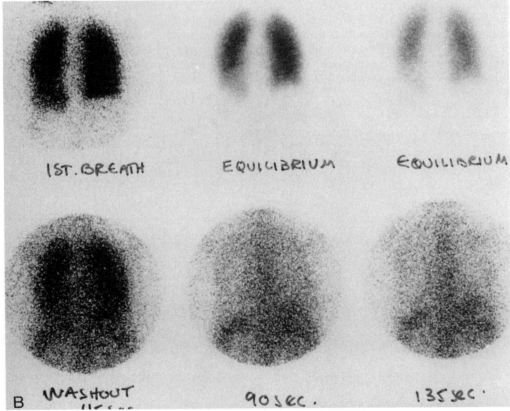

FIGURE 18A.6. High probability of pulmonary embolism. **A:** Chest radiograph shows pleuroparenchymal scarring at both bases and a mediastinum that is wide because of vascular ectasia. **B:** ^{133}Xe ventilation scan shows normal ventilation. In the washout phase (camera intensity purposely increased here), there is residual bone, liver, and spleen activity from a previous ^{67}Ga scan. Consequently a high-energy collimator was used for both ventilation and perfusion images. *(Figure continues.)*

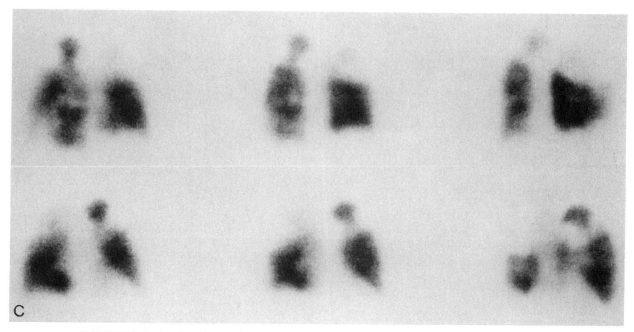

FIGURE 18A.6. *Continued.* **C:** Perfusion study shows large, bilateral mismatched defects. When a low-energy (^{99m}Tc) examination is performed on a patient with higher-energy tracer "on board" (^{67}Ga), it is imperative to collimate for the high-energy photons.

Table 18A.2. *Scintigraphic Reference Criteria for Pulmonary Emboli*

Biello criteria	Revised PIOPED criteria
High probability	**High probability (≥80%)**
Q substantially larger than CXR opacity, which shows some area of mismatch	Two or more large mismatched segmental perfusion defects or the equivalent in moderate or large and moderate mismatched defects[a]
Two or more large or moderate-sized mismatched defects, CXR normal in corresponding area	
Intermediate probability	**Intermediate probability (20% to 79%)**
Diffuse V/Q match	One moderate and one large mismatched segmental perfusion defects or the equivalent in moderate segmental perfusion defects
Matched Q and CXR	Single matched ventilation-perfusion defect with clear chest radiograph[b]
Single moderate V/Q mismatch (one segment or smaller) with CXR normal in area	Difficult to categorize as low or high, or not described as low or high
Low probability	**Low probability (≤19%)**
Small V/Q mismatches	Nonsegmental perfusion defects (e.g., cardiomegaly, enlarged aorta, enlarged hila, elevated diaphragm)
Q defect substantially smaller than CXR opacity	Any perfusion defect with a substantially larger chest radiographic abnormality
V/Q match no more than 50% of one lung field	Perfusion defects matched by ventilation abnormality[b] provided that there are (a) clear chest radiograph and (b) some areas of normal perfusion in the lungs
	Any number of small perfusion defects with a normal chest radiograph
Normal	**Normal**
Normal perfusion	No perfusion defects—perfusion outlines exactly the shape of the lungs seen on the chest radiograph (note that hilar and aortic impressions may be seen, and the chest radiograph and/or ventilation study may be abnormal)

[a]Two large mismatched perfusion defects are borderline for high probability. Individual readers may correctly interpret individual scans with this pattern as high probability. In general, it is recommended that more than this degree of mismatch be present for the high-probability category.
[b]Very extensive matched defects can be categorized as low probability. Single V/Q matches are borderline for low probability and should be considered for intermediate in most cases by most readers, although individual readers may correctly interpret individual scans with this pattern as low probability.
Q, perfusion; CXR, chest radiograph; V, ventilation.

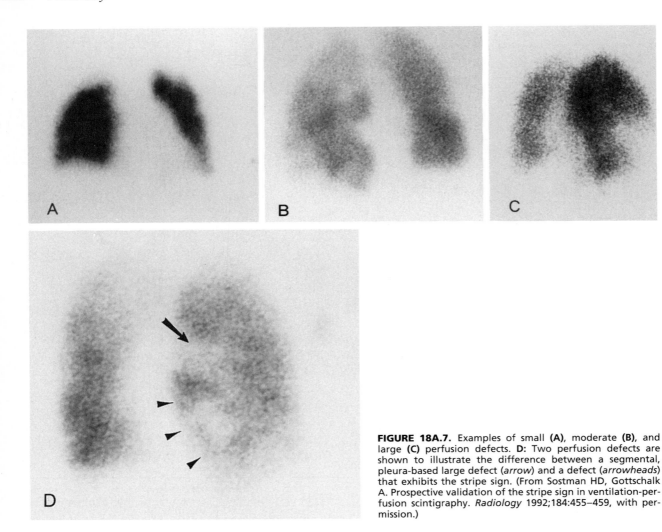

FIGURE 18A.7. Examples of small **(A)**, moderate **(B)**, and large **(C)** perfusion defects. **D:** Two perfusion defects are shown to illustrate the difference between a segmental, pleura-based large defect (*arrow*) and a defect (*arrowheads*) that exhibits the stripe sign. (From Sostman HD, Gottschalk A. Prospective validation of the stripe sign in ventilation-perfusion scintigraphy. *Radiology* 1992;184:455–459, with permission.)

75% of the area of a segment; and *large* means more than 75% of a segment. Figure 18A.7 shows examples of different sizes of perfusion defects. Different bronchopulmonary segments typically are of different sizes (Fig. 18A.8). In principle, one could attempt to individualize the rating of defect size to the particular segment in which the defect is thought to be located. In practice, however, most imaging specialists, including experts in the field, simply use an average, idealized segment and apply this size template to evaluation of defects in any location. A defect on a chest radiograph indicates a radiographic opacity in the region related to the perfusion or ventilation lesion. When a chest radiograph is called "normal," this also alludes to the chest radiographic appearance in the same region as the ventilation or perfusion defect. Finally, a lung zone is one third of a lung divided craniocaudally (upper, middle, and lower zones). Lung zones were used in the original PIOPED because all the centers used xenon as the ventilation agent. If aerosols are used, it is possible to match the ventilation defects to the perfusion defects on a segmental (or subsegmental) basis.

An example of a classic high-probability scan is shown in Fig. 18A.6. Examples of scans that should be interpreted as showing low or intermediate probability of PE are shown in Figs. 18A.9 through 18A.12.

Diagnostic Criteria: Newer Data and the PIOPED II Study

There are data to indicate that some experienced imaging specialists can achieve more accurate results using their own experience than with the reference criteria cited herein (55–57). Nevertheless, diagnostic reference criteria can be extremely useful, particularly for observers who do not have extensive and ongoing experience in interpreting V/Q studies. Use of reference criteria has been shown to reduce the number of indeterminate readings. In addition, if all the physicians in a group practice use the same reference criteria, standardization of V/Q scan interpretation is likely to improve. In the PIOPED, pairs of independent readers achieved high levels of prospective agreement (90% to 95%) for high probability and normal–near normal diagnoses but lesser agreement (70% to 75%) for intermediate and low probability. The implications of these findings for clinical interpretations are obvious. The good agreement between scan readers was achieved only after several practice sessions in which the description of findings and assignment of diagnostic categories were standardized. This discussion suggests that further refinement of diagnostic criteria is possible. There have been several recent attempts to do this. The PIOPED Nuclear Medicine Working Group

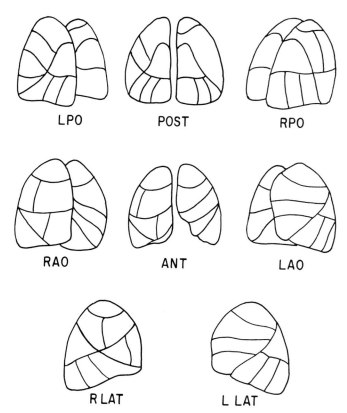

FIGURE 18A.8. Diagrammatic depiction of pulmonary segments. We use this as a reference for localizing perfusion defects. *LPO,* left posterior oblique; *POST,* posterior; *RPO,* right posterior oblique; *RAO,* right anterior oblique; *ANT,* anterior; *LAO,* left anterior oblique; *R LAT,* right lateral; *L LAT,* left lateral.

Table 18A.3. *Data on Mismatched Perfusion Defects in Patients with No History of Cardiopulmonary Disease*

Number of defects	Sensitivity (%)	Specificity (%)	PPV (%; 95% CI)
≥1	71	88	80 (74–86)
≥2	54	95	89 (83–95)
≥3	46	97	91 (85–97)
≥4	39	97	89 (81–97)
>5	32	98	92 (84–100)

Cumulative number of mismatched moderate or large-size perfusion defects compared with sensitivity, specificity, and positive predictive value (PPV) for pulmonary embolism in patients with no history of cardiopulmonary disease.
CI, confidence interval.
Data from Stein PD, Henry JW, Gottschalk A. Mismatched vascular defects. *Chest* 1993;104:1468–1472.

revised the PIOPED criteria as described earlier and shown in Table 18.2.

Articles by Stein et al. (58,59) help to make the criteria for high probability easier to apply and more sensitive. A subset of their data is shown in Tables 18A.3 and 18A.4. Their contribution has been to indicate (a) that the segmental equivalent concept (60) does not add a great deal to diagnostic accuracy and that the total number of large or moderate defects is the important finding and (b) that patients who have had cardiopulmonary disease must have more mismatched perfusion defects to achieve the same positive predictive value as patients who have no history of cardiopulmonary disease.

Despite these efforts to revise the diagnostic criteria, Hull and Raskob (60) point out that in their opinion, the low-probability criteria of PIOPED are still not acceptable. These authors argue that the 14% incidence of PE shown in PIOPED is too high.

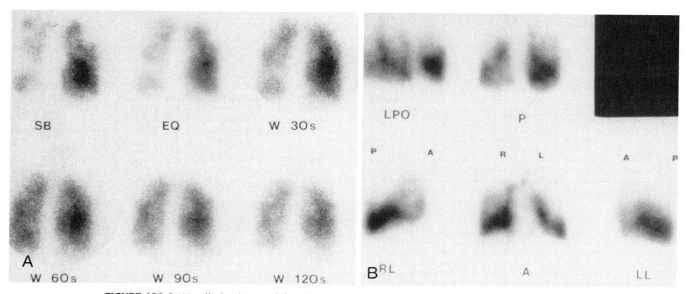

FIGURE 18A.9. Ventilation images **(A)** and perfusion images **(B)** in a patient with chronic obstructive pulmonary disease both show extensive abnormality involving most of the lungs but without areas of mismatch. Some segments with normal perfusion also are present. The revised PIOPED criteria (55) indicate this study would be categorized as having a low probability for pulmonary embolism (PE). With the PIOPED II criteria, this case would be interpreted as very low probably. Pulmonary angiographic findings were negative for PE in this case.

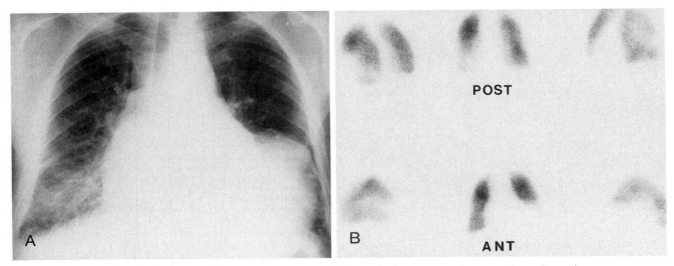

FIGURE 18A.10. The massive cardiomegaly and left ventricular aneurysm shown on this radiograph **(A)** account for the large perfusion defect in the left lung evident on the perfusion scintigram **(B)**. This defect is properly classified as nonsegmental. According to the PIOPED II criteria, this case is very low probability for pulmonary embolism. This patient did not have PE.

They indicate that "low probability" be considered "nondiagnostic." Dalen (61), expanding on this concept, indicated that the high-probability diagnosis is reliable and is sufficient to allow anticoagulant therapy to proceed. Similarly, a normal diagnosis on a V/Q scan is sufficient for withholding therapy provided there is no other source of thromboembolism (in other words, results of ultrasonography of the low extremities or other lower-extremity studies are normal). However, any other scan finding (intermediate probability or low probability) should be considered not enough information for a diagnosis, and the patient should undergo either low-extremity ultrasonography or pulmonary angiography.

In an effort to extract useful diagnoses from this "nondiagnostic" group, Stein and Gottschalk (62) using the PIOPED database collected a series of criteria each with a positive predictive value of less than 10% for PE. They introduced these criteria as a "very low probability" category (Table 18A.5). Gottschalk tested these very low probability criteria in the following way. The European prospective trial of spiral CT angiography (ESTI-

PEP) was set up such that each patient underwent V/Q scanning and spiral CT angiography (SCTA) and in some cases digital subtraction angiography. This prospective trial was organized by Herold at the University of Vienna. Schaeffer-Prokop and Prokop in Vienna, working from the complete ESTIPEP series, selected random ESTIPEP cases with normal or near-normal chest radiographic findings. The chest radiograph and the V/Q scan (or sometimes Q only) from these cases were sent to Gottschalk to interpret with no other information. Alderson had

Table 18A.4. *Data on Mismatched Perfusion Defects in Patients with a History of Cardiopulmonary Disease*

Number of defects	Sensitivity (%)	Specificity (%)	PPV (%; 95% CI)
≥1	63	86	68 (62–74)
≥2	51	93	77 (69–85)
≥3	44	95	80 (72–88)
≥4	40	96	84 (76–92)
≥5	37	98	89 (83–95)

Cumulative number of mismatched moderate or large-size perfusion defects compared with sensitivity, specificity, and positive predictive value for PE in patients who did have history of prior cardiopulmonary disease.
CI, confidence interval.
Data from Stein PD, Henry JW, Gottschalk A. Mismatched vascular defects. *Chest* 1993;104:1468–1472.

Table 18A.5. *Criteria for Very Low Probability Interpretation of Ventilation-Perfusion Lung Scan*

Criterion	No. of cases of pulmonary embolism	No. of patients, lungs, or lung zones or regions	PPV (%)
Nonsegmental perfusion abnormality	8	103[a]	8
Perfusion defect smaller than corresponding radiographic defect	3	40[a]	8
Matched ventilation-perfusion defects in two or three zones of a single lung (normal radiograph)	1	30[a]	3
One to three small segmental perfusion defects	1	68[b]	1
Triple matched defect in the upper or middle lung zone	1	27[c]	4
Stripe sign	6	85[d]	7

[a]Individual lungs were evaluated.
[b]Patients were evaluated.
[c]Lung zones were evaluated.
[d]Lung regions were evaluated.
PPV, positive predictive value.
From Stein PD, Gottschalk A. Review of criteria appropriate for a very low probability of pulmonary embolism on ventilation-perfusion lung scans. *Radiographics* 2000;20:99–105, with permission.

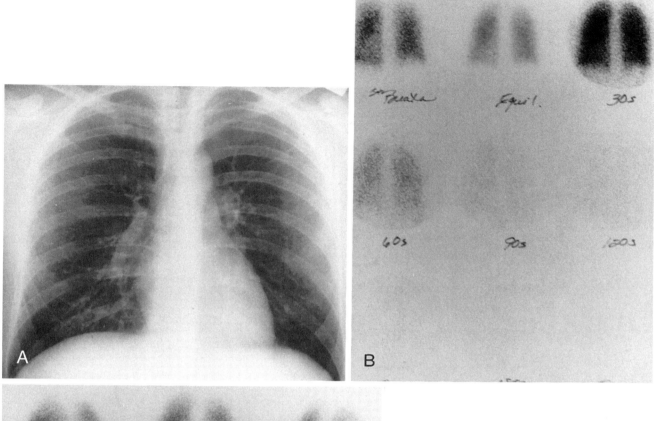

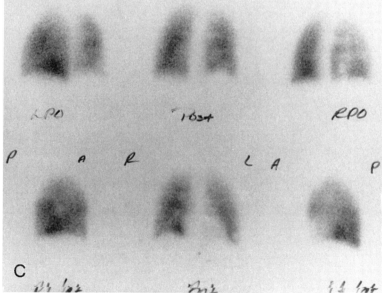

FIGURE 18A.11. A: Chest radiograph is normal except for prominence of the right descending pulmonary artery. **B:** Ventilation images are normal. **C:** Perfusion images show multiple small, segmental perfusion defects, particularly noticeable in the right lung. However, a single moderate segmental lesion also is present in the lateral segment of the right lung base. This patient had no cardiopulmonary disease; thus this case can be interpreted as high probability. If only the small segmental lesions were present, the case should be interpreted as low probability. At angiography, this patient had an embolus in the basal segments of the right lower lobe.

previously suggested that the V/Q scan was highly effective when the chest radiograph was "uncomplicated" (63). To test this concept, Gottschalk read the cases using the revised PIOPED criteria for high probability (two segments mismatched defect or their equivalent) to diagnose "PE present" or using the very-low-probability category coupled with normal findings to diagnose "PE absent." The purpose was to assess the validity of the very-low-probability criteria and to see whether a significant

number of definitive readings could be obtained for this group of patients. In the original PIOPED trial, the number of definitive readings with appropriate clinical assessment (high probability with PE or near-normal or normal probability with no PE) was quite reliable, but definitive readings were given for fewer than 30% of the total PIOPED patients. Gottschalk's readings from ESTIPEP were compared with SCTA or DSA reading if they were available. Of the 127 cases Gottschalk reviewed, 12 cases

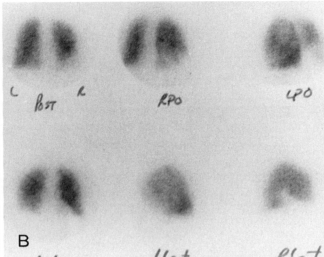

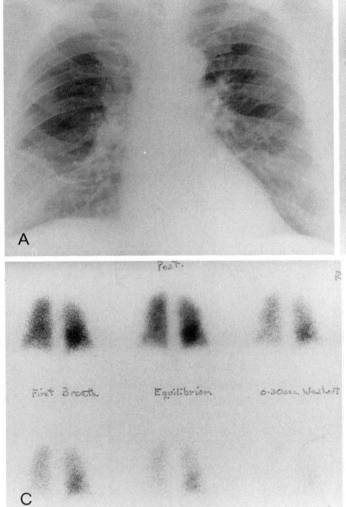

FIGURE 18A.12. An opacity at the right base on the chest radiograph **(A)** matches a perfusion defect on the perfusion scintigram **(B)**. A single area of ¹³³Xe retention **(C)** medial to the radiographic opacity is matched by a perfusion defect. This case shows a triple match in the right lower lung zone and an adjacent single matched ventilation-perfusion defect with regionally normal chest radiographic findings. This scan is properly classified as showing intermediate probability of pulmonary embolism. Angiography showed embolism in multiple basilar segments of the right lower lobe.

(9%) had no definitive SCTA reading (the three central SCTA readers for each case could not agree). Thirty cases also had DSA images, but this only increased the total with a diagnostic standard to 117. For most of the series, the SCTA acted as a reference standard because the reference standard DSA image was available for only a small number of patients. Gottschalk found that 9 V/Q scans could not be interpreted for technical reasons. This left 108 cases he could read that had a reference SCTA or DSA image. Readings (PE present or PE absent) were definitive for 89% of the interpretable V/Q scans. For cases with a definitive reading (PE present or PE absent), the sensitivity was 90%, and the specificity was 97%. These results suggested that the very-low-probability criteria were useful (Table 18A.6).

At the time of this writing, the PIOPED II is just beginning. The purpose of PIOPED II is to determine the extent to which SCTA can be used as a minimally invasive diagnostic test for pulmonary thromboembolism. It is a multicenter study involving Calgary, Cornell, Emory, Duke, Henry Ford, Massachusetts General Hospital, the University of Michigan, and Washington University. Each prospectively recruited patient in PIOPED II will undergo both a V/Q scan and SCTA. The aim of PIOPED II is to examine patients with suspected PE and ultimately determine the sensitivity and specificity of SCTA for the diagnosis of acute PE. The determination of PE status will be made with a combination of V/Q scintigraphy, venous ultrasonography of the lower extremities, pulmonary angiography, and venography. In some instances, a diagnosis of DVT (above the calf) by means

Table 18A.6. *Reliability of Definitive Readings*

V/Q reading	SCTA or DSA	
	PE present	PE absent
PE present	26	2
PE absent	3	65

Sensitivity, 90%; Specificity, 97%; Positive predictive value, 93%; Negative predictive value, 96%; Positive likelihood ratio, 30.0; Negative likelihood ratio, 0.11%; Accuracy, 95%.
V/Q, ventilation-perfusion; SCTA, spiral computed tomographic angiography; DSA, digital subtraction angiography.

of venous ultrasonography (in an area with no previous DVT) will be used as a surrogate for a diagnosis of acute PE. A high-probability finding on a V/Q scan of a patient with no previous PE will be considered diagnostic of acute PE. In addition, a normal V/Q scan result will be considered to exclude PE. All other V/Q scan readings will be evaluated, but the interpretation will be superseded by the results of low-extremity ultrasonography or pulmonary DSA. In general, when the result of venous lower-extremity ultrasonography is negative, the patient will undergo pulmonary DSA for assessment of the presence of acute PE. The only exception is a case in which lower-extremity ultrasonographic findings are normal and findings of lower-extremity spiral CT venography are abnormal. In this instance, the patient may undergo either lower-extremity contrast venography or DSA depending on the desire of the referring physician. The modification of V/Q scintigraphy criteria described earlier is not being used to determine PE status in PIOPED II. PIOPED II is being used as a prospective study to assess the validity of the new criteria. The PIOPED II diagnostic criteria for V/Q scans are listed in Table 18A.7. In general, the revised PIOPED criteria

Table 18A.7. *PIOPED II Ventilation-Perfusion (V/Q) Scan Criteria*

High scan probability
  Two or more large mismatched segmental defects or the equivalent in moderate or large and moderate defects
Intermediate-indeterminate scan probability
  One half to one and one half segmental equivalents
  Difficult to categorize as high or low
  Solitary moderate or large segmental size triple match in lower lobe (zone)
  Multiple opacities with associated perfusion defects
Low scan probability
  A single matched V/Q defect
  More than three small segmental lesions
  Probable pulmonary embolism mimic
    One lung mismatched (whiteout) with absent perfusion
    Solitary lobar mismatch
    Mass or other chest radiographic lesion causing all mismatch
  Moderate sized pleural effusion (greater than costophrenic angle but less than one third of pleural cavity with no other perfusion defect in either lung)
  Marked heterogeneous perfusion
Very low scan probability
  Nonsegmental lesion, e.g., prominent hilum, cardiomegaly, elevated diaphragm, linear atelectasis, costophrenic angle effusion with no other perfusion defect in either lung
  Perfusion defect smaller than radiographic lesion
  Two or more V/Q matched defects with regionally normal chest radiograph and some areas of normal perfusion elsewhere in the lungs
  One to three small segmental perfusion defects
  A solitary triple matched defect in the mid or upper lung zone confined to a single segment
  Stripe sign present around the perfusion defect (best tangential view)
  Pleural effusion of one third or more of the pleural cavity with no other perfusion defect in either lung
Normal perfusion scan
  No perfusion defect. Perfusion scan must outline the shape of the lungs seen on chest radiograph, which could be abnormal (e.g., scoliosis).

PIOPED, prospective investigation of pulmonary embolism diagnosis.

for high probability have been maintained. The intermediate-probability and low-probability criteria have been revised, and very-low-probability criteria have been added. The concept of stratifying the patients into those with and those without cardiopulmonary disease is not included in these criteria. However, appropriate clinical data to make this stratification are being gathered in the study, and the final outcome data will be used to assess the effectiveness of this stratification to see whether this clinical addition can be used to improve the diagnosis of "high probability."

The final PIOPED II V/Q scan criteria represent revisions such as those cited earlier evaluated with the combined wisdom of the PIOPED II nuclear medicine working group. This group includes the nuclear medicine physician responsible for PIOPED II at the eight participating clinical centers. The final interpretation of each V/Q scan will be done with techniques comparable with those used in the original PIOPED. Each central reader will receive a chest radiograph and a V/Q scan from one of the centers (not the reader's own) to interpret with no other data available. Using PIOPED II criteria, the reader will assess the V/Q scan. A second central reader will similarly assess the same V/Q scan. For purposes of the study, both readers must make a high-probability interpretation. If not, the V/Q scan is sent to a third central reader, and majority interpretation rules. A normal interpretation must have at least two central readers in agreement. Any reading other than normal or high probability will be considered "nondiagnostic" for purposes of the study, and the data will be saved for ultimate analysis. Each central reader has the ability to provide for each case an intuitive percentage probability that the V/Q scan indicates PE and to provide an idea of where in the category the reading lies. For example, if the interpretation is "intermediate probability" the central reader can indicate whether it is at the low, middle, or high end of that probability category. When PIOPED II is completed, it will be possible to evaluate the scan criteria and to determine whether stratification by cardiopulmonary disease or no cardiopulmonary disease is useful. These data together with the data to be collected about SCTA should determine how a center can best use these two imaging modalities.

Pulmonary Embolism Mimics

Numerous diseases can cause V/Q mismatch, but fortunately most of them are quite uncommon (11). The pathologic process of these lesions involves the pulmonary vessels, whether in the lumen, the vessel wall, or the perivascular tissues, and produces vascular occlusive physiologic findings. The most common cause of V/Q mismatch that is not acute PE is unresolved previous PE (Fig. 18A.13). One study (64) showed that as many as 35% of patients with acute PE have incomplete scintigraphic resolution. Data from the PIOPED study imply that previous PE is one of the most common causes of false-positive "high-probability" results on scans (the positive predictive value of a high-probability scan result was 91% among patients with no history of previous PE and only 74% among those with that history, [$P < .05$]). Other processes occurring in the pulmonary arterial lumen (embolism of material other than thrombus, in situ thrombosis or pulmonary artery tumor), processes involving the

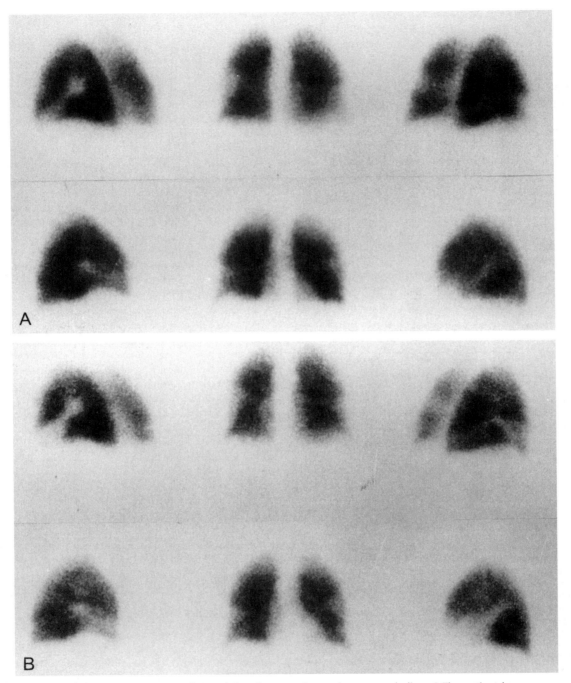

FIGURE 18A.13. Chronic perfusion defect from previous pulmonary embolism. **A:**The patient has a massive embolus with marked but incomplete resolution. **B:** Study obtained 18 months after **A** shows no change (except for lower display intensity). Findings on a chest radiograph and ventilation study at this time were entirely normal.

arterial wall (vasculitis, connective tissue disorder (Fig. 18A.14), tuberculosis, or irradiation), vascular anomalies (pulmonary arterial agenesis, peripheral coarctation (Fig. 18A.15), arteriovenous malformation, or surgical pulmonic-systemic shunts), and extrinsic compression of pulmonary arteries or veins (mediastinal or hilar carcinomas or fibrosis) can cause segmental or lobar perfusion deficits. In some of these pathologic entities, the perfusion deficits are matched by ventilatory or radiographic abnormalities, but a V/Q mismatch mimicking acute PE can be seen in all of them.

Despite the extensive list of possibilities, we have found that most PE mimics have one of three causes: (a) a chronic perfusion deficit from previous PE, (b) intravenous drug abuse, or (c) hilar or mediastinal involvement, usually by bronchogenic carcinoma.

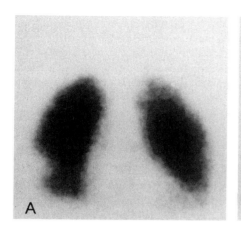
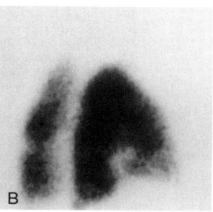

FIGURE 18A.14. Pulmonary embolism mimic. Anterior (**A**) and right posterior oblique (**B**) perfusion images of a patient with active systemic lupus erythematous. Chest radiograph showed only linear atelectasis and small pleural effusions. Findings on a ^{133}Xe ventilation study were normal. Multiple segmental perfusion defects are present. The study is a good example of a high-probability scan findings, but the findings at pulmonary angiography (performed because of the possibility of a pulmonary embolism mimic) were normal. Fortunately, this is a rare diagnostic problem.

Clues to the correct diagnosis often can be found on the chest radiograph, and the history is of paramount importance, because a chronic perfusion deficit from previous PE appears to be a common cause of false-positive scan results.

If the possibility of a PE mimic is present, it is essential to alert the referring physician to this fact. One also should obtain a baseline V/Q scan for all patients with PE whenever possible.

The ideal time to do so is approximately 3 months after the acute episode to avoid confusion in future interpretations.

Interpretive Pitfalls

Some physicians who interpret V/Q scans consider perfusion defects large or segmental only if perfusion is completely absent.

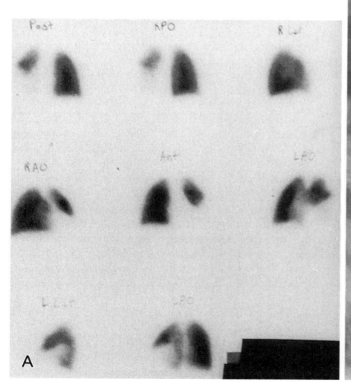
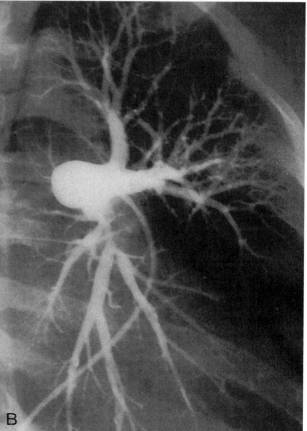

FIGURE 18A.15. A: Perfusion images show a large defect involving multiple segments of the left lung. Perfusion to the right lung is normal. **B:** Angiogram shows peripheral pulmonary artery coarctation, which accounts for the perfusion defect. There is no evidence of acute pulmonary embolism.

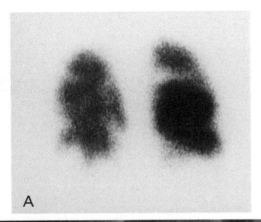

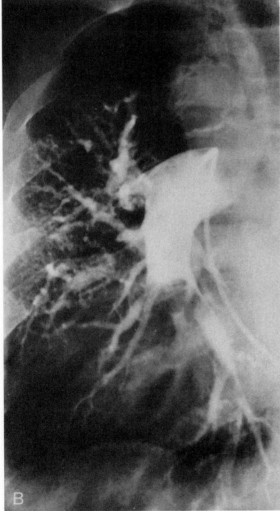

FIGURE 18A.16. Bilateral perfusion defects. **A:** Defects are evident on a posterior image. There is considerable retained perfusion in the left lower lobe (the down-but-not-out phenomenon). **B:** Left pulmonary angiogram printed in reverse to ease comparison with the scan shows extensive embolic occlusion of the lower-lobe arteries. Residual diminished perfusion does not exclude embolic occlusion in the segments involved.

This requirement will lead to erroneous results in the application of modern diagnostic criteria, in which only the area of the perfusion deficit is considered (Fig. 18A.16). The rationale for using decreased or absent perfusion as abnormal is that a partially occluding embolus often produces diminished rather than absent perfusion in the involved segments.

We caution against interpreting a lesion visible on only a single view of a perfusion series as an abnormal finding. We have found that this practice results in overcalling perfusion defects. The most common mistakes of this type are interpreting the defects caused by a prominent aortic arch or pulmonary hilum as due to PE. With an eight-view lung scan, almost any real lesion can be identified on at least two of the eight views.

It is worth reemphasizing that the chest radiograph can become a serious pitfall in the interpretation of V/Q scintigrams. A poor-quality radiograph may not show parenchymal opacities or pleural effusions that correspond to perfusion defects. Whenever possible, a conventional chest radiograph should be obtained, and it should be obtained as close as possible to the time of the V/Q scan.

It is difficult to make a diagnosis of recurrent PE with the V/Q scan alone. A central embolus, if present, can fragment over its resolution time (probably weeks), possibly causing a variety of perfusion scan patterns. Furthermore, differential clot lysis and varying pulmonary arterial pressures can cause changing scan patterns (65). Only when the lung scan has been stable for at least 3 months before an acute change can the diagnosis of recurrent PE be considered (Fig. 18A.13).

SUMMARY

It has been suggested on the basis of retrospective data that evaluation of patients with low- or intermediate-probability V/Q scans by means of lower-extremity ultrasonography is more cost-effective than is evaluation with pulmonary angiography (66). It also has been suggested that V/Q scintigraphy followed by serial impedance plethysmography is the most cost-effective diagnostic approach (67). Still other recent work has suggested that SCTA will prove cost-effective for evaluation of suspected PE (68,69).

These disparate conclusions illustrate the difficulties in evaluating, through direct clinical experiments with representative patient samples, all of the proposed clinical pathways for diagnostic evaluation of patients with suspected acute PE. Accordingly, direct experiments regarding cost-effectiveness in the management of venous thromboembolic disease are few, and fully comprehensive studies are lacking (and likely not practicable). Interesting studies have been conducted with decision analytic modeling (66–70). In these studies, however, some newer strategies were not directly compared, nor were newer data used regarding test characteristics and disease prevalence in different patient populations. The role of clinical judgment also was not factored in. One analysis of both cost and mortality and morbidity showed relatively small differences in mortality and morbidity despite almost twofold variations in cost.

Cost-effective practice requires that we do not use the full battery of imaging procedures now available for detecting venous thromboembolism in every patient. It is not yet clear which tests should be replaced, in which settings, for optimal patient outcomes and cost-effectiveness. It has been shown that perfusion scintigraphy can give normal and high-probability results as reliable as those obtained with the more expensive combined V/Q study (71), and it is less expensive than SCTA. In populations with a high prevalence of normal perfusion (e.g., 41% in the McMaster study [72] and 69% in the Leyenburg Hospital study [68]), it may be cost-effective to continue use of perfusion scintigraphy. Therefore one could propose a hybrid algorithm that combines the lower cost of perfusion scintigraphy with the higher overall accuracy and diagnostic yield of SCTA and ultrasonography. Of course, which clinical pathway is optimal depends on disease prevalence, test characteristics, costs of testing, costs of treatment, value of life, and many other factors. It is likely that different practice settings (e.g., rural clinic versus university hospital) will require different clinical pathways based on the prevalence of the target condition, the existence of comorbid conditions, test availability, and similar factors. Such implementations depend on clinical judgment and monitoring of both local results and the ongoing analysis of SCTA and other new technologies in the literature. Prospective evaluation of the cost-benefit performance of newer proposals for clinical pathways, compared with the "classic" model, should yield improved approaches to diagnostic evaluation. The availability of more definitive sensitivity and specificity measures of spiral CT pulmonary angiography will greatly aid such analyses. These should result from the PIOPED II study, which was recently funded by the National Heart Lung and Blood Institute.

REFERENCES

1. Morrell MT, Dunnill MS. The postmortem incidence of pulmonary embolism in a hospital population. *Br J Surg* 1968;55:347–352.
2. The PIOPED Investigators. Value of the ventilation/perfusion scan in acute pulmonary embolism. *JAMA* 1990;263:2753–2759.
3. Dalen JE, Alpert JS. Natural history of pulmonary embolism. *Prog Cardiovasc Dis* 1975;17:259–270.
4. Barritt DW, Jordan SC. Anticoagulant drugs in treatment of pulmonary embolism: controlled trial. *Lancet* 1960;1:1309–1312.
5. Moser KM, Fedullo PF, LitteJohn JK, et al. Frequent asymptomatic pulmonary embolism in patients with deep venous thrombosis. *JAMA* 1994;271:223–225.
6. Humphries JO, Bell WR, White RI. Criteria for the recognition of pulmonary emboli. *JAMA* 1976;235:2011–2012.
7. Bell WR, Simon TL, DeMets DS. The clinical features of submassive and massive pulmonary emboli. *Am J Med* 1977;62:355–359.
8. Pineda LA, Hathwar VS, Grant BJB. Clinical suspicion of fatal pulmonary embolism. *Chest* 2001;120:791–795.
9. Rodger MA, Jones G, Rasuli P, et al. Steady-state end-tidal alveolar dear space fraction and D-dimer: bedside tests to exclude pulmonary embolism. *Chest* 2001;120:115–119.
10. Landefeld CS, McGuire E, Cohen AM. Clinical findings associated with acute proximal deep venous thrombosis: a basis for quantifying clinical judgment. *Am J Med* 1990;88:382–388.
11. Pope CF, Sostman HD. Venous thrombosis and pulmonary embolism. In: Putman CE, Ravin CE, eds. *Textbook of diagnostic imaging.* Philadelphia: WB Saunders, 1988:584–604.
12. Hull R, Hirsh J, Sackett DL, et al. Clinical validity of a negative venogram in patients with clinically suspected venous thrombosis. *Circulation* 1981;64:622–625.
13. Redman HC. Deep venous thrombosis: is contrast venography still the diagnostic "gold standard"? *Radiology* 1988;168:277–278.
14. Bettmann MA, Robbins A, Braun SD, et al. Contrast venography of the leg: diagnostic efficacy, tolerance and complication rates with ionic and nonionic contrast media. *Radiology* 1987;165:113–116.
15. Lensing AWA, Prandoni P, Buller HR, et al. Lower extremity venography with iohexol: results and complications. *Radiology* 1990;177:503–505.
16. Lensing AWA, Prandoni P, Brandjes D, et al. Detection of DVT by real-time B-mode ultrasonography. *N Engl J Med* 1989;320:342–345.
17. Ginsberg JS, Caco CC, Brill-Edwards PA, et al. Venous thrombosis in patients who have undergone major hip or knee surgery: detection with compression US and impedance plethysmography. *Radiology* 1991;181:651–654.
18. Mattos MA, Londrey GL, Leutz DW, et al. Color-flow duplex scanning for the diagnosis and surveillance of acute DVT. *J Vasc Surg* 1992;15:366–376.
19. Vaccaro JP, Cronan JJ, Dorfman GS. Outcome analysis of patients with normal compression US examinations. *Radiology* 1990;175:645–649.
20. Davidson BL, Elliot CD, Lensing AWA, et al. Low accuracy of color Doppler US in the detection of proximal leg vein thrombosis in asymptomatic high risk patients. *Ann Intern Med* 1992;117:735–738.
21. Evans AJ, Sostman HD, Knelson MH, et al. Detection of DVT: prospective comparison of MRI with contrast venography. *Am J Roentgenol* 1993;161:131–139.
22. Evans AJ, Sostman HD, Witty LA, et al. Detection of DVT: prospective comparison of MRI and sonography. *J Magn Reson Imaging* 1996;1:44–51.
23. Cham MD, Yankelevitz DF, Shaham D, et al. Deep venous thrombosis: detection by using indirect CT venography. *Radiology* 2000;216:744–751.
24. Garg K, Kemp JL, Wojcik D, et al. Thromboembolic disease: comparison of combined CT pulmonary angiography and venography with bilateral leg sonography in 70 patients. *AJR Am J Roentgenol* 2000;175:997–1001.
25. Greenspan RH, Ravin CE, Polansky SM, et al. Accuracy of the chest radiograph in diagnosis of pulmonary embolism. *Invest Radiol* 1982;17:539–543.
26. Worsley DF, Alavi A, Aronchick JM, et al. Chest radiographic findings in patients with acute pulmonary embolism: observations from the PIOPED study. *Radiology* 1993;189:133–136.
27. Goodman LR, Curtin JJ, Mewissen MW, et al. Detection of pulmonary embolism in patients with unresolved clinical and scintigraphic diagnosis: helical CT vs angiography. *Am J Roentgenol* 1995;164:1369–1374.
28. Remy-Jardin MJ, Remy J, Petyt L, et al. Diagnosis of acute pulmonary embolism with spiral CT: comparison with pulmonary angiography and scintigraphy. *Radiology* 1996;200:699–706.
29. Sostman HD, Layish DT, Tapson VF, et al. Prospective comparison of helical CT and MR imaging in patients with clinically suspected pulmonary embolism. *J Magn Reson Imaging* 1996;6:275–281.
30. van Rossum AB, Treurniet FEE, Kieft GJ, et al. Role of spiral volumetric computed tomographic scanning in the assessment of patients with clinical suspicion of pulmonary embolism and an abnormal ventilation/perfusion lung scan. *Thorax* 1996;51:23–28.
31. Mayo JR, Remy-Jardin M, Muller NL, et al. Pulmonary embolism: prospective comparison of spiral CT with ventilation-perfusion scintigraphy. *Radiology* 1997;205:447–452.
32. Drucker EA, Rivitz SM, Shepard JO, et al. Acute PE: assessment of helical CT for diagnosis. *Radiology* 1998;209:235–241.
33. Ferretti GR, Bosson JL, Buffaz PD, et al. Acute pulmonary embolism: role of helical CT in 164 patients with intermediate probability at ventilation-perfusion scintigraphy and normal results at duplex US of the legs. *Radiology* 1997;205:453–458.
34. Goodman LR, Lipchik RJ, Kuzo RS, et al. Subsequent pulmonary embolism: risk after a negative helical CT pulmonary angiogram: prospective comparison with scintigraphy. *Radiology* 2000;215:535–542.
35. Harvey RT, Gefter WB, Hrung JM, et al. Accuracy of CT angiography versus pulmonary angiography in the diagnosis of acute pulmonary embolism. *Acad Radiol* 2000;7:786–797.

36. Qanadli SD, Hajjam M, Mesrolle B, et al. Pulmonary embolism detection: prospective evaluation of dual-section CT versus selective pulmonary angiography in 157 patients. *Radiology* 2000;217:447–455.

37. Baile EM, King GG, Muller NL, et al. Spiral computed tomography is comparable to angiography for the diagnosis of pulmonary embolism. *Am J Respir Crit Care Med* 2000;161:1010–1015.

38. Meaney JFM, Weg JG, Chenevert TL, et al. Diagnosis of pulmonary embolism with magnetic resonance angiography. *N Engl J Med* 1997; 336:1422–1427.

39. Gupta A, Frazer CK, Kumar A, et al. Acute pulmonary embolism: diagnosis with MR angiography. *Radiology* 1999;210:353–359.

40. Hurst D, Kazerooni EA, Stafford-Johnson D, et al. Diagnosis of pulmonary embolism: comparison of CT angiography and MR angiography in canines. *J Vasc Interv Ratiol* 1999;10:309–318.

41. McNeil BJ, Holman L, Adelstein J. The scintigraphic definition of pulmonary embolism. *JAMA* 1974;227:753–756.

42. Krasnow AZ, Isitman AT, Collier BD, et al. Diagnostic applications of radioaerosols in nuclear medicine. In: Freeman LM, ed. *Nuclear medicine annual 1993*. New York: Raven Press, 1993:123–193.

43. Hartmann IJC, Hagen PJ, Stokkel MPM, et al. Technegas Versus 81mKr Ventilation-perfusion scintigraphy: a comparative study in patients with suspected acute pulmonary embolism. *J Nucl Med* 2001; 42:393–400.

44. Alderson PO, Biello DR, Gottschalk A, et al. Tc-99m-DTPA aerosol and radioactive gases compared as adjuncts to perfusion scintigraphy in patients with suspected pulmonary embolism. *Radiology* 1984;153:515–521.

45. Ramanna L, Alderson PO, Berman D, et al. Comparison of Tc-99m-DTPA aerosol and radioactive gas ventilation studies in patients with suspected pulmonary embolism. *J Nucl Med* 1986;27:1391–1396.

46. Kotlyarov EV, Reba RC. The concept of using abnormal V/Q segment equivalents to refine the diagnosis of pulmonary embolism. *Invest Radiol* 1981;16:383(abst).

47. Wagner HN Jr, Lopez-Majano V, Langan JK, et al. Radioactive xenon in the differential diagnosis of pulmonary embolism. *Radiology* 1968; 91:1168–1174.

48. DeNardo GL, Goodwin DA, Ravasini R, et al. The ventilatory lung scan in the diagnosis of pulmonary embolism. *N Engl J Med* 1970; 282:1334–1336.

49. Alderson PO, Rujanavech N, Secker-Walker RH, et al. The role of 133-xenon ventilation studies in the scintigraphic detection of pulmonary embolism. *Radiology* 1976;120:633–640.

50. Neumann RD, Sostman HD, Gottschalk A. Current status of ventilation-perfusion imaging. *Semin Nucl Med* 1980;10:198–217.

51. Alderson PO, Biello DR, Sachariah KG, et al. Scintigraphic detection of pulmonary embolism in patients with obstructive pulmonary disease. *Radiology* 1981;138:661–666.

52. Biello DR, Mattar AG, McKnight RC, et al. Ventilation-perfusion studies in suspected pulmonary embolism. *Am J Roentgenol* 1979;133:1033–1037.

53. Carter WD, Brady TM, Keyes JW, et al. Relative accuracy of two diagnostic schemes for detection of pulmonary embolism by ventilation-perfusion scintigraphy. *Radiology* 1982;145:447–451.

54. Gottschalk A, Juni JE, Sostman HD, et al. Ventilation-perfusion scintigraphy in the PIOPED study: data collection and tabulation. *J Nucl Med* 1993;34:1109–1118.

55. Gottschalk A, Sostman HD, Juni JE, et al. Ventilation-perfusion scintigraphy in the PIOPED study: evaluation of the scintigraphic criteria and interpretations. *J Nucl Med* 1993;34:1119–1126.

56. Sullivan DC, Coleman RE, Mills SR, et al. Lung scan interpretation: effect of different observers and different criteria. *Radiology* 1983;149:803–807.

57. Freeman LM, Krynyckyi B, Zuckier LS. Enhanced lung scan diagnosis of pulmonary embolism with the use of ancillary scintigraphic findings and clinical correlation. *Semin Nucl Med* 2001;31:143–157.

58. Stein PD, Gottschalk A, Henry JW, et al. Stratification of patients according to prior cardiopulmonary disease and probability assessment based on the number of mismatched segmental equivalent perfusion defects. *Chest* 1993;104:1461–1467.

59. Stein PD, Henry JW, Gottschalk A. Mismatched vascular defects. *Chest* 1993;104:1468–1472.

60. Hull RD, Raskob GE. Low-probability lung scan findings: a need for change. *Ann Intern Med* 1991;114:142–143.

61. Dalen J. When can treatment be withheld in patients with suspected pulmonary embolism. *Arch Intern Med* 1993;153:1415–1418.

62. Stein PD, Gottschalk A. Review of criteria appropriate for a very low probability of pulmonary embolism on ventilation-perfusion lung scans. *Radiographics* 2000;20:99–105.

63. Alderson PO. Presentation to the Fleischner Society Post Graduate Course. Tuscon, Arizona, April 1999.

64. Paraskos VA, Adelstein SJ, Smith RE, et al. Late prognosis of acute pulmonary embolism. *N Engl J Med* 1973;289:55–58.

65. Alderson PO, Dzebolo NN, Biello DR, et al. Serial lung scintigraphy: utility in diagnosis of pulmonary embolism. *Radiology* 1983;149:797–802.

66. Beecham RP, Dorfman GS, Cronan JJ, et al. Is bilateral lower extremity compression sonography useful and cost-effective in the evaluation of suspected pulmonary embolism? *Am J Roentgenol* 1993;161:1289–1292.

67. Hull RD, Feldstein W, Stein PD, et al. Cost-effectiveness of pulmonary embolism diagnosis. *Arch Intern Med* 1996;156:68–72.

68. van Erkel AR, van Rossum AB, Bloem JL, et al. Spiral CT angiography for suspected pulmonary embolism: a cost-effectiveness analysis. *Radiology* 1996;201:29–36.

69. Paterson DI, Schwartzman K. Strategies incorporating spiral CT for the diagnosis of acute pulmonary embolism: a cost-effective analysis. *Chest* 2001;119:1791–1800.

70. Oudkerk M, van Beek EJR, van Putten WLJ, et al. Cost-effectiveness-analysis of various strategies in the diagnostic management of pulmonary embolism. *Arch Intern Med* 1993;153:947–954.

71. Stein PD, Terrin ML, Gottschalk A, et al. Value of V/Q scans vs. perfusion scans alone in acute pulmonary embolism. *Am J Cardiol* 1992;69:1239–1241.

72. Hull RD, Hirsh J, Carter CJ, et al. Pulmonary angiography, ventilation lung scan and venography for clinically suspected pulmonary embolism with abnormal perfusion lung scan. *Ann Intern Med* 1983;98:891–899.

Diagnostic Nuclear Medicine, Fourth Edition. Edited by M.P. Sandler, R.E. Coleman, J.A. Patton, F.J.Th. Wackers, A. Gottschalk. Lippincott Williams & Wilkins, Philadelphia 2003.

DETECTION OF DEEP VENOUS THROMBOSIS WITH 99MTC-LABELED PEPTIDES

RAYMOND TAILLEFER

Because of the clear link between acute deep venous thrombosis (DVT) and its life-threatening complication, pulmonary embolism, and because of other morbid sequelae, such as postphlebitic syndrome, the prompt diagnosis and appropriate management of acute DVT are important (1–4). Acute DVT is a common clinical condition with an estimated prevalence of 2 to 5 million cases per year in the United States (1,2). Furthermore, it has been shown that 70% to 90% of pulmonary emboli derive from acute DVT in the lower extremities (2,5). Unfortunately, the clinical diagnosis of DVT often is inaccurate. Acute DVT can be clinically silent; approximately 70% of patients with a confirmed case of pulmonary embolism have asymptomatic DVT (4). Conversely, acute DVT can be associated with nonspecific signs and symptoms. It has been shown that only 20% to 50% of patients with signs and symptoms that suggest DVT are confirmed to have acute DVT (6–8). There is a clear medical need for an objective and noninvasive method for accurate diagnosis of the presence of acute DVT.

Different imaging modalities have been proposed and evaluated (5,9). Contrast venography has been considered the standard of reference for the detection of DVT. The diagnostic imaging method used most frequently in the United States, however, is ultrasonography (10). Both imaging modalities have their limitations. Contrast venography is decreasingly used because it often is painful for the patient, can cause side effects, is relatively expensive, and is time-consuming to perform. The results may be technically inadequate or difficult to interpret in 10% to 30% of cases (1,11), and the reader cannot reliably differentiate acute, recurrent DVT from old, nonacute DVT in patients with a history of DVT (12). Because of these relative limitations, other noninvasive imaging methods have been or are used. These include impedance plethysmography and ultrasonography. Real-time B-mode ultrasonography with compression and pulsed-wave Doppler flow analysis (Duplex ultrasonography), increasingly used in combination with color Doppler flow imaging, is accepted to be highly sensitive and specific for detection of DVT

between the pelvis and knees in patients with localizing signs and symptoms and with no history of DVT in the affected extremity (13). However, this method is less accurate below the knee (13,14), in patients without localizing signs and symptoms (11,12), and in patients with a history of DVT (15–17). It has been reported that the presence of duplicate veins may lead to false-negative results (18). Ultrasonography is highly dependent on operator skill and experience, is technically difficult in evaluation of patients who are obese or who have markedly swollen limbs, and is not useful in evaluation of patients fitted with orthopedic casts (14).

Both contrast venography and ultrasonography are imaging procedures used to detect changes in venous anatomy due to the presence of an intraluminal thrombus that is sufficiently formed either to reduce vascular filling with contrast medium or to resist compression. An alternative approach to the diagnosis of acute DVT is to detect a molecular marker of acute DVT that is not present in old, organized (sometimes called "chronic") DVT. Several types of radiopharmaceuticals have been proposed for the diagnosis of acute DVT, and they have different principles or mechanisms of detection, the discussion of which is beyond the scope of this chapter. Recent advances in biotechnology allow the use of highly specific synthetic peptides or small molecular markers involved in the acute stages of DVT, formation of which can be labeled efficiently with ^{99m}Tc. A new radiopharmaceutical , ^{99m}Tc apcitide (Acutect; Diatide, Londonderry, NJ) previously known as ^{99m}Tc P280, has been approved by the U.S. Food and Drug Administration (FDA) for the clinical detection of acute DVT. This section briefly summarizes some of the clinical results and the radiopharmaceutical characteristics of this new imaging modality.

CLINICAL APPLICATIONS OF ^{99m}TC APCITIDE SCINTIGRAPHY IN THE DETECTION OF THROMBOEMBOLIC DISEASE

The initial imaging procedure used for the detection of acute DVT in clinical practice is ultrasonography. Although ultrasonography is highly sensitive and specific for detection of DVT between the pelvis and knees in patients with localizing signs

R. Taillefer: Department Of Nuclear Medicine, Hospital Hotel-Dieu De Montreal, Montreal, Quebec, Canada.

and symptoms and with no history of DVT in the affected extremity, this diagnostic method also has limitations. It is less accurate below the knee; in the evaluation of patients without localizing signs and symptoms, such as those with pulmonary embolism; and in the evaluation of patients with a history of DVT, in whom the presence of an old clot can decrease the specificity of the test.

In the evaluation of patients with signs and symptoms suggestive of acute DVT and with no history of DVT, ultrasonography remains the initial diagnostic modality of choice. However, if the findings at ultrasonography are normal or equivocal, ^{99m}Tc apcitide scintigraphy can be quite useful to confirm or establish the diagnosis, especially when there is a strong clinical suspicion of the presence of acute DVT. ^{99m}Tc apcitide scintigraphy can be particularly useful in the evaluation of obese patients, patients with trauma of the lower extremities, and patients with orthopedic casts, duplicate veins, or calf-vein thrombi. It also can be a useful alternative to contrast venography when that procedure is contraindicated or when it is technically difficult to perform or the images are difficult to interpret.

One of the most clinically useful indications for ^{99m}Tc peptide venous scintigraphy is in the diagnosis of acute DVT in patients with previous DVT who may have recurrent acute thrombosis superimposed on chronic venous disease. Unlike anatomic diagnostic procedures such as ultrasonography and contrast venography, ^{99m}Tc peptide scintigraphy can be highly specific for acute DVT because a molecular marker specific for acute DVT is involved. Therefore, in evaluation of patients with a history of DVT who have signs and symptoms of acute DVT, ^{99m}Tc peptide venous scintigraphy may be the initial diagnostic imaging modality of choice. Results of multicenter studies should confirm this indication.

Although ^{99m}Tc apcitide scintigraphy is not yet approved for detection of pulmonary embolism, it is likely that the role of ^{99m}Tc peptide venous scintigraphy will expand to concomitant detection of thrombus into the lung, if results of multicenter trials confirm a high diagnostic accuracy. In the mean time, ^{99m}Tc apcitide scintigraphy can be useful to patients with intermediate or indeterminate probability of pulmonary embolism at ventilation-perfusion scintigraphy of the lung and normal ultrasonographic findings in the lower extremities. Scintigraphy of the lower extremities and of the thorax can improve the diagnostic accuracy for detection of DVT and pulmonary embolism. In addition, ^{99m}Tc apcitide imaging is not limited to the lower extremities or to the lungs. It also can be used for detection of acute DVT of the upper extremities, especially in the care of hospitalized patients, who are prone to an increased incidence of acute DVT owing to use of indwelling catheters. Radionuclide thrombus imaging may be helpful in the detection of asymptomatic acute DVT in patients who are at high risk of this disorder, such as those undergoing high-risk surgical procedures.

Another interesting clinical possibility for imaging with ^{99m}Tc peptides involved in hemostasis is evaluation of arterial thrombus, especially coronary thrombus. This indication is under clinical investigation. ^{99m}Tc peptides in addition to ^{99m}Tc apcitide for detection of either venous or arterial thrombus are being evaluated (19–25).

^{99m}TC APCITIDE SCINTIGRAPHY
Clinical Results

Several clinical studies of the detection of thromboembolic disease have been performed with ^{99m}Tc-apcitide (26–30). A phase III multicenter clinical trial comparing ^{99m}Tc apcitide scintigraphy with contrast venography for imaging acute DVT is the most extensive one performed so far with this radiotracer. The results of this study have been reported (31) and are briefly summarized as follows. Two well-controlled clinical trials, referred to as *trial A* and *trial B,* were conducted with identical protocols. Each study was a prospective, multicenter, single-dose, within-patient comparative study of ^{99m}Tc apcitide scintigraphy and contrast venography, used as the standard of reference, for detecting and localizing acute DVT in the lower extremities. These studies were also designed to evaluate the safety and tolerance of a single intravenous administration of ^{99m}Tc apcitide to patients. A total of 280 patients were enrolled, and 34 North American and European institutions participated in the two trials.

Patients were to be within 10 days of onset of signs and symptoms of acute DVT or within 10 days after a surgical procedure associated with high risk of development of acute DVT. ^{99m}Tc apcitide scintigraphy and contrast venography were to be performed within 36 hours of one another. Each patient received approximately 20 mCi of ^{99m}T apcitide (70 to 100 μg of peptide) by means of intravenous injection. Anterior and posterior planar images of the pelvis, thighs, knees, and calves were obtained 10, 60, and 120 to 180 minutes after injection of ^{99m}Tc-apcitide. Images were required for a minimum of 750,000 counts over the pelvis and 300,000 counts over the lower regions. Contrast venography was performed according to the standard protocol at each institution.

The ^{99m}Tc apcitide images were read by three experienced readers blinded to all other patient information, including the results of contrast venography. The images were read from a computer screen with appropriate contrast adjustment. Complete sets of 10-, 60-, and 120- to 180-minute images were read for each patient. The criteria for acute DVT were asymmetric uptake of ^{99m}Tc apcitide in a deep vein relative to the corresponding contralateral deep venous segment or contiguous segments of the ipsilateral vein, which asymmetry persisted or intensified with time. In addition, the asymmetry was to be present in both anterior and posterior projections, if appropriate to the anatomic location of the vein (Figs 18B.1 through 18B.4). For each case, the following nine anatomical regions were evaluated: inferior vena cava, right and left iliac veins, and deep veins of the right and left thighs, knees, and calves. Each region was scored as positive or negative for acute DVT or as indeterminate. The final ^{99m}Tc apcitide result was defined as the majority result of the three readers. ^{99m}Tc apcitide images also were read by qualified personnel in the institutions in which they were acquired (referred to as institution-read ^{99m}Tc apcitide). The institutional readers had access to the patients' general clinical information but were not aware of the results of contrast venography. The contrast venograms were read by two experienced radiologists who were blinded to all other patient information, includ-

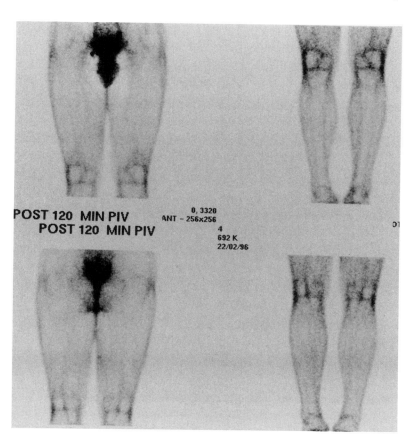

FIGURE 18B.1. ^{99m}Tc apcitide scintigraphic image obtained 120 minutes after administration of the radiotracer (*upper row,* anterior views; *lower row,* posterior views) to a normal patient without acute deep venous thrombosis (DVT). There is no asymmetric linear uptake in the projection of deep veins indicative of acute DVT in the calf, knee, or thigh. There is increased ^{99m}Tc apcitide uptake around the knees that increases over time. This is a normal variant secondary to synovial uptake.

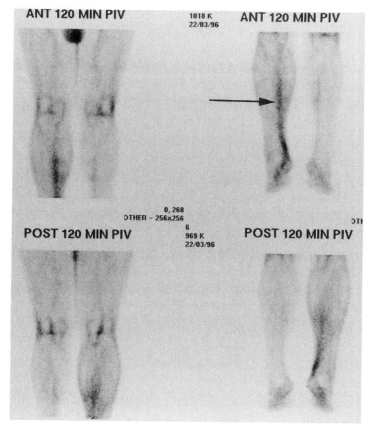

FIGURE 18B.2. Acute deep venous thrombosis (DVT) of the right calf confirmed with contrast venography. There is an increased asymmetric linear uptake of ^{99m}Tc apcitide in the right calf (*arrows*) corresponding to the DVT.

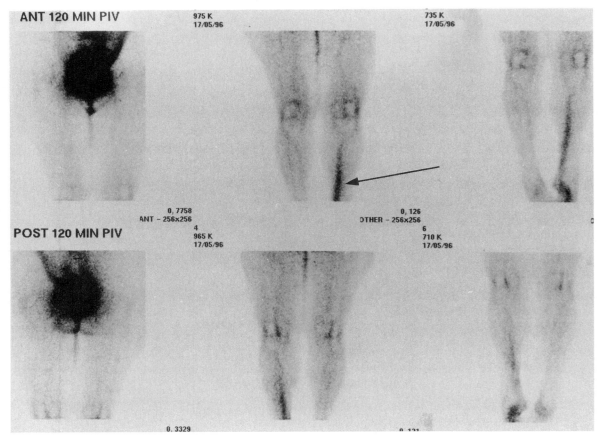

FIGURE 18B.3. Increased linear uptake of ^{99m}Tc apcitide (*arrows*) in the left calf corresponds to DVT proved at contrast venography.

ing the ^{99m}Tc apcitide results. For this blind reading, the final result was based on the consensus result of the two readers. When consensus was not reached, a third radiologist read the venograms, and the final result was the consensus of all three readers.

The blind reading was conducted according to the following standard criteria. For each case, the iliac, common femoral, superficial femoral, popliteal, peroneal, and posterior and anterior tibial veins were evaluated for intraluminal filling defects. An intraluminal filling defect was defined as an area of reduced or absent filling, at least partially surrounded by contrast medium and seen in at least two views, or lack of filling in a vein that had a cutoff with the configuration of a thrombus and wherein there was proximal filling. A study was defined as positive for DVT when an intraluminal filling defect was present. A study was defined as negative for DVT when all deep veins were visualized and there was no intraluminal filling defect. Venography was considered inadequate if there was a lack of filling of a region of the deep veins with no intraluminal filling defect in the same region. A ^{99m}Tc apcitide result was considered truly positive if results of ^{99m}Tc apcitide and venography were positive in the same anatomic region or in a contiguous region. A ^{99m}Tc apcitide result was considered truly negative if findings of both studies were negative in all regions. A ^{99m}Tc apcitide result was considered falsely positive if it was positive or indeterminate and

results of venography were negative. A ^{99m}Tc apcitide results was considered falsely negative if it was negative or indeterminate and the venographic result was positive.

Of the 280 patients, 37 were ineligible for efficacy evaluation, so the cases of 243 patients could be evaluated (123 women and 120 men; mean age, 59.6 years). The prevalence of a history of DVT or pulmonary embolism in this patient population was 24% (58 patients). Seventy percent of patients whose cases could be evaluated were taking some form of anticoagulant or antiplatelet medication, and 61.7% were being treated with heparin when ^{99m}Tc apcitide scintigraphy was performed. More than 90% of patients (91.8%, 223 or 243) underwent ^{99m}Tc apcitide scintigraphy and contrast venography within 36 hours of one another. Contrast venography was performed before ^{99m}Tc apcitide scintigraphy in the cases of 178 patients (73.2%).

When contrast venography was used as the "truth," blindly read ^{99m}Tc apcitide images of all patients whose cases could be evaluated in both trials combined had a sensitivity, specificity, and agreement rate of 73.4%, 67.5%, and 69.1%, respectively (47 true-positive results, 112 true-negative results, 54 false-positive results, and 17 false-negative results). When institution-read contrast venograms were used as the "truth," the corresponding values were 75.5%, 72.8%, and 74.0% for institution-read ^{99m}Tc apcitide imaging (83 true-positive results, 91 true-negative results, 34 false-positive results, and 27 false-negative re-

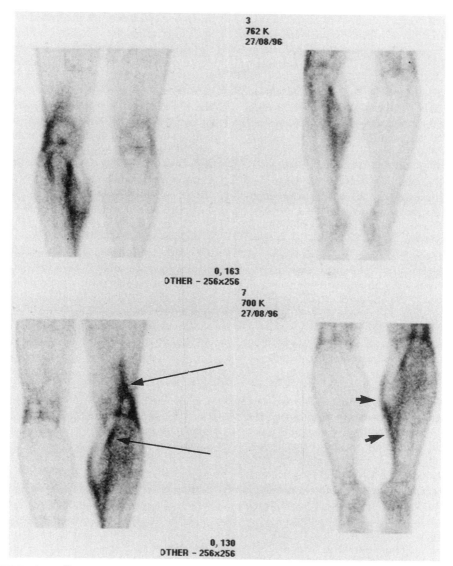

FIGURE 18B.4. [99mTc] apcitide scintigraphic image of a patient with both superficial (*arrowheads*) and deep (*arrows*) venous thrombosis of the right calf, popliteal, and distal femoral veins (*upper panel*, anterior views; *lower panel*, posterior views).

sults). When blindly read contrast venograms were used as the "truth," institution-read [99mTc] apcitide scintigraphy had a sensitivity of 81.3%, a specificity of 65.0%, and an agreement rate of 69.6% (52 true-positive results, 106 true-negative results, 57 false-positive results, and 12 false-negative results). In comparison with contrast to venography, [99mTc] apcitide scintigraphy had a sensitivity of 83.1%, a specificity of 76.8%, and an agreement rate of 78.4% in the detection of DVT of the calf. The corresponding values were 68.8%, 82.7%, and 80.0% for the detection of acute DVT of the knee. The values were 62.5%, 87.7%, and 83.4%, respectively, for the thigh. No patient had vena caval thrombus detected at venography, and only 6 patients had positive findings on venograms of the iliac region; none of which these was found with [99mTc] apcitide scintigraphy. The

anatomic distribution of disease in the study according to contrast venographic findings was 38% in the calf, 31% in the knee, 26% in the thigh, and 4% in the pelvis.

The complete patient populations included patients with a history of DVT or pulmonary embolism (24% of the total population) and patients who came to medical attention as long as 10 days from the onset of signs and symptoms. It is difficult to differentiate acute from nonacute DVT with contrast venography. Therefore in the complete trial populations, contrast venographic results may have been read as positive because of the presence of old, nonacute thrombus, whereas [99mTc] apcitide results would be expected to be negative in the absence of acute DVT. In the evaluation of patients who did not have a history of DVT or pulmonary embolism and who cam to medical attention within 3 days of the onset of signs and symptoms of acute DVT, it would be expected that results of contrast venography would be positive because of the presence of acute DVT and that of old, nonacute DVT. The sensitivity, specificity, and agreement rate of blindly read ^{99m}Tc apcitide images compared with those of blindly read venograms in the evaluation of patients with no history of DVT or pulmonary embolism and coming to medical attention within 3 days of the onset of signs and symptoms were 83.3%, 73.8%, and 76.7%. For institution-read ^{99m}Tc apcitide scintigraphy versus institution-read contrast venography, these values were 90.6%, 83.9%, and 87.3%. Thus in a patient population for whom positive results of contrast venography were likely to represent only acute disease, ^{99m}Tc apcitide scintigraphy was shown to be highly sensitive for the detection of acute DVT.

A comparison of ^{99m}Tc apcitide scintigraphy in the evaluation of patients who were or were not taking anticoagulation medication showed no discernible difference between the two groups. The agreement rate between ^{99m}Tc apcitide scintigraphy and contrast venography was 68% among patients taking no antiplatelet or anticoagulant, 70% among those taking at least one antiplatelet or anticoagulant, and 69% among patients taking heparin.

In designing a clinical trial to determine the efficacy of ^{99m}Tc apcitide (and that of other ^{99m}Tc peptides for the detection of acute DVT), the challenge is to find a way to definitively measure the "truth." Ultrasonography is used most often in clinical practice to diagnose acute DVT, but this method is not amenable to blind reading, has several limitations, and is not accepted as the standard of reference. Although contrast venography is used to assess venous anatomic features and not function, it is accepted as the standard of reference for thrombus detection. Therefore the ^{99m}Tc apcitide phase III clinical trials were designed to compare ^{99m}Tc apcitide scintigraphy with contrast venography as the "truth" for the detection of acute venous thrombosis. The primary efficacy endpoint, blindly read ^{99m}Tc apcitide scintigraphic images compared with blindly read contrast venograms, was chosen to remove any bias from the image evaluation. However, this also produced an artificial condition, because image evaluation in normal practice is performed with knowledge of all patient clinical information. In recognition of this factor, and of the known, relatively high interobserver variability in blindly read venograms (32,33), a target endpoint of agreement rate of 75% to 80% is certainly adequate. This range of agreement rate was achieved in this large multicenter trial.

Nonetheless, there remained the fundamental problem that the functional test, ^{99m}Tc apcitide scintigraphy, was being compared with the anatomic test, contrast venography. Thus the result of the anatomic test could be positive because of the presence of nonacute DVT, whereas the results of ^{99m}Tc apcitide scintigraphy would not be expected to be positive in the absence of acute thrombosis. To address this issue, analysis of data from a subset of patients who had no history of DVT or pulmonary embolism and who came to medical attention soon after (within 3 days of the onset of signs and symptoms of acute DVT) is certainly more adequate in the context of evaluating patients who definitely have acute DVT. In evaluation of these patients, one would expect that results of contrast venography would be positive only because of the presence of acute thrombus. The

analysis showed that, in the evaluation of these patients, ^{99m}Tc apcitide scintigraphy was effectively highly sensitive (90.6%) for the detection of acute DVT. According to these results, the negative predictive value of ^{99m}Tc apcitide scintigraphy was high (90% to 97%), indicating that negative results of a ^{99m}Tc apcitide study should be of value in excluding acute DVT. Although the positive predictive value was not as high as the negative predictive value, the true accuracy of contrast venography is unknown. It is possible that the apparently false-positive findings at ^{99m}Tc apcitide scintigraphy resulted from a greater sensitivity than that of contrast venography in the detection of acute thrombi, which do not produce a visible intraluminal filling defect on venograms. These limitations will always be present in any studies in which a functional test, such as imaging with ^{99m}Tc-labeled peptide scintigraphy, is compared with an anatomic test.

A subgroup of patients at our institution (26) participated in a prospective study to compare the diagnostic value of early and delayed imaging with ^{99m}Tc apcitide in evaluations of suspected acute DVT in which contrast venography was used as a standard of reference. Thirty-nine patients (17 women and 22 men) with signs and symptoms suggestive of acute DVT (within 10 days of onset) and scheduled for contrast venography were given an injection of approximately 20 mCi (740 MBq) of ^{99m}Tc apcitide within 36 hours of contrast venography. Both anterior and posterior planar images of the lower extremities (described earlier) were obtained 10, 60, and 120 minutes after the injection of ^{99m}Tc apcitide. The three sets of images initially were read randomly and separately by three experienced observers blinded to the clinical history, the site of acute DVT, and results of contrast venography. All the images from the three sets for a given patient were analyzed together during a second reading session. Conventional contrast venography was performed before ^{99m}Tc apcitide scintigraphy for 31 patients and after scintigraphy for 8 patients. Twenty-two patients were found to have acute DVT at contrast venography, and 17 had normal findings. Six cases of acute DVT were infrapopliteal. One patient did not complete the third set of images of ^{99m}Tc apcitide. The sensitivity of ^{99m}Tc apcitide imaging in the detection of acute DVT was 63.6% (14/22), 68.2% (15/22), 76.2% (16/21), and 86.4% (19/22) for images obtained 10, 60, 120 minutes after injection and for the 3 sets analyzed together. The specificity was 82.4% (14/17), 76.5% (13/17), 88.2% (15/17), and 88.2% (15/17) for images obtained 10, 60, 120 minutes after injection and the three sets of images together. Although the set of ^{99m}Tc apcitide images obtained 120 minutes after injection showed a good overall diagnostic accuracy, the combination of at least two sets of images provided the highest diagnostic accuracy in detection of acute DVT.

Having two different sets of ^{99m}Tc apcitide images allows for the use of an increased number of interpretation criteria for the presence of acute DVT. The asymmetry of increased deep venous ^{99m}Tc apcitide uptake should be seen in two or more imaging sessions, and early asymmetric radiotracer uptake should persist or be enhanced on delayed images. The use of at least two sets of ^{99m}Tc apcitide images includes not only spatial criteria on the location of an area of increased uptake but also temporal criteria on the changes of the uptake at two different time points.

A first set of images ideally should be obtained soon after administration of ^{99m}Tc apcitide. These early images can serve as a reference to assess the location of various deep veins of the lower extremities. Comparison of delayed images and early studies allows better evaluation of the evolution of increased deep venous uptake over time and therefore a better diagnosis of acute DVT. Although the set of ^{99m}Tc apcitide images obtained 120 minutes after injection provided the highest diagnostic accuracy for a single set of images, analysis of the three sets together resulted in better accuracy. Overall analysis did not show any statistical difference between the 10- and 60-minute, 10- and 120-minute, and 60- and 120-minute image combinations. Therefore the use of at least two sets of images, an initial set obtained soon after the injection and a second obtained 60 to 120 minutes later, provides the highest diagnostic accuracy for ^{99m}Tc apcitide scintigraphy in detection of acute DVT.

Although ^{99m}Tc apcitide has been approved by the FDA for detection of acute DVT, this radiopharmaceutical has been investigated for other possible clinical applications, such as detection of acute pulmonary embolism. Easton (34) reported the preliminary results of a study of the utility of ^{99m}Tc apcitide in demonstrating the presence of acute pulmonary emboli proved with either pulmonary angiography or spiral computed tomography. Ten consecutively recorded cases of proven pulmonary emboli were evaluated with planar, single photon emission tomographic, and blood-pool subtraction techniques. Seven of the ten cases exhibited increased ^{99m}Tc apcitide uptake in the same location as emboli seen at pulmonary angiography or spiral computed tomography. The author concluded that acute pulmonary embolism can be detected with ^{99m}Tc apcitide pulmonary imaging, which may be a valuable complement to evaluation of acute DVT. Detection of acute pulmonary embolism (Fig 18B.5) also has been accomplished with other ^{99m}Tc labeled peptides, such as ^{99m}Tc DMP 444, which is another ^{99m}Tc-labeled platelet glycoprotein IIb/IIIa complex (GpIIb-IIIa) receptor antagonist.

^{99m}Tc Apcitide Uptake Mechanisms

Both contrast venography and ultrasonography provide anatomic information about the vascular obstruction. Neither provides functional information that allows reliable differentiation between acute and chronic thrombus. This is particularly important in cases of recurrent DVT in which acute thrombus may be present along with chronic (organized) thrombus. Therefore there is an important and unmet diagnostic need for an objective diagnostic method that exploits a functional or biochemical difference between acute and nonacute DVT and allows accurate detection and localization of acute DVT. Because platelets are involved in acute but not nonacute thrombi, radiolabeled platelets have been investigated for imaging of thrombi (35–37). However, it was found that this method was of limited use to heparin-treated patients and that a long delay was necessary between injection and imaging (38). Because activated platelets are present in acute thrombi but not in old, organized, nonacute thrombi, the GpIIb-IIIa receptor is a molecular marker of acute thrombus. ^{99m}Tc apcitide is a small, synthetic peptide containing a binding region for binding to the GpIIb-IIIa receptor and a complex of the radionuclide ^{99m}Tc. In vitro studies have demon-

strated that ^{99m}Tc apcitide binds with a high affinity to GpIIb-IIIa receptors, does not bind appreciably to the vitronectin receptor on endothelial cells, and has an affinity for binding to activated human platelets that is three times greater than that for binding to resting platelets (39).

The utility of ^{99m}Tc apcitide in obtaining scintigraphic images of venous thrombi was demonstrated in a canine model of venous thrombosis. Venous thrombi 24 hours old were produced with an inserted embolization coil. ^{99m}Tc apcitide uptake by the thrombi was quantified by means of excision and counting. Thrombus uptake of ^{99m}Tc apcitide was significantly greater than that of ^{99m}Tc gluceptate, which served as a negative control. ^{99m}Tc apcitide thrombus-to-blood and thrombus-to-muscle ratios averaged 4.4 and 11.0, respectively. Additional in vivo studies with a canine model of arterial thrombosis showed that apcitide and bibapcitide inhibited thrombosis at doses much higher than the maximum dose for humans.

Because patients receiving ^{99m}Tc apcitide for the detection of DVT may be medicated with either aspirin or heparin, the possibility that aspirin and heparin may enhance the antiaggregatory action of ^{99m}Tc apcitide was examined. Oral administration of aspirin at a dose sufficient to block arachidonic acid–induced platelet aggregation did not affect the ability of ^{99m}Tc apcitide to inhibit adenosine diphosphate–induced aggregation of the platelets of humans. Heparin, at anticoagulating concentrations (0.2 to 0.6 U/mL) also did not enhance the antiaggregatory effect of ^{99m}Tc apcitide.

Pharmacokinetics of ^{99m}Tc Apcitide

The biodistribution, accumulation and elimination, and radiation dosimetry of ^{99m}Tc apcitide were determined in a phase I study performed with 10 healthy volunteers who were given injection of 100 μg of peptide radiolabeled with 10 mCi (370 MBq) of ^{99m}Tc. The renal system is the main pathway for elimination, and approximately 80% of the activity is eliminated through the kidneys. One third of the injected activity is eliminated within the first hour. The rest of the activity is cleared by the hepatobiliary system within normal gastrointestinal transit times. Blood clearance of ^{99m}Tc apcitide is rapid: 18% remains in the blood 30 minutes after injection; 11%, 1 hour after injection; and 0.5%, 24 hours after injection. When the data are fit to a two-compartment model, the half-time of the rapid phase is 15.6 minutes and the half-time of the slow component is 124.4 minutes. The rapid blood clearance and urinary excretion give low background activity that can allow thrombus localization. Radiation dose estimates for ^{99m}Tc apcitide studies showed that the critical organ was found to be the wall urinary bladder (0.3 rad/mCi), and the effective dose equivalent was 0.037 rem/mCi (0.01 mSv/MBq).

Technical Aspects

Patient preparation for ^{99m}Tc apcitide scintigraphy is minimal. Because the kidneys are the main route of excretion of ^{99m}Tc apcitide, patients should be well hydrated with oral or intravenous fluids, unless contraindicated, to facilitate voiding. Immediately before the study and during the first few hours after

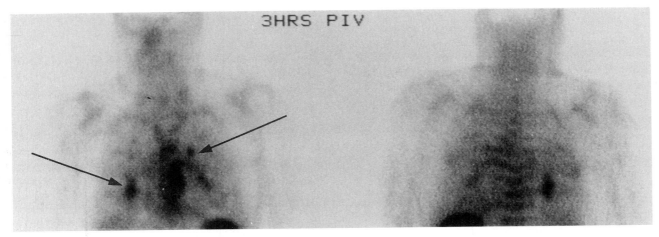

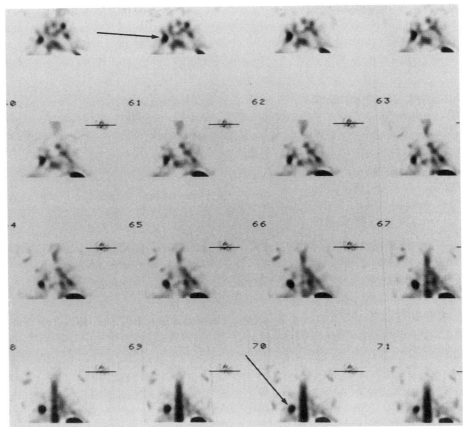

FIGURE 18B.5. Planar thoracic images (*left,* anterior view; *right,* posterior view) obtained at 3 hours after injection of 20 mCi (740 MBq) of ^{99m}Tc DMP 444 (another platelet glycoprotein IIb/IIIa complex receptor antagonist) into a patient with proven bilateral pulmonary emboli. Three foci of increased uptake (*arrows*) correspond to the sites of pulmonary emboli. Single photon emission computed tomographic images of the same patient show the most important site of embolism (*arrows*).

injection of the radiotracer, the patient should be encouraged to void frequently to empty the bladder. A dose of approximately 75 to 100 μg of peptide radiolabeled with 20 to 25 mCi (740 to 925 MBq) of ^{99m}Tc usually is administered into a peripheral vein of an upper extremity or can be injected into a pedal vein. An injection into the arm is advantageous in the care of patients with swollen legs. Injection into a pedal vein can be useful, if

the vein is accessible, for direct delivery of the radiotracer into the deep venous system to be evaluated. This can be particularly useful in the care of a patient with extensive acute DVT of one lower limb, whereas pedal injection into the extremity to be studied facilitates rapid uptake of the radiotracer by the clot and gives better delineation of the proximal part of the thrombus. Preferably, ^{99m}Tc apcitide should be administered through an indwelling venous catheter or with a butterfly administration set. Before image acquisition, tight clothing, stockings, or any lower extremity vascular compression devices should be removed to decrease the risk of vasculature constriction. ^{99m}Tc apcitide scintigraphy can be conducted with an orthopedic cast in place.

Previous clinical studies (26) have shown that at least two sets of planar images of the two lower extremities (both anterior and posterior views) including the pelvis, thighs, knees, and calves should be acquired to determine the presence of acute DVT. One set is started 10 to 15 minutes (early phase) and one set is started 60 to 90 minutes (delayed phase) after injection of ^{99m}Tc apcitide. Although many cases of acute DVT can be diagnosed with early images, better diagnostic accuracy is achieved by means of comparing delayed images with early images. A large-field-of-view single- or dual-head gamma camera equipped with either a low-energy all-purpose or a low-energy high-resolution parallel hole collimator is preferred. Planar images should be acquired for a minimum of 750,000 counts for images over the pelvis and a minimum of 500,000 counts for images over the lower regions. This can be conveniently accomplished with an image acquisition time of 5 minutes. Of course, if the clinical condition allows it, an image acquisition time of up to 10 minutes is preferable and results in improved counting statistics.

For accurate image interpretation, it is important to correctly position the patient with maintained alignment for all images acquired at all time points. To avoid motion during imaging, the patient should be comfortably positioned supine on the imaging table. The lower extremities should be symmetrically positioned to allow comparison of early and delayed images. It is useful to bind the feet together to stabilize the legs. Because external compression of the limbs can affect the diagnostic accuracy of the test, bedclothes, bedding, and pillows should be removed, and flexion of the knees should be avoided. Urinary drainage catheters should be positioned so that they drain freely and are out of the field of view. The urinary bladder also can be shielded. A masked or empty bladder is necessary for visualization of the iliac veins.

Experience from the phase III clinical trial has shown that the images should be presented digitally to allow appropriate contrast, brightness, and threshold image adjustment. Before image interpretation, it can be useful to review the clinical status of the patient, especially to avoid false-positive interpretations. Trauma, fractures, hip or knee replacement, cellulitis, arthritis, or varicosities can cause foci of increased ^{99m}Tc apcitide uptake, although these conditions usually have a typical pattern of distribution different from that of acute DVT.

Deep venous thrombi originate in regions of low flow in the deep venous system (usually of the lower extremities), frequently in a venous valve cusp or in a large venous sinus in the calf (40). Hypercoagulability and vascular endothelial irritation are believed to be comorbid factors (1). The initial process in thrombosis is platelet deposition, followed by proximal propagation of the initial thrombus, with incorporation of fibrin, red blood cells, and platelets. In the process of becoming incorporated into a thrombus, platelets become activated (41). One of the consequences of this phenomenon is that the GpIIb-IIIa receptors on the surface of the activated platelets become competent

to bind fibrinogen (42), which cross-links the platelets. The result is platelet aggregation. The thrombus can lyse or eventually become organized. Until it has lysed or become organized, the thrombus is susceptible to continued propagation, sometimes extending along the entire course of the deep venous system, and to detachment from the vessel wall and embolization. This is acute venous thrombosis, and it is this type of venous thrombus most likely to result in pulmonary embolism (43). Once it has become organized, a thrombus becomes stabilized and difficult to dislodge. This condition is sometimes called *chronic DVT,* but the term *nonacute DVT* is used to avoid confusion with the condition of chronic, recurrent acute DVT. During the process of thrombus organization, which can start within 48 hours, platelets and platelet residues undergo phagocytosis, and by the second week, the process has progressed to a fibrotic mass covered by smooth muscle cells that is eventually covered by new endothelium.

CONCLUSION

^{99m}Tc apcitide scintigraphy is a new type of diagnostic procedure in nuclear medicine. Since introduction of this technique to clinical practice, promising results have been reported. Further studies are needed to fully appreciate the clinical potential of ^{99m}Tc apcitide and related agents. The introduction of ^{99m}Tc apcitide scintigraphy will certainly expand the role of nuclear medicine in a diagnostic area in which nuclear medicine previously played a marginal role.

REFERENCES

1. Hirsh J, Hoak J. Management of deep vein thrombosis and pulmonary embolism. *Circulation* 1996;93:2212–2245.
2. Moser KM. Venous thromboembolism. *Am Rev Respir Dis* 1990;141: 235–249.
3. Dalen JE, Alpert JS. Natural history of pulmonary embolism. *Prog Cardiovasc Dis* 1975;17:259–270.
4. Anderson FA, Wheeler HB, Goldberg RT, et al. A population-based perspective of the hospital incidence and case facility rates of deep vein thrombosis and pulmonary embolism. *Ann Intern Med* 1991;151: 933–938.
5. Hull RD, Hirsh J, Carter C, et al. Diagnostic efficacy of impedance plethysmography for clinically suspected DVT: a randomized trial. *Ann Intern Med* 1985;102:21.
6. Wells RD, Hirsh J, Anderson DR, et al. Accuracy of clinical assessment of deep-vein thrombosis. *Lancet* 1995;345:1326–1330.
7. Stamatakis JD, Kakkar VV, Lawrence D, et al. The origin of thrombi in the deep veins of the lower limb: a venography study. *Br J Radiol* 1978;65:449–451.
8. Lensing AWA, Prandoni P. Distribution of venous thrombi in symptomatic patients. *Thromb Haemost* 1991;65:1730–1736.
9. Lensing AWA, Prandoni P, Brandjes D, et al. Detection of deep venous thrombosis by real-time B-mode ultrasonography. *N Engl J Med* 1989; 320:342.
10. Lensing AWA, Hirsh J, Buller HR. Diagnosis of venous thrombosis. In Coleman RW, Hirsh J, Marder VJ. Salzman EW, eds. *Hemostasis and thrombosis: basic principles and clinical practice.* Philadelphia: JB Lippincott, 1987:1297–1302.
11. Anand SS, Wells PS, Hunt D, et al. Does this patient have deep vein thrombosis? *JAMA* 1998;279:1094–1099.
12. Hull RD, Carter CJ, Jay RM, et al. The diagnosis of acute recurrent

deep vein thrombosis: a diagnostic challenge. *Circulation* 1983;67:901–906.

13. Cronan JJ. Venous thromboembolic disease: the role of ultrasound. *Radiology* 1993;186:619–630.

14. Rose SC, Zwiebel WJ, Nelson BD, et al. Symptomatic lower extremity deep venous thrombosis: accuracy, limitations, and role of color duplex flow imaging in diagnosis. *Radiology* 1990;175:639–644.

15. Lensing AWA, Doris I, McGrath FP, et al. A comparison of compression ultrasound with color Doppler ultrasound for the diagnosis of symptomless postoperative deep vein thrombosis. *Arch Intern Med* 1997;157:765–768.

16. Davidson BL, Elliott CG, Lensing AWA. Low accuracy of color Doppler ultrasound in the detection of proximal leg vein thrombosis in asymptomatic high-risk patients. *Ann Intern Med* 1992;117:735–738.

17. Cronan JJ, Leen V. Recurrent deep venous thrombosis: limitations of ultrasound. *Radiology* 1989;170:739–742.

18. Screaton NJ, Gillard JH, Berman LH, et al. Duplicated superficial femoral veins: a source of error in the sonographic investigation of deep vein thrombosis. *Radiology* 1998;206:397–401.

19. Seabold JE, Salisbury SM, Edell SL, et al. Does heparin therapy affect the results of ^{99m}Tc-DMP 444 scintigraphy for detection of acute deep vein thrombosis (DVT)? *J Nucl Med* 1999;40:152P (abst).

20. Ezov N, Nimrod B, Parizada B, et al. Recombinant polypeptides derived from the fibrin binding domain of fibronectin are potential agents for the imaging of blood clots. *Thromb Haemost* 1997;77:796–803.

21. Rosenthal L, Leclerc J. A new thrombus imaging agent: human recombinant fibrin binding domain labeled with 111In. *Clin Nucl Med* 1995;20:398–402.

22. Taillefer R, Lambert R, Boucher L, et al. ^{99m}Tc-Fibrin binding domain of fibronectin (FBD): a new radiopharmaceutical for detection of acute deep vein thrombosis (preliminary study). *J Nucl Med* 1999;40:11P (abst).

23. Knight LC, Baidoo KE, Romano JE, et al. 99mTc-labeled bitistatin for imaging pulmonary emboli and deep venous thrombi. *J Nucl Med* 1999;40:122P (abst).

24. Pallela VR, Thakur ML, Consigny PM, et al. Imaging vascular thrombosis with ^{99m}Tc-labeled fibrin binding peptide. *J Nucl Med* 1999;40:121P (abst).

25. Cyr JE, Nelson CA, Pearson DA, et al. ^{99m}Tc. radiolabeling and biological evaluation of a new GP IIb/IIIa receptor binding agent, P424. *J Nucl Med* 1999;40:198P (abst).

26. Taillefer R, Thérasse E, Turpin S, et al. Comparison of early and delayed imaging with ^{99m}Tc-apcitide (^{99m}Tc-P280) in detection of acute deep venous thrombosis: correlation with contrast venogram. *J Nucl Med* 1999; 40:2028–2035.

27. Muto P, Lastoria S, Varella P, et al. Detection of deep venous thrombosis with ^{99m}Tc-labeled synthetic peptide P280. *J Nucl Med* 1995;36:1384–1391.

28. Weiland FL, Carretta RF, Holder LE, et al. Tc-99m P280 detection of deep venous thrombosis (DVT) in patients with a prior history of DVT. *J Nucl Med* 1997;38:98(abst).

29. Taillefer R, Abdel-Nabi HH, Buxton-Thomas M, et al. Multicenter clinical trial comparing Tc-99m P280 to contrast venography for detection and localization of acute deep venous thrombosis. *J Nucl Med* 1997;38:98(abst).

30. Weiland FL, Carretta RF, Holder FE, et al. Safety and efficacy of Tc-99m P280 for the detection and localization of acute deep venous thrombosis. *J Nucl Med* 1997;38:98(abst).

31. Taillefer R, Edell S, Innes G, et al. Acute thromboscintigraphy with ^{99m}Tc-apcitide: results of the phase 3 multicenter clinical trial comparing ^{99m}Tc-apcitide scintigraphy with contrast venography for imaging acute deep venous thrombosis. *J Nucl Med* 2000;41:1214–1223.

32. McLaughlin MSF, Thomson JG, Taylor DW, et al. Observer variation in the interpretation of lower limb venograms. *Am J Roentgenol* 1979;132:227–229.

33. Hull R, Hirsh J, Sackett DL, et al. Clinical validity of a negative venogram in patients with clinically suspected venous thrombosis. *Circulation* 1981;64:622–625.

34. Easton EJ. Acutect and pulmonary embolism. *J Nucl Med* 1999;40:11P(abst).

35. Ezekowitz MD, Pope CF, Sostman HD, et al. 111In platelet scintigraphy in the diagnosis of acute venous thrombosis. *Circulation* 1986;73:668–674.

36. Clark-Pearson DL, Coleman RE, Siegal R, et al. 111In platelet imaging for the detection of deep venous thrombosis and pulmonary embolism in patients without symptoms after surgery. *Surgery* 1985;98:98–104.

37. Thakur ML, Welch MJ, Joyst JH, et al. 111In labeled platelets: studies in preparation and evaluation of in vitro and in vivo functions. *Thromb Res* 1976;9:345–357.

38. Seabold JE, Conrad GR, Kimball DA, et al. Pitfalls in establishing the diagnosis of deep venous thrombosis by 111In platelet scintigraphy. *J Nucl Med* 1988;29:1169–1180.

39. Lister-James J, Knight LC, Maurer AH, et al. Thrombus imaging with a technetium-99m–labeled, activated platelet receptor-binding peptide. *J Nucl Med* 1996;37:775–781.

40. Nicolaides AN, Kakkar VV, Field ES, et al. The origin of deep vein thrombosis: a venographic study. *Br J Radiol* 1971;44:653–663.

41. Coleman RW, Cook JJ, Niewiarowski S. Mechanisms of platelet aggregation. In: Coleman RW, Hirsh J, Marder VJ, et al., eds. *Hemostasis and thrombosis: basic principles and clinical practice,* 3rd ed. Philadelphia: JB Lippincott, 1994:508–523.

42. Marguerie GA, Plow EF, Edgington TS. Human platelets possess an inducible and saturable receptor specific for fibrinogen. *J Biol Chem* 1979;254:357–363.

43. Freiman DG. The structure of thrombi. In: Coleman RW, Hirsh J, Marder VJ, et al. eds. *Hemostasis and thrombosis: basic principles and clinical practice.* Philadelphia: JB Lippincott, 1987:1123–1135.

Diagnostic Nuclear Medicine, Fourth Edition. Edited by M.P. Sandler, R.E. Coleman, J.A. Patton, F.J.Th. Wackers, A. Gottschalk. Lippincott Williams & Wilkins, Philadelphia 2003.

19

SCINTIGRAPHIC STUDIES OF NONEMBOLIC LUNG DISEASE

BRUCE R. LINE

Although the use of scintigraphy in the evaluation of nonembolic disease is much less frequent than in the evaluation of thromboembolism, the diagnostic and technical challenges in nonembolic disease are far greater for practitioners of nuclear medicine. Over the past decades, scintigraphic evaluation of pulmonary function, inflammation, infection, and metabolic disorders has been developed and applied clinically. The initial portion of the chapter discusses the functional, technical, metabolic, and molecular principles that underlie these scintigraphic studies. This introduction is followed by a review of the clinical experience gained from applying these scintigraphic studies to nonembolic lung disease.

SCINTIGRAPHIC METHODS OF LUNG FUNCTION ASSESSMENT

Scintigraphic Patterns of Pulmonary Dysfunction

Respiratory gas transfer occurs under optimum conditions when the rates of capillary perfusion and alveolar ventilation are nearly matched. With mismatch, the ability of the alveolar-capillary unit to maintain its function declines. Thus the presence of parenchymal disease can be detected through the presence of local abnormalities in the distribution of ventilation or perfusion. Normal scintigraphic studies of the lung demonstrate homogeneous patterns of matched ventilation and perfusion, a pattern that is disturbed in the presence of lung disease. For the sake of simplicity, the myriad of pathologic conditions affecting the lung can be divided into four functional categories: the vascular occlusive state and the consolidative, obstructive, and restrictive states (Fig. 19.1). Each of these pathophysiologic conditions is associated with scintigraphically detectable distortions of ventilation and perfusion.

Vascular occlusive conditions include those caused by pulmonary emboli, neoplastic vascular compression, or pulmonary vasculitis. Ventilation is unaffected because occlusion in the pulmonary arterial tree usually leaves alveoli structurally intact (Fig.

19.1A). Nonetheless, airway pneumoconstriction can be caused either by substances released from emboli or by a reduction in alveolar carbon dioxide, a potent airway dilator. This response usually is transient and is not commonly found in scintigraphic studies (1). In the absence of this effect, ventilation is preserved in regions of vascular occlusion; that is, a functional ventilation-perfusion mismatch occurs.

The consolidative state (Fig. 19.1B) exists when pulmonary infarction occurs with pulmonary embolism (2), as well as in many types of infection and inflammatory lung disease. With inadequate supplies of oxygen for alveolar metabolism, pulmonary surfactant production can be inhibited, and alveolar collapse and atelectasis occur. Injury to the capillary bed increases capillary permeability, and leakage of intravascular fluid into the alveolar space worsens the abnormalities. Although the degree of ventilation or perfusion loss can vary, both usually are markedly reduced.

The obstructive state (Fig. 19.1C) exists in chronic lung diseases, such as emphysema, bronchitis, or bronchiectasis, and in acute asthmatic exacerbation. Destructive loss of alveolar walls and the capillary bed in emphysema increases alveolar volume and decreases the surface area for gas exchange. Partial airway obstruction can be caused by either loss of structural support or excessive bronchial secretions, bronchospasm, or foreign bodies, all of which increase resistance to airflow and decrease alveolar oxygen tension. The precapillary sphincters respond to alveolar hypoxia by constricting, thereby protecting the patient from large shunts of unoxygenated blood. This state is associated with increased regional lung volumes, reduced ventilation, and matched perfusion abnormalities. Reduced perfusion results from either loss of capillary bed or hypoxic vasoconstriction (Fig. 19.2).

The morphologic features of restrictive lung disease (Fig. 19.1D) are caused by chronic inflammation and fibrosis, which may eventually obliterate alveoli. Fibrotic alveolar stiffening, however, helps to keep the airways from collapsing. Because secretions are not excessive in this state, ventilation can be preserved or even increased through decreases in alveolar compliance. Because capillaries become entrapped by thickened and inflamed alveolar walls, regional ventilation usually is increased relative to perfusion (3).

B.R. Line: Diagnostic Radiology, Division of Nuclear Medicine, University of Maryland Medicine, Baltimore, MD.

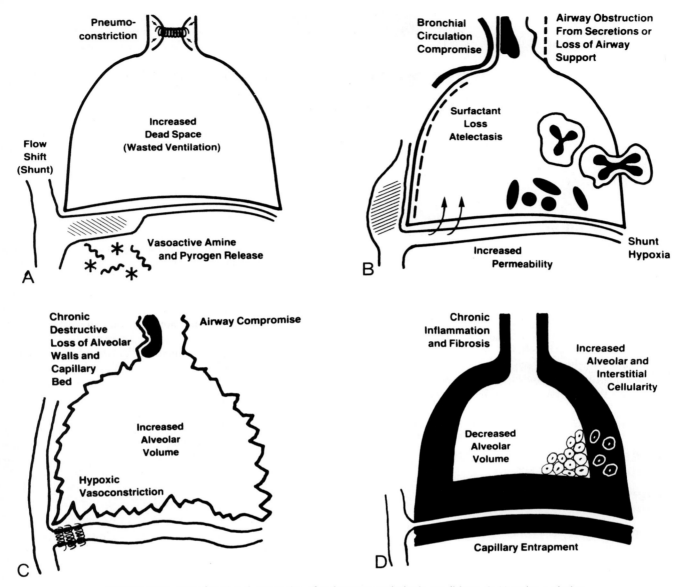

FIGURE 19.1. Four functional categories of pulmonary pathologic conditions. **A:** Vascular occlusive disease, here represented by pulmonary embolism, produces mechanical obstruction to blood flow and increased ventilatory dead space. **B:** Consolidative disease, caused either by pulmonary infection or by embolic infarction. In rare instances, bronchoconstriction occurs. **C:** Obstructive disease as found in pulmonary emphysema associated with increased lung volume, reduced ventilation, and perfusion abnormalities from loss of capillary bed or hypoxic vasoconstriction. **D:** Restrictive disease characterized by capillary entrapment and reduced alveolar volume secondary to chronic inflammation and fibrosis.

Ventilation-Perfusion Scans in Assessment of Regional Function

Physiologic Factors Affecting Lung Images

Perfusion Images

Pulmonary blood flow increases toward the bottom of the upright lung. Its gradient of change is determined by the relations between alveolar, capillary arterial, and capillary venous pressure (4). The upright lung can be divided into four contiguous physiologic zones (Fig. 19.3), beginning with the most apical (zone 1) and progressing to the most basal (zone 4). In zone 1, there is little blood flow because the alveolar pressure in the apex exceeds both capillary arterial and venous pressure. Slightly lower, in zone 2, capillary arterial pressure gradually increases above the alveolar pressure, and blood flow increases in proportion to the difference. Lower still, in zone 3, both capillary arterial and venous pressure are greater than alveolar pressure, causing full distention of the capillary. Here flow depends on the difference between the arterial and venous pressure alone. At the bottom of the lung, in zone 4, flow can be reduced by compression of the lung from abdominal viscera or perivascular fluid.

Gravitational effects on the lung cause the apex to base perfu-

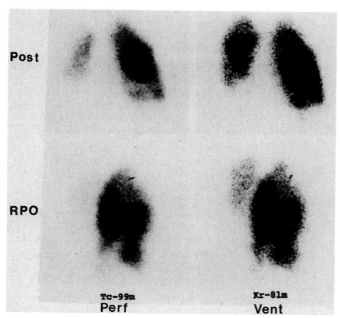

FIGURE 19.2. Obstructive airway disease. Selected ^{99m}Tc perfusion (*Perf*) and ^{81m}Kr ventilation (*Vent*) images illustrate the pattern of matching the ventilation and perfusion abnormalities present in obstructive airway disease. ^{81m}Kr studies show the regional distribution of tidal ventilation. In patients with airway disease, ^{81m}Kr images often reveal distributions of activity almost identical to those seen in the same perfusion view. Such close similarity is illustrated in the case of this patient, who had obstructive airway disease. The likelihood for such similarity is enhanced by the fact that the ^{81m}Kr image is obtained immediately after each perfusion image by having the patient inhale ^{81m}Kr in the same position in which the perfusion view was obtained (without moving the patient). *Post*, posterior; *RPO*, right posterior oblique.

sion gradient to be nearly homogeneous horizontally. Although nearly every disease affecting the lung disturbs regional perfusion, healthy persons have homogeneous blood flow patterns well into middle age. Fedullo et al. (5) found it very uncommon for either smokers or nonsmokers between 30 and 49 years of age to have abnormal perfusion scans.

Ventilation Images

The distribution of ventilation is altered by abnormal airway resistance or abnormal alveolar compliance. These abnormalities are important scintigraphically, because they determine the local rates of arrival or elimination of gases such as xenon or krypton as well as the extent of aerosol deposition (Fig. 19.4). For example, the regional clearance time of xenon is roughly proportional to the product of local compliance and airway resistance.

Compliance is expressed as the ratio of the change in lung volume to a change in distending pressure. Alveoli with low compliance due to stiffening by interstitial fluid or fibrosis have a small volume and exchange a large fraction of their volume with each respiration. Alveoli with increased compliance, as found in chronic obstructive pulmonary disease, usually have reduced wall integrity. They are larger than normal for a given transpulmonary pressure and exchange a smaller fraction of their internal volume during respiration. This fractional exchange (flow per unit alveolar volume) is an important physiologic determinant of oxygen–carbon dioxide exchanging capability and affects the rate of tracer arrival and clearance in ventilation images.

Regional airway resistance is the second major factor determining the distribution of lung ventilation. For a given change in inflation pressure, gas flow is inversely related to airway resistance (the higher the resistance, the lower is the flow). Increased airway resistance can be caused by any process that reduces airway diameter. Increased airway secretions, bronchospasm, the

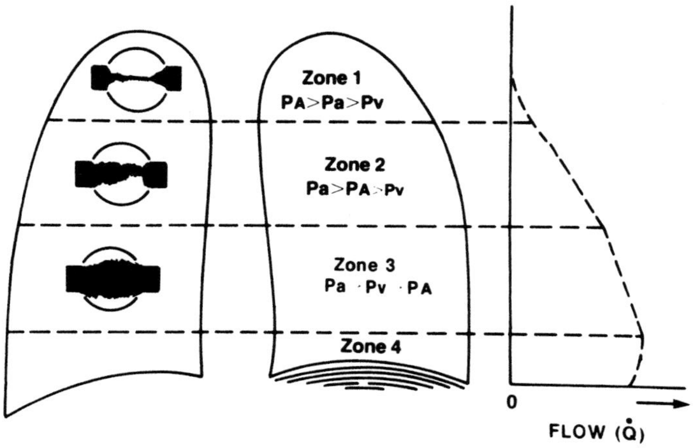

FIGURE 19.3. Effect of gravitational gradients on the distribution of pulmonary perfusion. Zones of perfusion in upright patients. The gradient of perfusion is determined by the relations between alveolar, arterial capillary, and venous capillary pressures.

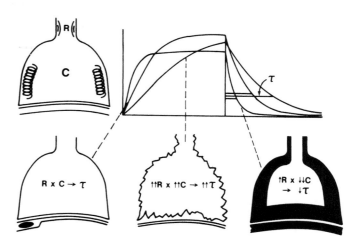

FIGURE 19.4. Morphologic factors affecting clearance time. The product of regional airway resistance (*R*) and alveolar compliance (*C*) is the clearance rate (τ). The normal or vascular occlusive states are characterized by normal xenon washout kinetics. In the obstructive state, however, the resistance and compliance of the alveolus increase owing to damage to the alveolar wall. This increases the time required for xenon clearance. In the restrictive state, the resistance of the airway increased slightly, but the overwhelming decrease in compliance due to alveolar stiffening causes the clearance time to decrease.

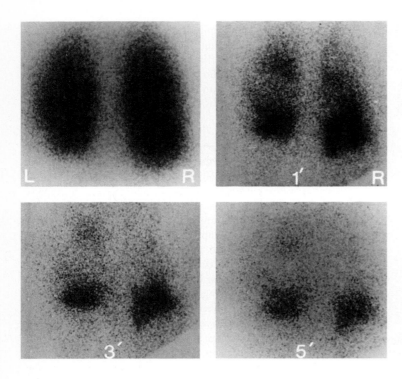

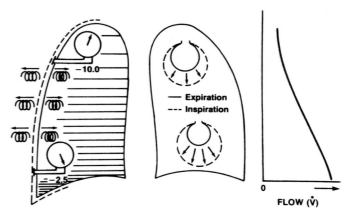

FIGURE 19.5. Xenon clearance in obstructive airway disease. Posterior wash-in (*top left*) and sequential (1-minute, 3-minute, and 5-minute) washout ^{133}Xe images of a patient with obstructive airway disease. In patients with obstructive airway disease, the clearance of xenon is slow and inhomogeneous. The inhomogeneity of clearance is the most reliable hallmark of obstructive airway disease because changes in minute ventilation and other variables affect overall clearance times more than the regional pattern of clearance does.

presence of foreign bodies, extrinsic airway compression, parenchymal strictures, and loss of supporting lung tissue that normally keeps the airway patent all can increase resistance to airflow.

The combined influences of regional compliance and resistance together affect the rate of tracer localization and removal. The product of the resistance and the compliance of a region is the time constant of the region. This time constant, or clearance time, is simply the time needed to exchange the volume of gas in the region once. It also is equal to 1.44 times the effective tracer half-life in the region. Time constants of 200 seconds or longer are common in regions of severe obstructive airway disease where both the airway resistance and alveolar compliance are increased because of damage to the alveolar wall. This increases the time required for gas turnover or tracer clearance (Fig. 19.5). In the restrictive state, the resistance of the airway is slightly increased, but the overwhelming decrease in compliance due to alveolar stiffening causes the clearance time to decrease. The normal or vascular occlusive states are characterized by normal airflow kinetics.

Regional ventilation normally increases gradually toward the bottom of the lung, following the influence of the intrapleural pressure gradient (Fig. 19.6). This gradient is formed by three factors: (a) the outward pull of the chest wall, (b) the opposing inward pull of the lung, and (c) the weight of the lung. Intrapleural pressure is most negative at the top of the lung and least negative at the bottom, where the weight of the lung is the greatest. Because alveoli at the top of the lung experience a greater distending pressure, they are larger at end-expiration than are those at the bottom of the lung. Therefore, the alveoli at the top of the lung fill to a lesser extent during inspiration than do those at the bottom. This causes ventilatory flow to increase

toward the lung base in a smooth pattern that is horizontally homogeneous. However, ventilatory flow no longer is homogeneous where the morphologic features of the alveoli are changed by alveolar disease.

Patient positioning has an important effect on the distribution of pulmonary function. In the upright position, intrapleural pressure becomes progressively more subatmospheric from the lung base (approximately −2.5 cm water), where the lung is compressed by its own weight, to the apex (−10 cm water), where the weight lung tends to pull the lung down and away from the parietal pleural surface. This apical negative pressure stretches the alveoli outward, making them larger and less compliant. These alveoli ventilate inefficiently compared with the

FIGURE 19.6. Gravity-induced gradient of ventilation in upright patients. Regional ventilation increases gradually toward the bottom of the lung following the influence of the intrapleural pressure gradient.

less distended alveoli in the lung base. These regional differences can be altered by means of changing the position of the patient. In healthy upright patients, the bases ventilate better than do the apices, but in the lateral decubitus position, the lower lung shows greater ventilation per unit volume than does the upper lung. When a patient is examined in the supine position, there is little apex-to-base gradient in alveolar size, but there is an anterior-posterior lung gradient, the lowermost alveoli being less distended and ventilating more efficiently.

Ventilation-perfusion mismatch occurs physiologically because capillary perfusion tends to be greater than the alveolar ventilation in dependent lung zones, and it decreases more rapidly than does ventilation toward the top of the lung. In the upright lung, for example, the V/Q ratio approximates values of 0.5 to 1 in the lower lobes and increases to approximately 3.5 in the apical zones. Because the gradients of these two flow rates tend to change smoothly and are homogeneous along horizontal planes, the V/Q ratio increases smoothly toward the top of the lung. Thus, as with ventilatory or perfusion distributions, pulmonary dysfunction is reflected by regionally inhomogeneous V/Q ratios.

Xenon Ventilation Studies

In a typical ^{133}Xe ventilation study, the patient is positioned with his or her back to the gamma camera. The patient inhales from a closed-loop lead-shielded delivery system that contains 400 to 800 MBq xenon and a carbon dioxide absorber. The patient initially breathes room air until comfortable with the device. Care is taken to ensure that there are no loose tubing connections or avenues of gas escape at the system-patient interface. Once xenon rebreathing is begun, an initial "first breath" image of 50,000 counts is obtained. Although some patients with obstructive airway disease do not reach equilibrium, 5-minute xenon rebreathing (wash-in phase) allows regions with time constants of 100 seconds or less to achieve at least 95% of the equilibrium value (6). During the wash-in, two 400,000-count equilibrium images are obtained. The patient then begins to breathe room air (washout phase). The room air is inhaled and expired into an exhaust system or through a charcoal trap. During washout, a sequence of 50,000-count images is obtained, each 30 to 60 seconds for a total of 5 to 8 minutes. Collection of washout images for a preset count ensures that the intensity of the images is proper and that regions with mild to moderate clearance abnormalities are evident in the later washout frames.

Ventilation compromise manifests as slow xenon clearance. Prolonged retention of xenon (beyond the third minute of washout) suggests obstructive airway disease. There is no absolute normal range of clearance times because the time required to clear a region of lung depends on the local lung volume and airflow. For example, increasing airflow by means of a change in either rate or depth of respiration decreases pulmonary clearance time (Fig. 19.7). Although it may be difficult to pick a clearance time that differentiates normal and abnormal regions, the normal lung appears homogeneous horizontally in regional volume, ventilation, and xenon clearance rate. Thus inhomogeneity of lung clearance during xenon washout is an indicator of dysfunctional lung (Fig. 19.5). The degree of ventilatory func-

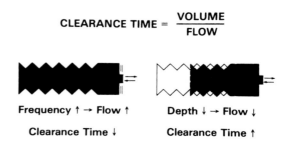

FIGURE 19.7. Patient factors affecting clearance time estimates. Clearance time is related to regional volume and flow rates and can be modified with changes in frequency or depth of respiration. For example, increasing airflow by means of changes in rate or depth of respiration decreases pulmonary clearance time.

tional abnormality in a lung region can be estimated from its clearance time constant with a modified Stewart-Hamilton equation (6,7) (Fig. 19.8). A clearance time can be estimated for each image pixel and assembled into an image of regional clearance time (Fig. 19.9). Patients with ventilatory dysfunction have wide distributions of clearance time with higher intensities in the clearance time image in regions associated with reduced airflow. The ventilation image can be used to assess the effect of clearance time abnormalities on regional tidal airflow and can

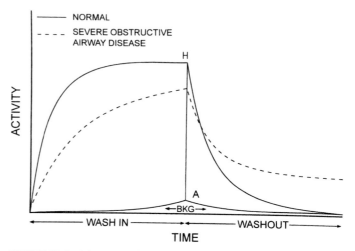

FIGURE 19.8. Schematics show xenon time versus activity curves from lung regions with theoretically normal and abnormal ventilation. Regions of normal ventilation (*solid lines*) are characterized by an exponential increase in activity during wash-in that eventually plateaus when equilibrium is reached (when the amount of activity entering the region with each breath is the same as that leaving the region). This is the height (*H*) in the diagram. During normal washout, a rapid, exponential decline in activity becomes somewhat slower during the later phases of clearance. Regional clearance can be quantified by means of dividing the counts at *H* by the area (*A*) under the washout curve. In patients with disease (*dashed lines*), the rate of increase in activity during wash-in is slower, and equilibrium is not reached by the time washout begins. Washout is slower, and the area under the washout curve is greater. Because the *H* reached at the end of the time allowed for wash-in is lower and the *A* is greater, the calculation of *H/A* indicates that regional air exchange is lower. If a patient with abnormal regions were allowed to continue breathing for many minutes, the regions may eventually come to equilibrium, but the radiation dose to the patient would be greatly increased. Therefore wash-in sequences usually are terminated after 3 to 5 minutes of breathing.

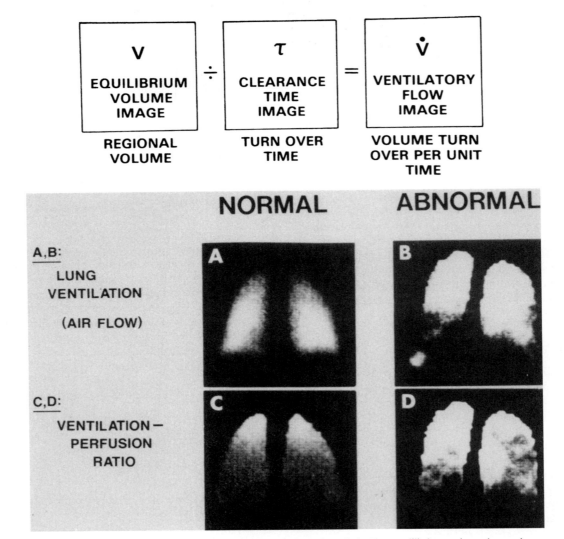

FIGURE 19.9. A: Regional clearance time and ventilation analysis. The equilibrium volume image is combined with the clearance time image to obtain the ventilation flow image, that is, the volume turnover per unit time. **B:** Functional images of lung ventilation and ventilation-perfusion ratios. The patient with normal findings shows the typical increase of V/Q ratios in the apices and an even decrease in the V/Q ratios through the lung bases. The patient with abnormal findings had pulmonary fibrosis and several areas of elevated V/Q ratios (*bright areas* on the functional images). These areas indicate regions where ventilation exceeds perfusion by an abnormal amount (areas of so-called dead-space ventilation). In the lung bases and midzones, of the patient with abnormal findings, the dark areas indicate regions of low V/Q ratios (areas with V/Q ratios much less than 1.0). These zones represents regions of so-called intrapulmonary shunting. (From Alderson PO, Line BR. Scintigraphic evaluation of regional pulmonary ventilation. *Semin Nucl Med* 1980;10:218–242, with permission.)

be compared directly with the static perfusion scan to evaluate regional V/Q matching (Fig. 19.9). The computed V/Q values are very crude estimates of the physiologic condition of the alveoli. They reflect the macroscopic V/Q relations from poorly defined cylinders of lung perpendicular to the camera face. Nonetheless, they can be used to assess ventilation-to-perfusion matching and provide information useful in evaluating the relative function of various portions of the lung.

Krypton Ventilation Studies

[81m]Kr is a relatively insoluble inert gas with a 13-second half-life. It decays to [81]Kr by isomeric transition, emitting 190-keV γ-rays (65%) and internal conversion electrons. The gas is obtained by means of elution of a generator that contains its 4.7-hour half-life parent [81]Rb. During [81m]Kr ventilation studies, patients breathe at their own rate from a reservoir that stores the [81m]Kr being eluted from the generator. The higher photon voltage of [81m]Kr allows [81m]Kr ventilation studies to follow ^{99m}Tc macroaggregated albumin perfusion scans. Given its short, 13.4-second half-life, [81m]Kr can be administered intermittently, so that ventilation images can be interdigitated with each of the six- to eight-view perfusion study images (Fig. 19.2). [81m]Kr studies can be easily performed on infants, children, uncooperative patients, or patients receiving mechanical ventilation. The rapid

disappearance of the tracer from the lungs also allows ventilation studies to be performed before and after medications are given or exercise is undertaken. The gas does not require expensive delivery systems, room monitors, ventilation ducts, fans, or charcoal traps. Its low dosimetric requirements and absence of gas waste disposal problems make ^{81m}Kr an attractive alternative to ^{133}Xe. Perhaps most important, the static distribution of ^{81m}Kr reflects the pattern of lung ventilation ($\dot{V}$). It is therefore directly comparable with the distribution of ^{99m}Tc microaggregated albumin perfusion ($\dot{Q}$) in evaluation of the regional ventilation-perfusion ratio ($\dot{V}/\dot{Q}$) (8–10).

Static ^{81m}Kr images reflect ventilation because of the mechanics of respiration and bulk airflow in the lung airways. Beyond the gases in the dead space, a significant fraction of the molecules inhaled into the alveoli with each breath are exhaled. This means that the radioactive species of ^{81m}Kr is primarily concentrated in the dead space, in the terminal conducting airways, and in the proximal respiratory zone. The molecules that occupy the more distal alveolar regions (90% of lung volume) have a much longer residence and a correspondingly lower specific activity. Hence the total count rate in the static ^{81m}Kr lung image is caused predominantly by ^{81m}Kr in the tidal volume. The faster the tidal volume is refreshed, the higher is its mean activity, and the higher is the lung image intensity.

Experimental evidence suggests that ^{81m}Kr does a good job reflecting $\dot{V}$ at all flow rates, even at the ventilatory turnover rates that occur among infants and children (11). On the basis of results of gated lung studies of ^{81m}Kr distributions over a range of respiratory frequencies, tidal volumes and alveolar turnover rates, Modell and Graham (11) found that both end-expiration and end-inspiration activities were linearly related to $\dot{V}$ for ventilatory turnover rates up to and exceeding 10 per minute.

Radioaerosol Inhalation Studies

Radioaerosols are very small droplets deposited in the lung by means of impaction in the central airways, sedimentation in more distal airways, and random contact with alveolar walls during diffusion in the air sacs (12). Radioaerosols have become widely used as a means for investigating regional ventilation, largely because of the introduction of small and efficient aerosol nebulizers. Nebulizers produce submicron aerosols that penetrate to the lung periphery, except where there is excessive airway turbulence from rapid, shallow breathing or partial airway obstruction. In these circumstances, there may be substantial degrees of central lung deposition that can lead to poor images of peripheral ventilation.

The radioaerosol most commonly used is ^{99m}Tc diethylenetriaminepentaacetic acid (DTPA), in part because of its rapid renal clearance. DTPA is a small, water-soluble chelate that is chemically inert and clears the lung through the alveolar-capillary membrane (13). Because of the low amounts deposited in the lung and the short pulmonary half-time (55 minutes) the radiation dose to patients from preperfusion DTPA aerosol scintigraphy is lower than that of either ^{81m}Kr or ^{133}Xe studies.

^{99m}Tc aerosol studies (Fig. 19.10) have proved a satisfactory alternative to ^{81m}Kr studies in the setting of pulmonary embolism screening (14) but are less accurate than ^{81m}Kr studies in defining regional ventilation (15). Aerosol activity usually is absent or diminished in areas of obstructive airway disease. Airway deposition patterns (central hotspots) are found in areas of nonlaminar airflow or turbulence because of mucous secretions, airway narrowing, or collapse. For example, aerosols accumulate at sites of obstructive bronchospasm, such as those present in active asthma. Aerosols are not commonly used to study regional ventilation associated with nonembolic lung disease because of the relatively nonlinear relation between ventilation, flow rate, and aerosol deposition.

Technegas and Pertechnegas are two other aerosolized forms of ^{99m}Tc. Technetium generator eluate that has been heated in a graphite crucible at 2,500°C in 100% argon produces ultrafine dispersion of hexagonal platelets of metallic technetium, each closely encapsulated with a thin layer of graphitic carbon (16, 17). Pertechnegas is generated under an atmosphere of 3% oxygen mixed in argon and does not appear to be encapsulated by carbon (18). Particle sizes are 100 to 200 nm and adhere to the walls of the alveoli on inhalation. These forms of ^{99m}Tc are much smaller than aerosols of ^{99m}Tc DTPA (~2 μm) and are closer to uniform size. They more closely approximate gas than does DTPA aerosol and penetrate farther into the lung. The predicted lung deposition is 37% in the alveolar region and 5% in the bronchial region (19).

Once inhaled, Technegas remains in the lungs for a long time, whereas Pertechnegas rapidly disappears. This difference in epithelial clearance after inhalation has been attributed to the presence of the carbon encapsulation of Technegas (18).

Assessment of Alveolar–Capillary Membrane Permeability

The primary use of radioaerosols in the evaluation of nonembolic lung disease is assessment of alveolar–capillary membrane permeability (20–22). The rate of aerosol clearance from the lung is accelerated in the presence of epithelial alveolar injury (Fig. 19.11). Furthermore, pulmonary capillary protein leaks can be evaluated by means of serial determination of the lung-heart radioactivity ratio (23,24).

The alveolar epithelium and capillary endothelium normally are separated by the connective tissue of the interstitial space. DTPA clearance is modulated primarily by alveolar epithelial permeability because the alveolar epithelium is the chief barrier to diffusion of solutes between the alveolar surface and the pulmonary capillaries (22). Several factors, however, influence the rate at which solutes leave the lung. One of the most important is determined by the site of aerosol deposition. Relatively rapid clearance occurs by means of transepithelial absorption if the aerosol lands on small airways or alveolar surfaces. Much slower clearance by mucociliary transport removes aerosol impacting on large airways. Where the aerosol lands is determined by regional airflow, by aerosol particle size, and by the rate and depth of ventilation. Larger aerosols have greater inertia and are more likely to impact on proximal airway walls. The submicron-sized aerosols used clinically are deposited primarily in small airways

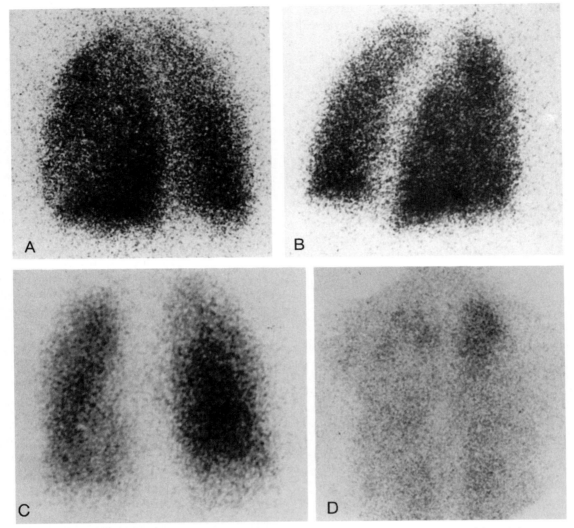

FIGURE 19.10. Radioaerosol detection of regional airway abnormality. Left **(A)** and right **(B)** posterior oblique ⁹⁹ᵐTc DTPA aerosol images and a ¹³³Xe study with a single-breath **(C)** and a 3-minute washout image **(D)**. Mild ¹³³Xe retention is present in both upper lobes. These mild airway abnormalities are detected as small deficits of aerosol deposition in the posterior aspects of both upper lobes **(A, B)**. Radioaerosol studies are nearly as sensitive as ¹³³Xe washout studies in detecting airway disease, and regions with especially mild airway abnormalities detected only with ¹³³Xe usually are associated with small or absent perfusion abnormalities. (From Alderson PO, Biello DR, Gottschalk A, et al: Comparison of ⁹⁹ᵐTc DTPA aerosol and radioactive gases as adjuncts to perfusion scintigraphy in patients with suspected pulmonary embolism. *Radiology* 153:515—521, 1984, with permission.)

and alveoli (80% or more). Maximum peripheral deposition occurs during quiet breathing, whereas rapid inhalation causes turbulent flow and more central deposition at airway bifurcations (Fig. 19.12). Although DTPA is removed from the lung by the pulmonary circulation, increasing pulmonary blood flow does not markedly increase DTPA clearance (25) because DTPA diffusion is slow in comparison with blood flow. The rate of diffusion is directly dependent on both the permeability of the epithelial wall and the surface area available for diffusional transfer. For example, exercise increases pulmonary clearance (26), probably through recruitment of the pulmonary microvascular bed and unfolding of alveolar septa. These factors increase the surface area for diffusion. Pulmonary clearance of DTPA has been found to increase during rapid, shallow ventilation with increased positive end-expiratory pressure (27). Egan et al. (28) showed that the alveolar epithelium becomes more permeable as inflation volume increases. The mechanism for the increase in DTPA clearance at a high lung volume may be the result of increased surface area for diffusion-increased permeability of the epithelium or changes in the functional integrity of the alveolar surfactant layer (29). Another determinant of solute transfer across the alveolar epithelial barrier relates to the size of the tracer molecule. As a first approximation, the rate of diffusion of a small molecule is inversely proportional to the square root of its molecular weight; the smaller the molecule, the faster it diffuses.

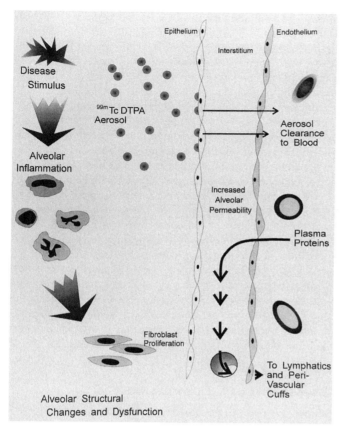

FIGURE 19.11. Clearance of ^{99m}Tc DTPA aerosol. Submicron-sized ^{99m}Tc-labeled aerosols enter the alveolus and settle onto the epithelial surface. The rate at which solutes pass into the interstitium and then into the blood depends on the alveolar epithelial wall integrity. Diffuse lung diseases that cause alveolar inflammation and loss of epithelial integrity result in increased clearance of aerosol. The epithelium is normally less permeable than is the endothelium. Plasma proteins that leave the lung capillaries normally do not enter the alveoli but pass down the interstitial space to the lymphatic vessels and perivascular cuff. (From Line BR. Scintigraphic studies of inflammation in diffuse lung disease. *Radiol Clin North Am* 1991;29:1095–1114, with permission.)

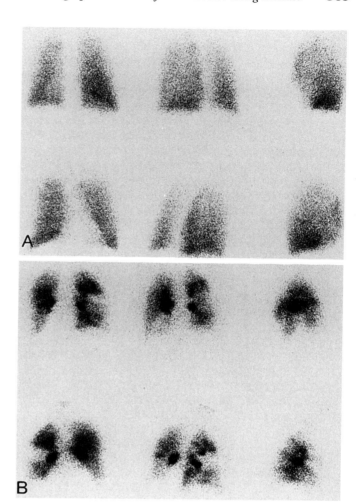

FIGURE 19.12. ^{99m}Tc DTPA aerosol pulmonary deposition patterns related in part to respiratory rate and tidal volume. **A:** Normal six-view ^{99m}Tc DTPA aerosol deposition pattern in a 59-year-old man who did not smoke and who had radiographically normal lungs. **B:** Images of a 26-year-old man with AIDS who had a normal ^{67}Ga scan 3 weeks earlier and a normal chest radiograph at the time of the radionuclide study. He was breathing rapidly and had a small tidal volume during administration of the aerosol. The irregular peripheral distribution and intense central foci are most likely sites of highly turbulent flow at airway bifurcations. (From Line BR. Scintigraphic studies of inflammation in diffuse lung disease. *Radiol Clin North Am* 1991;29:1095–1114, with permission.)

Because of its rapid disappearance from the lungs, Pertechnegas has been suggested as useful in measuring pulmonary epithelial permeability. Fanti et al. (30) conducted a study with nonsmokers who had no evidence of pulmonary disease. The investigators found a homogeneous distribution in the lungs and rapid Pertechnegas clearance through the alveolar-capillary barrier. Others investigators, however, have found that the disappearance from the lungs of inhaled Pertechnegas is similar to that of inhaled pertechnetate aerosol (TcO$_4$). Results of neither Pertechnegas nor TcO$_4$ inhalation studies can help differentiate smokers from nonsmokers according to clearance half-times (31).

Procedure to Determine Aerosol Clearance

To measure the pulmonary clearance rate of DTPA aerosol, the aerosol is breathed quietly for 1 to 2 minutes. Submicron-sized aerosols are generated with commercially available jet nebulizers

loaded with 30 to 50 mCi of ^{99m}Tc DTPA in 2 mL of saline solution. The nebulizer is driven by a compressed oxygen tank that delivers a flow rate of 10 L/minute (29). Although a dose of 30 to 50 mCi of ^{99m}Tc DTPA is administered as an aerosol, only 2 mCi of radionuclide typically is retained in the lungs. At this level, the lungs receive between 2 and 8 mrad; the average radiation exposure to the whole body is approximately 40 mrad (21).

The rate of pulmonary ^{99m}Tc DTPA clearance can be measured with either a sodium iodide probe or gamma camera. Care must be taken to properly prepare the patient for measurement. The patient should avoid deep breathing or vital capacity maneuvers before and during aerosol administration and scanning. The more rapid curvilinear clearance produced by several deep breaths may be caused by transiently increased epithelial permeability or reduced volume of liquid in the alveoli in some lung regions. Resting for 20 minutes before inhaling the aerosol of ^{99m}Tc DTPA is recommended to avoid alterations in clearance rates from deep breathing (32). During the first 30 minutes, the normal ^{99m}Tc DTPA pulmonary clearance curve can be modeled as a single compartment that empties exponentially with a mean half-time of 86 ± 26 minutes (29). Multicompartmental curves can occur when there are two or more populations of alveoli, one having significantly greater clearance than the others. Increased pulmonary aerosol clearance rates have been reported in a variety of diffuse lung diseases such as interstitial fibrotic disorders (21), adult respiratory distress syndrome (ARDS) (33), or opportunistic infections related to acquired immunodeficiency syndrome (AIDS) (34). Smoking of tobacco or physiologic factors such as inspiratory lung volume, posture, and exercise also influence epithelial lung clearance.

As a determinant of lung injury, there is much to recommend ^{99m}Tc DTPA studies with regard to ease of performance and noninvasiveness. The tracer is inexpensive, widely available, and associated with low radiation exposure of the patient. The ^{99m}Tc DTPA study can be completed within 1 hour. Furthermore, examinations the same radiopharmaceutical agent can provide information on regional ventilation and mucociliary clearance rates. However, there are several reasons why ^{99m}Tc DTPA clearance studies are not used widely as a means to assess lung injury. As experience with this method has increased, it has been criticized as being too nonspecific to be a clinically useful indicator of acute lung injury. For example, equivalent increases in ^{99m}Tc DTPA clearance have been reported in healthy persons breathing at high lung volumes and in patients with ARDS (33). There are enormous diagnostic, therapeutic, and prognostic differences between these conditions that are not reflected in DTPA clearance (35). In part, this lack of specificity can be related to the small size, and hence excessive sensitivity, of the DTPA molecule to changes in the alveolar epithelium. For example, clearance of ^{99m}Tc DTPA and that of ^{99m}Tc human serum albumin (HSA) both are equally affected by positive end-expiratory pressure and lung injury (36), but aerosols of ^{99m}Tc HSA have a clearance unchanged by lung inflation. Furthermore, deposition of ^{99m}Tc HSA within 15 minutes of administration of oleic acid increases the clearance rate of ^{99m}Tc HSA to an extent that correlates well with postmortem lung water volume. It is possible that in the future, non-DTPA aerosols may be used in procedures that are simple and noninvasive, have a low radiation dose, and provide a way to assess lung injury rapidly in diffuse lung diseases.

Assessment of Mucociliary Clearance

^{99m}Tc-radiolabelled macroaggregated albumin and sulfur colloid are inert and nonpermeable substances that can be delivered to the tracheobronchial surfaces as aerosols and used noninvasively to determine mucociliary clearance rates. During imaging studies spanning 60 to 120 minutes, subjects are asked to refrain from coughing and maintain a normal pattern of breathing. Clearance of the aerosolized particulates are assessed visually and by means of quantitative curve fitting. Time versus activity curves obtained over each lung are fit to two-compartment models to determine

the fast and slow components of the clearance process. The half-time of the fast compartment is used as a measure of mucociliary clearance (37). Using this approach, Pifferi et al. (38) demonstrated that patients with primary ciliary dyskinesia do not have increased clearance rates in response to local inflammation the way healthy persons do.

Mucociliary transport depends on several factors. The most important are ciliary activity, production of mucus, and differential airflow. Mucociliary impairment may be a reflection of airway inflammation, chronic obstructive pulmonary disease, or exacerbation of asthma. Even persons with asthma whose condition is stable have impaired mucociliary clearance compared with healthy persons (39). Reduced mucociliary clearance also can be demonstrated in patients who have undergone bronchial surgery, tracheobronchoplasty, or pulmonary irradiation (37,40).

Unfortunately, a number of practical difficulties have limited application of this technology to the research laboratory. To meaningfully compare mucociliary clearance on serial occasions, it is necessary to ensure similar initial deposition patterns. The closer to central the deposition pattern, the more rapidly are the deposited particles cleared because of the shorter path of these particles to the pharynx. Changing breathing patterns also complicate assessment of changes in mucociliary clearance.

Assessment of Inflammation

Inflammation, Injury, and ^{67}Ga Uptake in the Lung

In most diffuse lung diseases, injury is associated with inflammatory infiltration of the alveolar and interstitial spaces. Acute inflammation is primarily exudative. It is characterized by vasodilatation, increased vascular permeability, and emigration of polymorphonuclear leukocytes. Chronic inflammation is characterized by a predominantly mononuclear cell infiltrate (macrophages, lymphocytes, and plasma cells) and by a fibroblastic proliferative response that usually leads to parenchymal derangement and pulmonary dysfunction.

In many of the diffuse lung diseases (Table 19.1), ^{67}Ga scintigraphy is useful in evaluating the presence and extent of acute and chronic pulmonary inflammation. Whereas normal lung accumulates little ^{67}Ga, the isotope localizes in the pulmonary parenchyma of patients who have alveolitis. Using techniques for evaluation of the amount of localization, several investigators have suggested that the quantity and intensity of gallium uptake reflect the degree of inflammatory change in the lung. Others assert that gallium scintigraphy is helpful for identifying subclinical disease and for evaluating the response to treatment (41, 42).

There are important assumptions implicit in the use of ^{67}Ga scanning to stage the alveolitis of diffuse lung disease. First, it is assumed that ^{67}Ga is localized by a mechanism related to inflammation and the process of lung injury (Fig. 19.13). It is assumed that the amount of gallium localized in the lung is proportional to the degree of pulmonary injury. Finally, for localization to be of clinical significance it is assumed that the associated lung injury causes permanent dysfunction if the patient is not treated. It is unlikely that these assumptions are valid

Table 19.1. *Diffuse Nonmalignant Lung Diseases Showing* ^{67}*Ga Lung Uptake*

Infections
  Tuberculosis
  Atypical mycobacterial infection
  Pneumocystis carinii pneumonia
  Cytomegalovirus infection
  Actinomycosis
  Cryptococcal infection
  Aspergillosis
  Blastmycosis
  Filariasis
Drug reactions
  Amiodarone
  Bleomycin
  Busulfan
  Cyclophosphamide
  Methotrexate
  Nitrofurantoin
  Procarbazine
  Vincristine
Disorders of unknown origin
  Sarcoidosis
  Idiopathic pulmonary fibrosis
  Histiocytosis X
  Progressive systemic sclerosis
  Polymyosistis-dermatomyositis
  Mixed connective tissue disease
  Systemic lupus erythematosus
  Rheumatoid arthritis
  Lymphocytic interstitial pneumonitis
  Lymphomatoid granulomatosis
  Wegener granulomatosis
Organic and inorganic dusts
  Coal workers pneumoconiosis
  Silicosis
  Asbestosis
  Berylliosis
  Talc granulomatosis
Miscellaneous injuries
  Adult respiratory distress syndrome
  Postcardiopulmonary pump syndrome
  Radiation (direct or scatter)

From Line BR. Scintigraphic studies of inflammation in diffuse lung disease. *Radiol Clin North Am* 1991;29:1095–1114, with permission.

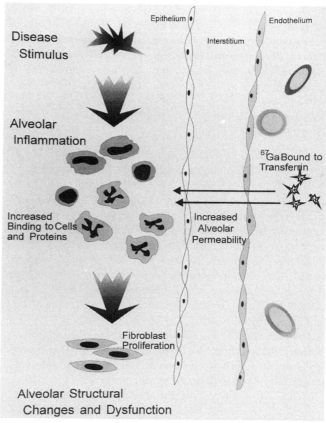

FIGURE 19.13. Possible factors influencing ^{67}Ga uptake. When a disease stimulus leads to alveolar inflammation, populations of activated alveolar effector cells release substances that increase alveolar permeability. The serum protein transferrin, which carries ^{67}Ga, leaks into the interstitial and alveolar spaces, where the isotope becomes localized by cells or other alveolar protein substances. ^{67}Ga does not localize in lung fibroblasts and does not reflect the degree of alveolar dysfunction caused by structural changes in the alveoli. (From Line BR. Scintigraphic studies of inflammation in diffuse lung disease. *Radiol Clin North Am* 1991;29:1095–1114, with permission.)

for all diffuse lung diseases, but for some, there is sufficient evidence to accept these premises as true.

The mechanisms of ^{67}Ga localization in regions of inflammation are not clearly defined. Many factors are known to contribute to ^{67}Ga uptake, and it is likely that their influence depends on the disease and the extent of injury. One important factor is that ^{67}Ga behaves as iron in vivo, being bound by transferrin after intravenous administration. The subsequent distribution of ^{67}Ga depends on its migration from the plasma to tissue proteins and cells that have a stronger affinity for the radionuclide (43). Thus erythema, hyperpermeability of the capillary endothelium, and the presence of gallium-binding cells in areas of inflammation may partially explain the localization of ^{67}Ga in the lung. The transferrin receptor on the surface of cells appears to be important in the localization of ^{67}Ga in lung cancer and in some diffuse lung diseases (44). Transferrin receptors have been identified in the membrane of alveolar macrophages

in idiopathic pulmonary fibrosis and in epithelioid cells of granuloma in sarcoidosis and pneumoconiosis (44).

The character of the injurious process in each of the diffuse lung diseases depends on both number and type of inflammatory cells and on the state of activation (45). Activated alveolar macrophages, for example, play an important role in perpetuating lung injury, including the release of neutrophil chemotactic factor, a mediator that attracts neutrophils with their potent oxidants and proteases. In other circumstances, macrophages may contribute to the formation of granuloma because of their role in activating T lymphocytes (45). Thus a positive result of a ^{67}Ga scan probably reflects, at least in part, the density of activated inflammatory cells in the lung parenchyma and, for some diseases, the numbers of activated macrophages in the lower respiratory tract. It is also of interest that 60% to 70% of inhaled ^{67}Ga aerosol is retained in the lungs for more than 96 hours by healthy nonsmokers (46). The predominant site of this localization is the alveolar macrophage. This finding suggests that lung injury may expose the population of resident alveolar macrophages to sufficient

^{67}Ga for external detection even in diseases not associated with increased numbers of activated macrophages. Thus increased permeability of the lung microvasculature and alveoli to ^{67}Ga-laden serum proteins in association with injury may be crucial to achieving detectable localization of a pulmonary tracer.

Imaging Technique and Quantification of Gallium Lung Uptake

^{67}Ga is a cyclotron-produced radionuclide that decays through electron capture. It generates γ emission in three principal energy peaks at 93 keV (41%), 185 keV (23%), and 300 keV (18%). Hence ^{67}Ga scintigraphy commonly is performed with a large-field-of-view gamma camera that has multiple energy peak acquisition capability and medium energy collimation. Imaging routinely begins 48 to 72 hours after intravenous injection of 3 to 5 mCi of ^{67}Ga citrate. Gallium is slowly removed from the bloodstream, hence pulmonary images obtained within the first 24 hours after injection may be clouded by a high blood pool background. This may result in diffusely increased lung activity even in healthy persons.

Although normal lung tissue does not accumulate appreciable levels of ^{67}Ga, localization does occur normally in other thoracic sites. Faint bronchial activity is common, and in children, ^{67}Ga activity can be seen in normal thymic tissue (47).

Gallium is physiologically absorbed by bone matrix and can be localized to a small extent by marrow. Activity usually is evident in the rib cage, spine, and scapulae. The lower end of each scapula may show a prominent concentration of activity because of the thickness of the bone at this site. In women, the normal faint localization of ^{67}Ga in breast tissue may be enhanced during pregnancy and menarche and during administration of cyclic estrogen or progestational agents; the enhancement can be particularly prominent in postpartum women.

Investigators began to estimate the degree of lung uptake of ^{67}Ga soon after it was recognized that ^{67}Ga localization may reflect the extent of pulmonary inflammatory disease (48,49). The simplest, albeit binary, means to detect increased gallium lung localization is to discern whether the heart is silhouetted against the lung. In a graded qualitative approach used by several investigators, scans are classified as negative when the pulmonary uptake does not exceed soft-tissue background (proximal upper limb), 1+ when soft-tissue uptake and lung uptake are equal, 2+ when lung uptake is greater than soft-tissue uptake but less than liver uptake, 3+ when lung uptake is equal to liver uptake, and 4+ when lung uptake is greater than liver uptake. Qualitative evaluations are simple to make and usually are adequate to gauge disease activity. Semiquantitative procedures also rely on internal reference regions to estimate the degree of uptake but extend the power of qualitative estimates. In these procedures localization size and intensity are taken into account to generate an "index" of lung activity. In one of the original semiquantitative procedures (48), the area of each region of increased ^{67}Ga uptake is estimated as a percentage of total lung area. The intensity of gallium uptake within each of these areas is graded on a scale of 0 to 4. The area and intensity factors from each area

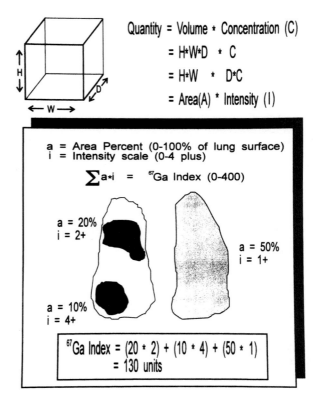

FIGURE 19.14. Semiquantitative assessment of ^{67}Ga uptake The quantity of ^{67}Ga localization is estimated according to the simple model of a container from which volume and concentration estimates can be derived. For scintigraphic images, volume and concentration are represented by image area and intensity estimates. The ^{67}Ga index is obtained by means of adding the products of area and intensity for each region of abnormal gallium uptake. The area index is expressed as a percentage of the entire lung surface area. The intensity index is determined on a scale of 0 to 4+, where 0 represents the background and 4+ is equivalent to the most intense body region. In the example shown, three areas of uptake with intensities above background are assigned area (*a*) and intensity (*I*) index values. The sum of the products of area and intensity yields a ^{67}Ga index of 130 index units. (From Line BR. Scintigraphic studies of inflammation in diffuse lung disease. *Radiol Clin North Am* 1991; 29: 1095-1114, with permission.)

are multiplied, and the sum of these products yields the gallium lung index (Fig. 19.14).

Evaluation of Metabolic Properties of the Lung

In addition to its function as an organ of external gas exchange, the lung serves as a metabolic regulator of substances circulating in the blood. The lung has been shown to modify many circulating vasoactive substances by means of activation, deactivation, or removal and storage for subsequent metabolism and release (50). It is possible to evaluate regional pulmonary amine metabolism by use of single-photon radiopharmaceuticals such as ^{123}I-amphetamine (51) or diamine (52). ^{123}I-metaiodobenzylguanidine (MIBG), which accumulates through active transport-dependent mechanisms, has been used to depict early, short-term disorders of pulmonary amine metabolism (52). For example, large and rapid decreases in MIBG lung activity have been found with bleomycin toxicity (53). Positron emission tomography (PET) can be used to quantitatively evaluate biologically important radiotracers, including carbon (^{11}C), nitrogen (^{13}N), and oxygen (^{15}O). Results of studies to measure amine clearance, glucose metabolism, and receptor localization can be quantified regionally with an accuracy unrivaled by any other noninvasive technique (54).

SPECIFIC DISEASE APPLICATIONS

Destructive Lung Disease

Over the years many studies have been conducted to apply V/Q scanning to nonembolic lung disorders. ^{133}Xe has been used to evaluate the extent of air trapping after smoke inhalation injury (55) or exposure to airway toxins. ^{81m}Kr and radioaerosols have been used to evaluate the restrictive lung disease of radiation fibrosis (56). Both perfusion and ventilation have been shown to decrease within minutes of pulmonary contusion (57), an example of posttraumatic consolidative lung disease.

Nonetheless, ventilation-perfusion (VQ) lung studies are not in routine use in the evaluation of nonembolic lung disease. Despite evidence to suggest that regional ventilation studies can be more sensitive to the presence of lung disease than are pulmonary function studies or radiographic assessment (58,59), there is little clinical enthusiasm for routine scanning. This lack of enthusiasm is due in part to the nonspecific nature of VQ scintigraphic abnormalities. VQ scans are not a satisfactory means to define the cause of a disease or the local cause of ventilation abnormalities. Similar findings can accompany airway secretions, atelectasis, bronchial obstruction, invasion or collapse, parenchymal destruction, inflammation, or edema. Abnormal study findings also may have little pathophysiologic importance. For example, diffuse ventilation abnormalities are found in 41% of middle-aged smokers with either mild or no respiratory symptoms. There is only a weak relation between an abnormal result of a ventilation scan and the deterioration of overall lung function (reduced forced expiratory volume in 1 second [FEV$_1$] and vital capacity, increased single-breath nitrogen slope and closing volume). There is no relation between the presence of chronic expectoration and an abnormal scan result (60). Although ventilatory dysfunction can be an early sign of disease, the extent of scintigraphic findings caused by age-related "normal" dysfunction is unknown. Other reasons for the lack of a routine use of VQ scintigraphy are logistical and economic, but perhaps the most important is the general utility of standard pulmonary function studies and chest radiography.

With the exception of studies performed before lung resection to predict postoperative lung reserve (61), VQ scans are rarely used in staging pulmonary disease (62) because of pulmonologists' reliance on results of pulmonary function tests and because of the relative (nonabsolute) nature of pulmonary scintigraphy. Unlike gallium lung scans or aerosol clearance studies, in which the acute process can be detected, in ventilation studies it is not possible to separate acute and controllable disease from chronic parenchymal processes. Similar arguments hold for serial assessment of pulmonary disease. As an indicator of overall change, there are too many circumstances in which regional function is either unreliable or too misleading to be useful in following

disease progression or response to therapy. Standard chest radiography and pulmonary function tests are not likely to be displaced by routine scintigraphy in such assessments. Nonetheless, ventilation studies have an important role in the care of certain patient populations, such as small children and infants, when lack of cooperation is an issue and when accurate results of pulmonary function tests are difficult to obtain (63).

Scintigraphic Studies in the Care of Children

Use of radioactive gases is a simple, safe, and unique method for evaluating regional lung function in children with pulmonary disease. Use of inert gases, such as ^{81m}Kr, provides high-quality images with low radiation exposure and requires little cooperation from the child. ^{81m}Kr ventilation and ^{99m}Tc perfusion scanning are particularly useful in examinations of small children, in which tests of overall pulmonary function cannot be performed because of lack of cooperation (63).

^{133}Xe scans have been used to screen children before bronchoscopic examination with the aim of establishing a more exact indication for bronchography (64). A study with another inhalation scintigraphic agent, ^{99m}Tc Technegas, has been found to be a reliable, nonhazardous procedure for preselecting young patients for directed bronchoscopy (65).

Bronchoplural Fistula and Foreign Body Aspiration

Fistulas following pneumonectomy and in the setting of empyema have been imaged with ^{133}Xe ventilation lung scanning (66). Because of its ease and simplicity, a ventilation study should be one of the first diagnostic tests performed when bronchopleural fistula is suspected.

Aspiration of a foreign body into the lower respiratory tract is an emergency that occurs mainly among young children, 70% of whom are younger than 4 years. It is a main cause of accidental death among children younger than 1 year. Although complete obstruction is relatively rare, foreign bodies can cause radiographic signs of obstructive emphysema, atelectasis, or elevation of the diaphragm. More commonly, however, the radiograph is of limited help, and fluoroscopy may be insensitive to the presence of small foreign bodies. In this setting, ^{133}Xe ventilation scanning has been found useful in the selection of patients for bronchoscopy (67) because it is rapidly performed and requires little patient cooperation.

Hyperlucent Lung

Swyer-James syndrome is thought to result from insults to the lung during childhood. These insults include radiation therapy, measles, pertussis, tuberculosis, adenoviral infection, and aspiration of a foreign body. These events initiate an inflammatory process that proceeds to bronchiolitis obliterans with eventual destruction of the lung parenchyma. The reduction in the pulmonary capillary bed causes significant reduction in the major pulmonary arteries and ultimately hypoplastic vasculature (68). The radiographic features of these pathologic changes are a small hyperlucent lung with an ipsilateral small hilum, diffuse air trapping, and segmental bronchiectasis.

Careful assessment of the VQ scan findings help in reliable differentiation between primary ventilatory causes of unilateral hyperlucent lung and Swyer-James syndrome (68). Swyer-James syndrome usually is associated with significantly reduced and irregular ventilation and perfusion to the affected lung. Primary acquired causes of hyperlucency due to bronchial obstruction (e.g., foreign body, intrabronchial neoplasm, mucous plug) or pulmonary artery occlusion (e.g., pulmonary artery stenosis, pulmonary arteritis, massive pulmonary embolism) can be differentiated because of the nearly complete loss of either airflow or blood flow to the affected lung on the scan. Thus the VQ scan can be important to patients with acute conditions, accurate assessment of which can preclude more invasive diagnostic procedures.

Pulmonary Vascular Disorders

Evaluation of Pulmonary Vascular Abnormality and Shunt

Congenital or postoperative lung perfusion abnormalities in patients with congenital heart defects may be asymptomatic and difficult to detect, especially if they are unilateral. These abnormalities often are amenable to correction with surgery or balloon angioplasty. Fewer than one half of patients with these disorders have chest radiographic findings that correspond to abnormalities evident at perfusion scintigraphy (69). Scans also can be used to quantitate relative pulmonary blood flow, information important in planning interventions not available from chest radiography or two-dimensional echocardiography (69). More than 80% of patients have perfusion abnormalities involving up to an entire lung after operations for transposition of the great arteries (70). In patients such as these, scans may be used in the postoperative period to assess capillary perfusion reserve. Scintigraphy also can be used to determine the severity of pulmonary parenchymal damage in patients with atrial septal defect. Patients with apically redistributed and mottled perfusion have a significant increase in pulmonary arteriolar resistance and a significant decrease in pulmonary to systemic blood flow ratio (71).

Severe hypoxia often is caused by an intrapulmonary shunt through a pulmonary arteriovenous fistula. These abnormalities are tiny and are difficult to depict angiographically. Hypoxemia induced by intrapulmonary shunts is associated with high intraoperative and postoperative risk and is a relative contraindication to liver transplantation (72). Thus calculation of the right-to-left shunt through a pulmonary arteriovenous malformation is important in assessing surgical risk. It is also used to gauge the potential benefit from therapeutic embolization or surgical resection.

^{99m}Tc albumin macroaggregates or microspheres have been used for measurement of cardiac output or its distribution among various organs, study of right to left intracardiac shunts, and the diagnosis of abnormalities of the great veins (72). The systemic distribution of labeled albumin particles can be used to determine shunt fraction because the particles do not normally traverse the pulmonary capillary bed. The right to left shunt fraction can be obtained by means of comparing radioactive

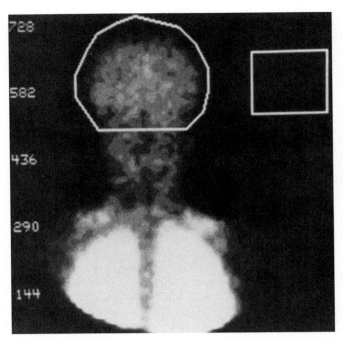

FIGURE 19.15. Calculation of intrapulmonary shunt index in a patient with high intrapulmonary shunting and localization of ^{99m}Tc macroaggregated albumin in the brain. Brain and background regions of interest are shown. Shunt index is determined with the background corrected percentage of activity in the brain relative to the lung (From Grimon G, Andre L, Bernard O, et al. Early radionuclide detection of intrapulmonary shunts in children with liver disease. *J Nucl Med* 1994; 35:1328–1332, with permission.)

counts in the right kidney (an index of systemic activity) to counts in the injected dose (or total lung counts) (73). Whole-body scanning has been used to calculate the right to left shunt fraction, but extrapulmonary activity may be falsely elevated because of the presence of unbound ^{99m}Tc or scatter from the lung region (72).

An index based on brain and pulmonary activity can be used to quantify the intrathoracic shunt (Fig. 19.15). Determination of brain activity avoids pulmonary scattering and possible salivary or thyroid activity. Cerebral activity is not increased by unbound ^{99m}Tc (72).

Evaluation of Hemoptysis and Hemorrhage

^{99m}Tc colloid and ^{99m}Tc red blood cells have been used to identify hemoptysis with techniques developed primarily to locate gastrointestinal bleeding (74). The minimum detectable rate of bleeding appears to be approximately 50 mL/24 hours. In patients with massive pulmonary hemorrhage, localized deposition of radionuclide can be found rapidly and confirmed with bronchoscopy. In this setting, lung scans provide clinically useful information regarding the bleeding site not available from the medical history, physical examination, or chest radiograph (75).

Pulmonary Hypertension

The diagnosis of primary pulmonary hypertension is made by means of exclusion and must be differentiated from thromboembolic pulmonary hypertension, which can be corrected surgically. Unfortunately, patients with chronic thromboembolic pulmonary hypertension commonly come to medical attention with progressive dyspnea, evidence of cor pulmonale, and no clear history of acute thromboembolism. Although perfusion scans in the evaluation for primary pulmonary hypertension can show certain abnormalities, such as nonsegmental, patchy defects of perfusion, the presence of segmental or larger perfusion defects should suggest the diagnosis of potentially correctable, large-vessel thromboembolic pulmonary hypertension rather than small-vessel, obliterative (primary, idiopathic) pulmonary hypertension (76). A retrospective review of the records of 15 patients with angiography- or biopsy-documented primary pulmonary hypertension showed that none of the patients had a segmental or larger perfusion defect. Such defects have been uniformly present in patients with large-vessel thromboembolic pulmonary hypertension (77).

Neoplastic Lung Disease

Lung cancer is the most frequent cause of cancer deaths among both men and women in the United States. The overall incidence is rising. Bronchogenic carcinoma now accounts for approximately 25% of all deaths of cancer and has an overall 5-year survival rate of only 13%. The diagnosis, staging, and follow-up management of lung cancer present a variety of radiographic challenges (78). The incidence of adenocarcinoma has increased over the past few decades, yet the incidence of squamous cell carcinoma has remained roughly stable. Worldwide approximately 80% to 85% of cases of lung cancer can be attributed to tobacco smoking. Changes in smoking prevalence precede those in lung cancer mortality by approximately 15 to 20 years (79). The highest survival rate is reported for adenocarcinoma, and small cell carcinoma has the worst prognosis. The survival rates for squamous cell and large cell carcinoma are intermediate (79).

It is likely that all bronchogenic carcinomas are derived from a pluripotential stem cell of epithelial origin. The term *bronchogenic carcinoma,* literally meaning a carcinoma of the bronchus, has come to represent any of the major cell types of lung cancer comprising squamous cell, small cell, large cell, adenosquamous, and adenocarcinoma. Together these account for more than 90% of all lung cancers. Other relatively rare primary lung neoplasms include sarcoma, mesothelioma, and carcinoid and mucoepidermoid cancers.

For clinical purposes, bronchogenic carcinoma usually is subdivided into two categories: small cell and non–small cell lung cancer. Twenty percent of malignant tumors of the lung are small cell lung cancer (SCLC). These tumors divide rapidly and are metabolically active. They are relatively sensitive to chemotherapy and radiation therapy. Unfortunately, they also are often widely disseminated by the time they come to medical attention. With systemic therapy, the mean survival time is less than 1 year, and the 5-year survival rate is an abysmal 10% (80). SCLC expresses the entire range of neuroendocrine cell markers and is believed to arise from pulmonary endocrine cells scattered throughout the tracheobronchial tree. Non–small cell lung cancer (NSCLC) is less metabolically active, less disseminated, and less responsive to chemotherapy or radiation therapy than is SCLC.

Squamous cell carcinoma almost always grows from the hilum, beginning with squamous metaplasia that progresses to dysplasia and carcinoma in situ and subsequently invades the basement membrane. Squamous cell carcinoma tends to spread locally, approximately 50% showing only intrathoracic spread at the time of diagnosis.

Adenocarcinoma usually is peripheral and is composed of mucin-producing glandular elements that may be associated with scarring. The prognosis usually is worse than that of squamous cell cancer, the lesion frequently manifesting with metastasis. Large cell carcinoma is composed of large polygonal cells that originate peripherally under the pleura. It tends to invade the lung tissue and the pleural space, sparing the bronchi. The prognosis and route of dissemination are the same as for adenocarcinoma.

Chest radiography with or without supplemental sputum cytologic examination can help detect lung cancer at an earlier stage than when these procedures are not performed, but chest radiographic screening has not been found to reduce the overall mortality of lung cancer. Radiologic detection of lung cancer occurs relatively late in the course of the disease. Given that the smallest detectable lesion is approximately 10 mm in diameter, by the time the diagnosis can be made, the tumor has undergone approximately 30 doublings in cell mass and has achieved a population of more than 1 billion cells. Depending on cell type, each doubling requires 30 to 180 days, so by the time of detection, the average cancer has been present for nearly 9 years. It is little surprise, therefore, that none of the current clinical, laboratory, radiographic, or scintigraphic technologies has been shown to have any impact on survival when used as a screening test for lung cancer (81). The utility of a cancer screening test depends ultimately on its ability to help detect early disease, but the cost of a program depends on both the expense of the test itself and the added cost and morbidity of false-positive results that lead to other unnecessary procedures. The requirement of adequate sensitivity and very high specificity is beyond the capabilities of current imaging technologies. Thus the role of imaging procedures is relevant only to cancer staging and follow-up studies after therapy.

Staging of Lung Cancer

Bronchogenic carcinoma is staged to estimate the anatomic extent of the cancer and thereby define the therapeutic approach and prognosis. The most broadly accepted staging system is that proposed by the 1986 American Joint Commission on Cancer. In this system TNM notation is used to codify cancer stage (I to IV) from the degree and distribution of disease at the primary tumor (T), in thoracic nodes (N), and at metastatic sites (M). The 5-year survival rates for stage I and II disease are 50% to 70% and 30% to 50% respectively, provided that the tumor does not extend beyond the lung and that the mediastinal nodes are uninvolved. In stage IIIa (extension beyond the lung parenchyma or ipsilateral mediastinal lymph nodes) the 5-year survival rate decreases to less than 20%. Disease in stage IIIb (contralateral mediastinal or hilar node involvement) or stage IV (distant metastasis) has much poorer outcome, a 5-year survival less than 5% (82). Mountain (83) reported on recent revisions in the TNM system and analyzed a collected database containing data on 5,230 patients. In this large group of patients, the distribution of the different histologic types was adenocarcinoma, 47.2%; squamous cell carcinoma, 33.9%; large cell carcinoma, 3.1%; SCLC, 11.9%; and carcinoma not specified, 3.9%.

The TNM lung cancer staging system has had its greatest effect on NSCLC. SCLC, however, is differentiated from other bronchopleural neoplasms by its great likelihood of the presence of covert and overt metastatic tumor when the patient comes to medical attention. For SCLC, the clinical performance status and the extent of tumor dissemination are the most important prognostic factors. A clinical, two-stage system proposed by the Veterans Administration Lung Group differentiates limited and extensive disease and has a higher prognostic strength than does TNM stage (84). Limited disease is defined as confined to the hemithorax, mediastinum, and ipsilateral supraclavicular space, whereas extensive disease has escaped these boundaries.

Radionuclides in Detection of Lung Neoplasia

Although radiography, computed tomography (CT) and magnetic resonance imaging (MRI) are still the methods of choice for the study of lung cancer, they have limitations in evaluating suspicious lung nodules, assessing mediastinal involvement, determining the viability of treated tumor, and making the diagnosis of relapse. Radionuclide procedures are focused on diagnosis, staging, restaging, and monitoring of therapy for lung cancer. These procedures take advantage of features of the disease, such as pathologic changes in tumor cell metabolism, increased tumor blood flow, and enhanced permeability of the tumor capillaries. They may also target specific cell surface receptors, uptake mechanisms, and intracellular binding sites (85). Many radiopharmaceuticals have been used for this, including gallium, monoclonal antibodies (MoAbs), somatostatin analogs, lipophilic cations, and positron tracers.

^{67}Ga citrate was one of the first tracers used to stage lung cancer. ^{67}Ga was first described as an oncologic tracer in 1969 by Edwards and Hayes (86). Over the years, it has been studied in several contexts but has not achieved a lasting clinical role. In early studies, it was reported to have high sensitivity and specificity in the detection of primary lung tumors and mediastinal disease, but subsequent investigations with larger populations were unable to substantiate the initial success. Unfortunately, gallium scintigraphy has been found too nonspecific. It also has been evaluated as a means to characterize lesions before and in response to radiation therapy. Although it has been confirmed that tracer uptake varies during treatment, uptake is not clearly related to treatment response (87). The use of tracer imaging in the evaluation of distant spread of lung cancer has been disappointing (88). It may show localization caused by tissue injury after radiation therapy or chemotherapy, it may localize in benign mediastinal processes such as thymic hyperplasia, and the results are positive in a broad cross-section of acute and chronic infections. Confounding results due to localization of ^{67}Ga in inflammatory diseases, a high blood pool background, and limited image resolution have caused imaging with ^{67}Ga to fall

out of use. At present, there is little to justify the use of this radiopharmaceutical in the evaluation of lung cancer.

Radiolabeled antibodies against tumor-associated antigens in lung cancer include MoAb 79IT/36 raised against human osteosarcoma; MoAb HMFG1 raised against human milk fat globule membranes, which reacts strongly with NSCLC; MoAb PO66 raised against NSCLC; MoAb NR-LU-10 raised against a cell membrane glycoprotein expressed on NSCLC and SCLC; and both MoAb ZCE025 and MoAb FO23C5 raised against carcinoembryonic antigen (CEA). Intact or whole MoAb immunoreagents have a prolonged intravascular half-life, high uptake in the reticuloendothelial system and sub-optimal penetration in tumor lesions. Smaller fragments of the whole antibody have been prepared to help address these problems. Radiolabeled MoAbs and fragments in the management of lung cancer have been evaluated in several multicenter trials. A number of studies have shown the clinical utility of MoAb imaging and report accuracy rates that compare favorably with those of CT. Limiting factors include high background uptake by normal tissues in addition to tumor and the inherent problems of detecting and localizing small lesions (89). Improved accuracy may result from image fusion or registration techniques that allow correlation with CT and MRI findings. For example, "fused" radiolabeled-antibody single positron emission CT (SPECT) with CT in the examination of patients with lung cancer has been shown to decrease the rate of false-positive results of SPECT and false-negative results of CT (90).

Studies of pulmonary lesions performed with radiolabeled antibodies have a sensitivity ranging from 68% to 100% depending on the antigen targeted, the radiolabel, and the antibody form. Lower sensitivities are generally found with tracers that clear the blood slowly or decay rapidly because of a low tumor target to blood background ratio (91). For example, blood pool activity in pulmonary vessels was more intense than in the lung tumors at 6 to 8 hours for an anti-CEA ^{99m}Tc Fab' antibody fragment in patients with NSCLC (91). Better imaging results were evident with CEA-specific ^{111}In F(ab')$_2$ (Fig. 19.16) (92). MoAb imaging has compared well with CT in the staging of primary tumors. In a study comparing CT with ^{111}In F(ab')$_2$ fragments of an anti-CEA antibody the MoAb study showed an accuracy of 78% for T3 disease and 86% for T4 disease. The accuracy of CT was 78% for T3 disease and 84% for T4 disease. To avoid high blood pool background activity, images typically were obtained approximately two blood half-lives after antibody administration (91).

Nonspecific factors may play a supportive role in tumor detection. For example, in one study, the target antigen was present in only 89% of the tumors in which the antibody localized (92). Nonspecific antibody uptake in histologically nonreactive tumors may be caused by anomalies in tumor angioarchitecture, enhanced transvascular leak in neoplastic capillaries, cross-reactivity with nontarget antigens, and nonspecific ^{111}In uptake by transferrin receptors of tumor cells (93). Interest in radiolabeled antibodies has declined because of the introduction of nonimmunologic technetium-labeled agents that are easier to use and less expensive than MoAbs and because of the small number of suitable MoAbs on the market.

Radiolabeled peptides have been used successfully to image

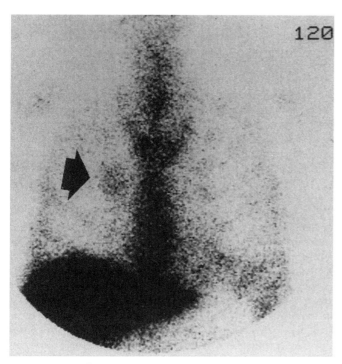

FIGURE 19.16. ^{111}In anti-CEA monoclonal antibody image shows squamous cell carcinoma of the right anterior bronchus. Anterior view of the thorax 120 hours after intravenous injection shows circumscribed uptake in the right hilar region. Left lower lobe activity is caused by the cardiac blood pool. The tumor to heart ratio was 1.02, and the tumor to lung ratio was 1.6 (From Biggi A, Buccheri G, Ferrigno D, et al. Detection of suspected primary lung cancer by scintigraphy with indium-111-anti-carcinoembryonic antigen monoclonal antibodies (type F023C5) *J Nucl Med* 1991;32:2064–2068, with permission.)

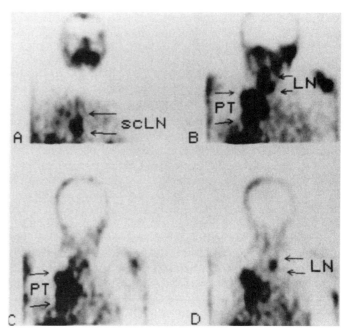

FIGURE 19.17. Localization of ^{123}I-Tyr-3-octreotide accumulation in small cell lung cancer. Coronal SPECT images of the head and thorax show positive image of the primary tumor and lymph-node metastatic lesion. **A:** Subcarinal lymph-node metastatic lesion (*scLN*). **B, C:** The primary tumor (*PT*; diameter, 8 cm) in the right upper lobe is delineated. **B, C, D:** Lymph-node metastatic lesion (*LN*) in the superior mediastinum. Activity in the *lower left* part of all images represents physiologic tracer uptake by the liver. (From Leitha T, Meghdadi S, Studnicka M, et al. The role of iodine-123-Tyr-3-octreotide scintigraphy in the staging of small-cell lung cancer. *J Nucl Med* 1993;34:1397–402, with permission.)

high-affinity somatostatin receptors on SCLC tumors (Fig. 19.17) (94). Among the lung cancers, SCLC tumors are relatively unique in this regard in that they stem from cells that express high-affinity somatostatin receptors and have the ability to synthesize peptide hormones through amine precursor uptake and decarboxylation (APUD cells). Somatostatin receptor scintigraphic studies have shown that 50% to 75% of SCLC tumors express receptors for somatostatin (95). Of the five known receptor subtypes, types 1 and 2 are those mainly found in SCLC (96). Somatostatin receptor imaging offers high sensitivity for the detection of primary tumors but has low sensitivity for metastatic lesions. This reduced sensitivity may occur because (a) metastatic lesions have a different type or a lower density of receptors or may lack them entirely (95,97) or (b) visualization is possible because receptors are present on inflammatory response cells surrounding the primary tumor that may not be present in metastatic lesions (95).

Pentavalent ^{99m}Tc dimercaptosuccinic acid [^{99m}Tc (V) DMSA] is a tracer developed as a general tumor imaging agent. At present its main clinical use is the study of medullary cancer of the thyroid. The mechanism of tumor uptake of this pharmaceutical is not clear, but Hirano et al. (98) suggested the mechanism is related to the similarity of this agent to phosphate molecules, which accumulate because of increased protein metabolism. The high blood pool activity makes it difficult to

evaluate small lesions, mediastinal tumor extension, or mediastinal involvement (98).

Other tracers, such as ^{201}Tl and ^{18}F-fluorodeoxyglucose (FDG), localize because of the increased metabolism of tumor tissue. ^{201}Tl is a potassium analog but has 5 times the affinity to the cell. It is therefore transported into the cell instead of potassium. This transportation may be regulated by sodium–potassium–adenosine triphosphatase (Na-K-ATPase) (99). It accumulates in a high percentage of lesions of primary lung cancer (100). Initial tumor localization is likely caused by a combination of increased relative blood flow and high metabolic activity. Other factors that can influence ^{201}Tl uptake by tumor cells include tumor viability and type, the cotransport system, the calcium ion channel system, vascular immaturity with leakage, and increased cellular membrane permeability. There is also a longer ^{201}Tl residence time in neoplastic tissue relative to normal or inflamed cells (100). Slower clearance of ^{201}Tl in adenocarcinoma and SCLC relative to squamous cell carcinoma has been described (100), but these differences have not been shown to be of clinical utility. Thallium SPECT has been found useful in the detection of mediastinal lymph-node metastatic lesions larger than 1.0 cm in diameter (101). It also has been used to differentiate benign from malignant lesions, assess lesion dedifferentiation, evaluate patient prognosis, and determine treatment response after radiation therapy or chemotherapy. Nonetheless, ^{201}Tl has relatively poor imaging characteristics compared with ^{99m}Tc, leading to similar types of evaluations with ^{99m}Tc hexakis-2-methoxy-isobutyl-isonitrile (^{99m}Tc sestamibi, or MIBI).

^{99m}Tc sestamibi is a lipophilic cation the in vitro uptake and retention of which involve passive diffusion across cell membranes, propelled by large negative transmembrane potentials (102). Several authors have used MIBI in the evaluation of primary tumors, and others have studied the rate of detection of mediastinal involvement (103). These results suggest the usefulness of MIBI imaging in lung cancer staging.

A relatively unique aspect of MIBI imaging is its potential for assessing multidrug resistance of tumors. Multidrug resistance is associated with increased expression of transmembrane P-glycoprotein on tumor cells that functions as an energy-dependent efflux pump for some anticancer drugs, such as doxorubicin, etoposide, paclitaxel, and the vinca alkaloids, and decreases the intracellular concentrations of these drugs (104). Because MIBI seems to be a suitable transport substrate as well, several studies have been performed to assess the role of MIBI in the prediction of clinical response of lung cancer to chemotherapy (105,106). Kostakoglu et al. (106) correlated MIBI washout rates and degree of MIBI accumulation with the expression of P-glycoprotein in tumour tissues in 46 patients with lung cancer. The investigators concluded that although MIBI washout rates do not seem to correlate with the P-glycoprotein density of tumor cells, the ability of tumors to accumulate MIBI correlates well with increased levels of P-glycoprotein expression.

^{99m}Tc tetrofosmin is another tracer designed for myocardial perfusion imaging. It is under investigation as a tumor-imaging agent. Although it is likely that its lipophilic cation may diffuse across the sarcolemmal and mitochondrial membranes, the mechanism of accumulation of this radiopharmaceutical in cancer tissue is still not well understood. The glucose analog FDG and PET have been highly successful in imaging all cell types of lung cancer (Fig. 19.18) (107). Elevated uptake of FDG has

been demonstrated in all lung cancer cell types, and this radiopharmaceutical is used for most PET studies of lung cancer (108). Malignant tumors have a markedly accelerated metabolism, especially glycolysis, DNA synthesis, and protein synthesis (109). Relative to normal tissue, tumor cells express more messenger RNA for the glucose transporter molecule that subsequently results in increased glucose uptake and metabolism. FDG behaves similarly to D-glucose in its transport through the cell membrane and phosphorylation by hexokinase in the glycolytic pathway. However, once FDG is phosphorylated, structural changes produced by a hexose-phosphate bond largely prevent FDG from being catabolized or transported back into the extracellular space. Thus increased uptake and accumulation of FDG occur within highly metabolic tumor cells (110).

Neoplastic cells also have increased amino acid utilization. Methionine labeled with ^{75}Se was initially studied in the evaluation of patients for lung cancer, but it has high β emissions, so only microcurie quantities can be used for imaging. The positron emitting radiopharmaceutical L-methyl ^{11}C methionine (MET) has far superior imaging characteristics, and its short half-life of 20 minutes allows it to be used in relatively large doses (111). Although uptake of both FDG and MET varies with tumor type, the reproducibility and utility of this finding are controversial (112). Selection of treatment based on the specific histologic type of the tumor per se has not been justified, because survival depends on resectability in toto and not on histologic features.

Another important property of tumor growth is DNA replication in neoplastic cells. ^{57}Co bleomycin binds firmly to DNA in the same way as Fe bleomycin, the cytotoxic form of bleomycin (113). The initial uptake of ^{57}Co bleomycin depends on tumor blood flow, tumor capillary permeability, and extracellular volume. Eight hours later, however, after blood and extracellular space concentrations decrease, tumor activity appears to reflect DNA binding and tumor cell kinetics (85,114). Rapidly growing tumors that have a poor prognosis also have a large

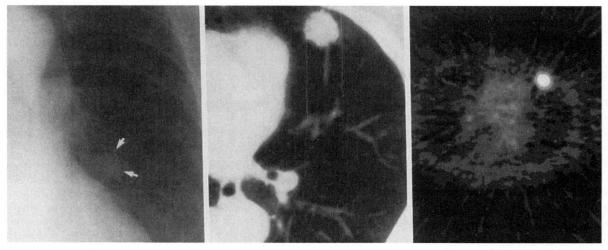

FIGURE 19.18. Asymptomatic adenocarcinoma in a 72-year-old woman. **A:** Posterior chest radiograph shows a 1.5-cm lingular nodule adjacent to the left border of the heart. Radiographs obtained previously were not available. **B:** CT scan of the nodule shows a homogeneous, irregularly marginated lesion. **C:** Axial FDG PET scan shows substantial uptake in the nodule. Biopsy showed adenocarcinoma. (From Patz EF Jr, Lowe VJ, Hoffman JM, et al. Focal pulmonary abnormalities: evaluation with F-18 fluorodeoxyglucose PET scanning. *Radiology* 1993;188:487–490, with permission.)

proportion of cells engaged in DNA synthesis. These tumors also appear to have high ^{57}Co-bleomycin uptake (114).

PET scanners are becoming widely available and are establishing an important clinical role because (a) the labeled compounds are biologically important, (b) the isotope half-life usually is short, and (c) the isotope tissue concentration can be determined quantitatively, accurately, and in many cases noninvasively (54). PET radionuclide imaging studies are of greatest practical importance in identifying pulmonary tumors, staging hilar and mediastinal nodes, and evaluating the treated patient for recurrence of disease. In lung cancer staging studies, whole-body imaging and attenuation correction are used to improve sensitivity to small lesions or lymph-node metastatic lesions in the central hilar or mediastinal regions. In attenuation-corrected studies, a semiquantitative parameter may be useful in characterization of the lesion (115,116). This parameter, the standard uptake value or standard uptake ratio (SUR) normalizes FDG accumulation in a region to the patient's body mass and the injected dose. Although this parameter depends on the time after injection and depends on the size of the lesion measured, it can be useful in differentiating benign from malignant tissue (117). Lung cancers generally have SUR values greater than 2.5, and benign lesions have values less than this. In one study, the SUR value of malignant lesions averaged 5.9 ± 2.7; benign masses had a mean SUR of 2.0 ± 1.7 (118). The SUR has been correlated with lesion doubling time (119) and the degree of cell differentiation. The SUR should be used with circumspection, however, given that sites of inflammation, contracting muscle, and urinary activity can easily exceed SUR values of 2.5 and given that bronchoalveolar cancer commonly has values less than 2.5. False-negative results of FDG PET occur in examinations of patients with pulmonary carcinoid and bronchoalveolar cancer, possibly because of the lower metabolic and growth rates of these diseases. These cancers have longer doubling times and less proliferative potential than other types of cancer (120).

Solitary Pulmonary Nodules

Many cases of lung carcinoma are initially encountered as solitary pulmonary nodules. These nodules are parenchymal lung lesions that are usually well defined and less than 4 cm in diameter. An estimated 130,000 new benign or malignant solitary pulmonary nodules are detected each year in the United States. Primary bronchogenic carcinoma and benign granuloma constitute more than 80% of pulmonary nodules, with approximately equal distribution in both categories (121). Less common diagnoses include hamartoma (6%), solitary metastatic lesion from non-lung primaries (5%), and bronchial adenoma (2%) (121).

The goal of evaluation of a solitary pulmonary nodule is to differentiate benign and malignant disease. Factors that increase the probability of malignancy include cigarette smoking, patient age greater than 35 years, irregular nodule margins, absence of calcification, and the size of the nodule (122). In a recent study of lung nodules larger than 3 cm in diameter, 98% of the nodules were malignant (123). The only two definite radiographic criteria for benign solitary pulmonary nodules are the presence of central, concentric, or stippled calcification, as seen on chest radiographs or CT scans, and stability of the nodule for more than 2 years (123). Plain radiography and CT are most com-

monly used to evaluate solitary pulmonary nodules, but most noncalcified solitary pulmonary nodules remain indeterminate (124). The typical pattern of dense central, laminated, or diffuse calcification, which almost excludes malignancy, occurs in only a small number of solitary pulmonary nodules (124).

FDG PET has been found highly accurate in differentiating benign from malignant focal pulmonary abnormalities seen on chest radiographs (Fig. 19.19) (110,123,124). In one series of 51 well-characterized pulmonary nodules, malignant lesions all exceeded a threshold value of FDG localization (standardized uptake ratio, 2.5). All nodules below the threshold were found to be benign disease (110). In a prospective study with 30 patients who had indeterminate solitary pulmonary nodules less than 3 cm in diameter, FDG differential uptake ratios produced positive and negative predictive values of approximately 90% (123).

The sensitivity of this FDG PET ranges between 82% and 100%, the specificity between 75% and 100%, and the accuracy between 79% and 94% (107,115,116,119,125,126). Specificity can vary with geographic area according to the prevalence of granulomatous disease. The negative predictive value of FDG PET is high, which makes it useful to reduce the number of pleural biopsies and limited thoracotomies for benign pleural disease.

Results of the foregoing studies suggest that FDG PET has a high degree of accuracy in differentiating benign from malignant pulmonary nodules larger than 1 cm in diameter. Quantitation is difficult, however, for lesions smaller than 1 cm in diameter because of limits in PET resolution, respiratory motion, and partial volume effects (110). Occasional false-positive results have been found in the evaluation of highly metabolic benign disease such as tuberculosis, histoplasmosis, aspergilloma, and abscesses (110,112,123). Analogous results that differentiate benign and malignant solitary pulmonary nodules have been found in studies comparing FDG and MET (127).

Evaluation of Mediastinal Lymph Nodes and Metastasis

Preoperative assessment of the mediastinal lymph nodes is mandatory because if mediastinal lymph-node metastatic lesions are present at the time of diagnosis, the 5-year survival rate after surgery decreases to less than 10% (107). Unfortunately, with regard to diagnostic imaging accuracy in presurgical staging, prospective data from the multi-institutional Radiologic Diagnostic Oncology Group trial showed that in evaluation for NSCLC, CT was only 52% sensitive and 69% specific, whereas MRI was 48% sensitive and 64% specific (128). The accuracy of CT also varies according to the mediastinal region examined; for example, the aortopulmonary window region is less accurately assessed than the paratracheal, subcarinal, and anterior mediastinal regions (81). The location of the primary cancer is one of the factors that can decrease the accuracy of anatomic staging. Squamous cell cancer, which often is centrally located, can cause postobstructive, reactive lymph-node enlargement and false-positive nodal assessment. Furthermore, it is often difficult to determine the size and extent of the primary tumor within the density caused by postobstructive collapse and reactive inflammation (91).

FDG PET imaging can provide information to enhance the

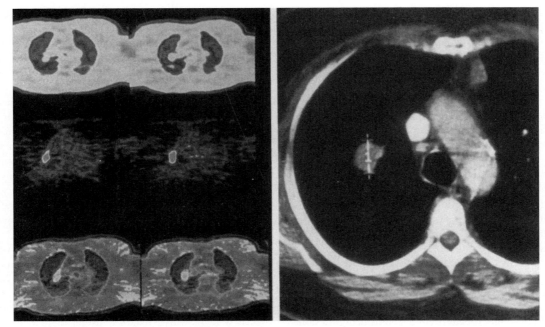

FIGURE 19.19. FDG PET scan **(A)** and CT scan **(B)** of a 50-year-old woman with a 2.0 cm × 1.5 cm nodule in the right lung found to be adenocarcinoma at thoracotomy. Intense metabolic activity is present in the nodule on the emission scans **(A,** *middle images*) obtained in the transaxial projection. *Top images* in **A** are transmission scans; *bottom images* in **A** are overlays. (From Gupta NC, Frank AR, Dewan NA, et al. Solitary pulmonary nodules: detection of malignancy with PET with 2-[F-18]-fluoro-2-deoxy-D-glucose. *Radiology* 1992;184:441–444, with permission.)

accuracy of presurgical staging (107). Most studies in this field conclude that the accuracy of PET in detecting mediastinal involvement is higher than that of CT or MRI (107,129–132). A prospective trial to compare FDG PET and CT in the evaluation of surgically confirmed disease, including a high percentage of mediastinal disease, showed that PET (82% sensitive, 81% specific, 81% accurate) was significantly better than CT (64% sensitive, 44% specific, 52% accurate) in the staging of mediastinal disease (Fig. 19.20) (107). Similarly, in a prospective study, the sensitivity of FDG PET for detecting distant metastases was 100% with a specificity of 94% and an accuracy of 96% (109). Vansteenkiste et al. (131) suggested that implementation of FDG PET would reduce the number of mediastinoscopies performed but not deny the patient the chance for curative resection based on results of imaging.

It is likely that the greater utility of PET relative to more conventional whole-body or planar scintigraphy is related to the high sensitivity of PET (20 to 50 times more sensitive than imaging with a conventional gamma camera) and tumor to blood background ratios that are often more than 10:1 (107). Like that of other radionuclides (^{67}Ga, ^{201}Tl), however, uptake of FDG is not specific for malignant lesions. False-positive results are caused mainly by inflammatory disease. Nonetheless, that FDG uptake is quantitated in PET may lead to greater specificity than can be achieved in the more qualitative γ emission studies. Because PET scans lack anatomic information, the highest accuracy is achieved when the metabolic information of PET and the anatomic information of CT are used together (107,131).

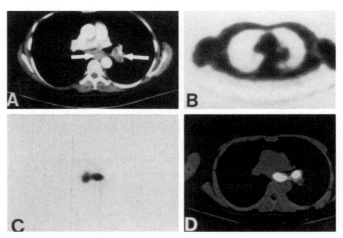

FIGURE 19.20. FDG PET scans of a patient with mediastinal node involvement from non–small cell lung cancer. **A:** Enlarged mediastinal lymph nodes (*arrows*) are present on a diagnostic contrast-enhanced CT scan. **B:** Transmission PET scan provides low-resolution anatomic image of thorax. **C:** Emission PET scan shows intense FDG uptake by the mediastinum 50 to 60 minutes after tracer injection. **D:** Anatometabolic fusion image shows intense FDG uptake by enlarged nodes. Metastatic (poorly differentiated) cancer was proved present in mediastinal nodes in this patient (From Wahl RL, Quint LE, Greenough RL, et al. Staging of mediastinal non-small cell lung cancer with FDG PET, CT, and fusion images: preliminary prospective evaluation. *Radiology* 1994;191: 371–377, with permission.)

Follow-up Evaluation after Cancer Therapy

The therapeutic effectiveness of radiation therapy and chemotherapy for cancer usually is evaluated on the basis of morphologic changes in tumor size. It is well known, however, that changes in tumor size do not necessarily indicate a therapeutic effect (133). Furthermore, anatomic imaging modalities provide important morphologic information but often do not help differentiate recurrent tumor and benign posttreatment inflammation or fibrosis (78).

FDG PET has been used to evaluate lung cancer after therapy in an effort to predict treatment response (133,134). Unfortunately, decreased FDG uptake with treatment does not necessarily indicate a good prognosis (133). Similar findings were obtained in a study with MET (135). It is probably too much to expect that uptake of FDG or MET can define the biologic characteristics of a tumor sufficiently to characterize prognosis. A host of factors beyond metabolic activity are important in this regard.

FDG PET imaging can be used to differentiate persistent or recurrent bronchogenic carcinoma from posttherapy fibrosis (Fig. 19.21). Quantitative analysis of FDG uptake is highly successful in separating these patient groups (78). Patients with residual radiographic abnormalities that are greater than 1 cm in diameter but normal findings on PET scans very likely are free of disease. However, apparent FDG activity in lesions smaller than 1 cm may be falsely low because of partial volume effects on PET images (78). False-positive results in this setting can be caused by inflammation due to infection or radiation therapy within the last 12 months. Postirradiation inflammatory changes have to subside for PET to provide an accurate quantitative assessment of tumor viability with less chance of false-positive results. Patz et al. (78) suggested that positive results of PET 2 months after treatment could be considered indicative of tumor, whereas Frank et al. (136) suggested a period of 4.5 months.

Other Radionuclide Studies in Lung Cancer

[67]Gallium scans have been evaluated with regard to uptake in the primary tumor, mediastinal uptake, and localization in distant metastatic disease. More than 90% of lesions of NSCLC take up [67]Ga. The overall accuracy for detecting a suspected primary tumor is 89% (137). The overall accuracy for mediastinal staging in the care of patients with peripheral lung cancer is 80%. The presence of a centrally located primary tumor causes the accuracy to decrease to 61% because of the difficulty in differentiating uptake of the primary lesion from that of mediastinal lymph nodes (137,138). Although gallium scans can help in identification of mediastinal node involvement, there is considerable controversy over the relation between the sensitivity and the specificity of the method. Two main factors limit the sensitivity of ^{67}Ga scintigraphy. Microscopic intranodal metastatic lesions may not increase the size of a node into the range (>1.5 to 2.0 cm) successfully resolved with ^{67}Ga scintigraphy. Second, in patients with primary paramediastinal tumors, gallium uptake by adjacent mediastinal nodes may not be separately identifiable owing to the proximity of the nodes to the primary tumor.

The accuracy of scanning for metastasis to distant organ exceeds 90%. Otherwise occult metastatic disease is identified in approximately 10% of patients (81). Because distant extrathoracic metastatic lesions are detected, ^{67}Ga scanning may help identify a small group of patients who can be spared an unneeded operation. [67]Ga scanning fails specifically for metastasis within the brain; thus it does not supplant CT of the brain, and it is less sensitive than bone scans in the detection of osseous metastasis. Because CT is currently used in the staging of most cases of lung cancer, the additional yield from ^{67}Ga scintigraphy has proved relatively low. Fewer than 10% of patients have significant findings at ^{67}Ga scintigraphy that were not suspected at CT. Most of these patients have clinical findings suggesting the presence of metastatic disease (139). Thus ^{67}Ga scintigraphy is no longer considered a primary imaging modality in the staging of pulmonary tumors (81).

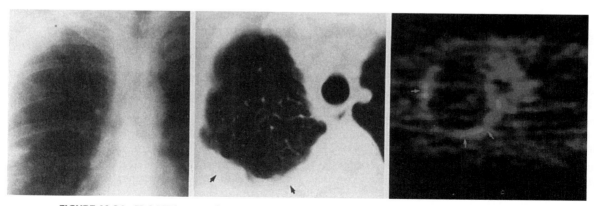

FIGURE 19.21. FDG PET images of a patient with recurrent bronchogenic carcinoma. **A:** Posteroanterior chest radiograph shows minimal right apical pleural thickening 12 months after right lower lobe resection for bronchoalveolar cell carcinoma. **B:** CT scan of the right apex shows thickening of the pleura, which suggests recurrent tumor (*arrows*). **C:** Axial FDG PET image of the right apex shows several small areas of distinctly increased FDG uptake (*arrows*). Results of percutaneous biopsy revealed recurrent tumor. (From Patz EF Jr, Lowe VJ, Hoffman JM, et al. Persistent or recurrent bronchogenic carcinoma: detection with PET and 2-[F-18]-2-deoxy-D-glucose. *Radiology* 1994;191:379–382, with permission.)

[201]Tl has been shown to localize in malignant pulmonary tumors. Tonami et al. (100) conducted a study with 170 patients who had a malignant pulmonary lesion larger than 20 mm in diameter on surgical specimens. Results of SPECT performed 3 hours after injection were positive in all of the 147 malignant pulmonary lesions and 16 of 23 (69.6%) benign pulmonary foci. The duration of the presence of ^{201}Tl in malignant tumors was shown significantly longer than that in benign disease. Although mediastinal blood pool activity clouded early images, mediastinal lymph-node metastatic lesions were detected on delayed scans. The smallest lesion was 1.5 cm in diameter (100). Although ^{201}Tl imaging provides insight into the metabolic nature of pulmonary and mediastinal masses, it remains unclear whether this modality can challenge the utility of CT.

Radionuclide studies of the brain, liver, and bones have been used to detect metastatic disease, but the results are rarely abnormal in examinations of patients without suggestive symptoms or signs of metastasis. Conversely, when clinical signs of metastatic disease are present, the results of liver scintigraphy often are false-negative (81). Given their greater accuracy and anatomic detail, CT scans of the brain and liver have essentially replaced the corresponding radionuclide studies. Bone scans have been shown to depict clinically unsuspected metastases in as many as 8% of patients and are useful for confirming the presence of metastatic disease in patients with clinical findings (81).

VQ studies have not been useful in tumor detection or in predicting the likelihood of resectability. Pulmonary scintigraphy is generally too nonspecific to assess the presence or extent of lung carcinoma. Mediastinal or hilar involvement, for example, is unsuspected scintigraphically in 50% of patients (140). Although VQ studies may allow tumor localization in a small number of patients with abnormal results of sputum cytologic examination and normal findings on chest radiographs, no specific patterns have been found (141). The frequency of inability to resect a tumor may increase when perfusion of the affected lung decreases to one third or less of the total pulmonary blood flow (142), but this finding is too unreliable to be considered a contraindication to surgical therapy (140).

Assessment of Postresection Pulmonary Reserve

Despite the limitations of scintigraphy in evaluating resectability, quantitative studies have an important role in determining whether the patient can undergo an operation. Considerable disability may result from hypercarbia and chronic ventilatory insufficiency if the patient's postoperative FEV_1 is less than 0.8 L (143,144). To avoid crippling surgery, the contribution of the involved lung to the overall function must be known (145). The good correlation between results of differential bronchospirometry and those of xenon radiospirometry (146) prompted the use of xenon in predictions of postoperative FEV_1 and forced vital capacity in the care of patients undergoing pneumonectomy. Quantitative differential perfusion scanning later was found to be as accurate as these two modalities in predicting postoperative lung function (145), presumably because of a close relation between unilateral ventilation and perfusion in patients with lung cancer. Split-field perfusion scanning rapidly became the procedure of choice because it was simple to perform and widely available (Fig. 19.22).

It has been suggested that for patients undergoing lung resection, preoperative evaluation should include total pulmonary function measurements. It is highly likely that the patient will tolerate removal of an entire lung if preoperative studies meet the following criteria:

FEV_1 is greater than 50% of forced vital capacity and is more than 2 L.

The maximum voluntary ventilation is greater than 50% of predicted value.

The ratio of residual volume to total lung capacity is less than 50%.

If these criteria are not satisfied, radionuclide split function studies are appropriate. Surgery usually is not performed if a postoperative FEV_1 less than 0.8 L is predicted (147). Split function studies are performed by means of summing the activity of each lung in anterior and posterior views. The postoperative FEV_1 is predicted by means of multiplying the preoperative value by the ratio of the counts in the lung that will remain to total lung activity (Table 19.2).

When pneumonectomy is avoidable, segmental resection or lobectomy has become the surgical procedure of choice. The operative mortality of lobectomy is approximately the same as that of pneumonectomy, but the 5-year survival rate is higher after lobectomy, presumably because of a lower incidence of respiratory disability.

Because of the difficulty of obtaining quantitative xenon ventilation measurements in multiple views, [81m]Kr scintigraphy and aerosol inhalation studies are attractive alternatives for estimating lobar ventilation. [81m]Kr imaging has been found to allow quantification of both regional ventilation and lobar V/Q ratios (148). Appropriate regions of interest are drawn to separate lobes of the lung by means of either [81m]Kr ventilation or ^{99m}Tc perfusion imaging. Regional quantitation may be best performed with lateral and oblique images, because lobar separation is more readily defined in these views. Although the interlobar planes are not as well defined in the posterior oblique views, they are less affected by counts from the opposite lung. Although the optimum method for extracting lobar data is not established, an average of the lobar counts obtained from the lateral and oblique views may be a reasonable compromise between the conflicting goals of optimum lobar separation and avoidance of contralateral activity.

The percentage of global function contributed by the selected lobe is determined as the ratio of counts in that lobe to total counts in the lung. The predicted postlobectomy FEV_1 may be determined as in the split function study, that is, by multiplying the preoperative FEV_1 by the lobar percentages of the ventilation or perfusion of the lung regions that will remain.

Inflammatory Lung Disease

The diffuse lung diseases encompass more than 150 causes disseminated throughout the lung parenchyma (149). Although some of these diseases develop rapidly because of the action of infectious or toxic agents, most of the disorders are chronic,

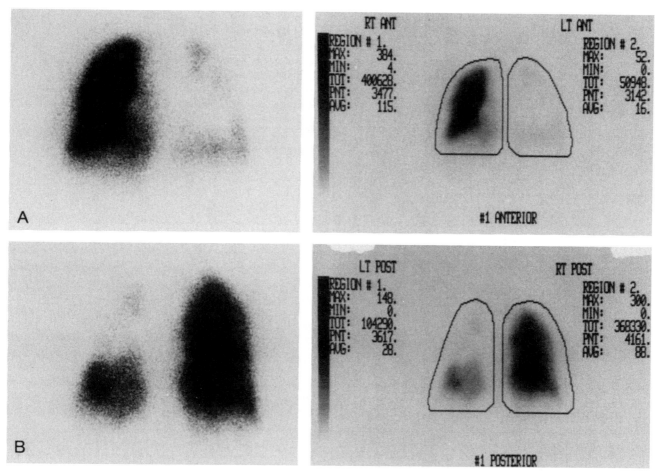

FIGURE 19.22. Radionuclide split function study before lung resection. Anterior **(A)** and posterior **(B)** perfusion images (*left*) and quantitative analyses (*right*) of a patient with a central carcinoma of the left lung. The importance of performing both anterior and posterior quantitative studies is illustrated by the fact that in the anterior view the relatively normal right lung contains nearly eight times as many total counts as the left lung. In the posterior projection, however, the right lung contains only three or four times as many counts. Quantitative data from both projections must be combined to allow accurate prediction of postoperative relative lung function. (From Alderson PO, Biello DR. Radionuclide studies of the pulmonary vasculature. In: Taveras JM, Ferucci JT, eds. *Radiology: diagnosis, imaging, intervention.* Vol 1. Philadelphia: JB Lippincott Co, 1986:11, with permission.)

Table 19.2. *Ventilation and Perfusion Scintigraphy for Estimating Lobar Ventilation*

	^{81m}K Ventilation ($\dot{V}$) (%)	^{99m}Tc MAA Perfusion ($\dot{Q}$) (%)	$\dot{V}/\dot{Q}$
Right lung	59.5	52.3	1.14
Left lung	40.5	47.7	.85
Left upper lobe	8.6	7.2	1.19
Left lower lobe	31.9	40.5	.79
Predicted FEV$_1$ (mL)	1.49	1.52	

The preoperative FEV$_1$ was 1.64 L. Before left upper lobectomy the predicted postoperative FEV$_1$ was calculated as follows:

PreOp FEV$_1$ × (100% − $\dot{V}$%$_{LUL}$) or preOp FEV$_1$ × (100% − $\dot{Q}$%$_{LUL}$)
MAA, macroaggregated albumin.

taking months to years to manifest themselves clinically. The delay is probably caused by the functional reserve of the lung, which allows it to sustain substantial injury before symptoms occur. Because of the possible disparity between injury and symptoms, it is useful to conceptualize each of the diffuse lung diseases as two overlapping processes. One of these is the active injurious process, and the other is a condition that is closer to static and represents the dysfunction resulting from injury. This distinction is important, because alveolar injury must be managed before it leads to irreversible structural deterioration. Unfortunately, results of pulmonary function tests and chest radiographs are strongly influenced by derangements of alveolar structure that may have little relation to the extent of ongoing injury (150).

To determine the appropriate therapy, it is necessary to characterize the cellular nature of the inflammation and to stage the degree of alveolar injury. Lung biopsy or bronchoalveolar lavage studies are essential tools for achieving these ends. Subsequent monitoring of the nature and extent of alveolitis, however, has been difficult because of the patients' poor acceptance of repeated lung biopsies and because of the limited value of lung function tests or chest radiographs as indicators of ongoing injury (151). Noninvasive tests that can be used to evaluate the "activity" of a diffuse pulmonary disease process include ^{67}Ga citrate lung scanning and ^{99m}Tc DTPA clearance studies. These tests are not markedly affected by the functional state of the lung parenchyma.

Uptake of ^{67}Ga in the lungs of patients who have active diffuse lung disease is common, even in the absence of gross radiographic changes. It has been observed in both acute and chronic diseases across a broad range of etiologic factors (Table 19.1). It is found in patients with acute disease secondary to bacterial, fungal, mycoplasmal, and opportunistic infections (152). ^{67}Ga uptake also occurs in pulmonary toxicity associated with chemotherapy and has been proposed for the early detection of interstitial pneumonitis associated with bleomycin or cyclophosphamide therapy (153,154). Drug addicts also may have normal findings on chest radiographs and intense accumulation of gallium in the lungs, which probably is related to hypersensitivity to talc associated with long-term intravenous injection of addictive drugs (152). Patients who have lung or mediastinal neoplasms who undergo scanning immediately after receiving radiation therapy may have diffuse ^{67}Ga lung uptake caused by transient radiation pneumonitis (87). Several disorders representative of granulomatous, infectious, toxic, idiopathic, and connective tissue diseases are discussed briefly to illustrate the variety of causes of diseases in which ^{67}Ga scanning has been useful clinically.

Open lung biopsy, bronchoalveolar lavage, and ^{67}Ga lung scanning are the three most widely used tests to monitor pulmonary inflammation in diffuse lung disease. Lung biopsy is the most sensitive and specific among these procedures, but only a small area of the lung is sampled and the procedure usually is limited to a single use during the course of the disease. Bronchoalveolar lavage may be performed repeatedly for assessment of the types, relative numbers, and activation of the effector cells present in the lower respiratory tract. ^{67}Ga scanning is the least invasive study and is used to assess the activity of disease in the entire lung as well as in extrapulmonary sites.

Many studies show relatively good correlation among these three assessments of disease activity in diffuse lung disease, but results can vary depending on the disease and the study design. The reasons for agreement and disagreement are poorly understood, but several factors may contribute to the findings. These factors include differences in the amount of lung sampled, differences in the timing or frequency of sampling, and differences in the aspect of the injury and inflammatory process sampled in each test. For example, comparisons between gallium scanning and either lavage or lung biopsy may suffer from differences in the site or the amount of lung examined. The cellular material obtained from saline lavage is derived from a relatively limited region of lung parenchyma. Because the distribution of disease lesions is not always diffuse and homogeneous, such a sample may not be representative. Another situation in which ^{67}Ga scanning and lavage differ is airway disease. Results of lavage analysis

are difficult to interpret in the presence of bronchitis (the cell samples recovered are contaminated by airway cells), and ^{67}Ga scanning is generally insensitive to inflammation limited to major airway tissue.

^{67}Ga localization is likely to be an early event in pulmonary inflammation and should be strongly influenced by factors that increase endothelial permeability and less strongly influenced by the cellularity of the inflammatory process. Furthermore, gallium localization is not a measure of pulmonary fibrosis, and it is unlikely to be highly predictive of disease outcome or prognosis. In combination with bronchoalveolar lavage or biopsy, gallium scanning appears useful as a tool to initially stage the alveolitis of many of the inflammatory diffuse lung diseases (45, 155). During the course of therapy, it may be valuable to determine the effectiveness of treatment in reducing alveolar inflammation. It may be of limited use, however, as a measure of the effect of therapy on the population of effector cells in the lower respiratory tract.

Sarcoidosis and Other Granulomatous Diseases

Sarcoidosis is a multisystem granulomatous disorder of unknown causation that frequently occurs with mediastinal or hilar adenopathy and pulmonary infiltration. The lower respiratory tract is the site most commonly associated with morbidity and mortality. At least 90% of patients who have sarcoidosis have pulmonary manifestations; 20% to 25% have a permanent loss of lung function, and 5% to 10% die of complications related to sarcoidosis (156).

Results of ^{67}Ga lung scanning are positive in most patients who have sarcoidosis and may be observed in both intrathoracic and extrathoracic lymph nodes and in other organs where there is active disease (Fig. 19.23) (155). In addition to being useful in assessing the magnitude of the alveolitis of the disease (157, 158), ^{67}Ga scans are of use in guiding lung biopsy and in choosing pulmonary segments for bronchoalveolar lavage (159). Gallium scanning appears to be valuable in follow-up studies of patients with sarcoidosis who are undergoing steroid therapy, and the results may be a more sensitive indicator of treatment response than are clinical symptoms, chest radiographs, and pulmonary function tests (159).

In the lung, the pattern is generally diffuse and often intense, but like the disease itself, uptake can have highly variable manifestations. Several patterns of gallium localization have been reported to be highly specific for sarcoidosis. In 605 consecutive gallium scans, right paratracheal with parahilar and infrahilar lymph node uptake was found only in patients who had sarcoidosis (160). These authors also found that the combination of symmetric parotid, lacrimal, and submandibular salivary gland localization also was strongly associated with sarcoidosis.

The limitations of chest radiography in the detection of sarcoid parenchymal disease are well recognized (161). It is clear that the classic radiographic groups of sarcoidosis do not necessarily represent sequential progression or activity of the disease. In a large combined study with untreated patients with sarcoidosis (159), ^{67}Ga lung uptake was found in 20% of one group of patients even though the lung was radiographically clear. Nearly one half (44%) of patients who had normal radiographs had

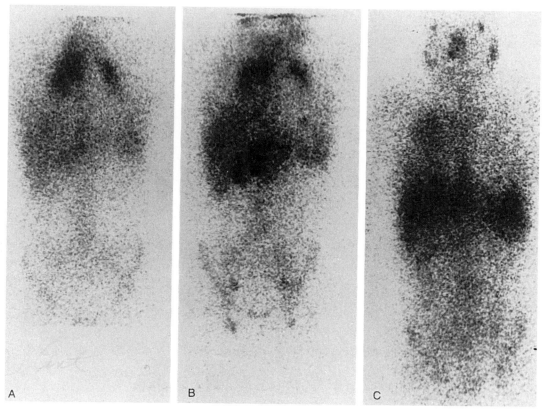

FIGURE 19.23. Scintigraphic pattern variation over a 16-month period in a patient with sarcoidosis. **A:** Anterior scintiscan of a 24-year-old woman shows uptake suggesting right peritracheal, hilar, and early paraaortic disease. **B:** Scintiscan obtained 5 months later shows a similar mediastinal pattern but also increased activity in the parenchyma of the right lower lobe and greater abdominal disease involving nodal sites in the paraaortic, inguinal, and femoral regions. **C:** Scintiscan obtained 16 months after **A.** The nodal uptake pattern has disappeared in all sites, but there is now marked involvement of the right pulmonary parenchyma. Parotid localization also is evident. (From Line BR. Scintigraphic studies of inflammation in diffuse lung disease. *Radiol Clin North Am* 1991;29:1095–1114, with permission).

positive scan results. Among patients examined 3 to 9 months later, the gallium lung scan was more sensitive to altered disease status than was the chest radiograph in 42% of untreated patients and in 46% of treated patients. No patient undergoing therapy had worse radiographic findings with an unchanged scan. Among 154 patients who underwent three to nine scans at intervals of 2 to 12 months, ^{67}Ga lung scanning was far more sensitive than was chest radiography in both detection of improvement and prediction of relapse. Among 20% of 481 untreated patients, gallium lung scanning appeared to be the only noninvasive method with which clinical activity could be detected. In contrast, in a group of 179 untreated patients who had negative results of ^{67}Ga lung scans, other signs of clinical activity (fever, weight loss, arthralgia, extrathoracic involvement) were present in 51 patients (30%).

The use of ^{67}Ga scans to monitor the progress of sarcoidosis has been judged impractical because the radiation exposure to the patient makes repetition more often than twice a year undesirable and because prednisone therapy inhibits ^{67}Ga uptake (162). Because many patients have positive results of scans as therapy is withdrawn (159), however, ^{67}Ga scintigraphy may be

valuable in defining a subset of patients at risk of continued alveolitis and in separating them from patients whose inflammatory stimulus has abated (Fig. 19.24). For example, there is rebound positivity of the gallium lung scan in approximately 40% of patients after discontinuation of steroids and in approximately 20% of patients after reduction of steroid therapy (159). The time at discovery of rebounds ranged from 1 month to 3 years. When scanning is used to monitor therapy, it is recommended that the ^{67}Ga dose be reduced from 3 to 5 mCi to 1.5 mCi, especially when the subjective scoring method is used. This reduces the cost and the radiation burden of follow-up imaging studies (159).

The relation between the degree of gallium localization and disease prognosis is controversial. Observation of 32 patients with sarcoidosis 3 or more years after the initial gallium scans showed no correlation between initial findings and later course (162). In another study, patients with sarcoidosis who had 28% or more T cells in the lavage analysis and a positive results of a gallium scan had clear deterioration in lung function over a 6-month period, unlike patients who had less than 28% T cells or a negative result of a gallium scan or both (42).

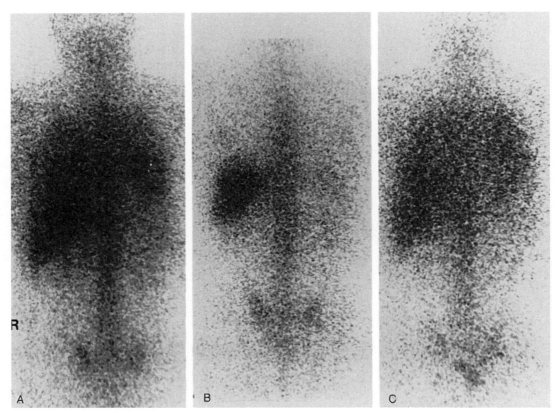

FIGURE 19.24. ^{67}Ga scans spanning a period of glucocorticoid therapy for sarcoidosis in a 47-year-old man. **A:** Posterior whole-body scintiscan shows diffuse pulmonary localization of ^{67}Ga nearly equivalent to that of the liver in intensity. **B:** Scintiscan obtained 7 months later while the patient was undergoing glucocorticoid therapy. Spine and liver localization is clearly more intense than that of the lung, which has a normal uptake pattern. **C:** Scintiscan obtained 4 months after the end of therapy shows diffuse intense localization consistent with reactivation of sarcoid alveolitis. (From Line BR. Scintigraphic studies of inflammation in diffuse lung disease. *Radiol Clin North Am* 1991;29:1095–1114, with permission).

Fibrotic Lung Diseases

Idiopathic Pulmonary Fibrosis

Idiopathic pulmonary fibrosis (IPF) is a fatal disorder characterized by parenchymal inflammation and interstitial fibrosis. Results of gallium scans are positive in approximately 70% of all patients who have IPF (48,163). The pattern usually is diffuse and confined to the lung parenchyma. Quantitative ^{67}Ga scan evaluations have been useful in staging of the activity of IPF and in evaluating response to therapy. Therapeutic intervention can suppress alveolar inflammation as measured by ^{67}Ga lung uptake and the number of inflammatory cells in lavage samples (48,164). The level of ^{67}Ga, however, has not been a consistent predictor of which patients' conditions will deteriorate. In one study, for example, the condition of patients with normal levels of uptake deteriorated and that of patients with high uptake was unchanged or improved (151). Other investigators found that patients' conditions deteriorated when the patient had higher ^{67}Ga lung uptake, especially when there was an associated increase in lavage neutrophil count (165).

Collagen Vascular Diseases

The interstitial process in many collagen vascular diseases (e.g., rheumatoid arthritis, systemic lupus erythematosus, polymyo- sitis-dermatomyositis, and overlap syndrome) is associated with alveolitis, in which inflammatory and immune effector cells are thought to mediate much of the lung parenchymal injury (150). ^{67}Ga scanning and bronchoalveolar lavage may be useful in assessment of progressive pulmonary fibrosis in collagen vascular disease (Fig. 19.25). For example, progressive systemic sclerosis (PSS), or scleroderma, is a disorder in which fibrous connective tissue is deposited in many organs. Respiratory insufficiency is a major cause of death among patients who have PSS. Results of ^{67}Ga scans are positive in three fourths of patients, showing diffuse, primarily lower zone uptake often independent of the pattern on the chest radiograph (166,167). In one study with a small group of patients with PSS, there was no consistent effect of glucocorticoid therapy on the result of the ^{67}Ga scan or proportion of cells in lavage fluid (167). In another study with patients who had various collagen vascular diseases, ^{67}Ga uptake occurred in the lung in 17 of 20 patients with progressive dyspnea but in none of 16 patients without progressive symptoms (168).

Pneumoconiosis

Pneumoconiosis is a group of chronic diseases of the lower respiratory tract that result from prolonged exposure to high concen-

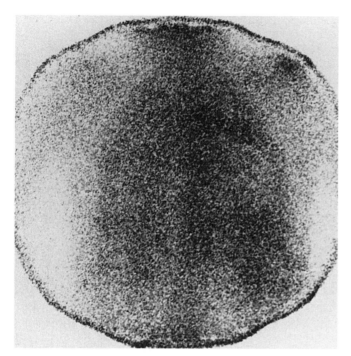

FIGURE 19.25. Diffuse pulmonary uptake in lung affected by progressive rheumatoid disease in a 68-year-old woman. Posterior scan of the thorax shows homogeneous 2 to 3+ intensity in the left lung and a more heterogeneous pattern on the right. The intensity of the lung approximates that of the liver. A focus of intense activity in the right shoulder was associated with acute symptoms of rheumatoid disease. (From Line BR. Scintigraphic studies of inflammation in diffuse lung disease. *Radiol Clin North Am* 1991;29:1095–1114, with permission).

trations of airborne inorganic dust, such as dusts of asbestos, coal, and silica. Studies of the diseases caused by these three dusts show that persons who do not smoke but who have such disorders have ongoing, active inflammation of the lower respiratory tract (169). Although ^{67}Ga uptake does not appear to be associated with increased percentages of lavage cell subpopulation, gallium does appear to be localized in the lung through enhanced protein-bound leakage into the bronchoalveolar milieu and through accumulation by macrophages at disease sites (170).

Gallium scanning can be used to detect the early stages of pneumoconiosis and to gauge the activity and progression of the disease (171). Siemsen et al. (171) reported a high incidence of positive results of gallium lung scans among 98 patients with silicosis. These investigators found that in 25% of their patients, ^{67}Ga accumulation was intense and more extensive than expected from the radiographic abnormalities. Nearly 90% of crocidolite-exposed workers who had asbestosis had increased gallium uptake in the lungs (172). In addition, pulmonary gallium uptake increased in almost one half of the crocidolite-exposed workers who do not have definite chest radiographic evidence of asbestosis. This finding suggested the presence of subclinical pulmonary inflammation (170). Although the disease findings in these workers did not meet the criteria for asbestosis, 85% of these patients had increased rigidity of the lung pressure volume curve. Several of these workers had evidence of macrophage al-

veolitis as detected with lung biopsy and lavage. Follow-up studies showed that most of these workers had asbestosis within 5 years (173). Hence asbestos-exposed individuals with equivocal or normal chest radiographs who have increased pulmonary gallium uptake or an abnormal lavage result appear at risk of development of asbestosis (172,173).

Pulmonary Drug Toxicity

There has been a rapid growth of the list of drugs and their injurious metabolites that have been implicated in lung injury. Reactive oxygen metabolites, for example, appear to play an important role in ARDS, emphysema, pulmonary oxygen toxicity, and radiation-induced pulmonary damage. Oxidant species include the superoxide anion, hydrogen peroxide, the hydroxyl radical, singlet oxygen, and hypochlorous acid. These molecules form within polymorphonuclear cells and phagocytic cells, including macrophages and monocytes. Toxic effects appear to occur through participation of these molecules in oxidation-reduction reactions and subsequent fatty-acid oxidation that may lead to membrane instability and inflammatory reactions (174).

Localization of ^{67}Ga in the pulmonary inflammation associated with cytotoxic or hypersensitivity injury has been reported for a large number of drugs. Amiodarone toxicity is a reasonable example of the use of ^{67}Ga in these disorders. Potentially lethal pulmonary toxicity may occur in 5% to 10% of patients receiving a daily dose of 400 to 800 mg of amiodarone for refractory arrhythmia. ^{67}Ga scintigraphy is reported to be sensitive to the presence of amiodarone pulmonary toxicity. Scan abnormalities often are intense, even when radiographic changes are subtle or nonspecific (175). Pulmonary toxicity and related ^{67}Ga uptake appear to be dose related, and resolution of scintigraphic and radiographic findings is observed when amiodarone is withheld (176). Thus abnormalities on ^{67}Ga images parallel the development of amiodarone pulmonary toxicity and may help to establish a diagnosis, especially when the chest radiographic findings are normal or ambiguous (176).

Adult Respiratory Distress Syndrome

ARDS is estimated to affect 150,000 persons each year and to be fatal for approximately one half of these patients (177). Radionuclide techniques used for the diagnosis and study of ARDS include the routine clinical procedures of perfusion lung scanning, gallium and white-cell imaging, PET-based indicator dilution methods for measuring extravascular lung water, and means of measuring protein accumulation, protein flux, and solute transfer (54). The techniques that reflect the rate of protein leak from the microvasculature and sensitive measures of rapidly reversible alveolar injury appear most promising. Although clinical usefulness remains to be documented, these methods may ultimately assist with the diagnosis of ARDS and with the evaluation of prognosis and therapy (178). Aerosol studies may be useful for evaluating patients with ARDS, because this disorder is associated with changes in alveolar-capillary permeability (20) that occur before radiographs and other forms of common clinical assessment are able to show the presence of the abnormality.

Infectious Lung Disease and Acquired Immunodeficiency Syndrome

Although ^{67}Ga has been described in association with all types of infectious etiologic factors, now its primary use in this regard is evaluation of patients who have AIDS and associated pneumonia. Worldwide, approximately 10 million persons are estimated to have infection with the human immunodeficiency virus (HIV). In the next decade, as many as 50% of these persons will have maladies related to HIV infection (179). Patients who have AIDS characteristically also have lymphocytopenia and are predisposed to opportunistic infection. The most common of these are *Pneumocystis carinii* pneumonia (PCP), disseminated *Mycobacterium avium–intracellulare* (MAI) infection, *Candida* esophagitis, toxoplasmosis, and cytomegalovirus (CMV), *Cryptococcus*, and herpes simplex infections.

^{67}Ga citrate scans play an important role in the clinical treatment of the patients with AIDS who have a fever or respiratory symptoms. In part this is because of the high prevalence of PCP among patients with AIDS and the high sensitivity (90% to 96%) of gallium scanning for PCP (180–182). Although diffuse interstitial infiltrates on chest radiographs may be present in early cases of PCP, subtle prolonged symptoms and normal findings on chest radiographs frequently occur. Unfortunately, chest radiographs have relatively low sensitivity for the detection of early lung disease in patients who have AIDS. Kramer et al. (181) found that 27 of 57 ^{67}Ga lung scans with abnormal findings were associated with normal chest radiographs. Conversely, normal findings on a gallium scan with abnormal findings on a chest radiograph often are associated with pulmonary Kaposi sarcoma (182). Kaposi sarcoma is a major manifestation of AIDS. In one review it was described as present (with or without other

manifestations of the syndrome) in one third of patients who had AIDS (183).

PCP has a variable presentation on gallium lung scans, ranging from no to total lung involvement and from minimal above background activity to greater than hepatic uptake (Fig. 19.26). Diffuse pulmonary uptake is the most common gallium scan pattern associated with PCP. Perihilar or nodal uptake is much less common but has been reported (181). In a study with 180 patients who had positive serologic results for HIV infection and had suspected pulmonary infection, the presence of a heterogeneous diffuse uptake pattern had an 87% positive predictive value for PCP, which was higher than that of any other pattern (184). The negative predictive value of a normal result of a ^{67}Ga lung scan for PCP was 96%. When scans with only nodal lung uptake also were considered negative for PCP, the negative predictive value increased to 98% (184). Kramer et al. (184) found a positive result of a ^{67}Ga lung scan to have a 93% positive predictive value for any pulmonary disease but commented that this value was probably low because of the difficulty in verifying disease in some patients. In another study, 20 patients with suspected PCP were evaluated with ^{67}Ga scans and fiberoptic bronchoscopy for initial diagnosis and response to therapy. ^{67}Ga localization was found in 100% of patients who had PCP, including those who had subclinical infection. Fiberoptic bronchoscopy demonstrated the presence of *P. carinii* in the bronchial washings of all of patients (19 patients), whereas only 13 of 16 patients (81%) were found to have *P. carinii* in lung tissue obtained by means of transbronchial biopsy (185).

Because gallium scanning is relatively expensive, requiring 48 to 72 hours to be completed, its use in the initial diagnosis of PCP generally should be restricted to patients who have normal

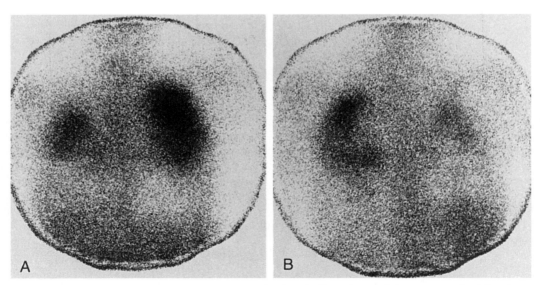

FIGURE 19.26. *Pneumocystic carinii* pneumonia (PCP) and effect of aerosol therapy. Anterior **(A)** and posterior **(B)** images of the thorax of a 45-year-old man with AIDS who was receiving prophylactic treatments of aerosolized pentamidine and had documented PCP infection involving primarily the upper lung zones. In **A,** the cardiac region is silhouetted by the lungs, a finding that suggests lower-intensity alveolitis in the lower lobes. The localization pattern is presumably caused by better delivery of aerosolized prophylactic drug to the lower lung regions. (From Line BR. Scintigraphic studies of inflammation in diffuse lung disease. *Radiol Clin North Am* 1991;29:1095–1114, with permission).

or atypical chest radiographs but suggestive clinical symptoms. A patient who has AIDS or who is at risk of AIDS who has typical symptoms and chest radiographic abnormalities suggestive of PCP do not need gallium scanning in addition to fiberoptic bronchoscopy to confirm the diagnosis (185). Because of the slow response to therapy and the high rate of recurrence, Ganz and Serafin (179) suggest that a baseline and a follow-up gallium scan may be useful to ascertain successful response to treatment and to detect early recurrences. PCP recurs in more than one half of patients within 18 months.

The effectiveness of gallium scanning among the HIV-seropositive population is the result of not only its sensitivity for PCP but also its utility in the detection of other opportunistic infections, inflammatory processes, and lymphomas that occur in these patients. When PCP is not present, other disease processes usually are documented. MAI, for example, causes widespread disease in 25% to 50% of patients with AIDS (186). Other granulomatous diseases that may mimic MAI infection include coccidioidomycosis, histoplasmosis, and tuberculosis. In mycobacterial lung infections, the gallium scintigraphic pattern may show increased activity associated with tuberculosis pleural effusion or tuberculosis lobar pneumonia or show patchy low-grade uptake along with hilar and nonhilar nodal uptake. The atypical mycobacterial infections manifest more frequently as extra hilar nodes, whereas tuberculosis tends to be more commonly limited to hilar uptake (179). In one study, the positive predictive value for MAI infection of gallium accumulation in intrathoracic regional lymph nodes was 90% (181). Only one patient had lymphadenopathy appreciated on the plain radiograph. Because MAI infection is common among AIDS patients, the finding of focal lymph node ^{67}Ga uptake (Fig. 19.27) should suggest MAI lymphadenitis (181). However, nodal gallium uptake along with normal lung activity has been seen in patients who have lymphoma (184,187) and possibly in those who have AIDS-related complex lymphadenopathy (187).

Siemsen et al. (158) reported high-intensity ^{67}Ga pulmonary uptake in 97% of patients with active tuberculosis. These investigators found a positive correlation between the extent of gallium accumulation and the extent of radiographic abnormality. All patients with active disease and a positive baseline result of a gallium scan who underwent repeated scanning 3 to 9 months

after tuberculostatic chemotherapy had disappearance or marked regression of gallium concentration (158). Although active disease is difficult to diagnose when extensive fibrotic areas appear on chest radiographs, reactivated tuberculous foci can be found with gallium imaging (158). Whole-body scanning appears to be a simple, useful means to locate active foci of extrapulmonary tuberculosis and can demonstrate the response to effective therapy (188).

Of the bacterial infections in patients who have AIDS, streptococcal pneumonia is the most common, but *Haemophilus influenzae* and *Salmonella typhi* also occur. The gallium scintigraphic pattern of localized lobar uptake without nodal uptake suggests bacterial infection rather than PCP or mycobacterial infection. When ^{67}Ga is localized in multiple pulmonary lobes as well as in bone, an aggressive bacterial infection such as actinomycosis or nocardia should be considered (189). In these aggressive bacterial infections, the results of needle biopsy often are negative.

Clinically significant pulmonary CMV infection is uncommon and usually occurs in conjunction with more aggressive PCP. Because of the difficulty in diagnosing CMV infection, the pattern of uptake seen on a whole-body gallium scan may be important. CMV infection is suggested by a pattern of low-grade lung uptake with perihilar prominence (184) associated with eye (retinitis), adrenal, and renal uptake at 48 hours or persistent colonic uptake when diarrhea persists and there are no obvious pathogens in several stool specimens (179).

FUTURE APPLICATIONS OF RADIONUCLIDE LUNG STUDIES

In the past, pulmonary nuclear medicine has been dominated by techniques that depict the distribution of pulmonary perfusion and ventilation, or V/Q balance, and these techniques have been used to detect pulmonary embolism, obstructive airway disease, carcinoma of the lung, and other pulmonary disorders in humans. With the development of emission tomography and the potential for new, function-oriented radiopharmaceuticals, nuclear medicine investigators are developing techniques for assessing alveolar-capillary permeability to specific molecules, for evaluation of pulmonary cell kinetics and the role of these cells in pulmonary disorders, and for evaluating various aspects of lung metabolism. The years ahead are likely to see major improvements in our ability to diagnose nonembolic pulmonary disorders.

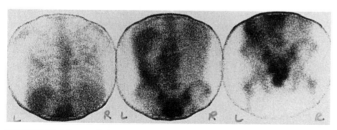

FIGURE 19.27. Nodal disease pattern in a patient with *Mycobacterium avium–intracellulare* infection. Posterior ^{67}Ga scans of the chest, abdomen, and pelvis of a 37-year-old man with AIDS. The patient had a history of *Pneumocystis carinii* pneumonia but had nodal uptake in the hilar zones and paraaortic region as well as splenic and marrow space prominence. The patient was subsequently found to have a disseminated *Mycobacterium avium–intracellulare* infection. (From Line BR. Scintigraphic studies of inflammation in diffuse lung disease. *Radiol Clin North Am* 1991;29:1095–1114, with permission).

REFERENCES

1. Kessler RM, McNeil BJ. Impaired ventilation in a patient with angiographically demonstrated pulmonary emboli. *Radiology* 1975;114:111–112.
2. Moser KM. Pulmonary embolism. *Am Rev Respir Dis* 1977;115:829–952.
3. Scadding JG. Diffuse pulmonary alveolar fibrosis. *Thorax* 1974;29:271–281.
4. West JB. Pulmonary function studies with radioactive gases. *Annu Rev Med* 1967;18:459–470.
5. Fedullo PF, Moser KM, Hartman MT, et al. Patterns of pulmonary

perfusion scans in normal subjects, III: the prevalence of abnormal scans in nonsmokers 30 to 49 years of age. *Am Rev Respir Dis* 1983; 127:776–779.

6. Bunow B, Line BR, Horton MR, et al. Regional ventilatory clearance by xenon scintigraphy: a critical evaluation of two estimation procedures. *J Nucl Med* 1979;20:703–710.

7. Secker-Walker RH, Hill RI, Markham J, et al. The measurement of regional ventilation in man: a new method of quantitation. *J Nucl Med* 1973;14:725–732.

8. Harf A, Pratt T, Hughes JMB. Regional distribution of Va/Q in man at rest and with exercise measured with krypton-81m. *J Appl Physiol* 1978;0:115–123.

9. Hughes JM. Short-life radionuclides and regional lung function. *Br J Radiol* 1979;52:353–370.

10. Meignan M, Simonneau G, Oliveira L, et al. Computation of ventilation-perfusion ratio with Kr-81m in pulmonary embolism. *J Nucl Med* 1984;25:149–155.

11. Modell HI, Graham MM. Limitations of Kr-81m for quantitation of ventilation scans. *J Nucl Med* 1982;23:301–305.

12. Stuart BO. Deposition of inhaled aerosols. *Arch Intern Med* 1973; 131:60–73.

13. Coates G, Dolovich M, Koehler D, et al. Ventilation scanning with technetium labeled aerosols. DTPA or sulfur colloid? *Clin Nucl Med* 1985;10:835–838.

14. Alderson PO, Biello DR, Gottschalk A, et al. Tc-99m-DTPA aerosol and radioactive gases compared as adjuncts to perfusion scintigraphy in patients with suspected pulmonary embolism. *Radiology* 1984;153: 515–521.

15. Susskind H, Brill AB, Harold WH. Quantitative comparison of regional distributions of inhaled Tc-99m DTPA aerosol and Kr-81m gas in coal miners' lungs. *Am J Physiol Imaging* 1986;1:67–76.

16. Burch WM, Sullivan PJ, McLaren CJ. Technegas: a new ventilation agent for lung scanning. *Nucl Med Commun* 1986;7:865–971.

17. Senden TJ, Moock KH, Gerald JF, et al. The physical and chemical nature of technegas. *J Nucl Med* 1997;38:1327–1333.

18. Isawa T, Lee BT, Hiraga K. High-resolution electron microscopy of technegas and pertechnegas. *Nucl Med Commun* 1996;17:147–152.

19. Lloyd JJ, Shields RA, Taylor CJ, et al. Technegas and pertechnegas particle size distribution. *Eur J Nucl Med* 1995;22:473–476.

20. Huchon GJ, Little JW, Murray JF. Assessment of alveolar–capillary membrane permeability of dogs by aerosolization. *J Appl Physiol* 1981; 51:955–962.

21. Rinderknecht J, Shapiro L, Krauthammer M, et al. Accelerated clearance of small solutes from the lungs in interstitial lung disease. *Am Rev Respir Dis* 1980;121:105–117.

22. Jones JG, Minty BD, Lawler P, et al. Increased alveolar epithelial permeability in cigarette smokers. *Lancet* 1980;1:66–68.

23. Sugerman HJ, Strash AM, Hirsch JI, et al. Sensitivity of scintigraphy for detection of pulmonary capillary albumin leak in canine oleic acid ARDS. *J Trauma* 1981;21:520–527.

24. Anderson RR, Holliday RL, Driedger AA, et al. Documentation of pulmonary capillary permeability in the adult respiratory distress syndrome accompanying human sepsis. *Am Rev Respir Dis* 1979;119: 869–877.

25. Rizk NW, Luce JM, Hoeffel JM, et al. Site of deposition and factors affecting clearance of aerosolized solute from canine lungs. *J Appl Physiol* 1984;56:723–729.

26. Meignan M, Rosso J, Leveau J, et al. Exercise increases the lung clearance of inhaled technetium-99m DTPA. *J Nucl Med* 1986;27: 274–280.

27. Evander E, Wollmer P, Jonson B. Pulmonary clearance of inhaled [99Tcm]DTPA: effects of ventilation pattern. *Clin Physiol* 1990;10: 189–199.

28. Egan EA, Nelson RM, Olver RE. Lung inflation and alveolar permeability to non-electrolytes in the adult sheep in vivo. *J Physiol (Lond)* 1976;260:409–424.

29. Coates G, O'Brodovich H. Measurement of pulmonary epithelial permeability with 99mTc-DTPA aerosol. *Semin Nucl Med* 1986;16: 275–284.

30. Fanti S, Compagnone G, Pancaldi D, et al. Evaluation of lung clearance of inhaled pertechnegas. *Ann Nucl Med* 1996;10:147–151.

31. Isawa T, Teshima T, Anazawa Y, et al. Inhalation of pertechnegas: similar clearance from the lungs to that of inhaled pertechnetate aerosol. *Nucl Med Commun* 1995;16:741–746.

32. Smith RJ, Hyde RW, Waldman DL, et al. Effect of pattern of aerosol inhalation on clearance of technetium-99m-labeled diethylenetriamine pentaacetic acid from the lungs of normal humans. *Am Rev Respir Dis* 1992;145:1109–1116.

33. Mason GR, Effros RM, Uszler JM, et al. Small solute clearance from the lungs of patients with cardiogenic and noncardiogenic pulmonary edema. *Chest* 1985;88:327–334.

34. Mason GR, Duane GB, Mena I, et al. Accelerated solute clearance in *Pneumocystis carinii* pneumonia. *Am Rev Respir Dis* 1987;135: 864–868.

35. Huchon GJ, Montgomery AB, Lipavsky A, et al. Respiratory clearance of aerosolized radioactive solutes of varying molecular weight. *J Nucl Med* 1987;28:894–902.

36. Peterson BT, Dickerson KD, James HL, et al. Comparison of three tracers for detecting lung epithelial injury in anesthetized sheep. *J Appl Physiol* 1989;66:2374–2383.

37. Kosuda S, Kubo A, Sanmiya T, et al. Assessment of mucociliary clearance in patients with tracheobronchoplasty using radioaerosol. *J Nucl Med* 1986;27:1397–1402.

38. Pifferi M, Caramella D, Bartolozzi C, et al. CT-guided radiolabelled aerosol studies for assessing pulmonary impairment in children with bronchiectasis. *Pediatr Radiol* 2000;30:632–637.

39. O'Riordan TG, Zwang J, Smaldone GC. Mucociliary clearance in adult asthma. *Am Rev Respir Dis* 1992;146:598–603.

40. Konrad F, Schreiber T, Brecht-Kraus D, et al. Mucociliary transport in ICU patients. *Chest* 1994;105:237–241.

41. Beaumont D, Herry JY, le Cloirec J, et al. Sensitivity of 67Ga-scanning in sarcoidosis: detection of biopsy proven pulmonary lesions radiographically undetectable. *Eur J Nucl Med* 1982;7:41–43.

42. Keogh BA, Hunninghake GW, Line BR, et al. The alveolitis of pulmonary sarcoidosis: evaluation of natural history and alveolitis-dependent changes in lung function. *Am Rev Respir Dis* 1983;128:256–265.

43. Hoffer PB, Huberty J, Khayam BH. The association of Ga-67 and lactoferrin. *J Nucl Med* 1977;18:713–717.

44. Tsuchiya Y, Nakao A, Komatsu T, et al. Relationship between gallium 67 citrate scanning and transferrin receptor expression in lung diseases. *Chest* 1992;102:530–534.

45. Crystal RG, Bitterman PB, Rennard SI, et al. Interstitial lung diseases of unknown cause: disorders characterized by chronic inflammation of the lower respiratory tract. *N Engl J Med* 1984;310:235–244.

46. Kennedy SM, Walker DC, Belzberg AS, et al. Macrophage accumulation of inhaled gallium-67 citrate in normal lungs. *J Nucl Med* 1985; 26:1195–1201.

47. Johnson PM, Berdon WE, Baker DH, et al. Thymic uptake of gallium-67 citrate in a healthy 4 year old boy. *Pediatr Radiol* 1978;7: 243–244.

48. Line BR, Fulmer JD, Reynolds HY, et al. Gallium-67 citrate scanning in the staging of idiopathic pulmonary fibrosis: correlation and physiologic and morphologic features and bronchoalveolar lavage. *Am Rev Respir Dis* 1978;118:355–365.

49. Siemsen JK, Grebe SF, Sargent EN, et al. Gallium-67 scintigraphy of pulmonary diseases as a complement to radiography. *Radiology* 1976;118:371–375.

50. Gillis CN. Metabolism of vasoactive hormones by lung. *Anesthesiology* 1973;39:626–632.

51. Touya JJ, Rahimian J, Grubbs DE, et al. A noninvasive procedure for in vivo assay of a lung amine endothelial receptor. *J Nucl Med* 1985;26:1302–1307.

52. Slosman DO, Brill AB, Polla BS, et al. Evaluation of [iodine-125]N,N,N'-trimethyl-N'-[2-hydroxy-3-methyl-5-iodobenzyl]-1,3-propanediamine lung uptake using an isolated-perfused lung model. *J Nucl Med* 1987;28:203–208.

53. Slosman DO, Polla BS, Donath A. 123I-MIBG pulmonary removal: a biochemical marker of minimal lung endothelial cell lesions. *Eur J Nucl Med* 1990;16:633–637.

54. Schuster DP. Positron emission tomography: theory and its application to the study of lung disease. *Am Rev Respir Dis* 1989;139:818–840.

55. Robinson NB, Hudson LD, Robertson HT, et al. Ventilation and perfusion alterations after smoke inhalation injury. *Surgery* 1981;90:352–363.

56. Alderson PO, Bradley EW, Mendenhall KG, et al. Radionuclide evaluation of pulmonary function following hemithorax irradiation of normal dogs with 60Co or fast neutrons. *Radiology* 1979;130:425–433.

57. Oppenheimer L, Craven KD, Forkert L, et al. Pathophysiology of pulmonary contusion in dogs. *J Appl Physiol* 1979;47:718–728.

58. Fazio F, Lavender JP, Steiner RE. 81mKr ventilation and 99mTc perfusion scans in chest disease: comparison with standard radiographs. *Am J Roentgenol* 1978;130:421–428.

59. Susskind H, Atkins HL, Goldman AG, et al. Sensitivity of Kr-81m and Xe-127 in evaluating nonembolic pulmonary disease. *J Nucl Med* 1981;22:781–786.

60. Barter SJ, Cunningham DA, Lavender JP, et al. Abnormal ventilation scans in middle-aged smokers: comparison with tests of overall lung function. *Am Rev Respir Dis* 1985;132:148–151.

61. Narabayashi I, Otsuka N. Pulmonary ventilation and perfusion studies in lung cancer. *Clin Nucl Med* 1984;9:97–102.

62. Ellis DA, Hawkins T, Gibson GJ, et al. Role of lung scanning in assessing the resectability of bronchial carcinoma. *Thorax* 1983;38:261–266.

63. Gordon I, Helms P, Fazio F. Clinical applications of radionuclide lung scanning in infants and children. *Br J Radiol* 1981;54:576–585.

64. Fein R, Thal W, Otto HJ, et al. Combined 113Xe/99mTC human serum albumin microspheres lung scintigraphy in children with recurrent and chronic bronchitis. *Z Erkr Atmungsorgane* 1988;171:135–142.

65. Kropp J, Overbeck B, Klumpp J, et al. Inhalation scintigraphy with an ultrafine aerosol in infants with functional bronchial stenoses. *Clin Nucl Med* 1993;18:223–226.

66. Moote D, Ehrlich L, Martin RH. Postpneumonectomy bronchopleural fistula imaged by ventilation lung scanning. *Clin Nucl Med* 1987;12:337–338.

67. Samuel J, Houlder AE. Use of Xe-133 gas in the detection of foreign bodies in the lower respiratory tract. *Clin Otolaryngol* 1987;12:115–117.

68. Miller MB, Caride VJ. Ventilation-perfusion scan in the acutely ill patient with unilateral hyperlucent lung. *J Nucl Med* 1988;29:114–117.

69. Tamir A, Melloul M, Berant M, et al. Lung perfusion scans in patients with congenital heart defects. *J Am Coll Cardiol* 1992;19:383–388.

70. Houzard C, Andre M, Guilhen S, et al. Perfusion lung scan in patients operated for transposition of the great arteries. *Clin Nucl Med* 1989;14:268–270.

71. Hayashida K, Nishimura T, Kumita S, et al. Scintigraphic determination of severity in pulmonary parenchymal damage in patients with atrial septal defect. *Eur J Nucl Med* 1990;16:713–716.

72. Grimon G, Andre L, Bernard O, et al. Early radionuclide detection of intrapulmonary shunts in children with liver disease. *J Nucl Med* 1994;35:1328–1332.

73. Chilvers ER, Peters AM, George P, et al. Quantification of right to left shunt through pulmonary arteriovenous malformations using 99Tcm albumin microspheres. *Clin Radiol* 1988;39:611–614.

74. Winzelberg GG, Wholey MH, Jarmolowski CA, et al. Patients with hemoptysis examined by Tc-99m sulfur colloid and Tc-99m-labeled red blood cells: a preliminary appraisal. *Radiology* 1984;153:523–526.

75. Haponik EF, Rothfeld B, Britt EJ, et al. Radionuclide localization of massive pulmonary hemorrhage. *Chest* 1984;86:208–212.

76. Fishman AJ, Moser KM, Fedullo PF. Perfusion lung scans vs pulmonary angiography in evaluation of suspected primary pulmonary hypertension. *Chest* 1983;84:679–683.

77. Lisbona R, Kreisman H, Novales DJ, et al. Perfusion lung scanning: differentiation of primary from thromboembolic pulmonary hypertension. *Am J Roentgenol* 1985;144:27–30.

78. Patz EF Jr, Lowe VJ, Hoffman JM, et al. Persistent or recurrent bronchogenic carcinoma: detection with PET and 2-[F-18]-2-deoxy-D-glucose. *Radiology* 1994;191:379–382.

79. Valanis BG. Epidemiology of lung cancer: a worldwide epidemic. *Semin Oncol Nurs* 1996;12:251–259.

80. Boring CC, Squires TS, Tong T, et al. Cancer statistics, 1994. *CA Cancer J Clin* 1994;44:7–26.

81. Ferguson MK. Diagnosing and staging of non–small cell lung cancer. *Hematol Oncol Clin North Am* 1990;4:1053–1068.

82. Mountain CF. A new international staging system for lung cancer. *Chest* 1986;89:225S–233S.

83. Mountain CF. Revisions in the international system for staging lung cancer. *Chest* 1997;111:1710–1717.

84. Leitha T, Meghdadi S, Studnicka M, et al. The role of iodine-123-Tyr-3-octreotide scintigraphy in the staging of small-cell lung cancer. *J Nucl Med* 1993;34:1397–1402.

85. Front D, Israel O, Even SE, et al. The concentration of bleomycin labeled with Co-57 in primary and metastatic tumors. *Cancer* 1989;64:988–993.

86. Edwards CL, Hayes RL. Tumor scanning with 67Ga citrate. *J Nucl Med* 1969;10:103–105.

87. van der Schoot JB, Groen AS, et al. Gallium-67 scintigraphy in lung diseases. *Thorax* 1972;27:543–546.

88. Abdel-Dayem HM, Scott A, Macapinlac H, et al. Tracer imaging in lung cancer. *Eur J Nucl Med* 1994;21:57–81.

89. Rusch V, Macapinlac H, Heelan R, et al. NR-LU-10 monoclonal antibody scanning: a helpful new adjunct to computed tomography in evaluating non-small-cell lung cancer. *J Thorac Cardiovasc Surg* 1993;106:200–204.

90. Kramer EL, Noz ME. CT-SPECT fusion for analysis of radiolabeled antibodies: applications in gastrointestinal and lung carcinoma. *Int J Rad Appl Instrum B* 1991;18:27–42.

91. Kramer EL, Noz ME, Liebes L, et al. Radioimmunodetection of non–small cell lung cancer using technetium-99m-anticarcinoembryonic antigen IMMU-4 Fab' fragment: preliminary results. *Cancer* 1994;73:890–895.

92. Biggi A, Buccheri G, Ferrigno D, et al. Detection of suspected primary lung cancer by scintigraphy with indium-111-anti-carcinoembryonic antigen monoclonal antibodies (type F023C5). *J Nucl Med* 1991;32:2064–2068.

93. Buccheri G, Biggi A, Ferrigno D, et al. Anti-CEA immunoscintigraphy might be more useful than computed tomography in the preoperative thoracic evaluation of lung cancer: a comparison between planar immunoscintigraphy, single photon emission computed tomography (SPECT), and computed tomography. *Chest* 1993;104:734–742.

94. Krenning EP, Bakker WH, Breeman WA, et al. Localisation of endocrine-related tumours with radioiodinated analogue of somatostatin. *Lancet* 1989;1:242–244.

95. Hochstenbag MM, Heidendal GA, Wouters EF, et al. In-111 octreotide imaging in staging of small cell lung cancer. *Clin Nucl Med* 1997;22:811–816.

96. Taylor JE, Theveniau MA, Bashirzadeh R, et al. Detection of somatostatin receptor subtype 2 (SSTR2) in established tumors and tumor cell lines: evidence for SSTR2 heterogeneity. *Peptides* 1994;15:1229–1236.

97. Berenger N, Moretti JL, Boaziz C, et al. Somatostatin receptor imaging in small cell lung cancer. *Eur J Cancer* 1996;32A:1429–1431.

98. Hirano T, Otake H, Yoshida I, et al. Primary lung cancer SPECT imaging with pentavalent technetium-99m-DMSA. *J Nucl Med* 1995;36:202–207.

99. Takekawa H, Itoh K, Abe S, et al. Thallium-201 uptake, histopathological differentiation and Na-K ATPase in lung adenocarcinoma. *J Nucl Med* 1996;37:955–958.

100. Tonami N, Yokoyama K, Shuke N, et al. Evaluation of suspected malignant pulmonary lesions with 201Tl single photon emission computed tomography. *Nucl Med Commun* 1993;14:602–610.

101. Tonami N, Shuke N, Yokoyama K, et al. Thallium-201 single photon emission computed tomography in the evaluation of suspected lung cancer. *J Nucl Med* 1989;30:997–1004.

102. Piwnica-Worms D, Kronauge JF, Chiu ML. Uptake and retention of hexakis (2-methoxyisobutyl isonitrile) technetium(I) in cultured

chick myocardial cells: mitochondrial and plasma membrane potential dependence. *Circulation* 1990;82:1826–1838.

103. Chiti A, Maffioli LS, Infante M, et al. Assessment of mediastinal involvement in lung cancer with technetium-99m-sestamibi SPECT. *J Nucl Med* 1996;37:938–942.

104. Luker GD, Fracasso PM, Dobkin J, et al. Modulation of the multidrug resistance P-glycoprotein: detection with technetium-99m-sestamibi in vivo. *J Nucl Med* 1997;38:369–372.

105. Bom HS, Kim YC, Song HC, et al. Technetium-99m-MIBI uptake in small cell lung cancer. *J Nucl Med* 1998;39:91–94.

106. Kostakoglu L, Kiratli P, Ruacan S, et al. Association of tumor washout rates and accumulation of technetium-99m-MIBI with expression of P-glycoprotein in lung cancer. *J Nucl Med* 1998;39:228–234.

107. Wahl RL, Quint LE, Greenough RL, et al. Staging of mediastinal non–small cell lung cancer with FDG PET, CT, and fusion images: preliminary prospective evaluation. *Radiology* 1994;191:371–377.

108. Knight SB, Delbeke D, Stewart JR, et al. Evaluation of pulmonary lesions with FDG-PET: comparison of findings in patients with and without a history of prior malignancy. *Chest* 1996;109:982–988.

109. Bury T, Dowlati A, Paulus P, et al. Whole-body 18FDG positron emission tomography in the staging of non–small cell lung cancer. *Eur Respir J* 1997;10:2529–2534.

110. Patz EF Jr, Lowe VJ, Hoffman JM, et al. Focal pulmonary abnormalities: evaluation with F-18 fluorodeoxyglucose PET scanning. *Radiology* 1993;188:487–490.

111. Waxman AD. The role of nuclear medicine in pulmonary neoplastic processes. *Semin Nucl Med* 1986;16:285–295.

112. Strauss LG, Conti PS. The applications of PET in clinical oncology. *J Nucl Med* 1991;32:623–648.

113. Fujimoto J. Radioautographic studies on the intracellular distribution of bleomycin-14C in mouse tumor cells. *Cancer Res* 1974;34:2969–2974.

114. Even SE, Bettman L, Iosilevsky G, et al. SPECT quantitation of cobalt-57–bleomycin to predict treatment response and outcome of patients with lung cancer. *J Nucl Med* 1994;35:1129–1133.

115. Lowe VJ, Hoffman JM, Delong DM, et al. Semiquantitative and visual analysis of FDG-PET images in pulmonary abnormalities. *J Nucl Med* 1994;35:1771–1776.

116. Patz EF Jr, Lowe VJ, Hoffman JM, et al. Focal pulmonary abnormalities: evaluation with F-18 fluorodeoxyglucose PET scanning. *Radiology* 1993;188:487–490.

117. Lowe VJ, Delong DM, Hoffman JM, et al. Optimum scanning protocol for FDG-PET evaluation of pulmonary malignancy. *J Nucl Med* 1995;36:883–887.

118. Duhaylongsod FG, Lowe VJ, Patz EF Jr, et al. Detection of primary and recurrent lung cancer by means of F-18 fluorodeoxyglucose positron emission tomography (FDG PET). *J Thorac Cardiovasc Surg* 1995;110:130–139.

119. Duhaylongsod FG, Lowe VJ, Patz EF Jr, et al. Lung tumor growth correlates with glucose metabolism measured by fluoride-18 fluorodeoxyglucose positron emission tomography. *Ann Thorac Surg* 1995;60:1348–1352.

120. Higashi K, Ueda Y, Seki H, et al. Fluorine-18-FDG PET imaging is negative in bronchioloalveolar lung carcinoma. *J Nucl Med* 1998;39:1016–1020.

121. Caskey CI, Zerhouni EA. The solitary pulmonary nodule. *Semin Roentgenol* 1990;25:85–95.

122. Lillington GA. Management of solitary pulmonary nodules. *Dis Mon* 1991;37:271–318.

123. Dewan NA, Gupta NC, Redepenning LS, et al. Diagnostic efficacy of PET-FDG imaging in solitary pulmonary nodules: potential role in evaluation and management. *Chest* 1993;104:997–1002.

124. Gupta NC, Frank AR, Dewan NA, et al. Solitary pulmonary nodules: detection of malignancy with PET with 2-[F-18]-fluoro-2-deoxy-D-glucose. *Radiology* 1992;184:441–444.

125. Conti PS, Lilien DL, Hawley K, et al. PET and [18F]-FDG in oncology: a clinical update. *Nucl Med Biol* 1996;23:717–735.

126. Lowe VJ, Duhaylongsod FG, Patz EF, et al. Pulmonary abnormalities and PET data analysis: a retrospective study. *Radiology* 1997;202:435–439.

127. Kubota K, Matsuzawa T, Fujiwara T, et al. Differential diagnosis of lung tumor with positron emission tomography: a prospective study. *J Nucl Med* 1990;31:1927–1932.

128. Webb WR, Gatsonis C, Zerhouni EA, et al. CT and MR imaging in staging of non–small cell bronchogenic carcinoma: report of the Radiologic Diagnostic Oncology Group. *Radiology* 1991;178:705–713.

129. Patz EF Jr, Lowe VJ, Goodman PC, et al. Thoracic nodal staging with PET imaging with 18FDG in patients with bronchogenic carcinoma. *Chest* 1995;108:1617–1621.

130. Scott WJ, Gobar LS, Terry JD, et al. Mediastinal lymph node staging of non–small-cell lung cancer: a prospective comparison of computed tomography and positron emission tomography. *J Thorac Cardiovasc Surg* 1996;111:642–648.

131. Vansteenkiste JF, Stroobants SG, De Leyn PR, et al. Mediastinal lymph node staging with FDG-PET scan in patients with potentially operable non–small cell lung cancer: a prospective analysis of 50 cases. Leuven Lung Cancer Group. *Chest* 1997;112:1480–1486.

132. Steinert HC, Hauser M, Allemann F, et al. Non–small cell lung cancer: nodal staging with FDG PET versus CT with correlative lymph node mapping and sampling. *Radiology* 1997;202:441–446.

133. Ichiya Y, Kuwabara Y, Otsuka M, et al. Assessment of response to cancer therapy using fluorine-18-fluorodeoxyglucose and positron emission tomography. *J Nucl Med* 1991;32:1655–1660.

134. Kim EE, Chung SK, Haynie TP, et al. Differentiation of residual or recurrent tumors from post-treatment changes with F-18 FDG PET. *Radiographics* 1992;12:269–279.

135. Kubota K, Yamada S, Ishiwata K, et al. Evaluation of the treatment response of lung cancer with positron emission tomography and L-[methyl-11C]methionine: a preliminary study. *Eur J Nucl Med* 1993;20:495–501.

136. Frank A, Lefkowitz D, Jaeger S, et al. Decision logic for retreatment of asymptomatic lung cancer recurrence based on positron emission tomography findings. *Int J Radiat Oncol Biol Phys* 1995;32:1495–1512.

137. Pannier R, Verlinde I, Puspowidjono I, et al. Role of gallium 67 thoracic scintigraphy in the diagnosis and staging of patients suspected of bronchial carcinoma. *Thorax* 1982;37:264–269.

138. Fosburg RG, Hopkins GB, Kan MK. Evaluation of the mediastinum by gallium-67 scintigraphy in lung cancer. *J Thorac Cardiovasc Surg* 1979;77:76–82.

139. MacMahon H, Scott W, Ryan JW, et al. Efficacy of computed tomography of the thorax and upper abdomen and whole-body gallium scintigraphy for staging of lung cancer. *Cancer* 1989;64:1404–1408.

140. Lipscomb DJ, Pride NB. Ventilation and perfusion scans in the preoperative assessment of bronchial carcinoma. *Thorax* 1977;32:720–725.

141. Katz RD, Alderson PO, Tockman MS, et al. Ventilation-perfusion lung scanning in patients detected by a screening program for early lung carcinoma. *Radiology* 1981;141:171–178.

142. Secker-Walker RH, Alderson PO, Wilhelm J, et al. Ventilation-perfusion scanning in carcinoma of the bronchus. *Chest* 1974;65:660–663.

143. Olsen GN, Block AJ, Swenson EW, et al. Pulmonary function evaluation of the lung resection candidate: a prospective study. *Am Rev Respir Dis* 1975;111:379–387.

144. Williams CD, Brenowitz JB. "Prohibitive" lung function and major surgical procedures. *Am J Surg* 1976;132:763–766.

145. Wernly JA, DeMeester TR, Kirchner PT, et al. Clinical value of quantitative ventilation-perfusion lung scans in the surgical management of bronchogenic carcinoma. *J Thorac Cardiovasc Surg* 1980;80:535–543.

146. DeMeester TR, Van Heertum RL, Karas JR, et al. Preoperative evaluation with differential pulmonary function. *Ann Thorac Surg* 1974;18:61–71.

147. Block AJ, Olsen GN. Preoperative pulmonary function testing. *JAMA* 1976;235:257–258.

148. Ciofetta G, Silverman M, Hughes JM. Quantitative approach to the study of regional lung function in children using krypton 81m. *Br J Radiol* 1980;53:950–959.

149. Krumpe PE, Lum CC, Cross CE. Approach to the patient with diffuse lung disease. *Med Clin North Am* 1988;72:1225–1246.

150. Crystal RG, Gadek JE, Ferrans VJ, et al. Interstitial lung disease:

current concepts of pathogenesis, staging and therapy. *Am J Med* 1981;70:542–568.

151. Pantin CF, Valind SO, Sweatman M, et al. Measures of the inflammatory response in cryptogenic fibrosing alveolitis. *Am Rev Respir Dis* 1988;138:1234–1241.

152. Bekerman C, Hoffer PB, Bitran JD, et al. Gallium-67 citrate imaging studies of the lung. *Semin Nucl Med* 1980;10:286–301.

153. Richman SD, Levenson SM, Bunn PA, et al. 67Ga accumulation in pulmonary lesions associated with bleomycin toxicity. *Cancer* 1975;36:1966–1972.

154. MacMahon H, Bekerman C. The diagnostic significance of gallium lung uptake in patients with normal chest radiographs. *Radiology* 1978;127:189–193.

155. Line BR, Hunninghake GW, Keogh BA, et al. Gallium-67 scanning to stage the alveolitis of sarcoidosis: correlation with clinical studies, pulmonary function studies, and bronchoalveolar lavage. *Am Rev Respir Dis* 1981;123:440–446.

156. Israel HL. Prognosis of sarcoidosis. *Ann Intern Med* 1970;73:1038–1039.

157. Heshiki A, Schatz SL, McKusick KA, et al. Gallium 67 citrate scanning in patients with pulmonary sarcoidosis. *Am J Roentgenol Radium Ther Nucl Med* 1974;122:744–749.

158. Siemsen JK, Grebe SF, Waxman AD. The use of gallium-67 in pulmonary disorders. *Semin Nucl Med* 1978;8:235–249.

159. Rizzato G, Blasi A. A European survey on the usefulness of 67Ga lung scans in assessing sarcoidosis: experience in 14 research centers in seven different countries. *Ann N Y Acad Sci* 1986;0:463–478.

160. Sulavik SB, Spencer RP, Weed DA, et al. Recognition of distinctive patterns of gallium-67 distribution in sarcoidosis. *J Nucl Med* 1990;31:1909–1914.

161. Young RL, Krumholz RA, Harkleroad LE. A physiologic roentgenographic disparity in sarcoidosis. *Dis Chest* 1966;50:81–86.

162. Israel HL, Gushue GF, Park CH. Assessment of gallium-67 scanning in pulmonary and extrapulmonary sarcoidosis. *Ann N Y Acad Sci* 1986;0:455–462.

163. Crystal RG, Fulmer JD, Roberts WC, et al. Idiopathic pulmonary fibrosis: clinical, histologic, radiographic, physiologic, scintigraphic, cytologic, and biochemical aspects. *Ann Intern Med* 1976;85:769–788.

164. Turner WM, Haslam PL. The value of serial bronchoalveolar lavages in assessing the clinical progress of patients with cryptogenic fibrosing alveolitis. *Am Rev Respir Dis* 1987;135:26–34.

165. Vanderstappen M, Mornex JF, Lahneche B, et al. Gallium-67 scanning in the staging of cryptogenetic fibrosing alveolitis and hypersensitivity pneumonitis. *Eur Respir J* 1988;1:517–522.

166. Baron M, Feiglin D, Hyland R, et al. 67Gallium lung scans in progressive systemic sclerosis. *Arthritis Rheum* 1983;26:969–974.

167. Rossi GA, Bitterman PB, Rennard SI, et al. Evidence for chronic inflammation as a component of the interstitial lung disease associated with progressive systemic sclerosis. *Am Rev Respir Dis* 1985;131:612–617.

168. Greene NB, Solinger AM, Baughman RP. Patients with collagen vascular disease and dyspnea: the value of gallium scanning and bronchoalveolar lavage in predicting response to steroid therapy and clinical outcome. *Chest* 1987;91:698–703.

169. Rom WN, Bitterman PB, Rennard SI, et al. Characterization of the lower respiratory tract inflammation of nonsmoking individuals with interstitial lung disease associated with chronic inhalation of inorganic dusts. *Am Rev Respir Dis* 1987;136:1429–1434.

170. Begin R, Cantin A, Drapeau G, et al. Pulmonary uptake of gallium-67 in asbestos-exposed humans and sheep. *Am Rev Respir Dis* 1983;127:623–630.

171. Siemsen JK, Sargent EN, Grebe SF, et al. Pulmonary concentration of Ga67 in pneumoconiosis. *Am J Roentgenol Radium Ther Nucl Med* 1974;120:815–820.

172. Hayes AA, Mullan B, Lovegrove FT, et al. Gallium lung scanning and bronchoalveolar lavage in crocidolite-exposed workers. *Chest* 1989;96:22–26.

173. Begin R, Cantin A, Berthiaume Y, et al. Clinical features to stage alveolitis in asbestos workers. *Am J Ind Med* 1985;8:521–536.

174. Freeman BA, Crapo JD. Biology of disease: free radicals and tissue injury. *Lab Invest* 1982;47:412–426.

175. van Rooij WJ, van der Meer SC, van Royen EA, et al. Pulmonary gallium-67 uptake in amiodarone pneumonitis. *J Nucl Med* 1984;25:211–213.

176. Zhu YY, Botvinick E, Dae M, et al. Gallium lung scintigraphy in amiodarone pulmonary toxicity. *Chest* 1988;93:1126–1131.

177. Rinaldo JE, Rogers RM. Adult respiratory-distress syndrome: changing concepts of lung injury and repair. *N Engl J Med* 1982;306:900–909.

178. Mishkin FS, Mason GR. Application of nuclear medicine techniques to the study of ARDS. *J Thorac Imaging* 1990;5:1–8.

179. Ganz WI, Serafini AN. The diagnostic role of nuclear medicine in the acquired immunodeficiency syndrome. *J Nucl Med* 1989;30:1935–1945.

180. Barron TF, Birnbaum NS, Shane LB, et al. Pneumocystis carinii pneumonia studied by gallium-67 scanning. *Radiology* 1985;154:791–793.

181. Kramer EL, Sanger JJ, Garay SM, et al. Gallium-67 scans of the chest in patients with acquired immunodeficiency syndrome. *J Nucl Med* 1987;28:1107–1114.

182. Woolfenden JM, Carrasquillo JA, Larson SM, et al. Acquired immunodeficiency syndrome: Ga-67 citrate imaging. *Radiology* 1987;162:383–387.

183. Fauci AS, Macher AM, Longo DL, et al. NIH conference: acquired immunodeficiency syndrome—epidemiologic, clinical, immunologic, and therapeutic considerations. *Ann Intern Med* 1984;100:92–106.

184. Kramer EL, Sanger JH, Garay SM, et al. Diagnostic implications of Ga-67 chest-scan patterns in human immunodeficiency virus–seropositive patients. *Radiology* 1989;170:671–676.

185. Tuazon CU, Delaney MD, Simon GL, et al. Utility of gallium-67 scintigraphy and bronchial washings in the diagnosis and treatment of *Pneumocystis carinii* pneumonia in patients with the acquired immune deficiency syndrome. *Am Rev Respir Dis* 1985;132:1087–1092.

186. Hawkins CC, Gold JW, Whimbey E, et al. Mycobacterium avium complex infections in patients with the acquired immunodeficiency syndrome. *Ann Intern Med* 1986;105:184–188.

187. Bitran J, Bekerman C, Weinstein R, et al. Patterns of gallium-67 scintigraphy in patients with acquired immunodeficiency syndrome and the AIDS related complex. *J Nucl Med* 1987;28:1103–1106.

188. Sarkar SD, Ravikrishnan KP, Woodbury DH, et al. Gallium-67 citrate scanning: a new adjunct in the detection and follow-up of extrapulmonary tuberculosis—concise communication. *J Nucl Med* 1979;20:833–836.

189. Zuckier LS, Ongseng F, Goldfarb CR. Lymphocytic interstitial pneumonitis: a cause of pulmonary gallium-67 uptake in a child with acquired immunodeficiency syndrome. *J Nucl Med* 1988;29:707–711.

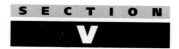

BONE

20

PRIMARY AND METASTATIC BONE DISEASE

MARTIN CHARRON
MANUEL L. BROWN

Bone scintigraphy is one of the most commonly performed nuclear medicine studies. The bone scan has been used for more than 30 years in evaluating primary bone tumors, metastatic bone tumors, and primary soft-tissue tumors. This chapter reviews the common scintigraphic findings in benign and malignant primary bone tumors and in metastatic disease and the efficacy of bone scintigraphy in evaluation for common malignant lesions.

Conventional radiographic examinations can often reveal the anatomic location of a lesion and its effect on normal bone and can lead to a suggestion as to its histologic type. Bone scintigraphy with ^{99m}Tc methylene diphosphonate (MDP) is a highly sensitive, widely available, and safe procedure. Because of its high degree of sensitivity, bone scintigraphy provides for the early detection of metastatic disease in the entire skeleton and involves a radiation dose to the patient that is comparable with that of conventional radiographic procedures. The clinical role of positron emission tomography (PET) in evaluation for bone metastasis is not yet defined; however, as described in this chapter, there is emerging evidence that this imaging method also may aid patient treatment in this area with the use of either [^{18}F]-fluorodeoxyglucose (FDG) or ^{18}F fluoride ion (1,2).

Whole-body bone scintigraphy is an excellent method for evaluating patients for suspected metastatic disease because most metastatic lesions manifest as areas of increased activity. In the evaluation of patients with primary bone tumors or of patients who have malignant lesions that become lytic, greater attention to detail is important to optimize the bone scan. In these cases, the diagnostic accuracy of bone scintigraphy is highly dependent on the technical quality of the study.

PATTERNS

There are several patterns of abnormality to be aware of in evaluation for neoplastic diseases. In benign osseous neoplasms, up-

take can vary from being quite faint if present at all, such as in fibrocortical defects or nongrowing bone islands, to markedly intense, as in giant cell tumors. Relatively intense focal uptake can be seen in osteoid osteoma, sometimes with a double-density sign, and several tumors can have a doughnut pattern of uptake with moderately increased uptake in the periphery of the lesion surrounding a relatively photopenic central area. Another pattern that can be seen in both benign and malignant disease is the extended pattern of abnormally increased radiopharmaceutical accumulation in the bones of an extremity, either in the bones adjacent to the primary lesion or more distally throughout the extremity (Fig. 20.1).

The patterns of uptake of benign tumors are shown in Table 20.1. Osseous metastatic disease usually occurs in sites of relatively increased blood flow, such as areas of active bone marrow. In a survey of the pattern of metastatic disease, Krishnamurthy et al. (3) found that metastatic lesions occur in the axial skeleton in approximately 80% of cases. The other lesions occurred in the extremities and skull. This distribution is similar for most soft-tissue tumors that metastasize to bone by the venous or lymphatic route. However, lung tumors that can metastasize by the arterial route can be isolated solitary lesions in the distal aspects of extremities. The most common manifestation of widespread metastatic disease is numerous asymmetric areas of increased uptake throughout the axial skeleton and, to a lesser extent, the appendicular skeleton (Fig. 20.2).

Boxer et al. (4) reviewed the records of a large series of patients with breast cancer who were eventually found to have disease metastatic to bone. In their series, 21% of the cases initially manifested as a solitary metastatic lesion of the bone, the most common site being a vertebra. In patients with known soft-tissue or primary bone tumors, the likelihood that any solitary area of increased uptake on a bone scan represents metastatic disease varies on a site by site basis. Several articles discuss solitary lesions (5–12). By combining the results of these articles, one can make some general statements concerning the importance of a solitary lesion. In a patient with a known soft-tissue or osseous malignant tumor, a solitary lesion in the pelvis or a vertebra is caused by metastatic disease 60% to 70% of the time. Lesions in the extremities or the skull are caused by metastatic disease 40% to 50% of the time. It is much less likely for a solitary rib lesion

M. Charron: Department of Radiology, University of Pennsylvania, and Division of Nuclear Medicine, Radiology, Children's Hospital of Philadelphia, Philadelphia, PA.

M.L. Brown: Radiology, Henry Ford Hospital, Detroit, MI.

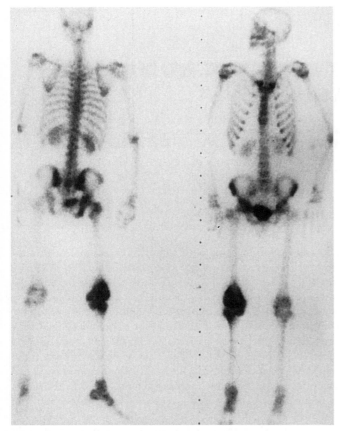

FIGURE 20.1. Intense uptake in a giant cell tumor of the distal right femur in an 18-year-old patient. Evident is the extended pattern of the abnormality with moderately increased uptake in the proximal tibia, mildly increased uptake in the proximal femur, and mildly increased uptake throughout the rest of the right leg and right ischium.

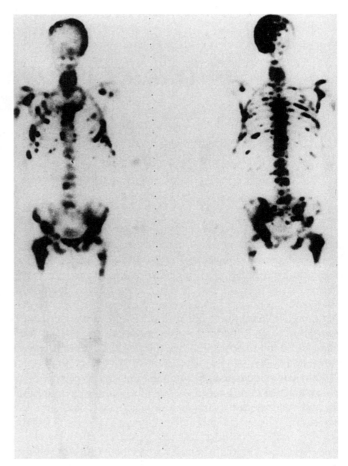

FIGURE 20.2. Prostate cancer. Numerous sites of markedly increased uptake throughout the axial skeleton, proximal appendicular skeleton, and skull in a patient with metastatic prostate cancer.

Table 20.1. *Appearance of Benign Tumors at Bone Scintigraphy*

Adamantinoma	++
Aneurysmal bone cyst	+++
Bone cyst	−/o
Bone island	o/+
Chondroblastoma	−++
Cortical desmoid	o/+
Enchondroma	o/+
Fibrous cortical defect	o/+
Fibrous dysplasia	+++
Giant cell tumor	+++
Hemangioma	▲
Hereditary multiple exostosis	▲
Multiple enchondromatosis	▲
Myositis ossificans	▲
Nonossifying fibroma	+
Osteoblastoma	+++
Osteoid osteoma	+++
Osteoma	▲
Solitary osteochondroma	▲

+, ++, +++, mild, moderate, intense; −, "cold"; ▲, variable; o, isointense.
Modified from Kech G, Christle JH, Mettler FA. Benign bone tumors and tumor conditions: In Mettler FA Jr, ed. *Radionuclide bone imaging and densitometry*. New York: Churchill-Livingstone, 1988;32, with permission.

to be caused by metastatic disease. In a study by Tumeh et al. (12), a single lesion in the rib was caused by metastatic disease in only 10% of cases. An isolated sternal lesion in a patient with known carcinoma of the breast has a much higher likelihood of being caused by metastatic disease (Fig. 20.3). In a study by Kwai et al. (8), almost 80% of these lesions were caused by metastatic disease. When a bone scan shows a solitary lesion in a patient with known malignant disease, especially if there is the possibility of recent trauma, it is important to assess the finding with plain-film radiography. If a plain radiograph does not show a benign cause for the uptake and there is a need for accurate assessment of the lesion, plain-film tomography, computed tomography (CT), or magnetic resonance imaging (MRI) and, when appropriate, biopsy may be needed (13,14).

Another pattern that results from metastatic disease is generalized increased uptake throughout the skeleton, a pattern called *superscan*. Superscan occurs when there is diffuse metastatic disease. It is often associated with relatively little, if any, accumulation of radiopharmaceutical in the kidneys. With modern gamma cameras, the bladder often is seen in patients with superscan. Superscan can be caused by metabolic bone disease.

Greenberg et al. (15) described the pattern of the flare phenomenon in metastatic disease. This occurs after therapeutic

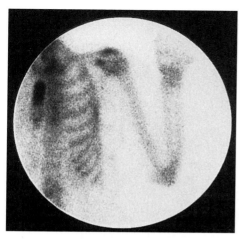

FIGURE 20.3. Breast cancer. Solitary site of intense uptake in the sternum represents metastatic disease in a patient with breast cancer.

intervention when the patient's clinical condition improves but serial bone scintigraphy shows increasing intensity in lesions or new lesions. Repetition of bone scintigraphy in several months shows marked improvement. The flare phenomenon has been described to occur among as many as 20% of patients, but the frequency of occurrence clearly depends on the type of tumor, the therapy, and the interval between the therapy and the bone scan (16–20). One study showed that the flare phenomenon is a good prognostic sign (21).

A pattern seen on images of some patients with disease metastatic to the lung is hypertrophic pulmonary osteoarthropathy (HPO). Diffuse and symmetric increased uptake in the diaphysis and metaphysis of tubular bones along the cortical margins produces distinctive parallel tracks. Ali et al. (22) reported the following distribution of HPO involvement among 48 patients: tibia and fibula, 95%; femur, 88%; radius and ulna, 85%; feet, 81%; scapula, 67%; mandible, 42%; clavicle, 33%; ribs, 2%; and pelvis, 2%. Of note, none of these 48 patients had increased spinal uptake. The scintigraphic findings of HPO frequently appear before radiographic abnormalities, correspond well with clinical manifestations, and may decrease after treatment.

BENIGN BONE TUMORS

One cannot differentiate a benign from a malignant bone tumor on the basis of scintigraphic findings. Samuels (23) stated that with [87]Sr bone scans, benign bone lesions often appear only slightly more intense than surrounding bone, whereas malignant lesions often have intense radionuclide concentration. Although this characterization is a reasonable generalization, the intensity of a lesion on a bone scan is not predictive of histopathologic outcome. Osteoid osteoma and benign giant cell (Fig. 20.1) tumors may have uptake as intense as that of any primary malignant bone tumor or metastatic lesion.

Uptake in benign tumors during bone scintigraphy has been well described by Keck et al. (24) (Table 20.1). A benign bone tumor usually is found when bone scanning is performed to

assess musculoskeletal pain or when the study is ordered to assess metastatic disease for a lesion that is initially thought malignant.

Adamantinoma (Ameloblastoma)

Adamantinoma is a rare tumor of unknown cell origin. Radiographically the lesion is large and radiolucent. The most common location is the midshaft of the tibia. Adamantinoma can occur in association with fibrous dysplasia or osteofibrous dysplasia. It is an uncommon, pluripotential neoplasm. A bone scan shows moderate uptake.

Aneurysmal Bone Cyst

Aneurysmal bone cysts are uncommon benign tumors of unknown causation. One half of cases involve the long bones. Most cases occur in children and adolescents. As many as one third of these lesions are linked to other benign or malignant processes. A bone scan typically reveals a doughnut pattern. Hyperemia can be absent despite the presence of increased uptake on the delayed image. Hudson (25) reported that 64% of aneurysmal bone cysts have the doughnut pattern of uptake (Fig. 20.4).

Bone Island

Bone islands are focal areas of mature lamellar bone located within normal cancellous bone. This common lesion may enlarge after puberty. It is devoid of malignant potential. Bone islands can have increased uptake (26,27) or normal uptake (28) on a bone scan.

Chondroblastoma

Chondroblastoma is an uncommon benign tumor that originates from cartilage and often involves the epiphysis of the lower extremities. Flat bones that can be involved include the talus and calcaneus. The lesion is highly cellular and composed of chondroblast-like cells with distinct outlines. Most exhibit intense uptake on bone scans (29–32).

Desmoplastic Fibroma

Desmoplastic fibroma of bone is a very rare, benign, but locally aggressive, tumor and is characterized by small fibroblasts, fibers of collagen, and absence of new bone. The location is usually the long bones, vertebrae, and pelvis (33). The lesion occurs most often during the first three decades of life and has no sex predilection. A bone scan shows increased uptake.

Enchondroma

Enchondroma is a common, benign, asymptomatic tumor located in the metaphyses, frequently of the hand (50%). It is composed of lobules of mature hyaline cartilage. A bone scan shows normal or mildly increased uptake. A rapid change with increased uptake suggests malignant transformation. A bone scan is recommended in the initial evaluation to search for other

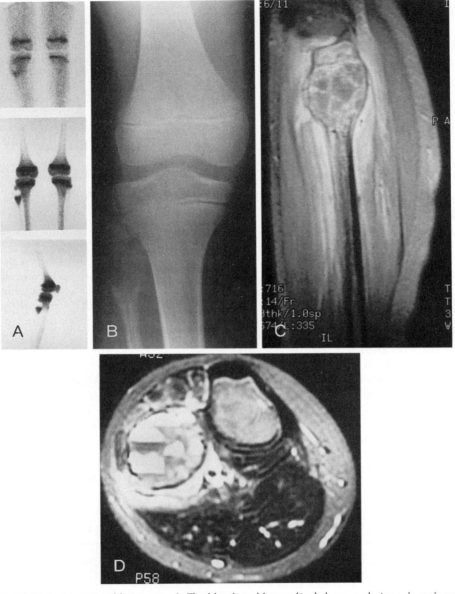

FIGURE 20.4. Aneurysmal bone cyst. **A:** The blood-pool image (*top*) shows a photopenic region surrounded by a rim of increased activity involving the proximal aspect of the right fibula. The delayed anterior (*middle*) and right lateral projection (*bottom*) also have a doughnut pattern. **B:** Plain radiograph of the right knee shows a lytic expansile lesion of the proximal end of the shaft of the right fibula with a pathologic fracture. **C, D:** Magnetic resonance image reveals a proximal fibular lesion consisting of multiple cavernous spaces containing fluid. The appearance is most suggestive of aneurysmal bone cyst.

lesions and as a baseline. Enchondromatosis or multiple enchondroma is a sporadic condition. It is usually first identified in infancy. Multiple enchondroma originates in the metaphyseal regions of tubular bones and in flat bones.

Epidermoid Cyst

An epidermoid cyst is a sharply delineated cystic tumor that has a lining of squamous epithelium filled with a spongy material.

If large enough, the center of the lesion is photopenic on a bone scan.

Fibrous Cortical Defect

A fibrous cortical defect is small, eccentric in location, and pure cortical rest of fibrous tissue. It originates from the periosteum and invades the underlying cortex. The lesion occurs in both children and adolescents and is rarely seen in patients younger than 2 years and almost never after the age of 14 years. One third of the pediatric population may have one or more of these lesions (34). Findings on plain radiographs usually are distinctive—a round, oval, or multiloculated lucency often with sclerotic edges. This common benign tumor rarely shows uptake of ^{99m}Tc MDP unless fractured (35).

Fibrous Dysplasia

This benign tumor of fibrous tissue involves either one or more bones and usually does not cause symptoms. The incidence of malignant transformation is less than 1%. The lesion usually is recognized before the patient is 20 years of age. The bone scan shows markedly intense, increased activity in all three phases. As many as 15% of lesions depicted on plain radiographs may not be detected on bone scans (36). In one series, 85% of patients with polyostotic fibrous dysplasia eventually had a pathologic fracture.

Giant Cell Tumor (Osteoclastoma)

Giant cell tumors constitute less than 5% of all primary bone tumors. Most of them are benign (90%) and have a high predilection to recurrence (~50%). Almost all giant cell tumors have increased uptake of ^{99m}Tc MDP (37), although minimal uptake may be seen (30,38,39). The hypervascular lesion can be identified in the angiographic phase, and a doughnut sign is seen approximately 50% of the time (40). Abnormal uptake often is found beyond the tumor margin, in the bone adjacent to the joint, and in other joints of the same extremity (Fig. 20.1).

Hemangioma

Hemangioma of bone is composed of many vascular channels of different sizes and can be cavernous, capillary, or venous. The common sites of involvement are the vertebrae and calvarium. Hemangioma can have increased perfusion in the angiogram phase and photopenia on the delayed images (41). On radiographs hemangiomas that involve the spine and are large have exaggerated vertical trabeculae or collapse of the vertebral body.

Osteoblastoma

Osteoblastoma is closely related to osteoid osteoma. There is considerable debate about whether the origin is infectious or neoplastic. Differentiation between osteoblastoma and osteoid osteoma is not histologic but is based on size. When the nidus is larger than 2 cm in diameter, the lesion is called *osteoblastoma.* When the nidus is smaller than 2 cm in diameter, it is called *osteoid osteoma.* CT scans are used for evaluation of the morphologic features of the tumor and the effects on adjacent structures. The lesion has well-marginated borders and is relatively lucent and expansile. A bone scan typically reveals intense accretion on the blood-pool and delayed images (42). Bone scans are especially useful in the detection of obscure lesions on plain radiographs, such as lesions that appear in the sacrum or small lesions in the spine (43–47).

Osteochondroma

Osteochondroma is an osseous projection from the surface of normal bone in areas where cartilage is present. It is not a true neoplasm and is a developmental defect of unknown causation. A bone scan cannot help differentiate benign from malignant osteochondroma, although intensity on a bone scan generally increases as a lesion undergoes malignant degeneration. Lack of uptake of ^{99m}Tc MDP almost excludes the possibility of malignant transformation of osteochondroma (48). Hereditary multiple exostosis is similar to solitary osteochondroma, except that the cartilage cap is thicker, the frequency of malignant transformation is higher, and inheritance is autosomal dominant. The lesions can appear anywhere in the skeleton, although they are more frequently located around the knee and wrist (Fig. 20.5).

Osteoid Osteoma

First described by Jaffe (49), osteoid osteoma is a painful, benign bone lesion characterized by a small nidus (usually less than 1 cm in diameter) of calcified osteoid tissue in a stroma of loose vascular connective tissue surrounded by a margin of dense sclerotic bone. The sensitivity of conventional skeletal radiography in the diagnosis of osteoid osteoma ranges from 55% to 90% (50–53). Forty percent of cases of osteoid osteoma occur in the femur and tibia and 10% in the spine. Osteoblastoma is more frequent in the spine.

Bone scanning is of great value in identification of the lesion,

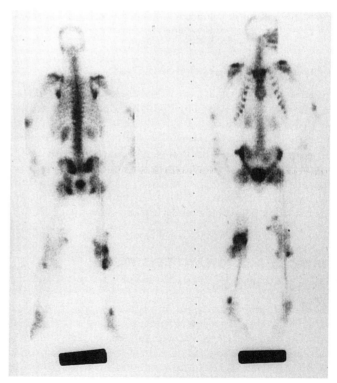

FIGURE 20.5. Osteochondromatosis. Young adult with multiple hereditary osteochondromatosis. Prominent lesions are present above the knee, on the right part of the pelvis, and on the right ankle.

especially in the spine and pelvis. With rare exception, osteoid osteoma avidly accumulates ^{99m}Tc MDP on the three phases of the bone scan. Thus the sensitivity of bone scanning is excellent. In a series of 20 patients with symptomatic osteoid osteoma, all 20 had positive results of bone scans, whereas only 11 had positive findings at radiography (54,55). Some patients come to medical attention with referred pain, and imaging should include at least one joint near and below the site of pain; for example, osteoid osteoma in the intratrochanteric region can cause pain referred to the knee or back. Helms et al. (56) described a double-density sign purportedly specific for osteoid osteoma. This sign consists of intense central uptake with less uptake in the sclerotic bone, findings that do not occur in cases of osteomyelitis or abscess. Pinhole imaging may be helpful, especially if the planar images do not contain enough information for a diagnosis.

Lee et al. (57) reported on their experience with radionuclide imaging, tetracycline fluorescence, and thermography in the preoperative staging of osteoid osteoma. They concluded that intraoperative radionuclide imaging is a reliable technique in confirming complete removal of the nidus with no increase in operating time.

Osteoma

Osteoma is a benign tumor that usually occurs in the calvarium, paranasal sinuses, and mandible. It usually is asymptomatic and does not undergo malignant degeneration. These lesions show evidence of extreme sclerosis on radiographs and measure approximately 2 cm in diameter. Gilday and Ash (35) reported one case of osteoma with intense accumulation of MDP.

Simple (Unicameral) Bone Cyst

Unicameral bone cyst is a true fluid-filled cyst walled off by fibrous tissue with varying amounts of hemosiderin. The recommended imaging approach is first to obtain a plain radiograph and then, if needed, to perform CT or MRI to define the content of the lesion. Bone scintigraphy is recommended if trauma is suspected. These lesions typically have abnormally increased activity after a fracture. An untraumatized cyst can be undetectable, but typically a bone scan discloses a slightly reactive margin surrounding a photopenic center, the doughnut sign.

PRIMARY MALIGNANT LESIONS

Chondrosarcoma

Chondrosarcoma is a tumor of cartilaginous origin. The typical radiographic appearance is a radiolucent, expansile, irregular lesion. The margin of the tumor with time can become ill defined with cortical destruction and invasion of the adjacent soft tissue. CT and MRI are useful to define the extent of the tumor, in both the bone and the soft tissue. The medullary form of chondrosarcoma shows patchy areas of moderately increased activity on a bone scan. The exostotic form of chondrosarcoma has high focal uptake. Chondrosarcoma in the spine is detected more

easily with bone scintigraphy than with routine radiography (58). One group (59) detected chondrosarcoma with ^{99m}Tc tetrofosmin. Another study (60) showed that FDG PET can be an objective and quantitative adjunct in the differential diagnosis and grading of chondrosarcoma.

Ewing Sarcoma

Ewing sarcoma often arises in the femur or pelvis and is the second most common malignant bone tumor among children and young adults. One half of cases occur between the ages of 10 and 20 years. The recommended approach to imaging involves obtaining plain radiographs, performing MRI for tumor extent, and obtaining a bone scan for evaluating metastatic sites. Ewing sarcoma often has very intense activity on the three phases of a bone scan. These findings of this highly vascular tumor can be similar to those of osteomyelitis. Uptake usually is homogeneous and has been contrasted to the patchy uptake found with osteosarcoma (61) (Fig. 20.6). Uptake in the soft tissue is less common in patients with Ewing sarcoma than in patients with osteosar-

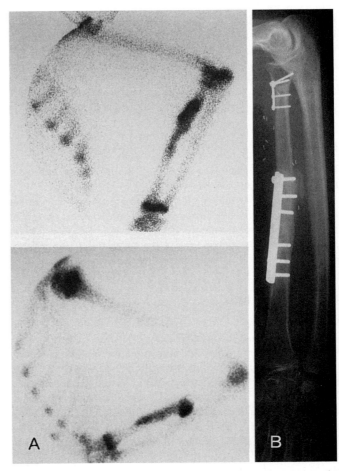

FIGURE 20.6. Ewing sarcoma. **A:** Bone scan (*top*) shows primary uptake in the Ewing sarcoma involving the left radius. Bone scan obtained 2 years later (*bottom*) shows similar uptake; however, this was secondary to postsurgical change. **B:** Plain radiograph reveals two orthopedic fixation devices with evidence of callous formation and orthotopic ossification.

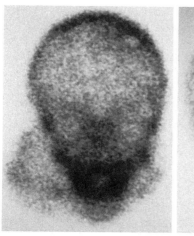
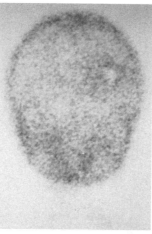

FIGURE 20.7. Eosinophilic granuloma. Vertex images (*left,* without lead shielding) show a photopenic region in the skull surrounded by a rim of faintly increased activity.

coma because of the lack of production of osteoid. Decreased uptake in the primary tumor is found 3 to 4 months after radiation therapy (62). Persistence of increased uptake after treatment suggests tumor recurrence, infection, or fracture. Bone marrow involvement can be evaluated with ^{99m}Tc sulfur colloid. However, results of bone marrow imaging are unreliable after chemotherapy or radiation therapy (63).

The sensitivity of bone scintigraphy in the detection of histiocytosis X has been reported to range from 35% to 94%. Bone scanning cannot be used reliably for screening. One report suggested that bone scintigraphy is more reliable for detection of recurrence during follow-up examinations (64). In addition, there are occasional instances of detection of lesions on bone scans that are not detected on plain radiographs; therefore the greatest sensitivity is probably achieved by the combination of radiographs and bone scans (64–67). Large lytic lesions can be photopenic on bone scans.

Eosinophilic granuloma, the benign form of histiocytosis, can express itself monostotically or polyostotically. A bone scan can show decreased, normal, or increased uptake (Fig. 20.7). Kumare and Balachandran (68) reported on a series of 24 lesions in seven patients. Radiography depicted 92% of the lesions, and a bone scan depicted 67%. ^{99m}Tc hexakis-2-methoxy-isobutyl-isonitrile (MIBI) imaging does not appear useful in the diagnosis of Ewing sarcoma (69).

Multiple Myeloma

Multiple myeloma is the most common primary bone tumor among adults. Several articles review the role of bone scintigraphy (70–74), ^{67}Ga (75), and FDG (76) in the diagnosis of multiple myeloma, and all show that plain radiograph radiography remains the primary method of evaluating skeletal involvement by myeloma. Although bone scintigraphy can show many of the lesions seen on radiographs, radiographs are more likely to show more extensive disease than do bone scans (73,74). Feggie et al. (77) found that bone scintigraphy occasionally is

helpful in the diagnosis of multiple myeloma in areas that are difficult to evaluate with routine radiography, such as in the ribs and sternum. A bone scan also should be considered when a patient with multiple myeloma has bone pain and normal findings on radiographs. Feggie et al. (77) also evaluated the role of bone marrow scintigraphy in the diagnosis of multiple myeloma. They documented marrow expansion; however, use of bone marrow scintigraphy did not improve diagnostic accuracy.

Osteosarcoma

Osteosarcoma constitutes one fifth of all primary malignant bone tumors. The peak incidence is during the second or third decade of life, and there is a second peak in the sixth decade. Osteosarcoma is known to occur after radiation therapy or chemotherapy (78). The recommended approach to the evaluation of patients for osteosarcoma involves obtaining plain radiographs and performing bone scintigraphy to detect metastasis and MRI to establish the extent of the primary lesion. A new coregistration technique has been applied to the combination of ^{201}Tl single photon emission computed tomography and MRI data for evaluating bone lesions and may provide additional anatomic information for localizing functional abnormalities. This may be valuable for defining targets for biopsy, planning surgical treatment, and using minimally invasive therapies (79). A bone scan typically reveals intense and expanded uptake (Fig. 20.8), and photopenic areas occasionally are found in the tumor. The extended pattern of increased uptake on a bone scan limits the usefulness of this modality for determination or the local extent of involvement.

Osteosarcoma that occurs in Paget disease manifests a pattern on bone scan very different from that of primary osteosarcoma. The appearance is a photopenic lesion surrounded by diffusely increased activity. The cold area represents the osteosarcoma, and the surrounding hot area is Paget disease. This pattern was found in 13 of 17 patients with osteosarcoma arising in pagetic bone (80). In contrast, primary osteosarcoma arising de novo tends to have markedly increased radioactivity.

Distant osseous metastatic lesions are found at initial staging in only approximately 2% of cases (81,82). Nevertheless, an initial bone scan may be important because the presence of metastatic disease greatly alters the choice of therapy. Osseous metastatic lesions have been found to occur at a rate of 1% per month 5 to 29 months after diagnosis with a decrease in the rate thereafter (83). Follow-up bone scans at intervals of approximately 6 months therefore are recommended. With the routine use of chemotherapy in the management of osteosarcoma, approximately 20% of patients have bone metastasis before lung metastasis (81,82,84). Bone scans also can depict soft-tissue metastatic lesions before the lesions appear on a chest radiograph (85–90). However, CT has the highest sensitivity for detection of pulmonary metastatic lesions.

Edeline et al. (91) described the usefulness of bone scans in 19 cases of pediatric osteosarcoma. Bone scans were performed before chemotherapy and were repeated halfway through the course of chemotherapy at 6 weeks. Sommer et al. (92) also studied the effect of preoperative chemotherapy on the uptake of ^{99m}Tc MDP in 30 patients with osteosarcoma and correlated

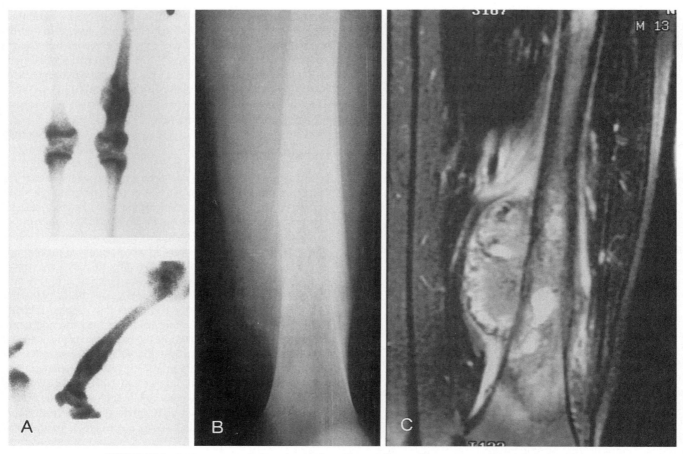

FIGURE 20.8. Osteosarcoma. **A:** Anterior (*top*) and lateral (*bottom*) bone scans of the left femur of a 13-year-old boy with osteosarcoma show intense uptake that extend into the soft tissue. **B:** Plain radiograph of the femur shows the lesion with a soft tissue mass. **C:** Magnetic resonance image of the left femur shows extensive marrow abnormally and a large mass extending into the soft tissue.

this with the surgical specimen. The overall accuracy in presurgical prediction of tumor regression was found greater than 90%, and it was found possible to localize areas of viable tumor larger than 1 cm in diameter. These authors concluded that ^{99m}Tc MDP bone scanning is a highly sensitive and specific modality for the accurate evaluation of tumor regression after treatment.

Menendez et al. (93) evaluated the ^{201}Tl scans of 16 patients with high-grade osteosarcoma or soft-tissue sarcoma to determine whether this technique can be used to ascertain accurately the amount of viable tumor and to predict the response to chemotherapy. They concluded that ^{201}Tl scintigraphy should be used concomitantly with other radiographic procedures in the diagnosis, planning of treatment, and follow-up management of sarcoma, because this technique appears to be able to help predict the response of high-grade osteosarcoma to preoperative chemotherapy. Rosen et al. (94) similarly reported that in the management of 24 cases osteosarcoma decreased uptake of ^{201}Tl correlated with a good response to preoperative chemotherapy. In one series (95), ^{201}Tl imaging for bone and soft-tissue tumors was better than three-phase bone scintigraphy alone but was not good enough to clearly differentiate malignant lesions from benign ones. ^{201}Tl scintigraphy performed in combination with

three-phase bone scintigraphy may be superior to either one of the two imaging procedures alone for the diagnosis of bone and soft-tissue tumors. A change in the tumor uptake of ^{201}Tl scintigraphy after preoperative chemotherapy can be precisely predictive of tumor necrosis in osteosarcoma (96–101). FDG PET is a promising tool for noninvasive evaluation of the response to neoadjuvant chemotherapy for osteosarcoma. This can affect the choice of surgical strategy, because a limb salvage procedure cannot be recommended to patients who do not respond to preoperative chemotherapy unless wide surgical margins can safely be achieved (102,103).

Rhabdomyosarcoma

Rhabdomyosarcoma is a malignant soft-tissue tumor of muscular origin and frequently involves the head and neck, the genitourinary tract, and the extremities. The recommended diagnostic approach includes plain radiography, ultrasonography, and MRI. Bone scanning is useful to define bone metastasis (Fig. 20.9) and occasionally soft-tissue uptake of the primary tumor.

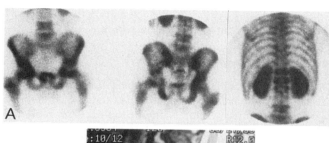

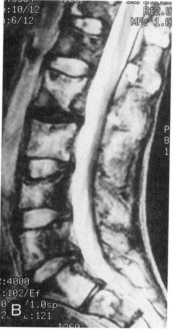

FIGURE 20.9. Rhabdomyosarcoma. **A:** Selected images from a bone scan of an 8-year-old with rhabdomyosarcoma show extensive abnormal uptake in the pelvis and spine. The inhomogeneous uptake in the spine may be related to tumor or previous radiation therapy. Chemotherapy caused the increased renal activity. **B:** Magnetic resonance image shows diffuse abnormality of the bone marrow within the spine most likely caused by diffuse bone marrow involvement of malignant growth.

METASTATIC LESIONS

Breast Cancer

Bone scanning is more sensitive for the early detection of metastatic disease in breast cancer than are routine skeletal surveys (104–106). Abnormalities on a bone scan can precede radiographic findings by 4 to 6 months (105–107). The role of bone scanning in staging breast carcinoma has been studied in a number of centers (108–111). These studies show a very low true-positive yield in the detection of stage I and II disease, which increases to approximately 14% in stage III disease. In a retrospective study of the records of almost 400 patients, Ahmed et al. (112) found a frequency of true-positive results of bone scans increasing from 2.5% for stage I disease to 16% for stage II disease. Coleman et al. (21) reported a true-positive yield of zero for stage I, 3% for stage II, 7% for stage III, and 47% for stage IV breast cancer. The efficacious use of bone scintigraphy must be considered in the initial staging of breast cancer. Patients with relatively small primary tumors (<2 cm in diameter) need

only preoperative scans when symptoms are present or laboratory values are worrisome for metastatic disease. Coleman et al. (21) recommend a baseline bone scan for all patients with stage II through IV disease.

There are also conflicting results regarding the utility of bone scanning in routine follow-up evaluation of patients with breast cancer. Front et al. (113) found metastatic disease on the bone scans of 32 patients without bone pain. Chaudary et al. (114) had similar findings. At least two studies (115,116) have shown much closer correlation between musculoskeletal pain and documented metastatic disease. In the study by Ahmed et al. (112), 27 patients underwent bone scans at the initial evaluation, but only eight of those had scan results considered positive for metastatic disease.

A substantial number of patients have metastatic disease as a solitary lesion (6). Patients with known breast cancer who have an isolated sternal lesion (Fig. 20.3) have a very high likelihood (approximately 80%) that the lesion is caused by metastatic disease (10).

The flare phenomenon can occur in patients who have breast cancer. In a study by Coleman et al. (21), 12 of 16 patients with lytic metastatic disease had evidence of worsening at bone scanning, which later showed improvement after successful therapy. This flare response was seen in patients who responded to therapy but not in nonresponders. Therefore, Coleman et al. concluded that the flare response was a common and not an unusual finding when successful systemic therapy has been administered.

Metastatic disease from breast carcinoma often starts in the bone marrow. Imaging tests to evaluate marrow as opposed to osseous involvement should be more sensitive for detecting early metastatic disease. This has been the case in several reports in the MRI literature. Duncker et al. (117), using a marrow scanning technique with a radiolabeled antigranulocyte monoclonal antibody (with normal marrow distribution), detected metastatic disease as defects in the bone marrow in 25 of 32 patients. Bone scanning performed at approximately the same time showed metastatic disease in only 53% of patients. In most (~70%) patients who had positive results of bone scans and of marrow scans, the marrow scans showed more lesions. The investigators concluded that bone marrow scintigraphy was a better test for the early detection of metastatic disease among patients with breast cancer than was conventional bone scintigraphy. A group from Grenoble, France (118), showed that in patients with asymptomatic breast cancer, a CA15-3 level less than 25 U/mL is strongly predictive of a negative bone scan result, whereas a high level suggests neoplastic bone involvement.

Head and Neck Tumors

An early study by Wolfe et al. (119) showed that there was a very low prevalence of bone metastasis at the time of initial staging in their series of 118 patients. Sham et al. (120) conducted a study with 132 patients who had nasopharyngeal carcinoma and no clinical evidence of distant metastatic disease. Their results showed a relatively low sensitivity and specificity of bone scanning, and they did not recommend the routine use of bone scintigraphy for the staging of nasopharyngeal carcinoma. Although Wolfe et al. (119), Sham et al. (120), and Brown and Leakos (121) found a relatively low yield for bone scintigraphy in the diagnosis of head and neck cancer, Sundram et al. (122) had different results. Their study included 143 patients at the time of staging and an additional 162 patients during follow-up evaluation because of bone pain or other suggestions of metastasis. They found a relatively high yield for the initial staging of nasopharyngeal carcinoma; 23% of patients had evidence of bony metastases. Bone scans obtained as part of the follow-up examinations had a 59% true-positive yield.

Lung Carcinoma

Bone scintigraphy is not required as a routine preoperative test in the care of patients with newly diagnosed lung cancer because of its relatively low yield (123). When the findings on a bone scan are positive, there is a very poor prognosis among patients with bronchogenic carcinoma. In a study by Gravenstein et al. (124), 46 patients had abnormal bone scans. In this group of patients, 40 were dead within 6 months, and another 4 died within 1 year. Similar results were found by Merric and Merric (125) who followed the cases of almost 600 patients with lung cancer. Their results showed that bone scintigraphy had a sensitivity of 89% and an accuracy of 78%. They also found that bone pain and abnormal bone scan results were independently associated with a significant reduction in survival for all cell types of lung cancer. Park et al. (126) found that the presence of more than two areas of abnormal uptake on a bone scan was a significant poor prognostic factor in the care of patients with lung cancer. Patients with only one or two abnormal areas at diagnosis did not have a change in overall survival rate.

Bone scintigraphy for lung cancer also can show evidence of hypertropic pulmonary osteoarthropathy. In bone scanning for lung cancer, it is important to image the entire body, including the distal extremities, because isolated peripheral lesions can occur in the hands and feet (127,128).

Lymphoma

Lymphoma is the third most common neoplasm among children. Hodgkin disease represents approximately 5% of cases of childhood malignant disease, and four histologic types are described and relate to prognosis. Bone scans in one series showed an average of 3.5 lesions per study among patients with Hodgkin and non-Hodgkin lymphoma when the results were positive; however, a bone scan result was considered positive in only 4% of cases. Skeletal pain, although specific, was very insensitive. Patients with Hodgkin disease had more frequent extremity lesions and fewer axial lesions than did those with non-Hodgkin lymphoma (129). Schecter et al. (130) reported that bone scanning was useful in the initial staging of Hodgkin lymphoma, with a 45% increase in detection of osseous involvement compared with conventional radiography. [67]Ga scintigraphy is essential in the evaluation of soft-tissue involvement. After therapy, ^{67}Ga scintigraphy has a clinical effect when radiologic abnormalities persist because the results can lead to avoidance of unnecessary complementary treatment or confirm the need to change

treatment modality (131). PET may provide more information about extranodal lymphoma than does incremental CT (132).

Neuroblastoma

Neuroblastoma is a highly malignant neural crest tumor and is the second most common solid malignant tumor of childhood. It is locally invasive and can metastasize to liver, skin, bone, and bone marrow.

Bone Scan

Bone scans are used in neuroblastoma to both detect bone metastasis and to reveal primary uptake in the soft-tissue tumor caused by microcalcification or macrocalcification. Heisel et al. (133) reported that 91% of primary tumors were diagnosed by means of bone scan compared with 72% by means of radiographic examination (Fig. 20.10). Photopenic lesions (Fig. 20.11) may be present on a bone scan and can be explained by impairment of blood flow or extensive destruction. MacDonald et al. (134) found that the scintigraphic appearance at diagnosis does not confer any prognostic information in the care of children with advanced neuroblastoma.

Metaiodobenzylguanidine

Metaiodobenzylguanidine (MIBG) structurally resembles the endogenous neurotransmitter hormone norepinephrine and the

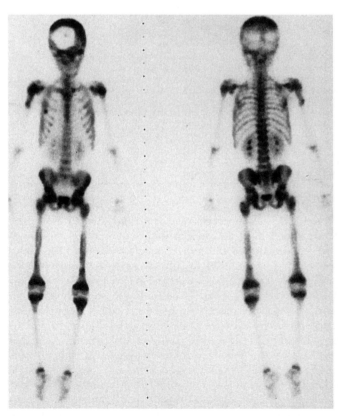

FIGURE 20.10. Neuroblastoma. Bone scan of an 8-year-old patient with stage IV neuroblastoma shows numerous areas of metastatic involvement of the bone and postsurgical change in the skull.

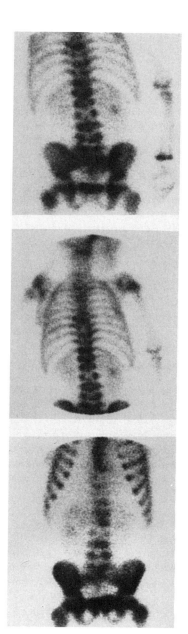

FIGURE 20.11. Neuroblastoma. Posterior bone images of the chest (*top*) and spine (*middle*) and the anterior image of the pelvis (*bottom*) show widespread metastatic disease in a 5-year-old patient with neuroblastoma. The pelvis is involved diffusely, and the areas of increased and decreased uptake show that the spine contains metastatic disease.

ganglion blocking drug guanethidine. In staging known neuroblastoma, MIBG scintigraphy can provide more information than can CT or MRI. After treatment, an abnormal focus of uptake represents evidence of viable tumor. Trocone et al. (135) conducted a study with 158 patients with different amine precursor uptake and decarboxylase (APUD) tumors. Sensitivity was greater than 80% in the diagnosis of both pheochromocytoma and neuroblastoma. The specificity was greater than 95%, and no false-positive results were found in tumors not originating from the neural crest. The investigators compared MIBG scanning and CT and concluded that MIBG scanning allowed

whole-body screening, gave fewer false-positive results, had exquisite specificity, and often allowed identification of the cause of the primary lesion. MIBG scanning was found reliable in initial staging, in the postoperative phase, and in monitoring of the response to different treatments. MIBG scintigraphy allows imaging of the functional aspect of these neoplastic lesions. Schmiegelow et al. (136) evaluated 145 MIBG scans performed on 96 children, including 71 with neuroblastoma and 25 with other neoplastic or nonneoplastic diseases. The MIBG studies had a sensitivity of 94% and a specificity of 88%.

Because bone scanning and MIBG scanning both are used to evaluate neuroblastoma, the accuracy of the two techniques has been compared for the same patients. Lumbroso et al. (137) obtained 115 whole-body MIBG and bone scans for 70 children. With cytologic findings as the standard of reference, the sensitivity of MIBG scanning for detection of the primary lesion was 73%; for involvement of the bone marrow, the sensitivity was 90%, and the specificity was 100%. In comparison, bone scans had a sensitivity of 78% and a specificity of 51%. The sensitivity of MIBG scanning was 10% greater than that of bone scanning for bone and bone marrow metastasis. However, in patients with normal findings on MIBG scans, the use of bone scans is recommended.

The advantages of bone scanning over MIBG imaging for the evaluation of neuroblastoma (138–142) are that (a) some patients have abnormal findings on a bone scan despite having normal findings of MIBG imaging, (b) imaging is completed 3 hours after injection, and (c) the radiation exposure is lower. The disadvantages of bone scanning are that (a) it has poor specificity for a single lesion, (b) the sensitivity is somewhat lower in the growth-plate area, and (c) the study is technically demanding to obtain the best results. The advantages of the MIBG scanning over bone scanning are (a) it has high intraobserver consistency, (b) some patients have abnormal findings despite having normal findings on a bone scan, (c) it allows accurate assessment of the viability of the tumor posttreatment, and (d) it allows evaluation of extraosseous involvement. The disadvantage of MIBG imaging are (a) the study takes 2 to 3 days, (b) it results in a higher radiation dose, and (c) it has poor sensitivity for metastatic liver disease. MIBG was approved by the U.S. Food and Drug Administration in 1994. Because of the data currently available, our recommendation is (a) if there is a question of sensitivity, namely, "Is there any lesion in the entire body?" use both MIBG and bone scans and (b) if the clinical question is, "Is there a local lesion?" CT or MRI is probably more sensitive. If the clinical question is one of specificity, namely, "Is a finding on a plain radiograph CT scan, or MR image viable tumor?" MIBG scanning is the proper study.

Prostate Cancer

One of the major indications for bone scintigraphy in the past has been staging and early detection of metastatic disease from carcinoma of the prostate. In a study in the 1970s, Shaffer and Pendergrass (143) found bone scanning more sensitive in the detection of early metastatic disease than were radiographs, clinical evaluation, and the laboratory studies that were available at that time. Their study with 219 patients with adenocarcinoma of the prostate showed that 47% of patients without pain had positive bone scan results, 39% of patients with normal acid phosphatase levels had positive bone scan results, and 23% of patients with normal alkaline phosphatase levels had positive bone scan results. Fifteen percent of patients with positive bone scan results had no bone pain, and both alkaline and acid phosphatase levels were normal. Other studies (144,145) also have demonstrated the high sensitivity of bone scintigraphy.

Bone scans have value as a means of prognostic stratification. Soloway et al. (146) performed semiquantitative grading of bone scans using an estimate that showed good correlation with survival. In this classification, the 2-year survival rates for extent of disease in classes I through IV were 94%, 74%, 68%, and 40%, respectively. This prognostic value also was shown in a European study (147). Bone scanning also is of use for prognosis after treatment (20,147). However, patients treated for cancer of the prostate may have the flare phenomenon (17,20,148).

Since the introduction of the prostate-specific antigen (PSA) assay, the role of bone scintigraphy in the initial evaluation of patients for prostate cancer, the evaluation of early metastatic disease, and follow-up evaluation of these patients during therapy has changed dramatically. Measurement of PSA is more specific than is measurement of prostatic acid phosphatase in the detection of early prostate cancer (149), but the serum level also is elevated in benign prostatic hyperplasia. In a large study from the Mayo Clinic, Chybowski et al. (150) found that PSA level correlated well with results of bone scintigraphy. The results showed that in the initial evaluation of patients, those who had a low PSA level had a very low likelihood of having positive bone scan results for metastatic disease. Among approximately 300 men with a PSA level of 20 ng/mL or less, only 1 patient had a positive bone scan result, yielding a negative predictive value of 99.7%. Similar results were reported by Freitas et al. (151). In this series patients who had a PSA level of 8 ng/mL or less rarely had positive bone scan results. The negative predictive value with this level of PSA was 98.5%. In another study from the Mayo Clinic, Oesterling et al. (152) did a retrospective review of 2,064 consecutively enrolled patients with prostate cancer. For that study the investigators used a PSA level of 10 mg/mL or less. For patients who met this criterion and had no skeletal symptoms, a bone scan did not appear to be necessary for initial staging. In this large series, the criteria of a low PSA and no skeletal symptoms occurred in only 39% of patients with newly diagnosed prostate cancer. In this time of cost containment, it is reasonable to conclude that bone scanning is not indicated in the evaluation of patients with newly diagnosed prostate cancer if the serum PSA level is in the lower range of abnormal (10 to 20 mg/mL) and if the patient does not have pain suggestive of metastatic disease.

The routine use of bone scintigraphy in the follow-up care of patients with prostate cancer also is declining because of the use of PSA assays. A study by Miller et al. (153) showed that all patients with bone metastasis had a PSA levels of 20 ng/mL or greater. Sissons et al. (154), however, concluded that although measurement of PSA level is appropriate follow-up care, bone scans are useful for the evaluation of patients with symptoms or when a change in management is contemplated. The use of PSA measurement to assess progression of metastatic disease,

although valuable in most cases, may not be as valuable in the care of patients who have undergone hormonal treatment. Leo et al. (155) conducted a study with a group of patients who had undergone antiandrogen therapy and compared their results with those of a group of patients with no previous therapy for prostate cancer. The investigators concluded that a serum PSA level in the normal range in prostate cancer patients who have been treated hormonally does not necessarily mean that the patient is free of disease or that the disease is stable.

In patients who have undergone radical prostatectomy, PSA levels decrease to zero. These patients do not need evaluation with bone scintigraphy until symptoms develop or PSA level increases (156).

Although bone scanning remains an important study in initial staging, detection of early metastatic disease, and evaluation during and after therapy for prostate cancer, the introduction of PSA testing has changed the appropriate use of bone scintigraphy. Bone scanning should be limited to patients who have either elevation of PSA level, patients who have symptoms, patients who have been hormonally treated, or patients whose care may be altered according to the results of bone scanning.

Renal Cell Carcinoma

Kim et al. (157) found bone scanning more sensitive than plain radiography for the detection of renal cell carcinoma metastatic to bone. Steinbacher et al. (158), however, found that 16% of 91 osteolytic lesions showed no radiopharmaceutical accumulation. If photon-deficient lesions are to be detected, much greater care must be taken to obtain a bone scan with high-resolution collimation and longer imaging times to obtain higher information density.

Bone scintigraphy, although sensitive for detection of disease, has only limited value in the care of patients with renal cell carcinoma. Lindner et al. (159) in a review of 231 charts found the cases of 71 patients who had metastasis at first presentation. In that study, there was no case in which the first diagnosis of metastatic disease was made with the bone scan. The data indicated that routine bone scintigraphy in the absence of clinical or laboratory findings suggestive of metastatic disease was not indicated. In a more recent study, Atlas et al. (160) found bone scanning not as good a prognostic indicator as preoperative serum alkaline phosphatase level.

With the relatively low yield in the preoperative setting (159, 161) and difficulties in detecting some lesions in the postoperative setting, bone scintigraphy should not be performed routinely in the care of patients with renal cell carcinoma. Bone scans should be used when patients have symptoms and findings on plain radiographs are normal or when a change in therapy depends on the results of a bone scan.

CONCLUSION

At this time, competing imaging modalities such as MRI, PET, and spiral CT impinge on the role of MDP bone scintigraphy. The strength of this technique remains the ability to image the entire body easily. However, it is also important to strive for a quality examination. This is critical when photopenic lesions are possible, because these lesions can be easily missed with bad technique. For primary tumors, when high-quality bone scans are coupled to plain radiographs, and the degree of uptake, the location of the lesion, and the age of the patient add to the radiographic appearance, differential diagnosis improves. In the care of patients with metastatic bone disease, bone scanning often is the easiest and most effective way to follow the course of disease. As such, it will be a mainstay in most nuclear medicine facilities for years to come.

REFERENCES

1. Cook GJ, Fogelman I. The role of positron emission tomography in the management of bone metastases. *Cancer* 2000;88[12 Suppl]: 2927–2933.
2. Kao CH, Hsieh JF, Tsai SC, et al. Comparison and discrepancy of 18F-2-deoxyglucose positron emission tomography and Tc-99m MDP bone scan to detect bone metastases. *Anticancer Res* 2000;20: 2189–2192.
3. Krishnamurthy GT, Tubis M, Hiss J, et al. Distribution pattern of metastatic bone disease: a need for total body skeletal image. *JAMA* 1977;237:2504.
4. Boxer DI, Todd CEC, Coleman R, et al. Bone secondaries in breast cancer: the solitary metastasis. *J Nucl Med* 1989;30:1318–1320.
5. Boyd CM, Ridout RG, Angtuaco TL, et al. Significance of the solitary lesion on bone scans of adults with primary extraosseous cancer. *Radiology* 1984;153:119(abst).
6. Brown ML. The role of radionuclides in the patient with osteogenic sarcoma. *Semin Roentgenol* 1989;24:185.
7. Corcoran RJ, Thrall JH, Kyle RW, et al. Solitary abnormalities in bone scans of patients with extraosseous malignances. *Radiology* 1976; 121:663.
8. Kwai AH, Stomper PC, Kaplan WD. Clinical significance of isolated scintigraphic sternal lesions in patients with breast cancer. *J Nucl Med* 1988;29:324.
9. Rappaport AH, Hoffer PB, Genant HK. Unifocal bone findings by scintigraphy: clinical significance in patients with known primary cancer. *West J Med* 1978;129:188–192.
10. Robey EL, Schellhammer F. Solitary lesions on bone scan in genitourinary malignancy. *J Urol* 1984;132:1000–1002.
11. Shirazi PH, Rayudu GVS, Fordham EW. Review of solitary 18F bone scan lesions. *Radiology* 194;112:369.
12. Tumeh SS, Beadle G, Kaplan WD. Clinical significance of solitary rib lesions in patients with extraskeletal malignancy. *J Nucl Med* 1985; 26:1140.
13. Fernandes DS, Aye RW, Garnett, DJ, et al. Target-specific rib biopsy using the gamma probe. *Am J Surg* 2000;179:389–390.
14. Eustace S, Tello R, DeCarvalho V, et al. A comparison of whole-body turboSTIR MR imaging and planar 99mTc-methylene diphosphonate scintigraphy in the examination of patients with suspected skeletal metastases. *Am J Roentgenol* 1997;169:1655–1661.
15. Greenberg EJ, Chu FCH, Dwyer AJ, et al. Effects of radiation therapy on bone lesions as measured by 67Ga and 85Sr local kinetics. *J Nucl Med* 1972;13:747.
16. Gillespie PJ, Alexander JL, Edelstyn GA. Changes in 87mSr concentrations in skeletal metastases in patients responding to cyclical combination chemotherapy for advanced breast cancer. *J Nucl Med* 1975;16: 191.
17. Pollen JJ, Witztum KF, Ashburn WL. The flare phenomenon on radionuclide bone scan in metastatic prostate cancer. *Am J Roentgenol* 1984;142:773–776.
18. Rossleigh MA, Lovegrove FTA, Reynolds PM, et al. Serial bone scans in the assessment of response to therapy in advanced breast carcinoma. *Clin Nucl Med* 1982;7:397–402.
19. Rossleigh MA, Lovegrove FTA, Reynolds PM, et al. The assessment

20. Levenson RM, Sauerbrunn BJL, Bates HR, et al. Comparative value of bone scintigraphy and radiography in monitoring tumor response in systemically treated prostatic carcinoma. *Radiology* 1983;146: 513–518.
21. Coleman RE, Rubens RD, Fogelman I. Reappraisal of the baseline bone scan in breast cancer. *J Nucl Med* 1988;29:1045–1049.
22. Ali A, Tetalman MR, Fordham EW. Distribution of hypertrophic pulmonary osteoarthropathy. *Am J Roentgenol* 1980;134:771–780.
23. Samuels LD. Diagnosis of malignant bone disease with strontium-87m scans. *Can Med Assoc J* 1971;104:411–413.
24. Keck G, Christie JH, Mettler FA. Benign bone tumors and tumorlike conditions. In: Mettler FA Jr, ed. *Radionuclide bone imaging and densitometry*. New York: Churchill-Livingstone, 1988:31–61.
25. Hudson TM Scintigraphy of aneurysmal bone cysts. *Am J Roentgenol* 1984;142:761.
26. Sickles EA, Genant HK, Hoffer PB. Increased localization 99mTc-pyrophosphate in a bone island: a case report. *J Nucl Med* 1976;17: 113–115.
27. Raback DL. Tc-99m-MDP bone scintigraphy and "growing" bone islands. *Clin Nucl Med* 1980;5:98–101.
28. Hall FM, Goldberg RP, Davies JA, et al. Scintigraphic assessment of bone island. *Radiology* 1980;135:737–742.
29. Murray IP. Bone scanning in the child and young adult. *Skeletal Radiol* 1980;5:1–14.
30. Simon M, Kirchner PT. Scintigraphic evaluation of primary bone tumors: comparison of technetium-99m phosphonate and gallium citrate imaging. *J Bone Joint Surg Am* 1980;62:758–764.
31. Humphry A, Gilday DL, Brown RG. Bone scintigraphy in chondroblastoma. *Radiology* 1980;13:497–499.
32. Ulreich S, Swartz G, Stier SA, et al. Benign chondroblastoma of the talus demonstrated by skeletal scanning. *Clin Nucl Med* 1978;3:62.
33. Giannestras NJ, Diamond JR. Benign osteoblastomas of the talus. *J Bone Joint Surg* 1958;40:469.
34. Blau RA, Kwick DL, Westphal RA. Multiple non-ossifying fibromas: a case report. *J Bone Joint Surg Am* 1988;70:299–304.
35. Gilday DC, Ash JM. Benign bone tumor. *Semin Nucl Med* 1976;1: 33–46.
36. Machida K, Makita K, Nishikawa J, et al. Scintigraphic manifestation of fibrous dysplasia. *Clin Nucl Med* 1986;11:426–429.
37. Levine E, De Smett AA, Neff JR. Role of radiologic imaging in management planning of GCT of bone. *Skeletal Radiol* 1984;12:79–89.
38. Goodgold HM, Chen DCP, Majd M, et al. Scintigraphic features of giant cell tumor. *Clin Nucl Med* 1984;9:526–530.
39. Veluvolu P, Collier BD, Isitman AT. Scintigraphic skeletal "doughnut" sign due to giant cell tumor of the fibula. *Clin Nucl Med* 1984; 9:631–634.
40. Van Nonstrand D, Madewell JE, McNiesh LM, et al. Radionuclide bone scanning in giant cell tumor. *J Nucl Med* 1986;27:329–338.
41. Williams AG, Mettler FA. Vertebral hemangioma, radionuclide, radiographic and CT correlation. *Clin Nucl Med* 1985;10:598.
42. Martin NL, Preston DF, Robinson RG. Osteoblastomas of the axial skeleton shown by skeletal scanning. *J Nucl Med* 1976;17:187.
43. Pettine KA, Klassen RA. Osteoid-osteoma and osteoblastoma of the spine. *J Bone Joint Surg* 1986;68:354–361.
44. Wells RG, Miller JH, Sty JR. Scintigraphic patterns in osteoid osteoma and spondylolysis. *Clin Nucl Med* 1987;12:39–44.
45. Dahlin DC. *Bone tumors*, 3rd ed. Springfield: Charles C Thomas, 1978:28–42.
46. Kroon HM, Schurmans J. Osteoblastoma: clinical and radiologic findings in 98 new cases. *Radiology* 1990;175:783–790.
47. Kenan S, Floman Y, Robin GC, et al. Aggressive osteoblastoma: a case report and review of the literature. *Clin Orthop* 1985;195:294–298.
48. Lange RH, Lange TH, Rao BK. Correlative radiographic, scintigraphic and histological evaluation of exostoses. *J Bone Joint Surg* 1984;66:1454–1459.
49. Jaffe HL. Osteoid osteoma a benign osteoblastic tumor composed of osteoid and atypical bone. *Arch Surg* 1935;31:709–728.

50. Radcliffe SN, Walsh HJ, Carty H. Osteoid osteoma: the difficult diagnosis. *Eur J Radiol* 1998;28:67–79.

51. Swee RG, McLeod Ra, Beabout JW. Osteoid osteoma: detection, diagnosis, and localization. *Radiology* 1979:130:117–123.

52. Smith FW, Gilday DL. Scintigraphic appearances of osteoid osteoma. *Radiology* 1980;137:191–195.

53. Omojola MF, Cockshott WP, Beatty EG. Osteoid osteoma: an evaluation of diagnostic modalities. *Clin Radiol* 1981;32:199–204.

54. Lisbona R, Rosethall L. Role of radionuclide imaging in osteoid osteoma. *Am J Roentgenol* 1979;132:77–80.

55. Rosenthall L, Lisbona R. Role of radionuclide imaging in osteoid osteoma. *Am J Roentgenol* 1979;132:77–80.

56. Helms C, Hattner R, Vogler J. Osteoid osteoma, radionuclide diagnosis. *Radiology* 1984;151:779.

57. Lee DH, Malawer MN. Staging and treatment of primary and persistent (recurrent) osteoid osteoma: evaluation of intraoperative nuclear scanning, tetracycline fluorescence, and tomography. *Clin Orthop* 1992;281:229–238.

58. Smith FW, Nandi MB, Mils K. Spinal chondrosarcoma demonstrated by Tc-99m–MDP bone scan. *Clin Nucl Med* 1980;7:111–112.

59. Buyukdereli G, Sargin O, Ozbarlas S. Tc-99m tetrofosmin imaging in chondrosarcoma. *Clin Nucl Med* 2000;25:64–65.

60. Aoki J, Watanabe H, Shinozaki T, et al. FDG-PET in differential diagnosis and grading of chondrosarcomas. *J Comput Assist Tomogr* 1999;23:603–608.

61. Nair N. bone scanning in Ewing's sarcoma. *J Nucl Med* 1985;26: 349–352.

62. McNeil BJ, Cassady JR, Geiser CF, et al. Fluorine-18 bone scintigraphy in children with osteosarcoma or Ewing's sarcoma. *Radiology* 1973;109:27–31.

63. Siddiqui AR, Oseas RS, Wellman HN, et al. Evaluation of bone marrow scanning with technetium-99m sulfur colloid in pediatric oncology. *J Nucl Med* 1979;20:379–386.

64. Crone-Munzebrock W, Brassow F. A comparison of radiographic and bone scan findings in histiocytosis X. *Skeletal Radiol* 1983;9:170–173.

65. Parker BR, Pinckney L, Etcubanas E. Relative efficacy of radiographic and radionuclide bone surveys in the detection of the skeletal lesions of histiocytosis X. *Radiology* 1980;134:377–380.

66. Siddiqui AR, Tashjian JH, Lazarus K, et al. Nuclear medicine studies in evaluation of skeletal lesions in children with histiocytosis X. *Radiology* 1981;140:787–789.

67. Schaub T, Ash JM, Gilday DL. Radionuclide imaging in histiocytosis X. *Pediatr Radiol* 1987;17:397–404.

68. Kumar R, Balachandran S. Relative roles of radionuclide scanning and radiographic imaging in eosinophilic granuloma. *Clin Nucl Med* 1980;5:538.

69. Bar-Sever Z, Cohen IJ, Connolly LP, et al. Tc-99m MIBI to evaluate children with Ewing's sarcoma. *Clin Nucl Med* 2000;25:410–413.

70. Watanabe N, Shimizu M, Kageyama M, et al. Multiple myeloma evaluated with 201Tl scintigraphy compared with bone scintigraphy. *J Nucl Med* 1999;40:1138–1142.

71. Ludwig H, Kumpan W, Sinzinger H. Radiography and bone scintigraphy in multiple myeloma; a comparative analysis. *Br J Radiol* 1982; 55:173.

72. Nilsson-Ehle H, Holmdahl C, Suurkiula M, et al. Bone scintigraphy in the diagnosis of skeletal involvement and metastatic calcification in multiple myeloma. *Acta Med Scand* 1982;211:427.

73. Woolfenden JM, Pitt MJ, Durie BGM, et al. Comparison of bone scintigraphy in radiography in multiple myeloma. *Radiology* 1980; 134:723.

74. Wahner HW, Kyle RA, Beabout JW. Scintigraphic evaluation of the skeleton in multiple myeloma. *Mayo Clin Proc* 1980;55:739–746.

75. De Rosa G, Pezzullo L, Del Vecchio S. Avid (67)Ga uptake in multiple myeloma relapsing after bone marrow transplant. *Haematologica* 2000;85:764.

76. el-Shirbiny AM, Yeung H, Imbriaco M, et al. Technetium-99m-MIBI versus fluorine-18-FDG in diffuse multiple myeloma. *J Nucl Med* 1997;38:1208–1210.

77. Feggie LM, Spanedda R, Scutellari PN, et al. Bone marrow scintigraphy in multiple myeloma: a comparison with bone scintigraphy and skeletal radiology. *Radiol Med (Torino)* 1988;76:311–315.

78. Freeman CRK, Gledhill R, Chevalier LM, et al. Osteogenic sarcoma following treatment with megavoltage radiation and chemotherapy for bone tumors in children. *Med Pediatr Oncol* 1980;8:35–382.

79. Wong TZ, Connolly LP, Treves ST. Registration of three-dimensional magnetic resonance and radionuclide skeletal images. *Clin Nucl Med* 1999;24:859–863.

80. Smith J, Botet JF, Yeh SD. Bone sarcomas in Paget disease: a study of 85 patients. *Radiology* 1984;152:583.

81. Goldstein H, McNeil BJ, Zufall E, et al. Changing indications for bone scintigraphy in patients with osteosarcoma. *Radiology* 1980;135: 177–180.

82. McKillop JH, Etcubnas E, Goris ML. The indications for and limitations of bone scintigraphy in osteogenic sarcoma. *Cancer* 1981;48: 1133–1138.

83. McNeil BJ, Hanley J. Analysis of serial radionuclide bone images in osteosarcoma and breast carcinoma. *Radiology* 1980;135:171–176.

84. McNeil BJ. Value of bone scanning in neoplastic disease. *Semin Nucl Med* 1984;14:277.

85. Teates CD, Brpwer AC, Williamson BJR. Osteosarcoma extraosseous metastases demonstrated on bone scans and radiographs. *Clin Nucl Med* 1977;2:298–302.

86. Samuels LD. Lung scanning with [87m]Sr in metastatic osteosarcoma. *Am J Roentgenol* 1968;104:766–769.

87. Flowers WM.[99m]Tc-polyphosphate uptake within pulmonary and soft-tissue metastases from osteosarcoma. *Radiology* 1974;112: 377–378.

88. Ghaed N, Thrall JH, Pinsky SM, et al. Detection of extraosseous metastases from osteosarcoma with ^{99m}Tc-polyphosphate bone scanning. *Radiology* 1974;112:373–375.

89. Hughes S. Radionuclides in orthopaedic surgery. *J Bone Joint Surg Br* 1980;62:141–150.

90. Siddiqui AR, Wellman HN, Weetman RM, et al. Bone scanning in management of metastatic osteogenic sarcoma. *Clin Nucl Med* 1979; 4:6–11.

91. Edeline V, Frouin F, Bazin JP, et al. Factor analysis as a means of determining response to chemotherapy in patients with osteogenic sarcoma. *Eur J Nucl Med* 1993;20:1175–1185.

92. Sommer HJ, Knop J, Heise U, et al. Histomorphometric changes of osteo sarcoma after chemotherapy: correlation with ^{99m}Tc methylene diphosphonate functional imaging. *Cancer* 1987;59:252–258.

93. Menendez LR, Fideler BM, Mirra J. Thallium-201 scanning for the evaluation of osteosarcoma and soft–tissue sarcoma: a study of the evaluation and predictability of the histological response to chemotherapy. *J Bone Joint Surg Am* 1993;75:526–531.

94. Rosen G, Loren GJ, Brien EW, et al. Serial thallium-201 scintigraphy in osteosarcoma: correlation with tumor necrosis after preoperative chemotherapy. *Clin Orthop* 1993;293:302–306.

95. Nishiyama Y, Yamamoto Y, Toyama Y, et al. Diagnostic value of Tl-201 and three-phase bone scintigraphy for bone and soft-tissue tumors. *Clin Nucl Med* 2000;25:200–205.

96. Kunisada T, Ozaki T, Kawai A, et al. Imaging assessment of the responses of osteosarcoma patients to preoperative chemotherapy: angiography compared with thallium-201 scintigraphy. *Cancer* 1999; 86:949–956.

97. Sumiya H, Taki J, Tsuchiya H, et al. Midcourse thallium-201 scintigraphy to predict tumor response in bone and soft-tissue tumors. *J Nucl Med* 1998;39:1600–1604.

98. Sato O, Kawai A, Ozaki T, et al. Value of thallium-201 scintigraphy in bone and soft tissue tumors. *J Orthop Sci* 1998;3:297–303.

99. Taki J, Sumiya H, Tsuchiya H, et al. Evaluating benign and malignant bone and soft-tissue lesions with technetium-99m-MIBI scintigraphy. *J Nucl Med* 1997;38:501–506.

100. Kawai A, Sugihara S, Kunisada T, et al. Imaging assessment of the response of bone tumors to preoperative chemotherapy. *Clin Orthop* 1997;337:216–225.

101. Imbriaco M, Yeh SD, Yeung H, et al. Thallium-201 scintigraphy for the evaluation of tumor response to preoperative chemotherapy in patients with osteosarcoma. *Cancer* 1997;80:1507–1512.

102. Schulte M, Brecht-Krauss D, Werner M, et al. Evaluation of neoadjuvant therapy response of osteogenic sarcoma using FDG PET. *J Nucl Med* 1999;40:1637–1643.

103. Nadel HR. Thallium-201 for oncological imaging in children. *Semin Nucl Med* 1993;23:243–254.

104. Citrin DL, Tormey DC, Carbone PP. Implications of the ^{99m}Tc diphosphonate bone scan on treatment of primary breast cancer. *Cancer Treat Rep* 1977;61:1249.

105. Galasko CSB. The detection of skeletal metastases from carcinoma of the breast. *Surg Gynecol Obstet* 1971;132:1019.

106. Sklaroff DM, Charkes ND. Bone metastases from breast cancer at the time of radical mastectomy. *Surg Gynecol Obstet* 1968;127:763.

107. Joo KG, Parthasarathy KL, Bakshi SP, et al. Bone scintigrams: their clinical usefulness in patients with breast carcinoma. *Oncology* 1979;36:94.

108. Hahn P, Vikterlof KJ, Rydman H, et al. The value of whole body bone scan in the preoperative assessment of carcinoma of the breast. *Eur J Nucl Med* 1979;4:207.

109. McNeil BJ, Pace PD, Gray EB, et al. Preoperative and follow-up bone scans in patients with primary carcinoma of the breast. *Surg Gynecol Obstet* 1978;147:745.

110. O'Connell MJ, Wahner HW, Ahmann DL, et al. Value of preoperative radionuclide bone scan in suspected primary breast carcinoma. *Mayo Clin Proc* 1978;53:221.

111. Wilson GS, Rich MA, Brennan MJ. Evaluation of bone scan in preoperative clinical staging of breast cancer. *Arch Surg* 1980;115:415.

112. Ahmed A, Glynn-Jones R, Ell PJ, et al. Skeletal scintigraphy in carcinoma of the breast: a 10-year retrospective study of 389 patients. *Nucl Med Commun* 1990;11:421.

113. Front D, Schneck SO, Frankel A, et al. Bone metastases and bone pain in breast cancer: are they closely associated? *JAMA* 1979;242:1747.

114. Chaudary MA, Maisey MN, Shaw PJ, et al. Sequential bone scans and chest radiographs in the postoperative management of early breast cancer. *Br J Surg* 1983;70:517.

115. Brand WN. Clinical value of bone scanning with fluorine-18. In: Goswitz FA, Andrew GA, Viamonte, eds. *Clinical uses of radionuclides: critical comparison with other techniques.* Oakridge, TN: US Atomic Energy Commission, 1972:156.

116. Schutte HE. The influence of bone pain on the results of bone scan. *Cancer* 1979;44:2039.

117. Duncker CM, Carrio I, Berna L, et al. Radioimmune imaging of bone marrow in patients with suspected bone metastases from primary breast cancer. *J Nucl Med* 1990;31:1450–1455.

118. Buffaz PD, Gauchez AS, Caravel JP, et al. Can tumour marker assays be a guide in the prescription of bone scan for breast and lung cancers? *Eur J Nucl Med* 1999;26:8–11.

119. Wolfe JA, Rowe LD, Lowry LD. The value of radionucleotide scanning in the staging of head and neck carcinoma. *Ann Otol Rhinol Laryngol* 1979;88:832–836.

120. Sham JS, Tong CM, Choy D, et al. Role of bone scanning in detection of subclinical bone metastases in nasopharyngeal carcinoma. *Clin Nucl Med* 1991;16:27–29.

121. Brown DH, Leakos M. The value of a routine bone scan in a metastatic survey. *J Otolaryngol* 1998;27:187–189.

122. Sundram FX, Chua ET, Goh AS, et al. Bone scintigraphy in nasopharyngeal carcinoma. *Clin Radiol* 1990;42:166–169.

123. Ramsdell JW, Peters RM, Taylor AT, et al. Multiorgan scans for staging lung cancer: correlation with clinical evaluation. *J Thorac Cardiovasc Surg* 1977;73:653.

124. Gravenstein S, Pelta MA, Pories W. How ominous is an abnormal scan in bronchogenic carcinoma? *JAMA* 1979;241:2523.

125. Merric MV, Merric JM. Bone scintigraphy in lung cancer: a reappraisal. *Br J Radiol* 1986;59:1185.

126. Park JY, Kim KY, Lee J, et al. Impact of abnormal uptakes in bone scan on the prognosis of patients with lung cancer. *Lung Cancer* 2000;28:55–62.

127. Kosuda S, Gokan T, Tamura K, et al. Radionuclide imaging of two

128. Lederer A, Fluckiger F, Wildling R, et al. A solitary metastasis in the trapezium bone. *Radiologe* 1990;30:79–80.

129. Orzel JA, Sawaf NW, Richardson ML. Lymphoma of the skeleton: scintigraphic evaluation. *Am J Roentgenol* 1988;150:1095–1099.

130. Schetecter JP, Jones SE, Woolfended JM, et al. Bone scanning in lymphoma. *Cancer* 1976;38:1142–1148.

131. Delcambre C, Reman O, Henry-Amar M, et al. Clinical relevance of gallium-67 scintigraphy in lymphoma before and after therapy. *Eur J Nucl Med* 2000;27:176–184.

132. Moog F, Bangerter M, Diederichs CG, et al. Extranodal malignant lymphoma: detection with FDG PET versus CT. *Radiology* 1998;206:475–481.

133. Heisel MA, Miller JH, Reid BS, et al. Radionuclide scan in neuroblastoma. *Pediatrics* 1983;71:206–209.

134. MacDonald WB, Stevens MM, Dalla Pozza L, et al. Gallium-67 and technetium-99m–methylene diphosphonate skeletal scintigraphy in determining prognosis for children with stage IV neuroblastoma. *J Nucl Med* 1993;34:1082–1086.

135. Troncone L, Rufini V, Montemaggi P, et al. The diagnostic and therapeutic utility of radiodinated metaiodobenzylguanidine (MIBG). *Eur J Nucl Med* 1990;16:325–335.

136. Schmiegelow K, Simes MA, Agertoft L, et al. Radio-iodobenzylguanidine scintigraphy of neuroblastoma: conflicting results, when compared with standard investigations. *Med Pediatr Oncol* 1989;17:127–130.

137. Lumbroso JD, Guermazi F, Hartmann O, et al. Meta-iodobenzylguanidine (MIBG) scans in neuroblastoma: sensitivity and specificity, a review of 115 scans. In: Evans AE, D'Angio GJ, Kdudson A, et al., eds. *Advances in neuroblastoma research.* New York: Alan R. Liss, 1988:689–705.

138. Shulkin BL, Shapiro B, Hutchinson RJ. Iodine-131-metaiodobenzylguanidine and bone scintigraphy for the detection of neuroblastoma. *J Nucl Med* 1992;33:1735–1740.

139. Parisi MT, Greene MK, Dykes TM, et al. Efficacy of metaiodobenzylguanidine as a scintigraphic agent for the detection of neuroblastoma. *Invest Radiol* 1992;27:768–773.

140. Englaro EE, Gelfand MJ, Harris RE, et al. I-131 MIBG imaging after bone marrow transplantation for neuroblastoma. *Radiology* 1992;182:515–520.

141. Gordon I, Peters AM, Gutman A, et al. Skeletal assessment in neuroblastoma: the pitfalls of iodine-123–MIBG scans. *J Nucl Med* 1990;31:129–134.

142. Gilday DL, Greenberg M. The controversy about the nuclear medicine investigation of neuroblastoma [Editorial]. *J Nucl Med* 1990;31:135.

143. Schaffer DL, Pendergrass HP. Comparison of enzyme, clinical radiographic, and radionuclide methods of detecting bone metastases from carcinoma of the prostate. *Radiology* 1976;121:431.

144. McGregor B, Tulloch AGS, Quinlan MF, et al. The role of bone scanning in the assessment of prostatic carcinoma. *Br J Urol* 1978;50:178.

145. O'Donogue EPN, Constable AR, Sherwood T, et al. Bone scanning and phosphatases in carcinoma of the prostate. *Br J Urol* 1978;50:172.

146. Soloway MS, Hardeman SW, Hickey D, et al. Stratification of patients with metastatic prostate cancer based on extent of disease on initial bone scan. *Cancer* 1988;61:195–202.

147. Lund F, Smith PH, Suciu S, for the EORTC Urological Group. Do bone scans predict prognosis in prostatic cancer? A report of the EORTC Protocol 30762. *Br J Urol* 1984;56:58–63.

148. Johns WD, Garnick MB, Kaplan WD. Leuprolide therapy for prostate cancer: an association with scintigraphic "flare" on bone scan. *Clin Nucl Med* 1990;15:485–487.

149. Stamey TA, Yang N, Hay AR, et al. Prostate-specific antigen as a serum marker for adenocarcinoma of the prostate. *N Engl J Med* 1987;317:909–916.

150. Chybowski FM, Keller JL, Bergstralh EJ, et al. Predicting radionuclide

bone scan findings in patients with newly diagnosed, untreated prostate cancer: prostate specific antigen is superior to all other clinical parameters. *J Urol* 1991;145:313.

151. Freitas JE, Gilvydas R, Ferry JD, et al. The clinical utility of prostate-specific antigen and bone scintigraphy in prostate cancer follow-up. *J Nucl Med* 1991;32:1387–1390.

152. Oesterling JE, Martin SK, Bergsralh EJ, et al. The use of prostate-specific antigen in staging patients with newly diagnosed prostate cancer. *JAMA* 1993;269:57–60.

153. Miller PD, Eardley I, Kirby RS. Prostate specific antigen and bone scan correlation in the staging and monitoring of patients with prostate cancer. *Br J Urol* 1992;70:295–298.

154. Sissons GRJ, Clements R, Peeling WB, et al. Can serum prostate-specific antigen replace bone scintigraphy in the follow-up of metastatic prostate cancer. *Br J Urol* 1992;65:861–864.

155. Leo ME, Bilhart DL, Bergstralh EJ, et al. Prostate-specific antigen in hormonally treated stage D2 prostate cancer: is it always an accurate indicator of disease status? *J Urol* 1991;145:802.

156. Terris MK, Kilnecke AS, McDougall IR, et al. Utilization of bone scans in conjunction with prostate-specific antigen levels in the surveillance for recurrence of adenocarcinoma after radical prostatectomy. *J Nucl Med* 1991;32:1713.

157. Kim EE, Bledin AG, Gutierrez C, et al. Comparison of radionuclide images and radiographs for skeletal metastases from renal cell carcinoma. *Oncology* 1983;40:284–286.

158. Steinbacher M, Rieden K, Bihl H, et al. Uptake behavior of bone metastases of hypernephroma in the 99mTc-MDP bone scintigram: a comparison with x-ray findings. *Rofo Fortschr Geb Rontgenstr Nuklearmed* 1987;146:555.

159. Lindner A, Goldman DG, deKernion JB. Cost effective analysis of prenephrectomy radioisotope scans in renal cell carcinoma. *Urology* 1983;22:127–129.

160. Atlas I, Kwan D, Stone N. Value of serum alkaline phosphatase and radionuclide bone scans in patients with renal cell carcinoma. *Urology* 1991;38:220–222.

161. Rosen PR, Murphy KG. Bone scintigraphy in the initial staging of patients with renal cell carcinoma [Concise Communication]. *J Nucl Med* 1984;25:289–291.

21

BENIGN BONE DISEASE

VASEEM U. CHENGAZI
ROBERT E. O'MARA

Scintigraphic imaging has become one of the most frequently performed procedures in nuclear medicine departments, mainly because of the ability to image the entire skeleton economically and with a low radiation dose to the patient. The wide availability of gamma cameras with steadily improving performance characteristics, a choice of radiopharmaceuticals, and the emergence of newer techniques such as iterative reconstruction of single photon emission computed tomography (SPECT) data and positron emission tomography (PET) will ensure a continued role for this modality as a highly sensitive method for detecting a wide variety of skeletal diseases. An astute nuclear medicine physician can improve the specificity of imaging by means of applying pattern recognition in a given clinical context to aid the referring physician in arriving at the correct diagnosis. The main indications for skeletal scintigraphy are neoplasm and trauma, which are discussed in Chapters 20 and 22. The role of PET of bone is discussed in Chapter 23. This chapter deals predominantly with benign disease in which skeletal imaging may play a significant role, including infection, metabolic disease, osteonecrosis, arthritis, and aftermath of irradiation of bone. In assessing these entities, one must be aware of the relation between chronologic evolution of a disease process under study and the scintigraphic appearance. In arriving at a conclusion, one must be able to incorporate information from processes such as the soft-tissue uptake of radiopharmaceuticals, underlying bone disease, or the sequelae of surgical intervention.

When used appropriately in a management algorithm, skeletal scintigraphy can be used for early recognition, assessment of the extent and activity status, and differential diagnosis of a disease process. It can also be used to identify sites for further evaluation with other radiographic techniques or with closed or open biopsy and to assess the efficacy of therapeutic regimens. This role in a given situation must be determined in relation to the complementary and sometimes competing roles of radiographic evaluation. Standard radiographic evaluations of bone excel in the demonstration of osseous structural detail, whereas

scintigraphy excels in the evaluation of function. Thus disease processes with a slow rate of mineral loss or gain become evident at a later stage in conventional radiography, whereas metabolically inactive lesions may not be visualized at scintigraphy. In addition, computed tomography (CT) is playing an increasing role in defining involvement of bone by disease. Magnetic resonance imaging (MRI) offers the best resolution of soft-tissue versus bone involvement of any imaging technique and the ability to visualize bone marrow changes and diseases that cause increased tissue water. MRI also has the advantage of not entailing radiation, a factor especially important in imaging pediatric patients.

More rapid imaging systems in both modalities are under active development, and the ability to visualize large parts or all of the skeletal system has become real. One possible algorithmic approach is presented in Fig. 21.1, whereby the role of skeletal scintigraphy is determined by the focality of symptoms. For localized symptoms, a standard direct radiograph can be obtained first. Despite its somewhat low sensitivity, direct radiography is inexpensive, quick, and readily available. If the findings are noncontributory, other imaging modalities can be used. For diffuse or multifocal symptoms, skeletal scintigraphy can be used first and be followed up by appropriate direct radiographic, CT, or MRI examinations directed at specifically identified areas. This suggested algorithm can be modified by advances in imaging and diagnostic techniques, such as screening for biochemical and metabolic markers, and must be adapted to each institution.

V. Chengazi: Department of Radiology, Division of Nuclear Medicine, University of Rochester, and Division of Nuclear Medicine, Strong Memorial Hospital, University of Rochester Medical Center, Rochester, NY.

R.E. O'Mara: Department of Radiology, Division of Nuclear Medicine, Strong Memorial Hospital, University Of Rochester Medical Center, Rochester, NY.

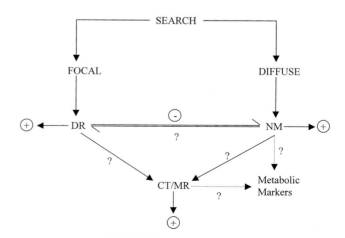

FIGURE 21.1. Focal symptoms.

Differences in available equipment, imaging times, and availability of personnel must be recognized.

INFECTION

Skeletal scintigraphy plays an important role in the evaluation of patients believed to have acute osteomyelitis. As with most osseous lesions, findings at bone imaging frequently are abnormal in the presence of acute osteomyelitis, whereas findings on conventional radiographic images are normal or equivocal. In infectious disease, in particular, radiographs tend to depict osseous abnormalities late in the course of the disease. Abnormal findings on bone scans occur early in the process and allow early institution of therapy. If the diagnosis of infection is in doubt, the imaging procedure may point to the area to be considered for biopsy and subsequent microbiologic studies. Satisfactory results are obtained only when the nuclear medicine physician is willing to pay great attention to technique. This includes willingness to tailor the study to the particular patient problem,

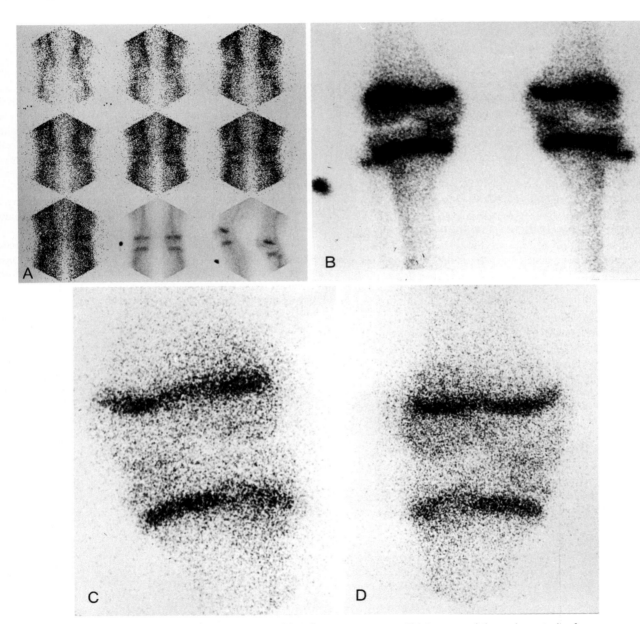

FIGURE 21.2. Perfusion study for possible inflammatory process. This is a normal three-phase study of a 10-year-old boy evaluated for possible osteomyelitis of the right knee. He had fever, and pain in the right knee for 4 days. Findings on radiographs were normal. **A:** Perfusion and immediate soft-tissue views show no abnormal changes. **B:** Delayed magnified views show the knees are symmetric and normal. **C, D:** Pinhole views of the knees also have normal findings. The lack of change in perfusion indicates that no infectious or inflammatory process is taking place in this child's leg. Detailed views, such as these, in several projections must be obtained if the bone scan is to be used properly.

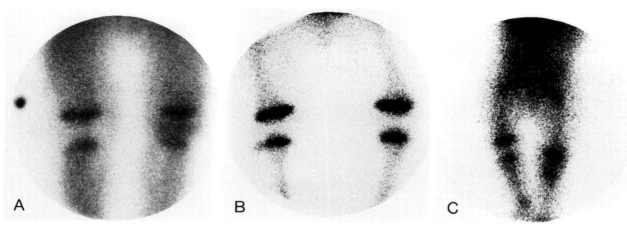

FIGURE 21.3. Soft-tissue infection. Bone scans of a 6-year-old boy with fever for 3 days and pain and swelling in the left knee for 2 days before the study. There is increased perfusion to the left leg and knee. **A:** Immediate soft-tissue views show increased soft-tissue activity in and around the knee joint. **B:** Two-hour delayed views of the knees show no focal changes of increased activity in the bones of the joint. At this time, the findings were considered consistent with cellulitis or septic arthritis of the knee rather than osteomyelitis. **C:** A twenty-four-hour gallium study shows diffusely increased activity around the soft tissues of the joint with no abnormal osseous localization. Culture of the joint aspirate revealed *Staphylococcus aureus.*

use of several projections and magnification views to adequately assess questionable areas, especially in young patients, and use of SPECT as an alternative approach to obtaining maximum information from imaging studies in the care of such patients.

In most centers, the standard approach to assess for osteomyelitis is to perform a three-phase procedure to examine perfusion, immediate soft-tissue blood pool, and delayed (2 to 4 hours) bone uptake. Almost any pathologic condition affecting bone causes increased perfusion in that area. The main advantage of a perfusion study is its high negative predictive value. Normal perfusion in the region under examination usually excludes the presence of an acute inflammatory process (Fig. 21.2). Increased

soft-tissue activity in the initial imaging phase occurs with cellulitis. Clearing of this activity to normal or slightly increased activity levels in a diffuse pattern in the same or distal areas on delayed images is the usual pattern when cellulitis alone is present. When soft-tissue inflammation and infection are present together, the resulting increased perfusion to an affected limb increases activity in that limb (Fig. 21.3). When soft-tissue infection alone is present, no focal, abnormally increased areas of activity are present in the bone, but a diffuse increase in the osseous structures may be observed, the so-called watershed effect. Osteomyelitis usually manifests as an area of focally increased activity on routine delayed images (Fig. 21.4). At times,

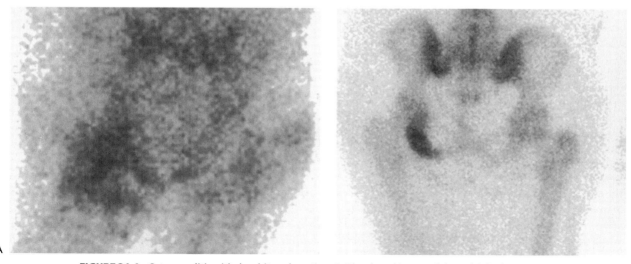

FIGURE 21.4. Osteomyelitis with decubitus ulceration. **A:** Blood pool image of the pelvis in the posterior projection shows abnormal vascularity caused by cellulitis in the left gluteal region. The central region of relative photopenia indicates necrosis. **B:** Delayed image of the same projection shows abnormally increased uptake in the underlying left ischium, a finding that suggests osteomyelitis.

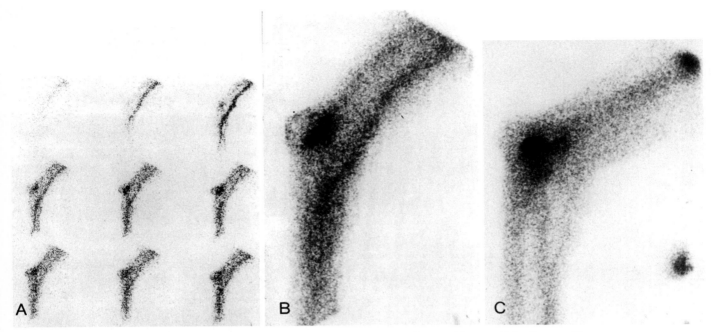

FIGURE 21.5. Osteomyelitis cellulitis. A 47-year-old had a 2-day history of fever and left elbow swelling and pain without trauma. Findings on radiographs were normal. **A:** Perfusion-phase image shows increased perfusion to the elbow, including the bursa. **B:** Blood-pool phase image shows increased activity in the bursa that indicates olecranon bursitis. **C:** Six-hour delayed view shows clearing of bursal soft-tissue activity with a focal increase in the olecranon. *Staphylococcus aureus* organisms were cultured from a specimen obtained by means of needle biopsy of the olecranon.

delay past the usual 2- to 4-hour period for delayed static imaging accentuates the difference between focal areas of increased activity and diffuse activity seen as a result of increased perfusion. These fourth and fifth phase studies usually are performed 6 to 8 hours after injection or 24 hours after injection (Fig. 21.5). When used in this manner, the routine skeletal imaging procedure has both high sensitivity and high specificity in the evaluation of osteomyelitis (1). In most situations, the sensitivity of bone scintigraphy for the detection of osteomyelitis approaches 90% with a likewise high specificity and overall accuracy. Despite this, plain-film radiography is the initial procedure of choice in cases in which osteomyelitis is suspected because of its low cost, ready availability, and lack of a total-body radiation dose. When the radiographic findings are normal or equivocal in the face of significant clinical suspicion, radionuclide imaging is indicated. One advantage of scintigraphy is the ability to image the entire skeleton, as in evaluation for multifocal osteomyelitis (Fig. 21.6).

Findings at routine bone imaging are not abnormal in all cases of osteomyelitis. Difficulty can be encountered at both ends of the age spectrum. Some experts regard the use of routine skeletal scintigraphy in the care of neonates as futile, whereas others report results similar to those stated earlier (2–5). Difficulty in diagnosis can be met at the other end of the age spectrum, in examinations of the elderly, especially those with peripheral vascular disease, as occurs with diabetes. In these patients, poor blood flow can make abnormal findings at best equivocal, particularly when superimposed on degenerative diseases of the joints or other underlying bone conditions, such as Charcot-type joints in the feet of patients with diabetes.

Frequently, osteomyelitis may not be acute but chronic, which results in rather poor uptake of the bone-seeking radiopharmaceutical, even in young patients (Fig. 21.7). In some instances, especially in the pediatric age group, the early increased pressure in the marrow space may result in decreased radionuclide accumulation and the appearance of a photon-deficient lesion at the site of infection. This sign usually occurs very early in the disease. Serial studies with routine bone-imaging agents or with secondary agents such as ^{67}Ga citrate or radiolabeled leukocytes may help achieve the diagnosis (6–9) (Fig. 21.8). Multifocal abnormal sites can be seen when osteomyelitis is caused by organisms such as *Salmonella typhi,* or they may be the result of viral infection (10) (Fig. 21.9). Addition of intervening antibiotic therapeutic regimens, whether complete or incomplete, may result in reduced intensity of activity in patients undergoing bone scintigraphic examinations for osteomyelitis.

Other Radiopharmaceuticals

[67]Ga citrate has been used to study both acute and chronic osteomyelitis, especially as backup in cases in which osteomyelitis is under clinical suspicion and findings on routine bone scans and radiographs are normal or equivocal. Early imaging 24 hours after injection may show abnormally increased activity at the site of suspected involvement. It is still important, however, to delay for a 48-hour image, especially of the axial skeleton and

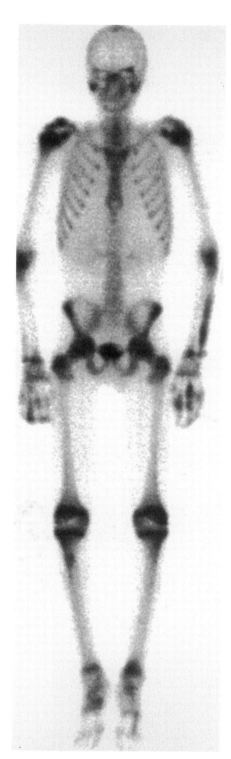

FIGURE 21.6. Multifocal osteomyelitis. Abnormal areas of irregularly increased uptake occur at several sites, including most notably the distal part of the ulna (left more than right), proximal part of the right tibia, several metacarpals bilaterally, and the left fourth metatarsal.

before reporting the results of the study as normal. Nonetheless, a ^{67}Ga study shows increased activity in areas of increased bone remodeling, such as fractures, surgical sites, neuropathic changes, arthritis, and pseudoarthrosis. One method proposed to increase sensitivity and specificity for the detection of osteomyelitis is to compare ^{67}Ga uptake in the suspect lesion with that on a routine bone scan (Fig. 21.10). The mismatch of greater increased ^{67}Ga uptake versus normal or increased activity of an agent used in routine bone imaging is an important finding. It indicates infectious involvement, especially in inviolate bone not affected by previous trauma, surgery, or another process (11,12).

^{111}In-labeled white blood cells (WBCs) have been used to study bone infection. Several studies have indicated sensitivity and specificity in the high 80% to low 90% range. Some authors believe results of an ^{111}In-WBC scan are abnormal before conventional radionuclide bone imaging and that the scans show a higher concentration in experimental joint inflammation than do ^{67}Ga scans (13–17). However, chronic infection and previous antibiotic therapy have been shown to reduce sensitivity (18).

Several techniques for labeling leukocytes with ^{99m}Tc have been proposed. The most common procedure is to label the leukocytes with ^{99m}Tc hexamethylpropyleneamine oxime (HMPAO). The sensitivity and specificity for ^{99m}Tc WBCs is similar to that for ^{111}In WBCs. It is to be expected that studies with either agent would have similar false-positive and false-negative results because both procedures entail use of use leukocytes to carry the radionuclide to the site of infection. Nonetheless, ^{99m}Tc WBC has advantages. The higher dose administered allows superior technical imaging, including SPECT. The possibility of labeling leukocytes with ^{99m}Tc HMPAO is more prevalent than is that of labeling with ^{111}In. Almost all hospitals have technetium generators available on a routine basis, whereas ^{111}In must be ordered for a specific patient study. However, both ^{111}In and ^{99m}Tc-WBCs have the limitation of requiring cell separation and labeling techniques. The procedure can take as long as 2 hours, and it must be ensured that the WBCs are separated with considerable skill to avoid cell damage and red blood cell labeling, especially with the ^{99m}Tc HMPAO technique. Newer kits may allow more rapid labeling.

Use of labeled leukocytes is not 100% specific in the diagnosis of acute infection. Sensitivity and specificity are reduced in the presence of chronic infection and soft-tissue sepsis (Fig. 21.11), especially sepsis adjacent to bones, of previous conditions such as fractures and tumors, and of previous treatment with antibiotics or steroids. Nonetheless, leukocyte labeling plays a strong role in either primary or secondary skeletal imaging in the diagnosis of infectious disease (19,20).

Early results with the use of radiolabeled antibodies show some promise in the study of infected bone. The first reports concern technetium- or iodine-labeled antigranulocyte antibodies, for which high sensitivity and specificity are reported (21–23). Unfortunately, these are produced from mouse antibodies, and adverse human antimouse antibody (HAMA) reactions have been reported. ^{111}In- and ^{99m}Tc-labeled human polyclonal immunoglobulin G has been introduced (24–26). Early results appear promising with high sensitivity and specificity. Because this class of agents is a human antibody, it does not produce the HAMA reaction that can occur with murine-based

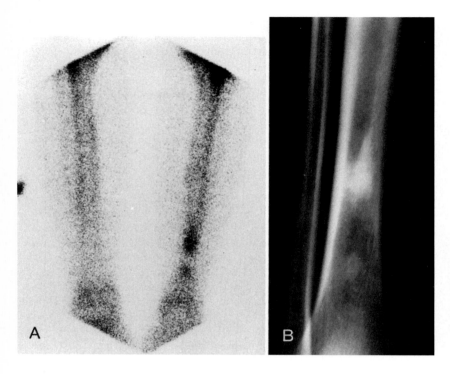

FIGURE 21.7. Chronic osteomyelitis. A 16-year-old female athlete had pain in the left lower leg 4 months before the examination. Radiographs at that time revealed a poorly defined density believed to represent a stress fracture. The patient was told to stay at rest for 6 weeks and had some relief of pain. When she resumed activity, the pain returned and increased. There was no radiographic change, and a cast was applied for 4 weeks. On removal of the cast, the pain immediately returned, and the bone imaging study was ordered. Results of the perfusion study were normal. **A:** Delayed view of the leg shows two sites of low-grade abnormally increased activity in the tibia. This was considered more consistent with a chronic osteomyelitis than with a fracture. **B:** Results of radiographic tomography confirmed the presence of two lesions. Biopsy showed changes that suggested chronic, indolent osteomyelitis. This condition can be difficult to diagnose with routine bone imaging or secondary studies, such as those performed with ^{67}Ga citrate or ^{111}In-labeled leukocytes.

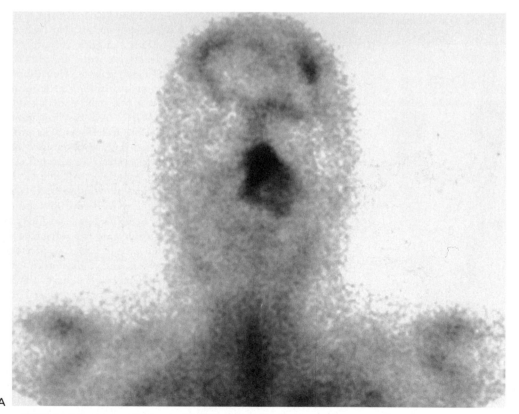

FIGURE 21.8. Images obtained with ^{99m}Tc white blood cells show osteomyelitis of the frontal bone after paranasal sinus surgery. **A:** Four weeks after surgery with abnormal uptake in the frontal bone. *(Figure continues.)*

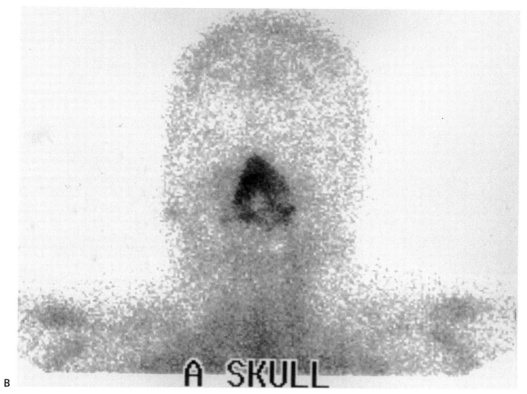

B

FIGURE 21.8. *Continued.* **B:** Resolution after an appropriate course of antibiotic therapy. Loss of intensity of uptake in the paranasal region is evident with healing of postsurgical changes.

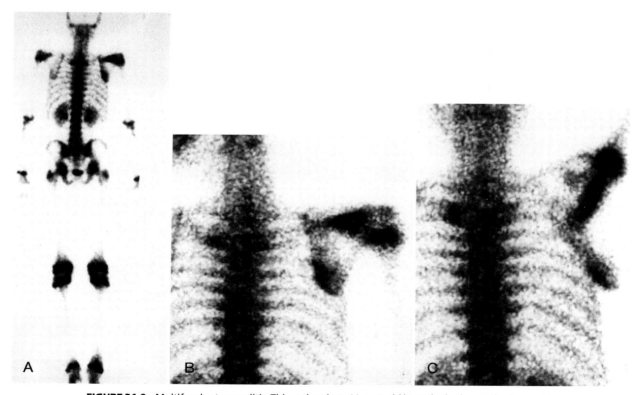

FIGURE 21.9. Multifocal osteomyelitis. This patient is an 11-year-old boy who had upper back, shoulder, and ankle pain during a viral pulmonary infection. **A:** Posterior total body view shows abnormally increased activity in the right distal tibia, right scapula, and third left costovertebral junction. **B, C:** Evidence on spot views of the posterior part of the chest with arms neutral and elevated confirms the abnormal sites in the left third rib and right scapula.

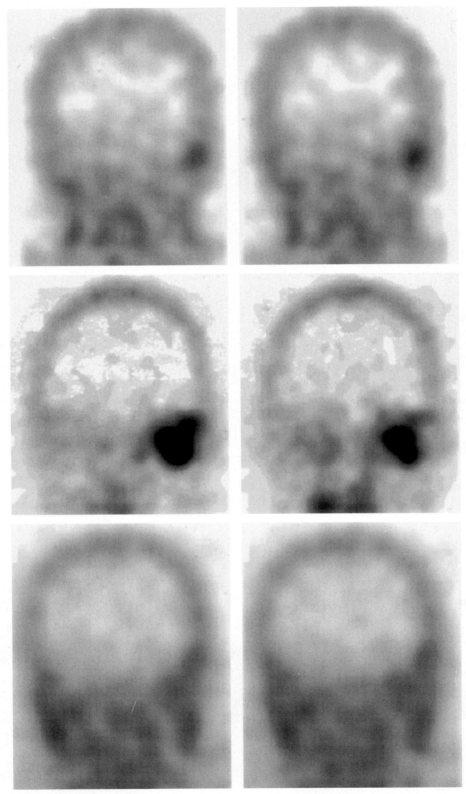

FIGURE 21.10. Left-sided malignant otitis externa with osteomyelitis. Selected coronal sections from SPECT studies of the skull show abnormal uptake imaged with ^{67}Ga citrate (*top row*) and ^{99m}Tc methylene diphosphonate (*middle row*) at initiation of antibiotic therapy. Repeated ^{67}Ga scan (*bottom row*) shows loss of abnormal uptake consistent with healing after 8 weeks of therapy.

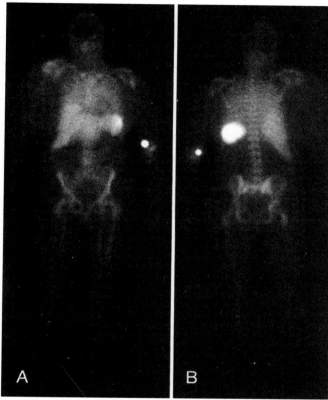

FIGURE 21.11. Septic arthritis. Anterior **(A)** and posterior **(B)** views of a 56-year-old woman undergoing hemodialysis who has a documented infection in the right arm (marked swelling) and septicemia. ^{99m}Tc white blood cell study shows abnormal activity in the right shoulder joint but not in the bones. No other abnormal areas are evident. *Klebsiella mobilis* (*Enterobacter aerogenes*) was cultured by means of needle aspiration from the joint.

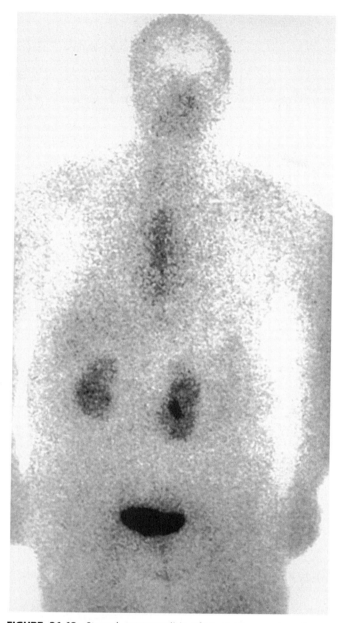

FIGURE 21.12. Sternal osteomyelitis after coronary artery bypass grafting. Image obtained with ^{99m}Tc ciprofloxacin shows lack of bone marrow uptake, which would be present on a white blood cell study. (Courtesy of Professor K. E. Britton, St. Bartholomew's Hospital, London, UK.)

antigranulocyte antibodies. This group of agents remains of considerable interest and promise depending on the outcome of studies.

A newer approach is imaging with radiolabeled antibiotics, such as ^{99m}Tc ciprofloxacin (Infecton). This agent is based on a quinolone antibiotic and has been shown to accumulate in the presence of active bacterial infection with a sensitivity somewhat better than and a specificity markedly better than that of radiolabeled WBC (Figs. 21.12, 21.13). Further experience with this agent is needed before its place in the imaging algorithm is fully ascertained (26a,26b).

Other Modalities

CT can be a valuable tool in the attempt to diagnose osteomyelitis. CT with bone windows gives excellent images of the bony cortex. It may well be used in many cases to determine the extent of bone infection and to guide biopsy for specimen retrieval and study.

MRI has the best resolution of soft-tissue involvement, as opposed to bone involvement, of any of the current radiographic techniques. Many studies have indicated that the sensitivity and specificity of MRI are quite high and may even exceed those of radionuclide studies. However, any process that replaces bone

marrow or causes increased tissue water, such as healing fractures, metabolic conditions, and tumors, can resemble osteomyelitis. Artifacts produced by orthopedic insertion of prosthetic devices can degrade images and reduce diagnostic accuracy. MRI is considerably more expensive than the radionuclide approach, and time on MRI units may not be available to examine a patient in an emergency.

Imaging Strategies

The plethora of radionuclide and radiologic imaging techniques demonstrates that except in very simple cases of acute peripheral

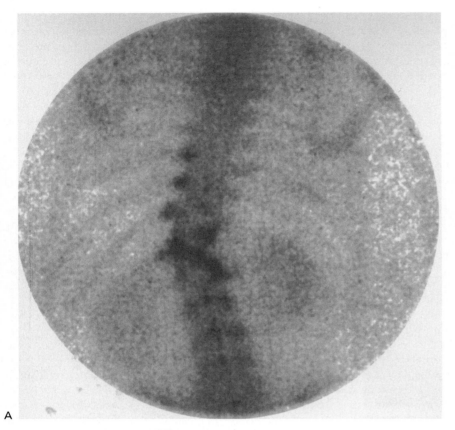

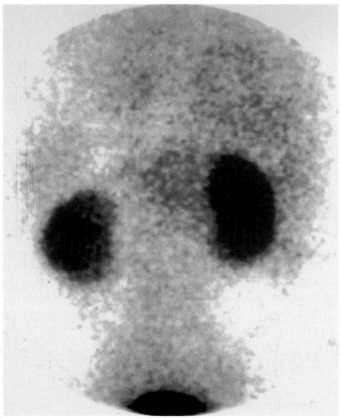

FIGURE 21.13. Tuberculous abscess. Image obtained with ^{99m}Tc methylene diphosphonate **(A)** shows abnormal uptake at site of angulation. Image obtained with ^{99m}Tc ciprofloxacin **(B)** shows increased uptake medial to the upper pole of the right kidney in the abscess. (Courtesy of Professor K. E. Britton, St. Bartholomew's Hospital, London, UK.)

osteomyelitis, the diagnosis of bone infection may be difficult to achieve without surgical intervention that can include bone biopsy, joint aspiration, and the like. Nonetheless, protocols have been developed to assist in the more complex cases of bone infection either directly or through pattern recognition. The following are descriptions of some protocols in use in our institution.

Evaluation of the diabetic foot remains a vexing problem (27). Osteomyelitis may be the result of direct extension of chronic soft-tissue infection in these patients. We have obtained our best results using combined ^{67}Ga and ^{99m}Tc methylene diphosphonate (MDP) studies in which the mismatch of increased ^{67}Ga activity versus normal or increased amounts of a routine bone imaging agent is an important finding that indicates infectious involvement (28). The combined use of radionuclide agents increases the cost to the point that the argument concerning the increased expense of CT or MRI imaging is no longer valid. With ^{67}Ga or leukocyte imaging it may not be possible to differentiate soft-tissue infection from underlying bone infection without a good-quality radiolabeled phosphonate bone scan (29, 30).

Axial, especially vertebral, infection may be difficult to diagnose with routine bone imaging and the combined use of radionuclides is needed (31,32). Radiolabeled leukocyte imaging may give poor results when WBCs are used alone because the agent normally distributes in the bone marrow as well as in areas of infection. Indeed, 10% to 30% of infected vertebral bodies may appear as a photon-deficient lesion on a leukocyte scan (33–35) (Fig. 21.14). It may be best to use a combination of leukocyte imaging with an agent such as ^{99m}Tc-labeled nanocolloid for demonstration of normal marrow distribution and any interruption in this pattern (36,37). When this technique is used, one must use ^{111}In WBC if dual-isotope imaging is to be performed; otherwise a 2-day study is needed. The demonstration of incongruent leukocyte and colloid images with increased leukocyte activity and decreased colloid uptake has a high diagnostic value. Our general practice is to perform an initial evaluation with MRI and then, if necessary, use radionuclide techniques for the detection of vertebral infection. Another approach to demonstrating incongruous marrow and leukocyte activity is to double-label leukocytes with ^{99m}Tc HMPAO and ^{111}In. The bone marrow can be detected on images obtained on the ^{99m}Tc photopeak 1 hour after injection and compared (both qualitatively and quantitatively) with images obtained 24 hours after injection on the ^{111}In photopeak.

Differentiation of septic arthritis from osteomyelitis with routine skeletal imaging alone can present a difficult problem (38). In most cases of septic arthritis, diffusely increased activity in the bones of the joint can be seen on delayed images, but perfusion in early soft-tissue uptake and early blood pool images may be limited to the soft tissues only. If a focal area of abnormally increased ^{99m}Tc phosphonate activity is not seen in the bones around the joint, the diagnosis of osteomyelitis cannot be established. Here, again, ^{67}Ga citrate imaging or, more commonly, radiolabeled WBC imaging can be helpful. In the presence of septic arthritis, these agents demonstrate activity patterns of a diffuse nature in the soft tissue in and around the joint with no

focal abnormality in bone. However, this can be difficult to ascertain without demonstration of exactly where the bone lies in relation to the soft-tissue infection and may necessitate combined imaging, such as ^{99m}Tc MDP–^{111}In WBC imaging. An ^{111}In WBC–^{99m}Tc MDP combined study is more specific than a ^{67}Ga–^{99}Tc MDP study and produces fewer equivocal results. Although the ^{111}In WBC–^{99m}Tc MDP combination decreases the number of false-positive results, abnormal findings still occur among patients with neuropathic joint disease, rheumatoid arthritis, gout, and even metastatic disease. Even with such combined efforts, differentiation can be difficult. Aspiration of the joint and culture of the contents remain an advantageous and rapid tool in this situation.

In examinations of pediatric patients, especially neonates, we use ^{99m}Tc MDP in the three- or four-phase mode for whole-body imaging. Others have recommended ^{99m}Tc WBC as the procedure of choice for the detection of osteomyelitis (39). Whole-body MRI may prove the procedure of choice because it does not involve radiation exposure of a child, although young infants may need sedation to prevent motion artifacts.

We usually evaluate surgical prostheses with ^{99m}Tc WBC as the first step, especially when the question is one of infection versus loosening (40,41) (Fig. 21.15). Routine phosphonate imaging techniques are rarely helpful in these situations because they continue to show abnormally increased uptake for a considerable period after surgical intervention. The newer types of prostheses can have a scintigraphic appearance different from that of older prostheses. Increased activity along the stem of a porous prosthesis can be seen as a normal change for as long as 2 to 3 years after surgery, depending on whether a weight-bearing bone is involved and the level of physical activity of the patient. Abnormal activity from loosening usually is located along the lateral border of the tip. Some leukocyte accumulation can occur postoperatively, and this can cause difficulty.

At times, combined procedures such as ^{99m}Tc MDP imaging and ^{111}In chloride or ^{111}In diethylenetriaminepentaacetic acid (DTPA) arthrography may be necessary. The results with these approaches are not strikingly different from those of contrast arthrography, although the radionuclide arthrogram may give better definition of the location of the metallic prosthesis. A combined ^{111}In WBC and ^{99m}Tc MDP bone scan can be performed in which the leukocyte label has relatively greater uptake in infected bone than in noninfected reactive bone (42). A similar approach for concordant or discordant pattern formation can be performed with a radiolabeled WBC and radiocolloid combination in which the discordant pattern is increased ^{111}In WBC uptake that is greater than the radiocolloid uptake. These techniques lead to higher specificity for the presence of infection in these complicated patterns (43).

Persons with sickle cell disease often have acute bone pain. Although this usually is a result of infarction, it can represent osteomyelitis. This clinical problem can be difficult to solve on a routine basis. Early in infarction, a routine phosphonate bone scan can show a photon-deficient lesion. A similar photon-deficient lesion is found with colloid marrow imaging in the early phase of infarction (44). As a result, increased activity on a routine phosphonate bone imaging study performed within days,

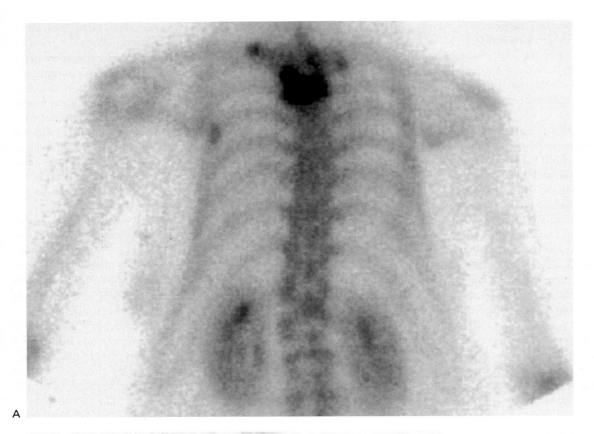

A

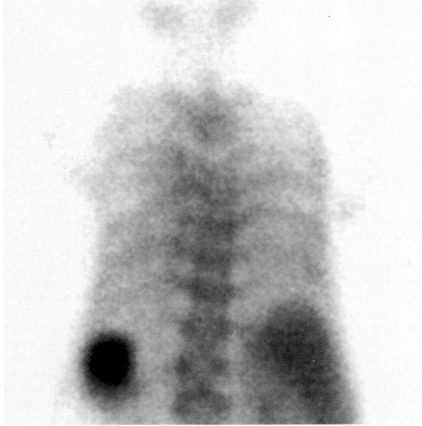

B

FIGURE 21.14. Osteomyelitis of the thoracic spine. Conventional bone scan shows intensely increased uptake (**A**) but white blood cell image shows photopenia (**B**). Biopsy showed *Staphylococcus aureus* was the causative organism.

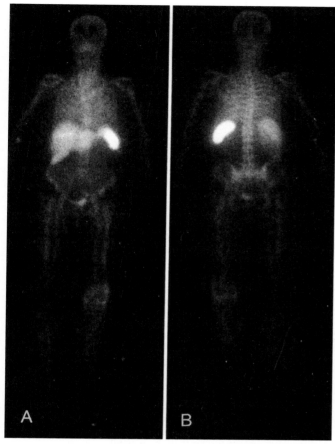

FIGURE 21.15. Infected prosthesis. ^{99m}Tc white blood cell (WBC) scan of an 81-year-old woman with a history of bilateral total-knee replacement 6 years earlier and increasing left knee pain. Radiographs were not helpful. ^{99m}Tc WBC study shows abnormal accumulation across the bone and prosthesis on the left and in adjacent soft tissue (**A**, anterior; **B**, posterior). An infected prosthesis was removed surgically.

or at most a week, of the onset symptom suggests infection. Likewise, normal colloid marrow distribution during this initial week after onset increases the likelihood of infection. However, phosphonate activity increases rapidly in a nonuniform manner in infarcts as the bone tries to repair itself and the infarct is revascularized. As a result, the increased phosphonate activity after the first week does not help differentiate osteomyelitis from infarction. Therefore at this time interval imaging with radiolabeled WBCs becomes an important tool to increase the sensitivity of diagnosis of infection (45).

Both ^{111}In and ^{99m}Tc WBCs as well as ^{67}Ga citrate can be used to assess the effects of therapy (Fig. 21.10). Abnormally increased uptake of these agents before therapy returns to normal after definitive antibiotic therapy (46–48). Uptake of ^{99m}Tc phosphonate is not useful to monitor therapy because uptake remains abnormal as a result of reparative bone formation even after definitive therapy has been completed and the infection eliminated. With the newer therapeutic administration advances, the patient no longer needs prolonged hospitalization. As a result, these procedures are much less frequently performed than they were a few years ago.

OSTEONECROSIS

Osteonecrosis (formally called *avascular* or *aseptic necrosis*) involves the death of both the osseous and marrow components of bone. Skeletal scintigraphy shows photon-deficient lesions at sites of osteonecrosis well in advance of radiographic changes (49,50). Although osteonecrosis can be detected in numerous skeletal locations, the greatest clinical experience has been gained in evaluation of lesions of the femoral head (51) (Fig. 21.16). In addition to idiopathic osteonecrosis (Legg-Calvé-Perthes disease), interruption of blood supply to the femoral head or another area occurs in conditions such as trauma, slipped capital femoral epiphysis, septic joint, and leukemia. Other causes include vasculitis, infarction (sickle cell disease, Gaucher disease), neoplasm, alcoholism, caisson disease, lupus erythematosus, steroid therapy, and impaired circulation, such as that associated with diabetes and frostbite. When skeletal scintigraphy is used as the primary diagnostic modality, correlation with the clinical condition is vital. Studies performed soon after the onset of clinical symptoms may demonstrate a photon-deficient lesion, whereas performed later after onset of symptoms may demonstrate increased activity around and at the site of necrosis, the sequelae of revascularization, or bone remodeling. If the bone contains marrow, both ^{99m}Tc phosphonate and ^{99m}Tc sulfur colloid imaging of the marrow can be used to diagnose osteonecrosis. Skeletal scintigraphy usually is preferred because many adults may not have sufficient active marrow in the bone area to be studied to provide adequate uptake of the colloidal agents. Attention to technique is vital here, as it always is in skeletal scintigraphy. The study should be tailored to the patient and should include magnification or pinhole views of the affected and contralateral site in the frog-leg position, or, preferably, SPECT of the hip or other bones under consideration (52–55). Some investigators believe the changes due to steroid therapy are the result of microfracture and may not be associated with initial decreased femoral head activity. This has not been our experience or that of others. It is important to document the findings at skeletal scintigraphy in relation to the onset of symptoms. When such patients undergo imaging soon after the advent of symptoms, a photon-deficient lesion in the femoral head may be seen. However, advancement to microfracture and revascularization is more rapid than in the usual idiopathic case.

In idiopathic osteonecrosis, or Legg-Calvé-Perthes disease, the earliest sign is the absence of activity most commonly seen in the superolateral portion of the femoral head and associated with normal findings on radiographs (56,57). The appearance of disease may then go through stages that include early revascularization within 4 months after onset. At this time, early radiographic changes can be seen, whereas a radionuclide study shows a lateral column of revascularization. The third stage after onset in uncomplicated cases is generally represented by diffuse zones of increased activity. The last stage shows a return to normal activity with no area of activity greater than that in the epiphysis (Fig. 21.17). In severe cases, the femoral head may never return to normal activity, but as remodeling occurs, increased tracer uptake may be seen for a prolonged time. MRI and CT can be used to study osteonecrosis with somewhat higher sensitivity of MRI for femoral osteonecrosis in adults. In pediatric cases, the

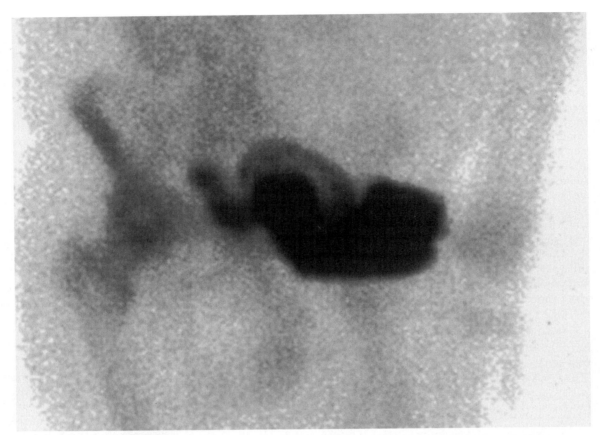

FIGURE 21.16. Osteonecrosis of the right femoral head imaged in the right anterior oblique projection in a patient who has undergone urinary diversion. A rim of increased uptake is present in the femoral head with the central photopenia of necrosis.

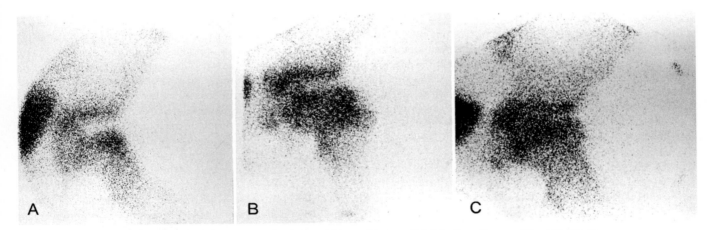

FIGURE 21.17. Pinhole views of a 9-year-old boy with Legg-Calvé-Perthes disease of the left hip. **A:** Study obtained 2 weeks after the onset of pain in this hip shows lack of activity in the superior lateral portion of the femoral head. **B:** Study obtained 10 months after **A** shows base filling. **C:** Image obtained 26 months after the onset of symptoms shows revascularization and remodeling of the femoral head. This is the common pattern in this disease.

relation is similar; despite greater expense, MRI has the advantage of no radiation exposure (58).

Spontaneous osteonecrosis is an idiopathic disorder of knee that occurs among elderly patients with a rapid onset of pain. Although it usually involves the medial femoral condyle, multifocal involvement can occur. Abnormally increased ^{99m}Tc phosphonate activity precedes radiographic abnormality. This condition may be related to nontraumatic osteonecrosis of underlying conditions, as described earlier. This disorder and a similar rare disorder, regional migratory osteoporosis, can involve multiple sites, most commonly the femoral condyles, the femoral or humeral heads, and the talus.

Osteochondritis includes ischemic necrosis and repair of many bones, including the medial femoral condyle (osteochondritis dissecans), the talus, the humerus, the carpal and tarsal navicular bones, the lunate bones, the tibial tuberosity, and the heads of the second and third metatarsals. Although skeletal radiographs frequently have diagnostic findings evident at the time of clinical presentation, skeletal scintigraphy may show increased activity before the appearance of the radiographic abnor-

mality (59). These entities almost invariably manifest as a focus of increased activity even when imaging is performed soon after the onset of symptoms, when one might expect focal photopenic defects.

Bone imaging has not been shown to be an accurate indicator of complete healing in patients with osteonecrosis (60). Studies of resolving femoral neck fractures indicate that imaging may be a means for discriminating between patients who heal normally and those who will have avascular aseptic necrotic complications and need a prosthesis (Fig. 21.18). The findings on skeletal images depend on when the study is performed after the initiating insult, the quality of repair mechanisms, and morphologic changes in the bone or joint. Traumatic osteonecrosis occasionally is found next to a fracture and may prove difficult to image completely without specialized techniques such as SPECT, because the activity related to healing at the fracture site can obscure adjacent findings in planar projections (39,61, 62).

In patients with sickle cell anemia as the underlying cause of infarction, it is again important to relate the time of bone imag-

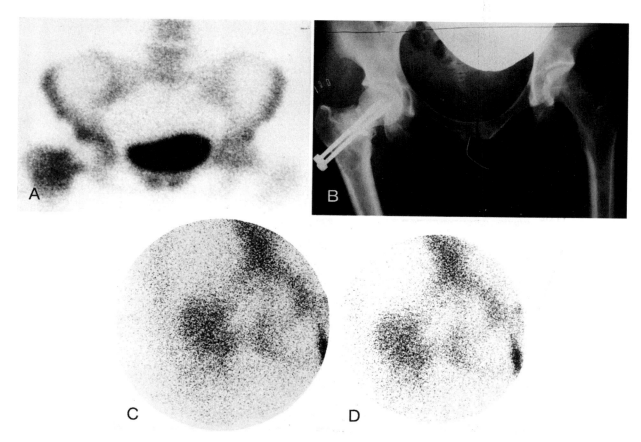

FIGURE 21.18. Fracture of femoral neck. **A:** Anterior view of the pelvis of a 22-year-old woman approximately 7 hours after fracture of the femoral neck in a car accident. The photopenic area in the head is a sign of interruption of the vascular supply to the femoral head. Although such photon-deficient areas also are seen with the pressure effect of intracapsular hemorrhage, infection, and the like, it is important to alert the surgeon so that he or she may better plan the operative repair. **B:** Frontal radiographs of the pelvis 1 week after **A** show hip pins. A pedicled flap graft was performed in an attempt to restore vascularity to the femoral head. **C:** Pinhole magnification views of the right hip obtained at the time of **B** show activity in the superior lateral portion that is presumed to be in the flap and not in the femoral head. **D:** Views 2 months after **B** and **C** show a nonviable femoral head. At this time, a prosthesis was installed.

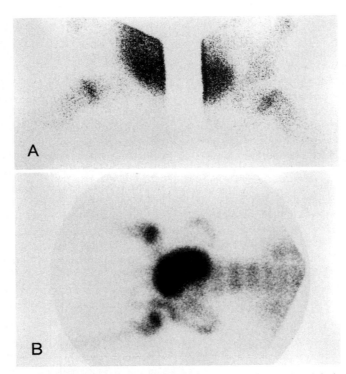

FIGURE 21.19. Bone infarction associated with sickle cell anemia. **A:** Anterior pinhole collimator views of the hips of an 18-month-old child who had been irritable for 3 days and had refused to move her right leg for 4 days. Absence of activity in both femoral heads is evident. This is one time when relying on pinhole views alone without scout views of the skeleton can lead one astray. **B:** Anterior view of the lower spine and pelvis shows a large photon-deficient area in the right hemipelvis that is difficult to appreciate on the pinhole magnification view. This represents bone infarction due to sickle cell crisis.

ing to the chronology of the clinical events. Soon after infarction, a photon-deficient lesion may be present on the bone scan (Fig. 21.19). (Bone marrow imaging gives a similar finding if the insult occurs in a part of the skeleton containing marrow.) Later, as the bone repairs itself, increased activity is found. Because osteomyelitis is a frequent complication at these sites, radiolabeled leukocyte imaging may be necessary to differentiate the two entities. MRI of symptomatic areas is playing an increasing role in the evaluation of these patients, especially those in the pediatric age group.

Bone imaging techniques can be used to assist the surgeon in delineating the level of the loss of vascularity and viability of bone in conditions such as frostbite and diabetes. In such instances, routine bone imaging can be combined with (a) marking of the patient's skin at the level of reasonable bone activity by use of external radioactive markers and a persistence scope when imaging the patient or (b) a transmission image of the leg associated with dermal marking at that time (Fig. 21.20). Both techniques greatly assist the surgeon if amputation is planned.

ARTHRITIS

Although it is not commonly used, skeletal imaging can be of assistance in the diagnosis of arthritis (63–65). However, because bone scanning is a nonspecific procedure (Fig. 21.21), pattern recognition (Fig. 21.22) as well as interpretation in the

clinical context plays an important role in differentiation of the variety of causes of arthritis, such as rheumatoid, degenerative, or osteoarthritis; inflammatory, psoriatic, gouty arthritis; Reiter syndrome; ankylosing spondylitis; lupus erythematosus; sarcoidosis; and regional migratory osteoporosis (Figs. 21.23 through 21.25). The ability to obtain total-body views allows rapid and more economical multiple joint evaluation than does conventional radiographic evaluation. Skeletal scintigraphy can show a diffuse periarticular increase that reflects increased perfusion of the soft tissues in arthritis that affects soft tissue and cartilage. It also represents osteoblastic activity in subchondral bone and on occasion shows focal abnormal findings before the patient reports joint pain or radiographic changes are present. A routine bone scan can be combined with studies performed after injection of ^{99m}Tc pertechnetate or albumin to allow differentiation between inflammatory, proliferative arthropathy, such as rheumatoid arthritis, and degenerative osteoarthritis. The latter is not associated with increased soft-tissue uptake of ^{99m}Tc pertechnetate or albumin. It must be remembered that although abnormal ^{99m}Tc pertechnetate uptake is sensitive and specific for the presence of synovitis, it says nothing about the etiologic factor. Other forms of inflammatory arthritis, including gout and sarcoidosis, may be associated with dramatic uptake of radiolabeled leukocytes, antibodies, and ^{67}Ga citrate. As a result, differentiation from osteomyelitis in periarticular bone can be difficult or impossible with scintigraphy alone (Fig. 21.26).

When patients undergo evaluation for peripheral arthritic

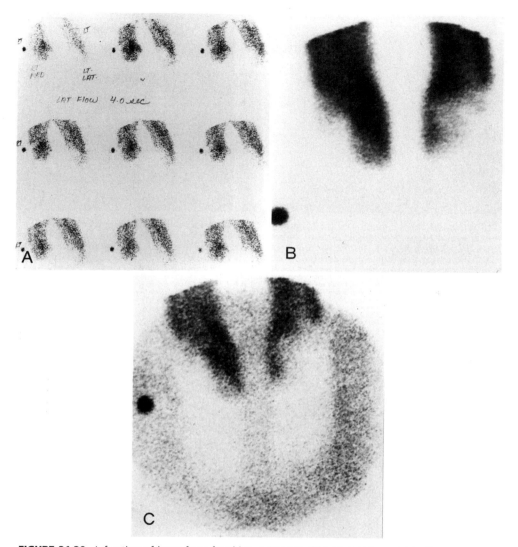

FIGURE 21.20. Infarction of bone from frostbite. A 27-year-old man was brought to the emergency department after spending a night exposed to a northern climate. **A:** Perfusion study shows bilateral lack of perfusion of the ankles and feet. **B:** Delayed static images in the plantar projection show lack of osseous activity. **C:** Outline of the feet allows determination of the level of activity by means of a transmission scan with the source behind the feet and face of the collimator. (Courtesy of Dr. Herman Wallinga, The Genesee Hospital, Rochester, NY.)

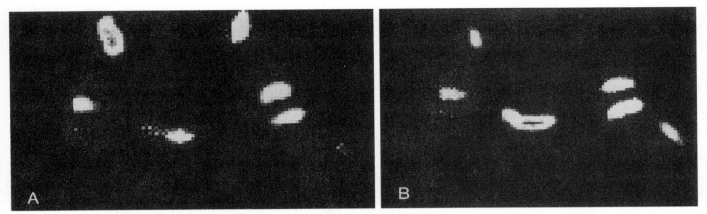

FIGURE 21.21. Rheumatoid arthritis. Coronal SPECT views (**A** and **B**) show the hips of an 18-year-old woman with known rheumatoid arthritis. She reported pain in the left hip. Findings on conventional radiographs were normal. Despite abnormally increased activity in the left hip, including the greater trochanter (also abnormal on the perfusion and blood pool phases), this case illustrates the problem of nonspecificity in skeletal scintigraphy. Similar findings are found with trauma, tumor, infection, and trochanteric bursitis.

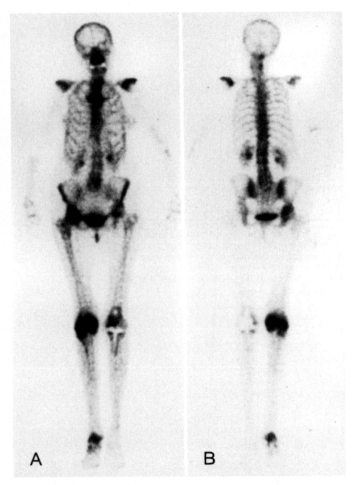

FIGURE 21.22. Degenerative arthritis. Total body anterior (**A**) and posterior **B** views of a 67-year-old woman with pain in several joints for years. Nonsymmetric, diffuse joint involvement is evident, especially in weight-bearing or motion-stressed joints. The patient had undergone prosthetic knee replacement 4 years earlier.

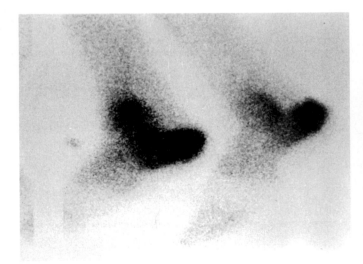

FIGURE 21.23. Reiter syndrome. Lateral and medial views of both ankles and both feet of a 30-year-old man with uveitis and prostatitis. He reported pain in the left heel and back. This study exhibited an inflammation index (ratio of activity over the rear of the calcaneus to an equal sized area at the junction of the mid and lower third of the tibia) of 14.8. Diffusely abnormal activity also was found in the back. These findings are consistent with the diagnosis of Reiter syndrome.

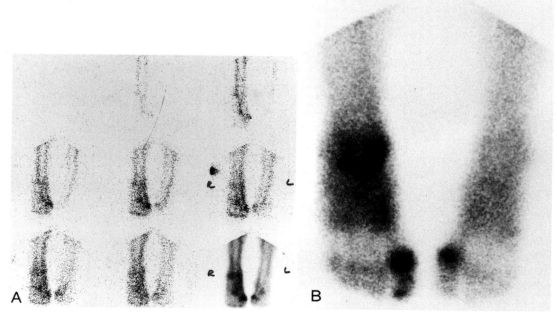

FIGURE 21.24. Gouty arthritis. A 60-year-old man was admitted to the hospital after a myocardial infarction. On the fifth day of hospitalization, he began to report severe pain in both great toes that was much worse on the right. A bone scan was performed to investigate the possibility of vascular compromise in the lower extremities. **A:** Perfusion and immediate soft-tissue phases show marked increased perfusion to the right ankle and foot with focal increased perfusion to the hallux valgus deformity in the left foot. **B:** Delayed skeletal image shows abnormal foci of activity around the great toes and right ankle. Marked elevation of the serum urate levels led to the final diagnosis of gouty arthritis.

problems, three-phase bone scanning usually is performed. The perfusion and early blood-pool images may allow identification of synovial involvement and avoid the need for a combined ^{99m}Tc pertechnetate and albumin study. Individual joints must be studied with high-resolution views or SPECT for complex joints. The pattern of distribution of abnormality on the delayed images may be typical of the type of arthritis involved and allow for diagnostic separation. Normal results of skeletal imaging indicate lack of active arthritic involvement. Despite the sensitivity of skeletal scintigraphy, most rheumatologists perform an evaluation with only a combination of clinical history, physical examinations, and conventional laboratory and radiographic studies.

Quantitative methods of studying individual joints have met with mixed success, and none has become widely accepted (66–68). Little is known about normal and abnormal quantitative values for regions other than the sacroiliac and temporomandibular joints (69,70). The quantitative indices usually are calculated as the ratio of activity in areas such as the sacroiliac joint compared with normal sacrolumbar or iliac bone activity. The technique is quite dependent on the imaging position of the patient as well as patient age and chronologic status of the disease (Fig. 21.27). This approach remains somewhat controversial, with mixed results from a variety of investigators. Profile slice counting and separate regions of interest have been proposed. We prefer the region of interest method because the pattern of sacroiliitis ranges from focal involvement early to later involvement of the entire joint. Another reason for preferring separate regions of interest is the difficulty that can be met in counting over the sacral tubercle when it appears as an anatomic variant.

Similar applications have been made to other regions, such as the temporomandibular joint. SPECT imaging improves the sensitivity of detection and quantification of bony involvement.

Ankylosing spondylitis is a chronic soft-tissue inflammatory process that usually involves the sacroiliac and vertebral joints but also can involve peripheral joints, the sternum, and the costochondral junctions. Involvement of peripheral joints frequently is confused with rheumatoid arthritis. Progression of the disease can lead to debilitating conditions with osseous ankylosis and fusion of the vertebral bodies that result in rigidity of the spine that can lead to fracture. Bone imaging is successful in early detection of such spinal fractures (71). This condition usually manifests as a pattern of focal increased activity in a vertebral body superimposed on the more diffusely increased activity resulting from ankylosing spondylitis.

When joint replacement is considered necessary, bone imaging can be used to show the areas of greatest involvement. SPECT findings are predictive of compartmental involvement in cases of arthritis involving the knees (72,73). Contrast arthrography or routine radiographic study is far less accurate in the prediction of compartmental involvement.

METABOLIC DISEASE

The exact role of bone imaging in evaluating metabolic bone disease is still unclear because many varieties of such disease have similar scintigraphic findings (74,75). A variety of quantification techniques have been suggested that do offer useful information

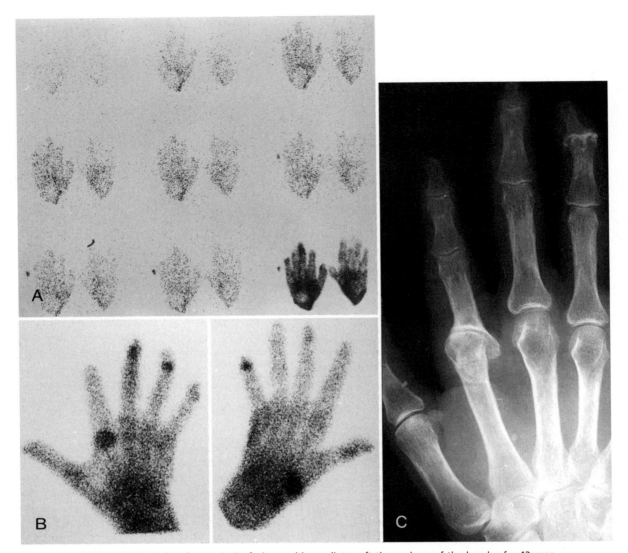

FIGURE 21.25. Scleroderma. **A:** Perfusion and immediate soft-tissue views of the hands of a 42-year-old woman with known scleroderma. **B:** Delayed bone views show focal joint abnormalities in diffuse joints of the hand that correspond quite well to the radiograph, **(C)** indicating which joints are actively involved. This patient was being evaluated for possible osteomyelitis of the tip of the right index finger, which is, in fact, normal.

(76–80). These range from highly technical total-body calculations involving sophisticated whole-body counting equipment to more practical approaches for smaller, clinically oriented community hospitals. The latter approaches involve determination of the percentage of an injected dose of ^{99m}Tc MDP retained in the skeletal system based on calculations derived from simple scintillation detectors or a gamma camera. Bone absorption studies that involve single or dual photopeaks have been used, as have CT and neutron activation analysis. Focal quantification, such as the 24-hour to 4-hour ratio of ^{99m}Tc MDP uptake over lesions as opposed to areas that are not lesions or such as SPECT calculations of skull uptake of ^{99m}Tc MDP, has been proposed. All of these techniques have been used with reasonable success in the evaluation of patients for acromegaly, hyperthyroidism, primary hyperparathyroidism, renal osteodystrophy, os-

teonecrosis, osteoporosis, osteomalacia, and other diseases of calcium metabolism (81–83). The lack of full acceptance of such procedures in the study of these conditions is the result of technical difficulties. The variety of quantification techniques already introduced produces different numerical values for subjects with normal findings and those with abnormal findings depending on the laboratory in which the techniques are used. Some techniques measure trabecular bone, some measure cancellous bone, and some measure both. The techniques also require exact standardization of the application among patients within an individual laboratory. Many technical factors affect the quality of the results, including choice of radiopharmaceutical, choice of collimator and camera system, time of imaging after injection, information density on the images, computer and display options, matrix size, region of interest, profile selections, total body

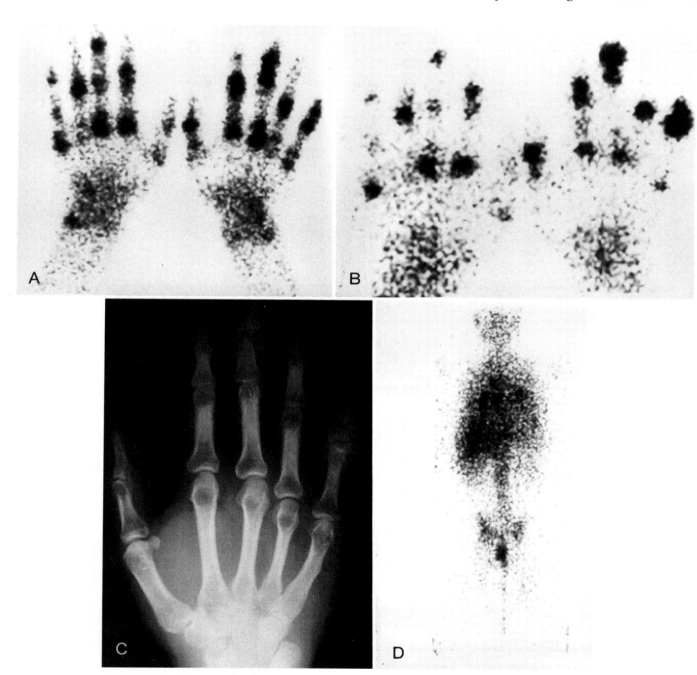

FIGURE 21.26. Sarcoidosis. **A:** Delayed views from three-phase bone scan of a 32-year-old man with increasing weakness and pain in his fingers for 2 months. A similar pattern was seen during the perfusion and immediate phases. **B:** Similar projection from a ^{67}Ga citrate study 72 hours later. **C:** Magnification radiograph of the right hand shows destruction of the third and fifth distal interphalangeal (DIP) joints. **D:** Anterior total body views from 72-hour ^{67}Ga study show an increase in diffuse pulmonary activity and abnormal activity in hilar and mediastinal nodes. Sarcoid was confirmed by means of biopsy of the fifth DIP joint.

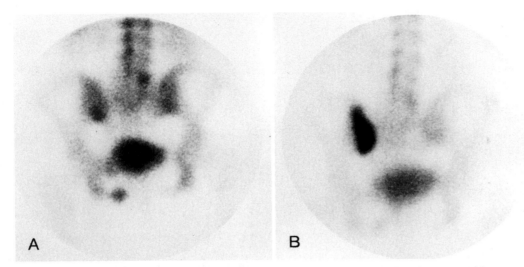

FIGURE 21.27. Sacroiliitis. Posterior views of the lower lumbar spine and pelvis of a 37-year-old woman with symptoms suggesting sacroiliitis. **A:** The initial study shows diffuse abnormal activity throughout the thoracolumbar spine as a result of the patient's severe scoliosis. A focal area of increased uptake in the inferior aspect of the left sacroiliac joint is a sign of early sacroiliitis. **B:** Six months later, the pain has worsened despite therapy. Skeletal image shows involvement of the entire sacroiliac area. This pattern illustrates the usual development of sacroiliitis.

counting, standard background subtraction techniques, and calculation of normal ranges determined by age and sex.

A routine radionuclide bone scan does not give a good measure of absolute bone uptake. Abnormally increased uptake can be suggested by an increase in the bone to soft-tissue ratio, but only when this ratio is markedly elevated. One of the two best measures that have achieved some clinical use is quantitation of retained phosphonate skeletal activity after 24 hours (84). Such measurements improve the detection of metabolic disease over qualitative or visual evaluation of total body scans. Of the many metabolic disorders, only osteoporosis is associated with normal levels of retention. All others are associated with increased retention.

The second quantification method for evaluation is bone densitometry as used in the study of osteoporosis. This condition increases with normal aging but also is found as a component of many diseases. Accurate and early diagnosis is essential to involve the patient in therapy to prevent fractures. Numerous techniques for the measurement of bone density are used, but all rely on measuring the difference in attenuation of photons of a specific energy by soft tissue and bone in comparison with standards (85–89). The most commonly used measurement of bone mineral mass is single-photon absorptiometry with scanning across the radius, calcaneus, a vertebra, or even the hip. Other techniques include dual-photon absorptiometry, dedicated x-ray absorptiometry, or quantitative CT involving both single- and dual-energy techniques (see Chapter 33).

Qualitative imaging of the variety of metabolic diseases may suggest their presence. The degree of activity between bone and soft tissues changes with increased activity in the bone. Scan findings can range from increased uptake at the costochondral junction (beading), mandible, skull, sternum, ribs, and the jux-

taarticular areas of the long bones (Fig. 21.28). Renal activity can be decreased or absent, resulting in a "superscan" appearance. In hyperparathyroidism, soft-tissue activity can be found in the lungs, stomach, and elsewhere because of metastatic calcifications. Focal areas of increased osseous activity can be seen at the sites of brown "tumors." Focal increases also can be seen at the

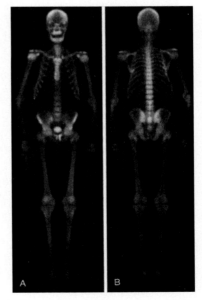

FIGURE 21.28. Hyperparathyroidism. Anterior **(A)** and posterior **(B)** total-body images in a 39-year-old male renal transplant patient complaining of back and right shoulder pain. Note the diffusely increased activity in bones and the lack of soft tissue and renal activity.

pseudofractures (of osteomalacia) and fractures of osteogenesis imperfecta. Multiple benign compression fractures of the spine are common among patients with osteoporosis.

Imaging techniques can be useful in assessing a variety of conditions such as renal migratory osteoporosis, hypertropic pulmonary osteoarthropathy, reflex sympathetic dystrophy, Paget disease, or any osteosclerotic condition with increased bone metabolism, such as melorheostosis and poikilocytosis (90–94).

Hypertrophic osteoarthropathy, which usually is caused by pulmonary disease, is evident before radiographic changes can be seen (95) (Fig. 21.29). This disorder usually produces a fairly characteristic appearance on scintigraphic studies. The pattern consists of a generalized increase in cortical activity in the long bones and focal sites of increased activity in the periarticular regions of the long bones, phalanges, scapula, and clavicle.

Reflex sympathetic dystrophy is another condition in which skeletal scintigraphic changes are seen before radiographic evidence of the condition is present. This is true whether the sympathetic dystrophy is the result of trauma or vascular compromise or is idiopathic. It is important to relate study findings to the duration of symptoms. Increased perfusion and early blood-pool activity usually are evident only in the first 2 to 3 months after onset of the process. Delayed static images reveal diffuse periarticular activity in the affected extremity for no more than 1 year

after the beginning of symptoms. This radionuclide diagnosis is less accurate because the images can return to normal or even show reduced activity.

Paget disease (osteitis deformans) is frequently seen among middle-aged and older persons. Bone scan changes usually precede radiographic abnormalities (96). Paget disease usually is polyostotic, only 20% to 30% of early cases being monostotic (Fig. 21.30). Increased activity can be present in the early osteolytic phase as well as in the later osteoblastic phase (97). In the early osteolytic stage (circumscripta), perfusion and blood-pool images can precede changes in delayed static bone images (98). Uptake is most intense at the edge of a lytic lesion (99). In the later, osteoblastic phase, one can see diffuse involvement at several bony sites. This involvement can be unilateral and cause apparent expansion of the bone of the extremities and the ribs and clavicle. In long bones, the abnormal activity pattern invariably extends to at least one end of the bone. Calvarial activity can be intense and range from focal to diffuse involvement (100) (Fig. 21.31).

At times the polyostotic nature of Paget disease can make it difficult to differentiate this disorder from metastasis on scans or radiographs. Although the scan patterns described earlier make the diagnosis of Paget disease more likely, one may eventually have to resort to biopsy for differentiation. Serial studies of

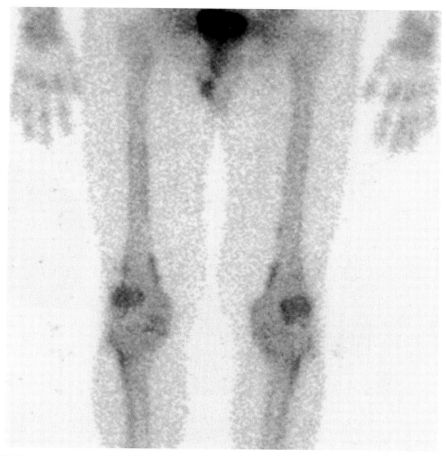

FIGURE 21.29. Hypertrophic pulmonary osteoarthropathy. Image shows characteristically increased uptake in a cortical pattern in the distal portions of the femurs.

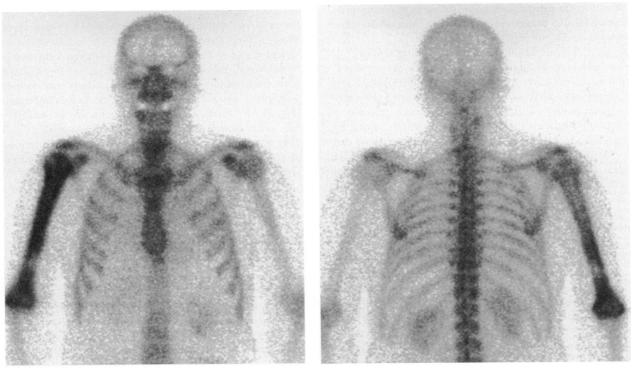

FIGURE 21.30. Anterior **(A)** and posterior **(B)** projections show monostotic Paget disease affecting the right humerus. Abnormal activity extends to the ends of the bone.

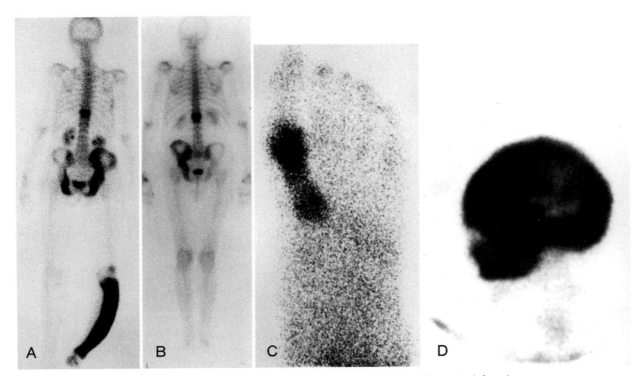

FIGURE 21.31. Paget disease has many faces. It can be monostotic or polyostotic, deform bone or not, and have uneven uptake, as in osteitis circumscripta. **A:** Posterior view shows marked increased activity in several bones in a 54-year-old woman. **B:** Posterior projection shows much less deformity of the spine and pelvis of a 68-year-old man. **C:** Plantar view of a 57-year-old man with pain in the left leg and foot. This was the only site of abnormality in this patient. **D:** Lateral view of the skull of a 57-year-old woman with diffuse but uneven activity in the skull with sparing of the mandible. This was the only abnormal site in this patient.

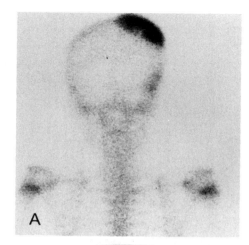

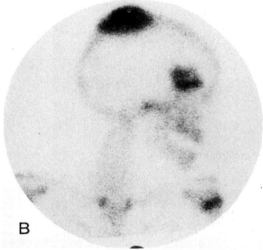

FIGURE 21.32. Polyostotic fibrous dysplasia. **A:** Posterior view of the skull shows markedly increased activity at the site of what was thought to be monostotic fibrous dysplasia in the posterior region in an 11-year-old boy. Lateral views of the skull **(B)** show a second site in the skull that may be faintly visualized in the posterior view. This places the disorder into the category of polyostotic fibrous dysplasia.

the activity pattern in Paget disease may allow differentiation of the development of sarcoma, which occurs among approximately 1% of patients (101). Early sarcomatous degeneration usually occurs as an even further increase in the already dramatic focal activity changes. Later changes can manifest as photon-deficient lesions, presumably caused by interruption of the blood supply and bone necrosis.

A diphosphonate, disodium etidronate, is a commonly used drug in the therapy for Paget disease. Serial bone scans can be used to monitor the effectiveness of the therapeutic regimen, This is important finding because therapeutic doses of this drug can be toxic. Successful therapy usually is seen as a decrease in radionuclide activity (102,103). Quantitative study can be used for assessing the effect of this therapy for Paget disease and in therapy for fibrous dysplasia, eosinophilic granuloma, and histiocytosis X (when the results are abnormal). Fibrous dysplasia and other types of bone dysplasia are conditions in which the scan results can be quite abnormal in the face of normal radiographic

findings. It is important to determine whether the condition is polyostotic or monostotic for therapeutic regimens to be begun (Fig. 21.32). Skeletal scintigraphy allows a rapid, safe, reliable, and economical study of the entire skeleton in such patients. Unlike Paget disease, fibrous dysplasia in a long bone frequently does not reach the end of the bone, a minor differentiating point.

Other dysplastic conditions of bone can manifest in a variety of patterns. Such patterns range from dense and uneven distribution in a single bone, usually the femur, which occurs with melorheostosis, to widespread punctate-increased activity in poikilocytosis, to the marked skeletal deformity and multiple fractures of osteogenesis imperfecta (104–106).

MISCELLANEOUS CONDITIONS

Irradiated Bone

Localization of bone-seeking radiopharmaceuticals usually is decreased at radiation therapy portals (Fig. 21.33). However, increased activity can be seen if bone imaging is performed soon

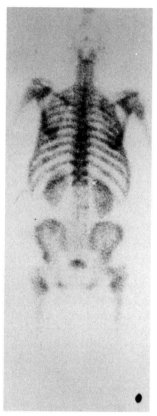

FIGURE 21.33. Decreased activity at radiation therapy portal. A 23-year-old man with testicular seminoma treated with a radiation therapy portal 7 months earlier reported back pain. Posterior image shows photon-deficient regions in the lumbar spine that correspond to the portal. The activity in the rest of the thoracic spine and rib case poses a problem. Quantitation of this activity by means of ratioing selected areas of interest to the tibia frequently assists in determining whether the activity is caused by sparing or actual increased uptake. In this case, uptake was within normal limits. The back pain disappeared without any further therapy.

after completion of radiation therapy (107,108). Numerous factors influence the localization of bone-seeking radiopharmaceuticals in irradiated portions of bone. These include the amount and rate of delivery of the radiation, the time between the treatment and the imaging study, and the type of irradiated tissue. In animal experiments and some clinical situations, bone imaging reveals increased activity over the treatment portal for the first few weeks after cessation of radiation therapy. Within 2 to 3 months, the activity pattern in the treated area decreases, giving a photopenic pattern at the site of irradiation. In one clinical study, 14 of 20 patients examined 4 to 6 months after treatment had such photopenic defects on bone images (109). No changes were seen in regions that received less than 2,000 rad, and the mean dose delivered was 3,750 rad. The causes of such defects are unclear but usually are assumed the result of vasculitis and hyalinization of small vessels (osteonecrosis). The normal activity pattern can return within 12 months but more commonly takes several years. An increase in radionuclide uptake can be observed in soft tissue included in the radiation portal.

Because of the presence of a photopenic area in bone within the radiation portal, it often is difficult to decide whether activity in bones adjacent to the portal is normal or abnormal. Quantification techniques involving the calculation of abnormal to normal bone ratios can aid in solving this clinical problem.

Grafted Bone

The use of bone grafting has increased with the development of better surgical techniques and the ability to preserve viable bone. The three-phase bone scan is an excellent noninvasive method of monitoring viability in grafts. Autologous grafts with accompanying microvascularization produce a pattern that shows uniform perfusion, blood pool, and delayed activity throughout the graft immediately after surgery (110). Early in the postsurgical phase this activity pattern can increase over the surrounding bone, but it becomes closer to uniform with the surrounding bone within 12 to 18 months as the graft is assimilated and healing is completed (38) (Fig. 21.34).

Most allografts are not well microvascularized at the time of surgical insertion and rely on reestablishment of blood flow from surrounding vessel attachment (111,112). In the immediately postsurgical phase, the graft can appear as a photon-deficient area. Repeated examinations are necessary for full evaluation. These images show progressively increased perfusion, blood pool, and delayed uptake that begins at the edges of the graft and migrates centrally as revascularization progresses. This sequential change follows the time curve in which osteoblastic cells repopulate the graft from the peripheral portions. Skeletal scintigraphy is more sensitive than is plain radiography, CT, or MRI in monitoring this revascularization process. Magnification and SPECT images may be necessary to separate peripheral osseous activity from adjacent normal bone and soft-tissue activity for full evaluation.

Soft-tissue Accumulation

In healthy persons, the soft-tissue structures readily visualized usually are the kidney and the bladder. The soft-tissue back-

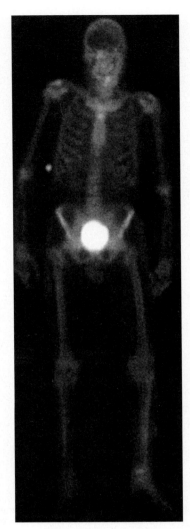

FIGURE 21.34. Bone graft. Image obtained 3 months after a 42-year-old man underwent radiation therapy and surgical excision of squamous cell carcinoma of the mouth that involved the left mandible. An autograft from the left fibula was used to reconstruct the mandible. Anterior total body view shows activity in the left mandibular graft that indicates viability and activity in the left fibula at the site from which the graft was removed.

ground usually is slight, especially in younger persons. Young persons not only have good renal function and thereby excrete a large portion (40% to 50%) of the injected dose, resulting in efficient clearance of activity from soft tissues, but also have high blood flow and metabolic activity in bone. With aging, generalized soft-tissue background often increases, presumably as a result of the reduction in bone metabolism, osseous blood flow, and decreasing renal function. Diminished renal uptake can be seen in so-called superscan, but this phenomenon is associated with low soft-tissue background activity and increased skeletal uptake, which reduces the amount of tracer available for renal excretion. The genitourinary system should be inspected in every bone imaging procedure to evaluate for space-occupying lesions in the kidney or bladder as well as distortion or displacement of these structures by extrarenal and extravesicular masses.

A rough estimate of renal function can also be made on these studies. Diffusely increased activity within the kidneys in a cortical pattern can be seen in conditions such as amyloidosis and sarcoidosis, after radiation therapy or chemotherapy, and in a pelvocalyceal and ureteric pattern in obstructive disorders.

The presence of abnormal activity in soft tissue usually is the result of increased blood flow, calcification, irradiation, changes in endocrine function, tissue necrosis, or direct interaction with injected pharmaceuticals such as iron dextran (Fig. 21.35). Tumors such as neuroblastoma, lymphoma, and carcinoma lung frequently exhibit soft-tissue accumulation. Occasional soft-tissue activity patterns can be seen with other tumors, but this is a much less common event (Fig. 21.36). Nonosseous uptake resulting from infarction or another vascular insult, including injury to the heart, brain, gastrointestinal tract, and muscle, can be seen in soft tissue. Bone imaging is one of the most sensitive indicators of rhabdomyolysis (Fig. 21.37). The cause of rhabdo-

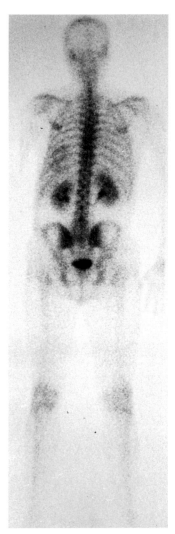

FIGURE 21.36. Soft-tissue activity with carcinoma of the colon. Posterior total body image from study performed on a 46-year-old man with known carcinoma of the colon, now being evaluated for back pain. Abnormal increased activity in the liver is evident. Routine liver images showed multiple defects. Biopsy showed metastatic adenocarcinoma of the colon.

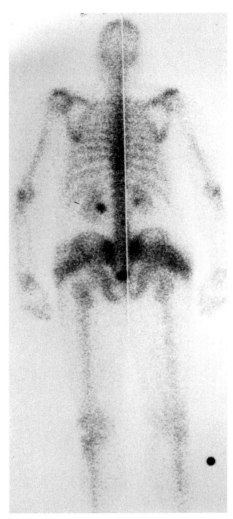

FIGURE 21.35. Soft-tissue activity with iron dextran injection. Posterior total body view from a ^{99m}Tc MDP study performed on a 57-year-old man with iron-deficiency anemia and back pain. He had been receiving intramuscular injections of iron dextran in both buttocks. Soft-tissue activity in the buttocks corresponds to the injection sites.

myolysis includes trauma, especially among runners, frostbite, and alcohol abuse. Intense increased perfusion of blood pool and delayed accumulation can be seen in myositis ossificans (heterotopic bone formation) long before radiographic evidence of this process is found (Fig. 21.38). A three-phase bone scan can be used to assist the surgeon in planning when to surgically excise sites of heterotopic bone formation. Thus surgery can be delayed until these areas have lost increased perfusion and delayed avidity for bone-seeking radiopharmaceuticals. Attempts at surgical removal before this happens usually result in recurrence of the process. Increased amounts of bone-seeking radionuclides can be found in areas of inflammation and abscesses (Figs. 21.39, 21.40). Increased activity in the breast can be seen in healthy women, particularly perimenstrually or during hormonal replacement. It also can be found in patients with carcinoma of the breast, mastitis, trauma, or fibrocystic disease. In

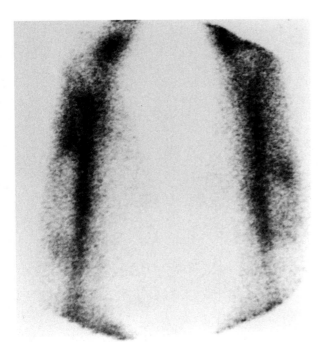

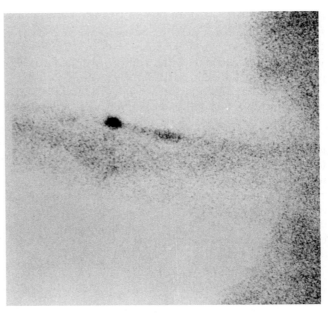

FIGURE 21.37. Rhabdomyolysis due to frostbite. Posterior views of the legs from routine bone imaging study show rhabdomyolysis of the calf muscles caused by exposure and frostbite. (Courtesy of Dr. Herman Wallinga, The Genesee Hospital, Rochester, NY.)

FIGURE 21.39. Soft-tissue activity in thrombophlebitis. Left upper extremity 1 hour after injection of ^{99m}Tc MDP into the antecubital fossa of a 51-year-old female. Slight extravasation is evident in the injection site, followed by the linear activity along the basilic vein. This is the result of thrombophlebitis of this vein after placement and removal of a central venous pressure catheter.

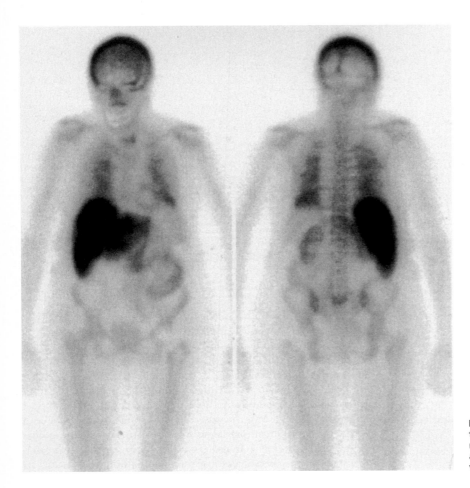

FIGURE 21.38. Extensive soft-tissue calcification due to persistent hypercalcemia. Anterior (*left*) and posterior (*right*) projections show intense uptake in the liver and in the pleural cavities. Ring-like outline of the left ventricle is evident.

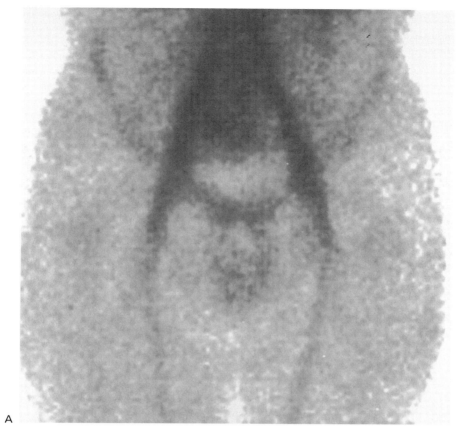

A

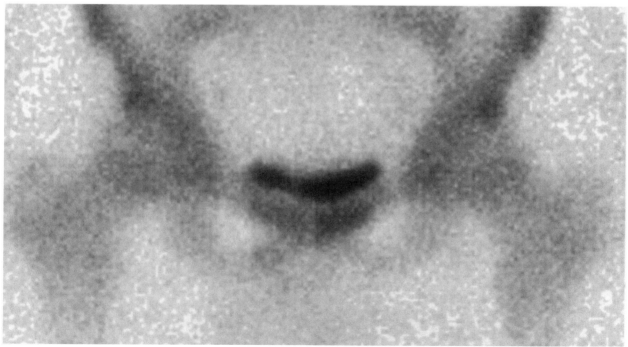

B

FIGURE 21.40. Osteitis pubis. Images show increased blood pool **(A)** and increased uptake **(B)** in both pubic bones distinct from bladder activity in the anterior projection.

Table 21.1. *Soft-Tissue Accumulation of Bone-Seeking Radiopharmaceuticals*

Locations of normal accumulation
    Kidney
    Ureter
    Bladder
    Breast
    Cartilage rib, thyroid cricoid
    Urine and salivary contamination
Abnormal accumulation
    Granuloma, fungal infection
    Inflammation, cellulitis
    Abscess
    Thrombophlebitis, vasculitis
    Tumors
        Lung, lymphoma, neuroblastoma, breast, ovary, hemangioma, osteosarcoma, thyroid, fibroid, etc.
        Soft-tissue metastasis from colon, pancreas, ovary, etc.
    Radiation treatment ports
    Infarction: myocardial cerebral, muscle, gastrointestinal, splenic
    Fluid collections: effusion, ascites, edema, lymphedema
    Myositis ossificans, heterotopic bone formation
    Rhabdomyolysis, polymyositis, muscle trauma
    Healing wound
    Amyloidosis: heart, liver, kidneys, para-articular stomach
    Hyperthyroidism
    Scleroderma
    Dermatomyositis
    Sickle cell disease
    Uremia
    Fat necrosis
    Hepatic necrosis
    Hematoma
    Paraplelgic states
    Pseudogout
    Hypervitaminosis D, tretinoin toxicity
    Postoperative heterotopic calcification and bone formation
    Hypercalcemia
    Hemochromatosis
    Sarcoid
    Obesity
    Pulmonary microlithiasis
    Renal microlithiasis
    Calcified aneurysms
    Pseudoxanthoma elasticum
    Heart valve calcification
    Cutaneous calcinosis universalis
    Venous stasis or obstruction
    Adriamycin toxicity
    Congestive heart failure
    Dehydration
    Aftermath of sympathectomy
    Lymphedema
    Fibrocystic disease
    Iron dextran injection sites
Artifactual accumulation due to faculty preparation
    Thyroid, gastrointestinal tract, salivary glands with free pertechnetate
    Liver or spleen with colloid formation
    Biliary system
    Renal
    Excess iron and blood (multiple transfusions)
Intraarterial injection, injection sites, and lymph nodes after extravasation

men, breast activity usually is associated with gynecomastia. Diffuse abnormal activity can be seen in body cavities, such as the thorax, with pleural effusions, and in the abdomen with ascites.

Diffusely abnormal soft-tissue activity can be seen in diseases such as hypoparathyroidism or hyperparathyroidism, scleroderma, polymyositis, and sickle cell disease long before they are evident on radiographs. Activity within the stomach can be the result of improper formulation of the bone-seeking complexes or a delay between preparation and injection as a result of oxidation of the radiopharmaceutical. It also can be the result of gastritis, sarcoidosis, amyloidosis, trauma, antacid abuse, hyperparathyroidism, dialysis, and tretinoin toxicity. One must always be sure that previous nuclear medicine procedures are not causing apparent soft-tissue uptake on bone scans.

A list of conditions that cause soft-tissue localization is given in Table 21.1. This is at best a partial list and is constantly being enlarged. However, it is important that these causes of soft-tissue localization of bone-seeking radiopharmaceuticals be kept in mind when bone imaging studies are reviewed so that mistakes in interpretation are not made. Proper attention to soft-tissue activity patterns can lead to a diagnosis.

SUMMARY

The use of bone imaging has advanced to its present position by virtue of the diagnostic information that it provides about a variety of bone diseases, including benign disease. Further developments in radiopharmaceuticals and analysis contribute to the evolution of the role of skeletal scintigraphy. Skeletal imaging is a valuable tool in the study of benign diseases provided good communication is maintained between the referring clinician and nuclear medicine physician to tailor the procedure to answer a given clinical question. The exact role of radionuclide bone imaging in relation to other imaging procedures, such as plain-film radiography, CT, and MRI continues to evolve as progress is made in the development and application of all these modalities. Nuclear medicine physicians must remain knowledgeable about the advantages and disadvantages of the imaging processes applicable to care of an individual patient so that the best clinical decisions can be made while increasingly tight resources are used most economically. Attention to technical factors is important, as is continuing effort to increase knowledge concerning the patterns of benign disease that can be seen with skeletal scintigraphy.

REFERENCES

1. O'Mara RE, Wilson GA, Burke AM. The role of nuclear imaging in osteomyelitis. In: Raynaud C, ed. *Nuclear medicine and biology: proceedings of the Third World Congress of Nuclear Medicine and Biology.* Vol. I. Paris: Pergamon Press, 1982:1094.
2. Ash JM, Gilday DL. Futility of bone scanning in neonatal osteomyelitis [Concise Communication]. *J Nucl Med* 1980;21:417.
3. Gilday DL, Paul DJ, Paterson J. Diagnosis of osteomyelitis in children by combined blood pool and bone imaging. *Radiology* 1975;117:331.
4. Bressler EL, Conway JJ, Weiss SC: Neonatal osteomyelitis examined by bone scintigraphy. *Radiology* 1984;685–688.

5. Bressler EL, Conway JJ, Weiss SC. Neonatal osteomyelitis examined by bone scintigraphy. *Radiology* 1984;152:685–688.
6. Graham GD, Lundy MM, Frederick RJ, et al. Scintigraphic detection of osteomyelitis with 99m-Tc MDP and 67-Ga citrate. *J Nucl Med* 1983;24:1019.
7. Handmaker H, Giammona ST. Improved early diagnosis of acute inflammatory skeletal articular diseases in children: a two radiopharmaceutical approach. *Pediatrics* 1984;73:661.
8. Rosenthall L. Radionuclide investigation of osteomyelitis. *Curr Opin Radiol* 1992;4:62.
9. Keenan AM, Tindel NL, Alavi A. Diagnois of pedal osteomyelitis in diabetic patients using current scintigraphic techniques. *Arch Intern Med* 1989;149:2262.
10. Howman-Giles R, Uren R. Multifocal osteomyelitis in childhood: review by radionuclide bone scan. *Clin Nucl Med* 1992;17:274.
11. Rosenthall L, Kloiber R, Damtew B, et al. Sequential use of radiophosphate and radiogallium imaging in the differential diagnosis of bone, joint and soft tissue infection: quantitative analysis. *Diagn Imaging* 1982;51:249–258.
12. Wellman HN, Siddiqui AR, Mail JT, et al. Choice of radiotracer in the study of bone or joint infection in children. *Ann Radiol (Paris)* 1983;26:411–420.
13. Wellman HN, Georgi P, Sinn H, et al. Scintimaging of skeletal infectious processes with a new leukocyte labeling technique utilizing In-111 acetylacetone. *J Nucl Med* 1981;22:27.
14. Raptopoulis V, Doherty PW, Goss TP, et al. Acute osteomyelitis: advantage of white cell scans in early detection. *Am J Roentgenol* 1982;139:1077.
15. McDougall IR, Raumert JE, Lantieri RL. Evaluation of 111-In leukocyte whole-body scanning. *Am J Roentgenol* 1979;133:849.
16. Guze BH, Webber MM, Hawkins RA, et al. Indium-111 white blood cell scans: sensitivity, specificity, accuracy, and normal patterns of distribution. *Clin Nucl Med* 1990;5:8.
17. Schauwecker DS. Osteomyelitis. Diagnosis with In-111 labeled leukocytes. *Radiology* 1989;171:141.
18. Datz FL, Thorne DA. Effect of antibiotic therapy on the sensitivity of indium-111 labeled leukocyte scans. *J Nucl Med* 1986;27:1849–1953.
19. Peters AM. The utility of ^{99m}TcHMPAO-leukocytes for imaging infection. *Semin Nucl Med* 1994;24:2:110.
20. Schauwecker DS. The scintigraphic diagnosis of osteomyelitis. *Am J Roentgenol* 1992;158:9.
21. Lind P, Langsteger W, Koltringer P, et al. Immunoscintigraphy of inflammatory process with a technetium-99m-labeled monoclonal antigranulocyte antibody (Mab BW 250/183). *J Nucl Med* 1990;31:417–423.
22. Seybold K, Locher JT, Cossemans C, et al. Immunoscintigraphic localization of inflammatory lesions: clinical experience. *Eur J Nucl Med* 1988;13:587–593.
23. Kroiss A, Bock F, Perneczyk G, et al. Clinical application of Tc-99m-labeled granulocytes antibody in bone and joint disease. *Prog Clin Biol Res* 1990;355:337.
24. Hotze AL, Briele B, Overbeck B, et al. Technetium-99m-labeled antigranulocyte antibodies in suspected bone infections. *J Nucl Med* 1992;33:526.
25. Oyen WJ, Claessens RA, van Horn JR, et al. Scintigraphic detection of bone and joint infections with indium-111-labeled nonspecific polyclonal human immunoglobulin G. *J Nucl Med* 1990;31:403.
26. Fischman AJ, Rubin RH, Khaw BA, et al. Detection of acute inflammation with In-111 labeled nonspecific polyclonal IgG. *Semin Nucl Med* 1988;18:335–334.26a. Vinjamuri S, Hall AV, Solanki KK, et al. Comparison of 99m-Tc-Infecton imaging with radiolabelled white-cell imaging in the evaluation of bacterial infection. *Lancet* 1996;347:233–235.26b. Sonmezoglu K, Sonmezoglu M, Halac M, et al. Usefulness of (99m)Tc-ciprofloxacin (Infecton) scan in diagnosis of chronic orthopedic infections: comparative study with (99m)Tc-HMPAO leukocyte scintigraphy. *J Nucl Med* 2001;42:567–574.
27. Littenberg B, Mushlin AI. Technetium bone scanning in the diagnosis of osteomyelitis: a meta-analysis of test performance: diagnostic technology assessment consortium. *J Gen Intern Med* 1992;7:158–164.
28. Splittgerber GF, Spiegelhoff DR, Buggy BP. Combined leukocyte and bone imaging used to evaluate diabetic osteoarthropathy and osteomyelitis. *Clin Nucl Med* 1989;14:156–160.
29. Gandsman EJ, Deutsch SD, Kahn CB, et al. Differentiation of Charcot joint from osteomyelitis through dynamic bone imaging. *Nucl Med Commun* 1990;11:45–53.
30. Zeiger LA, Fox IM. Use of indium-111-labeled white blood cells in the diagnosis of diabetic foot infections. *J Foot Surg* 1990;29:46–51.
31. Choong K, Monaghan P, McGaigan L, et al. Role of bone scintigraphy in the early diagnosis of discitis. *Ann Rheum Dis* 1990;49:932–934.
32. Nolla-Sole JM, Mateo-Soria L, Rozadilla-Sacanall A, et al. Role of technetium-99m diphosphonate and gallium-67 citrate bone scanning in the early diagnosis of infectious spondylodiscitis: a comparative study. *Ann Rheum Dis* 1992;51:665–657.
33. Whalen JJL, Brown ML, McLeod R, et al. Limitations of indium leukocyte imaging for the diagnosis of spine infections. *Spine* 1991;16:193–197.
34. Eisenberg B, Powe JE, Alavi A. Cold defects in In-111-labeled leukocyte imaging of osteomyelitis in the axial skeleton. *Clin Nucl Med* 1991;16:103–106.
35. Jacobson AF, Gilles CP, Cerqueira MD. Photopenic defects in marrow containing skeleton on indium-111 leukocyte scintigraphy: prevalence at sites suspected of osteomyelitis and as an incidental finding. *Eur J Nucl Med* 1992;19:858–864.
36. King AD, Peters AM, Stuttle AW, et al. Imaging of bone infection with labelled white blood cells: role of contemporaneous bone marrow imaging. *Eur J Nucl Med* 1990;17:148–151.
37. Palestrao CJ, Roumanas P, Swyer AJ, et al. Diagnosis of musculoskeletal infection using combined In-111 labeled leukocyte and Tc-99m SC marrow imaging. *Clin Nucl Med* 1992;17:269–273.
38. Kim EE, Haynie TP, Podoloff DA, et al. Radionuclide imaging in the evaluation of osteomyelitis and septic arthritis. *Crit Rev Diagn Imaging* 1989;29:257–305.
39. Lantoo T, Kaukonen JP, Kokkola A, et al. Tc-99m HMPAO labeled leukocytes superior to bone scan in the detection of osteomyelitis in children. *Clin Nucl Med* 1992;17:7–10.
40. Copping C, Dalgiesh SM, Dudley NJ, et al. The role of ^{99m}Tc-HMPAO white cell imaging in suspected orthopaedic infection. *Br J Radiol* 1992;65:309–312.
41. Verlooy H, Mortelmans L, Verbruggen A, et al. Tc-99m HM-PAO labelled leucocyte scanning for detection of infection in orthopedic surgery. *Prog Clin Biol Res* 1990;355:181–187.
42. Bessette PR, Hanson MJ, Czarnicki DJ, et al. Evaluation of postoperative osteomyelitis of the sternum comparing CT and dual Tc-99m MDP bone and In-111 WBC SPECT. *Clin Nucl Med* 1993;18:197–202.
43. Al–Sheikh W, Sfakianakis GN, Hourani M, et al. A prospective comparative study of the sensitivity and specificity in In-111 leukocyte, gallium 67-citrate and bone scintigraphy and roentgenograms in the diagnosis of osteomyelitis with and without orthopedic prosthesis. *J Nucl Med* 1982;23:29.
44. Kim HC, Alavi A, Russell MD, et al. Differentiation of bone and bone marrow infarcts from osteomyelitis in sickle cell disorders. *Clin Nucl Med* 1989;14:249–254.
45. Fernandez-Ulloa M, Vasavada PJ, Black RR. Detection of acute osteomyelitis with indium-111-labeled white blood cells in a patient with sickle cell disease. *Clin Nucl Med* 1989;14:97–100.
46. Kolyoas E, Rosenthal L, Ahronheim GA, et al. Serial 67-Ga-citrate imaging during treatment of acute osteomyelitis in childhood. *Clin Nucl Med* 1978;3:461.
47. Graham GD, Lundy MM, Moreno AJ, et al. The role of Tc-99m MDP and Ga-67 citrate in predicting the cure of osteomyelitis. *Clin Nucl Med* 1983;8:344.
48. Newman, LG, Waller J, Palestro CJ, et al. Unsuspected osteomyelitis in diabetic foot ulcers: diagnosis and monitoring by leukocyte scanning with indium-111 oxyquinoline. *JAMA* 1991;266:1246–1251.
49. Bauer G, Weber DA, Ceder L, et al. Dynamics of Tc-99m methylene-diphosphonate imaging of the femoral head following hip fracture. *Clin Orthop* 1980;152:85.

460 *Bone*

50. Gregg PJ, Walder DN. Scintigraphy versus radiography in early diagnosis of experimental bone necrosis with special reference to caisson disease of bone. *J Bone Joint Surg Br* 1980;62:214.
51. Uren RF, Howman-Giles R. The cold hip sign on bone scan: a retrospective review. *Clin Nucl Med* 1991;16:553–556.
52. Danigelis JA. Pinhole imaging in Legg-Perthes disease: further observations. *Semin Nucl Med* 1976;17:184.
53. Murray IP, Dixon J. The role of single photon emission computed tomography in bone scintigraphy. *Skeletal Radiol* 1989;18:493.
54. Krasnow AZ, Collier SD, Peck DC, et al. The value of oblique angle reorientation in SPECT bone scintigraphy of the hips. *Clin Nucl Med* 1990;15:287.
55. Kim KY, Lee SH, Moon DH, et al. The diagnostic value of the triple-head single photon emission computed tomography (3H-SPECT) in avascular necrosis of the femoral head. *Int Orthop* 1993;17:132–138.
56. Conway JJ, Weiss SC, Maldonadov U. Scintigraphic patterns in Legg-Calve-Perthes disease. *Radiology* 1983;149P:102.
57. Lausten GA, Christensen SB. Distribution of 99mTc-phosphate compounds in osteonecrotic femoral heads. *Acta Orthop Scand* 1989;60:419–423.
58. Alavi A, Mitchell M, Kundelh H, et al. Comparison of RN, MRI, and XCT imaging in the diagnosis of avascular necrosis of the femoral head. *J Nucl Med* 1986;27:1952.
59. Cahill BR, Phillips MR, Navarro R. The results of conservative management of juvenile osteochondritis dissecans using joint scintigraphy: a prospective study. *Am J Sports Med* 1989;17:601–605.
60. Sutherland AD, Savage JP, Paterson DC, et al. The nuclide bone scan in the diagnosis and management of Perthes' disease. *J Bone Joint Surg* 1980;147:221.
61. Mortensson W, Rosenborg M, Gretzer H. The role of bone scintigraphy in predicting femoral head collapse following cervical fractures in children. *Acta Radiol* 1990;31:291–292.
62. Stromquist B. Femoral head vitality after intracapsular hip fracture: 490 cases studied by intravital tetracycline labeling and Tc-MDP radionuclide imaging. *Acta Orthop Scand* 1983;54[Suppl 200].
63. Hoffer PB, Genant HK. Radionuclide joint imaging. *Semin Nucl Med* 1976;6:121.
64. Weissberg DL, Resnick D, Taylor A, et al. Rheumatoid arthritis and its variants: analysis of scintiphotographic, radiographic and clinical examinations. *Am J Roentgenol* 1978;131:665.
65. Greyson ND. Radionuclide bone and joint imaging in rheumatology. *Bull Rheum Dis* 1980;30:1034.
66. Khalkhali I, Stadalnik RC, Weisner KB, et al. Bone imaging of the heel in Reiter's syndrome. *Am J Roentgenol* 1979;132:110.
67. Sewell JR, Balck CM, Chapman AH, et al. Quantitative scintigraphy in diagnosis and management of plantar fasciitis. *J Nucl Med* 1980;21:633.
68. Ho G Jr, Sadovnikoff N, Malhotra CM, et al. Quantitative sacroiliac joint scintigraphy: clinical assessment. *Arthritis Rheum* 1979;22:837.
69. Domeij-Nyberg B, Kjallman M, Nylen O, et al. The reliability of quantitative bone scanning in sacroiliitis. *Scand J Rheumatol* 1980;9:77.
70. Katzberg RW, O'Mara RE, Tallent RH, et al. Radionuclide skeletal imaging and single photon emission computed tomography in suspected internal derangements of the temporomandibular joint. *J Oral Maxillofac Surg* 1984;42:782.
71. Resnick D, Williamson S, Alazraki N. Focal spinal abnormalities on bone scans in ankylosing spondylitis. *Clin Nucl Med* 1981;6:213.
72. Thomas RH, Resnick D, Alazraki NP, et al. Compartmental evaluation of osteoarthritis of the knee. *Radiology* 1975;116:585.
73. Collier BD, Johnson RP, Carrera GF, et al. Chronic knee pain assessed by SPECT: comparison with other modalities. *Radiology* 1985;157:795.
74. McAfee JG. Radionuclide imaging in metabolic and systemic skeletal diseases. *Semin Nucl Med* 1987;17:334.
75. Clarke SE, Fogelman I. Bone scanning in metabolic and endocrine bone disease. *Endocrinol Metab Clin North Am* 1989;18:977–993.
76. Fogelman I, Bessent RG, Gordon D. A critical assessment of bone scan quantitation (bone to soft tissue ratios) in the diagnosis of metabolic bone disease. *Eur J Nucl Med* 1981;6:93.
77. Fogelman I, Hay ID, Citrin DL, et al. Semiquantitative analysis of the bone scan in acromegaly: correlation with human growth hormone values. *Br J Radiol* 1980;53:974.
78. Worth DP, Smye SW, Robinson PJ, et al. Quantitative bone scanning in the diagnosis of aluminum osteomalacia. *Nephrol Dial Transplant* 1989;4:721–724.
79. Rubini G, Lauriero F, Rubini D, et al. 99mTc-MDP global skeletal uptake and markers of bone metabolism in patients with bone diseases. *Nucl Med Commun* 1993;14:567-572.
80. Reschini E, Ulivieri FM, Ortolani S. Clinical experience with two simple methods of measurement of 99mTc-methylene diphosphonate body retention in bone disease. *J Nucl Biol Med* 1991;35:123–130.
81. Novikov AI, Ermolenko AE, Ermakova IP, et al. Dynamic scintigraphy with sodium 1-hydroxy-ethane-1,1 diphosphonate for the differential diagnosis of osteomalacia in patients in the terminal stage of chronic kidney failure. *Urol Nefrol (Mosk)* 1990;Mar-Apr:11–15.
82. Ohashi K, Smith HS, Jacobs MP. "Superscan" appearance in distal renal tubular acidosis. *Clin Nucl Med* 1991;16:318–320.
83. Kitamura N, Wada S, Hayama K, et al. Study on renal osteodystrophy using 2-compartment model analysis of bone scintigraphy: clinical significance of K index. *Shigaku* 1989;77:983–995.
84. Israel O, Kleinhaus U, Keren R, et al. The 24 hour/4 hour ratio (T/F ratio) of Tc-99m MDP uptake in patients with bone metastases and degenerative changes. *J Nucl Med* 1984;25:77.
85. Isaia GC, Salamano G, Mussetta M, et al. Photon densitometry in the diagnosis of osteoporosis. *Minerva Endocrinol* 1991;16:93–99.
86. Valkema R, Verheij LF, Blokland JA, et al. Limited precision of lumbar spine dual-photon absorptiometry by variations in the soft-tissue background. *J Nucl Med* 1990;31:1774–1781.
87. Fogelman I. An evaluation of the contribution of bone mass measurements to clinical practice. *Semin Nucl Med* 1989;19:62–68.
88. Ryan PJ, Evans P, Gibson T, et al. Osteoporosis and chronic back pain: a study with single-photon emission computed tomography bone scintigraphy. *J Bone Miner Res* 1992;7:1455–1460.
89. Bergot C, Laval-Jeantet AM, Laval-Jeantet MH, et al. Measurement of vertebral bone density. Quantitative tomodensitometry or dual-photon absorptiometry? *J Radiol* 1993;74:195–204.
90. Iancu TC, Almagor G, Friedman E, et al. Chronic familial hyperphosphatasemia. *Radiology* 1978;129:669.
91. O'Mara RE, Pinals RS. Bone scanning in regional migratory osteoporosis. *Radiology* 1970;97:579.
92. Bray ST, Partain CL, Teates CD, et al. The value of the bone scan in idiopathic regional migratory osteoporosis. *J Nucl Med* 1979;20:1268.
93. Kozin F. Soin JS, Ryan LM, et al. Bone scintigraphy in the reflex sympathetic dystrophy syndrome. *Radiology* 1981;138:437.
94. Ali A, Tetalmin MR, Fordham EW, et al. Distribution of hypertrophic pulmonary osteoarthropathy. *Am J Roentgenol* 1980;134:771.
95. Vaquer RA, Dunn EK, Bhat S, et al. Reversible pulmonary uptake and hypertrophic pulmonary osteoarthropathic distribution of technetium-99m methylene diphosphonate in a case of *Pneumocystis carinii* pneumonia. *J Nucl Med* 1989;30:1563–1567.
96. Lavender JP, Evans MA, Arnot R, et al. A comparison of radiography and radioisotope scanning in the detection of Paget's disease and in the assessment of response to human calcitonin. *Br J Radiol* 1977;50:243.
97. Wioland M, Bonnerot V. Diagnosis of partial and total physeal arrest by bone single-photon emission computed tomography. *J Nucl Med* 1993;34:1410–1415.
98. Chaudhuri TK, Fink S. Radionuclide imaging in osteitis deformans. *Am J Physiol Imaging* 1990;5:42–45.
99. Boudreau RJ, Llisbona R, Hadjiipavlou A. Observations on serial radionuclide blood flow studies in Paget's disease. *J Nucl Med* 1981;22:510.
100. Brixen K, Hansen HH, Mosekilde L, et al. SPECT bone scintigraphy in assessment of cranial Paget's disease. *Acta Radiol* 1990;31:549–550.
101. Patel U, Gallacher SJ, Boyle IT, et al. Serial bone scans in Paget's disease: development of new lesions, natural variation in lesion intensity and nature of changes seen after treatment. *Nucl Med Commun* 1990;11:747–760.

102. Ryan PJ, Gibson T, Fogelman I. Bone scintigraphy following intravenous pamidronate for Paget's disease of bone. *J Nucl Med* 1992;33:1589–1593.
103. Weber DA. The quantitative measurement of the response to treatment. *Int J Radiol Oncol Biol Phys* 1976;1:1221.
104. Davis DC, Skylawer R, Cole RL. Melorheostosis on three-phase bone scintigraphy: case report. *Clin Nucl Med* 1992;17:561–564.
105. Mahoney J. Acong DM. Demonstration of increased bone metabolism in melorheostosis by multiphase bone scanning. *Clin Nucl Med* 1991;16:847–848.
106. Adams BK, Smuta NA. The detection of extramedullary hematopoiesis in a patient with osteopetrosis. *Eur J Nucl Med* 1989;15:803–804.
107. King MA, Weber DA, Casarett GW, et al. A study of irradiated bone, II: changes in Tc-99m pyrophosphate bone imaging. *J Nucl Med* 1980;21:22.
108. King MA, Casarett GW, Weber DA, et al. A study of irradiated bone, III: scintigraphic and radiographic detection of radiation induced osteosarcomas. *J Nucl Med* 1980;21:426.
109. Hattner RS, Hartmeyer J, Wara WM. Characterization of radiation-induced photopenic abnormalities on bone scans. *Radiology* 1982;145:161.
110. Dee P, Lambruschi PG, Hiebert JM. Use of ^{99m}Tc-MDP bone scanning in the study of vascularized bone implants. *J Nucl Med* 1981;22:522.
111. Stevenson JS, Bright RW, Dunson GL, et al. Technetium-99m phosphate bone imaging: a method of assessing bone graft healing. *Radiology* 1974;110:391.
112. Velasco JG, Vega A, Leisorek A. The early detection of free bone graft viability with ^{99m}Tc: a preliminary report. *Br J Plast Surg* 1976;29:344.

22

ATHLETIC INJURIES

LAWRENCE E. HOLDER

Athletic injuries often are considered a subset of traumatic injury. Understanding the mechanisms of injury, which often are related to the actions and activities of a particular sport, allows for a more specific differential diagnosis. Placing the demonstrated blood flow, relative vascularity, and metabolic activity into the context of the athlete's training regimen, level of participation (professional, college, high school, recreational), and short- and long-term goals allows the nuclear physician to participate with the treating physician in patient care. Even if a specific diagnosis cannot be made, therapy often can be started if the site of increased bone turnover can be precisely located and its degree of metabolic activity estimated. Appropriate additional anatomic imaging correlation can then be suggested (1–3).

PATHOPHYSIOLOGIC AND BIOMECHANICAL CONSIDERATIONS

Three-phase Bone Imaging

Three-phase bone imaging (TPBI) in sports medicine is important because there usually is clinical uncertainty as to the cause of the symptoms. Information about blood flow, vascularity, and metabolic activity allows for differential diagnosis and for the provision of physiologic information, which even without a specific diagnosis, can direct appropriate therapy (1,4,5). Rupani et al. (5) and Deutcsch and Gandsman (6) described three phases to help date an injury. They expanded the earlier observations of Matin (7) regarding the relation of fracture healing demonstrated on delayed bone images to the time after injury when imaging was performed. In general, spatial resolution should take precedence over temporal resolution in choosing acquisition parameters for the radionuclide angiography. Spatial resolution considerations also necessitate use of the highest-resolution collimators possible for delayed images. Single photon emission computed tomography (SPECT) is used when needed to further define the location of an abnormal focus of increased tracer (8–10), which is critical in the effort to determine a specific cause.

Periostitis and Shin Splints

Shin splints, or medial tibial stress syndrome (11–14), has been defined as disruption of the Sharpey fiber-periosteum interface. It is caused by abnormal excursion of the soleus muscle-tendon complex. Pathologic and scintigraphic changes represent periostitis. Other periosteal lesions, such as periostitis resulting from a direct blow to the shin by a lacrosse stick, for example, should not be confused with the shin splints lesion causing pain in the leg.

Biomechanical Stress Lesions

Biomechanical stress lesions are the sports medicine equivalent of the repetitive stress syndromes, such as carpal tunnel syndrome, which affect the musculoskeletal system as the result of a wide range of activities (2,15). In some cases these lesions represent enthesopathy or other more generic type stress responses of bones and joints, simply with a sports activity–related etiologic factor. An enthesis is the site of insertion of a tendon, ligament, or articular capsule into bone. Resnick and Niwayama (16) suggested that alteration at these sites be called *enthesopathy*.

Avulsion Fracture

Avulsion fractures are caused by the pull of a muscle or tendon and usually occur in younger, skeletally immature patients whose apophyseal attachments are less strong than the tendon-bone interfaces. Even after the physis appears closed radiographically, there is a relative weakness at this site for several years, and avulsion fractures are occasionally seen after fusion of the apophysis. In the athletic setting, avulsion injuries also occur in the mature skeleton because of very strong concentrations of force associated with overstretched muscle-tendon complexes.

Avascular Necrosis

Sudden disruption of the blood supply to areas of bone without adequate collateral blood supply is an obvious cause of avascular necrosis, as illustrated by the football injury sustained by Heisman trophy winner Bo Jackson. Less obvious, often repetitive microtraumatic episodes also result in avascular injuries to bone (17) (see Chapter 21).

L.E. Holder: Department of Radiology, University of Florida, Shands-Jacksonville, Jacksonville, FL.

Bone Bruise

Bone bruise is a nonspecific term most often used in the athletic setting to describe a focal, traumatic painful injury to bone. It does not have the clinical or imaging findings associated with more established or accepted lesions or syndromes, such as shin splints or stress fracture. Initially, a tiny focal area of increased tracer accumulation on a delayed bone scan was postulated to represent repair associated with minimal intraosseous bleeding or periosteal elevation (4). During magnetic resonance imaging (MRI), a geographic, nonlinear area of bone marrow signal abnormality involving subcortical bone on T1-weighted or fat-suppressed T2-weighted images also has been called a bone bruise (18–20). Postulation regarding the underlying pathophysiologic process have included bleeding, edema, hyperemia, or microfractures. A radionuclide bone scan is used to determine the physiologic significance of nonspecific anatomic findings seen with other imaging modalities and to detect foci of abnormal metabolism when such anatomic imaging modalities do not show lesions.

Stress Fractures

Stress fractures in the athletic setting are most often fatigue fractures associated with cyclic loading of normal bone. As the biomechanics become more understood, older, more situational subcategories, such as *novice syndrome* or *overuse syndrome,* are used less often (4). Acute damage to a small number of osteonal units can occur as the applied stress exceeds the inherent strength of the bone or when loading initiates appropriate remodeling but continues or increases before remodeling is complete, fatigue fracture occurring during the process.

Tendonitis, Strains, Myositis, Bursitis

Primary soft-tissue processes occasionally are found during TPBI when they are associated with increased perfusion or vascularity, which can be seen on phase I or phase II images. Most often, however, these lesions are detected because of secondary changes to associated or underlying bone that produce focal areas of increased tracer uptake on delayed images. The exact cause of such uptake is uncertain (2). Some authors suggest that more intense diffuse uptake around the lateral ligaments of the ankle is related to more severe injury and may warrant more aggressive therapy (21). Direct localization of labeled bone tracers in injured muscle, whether in the process of resolving or progressing to myositis ossificans or heterotopic bone formation, is a common finding in the evaluation of athletes for pain. Baker (22) reviewed clinical concepts in the diagnosis and management of musculotendinous injuries. He defined *strain* as a stretch or tear of a musculotendinous unit. A first-degree strain involves minimal stretching; second-degree strain indicates partial tearing; and third-degree strain indicates complete disruption of a portion of this unit. The bleeding and pathophysiologic sequelae underlie tracer uptake in the injured muscle. Early work by Siegel et al. (23), which still appears valid, suggested that uptake of ^{99m}Tc diphosphonate in acutely damaged skeletal muscle is directly related to the deposition of calcium salts within the injured muscle fibers.

A bursa is a synovial membrane sac located around a joint or at a bony prominence where muscle or tendon movement occurs. When inflamed, the bursa is a source of pain. Most episodes of bursitis are not imaged immediately, but when bursitis is detected on delayed bone scans as a focus of abnormal increased activity in the subadjacent bone, it can be implicated as a source of pain. The mechanism of tracer uptake in calcific bursitis is probably similar to that in lesions such as myositis or calcifying hematoma, whereas the pathophysiologic mechanism of direct bone uptake is not understood but is probably similar to the increased delayed activity associated with tendonitis (3).

ANKLE AND FOOT

Navicular Stress Fracture

All types of injury involving the navicular bone, but especially stress fractures, often are symptomatic for months before the diagnosis is considered (24,25). Running with abrupt stops and starts, as by athletes such as basketball players and racket sports participants, directs posterior to anterior force through the navicular bone. On delayed images, intense focal uptake involving the entire navicular bone is characteristic (Fig. 22.1). Increased radionuclide angiographic and -pool activity in more acute cases reflecting the stage of healing or, paradoxically, in later cases, reflect nonunion and inflammatory stress change. SPECT for anatomic localization can be helpful (26). Plain radiographs obtained in the anatomic anteroposterior projection (27) can be helpful, but computed tomography (CT) or MRI is more sensitive in confirming the presence of the fracture (28,29)

Calcaneal Stress Fracture

Calcaneal stress fracture often is first diagnosed when the foot is imaged for unexplained pain. Focal linear increased tracer accumulation, often necessitating computer manipulation of images for optimal definition, is most often located in the superior midportion of the calcaneus (2,4,30).

Metatarsal Stress Fracture

Most commonly occurring in the second, third, and fourth metatarsals, stress fractures are similar to those in other long cortical bones (5). Particularly when background-subtracted delayed images are obtained, the uptake is focal and fusiform. In the first metatarsal, where much of the weight bearing affects cancellous bone rather than cortical bone, the abnormal activity on bone scans often is more horizontal or perpendicular to the direction of stress (4,31). Because of differences in management between fractures of the tuberosity of the fifth metatarsal and of the metatarsal shaft within 1.5 cm of the tuberosity (32), it is important to locate precisely the site of the fracture.

Stubbing Injuries to the Hallux

Stubbing injuries to the hallux, as reported by Jahss (33) in 1981, are less common than capsular and tendon injuries to

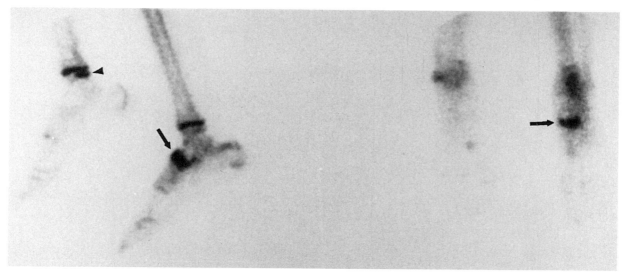

FIGURE 22.1. Navicular stress fracture. Delayed plantar (*right*) and right medial, left lateral (*left*) images. Moderately intense, focal, increased tracer accumulation defines the entire navicular bone (*arrows*). Physeal activity in the distal fibula is most apparent on the left lateral view (*arrowhead*).

the metatarsophalangeal joint, which often are called *turf toe,* referring to a sprain of the metatarsophalangeal joint occurring as a result of an injury on one of the newer artificial playing surfaces (34). A turf toe is swollen and tender but usually is stable to stress. A stubbing fracture tends to occur more often when a youngster is running barefoot. When Salter type I fractures do occur, they should be considered compound and prophylactically managed with antibiotics (35). TPBI, which confirms the presence of active bone disease, may have to be supplemented by ^{67}Ga citrate or ^{99m}Tc or ^{111}In white blood cell imaging for further differential diagnosis if there is a reason not to give antibiotics (35).

Os Trigonum Syndrome

The os trigonum is an accessory ossicle located at the posterior aspect of the talus (36). When posterior ankle pain is present, especially if the pain increases with flexion of the great toe, the diagnostic considerations of the visualized ossicle are a normal os trigonum, fracture of the posterior process of the talus, a bruised ossicle, and disruption of fibrous fusion of the ossicle. Focal increased uptake of tracer in the os trigonum on delayed images suggests that whatever the underlying cause, this ossicle is the source of pain (2). Surgical removal often is necessary for relief of pain.

Tibiotalar Impingement Syndrome

As described by Black and Brand (37), repetitive trauma occurs when an athlete "drives" off a planted foot, and the anterior edge of the distal tibia impinges against the neck of the talus. O'Donoghue (38) postulated that spur formation was the result of direct trauma during forcible dorsiflexion of the foot on the leg. Abnormally increased uptake of tracer on delayed images localizes to the osseous spurs indicates that active repair is taking

place and indirectly implies that the spur is the source of pain (Fig. 22.2).

Retrocalcaneal Bursitis

The retrocalcaneal recess often called the *preachilles bursa* is the radiolucent triangle at the inferior end of the preachilles fat pad located between the posterior aspect of the calcaneus and the Achilles tendon. On delayed scintigraphic images, increased ac-

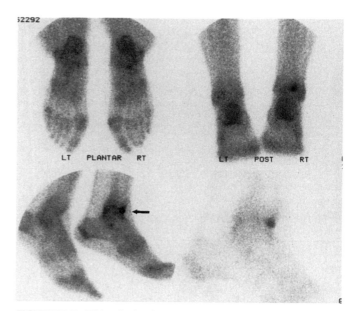

FIGURE 22.2. Tibiotalar impingement syndrome. Delayed images, including a magnified right lateral view (*lower right*), show a tiny focus of moderately increased tracer accumulation associated with a hypertrophic spur at the anterior lip of the right tibia (*arrow*). (From Holder LE. Bone scintigraphy in skeletal trauma. *Radiol Clin North Am* 1993; 31:739–781, with permission.)

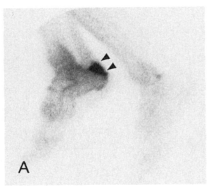

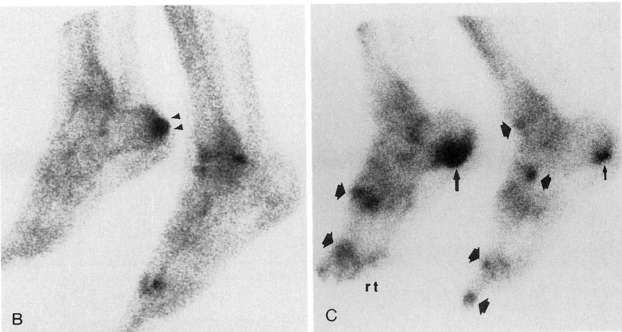

FIGURE 22.3. **A:** Retrocalcaneal bursitis. Delayed lateral view shows focally intense tracer accumulation in the retrocalcaneal bursa and underlying bone surface of the calcaneus (*arrowheads*). **B:** Lateral Achilles tendonitis. Delayed lateral view shows round, focally increased accumulation of tracer in the posterior calcaneus at the junction of the middle and lower thirds at the insertion of the Achilles tendon (*arrowheads*). **C:** Plantar fasciitis. Delayed lateral views show focally increased accumulation of tracer in the posteroinferior portion of the calcaneus at the level of the medial tuberosity, right foot (*large arrow*). *Small arrows* point to areas of nonspecific stress changes. (From Holder LE. Bone scintigraphy in skeletal trauma. *Radiol Clin North Am* 1993;31:739–781, with permission.)

tivity, possibly due to calcification, can be seen in the inflamed bursa itself or, more commonly, in the adjacent posterosuperior aspect of the calcaneus (4) (Fig. 22.3). When combined with inflammation of the superficial bursa dorsal to the Achilles tendon and Achilles tendonitis itself, the diagnosis of regional bursitis (Haglund disease) can be considered (3,39).

Achilles Tendonitis

The Achilles tendon, anatomically called the *calcaneal tendon,* inserts into the middle part of the posterior surface of the calcaneus. Most often this insertion is visualized on delayed images as a focal area of increased tracer accumulation involving the bone (4). Posttraumatic calcification within the substance of the

Achilles tendon at the site of previous rupture occasionally shows mildly increased tracer accumulation. Calcifications seen on radiographs at the insertion site, which do not take up tracer, are common among patients without symptoms. These are thought to result from previous trauma and when not metabolically active by inference are no longer associated with the production of pain (4) (Fig. 22.3).

Plantar Fasciitis

Plantar fasciitis is traumatic inflammation secondary to a strain or tear of the long plantar ligament or aponeurosis. The more typical pain, as well as the abnormal focal increased tracer accumulation seen on delayed images, is located at the fascial origin at the medial tuberosity of the calcaneus (Fig. 22.3). Although a calcaneal spur can be present, it is not enough evidence to confirm a diagnosis. A radionuclide bone scan occasionally shows abnormal tracer uptake on the angiographic and blood-pool phases, but most often imaging is performed for patients with chronic symptoms and when findings in the first two phases are normal (4).

Osteochondral Fracture of the Talar Dome

Osteochondral fractures of the talar dome should be suspected in athletes who continue to have pain and disability after a "routine ankle sprain." Focal increased accumulation of tracer, often subarticular but also involving the entire posterior half of the talus, is seen on delayed images (40). MRI of patients whose plain radiographs have normal findings (41), even in retrospect, can provide confirmation and allow fracture staging.

Lisfranc Fracture

The original reports of fracture-dislocation of the tarsometatarsal joint described the injury among cavalry officers and subsequently among patients involved in motor vehicle and industrial accidents. Sports-related Lisfranc fractures occur as a result of combined forced plantar flexion and rotation, with or without adduction of the forefoot (42). The injury is primarily soft-tissue disruption of the ligamentous support of the articulation but can include a fracture. Radionuclide bone imaging is important because in many of these patients the fracture is not seen during the initial evaluation, and the patient is evaluated later for pain of possibly osseous origin and of uncertain causation.

Cuneiform and First Metatarsal Base Stress Fractures

Because a large proportion of body weight passes through the base of the first metatarsal, this bone is susceptible to stress fractures of the compression type (43,44). Although abnormal activity on routine delayed images usually can be localized to the specific tarsal bone or metatarsal base, because of the intensity of activity present in acute fractures, background subtracted images may be necessary for precise localization.

Reflex Sympathetic Dystrophy

Reflex sympathetic dystrophy (RSD) is a pain syndrome described as an excessive or exaggerated response to injury to an extremity. It manifests with four almost constant characteristics: (a) intense or unduly prolonged pain, (b) vasomotor disturbances, (c) delayed functional recovery, and (d) various associated trophic changes. RSD is less common after athletic injury but should be kept in mind when healing is prolonged or pain is out of proportion to that expected. Findings in the foot are similar to those in the hand—diffuse increased tracer uptake throughout the hindfoot, midfoot, and forefoot with juxtaarticular accentuation of tracer uptake. (45,46).

LEG

Tibial Stress Fracture

Tibial stress fractures are most commonly detected on delayed bone scans as solitary, focal, fusiform, longitudinally oriented areas of increased uptake involving the posterior medial cortex (Fig. 22.4) (5,47). Depending on the time of injury in relation to the age and severity of the stress fracture, the findings on the radionuclide angiogram may be abnormal for 2 to 4 weeks, with a mean of 2.9 weeks; the blood-pool or tissue-phase images may be abnormal for 1 to 8 weeks, with a mean of 5.2 weeks; and the delayed images may be abnormal for 3 to 36 weeks, with a mean of 11 weeks (5). Although there has been intermittent controversy about the specific scintigraphic pattern and its relation to other bone stress lesions (48,49), most authors agree with this classification (50,51). The specific location of the stress fracture is related to the biomechanics in the individual patient (5,52–55) (Fig. 22.5). Rosen et al. (56) and Rupani et al. (5) have emphasized the multiplicity of lesions. Both groups note that many of the second and third lesions were asymptomatic.

Fibular Stress Fracture

Fibular stress fractures are much less common than are tibial stress fractures. They occur most often in the lower third of the bone, possibly secondary to stress resulting from powerful contraction of the flexor muscles of the ankle and foot that

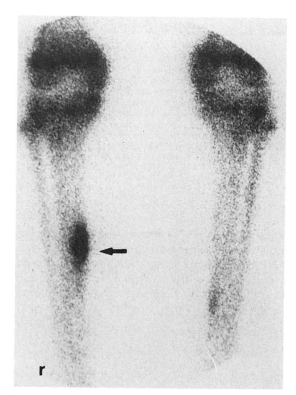

FIGURE 22.4. Tibial stress fracture. Delayed anterior image shows focal fusiform increased tracer uptake in the middle third of the medial tibial cortex (*arrow*). The medial view (*not shown*) showed a posterior cortical location of activity.

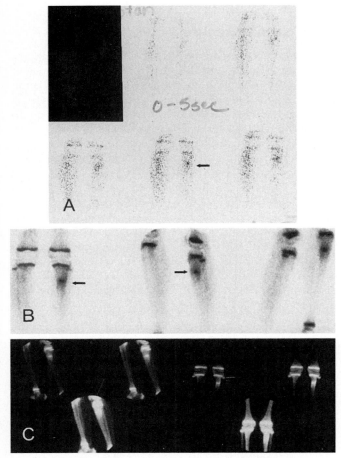

FIGURE 22.5. Proximal tibial stress fracture. **A:** Radionuclide angiogram shows minimal increased tracer uptake in the proximal left tibia (*arrow*). **B:** Blood-pool images. Anterior, left lateral, right medial views show moderately intense focal, increased tracer uptake in the proximal left tibia (*arrow*). **C:** Delayed images, triple-lens Polaroid display. Anterior (*right*) and left lateral, right medial (*left*) images show linear, intense increased activity in the proximal tibia somewhat posteromedially. Blood-pool and delayed images show increased vascularity and metabolic activity associated with the normal physis activity of the femur, tibia, and fibula. (From Holder LE. Bone scintigraphy in skeletal trauma. *Radiol Clin North Am* 1993;31:739–781, with permission.)

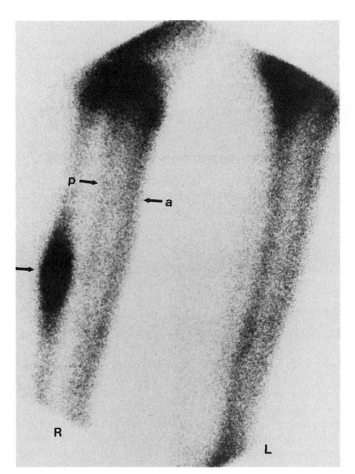

FIGURE 22.6. Fibular stress fracture. Lateral view of right leg (*R*) and simultaneously obtained medial view of left leg (*L*) show a focal fusiform area of increased tracer in fibula (*arrow*). Definition of the anterior (*a*) and posterior (*p*) tibial cortices is evident. (From Holder LE, Matthews LS. The nuclear physician and sports medicine. In: Freeman LM, Weissman HS, eds. *Nuclear medicine annual 1984*. New York: Raven Press, 1984:81–140, with permission.)

approximate the fibula to the tibia (5,57,58). Most investigators agree that excessive muscular force on the proximal fibula is the underlying mechanism. The focal fusiform increased tracer uptake on delayed images usually involves the posterior cortex. Even with good imaging technique, however, the smaller size of the fibula does not always allow separation of the anterior and posterior cortices, as occurs with tibial stress fractures (Fig. 22.6).

Shin Splints

The clinical entity shin splints, sometimes called *medial tibial stress syndrome,* is characterized by the findings of exercise-induced pain and tenderness to palpation along the posteromedial border of the tibia (11–13). Findings on radionuclide angiographic and blood-pool images are almost always normal in these patients. On delayed images, tibial lesions involve the posterior cortex, are longitudinally oriented, and usually are long, involving one third of the length of the bone. These images most often show varying tracer uptake along the length of the affected area (11) (Fig. 22.7). Results of cadaveric, electromyographic, and muscle stimulation studies emphasize the relation of this syndrome to the soleus muscle and its investing fascia (12).

Myositis Ossificans

Traumatic myositis ossificans usually results from blunt trauma to large muscle groups (59). The process usually is self-limited because the calcific deposits in the soft tissues eventually mature. Pain may persist, however, owing to mechanical irritation or increased compartmental pressure. Radionuclide bone imaging is used to assess and confirm maturation of these masses. When the mass is mature, the metabolic activity on delayed images is similar in intensity to that of normal bone.

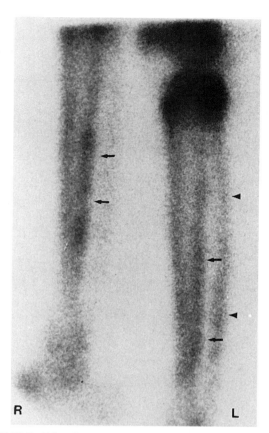

FIGURE 22.7. Shin splints. Delayed-image left lateral and right medial views show the abnormality is longer than in a stress fracture and often demonstrates varying intensity of tracer accumulation along its length. Shin splints are particularly evident on the right medial view (*arrows*). Fibular is particularly evident in the left lateral view (*arrowheads*).

Interosseous Membrane Hemorrhage

Patients with severe rotational ankle trauma can injure the interosseous membrane between the tibia and fibula, and hemorrhage (60) and often calcification of the interosseous membrane (61) develop. Increased radiotracer activity on all three phases of the study again demonstrates the degree of metabolic activity and/or maturation present (61).

KNEE AND THIGH

Quadriceps Mechanism Injury

Common to all quadriceps mechanism injuries is strong contraction of the quadriceps muscle opposed by forced flexion of the knee. Composed of the quadriceps femoris muscle and tendon, the patella, and the patellar tendon, the specific site of injury often is related to patient age (62). In adults, focal increased activity on delayed images at the origin at the inferior pole of the patella is called *patellar tendonitis* (Fig. 22.8). In children, focal increased activity on delayed images at the tibial tubercle insertion of the patellar tendon is most common.

Anterior Knee Pain

Dye et al. (63,64) use radionuclide bone imaging as part of the routine evaluation of patients with unexplained knee pain. Focal uptake seen on delayed images can be associated with abnormal cartilage and subarticular bone. Although attempts at specificity have been made, the findings in general remain nonspecific, and MRI is now the first imaging modality used in this clinical setting (65). Chondromalacia of the patella (66) and subchondral bone changes secondary to chronic meniscal tears (67) are two examples of attempts at specificity. RSD in the knee, although not rigorously documented, has been described as having diffuse increased uptake in all three compartments (68,69). In postpatellectomy syndrome, patients have more focal increased uptake in the femoral groove. RSD is discussed in more detail in Chapter 21.

Painful Bipartite Patella

One of the more common indications for TPBI in the athletic setting is to evaluate the physiologic significance of an anatomic lesion identified on radiographs. Bipartite patella, with the accessory ossification center located at the supralateral pole, is not an uncommon radiologic finding among adolescents (70). Focal increased tracer accumulation at the site of the osseous fragmentation suggests that these fragments are mobile and the source of pain.

Stress Fracture of the Femoral Shaft

Stress fractures of the proximal medial shaft of the femur in runners demonstrate focal, fusiform increased activity on delayed images that involves the medial cortex of the femur (71–73) (Fig. 22.9). It is difficult to differentiate by means of scintigraphy true femoral shaft stress fractures from adductor avulsion-type injuries, although stress fractures early in their course tend to have increased flow and blood-pool activity on the first two phases of radionuclide angiography.

Adductor Avulsion Fracture

Adductor avulsion injuries tend to occur when the groin muscles are being stretched. Patients often remember exactly when the first pain occurred (74). Activity on delayed images can be more focal and less fusiform than often is seen with the femoral shaft stress fracture. The mechanism of injury, however, and anatomic localization help relate the focus of uptake to a particular muscle or tendon and allow the characteristics of uptake to be related to the mechanism of injury (74,75) (Fig. 22.9).

Soft-tissue Injury

Soft-tissue injuries usually are clinically obvious or suspected and are evaluated with ultrasonography or MRI. If located in deeper structures, however, the injury often is encountered incidentally when imaging is performed to evaluate nonspecific pain of possibly osseous origin. Hematoma before any calcification can appear as a photon-deficient area on both blood-pool and

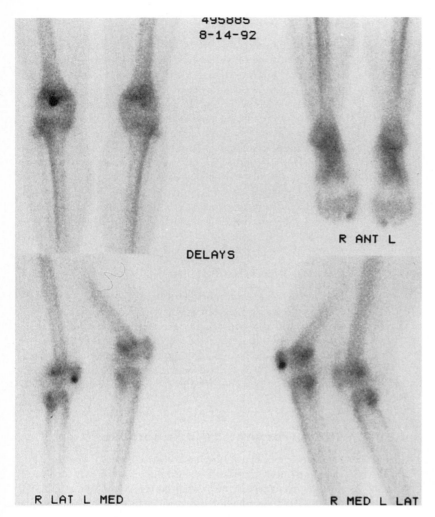

495885
8-14-92

R ANT L

DELAYS

R LAT L MED

R MED L LAT

FIGURE 22.8. Patellar tendonitis. Delayed images show focal, mild to moderately intense increased tracer uptake in the inferior pole of the right patella. In simultaneous acquisition of a medial view of one knee and the contralateral lateral view, it is difficult to image the true anatomic position of both knees. (From Holder LE. Bone scintigraphy in skeletal trauma. *Radiol Clin North Am* 1993; 31:739–781, with permission.)

delayed images with a rim of increased vascularity on the blood-pool images as well as occasional activity surrounding the hematoma on delayed images. For example, Martire (60) reported on a long-distance runner with right calf pain who had a ruptured popliteal cyst. The cyst was identified at delayed imaging as a photon-deficient area with a rim of slight increased activity.

PELVIS AND HIPS
Pubic Symphysitis

Pubic symphysitis is common among runners. Koch and Jackson (76) postulated that avulsion of the adductor and rectus abdominis muscles are the cause. The symptoms often are vague and referred to the lower abdomen or groin, occasionally with perineal radiation. When the appropriate athletic history is present, the diagnosis most often is confirmed when pain is present over the pubis. Delayed radionuclide images show increased activity involving varying portions of one or both pubic bones at the symphysis. This increased activity most often obliterates the central area of relative photon deficiency that in the normal situation

represents the fibrocartilaginous symphysis (4). Stress fractures of the pubic ramus are thought to be produced by the tensile forces resulting from strong muscle pulls on the lateral part of the pubic ramus and ischium as the hip is extended (77,78).

Avulsion Injuries

Fernbach and Wilkinson (79) discussed the entire range of apophyseal avulsion fractures of the pelvis and proximal femur that occur among adolescents engaged in active sports. Fernandez-Ulloa et al. (78) reviewed the anatomic and physiologic characteristics of the pelvic and hip regions and emphasized the importance of these characteristics to scintigraphy (Fig. 22.10). In this area, symmetric patient positioning for imaging is most important because even slight rotation can produce asymmetric anterior iliac crest activity. The degree of metabolic activity associated with enthesopathy and by inference the role of enthesopathy as the site or origin of pain can be ascertained with TPBI. The abnormality is demonstrated by means of focal tracer accumulation on delayed images.

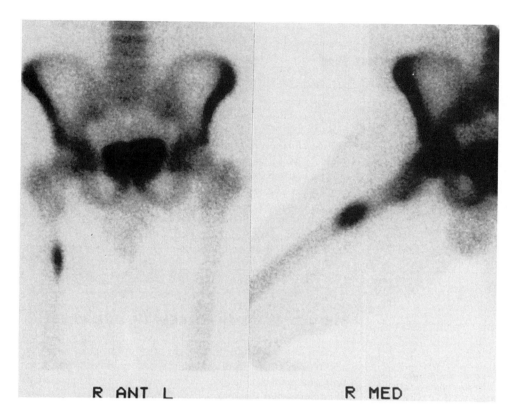

R ANT L   R MED

FIGURE 22.9. Adductor avulsion versus femoral shaft stress fracture in a 16-year-old patient. Delayed images show abnormal medial uptake of tracer is not as linear as it is in a typical shin splints–type lesion, nor is it quite as fusiform as usual in stress fractures. The history strongly suggested adductor avulsion. (From Holder LE. Bone scintigraphy in skeletal trauma. *Radiol Clin North Am* 1993;31: 739–781, with permission.)

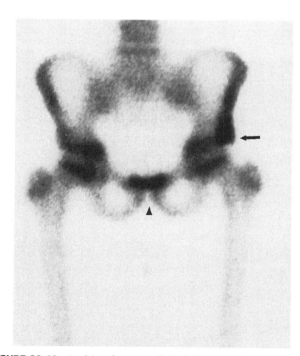

FIGURE 22.10. Avulsion fracture of the left rectus femoris. Delayed anterior image shows very intense focal activity associated with the apophysis for the rectus femoris muscle at the anteroinferior iliac spine (*arrow*). The normal photon deficiency associated with the fibrocartilage at the symphysis is evident (*arrowhead*). (From Holder LE. Bone scintigraphy in skeletal trauma. *Radiol Clin North Am* 1993;31:739–781, with permission.)

Epiphyseal and Physeal Injuries

Epiphyseal and physeal injuries that tend to occur among adolescent athletes have been well-reviewed by Resnik (80). Although MRI can depict unossified cartilage in an immature skeleton, radionuclide bone imaging has an important place in differential diagnosis. In the evaluation of patients with slipped capital femoral epiphysis, which occurs predominantly during the adolescent growth spurt, physeal activity on blood-pool and especially on delayed images is more intense, broader, and thicker than it is on the normal side (4).

Stress Fracture of the Femoral Neck

Stress fracture of the femoral neck in athletes usually occurs in the medial aspect at the point of maximum compression stress (4,81,82). Because athletes tend to play through what they consider minor pain, many patients with stress fractures of the femoral neck have preexistent radiographic evidence of such a fracture. Bone scintigraphy is performed to document the age of the lesion so that appropriate therapeutic advice can be provided (Fig. 22.11). Most authors report essentially 100% sensitivity in the detection of symptomatic stress fractures of the femoral neck and other bones (4,5).

SPINE

Although CT or MRI is currently used before radionuclide bone imaging in evaluation for low back pain, when unexplained pain

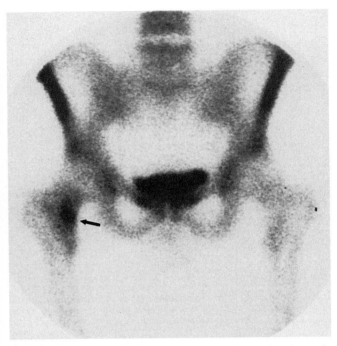

FIGURE 22.11. Stress fracture of the femoral neck. Delayed anterior image shows intense round focal area of increased tracer uptake in the distal medial aspect of the femoral neck. (From Holder LE. Bone scintigraphy in skeletal trauma. *Radiol Clin North Am* 1993;31:739–781, with permission.)

of possibly osseous origin persists, TPBI with planar and SPECT techniques usually is performed (2,4,83–86). An alternative is to identify a radiographic lesion such as a pars interarticularis defect with CT or MRI. A radionuclide bone scan is performed to evaluate the metabolic activity or physiologic significance of the anatomic lesion (5,84,85–88). Collier et al. (86), Bellah et al. (83) and others have discussed the important role of SPECT (Fig. 22.12). Most authors consider bone scintigraphy valuable in the evaluation of athletes with low back pain. The common etiologic factor in athletic injuries appears to be the hyperextended position, which places increased stress on the posterior elements of the spine. Pedicle stress fractures, stress lesions of the spinous processes, and stress associated with lamina defects have all been reported. Sports-related injuries in the thoracic and cervical spine are most often related to direct trauma and are evaluated and considered similarly to traumatic lesions in other areas.

SHOULDER, UPPER EXTREMITY, AND CHEST

Various degrees of separation of the acromioclavicular joint usually are recognized from the clinical history, physical examination, and plain radiographs. When imaging is performed as part of an evaluation for unexplained shoulder pain, delayed images show increased tracer accumulation on both the acromion and clavicular sides with obliteration of the normal photon deficiency of the joint space. This finding is nonspecific but provides objective evidence that the pain is probably coming from the acromi-

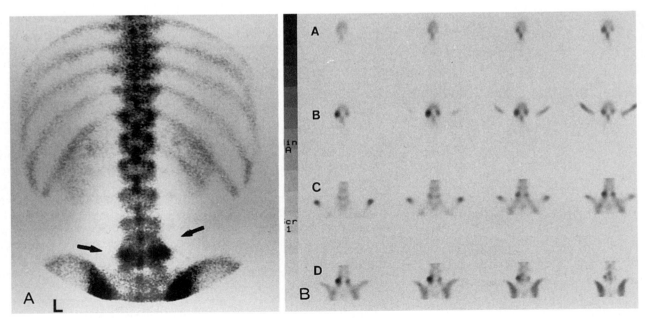

FIGURE 22.12. Bilateral spondylolisthesis. **A:** Posterior planar image shows bilateral increased activity (*arrows*) is greater on the right than on the left (*L*). Posterior oblique views (*not shown*) were highly suggestive of a pars interarticularis location. **B:** SPECT images show sequential reconstructed 1-pixel, 6-mm-thick transaxial sections (*rows A and B*) and coronal sections with increased contrast and further localized abnormal tracer uptake (*rows C and D*). (From Holder LE. Bone scintigraphy in skeletal trauma. *Radiol Clin North Am* 1993;31:739–781, with permission.)

oclavicular joint. The appearance of the uptake in middle-aged racket sport participants is no different from that in acromioclavicular arthritis secondary to non–sports-related causes. Osteolysis of the distal clavicle similarly occurs in sports related trauma (89,90). Stress fractures of the first rib have occurred in a variety of athletes, and the topic is reviewed by Gurtler et al. (91). Fatigue fractures of the medial aspect of the clavicle (92) also have been reported. Stress injuries to the humerus, including stress fractures, avulsion, and periostitis, often occur among gymnasts, weight lifters, and baseball pitchers (60,93). Patel (94) in a review emphasized a multimodality approach to the evaluation of athletic injuries in the shoulder and upper extremity.

Myositis

Myositis ossificans of the arm is less common than that of the thigh. The classic triad of local pain, a hard palpable mass in the muscle, and flexion contracture of the muscle is present only occasionally (95,96). Tackler's exostosis results from contusions and strains of the outer aspect of the mid humerus with the

development of a myositis mass. When heterotopic bone formation results and surgical removal is being considered for relief of pain, radionuclide bone imaging is used to document maturation of the process (4,95) (Fig. 22.13). Uptake in mature heterotopic bone formation on delayed images is similar in intensity to uptake in other portions of the humerus (normometabolic).

ELBOW AND FOREARM

The osseous changes resulting from the many types of elbow stress in sports activities include bony hypertrophy, loose bodies, traction spur formation, osteochondral irregularities, and epiphyseal and apophyseal changes. These lesions often are seen on plain radiographs (2,5,97,98). TPBI has been used to detect abnormally increased metabolic activity and, by implication, to determine the physiologic significance of these changes. For imaging of the elbow, computer-manipulated, background-subtracted images or creative positioning, such as the acute flexion

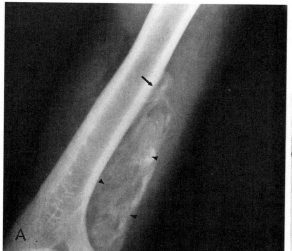
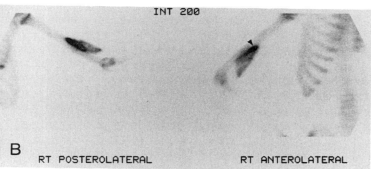
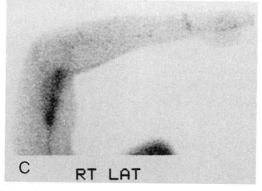

FIGURE 22.13. Myositis ossificans of the upper extremity. **A:** Plain radiograph shows ossification in the anteromedial muscle of the forearm (*arrowheads*). At the upper portion of the mass is a tiny focus of periosteal new bone (*arrow*). **B:** Delayed oblique images show separation of most of this activity from the bone and its shape, which corresponds to the ossification on the radiograph. The *upper area,* which is more focally intense, may represent an associated avulsion (*arrowhead*). **C:** Blood-pool lateral view shows increased vascularity of heterotopic bone formation, which suggests further that the lesion is not mature.

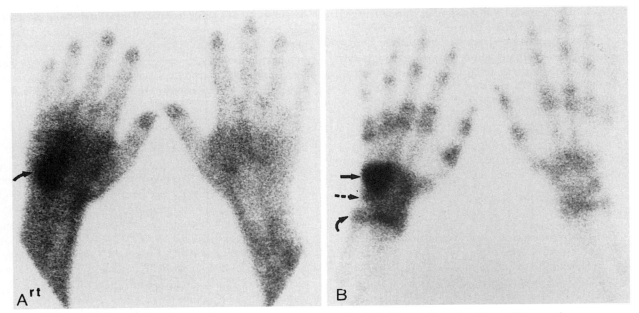

FIGURE 22.14. Fracture of the hook of the hamate. **A:** Blood-pool image shows focal area of increased tracer accumulation in the general area of the hamate (*arrow*). **B:** Delayed image shows a focal increase in tracer accumulation localized to the hamate (*short, straight arrow*). Distal ulna (*curved arrow*) and pisiform (*broken arrow*) are on the ulnar side of the proximal carpal row. In this relatively acute fracture, the intensity of activity blurs the margins of the individual carpal bone. (From Holder LE, Matthews LS. The nuclear physician and sports medicine. In: Freeman LM, Weissman HS, eds. *Nuclear medicine annual 1984.* New York: Raven Press, 1984:81–140, with permission.)

view (99), often are necessary to define the precise focus of greatest activity.

Medial epicondylitis (Little League elbow) and lateral epicondylitis (tennis elbow) usually are clinically obvious. When the degree of inflammation is marked owing to any cause, the radionuclide angiographic and blood-pool phases of the study can have positive results (2). During imaging, the most sensitive indicator of abnormality is focal uptake on delayed images. Torg and Moyer (100) described a stress fracture through the epiphyseal plate in an adolescent baseball pitcher and discussed King's original description of the mechanics of pitching.

Stress Fracture

Stress fractures in the diaphysis of the ulna have been reported by a variety of authors. Most postulate repeated flexor muscle activity as the etiologic factor (101–104). Lesions have been identified in tennis players, weight lifters, and baseball and softball players. Delayed images show focal fusiform increased tracer occasionally localized to one portion of the cortex, but more often the activity tends to be circumferential.

WRIST AND HAND

Athletic injuries to the wrist and hand are commonly encountered in sports medicine practice (104). Occult fracture, stress fracture, bone bruise, or even less specific subchondral or periosteal injury can cause focal tracer uptake. The location of uptake, clinical symptoms, and therapeutic considerations dictate the

need for additional anatomic imaging. Some authors have described focal uptake in areas such as the distal part of the radius as a stress fracture even without plain radiographic or CT confirmation (105). I prefer the term *bone bruise* or *nonspecific stress response* if the history is longer than 2 weeks and there is no plain radiographic correlation (1,2,106). Other authors have reported that fractures usually can be found if more advanced imaging modalities such as CT are used to evaluate regions of focal abnormal tracer uptake on bone scans (107). The scaphoid, lunate, trapezium, and distal radius are most commonly involved.

Stark et al. (108) described tennis players, golfers, and baseball players who fractured the hook of the hamate with the butt end of a racket, club, or bat by means of striking it during a swing. Although carpal tunnel radiography was described as being extremely sensitive, I have found that radionuclide bone imaging to identify the site of injury supplemented by CT for anatomic detail is necessary for some fractures of the hook and most fractures of the base of the hamate. Delayed images show a focal increase in tracer accumulation. Radionuclide angiographic or and blood-pool images may be abnormal if the fracture is acute (Fig. 22.14).

Reflex sympathetic dystrophy as a posttraumatic sequela of athletic injury is less common than it is after work-related injuries (47,109–110). Avascular necrosis of the lunate is also a common lesion that can occur in the athletic setting (111). These syndromes are discussed in Chapter 21.

REFERENCES

1. Holder LE. Clinical radionuclide bone imaging. *Radiology* 1990;176: 607–614.

2. Holder LE. Bone scintigraphy in skeletal trauma. *Radiol Clin North Am* 1993;31:739–781.
3. Pavlov H. Athletic injuries. *Radiol Clin North Am* 1990;28:435–443.
4. Holder LE, Matthews LS. The nuclear physician and sports medicine. In: Freeman LM, Weissman HS, eds. *Nuclear medicine annual: 1984.* New York: Raven Press, 1984:81–140.
5. Rupani HD, Holder LE, Espinola DA, et al. Three-phase radionuclide bone imaging in sports medicine. *Radiology* 1985;156:187–196.
6. Deutsch SD, Gandsman EJ. The use of bone scanning for the diagnosis and management of musculoskeletal trauma. *Surg Clin North Am* 1983;63:567–583.
7. Matin P. The appearance of bone scans following fractures, including immediate and long-term studies. *J Nucl Med* 1979;20:1227–1231.
8. Holder LE, Fogelman I, Collier DC. *Atlas of planar and SPECT bone imaging,* 2nd ed. London: Martin Dunitz, 2000.
9. Sarikaya I, Sarikaya A, Holder LE. The role of single photon emission computed tomography in bone imaging. *Semin Nucl Med* 2001;31:3–16.
10. Van de Wall H, Storey G, Frater C, et al. Importance of positioning and technical factors in anatomic localization of sporting injuries in scintigraphic imaging. *Semin Nucl Med* 2001;31:17–27.
11. Holder LE, Michael RH. The specific scintigraphic pattern of "shin splints in the lower leg" [Concise Communication]. *J Nucl Med* 1984;24:865–869.
12. Michael RH, Holder LE. The soleus syndrome: a cause of medial tibial stress (shin splints). *Am J Sports Med* 1985;13:87–94.
13. Mubarak SJ, Gould RN, Lee YF, et al. The medial tibial stress syndrome (a cause of shin splints). *Am J Sports Med* 1982;10:201–205.
14. Batt ME, Ugalde V, Anderson MW, et al. A prospective controlled study of diagnostic imaging for acute shin splints. *Med Sci Sports Exerc* 1998;30:1564–1571.
15. Lawson JP. Not-so-normal variants. *Orthop Clin North Am* 1990;21:483–495.
16. Resnick D, Niwayama G. Entheses and enthesopathy. *Radiology* 1983;146:1–9.
17. Brower AC. The osteochondroses. *Orthop Clin North Am* 1983;14:99–117.
18. Mink JH, Deutsch AL. Occult cartilage and bone injuries of the knee: detection, classification and assessment with MR imaging. *Radiology* 1989;170:823–829.
19. Miller MD, Osborne JR, Gordon WT, et al. The natural history of bone bruises: a prospective study of magnetic resonance–imaging detected trabecular microfractures in patients with isolated medial collateral ligament injuries. *Am J Sports Med* 1998;26:15–19.
20. Lal NR, Jamadar DA, Doi K, et al. Evaluation of bone contusions with fat-saturated fast spin-echo proton-density magnetic resonance imaging. *Can Assoc Radiol J* 2000;51:182–185.
21. Maurice H, Watt I. Technetium-99m hydroxymethylene diphosphonate scanning of acute injuries to the lateral ligaments of the ankle. *Br J Radiol* 1989;62:31–34.
22. Baker BE. Current concepts in the diagnosis and treatment of musculotendinous injuries. *Med Sci Sports Exerc* 1984;16:323–327.
23. Siegel BA, Engel WK, Derrer EC. Localization of technetium-99m diphosphonate in acutely injured muscle. *Neurology* 1977;27:230–238.
24. Goergen TG, Venn-Watson EA, Rossman DJ, et al. Tarsal navicular stress fractures in runners. *Am J Roentgenol* 1981;136:201–203.
25. Torg JS, Pavlov H, Cooley LH, et al. Stress fractures of the tarsal navicular. *J Bone Joint Surg Am* 1982;64:700–712.
26. Groshar D, Gorenberg M, Ben-Haim S, et al. Lower extremity scintigraphy: the foot and ankle. *Semin Nucl Med* 1998;28:62–77.
27. Pavlov H, Torg JS, Freiberger RH. Tarsal navicular stress fractures: radiographic evaluation. *Radiology* 1983;148:641–645.
28. Kiss ZS, Khan KM, Fuller PJ. Stress fractures of the tarsal navicular bone: CT findings in 55 cases. *Am J Roentgenol* 1993;160:111–115.
29. Eustace S, Adams J, Assaf A. Emergency MR imaging of orthopedic trauma: current and future directions. *Radiol Clin North Am* 1999;37:975–974.
30. Weissman BNW, Sledge CB, eds. *Orthopedic radiology.* Philadelphia: WB Saunders, 1986:50–54.
31. Levy JM. Stress fractures of the first metatarsal. *Am J Roentgenol* 1978;130:679–681.
32. Delee JC, Evans JP, Julian J. Stress fracture of the fifth metatarsal. *Am J Sports Med* 1983;11:349–353.
33. Jahss MH. Stubbing injuries to the hallux. *Foot Ankle* 1981;1:327–332.
34. Coker TP, Arnold JA, Weber DL. Traumatic lesions of the metatarsophalangeal joint of the great toe in athletes. *Am J Sports Med* 1978;6:326–335.
35. Pinckney LE, Currarino G, Kennedy LA. The stubbed great toe: a cause of occult compound fracture and infection. *Radiology* 1981;138:375–377.
36. Johnson RP, Collier BD, Carrera GF. The os trigonum syndrome: use of bone scan in the diagnosis. *J Trauma* 1984;8:761–764.
37. Black HM, Brand RL. Injuries of the foot and ankle. In: Scott WN, Missonson W, Nicholas JA, eds. *Principles of sports medicine.* Baltimore: Williams & Wilkins, 1984:356–358.
38. O'Donoghue DH. Impingement exostoses of the talus and tibia. *J Bone Joint Surg Am* 1957;39:835–852.
39. Pavlov H, Heneghan MA, Hersh A, et al. The Haglund syndrome: initial and differential diagnosis. *Radiology* 1982;144:83–88.
40. Urman M, Ammann W, Sisler J, et al. The role of bone scintigraphy in the evaluation of talar dome fractures. *J Nucl Med* 1991;32:2241–2244.
41. Anderson IF, Crichton KJ, Grattan-Smith T, et al. Osteochondral fractures of the dome of the talus. *J Bone Joint Surg Am* 1989;71:1143–1152.
42. Curtis MJ, Myerson M, Szura B. Tarsometatarsal joint injuries in the athlete. *Am J Sports Med* 1993;21:497–502.
43. Meurman KOA, Elfving S. Stress fracture of the cuneiform bones. *Br J Radiol* 1980;53:157–160.
44. Marymont JH Jr, Mills GQ, Merritt WD III. Fracture of the lateral cuneiform bone in the absence of severe direct trauma. *Am J Sports Med* 1980;8:135–136.
45. Holder LE, Cole LA, Myerson MS. Reflex sympathetic dystrophy in the foot: clinical and scintigraphic criteria. *Radiology* 1992;184:531–535.
46. Fournier RS, Holder LE. Reflex sympathetic dystrophy: diagnostic controversies. *Semin Nucl Med* 1998;28:116–123.
47. Roub LW, Gumerman LW, Hanley EN, et al. Bone stress: a radionuclide imaging perspective. *Radiology* 1979;132:431–438.
48. Zwas ST, Elkanovitch R, Frank G. Interpretation and classification of bone scintigraphic findings in stress fractures. *J Nucl Med* 1987;28:452–457.
49. Matheson GO, Clement DB, McKenzie DC, et al. Stress fractures in athletes: a study of 320 cases. *Am J Sports Med* 1987;15:46–58.
50. Matin P. Bone scintigraphy in the diagnosis and management of traumatic injury. *Semin Nucl Med* 1983;13:104–122.
51. Goldfarb CF. Interpretation and classification of bone scintigraphic findings in stress fractures [Letter]. *J Nucl Med* 1988;29:1150–1151.
52. Daffner RH, Martinez S, Gehweiler JA Jr, et al. Stress fractures of the proximal tibia in runners. *Radiology* 1982;142:63–65.
53. Blank S. Transverse tibial stress fractures: a special problem. *Am J Sports Med* 1987;15:597–602.
54. Hulkko A, Orava S. Stress fractures in athletes. *Int J Sports Med* 1987;8:221–226.
55. Elba CSCE, Etchebehere M, Gamba R, et al. Orthopedic pathology of the lower extremities: scintigraphic evaluation in the thigh, knee and leg. *Semin Nucl Med* 1998;28:41–61.
56. Rosen PR, Micheli LJ, Treves S. Early scintigraphic diagnosis of bone stress and fractures in athletic adolescents. *Pediatrics* 1987;70:11–15.
57. Devas MB, Sweetnam R. Stress fractures of the fibula: a review of 50 cases in athletes. *J Bone Joint Surg Am* 1956;59:869–874.
58. Symeonides PP. High stress fractures of the fibula. *J Bone Joint Surg Br* 1980;62:192–193.
59. Lipscomb AB, Thomas ED, Johnston RK. Treatment of myositis ossificans in athletes. *Am J Sports Med* 1976;4:111–120.
60. Martire JR. The role of nuclear medicine bone scans in evaluating pain in athletic injuries. *Clin Sports Med* 1987;6:713–737.
61. Whiteside LA, Reynolds FC, Ellsasser JC. Tibulo-fibular synostosis

and recurrent ankle sprains in high performance athletes. *Am J Sports Med* 1978;6:204–208.

62. Nance EP Jr., Kaye JJ. Injuries of the quadriceps mechanism. *Radiology* 1982;142:301–307.
63. Dye SF, Chew MH. The use of scintigraphy to detect increased osseous metabolic activity about the knee. *J Bone Joint Surg Am* 1993; 75:1388–1406.
64. Dye SF, Boll DA. Radionuclide imaging of the patellofemoral joint in young adults with anterior knee pain. *Orthop Clin North Am* 1986; 17:249–262.
65. Munshi M, Davidson M, MacDonald PB, et al. The efficacy of magnetic resonance imaging in acute knee injuries. *Clin J Sport Med* 2000; 10:34–39.
66. Kohn HS, Guten GN, Collier BD, et al. Chondromalacia of the patella: bone imaging correlated with arthroscopic findings. *Clin Nucl Med* 1988;13:96–98.
67. Collier BD, Johnson RP, Carrera GF, et al. Chronic knee pain assessed by SPECT: comparison with other modalities. *Radiology* 1985;157: 795.
68. International Association for the Study of Pain, Subcommittee on Taxonomy. Classification of chronic pain. *Pain* 1987;3[Suppl]: 29–30.
69. Katz MM, Hungerford DS. Reflex sympathetic dystrophy affecting the knee. *J Bone Joint Surg Br* 1987;69:797–803.
70. Ogden JA, McCarthy SM, Jokl P. The painful bipartite patella. *J Pediatr Orthop* 1982;2:263–269.
71. Lombardo SJ, Benson DW. Stress fractures of the femur in runners. *Am J Sports Med* 1982;10:219–227.
72. Blatz DJ. Bilateral femoral and tibial shaft stress fractures in a runner. *Am J Sports Med* 1981;322–325.
73. Butler JE, Brown SL, McConnell BG. Subtrochanteric stress fractures in runners. *Am J Sports Med* 1982;10:228–232.
74. Rockett JF, Freeman BL. Scintigraphic demonstration of pectineus muscle avulsion injury. *Clin Nucl Med* 1990;15:800–803.
75. Charkes ND, Siddhivarn N, Schneck CD. Bone scanning in the adductor insertion avulsion syndrome ("thigh splints"). *J Nucl Med* 1987;28:1835–1838.
76. Koch RA, Jackson DW. Pubic symphysitis in runners: a report of two cases. *Am J Sports Med* 1981;9:62–63.
77. Pavlov H, Nelson TL, Warren RF, et al. Stress fractures of the pubic ramus: a report of twelve cases. *J Bone Joint Surg Am* 1982;64: 1020–1025.
78. Fernandez-Ulloa M, Klostermeier TT, Lancaster KT. Orthopedic nuclear medicine: the pelvis and hip. *Semin Nucl Med* 1998;28:25–40.
79. Fernbach SK, Wilkinson RH. Avulsion injuries of the pelvis and proximal femur. *Am J Roentgenol* 1981;137:581–584.
80. Resnik CS. Diagnostic imaging of pediatric skeletal trauma. *Radiol Clin North Am* 1989;27:1013–1022.
81. Erne P, Burckhardt A. Femoral neck fatigue fracture. *Arch Orthop Trauma Surg* 1980;97:213–220.
82. El-Khoury GY, Wehbe MA, Bonfiglio M, et al. Stress fractures of the femoral neck: a scintigraphic sign for early diagnosis. *Skeletal Radiol* 1981;6:271–273.
83. Bellah RD, Summerville DA, Treves ST, et al. Low-back pain in adolescent athletes: detection of stress injury to the pars interarticularis with SPECT. *Radiology* 1991;180:509–512.
84. Papanicolaou N, Wilkinson RH, Emans JB, et al. Bone scintigraphy and radiography in young athletes with low back pain. *Am J Roentgenol* 1985;145:1039–1044.
85. Jackson DW, Wiltse LL, Dingeman RD, et al. Stress reactions involving the pars interarticularis in young athletes. *Am J Sports Med* 1981; 9:304–312.
86. Collier BD, Johnson RP, Carrera GF, et al. Painful spondylolysis or

87. Traughber PD, Havlina JM Jr. Bilateral pedicle stress fractures: SPECT and CT features. *J Comp Assist Tomogr* 1991;15:338–340.
88. Jackson DW, Wiltse LL, Cirincione RJ. Spondylolysis in the female gymnast. *Clin Orthop* 1976;117:68–73.
89. Cahill BR. Osteolysis of the distal part of the clavicle in male athletes. *J Bone Joint Surg Am* 1982;64:1053–1058.
90. Matthews LS, Simonson BG, Wolock BS. Osteolysis of the distal clavicle in a female body builder: a case report. *Am J Sports Med* 1993; 21:150–152.
91. Gurtler R, Pavlov H, Torg JS. Stress fracture of the ipsilateral first rib in a pitcher. *Am J Sports Med* 1985;13:277–279.
92. Kaye JJ, Nance EP Jr, Green NE. Fatigue fracture of the medial aspect of the clavicle. *Radiology* 1982;144:89–90.
93. Fulton MN, Albright JP, El-Khoury GY. Cortical desmoid-like lesion of the proximal humerus and its occurrence in gymnasts (ringman's shoulder lesion). *Am J Sports Med* 1979;7:57–61.
94. Patel M. Upper extremity radionuclide bone imaging: shoulder, arm, elbow, and forearm. *Semin Nucl Med* 1998;28(1):3–13.
95. Huss CD, Puhl JJ. Myositis ossificans of the upper arm. *Am J Sports Med* 1980;8:419–424.
96. Tondeur M, Haentjens M, Piepsz A, et al. Muscular injury in a child diagnosed by ^{99m}Tc-MDP bone scan. *Eur J Nucl Med* 1989;15: 328–329.
97. Slocum DB. Classification of elbow injuries from baseball pitching. *Tex Med* 1968;64:48–53.
98. Gore RM, Rogers LF, Bowerman J, et al. Osseous manifestations of elbow stress associated with sports activities. *Am J Roentgenol* 1980; 134:971–977.
99. Fink-Bennett D, Carichner S. Acute flexion of the elbow: optimal imaging position for visualization of the capitellum. *Clin Nucl Med* 1986;11:667–668.
100. Torg JS, Moyer RA. Non-union of a stress fracture through the olecranon epiphyseal plate observed in an adolescent baseball pitcher. *J Bone Joint Surg Am* 1977;59:264–265.
101. Mutoh Y, More T, Suzuki Y. Stress fractures of the ulna in athletes. *Am J Sports Med* 1982;10:365–367.
102. Hamilton HK. Stress fracture of the diaphysis of the ulna in a body builder. *Am J Sports Med* 1984;12:405–406.
103. Rettig AC. Stress fracture of the ulna in an adolescent tournament tennis player. *Am J Sports Med* 1983;11:103–106.
104. Linscheid RL, Dobyns JH. Athletic injuries of the wrist. *Clin Orthop* 1985;198:141–151.
105. Loosli AR, Leslie M. Stress fractures of the distal radius: a case report. *Am J Sports Med* 1991;19:523–524.
106. Pin PG, Semenkovich JW, Young VL, et al. Role of radionuclide imaging in the evaluation of wrist pain. *J Hand Surg [Am]* 1988;13: 810–814.
107. Tiel-van Buul MM, vanBeek EJ, Dijkstra PF, et al. Significance of a hot spot on the bone scan after carpal injury: evaluation by computed tomography. *Eur J Nucl Med* 1993;20:159–164.
108. Stark HH, Jobe FW, Boyes JH, et al. Fracture of the hook of hamate in athletes. *J Bone Joint Surg Am* 1977;59:575–582.
109. Holder LE, Mackinnon SE. Reflex sympathetic dystrophy in the hands: clinical and scintigraphic criteria. *Radiology* 1984;152: 517–522.
110. Mackinnon SE, Holder LE. The use of three-phase radionuclide scanning in the diagnosis of reflex sympathetic dystrophy. *J Hand Surg [Am]* 1984;9:556–563.
111. Sowa DT, Holder LE, Patt PG, et al. Application of magnetic resonance imaging to ischemic necrosis of the lunate. *J Hand Surg [Am]* 1989;14:1008–1016.

Diagnostic Nuclear Medicine, Fourth Edition. Edited by M.P. Sandler, R.E. Coleman, J.A. Patton, F.J.Th. Wackers, A. Gottschalk. Lippincott Williams & Wilkins, Philadelphia 2003.

23

PET IMAGING OF THE SKELETAL SYSTEM

RANDALL A. HAWKINS
CARL K. HOH
MICHAEL E. PHELPS

Imaging bone metabolic activity with gamma-camera systems and ^{99m}Tc-methylene diphosphonate (MDP) and related radiopharmaceuticals is one of the most common and important techniques employed in nuclear medicine. Other chapters deal extensively with the various methods and techniques employed in the scintigraphic evaluation of the skeletal system. In addition to single photon emitters, positron emitting radiopharmaceuticals, including [^{18}F]fluoride ion, and other radiopharmaceuticals, including 2-[^{18}F]fluoro-2-deoxy-D-glucose (FDG), have been employed for evaluation of the skeletal system (1–8). In fact, [^{18}F]fluoride ion was at one time the standard bone scanning agent (9–15), but it was replaced for routine clinical use in the 1970s by ^{99m}Tc-labeled bone-seeking radiopharmaceuticals, because of the more optimal physical characteristics of ^{99m}Tc for gamma-camera systems.

Positron emission tomography (PET), like single photon emission computed tomography (SPECT) produces tomographic images reflective of the tissue distribution of administered radiopharmaceuticals. Because of the more physically precise methods for photon attenuation correction with PET, compared with single photon gamma-camera techniques, one potential advantage of PET bone imaging is greater quantitative precision. In addition, because PET systems in general have better resolution than most gamma-camera or SPECT systems (15), it is possible to obtain images of the skeletal system of higher resolution with PET than with SPECT.

With modern PET systems, however, there is a relatively limited amount of experience with PET bone imaging. Most of the reported investigations have focused on evaluation of musculoskeletal malignancies with the PET FDG technique, but some studies have also been performed with [^{18}F]fluoride ion (1–6, 8).

RADIOPHARMACEUTICALS AND KINETIC MODELS

The fundamental biologic information produced by PET, like other nuclear medicine methods, is dependent on the radiopharmaceutical employed. Reviews of PET radiopharmaceuticals are available (1,11,17,18), but to date the positron emitting radiopharmaceuticals of most relevance to bone are [^{18}F]fluoride ion and FDG.

Blau et al. (13) were the first to perform bone imaging with [^{18}F]fluoride ion. Following their initial work, [^{18}F]fluoride ion became the standard nuclear medicine bone scanning agent (9–14).

Because of interest in fluoride as a potential therapeutic agent for osteoporosis and because of the role of fluoride in preventing dental caries, there is a large literature on the metabolism and pharmacokinetics of fluoride (19). In vitro studies have demonstrated that fluoride ion exchanges with the hydroxyl ion in the bone mineral hydroxyapatite crystal $Ca_{10}(PO_4)_6(OH)_2$ to form fluoroapatite: $Ca_{10}(PO_4)_6(F)_2$ (20). Because PET studies of bone with [^{18}F]fluoride ion use tracer quantities of fluoride ion, the direct pharmacologic effects of macroscopic (as opposed to tracer) quantities of fluoride ion on both bone cells and bone crystals (19) do not have to be considered when interpreting PET [^{18}F]fluoride ion studies. However, kinetic PET [^{18}F]fluoride ion studies are an excellent way to map the distribution of fluoride ion transport and trapping in bone, based on the tracer principle.

Studies have shown that there is a high initial extraction fraction of [^{18}F]fluoride ion in its transit through bone (21,22). Based on the assumption that the initial extraction fraction approximated 100%, Reeve et al. (23) estimated skeletal blood flow in humans with a plasma clearance method alone (i.e., without PET imaging) with [^{18}F]fluoride ion. Using this clearance method, Wooton et al. (24) found a positive correlation between decreases in skeletal blood flow and decreases in alkaline phosphatase in patients with Paget's disease treated with calcitonin.

Charkes et al. (25–27) were the first to develop an in vivo pharmacokinetic model of [^{18}F]fluoride ion distribution using

R.A. Hawkins: Department of Radiology, UCSF Medical Center, San Francisco, CA.
C.K. Hoh: Department of Radiology, UCSD Medical Center, San Diego, CA.
M.E. Phelps: Department of Molecular and Medical Pharmacology, UCLA School of Medicine, Los Angeles, CA.

compartmental modeling techniques and animal tissue sampling data. The kinetic approaches described later for PET studies of [^{18}F]fluoride ion distribution are similar in concept to those originally developed by Charkes et al., but are based on direct imaging of the kinetics of bone uptake of [^{18}F]fluoride ion with a PET system. Although many elegant studies of in vivo pharmacokinetics of compounds have been performed with plasma and tissue sampling methods alone (28), PET and other imaging methods make it possible to "sample" (image) tissue noninvasively. When coupled with plasma measurements of radionuclide concentrations as a function of time, it becomes possible to apply a wide variety of mathematic models to PET data (15).

In addition to [^{18}F]fluoride ion, the other primary positron emitting radiopharmaceutical used in PET bone imaging applications is FDG (1,7,11). FDG, like glucose, is transported across capillary membranes via a carrier mediated transport process, in the direction of a concentration gradient (facilitated diffusion). Both FDG and glucose are then phosphorylated by hexokinase, but because the phosphorylation product FDG-6-PO$_4$ cannot be metabolized further through the glycolytic cycle (29), it accumulates in cells, unlike glucose-6-PO$_4$, which undergoes further metabolism through the glycolytic and Krebs cycle to be eventually metabolized to CO$_2$ and H$_2$O. Because deoxyglucose competes with glucose for both capillary transport and phosphorylation by hexokinase, Sokoloff et al. (30) were able to develop a mathematic model relating the net transport of ^{14}C deoxyglucose (DG) and accumulation of DG-6-PO$_4$ in tissue to glucose transport and metabolism based on Michaelis-Menten kinetics. The original Sokoloff deoxyglucose method, developed in rats for autoradiography, was extended to humans by Reivich, Phelps, and colleagues (31–33) using PET and FDG.

The intent of the FDG (and DG) model is to produce a measurement of tissue glucose metabolic rates with a single time measurement of tissue radionuclide concentration (i.e., ^{18}F, distributed between unphosphorylated FDG and FDG-6-PO$_4$) (Fig. 23.1). It is also necessary to measure the time course of FDG in the plasma space (the input function). In addition, if one desires an absolute measurement of tissue glucose metabolism in μmol/minute/g of tissue, it is necessary to also measure or arbitrarily assign a numerical value to a term in the FDG model known as the *lumped constant* (LC) (31–33). The LC is in essence a calibration term related to the fact that glucose and FDG have differential affinities (K$_m$ and V$_{max}$ values) for the glucose transporter protein and for hexokinase. Although numerical val-

ues for these affinity terms are available for glucose and FDG in some tissues, such as mammalian brain, in most human tissue, including bone and tumor tissues, the values are either unknown or approximations from related tissues are used.

Because the total amount of ^{18}F in tissue at any point in time (distributed between FDG and FDG-6-PO$_4$) is approximately linearly related to tissue glucose utilization, semiquantitative PET methods using ratios of tissue uptake are often employed (34).

As an alternative to the classic autoradiographic FDG model, it is also possible to perform kinetic FDG studies to directly measure FDG transport (forward, K$_1$ and reverse, k$_2$) and phosphorylation (k$_3$) and dephosphorylation (k$_4$) rate constants, as opposed to assuming population values for these rate constants in single time imaging studies with the autoradiographic model. The units most commonly used for these rate constants are mL/minute/g for K$_1$, and minute^{-1} for k$_2$, k$_3$, and k$_4$, respectively. Although this results in a simple expression for tissue glucose metabolic rates (Eq. 1), it is still necessary to assign a value to the LC if an absolute value (in units of μmol/minute/g tissue) is desired.

$$\text{Metabolic Rate Glucose} = \frac{K_1 \times k_3}{k_2 + k_3} \times \left(C_p/LC \right)$$

where K$_1$, k$_2$, and k$_3$ are the rate constants described previously; Cp is the plasma glucose concentration; and LC is the lumped constant. The reader is referred to more detailed discussions in the literature for a full discussion of the assumptions and methods used to measure tissue glucose metabolic rates with this method (1,30–35).

Most quantitative studies with the FDG method have been performed in brain and heart studies. Because of the potential to better biochemically characterize neoplasms based on numeric estimates of metabolism and because of interest in monitoring interventions in cancer, such as chemotherapy by serially measuring changes in metabolic parameters as opposed to relying on the more delayed end point of tumor volume changes, there is increasing interest in developing appropriately validated methods for quantitative PET FDG imaging in many tumor systems, including primary and metastatic bone tumors.

Although the mechanism of [^{18}F]fluoride ion uptake in bone, described earlier, is different than the biochemical mechanisms underlying FDG transport and phosphorylation, both processes have in common a tissue phase distributed between two kinetically discrete compartments—for FDG: (a) free FDG and (b) "metabolically trapped" FDG-6-PO$_4$; for [^{18}F]fluoride ion: (a) unbound and (b) hydroxyapatite crystal related bound [^{18}F]fluoride ion. Based on this similarity in tissue distribution kinetics, Hawkins et al. (36) employed the same three compartment model configuration illustrated in Fig. 23.1 to evaluate the kinetics of [^{18}F]fluoride ion uptake in bone with PET. These methods again illustrate that with PET, as with other digital tomographic imaging techniques such as SPECT, magnetic resonance imaging (MRI), and computed tomography (CT), the "output" of the studies fall into two categories: images and numeric results. A valuable characteristic of PET is the high resolution and quantitative precision of the method. This characteristic facilitates development of appropriate numeric descriptions of the results

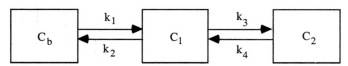

FIGURE 23.1. Three-compartment model configuration used for both the FDG (23–26,28) and [^{18}F]fluoride ion models (29). K$_1$ and k$_2$ refer to forward and reverse transport rate constants for both FDG and [^{18}F]fluoride ion, whereas k$_3$ and k$_4$ refer to rate constants for uptake and release from a metabolically trapped space in tissue for both agents. For FDG, these rate constants refer to the hexokinase and phosphatase catalyzed phosphorylation and dephosphorylation of FDG and FDG-6-PO$_4$ respectively, whereas for [^{18}F]fluoride ion k$_3$ and k$_4$ are rate constants for uptake and release from hydroxyapatite crystal related binding space in bone (29).

that may have practical clinical significance, as well as producing better insight into biochemical processes.

PET METHODS FOR BONE IMAGING

With both [^{18}F]fluoride ion and FDG, there are several methods one may use for acquiring PET bone images, including:

1. Standard transaxial attenuation corrected images at a preselected time after injection of [^{18}F]fluoride ion or FDG
2. Serial transaxial attenuation corrected images beginning simultaneously with injection of [^{18}F]fluoride ion or FDG (kinetic studies)
3. Whole-body images

Most PET systems contain rings of detectors, analogous to CT scanners in design (15). The axial field of view of such devices is defined by the number of detector rings and by the axial field of view of each ring, as well as by the acquisition and image reconstruction strategy employed. Some PET systems use two-dimensional detector systems similar to gamma-camera designs, but all PET systems, like other imaging devices, have a defined axial field of view.

If a patient is imaged in a given bed position within a PET scanner, the data may be corrected for tissue attenuation with a transmission scan method using a ^{68}Ga/^{68}Ge transmission source, and a set of transaxial images generated either in static mode (method 1) or kinetic mode (method 2). These acquisition sequences are the "gold standard" for PET acquisitions. Because a strength of PET, as compared with SPECT, is a more accurate retrieval of voxel count density based on more accurate attenuation correction methods (37), both methods 1 and 2 produce images of high resolution and quantitative precision.

A relative limitation of methods 1 and 2, however, is the axial field of view of the methods. The situation is very much analogous to SPECT. Although SPECT bone imaging is a very useful method for generating more anatomically precise cross-sectional bone scan images than planar gamma-camera methods, SPECT is not convenient for total skeletal surveys, because the acquisition time for serial SPECT image sets that include the whole body are inconveniently long.

Because many potential applications of [^{18}F]fluoride ion and FDG PET bone imaging involve patients with malignancies and potentially widespread skeletal and nonskeletal metastases, Dahlbom et al. (37) developed a whole-body PET imaging method that produces tomographic and nontomographic (projection) image sets of the whole body. The method is based on sequential acquisitions of standard transaxial PET image data sets at discrete locations in the body, followed by acquisitions at other body locations until the entire body (or more limited regions of interest) has been included in the data set. Standard transaxial images are reconstructed with filtered backprojection methods, and coronal and sagittal tomographic images are extracted from the stack of transaxial images via a sorting operation. In addition, two-dimensional projection images, analogous to two-dimensional raw data sets with SPECT, are generated by appropriate sampling and sorting of the raw sinographic data. The end result is a whole-body image set consisting of transaxial, coronal, and

sagittal tomographic images, together with two-dimensional projection images at various angles around the body. The data sets are now routinely corrected for photon attenuation with transmission scans.

Refinements of the whole-body PET method, that have increased both its quantitative precision and clinical utility, include development of practical attenuation correction approaches (38) and application of alternative reconstruction methods such as the three-dimensional method (39). The three-dimensional reconstruction method makes it possible to use a much higher fraction of coincident events in the image reconstruction process, essentially by including coincident events between detector planes, as well as within individual or directly adjacent detector planes. This technique has the effect of significantly increasing the count rate efficiency of the PET system, with a potential result being a decrease in acquisition time by up to a factor of four or more.

CLINICAL EXAMPLES OF PET BONE IMAGING
Normal Patterns

Fig. 23.2 includes examples of [^{18}F]fluoride ion images acquired with the whole-body PET method. Selected two-dimensional projection, as well as transaxial, coronal, and sagittal images, are included. Note that the relative body distribution of the [^{18}F]fluoride ion is very similar to the distribution of ^{99m}Tc MDP compounds, as expected based on the distribution and metabolism of the agent as discussed earlier.

In addition, because a single whole-body PET study can produce a large number of tomographic and projection images, it is very helpful to view such images on a workstation equipped with appropriate volume viewing software. Such display options are available on a variety of nuclear medicine workstations and, with the standardization of image file formats into DICOM and other standard file formats, display and viewing of such data sets on workstations designed for general imaging environments as part of larger picture archival communication systems (PACS) will become progressively easier and more routine.

Another advantage of workstation viewing strategies for whole-body PET [^{18}F]fluoride ion and FDG bone studies is the ease of appropriate contrast adjustment (windowing) of images. Although FDG uptake in normal bone is low, normal bone marrow uptake produces a visible signal on appropriately windowed FDG images. This uptake will be most evident in hematopoietically active marrow spaces, such as the vertebral bodies and proximal femoral shafts.

Pathologic Conditions

PET bone imaging with [^{18}F]fluoride ion produces the expected findings of increased tracer uptake in the range of pathologic conditions known to also cause increased uptake of ^{99m}Tc MDP and related compounds: neoplastic, inflammatory, traumatic, and other processes known to result in an acceleration of osteoblastic activity and bone blood flow.

In a series of 19 patients, with a range of malignant and benign skeletal conditions, Hoh et al. (2) found that the tomo-

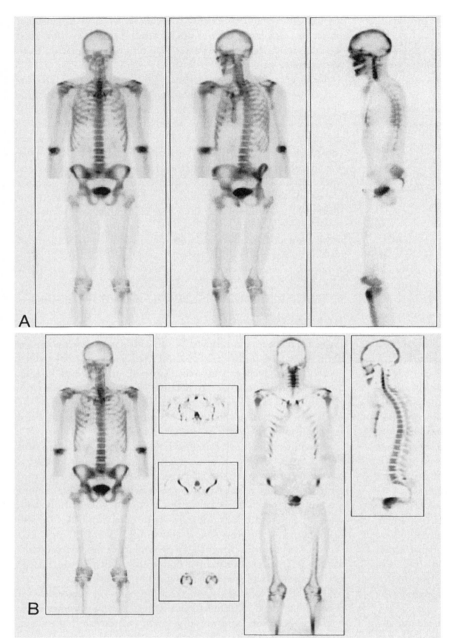

FIGURE 23.2. A: Projection images of [^{18}F]fluoride ion using whole-body PET technique in a normal volunteer. Illustrated are three different angular views of [^{18}F]fluoride ion distribution *(anterior on left, left anterior oblique in center,* and *lateral on right). Note that the lack of attenuation correction produces differential relative attenuation in the femurs and spine, most evident in the lumbar region, on the lateral as opposed to the anterior views. There is physiologic excretion of [^{18}F]fluoride ion into the bladder. The hands were not included in the acquisition sequence acquired over the upper body; acquisitions over the upper and lower body were photographically combined for this illustration. This image and other illustrations in this chapter were acquired on a Siemens 931-08 tomograph. This device has eight detector rings, and produces 15 simultaneous transaxial images, spaced at 6.75 mm per plane (2). (From Hoh CK, Hawkins RA, Dahlbom M, et al. Whole-body skeletal imaging with [^{18}F]fluoride ion and PET. J Comp Asst Tomogr* 1993;17:34–41, with permission.) **B:** Projection *(left)* and tomographic images *(right three columns)* of [^{18}F]fluoride ion distribution in a normal volunteer, illustrating the range of tomographic display options available with this technique. The second column of images includes three transaxial images at the approximate levels of the midthoracic spine, pelvis, and knees, respectively. Single coronal *(second from right)* and sagittal *(far right)* tomographic image sections are also included. Note the excellent delineation of the vertebral bodies and spinous processes, the tibial plateaus, and other bone structures.

graphic (transaxial, coronal, and sagittal) [^{18}F]fluoride ion images had a 13% higher sensitivity for lesion detection than did the projection image set. Given that a fundamental advantage of any form of tomography is higher in-plane contrast (15), this result is not surprising. The primary utility of projection whole-body images, both [^{18}F]fluoride ion and FDG, is to help the observer become appropriately oriented in three dimensions relative to the distribution of abnormalities. Specific lesions may only be visible, however, on the tomographic image set. Fig. 23.3, which contains [^{18}F]fluoride ion images of a patient with polyostotic fibrous dysplasia and metastatic osteogenic sarcoma, illustrates better delineation of a pathologic focus on a tomographic, as compared with projection, image (40).

Because accelerated osteoblastic activity and bone blood flow are sensitive, but nonspecific, indicators of pathology, it is logical to expect that images of a different process, such as tissue glucose utilization mapped with FDG, should produce a different view of bone pathology. A feature shared by many aggressive neoplasms is an acceleration of their glycolytic rates (41). Because bone (cortical and trabecular) has relatively low glucose utilization rates, compared to tissues such as the brain, heart, and striated muscle, whole-body PET FDG images in patients with skeletal primary or metastatic neoplasms often illustrate dramatic focal abnormalities that have very high contrast compared with the background normal bone FDG uptake pattern. This finding is illustrated in Fig. 23.4, in which skeletal metastases from a

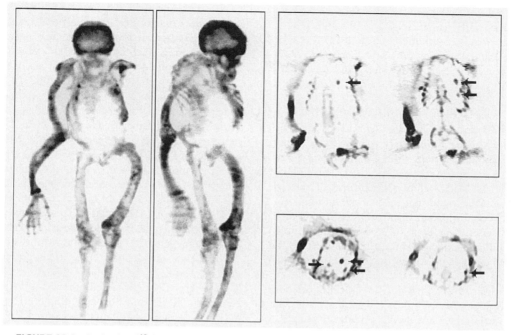

FIGURE 23.3. Projection [¹⁸F]fluoride ion bone images (*left two images*), coronal tomographic (*upper right images*), and transaxial tomographic (*lower right images*) in a patient with polyostotic fibrous dysplasia who had previously undergone an amputation of the left upper extremity for an osteosarcoma. Arrows on the tomographic images identify foci uptake in the lung fields consistent with metastatic osteogenic sarcoma deposits. These foci are more evident on the tomographic, as opposed to the projection planar, images. Note the dramatic distortion of skeletal anatomy and diffusely increased uptake of [¹⁸F]fluoride ion consistent with widespread fibrous dysplasia. (From Tse N, Hoh C, Hawkins R, et al. Positron emission tomography diagnosis of pulmonary metastases in osteogenic sarcoma. *Am J Clin Oncol* 1994;17:22–25, with permission.)

patient with primary carcinoma of the breast were detected with this method.

Whole-body and standard transaxial PET FDG imaging for cancer detection, staging, and treatment monitoring is becoming a major focus of both research and clinical use of PET. Review articles on this subject are available in the literature (1,17,18, 42,43). Specifically related to skeletal disease, several investigators have demonstrated that PET FDG imaging is useful for detecting and characterizing various types of primary and metastatic disease. A fundamental potential utility of the method is

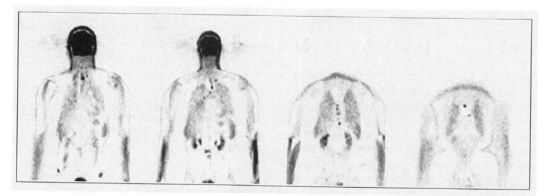

FIGURE 23.4. Four separate coronal PET FDG whole-body images (upper body region) in a patient with metastatic breast carcinoma. Note scattered areas of increased FDG uptake in the upper and midthoracic spine on all four images. Appropriate correlation of such images with plain films, as well as interactive windowing of images (see text), facilitates localization of individual lesions on images sets such as this. Note the very intense uptake of FDG in the brain (*left two images*) that, because of contrast setting, exceeds the upper limit of the gray scale. Note also the physiologic uptake of FDG in muscles, kidney, and bladder. There is only minimal FDG uptake in the heart on this study, because it was acquired in a fasting state.

differentiating benign from malignant causes of increased uptake on osteoblastic bone scans, either PET [^{18}F]fluoride ion or gamma-camera MDP studies. Although increased FDG uptake in bone is not pathognomonic for cancer [inflammatory processes may also produce increased FDG uptake and subcutaneous injections of FDG may result in significantly increased uptake in normal lymph nodes (44,45)], it is likely that the specificity of FDG will be higher than MDP or [^{18}F]fluoride ion for bone cancer detection, as indicated by initial studies. By using FDG, one is changing the primary cellular focus of the images from the osteoblastic system with [^{18}F]fluoride ion and MDP to cells with high glycolytic rates (i.e., cancer) with FDG. In a study of 25 patients with various types of musculoskeletal disorders, Adler et al. (46) found that by quantifying FDG uptake in lesions, they could more accurately differentiate benign from malignant processes. Kern et al. (47) in an earlier preliminary study, also found a good correspondence between FDG uptake and grade of malignancy in human musculoskeletal tumors.

These different mechanisms of FDG and [^{18}F]fluoride ion uptake also can produce uncoupling of [^{18}F]fluoride ion and FDG uptake (1) in primary or metastatic bone tumors successfully responding to treatment and in which a persistent osteoblastic response (resulting in increased uptake on a PET [^{18}F]fluoride ion or gamma-camera MDP bone scan) may indicate ongoing normal bone repair once the tumor, characterized by increased FDG uptake, has become suppressed. This characteristic of FDG imaging could make it particularly useful in patients with bone cancers in whom increased uptake of a bone-seeking tracer (e.g., MDP or [^{18}F]fluoride ion) may occur during treatment secondary to accelerated bone metabolism and repair (the FLARE response) that, in some cases, may be difficult to distinguish from progression of cancer itself.

QUANTITATIVE METHODS

Quantitative applications of PET bone imaging to date have been relatively limited. The primary potential application of quantitative PET FDG imaging in bone relates to disease characterization and treatment monitoring, as discussed in previous reviews (1,34). In addition, quantitative PET FDG kinetic studies can help elucidate normal metabolic processes, such as bone marrow-stimulating growth factors (GMCSF) effects on hematopoietically active marrow uptake of FDG (48). GMCSF is one of a family of glycoprotein cytokines that stimulates bone marrow production of granulocytes and macrophages and is of significant therapeutic importance in some cancer patients with suppressed bone marrow (49,50). Yao et al. (48) using dynamic PET FDG imaging, demonstrated that bone marrow FDG uptake (glucose metabolic rate) increased by up to threefold during 3 to 10 days of GMCSF therapy and progressively declined following therapy. Because these types of therapeutically induced alterations in bone marrow metabolic activity occur relatively uniformly in the hematopoietically active marrow spaces, differentiating such effects from discrete foci in increased FDG uptake in bone, secondary to metastatic disease (Fig. 23.4), should usually be straightforward with appropriate review of the images.

An additional form of quantification in bone for which there is a potential role for PET is in better defining and noninvasively measuring trabecular and cortical bone metabolic activity. Single photon emitters, such as ^{99m}Tc MDP, were previously used to evaluate generalized bone metabolism and were applied to specific disorders such as hyperparathyroidism, both with planar and SPECT methods (51–54). Such methods have not been widely used, partially because the challenge of absolute voxel quantification of signal secondary to accurate correction for tissue attenuation effects remains to be accurately solved. New generation SPECT systems, equipped with transmission sources for attenuation correction, as well as combined SPECT/CT systems, may result in renewed interest in utilization of single photon bone-seeking tracers for quantitative bone metabolic studies.

Using a kinetic PET acquisition sequence with [^{18}F]fluoride ion and the three compartment kinetic model illustrated in Fig. 23.1, Messa et al. (55) evaluated the utility of quantitative PET [^{18}F]fluoride ion kinetic studies in the evaluation of patients with one form of metabolic bone disease—renal osteodystrophy. Using kinetically determined estimates of net [^{18}F]fluoride ion transport (K in units of mL/minute/mL tissue) defined as $k^*_1k_3/(k_2 + k_3)$ (36,55), they measured [^{18}F]fluoride ion uptake in normal volunteers and in eight patients with renal osteodystrophy and compared the results to bone biopsy indicators of bone metabolic activity acquired from the renal osteodystrophy group.

Bone histomorphometry is a well-characterized tissue biopsy technique in which a variety of indices of bone mass, growth, and mineralization are measured quantitatively from biopsy samples. With oral tetracycline labeling, bone growth can be accurately measured with appropriate biopsy specimens. The literature contains additional details about the methodology of histomorphometry (56–58). Messa et al. (55) found a very good correlation between the PET index (K value) of bone metabolic activity obtained with dynamic [^{18}F]fluoride ion imaging and the histomorphometric index of bone formation rate. There was also a good correlation with K and serum alkaline phosphatase and parathyroid hormone levels (r > 0.8 in each case). Although this initial series requires validation in larger groups of patients, it illustrates the potential of quantitative PET bone imaging to better define metabolic characteristics of bone, some of which, such as bone formation rate, may otherwise be available only from direct tissue assay techniques. Other applications of [^{18}F]fluoride ion kinetic studies, including evaluations of kinetics between humeral and vertebral body bone (59) and allogenic bone graft viability (60), have been reported. Piert et al. (61) have also investigated the physiologic range of bone blood flows over which [^{18}F]fluoride ion kinetic studies can reliably estimate bone blood flow.

SUMMARY

Imaging the skeletal system with positron emitting radiopharmaceuticals is both a relatively old and also a new, evolving technique. Although clinical bone scanning with [^{18}F]fluoride ion was appropriately supplanted by gamma-camera methods using ^{99m}Tc diphosphonate-related compounds in the 1970s, because of the better sensitivity of gamma-cameras for 140 keV photons from ^{99m}Tc compared with 511 KeV annihilation photons from positron emitters, modern PET scanners make qualitative and quantitative imaging with [^{18}F]fluoride ion, FDG, and other radiopharmaceuticals practical and, in the appropriate setting, clinically useful.

Gamma-camera and SPECT (including SPECT/CT) methods are becoming progressively more sophisticated and precise. In situations in which the higher resolution and better quantitative precision of PET are required, [^{18}F]fluoride ion imaging and quantitative studies should have a role. These situations include both quantitative metabolic studies, such as the renal osteodystrophy work of Messa et al. (55) and other applications (59,60,61) and whole body studies in patients, in whom the resolution of a state-of-the-art PET system is needed to definitively detect or localize a lesion.

The major clinical role of PET bone imaging will probably be in the field of oncology, because of the greater specificity of FDG and other agents for mapping and detecting cancers than the highly sensitive, but nonspecific, bone scanning methods based on osteoblastic tracers MDP and [^{18}F]fluoride ion. Although the range of processes evaluated with PET will increase in the future, transaxial and whole-body methods with existing agents FDG and [^{18}F]fluoride ion indicate that it has an appropriate role to play in clinical medicine.

REFERENCES

1. Hawkins RA, Hoh C, Glaspy J et al. The role of positron emission tomography in oncology and other whole-body applications. *Sem Nucl Med* 1992;22:268–284.
2. Hoh CK, Hawkins RA, Dahlbom M et al. Whole body skeletal imaging with [^{18}F]fluoride ion and PET. *J Comp Asst Tomogr* 1993;17:34–41.
3. Hoh CK, Hawkins RA, Glaspy JA et al. Cancer detection with whole-body PET using 2-[^{18}F]fluoro-2-deoxy-D-glucose. *J Comp Asst Tomogr* 1993;17:582–589.
4. Cook GJR, Fogelman I. Detection of bone metastases in cancer-patients by F-18-flouride and F-18-flourodeoxyglucose positron emission tomography. *Q J Nucl Med* 2001;45:47–52.
5. Schirrmeister H, Guhlman A, Elsner K et al. Sensitivity in detecting osseous lesions depends on anatomic localization: planar bone scintigraphy verses F-18 PET. *J Nucl Med* 1999;40:1623–1629.
6. Hoegerle S, Juengling F, Otte A et al. Combined FDG and [F-18] fluoride whole-body PET: a feasible two-in-one approach to cancer imaging? *Radiology* 1998;209:253–258.
7. Moog F, Kotzerke J, Reske SN. FDG PET can replace bone scintigraphy in primary staging of malignant lymphoma. *J Nucl Med* 1999;40: 1407–1413.
8. Schirrmeister H, Guhlman A, Kotzerke J et al. Early detection and accurate description of extent of metastatic bone disease in breast cancer with fluoride ion and positron emission tomography. *J Clin Onc* 1999; 17:2381–2389.
9. French RJ, McCready VR. The use of ^{18}F for bone scanning. *Br J Radiol* 1967;40:655–661.
10. Spencer R, Herbert R, Rish MW et al. Bone scanning with ^{85}Sr, ^{87m}Sr and ^{18}F. Physical and radiopharmaceutical considerations and clinical experience in 50 cases. *Br J Radiol* 1967;40:641–654.
11. Moon NF, Dworkin HJ, LaFluer PD. The clinical use of sodium fluoride F-18 in bone photoscanning. *JAMA* 1968;204:974–980.
12. Harmer CL, Burns JE, Sams A et al. the value of fluorine-18 for scanning bone tumours. *Clin Radiol* 1969;20:204–212.
13. Blau M, Nagler W, Bender MA. Fluorine-18: a new isotope for bone scanning. *J Nucl Med* 1962;3:332–334.
14. Weber DA, Keys JW Jr, Landman S et al. Comparison of Tc-99m polyphosphate and F-18 for bone imaging. *Am J Roentgenol Radium Ther Nucl Med* 1974;121:184–190.
15. Sorenson JA, Phelps ME, eds. *Physics in nuclear medicine*, 2nd ed. Orlando, FL: Grune & Stratton, 1987.
16. Fowler JS, Wolf AP. Positron emitter-labeled compounds: priorities and problems. In: Phelps M, Mazziotta J, Schelbert H, eds. *Positron emission tomography and autoradiography: principles and applications for the brain and heart.* New York: Raven Press, 1986:391–450.
17. Gambhir SS, Czernin J, Schwimmer J et al. A tabulated summary of the FDG PET literature. *J Nucl Med* 2001;42(Suppl):1S–93S.
18. Bar-Shalom R, Valdivia AY, Blaufox MD. PET imaging in oncology. *Sem Nucl Med* 2000;30:150–185.
19. Murray TM, Singer FR, eds. Proceedings of the international workshop on fluoride and bone. *J Bone Miner Res* 1990;5(Suppl 1).
20. Grynpas MD. Fluoride effects on bone crystals. In: Murray TM, Singer FR, eds. Proceedings of the international workshop on fluoride and bone. *J Bone Miner Res* 1990;5(Suppl 1):S169–S175.
21. Van Dyke D, Anger HO, Yano Y et al. Bone blood flow shown with ^{18}F and the positron camera. *Am J Physiol* 1965;209:65–70.
22. Wooton R, Dore C. The single-passage extraction of ^{18}F in rabbit bone. *Clin Phys Physiol Meas* 1986;7:333–343.
23. Reeve J, Arlot M, Woton R et al. Skeletal blood flow, iliac histomorphometry, and strontium kinetics in osteoporosis: a relationship between blood flow and corrected apposition rate. *J Clin Endocrinol Metab* 1988; 66:1124–1131.
24. Wooton R, Reeve J, Spellacy E et al. Skeletal blood flow in Paget's disease of bone and its response to calcitonin therapy. *Clin Sci Molec Med* 1978;54:69–74.
25. Charkes ND, Brookes M, Makler PT. Studies of skeletal tracer kinetics. II. Evaluation of a five-compartment model of [^{18}F]fluoride kinetics in rats. *J Nucl Med* 1979;121:1150–1157.
26. Charkes ND, Makler PT Jr, Phillips C. Studies of skeletal tracer kinetics. I. Digital computer solution of a five-compartment model of [^{18}F]fluoride kinetics in humans. *J Nucl Med* 1978;19:1301–1309.
27. Charkes ND. Skeletal blood flow: implications of bone-scan interpretation. *J Nucl Med* 1980;21:91–98.
28. Lassen NA, Perl W. *Tracer kinetic methods in medical physiology.* New York: Raven Press, 1979.
29. Gallagher BM, Fowler JS, Gutterson NI et al. Metabolic trapping as a principle of radiopharmaceutical design: some factors responsible for the biodistribution of [^{18}F]2-deoxyglucose. *J Nucl Med* 1980;19: 1154–1161.
30. Sokoloff L, Reivich M, Kennedy C et al. The [^{14}C]deoxyglucose method for the measurement of local cerebral glucose utilization: theory, procedure, and normal values in the conscious and anesthetized albino rat. *J Neurochem* 1977;28:897–916.
31. Phelps ME, Huang SC, Hoffman EJ et al. Tomographic measurements of local cerebral glucose metabolic rate in humans with (F-18)-2-fluoro-2-deoxy-D-glucose: validation of method. *Ann Neurol* 1979;6: 371–388.
32. Reivich M, Kuhl D, Wolf A et al. The [^{18}F]fluorodeoxyglucose method for the measurement of local cerebral glucose utilization in man. *Circ Res* 1979;44:127–137.
33. Huang SC, Phelps ME, Hoffman EJ et al. Noninvasive determination of local cerebral metabolic rate of glucose in man. *Am J Physiol* 1980; 238:E69–E82.
34. Hawkins RA, Choi Y, Huang SC et al. Quantitating tumor glucose metabolism with FDG and PET. *J Nucl Med* 1992;33:339–344.
35. Hawkins RA, Phelps ME, Huang SC. Effects of temporal sampling, glucose metabolic rate and disruptions of the blood brain barrier (BBB) on the FDG model with and without a vascular compartment: studies in human brain tumors with PET. *J Cereb Blood Flow Metab* 1986;6: 170–183.
36. Hawkins RA, Choi Y, Huang SC et al. Evaluation of the skeletal kinetics of fluorine-18-fluoride ion with PET. *J Nucl Med* 1992;33: 633–642.
37. Dahlbom M, Hoffman EJ, Hoh CK et al. Evaluation of a positron emission tomography scanner for whole body imaging. *J Nucl Med* 1992;33:1191–1199.

38. Meikle SR, Dahlbom M, Cherry SR et al. Attenuation correction in whole body PET. *J Nucl Med* 1992;33:826(abst).

39. Cherry SR, Dahlbom M, Hoffman EJ. High sensitivity, total body PET scanning using 3-D data acquisition and reconstruction. *IEEE Trans Nucl Sci* 1992;39:1088–1092.

40. Tse N, Hoh C, Hawkins R et al. Positron emission tomography diagnosis of pulmonary metastases in osteogenic sarcoma. *Am J Clin Oncol* 1994;17:22–25.

41. Warburg O. On the origin of cancer cells. *Science* 1956;123:309–314.

42. Ott RJ. The applications of positron emission tomography to oncology. *Br J Cancer* 1991;63:343–345(editorial).

43. Strauss LG, Conti PS. The applications of PET in clinical oncology. *J Nucl Med* 1991;32:623–648.

44. Gold RH, Hawkins RA, Katz RD. Imaging osteomyelitis—from plain films to MRI: a pictorial essay. *AJR* 1991;157:365–370.

45. Wahl RL, Kaminski MS, Ethier SP et al. The potential of 2-deoxy-2[^{18}F]fluoro-d-glucose (FDG) for the detection of tumor involvement in lymph nodes. *J Nucl Med* 1990;31:1831–1835.

46. Adler LP, Blair HF, Makley JT. Noninvasive grading of musculoskeletal tumors using PET. *J Nucl Med* 1991;32:1508–1512.

47. Kern KA, Brunetti A, Norton JA et al. Metabolic imaging of human extremity musculoskeletal tumors by PET. *J Nucl Med* 1988;29:181–186.

48. Yao WJ, Hoh CK, Hawkins RA et al. Bone marrow glucose metabolic response to GMCSF by quantitative FDG PET imaging. *J Nucl Med* 1994;35:8P(abst).

49. Gasson JC. Molecular physiology of granulocyte-macrophage colony stimulating factor. *Blood* 1991;7:1131–1145.

50. Demetri GD, Antman KH. Granulocyte-macrophage colony-stimulating factor (GM-CSF): preclinical and clinical investigations. *Sem Oncol* 1992;19:362–385.

51. Fogelman I, Bessent RG, Turner JG et al. The use of whole-body retention of ^{99m}Tc-diphosphonate in the diagnosis of metabolic bone disease. *J Nucl Med* 1978;19:270–275.

52. Fogelman I, Bessent RG, Beastall G et al. Estimation of skeletal involvement in primary hyperparathyroidism. *Ann Intern Med* 1980;92:65–67.

53. Front D, Israel O, Jerushalmi J et al. Quantitative bone scintigraphy using SPECT. *J Nucl Med* 1989;30:240–245.

54. Israel O, Front D, Hardoff R et al. *In vivo* SPECT quantitation of bone metabolism in hyperparathyroidism. *J Nucl Med* 1991;32:1157–1161.

55. Messa C, Goodman WG, Hoh CK et al. Bone metabolic activity measured with positron emission tomography and [^{18}F]fluoride ion in renal osteodystrophy: correlation with bone histomorphometry. *J Clin Endocrinol Metab* 1993;77:949–955.

56. Parfitt AM, Drezner MK, Glorieux FH et al. Bone histomorphometry: standardization of nomenclature, symbols and units: report of the ASBMR histomorphometry nomenclature committee. *J Bone Mine Res* 1987;2:595–610.

57. Goodman WG, Coburn JW, Slatopolsky E et al. Renal osteodystrophy in adults and children. In: Favus MJ, ed. *Primer on the bone metabolic diseases and disorders of mineral metabolism,* 1st ed. Kelseyville, CA: American Society of Bone and Mineral Research, 1990:200–212.

58. Recker RR. Bone biopsy and histomorphometry in clinical practice. In: Favus MJ, ed. *Primer on the bone metabolic diseases and disorders of mineral metabolism,* 1st ed. Kelseyville, CA: American Society of Bone and Mineral Research, 1990:101–104.

59. Cook GJR, Lodge MA, Blake GM et al. Differences in skeletal kinetics between vertebral and humeral bone measured by ^{18}F-fluoride positron emission tomography in postmenopausal women. *J Bone Mine Res* 2000;15:763–769.

60. Piert M, Winter E, Becker GA et al. Allogenic bone graft viability after hip revision arthroplasty assessed by dynamic [^{18}F]fluoride ion positron emission tomography. *Eur J Nucl Med* 1999;26:615–624.

61. Piert M, Zittel TT, Machulla H-J et al. Blood flow measurements with [^{15}O]H$_2$O and [^{18}F]fluoride ion PET in porcine vertebrae. *J Bone Mine Res* 1998;13:1328–1336.

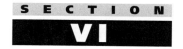

GASTROENTEROLOGY

24

ESOPHAGEAL TRANSIT, GASTROESOPHAGEAL REFLUX, AND GASTRIC EMPTYING

JEAN-LUC C. URBAIN
MARIE-CHRISTIANE M. VEKEMANS
LEON S. MALMUD

SCINTIGRAPHIC EVALUATION OF ESOPHAGEAL TRANSIT

The esophagus is a 20-cm long muscular tube that extends from the cricoid cartilage to the stomach. Histologically, the proximal third of the esophagus consists of striated muscle, the distal third is composed of smooth muscle, and the middle portion is a transitional mixture of the two. Anatomically, three areas can be identified: the upper esophageal sphincter, the body, and the lower esophageal sphincter. The coordinated function of these structures conveys swallowed material from the mouth to the stomach and clears residual substances.

Esophageal motility follows a precisely coordinated pattern. First, a pharyngeal contraction transfers the bolus through a relaxed upper esophageal sphincter into the esophagus. The sphincter then contracts, and a primary peristaltic wave propels the food bolus aborally into the stomach through a relaxed lower esophageal sphincter. Secondary peristaltic waves occur in the esophageal body in response to residual food or refluxed gastric content. Tertiary nonperistaltic contractions induced by intramural reflex mechanisms can also be seen as a variant phenomenon. The so-called deglutitive inhibition phenomenon refers to the complete inhibition of the contractile activity induced by a first swallow when a second swallow is initiated. This effect can last for 20 to 30 seconds and must be taken into account if performing a multiple swallow acquisition test.

Test Procedure

Test procedures vary depending on the radionuclide used, the type of bolus and its consistency, the position of the subject, the acquisition protocol, and the method of data processing and analysis.

J.L.C. Urbain: Department of Molecular and Functional Imaging, Cleveland Clinic Foundation, Cleveland, OH.
M.C.M. Vekemans: Cheh, Hornu, Belgium.
L.S. Malmud: Temple University Hospital, Philadelphia, PA.

Acquisition Protocol

The esophageal transit test should be performed after a 4 to 6 hour fast (1) and after withdrawal of any medication likely to interfere with esophageal motility.

Bolus Material

Solid food boluses are theoretically more physiologic in the assessment of esophageal transit (2–6); however, they usually disperse along the length of the esophagus and are practically inadequate for esophageal transit studies. In contrast, liquid boluses are homogeneous and provide more reproducible results. Water is the most common medium employed. It is usually given in the form of a bolus of 10 to 20 mL. Gelatin, a semisolid nutrient containing mainly water, is occasionally used as an alternative (7).

Radiopharmaceuticals

^{99m}Tc-sulfur colloid is usually preferred to label boluses, because it is inexpensive, easy to prepare, and neither absorbed nor secreted by the esophageal mucosa (8) and has optimal physical characteristics for imaging. Limitations to the use of ^{99m}Tc tracers include the radiation exposure and scattered activity from the stomach, particularly when using multiple radiolabeled boluses.

^{81m}Kr has been used as an alternative in water or glucose solution. Its short half-life of 13 seconds permits the use of several millicuries per test, while keeping a low radiation burden. It produces a better counting statistic, but cannot adequately visualize esophageal retention in patients with stasis.

Patient Positioning

The supine position is preferred for the early characterization of the esophageal motor disorders because it eliminates the effect of gravity (9). The erect position, however, is more physiologic and is used to evaluate the effectiveness of medical or surgical treatment of achalasia or scleroderma (10). When performing the test in both positions sequentially, the upright position is performed first in anticipation of more rapid clearance of the radioactivity from the esophagus (11).

Ideally, a ^{57}Co marker should be placed over the cricoid cartilage to facilitate the identification of the upper esophageal sphincter. The patient is then positioned to visualize the mouth, esophagus, and gastric fundus in the same field of view. Anterior imaging is usually performed with the assumption that the attenuation along the length of the esophagus is uniform (12).

Acquisition Procedure

When gelatin or a solid food is used, a spoon with ± 10 g of medium is administered. Liquid is usually given in a 10-mL bolus labeled with 150 to 500 µCi of ^{99m}Tc-sulfur colloid or albumin colloid (or alternatively up to 8 mCi of ^{81m}Kr) and given to the patient with a syringe or a straw. Patients are instructed to retain the bolus in the mouth and to swallow the entire bolus in one gulp; two or three practice swallows with unlabeled material help the patient to understand the procedure. The multiple-swallow technique is preferred over the single swallow test because of the considerable intraindividual variations in esophageal emptying in normals (13–15) and patients (16). Four to six swallows followed by multiple dry swallows at 20 to 30 second intervals are usually adequate (17).

Acquisition Parameters

A high-speed framing rate is required to image esophageal transit. Typically, two sets of 64×64 matrix dynamic images are acquired for a total of ± 2 minutes. During the first step, 0.25-second images are obtained to evaluate the oropharyngeal transit; for the second step, images of 1 second each are acquired to characterize the esophageal transit. Delayed images at 5, 10, and 15 minutes are useful in patients with significant stasis of radioactivity in the esophagus.

Data Processing—Data Analysis

The basic analysis of esophageal transit resides in the generation of time-activity curves using a global esophageal region of interest, ranging from the cricoid to the gastroesophageal junction, and separate regions outlined around the proximal, middle, and distal esophagus and the stomach.

Global esophageal transit is determined based on the amount of residual activity in the esophagus using the formula $C(t) = E\ max - E(t)/E\ max$, where $C(t)$ represents the percentage of esophageal emptying at time t, $E\ max$, the maximal count rate in the esophagus, and $E(t)$, the esophageal count rate at time t (18).

Four parameters can be derived from the segmental time-activity curves (Fig. 24.1) (11): (a) the esophageal transit time is the time interval between the peak activity of the proximal esophageal curve and the peak activity of the distal esophageal curve, (b) the segmental emptying time characterizes the time required for more than an arbitrary percentage of the maximal radioactivity in each region of interest to be eliminated, (c) the global esophageal emptying time represents the time from entry of the bolus in the proximal esophagus to the clearance of more than 90% from the entire esophagus, and (d) the esophagogastric transit time is defined as the time interval between peak activity of the proximal esophageal curve and maximal gastric activity (11).

Condensed Images

Summing all computer frames during the transit of the bolus, Kjellén, Svedberg, and Tibbling (19) introduced the concept of a "topographic picture" of the esophagus. A refined approach was proposed by Svedberg (20) and Klein and Wald (21) using the "condensed picture."

The condensed image consists of the summation of the activity in the pixel rows into a single column for each frame of the swallowing test data series, and the creation of a single image in which the vertical axis shows the spatial distribution of the radioactivity from the mouth to the stomach and the horizontal axis is temporal (Fig. 24.2). With this approach, a complete dynamic sequence is displayed in one single image, facilitating qualitative assessment of radionuclide esophageal transit and improving diagnostic ability (22). To integrate the dynamic sequences after each bolus swallow, Tatsch (18), in 1991, introduced the "pseudogating" technique of condensed esophageal images (Fig. 24.3). This technique has the advantage of displaying into one single image the average esophageal transit of multiple boluses and dry swallows. Its major built-in disadvantage resides in the sum of dynamic sequences that are not necessarily in phase with the swallows. This approach was further validated with manometry (23).

Parametric esophageal multiple swallows scintigraphy (PES) images have been used to evaluate esophageal motility disorders in patients with dysphageal symptoms and psychiatric disorders (24,25).

Interpretation

Visual inspection of dynamic sequences allows for the assessment of the completeness of bolus ingestion, for the assessment of progression of the bolus through the esophagus, and for the identification of bolus stasis in any portion of the esophagus. Episodes of reflux or any abnormal extraluminal focus of activity can also be detected.

In normal subjects, passage of the bolus from the pharynx into the esophagus takes less than 0.5 to 1 second. Esophageal transit time for water or semisolid boluses varies from 5.5 ± 1.1 to 9.5 ± 1.5 seconds, depending on the definition and calculation methods used (3,15,26–28). Because of the compression by the aortic arch or tracheal bifurcation, a slowing of bolus progression can be observed at the midportion of the esophagus. Abnormal esophageal motility caused by aging (the so-called presbyesophagus) and delayed esophageal transit in obese patients with reflux (29) have been described.

Esophageal motility disturbances are classically categorized into primary or secondary disorders depending on the pathophysiologic mechanisms. Disruption of the anatomy of the esophageal tube can also result in transit abnormalities. In this

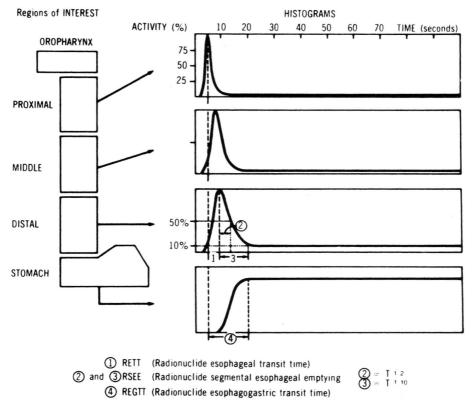

FIGURE 24.1. Parameters that can be derived from an esophageal transit study. Regions of interest around the entire esophagus; its proximal, middle, and distal segments; and the stomach allow for the determination of the esophageal transit time. The segmental emptying time, the global esophageal emptying time, and the esophagogastric transit time. (From Taillefer R, Beauchamp G. Radionuclide esophagogram. *Clin Nucl Med* 1984;9:465–483, with permission.)

chapter, we review the most common diseases that affect esophageal transit.

Primary Esophageal Motility Disorders

Achalasia

Achalasia is characterized by a loss of peristalsis in the esophageal body and a failure of the lower esophageal sphincter to relax. The esophageal transit test shows a marked and prolonged retention of the radioactive bolus in the distal segment of the esophagus with very little activity in the stomach. The condensed image may also demonstrate a chaotic movement of the activity (Fig. 24.4**B**).

Although the sensitivity of the test is high (2,18,30,31), endoscopy or radiographic techniques are the primary diagnostic tests of this disease because they permit exclusion of anatomic abnormalities or obstructive lesions, such as cancer. Quantitative evaluation of the effectiveness of pneumatic dilatation is the principal indication for esophageal transit scintigraphy (32).

Diffuse Esophageal Spasm

Diffuse esophageal spasm syndrome is characterized by spastic activity of the lower two thirds of the esophagus with intermittent chest pain and/or dysphagia. Typically, the radionuclide

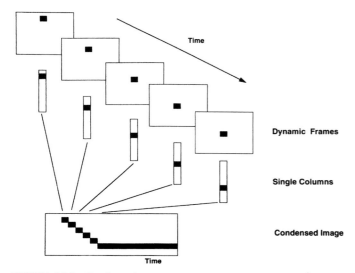

FIGURE 24.2. Condensed image representation. For each dynamic frame of the swallow set, the esophagus is represented by a single column. Columns are then added together to generate a single condensed image. On the condensed image, the spatial distribution of the radioactivity in the esophagus over time is represented by the vertical axis.

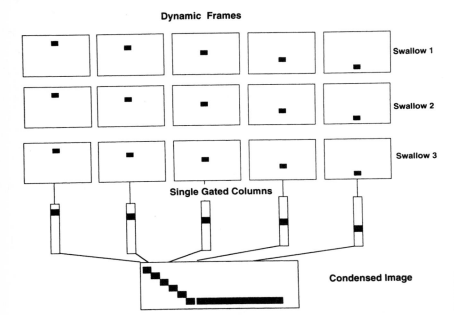

FIGURE 24.3. Gated esophageal condensed image. In the gated technique, columns of the same numbered frame of the swallow sets are added together and a single composite condensed image is generated.

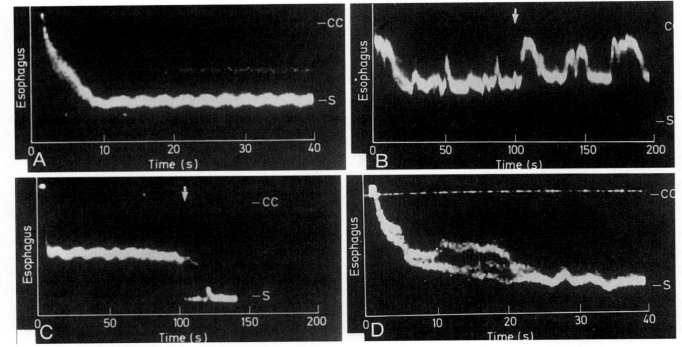

FIGURE 24.4. Esophageal condensed images. **A:** In normal subjects, the bolus transit quickly and smoothly through all segments. **B:** In achalasia, there is a marked and prolonged retention of the bolus in the distal segment of the esophagus with very little activity in the stomach. Episodes of retrograde motion are often observed. **C:** In patients with scleroderma a stagnation of the bolus in the lower portion of the esophagus is characteristic. The administration of water (*arrow*) can clear out the activity into the stomach by forcing the bolus through the hypokinetic segment. **D:** Patients with gastroesophageal reflux demonstrate retrograde movements of activity from the stomach into the esophagus. (From O'Conner MK, Byrne PJ, Keeling P et al. Esophageal scintigraphy: applications and limitations in the study of esophageal disorders. *Eur J Nucl Med* 1988;14:131–136, with permission.)

transit test demonstrates a prolonged transit time associated with decreased segmental esophageal emptying, periods of esophageal retrograde movements, and fragmentation of the radioactive bolus. Time-activity curves show multiple peaks of activity in all esophageal segments. Sensitivity of esophageal transit in this disorder is about 77% (33,34).

Nutcracker Esophagus
The nutcracker esophagus is characterized by high amplitude peristaltic contractions in the esophageal body occurring simultaneously with noncardiac chest pain and/or dysphagia (35). Typical scintigraphic findings consist in a prolonged retention of activity in the distal esophagus and a mild distal to midesophagus esophageal reflux.

The sensitivity of esophageal transit scintigraphy in detecting nutcracker esophagus depends on the cutoff value used for the amplitude of the mean distal esophagus contractions and the scintigraphic criteria used to assess the transit delay (36,37).

Nonspecific Motor Disorders
Abnormal manometric patterns that do not fit established criteria for diffuse esophageal spasm, achalasia, or scleroderma are considered nonspecific motor disorders of the esophagus. Manometric abnormalities include peristaltic contractions of low amplitude or prolonged duration, waveforms with multiple peaks or followed by repetitive waves, and/or sustained increase in the baseline esophageal pressure. The most common scintigraphic finding is a prolonged esophageal transit time with an incoordinated pattern. Sensitivity of the esophageal scintigraphic transit test in this disparate entity is variable.

Neuromuscular and Connective Tissue Disorders

Abnormal esophageal motility has been described in all connective tissue disorders, which involve either the smooth muscle, such as scleroderma, systemic lupus erythematosus, and Raynaud's disease, or the striated muscle, such as dermatopolymyositis (38).

In progressive systemic sclerosis, esophageal involvement is frequent, but often asymptomatic, in early stages of the disease. Esophageal transit scintigraphy has been employed to detect early involvement of the esophagus and to evaluate the impairment of the esophageal function.

The esophageal transit pattern is characteristic and demonstrates stagnation of the bolus in the lower two thirds of the esophagus (Fig. 24.4C). The sensitivity of scintigraphy in this disease is approximately 88% (39–43). Excellent correlation exists among scintigraphy, manometry, and the patient's symptoms (43). Abnormal esophageal motility has also been described in neuromuscular diseases such as myotonic dystrophy or myasthenia gravis.

Other Conditions
Tumors of the Esophagus
Evaluation by endoscopy is mandatory in patients with suspicion of tumors of the esophagus. Scintigraphically, tumors appear as areas of decreased radioactivity with stenotic lesions and are associated with delayed esophageal transit. In some instances, the esophageal lumen is enlarged above the stenosis. Esophageal transit scintigraphy is the only available tool for the quantitative evaluation of therapeutic approaches such as laser therapy or prosthesis placement and radiation therapy (25).

Zenker's Diverticulum
Zenker's diverticulum is an acquired pharyngoesophageal outpouch located above the upper esophageal sphincter. Classically, scintigraphic findings consist of an ovoid or spheric area of persistent esophageal retention of radioactivity at the level of the upper esophagus.

Esophageal Surgery
Radionuclide esophageal transit is the only test that allows for the physiologic quantitative evaluation of esophageal transit before and after surgical treatment for hiatal hernia and reflux.

Miscellaneous
An abnormal esophageal transit test is observed in about 50% of patients with gastroesophageal reflux (8,18,26,44). Diabetes mellitus, chronic alcoholism (45), infection, systemic illnesses, and trauma may also lead to secondary motor disorders of the esophagus. In cervical vertebropathy, a prolongation of the total esophageal transit time can be observed (46).

SCINTIGRAPHIC EVALUATION OF ESOPHAGEAL REFLUX

Gastroesophageal reflux scintigraphy was introduced in 1976 by Fisher et al. (47) to quantitate gastroesophageal reflux and to assess the effectiveness of medical and surgical treatment (48–54). The availability and accuracy of endoscopy, the Bernstein test, esophageal manometry, and 24-hour pH monitoring have made gastroesophageal reflux scintigraphy almost obsolete in adults. However, because of its physiologic and noninvasive character, scintigraphy has gained wide acceptance in the detection and evaluation of gastroesophageal reflux in infants and children.

Test Procedure
Acquisition Protocol

The patient is studied after an overnight fast and positioned supine under the camera to avoid the effect of gravity. Two additional aggravants of reflux are used to enhance the sensitivity of the test: (a) an acid load to the stomach can be given to decrease the tone of the lower esophageal sphincter, and (b) an inflatable abdominal binder placed around the lower abdomen is used to increase the pressure gradient across the lower esophageal sphincter.

Three hundred mL of acidified orange juice containing 300 μCi of ^{99m}Tc-sulfur colloid and consisting of 150 mL orange juice and 150 mL 0.1N hydrochloric acid are administered orally to the patient in the upright position, and a first static

30-second exposure image is acquired to ensure complete clearance of the radiolabeled material from the esophagus. If needed, 30 mL of water are given to clear any residual activity. Dynamic images are then acquired in the supine position, at baseline and at each 20 mm Hg pressure gradient from 0 to 100 mm Hg.

In infants and children, the study is performed using infant formula, milk, or pudding, and the examiner's hand is used to create pressure on the abdomen. Positions and circumstances during which reflux occurs can be determined scintigraphically as can the rate of gastric emptying (55,56). A possible relationship between gastroesophageal reflux and sudden infant death syndrome (57,58), as well as various respiratory diseases (59–61), has been evoked.

Giving ^{99m}Tc-sulfur colloid or, preferably, ^{111}In-DTPA in a liquid meal to the child at bedtime, and scanning the lungs the next day, can provide objective and direct evidence of pulmonary aspiration of refluxed gastric material (62).

Visual Description, Data Processing, and Interpretation

In healthy subjects, gastroesophageal reflux of radioactivity cannot be seen even by increasing pressure up to 100 mm Hg. In patients with reflux, an increase in the amount of reflux material is observed as the gradient across the lower esophageal sphincter is increased.

Reflux can be quantified at each step, using regions of interest over the esophagus and stomach using the formula $R = E(t) - E(b) \times 100/Go$, where R is the percentage of reflux material into the esophagus; $E(t)$, the esophageal counts at time t; $E(b)$, the paraesophageal background counts; and Go, the gastric counts at the beginning of the study. In practice, reflux $\geq 4\%$ is considered abnormal. This value coincides with the visibility of refluxed radioactivity on the gamma-camera screen. Overall sensitivity of the technique is in the range of 88% to 91%.

Reflux is also nicely documented on condensed images by a rebound of activity above the gastroesophageal junction line (Fig. 24.4**D**).

GASTRIC EMPTYING SCINTIGRAPHY

Anatomically, the stomach can be divided into three regions: the fundus, the corpus, and the antrum.

Physiologically, the human stomach consists of two functionally integrated, but electromechanically distinct, portions. The proximal stomach, which encompasses the fundus and the proximal corpus, functions as a reservoir for solid and liquid food and controls the emptying of liquids. The distal stomach, which includes the mid and distal corpus and the antrum, is characterized by peristaltic contractions at a rate of approximately 3 per minute. These contractions break down solid food into small particles and mix them with gastric secretions to form a semiliquid juice that is then emptied into the duodenum. The rate of gastric emptying is determined by many factors, including the volume; physical state; caloric content; caloric density; concentration of the nutrients; the meal distribution; and its salinity, acidity, and viscosity.

Emptying of Liquids

Saline, neutral, iso-osmolar, and calorically inert solutions empty in a single exponential manner as a function of volume (63,64). When the stomach is filled with a nutrient solution, the shape of the emptying curve becomes more linear (65) or may even consist of two linear phases: an initial rapid and a slower late phase (66). Osmolytes, acids, fatty acids (particularly medium-chains), carbohydrates, and proteins activate receptors along the small bowel and control gastric emptying by feedback mechanisms (67–71).

Emptying of Solids

Emptying-time course for solid food is sigmoidal in shape and characterized by an initial lag phase during which no or little solid emptying occurs; followed by a linear phase with a constant emptying rate; and a late, much slower phase. Physical characteristics of solid food, antral contractions, and antroduodenal coordination determine the lag phase duration and emptying rate. Both the lag phase and emptying time are increased by high caloric meals (72,73). Increasing the volume of solid food speeds up gastric emptying. This effect is overridden by intestinal inhibition, as additional calories enter the small intestine (74).

Emptying of a Solid-Liquid Test Meal

Liquids, in the presence of solids, empty much more rapidly than solids, but at a slower rate than if given alone (72,75). The *solid-liquid discrimination* appellation refers to the rapid emptying of water from the stomach while solids are retained; it is predominantly related to the sieving effect of solid particles by the pylorus and the antroduodenal coordination (76).

Emptying of Fat

Fat relaxes the fundus, lowers the intragastric pressure, increases the reservoir capacity, inhibits antral motility, and increases pyloric contraction (77). Fat slows the emptying of all constituents of a mixed meal (78) and is emptied at a slower rate than solids (79).

Test Procedure

Acquisition Protocol

Gastric emptying should to be evaluated following at least a 12-hour overnight fast (80,81). Subjects should refrain from smoking (82), and no medication likely to interfere with gastric emptying should be taken before the test. Diabetic patients should be studied early in the morning following administration of their insulin dose.

Test Meal—Test Meal Labeling

Among the various radionuclides and radiopharmaceuticals that have been used for labeling meals, both ^{99m}Tc-sulfur colloid and ^{111}In-DTPA have emerged as the tracers of choice because of their short half-lives, better imaging characteristics, low radiation burdens, and strong binding to food.

The first meal used to evaluate gastric emptying consisted of porridge, milk, bread and butter, and scrambled eggs, mixed with ^{51}Cr (83). Chicken liver, labeled in vivo with ^{99m}Tc-sulfur colloid, was introduced in 1976 to insure radiotracer binding to the solid food (84); it is the most stable test meal in gastric juice (85,86).

The dual-isotope scanning method, introduced in 1976 by Heading et al. (75), for the simultaneous measurement of ^{99m}Tc solid and ^{111}In-DTPA liquid emptying, had rapidly gained widespread clinical and investigational acceptance. With time however, it appeared that the liquid constituent of a test meal is less sensitive than the solid phase to detect gastric-emptying impairment (66,87,88).

Numerous solid foods, including whole eggs, egg whites, chicken liver, liver paté, hamburgers, fibers, and nondigestible particles, have been used with or without a liquid component, usually water. Because of the availability, low cost, and stability of ^{99m}Tc-sulfur colloid in gastric juice and the ready availability of eggs, radiolabeled eggs are now used in most nuclear medicine departments. Our standardized test meal consists of one scrambled egg, two slices of regular white bread (weighing ± 50 g each), and 150 mL of tap water and contains approximately 230 calories with 35% fat, 47% carbohydrate, and 18% protein. The egg is mixed with 0.5 to 1.0 mCi ^{99m}Tc-sulfur colloid, cooked until firm in a Teflon-coated pan, and given to the patient as an egg sandwich. For dual-isotope solid-liquid emptying studies, water is labeled with 75 μCi of ^{111}In-DTPA. Ingestion of the radiolabeled test meal should optimally be completed within 10 minutes.

Acquisition Procedure

To reproduce physiologic conditions, the patient is positioned sitting or standing in front of the gamma-camera. A ^{99m}Tc or ^{57}Co marker taped over the xiphoid process or the iliac crest helps to reposition the subject for the serial sets of images.

Dual Phase Emptying Test Meal

Immediately after ingestion of the ^{99m}Tc-radiolabeled solid phase of the meal, an initial 1-minute image of the stomach is acquired in the 140 keV $\pm 20\%$ ^{99m}Tc window using a medium-energy parallel hole collimator. The patient then ingests the liquid phase, labeled with ^{111}In-DTPA, and a second 1-minute picture is taken in the ^{99m}Tc window to calculate the downscatter percentage of ^{111}In into the ^{99m}Tc window. A third 1-minute picture is subsequently acquired on the 247 keV ^{111}In peak $\pm 20\%$ window. Pictures of the stomach are then taken in both windows every 10 minutes for 1 hour and every 15 to 20 minutes for up to 2 hours, if needed, until 50% emptying. Recently, it has been shown that extending gastric-emptying scintigraphy from 2 to 4 hours may detect more patients with gastroparesis. (89). Because exercise accelerates gastric emptying, the patient should remain seated between images.

Single Label Test Meal

When using a single radionuclide to label either the liquid or solid component of the meal, images are taken using the appro-priate radionuclide peak and collimator, following similar time intervals as for the dual-labeled meal.

Imaging

To allow for the correction of the increase of counts as the food moves from the more posterior fundus to the more anterior antrum, geometric mean data are obtained from simultaneous anterior and posterior static images (dual-headed system) or from anterior, immediately followed by posterior views (single-head system), using a 64 × 64 or 128 × 128 pixel matrix (90–93). Other correction methods have been advocated and use either an additional lateral view of the stomach (63), a left anterior oblique (LAO) projection (94–97), or the peak-to-scatter ratio (98).

To obtain information on antral motility, 64 × 64 pixel matrix dynamic images are taken at a rate of 1 frame per second for 4 minutes after each set of static images (99–102).

Visual Description—Data Processing

Visual Description

Immediately after meal completion, the test meal is usually retained in the proximal stomach. The water component of the meal distributes uniformly throughout the stomach before being emptied into the duodenum. In contrast, solid food moves progressively from the proximal to the distal stomach where it is ground into small particles before emptying (Fig. 24.5**A**).

Data Processing

The geometric mean of the gastric counts, i.e., the square root of the product of the anterior activity multiplied by the posterior activity in the stomach, is calculated at each imaging interval. Counts are corrected for radionuclide decay and normalized to 100% based on total gastric counts obtained immediately following ingestion of the meal. This is defined as $t = 0$ minutes. Data are then plotted as percentage retention versus time.

Liquid emptying typically follows a single exponential pattern, whereas solid emptying is sigmoidal in shape and characterized by an initial shoulder with little emptying called the lag phase (Tlag), followed by a linear phase and a much slower phase when the stomach is almost emptied (Fig. 24.6).

Data Analysis

The simplest method to evaluate gastric emptying is the determination on the gastric-emptying curve of the time required for 50% emptying (half-emptying time or $T_{1/2}$). This parameter does not fully characterize gastric emptying. Gastric-emptying data are more completely analyzed using mathematic functions that reflect the time course of emptying and, eventually, gastric-emptying physiology.

Two functions have been shown to adequately fit biphasic solid gastric-emptying data: the power exponential function $y = (e^{-kt})^B$ (103) and a modified power exponential function $y(t) = 1 - (1 - e^{-kt})^B$ (104). In both, $y(t)$ is the fractional meal retention at time t, k is the gastric-emptying rate in min-

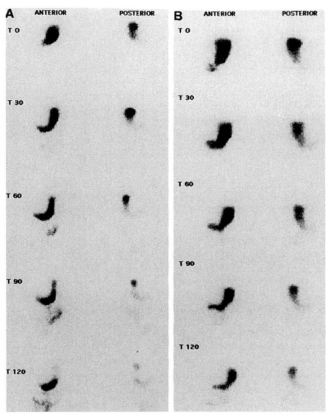

FIGURE 24.5. Gastric-emptying study of solids. Anterior and posterior images of the stomach are shown 0, 30, 60, 90, and 120 minutes after meal completion (TO) in a normal subject **(A)** and in a patient with diabetic gastroparesis **(B)**. In normal subjects, the test meal is initially retained in the proximal stomach and then moves progressively to the distal stomach where it is ground into small particles before emptying. In patients with diabetic gastroparesis, a significant retention of food is observed in the proximal portion of the stomach, and the filling of the distal stomach is delayed.

utes^{-1} and *B* is the extrapolated *y*-intercept from the terminal portion of the curve. Four parameters can be derived from these two functions: the *B* value, the Tlag (in minutes), the emptying rate (in percent of emptying per minute), and the half-emptying time ($T_{1/2}$)(in minutes). The *B* parameter determines the shape of the curve. Solid curves have usually an initial lag phase and *B* is greater than one. A value of *B* less than one indicates initial rapid emptying followed by a second slower emptying phase. This is the pattern often seen in patients after antrectomy or following ingestion of some liquid meals. Numerically, the lag phase, Tlag, is equal to Ir *B/k* (modified power exponential function) and to $[(B - 1)/B]^{1/B}/k$ (Elashoff function). Mathematically, it represents the time at which the second derivative of the function equals zero and coincides with the antral filling peak (Fig. 24.7). Liquid emptying curves are described by the single exponential function $y(t) = e^{-kt}$, where $y(t)$ is the fractional meal retention at time *t* and *k* is the emptying rate in minutes^{-1}.

Gastric Motility And Scintigraphy

Time activity curves generated from antral regions of interest display a sinusoid pattern that reflects the rhythmic mechanical activity of the antrum. Antral activity curves can be analyzed using the autocorrelation technique (99) and the Fourier transform function (99–102,105) to determine the frequency and the amplitude of gastric contractions (Fig. 24.8**A**). Fourier analysis of condensed gastric images is also used to evaluate gastric motility (106).

In normal subjects, gastric contractions occur at a rate of about three per minute, and the frequency and amplitude of those contractions can be correlated with the emptying of food (105). In diabetic gastroparesis, delayed gastric emptying is related to a retention of food in the proximal stomach, as well as to a decrease in the amplitude of antral contractions (99) (Fig. 24.8**B**). In functional dyspepsia, the amplitude of gastric con-

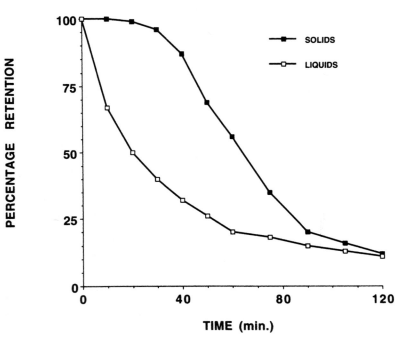

FIGURE 24.6. Gastric-emptying curves for solids and liquids. In normal subjects, solid emptying is sigmoidal in shape with an initial shoulder with no or little emptying (the lag phase), followed by a linear phase with constant emptying rate, and a much slower phase when the stomach is nearly empty. Liquid curve follows an exponential pattern.

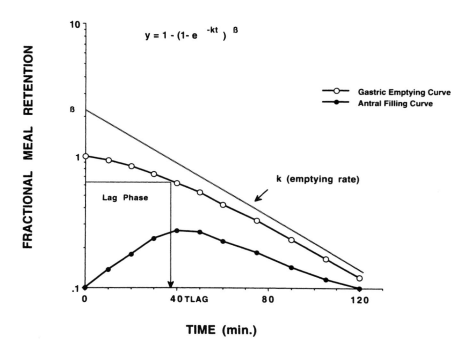

FIGURE 24.7. Modified power exponential fitting function. The modified power exponential function characterizes the three portions of a solid emptying curve: the lag phase (TLAG), which is numerically equal to ln B/k and corresponds to the inflection point of the total gastric-emptying curve and to the peak antral filling, the emptying rate (k), and half-emptying time.

tractions is increased regardless of the emptying rate (100,102) (Fig. 24.8**C**).

Reproducibility

Interindividual and intraindividual variations of gastric half-emptying time can be significant in normal subjects and patients with gastroparesis (63,66,107–110). This explains the broad range usually observed in normal subjects and emphasizes the need to carefully standardize the acquisition parameters, especially when the effects of a drug are being assessed.

Interpretation

In this section, we review the most frequent causes of gastric motility impairment and describe their gastric-emptying pattern.

Medical Disorders and Diseases

Diabetes
Delayed gastric emptying in symptomatic and asymptomatic diabetics (66,111–115) is mainly accounted for by a prolonged lag phase (66,116), an impairment of the proximal stomach function, and a reduction in the antral motor activity (99,113) (Fig. 24.9**B**). A markedly prolonged linear gastric emptying of solids (up to several hours) and a delayed emptying of liquids characterize advanced diabetic gastroparesis (66,114,115,117, 118). In patients with type II diabetes of recent onset, an accelerated gastric emptying for solids was recently described (119). The delayed in gastric emptying in type II diabetes could be related to higher postprandial level of glucose and glucagon (120).

Functional Dyspepsia
The clinical description of functional dyspepsia includes a constellation of symptoms such as abdominal pain or discomfort,

early satiety, fullness, distension, bloating, nausea, vomiting, belching, and epigastric or retrosternal burning. Dyspepsia is categorized as either organic or functional (idiopathic), based on the presence or the absence of underlying structural and/or biochemical abnormalities. Idiopathic dyspepsia occurs more commonly in women younger than the age of 50, but no correlation between the occurrence of symptoms and the menstrual cycle has been found. The pathophysiology of functional dyspepsia remains unclear. Antral hypomotility is observed in 25% to 70% of patients (121–123). However, a hypermotility pattern has also been described. In this case, an antropyloric dyscoordination motility pattern could be responsible for the delay in solid food emptying (100,102). Liquid emptying appears to be normal in these patients.

Anorexia Nervosa
About 80% of anorectic patients display a delayed gastric emptying for solids, while liquid emptying remains normal (124). Hypersensitivity of small intestinal nutrient receptors resulting from chronic food deprivation might explain the persistent delay in gastric emptying after oral renutrition of these patients.

Gastritis
In chronic gastritis, emptying of liquids is usually normal, whereas emptying of solids is delayed. Stasis of both liquids and solids has been described in atrophic gastritis, whereas in pernicious anemia delayed gastric emptying for solids only is observed (125,126).

Gastroesophageal Reflux
Gastric retention of acid and food favors gastroesophageal reflux in adults (127,128). More than 60% of patients with gastroesophageal reflux have delayed gastric emptying of solids. Liquids may be emptied normally or with a delay, depending on the test meal (127,129–131). In infants, a fundic disorder pro-

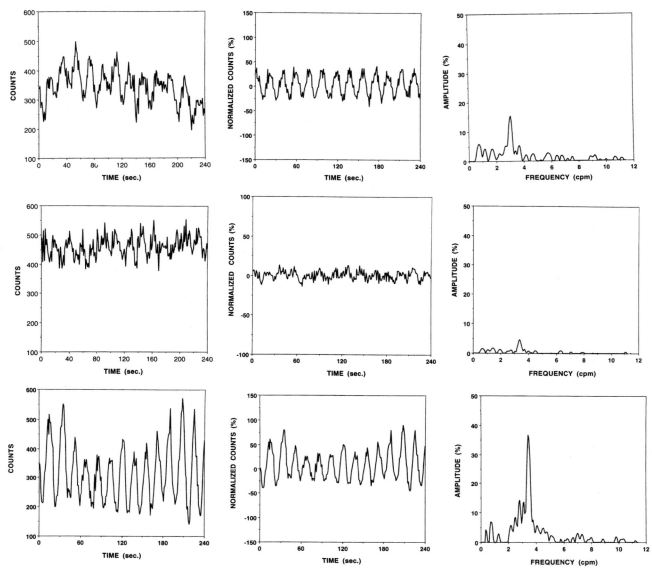

FIGURE 24.8. Antral time activity curves processing. The processing of dynamic antral time activity curves is shown in this figure for a healthy control (*top row*), a patient with diabetic gastroparesis (*middle row*) and a patient with functional dyspepsia (*lower row*). *Left column:* Four-minute raw antral time-activity curves. *Middle column:* Curves are normalized to their respective mean count. *Right column:* The autocorrelation function and the Fourier transform are then applied to determine the dominant frequency and the amplitude. In all subjects, the dominant frequency of the antral contractions is about three cycles per minute. The amplitude is the variable parameter of the contraction with a decrease in diabetic gastroparesis and an increase in functional dyspepsia.

ducing a rapid rise in the intragastric pressure is responsible for gastroesophageal reflux and gastric retention (132,133).

Acid-Peptic Diseases
Gastric Ulcer. Transient slow emptying has been observed in patients with an ulcer of the proximal stomach (83,131–133). Antral hypomotility, abnormalities of the interdigestive migrating motor complex, and increased concentration of bile salts are possible causes of gastric stasis. Suppression of gastric acid secretion with gastric acid suppressants is associated with delayed gastric emptying but increased antral motility (134).

Duodenal Ulcer. No definite conclusion can be found in the literature on gastric emptying in this disorder. Solid emptying has been found delayed by some authors (135,136) whereas others have reported a faster solid (82,137,138) or liquid emptying (130,139,140). Normal solid and liquid emptying has also been described (141,142).

Zollinger-Ellison Disease. Zollinger-Ellison disease has been unequivocally associated with rapid gastric emptying of both solids and liquids. A defective inhibitory mechanism of gastric

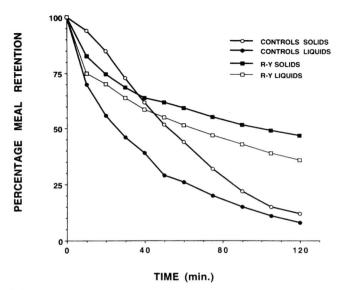

FIGURE 24.9. Gastric-emptying curves in patients Roux-en-Y diversion. In the Roux-en-Y gastrojejunostomy with vagotomy, both solid and liquid emptying follow a biexponential pattern with an early rapid emptying of the food from the stomach pouch and a slower emptying phase. No lag phase is observed for solids.

emptying resulting from extensive inflammation of gastric mucosa may be responsible (143,144).

Connective Tissue Disorders

Delayed gastric emptying of solids and liquids is present in 50% of patients with progressive systemic sclerosis (4,145). In systemic lupus erythematosus, polymyositis, and dermatomyositis, delayed gastric emptying, when present, may be asymptomatic. Antral hypomotility and impaired fasting motor activity are possible pathophysiologic factors (38).

Various

In patients with HIV the overall gastric emptying, but not lag phase, is delayed without any significant correlation with symptoms, autonomic dysfunction, or small intestinal motility (146). Patients with primary hypothyroidism also have a delayed gastric emptying. This delay does not correlate with thyroid-stimulating hormone (147).

Surgical Procedures

Gastric-emptying pattern may be affected in several different ways, depending on the type of operation. As a rule of thumb, proximal gastric vagotomy impairs the reservoir function and the emptying of liquids, whereas truncal or selective vagotomy affects both proximal and distal stomach and alters emptying of both solids and liquids. Antral removal suppresses the grinding and sieving of solid food, which is emptied faster into the small bowel.

Vagotomy

Highly Selective or Proximal Gastric Vagotomy. Following proximal gastric vagotomy, liquid emptying shows a biexponen-

tial pattern with an initial rapid emptying with up to 50% emptied within the first 10 minutes followed by a normal rate (148, 149). Solid gastric emptying, which may be slightly delayed initially, usually returns to normal within a few weeks or months (136,150,151). In some instances, prolongation of the solid lag phase persists for many months after surgery (152,153).

Truncal and Selective Vagotomy. Solid food emptying is transiently delayed, but this delay may persist in 20% to 25% of the patients (154–156). Liquid hypertonic solutions empty in an accelerated fashion, because of the loss of fundal relaxation and weakened duodenal feedback mechanisms (157–159).

Drainage Procedures. Pyloroplasty accelerates gastric emptying of solids and allows the passage of larger size particles in the small bowel (160). Following vagotomy and pyloroplasty, liquids empty precipitously, particularly in the erect position, and solid emptying is moderately delayed (161).

Gastrectomy

Proximal gastrectomy accelerates gastric emptying (162). After distal gastrectomy, solid emptying is accelerated and larger particles are allowed to pass into the small bowel (160,163–165). Liquid emptying is usually normal or rapid in this instance (148, 163,166). The combination of truncal vagotomy and distal gastrectomy accelerates gastric emptying of liquids (157,159), whereas solid emptying is retarded (164,167). Total or subtotal gastrectomy associated with truncal vagotomy results in an initial precipitous emptying followed by an exponential course for solids (168). In the Roux-en-Y diversion with vagotomy, gastric emptying of solids and liquids follows a biexponential curve characterized by an early rapid emptying of the remnant gastric pouch, followed by a very slow evacuation phase (153,164,169) (Fig. 24.9).

Intrathoracic Stomach

Emptying of the intrathoracic stomach is much slower than normal esophageal transit and is characterized by an early phase of rapid gastric evacuation (within the first 10 minutes after the meal), followed by a later slower phase (170,171). Gastroesophageal reflux may also occur with a high incidence, especially if the stomach is entirely intrathoracic (172–174).

Gastrokinetic Compounds

The increased interest in gastric-emptying procedures over the past two decades is partially explained by the availability of specific and effective gastrokinetic compounds. Numerous therapeutic trials have been conducted using scintigraphy to assess their effects on gastric emptying.

Metoclopramide increases both the frequency and amplitude of antral contractions and accelerates emptying of solids and liquids (113,175–178).

Domperidone inhibits the stomach's receptive relaxation reflex, increases antral motility, and improves antroduodenal coordination and, as a result, accelerates gastric emptying (124,179).

Cisapride is a prokinetic agent without antidopaminergic properties, which improves gastric emptying of solids and liquids in diabetics (114), in patients after gastric surgery, and in patients with idiopathic gastroparesis (180).

Erythromycin, a macrolide antibiotic, abolishes the solid-liquid discrimination in normals and in diabetics with gastroparesis and functional dyspepsia and dramatically increases gastric emptying of both solids and liquids (115,181). Erythromycin is a motilin agonist (182–184), which initiates Phase III of the interdigestive motor complex (185–188) and generates powerful antral contractions (189).

Recently, the gastrointestinal peptide motilin has been used successfully to improve gastric emptying of solids and liquids in diabetic gastroparesis (190), opening the avenue for the endocrine treatment of gastric stasis with physiologic compounds.

REFERENCES

1. Diamant NE, Akin AN. Effect of gastric contractions on the lower esophageal sphincter. *Gastroenterology* 1972;63:38–44.
2. Gross R, Johnson LF, Kaminski RJ. Esophageal emptying in achalasia quantitated by a radioisotope technique. *Dig Dis Sci* 1979;24:945–949.
3. DeVincentis N, Lenti R, Pona C et al. Scintigraphic evaluation of the esophageal transit time for the noninvasive assessment of esophageal motor disorders. *J Nucl Med* 1984;28:137–142.
4. Maddern GJ, Horowitz M, Jamieson GG et al. Abnormalities of esophageal and gastric emptying in progressive systemic sclerosis. *Gastroenterology* 1984;87:922–926.
5. Eriksen CA, Holdsworth RJ, Sutton D et al. The solid bolus esophageal transit test: its manometric interpretation and usefulness as a screening test. *Br J Surg* 1987;74:1130–1133.
6. Sutton D, Eriksen C, Kennedy N et al. Investigation of esophageal motility using a solid bolus egg transit technique: results of two studies. *Nucl Med Commun* 1988;9:158–159.
7. Bosch A, Dietrich R, Lanaro AE et al. Modified scintigraphic technique for the dynamic study of the esophagus. *Int J Nucl Med Biol* 1977;4:195–199.
8. Taillefer R, Beauchamp G, Devito M et al. Radionuclide esophagogram (Tc-99m-sulfur colloid) in experimental esophagitis: manometric and histopathologic correlations. *J Nucl Med* 1983;24:100(abst).
9. Hellemans J, Vantrappen G. Physiology. In: Van Trappen G, Hellemans J, eds. *Diseases of the esophagus.* Berlin: Springer-Verlag, 1974:40–102.
10. Lamki L. Radionuclide esophageal transit (RET) study. The effect of body posture. *Clin Nucl Med* 1985;10:108–110.
11. Taillefer R, Beauchamp G. Radionuclide esophagogram. *Clin Nucl Med* 1984;9:465–483.
12. Klein HA, Wald A. Esophageal transit scintigraphy. In: Freeman LM, Weissmann HS, eds. *Nuclear medicine annual.* New York: Raven Press, 1988:79–124.
13. Ham HR, Georges B, Froideville JL et al. Oesophageal transit of liquid: effects of single or multiple swallows. *Nucl Med Commun* 1985;6:263–267.
14. Sand A, Ham H, Piepsz A. Oesophageal transit patterns in healthy subjects. *Nucl Med Commun* 1986;7:741–745.
15. Klein HA, Wald A. Normal variation in radionuclide esophageal transit studies. *Eur J Nucl Med* 1987;13:115–120.
16. Tatsch K, Schroettle W, Kirsch CM. Multiple swallow test for the quantitative and qualitative evaluation of esophageal motility disorders. *J Nucl Med* 1991;32:1365–1370.
17. Bartlett RJV, Parkin A, Ware FW et al. Reproducibility of oesophageal transit studies: several "single swallows" must be performed. *Nucl Med Commun* 1987;8:317–326.
18. Tolin RD, Malmud LS, Reilley J et al. Esophageal scintigraphy to quantitate esophageal transit (quantitation of esophageal transit). *Gastroenterology* 1979;76:1402–1408.
19. Kjellén G, Svedberg JB, Tibbling L. Computerized scintigraphy of oesophageal bolus transit in asthmatics. *Int J Nucl Med Biol* 1981;8:153–158.
20. Svedberg JB. The bolus transport diagram: a functional display method applied to oesophageal studies. *Clin Phys Physiol Meas* 1982;3:267–272.
21. Klein HA, Wald A. Computer analysis of radionuclide esophageal transit studies. *J Nucl Med* 1984;25:957–964.
22. Klein HA. Applications of condensed dynamic images. *Clin Nucl Med* 1986;11:178–182.
23. Tatsch K, Voderholzer WA, Weiss MJ et al. Simultaneous assessment of bolus transport and contraction parameters in multiple-swallow investigations. *J Nucl Med* 1992;33:1291–1300.
24. Roland J, Dhaenen H, Ham HR et al. Esophageal motility disorders in patients with psychiatric disease. *Eur J Nucl Med* 1996;31:131–135.
25. Brandt-Mainz K, von Mallek D, Pottgen C et al. Parametric oesophageal multiple swallow scintigraphy for validation of dysphageal symptoms during external beam irradiation of mediastinal tumours. *Eur J Nucl Med* 2001;28:313–319.
26. Russell COH, Hill LD, Holmes ER III et al. Radionuclide transit: a sensitive screening test for esophageal dysfunction. *Gastroenterology* 1981;80:887–892.
27. Kjellén G, Svedberg JB. Solid-bolus passage in patients with pathological oesophageal acid clearing. *Scand J Gastroenterol* 1983;18:183–187.
28. Llamas-Elvira JM, Martinez-Parades M, Sopena-Monforte R et al. Value of radionuclide oesophageal transit in studies of functional dysphagia. *Br J Radiol* 1986;59:1073–1078.
29. Mercer CD, Rue C, Hanelin L et al. Effect of obesity on esophageal transit. *Am J Surg* 1985;149:177–181.
30. O'Connor MK, Byrne PJ, Keeling P et al. Esophageal scintigraphy: applications and limitations in the study of esophageal disorders. *Eur J Nucl Med* 1988;14:131–136.
31. Rozen P, Gelfond M, Zaltzman S et al. Dynamic, diagnostic, and pharmacological radionuclide studies of the esophagus in achalasia: correlation with manometric measurements. *Radiology* 1982;144:587–590.
32. Holloway RH, Krosin G, Lange RC et al. Radionuclide esophageal emptying of a solid meal to quantitate results of therapy in achalasia. *Gastroenterology* 1983;84:771–776.
33. Blackwell JN, Hannan WJ, Adam RD et al. Radionuclide transit studies in the detection of oesophageal dysmotility. *Gut* 1983;24:421–426.
34. DeCaestecker JS, Blackwell JN, Adam RD et al. Clinical value of radionuclide oesophageal transit measurement. *Gut* 1986;27:659–666.
35. Benjamin SB, Gerhardt DC, Castell DO. High amplitude, peristaltic esophageal contractions associated with chest pain and/or dysphagia. *Gastroenterology* 1979;77:478–483.
36. Benjamin SB, O'Donnell JK, Hancock J et al. Prolonged radionuclide transit in "Nutcracker esophagus." *Dig Dis Sci* 1983;28:775–779.
37. Drane WE, Johnson DA, Hagan DP et al. "Nutcracker" esophagus: diagnosis with radionuclide esophageal scintigraphy versus manometry. *Radiology* 1987;163:33–37.
38. Horowitz M, McNeil JD, Collins GJ et al. Abnormalities of gastric and esophageal emptying in polymyositis and dermatomyositis. *Gastroenterology* 1986;90:434–439.
39. Garg A, Prakash K, Gopinath PG et al. Radionuclide oesophageal transit time in progressive systemic sclerosis. *Indian J Med Res* 1984;79:110–113.
40. Carette S, Lacourciere Y, Lavoie S et al. Radionuclide esophageal transit in progressive systemic sclerosis. *J Rheumatol* 1985;12:478–481.
41. Davidson A, Russell C, Littlejohn GO. Assessment of esophageal abnormalities in progressive systemic sclerosis using radionuclide transit. *J Rheumatol* 1985;12:72–77.
42. Drane WE, Karvelis K, Johnson DA et al. Progressive systemic sclerosis: radionuclide esophageal scintigraphy and manometry. *Radiology* 1986;160:73–76.
43. Akesson A, Gustafson T, Wollheim F et al. Esophageal dysfunction and radionuclide transit in progressive systemic sclerosis. *Scand J Rheumatol* 1987;16:291–299.

44. Lundell L, Myers JC, Jamieson GG. Is motility impaired in the entire upper gastrointestinal tract in patients with gastro-oesophageal reflux disease? *Scand J Gastroenterol* 1996;31:131–135.
45. Russell CO, Gannan FR, Coatsworth J et al. Relationship among esophageal dysfunction, diabetic gastroenteropathy, and peripheral neuropathy. *Dig Dis Sci* 1983;28:289–293.
46. Hep A, Vanaskova E, Tosnerova V et al. Radionuclide oesophageal transit scintigraphy—a useful method for verification of oesophageal dysmotility by cervical vertebropathy. *Eur J Nucl Med* 2001;28:313–319.
47. Fisher RS, Malmud LS, Roberts GS et al. Gastroesophageal (GE) scintiscanning to detect and quantitate GE reflux. *Gastroenterology* 1976;70:301–308.
48. Malmud LS, Fisher RS. Quantitation of gastroesophageal reflux before and after therapy using the gastroesophageal scintiscan. *South Med J* 1978;71(Suppl 1):10–15.
49. Devos PG, Forget P, DeRoo M et al. Scintigraphic evaluation of gastroesophageal reflux (GER) in children. *J Nucl Med* 1979;20:636.
50. Malmud LS, Charkes ND, Littlefield J et al. The mode of action of alginic acid compound in the reduction of gastroesophageal reflux. *J Nucl Med* 1979;20:1023–1028.
51. Menin RA, Malmud LS, Petersen RP et al. Gastroesophageal scintigraphy to assess the severity of gastroesophageal reflux disease. *Ann Surg* 1980;191:66–71.
52. Malmud LS, Fisher RS. The evaluation of gastroesophageal reflux before and after medical therapies. *Semin Nuc Med* 1981;11:205–215.
53. Malmud LS, Fisher RS. Radionuclide studies of esophageal transit and gastroesophageal reflux. *Semin Nucl Med* 1982;12:104–115.
54. Malmud LS, Fisher RS. Scintigraphic evaluation of gastroesophageal reflux. In: Wahner HW, ed. *Nuclear medicine: quantitative procedures.* Boston: Little, Brown and Company, 1983:147–170.
55. Hillemeier AC, Lange R, McCallum RW. Delayed gastric emptying in infants with gastroesophageal reflux. *J Pediatr* 1981;98:190–193.
56. DiLorenzo C, Piepz A, Ham A et al. Gastric emptying with gastroesophageal reflux. *Arch Dis Child* 1987;62:449–453.
57. Leape LL, Holder TM, Franklin JD et al. Respiratory arrest in infants secondary to gastroesophageal reflux. *Pediatrics* 1977;60:924–928.
58. Herbst JJ, Book LS, Bray PF. Gastroesophageal reflux in the "near miss" sudden infant death syndrome. *J Pediatr* 1978;92:73–75.
59. Davis MV. Relationship between pulmonary disease, hiatal hernia and gastroesophageal reflux. *NYS J Med* 1972;72:935–938.
60. Euler AP, Byrne WJ, Ament ME et al. Recurrent pulmonary disease in children: a complication of gastroesophageal reflux. *Pediatrics* 1979;63:47–51.
61. Foglia RP, Fonkalsrud EW, Ament ME et al. Gastroesophageal fundoplication for the management of chronic pulmonary disease in children. *Am J Surg* 1980;140:72–77.
62. Ghaed N, Stein MR. Assessment of a technique for scintigraphic monitoring of pulmonary aspiration of gastric contents in asthmatics with gastroesophageal reflux. *Ann Allergy* 1979;42:306–308.
63. Collins PJ, Horowitz M, Cook DJ et al. Gastric emptying in normal subjects: a reproducible technique using a single scintillation camera and computer system. *Gut* 1983;24:1117–1125.
64. Smith JL, Jiang CL, Hunt JN. Intrinsic emptying pattern of the human stomach. *Am J Physiol* 1984;246:R959–R962.
65. McHugh PR, Moran TH. Calories and gastric emptying: a regulatory capacity with implications for feeding. *Am J Physiol* 1979;236(5):R254–R260.
66. Loo FD, Palmer DW, Soergel KH et al. Gastric emptying in patients with diabetes mellitus. *Gastroenterology* 1984;86:485–494.
67. Hunt JN. The site of receptors slowing gastric emptying in response to starch in test meals. *J Physiol* 1960;134:270–276.
68. Hunt JN, Knox MTA. A relation between the chain length of fatty acids and the slowing of gastric emptying. *J Physiol* 1968;194:327–336.
69. Burn-Murdoch RA, Fisher MA, Hunt JN. The slowing of gastric emptying by proteins in test meals. *J Physiol* 1978;274:477–483.
70. Gulsrud PO, Taylor IL, Watts HD et al. How gastric emptying affects glucose tolerance and symptoms after truncal vagotomy with pyloroplasty. *Gastroenterology* 1980;78:1463–1471.
71. Brener W, Hendrix TR, McHugh PR. Regulation of the gastric emptying of glucose. *Gastroenterology* 1983;85:76–82.
72. Moore JG, Christian PE, Coleman RE. Gastric emptying of varying meal weight and composition in man. Evaluation by dual liquid and solid phase isotopic method. *Dig Dis Sci* 1981;26:16–22.
73. Urbain JL, Siegel JA, Mortelmans L et al. Effect of solid-meal caloric content on gastric emptying kinetics of solids and liquids. *Nuklear Medizin* 1989;28:120–123.
74. Moore JG, Christian PE, Brown JA et al. Influence of meal weight and caloric content on gastric emptying of meals in man. *Dig Dis Sci* 1984;29:513–519.
75. Heading RC, Tothill P, McLoughlin GP et al. Gastric emptying rate measurement in man. A double isotope scanning technique for simultaneous study of liquid and solid component of a meal. *Gastroenterology* 1976;71:45–50.
76. Meyer JH. Motility of the stomach and gastroduodenal junction. In: Johnson LR, ed. *Physiology of the gastrointestinal tract.* New York: Raven Press, 1987:613–629.
77. Keinke O, Ehrlein HJ. Effect of oleic acid on canine gastroduodenal motility, pyloric diameter and gastric emptying. *Q J Exp Physiol* 1983;68:675–686.
78. Cortot A, Phillips SF, Malagelada J-R. Parallel gastric emptying of nonhydrolyzable fat and water after a solid-liquid meal in humans. *Gastroenterology* 1982;82:877–881.
79. Jian R, Vigneron N, Najean Y et al. Gastric emptying and intragastric distribution of lipids in man. A new scintigraphic method of study. *Dig Dis Sci* 1982;27:705–711.
80. Goo RH, Moore JG, Greenberg E et al. Circadian variation in gastric emptying of meals in man. *Gastroenterology* 1987;93:515–518.
81. Trout DL, King SA, Bernstein PA et al. Circadian variation in the gastric emptying response to eating in rats previously fed once or twice daily. *Chronobiol Int* 1991;8:14–24.
82. Johnson RD, Horowitz M, Maddox AF et al. Cigarette smoking and rate of gastric emptying: effect on alcohol absorption. *Br Med J* 1991;302:20–23.
83. Griffith GH, Owen GM, Kirkman S et al. Measurement of rate of gastric emptying using chromium-51. *Lancet* 1966;1:1244–1245.
84. Meyer JH, MacGregor IL, Gueller R et al. ^{99m}Tc-tagged chicken liver as a marker of solid food in the human stomach. *Am J Dig Dis* 1976;21:296–304.
85. Knight LC, Malmud LS. Tc-99m-ovalbumin labeled eggs: comparison with other solid food markers *in vitro. J Nucl Med* 1981;22:P28.
86. Knight LC, Fisher RS, Malmud LS. Comparison of solid food markers in gastric emptying studies. In: *Nuclear medicine and biology advances: proceedings of the Third World Congress of nuclear medicine and biology.* Paris, New York: Pergamon Press, 1982:2407–2410(3).
87. Urbain J-LC, Siegel JA, Charkes ND et al. The two-component stomach: effects of meal particle size on fundal and antral emptying. *Eur J Nucl Med* 1989;15:254–259.
88. Urbain J-LC, VanDenMaegdenbergh V, Siegel JA et al. The dual phase gastric emptying: is labeling of liquid useful? *Eur J Nucl Med* 1989;8:A532–533.
89. Guo JP, Maurer AH, Fisher RS et al. Extending gastric emptying scintigraphy from two to four hours detects more patients with gastroparesis. *Dig Dis Sci* 2001;46:24–29.
90. Tothill P, McLoughlin GP, Heading RC. Techniques and errors in scintigraphic measurements of gastric emptying. *J Nucl Med* 1978;19:256–261.
91. Tothill P, McLoughlin GP, Holt S et al. The effect of posture on errors in gastric emptying measurements. *Phys Med Biol* 1980;25:1071–1077.
92. Christian PE, Moore JG, Sorenson JA et al. Effects of meal size and correction technique on gastric emptying time: studies with two tracers and opposed detectors. *J Nucl Med* 1980;21:883–885.
93. Moore JG, Christian PE, Taylor AT et al. Gastric emptying measurements: delayed and complex emptying patterns without appropriate correction. *J Nucl Med* 1985;26:1206–1210.
94. Collins PJ, Horowitz M, Shearman DJC et al. Correction for tissue attenuation in radionuclide gastric emptying studies: a comparison of a lateral image method and a geometric mean method. *Br J Radiol* 1984;57:689–695.

95. Fahey FH, Ziessman HA, Collen MJ et al. Left anterior oblique projection and peak-to-scatter ratio for attenuation compensation of gastric emptying studies. *J Nucl Med* 1989;30:233–239.

96. Roland J, Dobbeleir A, Ham HR et al. Continuous anterior acquisitions in gastric emptying: comparison with the mean. *Clin Nucl Med* 1989;14:881–884.

97. Maurer AH, Knight LC, Krevsky B. Proper definitions for lag phase in gastric emptying of solid foods. *J Nucl Med* 1992;33:466–467.

98. Meyer JH, VanDeventer G, Graham LS et al. Error and corrections with scintigraphic measurement of gastric emptying of solid foods. *J Nucl Med* 1983;24:197–203.

99. Urbain J-LC, Vekemans M-C, Bouillon R et al. Characterization of gastric antral motility disturbances in diabetes using the scintigraphic technique. *J Nucl Med* 1993;34:576–581.

100. Urbain J-LC, et al. Characterization of gastric emptying pathophysiology in idiopathic dyspepsia using scintigraphy. *J Nucl Med* 1993;34:10P.

101. Urbain J-LC, Vekemans MC, Parkman H et al. Evaluation of the effect of gastrokinetic compounds on antral motor activity and gastric emptying using the radiogastrogram technique. *J Nucl Med* 1994;35:A684.

102. Urbain J-LC, Vekemans MC, Parkman H et al. Characterization of gastric antral motility in functional dyspepsia using digital antral scintigraphy. *J Nucl Med* 1995,36:1579–1586.

103. Elashoff JD, Reedy TJ, Meyer JH. Analysis of gastric emptying data. *Gastroenterology* 1982;83:1306–1312.

104. Siegel JA, Wu RK, Knight LC et al. Radiation dose estimates for oral agents used in upper gastrointestinal disease. *J Nucl Med* 1983;24:835–837.

105. Urbain J-LC, VanCutsem E, Siegel JA et al. Visualization and characterization of gastric contractions using a radionuclide technique. *Am J Physiol* 1990;259:G1062–G1067.

106. Linke R, Muenzing W, Hahn K et al. Evaluation of gastric motility by Fourier analysis of condensed images. *Eur J Nucl Med* 2000;27:1531–1537.

107. Chaudhuri TK, Greenwald AJ, Heading RC et al. A new radioisotopic technic for the measurement of gastric emptying time of solid meal. *Am J Gastroenterol* 1976;65:46–51.

108. Scarpello JHB, Barber DC, Hague RV et al. Gastric emptying of solid meals in diabetics. *Br Med J* 1976;2:671–673.

109. Carryer PW, Brown ML, Malagelada J-R et al. Quantification of the fate of dietary fibers in humans by a newly developed radiolabeled fiber marker. *Gastroenterology* 1982;82:1389–1394.

110. Brophy CM, Moore JG, Christian PE et al. Variability of gastric emptying measurements in man employing standardized radiolabeled meals. *Dig Dis Sci* 1986;31:799–806.

111. Campbell IW, Heading RC, Tothill P et al. Gastric emptying in diabetic autonomic neuropathy. *Gut* 1977;18:462–467.

112. Fox S, Behar J. Pathogenesis of diabetic gastroparesis: a pharmacologic study. *Gastroenterology* 1980;78:757–763.

113. Malagelada J-R, Rees WDW, Mazzotta LJ et al. Gastric motor abnormalities in diabetic and postvagotomy gastroparesis: effect of metoclopramide and bethanechol. *Gastroenterology* 1980;78:286–293.

114. Horowitz M, Maddox A, Harding PE et al. Effect of cisapride on gastric and esophageal emptying in insulin-dependent diabetes mellitus. *Gastroenterology* 1987;92:1899–1907.

115. Urbain J-LC, Vantrappen G, Janssens J et al. Intravenous erythromycin dramatically accelerates gastric emptying in gastroparesis diabeticorum and normals and abolishes the emptying discrimination between solids and liquids. *J Nucl Med* 1990;31:1490–1493.

116. Urbain J-LC, Siegel JA, Buysschaert M et al. Characterization of the early pathophysiology of diabetic gastroparesis. *Dig Dis Sci* 1987;32:930(A31).

117. Wright RA, Clemente R, Wathen R. Diabetic gastroparesis: an abnormality of gastric emptying of solids. *Am J Med Sci* 1985;289:240–242.

118. Horowitz M, Harding PE, Maddox A. Gastric and esophageal emptying in insulin-dependent diabetes mellitus. *J Gastroenterol Hepatol* 1986;1:97–113.

119. Phillips WT, Schwartz JG, McMahan CA. Rapid gastric emptying in patients with early non-insulin dependent diabetes mellitus. *N Engl J Med* 1991;324:130–131.

120. Fischer H, Heidemann T, Hengst K et al. Disturbed gastric motility and pancreatic hormone release in diabetes mellitus. *J Physiol Pharmacol* 1998;49:529–541.

121. Narducci F, Bassotti G, Granata MT et al. Functional dyspepsia and chronic idiopathic gastric stasis. Role of endogenous opiates. *Arch Int Med* 1986;146:716–720.

122. Kerlin P. Postprandial antral hypomotility in patients with idiopathic nausea and vomiting. *Gut* 1989;30:54–59.

123. Malagelada JR. Where do we stand on gastric motility? *Scand J Gastroenterol* 1991;175P:42–51.

124. McCallum RW, Grill BB, Lange RC et al. Definition of a gastric emptying abnormality in patients with anorexia nervosa. *Dig Dis Sci* 1985;30:713–722.

125. Halvorsen L, Dotevall G, Walan A. Gastric emptying in patients with achlorhydria or hyposecretion of hydrochloric acid. *Scand J Gastroenterol* 1973;8:395–399.

126. Frank EB, Lange R, McCallum RW. Abnormal gastric emptying in patients with atrophic gastritis with or without pernicious anemia. *Gastroenterology* 1981;80:1151.

127. McCallum RW, Berkowitz DM, Lerner E. Gastric emptying in patients with gastroesophageal reflux. *Gastroenterology* 1981;80:285–291.

128. Holloway RH, Hongo M, Berger K et al. Gastric distention: a mechanism for postprandial gastroesophageal reflux. *Gastroenterology* 1985;89:779–784.

129. Behar J, Ramsby G. Gastric emptying and antral motility in reflux esophagitis. *Gastroenterology* 1978;74:253–256.

130. Csendes A, Henriquez A. Gastric emptying in patients with reflux esophagitis or benign strictures of the esophagus secondary to reflux compared to controls. *Scand J Gastroenterol* 1978;13:205–207.

131. Maddern GJ, Chaterton BE, Collins PJ et al. Solid and liquid gastric emptying in patients with gastro-oesophageal reflux. *Br J Surg* 1985;72:344–347.

132. Rock E, Malmud L, Fisher RS. Motor disorders of the stomach. *Med Clin North Am* 1981;65:1269–1289.

133. Minami H, McCallum RW. The physiology and pathophysiology of gastric emptying in humans. *Gastroenterology* 1984;86:1592–1610.

134. Lin DS. Abnormal rates of gastric emptying. *Semin Nucl Med* 1985;15:70–71.

135. Parkman HP, Urbain J-LC, Knight LC et al. Effect of gastric acid suppressants on human gastric motility. *Gut* 1998;42:243–250.

136. Mistiaen W, VanHee R, Blockx P et al. Gastric emptying for solids in patients with duodenal ulcer before and after highly selective vagotomy. *Dig Dis Sci* 1990;35:310–316.

137. Fordtran JS, Walsh JH. Gastric acid secretion rate and buffer content of the stomach after eating. Results in normal subjects and in patients with duodenal ulcer. *J Clin Invest* 1973;52:645–657.

138. Geurts WJC, Winckers EKA, Wittebol P. The effects of highly selective vagotomy on secretion and emptying of the stomach. *Surgery* 1977;145:826–836.

139. Rotter JI, Rubin R, Meyer JH. Rapid gastric emptying—an inherited physiologic defect in duodenal ulcer. *Gastroenterology* 1979;76:1229(abst).

140. Parr NJ, Grime S, Critchley M et al. Abnormal pattern of gastric emptying of liquid in chronic duodenal ulcer. *Digestion* 1988;40:237–243.

141. George JD. Gastric acidity and motility. *Am J Dig Dis* 1968;13:376–383.

142. Cobb JS, Bank S, Marks IN. Gastric emptying after vagotomy and pyloroplasty: relation to some postoperative sequelae. *Am J Dig Dis* 1971;16:207–215.

143. Dubois A, VanEerdewegh P, Gardner JD. Gastric emptying and secretion in Zollinger-Ellison syndrome. *J Clin Invest* 1977;59:255–263.

144. Harrison A, Ippoliti A, Cullison R. Rapid gastric emptying in Zollinger-Ellison syndrome (ZES). *Gastroenterology* 1980;78:A1180(abst).

145. Peachey RD, Creamer B, Pierce JN. Sclerodermatous involvement of the stomach and small and large bowel. *Gut* 1969;10:285–292.

146. Neild PJ, Nijran KS, Yazaki E et al. Delayed gastric emptying in human immunodeficiency virus infection: correlation with symptoms, autonomic function, and intestinal motility. *Dig Dis Sci* 2000; 45:1491–1499.
147. Kahraman H, Kaya N, Demircali A et al. Gastric emptying time in patients with primary hypothyroidism. *Eur J Gastroenterol Hepatol* 1997;9:901–904.
148. Wilbur BG, Kelly KA. Effect of proximal gastric, complete gastric, and truncal vagotomy on canine gastric electric activity, motility and emptying. *Ann Surg* 1973;178:295–303.
149. Lavigne ME, Wiley ZD, Martin P et al. Gastric, pancreatic and biliary secretion and the rate of gastric emptying after parietal cell vagotomy. *Am J Surg* 1979;138:644–651.
150. Lopasso FP, BrunodeMello J, Meneguetti J et al. Study of gastric emptying in patients with duodenal ulcer before and after proximal gastric vagotomy. The use of solid and digestible particles labeled with Tc-99m. *Surg Gastroenterol* 1982;1:321–326.
151. Wilkinson AR, Johnston D. Effect of truncal, selective and highly selective vagotomy on gastric emptying and intestinal transit of food-barium meal in man. *Ann Surg* 1973;178:190–193.
152. Sheiner HJ, Quinlan MF, Thompson IJ. Gastric motility and emptying in normal and post-vagotomy subjects. *Gut* 1980;21:753–759.
153. Urbain J-LC, Penninckx F, Siegel JA et al. Effect of proximal vagotomy and Roux-en-Y diversion on gastric emptying kinetics in asymptomatic patients. *Clin Nucl Med* 1990;15:688–691.
154. Dragstedt LR, Schafer PW. Removal of the vagus innervation of the stomach in gastroduodenal ulcer. *Surgery* 1945;17:742–749.
155. Edwards LW, Herrington J. Vagotomy and gastroenterostomy—vagotomy and conservative gastrectomy: a comparative study. *Ann Surg* 1952;137:873–883.
156. Roman C, Gonella J. Extrinsic control of digestive tract motility. In: Johnson LR, ed. *Physiology of the gastrointestinal tract*. New York: Raven Press, 1981:289–334.
157. McKelvey STD. Gastric incontinence and postvagotomy diarrhoea. *Br J Surg* 1970;57:741–747.
158. Hinder RA, Horn BKP, Bremner CG. The volumetric measurement of gastric emptying and gastric secretion by a radioisotope method. *Dig Dis Sci* 1976;21:940–945.
159. Kelly KA. Effect of gastric surgery on gastric motility and emptying. In: Akkermans LMA, Johnson AG, Read NW, eds. *Gastric and gastro-duodenal motility*. East Sussex, UK: Praeger, 1984:241–262.
160. Meyer JH, Thomson JB, Cohen MB et al. Sieving of solid food by the canine stomach and sieving after gastric surgery. *Gastroenterology* 1979;76:804–813.
161. Wittebol P, Haarman HJ, Hoekstra A. Gastric emptying after gastric surgery. *Dig Surg* 1988;5:160–166.
162. Gustavsson S, Kelly KA. Effect of gastric and small bowel operations. In: Kummar D, Gustavsson S, eds. *Gastrointestinal motility*. London: John Wiley and Sons, 1988:291–310.
163. Hinder RA, San-Garde BA. Individual and combined roles of the pylorus and the antrum in the canine gastric emptying of a liquid and a digestible solid. *Gastroenterology* 1983;84:281–286.
164. Vogel SB, Vair DB, Woodward ER. Alterations in gastrointestinal emptying of 99m-Technetium labeled solids following sequential antrectomy, truncal vagotomy and Roux-en-Y gastroenterostomy. *Ann Surg* 1983;198:506–515.
165. Pasma FG, Akkermans LMA, Oei HY. Gastric emptying in asymptomatic partial gastrectomy (BII) patients. In: Roman C, ed. *Gastrointestinal motility: proceedings of the 9th International Symposium on gastrointestinal motility*. Lancaster: MTP Press, 1984:143–148.
166. Dozois RR, Kelly KA, Code CF. Effect of distal antrectomy on gastric emptying of liquids and solids. *Gastroenterology* 1971;61:675–681.
167. Yamagishi T, Debas HT. Control of gastric emptying: interaction of the vagus and pyloric antrum. *Ann Surg* 1978;187:91–94.
168. MacGregor IL, Martin P, Meyer JH. Gastric emptying of solid food in normal man and after subtotal gastrectomy and truncal vagotomy with pyloroplasty. *Gastroenterology* 1977;72:206–211.
169. Hocking MP, Vogel SB, Falasca CA et al. Delayed gastric emptying of liquids and solids following Roux-en-Y biliary diversion. *Ann Surg* 1981;194:494–501.
170. Mannell A, Hinder RA, Sun-Garde DA. The thoracic stomach: a study of gastric emptying, bile reflux and mucosal change. *Br J Surg* 1984;71:438–441.
171. Hölscher AH, Voit H, Buttermann G et al. Function of the intrathoracic stomach as esophageal replacement. *World J Surg* 1988;12:835–844.
172. Borst HG, Dragojevic D, Stegmann T et al. Anastomotic leakage, stenosis, and reflux after esophageal replacement. *World J Surg* 1978;2:861–866.
173. Pichlmaier H, Müller JM, Wintzer G. Oesophagusersatz. *Chirurg* 1978;49:65–71.
174. Skinner DB. Invited commentary to complications following esophageal resection. *World J Surg* 1978;2:865–866.
175. Hancock BD, Bowen-Jones E, Dixon R et al. The effect of metoclopramide on gastric emptying of solid meals. *Gut* 1974;15:462–467.
176. Metzger WH, Cano R, Sturdevant RAL. Effect of metoclopramide in chronic gastric retention after gastric surgery. *Gastroenterology* 1976;71:30–32.
177. Snape WJ, Battle WM, Schwartz SS et al. Metoclopramide to treat gastroparesis due to diabetes mellitus. A double-blind, controlled trial. *Ann Int Med* 1982;96:444–446.
178. McCallum RW, Ricci DA, Rakatansky H et al. A multicenter placebo-controlled clinical trial of oral metoclopramide in diabetic gastroparesis. *Diabetes Care* 1983;6:463–467.
179. Horowitz M, Harding PE, Chatterton BE et al. Acute and chronic effects of domperidone on gastric emptying in diabetes autonomic neuropathy. *Dig Dis Sci* 1985;30:1–9.
180. Urbain J-LC, Siegel JA, Debie N et al. Effect of Cisapride on gastric emptying in dyspeptic patients. *Dig Dis Sci* 1988;33:779–783.
181. Urbain J-LC, Bouillon M, Muls E et al. Effect of long-term oral erythromycin on gastric emptying and blood glucose control in patients with diabetic gastroparesis. *J Nucl Med* 1991;32:931.
182. Kondo Y, Torii K, Omura S et al. Erythromycin and its derivatives with motilin-like biological activities inhibit the specific binding of ^{125}I-motilin to duodenal muscle. *Bioch Biophys Res Commun* 1988;150:877–882.
183. Depoortere I, Peeters TL, Matthijs G et al. Macrolide antibiotics are motilin receptor agonists. *Hepato-Gastroenterol* 1988;35:198.
184. Peeters T, Matthijs G, Depoortere I et al. Erythromycin is a motilin receptor agonist. *Am J Physiol* 1989;257:G470–G474.
185. Itoh Z, Honda R, Hiwatashi K et al. Motilin-induced mechanical activity in the canine alimentary tract. *Scand J Gastroenterol* 1976;11(Suppl 39):93–110.
186. Itoh Z, Nakaya M, Suzuki T et al. Erythromycin mimics exogenous motilin in gastrointestinal contractile activity in the dog. *Am J Physiol* 1984;247:G688–G694.
187. Zara GP, Thompson HH, Pilot MA et al. Effects of erythromycin on gastrointestinal tract motility. *J Antimicrob Chemother* 1985;16:A175–A179.
188. Tomomasa T, Kuroume T, Arai H et al. Erythromycin induces migrating motor complex in human gastrointestinal tract. *Dig Dis Sci* 1986;31:157–161.
189. Annese V, Janssens J, Vantrappen G. Erythromycin accelerates gastric emptying by inducing antral contractions and improving antroduodenal coordination. *Gastroenterology* 1992;102:823–828.
190. Peeters TL, Muls E, Janssens J et al. Effect of motilin on gastric emptying in patients with diabetic gastroparesis. *Gastroenterology* 1992;102:97–101.

Diagnostic Nuclear Medicine, Fourth Edition. Edited by M.P. Sandler, R.E. Coleman, J.A. Patton, F.J.Th. Wackers, A. Gottschalk. Lippincott Williams & Wilkins, Philadelphia 2003.

25

CHOLESCINTIGRAPHY: CORRELATION WITH OTHER HEPATOBILIARY IMAGING MODALITIES

HARVEY A. ZIESSMAN
ROBERT K. ZEMAN
ESMA A. AKIN

Cholescintigraphy with ^{99m}Tc-iminodiacetic acid (IDA) radio-pharmaceuticals is a valuable hepatobiliary imaging method that stands independently on its own merits. However, it is important to understand the relationship of cholescintigraphy to anatomic biliary imaging methods. Choosing the first of several noninvasive tests for optimal evaluation of a sick patient is a common clinical dilemma. Other times, the best single test for a given clinical setting must be selected. If multiple tests have already been performed, the various results must be correlated and apparent discordant information explained. This can be accomplished by understanding the strengths and limitations of the various available modalities. This chapter focuses on the interrelationship between cholescintigraphy and other biliary imaging techniques (1).

ACUTE CHOLECYSTITIS

Acute Calculous Cholecystitis

Cholescintigraphy has had its greatest diagnostic impact in the patient with suspected acute cholecystitis (1–8) (Fig. 25.1). The magnitude of the problem is highlighted by the fact that cholelithiasis is the most common single indication for abdominal surgery in North America (9). The surgeon and internist are faced with many tests in the evaluation of suspected acute cholecystitis. Although the combination of steady colicky pain, increased leukocyte count, and fever represent a typical triad of symptoms, diagnostic error rates approaching 20% have been reported when

H.A. Ziessman: Department of Radiology, Division of Nuclear Medicine, Georgetown University Hospital, Washington, DC.
R.K. Zeman: Department of Radiology, George Washington University School of Medicine and Radiology, George Washington University Hospital, Washington, DC.
E.A. Akin: Department of Radiology, George Washington University School of Medicine, and Division of Nuclear Medicine, George Washington University Hospital, Washington, DC.

cholecystectomy is performed based solely on clinical findings (10,11). Although the role of early cholecystectomy is controversial, early diagnosis is essential to make informed therapeutic decisions (12,13). Complications such as gallbladder perforation, bile leakage, or pericholecystic abscesses, must be detected early. Their presence is often life threatening and will influence the surgeon's choice between open and laparoscopic cholecystectomy (14–16).

Before the advent of cholescintigraphy and ultrasonography, intravenous cholangiography was the only noninvasive procedure that could determine patency or obstruction of the cystic duct. Indeterminate results were frequent, approaching 40% in some series (17,18), and were especially likely when serum bilirubin was 2 to 4 mg/dL. False-positive results with failure of gallbladder visualization in the absence of biliary disease were commonplace (19). Hepatorenal side effects and serious contrast reactions too often resulted (20).

Cholelithiasis and acute cholecystitis are intimately related. Acute cholecystitis is associated with gallstones in more than 90% of cases. Real-time ultrasonography is the screening examination of choice for the detection of cholelithiasis, with a sensitivity and specificity in excess of 90% (21–29). It is far more sensitive in the detection of small stones (<5 mm) than oral cholecystography (OCG) (30). Cholelithiasis has a varied sonographic spectrum. A discrete echogenic focus within the gallbladder that shadows and moves to dependent position predicts the presence of gallstones in 98% of cases. A contracted shadowing gallbladder ("double-arc sign") and multiple small stones casting confluent shadows ("gravel") are also highly predictive of cholelithiasis (31,32).

Sludge or viscous bile differs in appearance from stones and can appear echogenic but does not cast an acoustic shadow. Sludge moves slowly along the dependent gallbladder wall with changing patient position. Its detection per se does not imply the presence of discrete calculi within the gallbladder, but it does represent lithogenic bile (33,34). Patients with chronic understimulation of the gallbladder, e.g., hyperalimentation, will often

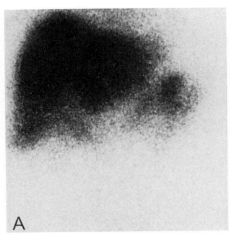 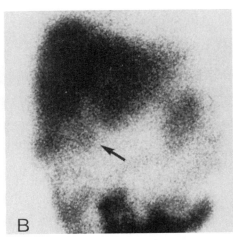 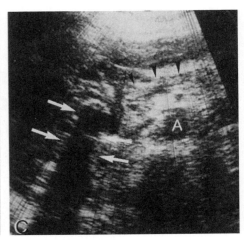

FIGURE 25.1. Acute cholecystitis. **A:** ^{99m}Tc-iminodiacetic acid (IDA) scintigraphy, 45-minute image. The gallbladder has failed to visualize. **B:** ^{99}Tc-IDA scintigraphy 4-hour image. Persistent failure of gallbladder visualization compatible with acute cholecystitis is present. The *arrow* indicates the gallbladder fossa. **C:** Sonogram, transverse scan. Marked shadowing (*arrows*) is seen extending from the gallbladder fossa. The gallbladder itself is not visualized. The pancreas is well demonstrated (*arrowheads*). (*A* = aorta.)

develop sludge. If not treated with periodic cholecystokinin (CCK) injections, sludge can progress to stones.

The sonographic criteria for acute cholecystitis are more complex than for cholelithiasis. Many sonographic findings have been reported as useful in the detection of acute cholecystitis (35–43): cholelithiasis, gallbladder distension, gallbladder wall thickening, intramural sonolucency, sludge, and maximum tenderness over the gallbladder (sonographic Murphy's sign) (37). Stones, intramural sonolucency, and the sonographic Murphy's sign are required to make the diagnosis of acute cholecystitis. Using these composite criteria, accuracy for the detection of acute cholecystitis has been reported to rival that of cholescintigraphy (43). However, relying on a single or less specific sonographic finding is not reliable (37).

A new sonographic criterion of acute cholecystitis has recently been suggested (44). Increased blood flow on power Doppler scans suggests the presence of hyperemia resulting from acute inflammation. In the past, color-flow ultrasound was not sufficiently sensitive to detect subtle increases in flow, but power Doppler can. This finding may be added to the composite sonographic criteria for acute cholecystitis and enhance the accuracy of ultrasound.

The presence of stones, even in the setting of suspected acute cholecystitis, is not by itself a specific indicator of acute inflammation. Although most patients with acute cholecystitis will have gallstones, so do 10% of men and 20% of women older than 55 years of age (45). Causes for false-positive examinations include shadowing from adjacent bowel gas or apparent shadowing from acoustic artifacts at the gallbladder neck. False-negative sonographic examinations may occur because of the tomographic nature of the technique and are particularly a problem in the gallbladder neck (ampullary pouch), which may not be imaged when it resides high in the porta hepatis.

Intramural lucency or hypoechoicity, is the second important criteria and has proven to be a reasonable indicator of acute

inflammation (Fig. 25.2). Sonolucency is truly intramural and represents subserosal edema (42). The area of lucency may be focal or continuous and circumferentially involve the gallbladder. Focal inflammation and the presence of striate lucency ("striped" appearance) are more specific for acute inflammation than a single, diffuse layer of edema (46,47). The latter as well as wall thickening without lucency has been reported in hepatitis, ascites, hypoalbuminemia, and other diseases, because of edema or lymphatic obstruction.

The sonographic Murphy's sign is reported to be quite accurate in one series, as high as 88%, in distinguishing acute cholecystitis from chronic cholecystitis or nongallbladder pathology (37). However, there are many pitfalls related to its use. It requires a cooperative, communicative patient who has not received recent analgesia. The differentiation of focal from diffuse pain is sometimes not straightforward. Laing et al. (37) found the overall sensitivity (94%) and specificity (85%) of sonography not quite as high as radionuclide imaging but close. Others have had similar experience (43). There have been few direct comparisons between ultrasound and cholescintigraphy. In those studies, cholescintigraphy had greater accuracy (6,48,49).

Gallbladder distension greater than 5 cm in anteroposterior diameter is abnormal (38) and can occasionally be present in acute cholecystitis. However, distension is neither a specific or reliable indicator of acute cholecystitis (38). Conditions associated with the lack of stimulation to gallbladder emptying, e.g., prolonged fasting, postoperative conditions, postvagotomy, partial biliary obstruction, and various metabolic disorders, may result in increased gallbladder size. With stasis, the gallbladder may retain sludge or static bile, which may not be a result of inflammation and is not a reliable indicator of acute cholecystitis. Gallbladder wall thickening without intramural sonolucency is also not specific for acute gallbladder inflammation (39–41).

Cholescintigraphy is the best single test with the clearest criterion for the diagnosis of acute cholecystitis (6,43,48–51). Failure of gallbladder visualization in the presence of normal hepatic

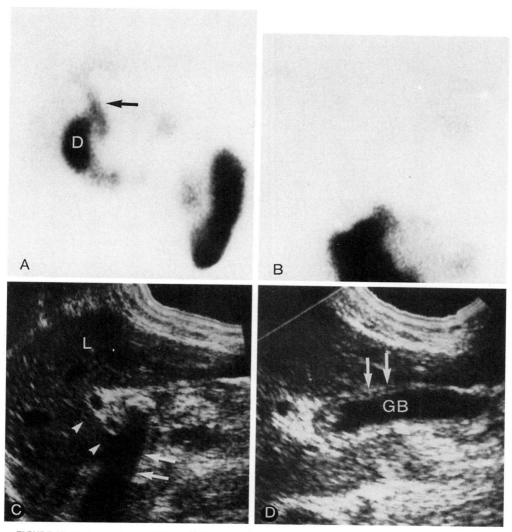

FIGURE 25.2. Acute cholecystitis. **A:** ^{99m}Tc-iminodiacetic acid (IDA) scintigraphy, 1-hour oblique image. The common bile duct (*arrow*) and duodenum (*D*) are identified, but the gallbladder is not visualized. **B:** ^{99m}Tc-IDA scintigraphy, 2-hour image. Persistent failure of gallbladder visualization is noted, suggesting the diagnosis of acute cholecystitis. **C:** Sonogram, sagittal scan. Dense shadowing is seen (*arrows*) from a large calculus in the gallbladder neck. The main and left portal vein branch (*arrowheads*) are also seen. *L*, liver. **D:** Sonogram, sagittal scan. A thin band of sonolucency (*arrows*) suggesting intramural edema is present and compatible with the inflammation of acute cholecystitis. (*GB* = gallbladder.) (From Zeman RK, Burrell MI. Gallbladder and bile duct imaging: a clinical radiologic approach. New York: Churchill Livingstone, 1987, with permission.)

uptake and biliary excretion reliably indicates cystic duct obstruction and acute cholecystitis, whereas normal gallbladder visualization almost always excludes the disease. False-positive scans may occur in patients who have experienced prolonged fasting or on total parenteral nutrition (Fig. 25.3), and are presumably related to bile stasis within the gallbladder preventing radiotracer entry. The use of CCK to preempty the gallbladder and morphine-augmented cholescintigraphy have reduced the frequency of false-positive studies (52).

Cholescintigraphy can differentiate the pain of low-grade biliary obstruction from acute or chronic cholecystitis (53) (Fig. 25.4). Obstruction may coexist in patients with acute cholecystitis because of passage of small stones into the bile duct or because

of the Mirizzi syndrome (fistulous tract between the cystic and common hepatic ducts and/or edema of the common hepatic duct). Obstruction by small stones may not result in sonographic evidence of biliary dilation. Scintigraphy can detect delayed biliary excretion of radiotracer before the development of anatomic findings and may suggest the need for endoscopic retrograde cholangiopancreatography (ERCP) before cholecystectomy if there are signs of high-grade biliary obstruction (53). Before laparoscopic intraoperative cholangiography and ERCP, retained stones were difficult to assess and treat. With current equipment and skills, it is straightforward to detect stones on intraoperative cholangiograms and to perform ERCP and mechanical lithotripsy (postcholecystectomy) to extract retained

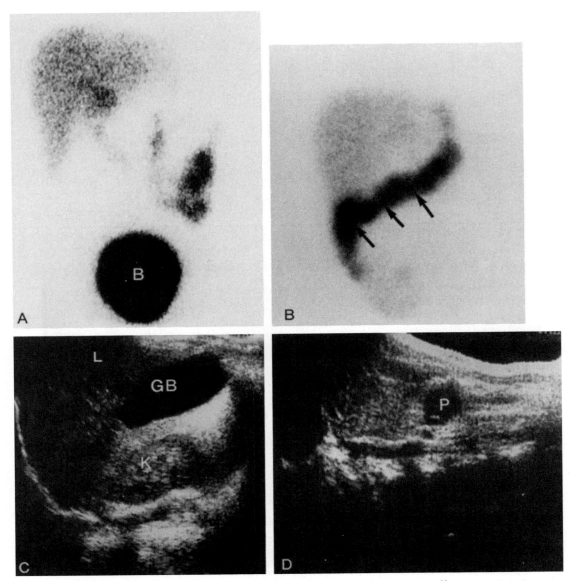

FIGURE 25.3. Traumatic pancreatitis causing failure of gallbladder visualization. **A:** ^{99m}Tc-iminodiacetic acid (IDA) scintigraphy, 4-hour image. Uptake is not identified within the gallbladder. *B*, bladder. **B:** ^{99m}Tc-IDA scintigraphy, 24-hour image. Persistent gallbladder nonvisualization is noted. Much activity is identified within the colon (*arrows*). **C:** Sonogram, oblique scan. The gallbladder (*GB*) is markedly distended. *K*, kidney; *L*, liver. **D:** Sonogram, sagittal scan. The pancreas (*P*) is enlarged and sonolucent, suggestive of acute pancreatitis. This was operatively confirmed. The gallbladder was distended. Cholecystectomy was performed but no evidence of gallbladder disease was ultimately found. Presumably this represents a rare occurrence of false-positive cholescintigraphy resulting from pancreatitis. (From Zeman RK, Burrell MI. Gallbladder and bile duct imaging: a clinical radiologic approach. New York: Churchill Livingstone, 1987, with permission.)

stones. Thus, it is now unusual to perform cholescintigraphy as a primary test to diagnose biliary obstruction pre-operatively. Obstruction is more likely seen as an incidental finding on scintigrams performed for acute cholecystitis.

Acute Acalculous Cholecystitis

Acute acalculous cholecystitis is a life-threatening illness occurring in hospitalized patients with extensive burns, multiple traumatic injuries, shock, or sepsis. It is associated with a high mor-

bidity and mortality because of its often atypical presentation. Mechanisms for acute acalculous cholecystitis include cystic duct obstruction from inflammatory debris, edema, and inspissated bile, or direct inflammation of the gallbladder wall by infection, ischemia, or toxins.

Inflammation limited to the gallbladder wall, but with cystic duct patency, could result in a false-negative cholescintigraphic study. Case reports and one published study have suggested an increased false-negative rate for the diagnosis of acute acalculous cholecystitis (54). However, critical analysis of that paper and

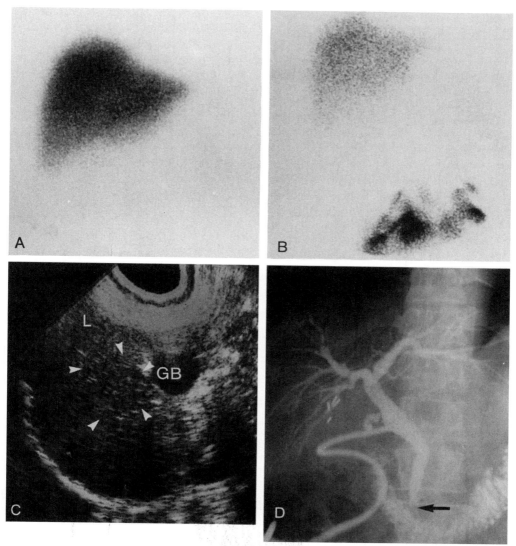

FIGURE 25.4. Acute common bile duct obstruction with minimal bile duct dilatation. This patient presented with pain but no clinical evidence of jaundice. **A:** ^{99m}Tc-iminodiacetic acid (IDA) scintigraphy, 6-hour image. Total obstruction is present with no evidence of intestinal activity. **B:** ^{99m}Tc-IDA scintigraphy, 24-hour image. Intestinal activity is present with some residual liver uptake. **C:** Sonogram, sagittal scan. Subtle intrahepatic biliary dilatation (*arrowheads*) is present, suggestive of mild obstruction. *GB*, gallbladder; *L*, liver. **D:** Immediate postoperative cholangiogram. A small stone causing biliary obstruction is seen lodged at the ampullar (*arrow*).

many subsequent studies have shown an overall good sensitivity for cholescintigraphy for the diagnosis of acute acalculous cholescintigraphy (>90%) (54–60). However, this is slightly lower than reported with the calculous form of the disease (95% to 98%). If the clinical suspicion is high and a false-negative study suspected (gallbladder filling), CCK can be helpful. Good contraction of the gallbladder rules out cholecystitis. Poor contraction would be consistent with either acute or chronic acalculous cholecystitis.

Prolonged fasting, parenteral nutrition, and concomitant serious illnesses all increase the incidence of a false-positive studies for acute cholecystitis (gallbladder nonvisualization) (61–63). These factors are very likely to be present in patients suspected of having acute acalculous cholecystitis. To minimize this potential

problem, CCK should be infused before starting a cholescintigraphic study in patients fasting for greater than 24 hours to empty the gallbladder of viscous concentrated bile that might prevent radiotracer entry. However, CCK may be ineffective in patients with chronic cholecystitis, in other diseases associated with gallbladder dysfunction, and for patients on various therapeutic drugs that inhibit gallbladder contraction (Table 25.1).

Other scintigraphic findings can increase diagnostic certainty that gallbladder nonvisualization is due to acute cholecystitis. Increased blood flow to the gallbladder fossa may be seen with acute cholecystitis (64). More commonly, increased pericholecystic hepatic uptake ("rim sign") is a very specific finding for acute cholecystitis and occurs when severe inflammatory or gangrenous changes are present (65,66). Finally, a radiolabeled leu-

Table 25.1. *Drugs and Diseases that Adversely Affect Gallbladder Contraction*

Drugs	Diseases
Morphine	Diabetes
Atropine	Pregnancy
Calcium blockers	Sprue
Octreotide	Achalasia
Progesterone and oral contraceptives	Irritable bowel syndrome
Indomethacin	Truncal vagotomy
Histamine$_2$ receptor agonists	Pancreatic insufficiency
Theophylline	Sickle cell disease
Glucagon	
Erythromycin	
Benzodiazepine	
Alcohol	

kocyte study can be performed. The white blood cells will localize in the inflamed gallbladder wall (67).

Sonography and/or computed tomography (CT) can be useful in confirming the diagnosis of acute cholecystitis. Findings suggestive of acute inflammation on sonography or CT, e.g., intramural lucency, increase the certainty that gallbladder nonvisualization on scintigraphy is due to acute cholecystitis. Ultrasound could be used for patients fasting greater than 24 hours, to demonstrate if the gallbladder indeed contracts when CCK is administered before the scintigraphic study. If the gallbladder does not contract, the patient is at increased risk for a false-positive study. On the other hand, a contracting gallbladder would be strong evidence against acute cholecystitis.

Recommendations

Both cholescintigraphy and sonography can be useful in the evaluation of acute cholecystitis. The choice depends largely on local and emergency availability, the clinical setting, and the type of information that is desired by the surgeon. The cost and technical expertise required to perform either sonography or hepatobiliary imaging are relatively comparable at most centers. Scintigraphy has somewhat greater overall accuracy than ultrasound and is the only technique that will confirm the pathophysiologic abnormality of cystic obstruction and gallbladder dysfunction. When the clinical index of suspicion for acute cholecystitis is high, scintigraphy should be used as the primary evaluation. It allows detection of acute cholecystitis and early or low-grade biliary obstruction in the absence of dilated ducts.

When the referring physician is uncertain of the diagnosis, sonography may be preferred because of its greater ability to detect non-gallbladder disease. Sonographic detection of cholelithiasis or other changes of chronic cholecystitis can be valuable in the patient with colic. A CT can be obtained in lieu of ultrasound in the setting of an acute abdomen or when gastrointestinal symptoms predominate over signs or symptoms of biliary disease.

Laparoscopic cholecystectomy is now a common surgical procedure not only for cholelithiasis but also for acute cholecystitis (68). Debate exists as to the value of early surgery versus surgery after inflammation has subsided. Although the latter appears

safer, there may be more adhesions, making the gallbladder more difficult to remove laparoscopically. Careful attention must be paid to recognition of complications of acute cholecystitis when reviewing cholescintigraphy and ultrasound images. Although some surgeons may approach gangrenous cholecystitis laparoscopically, the less experienced should opt for an open approach (Fig. 25.5). If gallbladder perforation, pericholecystic abscess, or gallbladder empyema is present, the open approach is also prudent (16). In a very toxic patient with acute cholecystitis, many surgeons will request ultrasound or CT in the face of positive scintigraphy to make certain that a pericholecystic abscess is not present. Evidence of low-grade biliary duct obstruction on cholescintigraphy or dilated ducts on ultrasound should result in an intraoperative cholangiogram or postoperative ERCP to exclude stones. The radiologist, nuclear physician, and surgeon must develop a relationship that recognizes each other's strengths and limitations.

CHRONIC CHOLECYSTITIS

Conventional cholescintigraphy is usually normal in chronic cholecystitis. Scintigraphic findings associated with chronic cholecystitis include gallbladder filling defects, delayed gallbladder visualization, delayed biliary-to-bowel transit, or rarely nonfilling of the gallbladder. However, these findings are uncommon and nonspecific (< 5%). Ultrasound's high sensitivity for gallstone detection makes it the study of choice for the diagnosis of chronic cholecystitis.

Patients with symptomatic chronic cholecystitis have poorly contracting gallbladders in response to a fatty meal or CCK, whereas patients with asymptomatic cholelithiasis usually have gallbladders that contract normally (69). In some cases, a surgeon may suspect that a patient's pain and cholelithiasis are not related. CCK cholescintigraphy can be useful in this setting. Patients with cholelithiasis and related biliary colic will have reduced gallbladder contractility.

Chronic Acalculous Cholecystitis

Evaluation of gallbladder contraction has proven most useful in the diagnosis of chronic *acalculous* cholecystitis. The acalculous form of chronic cholecystitis has been referred to in the medical literature by various names, including acalculous biliary disease, gallbladder dyskinesia, and gallbladder spasm. The patient's symptomatology and gallbladder histopathology are identical to that seen with the calculous form of the disease, except for the absence of stones. Because the imaging diagnosis of chronic cholecystitis relies heavily on the finding of cholelithiasis by ultrasound or OCG, surgeons are reluctant to operate without objective confirmation of disease. CCK-stimulated cholescintigraphy allows that confirmation.

Early investigations attempted to diagnose chronic acalculous cholecystitis with fatty meal or CCK-stimulated OCG but had mixed clinical results (70–74), likely resulting from the different CCK infusion methodologies used and the subjective methods for estimating gallbladder contraction. In the early 1980s, investigators began using cholescintigraphy (75). Many published in-

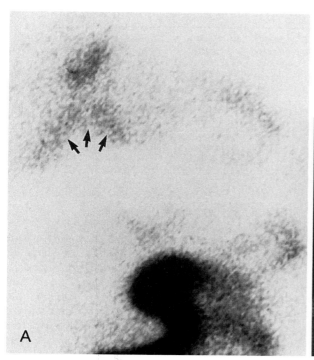

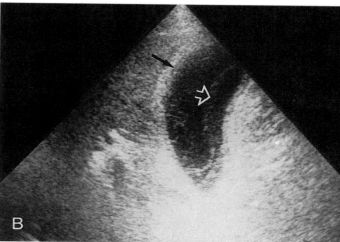

FIGURE 25.5. Gangrenous cholecystitis. **A:** ^{99m}Tc-iminodiacetic acid scintigraphy, 2-hour view shows a rim of increased tracer activity where the liver abuts the superior edge of the gallbladder (*arrows*). This finding is very suggestive of gangrenous cholecystitis with perihepatitis. **B:** Oblique sonogram shows gallbladder wall sonolucency (*arrow*) and an echogenic band protruding into the gallbladder lumen (*open arrow*). The latter is characteristic of sloughed gallbladder mucosa and occurs in patients with severe inflammation such as in gangrenous cholecystitis.

vestigations have since found CCK cholescintigraphy accurate for confirming or excluding the clinical diagnosis of chronic acalculous cholecystitis (75–83). Although most are retrospective, a particularly convincing prospective randomized study was reported by Yap et al. (78). They investigated 103 patients suspected of having the disease. Patients with a low gallbladder ejection fraction (GBEF) (<40%) were randomized into one of two groups, cholecystectomy or medical treatment. After follow-up of 13 to 54 months (mean 34), 91% of cholecystectomized patients had resolution of their symptoms and all but one showed histopathologic evidence of chronic cholecystitis. All medically treated patients continued to be symptomatic.

Although a fatty meal might be considered more physiologic than infusing CCK, the results are dependent on the adequacy of gastric emptying and the duodenal release of endogenous CCK. CCK infusion takes less time, is more reproducible, and easily standardized.

In the reported investigations (76–83), patients had been well worked up, other diseases were excluded, and the patients were followed clinically for months to years before CCK cholescintigraphy. The diagnosis of chronic acalculous cholecystitis should not be made in patients without adequate workup or follow-up or in the wrong clinical setting, e.g., during an acute illness. Many acute and chronic diseases, as well as drugs, can adversely affect gallbladder function (Table 25.1).

Proper methodology for CCK infusion is critical when evaluating gallbladder function. Bolus infusions of CCK cause spasm of the gallbladder neck and result in poor contraction. Short infusions of 1 to 3 minutes can produce similar results. One third of normal subjects have poor gallbladder contraction with a 1- to 3-minute infusion of sincalide (Kinevac), 0.01 to 0.02 µg/kg, but have normal contraction with a 30- to 60-minute infusion (84,85). Normal GBEF values are very dependent on the method of infusion. Importantly, clinically useful normal values cannot be established for 1- to 3-minute infusions because of the wide variability of individual response, however, normal values have been established for a 30- to 60-minute infusion (78,84,85) (Table 25.2). Finally, 1- to 3-minute infusions result in adverse symptoms of abdominal cramping and nausea in up to 50% of subjects, whereas the longer infusions do not cause the adverse symptoms (84,86).

Attempts have been made to use sonography in a manner similar to CCK cholescintigraphy (87,88). These studies show fair correlation between the two techniques. Reproducibility and accuracy is better with cholescintigraphy (69,70,89,90). Physiologically, different parameters are being measured. Sonography uses geometric assumptions to calculate an absolute gallbladder volume; cholescintigraphy uses radiotracer methodology to quantify relative volume changes. The radionuclide method is generally considered the method of choice. Unlike sonography, CCK cholescintigraphy is not operator-dependent and acquisition is continuous, is easily standardized, and has superior accuracy. One retrospective study reported that real-time ultrasound predicted histologic changes of chronic cholecystitis in 62% of

Table 25.2. *Normal Values for CCK Cholescintigraphy*

Reference	Dose	Infusion Length	Number of Subjects	Normal Values	Normals with GBEF <35%
Recommended methods					
84	0.02 μg/kg	30 min	23	>30%	2/23 (9%)
78	0.02 μg/kg/h	45 min[a]	40	>40%	0/40 (0%)
85	0.01 μg/kg/h	45 min	20	>33%	1/20 (5%)
85	0.01 μg/kg/h	60 min	20	>40%	1/20 (5%)
Methods not recommended					
84	0.02 μg/kg	3 min	23	>0%	8/23 (35%)
85	0.01 μg/kg	3 min	20	>17%	6/20 (30%)

Note: CCK, Cholecystokinin; GBEF, gallbladder ejection fraction.
[a]Computer acquired and quantified at 60 min.

patients with chronic acalculous cholecystitis, considerably poorer than the 89% predicted by scintigraphy (70).

MEDICAL VERSUS SURGICAL JAUNDICE

Jaundice represents a single and rather late-occurring manifestation of biliary obstruction. Other laboratory parameters, e.g., elevation of the serum alkaline phosphatase, usually occur earlier in the natural history of biliary obstruction and may be more specific for that diagnosis. In general, patients presenting with cholangitis and colicky pain often have benign causes of biliary obstruction such as choledocholithiasis or benign biliary strictures. Clinical and laboratory parameters often allow the physician to discern patients with medical jaundice from those with surgical jaundice. However, in many cases, this differentiation is not possible, and noninvasive imaging modalities are then useful to increase the likelihood of making the correct diagnosis.

Cholescintigraphy has achieved some success for evaluation of possible biliary obstruction (53,91–100). However, its some-

what limited use stems from a disappointing early experience with ^{99m}Tc dimethyl-IDA acid (HIDA) (3,96), which offered only slight advantage over intravenous cholangiographic agents for assessing common duct obstruction versus patency in the presence of jaundice. HIDA was not useful at serum bilirubin values in excess of 5 mg/dL. However, ^{99m}Tc disofenin (diisopropyl-IDA) and ^{99m}Tc mebrofenin (bromotrimethyl-IDA), the radiopharmaceuticals used today, have high hepatic extraction (90% and 98%), allowing biliary visualization at serum bilirubin levels of 20 mg/dL or higher (98–103) and thus compete favorably with other biliary imaging modalities in the jaundiced patient. Before these tracers, the diagnosis of biliary obstruction depended solely on the presence of dilated ducts detected by noninvasive cross-sectional techniques such as CT or sonography, followed by a confirmatory invasive test such as ERCP or percutaneous transhepatic cholangiography (PTC) (104,105).

Ultrasonography

In suspected biliary obstruction, most patients are screened with real-time ultrasonography. Biliary anatomy can be well defined.

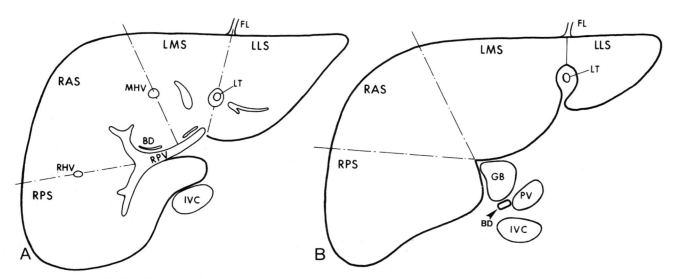

FIGURE 25.6. Normal sonographic biliary anatomy. Sagittal sonogram demonstrates the common bile duct (*BD, curved arrow*) diving posteriorly toward the inferior vena cava (*IVC*). The duct lies just anterior to the portal vein (*PV*). This is an important, relatively constant relationship. (*L* = liver.)

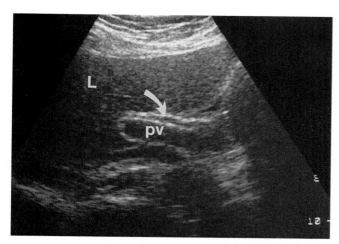

FIGURE 25.7. Normal common hepatic duct shows a normal caliber common hepatic duct (*curved arrow*). The duct normally passes directly anterior to the right portal vein (*pv*). This view has become the standard view that is used to measure the common hepatic duct size and should be part of every biliary sonogram. (*L* = liver.)

The normal intrahepatic biliary tree is composed of many barely visible 1-mm peripheral biliary ductules (106,107) that converge on centrally larger ducts, joining in the porta hepatis (hepatoduodenal ligament). The anatomy of this area has complex three-dimensional (3D) relationships and variability (108–115) (Fig. 25.6). Generally, the common hepatic duct lies anterior and lateral to the portal vein. The right hepatic artery usually passes behind the right hepatic duct but occasionally passes anterior to it (116). By "tracing out" the bile duct, in the right anterior oblique position (117,118), it can be seen diving posteriorly from the hepatoduodenal ligament into the pancreatic substance as it passes caudally (Fig. 25.7). The normal-sized bile duct is seen in up to 96% of patients (118).

The traditional criterion for the diagnosis of biliary obstruction is intrahepatic and extrahepatic biliary dilatation (119) (Fig.

25.8). Dilated intrahepatic ducts appear as multiple fluid-filled parallel channels or as stellate branching structures surrounded by the normally homogeneous hepatic parenchyma (120–122). Dilated ducts are differentiated from vessels by following their pattern of convergence. Biliary radicles also have greater through transmission and acoustic enhancement than their vascular counterparts (123). Doppler and color-flow imaging should show no signal from bile ducts and a continuous venous signal from portal vein branches. The upper limits of normal for the common hepatic duct size is now considered to be 6 mm, regardless of the presence or surgical absence of the gallbladder (124–128).

Dilation of the extrahepatic biliary ducts is easily identified (Fig. 25.9). There are potential pitfalls related to the use of biliary dilatation as the sole criterion for the diagnosis of obstruction. Dilation is most prevalent in obstruction of several days duration or greater and especially occurs secondary to malignant etiologies (129). Ducts may not be dilated in early obstruction. Although the degree of dilatation is not directly proportional to the serum bilirubin level, the largest dilated ducts tend to occur in deeply jaundiced patients (130). Several series have shown that benign causes of low-grade obstruction often do not cause significant dilatation of the biliary tract (53,131,132). Depending on patient selection, sonographic sensitivities for the diagnosis of biliary obstruction have ranged from 80% to 99% (121,122,125,129,130,133). Sonography can also provide information regarding the level and nature of an obstructing process in most instances (121,122,130,133–137) (Fig. 25.9). The type of pathology causing obstruction will influence the accuracy of sonography; a large pancreatic mass is much easier to see than a small intraluminal common duct stone. Ultrasound may also be used to assist in guidance for percutaneous decompression of the biliary tract.

CCK or a fatty meal in conjunction with ultrasonography has been used to evaluate the borderline or marginally dilated bile duct (138,139). This technique can result in a quasifunc-

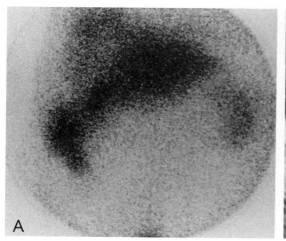 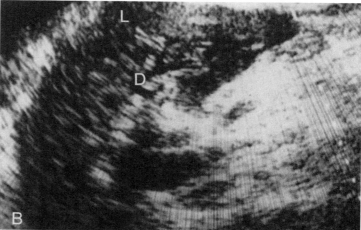

FIGURE 25.8. Klatskin tumor (cholangiocarcinoma) producing biliary obstruction. The patient was deeply jaundiced. **A:** 99mTc-iminodiacetic acid (IDA) scintigraphy, 4-hour image. Total obstruction is present. There is no biliary excretion **B:** Sonogram, oblique scan. Intrahepatic biliary dilatation is present. Note the stellate appearance of dilated ducts (*D*). *L* = liver. (*Figure continues.*)

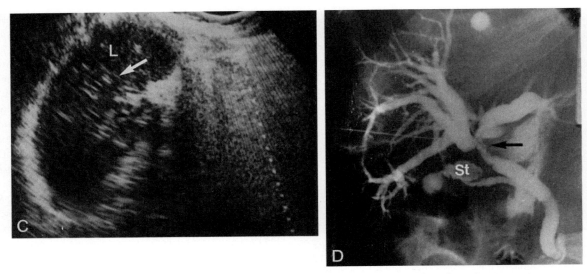

FIGURE 25.8. *Continued.* **C:** Sonogram, transverse scan. Sonography in another plane demonstrates the parallel channel appearance of dilated ducts (*arrows*). *L* = liver. **D:** Percutaneous transhepatic cholangiogram. A focal structure at the bifurcation (*arrow*) compatible with cholangiocarcinoma is causing obstruction of the right and left hepatic ducts. Incidentally noted is a stone (*St*) in the neck of the gallbladder.

tional evaluation. CCK stimulates bile flow, causes gallbladder contraction, and relaxes the sphincter of Oddi. The normal bile duct responds to a fatty meal or CCK by remaining the same or decreasing in size. If there is no obstruction, the duct should not dilate from the increased bile flow. When partial obstruction is present, the normal-sized or borderline duct will dilate. "Stressing" the biliary tract in this manner has improved the reliability of using ductal dilatation as a criterion of partial biliary obstruction in several series (138,139).

Computed Tomography

Many of the concepts regarding sonography also apply to CT evaluation of the biliary tract. Since the advent of helical (spiral) techniques, CT has improved dramatically for assessing pancreatic and biliary disorders (140,141). With CT, normal intrahepatic bile ducts are seldom visualized but the normal extrahepatic biliary tree is seen in almost 95% of cases (142,143) (Fig. 25.10). Intravenous contrast to opacify the major arterial and

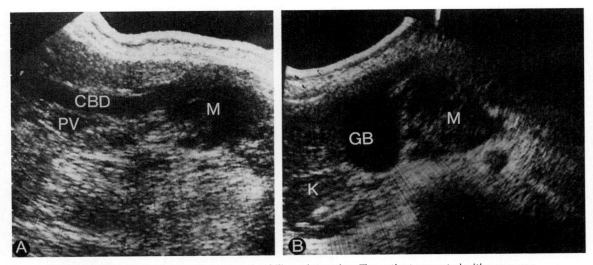

FIGURE 25.9. Pancreatic carcinoma causing biliary obstruction. The patient presented with vague constitutional symptoms but was not yet jaundiced at the time of imaging. **A:** Sonogram, oblique scan. A dilated common bile duct (*CBD*) is seen entering a large mass (*M*) in the head of the pancreas. *PV* = portal vein. **B:** Sonogram, transverse scan. Again noted is the large pancreatic mass (*M*) next to a moderately distended gallbladder (*GB*). (*K* = kidney.) (From Zeman RK, Taylor KJW, Burrell MI et al. Ultrasound demonstration of anicteric dilatation of the biliary tree. *Radiology* 1980;134:689, with permission.)

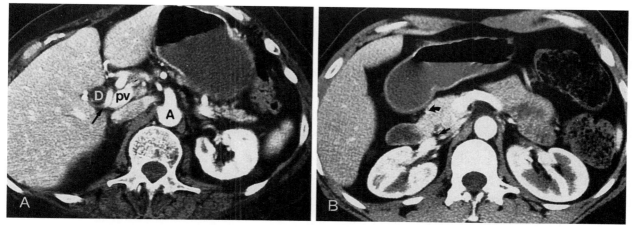

FIGURE 25.10. Computed tomography (CT) of the common hepatic duct and common bile duct. **A:** Contrast-enhanced CT scan shows a mildly dilated common hepatic duct (*D*) just anterior to the hepatic artery (*arrow*) and right portal vein (*pv*). *A* = aorta. **B:** This contrast-enhanced CT scan is obtained several centimeters caudad to that in **A.** The common bile duct (*arrow*) has migrated posteriorly as it descends through the pancreatic substance. The gastroduodenal artery (*curved arrow*) can also be appreciated because of its contrast enhancement. The duct may be seen in over 95% of patients, even when it is of normal caliber.

venous branches is essential for evaluation of the biliary tract. The ducts do not enhance with contrast, but rather stand out as negative, tubular defects against the hepatic parenchyma. Usually 150 mL of 60% or its equivalent concentration of contrast is injected at a rate of 3 mL/second or higher. Opacification of the normal biliary tree using cholangiographic agents is also possible for visualizing biliary anatomy on helical CT (144), but is of limited value for seeing the ducts in the jaundiced patient (145,146). Although data is limited on the normal size for the biliary tree, the same numbers used for sonography are applicable

to CT (147). The inside ductal diameter is best measured in the anteroposterior dimension along a straight segment of duct to minimize measurement errors that arise when the duct turns transversely within a single section just below the porta hepatis.

Evidence suggests similar sensitivity and specificity in diagnosing biliary obstruction using sonography or CT (148—152). Both allow the level and nature of obstruction to be categorized in most, but not all, cases (Figs. 25.11 and 25.12). Pedrosa et al. (153,154), studied 69 patients with biliary obstruction with high-quality conventional CT and showed that the level of ob-

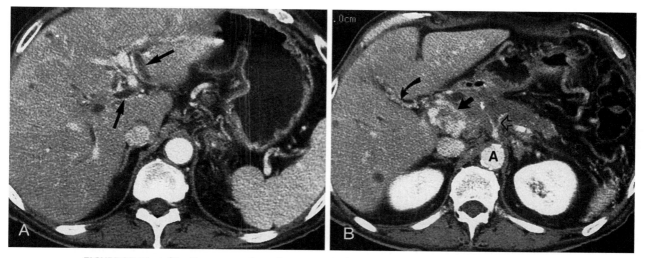

FIGURE 25.11. Infiltrative pancreatic carcinoma causing biliary obstruction. **A:** Contrast-enhanced computed tomography (CT) section through the liver shows dilated intrahepatic ducts (*arrows*). Because the ducts do not enhance with contrast, they appear as water density tubular structures. **B:** Enhanced CT section caudad to **A** shows diffuse, low-attenuation tumor replacing the pancreas. The celiac axis and its branches (*open arrow*) are encased by the tumor. The native portal vein exhibits cavernous transformation (*arrow*), and varices are present in the gallbladder fossa (*curved arrow*). The portal venous vascular changes have occurred because the portal vein was occluded by the tumor below this level. (*A* = aorta.)

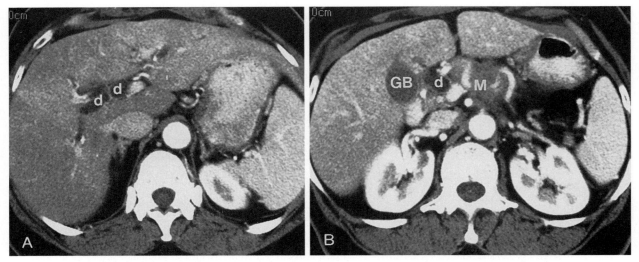

FIGURE 25.12. Pancreatic carcinoma causing biliary obstruction. **A:** Contrast-enhanced computed tomography (CT) scan obtained through the liver shows dilated intrahepatic ducts (*d*) indicative of biliary obstruction. **B:** Enhanced CT section several centimeters caudad to A displays a solid pancreatic mass (*M*) that is partially obstructing the hepatic and splenic arteries. The common bile duct (*d*) is also amputated by the mass. When vascular involvement is present as in this case, the tumor is not resectable. (*GB* = gallbladder.)

struction could be accurately determined in 97% of patients by counting the number of "rings" (cross sections obtained through the duct) extending below the porta hepatis and correlating this with anatomy of adjacent structures. By scrutinizing the appearance of the rings, intraluminal ductal contents, and the presence of any surrounding mass, the etiology of obstruction can be determined in up to 94% of patients. Baron (155) further refined these criteria and showed the importance of recognizing a subtle high-attenuation "bulls-eye" appearance in the duct as indicative of common bile duct (CBD) stones. Helical CT is a volumetric technique and slices can be reconstructed anywhere along the acquisition. This technique has improved the ability to detect small tumors and stones compared with conventional CT and allows creation of overlapping sections that may be used for 3D rendering of the vascular and biliary structures (156). CT following intravenous cholangiographic contrast or ERCP instillation of contrast is useful in selected cases (157).

Magnetic Resonance Imaging (MRI) and Magnetic Resonance Cholangiopancreatography (MRCP)

Conventional MRI is not currently used as a screening technique. It is extremely accurate at detecting malignant causes of biliary obstruction and rivals the detail of contrast-enhanced helical CT. It is generally reserved for assessing the pancreaticobiliary system in patients with allergies or renal dysfunction in whom iodinated contrast for CT is contraindicated (158,159).

MRCP, however, has become a widely available screening technique for the various etiologies of biliary obstruction, including stone disease. MRI can demonstrate dilated ducts as tubular structures with high signal on T2-weighted scans. Using gradient echo techniques, very rapid T2-weighted scans may now be obtained, which, when viewed in a coronal plane, mimic the ap-

pearance of a contrast cholangiogram (160). Most groups now use a two-dimensional (2D) or 3D fast spin-echo sequence that allow data acquisition during a single breath-hold.

One of the initial shortcomings of MRCP was its inability to accurately diagnose benign causes of biliary obstruction such as choledocholithiasis. The relative insensitivity of anatomic, noninvasive imaging techniques occurs because stones may be small and not produce significant ductal dilation. MRCP has become a highly accurate method for detecting choledocholithiasis. Sensitivities ranging from 89% to 93% and specificities of 90% to 99% have been reported (161,162). Stones appear as low signal-intensity filling defects surrounded by bright, high signal bile and can be seen regardless if dilatation is present or absent.

MRCP is sensitive for detecting the presence and level of biliary ductal obstruction in patients with malignant disease and is comparable to ERCP. (163) Clinically useful information regarding lesion characterization and staging can also be obtained by including a complete conventional precontrast and postcontrast MR study of the abdomen (164).

As on ERCP, neoplasms of the hepatic duct or biliary bifurcation (Klatskin tumor) produce an abrupt transition zone with dilatation of the bile ducts proximal to the obstruction (Fig. 25.13). If a hilar cholangiocarcinoma has isolated the right and left ductal system, it is unlikely to be resectable (164). Even if the ductal anatomy is conducive to resection, T1- and T2-weighted images after contrast administration are needed to accurately assess the lesion extent, detect hilar lymphadenopathy, and determine if vascular invasion is present.

The typical appearance on cholangiography of pancreatic head lesions is abrupt obstruction at the level of the head of the pancreas with the "double duct" sign because of biliary and pancreatic ductal dilatation and evidence of a mass in the head of the pancreas. On T1-weighted images, pancreatic tumors are

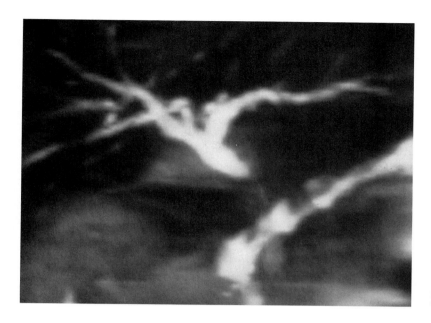

FIGURE 25.13. Magnetic resonance cholangiopancreatography of cholangiocarcinoma. T2-weighted turbo spin-echo image shows abrupt transition zone in the mid-common hepatic duct. The finding is suggestive of cholangiocarcinoma without involvement of the bifurcation.

hypointense relative to the surrounding parenchyma; lesion detection can be improved with fat-suppression techniques in which normal pancreas will be very bright compared with a pathologic process. (165). On dynamic gadolinium-enhanced studies, pancreatic adenocarcinoma enhances less than normal surrounding parenchyma. Distinguishing pancreatic cancer from focal chronic pancreatitis even with the inclusion of pancreatic T1- and T2-weighted images can be difficult. Although cancer more likely results in the double duct sign or a high-grade "rat-tailed" stricture than pancreatitis on MRCP, these signs are not infallible. Ultimately, biopsy will be needed to confirm the diagnosis. If cancer is proven, MRCP offers the advantage of staging the tumor because it will show the size of the mass, assess vascular encasement, and detect the hepatic metastases and the extent of lymph node involvement.

Ampullary carcinoma arising in the ampulla of Vater can mimic tumors of the head of the pancreas. It usually presents as a hypointense mass on T1-weighted images and involves both the CBD and pancreatic duct. One caveat is that small ampullary tumors might not be detected with MRCP; therefore, patients with suspected pancreaticobiliary disease but a normal MRCP should undergo ERCP because early detection is important because resection may be curative. (166)

MRCP is not a replacement for direct cholangiography; patients in need of intervention, such as biopsy or decompression of the bile ducts, still need to undergo these more invasive procedures. However, as a diagnostic modality, MRCP is comparable to ERCP and PTC for the detection of a variety of benign and malignant processes.

Contrast Cholangiography

PTC and ERCP have long been viewed as competitive procedures (167,168) and the only definitive way to diagnose biliary abnormalities (134). Both techniques allow conventional iodine-based radiographic contrast to be instilled into the biliary tree,

PTC by the antegrade route and ERCP by the retrograde route. The "skinny" 22-gauge Chiba needle is responsible for the success of PTC and its low complication rate (169–175). Fluoroscopic monitoring has allowed a virtually unrestricted number of needle passes and results in successful opacification of nearly 100% of dilated and nondilated bile ducts. This success rate represents a significant improvement over the early days of transhepatic cholangiography when relatively traumatic 16- and 18-gauge needles were used (176). ERCP likewise has evolved into a highly successful procedure, with less than 5% of cases concluding with inability to cannulate the relevant duct (177–181).

PTC and ERCP do not rely on intrahepatic or extrahepatic dilatation solely to make the diagnosis of obstruction. Greater emphasis is placed on the actual visualization of a pathologic obstructing process. Whether the biliary tree is studied from above or below, accurate diagnosis requires contrast material to be on both the proximal and distal sides of an obstructing lesion to fully categorize the intraluminal ductal appearance. Stones can occasionally mimic tumors and vice versa, if one does not adhere strictly to this rule. Both techniques may be used to guide subsequent biliary drainage procedures. Not only may catheters be placed in conjunction with PTC for establishing biliary drainage (182,183), but nasobiliary stents and internal biliary endoprostheses also may be placed via ERCP and the retrograde approach (184–186).

These invasive procedures have potential complications. PTC has a 3.4% reported complication rate in one multiinstitutional survey (187). Sepsis is a potentially life-threatening complication because of the creation of multiple biliary-venous fistulas at the time of needle and/or catheter introduction. ERCP has up to a 5% complication rate, largely stemming from endoscopic complications, as well as from contrast injection into the potentially obstructed biliary tree or pancreatic duct (188,189). ERCP requires greater technical expertise, specialized equipment, and greater expense to the patient. It is generally viewed as less traumatic because it does not involve traversing the liver parenchyma with needles. The relative merits, indications, and contraindications of the two techniques are beyond the scope of this chapter, but local expertise and availability often become the decisive factors.

Cholescintigraphy

With highly accurate noninvasive tomographic tests that provide information regarding the level and nature of obstruction and invasive tests that often precede heroic therapeutic procedures, what is the need for hepatobiliary scintigraphy? To a large extent, the need for scintigraphy is due to reliance on ductal dilatation as the only noninvasive indicator of obstruction. Patients with early, low-grade, or intermittent biliary obstruction may not demonstrate dilated ducts. Likewise, clinical and laboratory examinations in these patients may be unrewarding because obstruction in the absence of jaundice is a common occurrence (190–192). Thus, it is not surprising that there can be discord-

ance between the functional scintigraphic and the morphologic techniques, such as ultrasound or CT (193–198).

Discrepancy between the results of functional and anatomic imaging procedures was commonly seen in a study of 139 patients with suspected early or low-grade biliary obstruction (53). This study population was deliberately skewed to evaluate patients whose liver function tests were not conclusive or who had mild liver function abnormalities that when coupled with clinical symptoms were suggestive of biliary obstruction. Of 125 patients with a final diagnosis accurately established, 29 (23%) had discordant sonography and scintigraphy, i.e., one examination suggested biliary obstruction and the other did not. Thirteen patients had early obstruction (secondary to neoplasm) or low-grade obstruction (secondary to choledocholithiasis or benign strictures) (Figs. 25.4 and 25.14). These patients did not have sonographic evidence of ductal dilatation. Others have similarly reported that choledocholithiasis may not result in ductal dilatation (131,132). Abnormal biliary clearance of the radiopharma-

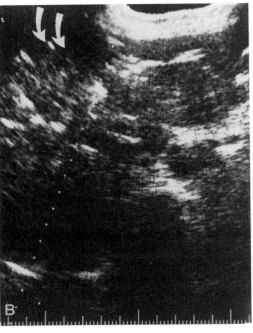

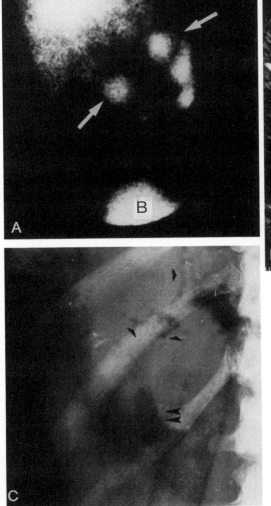

FIGURE 25.14. Refluxed biliary air following biliary bypass making sonographic evaluation of liver and biliary tree impossible. **A:** ^{99m}Tc-iminodiacetic acid scintigraphy, 40-minute image. Normal gut excretion is observed (*arrows*). On delayed views virtually no retained hepatobiliary activity was observed. *B* = bladder. **B:** Sonogram, transverse scan. Multiple echogenic foci, with irregular shadowing are scattered throughout the liver (*curved arrows*). This represents air within biliary ductules, making their assessment impossible. **C:** Plain film. Confirms the presence of air within the common duct (*double arrowheads*) and intrahepatic bile ducts (*single arrowheads*). (From Zeman RK, Lee C, Stahl RS et al. Ultrasonography and hepatobiliary scintigraphy in the assessment of biliary-enteric anastomoses. *Radiology* 1982;145:109–115, with permission.)

ceutical was demonstrated by cholescintigraphy in all 13 cases, indicating that functional abnormalities may precede morphologically evident disease. Seven additional patients demonstrated ductal dilation on sonography, yet had normal biliary clearance on scintigraphy. These patients all proved to have dilated bile ducts from prior common duct exploration or chronic passage of stones. Thus, functional and anatomic changes in the biliary tract clearly must be considered independent. Imaging discordance occurs in a significant number of patients.

The cholescintigraphic findings suggestive of obstruction deserve emphasis (53,199). Although delayed biliary-to-bowel transit is a common sign of partial common duct obstruction, it is neither sensitive nor specific. Approximately 20% of normal subjects have delayed biliary-to-bowel transit beyond 60 minutes. On the other hand, as many as 50% of patients with partial common duct obstruction have biliary-to-bowel transit by 60 minutes. The most important scintigraphic finding in partial common duct obstruction is delayed clearance of the common duct. Other findings commonly seen include segmental duct narrowing with prominent radiopharmaceutical retention above this site, persistent biliary pooling after delayed imaging or CCK infusion, and poor gallbladder contraction after CCK infusion (53,199).

Recommendations

Noninvasive anatomic procedures such as ultrasound or CT are the best initial screening procedures for most patients with suspected surgical jaundice. MRCP is rapidly gaining ground and is evolving into a primary screening technique. The presence of jaundice implies that the patient may be relatively late in the natural history of the obstructive process (147). With long-standing jaundice associated with weight loss, back pain, anemia, or other signs of chronicity, CT is often the first technique used to evaluate the patient. In this setting, pancreatic carcinoma is likely, and CT is better than ultrasound for tumor staging. The vast majority of patients with biliary dilatation detected in the presence of jaundice will have biliary obstruction.

Scintigraphy, however, should be considered in the patient whose symptoms are suggestive of biliary obstruction, but who is not clearly jaundiced and has only mild liver function abnormalities. In this setting, scintigraphy may show low-grade obstruction or segmental (focal) intrahepatic obstruction. The patient with suspected choledocholithiasis and colicky right upper quadrant pain may be a prime candidate for scintigraphy to distinguish the pain pattern resulting from choledocholithiasis from cholecystitis. The patient with prior bouts of jaundice or following common duct exploration in whom a dilated, atonic, but nonobstructed duct is suspected, also must be considered a candidate for cholescintigraphy. In these patients demonstration of normal drainage can avert needless, additional evaluation.

POSTOPERATIVE BILIARY TRACT
Biliary Diversion

Cholescintigraphy is very useful for evaluating the postoperative biliary tract, specifically following the creation of biliary-enteric

anastomoses. Evaluation of the acute and immediate complications of surgery, as well as long-term follow-up for biliary patency, is possible. Although percutaneous and retrograde drainage of the biliary tree has achieved considerable popularity, surgical diversion of the biliary tract remains an alternative in conjunction with curative resection of tumors or for benign strictures inaccessible by other methods (200–204).

There are many surgical techniques for biliary diversion. It is essential for those involved in imaging of the postoperative biliary tract understand the postoperative anatomy in each patient. Biliary scintigraphy can be helpful for all types of biliary-enteric anastomoses, but is most valuable in the evaluation of patients with prior choledochojejunostomy or intrahepatic cholangiojejunostomy (205,206). Choledochojejunostomy is a direct anastomosis of the extrahepatic portion of the CBD or common hepatic duct to a Roux-en-Y loop of jejunum. This procedure requires a long segment of nondiseased duct to be available for creation of a mucosa-to-mucosa anastomosis and is commonly used in liver transplants. The intrahepatic cholangiojejunostomy and its modifications is a more complex procedure, requiring direct anastomosis between small bowel and intrahepatic ducts, which must be dissected out individually from deep within the hepatic substance, usually the left lobe. This operation is traditionally reserved for those patients with little or no chance for the creation of a choledochojejunostomy because of stricture formation (benign or malignant) extending to involve the suprapancreatic CBD or the porta hepatis itself.

Other commonly performed procedures include choledochoduodenostomy, cholecysto-duodenostomy, and cholecystojejunostomy. The latter two procedures are still used frequently in benign disease states, but are now rarely used for the treatment of malignant strictures, especially pancreatic carcinoma, because of the likelihood of early tumor obstruction of the cystic duct.

Many complications may befall the postoperative patient after the creation of biliary diversion (207). Biliary leakage is among the most common immediate complications. Cholescintigraphy is well established in the detection of biliary leakage (208,209). Before percutaneous drainage of bilomas, cholescintigraphy can ensure that central biliary obstruction is not present. If it is present, percutaneous decompression would probably be ineffective. The major nonacute problem seen in the postoperative patient is symptoms and/or laboratory evidence suggesting recurrent obstruction. Unfortunately, the findings are often ambiguous in the patient who has had biliary obstruction previously relieved by diversion (210,211). Serum alkaline phosphatase is often persistently elevated even with a normal postoperative biliary tract (212). Likewise, cholangitis may occur for many reasons in the postoperative patient, especially in areas of segmental biliary obstruction not bypassed at the time of original surgery. Therefore, cholangitis may not necessarily represent recurrent or treatable obstruction.

Before biliary scintigraphy, sonography and invasive procedures, e.g., PTC or ERCP, were used to evaluate the postoperative biliary tract (210–212). Contrast cholangiography, the most direct and definitive method to evaluate the biliary tract, has limitations. If a long Roux-en-Y loop is created as part of the anastomosis, it may be impossible to reach the biliary tract via the retrograde endoscopic route. PTC can be used to visualize the biliary tree, but is an invasive procedure with associated morbidity. A role for the noninvasive study exists to establish which patients will benefit from cholangiography.

In the postoperative patient, sonography has received mixed reviews. Nondiagnostic examinations are frequent, occurring in up to 67% of patients (121), usually resulting from gas in the anastomotic bowel segment or refluxed biliary air (Fig. 25.15), a finding that does not guarantee biliary tract patency. Refluxed biliary air gives rise to spurious high-level echoes and shadowing within the liver, making it impossible to diagnose biliary dilatation. Furthermore, persistent biliary dilatation of the postbiliary diversion ducts may be present even when biliary obstruction has been adequately relieved by surgery. In one study, 5 of 23 patients had a persistently dilated biliary tree, yet did not have recurrent obstruction (206). Loss of bile duct tone and longstanding dilatation can be permanent, even if obstruction is later successfully relieved (213).

Cholescintigraphy is very accurate and has great clinical impact in the management of the postoperative patient (206,209, 214). However, there is debate over the merits of MRCP versus scintigraphy. Cholescintigraphy is the only noninvasive technique that can distinguish obstructed dilated ducts from those that are just persistently dilated (Fig. 25.16). MRCP has shown sensitivities and specificities of almost 100% in visualizing the postoperative stricture and detecting obstruction when new dilatation is present (215,216). We suggest the following approach to our surgeons. Baseline scintigraphy and sonography several weeks after surgery gives the greatest sensitivity for detecting future subtle changes in duct size or deterioration in biliary drainage. If the ducts remain dilated postoperatively, scintigraphy should be used for long-term follow-up. If the dilatation is associated with ongoing signs of obstruction and poor drainage on cholescintigraphy, further investigation with MRCP or invasive means is needed. If the patient's biliary tract decompresses

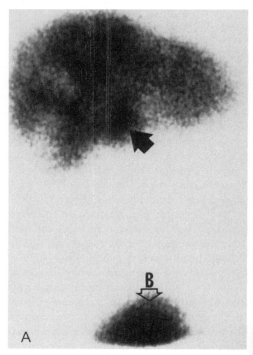
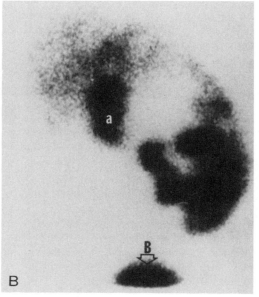
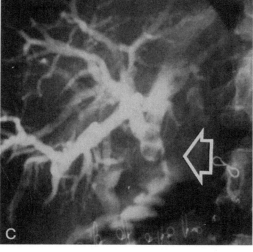
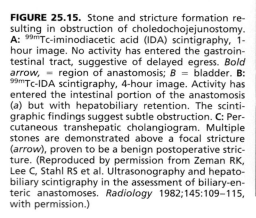

FIGURE 25.15. Stone and stricture formation resulting in obstruction of choledochojejunostomy. **A:** ⁹⁹ᵐTc-iminodiacetic acid (IDA) scintigraphy, 1-hour image. No activity has entered the gastrointestinal tract, suggestive of delayed egress. *Bold arrow,* = region of anastomosis; *B* = bladder. **B:** ⁹⁹ᵐTc-IDA scintigraphy, 4-hour image. Activity has entered the intestinal portion of the anastomosis (*a*) but with hepatobiliary retention. The scintigraphic findings suggest subtle obstruction. **C:** Percutaneous transhepatic cholangiogram. Multiple stones are demonstrated above a focal stricture (*arrow*), proven to be a benign postoperative stricture. (Reproduced by permission from Zeman RK, Lee C, Stahl RS et al. Ultrasonography and hepatobiliary scintigraphy in the assessment of biliary-enteric anastomoses. *Radiology* 1982;145:109–115, with permission.)

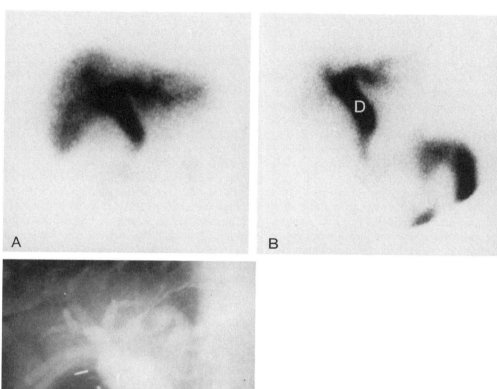

FIGURE 25.16. Postcholecystectomy syndrome in middle-aged female with recurrent abdominal pain following cholecystectomy. **A:** ^{99m}Tc-iminodi-acetic acid (IDA) scintigraphy, 1-hour image. There is marked retention of biliary activity and absence of intestinal visualization. **B:** ^{99m}Tc-IDA scintigraphy, 2-hour image. Persistent biliary activity is noted representing an extremely abnormal drainage pattern. *D* = common bile duct. **C:** Endoscopic retrograde cholangiopancreatogram. Marked dilatation of the common duct (*D*) and intrahepatic bile ducts is present. Delayed drainage of contrast was also noted. The patient obtained dramatic clinical improvement following endoscopic papillotomy.

back to normal size and is free of air, sonography can be used alone as a means for follow-up (217). If duct size is normal, but large amounts of biliary air are present, MRCP can be used for follow-up. Percutaneous transhepatic cholangiography may ultimately be needed to document the nature of an obstructing lesion, but by the proper use of scintigraphy, sonography, and MRCP many patients can be spared this invasive procedure.

Postcholecystectomy Syndrome

Evaluation of the postcholecystectomy biliary tract poses problems similar to those discussed for evaluation of jaundice and biliary diversion. Following cholecystectomy, recurrent abdominal pain or liver function abnormalities may result from many causes, e.g., common duct stricture, recurrent or retained common duct stones, stone formation in a prominent cystic duct, and sphincter of Oddi dysfunction (218–220). The postchole-

cystectomy patient also continues to be at risk for the many causes of biliary obstruction that plague the unoperated patient.

Sphincter of Oddi dysfunction is the cause for pain in 14% of patients with the postcholecystectomy pain syndrome (221). The pain is caused by a motility disorder of the papillary region resulting in either a fixed (papillary stenosis) or intermittent (biliary dyskinesia) partial obstruction, but without an obvious mechanical etiology, e.g., stricture or retained stone. The sphincter may show increased resting pressures or increased frequency or amplitude of phasic contractions on manometry. Biliary dyskinesia, in contrast to stenosis, may be responsive to sphincter relaxants, e.g., amyl nitrite or CCK. Proposed mechanisms for sphincter dysfunction include damage from prior passage of stones or traumatic duct exploration, although a congenital or development abnormality may be the cause in some patients. Treatment requires endoscopic sphincterotomy (222). Pharmacologic therapies are under investigation (223).

A clinical classification that emphasizes the wide spectrum of this disease is gaining acceptance (224). Type I patients have abnormal liver function studies, a dilated CBD, and slow drainage of contrast at ERCP. They likely have an organic structural alteration of the papillary region. Type II patients have only one or two of these features, whereas type III patients are those with suggestive pain, but normal duct diameter, drainage time, and liver chemistries. Type I patients are the easiest to diagnose and do not need scintigraphy or sphincter of Oddi manometry. Sphincter ablation is appropriate treatment. Type II and III patients require confirmatory scintigraphic or manometry to justify the risks of sphincter ablation (225).

Before 1970, exploratory laparotomy and inability to pass a Bakes dilator greater that 3 mm in diameter were the criteria used to establish the presence of sphincter of Oddi stenosis. Fiberoptic endoscopy and ERCP made it possible to determine whether a specific anatomic cause of biliary obstruction was present (224–226). In the presence of nonspecific dilatation of the bile duct on ERCP (no stone or fibrosis), delayed drainage of contrast material beyond 45 minutes is considered abnormal and suggestive, although nonspecific, for the diagnosis of sphincter stenosis (226). Endoscopic sphincter of Oddi manometry can document abnormal sphincter tone and dynamics and has become the gold standard (222,226). However, manometry requires technical expertise not widely available and is difficult to perform in many patients because narcotics cannot be given before or during cannulation. Manometry is also prone to subjective interpretative errors and its reproducibility has been questioned (227). Pancreatitis is a serious complication with a higher frequency than seen with diagnostic ERCP. A noninvasive alternative is desirable.

Although other manometric abnormalities in addition to elevation of basal sphincter pressure have been described with sphincter dysfunction, they are less reproducible. Only elevated basal pressure is associated with therapeutic benefit after papillotomy (222). A finding often described as characteristic of sphincter dysfunction is a "paradoxical" response to CCK, i.e., a rise rather than the expected fall in basal sphincter pressure. However, in all endoscopic and animal investigations, CCK has always been administered as a rapid intravenous infusion, a method known to cause spasm in normal individuals (228). When infused in a more physiologic manner as a slower infusion, this paradoxic response has not been seen (229,230).

Real-time ultrasound has been used for evaluating the postcholecystectomy biliary tract (126,127). Because sonography provides anatomic information, it depends on duct size to diagnose an abnormality. However, significant pathology may be present in the absence of significant ductal dilatation. Follow-up sonography is most beneficial if the prior bile duct diameter is known from surgery or baseline studies. Unfortunately, this is often not available.

Cholescintigraphy can have an important impact on the evaluation of the postcholecystectomy patient. The radionuclide method provides a physiologic assessment of duct drainage that correlates well with contrast washout from the biliary tract observed on ERCP (231,232). In a prospective study of 30 patients with the postcholecystectomy syndrome, qualitative image interpretation with ^{99m}Tc-IDA allowed detection of patients with anatomic causes of obstruction and sphincter of Oddi stenosis

(231). The most prevalent scintigraphic pattern was that of retention of ductal activity without evidence of washout by 2 hours after injection (Fig. 25.17). Delayed biliary-to-bowel transit was a less sensitive diagnostic criteria. Resolution of this abnormal pattern was seen in patients on follow-up studies after sphincterotomy.

Recent cholescintigraphic studies have used quantitative parameters of uptake and clearance to diagnose obstruction (229, 230,233–236). Regions-of-interest (ROIs) drawn on computer-acquired studies are used to generate time-activity curves from which quantitative parameters are derived (Fig. 25.18). Results have been generally good, with sensitivities between 83% to 100% and specificities of 81% to 85% (234,236,238,239). However, various ROIs (liver alone, liver with bile ducts, bile duct alone, liver hilum, etc.) and different quantitative parameters (T max, T 1/2, percent emptying at 45 and 60 minutes, etc.) have been recommended by investigators. Quantification has been particularly useful for confirming the effectiveness of therapy.

The diagnostic efficacy of quantitative cholescintigraphy and fatty meal sonography was evaluated in postcholecystectomy patients (203,230,237). Results were correlated with ERCP and manometry. The rationale for fatty meal sonography is that the CCK-induced increased bile flow through the common duct may unmask a partial obstruction by increasing common duct pressure and diameter proximal to the obstruction. In 56 patients, ^{99m}Tc-IDA and ultrasound had a 67% sensitivity; specificity was 85% for cholescintigraphy and 100% for sonography (230).

One report has shown excellent results with CCK-augmented cholescintigraphy for detecting sphincter of Oddi dysfunction in postcholecystectomy patients (238). Manometry was the standard. CCK was used to increase bile flow and stress the capacity of the bile ducts. They used a diagnostic semiquantitative scoring method that combined both image analysis and quantitative parameters. In 26 selected patients, the scintigraphic score separated all obstructed from nonobstructed patients. Another investigation reported good results (83% sensitivity, 81% specificity) using morphine-augmented cholescintigraphy (239).

An increasing body of evidence confirms the utility of cholescintigraphy for making this diagnosis. However, these studies are limited by the number of patients studied and the adequacy of the gold standard used. Although manometry and ERCP are often the standard for comparison, the true standard should be the patient's clinical response to treatment confirmed objectively by a return to normal of the diagnostic parameters found to be abnormal preoperatively. This type of data is very limited (229, 240). Further prospective studies are needed to better define the relative accuracy of ultrasonography, scintigraphy, ERCP, and manometry, using outcome results with patients classified clinically (types I to III).

Recommendations

With more confirmatory data, one could postulate various clinical imaging approaches. Cholescintigraphy could be used as a screening test to detect patients with partial biliary obstruction. This approach would capitalize on the sensitivity of cholescintigraphy. If it was positive, ERCP would be used to look for stones

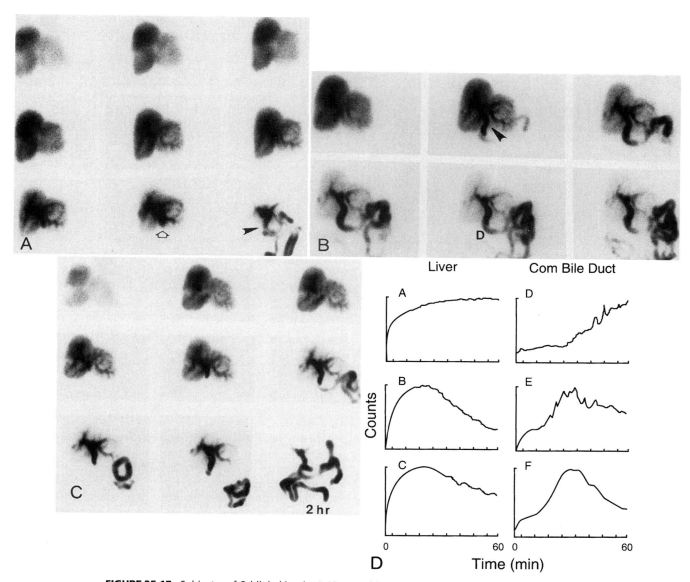

FIGURE 25.17. Sphincter of Oddi dyskinesia. A 46-year-old woman postcholecystectomy with recurrent abdominal pain. ERCP excluded mechanical obstruction. Manometry revealed elevated sphincter of Oddi pressure of 48 mm Hg. Presphincterotomy and postsphincterotomy cholescintigraphy was performed. **A:** Preoperative study. Sequential images over 60 minutes show prominent intrahepatic biliary retention and focal retention in the region of the common hepatic duct (*open arrowhead*). A 2-hour image shows that the obstruction is at the level of the sphincter of Oddi (*closed arrowhead*). **B:** Repeat preoperative study, but with continuous cholecystokinin (CCK) (sincalide) infusion. At 60 minutes there is retained activity in a prominent common duct (*arrowhead*), but normal biliary-to-bowel transit into the duodenum (*D*). The 2-hour image (not shown here) was unchanged. **C:** Postsphincterotomy study. Although there is still prominent radiotracer retention within the common duct, hepatic clearance and biliary-to-bowel transit have improved significantly from the baseline study (A) and, interestingly, looks similar to the preoperative study with CCK (B). **D:** Time-activity curves for the three foregoing studies derived from regions-of-interest drawn for the liver (A, B, C) and the common bile duct (D, E, F). The preoperative study shows very delayed liver uptake and clearance (A) and a progressively rising common duct curve (D). The preoperative study with CCK infusion shows significant improvement with a much earlier time-to-peak and significantly improved clearance (downslope) for both the liver (B) and common duct (E). The postsphincterotomy curves (C, F) are remarkably similar to the CCK preoperative study.

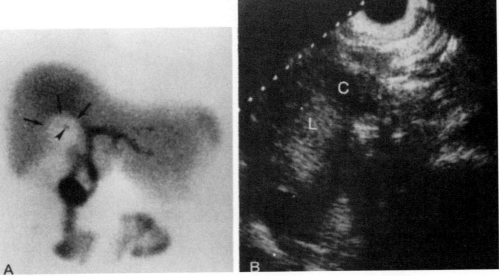

FIGURE 25.18. Hematoma with small central bile leak. The patient had sustained a gunshot wound. **A:** ^{99m}Tc-iminodiacetic acid scintigraphy, 40-minute image. A parenchymal defect is identified (*arrows*) with central biliary leakage (*arrowhead*). **B:** Sonogram, transverse scan. A large focal collection (*C*) can be seen just above the gallbladder fossa. This could represent blood, bile, or sterile or infected fluid. *L* = liver. Only scintigraphy can noninvasively determine the presence of bile leakage.

or stricture and as a guide to sphincterotome placement. Delayed ERCP views to determine contrast drainage after ERCP could be eliminated, allowing for papillotomy to be performed at one sitting without having to remove the endoscope (231). Manometry could be reserved for borderline cases or when clinical suspicion exists in the face of negative cholescintigraphy. Another approach would be to reserve cholescintigraphy until after ERCP and a mechanical etiology has been excluded. The specificity for diagnosis of sphincter dysfunction in this select group of patients would likely be high.

TRAUMA

Hepatic injury is the second most common injury following blunt or penetrating abdominal trauma (241). Blunt and penetrating trauma are managed differently. Penetrating injuries that may involve the liver or biliary tree are immediately explored (242). Blunt injuries are explored if there is hemodynamic instability, abnormal peritoneal lavage fluid, CT findings suggestive of major hepatic disruption, or evidence for viscous perforation (243,244). Coexistent biliary and hepatic injury occurs often but may not be initially detected even if immediate exploratory laparotomy is performed. The conservative approach of ligating medium-sized and larger vessels, debriding devitalized tissues, and draining the surgical bed are preferred to suturing large areas of liver parenchyma and attempting to ligate every small vessel and bile duct (245). This approach results in a low complication rate, but may result in space-occupying lesions and delayed biliary leakage, which can be identified with noninvasive imaging.

The evaluation of trauma requires interplay between biliary scintigraphy and the other anatomic imaging modalities. There are many possible posttraumatic lesions that must be differentiated, including hepatic laceration, hepatic hematoma, bile duct transection, extrahepatic biliary leakage, intrahepatic biloma formation, and gallbladder perforation. Secondary and remote effects of trauma, such as traumatic pancreatitis, acalculous cholecystitis, and secondary hematoma infection with subsequent liver abscess formation, may occur.

Space-occupying posttraumatic liver lesions have been evaluated by ^{99m}Tc-sulfur colloid liver scintigraphy, however, sonography and CT are the usual methods to detect liver parenchymal injuries such as hematoma and biloma formation (246–249). However, only biliary scintigraphy can demonstrate communication between the biliary tree and space-occupying lesions that represent biloma formation (250–255) (Fig. 25.19). Cholescintigraphy can also identify space-occupying lesions, e.g., hematoma and abscess, as effectively as ^{99m}Tc-sulfur colloid scintigraphy (250,256) when careful analysis of the early parenchymal images is performed.

Biliary leakage is common following penetrating and blunt trauma. In a series of 21 patients with suspected noniatrogenic biliary trauma, 33% had biliary leakage (250). Leakage initially may be occult and only suspected after clinical deterioration or discharge of bilious material from surgical drains, often occurring days after injury. As a hematoma resolves, tamponade of injured bile ducts lessens. Cholescintigraphy can follow the rate of biliary leakage and assess healing in patients treated conservatively. Cholangiography may be reserved for patients who have persistent, severe, or increasing leakage. If biliary excretion into the gastrointestinal tract decreases, suggesting partial obstruction, a coexistent central biliary injury must be considered (Fig. 25.20). ERCP or PTC must be performed in this setting.

If biliary excretion by normal pathways into the gastrointesti-

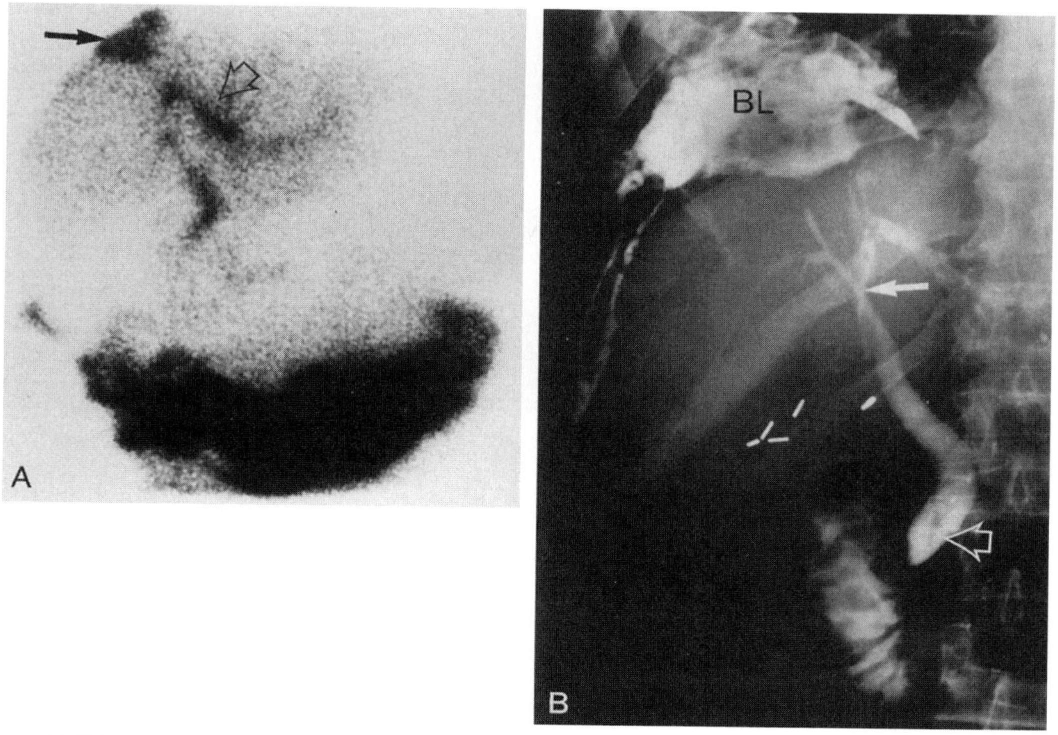

FIGURE 25.19. Persistent biliary leakage because of concomitant large bile duct injury. **A:** ^{99m}Tc-iminodiacetic acid scintigraphy, 4-hour image. A focal bile leak (*arrow*) is identified over the dome of the liver. In addition, there is pooling of activity within the common bile duct and left hepatic duct (*open arrow*). **B:** Endoscopic retrograde cholangiopancreatogram. The presence of a large bile leak (*BL*) is confirmed. Also identified is a stricture the common bile duct just below the bifurcation (*arrow*). A low-grade distal stricture (*open arrow*) with bile duct cast (poorly seen) is also present. Without corrective biliary surgery, biliary leakage would continue indefinitely as the obstructed biliary tree decompresses into the biloma.

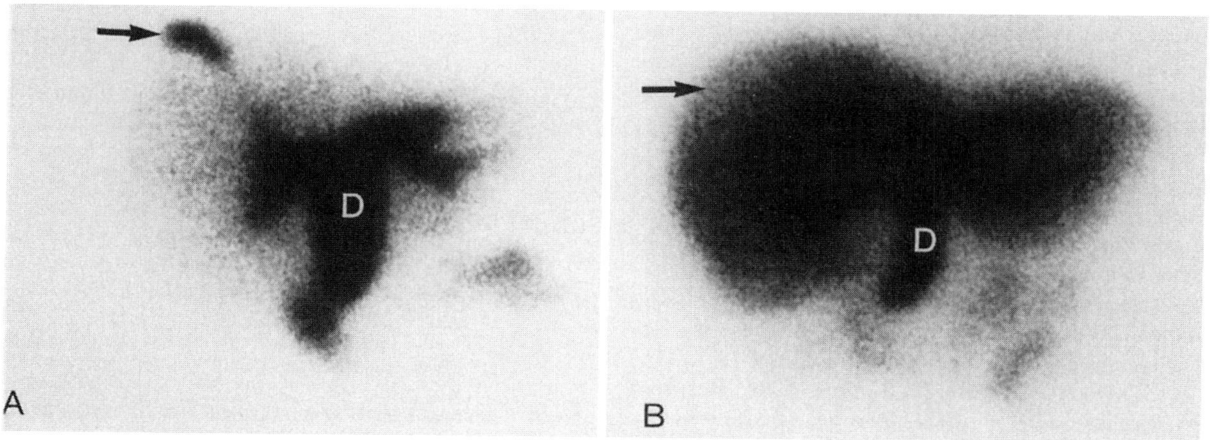

FIGURE 25.20. Biloma with subsequent superinfection and abscess formation. The patient sustained a knife wound to the right upper quadrant. **A:** ^{99m}Tc-iminodiacetic acid (IDA) scintigraphy, 1-hour image (13 days after injury). On this image, extrahepatic leakage of isotope (*arrow*) is compatible with a contained biloma. *D* = prominent duct activity. **B:** ^{99m}Tc-IDA scintigraphy, 40-minute image (10 weeks after injury). A focal photopenic area (*arrow*) is identified on this scan. Bile duct (*D*) activity is prominent caused by a long-standing choledochal cyst unrelated to the patient's current injury. Despite diminished leakage, the persistent defect and clinical deterioration prompted further evaluation. *(Figure continues.)*

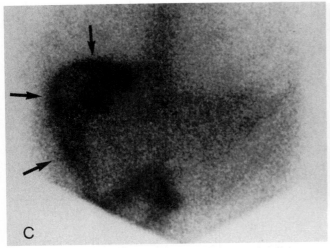

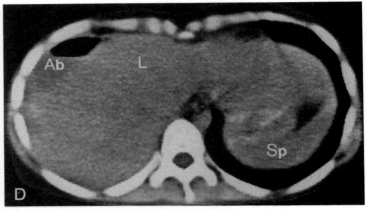

FIGURE 25.20. *Continued.* **C:** ^{67}Ga scan, 24-hour image. Increased uptake is noted surrounding the hepatic periphery (*arrows*). Inflammation or frank abscess was considered. **D:** Computed tomogram through the superior portion of the liver confirms the presence of an abscess (*Ab*). This collection also extended inferiorly on other sections. Thus, despite diminution in biliary leakage, the presence of a persistent defect and clinical deterioration must be considered suggestive of secondary abscess formation. *L* = liver; *Sp* = spleen. (From Zeman RK, Lee C, Stahl RS et al. Strategy for the use of biliary scintigraphy in noniatrogenic biliary trauma. *Radiology* 1984;151:771, with permission.)

nal tract is not maintained, bile may preferentially flow into a contained biloma, resulting in an abscess or chronic biliary fistula. Percutaneous stenting of the biliary injury or surgical repair is mandatory if leakage occurs with coexistent distal obstruction. If biloma formation is present, but coexists with relatively normal biliary excretion, a conservative approach may be used. Placing a short stent in the distal CBD will usually reduce biliary leakage even without stenting the actual injured area. Percutaneous drainage of the biloma can be reserved for patients in whom clinical deterioration or superinfection is suggested (257,258). Not all patients with small bilomas need percutaneous drainage; small amounts of biliary leakage are common following injury.

The interplay between cross-sectional techniques and biliary scintigraphy is important in following the resolution of a space-occupying process. Regardless of the nature of a space-occupying lesion, diminution in size following injury is desirable. In the patient with biloma formation who is not clinically improving despite diminished biliary leakage on scintigram, secondary abscess formation must be considered (Fig. 25.21). Likewise, detecting a persistent parenchymal defect that is not diminishing in size on the scintigraphic study also suggests the need for cross-sectional imaging. Sonography and CT are used to follow progress in the posttraumatic liver (246–249). With a persistent parenchymal defect and clinical deterioration, percutaneous aspiration of the lesion must be considered to diagnose liver abscess.

Posttraumatic pancreatitis (Fig. 25.3) and other inflammatory processes adjacent to the biliary tree may cause scintigraphic abnormalities of delayed biliary egress, transiently, or failure of gallbladder visualization. Cross-sectional techniques may be used to explain and add specificity to the scintigraphic findings by confirming the extrabiliary nature of the pathology. There are many systemic manifestations of severe trauma, such as acalcu-

lous cholecystitis and changes following total parenchymal nutrition, that also must be considered in the trauma patient because they may cause gallbladder nonvisualization on the scintigraphic study (61,259–261).

SUMMARY

This chapter has reviewed selective biliary disorders discussing the importance of biliary scintigraphy and its relationship to the anatomic cross-sectional imaging techniques. Interaction and interplay between the various imaging modalities allows for a greater understanding of the strengths and limitations of each method, and maximizes cost-effective patient care.

REFERENCES

1. Zeman RK, Burrell MI. *Diagnostic imaging of the gallbladder and bile ducts. A clinical-radiologic approach.* New York: Churchill-Livingstone, 1987.
2. Weissmann HS, Frank MS, Bernstein LM et al. Rapid and accurate diagnosis of acute cholecystitis with 99mTc-HIDA cholescintigraphy. *AJR* 1979;132:523.
3. Rosenthal L, Shaffer EA, Lisbona R et al. Diagnosis of hepatobiliary disease by 99mTc-HIDA cholescintigraphy. *Radiology* 1978;126:467.
4. Pare P, Shaffer EA, Rosenthal L. Nonvisualization of the gallbladder by 99mTc-HIDA cholescintigraphy as evidence of cholecystitis. *Can Med Assoc J* 1978;118:384.
5. Suarez CA, Block F, Bernstein D et al. The role of HIDA/PIPIDA scanning in diagnosing cystic duct obstruction. *Ann Surg* 1980;191:391.
6. Zeman RK, Burrell MI, Cahow CE et al. Diagnostic utility of cholescintigraphy and ultrasonography in acute cholecystitis. *Am J Surg* 1981;141:446.
7. Cheng TM, Davis MA, Seltzer SE et al. Evaluation of hepatobiliary

imaging by radionuclide scintigraphy, ultrasonography, and contrast cholangiography. *Radiology* 1979;133:761.

8. Fonseca C, Greenberg D, Rosenthal L et al. Assessment of the utility of gallbladder imaging with 99mTc-HIDA. *Clin Nucl Med* 1978;3:437.
9. Schein CJ. *Acute cholecystitis.* New York: Harper and Row, 1972.
10. Essenhigh DM. Management of acute cholecystitis. *Br J Surg* 1966;53:1032.
11. Halasz NA. Counterfeit cholecystitis. A common diagnostic dilemma. *Am J Surg* 1975;130:189.
12. Cole WH. Gallbladder disease. *Surg Clin North Am* 1978;58:917.
13. Lahtiner J, Alhava EM, Aukee S. Acute cholecystitis treated by early and delayed surgery. A controlled clinical trial. *Scand J Gastroenterol* 1978;13:673.
14. Isch JH, Finneran JC, Nahrwold DL. Perforation of the gallbladder. *Am J Gastroenterol* 1971;55:451.
15. National Institute of Health Consensus Conference statement on gallstones and laparoscopic cholecystectomy. *Amer J Surg* 1993;165:390.
16. Frazee RC, Robert JW, Symmond R. What are the contraindications for laparoscopic cholecystectomy? *Am J Surg* 1992;164:491.
17. Johnson HC, McLaren JR, Weens HS. Intravenous cholangiography. *Am J Surg* 1954;140:600.
18. Harrington OB, Beall AC, Noon G et al. Intravenous cholangiography in acute cholecystitis. *Arch Surg* 1964;88:585.
19. Eckelberg ME, Carlson HC, McIlrath DC. Intravenous cholangiography with intact gallbladder. *AJR* 1970;110:235.
20. Ansell G. Adverse reactions to contrast agents. *Invest Radiol* 1970;5:374.
21. Goldberg BB, Harris K, Brooker W. Ultrasonic and radiographic cholecystography: a comparison. *Radiology* 1974;111:405.
22. Leopold G, Amberg J, Gosink BB et al. Gray scale ultrasonic cholecystography: a comparison with conventional radiographic techniques. *Radiology* 1975;121:445.
23. Bartrum RJ, Crow HI, Foote SR. Ultrasonic and radiographic cholecystography. *N Engl J Med* 1977;296:538.
24. Crade M, Taylor KJW, Rosenfield AT et al. Surgical and pathologic correlation of cholecystosonography and cholecystography. *AJR* 1978;131:227.
25. Detweiler RP, Kim DS, Longerbeam JK. Ultrasonography and oral cholecystography: a comparison of their use in the diagnosis of gallbladder disease. *Arch Surg* 1980;115:1096.
26. McIntosh DMF, Penney HF. Gray scale ultrasonography as a screening procedure in the detection of gallbladder disease. *Radiology* 1980;136:725.
27. Cooperberg PL, Pon MS, Wong P et al. Real-time high resolution ultrasound in the detection of biliary calculi. *Radiology* 1979;131:789.
28. Krook PM, Allen FM, Bush WH et al. Comparison of real-time cholecystosonography and oral cholecystography. *Radiology* 1980;135:145.
29. Anderson JC, Harned RK. Gray scale ultrasonography of the gallbladder: an evaluation of accuracy and report of additional ultrasound signs. *AJR* 1977;129:975.
30. Garra BS, Davros WJ, Lack EE et al. Visibility of gallstone fragments at ultrasound and fluoroscopy. Implications for monitoring of gallstone lithotripsy. *Radiology* 1990;174:343.
31. Raptopoulos V, D'Orsi C, Smith E et al. Dynamic cholecystosonography of the contracted gallbladder: the double arc shadow sign. *AJR* 1982;138:275.
32. Simeone JF, Ferrucci JT. New trends in gallbladder imaging. *JAMA* 1981;246:380.
33. Lee SP, Nicholls JF. Nature and composition of biliary sludge. *Gastroenterology* 1986;90:677.
34. Simeone JF, Mueller PR, Ferrucci JT et al. Significance of nonshadowing focal opacities at cholecystosonography. *Radiology* 1980;137:181.
35. Zeman RK, Garra BS. Gallbladder imaging: The state-of-the-art. *Gastroent Clin N Am* 1991;2:127.
36. Stoller JL, Cooperberg PL, Simpson WM. Diagnostic ultrasonography in acute cholecystitis. *Can J Surg* 1979;22:374.
37. Laing FC, Federle MP, Jeffery RB et al. Ultrasonic evaluation of patients with acute right upper quadrant pain. *Radiology* 1981;140:449.
38. Raghavendra BN, Feimer HD, Subramanyam BR et al. Acute cholecystitis: sonographic-pathologic analysis. *AJR* 1981;137:327.
39. Marchal G, Crolla D, Baert AL et al. Gallbladder wall thickening: a new sign of gallbladder disease visualized by gray scale cholecystosonography. *J Clin Ultrasound* 1978;6:177.
40. Mindell HJ, Ring AB. Gallbladder wall thickening: ultrasonic findings. *Radiology* 1979;133:699.
41. Crade M, Taylor KJW, Viscomi GN. Need for care in assessing gallbladder wall thickening. *AJR* 1980;135:423.
42. Marchal GJF, Casaer M, Baert AL et al. Gallbladder wall sonolucency in acute cholecystitis. *Radiology* 1979;133:429.
43. Ralls PW, Colletti PM, Lapin SA et al. Real-time sonography in suspected acute cholecystitis. *Radiology* 1985;155:767.
44. Uggowitzer M, Kugler C, Schramayer G et al. Sonography of acute cholecystitis: comparison of color and power Doppler sonography in detecting a hypervascularized gallbladder wall. *AJR* 1997;168:707.
45. Friedman GD, Kannel WB, Dawber TR. The epidemiology of gallbladder disease: observations in the Framingham Study. *J Chron Dis* 1966;19:273.
46. Cohan RH, Mahony BS, Bowie JD et al. Striated intramural gallbladder lucencies on US studies. Predictors of acute cholecystitis. *Radiology* 1987;164:31–35.
47. Teefey SA, Baron RL, Bigler SA. Sonography of the gallbladder. Significance of striated (layered) thickening of the gallbladder wall. *AJR* 1991;156:945.
48. Freitas JE, Mirkes SH, Fink-Bennett DM et al. Suspected acute cholecystitis: comparison of hepatobiliary scintigraphy versus ultrasonography. *Clin Nucl Med* 1982;7:364.
49. Samuels BI, Freitas JE, Bree RL et al. A comparison of radionuclide hepatobiliary imaging and real-time ultrasound for the detection of acute cholecystitis. *Radiology* 1983;147:207.
50. Worthen NJ, Uszler JM, Funamura JL. Cholecystitis: prospective evaluation of sonography and 99mTc-IDA cholescintigraphy. *AJR* 1981;137:973.
51. Ralls RW, Colletti PM, Halls JM et al. Prospective evaluation of 99mTc-IDA cholescintigraphy and gray-scale ultrasound in the diagnosis of acute cholecystitis. *Radiology* 1982;144:369.
52. Kim EE, Pjura G, Lowry P et al. Morphine augmented cholescintigraphy in the diagnosis of acute cholecystitis. *AJR* 1986;147:1177.
53. Zeman RK, Lee C, Jaffe MH et al. Hepatobiliary scintigraphy and sonography in early biliary obstruction. *Radiology* 1984;153:793.
54. Shuman WP, Rogers JV, Rudd TG et al. Low sensitivity of sonography and cholescintigraphy in acalculous cholecystitis. *AJR* 1984;142:531.
55. Cornelius EA. Sensitivity of sonography and cholescintigraphy in acalculous cholecystitis. *AJR* 1984;143:1121.
56. Weissman HS, Berkowitz D, Fox MS et al. The role of technetium-99m iminodiacetic acid (IDA) cholescintigraphy in acute acalculous cholecystitis. *Radiology* 1983;146:177.
57. Savoca PE, Longe WE, Zucker KA et al. The increasing prevalence of acalculous cholecystitis in outpatients. *Ann Surg* 1990;211:433.
58. Rammana L, Brachman MB, Tanesescu DE et al. Cholescintigraphy in acute acalculous cholecystitis. *Am J Gastroenterol* 1984;79:650.
59. Swayne LC. Acute acalculous cholecystitis: sensitivity in detection using technetium-99m iminodiacetic acid cholescintigraphy. *Radiology* 1986;160:33.
60. Mirvis SE, Vainright JR, Nelson AW. The diagnosis of acute acalculous cholecystitis. Comparison of sonography, scintigraphy, and CT. *AJR* 1986;147:1171.
61. Kalff V, Froelich JW, Lloyd R et al. Predictive value of an abnormal hepatobiliary scan in patients with severe intercurrent illness. *Radiology* 1983;146:191.
62. Drane WE, Nelp WB, Rudd TG. The need for routine delayed radionuclide hepatobiliary imaging in patients with intercurrent illness. *Radiology* 1984;151:763.
63. Fig LM, Stewart RE, Wahl RL. Morphine-augmented hepatobiliary scintigraphy in the severely ill: caution is in order. *Radiology* 1990;175:473–476.

64. Colletti PM, Ralls PW, Siegel ME et al. Acute cholecystitis: diagnosis with radionuclide angiography. *Radiology* 1987;163:615.

65. Bushnell DL, Perlman SB, Wilson MA et al. The rim sign: association with acute cholecystitis. *J Nucl Med* 1982;27:353.

66. Meekin GK, Ziessman HA, Klappenbach RS. Prognostic value and pathophysiologic significance of the rim sign in cholescintigraphy. *J Nucl Med* 1987;28:1679.

67. Datz FL. Utility of indium-111-labeled leukocyte imaging in acute acalculous cholecystitis. *AJR* 1986; 147:813–814.

68. Wilson RG, Macintyre IM, Nixon SJ et al. Laparoscopic cholecystectomy as a safe and effective treatment for severe acute cholecystitis. *BMJ* 1992;305:394.

69. Fisher RS, Stelzer F, Rock E et al. Abnormal gallbladder emptying in patients with gallstones. *Dig Dis Sci* 1982;27:1019.

70. Brugge WR, Brand DL, Atkins HL et al. Gallbladder dyskinesia in chronic acalculous cholecystitis. *Dig Dis Sci* 1986;31:461.

71. Nora PF, McCarthy W, Sanez N. Quantitative gallbladder imaging following cholecystokinin. *Arch Surg* 1974;108:507.

72. Goldberg HI. Cholecystokinin cholecystography. *Sem Roentgenol* 1976;11:175.

73. Nathan MH, Newman A, Murra DJ. Cholecystokinin cholecystography. *AJR* 1970;110:246.

74. Dunn FH. Christensen EC, Reynolds J et al. Cholecystokinin cholecystography. *JAMA* 1974;228:997.

75. Topper TE, Ryerson TW, Nora PF. Quantitative gallbladder imaging following cholecystokinin. *J Nucl Med* 1980;21:694.

76. Pickleman J, Peiss RL, Henkin R et al. The role of sincalide cholescintigraphy in the evaluation of patients with acalculous gallbladder disease. *Arch Surg* 1985;120:693.

77. Fink-Bennett D, DeRidder P, Kolozsi WZ et al. Cholecystokinin cholescintigraphy: detection of abnormal gallbladder motor function in patients with chronic acalculous gallbladder disease. *J Nucl Med* 1991;32:1695.

78. Yap L, Wycherley AG, Morphett AD et al. Acalculous biliary pain: cholecystectomy alleviates symptoms in patients with abnormal cholescintigraphy. *Gastroenterology* 1991;101:786.

79. Zech ER, Simmons LB, Kendrick RR et al. Cholecystokinin enhanced hepatobiliary imaging with ejection fraction calculation as an indicator of disease of the gallbladder. *Surg Gyn Ob* 1991;172:21.

80. Misra DC, Blossom GB, Finnk-Bennett D et al. Surgical therapy for biliary dyskinesia. *Arch Surg* 1991;126:957.

81. Halverson JD, Garner BA, Siegel BA et al. The use of hepatobiliary scintigraphy in patients with acalculous biliary colic. *Arch Int Med* 1992;152:1305.

82. Middleton GW, Williams JH. Is gallbladder ejection fraction a reliable predictor of acalculous gallbladder disease. *Nucl Med Commun* 1992; 13:894.

83. Sorenson MK, Fancherr S, Lang NP et al. Abnormal gallbladder nuclear ejection fraction predicts success of cholecystectomy in patients with biliary dyskinesia. *Am J Surg* 1993;166:672.

84. Ziessman HA, Fahey FH, Hixson DJ. Calculation of a gallbladder ejection fraction: advantage of continuous sincalide infusion over the three-minute infusion method. *J Nucl Med* 1992;33:537.

85. Ziessman HA, Agarwal A, ZaZa A. CCK cholescintigraphy: optimal methodology for sincalide infusion. *Radiology* 2001;221:404–410.

86. Sarva RP, Shreiner DP, Van Thiel D et al. Gallbladder function: methods for measuring filling and emptying. *J Nucl Med* 1985; 26: 140–146.

87. Masclee AM, Hopman WPM, Corstens FHM et al. Simultaneous measurement of gallbladder emptying with cholescintigraphy and US during infusion of physiologic doses of cholecystokinin: a comparison. *Radiology* 1989;173:407.

88. Radberg G, Asztely M, Moonen M et al. Contraction and evacuation of the gallbladder studied simultaneously by ultrasonography and Tc-99m labeled diethyl-iminoacetic acid scintigraphy. *Scand J Gastroenterol* 1993;28:709–913.

89. Donald JJ, Fache JS, Buckley AR et al. Gallbladder contractility: variation in normal subjects. *AJR* 1991;157:753.

90. Krishnamurthy GT, Bobba VR, Kingston E. Radionuclide ejection

91. Nielsen SP, Trap-Jensen J, Lindenberg J et al. Hepatobiliary scintigraphy and hepatography with Tc-99m diethyl-acetanilido-iminodiacetate in obstructive jaundice. *J Nucl Med* 1978;19:452.

92. Rosenthall L. Cholescintigraphy in the presence of jaundice. *Semin Nucl Med* 1982;12:53.

93. Klingensmith WC III, Johnson ML, Kuni CC et al. Complementary role of Tc-99m-diethyl-IDA and ultrasound in large and small duct obstruction. *Radiology* 1981;138:177.

94. Klingensmith WC III, Kuni CC, Fritzberg AR. Cholescintigraphy in extrahepatic biliary obstruction. *AJR* 1982;139:65.

95. Pauwels S, Piret L, Schoutens A et al. Tc-99m-diethyl-IDA imaging: clinical evaluation in jaundiced patients. *J Nucl Med* 1980;21:1022.

96. Fonseca C, Rosenthall L, Greenberg D et al. Differential diagnosis of jaundice by 99mTc-IDA hepatobiliary imaging. *Clin Nucl Med* 1979;4:135.

97. Nadel M, Sorenson TIA, Jerichau IJ et al. Hepatobiliary scintigraphy with 99mTc-labelled diethyl acetanilide imino diacetic acid in the differential diagnosis of jaundice. *Dan Med Bull* 1980;27:278.

98. Weissmann HS, Frank M, Rosenblatt R et al. Cholescintigraphy, ultrasonography, and computerized tomography in the evaluation of biliary tract disorders. *Semin Nucl Med* 1979;9:22.

99. Scott BB, Evans JA, Unsworth J. The initial investigation of jaundice in a district general hospital: a study of ultrasonography and hepatobiliary scintigraphy. *Br J Radiol* 1980;53:557.

100. Seltzer SE, Jones B. Imaging the hepatobiliary system in acute disease. *AJR* 1980;135:407.

101. Hernandez M, Rosenthall L. A cross-over study comparing the kinetics of Tc-99m labelled diethyl and diisopropyl-IDA. *Clin Nucl Med* 1980;5:352.

102. Stadalnik RC, Matolo NM, Jansholt A et al. Clinical experience with 99mTc-disofenin as a cholescintigraphic agent. *Radiology* 1981;140: 797.

103. Wistow BW, Subramanian G, Gagne GM et al. Experimental and clinical trials of new 99mTc-labeled hepatobiliary agents. *Radiology* 1978;128:793.

104. Berk RN, Cooperberg PL, Gold RP et al. Radiography of the bile ducts. *Radiology* 1982;145:1.

105. Ferrucci JT, Adson MA, Mueller RP et al. Advances in the radiology of jaundice: a symposium and review. *AJR* 1983;141:1.

106. Taylor KJW, Carpenter DA, McCready VR. Gray scale echography in the diagnosis of intrahepatic disease. *J Clin Ultrasound* 1973;1: 284.

107. Reid MH. Visualization of the bile ducts using focused ultrasound. *Radiology* 1976;118:155.

108. Goldberg BB. Ultrasonic cholangiography-gray-scale B-scan evaluation of the common bile duct. *Radiology* 1976;118:401.

109. Taylor KJW, Carpenter DA. Anatomy and pathology of the porta hepatis demonstrated by gray scale ultrasonography. *J Clin Ultrasound* 1975;3:117.

110. Weill F, Eisenscher A, Aucant A et al. Ultrasonic study of the venous patterns in the hypochondrium: an anatomical approach to differential diagnosis of obstructive jaundice. *J Clin Ultrasound* 1975;3:23.

111. Perlmutter GS, Goldberg BB. Ultrasonic evaluation of the common bile duct. *J Clin Ultrasound* 1976;4:107.

112. Sample WF. Techniques for improved delineation of normal anatomy of the upper abdomen and high retroperitoneum with gray scale ultrasound. *Radiology* 1979;124:197.

113. Filly RA, Laing FC. Anatomic variation of portal venous anatomy in the porta hepatis; ultrasonographic evaluation. *J Clin Ultrasound* 1978;6:83.

114. Marks WM, Filly RA, Callen PW. Ultrasonic anatomy of the liver: a review with new applications. *J Clin Ultrasound* 1979;7:137.

115. Sexton CC, Zeman RK. Correlation of computed tomography, sonography and gross anatomy of the liver. *AJR* 1983;141:711.

116. Willi UV, Teele RL. Hepatic arteries and the parallel-channel sign. *J Clin Ultrasound* 1979;7:125.

117. Behan M, Kazam E. Sonography of the common bile duct: value of the right anterior oblique view. *AJR* 1978;130:701.

fraction: a technique for quantitative analysis of motor function of the human gallbladder. *Gastroenterol* 1982;80:482.

118. Parulekar SG. Ultrasound evaluation of common bile duct size. *Radiology* 1979;133:703.

119. Taylor KJW, Rosenfield AT, deGraaf CS et al. Factors affecting the recognition of the dilated biliary tree in the jaundice patient. In: White DN, ed. *Ultrasound in medicine*, vol 4. New York: Plenum Press, 1978:125.

120. Conrad MR, Landay MJ, James JO. Sonographic parallel channel sign of biliary tree enlargement in mild to moderate obstructive jaundice. *AJR* 1978;130:279.

121. Sample WF, Sarti DA, Goldstein LL et al. Gray-scale ultrasonography of the jaundiced patient. *Radiology* 1978;128:719.

122. Malini S, Sabel J. Ultrasonography in obstructive jaundice. *Radiology* 1977;123:429.

123. Taylor KJW, Rosenfield AT, deGraaf CS. Anatomy and pathology of the biliary tree as demonstrated by ultrasound. In: Taylor KJW, ed. *Clinics in diagnostic ultrasound*, vol 1, Diagnostic ultrasound in GI disease. New York: Churchill Livingstone, 1979:109.

124. Weill F, Eisencher A, Zeltner F. Ultrasonic study of the normal and dilated biliary tree: the "shotgun" sign. *Radiology* 1978;127:221.

125. Cooperberg, PL. High-resolution real time ultrasound in the evaluation of the normal and obstructed biliary tract. *Radiology* 1978;124:477.

126. Graham MF, Cooperberg PL, Cohen MM et al. The size of the normal common hepatic duct following cholecystectomy: an ultrasonographic study. *Radiology* 1980;135:137.

127. Mueller PR, Ferucci JT, Simeone JF et al. Postcholecystectomy bile duct dilatation: myth or reality? *AJR* 1981;136:355.

128. Sauerbrei EE, Cooperberg PL, Gordon P et al. Discrepancy between radiographic and sonographic bile duct measurements. *Radiology* 1980;137:751.

129. Lapis JL, Orlando RC, Mittelstaedt CA et al. Ultrasonography in the diagnosis of obstructive jaundice. *Ann Intern Med* 1978;89:61.

130. Taylor KJW, Rosenfield AT, Spiro HM. Diagnostic accuracy of gray scale ultrasonography for the jaundiced patient. *Arch Intern Med* 1979;139:60.

131. Cronan JJ, Mueller PR, Simeone JF et al. Prospective diagnosis of choledocholithiasis. *Radiology* 1983;146:467.

132. Gross BH, Harter LP, Gore RM et al. Ultrasonic evaluation of common bile duct stones: prospective comparison with endoscopic retrograde cholangiopancreatography. *Radiology* 1983;146:471.

133. Neiman HL, Mintzer RA. Accuracy of biliary duct ultrasound: comparison with cholangiography. *AJR* 1977;129:979.

134. Gold RP, Casarella WJ, Stern G et al. Transhepatic cholangiography: the radiological method of choice in suspected obstruction jaundice. *Radiology* 1979;133:39.

135. Koenigsberg M, Wiener SN, Walzer A. The accuracy of sonography in the differential diagnosis of obstructive jaundice: a comparison with cholangiography. *Radiology* 1979;133:157.

136. Laing FC, Jeffrey RB, Wing VW et al. Biliary dilatation: defining the level and cause by real-time US. *Radiology* 1986;160:39.

137. Haubek A, Pederson JH, Burcharth F et al. Dynamic sonography in the evaluation of jaundice. *AJR* 1981;136:1071.

138. Simeone JF, Mueller PR, Ferrucci JT et al. Sonography of the bile ducts after a fatty meal: an aid in detection of obstruction. *Radiology* 1982;143:211.

139. Darweesh RMA, Dodds WJ, Hogan WJ et al. Fatty meal sonography for evaluating patients with suspected partial common duct obstruction. *AJR* 1988;151:63.

140. Zeman RK, Fox SH, Silverman PM et al. Helical (spiral) CT of the abdomen. *AJR* 1993;160:719.

141. Dupuy DE, Costello P, Ecker CP. Spiral CT of the pancreas. *Radiology* 1992;183:815.

142. Clark LR, Jacobs NM, Zeman RK et al. Enhanced pancreatic CT imaging utilizing a geometric magnification technique. *Invest Radiol* 1985;20:531.

143. Zeman RK, Zeiberg AS, Davros WJ et al. Routine helical CT of the abdomen: image quality considerations. *Radiology* 1993;189:395.

144. Brink JA, Heiken JP, Balfe DM et al. Noninvasive cholangiography with spiral CT. *Radiology* 1992;185(P):141.

145. Gold JA, Zeman RK, Schwartz A. Computed tomographic cholangiography in a canine model of biliary obstruction. *Invest Radiol* 1979;14:498.

146. Greenberg M, Greenberg BM, Rubin JM. CT cholangiography: a new technique for evaluating the head of the pancreas and the distal biliary tree. *Radiology* 1982;144:363.

147. Zeman RK, Burrell MI, Gold JA et al. The intrahepatic and extrahepatic bile ducts in surgical jaundice: diagnostic and therapeutic implications. *CRC Crit Rev Diagn Imaging* 1984;21:1.

148. Stanley RJ, Sagel SS, Levitt RG. Computed tomography of the body: early trends in application and accuracy of the method. *AJR* 1976;127:53.

149. Havrilla TR, Haaga JR, Alfidi RJ et al. Computed tomography and obstructive biliary disease. *AJR* 1977;128:765.

150. Levitt RG, Sagel SS, Stanley RJ et al. Accuracy of computed tomography of the liver and biliary tract. *Radiology* 1977;124:123.

151. Shimizu H, Ida M, Takayama S et al. The diagnostic accuracy of computed tomography in obstructive biliary disease: a comparative evaluation with duct cholangiography. *Radiology* 1981;138:411.

152. Stanley RJ, Sagel SS, Levitt RG. Computed tomography of the liver. *Radiol Clin North Am* 1977;15:331.

153. Pedrosa CS, Casanova R, Rodriquez R. Computed tomography in obstructive jaundice. Part I: the level of obstruction. *Radiology* 1981;139:627.

154. Pedrosa CS, Casanova R, Lezanu AJ et al. Computed tomography in obstructive jaundice. Part II: the cause of obstruction. *Radiology* 1981;139:635.

155. Baron RL. Common bile duct stones: reassessment of criteria for CT diagnosis. *Radiology* 1987;162:419.

156. Zeman RK, Davros WJ, Berman P et al. Three-dimensional models of the abdominal vasculature based on helical CT: usefulness in patients with pancreatic neoplasms. *AJR* 1994;162:1425.

157. Princenthal R, Burrell MI, Zeman RK et al. CT studies of the biliary tract after PTC or ERCP: a new imaging technique. *Radiology* 1983;149(P):175.

158. Low RN, Sigeti JS, Francis IR et al. Evaluation of malignant biliary obstruction: efficacy of fast multiplanar spoiled gradient-recalled MR imaging vs spin-echo MR imaging, CT, and cholangiography. *AJR* 1994;162:315.

159. Muller MF, Meyenberger C, Bertschinger P et al. Pancreatic tumors: evaluation with endoscopic US, CT, and MR imaging. *Radiology* 1994;190:745.

160. Morimoto K, Shimoi M, Shirakawa T et al. Biliary obstruction: evaluation with three-dimensional MR cholangiography. *Radiology* 1992;183:578.

161. Alcarez MJ, De la Morena EJ, Polo A et al: A comparative study of magnetic resonance cholangiography and direct cholangiography. *Rev Esp Enferm Dig* 2000;92:427.

162. Varghese JC, Farrell MA, Courtney G et al: A prospective comparison of magnetic resonance cholangiopancreatography with endoscopic retrograde cholangiopancreatography in the evaluation of patients with suspected biliary tract disease. *Clin Radiol* 1999;54:513.

163. Georgeopoulous SK, Schwartz LH, Jarnagin WR et al: Comparison of magnetic resonance and endoscopic retrograde cholangiopancreatography in malignant pancreaticobiliary obstruction. *Arch Surg* 1999;134:1002.

164. Pavone P, Laghi A, Passariello R: MR cholangiopancreatography in malignant biliary obstruction. *Sem Ultrasound CT MRI* 1999;20:317.

165. Mitchell DG, Vinitsky S, Sapanaro S et al: Liver and pancreas: Improved spin-echo T1. contrast by shorter echo time and fat suppression at 1.5T. *Radiology* 1991;178:67.

166. Geier A, Nguyen HN, Gartung C et al: MRCP and ERCP to detect small ampullary carcinoma. *Lancet* 2000;356:04.

167. Berk RN, Ferrucci JT, Goldstein HM et al. Diagnostic imaging of the liver and bile ducts. *Invest Radiol* 1978;13:265.

168. Elias E, Hamlyn AN, Jain S et al. Randomized trial of percutaneous transhepatic cholangiography with the Chiba needle versus endoscopic retrograde cholangiography for duct visualization in jaundice. *Gastroenterology* 1976;71:439.

169. Okuda K, Tanikawa K, Emura T et al. Nonsurgical, percutaneous

transhepatic cholangiography-diagnostic significance in medical problems of the liver. *Dig Dis* 1974;19:21.

170. Pereiras R, Chiprut RO, Greenwald RA et al. Percutaneous transhepatic cholangiography with the skinny needle: a rapid, simple, and accurate method in the diagnosis of cholestasis. *Ann Intern Med* 1977; 86:526.

171. Hinde GDFB, Smith PM, Craven JL. Percutaneous cholangiography with the Okuda needle. *Gut* 1977;18:610.

172. Jain S, Long RG, Scott J et al. Percutaneous transhepatic cholangiography using the "Chiba" needle—80 cases. *Br J Radiol* 1977;50:175.

173. Mintzer RA, Neiman HL. Chiba needle percutaneous transhepatic cholangiography. *Gastrointest Radiol* 1977;1:315.

174. Ariyama J, Shirakabe H, Ohashi K et al. Experience with percutaneous transhepatic cholangiography using the Japanese needle. *Gastrointest Radiol* 1978;2:359.

175. Mueller PR, Harbin WP, Ferrucci JT et al. Fine-needle transhepatic cholangiography: reflections after 450 cases. *AJR* 1981;136:85.

176. Jaques PF, Mauro MA, Scatliff JH. The failed transhepatic cholangiogram. *Radiology* 1980;134:33.

177. Oi I. Fiberduodenoscopy and endoscopic pancreatocholangiography. *Gastrointest Endosc* 1970;17:59.

178. Tagagi K, Ikeda S, Nakagawa Y. Retrograde pancreatography and cholangiography by fiberduodenoscope. *Gastroenterology* 1970;59: 445.

179. Vennes JA, Silvis SE. Endoscopic visualization of bile and pancreatic ducts. *Gastrointest Endosc* 1972;18:149.

180. Cotton PB. Progress report: cannulation of the papilla of Vater by endoscopy and retrograde cholangiopancreatography (ERCP). *Gut* 1972;13:1014.

181. Kessler RE, Falkenstein DB, Clemett AR et al. Indications, clinical value, and complications of endoscopic retrograde cholangiopancreatography. *Surg Gynecol Obstet* 1976;142:856.

182. Ring EJ, Oleaga JA, Freiman DB et al. Therapeutic applications of catheter cholangiography. *Radiology* 1978;128:333.

183. Ferrucci JT Jr, Mueller PR, Harbin W. Percutaneous transhepatic biliary drainage technique, results, and applications. *Radiology* 1980; 135:1.

184. Wurbs D, Classen M. Transpapillary long-standing tube for nasobiliary drainage. *Endoscopy* 1977;9:186.

185. Riemann JF, Lux G, Rosch W et al. Nonsurgical biliary drainage-technique, indications and results. *Endoscopy* 1981;13:157.

186. Geenen JE, Hogan WJ, Shaffer RD et al. Endoscopic electrosurgical papillotomy and manometry in biliary tract disease. *JAMA* 1977;237: 8075.

187. Harbin WP, Mueller PR, Ferrucci JT. Transhepatic cholangiography: complications and use patterns of the fine-needle technique. *Radiology* 1980;135:15.

188. Zimmon DS, Falkenstein DB, Riccobono C et al. Complications of endoscopic retrograde cholangiopancreatography: analysis of 300 consecutive cases. *Gastroenterology* 1975;69:303.

189. Bilbao MK, Dotter CT, Lee TG et al. Complications of endoscopic retrograde cholangiopancreatography (ERCP): a study of 10,000 cases. *Gastroenterology* 1976;70:314.

190. Zeman RK, Taylor KJW, Burrell MI et al. Ultrasound demonstration of anicteric dilation of the biliary tree. *Radiology* 1980;134:689.

191. Weinstein DP, Weinstein BJ, Brodmerkel GJ. Ultrasonography of biliary tract dilation without jaundice. *AJR* 1979;132:729.

192. Weinstein BJ, Weinstein DP. Biliary tract dilatation in the nonjaundiced patient. *AJR* 1980;134:899.

193. Zeman RK, Taylor KJW, Rosenfield AT et al. Acute experimental biliary obstruction in the dog: sonographic findings and clinical implications. *AJR* 1981;136:965.

194. Klingensmith WC III, Whitney WP, Spitzer UM et al. Effect of complete biliary tract obstruction on serial hepatobiliary imaging in an experimental model (concise communication). *J Nucl Med* 1981; 22:866.

195. Muhletaler CA, Gerlock AJ, Fleischer AC et al. Diagnosis of obstructive jaundice with nondilated bile ducts. *AJR* 1980;134:1149.

196. Beinart CB, Efremidis J, Cohen B et al. Obstruction without dilatation: importance in evaluating jaundice. *JAMA* 1981;245:353.

197. Thomas JL, Zornoza J. Obstructive jaundice in the absence of sonographic biliary dilatation. *Gastrointest Radiol* 1980;5:357.

198. Floyd JL, Collins TL. Discordance of sonography and cholescintigraphy in acute biliary obstruction. *AJR* 1983;140:501.

199. Krishnamurthy GT, Lieberman DA, Brar HS. Detection, localization, and quantitation of degree of common bile duct obstruction by scintigraphy. *J Nucl Med* 1985;26:726.

200. Longmire WP, Lippman HN. Intrahepatic cholangiojejunostomy—an operation for biliary obstruction. *Surg Clin North Am* 1956;36:849.

201. Madden JL, Chun JY, Kandalaft S et al. Choledochoduodenostomy: an unjustly maligned surgical procedure. *Am J Surg* 1970;119:45.

202. Warren KW, Jefferson MF. Prevention and repair of strictures of the extrahepatic bile ducts. *Surg Clin North Am* 1973;53:1169.

203. Bismuth H, Corlette MB. Intrahepatic cholangioenteric anastomosis in carcinoma of the hilus of the liver. *Surg Gynecol Obstet* 1975;140: 170.

204. Cameron JL, Gayler BW, Harrington DP. Modification of the Longmire procedure. *Ann Surg* 1978;187:379.

205. Cahow CE. Intrahepatic cholangiojejunostomy: a new simplified approach. *Am J Surg* 1979;137:443.

206. Zeman RK, Lee C, Stahl RS et al. Ultrasonography and hepatobiliary scintigraphy in the assessment of biliary-enteric anastomoses. *Radiology* 1982;145:109.

207. Bowers RM. Morbid conditions following choledochojejunostomy. *Ann Surg* 1964;159:424.

208. Weissmann HS, Chun KJ, Frank M et al. Demonstration of traumatic bile leakage with cholescintigraphy and ultrasonography. *AJR* 1979; 133:843.

209. Weissmann HS, Gliedman ML, Wilk PJ et al. Evaluation of the postoperative patient with 99mTC-IDA cholescintigraphy. *Semin Nucl Med* 1982;12:27.

210. Papp J, Tulassay Z, Bielawski J. Diagnostic value of endoscopic retrograde cholangio-pancreatography in biliodigestive anastomosis. *Acta Hepatogastroenterol* 1977;24:41.

211. Gold PR, Price JB. Thin needle cholangiography as the primary method for the evaluation of the biliary-enteric anastomosis. *Radiology* 1980;136:309.

212. Classen M, Fruhmorgen P, Kozu T. Endoscopic radiologic demonstration of biliodigestive fistulas. *Endoscopy* 1971;3:138.

213. Vogel VH, Segebrecht P, Schreiber MW. Postoperative retonisierung dilatierter gallenwege. *Fortschr Rontgenstr* 1980;132:522.

214. Rosenthall L, Fonseca C, Arzoumanian A et al. 99mTc-IDA hepatobiliary imaging following upper abdominal surgery. *Radiology* 1979; 130:735.

215. Pavone P, Laghi A, Catalano C et al. MRCP in the examination of patients with biliary-enteric anastomoses. *AJR* 1997;169:807–811.

216. Fulcher AS, Turner MA. Orthotopic liver transplantation: evaluation with MR cholangiography. *Radiology* 1999;211:715–722.

217. Wilson SR, Toi A. Sonography accurately detects biliary obstruction in patients with surgically created biliary-enteric anastomosis. *AJR* 1990;155:789.

218. Grage TB, Lober PH, Imamoglu K et al. Stenosis of the sphincter of Oddi: a clinicopathologic review of 50 cases. *Surgery* 1960;48:304.

219. Cattell RB, Colcock BP, Pollack JL. Stenosis of the sphincter of Oddi. *N Engl J Med* 1957;256:429.

220. Zimmon DS, Ferrara TP, Clemett AR. Radiology of papilla of Vater stenosis. *Gastrointest Radiol* 1978;3:343.

221. Steinberg WM. Sphincter of Oddi dysfunction: a clinical controversy. *Gastroenterology* 1988;95:1409.

222. Geenen JE, Hogan WJ, Dodds WJ et al. The efficacy of endoscopic sphincterotomy after cholecystectomy in patients with sphincter of Oddi dysfunction. *N Eng J Med* 1989;320:82.

223. Sand J, Nordback I, Koskinen M et al. Nifedipine for suspected type II sphincter of Oddi dyskinesia. *Am J Gastro* 1993;88:530.

224. Hogan WJ, Geenen JE, Dodd WJ. Dysmotility disturbances of the biliary tract: classification, diagnosis and treatment. *Semin Liver Dis* 1987;7:302.

225. Ruffolo TA, Lehman GA. HIDA imaging in postcholecystectomy

syndrome—clinical value or romancing the stone? *Am J Gastro* 1991; 86:1092.

226. Geenen JE, Hogan WJ. Endoscopic access to the papilla of Vater. *Endoscopy* 1980;(Suppl):47.

227. Thune A, Scicchitano J, Roberts-Thomson I et al. Reproducibility of endoscopic sphincter of Oddi manometry. *Dig Dis Sci* 1991;36:1401.

228. Venu RP, Greenen JE. Diagnosis and treatment of disease of the papilla. *Clin Gastroenterology* 1986;15:439.

229. Shaffer EA, Hershfield NB, Logan HK et al. Cholescintigraphic detection of functional obstruction of the sphincter Oddi. Effect of papillotomy. *Gastroenterology* 1986;90:728.

230. Darweesh RMA, Dodds WJ, Hogan WJ et al. Efficacy of quantitative hepatobiliary scintigraphy and fatty-meal sonography for evaluating patients with suspected partial common duct obstruction. *Gastroenterol* 1988;94:779.

231. Zeman RK, Dobbins J, Gorelick F et al. Biliary scintigraphy and endoscopic retrograde cholangiographiopancreatography (ERCP) in the evaluation of post-cholecystectomy syndrome. *Radiology* 1985; 156:567.

232. Lee RGL, Gregg JA, Korxhetz AM et al. Sphincter of Oddi stenosis: diagnosis using hepatobiliary scintigraphy and endoscopic manometry. *Radiology* 1985;156:793.

233. Pace RF, Chamberlain MJ, Passi RB. Diagnosing papillary stenosis by technetium-99m HIDA scanning. *Can J Surg* 1983;26:191.

234. Kloiber R, AuCoin R, Hershfield NB et al. Biliary obstruction after cholecystectomy: diagnosis with quantitative cholescintigraphy. *Radiology* 1988;169:643.

235. Grimon G, Buffet C, Andre L et al. Biliary pain in postcholecystectomy patients without biliary obstruction. *Dig Dis Sci* 1991;36: 317.

236. Corazziari E, Cicala M, Habib FI et al. Hepatoduodenal bile transit in cholecystectomized subjects. Relationship of sphincter of Oddi function and diagnostic value. *Dig Dis and Sci* 1994;39:1985–1993.

237. Simeone JF, Butch RJ, Mueller PR et al. The bile ducts after a fatty meal: further sonographic observations. *Radiology* 1985;154:763.

238. Sostre S, Kaloo AN, Spiegler EJ et al. A noninvasive test of sphincter of Oddi dysfunction in postcholecystectomy patients: the scintigraphic score. *J Nucl Med* 1992;33:1216.

239. Thomas PD, Turner JG, Dobbs BR et al. Use of ^{99m}Tc-DISIDA biliary scanning with morphine provocation for the detection of elevated sphincter of Oddi basal pressure. *Gut* 2000;46:838–841.

240. Roberts-Thomson IC, Toouli J, Blanchett W et al. Assessment of bile flow by radioscintigraphy in patients with biliary-type pain after cholecystectomy. *Aust NZ J Med* 1986;16:788.

241. Dickerman RM, Dunn EL. Splenic, pancreatic, and hepatic injuries. *Surg Clin North Am* 1981;61:3.

242. Smith L. The Sir Ernest Finch Memorial Lecture: injuries of the liver, biliary tree and pancreas. *Br J Surg* 1978;65:673.

243. Defore W, Mattox K, Jordan G et al. Management of 1,590 consecutive cases of liver trauma. *Arch Surg* 1976;111:493.

244. Longmire WP, McArthur MS. Occult injuries of the liver, bile duct and pancreas after blunt abdominal trauma. *Am J Surg* 1973;125: 661.

245. Trunkey DD, Shires GT, McClelland R. Management of liver trauma in 811. consecutive patients. *Ann Surg* 1974;179:722.

246. Esensten M, Ralls PW, Colletti P et al. Post-traumatic intrahepatic biloma: sonographic diagnosis. *AJR* 1983;140:303.

247. Wicks JD, Silver TM, Bree RL. Gray scale features of hematomas: an ultrasonic spectrum. *AJR* 1978;131:977.

248. Federle MP, Goldberg HI, Kaiser JA et al. Evaluation of abdominal trauma by computed tomography. *Radiology* 1981;138:637.

249. Toombs BD, Sandler CM, Rauschkolb EN et al. Assessment of hepatic injuries with computed tomography. *J Comput Assist Tomogr* 1982;6:72.

250. Zeman RK, Lee C, Stahl RS et al. Strategy for the use of biliary scintigraphy in non-iatrogenic biliary trauma. *Radiology* 1984;151: 771.

251. Sty JR, Starshak RJ, Hubbard AM. Radionuclide hepatobiliary imaging in the detection of traumatic biliary tract disease in children. *Pediatr Radiol* 1982;12:115.

252. Caride VJ, Gibson DW. Noninvasive evaluation of bile leakage. *Surg Gynecol Obstet* 1982;154:517.

253. Christensen PB, Oestek-Joergensen E, Schoubye J et al. Scintigraphy with 99mTc-C2, 6-diethylacentanilides acid as a diagnostic test in traumatic lesions of the liver and biliary tract. *Gastrointest Radiol* 1981; 6:43.

254. Kuni CC, Klingensmith WC, Koep LJ et al. Communication of intrahepatic cavities with bile ducts: demonstration with Tc-99-m diethyl IDA imaging. *Clin Nucl Med* 1980;5:349.

255. Sty JR, Babbitt DP, Squires W. Tc-99m IDA hepatobiliary imaging: a fractured liver. *Clin Nucl Med* 1979;4:493.

256. Brown ML, Freitas JE, Wahner HW. Useful hepatic parenchymal imaging in hepatobiliary scintigraphy. *AJR* 1981;136:893.

257. Kuligowska D, Schlesinger A, Miller KB et al. Bilomas: a new approach to the diagnosis and treatment. *Gastrointest Radiol* 1983;8: 237.

258. Mueller PR, Ferrucci JT, Simeone JF et al. Detection and drainage of bilomas: special considerations. *AJR* 1983;140:715.

259. Shuman WP, Gibbs P, Rudd TG et al. PIPIDA scintigraphy for cholecystitis: false-positives in alcoholism and total parenteral nutrition. *AJR* 1982;138:1.

260. Serafini AN, Al-Sheikh W, Barkin JS et al. Biliary scintigraphy in acute pancreatitis. *Radiology* 1982;144:591.

261. Edlund G, Kempi V, van der Linden W. Transient nonvisualization of the gallbladder by Tc-99m HIDA cholescintigraphy in acute pancreatitis (concise communication). *J Nucl Med* 1982;23:117.

Diagnostic Nuclear Medicine, Fourth Edition. Edited by M.P. Sandler, R.E. Coleman, J.A. Patton, F.J.Th. Wackers, A. Gottschalk. Lippincott Williams & Wilkins, Philadelphia 2003.

26

SCINTIGRAPHIC DETECTION AND LOCALIZATION OF GASTROINTESTINAL BLEEDING SITES

ABASS ALAVI
DANIEL WORSLEY
HONGMING ZHUANG

Successful management of patients with acute gastrointestinal (GI) bleeding depends on accurate localization of the bleeding site. In cases of massive GI hemorrhage, it is important to identify the bleeding site rather than the specific cause soon after the onset so that appropriate angiographic or surgical interventions are initiated. The clinical symptoms and signs of acute GI bleeding are relatively clearcut but nonspecific in localizing the site of hemorrhage. Patients with hematemesis usually have an upper GI bleeding site proximal to the ligament of Treitz. Common causes of upper GI bleeding are esophageal varices, Mallory-Weiss tears, peptic ulcer disease, esophagitis, gastritis, and neoplasms. Melena, passage of black tarry stool per rectum, commonly occurs in patients with upper GI bleeding. However, hemorrhage distal to the ligament of Treitz might also cause this finding. Hematochezia, the passage of the bright red blood per rectum, occurs often in patients with bleeding site distal to the ligament of Treitz. However, acute bleeding from the esophagus, stomach, or duodenum with rapid transit through the GI tract may also result in hematochezia. The most common causes of GI bleeding in adults within the small bowel distal to the ligament of Treitz are inflammatory mucosal lesions related to Crohn's disease or infection and neoplasms. In children, other causes of small bowel bleeding include Meckel's diverticulum, intussusception, and Henoch-Schönlein purpura. The most common causes of bleeding in the colon are diverticular disease, angiodysplasia, inflammatory bowel disease, neoplasms, arteriovenous malformations, and arterioenteric fistulas. Because of the lack of specificity of the clinical findings in localizing the site

of the GI bleeding, endoscopy and radiologic studies are often used for this purpose.

Flexible endoscopic examination of the esophagus, stomach, and duodenum is of considerable value in the diagnosis and management of patients with upper GI bleeding. However, endoscopy of the colon is associated with significant morbidity and is of limited success in localizing the bleeding site in patients with active hemorrhage (1). In addition, bleeding sites in the small bowel cannot be successfully visualized with current endoscopic techniques. Radiographic barium studies have no role in the evaluation of patients with acute GI bleeding. Visceral angiography of the GI tract has long been used both in the diagnosis and treatment of GI bleeding. Animal studies have demonstrated evidence of hemorrhage in the small bowel at a rate as low as 0.5 mL per minute using angiographic techniques (2). The successful localization of GI bleeding with angiography depends not only on the rate but also on the type of bleeding and the time of the examination. Arterial or capillary bleeding can be readily detected with angiography, whereas demonstration of venous bleeding is very difficult with this technique. Timing of the study is also of paramount importance in the angiographic localization of sites of GI bleeding. Patients must be actively bleeding while the contrast is administered into the artery that supplies the site of hemorrhage for successful results. However, GI bleeding, particularly in the lower GI tract, is often intermittent and, therefore, the bleeding sites are often undetected with angiographic techniques. Pharmacologic enhancement of the bleeding diathesis before angiography, with heparin, intraarterial vasodilators, or thrombolytic agents in selected patients may improve the diagnostic performance of the procedure with minimal complications (3,4).

The ability of the scintigraphic techniques to view the entire abdomen offers an important advantage over endoscopy or visceral angiography. Early work with radionuclides for the localization of sites of GI bleeding used an *in vivo* nonimaging technique with a Geiger counter (5). This research was succeeded by scintigraphic techniques predominantly using ^{99m}Tc-sulfur colloid

A. Alavi: Division of Nuclear Medicine, University of Pennsylvania Medical Center, Philadelphia, PA.

D. Worsley: Division of Nuclear Medicine, Department of Radiology, Vancouver General Hospital, University of British Colombia, Vancouver, BC.

H. Zhuang: Department of Radiology, Division of Nuclear Medicine, University of Pennsylvania, Philadelphia, PA.

and ^{99m}Tc-labeled red blood cells (6–12). Researchers have used other radiopharmaceuticals to detect and localize sites of GI bleeding including ^{99m}Tc-labeled heat treated red blood cells and ^{111}In-labeled red blood cells (13–20). However, scintigraphic techniques using ^{99m}Tc-sulfur colloid and ^{99m}Tc-labeled red blood cells are most commonly used in clinical practice and are the focus of this chapter.

[99M]TC-SULFUR COLLOID TECHNIQUE

Theoretical Considerations

The ^{99m}Tc-sulfur colloid technique is based on these theoretical considerations: When a radioactive agent cleared by a specific organ (e.g., the liver, spleen, and marrow) is injected intravenously into a patient with active bleeding, a fraction of the injected activity will extravasate at the bleeding site and be eliminated from the circulation. This phenomenon is repeated each time the blood recirculates, adding another, but smaller, fraction to the activity already at the site of the hemorrhage. Because of continued clearance of the radioactive agent from the vascular system by the target organ, a contrast is eventually reached between the site of the bleeding and surrounding background (Fig. 26.1). The relationship between the activity at a bleeding site and the background activity (i.e., activity in the vascular system) is graphically described in Fig. 26.2. Immediately after the intravenous administration of the radioactive agent, the background activity decreases exponentially while the activity at the bleeding site increases exponentially. A contrast begins to develop between the bleeding site and the background when these two curves cross. Maximum contrast occurs at the completion of the extraction of the intravascular activity by the target organ.

[99m]Tc-sulfur colloid is considered to be the most favorable agent available for this purpose. In normal individuals, ^{99m}Tc-sulfur colloid administered intravenously is cleared from the circulation by the reticuloendothelial cells in the liver, spleen, and bone marrow with a half-time of 2.5 to 3.5 minutes. By 12 to 15 minutes most of the injected activity is cleared from the vascular system (background). In patients with diffuse liver disease, the rate of clearance of the particles is decreased. In these patients, a maximum contrast between the bleeding site and the background may not be achieved within the first 12 to 15 minutes of the administration of the radiopharmaceutical.

Imaging Techniques

No patient preparation is required. Using a large field-of-view camera, the patient is positioned with the entire lower abdomen (excluding the upper half of the liver) within the field of view. Flow images (5 seconds per frame) are obtained following intravenous administration of 370 to 550 mBq of ^{99m}Tc-sulfur colloid (children 7.4 MBq/kg, minimum activity 74 MBq). If necessary, the patient is repositioned so that the inferior half of the liver and spleen are at the top of the field of view. Sequential images are then acquired in a cine format every 2 minutes for 20 minutes (Fig. 26.3). If a bleeding site is detected, further imaging is necessary to determine the progression of activity and define the anatomic location of the bleeding site (Figs. 26.4

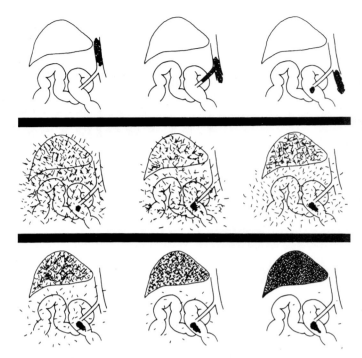

FIGURE 26.1. Theoretical basis of sulfur colloid technique. An agent cleared by an organ such as the liver is injected intravenously. At the bleeding site, a fraction of the injected activity extravasates and is eliminated from the circulation. This phenomenon is repeated each time the blood recirculates. Because of rapid clearance of the radioactive agent by the target organ, eventually a contrast is reached between the bleeding site and the surrounding background. (From Alavi A, Ring EJ. Localization of gastrointestinal bleeding: superiority of ^{99m}Tc sulfur colloid compared with angiography. *AJR* 1981;137:741–748, with permission.)

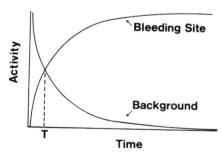

FIGURE 26.2. Graphical presentation of theoretical considerations described in Fig. 26.1. The background activity decreases exponentially immediately after intravenous administration of this agent. The activity at the bleeding site increases exponentially in the opposite direction. A contrast is reached between the bleeding site and the surrounding background activity when the two curves cross (7). (From Alavi A, Ring EJ. Localization of gastrointestinal bleeding: superiority of ^{99m}Tc sulfur colloid compared with angiography. *AJR* 1981;137:741–748, with permission.)

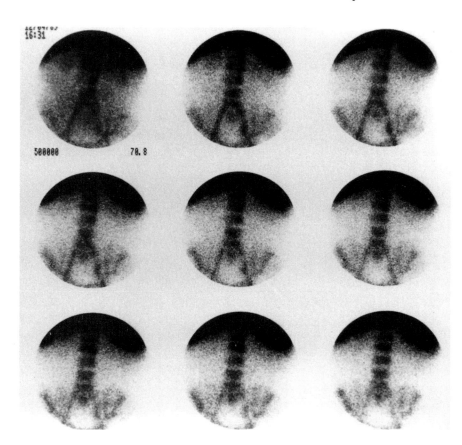

FIGURE 26.3. ^{99m}Tc-sulfur colloid bleeding study. Normal study (0 to 9 minutes). Sulfur colloid is distributed in the reticuloendothelial cells of the liver, spleen, and marrow after its removal from the intravascular space. The majority of the activity is sequestered in the liver. Optimally, the inferior aspect of the liver is positioned at the superior portion of the image so that most of the hepatic and splenic activity is not in the field of view. The remainder of the activity can be noted in the marrow of the lumbar spine and pelvis. No other areas of activity are present. There is no evidence of active gastrointestinal hemorrhage. (From Alavi A, Ring EJ. Localization of gastrointestinal bleeding: superiority of ^{99m}Tc sulfur colloid compared with angiography. *AJR* 1981;137:741–748, with permission.)

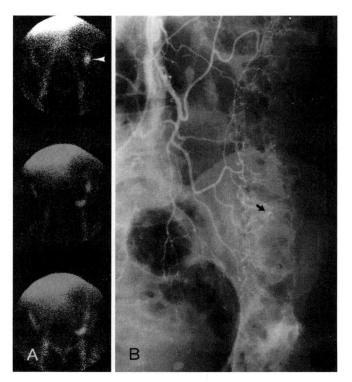

FIGURE 26.4. Low rate sigmoid bleed. **A:** Within a few minutes of intravenous administration of ^{99m}Tc-sulfur colloid the scan shows evidence of extravasation in the left lower quadrant area (*top*). Later the activity moves along the iliac crest corresponding to the direction of the sigmoid colon (*middle* and *bottom*). **B:** Contrast angiogram of the inferior mesenteric artery reveals a small extravasation of the contrast medium (*arrow*) at the junction of the descending colon and the sigmoid colon. (From Alavi A. Detection of gastrointestinal bleeding with ^{99m}Tc-sulfur colloid. *Semin Nucl Med* 1982;12:126–138, with permission.)

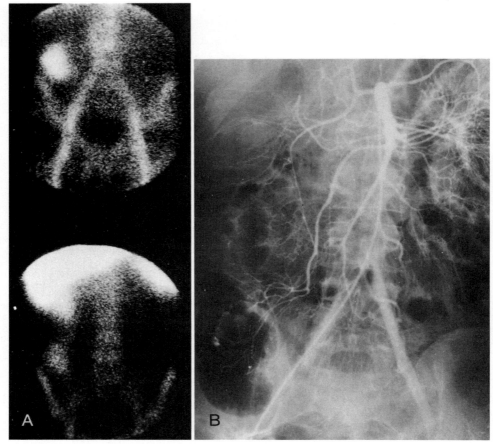

FIGURE 26.5. Lesion resulting from ischemia. **A:** ^{99m}Tc-sulfur colloid scan obtained within approximately 3 minutes after injection (*top left*) shows a bleeding site (*arrow*). The activity gradually moves up toward the liver. Based on these images the site of bleeding was diagnosed to be in the cecum. **B:** Angiogram of the superior mesenteric immediately after completion of the scan shows extravasation of the contrast medium in the cecal region. The site of extravasation corresponds exactly to the area seen on the scan. (From Alavi A, Ring EJ. Localization of gastrointestinal bleeding: superiority of ^{99m}Tc sulfur colloid compared with angiography. *AJR* 1981;137:741–748, with permission.)

to 26.7). If no bleeding site is found, the patient should be repositioned for a left anterior oblique view to minimize hepatic activity, and a 2-minute static image acquired. Finally, if the study continues to be negative, an anterior image for 2 minutes should be obtained to allow any activity concealed by the liver and spleen to advance within the lumen of the GI tract away from these high-activity organs. If the patient has a bowel movement during the examination, the stool should be imaged. It may be the only positive finding in a patient with rectal or rectosigmoid junction bleeding (Figs. 26.8 to 26.11). It is advisable to perform a rectal examination on every patient with negative scan and image the extracted blood for extravasated radioactive blood. This finding may be the only evidence for bleeding in the rectum. If the initial ^{99m}Tc-sulfur colloid bleeding study is negative and there is a suspicion of further bleeding, a repeat study can be performed at any time following the preceding examination (Fig 26.12). Before the injection of a second dose of ^{99m}Tc-sulfur colloid a static image, which can be subtracted from subsequent images, should be obtained. Alternatively, covering the liver and spleen with a lead apron may assist in decreasing the counts from these organs.

Interpretation

The rapid clearance of activity from the vascular space with ^{99m}Tc-sulfur colloid enhances the visualization of extravasated activity. Bleeding sites are best demonstrated within 10 to 15 minutes after injection and are seen as extravasated activity that changes configuration with time. Activity may move in both antegrade and retrograde directions. Focal activity that remains fixed and does not change configuration with time most likely represents an ectopic or accessory spleen and is unlikely to represent a site of GI bleeding (21). Other false-positive interpretations may be related to extramedullary hematopoiesis, focal bone marrow activity, Paget's disease, or increased activity within transplanted kidneys (22–24).

^{99M}TC-LABELED RED BLOOD CELL METHOD

Labeled intravascular tracers such as ^{99m}Tc-labeled red blood cells, have also been shown to be useful in determining sites of lower GI bleeding. In patients with intermittent GI bleeding,

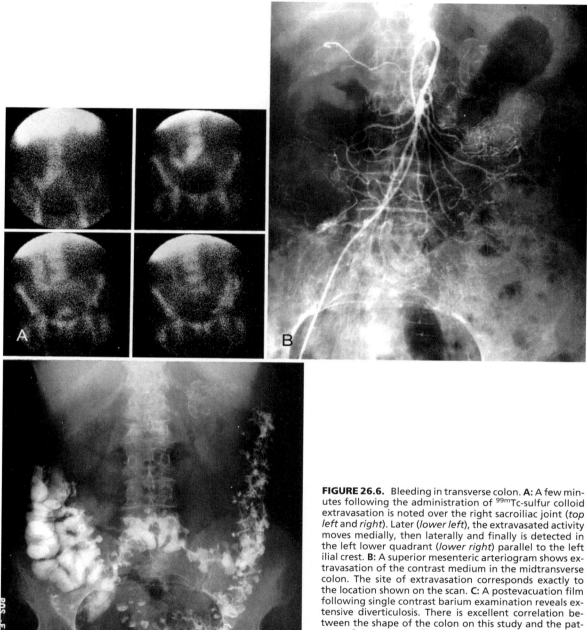

FIGURE 26.6. Bleeding in transverse colon. **A:** A few minutes following the administration of ^{99m}Tc-sulfur colloid extravasation is noted over the right sacroiliac joint (*top left* and *right*). Later (*lower left*), the extravasated activity moves medially, then laterally and finally is detected in the left lower quadrant (*lower right*) parallel to the left ilial crest. **B:** A superior mesenteric arteriogram shows extravasation of the contrast medium in the midtransverse colon. The site of extravasation corresponds exactly to the location shown on the scan. **C:** A postevacuation film following single contrast barium examination reveals extensive diverticulosis. There is excellent correlation between the shape of the colon on this study and the pattern of movement of the extravasated activity on the scan. (From Alavi A, Ring EJ. Localization of gastrointestinal bleeding: superiority of ^{99m}Tc sulfur colloid compared with angiography. *AJR* 1981;137:741–748, with permission.)

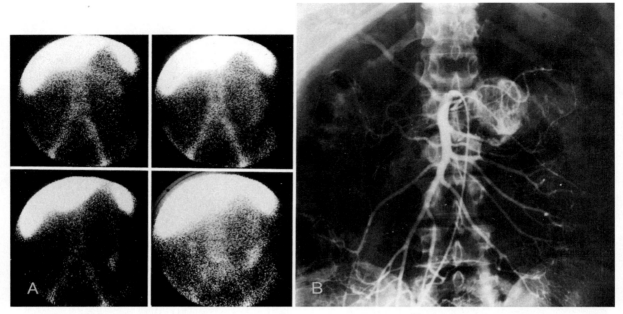

FIGURE 26.7. Small bowel hemorrhage. **A:** Soon after the injection of ^{99m}Tc-sulfur colloid an area of intense activity (blood pool) is seen in the left upper quadrant (*top left*). With time, extravasated blood is seen at the same site (*top right*), then moving caudally (*lower left*), and finally seen on the right side (*lower right*). This is a typical appearance for small bowel hemorrhage. **B:** A superior mesenteric arteriogram shows a vascular lesion in the jejunum corresponding to the site seen on the scan. The appearance of this lesion in the angiogram is most consistent with a leiomyoma of the bowel. This diagnosis was confirmed by histopathologic examination.

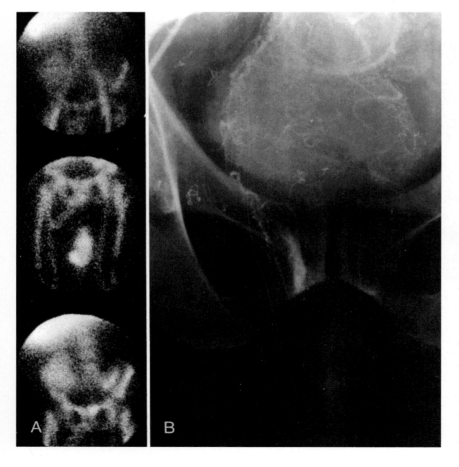

FIGURE 26.8. Bleeding site in rectum. **A:** Very shortly after the administration of ^{99m}Tc-sulfur colloid, a faint uptake is noted in the right lower quadrant corresponding to the site of the transplanted kidney (*top*). No other abnormal activity is noted in the rest of the abdomen. Intense activity is detected in the clots discharged from the rectum into a bedpan (*middle*). An image of the lower abdomen reveals activity in the left lower quadrant area parallel to the left iliac crest (*bottom*). **B:** Selective angiography of the inferior mesenteric artery following the performance of the scan shows extravasation of the contrast medium into the rectal cavity. This confirms the scintigraphic interpretation. The cause of the hemorrhage could not be determined even by endoscopy or direct examination in the operating room. (From Alavi A, Ring EJ. Localization of gastrointestinal bleeding: superiority of ^{99m}Tc sulfur colloid compared with angiography. *AJR* 1981;137:741–748, with permission.)

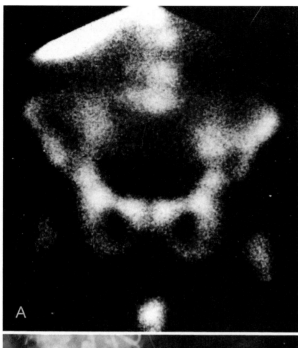

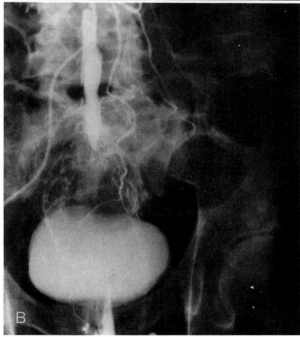

FIGURE 26.9. Rectal bleeding site. **A:** The image was obtained at the completion of a study on a patient who previously had an inconclusive rectosigmoidoscopy and negative arteriography. The scan shows the extravasated blood below the perineum. This indicated that the bleeding site was in the rectum, which was confirmed by repeated arteriography. **B:** After completion of the scan, an inferior mesenteric arteriogram shows extravasation of the contrast medium superimposed on the pubic bone. This confirms the findings on the scan. Unfortunately, because of reliance on rectosigmoidoscopic diagnosis, the first arteriogram did not include this area and therefore did not demonstrate the site of hemorrhage. This scan was crucial on the management of this patient. (From Alavi A, McLean GK. Radioisotopic detection of gastrointestinal bleeding: an integrated approach to the diagnostic and therapeutic modalities. In: Freeman LM, Weissman H, eds. *Nuclear medicine annual 1980.* New York: Raven Press, 1980:177–218, with permission.)

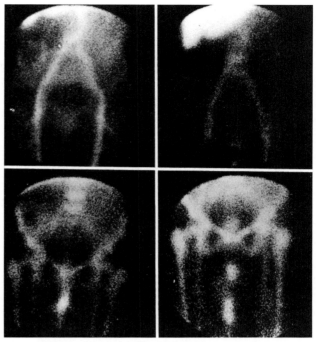

FIGURE 26.10. Rectal hemorrhage. Typical pattern of hemorrhage in the rectal area as detected by the scan. Rectosigmoidoscopy was done before scintigraphy and was reported to show hemorrhage above the sigmoid colon. A repeated examination revealed a small ulcer in the rectum that was treated successfully with silver nitrate application.

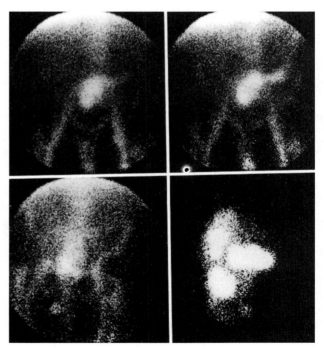

FIGURE 26.11. Bleeding sigmoid lesion. A positive scan with bleeding site in the sigmoid colon (*top left*) that moves in a retrograde fashion into the descending colon (*top right*) and forward into the rectum (*lower left*), and finally into the bedpan (*lower right*). This patient was treated successfully by intravenous administration of vasopressin without further investigation with other modalities. (From Alavi A. Detection of gastrointestinal bleeding with ^{99m}Tc-sulfur colloid. *Semin Nucl Med* 1982;12:126–138, with permission.)

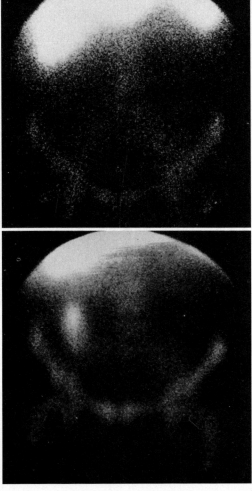

FIGURE 26.12. Intermittent hemorrhage demonstrated by ^{99m}Tc-sulfur colloid scan. *Top:* No evidence of hemorrhage in a patient with lower GI bleeding. *Bottom:* A repeat scan 1 hour later following a bloody bowel movement shows an area of hemorrhage in the cecal region.

^{99m}Tc-labeled red blood cells offer a longer time window for imaging compared with ^{99m}Tc-sulfur colloid. However, images obtained at later times following the injection can be misleading with regard to the site of hemorrhage because of antegrade and retrograde movement of activity within the lumen of the GI tract (25,26). The minimum detectable bleeding rates for ^{99m}Tc-labeled red blood cells is somewhat larger compared with ^{99m}Tc-sulfur colloid techniques in animal models (27). Therefore, the time required to visualize low rates of bleeding with ^{99m}Tc-labeled red blood cells is considerably longer as compared with ^{99m}Tc-sulfur colloid.

Imaging Technique

The highest possible labeling efficiency can be achieved only by using the *in vitro* techniques (28,29). *In vivo* labeling of red blood cells can be achieved using a kit that contains stannous

chloride. This approach does not require handling of blood products and is widely used for blood pool imaging of the heart (30). With the *in vivo* technique, the labeling efficiency is significantly lower than that achievable with *in vitro* techniques (70% vs. 95%, respectively). Because of the low labeling efficiency with *in vivo* technique, free pertechnetate secreted from the stomach and small bowel may cause false-positive results. Once the blood is labeled, the patient is positioned under the gamma-camera with most of the abdomen within the field of view. Flow images are obtained (5 seconds per frame) following the intravenous administration of 700 to 800 MBq of ^{99m}Tc-labeled red blood cells (Fig. 26.13**A**). Then 15- to 30-second dynamic images (approximately 500,000 counts per image) are acquired for 60 to 90 minutes (Fig. 26.13**B** and **C**). If the bleeding site is detected, further imaging is recommended to determine the progression of activity and determine the anatomic location of the bleeding site. A nuclear enema can be performed to define the colonic anatomy and assist in the interpretation of a positive study (31). If no bleeding focus is localized, additional images may be acquired for up to 24 hours.

Interpretation

Cinematic display of acquired data is necessary to optimize image interpretation (32). Serial image subtraction, using data from early images in the study, is an additional, relatively simple technique that can be performed to enhance detection of activity that changes with time (33). As with ^{99m}Tc-sulfur colloid, the diagnosis of GI bleeding is made when extravasated activity is noted within the bowel lumen that changes with time (Figs. 26.14 to 26.17). The distribution and intensity of extravasated activity will change with time because of retrograde and antegrade transit within the bowel lumen. False-positive studies have been reported related to genitourinary tract (GU) activity and free pertechnetate within the GU tract (34–36). Focal accumulation of ^{99m}Tc red cells related to hepatic hemangioma or esophageal or mesenteric varices will not change configuration during the length of the study and, therefore, should not be confused with sites of GI bleeding (37–39).

DISCUSSION

Advocates for ^{99m}Tc-sulfur colloid imaging and ^{99m}Tc-labeled red blood cell imaging techniques have described the relative merits of each technique (10,40–42). The major disadvantage of the ^{99m}Tc-sulfur colloid method relates to the intermittent nature of GI bleeding and the necessity of the injection of the radiotracer while the patient is actively bleeding. Two studies in which both techniques were performed in the same patient are reported in the literature (41,42). Both studies report very high sensitivity and specificity for ^{99m}Tc-labeled red blood cells and relatively poor sensitivity for the ^{99m}Tc-sulfur colloid. The conclusion from these studies was that intravascular markers such as ^{99m}Tc-labeled red blood cells have a higher sensitivity in detecting GI bleeding, because of the intermittent nature of the process. Unfortunately, the initial enthusiasm for the ^{99m}Tc red blood cell technique has not been substantiated by recent

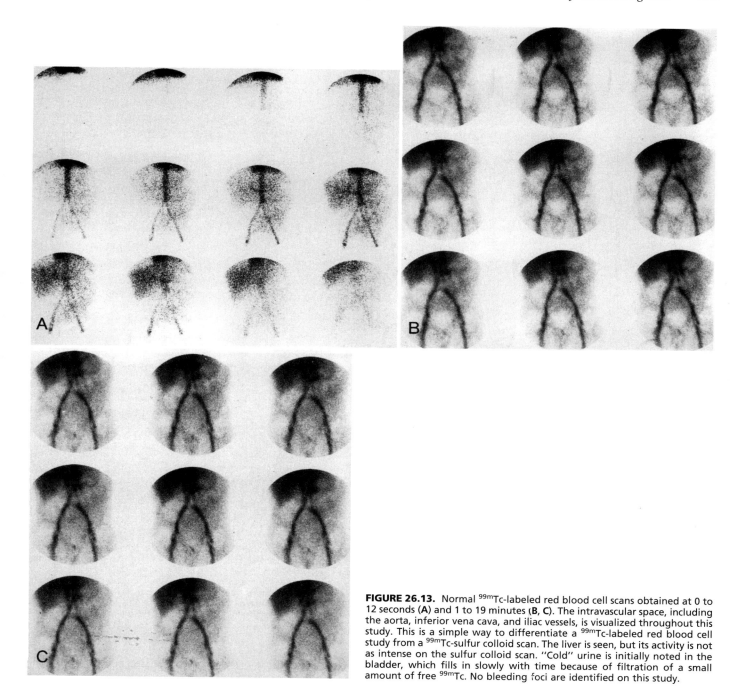

FIGURE 26.13. Normal ^{99m}Tc-labeled red blood cell scans obtained at 0 to 12 seconds (**A**) and 1 to 19 minutes (**B, C**). The intravascular space, including the aorta, inferior vena cava, and iliac vessels, is visualized throughout this study. This is a simple way to differentiate a ^{99m}Tc-labeled red blood cell study from a ^{99m}Tc-sulfur colloid scan. The liver is seen, but its activity is not as intense on the sulfur colloid scan. "Cold" urine is initially noted in the bladder, which fills in slowly with time because of filtration of a small amount of free ^{99m}Tc. No bleeding foci are identified on this study.

studies. In two large series, the authors questioned the merit of ^{99m}Tc-labeled red blood cell technique in localizing the bleeding sites for surgical intervention (43–44). In fact, one report advocates abandoning its routine use as a screening test before angiography. Obviously, this may be an extreme view of the test, and at least some of the inaccuracies encountered can be attributed to the improper interpretation of the results acquired. A decade before these publications appeared in the literature, it was predicted that careless use of this method might result in mismanagement of patients with GI bleeding (10). It is well established

that if the bleeding is detected only with later imaging, the site of extravasation may be easily misrepresented. In patients with hemorrhage, the transit of intestinal contents, including the extravasated blood, is accelerated. We have encountered patients who could have been diagnosed as having a bleeding site in the sigmoid colon instead of the hepatic flexure or the transverse colon if imaging had been delayed for only 10 to 15 minutes. We have undertaken a similar study in our institution comparing ^{99m}Tc-sulfur colloid scans with ^{99m}Tc red blood cell images in the first 60 minutes after the administration of the radiotracer.

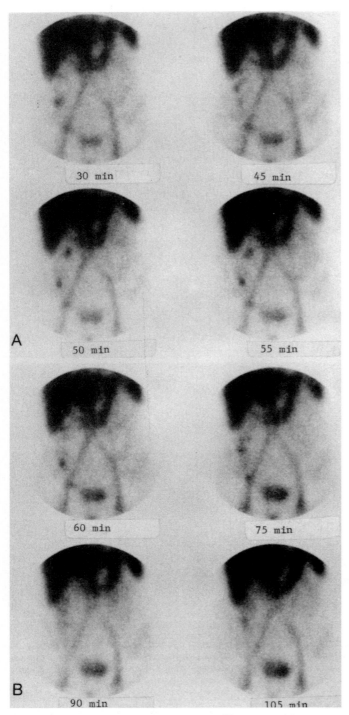

FIGURE 26.14. Cecal bleeding detected by ^{99m}Tc-labeled red blood cells. **A:** An image obtained at 20 minutes shows a point of faint extravasation in the right lower quadrant area. The intensity of this activity increases with time. **B:** No significant changes are seen on images obtained at 54 and 56 minutes. The negative defect seen on these images probably represents a nonradioactive clot in the same location. (Photo courtesy of Jerome Jacobstein, M.D., Graduate Hospital, Philadelphia.)

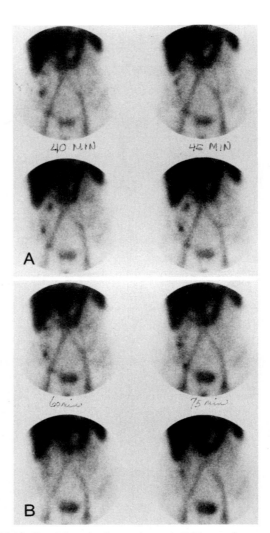

FIGURE 26.15. Right colon hemorrhage. **A:** Evidence of extravasation is seen in the right colon on image obtained at 30 minutes. Later images acquired at 45, 50, and 55 minutes show a slight change in the appearance of the activity in the lumen of the bowel. **B:** Images obtained at 60, 75, 90, and 105 minutes reveal no significant progression of the extravasated blood in the lumen of the colon. Note intense visualization of the stomach on all images obtained on this patient. (Photo courtesy of Jerome Jacobstein, M.D., Graduate Hospital, Philadelphia.)

In contrast to the previously described reports, no significant difference in performance was noted between the two techniques.

In a retrospective review of 359 GI bleeding studies in our center, we compared the performance of the two techniques in a similar population of patients. One hundred ninety-three patients underwent ^{99m}Tc-sulfur colloid imaging, which lasted 30 minutes, and 138 were examined with ^{99m}Tc-labeled red blood cell imaging for 60 minutes. In addition, in 28 patients ^{99m}Tc-sulfur colloid imaging was followed by up to several hours of ^{99m}Tc-labeled red blood cell continuous scanning. We noted that the detection rate of the sites of bleeding was similar between the two methods: Among 193 scans with ^{99m}Tc-sulfur colloid, 47 (24.4%) successfully identified the bleeding sites. In 138 examined with ^{99m}Tc-labeled red blood cell, 38 (27.5%) were

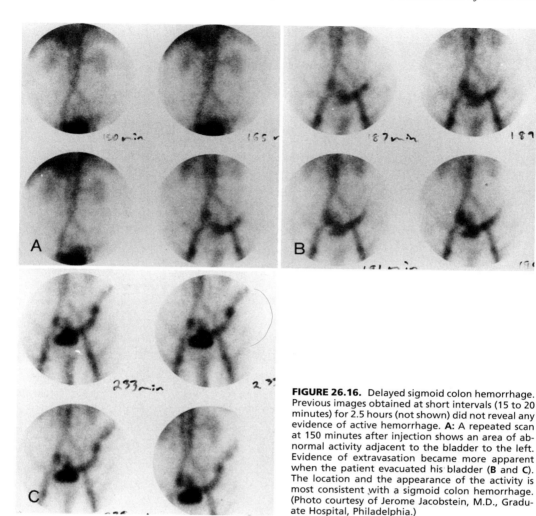

FIGURE 26.16. Delayed sigmoid colon hemorrhage. Previous images obtained at short intervals (15 to 20 minutes) for 2.5 hours (not shown) did not reveal any evidence of active hemorrhage. **A:** A repeated scan at 150 minutes after injection shows an area of abnormal activity adjacent to the bladder to the left. Evidence of extravasation became more apparent when the patient evacuated his bladder (**B** and **C**). The location and the appearance of the activity is most consistent with a sigmoid colon hemorrhage. (Photo courtesy of Jerome Jacobstein, M.D., Graduate Hospital, Philadelphia.)

successful in identifying the site of hemorrhage. Although it appeared that ^{99m}Tc-labeled red blood cell imaging had slightly higher sensitivity than ^{99m}Tc-sulfur colloid imaging (27.5% vs. 24.4%), the difference is not statically significant ($p = 0.71$). In 28 patients scanned with ^{99m}Tc-sulfur colloid first and followed immediately by ^{99m}Tc-labeled red blood cell examination, 4 (14.8%) additional positive results were noted by red blood cell imaging. Among these 4 positive results, only one occurred within 1 hour of the beginning of the red blood cell study. Obviously, it is impractical to image a patient for a extended period on a routine basis because of the practical reasons and the low yield from such prolonged and labor intensive examination. Interestingly, there was a significant difference ($p = 0.009$) in the proportion of positive results between the studies performed at regular working hours (30.7%, 71 of 231) and those during evening and night shifts (14.1%, 18 of 128). The reason for the low rate of success for detecting the sites of bleeding during on-call studies is likely due to the length of time between the request and the initiating of the scan. In this population, the shortest time interval between the time the scan was requested and the time the scan was performed was approximately 25 minutes and

50 minutes for ^{99m}Tc-sulfur colloid imaging and for ^{99m}Tc-labeled red blood cell scan, respectively, when the studies were done at regular working hours. However, this time interval increased to about 2 hours for most on-call studies because of logistical reasons. Considering the similar sensitivity of the two techniques, ^{99m}Tc-sulfur colloid imaging was the study of choice during off hours because of its technical simplicity, which provides expeditious results for optimal patient care and for effective use of resource available. The majority of ^{99m}Tc-sulfur colloid imaging (98 of 193) were performed off hours. In contrast, only 21.7% (30 of 138) of the ^{99m}Tc-labeled red blood cell scans were done at late shifts. When the study results during the regular working hours were compared, ^{99m}Tc-sulfur colloid imaging appeared to have slightly higher sensitivity (34.7%, 33 of 95) than ^{99m}Tc-labeled red blood cell scan (31.5%, 34 of 108) although statistically there was insignificant difference ($p = 0.84$) between the two. Similarly, the sensitivity of ^{99m}Tc-sulfur colloid imaging at off hours was 14.3% (14 of 98), which was almost identical to ^{99m}Tc-labeled red blood cell scans performed at late shift (13.3%, 4 of 30). The simplicity of performing ^{99m}Tc-sulfur colloid imaging compared with ^{99m}Tc-labeled red blood

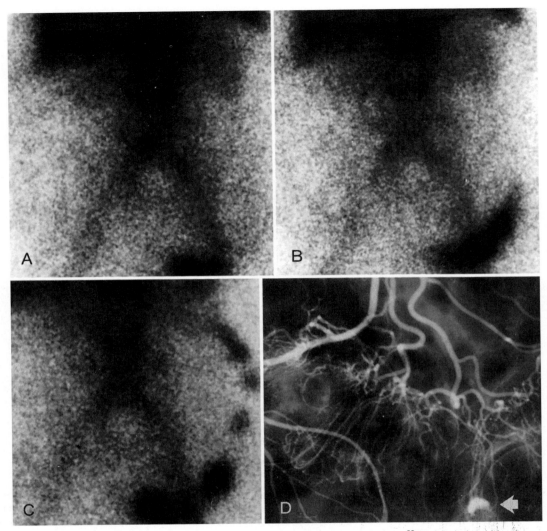

FIGURE 26.17. Sigmoid bleed. Patient with a bleeding sigmoid diverticulum, ^{99m}Tc-labeled red blood cell scans obtained at 15 (**A**), 30 (**B**), and 60 (**C**) minutes after its administration, show early localization in the sigmoid colon. With time there is retrograde transport of radioactive blood to the splenic flexure. **D:** Magnification view of an angiogram demonstrates extravasation into the bleeding diverticulum (*arrow*).

cell scans provides potential advantage over ^{99m}Tc-labeled red blood cell imaging for at least emergency studies at late shifts.

We analyzed 76 positive ^{99m}Tc-sulfur colloid scans to determine the speed with which extravasated blood moves in the GI tract. In each case, the site of hemorrhage was visualized within the first 10 minutes. The transit of extravasated blood was determined in the following segments of the GI tract: jejunum, ileum, ascending colon, transverse colon, descending colon, and rectosigmoid colon. Within 10 minutes after administration, in 37 patients a large portion of one segment of the bowel was visualized (Fig. 26.18). Within the same time interval, 19 patients had two segments, 9 had three segments, and 3 had four segments of the GI tract outlined. In 8 patients, the activity within the lumen of the bowel disappeared minutes after visualization. Seven of these 8 patients suffered from small bowel hemorrhage. In general, the slowest transit occurred with bleeding in the rectosigmoid colon and the fastest in the small bowel.

These data indicate that the transit of intestinal contents is significantly accelerated in patients with GI bleeding. Therefore, early and frequent images of the abdomen must be obtained after the administration of the radiotracer for accurate localization of the site of hemorrhage (Figs. 26.19 to 26.20).

Extravasated blood moves in both antegrade and retrograde fashion soon after it enters into the lumen of the bowel. This phenomenon is often seen with both ^{99m}Tc-sulfur colloid and blood pool imaging. Therefore, if a large segment of the large bowel is outlined on delayed images the true site cannot be determined from those images. For example, if the whole transverse, descending, and sigmoid colons are visualized on delayed images, the site of bleeding could be located anywhere from the duodenum to the rectum.

With intravascular indicators, structures with significant vascular volume, such as varices and arteriovenous malformations, and organs with significant blood pool, such as the liver, spleen,

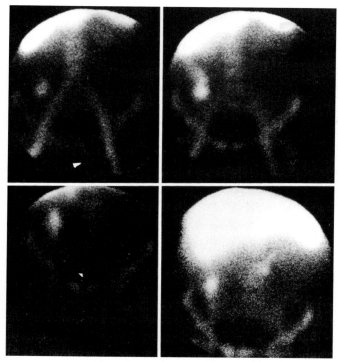

FIGURE 26.18. Clearcut cecal bleeding. These images demonstrate a bleeding point in the cecum with visualization of the transverse colon on the later scan. A right hemicolectomy was performed without angiographic confirmation. This resulted in complete cessation of lower GI hemorrhage.

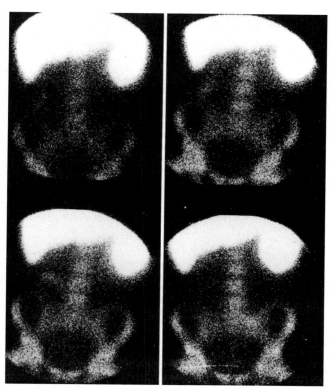

FIGURE 26.20. Transient visualization of small bowel hemorrhage. Similar to Fig. 26.19, this study shows transient activity in the right flank that disappears with time. This was interpreted to represent a small bowel hemorrhage.

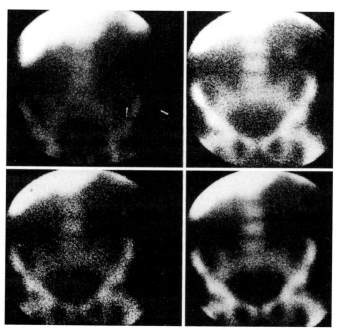

FIGURE 26.19. Transient visualization of small bowel hemorrhage. An area of faint activity is seen in the left upper quadrant area (*top right*) that later becomes more faint and finally disappears. This pattern is commonly seen with small bowel hemorrhage.

and kidneys, may interfere with visualization of the bleeding site or be interpreted erroneously as the site of hemorrhage.

When *in vivo* ^{99m}Tc-labeled red blood cells are used to detect the bleeding site, only 60% to 70% of the injected activity (^{99m}Tc pertechnetate) will be tagged to the red blood cells (45). Of the remaining 30% to 40%, a significant fraction is seen in the stomach, small and large bowels, kidneys, and bladder. The presence of these activities may result in false-positive and false-negative results. Using modified *in vivo* techniques, the percentage of unbound activity is decreased although not eliminated (46). Interestingly, even with high *in vitro* labeling efficacy with kits available for this purpose, kidney and bladder are often visualized with this approach.

The diagnostic evaluation and management of patients with GI bleeding is not uniform. However, the objective of diagnostic imaging, including scintigraphy, is to confirm and localize the site of GI bleeding. A summary of studies performed to determine the accuracy of ^{99m}Tc red blood cell imaging in localizing sites of GI bleeding is found in Table 26.1 (43–44,47–51). Results vary substantially, which probably relate to patient selection and referral bias. For example, in the three larger series, the proportion of patients in which the diagnosis was confirmed ranged from only 42% to 49% (43,44,51). Included in these series were patients in whom the diagnosis of bleeding was confirmed only on late (24-hour) imaging. Although late imaging provides objective evidence for the presence or absence of continued bleeding, the site of bleeding could not be reliably deter-

Table 26.1. *Accuracy of ^{99m}Tc-RBC Technique in Accurately Localizing the Site of Hemorrhage*

Reference	Number of Patients	Number of Abnormal Studies	Confirmed Diagnosis (%)	Correct Localization (%)[a,b]	Incorrect Location or False Negative (%)
43	76	26	16 (62)	15 (94)	1 (6)
45	162	98	46 (47)	24 (52)	22 (48)
46	203	52	22 (42)	9 (40)	13 (59)
47	59	45	32 (71)	28 (88)	4 (13)
44	41	31	30 (97)	29 (97)	1 (3)
48	100	62	58 (94)	48 (83)	10 (17)
49	153	90	44 (49)	33 (75)	11 (25)

[a]In most patients the "supposedly" correct site was shown by nonangiographic techniques.
[b]Accuracy of the ^{99m}Tc-RBC technique varies from 40% to 94%.

mined based solely on late images (25,26). A positive scintigraphic study followed by a negative visceral angiogram is well recognized and is usually due to intermittent or venous bleeding. In addition, several series have included patients with upper GI bleeding (52). In these patients, upper GI endoscopy would have been expected to identify the bleeding sites, because scintigraphy has a very limited role in the evaluation of patients with upper GI bleeds. In a subset of patients in whom upper GI bleeding was excluded and the ^{99m}Tc-labeled red blood cell scan was positive within 2 hours, the accuracy of localization of scintigraphy was 100% (51).

One major deficiency of almost all the reported studies is the lack of comparison between scintigraphic and angiographic findings. Instead of confirmation by angiographic evidence for the site of active hemorrhage, most authors have selected other indirect criteria for this purpose, including demonstration of common lesions such as diverticula and polyps as visualized on barium or endoscopic examinations. These lesions are very often detected on routine examination of patients who have no clinical evidence of hemorrhage. Therefore, confirmation of hemorrhage can be achieved only by demonstration of extravasation of blood by angiographic or endoscopic procedures.

Relative Usefulness as Screening Test

A large number of negative results will be observed in patients studied with either ^{99m}Tc-sulfur colloid or ^{99m}Tc-labeled red blood cell techniques. This indicates that a majority of patients with lower GI hemorrhage will have stopped bleeding before they are referred to the nuclear medicine laboratory. The time interval between the bleeding episodes and the duration of the hemorrhage varies considerably among patients. Most episodes of bleeding last for a few hours followed by a cessation period of several hours. A coordinated effort between the clinicians and the nuclear medicine staff is essential for successful detection and localization of the site of hemorrhage. The most effective approach is to scan the patient soon after one or two large bloody bowel movements. Whenever a bleeding episode is suspected, a repeated study should be carried out. Higher radiation exposure from repeated injections of either ^{99m}Tc-sulfur colloid or ^{99m}Tc-labeled red blood cells may be considered a disadvantage. How-

ever, most patients with lower GI bleeding are in their 60s and 70s. Therefore, theoretical risks from radiation exposure, which are expected to occur many years later, are minimal compared with those posed by the hemorrhage and the events that may follow. Also, the radiation exposure from repeated nuclear scans is lower than that received during visceral arteriography. Delayed localization of the bleeding site usually results in multiple blood transfusions. The probability of developing blood-borne infections increases as the number of transfusions increases. Blind surgery without accurate localization of the bleeding site carries considerable risks.

Reports indicate that attempts to localize the site of hemorrhage in the upper GI tract on a routine basis do not significantly affect the outcome (53–57). In one report, hospital deaths, recurrence of bleeding, number of blood transfusions, early death after recurrent hemorrhage, and duration of hospital stay were identical between the control group and those who underwent early endoscopy to localize the site of hemorrhage (58). These data suggest that after the diagnosis of upper GI bleeding is established, aggressive workup to localize the site should be postponed until surgical or other major interventions are contemplated. At this time upper GI endoscopy is considered the most reliable examination to visualize the site of bleeding. Angiography is used mainly to stop the hemorrhage.

In a series of 82 patients with positive ^{99m}Tc-sulfur colloid scans, GI hemorrhage was noted to occur with these frequencies at four anatomic sites: jejunum 28%, ileum 11%, right colon 21%, and left colon 40%. These data contradict two previous reports that showed significantly higher incidence of hemorrhage in the right colon than in the left (59). The latter data were obtained using contrast visceral angiography. These findings have led some surgeons to perform right hemicolectomy when examinations carried out failed to localize the site of hemorrhage. Obviously, this practice should be discouraged and every attempt must be made to demonstrate the site of bleeding before any major surgical intervention is planned.

The performance of either a ^{99m}Tc-sulfur colloid or ^{99m}Tc-labeled red blood cell scan of the abdomen as a screening examination for detection and localization of bleeding sites in the large and small bowel offers several attractive advantages. The studies are relatively simple and can be performed rapidly. The proce-

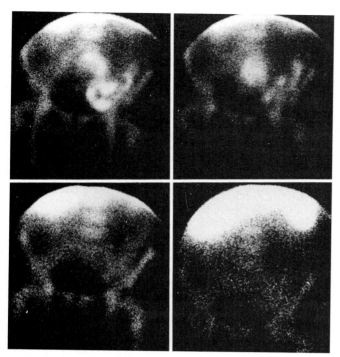

FIGURE 26.21. Positive scan and negative angiogram. ^{99m}Tc-sulfur colloid scan in a patient with active rectal bleeding reveals an S-shaped activity in the left lower quadrant (*top left*). This scintiphoto was obtained 3 minutes after injection. At 6 minutes this activity is fragmented into separate areas in the same location (*top right*). At 10 minutes a line of activity is seen in the left flank (very likely the descending colon) (*bottom left*). The last image was obtained at 20 minutes after the patient has a blood bowel movement (*bottom right*). Based on these findings, the site of hemorrhage was thought to be in the sigmoid colon. The arteriogram done immediately following the scan was within normal limits. (From Alavi A, Ring EJ. Localization of gastrointestinal bleeding: superiority of ^{99m}Tc sulfur colloid compared with angiography. *AJR* 1981;137:741–748, with permission.)

dures are totally noninvasive and can be obtained at bedside if necessary. The cost is low and one person can perform it with the instruments and radiopharmaceuticals available at most institutions. It may even be performed in the operating room in the course of a laparotomy to locate the site of the hemorrhage (60). Sensitivity is high and the procedure can be easily repeated, an especially important point in patients with intermittent bleeding (Fig. 26.21).

Use as Guide to Invasive Examinations

The performance of multiple invasive examinations, each having a high probability of negative results, is extremely undesirable, although it may be considered preferable to an undirected exploratory laparotomy. Properly integrated into clinical management, the radioisotopic screening procedure can be extremely helpful in guiding invasive examinations in terms of timing and localizing the area of interest.

If the site of the hemorrhage cannot be determined from images obtained after intravenous administration of the tracer, an enema with either ^{99m}Tc-sulfur colloid or ^{99m}Tc-DTPA may help localize the site. This is infrequently necessary with either ^{99m}Tc-sulfur colloid or ^{99m}Tc-labeled red blood cell studies (61).

ROLE OF NUCLEAR PROCEDURES IN CONSERVATIVE MANAGEMENT OF GASTROINTESTINAL BLEEDING

The advances made in the localization of bleeding sites with angiography, endoscopy, and nuclear medicine procedures have resulted in improvement in the conservative management of patients. Surgery is used as a last resort when these measures fail to stop the bleeding. Endoscopy is being used to provide treatment in selected cases of upper GI hemorrhage (62,63). Successful cessation of hemorrhage has been achieved by electrocoagulation of a variety of lesions such as gastritis and Mallory-Weiss tears. However, at this point endoscopic treatment of GI bleeding is considered investigational (64).

The use of angiography in the management of patients with GI bleeding has been of great value (65–69). In most patients, conservative angiographic techniques succeed in controlling bleeding. Vasopressin has been the most extensively used of all the agents to stop hemorrhage. Because of its widespread application, this approach is discussed in detail. However, alternate modes of therapy are mentioned only briefly.

Initially, embolic therapy was reserved for patients who failed to respond to vasoconstrictive agents (70). However, with more experience, this approach is being used more commonly as a primary hemostatic modality. This therapeutic modality requires precise angiographic localization of the site of bleeding. The catheter should be placed as close as possible to the area of bleeding. Although initially this approach was used to stop bleeding in gastric and duodenal lesions, because of their rich submucosal collateral network, embolization appears to be well tolerated in the distal bowel as well. A variety of agents have been used for short- and long-term occlusion of the vessels. Four of these, autogenous clots, Gelfoam (71), Ivalon (polyvinyl alcohol) (72), and steel coils (73,74) are used more commonly. Occlusions made with autogenous clots and Gelfoam are temporary, whereas Ivalon and steel coils create permanent closures of the vessel.

Balloon catheters also have been used to produce or help in the production of vascular constriction (75). Several approaches have been used to achieve this goal. Balloon catheter occlusion can be used as a temporary measure to stop bleeding or may be left in place permanently (76,77).

Vasopressin

Vasopressin is a polypeptide hormone that has found wide clinical acceptance as a therapeutic vasoconstricting agent because of its safety and reliability. Infusions of vasopressin produce significant and sustained reduction of splanchnic blood flow. Because of its direct action and rapid clearance, a dose of vasopressin can be adjusted to produce varying degrees of vasoconstriction and, consequently, an easily controllable and reversible ischemic effect. Vasopressin has remained the drug of choice for vasoconstrictive therapy (i.e., pharmacotherapy) of GI bleeding since its introduction as an intraarterial agent (78).

Basic Pharmacology

Vasopressin is supplied as an aqueous solution of an extract of the posterior pituitary gland. It consists almost exclusively of a pressor agent and is substantially free of oxytoxic activity. The hormone has a direct action on the smooth muscle of the splanchnic vascular bed and the GI tract. It causes an intense arteriolar and capillary vasoconstriction (79,80). In humans and other primates, vasopressin constricts arteries of all sizes—as the dose is steadily increased, the vasoconstrictor effect progresses from the distal small arteries to the more proximal larger vessels (81).

Rate and Route of Administration

Most of the recent controversy over vasopressin therapy has centered about its rate and route of administration. The high doses (i.e., 20 U given intravenously over 20 minutes) produce serious cardiac side effects and tachyphylaxis. Vasopressin was not widely employed clinically for the control of GI hemorrhage until the 1960s when Nussbaum, Baum, and colleagues (65,78, 82) reported control of bleeding esophageal varices with the use of selective superior mesenteric arterial infusions of vasopressin at low dose rates. Soon thereafter it was found that arterial bleeding also could be controlled by low-dose infusions of vasopressin (69). Selective infusion pharmacotherapy now has been used to control hemorrhage in all portions of the GI tract (68,83,84).

Intraarterial Vasopressin Infusion

Once the selective angiogram has accurately demonstrated the site of bleeding, a catheter is placed in the appropriate position and infusion through it is begun at a rate of 0.2 U vasopressin per minute. The drug is delivered as a diluted solution (using either normal saline or 5% dextrose in water solution as a diluent). The diluted drug is delivered continuously by an infusion pump at a rate of at least 0.5 m/minute. Follow-up arteriograms may be obtained at 15 to 20 minutes and accurately reflect the appropriateness of the dose of vasoconstrictor. If the drug is effective and the dose is appropriate, the follow-up arteriogram will show no extravasation. Thereafter, infusion is continued from 24 to 36 hours and then halved and continued for another 24 hours. If by clinical criteria, all hemorrhage has ceased, the catheter is kept in for an additional 8 to 12 hours and then withdrawn.

Any evidence of continued extravasation on the posttherapy arteriogram requires further treatment, even if the rate of extravasation is decreased in comparison with the pretherapy study. Generally, the rate is increased to 0.4 U/minute and the arteriogram is repeated to gauge efficacy of the increased dose. If this dose of vasospasm is successful in controlling bleeding, it is maintained for 12 to 24 hours and then tapered over the next 2 to 3 days. Any evidence of continued extravasation at a dose of 0.4 vasopressin per minute is an indication for discontinuation of the infusion. It has generally been found clinically that persistence of extravasation at dose rates of 0.4 U/minute indicates that infusion pharmacotherapy is unlikely to establish hemostasis and some other form of therapy should be employed.

Infusions of vasopressin at rates of 0.2 to 0.4 U/minute have been widely regarded as safe and unlikely to cause organ infarction. However, if the posttherapy arteriogram shows any evidence of "beading" of major vessels or poor washout of contrast medium, the patient may be excessively sensitive to the drug. The rate of infusion should be reduced by 50% and the arteriogram repeated after 15 to 20 minutes. If intense vasoconstriction persists even at the reduced dose rate, vasopressin therapy should be discontinued.

Intravenous Vasopressin Infusion

It has been shown that systemic infusions of vasopressin at rates comparable to those used in the superior mesenteric artery are equally effective in controlling variceal bleeding and could be used without added side effects or tachyphylaxis (85). Therefore, low-dose systemic vasopressin has become standard first-line therapy for variceal bleeding in many centers.

Vasopressin is given intravenously at the same dose levels that were used for intraarterial therapy. Delivering vasopressin intravenously is much simpler than the intraarterial routes and selective catheterization of mesenteric arteries is not required. However, vasopressin should be given through a large central venous line, rather than a peripheral line, because extravasation into local tissues can cause intense vasoconstriction with subsequent necrosis and sloughing of tissue. Monitoring the effectiveness of vasopressin given intravenously poses more difficulties than monitoring vasopressin given by the intraarticular route. For obvious reasons, direct assessment of the vasoconstrictor on the mesenteric vasculature is not possible. Clinical criteria can be used to evaluate the efficacy of therapy. However, these criteria may be misleading. The clinical introduction of scintigraphy for the detection of bleeding provides the clinician with a safe and reliable method of estimating the effectiveness of vasopressin therapy (86,87).

Side Effects of Vasopressin

When given in large doses, vasopressin produces a significant reduction in cardiac output probably secondary to a diminution in coronary arterial blood flow (88). Cardiac arrhythmias also have been associated with the administration of large doses of the drug (88). Even at low doses, a small number of patients may develop a non-dose-dependent cardiotoxic effect. Hypertension, bradycardia, and a variety of arrhythmias may be seen. These side effects are especially common if vasopressin is used selectively in a vessel supplying part of the adrenal gland. Almost all patients will develop a systemic antidiuretic hormone effect after variable periods; water retention and electrolyte imbalance are managed with diuretics and electrolyte replacement. Minor abdominal cramping and diarrhea are extremely common and represent insignificant pharmacologic effects of vasopressin therapy. These symptoms arise from the direct effect of vasopressin on the smooth muscle of the GI tract.

Scintigraphy as an Aid in Therapy

The introduction of scintigraphic technique has opened a new dimension in the evaluation and management of patients with

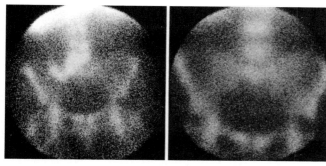

FIGURE 26.22. Follow-up examination after intravenous vasopressin infusion. The image on the left shows extravasation in the transverse colon. The image on the right, obtained after administration of vasopressin, shows no evidence of active hemorrhage.

GI bleeding. Because these examinations are completely noninvasive, one may administer the pharmacologic agents intravenously to simplify the management of these patients (86,87). Immediately following the demonstration of the bleeding site with scan, an initial trial of intravenous vasopressin is initiated to stop the hemorrhage. Approximately 1 hour following the initiation of this therapy, the patient is rescanned to evaluate the effect of the administered vasopressin. This is achieved by positioning the patient under the camera and obtaining an initial image of the abdomen. This ensures that the previously extravasated activity has been cleared from the lumen of the bowel and will not create a difficulty in the interpretation of the later images. In patients with GI bleeding, the peristaltic movement of the GI tract is often accelerated, and this results in rapid and complete propulsion of the extravasated radiopharmaceuticals along with the bloody bowel movements. This is enhanced further following the administration of vasopressin.

Following the initial images, another dose of either ^{99m}Tc-sulfur colloid or ^{99m}Tc-labeled red blood cells is administered intravenously, and serial images of the abdomen are obtained. If these images reveal cessation of the hemorrhage, the intravenous vasopressin infusion is continued as indicated above (Figs. 26.22 and 26.23). After the cessation of hemorrhage for more than 2 days, barium studies and/or endoscopy are performed to determine the underlying cause of bleeding. If the bleeding does not stop after the intravenous administration of vasopressin, angiography is performed to administer this agent intraarterially. If intraarterial vasopressin administration fails to stop the hemorrhage and the patient continues to bleed, surgery is recommended as a last resort in a majority of these patients.

Pediatric Applications—Meckel's Diverticulum

Meckel's diverticulum is a remnant of the vitelline duct, which normally obliterates by the fifth to ninth week of intrauterine life (89) but persists in 1.5% to 3% of the population. It is located on the antimesenteric border of the ileum approximately 50 to 80 cm from the ileocecal valve. Complications occur in 10% to 20% of the patients, and 80% of symptomatic patients are under the age of 15 (90). The most common complication

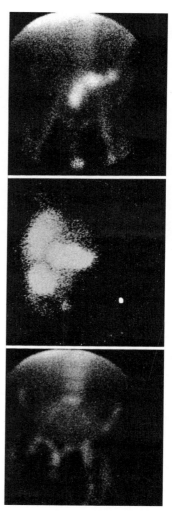

FIGURE 26.23. Cessation of hemorrhage following intravenous infusion of vasopressin. The top image shows evidence of hemorrhage in the sigmoid colon whereas the mid-image reveals radioactive blood in the stool. The lower image obtained after the intravenous administration of vasopressin shows evidence for complete cessation of the hemorrhage.

in children is lower GI bleeding caused by ulceration of the ileal mucosa by the adjacent ectopic acid-secreting gastric mucosa (91).

Routine small bowel barium studies are insensitive for demonstrating Meckel's diverticulum, probably because they are not well filled, especially when the ostium of the diverticulum is narrow (92). Small bowel enterolysis studies are more sensitive because compression radiographs increase the pressure (93). Angiographic diagnosis depends on hypervascularity of the lesion or demonstration of a remnant of the right vitelline artery (94–96). With an overall accuracy rate of more than 90%, Meckel's scintigraphy using ^{99m}Tc pertechnetate is the study of choice for demonstrating the presence of ectopic gastric mucosa in a Meckel's diverticulum (97). Fig. 26.24 shows selected images from sequential views of the abdomen obtained 30 minutes after the intervenous injection of 10 mg ^{99m}Tc pertechnetate. The focus of abnormal activity noted in the right midabdomen in the 15-

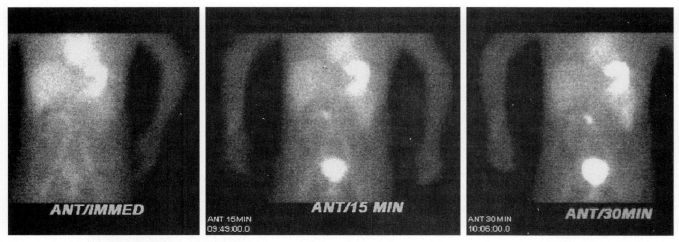

FIGURE 26.24. Images of a positive Meckel's diverticulum. The initial image does not reveal any abnormal uptake in the abdomen. However, a focus of activity is seen in right middle abdomen 15 minutes after injection which becomes more apparent in the 30 minute image. This is a typical finding for a Meckel's diverticulum.

minute image is secondary to a Meckel's diverticulum (confirmed at surgery).

The use of pentagastrin and cimetidine has been reported to enhance the sensitivity of Meckel's imaging (98–100). Pentagastrin may act by increasing acid production and tracer uptake, but acid production may be undesirable for the patient. By blocking secretion from the cells, cimetidine induces prolonged and increased uptake of the tracer by the gastric mucosa and might be useful in this case.

SUMMARY

The diagnosis of lower GI bleeding is usually easy to make. In contrast, localizing the site of bleeding may be extremely difficult. Using the techniques described earlier, the diligent nuclear physician may be able to detect the bleeding site precisely. However, if the cautions details are not observed, the tracer studies will show GI bleeding, but not the true bleeding site. This must be understood and carefully avoided. Done correctly, these tests

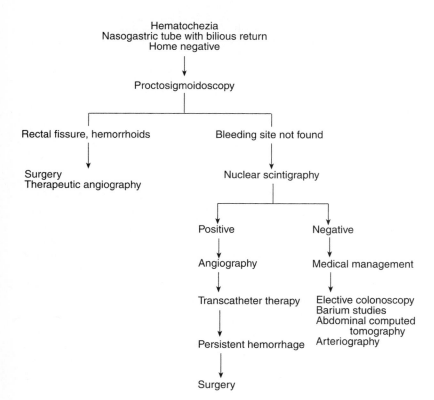

FIGURE 26.25. Algorithm for the diagnosis and treatment of lower gastrointestinal hemorrhage.

can have a major impact on patient care. Fig. 26.25 describes recommended algorithms for the diagnosis and treatment of patients with lower GI hemorrhage. As noted, nuclear studies should play a major role in this process. A prospective study comparing nuclear medicine GI bleeding study results with those of visceral angiography may further define the role of this procedure in patients with hemorrhage.

REFERENCES

1. Habr-Gama A, Waye JD. Complications and hazards of gastrointestinal endoscopy. *World J Surg* 1989;13:193–201.
2. Nusbaum M, Baum S. Radiologic demonstration of unknown sites of gastrointestinal bleeding. *Surg Forum* 1963;14:374–375.
3. Rosch J, Keller FS, Wawrukiewicz AS et al. Pharmacoangiography in the diagnosis of recurrent massive lower gastrointestinal bleeding. *Radiology* 1982;145:615–619.
4. Koval G, Benner KG, Rosch J et al. Aggressive angiographic diagnosis in acute lower gastrointestinal hemorrhage. *Dig Dis Sci* 1987;32:248–253.
5. McKibbin B, Watson BW. Localization of intestinal bleeding using a miniature geiger counter. *Gut* 1963;4:82–87.
6. Alavi A, Dann RW, Baum S et al. Scintigraphic detection of acute gastrointestinal bleeding. *Radiology* 1977;124:753–756.
7. Alavi A. Scintigraphic demonstration of acute gastrointestinal bleeding. *Gastrointest Radiol* 1980;5:205–208.
8. Bunker SR, Brown JM, McAuley RJ et al. Detection of gastrointestinal bleeding sites. Use of *in vitro* technetium Tc99m-labeled RBCs. *JAMA* 1982;247:789–792.
9. McKusick KA, Froelich J, Callahan RJ et al. [99m]Tc red blood cells for detection of gastrointestinal bleeding. *AJR* 1981;137:1113–1118.
10. Alavi A, McLean GK. Studies of GI bleeding with scintigraphy and the influence of vasopressin. *Semin Nucl Med* 1981;11:216–223.
11. Winzelberg GG, Froelich JW, McKusick KA et al. Radionuclide localization of lower gastrointestinal hemorrhage. *Radiology* 1981;139:465–469.
12. Winzelberg GG, McKusick KA, Strauss HW et al. Evaluation of gastrointestinal bleeding by red blood cells labeled *in vivo* with technetium-99m. *J Nucl Med* 1979;20:1080–1086.
13. Miskowiak J, Nielsen SL, Munck O et al. Abdominal scintiphotography with 99m-technetium-labeled albumin in acute gastrointestinal bleeding. An experimental study and case report. *Lancet* 1977;2:852–854.
14. Owunwanne A, Al-Wafai I, Vallgren S et al. Comparison of four technetium-99m radiopharmaceuticals for detection and localization of gastrointestinal bleeding in a sheep model. *Am J Physiol Imaging* 1988;3:192–196.
15. Abdel-Dayem HM, Mahajan KK, Ericsson S et al. Evaluation of technetium-99m DTPA for localization of site of acute upper gastrointestinal bleeding. *Clin Nucl Med* 1986;11:788–791.
16. Abdel-Dayem H, Mahajan K, Owuwanne A et al. The use of 99mTc-DTPA for detection and localization of site of acute gastrointestinal bleeding. *Eur J Nucl Med* 1988;14:98–104.
17. Owunwanne A, Al-Wafai I, Vallgren S et al. Evaluation of ^{99m}Tc mercaptoacetyltriglycine for the detection and localization of gastrointestinal bleeding in an experimental animal model. *Nucl Med Commun* 1988;9:369–372.
18. Schmidt KG, Rasmussen JW, Grove O et al. The use of indium-111-labeled platelets for scintigraphic localization of gastrointestinal bleeding with special reference to occult bleeding. *Scand J Gastroenterol* 1986;21:407–414.
19. Winzelberg GG, Castronovo FP, Callahan RJ et al. [111]In in oxine labeled red cells for detection of simulated lower gastrointestinal bleeding in an animal model. *Radiology* 1980;135:455–461.
20. Som P, Oster ZH, Atkins HL et al. Detection of gastrointestinal blood loss with ^{99m}Tc-labeled, heat-treated red blood cells. *Radiology* 1981;138:207–209.
21. Heyman S, Sunaryo FP, Ziegler MM. Gastrointestinal bleeding: an accessory spleen causing a false-positive Tc-99m-sulfur colloid study. *Clin Nucl Med* 1982;7:38–40.
22. Rowe DM, Schauwecker DS, Park HM. Focal bone marrow activity. A false positive on a sulfur colloid bleeding study. *Clin Nucl Med* 1985;10:295–296.
23. Veluvolu P, Isithman AT, Collier BD et al. False-positive technetium-99m sulfur colloid gastrointestinal bleeding study due to Paget's disease. *Clin Nucl Med* 1988;13:465–466.
24. Lecklitner ML. Pitfalls of gastrointestinal bleeding studies with ^{99m}Tc sulfur-colloid. *Semin Nucl Med* 1986;16:155–156.
25. Jacobson AF, Cerqueira MD. Prognostic significance of late imaging results in technetium-99m-labeled red cell gastrointestinal bleeding studies with early negative images. *J Nucl Med* 1992;33:202–207.
26. Jacobson AF. Delayed positive gastrointestinal bleeding studies with technetium-99m-red blood cells; utility of a second injection. *J Nucl Med* 1991;32:330–332.
27. Thorne DA, Datz FL, Remley K et al. Bleeding rates necessary for detecting acute gastrointestinal. *J Nucl Med* 1987;28:514–520.
28. Srivastava SC, Chervu LR. Radionuclide-labeled red blood cells: current status and future prospects. *Semin Nucl Med* 1984;14:68–82.
29. Landry A, Jr., Hartshorne MF, Bunker SR et al. Optimal technetium-99m RBC labeling for gastrointestinal hemorrhage study. *Clin Nucl Med* 1985;10:491–493.
30. Srivastava SC, Straub RF. Blood cell labeling with Tc-99m: progress and prospective. *Semin Nucl Med* 1990;20:41–51.
31. Bunker SR, Lull RJ, Jackson JH et al. The nuclear enema: a technique for scintigraphically demonstrating colonic anatomy. *Radiology* 1982;145:213.
32. Maurer AH, Rodman MS, Vitti RA et al. Gastrointestinal bleeding: improved localization with cine scintigraphy. *Radiology* 1992;185:187–192.
33. Patton DD, McNeill GC, Edelman K. Cine scintigraphy for gastrointestinal bleeding. *Radiology* 1993;187:582.
34. Abello R, Haynie TP, Kim EE. Pitfalls of a ^{99m}Tc-RBC bleeding study due to gallbladder and ileal-loop visualization. *Gastrointest Radiol* 1991;16:32–24.
35. McIntyre AS, Kamm MA. A case of factitious colonic bleeding. *J R Soc Med* 1990;83:465–466.
36. Lecklitner ML, Hughes JJ. Pitfalls of gastrointestinal bleeding studies with ^{99m}Tc-labeled RBCs. *Semin Nucl Med* 1986;16:151–154.
37. Moreno AJ, Byrd BF, Berger DE et al. Abdominal varices mimicking an acute gastrointestinal hemorrhage during technetium-99m red blood cell scintigraphy. *Clin Nucl Med* 1985;10:248–251.
38. Mountz JM, Ripley SD, Gross MD et al. The appearance of a large mesenteric varix on a technetium-99m red blood cell gastrointestinal bleeding study. *Clin Nucl Med* 1986;11:229–232.
39. Lecklitner ML. Hepatic cavernous hemangioma: a potential pitfall during evaluation of gastrointestinal bleeding with ^{99m}Tc-labeled erythrocytes. *Eur J Nucl Med* 1985;10:178–180.
40. Alavi A, Ring EJ. Localization of gastrointestinal bleeding: superiority of ^{99m}Tc sulfur colloid compared with angiography. *AJR* 1981;137:741–748.
41. Bunker SR, Lull RJ, Tanasescu DE et al. Scintigraphy of gastrointestinal hemorrhage: superiority of ^{99m}Tc red cells over ^{99m}Tc sulfur colloid. *AJR* 1984;143:543–548.
42. Siddiqui AR, Schauwecker DS, Wellman HN et al. Comparison of technetium-99m sulfur colloid and *in vitro* labeled technetium-99m RBCs in the detection of gastrointestinal bleeding. *Clin Nucl Med* 1985;10:546–549.
43. Bentley DE, Richardson JD. The role of tagged red blood cell imaging in the localization of gastrointestinal bleeding. *Arch Surg* 1991;126:821–824.
44. Hunter JM, Pezim ME. Limited value of technetium-99m-labeled red cell scintigraphy in localization of lower gastrointestinal bleeding. *Am J Surg* 1990;159:504–506.
45. Alavi A, Dann R, Staum M. Efficiency of *in vivo* technetium-99m red cell labeling. Presented at the World Federation of Nuclear Medi-

cine and Biology meeting, Washington, DC, September 17–21, 1978.

46. Froelich JW, Callahan RJ, Leppo J et al. Time course of *in vivo* labeling of red blood cells. *J Nucl Med* 1980;21:94.

47. Orecchia PM, Hensley EK, McDonald PT et al. Localization of lower gastrointestinal hemorrhage. Experience with red blood cells labeled *in vitro* with technetium Tc-99m. *Arch Surg* 1985;120:621–624.

48. Nicholson ML, Neoptolemos JP, Sharp JF et al. Localization of lower gastrointestinal bleeding using *in vivo* technetium-99m labeled red blood cell scintigraphy. *Br J Surg* 1989;76:358–361.

49. Gupta S, Luna E, Kingsley S et al. Detection of gastrointestinal bleeding by radionuclide scintigraphy. *Am J Gastroenterol* 1984;79:26–31.

50. Winzelberg GG, McKusick KA, Froelich JW et al. Detection of gastrointestinal bleeding with ^{99m}Tc-labeled red blood cells. *Semin Nucl Med* 1982;12:139–146.

51. Dusold R, Burke K, Carpenter W et al. The accuracy of technetium-99m-labeled red cell scintigraphy in localizing gastrointestinal bleeding. *Am J Gastroenterol* 1994;89:345–348.

52. Voeller GR, Bunch G, Britt LG. Use of technetium-labeled red blood cell scintigraphy in the detection and management of gastrointestinal hemorrhage. *Surgery* 1991;110:799–804.

53. Sandlow LJ, Becker GH, Spelberg MA et al. A prospective randomized study of the management of upper gastrointestinal hemorrhage. *Am J Gastroenterol* 1974;61:282–289.

54. Morris DW, Levine GM, Soloway RD et al. Prospective randomized study of diagnosis and outcome in acute upper gastrointestinal bleeding: endoscopy versus conventional radiography. *Am J Digest Dis* 1975;20:1103–1109.

55. Keller RT, Logan GM Jr. Comparison of emergent endoscopy and upper gastrointestinal series radiography in acute upper gastrointestinal hemorrhage. *Gut* 1976;17:180–184.

56. Dronfield MW, McIllmurray MB, Ferguson R et al. A prospective, randomized study of endoscopy and radiology in acute upper-gastrointestinal-tract bleeding. *Lancet* 1977;1:1167–1169.

57. Graham DY. Limited value of early endoscopy in the management of acute upper gastrointestinal-tract bleeding. A randomized, controlled trial. *N Engl J Med* 1981;304:925–992.

58. Peterson WL, Barnett CC, Smith HJ et al. Routine early endoscopy in upper-gastrointestinal-tract bleeding. A randomized, controlled trial. *N Engl J Med* 1981;304:925–929.

59. Casarella WJ, Galloway SJ, Taxin RN et al. "Lower" gastrointestinal tract hemorrhage: new concepts based on arteriography. *AJR* 1974;121:357–368.

60. Alavi A, Dann RW, Baum S. Radioisotopic localization of acute gastrointestinal bleeding site during exploratory laparotomy. *J Nucl Med* 1977;198:636(Abst).

61. Athanasoulis CA, Baum S, Rosch J et al. Mesenteric arterial infusions of vasopressin for hemorrhage from colonic diverticulosis. *Am J Surg* 1975;1129:212–216.

62. Youmans CR. Cystoscopic control of gastric hemorrhage. *Arch Surg* 1970;100:721–723.

63. Papp JP. Endoscopic electrocoagulation of upper gastrointestinal hemorrhage. *JAMA* 1976;236:2076–2079.

64. Dwyer RM, Haverback BJ, Bass M et al. Laser-induced hemostasis in the canine stomach: use of a flexible fiberoptic delivery system. *JAMA* 1975;231:486–489.

65. Nussbaum M, Baum S, Blakemore WS. Clinical experience with the diagnosis and management of gastrointestinal hemorrhage by selective mesenteric catheterization. *Ann Surg* 1969;170:506–514.

66. Conn HO, Ramsby GR, Storer EH. Selective intraarterial vasopressin in the treatment of upper gastrointestinal hemorrhage. *Gastroenterology* 1972;63:634–645.

67. Rosch J, Gary RK, Grollman JH et al. Selective arterial drug infusions in the treatment of acute gastrointestinal bleeding. *Gastroenterology* 1970;59:341–349.

68. Baum S, Rosch J, Dotter CT et al. Selective mesenteric arterial infusions in the management of massive diverticular hemorrhage. *N Engl J Med* 1973;288:1269–1272.

69. Baum S, Nusbaum M. The control of gastrointestinal hemorrhage by selective mesenteric arterial infusion of vasopressin. *Radiology* 1974;98:497–505.

70. Rosch J, Dotter CT, Brown MJ. Selective arterial embolization: a new method for control of acute gastrointestinal bleeding. *Radiology* 1972;102:303–306.

71. Barth KH, Strandberg JD, White RI. Long-term follow-up of transcatheter embolization with autologous clot. Oxycel and Gelfoam in domestic swine. *Invest Radiol* 1977;12:273–380.

72. White RI, Strandberg JD, Gross GS et al. Therapeutic embolization with long-term occluding agents and their effects on embolized tissues. *Radiology* 1977;125:677–687.

73. Gianturco C, Alderson JH, Wallace S. Mechanical devices for arterial occlusion. *AJR* 1975;124:428–435.

74. Anderson JH, Wallace S, Gianturco C et al. "Mini" Gianturco stainless steel coils for transcatheter vascular occlusion. *Radiology* 1979;132:301–303.

75. Wholey MH, Stockdale R, Hung TK. A percutaneous balloon catheter for the immediate control of hemorrhage. *Radiology* 1970;95:65–71.

76. Wholey MH. The technology of balloon catheters in interventional angiography. *Radiology* 1977;125:671–676.

77. White RI, Kaufman SL, Barth KH et al. Embolotherapy with detachable silicone balloons: technique and clinical results. *Radiology* 1979;131:619–627.

78. Nussbaum M, Baum S, Sakaiyalak P et al. Pharmacologic control of portal hypertension. *Surgery* 1967;62:299–310.

79. Morello DC, Klein NE, Wolferth CC et al. Management of diffuse hemorrhage from gastric mucosa. *Am J Surg* 1976;123:160–164.

80. Chuang VP, Reuter SR, Cho KJ et al. Alterations in gastric physiology caused by selected embolization and vasopressin infusion of the left gastric artery. *Radiology* 1976;120:533–536.

81. Ring EJ, Oleaga JA, Freiman DB et al. Comparison of the effect of vasopressin infusions on the mesenteric arteries of different species. *Invest Radiol* 1978;13:138–142.

82. Nussbaum M, Baum S, Kuroda K et al. Control of portal hypertension by selective mesenteric arterial drug infusion. *Arch Surg* 1968;97:1005–1013.

83. Athanasoulis CA, Baum S, Waltman AC et al. Control of acute gastric mucosal hemorrhage: intra-arterial infusion of posterior pituitary extract. *N Engl J Med* 1974;290:597–603.

84. Waltman AC, Greenfield AJ, Novelline RA et al. Pyloroduodenal bleeding and intra-arterial vasopressin: clinical results. *AJR* 1979;133:643–646.

85. Johnson WC. Control of varices by vasopressin: prospective radiological study. *Ann Surg* 1977;186:369–376.

86. Alavi A, McLean GK. Radioisotopic detection of gastrointestinal bleeding: an integrated approach to the diagnostic and therapeutic modalities. In: Freeman LM, Weissman H, eds. *Nuclear medicine annual 1980*. New York: Raven Press, 1980:177–218.

87. Alavi A, McLean GK. Studies of GI bleeding with scintigraphy and the influence of vasopressin. *Semin Nucl Med* 1981;11:216–223.

88. Drapanas T, Crowe CP, Shim WKT et al. The effect of Pitressin on cardiac output and coronary, hepatic and intestinal blood flow. *Surg Gynecol Obstet* 1961;133:484.

89. Vane DW, West KW, Grosfeld JL. Vitelline duct anomalies: experience with 217 childhood cases. *Arch Surg* 1987;122:542.

90. Lüdtke FE, Menda V, Köhler H et al. Incidence and frequency of complications and management of Meckel's diverticulum. *Surg Gynecol Obstet* 1989;169:537.

91. Rutherford RB, Akers DR: Meckel's diverticulum: a review of 148 pediatric patients, with special reference to the pattern of bleeding and to mesodiverticular vascular bands. *Surgery* 1966;59:618.

92. Maglinte DDT, Jordan LG, Van Hove ED et al: Chronic gastrointestinal bleeding from Meckel's diverticulum: radiologic considerations. *J Clin Gastroenterol* 1981;3:47.

93. Magline DDT, Elmore MF, Isenberg M et al. Meckel diverticulum: radiologic demonstration by enterolysis. *AJR* 1980;134:925.

94. Klein HJ, Alfidi RJ, Meaney TF et al. Angiography in the diagnosis of chronic gastrointestinal bleeding. *Radiology* 1971;98:83.

95. Bree RL, Reuter SR. Angiographic demonstration of a bleeding Meckel's diverticulum. *Radiology* 1973;108:287.

96. Muroff LR, Casarella WJ, Johnson PM. Preoperative diagnosis of Meckel's diverticulum: angiographic and radionuclide studies in an adult. *JAMA* 1974;229:1900.

97. Sfakianakis GN, Conway JJ. Detection of ectopic gastric mucosa in Meckel's diverticulum and in other aberrations by scintigraphy: I: pathophysiology and 10-year clinical experience. *J Nucl Med* 1981; 22:647.

98. Treves S, Grand RJ, Eraklis AJ. Pentagastrin stimulation of technetium-99m uptake by the ectopic gastric mucosa in a Meckel's diverticulum. *Radiology* 1978;128:771.

99. Petrokubi RJ, Baum S, Rohrer GV. Cimetidine administration resulting in improved pertechnetate imaging of Meckel's diverticulum. *Clin Nucl Med* 1978;3:385.

100. Diamond RH, Rothstein RD, Alavi A. The role of cimetidine-enhanced technetium-99m-pertechnetate imaging for visualizing Meckel's diverticulum. *J Nucl Med* 1991;32:1422.

Diagnostic Nuclear Medicine, Fourth Edition. Edited by M.P. Sandler, R.E. Coleman, J.A. Patton, F.J.Th. Wackers, A. Gottschalk. Lippincott Williams & Wilkins, Philadelphia 2003.

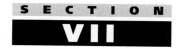

S E C T I O N
VII

HEMATOLOGY

27

BLOOD VOLUME AND VITAMIN B₁₂ GASTROINTESTINAL ABSORPTION

MYRON POLLYCOVE
MATHEWS B. FISH
MARY TONO

BLOOD VOLUME

Blood volume determinations require accurate individual measurements of red cell volume (RCV) and plasma volume (PV) normalized for correspondence to lean tissue mass. Disregard of these requirements has led to clouding of the diagnostic value of routine blood volume measurements and an erroneous assessment of their value.

Basic Concepts

The sensitivity, accuracy, and precision with which radiotracers can be measured have made them the labels of choice for measurement of RCV and PV. Tracers usually furnish precise, reproducible measurements of blood volumes, but these measurements may not agree accurately with the patient's volumes. Good precision indicates little variation in measurements, without regard to their agreement with the actual volumes; that is, their accuracy (1) with respect to the patient. Lack of accuracy in blood volume measurements has resulted in their disuse not lack of precision.

Total blood volume (TBV) is assumed to be the summation of RCV and PV, estimated by the use of labeled red cells and labeled proteins (2). Consequently, underestimation of TBV occurs in some patients with leukemia, in whom the volume of circulating leukocytes becomes a significant fraction of the total cells present (2,3).

The fundamental rule involved in exchangeable pool measurement, such as RCV and PV, is the dilution principle. After a known amount of material has been injected into an appropriate pool and has been equilibrated, a sample is taken from which

the unknown pool volume may be calculated according to the conservation-of-mass formula.

$$A_i = V_i C_i = V_p C_p \qquad [1]$$

or

$$V_p = V_i C_i / C_p \qquad [2]$$

in which A_i, V_i, and C_i are the amount, volume, and concentration of the radioactivity injected and C_p is the measured concentration of radioactivity after dilution by the volume of the unknown pool, V_p.

Kinetics and Physiology

Equilibration and Loss of Tracer

The basic assumptions that are made in applying isotope dilution analysis to blood volume measurements are

1. The amount or volume of the unknown does not change significantly during measurement.
2. The specific activity of the sample changes by a factor of two or more, as compared with the dose.
3. The rate of mixing is much greater than the rate at which the radiotracer leaves the body compartment.

The performance of blood volume measurements requires that

1. The radiotracer must be relatively stable, nonantigenic, small in volume, sterile, and nonpyrogenic.
2. The amount of free radionuclide must be known, so correction for this unbound activity can be made.
3. The specific activity of the radiotracer in the dose, standard, and postinjection samples must be easily measurable with available detector system.
4. The physiologic and chemical conditions of the whole procedure must be understood.
5. Equilibrium (uniform distribution or mixing) must be attained before samples are withdrawn from the pool. Attempts to shorten the procedure by circumventing equilibration before sampling leads to unknown and, at times, major errors.

M. Pollycove: U.S. Nuclear Regulatory Commission, Rockville, MD.

M.B. Fish: Department of Nuclear Medicine, Sacred Heart General Hospital, Oregon Medical Laboratory, Eugene, OR.

M. Tono: Department of Nuclear Medicine, University of California, San Francisco General Hospital, San Francisco, CA.

Invalid Calculations of Volume from Another Volume Measurement

If a constant relationship between body hematocrit [RCV ÷ (RCV + PV)] and venous hematocrit could be assumed, then either the PV or the RCV, and therefore the TBV, could be calculated from one measurement of RCV or PV, respectively. The use of this invalid assumption to circumvent either additional measurement can result in grossly inaccurate calculated blood volumes.

Normalization of Volume Measurements

After accurate volumes of plasma and red cells are measured, expressed in milliliters, the problem still remains of interpreting their significance for the patient being studied. Meaningful interpretation of these measurements requires careful consideration of the clinical status of the patient for appropriate normalization of the measured volumes.

In the performance of accurate blood volume measurements, four critical components must be clearly understood:

1. Mixing and equilibration must be complete before any measurements are taken.
2. Suitable extrapolation is required for PV and, in certain circumstances, for RCV measurement.
3. The variability of the body hematocrit/venous hematocrit ratio requires simultaneous independent measurements of both PV and RCV.
4. Proper normalization of volumes in accordance with the clinical status of the patient is necessary.

Equilibration and Extrapolation

Sterling (4) commented on the rapid initial decline in measured plasma ^{131}I-labeled albumin concentration ($T_{1/2}$ = 0.6 days) that was attributed to the extravascular exchangeable albumin pool. A greater methodologic concern is the variable duration of the initial mixing period required to establish completely uniform distribution of the albumin molecules throughout the entire PV. In many ill patients, this mixing period is prolonged far beyond the usual mixing period observed in normal persons.

One of the usual conditions occurring in a "rule out hypovolemia" request is shock. Noble and Gregersen (5) found that shock prolonged the mixing time of labeled albumin; the mean value was 14.0 minutes, compared with the mean normal mixing time of 7 minutes (6). Berson and Yalow (7) found the mixing of ^{131}I-labeled albumin to be virtually complete within 10 minutes after injection. They measured the rate at which activity was lost from the pool space of circulation of ^{32}P-labeled red cells and ^{131}I-labeled albumin to be on the order of 1% or less per 15 minutes during the rapid initial phase of decline. Therefore, samples drawn at 10 or 15 minutes extrapolated corrections to zero time are unnecessary (7).

Figure 27.1 illustrates however, that this assumption of a "normal" and predictable rate of mixing may be incorrect, even in the absence of congestive failure, edema, increased blood viscosity, splenomegaly, or shock. In these conditions, mixing may be greatly prolonged. When sampling times are delayed beyond

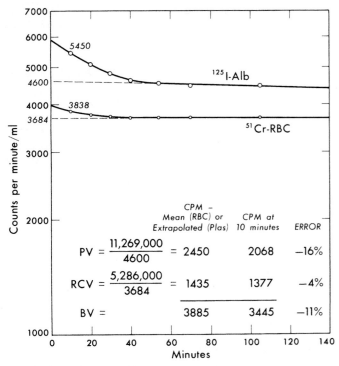

FIGURE 27.1. Accuracy of blood volume results. Serial blood sampling demonstrates that ^{125}I-labeled albumin (^{125}I-Alb) equilibration in the plasma volume requires 48 minutes, and 40 minutes are required for ^{51}Cr-labeled red normal blood cell (^{51}Cr-RBC) equilibration in the red cell volume. This 72-year-old man with normal blood pressure and pulse was neither in congestive heart failure nor edematous. If 10-minute samples were used to calculate volumes, the results would be very inaccurate.

15 minutes, extrapolation to zero time is necessary to correct for the progressive loss of albumin from the plasma pool.

Mixing of labeled red cells is also subject to wide variations. Although mixing normally is complete within 20 minutes (8), in patients with polycythemia or splenomegaly complete equilibration of labeled red cells may require as much as 60 minutes (9).

Another area of misunderstanding may arise when a plasma protein other than albumin is used to measure PV. The use of ^{113m}In transferrin to measure PV results in volume measurements that differ from the volume measurements obtained with albumin. ^{113m}In transferrin was studied in comparison with either ^{131}I immunoglobulin (IgG) or ^{125}I albumin volumes (10). Another study with multiple sampling for an hour demonstrated that the macromolecular ^{125}I fibrinogen volume also averaged 94.5% of the ^{131}I albumin volume (11). The volume in which a labeled plasma protein is distributed is not necessarily the volume of albumin distribution.

Body Hematocrit/Venous Hematocrit Ratio

The body hematocrit/venous hematocrit (f-cell) ratio has been used widely to circumvent simultaneous measurements of both RCV and PV. Because it is well known that the ratio of red cells to the sum of plasma plus red cells in peripheral venous blood (peripheral hematocrit) is usually higher than the ratio of red cells to plasma plus red cells in the total volume of circulating blood (body hematocrit) (1), the body hematocrit/peripheral hematocrit ratio, or f-cell ratio, has been used to calculate one volume from measurement of the other, so as to avoid measurement of the second volume.

The f-cell ratio is based on a number of assumptions that are not warranted in a highly heterogeneous population of ill patients. Although mean f-cell ratios of 0.86 to 0.92 have been found in normal subjects (7,12–18), in hospitalized patients and patients with severe anemia mean ratios of 0.86 (15,19) and 0.83 (15) have been reported.

With the use of accurate methodology and completely automated instrumentation, it costs little more to obtain multiple samples, label red cells, and calculate blood volumes that relate to the patient. The value of the resulting improvement in accuracy of the measurements obtained is highly significant. With the use of appropriate methodology, the time-consuming procedure of washing labeled red cells is avoided, and simultaneous measurements of both RCV and PV can be accomplished easily in a minimum amount of time.

To our knowledge, only three published blood volume studies have reported data for more than 100 patients. In the series of 336 patients of Fairbanks and Tauxe (19), the f-cell ratio range for 95% of the cases studied was 0.720 to 1.005, with a median of 0.860 for men and 0.887 for women. This broad range applied to all disease groups, including marked polycythemia. Because of the "error of variability inherent in the method," Fairbanks and Tauxe (19) concluded that the use of the f-cell ratio could only be "expected to provide erroneous results in a large proportion of studies."

Figure 27.2 shows a histogram of f-cell ratios calculated from measurements of 224 patients (mean = 0.89 ±0.14, 2 SD). These data have been collected in the Nuclear Medicine Department of San Francisco General Hospital (20). Although the

Table 27.1. *Cobalamin Body Content and Kinetics*

Daily dietary intake	5–30 μg
Daily absorption	1–4 μg
Daily loss	1–4 μg
Total body stores	5000 μg
Liver stores	1500 μg
Plasma level	200–900 pg/ml

mean f-cell ratio agrees with the accepted numbers of 0.89 to 0.92, this means ratio should not be applied to patients because of the wide range of f-cell ratios found in patients during our study (0.62 to 1.13). This is especially true in patients with shock and hypovolemia (mean f = 0.85 ±0.15, 2 SD). It is useful to consider the magnitude of errors that can be generated when one volume is calculated from the measurement of the other volume, assuming an f-cell ratio of 0.915. The calculated volumes shown in Table 27.1 were performed on two patients in our series, one with a very high f-cell ration of 1.13 and the other with a very low f-cell ration of 0.62. From these data we conclude that it is time to abandon the use of the f-cell ratio for calculating blood volumes. A similar conclusion was reached by Najean and Deschrywer (18) in their study of 329 cases.

Method of Blood Volume Measurement

The method for the measurement of blood volume that is used in the Nuclear Medicine Department at San Francisco General Hospital is similar to that described by Wood and Levitt (21), but with some modifications (22). This method was adopted to fulfill the aforementioned four major requirements for the accurate measurement of blood volumes. The procedure is quick, economical and allows consistently accurate measurements of RCV, PV, and TBV.

Fifteen milliliters of blood are taken from a patient, of which 5 mL are put aseptically into a Vacutainer tube containing 1 mL high citrate/low glucose (ACD) solution and 10 mL are put into a heparinized Vacutainer tube for preinjection background. Both tubes are mixed thoroughly. Under aseptic conditions, 100 μCi (3,700 kBq) of ^{51}Cr sodium chromate is put into the ACD tube, which then is incubated for 10 minutes at 39°C in a water bath. After the incubation period, 50 mg ascorbic acid is added to reduce hexavalent chromium to the trivalent state. A 15-microcurie (555 kBq) ^{125}I-labeled human serum albumin solution is prepared with saline. Adequate volume (1.5 to 5 ml) is prepared for the standard and dose of 10 μCi (370 kBq).

With a precalibrated syringe, 10 μCi (370 kBq) of ^{125}I are injected into a free-flowing intravenous line (clamp during injection, then flush for 30 seconds). Exact volume and time are noted. With a 5-mL precalibrated syringe, an exact volume of a well-mixed sample of ^{51}Cr-labeled blood is injected in a similar manner. Time of injection is noted. Approximately 1 mL of ^{51}Cr-labeled blood is saved for the standard. Postinjection samples (8 to 10 mL) are taken routinely at approximately 30, 45, and 60 minutes in heparinized Vacutainer tubes. Exact sampling time is noted. It is imperative that the vein used to collect the

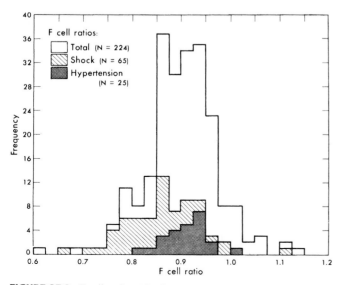

FIGURE 27.2. F-cell ratios. Distribution of f-cell ratios (body hematocrit/venous hematocrit) in 224 patients, 65 of whom were in shock and 25 of whom were hypertensive.

postinjection samples be different (preferably the opposite extremity) from the one in which the initial injections are made. The sampling procedure is prolonged for all cases in which poor mixing is suspected.

Microhematocrits are obtained in triplicate on all blood samples, including the ^{51}Cr-labeled dose. Approximately 2 mL of whole blood from samples taken at 0, 30, 45, and 60 minutes are aliquoted into corresponding counting vials (WB). Three drops of triton borate are added to the counting vials to hemolyze the red cells. The blood samples then are centrifuged, and 2 mL of plasma are aliquoted into corresponding counting vials (Pl). A 1:1,000 dilution of ^{51}Cr-labeled whole blood, ^{51}Cr-labeled plasma, and, ^{125}I-labeled human serum albumin is made by diluting 50 µL of each to 50 mL with water; 2-mL aliquots of each dilute standard are placed into corresponding counting vials. Thus, vials are prepared for counting as follows:

1. Water
2. Preinjection WB
3. Preinjection "0" Pl
4. Postinjection sample no. 1 WB
5. Postinjection sample no. 2 Pl
6. Postinjection sample no. 2 WB
7. Postinjection sample no. 2 Pl
8. Postinjection sample no. 3 WB
9. Postinjection sample no. 3 Pl
10. ^{51}Cr standard WB (1:1,000)
11. ^{51}Cr standard Pl (1:1,000)
12. ^{125}I standard (1:1,000)

The previously listed vials are counted in a well counter with two pulse-height analyzers, one on the ^{51}Cr peak and the other on the ^{125}I peak. All counted volumes are 2 mL, and each is counted for 2 minutes to obtain at least 4,000 counts in vials 4 to 12. Net counts per minute per milliliter are obtained on all vials by subtracting the appropriate background counts.

Calculations

^{51}Cr-Labeled Red Blood Cell Counts Per Minute (^{51}Cr RBC cpm) Injected

$$[WB \text{ dose std. (cpm/ml)}] - [\text{plasmacrit} \times Pl \text{ dose std. (cpm/ml)}] \times 10^3 \times \text{volume injected}$$

Counts Per Minute Per Milliliter of Red Cell Mass (Samples 1 to 3)

$$\frac{[WB(cpm/ml) - [\text{plasmocrit} \times Pl(cpm/ml)]}{Hct_v}$$

where Hct_v is venous microhematocrit uncorrected for trapped plasma.

Red Cell Volume

$$RCV = \frac{^{51}Cr \text{ RBC cpm injected}}{\text{avg. cpm/ml red cell mass}} \quad [3]$$

Avg. cpm/ml red cell mass is the average of the three samples, but

if the patient is receiving blood, a zero-intercept extrapolation is done on semilog graph paper.

Plasma Volume

$$PV = \frac{^{125}I \text{ std. (cpm/ml)} \times 10^3 \times \text{vol. Injected}}{\text{zero-intercept value}} \quad [4]$$

in which the zero intercept is obtained routinely by extrapolation of the three plasma samples; net counts per minute per milliliter on semilog graph paper.

Total Blood Volume
TBV = RCV + PV

Body Weight Adjustments
Values are reported in milliliters and in milliliters per kilogram, in which kilogram is the adjusted "ideal weight," as taken from the Metropolitan Life Insurance Table, 1959. Using height and body frame size (small, medium, or large bone) adjustment is made for the presence of ascites or edema, obesity (20), malnutrition, lack of normal fat in highly trained athletes, absent extremities, or pregnancy.

1. If the weight of the patient (not ascitic, edematous, or an amputee) is within the ideal range for his or her height and body frame, the patient's actual weight is used.
2. If the patient is obese, then 25% or 40% of the overweight is added to his or her ideal weight, respectively, to account for the added lean body mass and corresponding associated fat.
3. If the patient is a highly trained athlete, 10% to 15% of actual weight is added to measured weight so as to adjust for lack of normal fat. If the patient is emaciated, the measured weight is used, because the loss of lean tissue mass in wasting disease is roughly proportional to the loss of fat. We use the normal values shown in Table 27.2.

COBALAMIN MALABSORPTION

Excluding the extremely rare case of inadequate dietary intake (10), cobalamin deficiency is the result of defective absorption. Reviews of the gastric, luminal, and mucosal conditions and related pathophysiology of cobalamin malabsorption (23–27) are summarized in Table 27.2.

The gastric causes of cobalamin malabsorption are due to the lack of intrinsic factor (IF) and impaired intragastric release of food-bound cobalamin. An important cause of cobalamin malabsorption and severe deficiency is pernicious anemia. This condition is an autoimmune gastritis of late middle age and older adults with loss of acid and IF-secreting parietal cells of the fundus and body of the stomach. Total gastrectomy and complete destruction of gastric mucosa by corrosives also produce cobalamin malabsorption because of lack of IF. Some patients, usually many years after subtotal gastrectomy or gastrojejunostomy with or without vagotomy for peptic ulcer disease, will demonstrate cobalamin malabsorption and deficiency resulting

Table 27.2. *Causes of Cobalamin Malabsorption*

Gastric conditions	Pathophysiology
Pernicious anemia	Lack of IF
Total gastrectomy	Lack of IF
Other gastric surgery	Impaired gastric release of food protein-bound cobalamin and, in some, a decrease of IF
Atrophic gastritis, hypochlorhydria, and achlorhydria	Impaired gastric release of food protein-bound cobalamin
Histamine H_2-receptor antagonist and omeprazole	Impaired gastric release of food protein-bound cobalamin
Hereditary (Juvenile pernicious anemia)	Lack of adequate functioning IF

Intestinal luminal conditions	Pathophysiology
Pancreatic insufficiency	Impaired protease release of HC-cobalamin to IF
Zollinger-Ellison syndrome	Decreased intestinal pH resulting in impaired protease release of HC-cobalamin to IF and decreased binding of IF-cobalamin to IFCR
Bacterial overgrowth and fish tapeworm	Competition by organisms for uptake of cobalamin

Ileal mucosal conditions	Pathophysiology
Ileal resection and bypass	Decreased number of available IFCR receptors
Ileal disease	Decreased numbers of IFCR receptors
Cobalamin deficiency	Decreased number of functioning ileal enterocytes
Hereditary (Immersland-Grasbeck)	Impaired uptake or processing of IF-cobalamin by ileal enterocyte
Hereditary (TC II deficiency)	Impaired enterocyte release of cobalamin
Drugs (PAS, neomycin, colchicine)	Impaired enterocyte uptake and or processing of IF-cobalamin

IF, intrinsic factor.

from diminished IF secretion. This deficiency results from atrophy of the gastric remnant. Some patients who become cobalamin deficient exhibit normal absorption of crystalline vitamin B_{12}, but abnormally decreased absorption of food protein-bound vitamin B_{12} (28,29). Because these patients demonstrate marked hypochlorhydria or achlorhydria, it is felt that this malabsorption of cobalamin is due to diminished peptic digestion of ingested food protein with impaired release of food protein-bound cobalamin. A similar mechanism of cobalamin malabsorption has been noted especially in the elderly with intact stomachs that demonstrate achlorhydria or severe hypochlorhydria (30, 31). In addition, food-bound cobalamin malabsorption has been noted in drug induced achlorhydria associated with the use of histamine H_2-receptor antagonists [antagonists (32) and omeprazole (33)], as well as in patients who have had a gastric bypass procedure (Roux-en-Y gastrojejunostomy) for morbid obesity (34). The intestinal luminal conditions that result in cobalamin malabsorption are varied and as a group are an infrequent cause of cobalamin deficiency.

The receptors to which the IF-cobalamin complex bind are located in the distal ileum. Cobalamin malabsorption is uni-

formly observed after resection or bypass of more than 100 cm of the terminal ileum, but is quite often noted after other surgery, including the construction of ileocolic neobladders. Cobalamin malabsorption may result from conditions affecting more than 50 cm of the distal ileum. Because celiac disease tends to involve the proximal small intestine to a greater extent, cobalamin deficiency is uncommon with this disorder. Cobalamin deficiency severe enough to cause megaloblastic anemia may result in intestinal malabsorption of cobalamin because of impaired proliferation and replacement of the ileal mucosal enterocytes (35).

There are patients in whom cobalamin malabsorption is due to genetic causes (Table 27.2). These disorders are rare, are manifest at a young age, are inherited as autosomal recessive traits, and involve the cobalamin transport proteins IF, IFCR, and TCII (23).

Measurement of Cobalamin Absorption

Using radiolabeled vitamin B_{12}, a variety of methods have been developed to measure the gastrointestinal absorption of cobalamin. These techniques involved the quantification of activity in the whole body (36,37), liver (38), stool (37,39), blood (37, 40,41), or urine (42) after an oral test dose of the radiolabeled vitamin. Each of these approaches is associated with certain advantages and disadvantages when applied to different clinical and investigative situations. In the rare case in which adequate urine collections cannot be obtained, a method using either stool, blood, liver, or whole body measurements may be useful.

Of the radioisotopes of cobalt that have been used to label vitamin B_{12}, ^{57}Co and ^{58}Co are the most useful (43). They result in a low tissue radiation absorbed dose for the amount of activity administered, and their γ-ray emissions are separated adequately (^{57}Co: 122 and 136 keV; ^{58}Co: 511 and 810 keV) to allow for simultaneous scintillation counting.

The urinary excretion technique (Schilling test) is the most commonly employed procedure for evaluating cobalamin absorption. The major advantages of this procedure include good diagnostic accuracy, ease of handling and counting of the urine specimen, and the usual relative ease of obtaining a complete 24-hour collection. The Schilling test requires a parenteral injection of a pharmacologic amount (1 mg) of unlabeled vitamin B_{12} given within 6 hours (44) after the oral test dose to saturate cobalamin plasma and tissue binding sites, resulting in urinary excretion via glomerular filtration of approximately one third of the absorbed radiolabeled vitamin B_{12}. Therefore, the results of the Schilling test represent an index rather than an absolute measurement of gastrointestinal absorption. The pharmacologic amount of vitamin B_{12} used as a flushing dose results in a reticulocyte response in patients with either vitamin B_{12}-deficiency or folic acid-deficient megaloblastic anemia, obviating the opportunity of performing a diagnostic trial with physiologic amounts of one of these vitamins. Complete urine collections are required for accurate results. Whereas a 24-hour collection is adequate for patients with normal or near-normal renal function, a 48- to 72-hour collection is necessary for patients with significantly impaired renal function (45).

Because IF deficiency as noted in pernicious anemia is a very common cause of cobalamin malabsorption, evaluation of the absorption of free vitamin B_{12} and vitamin B_{12} with IF is usually among the initial diagnostic procedures used in patients with suspected cobalamin malabsorption. Testing of the absorption of vitamin B_{12} with IF may be performed sequentially after initial testing of vitamin B_{12} absorption, or the effect of exogenous IF may be assessed simultaneously with determination of the absorption of the unbound vitamin alone (37,46,47). The sequential method uses ^{57}Co-labeled vitamin B_{12} for each of the studies. IF is given with the second dose of labeled vitamin B_{12}. There must be a delay period between each phase of the sequential study of at least 3 days (43). The second approach involves the simultaneous oral administration of ^{57}Co-labeled vitamin B_{12} and ^{58}Co-labeled vitamin B_{12}-IF complex. Only a single, timed urine is required. Quantitation of both the ^{57}Co and ^{58}Co content in the single specimen can be accomplished accurately by a variety of dual radionuclide counting techniques on readily available equipment. Furthermore, this approach allows for calculation of the ratio of the absorbed IF-bound vitamin B_{12} to free vitamin B_{12}. This ratio is quite useful in the detection of IF deficiency, assists in the interpretation of borderline quantitative results, and can often provide diagnostic information regarding possible IF deficiency when specimen collection is adequate.

Obtaining useful and consistent results in a high percentage of patients studied by using either the sequential or combined methods requires careful attention to a number of procedural details including:

1. The patient's renal function must be assessed before performing the study. If the renal function is significantly decreased (creatinine 2.5 ml/dL or blood urea nitrogen 50 mg/dL) a second 24-hour urine collection (24 to 28 hours) is required.
2. The patient must be fasting overnight before the study and remain fasting for at least 2 hours after oral administration of the test dose. The patient should be specifically questioned to confirm a fasting state. The amount of vitamin B_{12} in a meal can significantly affect the fractional absorption of the test dose.
3. The patient should not receive parenteral vitamin B_{12} for at least 3 days before the study. Biliary excretion of some of this vitamin B_{12} into the gastrointestinal tract may significantly affect the fractional absorption of the test dose.
4. A blood specimen for determination of cobalamin and folate levels should be obtained before the study if measurement of these parameters was not performed. The flushing dose of vitamin B_{12} precludes accurate posttest measurement of serum cobalamin and possibly serum and red blood cell folate levels. Knowledge of the level of these vitamins may be helpful in overall interpretation of the patient's results.
5. The amount of vitamin B_{12} used in the test dose(s) must not saturate the limited IF-mediated mechanism for cobalamin absorption. The amounts that have been used range from 0.5 to 2.0 µg. Because the fractional absorption of the test dose is inversely related to the amount given within the range noted previously, a constant amount should be used for all studies. This amount should be the same as the amount used to establish the normal or reference range. The use of 1.0 µg or less has resulted in the best diagnostic separation of

normal individuals and patients with abnormal vitamin B_{12} absorption (38).

6. Although the flushing dose of vitamin B_{12} may be given at any time within 6 hours after oral administration of the test dose, giving the flushing dose at 2 hours provides a practical means of enforcing the fasting state for the requisite period after the test dose is given.
7. An evaluation of the patient's ability to collect an adequate 24-hour urine collection should be made before initiating the study. Depending on the clinical situation, an indwelling or condom catheter may be required. If the patient appears to be able to collect a 24-hour specimen, he or she must be carefully instructed, and the importance of having a complete collection must be strongly stressed.
8. Adequacy of the 24-hour urine collection should be assessed by comparing the measured urinary creatinine excretion to the expected urinary creatinine excretion based on the body weight. Because creatinine excretion correlates best with body muscle mass (48), the body weight should be an adjusted ideal weight as taken from the Metropolitan Life Insurance Table (1959). Using sex, height, and body frame size, an adjustment is made for obesity and ascites (49). Data obtained from 100 consecutive Schilling tests suggest that creatinine excretion values of greater than 18 mg/kg/24 hours for men and greater than 12 mg/kg/24 hours for women are associated with diagnostically adequate urine collections (50).
9. Every effort should be made to avoid contamination of the urine specimen, standards, and equipment with other radionuclides, especially ^{99m}Tc. ^{99m}Tc is used frequently and in multi-millicurie amounts. Its photon energy is similar to that of ^{57}Co. If the particular results or clinical situation suggests the possibility of ^{99m}Tc contamination, recounting of the specimens at 24 or 48 hours will readily clarify the situation. Methods for the sequential determination of the gastrointestinal absorption of vitamin B_{12} with and without IF and the simultaneous determination of the gastrointestinal absorption of free and IF-bound vitamin B_{12} are detailed later.

Sequential Determination of Gastrointestinal Absorption of Vitamin B_{12} with and without Exogenous IF

Pretest Information

Obtain the diagnosis and reason for study, hematologic findings, and blood cobalamin and folate levels if available. Check the status of the patient's renal function. Is the patient able to collect a 24-hour specimen? Has the patient been receiving parenteral vitamin B_{12}? If so, when was the last dose?

Patient Preparation

No vitamin B_{12} injection is given for at least 3 days before the test. The patient is to fast overnight.

Procedure

1. Verify fasting state.
2. Obtain patient's height and weight.

3. Administer test dose consisting of ^{57}Co-labeled vitamin B$_{12}$ containing 0.5 to 1.0 μg of the vitamin and 0.5 to 1.0 μCi (18.5 to 37 kBq) activity in capsular form (Rubratope-57 Diagnostic Kit, Squibb Diagnostic, New Brunswick, NJ).

4. Instruct the patient to collect all urine for a period of 24 hours after oral administration of test material. If there is a significant impairment of renal function have patient collect a second (24 to 48 hours) complete 24-hour specimen. The urine collection bottles should each contain 5 mL of toluene as a preservative.

5. Administer vitamin B$_{12}$ 1 mg intramuscularly at 2 hours after administration of test material. Patient may now eat.

6. *Specimen and standard preparation.* (If there is more than one 24-hour collection, handle each separately.)

   a. Mix specimen and measure and record total urine volume. Reserve a small amount of urine for creatinine determination.

   b. Aliquot 1 L of specimen into counting bottle. If the 24-hour collection is less than 1 L, add water to make a final volume of 1 L. Mix.

   c. Add 1.0 mL of ^{57}Co standard provided with test kit containing 2% of the activity of the oral ^{57}Co-labeled vitamin B$_{12}$ dose to 1 L of water in counting bottle. Mix.

   d. A counting bottle containing 1 L of water is used as a background sample.

7. *Counting specimens and standards.* Select an instrument with a detector suitable for the large counting bottle used and a γ-spectrometer to allow the selective counting of the main γ-photon peak of ^{57}Co. Count the background, standard, and patient sample bottles.

8. *Calculations.*

$$\% \ ^{57}\text{Co excretion} = \frac{2 \times U \times a}{X}$$

where X is the net ^{57}Co standard counts, a is the net ^{57}Co counts in urine, and U is the urine aliquot correction factor (total urine volume/urine volume counted). The constant 2 represents the fact that each 1.0 mL of standard contains 2% of the radioactivity in the test dose.

9. If the percentage urinary excretion is less than 9%, the test is repeated as described earlier except that a capsule of IF concentrate (INFXI unit) is administered orally with the ^{57}Co-labeled vitamin B$_{12}$ test dose. Such repeat testing can be performed 3 to 5 days following the day of the initial test dose.

Simultaneous Determination of Gastrointestinal Absorption of Free and IF-Bound Vitamin B$_{12}$

Obtain the diagnosis and reason for study and obtain hematologic findings and blood cobalamin and folate levels, if available. Check the status of the patient's renal function. Is the patient able to collect a 24-hour specimen? Has the patient been receiving parenteral vitamin B$_{12}$? If so, when was the last dose?

Patient Preparation

No vitamin B$_{12}$ injection is given for at least 3 days before the test. The patient is fasted overnight.

Procedure

1. Verify fasting state. Obtain specimen for blood vitamin B$_{12}$ and folate levels if there were no pretest measurements.

2. Obtain patient's height and weight.

3. Administer test dose consisting of two capsules:

   a. ^{58}Co-labeled vitamin B$_{12}$ that is provided in a capsule containing 0.25 μg of the vitamin and approximately 0.8 μCi (29.6 kBq) activity (Dicopac Kit, Medi-Physics, Inc., Arlington Heights, IL 60005).

   b. ^{57}Co-labeled vitamin B$_{12}$ bound to human gastric juice IF that is provided in a capsule containing 0.25 μg of the vitamin and approximately 0.5 μCi (18.5 kBq) of activity (Dicopac Kit). Give capsules separately, ensuring that each is swallowed. The patient is told to remain fasting.

4. Instruct the patient to collect all urine for a period of 24 hours after oral administration of test material. If there is significant impairment of renal function have patient collect a second (24 to 48 hours) complete 24-hour specimen. The urine collection bottles should contain 5 mL of toluene as a preservative.

5. Administer vitamin B$_{12}$ 1 mg intramuscularly 2 hours after administration of test material. The patient may now eat.

6. *Specimen and standard preparation.* (f there is more than one 24-hour collection, handle each separately.)

   a. Mix specimen and measure and record total urine volume. Reserve a small amount of urine for creatinine determination.

   b. Aliquot 1 L of specimen into counting bottle. If the 24-hour collection is less than 1 L, add water to make a final volume of 1 L. Mix.

   c. Add 1.0 mL of the ^{57}Co standard provided with the test kit containing 2% of the activity of the oral ^{57}Co-labeled vitamin B$_{12}$ dose to 1 L of water in a counting bottle. Mix.

   d. Add 1.0 mL of the ^{58}Co standard provided with the test kit containing 2% of the activity of the oral ^{58}Co-labeled vitamin B$_{12}$ dose to 1 L of water in a counting bottle. Mix.

   e. A counting bottle containing 1 L of water is used as a background sample.

7. *Counting specimens and standards.* Select an instrument with a detector suitable for the large counting bottles used, and a gamma-spectrometer to allow the selective counting of the main γ-photon peaks of each radionuclide. If the instrument has a multichannel analyzer, count data in the ^{57}Co and ^{58}Co photopeak windows, which can be obtained simultaneously. An instrument with a single channel analyzer requires first counting all samples at the photopeak settings of one of the radionuclides, then recounting all samples after changing the photopeak settings to those of the other radionuclide. Typical window settings used are 50 to 200 keV for the 122- and 136-keV photons of ^{57}Co, and 400 to 1,000 keV for the 511- and 810-keV photons of ^{58}Co.

8. *Calculations.* While using settings as noted earlier, the counts in the ^{58}Co window will reflect only ^{58}Co, whereas the counts in the ^{57}Co window will result from the ^{57}Co photons and downscatter photons of ^{58}Co. This contribution of counts

from ^{58}Co to the ^{57}Co window is taken into account in the following calculations. Because each standard contains 2% of the administered dose, the calculations are

$$\% \ ^{58}Co \ \text{excretion} \left(\text{free vitamin B}_{12} \right) = \frac{2 \times U \times b}{Z}$$

$$\% \ \text{Co-57 excretion} \left(\text{intrinsic factor-bound vitamin B}_{12} \right)$$

$$= \frac{2 \times U \times \left[\dfrac{a - b \times Y}{Z} \right]}{X}$$

where Z is the net counts ^{58}Co standard in ^{58}Co window, Y is the net counts ^{58}Co standard in ^{57}Co window, X is the net counts ^{57}Co standard in ^{57}Co window, b is the net counts in urine specimen in ^{58}Co window, a is the net counts in the urine specimen in ^{57}Co window, and U is the urine volume correction factor (total urine volume/urine volume counted).

If there is a second 24-hour urine collection, obtain by appropriate addition the total percentage ^{58}Co and percentage ^{57}Co excretion for the 48-hour period. Using these values, compute the ratio of absorbed IF-bound vitamin B$_{12}$ to absorbed free vitamin B$_{12}$.

Clinical Application and Interpretation

The appropriate clinical use of vitamin B$_{12}$ absorption measurements is to determine the mechanism of cobalamin malabsorption in patients with documented cobalamin deficiency or suspected cobalamin deficiency; dietary deficiency is very rare (51).

A number of studies in recent years have indicated that the spectrum of manifestations of cobalamin deficiency is quite broad and the relative coexistence of these manifestations is more varied than previously

Megaloblastic anemia is a manifestation of a severe degree of cobalamin deficiency. The degree of cobalamin deficiency is related to the cause and the severity and duration of the cause. Accordingly, the incidence of megaloblastic anemia is higher in those conditions associated with IF deficiency and ileal mucosal abnormalities and lower in intestinal luminal conditions and

Table 27.3. *Causes of Megaloblastic Anemia*

Cobalamin deficiency (see Table 27.2)
Folic acid deficiency
   Dietary deficiency
   Dietary deficiency with increase requirements
      Pregnancy, infancy
      Chronic hemolysis
   Intestinal malabsorption
      Extensive (jejunal) resection
      Gluten-sensitive enteropathy, tropical sprue
      Anticonvulsants
Inherited disorders of DNA synthesis
Drug-induced disorders of DNA synthesis
   Chemotherapeutic agents
Myelodysplastic and leukemic states
   Myelodysplasia associated with sideroblastic anemias and pre-
      leukemic states
   Erythroleukemia

Table 27.4. *Interpretive Ranges of Serum Cobalamin, Serum Folate, and RBC Folate Levels*

	Serum vitamin B (pg/mL)	Serum folate (ng/mL)	RBC folate[a] (ng/mL)
Normal range[b]	200–900	2.5–20.0	>175
Indeterminate range[b]	160–200	1.9–2.5	125–175
Low range[b]	<160	<1.9	<125

[a]RBC, red blood cell folate.
[b]Values are dependent upon method and laboratory.

conditions associated with impaired release of food-bound cobalamin (Table 27.2).

Although megaloblastic anemia is a major manifestation of cobalamin deficiency, identical hematologic abnormalities are found in folic acid deficiency and other conditions (26,27). The causes of megaloblastic anemias are outlined in Table 27.3.

Although the findings of dorsal and lateral column spinal cord involvement coupled with peripheral neuropathy (subacute combined degeneration) are highly suggestive of cobalamin deficiency (52), the neuropsychiatric manifestations of cobalamin deficiency are protean and also include isolated neuropathy and myelopathy, optic neuritis, dementia, depression, psychosis, and behavioral disturbances (53–57). Approximately one third of those patients exhibiting any of these neuropsychiatric conditions as a result of cobalamin deficiency show no hematologic abnormalities (58,59).

Serum folate and red blood cell folate levels should also be performed if the differential diagnosis includes folic acid deficiency. These vitamin levels are determined routinely by standard radioassay and enzyme assay techniques. Interpretative ranges of these analytes are shown in Table 27.4.

Along with this broadened definition of cobalamin deficiency, one must account for those conditions which, on occasion, may be associated with falsely low serum cobalamin levels without cobalamin deficiency and falsely normal serum cobalamin levels in patients with cobalamin deficiency (26,27) (Table 27.5). Because the serum folate level is quite sensitive to short-term changes in dietary folate (60), depressed serum levels in the absence of tissue deficiency may often be noted in chronically ill individuals. False-low serum folate levels may also be noted with a variety of acute and chronic small bowel disorders, anti-

Table 27.5. *Causes of Falsely Low and Falsely Normal Serum Cobalamin Levels*

Falsely low serum cobalamin level without cobalamin deficiency
   Folate deficiency
   Myeloma
   Aplastic anemia
   Pregnancy
   Oral contraceptives
   Transcobalamin I deficiency
Falsely normal serum cobalamin level with cobalamin deficiency
   Liver disease
   Chronic myelogenous leukemia
   Transcobalamin II deficiency
   Recent vitamin B$_{12}$ injection

Table 27.6. *Schilling Test Results in Normal Subjects and Patients with Cobalamin (Cbl) Malabsorption*

Groups	% Dose excreted		
	B$_{12}$	B$_{12}$ with IF	B$_{12}$-IF/B$_{12}$ ratio
Normal subjects	10–40	10–40	0.7–1.2
Food-bound Cbl malabsorption	10–40	10–40	0.7–1.2
Intrinsic factor deficient Cbl malabsorption	0–9	6–15	>1.4
Intestinal luminal and ileal mucosal Cbl malabsorption	0–9	0–9	0.7–1.2

IF, intrinsic factor.

convulsant therapy, hemolytic disorders, pregnancy, and infancy (26,27). Although the red cell folate is a better index of tissue folate stores, it is usually depressed in cobalamin deficiency (26, 27).

Although the blood levels of these vitamins are useful in defining the appropriate vitamin deficient state, particularly when it is of marked degree, there are limitations when these assays are applied to a broad range of deficiencies. For this larger spectrum of patients, urine and serum methylmalonic acid and homocysteine measurements are more sensitive and accurate than serum cobalamin levels in the diagnosis of cobalamin deficiency (58,60,61). Currently, however, accurate methylmalonic acid and homocysteine measurements require sophisticated technology, are performed routinely by a limited number of laboratories, and are relatively expensive.

The primary use of vitamin B$_{12}$ absorption studies is to determine the mechanism of cobalamin malabsorption in patients with demonstrated cobalamin deficiency. Such information, when combined with clinical and other laboratory findings, aids in the diagnosis of the specific causative condition (Table 27.2). The approved and commercially available reagents for the determination of cobalamin absorption include free (crystalline) radiolabeled vitamin B$_{12}$, radiolabeled vitamin B$_{12}$-IF complex, and IF. The range of results obtained by using these materials with the urinary excretion method (Schilling test) is shown in Table 27.6. The vitamin B$_{12}$ with IF/vitamin B$_{12}$ urinary excretion ratio is more valid when using the simultaneous dual radioisotope procedure, as compared with the sequential procedure, when fluctuation in cobalamin absorption status and completeness of urine collection must be taken into account.

SUMMARY

The measurement of cobalamin absorption using radiolabeled vitamin B$_{12}$ continues to be indispensable in the determination of the mechanism of cobalamin malabsorption. Careful attention to procedural details greatly aids in obtaining useful results in a large majority of the patients studied. Optimal interpretation of test results involves the use of appropriate physiologic and technical knowledge, a familiarity with causes of cobalamin deficiency and its manifestations, and an evaluation and synthesis of the pertinent clinical and laboratory data in the patient.

REFERENCES

1. Millison PL. *Blood transfusion in clinical medicine.* London: Blackwell Scientific Publications, 1983:65–92.
2. International Committee for Standardization in Hematology. Recommended methods for measurement of red-cell and plasma volume. *J Nucl Med* 1980;21:793.
3. Pierson RN Jr, Lin DH. Measurement of body compartments in children: whole-body counting and other methods. *Semin Nucl Med* 1972; 2:373.
4. Sterling K. Turnover rate of serum using ^{131}I. *J Clin Invest* 1951;30: 1228.
5. Noble RP, Gregerson MI. Mixing time and disappearance of T-1824 in shock. *J Clin Invest* 1946;25:158.
6. Gregersen MI. A practical method for the determination of blood volume with the dye t-1824. *J Lab Clin Med* 1944;29:1226.
7. Berson SA, Yalow RS. The use of K42 or P32 labeled erythrocytes and I131 tagged human serum albumin in simultaneous blood volume determinations. *J Clin Invest* 1952;31:572.
8. Tuckerman J, Finnerty FA Jr. Dilution curves of simultaneously administered I ^{131}-human serum albumin and Cr^{51}-labeled erythrocytes in patients with various types of edema. *Circ Res* 1961;9:1010.
9. Powsner ER, Raeside DE. *Diagnostic nuclear medicine.* New York: Grune & Stratton, 1971:311.
10. Wochner RD, Adatepe M, Van Amburg A et al. New method for estimation of plasma volume with the use of the distribution space of transferring-113m-indium. *J Lab Clin Med* 1970;75:711.
11. Bent-Hansen L. Initial plasma disappearance and distribution volume of I-131 albumin and I-125 fibrinogen in man. *Acta Physical Scand* 1989;136:455.
12. Gregersen MI, Rawson RA. Blood volume. *Physiol Rev* 1959;39: 307.
13. Chaplin H, Mollison PL, Vetter H. The body/venous hematocrit ratio: its constancy over a wide hematocrit range. *J Clin Invest* 1953;32:1309.
14. Donohue DM, Motulsky AG, Giblett ER et al. The use of chromium as a red cell tag. *Br J Haematol* 1955;1:249.
15. Loria A, Sanchez-Medal L, Kauffer N et al. Relationship between body hematocrit and venous hematocrit in normal, splenomegalic and anemic states. *J Lab Clin Med* 1962;60:396.
16. Moens RS, Busset R, Collet RA et al. Utilisation de l'albumine-I^{131}(RI-HSA) pour la determination du volume plasmatique et du volume sanguine chez le sujet normal. *J Suisse Med* 1962;92:1660.
17. Norberg B, Andersson E. Experiences with simultaneous determinations of erythrocyte and plasma volumes. *Scan J Clin Lab Invest* (Suppl) 1965;17:174(abst).
18. Najean Y, Deschrywer F. The body venous haematocrit ratio and its use for calculating total blood volume from fractional volumes. *Eur J Nucl Med* 1984;9:558.
19. Fairbanks VF, Tauxe WN. Plasma and erythrocyte volumes in obesity, polycythemia, and related conditions. In: Bergner PEE, Lushbaugh CC, eds. *Compartments, pools, and spaces in medical physiology.* Oak Ridge, TN: US Atomic Energy Commission, 1967:283.
20. Wright RR, Tono M, Pollycove M. Blood volume. *Semin Nucl Med* 1975;5:63.
21. Wood CA, Levitt SH. Simultaneous red cell mass and plasma volume determinations using ^{51}Cr tagged red cells and ^{125}I labeled albumin. *J Nucl Med* 1972;13:60.
22. Paix D. Letter to the editor. *J Nucl Med* 1965;6:717.
23. Schjonsby H. Vitamin B$_{12}$ absorption and malabsorption. *Gut* 1989; 30:1686–1691.
24. Festen HPM. Intrinsic factor secretion and cobalamin absorption; physiology and pathophysiology in the gastrointestinal tract. *Scan J Gastroenteral* 1991;188(Suppl):1–7.
25. Seetharam B, Ramanujam KS, Seetharam S et al. Normal and abnormal physiology of intrinsic factor mediated absorption of cobalamin (vitamin B$_{12}$). *Indian Biochem Biophys* 1991;28:324–330.
26. Babior BM. The megaloblastic anemias. In: Beutler E, Lichtman MA, Coller BS et al., eds. *Williams hematology,* 6th ed. New York: McGraw-Hill, 2001:425–445.

27. Jandl JH. Megaloblastic anemias. In: Jandl JH, ed. *Blood, textbook of hematology,* 2nd ed. Boston: Little, Brown and Company, 1996: 251–288.

28. Beck WS. Diagnosis of megaloblastic anemia. *Annu Rev Med* 1991; 42:311-322.

29. Lee GR. Megaloblastic and nonmegaloblastic macrocytic anemias. In: Lee GR, Bithell TC, Foerster J et al., eds. *Wintrobes clinical hematology,* 9th ed. Philadelphia: Lea & Febiger 1993:747–790.

30. Doscherholmen A, Swaim WR. Impaired assimilation of egg [57]Co vitamin B$_{12}$ in patients with hypochlorhydria and achlorhydria and after gastric resection. *Gastroenterology* 1973;64:913–919.

31. Streeter AM, Duraiappah B, Boyle R et al. Malabsorption of vitamin B$_{12}$ after vagotomy. *Ann I Surg* 1974;128:340–343.

32. Carmel R, Sinow RM, Siegel ME et al. Food cobalamin malabsorption occurs frequently in patients with unexplained low cobalamin levels. *Arch Intern Med* 1988;148:1715–1719.

33. Miller A, Furlong D, Burrows BA, Slingerland DW. Bound vitamin B absorption in patients with low serum B$_{12}$ levels. *Am J Hem* 1992; 40:163–166.

34. Force RW, Nakata MC. Effect of histamine H/2-receptor antagonists on vitamin B$_{12}$ absorption. *Ann Pharmacother* 1992;26:1283–1286.

35. Kittang E, Echjonsby H. Effect of gastric anacidity on the release of cobalamins from food and their subsequent binding to R-protein. *Scan J Gastroenterol* 1987;22:1031–1037.

36. Yale CE, Gohdes PN, Schilling RF. Cobalamin absorption and hematologic status after two types of gastric surgery for obesity. *Am J Hem* 1993;42:63–66.

37. Herbert V. Transient (reversible) malabsorption of vitamin B$_{12}$. *Br J Haematol* 1969;17:213–219.

38. Cottrall MF, Wells DG, Trott NG et al. Radioactive vitamin B$_{12}$ absorption studies: comparison of the whole body retention, urinary excretion and 9-hour plasma levels of radioactive vitamin B$_{12}$. *Blood* 1971; 38:604–613.

39. Fish MB, Pollycove M, Wallerstein RO et al. Simultaneous measurement of free and intrinsic factor (IF) bound vitamin B$_{12}$ (B$_{12}$) absorption: absolute quantitation with incomplete stool collection and rapid relative measurement using plasma B$_{12}$(IF):B$_{12}$ absorption ratio. *J Nucl Med* 1973;14:568–575.

40. Fone DJ, Cooke WT, Megmell MJ et al. [58]CO B$_{12}$ absorption (hepatic surface count) after gastrectomy, ileal resection and in coeliac disorders. *Gut* 1961;2:218–224.

41. Pollycove M, Apt L. Absorption, elimination and excretion of orally administered B$_{12}$ in normal subjects and in patients with pernicious anemia. *N Engl J Med* 1956;255:207–212.

42. Nelp WB, McAfee JG, Wagner HN. Single measurement of plasma radioactive vitamin B$_{12}$ as a test for pernicious anemia. *J Lab Clin Med* 1963;61:158–165.

43. McIntyre PA, Wagner HN. Comparison of the urinary excretion and 8-hour plasma test for vitamin B$_{12}$ absorption. *J Lab Clin Med* 1966; 68:966–971.

44. Schilling RF. Intrinsic factor studies II. The effect of gastric juice in the urinary excretion of radioactivity after oral administration of radioactive vitamin B$_{12}$. *J Lab Clin Med* 1953;42:860–866.

45. McIntyre PA. Use of radioisotope techniques in the clinical evaluations of patients with megaloblastic anemia. *Semin Nucl Med* 1975;5:79–94.

46. Gräsbeck R, Guëant JL. Mechanism of cobalamin absorption: intrinsic factor and its receptor. *J Nutr Sci Vitaminol* 1992;Spec No:110–113.

47. Rath CE, McCurdy PR, Duffy BJ. Effect of renal disease on the Schilling test. *N Engl J Med* 1957;256:111–114.

48. Latz JH, DeMase J, Donaldson RM. Simultaneous administration of gastric juice bound and free radioactive cyanocobalamin: rapid procedure for differentiating between intrinsic factor deficiency and other causes of vitamin B$_{12}$ malabsorption. *J Lab Clin Med* 1963;61: 266–271.

49. Bell TK, Bridges JM, Nelson MG. Simultaneous free and bound radioactive vitamin B$_{12}$ urinary excretion test. *J Clin Pathol* 1965;18: 611–613.

50. Digiogio J. Non-protein nitrogenous constituents. In: Henry RJ, Cannon DC, Winkelman JW, eds. *Clinical chemistry principles and technics,* 2nd ed. New York: Harper & Row, 1974.

51. Wright RR, Tono M, Pollycove M. Blood volume. *Semin Nucl Med* 1975;5:63–78.

52. Fish MB. unpublished data.

53. Forbes GB. *Human body composition—growth, aging, nutrition, and activity.* New York: Springer-Verlag, 1987.

54. Arias IM, Apt L, Pollycove M. Absorption of radioactive vitamin B$_{12}$ in non-anemic patients with combined system disease. *New Engl J Med* 1955;253:1005–1010.

55. Beck WS. Neuropsychiatric consequences of cobalamin deficiency. *Adv Int Med* 1991;36:33–53.

56. Fine EJ, Soria ED. Myths about vitamin B$_{12}$ deficiency. *South Med J* 1991;84:1475–1481.

57. Dommisse J. Subtle vitamin B$_{12}$ deficiency and psychiatry: a largely unnoticed but devastating relationship. *Med Hypothesis* 1991;34: 131–140.

58. Allen RH, Stabler SP, Savage DG et al. New approaches to the diagnosis of cobalamin (Cbl, vitamin B$_{12}$) deficiency in neuropsychiatric disorders. *J Nutr Sci Vitaminol* 1992;Spec No:130–133.

59. Regland B, Gottfries CB, Lindstadt G. Dementia patients with low serum cobalamin concentration: relationship to atrophic gastritis. *Aging Clin Exp Res* 1992;4:35–41.

60. Stabler SP, Allen RH, Savage DG et al. Clinical spectrum and diagnosis of cobalamin deficiency. *Blood* 1990;76:871–881.

61. Lindenbaum J, Healton EB, Savage DG et al. Neuropsychiatric disorders caused by cobalamin deficiency in the absence of anemia or macrocytosis. *N Engl J Med* 1988;318:1720–1728.

28

BONE MARROW SCINTIGRAPHY

MIJIN YUN
CHUN KIM
JOSEPH SAM
DIETER MUNZ
AND ABASS ALAVI

RADIOTRACERS, BIODISTRIBUTION, AND IMAGE ACQUISITION

Several radiotracers methodologies have been used for bone marrow scintigraphy (BMS). These techniques are divided into four scintigraphic categories depending on the target cell type: (a) reticuloendothelial (RE) imaging, (b) erythropoietic imaging, (c) granulopoietic imaging, and (d) unknown (1). ^{99m}Tc labeled colloids are taken up by the reticuloendothelial system (RES). Erythropoietic marrow can be visualized with ^{52}Fe. ^{99m}Tc labeled monoclonal antibodies are directed against nonspecific cross-reacting antigen 95 (NCA-95) and have been used clinically for imaging granulopoietic marrow in man (2). In addition, ^{111}In-chloride was briefly used as a marrow imaging agent. Its exact target cell has not been identified yet (1). Some investigators have used radiolabeled leukocytes as a bone marrow scanning agent (3).

The distributions of the hematopoietic system and RES are similar in normal individuals and in most disease states (4). This has been confirmed by simultaneous imaging with radioactive iron and radiocolloids (5). Therefore, from a practical perspective, any tracer may be used for routine studies, and the choice of the tracer can be based on availability, as well as the clinical situation. However, in some circumstances, such as aplastic anemia secondary to chemotherapy, dissociation between RE and erythroblastic function may occur (5). On the other hand, in patients with expansion of the marrow resulting from hemolytic anemia, this dissociation has not been seen. In these patients, radiocolloids appear to be the agents of choice in demonstrating the extent of marrow expansion, as well as the pattern of distribution (Fig. 28.1).

M. Yun: Department of Radiology, Yonsei University and Medical Center, Seoul, Korea.

C. Kim: Division of Nuclear Medicine, Department of Radiology, Mount Sinai School of Medicine, New York, NY.

J. Sam: Department of Radiology, Hospital of the University of Pennsylvania, Philadelphia, PA.

D. Munz: Department of Nuclear Medicine, Department of Radiology, Mount Sinai School of Medicine, New York, NY.

A. Alvai: Division of Nuclear Medicine, University of Pennsylvania Medical Center, Philadelphia, PA.

Depending on the availability of equipment, anterior and posterior whole-body views or multiple spot views of the entire skeleton should be obtained regardless of the tracer used. If multiple spot views are to be taken, it is preferable to begin imaging with a posterior pelvic view for desired counts to avoid the liver and spleen in the field of view. The acquisition time of this image is then used as "preset time" setting for recording the spot views of the rest of the body containing hematopoietic marrow (6). Alternatively, all images can be acquired for a fixed time that is routinely used in a particular laboratory. An appropriate collimator should be selected for each radionuclide: a low-energy (preferably high-resolution) collimator for ^{99m}Tc, a medium-energy collimator for ^{111}In, and a high-energy collimator for ^{52}Fe (if a gamma camera is used). Imaging procedures for the ^{99m}Tc-colloid and Tc-anti-NCA-95 antibody (Tc-NSAb) studies are discussed in more detail, because other tracers are not commonly used for BMS currently.

Colloids

Colloids are rapidly cleared from the blood by phagocytic cells in the RES, which include Kupffer cells in the liver, phagocytic cells in the spleen, and phagocytic reticulum cells in the bone marrow. The introduction of radioactive colloidal agents in 1969 made visualization of RE activity possible. ^{198}Au colloid was the first tracer used for BMS until ^{99m}Tc tagged colloids became available (7). ^{198}Au emits β rays and high-energy γ rays that are suboptimal for imaging. The introduction of ^{99m}Tc-colloids has made RE imaging feasible because the radiation dose is acceptable and the images are of good quality (8). In addition, it does not require sophisticated preparation.

^{99m}Tc-sulfur colloid (Tc-SC) is most commonly used in the United States. The size of the Tc-SC particles range from 100 to 1,000 nm. In normal adults, about 5% of the injected activity will be distributed in the RE cells of the marrow, and the remainder will be taken up by the liver (80% to 85%) and spleen (10%) (9). In most Tc-SC studies, bone marrow in the lower thoracic spine, upper lumbar spine, lower ribs, or lower sternum can not be properly evaluated because of the presence of intense activity in the liver and the spleen (Fig. 28.2).

The nanometer-sized colloid (nanocolloid) agents include ^{99m}Tc-nanocolloid (Tc-NC) that is produced from microaggre-

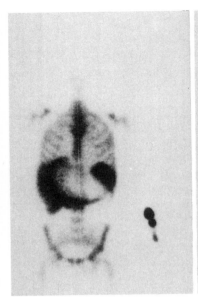
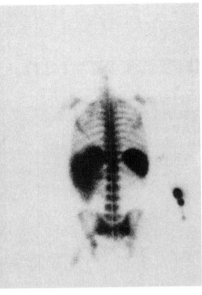

FIGURE 28.1. Normal marrow distribution. Anterior and posterior whole-body ^{99m}Tc-sulfur colloid scan demonstrates a normal pattern of bone marrow distribution. Intense activity is seen in the spine, ribs, and pelvis. Minimal marrow activity is noted in proximal upper and lower extremities. Also, significant reticuloendothelial uptake is visualized in the liver and spleen. Lower thoracic and upper lumbar spine marrow activity is clearly visualized because of the presence of a large mass in the left lobe of the liver. (From Fordham E, Amjal A. Radionuclide imaging of bone marrow. *Semin Hematol* 1981; 18:222–239, with permission.)

gated human serum albumin and ^{99m}Tc antimony sulfide colloid. These agents can also be used for lymphoscintigraphy and are commercially available in Europe. The diameter of Tc-NC particles is generally less than 80 nm, compared with 100 to 1,000 nm of Tc-SC (10). Nanocolloids are known to have a relative selectivity for bone marrow (15% to 20%) with relatively less hepatic and splenic uptake when compared with large-sized colloids (Fig. 28.3). However, it has been reported that scans using Tc-NC agents (Microlite, Dupont-NEN) show slightly higher background-to-bone-marrow ratio and more urinary activity than scans with Tc-SC (11). In a quantitative animal study, Tc-NC (nanocoll, Solco, Basle, Switzerland) showed lower relative and absolute uptake in the liver and spleen compared with the large-sized colloid (Albu-Res, Solco, Basle, Switzerland), whereas the bone marrow activity relative to the activity of kidneys, heart, lungs, intestines, and peripheral blood is higher for the large-sized colloid than for the nanocolloid. The latter has also been confirmed in humans (12). It has been suggested that large-sized colloid should be used for spot examination of a specific marrow region away from the liver and spleen, whereas nanocolloid should be used when examining structures close to the liver and spleen, as well as for depiction of the entire bone marrow.

About 5 to 20 mCi (185 to 740 MBq) of Tc-SC or small-sized colloid can be injected safely (1). Images of the marrow can be obtained 20 to 30 minutes after the intravenous administration. If a high target-to-background ratio is desired, it is advisable to wait 45 to 60 minutes before imaging to decrease the background activity. Shielding of the liver and spleen may be helpful in evaluating the anterior thorax, posterior thoracic, and lumbar spine on ^{99m}Tc-colloid studies.

The scans should be evaluated for homogeneity and intensity of activity in normal marrow, the presence and extent of peripheral marrow expansion, central marrow depletion, and focal marrow defects. Several schemes for grading of BMS findings have been proposed (13).

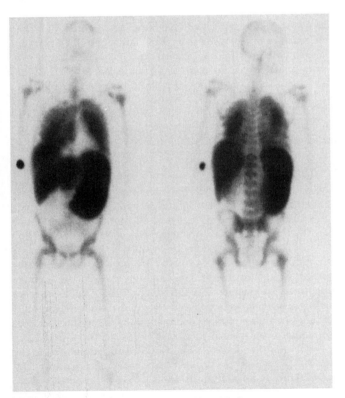

FIGURE 28.2. Peripheral marrow expansion. Moderate marrow expansion seen in this patient with β-thalassemia, Significant splenomegaly and lung uptake of ^{99m}Tc-sulfur colloid particles are noted. (From Fordham E, Amjal A. Radionuclide imaging of bone marrow. *Semin Hematol* 1981:18:222–239, with permission.)

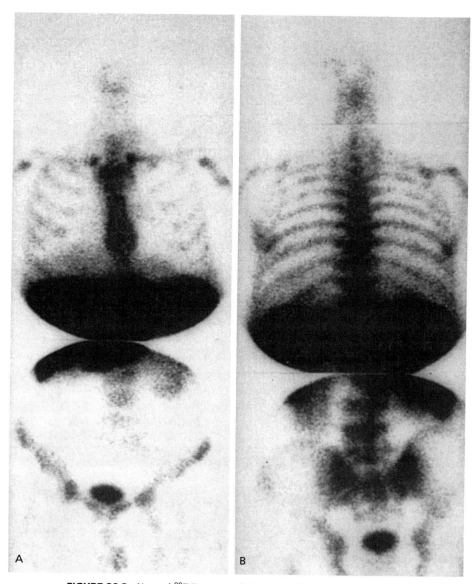

FIGURE 28.3. Normal ^{99m}Tc-nanocolloid scans. **A:** Anterior. **B:** Posterior.

The liver and spleen can also be imaged if clinically indicated or as a routine adjunct to marrow imaging. It is preferable to image the liver and spleen before marrow imaging, because a high target-to-background ratio is more important for the latter. Routine single photon emission computed tomography (SPECT) imaging of the liver at the time of bone marrow examination has been shown to be useful (14). Alternatively, some investigators acquire posterior images of the lumbar and pelvic marrow during routine radiocolloid liver scanning (15). Finally, some groups have performed an additional dynamic study of a selected marrow region (usually the sacrum and pelvis) from the time of injection and up to 40 minutes later (13,16).

Radioactive Iron

^{52}Fe is ideal for the assessment of erythropoietic marrow (5). ^{52}Fe is produced by a ^{55}Mn (p, 4n) ^{52}Fe reaction in a cyclotron

(17). ^{52}Fe decays by positron emission and by electron capture to ^{52m}Mn with a half-life of 8.2 hours. ^{52m}Mn decays with a half-life of 21.3 minutes, also by positron emission. This makes it relatively expensive and less widely available, although its half-life of 8.2 hours allows for transporting the radiotracer over greater distances and for imaging to be performed up to 24 hours after administration of the tracer. In addition to the two 511-keV photons produced by annihilation of the positron, ^{52}Fe emits a principal photon with an energy of 165 keV. The administered dose is limited to 100 to 200 μCi because of its relatively high radiation burden to the marrow (2.5 rads/100 μCi). Images of inferior quality are obtained using a regular scintillation camera equipped with a high-energy collimator. Positron emission tomography (PET) scanners can be used to produce images of high quality with ^{52}Fe (18). Approximately two thirds of the emitted 511-keV γ rays originate from ^{52m}Mn, a daughter product of ^{52}Fe. Fortunately, ^{52m}Mn appears to remain at the site of

^{52}Fe localization in the marrow and, therefore, does not adversely affect the images (18).

Quantitative assessments of erythropoiesis in areas of bone marrow expansion have been performed with ^{52}Fe (17). ^{52}Fe does not accumulate in the liver or spleen, which allows the detection of marrow abnormalities in the thoracic and lumbar areas. Marrow scanning with ^{52}Fe has also been used in the investigation of mass lesions that may represent extramedullary hematopoiesis (19). Another iron radionuclide, ^{59}Fe, is not suitable for imaging because of its high photon energy (1.099 and 1.292 MeV) and long half-life (45 days). However, these properties make this isotope suitable for nonimaging ferrokinetic studies of erythropoietic bone marrow activity.

^{111}In-Labeled Tracers

^{111}In-chloride is a marrow agent that is cyclotron-produced and has a half-life of 2.8 days. It decays by electron capture with high photon yields and emits photons with energies of 173 and 247 keV. After intravenous injection, ^{111}In binds rapidly to serum transferrin and is eliminated from the plasma with a half-life of 5 hours (1). Approximately 30% of ^{111}In is found in the bone marrow, 20% in the liver, 7% in the kidneys, and 1% in the spleen (1). The rest is distributed throughout the body fluids without specific tissue accumulation. The exact cellular and subcellular distribution of ^{111}In in bone marrow is not known (1). Despite the strong affinity of ^{111}In for transferrin (20), only 4% of the injected activity appears in circulating erythrocytes after 8 to 10 days as compared with 80% of iron (21). For BMS, 1 to 5 mCi (37 to 185 MBq) of ^{111}In-chloride is injected intravenously, and images are obtained 24 to 48 hours later.

In patients with normal bone marrow, the distribution of ^{111}In is similar to that of ^{99m}Tc-labeled colloids (1). This tracer has been occasionally helpful in demonstrating extramedullary hematopoiesis or hematopoietic cellularity in the sacrum (22). The mechanism of uptake of this radiopharmaceutical is different from the radionuclides of iron (23). In contrast to ^{52}Fe images, ^{111}In scans show soft tissue uptake in the genitals, liver, spleen, and kidneys and appear to have skeletal uptake (19). Hepatic and splenic uptake of ^{111}In does not reflect erythropoiesis (24). Numerous reports have indeed demonstrated disparity between ^{111}In activity and ^{52}Fe activity or erythropoietic cellularity in various conditions. Bone marrow irradiated with 500 rads failed to accumulate iron as expected but had unimpaired ^{111}In uptake (1). There was no correlation between the erythrocyte cellularity of the marrow and the indium bone marrow scan grade in patients with chronic renal disease (25). It was also shown that the distribution of ^{111}In and ^{52}Fe was different in most patients with a variety of hematologic disorders (26).

Despite some good results with this agent in the past (24, 27), the relatively high radiation dose and poor image quality compared with that obtained with ^{99m}Tc compounds precludes its routine use in patients with benign disorders. Furthermore, the almost negligible incorporation into erythrocytes precludes its use for the assessment of erythropoietic marrow activity.

Labeled Antibodies

NCA-95 is a glycoprotein subunit of the carcinoembryonic antigen (CEA) with a molecular weight of 95 kD. It is produced during differentiation of granulopoiesis, and is expressed in the cytosol and on the cell surface after the developmental stage of the promyelocytes (28). Immunohistochemical and fluorescence-activated cell sorter studies revealed that promyelocytes take up only small amounts of ^{99m}Tc BW 250/183 (an IgG1 isotype anti-NCA-95 monoclonal antibody) following intravenous administration of the radiotracer. In contrast, marrow myelocytes and metamyelocytes were more intensely stained than bone marrow granulocytes (29). The antibody does not activate complement or result in complement-mediated lysis. *In vitro* studies of phagocytosis and the killing of microorganisms, pinocytosis of colloidal gold, superoxide anion production, and lysosomal enzyme secretion indicate that binding of the antibodies to the NCA-95 associated epitope does not impair or inhibit granulocyte-specific functions. A sham dialysis model demonstrated viability of ^{99m}Tc BW 250/183-labeled granulocytes *in vivo*. Furthermore, 1-mg doses of ^{99m}Tc BW 250/183 do not alter peripheral granulocyte counts (30). Granulocyte counts in peripheral blood have no obvious effect on the biokinetics of ^{99m}Tc BW 250/183 or antibody-labeled neutrophilic granulocytes. However, repeated injections of these antibodies can induce human antimurine antibodies (HAMAs) in approximately 5% of patients. HAMA-murine monoclonal antibody complexes are phagocytosed by the RES and alter the biodistribution of the monoclonal antibody, with increased hepatic and/or splenic uptake, resulting in nondiagnostic scans (31). Overall, BMS using antigranulocyte monoclonal antibody is safe with a low incidence of side effects and rare HAMA production limiting repeated use of the antibody (32).

Within 5 to 15 minutes after intravenous administration of ^{99m}Tc BW 250/183, 5% to 33 % of the injected radioactivity is bound to granulocytes. The remainder is in the circulating blood as labeled IgG1 and a small percentage (< 10%) of labeled smaller molecules (metabolites) and pertechnetate. The latter two molecules appear in urine (33). Because human red bone marrow harbors 50- to 100-fold more granulopoietic cells than granulocytes in peripheral blood, anti-NCA-95 antibodies are taken up primarily in active red marrow after intravenous administration (34). Tc-NSAb has been successfully used to image granulopoietic bone marrow in humans (35). In support of this concept, immunohistology and flow cytometry studies in humans have shown selective staining of the granulopoietic cells both after *in vitro* incubation and after intravenous injection of Tc-NSAb (29). The uptake of ^{99m}Tc BW 250/183 in human red marrow represents granulopoietic activity and, in most cases, the overall hematopoietic status. Compared with that of ^{99m}Tc-NCs, the marrow uptake of ^{99m}Tc BW 250/183 is approximately two to four times higher (6). In addition, BMS using ^{99m}Tc BW 250/183 shows only faint activity in the liver and spleen without obscuring the lower ribs and thoracolumbar spine. Since it was introduced as a novel radiopharmaceutical in the late 1980s, ^{99m}Tc-NSAb has provided the highest image quality for BMS (Fig. 28.4) (36).

The activity administered per patient ranges between 185

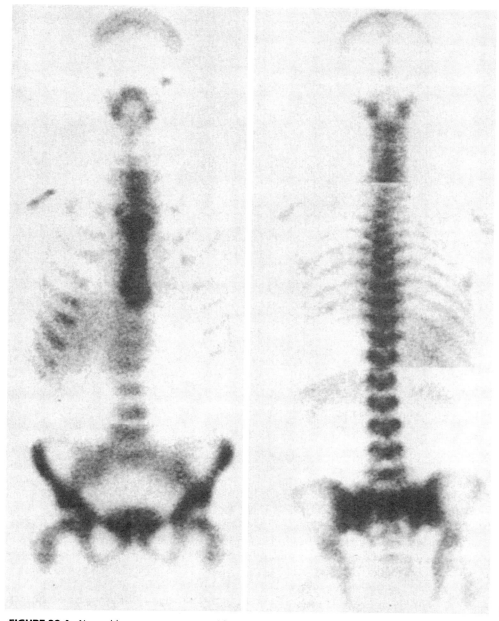

A   B

FIGURE 28.4. Normal bone marrow scans with Tc-anti-nonspecific cross-reacting antigen 95 antibody.
A: Anterior. **B:** Posterior.

to 740 mBq (protein dose, 100 to 400 mg). Because of the slow blood clearance of Tc-NSAb, imaging is usually performed 3 to 4 hours after injection (28). Overlapping spot views or whole-body scans covering the entire hematopoietic marrow should be recorded. The usual imaging time for a whole marrow scan is 45 to 60 minutes. In contrast to colloid imaging, shielding of the liver and spleen is not necessary, because these organs have only limited Tc-NSAb uptake as discussed previously (35). Evaluation of the marrow is done as described for ^{99m}Tc-colloid scans. The radiation exposure to the red marrow amounts to about 0.029 mSv/mBq, to the liver 0.022 mSv/mBq, and to the spleen 0.029 mSv/mBq. The effective dose equivalent is reported to be 0.011 mSv/mBq.

Other Tracers

Leukocytes [white blood cells (WBCs)] or granulocytes labeled with either ^{111}In or ^{99m}Tc are primarily used for localization of infection and not for BMS because the procedure is labor intensive and carries the risks of handling blood. However, these agents are reasonably good bone marrow imaging tracers (3). Although bone marrow activity presumably represents the RES distribution, a study showed that Tc-WBC activity correlated better with hematopoietic cellularity than ^{111}In-chloride activity (3). Although there is considerable liver activity when using labeled leukocytes, it is significantly less than that of colloid agents, so that the spine is usually not obscured (37) (Fig. 28.5). In a

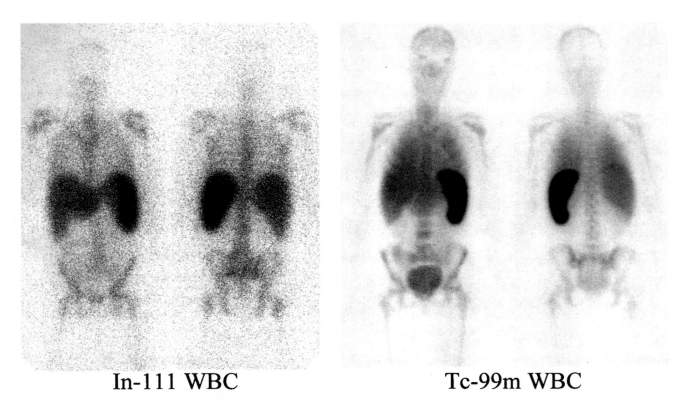

In-111 WBC   Tc-99m WBC

FIGURE 28.5. In-white blood cell (WBC) (*left*) and Tc-WBC (*right*) scans. The spine is not usually obscured.

study using tomographic technique, the bone-marrow-to-liver activity ratio for ^{111}In granulocytes was higher than that for Tc-NC. However, the activity ratios between bone marrow and spleen, as well as between bone marrow and tissue background, were not higher (37).

Compared with In-WBC images performed 18 to 24 hours after injection, Tc-WBC images usually show high pulmonary activity when obtained 2 to 6 hours after injection. Tc-WBC images also show some degree of intestinal, renal, and bladder activity. Nevertheless, Tc-WBC images show far better detail of the bone marrow (Fig. 28.5). The critical organ is the spleen. Diffusely decreased or absent bone marrow activity can be artifactually caused by rapid accumulation of the cells in inflammation site even in the absence of bone marrow disorders (38).

[18]F-fluorodeoxyglucose (FDG) is a positron emitter, an analogue of glucose that is transported into cells by various glucose transporters. It is then phosphorylated by hexokinase and trapped within the cell in proportion to the glycolytic rate of the cell (39). In 1930, Warburg et al. (40), found a higher rate of glycolysis (aerobic and anaerobic) in tumor cells. The increased glycolysis in tumor cells has been linked to increased activity of glycolytic enzymes and increased membrane glucose transport (41). Elevated FDG uptake has also been noted in a variety of physiologic variants and nonmalignant pathologic disease entities such as infection and inflammation (42). Thus, FDG provides the possibility of measuring glycolytic metabolism. FDG PET detects lesions based on their degree of disease activity rather than altered anatomy, whereas the other tracers for BMS image the distribution of functional bone marrow and marrow

involvement is seen as areas of absent or decreased activities. It also provides detection of lesions outside of the marrow with higher resolution, better anatomic localization, and a more precise quantification of tumor activity than these revealed by conventional BMS. Although FDG PET is not a tracer specific for BMS, it has become popular as a new approach to detect bone marrow involvement in malignant diseases.

Between 60 and 90 minutes after intravenous administration, FDG PET images provide reasonably high target-to-background ratios to detect malignant tumors and any lesions with increased glucose metabolism (42). Physiologic distribution of FDG occurs in the brain, liver, spleen, skeletal muscle, thyroid, salivary gland, thymus (especially in children), and digestive tract with variable intensity and frequency. The myocardium uses primarily free fatty acids in the fasting state, but glucose utilization is increased following glucose load, hypoxia, or ischemia. Myocardial FDG uptake is variable from intense to absent depending on the substrate availability in plasma, the hormonal milieu, and the cardiac workload. The urinary tract demonstrates significant activity because FDG is excreted via the kidneys. FDG distribution in the bone marrow is normally seen in regions of hematopoietically active sites and can vary according to the patient's age and marrow function (42).

CLINICAL APPLICATIONS

Diseases affecting the bone marrow can be categorized into the following pathologic processes: marrow replacement by malignant and benign entities; overproliferation of marrow components, which can be either malignant or benign; depletion of normal marrow components; and vascular abnormalities of the marrow, most notably seen in sickle cell anemia, which display a combination of the previously mentioned processes.

Marrow Replacement Disorders

Marrow replacement disorders are characterized, in general, by focal replacement of normal marrow components with abnormal cells, including metastatic neoplastic process; lymphomatous infiltrates; inflammatory cells resulting from infection (osteomyelitis); and RE cells resulting from various lysosomal storage disorders, typified by Gaucher's disease. As such, these disorders typically demonstrate focal areas of increased radiotracer accumulation, resulting from reactive bone formation, on bone scintigraphy; focal defects on BMS; and areas of abnormally decreased signal intensity (SI) on T1-weighted images (T1WI) and increased SI on T2-weighted images (T2WI).

Skeletal Metastases from Solid Tumors

Skeletal metastases occur almost invariably in the distribution of hematopoietic bone marrow and bones rich in red marrow. Bone marrow is the primary site of skeletal metastasis either by direct invasion or hematogenous dissemination, the latter being much more common (43). Skeletal metastasis from carcinomas of the breast, lung, prostate, thyroid, and kidney is common in adults, and neuroblastoma and Ewing's sarcoma is common in children (44).

Bone scan has been the screening method of choice for evaluation of most skeletal metastases. Metastases with a paucity of reactive bone formation or poor blood supply can be easily missed, as well as metastasis limited to the bone marrow. Because of its potential advantage to detect marrow involvement earlier than bone scintigraphy, BMS has been used for diagnosis of skeletal metastases. On BMS, focal marrow defects turned out to be the major criterion for marrow involvement from malignancies (45). The degree of peripheral marrow expansion increases with increasing numbers of skeletal metastases; however, it appears unreliable for establishing the diagnosis of metastases to the central skeleton (46). Marrow expansion was seen in 50% of patients without metastases versus 75.6% of patients with metastases.

Although BMS using large colloids is less than satisfactory (47), Tc-NC BMS appears feasible for detecting bone marrow metastasis earlier and, in general, for detecting more lesions than on bone scan in breast or lung cancers (45). In patients with metastatic prostate cancer, studies using Tc-NC appeared less sensitive than bone scan, although it might be helpful in evaluating equivocal cases, evaluating the responses to therapy, or identifying those patients at risk from myelosuppressive therapy (48).

The emergence of Tc-NSAb made BMS more promising in evaluation of bone marrow involvement by malignancies. Direct comparison of Tc-NSAb and Tc-NC was performed in 41 patients with various malignancies (6). Although both techniques were better than bone scan, Tc-NSAb showed more marrow lesions than Tc-NC scans. Compared with bone scan, Tc-NSAb has been shown to detect more and/or earlier metastatic lesions in patients with cancers of the breast, lung, prostate, kidney, or bladder (28). In contrast to most other reports, in a prospective study comparing bone scan, BMS with Tc-NSAb, and magnetic resonance imaging (MRI) in patients with solid malignant tumors, Tc-NSAb appeared to have little value in the detection of bone metastases (49). The major disadvantages of Tc-NSAb were nonspecific nature of bone marrow defects, low spatial resolution, and evaluation of only those portions of the skeleton containing red marrow. Bone marrow defects on BMS are not specific for metastases. Other benign diseases such as focal fatty degeneration of the marrow, focal necrosis, Paget's disease, bone infarction, and some benign tumors including hemangioma or lipoma may also cause defects (49). The lack of specificity was also seen in a study attempting to use BMS to improve the specificity of bone scans, which are equivocal for metastasis. Marrow defects concordant with bone scan lesions increased the likelihood of metastasis with a specificity of 79% but resulted in a false-positive rate of 21%, necessitating further investigation to exclude benign causes. Furthermore, BMS is unlikely to detect metastasis in the peripheral skeleton without marrow expansion or in the areas devoid of hematopoietic marrow such as previous radiation fields (49). In addition to focal marrow metastasis, BMS is of some value in identifying patients with diffuse bone marrow metastases (50). BMS can also exclude diffuse marrow infiltration in patients with an equivocal bone scan showing features of metabolic bone disease or of a near "super scan" (28). In these situations, BMS, even with a suboptimal agent such as Tc-SC, may be sufficient to diagnose or exclude diffuse marrow metastasis.

MRI is known to be more accurate than bone scan for the detection of skeletal metastases (51). Typically, metastases appear as focal, often multiple areas of low SI on T1WI that are hypointense to muscle or intervertebral disc; notable exceptions are metastatic melanoma and hemorrhagic metastases, which may display increased SI on T1WI resulting from deposits of paramagnetic melanin and extracellular hemoglobin, respectively. On T2WI, metastases are usually hyperintense but, in the presence of osteoblastic bony proliferation, may display variably decreased SI. Indeed, the appearance of metastases on magnetic resonance (MR) imaging is not specific and the importance of comparison with other imaging studies to exclude benign processes, such as bone islands, Paget's disease, and other causes of osteosclerosis, cannot be overemphasized. Most of the studies comparing bone scintigraphy with MRI for the detection of skeletal metastasis used planar bone scintigraphy and not SPECT imaging. In fact, when SPECT imaging was used, bone scintigraphy produced excellent results that were comparable to and complementary with MRI in detecting vertebral metastasis (52). MRI can be used to clarify an abnormal BMS by excluding potential false positives such as degenerative changes, hemangioma, or lipoma (49). Furthermore, MRI can occasionally be used to discriminate pathologic from osteoporotic vertebral fractures. MR findings that suggest that a fracture is the result of metastasis include diffuse abnormal SI throughout the entire vertebral body, extension of the abnormal SI into the posterior elements, and the presence of a paravertebral soft tissue component. Unfortunately, such features are not universally present, and MR cannot consistently differentiate changes associated with treatment or fracture from malignant tumors (53). Focal hematopoietic hyperplasia also makes a false-positive finding on MRI (54). In contrast to metastases in the spine and pelvis, MRI may not be as useful as bone scan in detecting skull, costal, or peripheral metastases (55). During the postoperative follow-up of breast cancer patients, decision on which modality to use can be further guided by consideration of malignant features, such as proliferative activity and hormonal receptor status (56). Bone scan sufficiently reflected foci in patients with estrogen receptor (ER) positive breast cancers or cancers with low proliferation, whereas bone scan was false negative in patients with ER negative or highly proliferative cancers, showing that MRI was useful in diagnosing such patients. Recent preliminary reports suggested another promising value of whole-body MRI using faster MR sequences to facilitate accurate evaluation of metastatic disease to the liver, brain, and bone, comparing favorably with conventional, multimodality staging strategies in patients with breast cancer (57).

Using FDG PET imaging as a new competing modality, some studies have provided promising results in the detection of skeletal metastases. Compared with bone scan, FDG PET in 145 patients with malignancies of various types was found reasonably sensitive and specific on a lesion by lesion basis (58). However, the performance of FDG PET may vary depending on the histology or metabolic grade of tumor. In patients with non-small cell lung cancer, FDG PET has been shown to be more accurate than bone scan (59). Bone scan may be of value in selected cases when PET can detect, but not precisely localize, a lesion to the skeleton (60). FDG PET has been shown to be superior to bone scan in the detection of osteolytic breast cancer metastases. Increased FDG uptake may reflect hypoxia induced increased glycolysis in these aggressive and highly destructive lesions that may have an inadequate blood supply (61). In contrast, osteoblastic metastases show lower FDG uptake and are often undetectable by FDG PET (62). A similar observation has been made in patients with prostate cancer, which predominantly causes sclerotic metastases. A lower sensitivity of FDG PET has been reported for the detection of skeletal metastases compared with bone scan (63). The lower sensitivity of sclerotic metastases might be associated with a slower glycolytic tumor metabolism or lower volumes of viable tumor tissue in the lesions (64). In a study of osseous metastases from malignant primary bone tumors, FDG PET was less sensitive than bone scan in patients with osteosarcoma but was superior to bone scan in patients with Ewing's sarcoma (65).

Traditionally, whole-body bone scan is considered to be the imaging modality of choice in the initial survey for skeletal metastasis, because of its high sensitivity, low cost, availability, and capacity to evaluate the entire skeleton. BMS has a high sensitivity and provides additional information on the distribution of functional hematopoietic marrow but suffers from a lack of specificity. In contrast to bone scan or BMS, both FDG PET and MRI have the advantage of providing information on the primary tumor, lymph nodes, and distant metastases in a single study. FDG PET appears to be particularly useful when MRI cannot differentiate changes related to treatment from residual or recurrent tumor. The relative value of FDG PET or MRI in diagnosing osseous metastases has not yet been completely elucidated. Each modality provides unique information regarding anatomy and disease activity. Therefore, understanding the strengths and weaknesses of these imaging modalities is essential for the optimal evaluation of these challenging patients.

Hodgkin's Disease and Non-Hodgkin's Lymphoma

Malignant lymphoma is a heterogeneous group of diseases characterized by a malignant proliferation of cells of the lymphoid system. It includes two separate disorders, Hodgkin's disease (HD) and the more common non-Hodgkin's lymphoma (NHL). HD typically involves the lymph nodes of young adults. The disease usually spreads predictably from the affected lymph nodes to the next along the lymphatics. Bone marrow involvement by HD is rare at presentation and is seen in 5% to 32% of patients over the course of the illness. Marrow involvement at diagnosis is most common with a histologic pattern of lymphocyte depletion or mixed cell type. It can be focal, multifocal, or diffuse infiltration, and focal lesions are more likely to be seen in the bone marrow distant from the iliac crests (66). NHL is a heterogeneous group of malignancies that afflicts an older patient population and has a variety of clinical presentations and clinical outcomes. NHL commonly first involves lymph nodes or other lymphatic tissues. The histologic pattern of tumor cell growth may be either follicular (nodular) or diffusely infiltrative. The spread is unpredictable, and patients often present with widespread systemic disease. The frequency and pattern of bone marrow involvement is variable from focal to diffuse depending on the grade and cell type. It is found in about 50% to 80% of patients with low grade and 25% to 40% with high grade at diagnosis (67). Compared with low grade, high-grade NHL appears to be more often associated with focal marrow infiltration other than the iliac crest (68). The prognostic significance of marrow involvement appears to be less clear with stage III or IV NHL than with clinical stage I and II disease (66).

Detection of bone marrow infiltration is important for staging and treatment decision in lymphoma patients and it is also considered to have a prognostic value (69). Random bone marrow biopsy of the iliac crest is prone to sampling error, and a biopsy negative for tumor does not exclude tumor involvement especially with evidence for diseases on imaging studies (70). Therefore, whole-body imaging has been a useful adjunct to blind biopsy in the complete assessment of the bone marrow. Although bone scan has been used to evaluate bone involvement of malignant lymphoma, it has a limited value for the detection of bone marrow disease and is typically used to exclude osseous metastases in malignant disease (71) (Fig. 28.6). Using iliac crest biopsy as a gold standard, an inferior sensitivity of BMS using nanocolloid was shown compared with MRI in patients with HD or low-grade NHL (70). BMS with antigranulocyte monoclonal antibody improves the sensitivity and diagnostic accuracy of BMS for the assessment of bone marrow involvement (72). Using unifocal or multifocal defects as the scintigraphic criterion for bone marrow involvement, the findings on Tc-NSAb agreed with iliac or sternal marrow biopsy or aspiration cytology in 31 of the 36 patients with malignant lymphoma. The Tc-NSAb

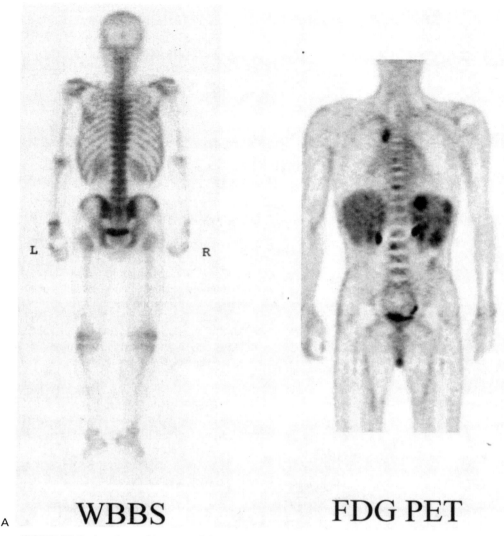

WBBS   FDG PET

A   B

FIGURE 28.6. A patient with non-Hodgkin's lymphoma, stage IV. **A:** Posterior whole-body view of the bone scan shows no definite evidence of abnormally increased bone uptake in the entire skeleton. **B:** Coronal view of the fluorodeoxyglucose positron emission tomography (FDG PET) shows increased uptake in the posterior mediastinum, spleen, and thoracic and lumbar spine. Bilateral iliac crest biopsies reveal lymphomatous involvement that is congruent with the FDG PET findings.

scans showed more widespread involvement of the skeletal system than bone scans (28). Diagnostic accuracy of BMS using ^{99m}Tc BW 250/183 and MRI was compared with that of iliac crest biopsy in 32 patients with malignant lymphoma (32). A low sensitivity of blind iliac crest biopsies to identify bone marrow infiltration in high-grade NHL and HD was shown in this study. Both imaging modalities showed a high rate of detection of bone marrow infiltration in patients with biopsies negative for tumor. The sensitivity of ^{99m}Tc BW 250/183 for the detection of lymphomatous marrow involvement was comparable to MRI.

MR findings of lymphomatous involvement of the skeleton are similar to those of other neoplastic metastases. One typically finds multiple foci of abnormally decreased SI on T1WI and increased SI on T2WI. Again, the high contrast provided by Short Tau Inversion Recovery (STIR) imaging can provide a clear-cut depiction of lymphomatous marrow involvement. Al-

though there have been a few reports in the literature of whole-body MRI for the detection of lymphomatous involvement of the bone marrow, the use of MR as a whole-body screening modality, as in the evaluation of osseous metastases, will have to await significant advances in magnet and receiver coil design. Similarly, some have investigated the use of magnetic resonance spectroscopy (MRS) to evaluate lymphomatous involvement in other parts of the body, primarily the brain, but these techniques have not been proven useful in studies with large patient populations nor are they widely available for routine clinical use (73).

FDG PET has been proposed as a new approach for the evaluation of bone marrow in lymphoma patients (69). The FDG PET and unilateral iliac crest biopsies were compared in 50 lymphoma patients and agreed in 39 patients; they were concordantly positive for tumor in 13 and concordantly negative for tumor in 26 patients (74). The study suggested a potential

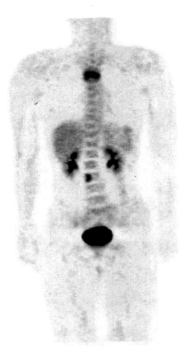

FIGURE 28.7. A 22-year-old patient with newly diagnosed Hodgkin's lymphoma and iliac crest bone marrow biopsy negative for tumor. Coronal view of the fluorodeoxyglucose positron emission tomography (FDG PET) demonstrates increased uptake in the T3 and L3 vertebrae that are proven to be lymphomatous involvement on the magnetic resonance images and follow-up FDG PET scan.

note for FDG PET to reduce the need for staging marrow biopsy. In a prospective study of 78 patients with untreated lymphoma, FDG PET provided additional information in patients with high-grade NHL and HD (69) (Fig 28.7). Complimentary results of both FDG PET and bone marrow biopsy were found in the group of patients with lower grade NHL. False-negative findings on FDG PET can occur in patients with a low density of marrow infiltration or involvement by some low-grade NHL with low or absent FDG uptake in their primary disease (69). Cytokine-induced diffusely increased bone marrow uptake on FDG PET can simulate generalized marrow metastasis or mask focal metastases in the marrow (75). Moreover, a recent report suggested less promising results regarding the role of FDG PET in lymphoma patients (76). FDG PET showed a higher overall negative predictive value than a positive predictive value (83.8% vs. 66.6%) in the detection of bone marrow involvement. At present, the role of FDG PET is controversial and must be further validated.

Bone marrow expansion is nonspecific and is observed in 33% to 81% of patients with malignant lymphoma (13). It appears difficult to differentiate marrow expansion resulting from benign causes from that resulting from malignant infiltration (70). Occasionally, central marrow depletion or even absent marrow radiocolloid uptake has been reported during the fulminant course of high-grade NHL (13).

Benign Marrow Replacement Disorders

Osteomyelitis

Osteomyelitis is a common clinical entity, with infection of the cortical bone and the bone marrow occurring through any of three routes: hematogenous spread; contiguous spread from adjacent source of infection, such as sinusitis or a cutaneous infection; and direct implantation, which may be iatrogenic or resulting from a penetrating injury. Patients of all ages are affected by osteomyelitis, and variation in the vascular anatomy of tubular bones with age results in characteristic patterns of infection in these bones. In infants and skeletally mature adults diaphyseal and metaphyseal vessels cross the growth plate allowing for spread of infection to the epiphysis. In contrast, vessels in children and adolescents do not cross the open growth plate, resulting in a metaphyseal predilection for hematogenously spread osteomyelitis in these patients.

As with other disorders of the bone marrow, conventional radiography of osteomyelitis is relatively insensitive for early detection of this disorder. It often takes several weeks, and a loss of 30% to 50% of bone density, before manifestations characteristic of osteomyelitis appear on plain films. Early findings are nonspecific and include soft tissue swelling, loss of fat planes, and joint effusions. Late findings include bone resorption, trabecular destruction, periostitis and ultimately involucrum, cloaca, and sequestrum formation.

Tc-NC and Tc-NSAb have been used for localization and assessment of disease activity in skeletal inflammatory disorders. The mechanisms include nanocolloid extravasation and conceivably phagocytosis by tissue macrophages or *in vivo* labeling of granulocytes infiltrating the inflammatory sites (77). It is worthwhile to note that subacute and chronic spondylitis, spondylodiscitis, and vertebral osteomyelitis usually cause clearly defined radiocolloid or Tc-NSAb marrow uptake defects in the corresponding vertebral bodies or the vertebrae adjacent to the inflamed intervertebral disc (78).

In the peripheral skeleton devoid of hematopoietic bone marrow, active osteomyelitis has been detected with a sensitivity of 80% to 90%, using Tc-NC or Tc-NSAb (78). Bone marrow expansion and/or defects have been observed with radiocolloid scintigraphy in 75% of patients with acquired immune deficiency syndrome (AIDS) (79). In a small series of patients, BMS using Tc-NSAb has been found to have a sensitivity of 95% and a specificity of 85% for detecting acute soft tissue inflammations and osteomyelitis of the appendicular skeleton (80).

Combined WBC/Tc-SC imaging has been successfully used by a number of investigators for diagnosing musculoskeletal infection in patients with marrow altering conditions (81). This technique appears to overcome certain inherent limitations of labeled WBC imaging alone. A potential limitation is the inability of this technique to consistently discriminate labeled WBC uptake in infection from normal uptake in normal bone marrow or macrophages at the site. This limitation may be further complicated by the heterogeneous distribution of bone marrow, a variability that may be exaggerated by certain underlying conditions. Several pathologic processes such as tumor, radiation therapy, trauma, Paget's disease, sickle cell disease, Gaucher's disease, and orthopedic implants can also produce alterations in the pattern of marrow activity on WBC images (81). Combined WBC and marrow imaging makes use of the fact that the skeletal activity normally present on both labeled WBC and Tc-SC images reflects radiotracer uptake by marrow or infiltrating cell with RES activity (Fig. 28.8). Conditions other than infection produce similar patterns of uptake on both studies (congruent

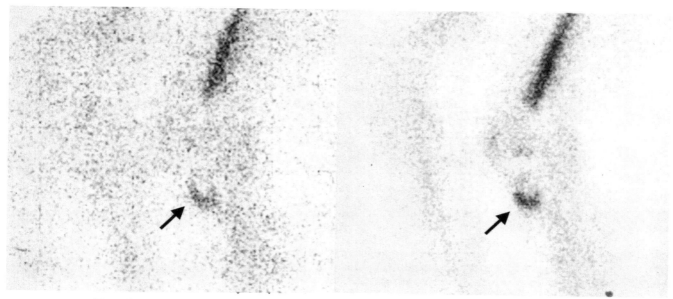

In-111 WBC

Tc-99m sulfur colloid

FIGURE 28.8. Scan after left knee prosthesis. There is congruent, focal increased activity on ^{111}In white blood cells and ^{99m}Tc-sulfur colloid images in the vicinity of the left knee prosthesis indicating active marrow in this region rather than infection.

images). Infection, however, results in opposite findings on these two radiotracers. While stimulating uptake of labeled leukocytes, infections can decrease the uptake of Tc-SC (82). The net result of these opposite effects is an incongruent WBC and marrow image (Fig. 28.9).

Several investigators have used Tc-NC for direct localization and assessment of activity in skeletal inflammatory diseases. Because the proposed mechanism of nanocolloid activity at sites of infection is a leak into the extravascular space, Tc-SC may

theoretically be superior to Tc-NC when combined WBC and marrow imaging is used. Large-sized particles are less likely to extravasate. Further studies may be necessary to clarify these issues.

Numerous studies have demonstrated the utility of MR imaging in the diagnosis and characterization of osteomyelitis, with sensitivities and specificities as high as 88% and 93%, respectively (83). As with other marrow replacement disorders, the edema and inflammatory cell infiltrate of osteomyelitis produce

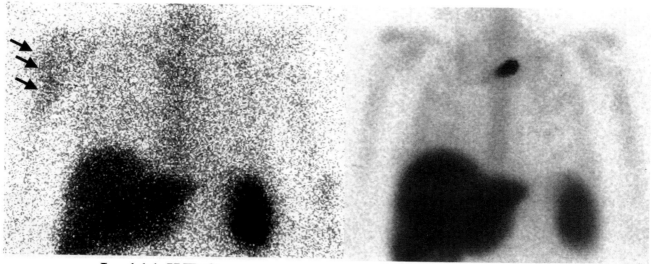

In-111 WBC

Tc-99m sulfur colloid

FIGURE 28.9. There is increased In-white blood cell activity (*arrows*) around the right shoulder prosthesis, which is unmatched on the Tc-sulfur colloid marrow scan indicating infection.

areas of decreased SI on T1WI and increased SI on T2-weighted and STIR imaging. In fact, some authors have noted that high sensitivity of STIR imaging tends to overestimate the extent of infection and that fat-suppressed contrast-enhanced MR images provide a more accurate assessment of the areas involved (84). MRI is also very sensitive in the detection of other signs of osteomyelitis, including cellulitis, sinus tracts, and soft tissue and intraosseous abscesses. MR may also detect chronic changes including involucrum, sequestrum, and cloaca formation, although these are usually better depicted by computed tomography (CT).

Gaucher's Disease

Gaucher's disease is a rare autosomal recessive lyosomal storage disorder resulting from deficiency of β-glucocerebrosidase leading to accumulation of glucosylceramide within histiocytes, so-called Gaucher cells, and in the RES. The disease typically involves the liver, spleen, bone marrow, and lymph nodes of Ashkenazi Jews. In the bone marrow, there is resultant necrosis, fibrosis, and remodeling causing the classic "Erlenmeyer flask" deformity of the distal femoral metaphyses. BMS may be used to evaluate the extent of marrow involvement and to follow the response to therapy. On MRI one again finds patchy, heterogeneously decreased SI on T1WI but also on T2WI and STIR images resulting from T2-shortening effects of the deposited glucosylceramide. MR is also useful for demonstrating areas of marrow infarction, which these patients are prone to develop in the acute and subacute phases of disease. The marrow infarction may appear as areas of well-demarcated low SI on T1WI with increased intensity on T2W and STIR sequences because of resultant edema. With time, these areas are replaced with fibrosis, which are of low SI on T1W, T2W, and STIR images.

Malignant Myeloproliferative Disorders

Myeloproliferative diseases are a family of disorders characterized by increased and ineffective hematopoietic cell proliferation in a clonal manner (85). The bone marrow displays varying degrees of hyperplasia, dysplasia, and fibrosis (44). Accordingly, in the early stages of these disorders it may be difficult to detect significant changes on BMS with either RE or hematopoietic agents and MR images. As the axial skeletal marrow begins to fail, peripheral expansion of marrow is noted with time on the BMS (Fig. 28.10). Finally, with the failure of the expanded peripheral marrow, splenic uptake of ^{52}Fe becomes apparent (Fig. 28.11). Lack of correlation between the presence and the degree of splenomegaly and the ^{52}Fe uptake suggests that splenomegaly precedes splenic erythropoiesis by a long time interval. Hepatic uptake of ^{52}Fe is nonspecific and is observed when there is complete hematopoietic failure (aplastic anemia) or when iron stores are saturated (e.g., following repeated blood transfusions). On MRI, there is apparent expansion or an abnormal distribution of the red marrow with diffuse or focal areas of decreased SI on T1WI. On occasion, there is sufficient replacement of fat cells to produce areas of decreased SI on T1WI that are lower than muscle or intervertebral disc, such that the disorder can be diagnosed without relying on abnormalities in red and yellow marrow distribution.

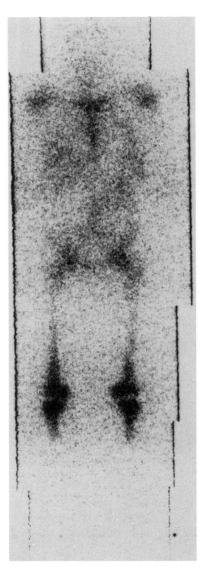

FIGURE 28.10. Polycythemia vera with peripheral marrow expansion. In this patient with a long history of polycythemia vera striking marrow activity is seen in the knee area indicating bone marrow expansion. Central marrow uptake of ^{52}Fe is somewhat reduced and some splenic activity is noted. (From Fordham E, Amjal A. Radionuclide imaging of bone marrow. *Semin Hematol* 1981;18:222–239, with permission.)

Multiple Myeloma

Multiple myeloma is the most common primary osseous malignancy in adults and is characterized by a monoclonal proliferation of plasma cells. Although multiple myeloma may be diagnosed by detecting large amounts of monoclonal immunoglobulins in the serum or urine, these are not universally present. Conventional radiographs may demonstrate lytic lesions and may be used for staging myeloma but are notoriously insensitive. Most investigators have found peripheral expansion on radiocolloid marrow scans (14). Focal defects in the axial skeleton have been observed in 40% to 50% of these patients (47). In a series of 10 patients with multiple myeloma, homogeneous peripheral expansion was seen in 8 patients, and expansion with focal marrow defects was

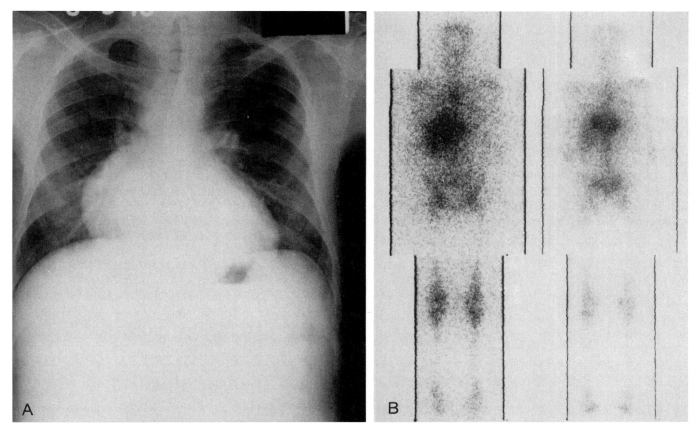

FIGURE 28.11. Intrathoracic extramedullary hematopoiesis. Chest x-ray film of this patient with long-standing thalassemia shows a large posterior mediastinal mass as a retrocardiac double destiny **A:** ^{52}Fe images show marked peripheral marrow expansion with normal central pattern. Intense concentration of this tracer in the posterior mediastinal mass is consistent with the diagnosis of extramedullary hematopoiesis **(B).** (From Fordham E, Amjal A. Radionuclide imaging of bone marrow. *Semin Hematol* 1981;18: 222–239, with permission.)

seen in the other two patients (86). Bone marrow expansion has also been observed on Tc-NSAb scans in 6 of 10 patients, whereas focal defects were found in 60% (87). BMS revealed significantly more extensive skeletal involvement when compared with bone scan (19.7% vs. 4.7%, $p < 0.001$). It has been reported that radiocolloid marrow scans may demonstrate cold lesions that precede radiographically observable lytic lesions by several months (47). However, no systematic studies to examine the temporal relation between marrow scans and radiographic findings have been performed. Focal defects on BMS are nonspecific. Although bone marrow expansion may be secondary to involvement of the central marrow by multiple myeloma, it may be seen as a purely "reactive expansion" that is often seen in nonmalignant diseases (1). The MRI appearance of multiple myeloma is nonspecific. As with many other marrow disorders, one typically finds decreased SI on T1WI and increased SI on T2WI and STIR imaging. However, myeloma patients can display a number of different patterns of distribution of these lesions. Many patients with biopsy proven myeloma have a normal marrow appearance. Some patients with early disease can display a so-called salt and pepper pattern with innumerable tiny foci of abnormal signal distributed diffusely throughout the marrow. Other patients, usually with more advanced disease, may demonstrate a multifocal distribution of areas

of decreased SI on T1WI and increased SI on T2WI. Finally, patients with very advanced disease can show diffuse infiltration with a SI that is homogeneously decreased on T1WI and homogeneously increased on T2WI. Interestingly, these patterns of marrow involvement do not appear to correlate with the interstitial, nodular, and diffuse patterns of marrow involvement noted on microscopic evaluation of the marrow.

Leukemia

Highly variable patterns on BMS are observed in leukemia, especially in acute forms of the disease (1). Normal scan can be seen early in disease or with mild involvement of disease. Occasionally, diffusely decreased radiocolloid marrow uptake and focal defects have been noted in acute and chronic myelogenous or lymphocytic leukemia (28). A variable degree of peripheral bone marrow expansion can occur when the associated anemia causes sufficient hematopoietic stimulation (1). False-negative findings on radiocolloid BMS were often found in the early stages of chronic lymphocytic leukemia (70). In patients with chronic myeloid leukemia, progression to myelofibrosis may be documented by BMS (28). Prolonged blood clearance of ^{123}I-labeled

NSAb has been observed in one patient with acute myeloid leukemia (88). In myelogenous leukemia, BMS using Tc-NSAb should be interpreted with caution because the expression of target antigen on the neoplastic myeloid cells is variable (89). Findings of normal or even increased uptake can be seen in chronic myeloid leukemia patients. In contrast, markedly decreased uptake was found in acute lymphocytic leukemia patients because of the lack of antibody binding sites on the lymphoid cells. MRI findings in leukemia are again nonspecific and are identical to metastatic involvement of the marrow. Leukemic infiltrates result in areas of decreased SI on T1WI and increased SI on T2WI. Fat suppressed Fast Spin Echo (FSE) and STIR imaging are often useful in discriminating leukemic foci, because of their higher SI on these sequences compared with normal hematopoietic marrow.

Benign Myeloproliferative Diseases

Myelodysplastic Syndrome

Myelodysplastic syndrome (MDS) is characterized by ineffective hematopoiesis or increased Intramedullary destruction of mature hematopoietic cells (44). Peripheral blood analysis shows normocytic anemia often associated with neutropenia, thrombocytopenia, and/or monocytosis. On BMS using TC-NSAb, findings of generalized, small defects or heterogeneous uptake with areas of decreased and increased uptake have been seen (28). Focal accumulation of blasts to which the antibody does not bind might be the cause of the small focal defects in the bone marrow.

Polycythemia Vera

Polycythemia vera is a neoplastic stem cell disorder associated with excessive proliferation of erythroid, and to a lesser degree, granulocytic and megakaryocytic precursors (85). In the early stages of polycythemia vera, the findings on BMS may be normal or show only minimal peripheral expansion. About 20% of cases ultimately progress to a "spent" phase with poor prognosis, characterized by progressive anemia, marrow fibrosis, and splenomegaly (44). With progression to myelofibrosis and myeloid metaplasia, peripheral expansion of bone marrow on BMS has been shown on ^{52}Fe PET (32), radiocolloids (1), and Tc-NSAb (28) (Fig. 28.10). Tc-NSAb uptake in the spleen can be moderately increased, probably related to myeloid metaplasia of the red pulp (neoplastic extramedullary hematopoiesis) (44). At this stage, the findings of marrow depletion and extramedullary hematopoiesis are similar to that of osteomyelofibrosis (28). However, systematic follow-up BMS studies in polycythemia vera to demonstrate its natural course have not been reported. In contrast, it was reported that the scan findings are normal in stress erythrocytosis (90).

Idiopathic Myelofibrosis

Idiopathic myelofibrosis is a chronic and progressive clonal hematopoietic disorder in which bone marrow fibrosis and extramedullary hematopoiesis are the typical findings (85). It prefer-

entially involves the central flat bones and proximal long bones and often causes osteosclerosis, or the thickening of bony trabeculae (44). Splenomegaly is present in all patients and may be massive in some patients. Hepatomegaly is seen in about 50% to 75% of patients but is not observed without splenomegaly. On radiocolloid BMS, normal patterns can be seen in the early stages of the disease and deficient marrow uptake is noted in advanced cases (28). The findings of massive splenomegaly, moderate hepatomegaly, and peripheral bone marrow expansion are usually observed (1). BMS using Tc-NSAb has shown decreased or, in advanced stages, even deficient central activity with marked peripheral expansion and massively increased uptake in the spleen, perhaps related to extramedullary hematopoiesis (28). In a validation study of Tc-NSAb against ^{52}Fe, Tc-NSAb was well correlated with ^{52}Fe in the evaluation of the hematopoietic bone marrow with some limitations (91). The extent of extramedullary hematopoiesis in the spleen could be difficult to define on Tc-NSAb scan. Normal colloid or ^{111}In scans despite mild to severe disease has also been reported (1). Therefore, ^{52}Fe scans or ferrokinetic studies might be required to accurately evaluate the severity of disease in the bone marrow and extramedullary hematopoiesis in specific situations. Bone scans may show a superscan pattern with diffusely increased skeletal uptake probably as a response to osteosclerosis.

Extramedullary Hematopoiesis

In patients with mass lesions in whom extramedullary hematopoiesis is considered, BMS with ^{52}Fe may obviate the need for surgical biopsy. Intense uptake of this agent indicates the presence of active red cell production at the abnormal site (Fig. 28.11). Patients with hypersplenism who are considered for splenectomy may benefit from BMS with ^{52}Fe. Scintigraphy may allow the presence and the degree of erythropoiesis to be determined before surgical intervention. In patients with considerable marrow activity in the spleen and clinically tolerable hypersplenism, splenectomy may produce deleterious effects.

Marrow Depletion

Aplastic Anemia

Aplastic anemia is characterized by marked hypocellularity of bone marrow and pancytopenia. Hypocellular bone marrow usually reveals homogeneously reduced or absent uptake on BMS using any marrow agents (1). Heterogeneous, patchy uptake of Tc-NSAb or ^{111}In can be seen during or after treatment suggesting marrow regeneration and residual marrow damage (92). Discrepancy between the RE or granulopoietic and erythropoietic agents is often seen, most consistently in aplastic anemia patients (93). Despite the lack of erythropoietic activity, considerable RE is seen on BMS in some patients with aplastic or hypoplastic anemia (5) (Fig. 28.12). In such patients, because of the systemic nature of the disorder, no extramedullary hematopoiesis is noted in any organ (28). With recovery, BMS may show normal uptake pattern several months earlier than that seen on bone marrow sampling or on peripheral blood counts (1). Therefore, BMS may be useful in detecting early changes in bone marrow function following treatment or spontaneous recovery.

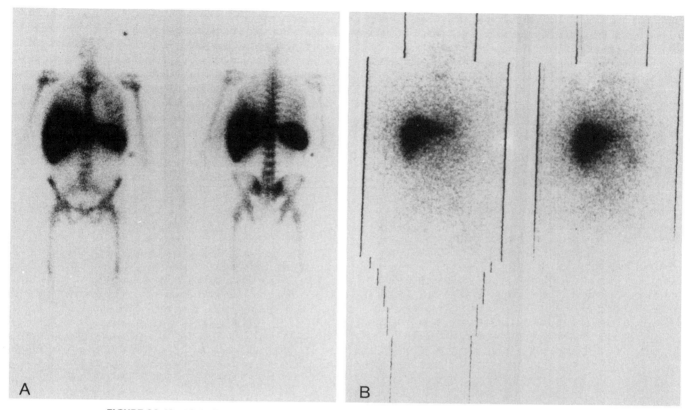

FIGURE 28.12. Dissimilar reticuloendothelial (RE) and erythropoietic marrow distribution. In this patient with hypoplastic marrow (proven on histologic marrow examination), RE images show significant marrow activity in the spine, ribs, pelvis, and both upper and lower extremities **(A)**. ^{52}Fe scintigrams reveal no central or peripheral marrow activities. The hepatic uptake of ^{52}Fe does not imply erythropoiesis in that organ **(B)**. (From Fordham E, Amjal A. Radionuclide imaging of bone marrow. *Semin Hematol* 1981; 18:222–239, with permission.)

Marrow Depletion Resulting from Chemotherapy or Radiation Therapy

Hypermetabolic bone marrow and/or extramedullary hematopoiesis resulting from cytokine therapy has been reported with ^{201}Tl-chloride, ^{99m}Tc-methylene diphosphonate (MDP), ^{99m}Tc-SC, ^{67}Ga-citrate, and FDG PET scan imaging (94). Cytokine-induced diffusely increased bone marrow uptake on FDG PET can simulate generalized marrow metastasis. The timing of the FDG PET study relative to cytokine therapy is an important clue for the differentiation of the two conditions. In case of hypermetabolic marrow, there is a rapid decrease of bone marrow metabolic rates 3 to 5 days after discontinuation of cytokine, although it can be higher than the baseline level for up to 4 weeks (75). It is also conceivable that the increased background FDG uptake in the bone marrow by cytokine therapy makes it difficult to assess focal marrow metastasis and its response to treatment. It has been suggested that FDG PET be delayed for 5 days after the completion of cytokine therapy so that FDG uptake in the bone marrow declines almost to the baseline level (75). Clearly defined tracer uptake defects with sharp borders in hematopoietic bone marrow are found at the radiation ports after irradiation (95). Decreased marrow activity secondary to radiation therapy can be readily identified on either RE or hematopoietic scans. Marrow regeneration may be noted within a few months after the radiation exposure with normal marrow distribution seen as early as 1 year (19). In one study, significant dissociation was noted between the RE and hematopoietic distribution in the irradiated area (5). This discrepancy was not observed in another study (19).

Vascular Abnormalities of Bone Marrow Avascular Necrosis of the Hip

Avascular necrosis (AVN) or osteonecrosis (ON) is a disease affecting patients of all ages, usually related to trauma but also associated with hemoglobinopathies, steroid use and hypercortisolism, alcoholism, pancreatitis, Gaucher's disease, and obesity. The femoral head is the most common site of involvement. BMS has been used to detect AVN because the bone marrow cells first die after a vascular insult to the bone (1). However, the detection of infarct in the femoral heads can be difficult in patients without hematologic disorders who do not have peripheral marrow expansion (96). In addition, absent radiocolloid uptake in the femoral heads has been observed in 45% of adults and makes this technique unreliable for detection of infarct (97). Both MRI and bone SPECT are known to be extremely sensitive for the diagnosis of AVN of the femoral head, 85% to 100% sensitivity with MRI and 85% to 97% sensitivity with bone SPECT (98). On bone scan, a photopenic defect is the earliest sign of AVN after the initial vascular event, followed by increased uptake resulting from reparatory process around the infarct process over a period of weeks to months.

MR has been shown to be more specific than bone scintigraphy in the diagnosis of ON (99,100). Furthermore, MR allows the detection and characterization of joint effusions, marrow edema or conversion, cartilage destruction, and other structural

alterations. Thus, MR has become the modality of choice for imaging this disorder. A staging system for AVN that relies on clinical symptomatology and radiographic findings has been developed by Ficat and Arlet (101). Stage 0 disease is characterized by normal radiographs and no clinical findings; it represents disease incidentally noted on MR or biopsy. In Stage I disease, patients are symptomatic but radiographs remain unremarkable. In Stage II disease, one finds subchondral sclerosis and osteopenia, but the femoral head retains its normal rounded contour. Late in this stage, one may find a "crescent sign," which refers to a crescentic area of lucency just under the articular surface that signals impending articular collapse. Articular collapse with flattening of the femoral head is characteristic of Stage III disease. As degenerative changes develop because of the altered mechan-

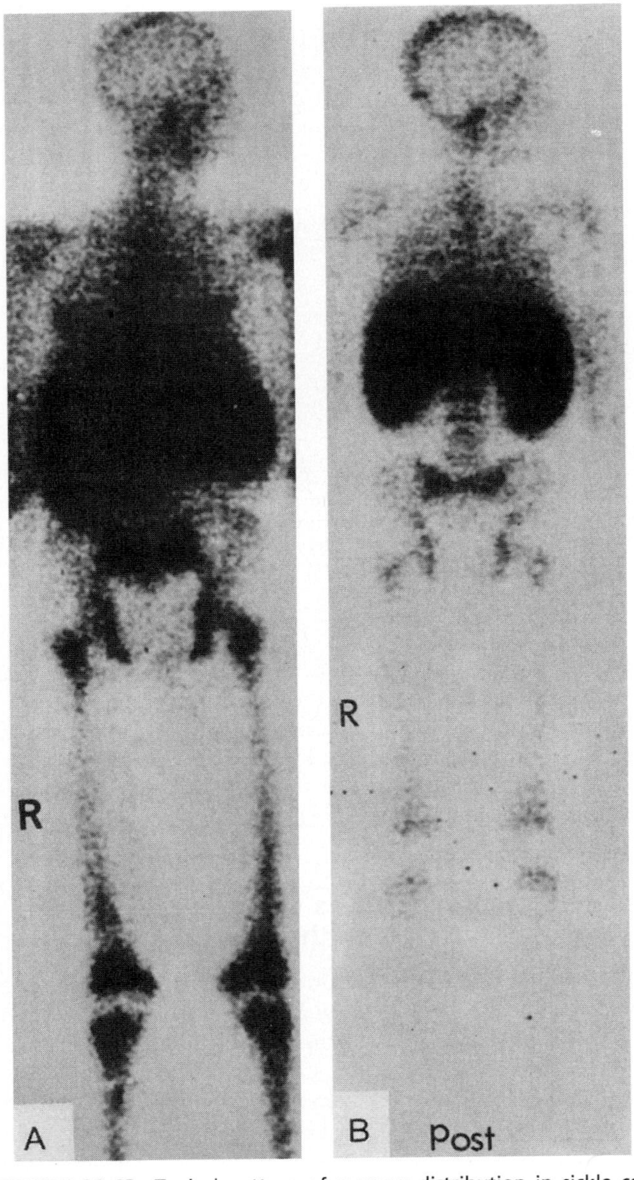

FIGURE 28.13. Typical pattern of marrow distribution in sickle cell anemia and sickle thalassemia. **A:** Bone marrow scan of a patient with sickle cell anemia reveals expansion of the marrow to the skull and long bones. This expansion is symmetric in the long bones. **B:** Bone marrow scan in sickle thalassemia shows less expansion of the marrow to the extremities. The spleen is moderately enlarged. (From Alavi A, Bond JP, Kuhl DE et al. Scan detection of bone marrow infarct in sickle cell disorders. *J Nucl Med* 1974;15:1003–1007, with permission.)

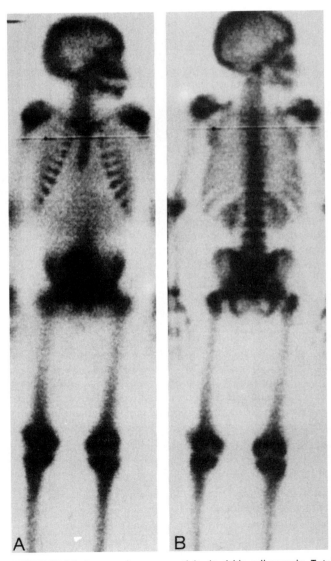

FIGURE 12.14. Increased osseous activity in sickle cell anemia. Total body bone scans of a patient with sickle cell anemia reveal extensive uptake of the bone-seeking agent throughout the skeleton. This is especially apparent in the lower extremities. This intense activity very likely represents increased blood flow to the skeleton because of the significantly expanded marrow in these patients.

ics, the AVN is categorized as stage IV. On MR, early infarcts appear as a rim of low SI on T1WI and are felt to represent repair at the infarct periphery. In 65% to 80% of cases, a "double line" sign will be present, consisting of outer low and inner high linear SI on T2WI. Mitchell et al. (102–105) have proposed a staging system based on the MR signal characteristics of the lesion. In this scheme, Stage A lesions display high SI on T1WI and low SI on T2SI, which corresponds to the signal characteristics of fat. In Stage B disease, one notes high SI on both T1WI and T2WI, corresponding to subacute blood. Stage C disease is typified by lesions with signal characteristics of edema, that is, low SI on T1WI and high SI on T2WI. Finally, stage D lesions have the appearance of bony fibrosis with low SI on both T1- and T2-weighted pulse sequences.

Hemolytic Disorders

BMS is usually normal without peripheral expansion in acute hemolytic disorders. Peripheral expansion occurs in chronic hemolytic anemias such as sickle cell disease and hereditary spherocytosis (1). In patients with hereditary spherocytosis, extramedullary hematopoiesis has been detected with ^{52}Fe PET and ^{111}In-chloride (106).

Sickle Cell Disease

Bone and joint complaints are common among patients with several types of sickle cell hemoglobinopathies. Usually they are transient, occur with a crisis, and resolve rapidly, producing no x-ray changes. These symptoms are often due to bone marrow infarction with or without secondary involvement of the bone structures. Typical AVN or bone infarction occurs almost invariably in fatty marrow. Sickle cell anemia is unusual in that marrow infarction occurs in areas of active hematopoiesis (107). The slow sinusoidal circulation in hematopoietic marrow provides an ideal environment for marrow ischemia and infarction in patients with sickle cell disorder. The diagnosis of marrow infarction remains difficult because of the lack of specific clinical signs or chemical parameters (108). At present, BMS would be the most sensitive and cost effective for early detection and evaluation of the extent of damage to the bone marrow. These tests appear to provide a specific pattern in patients with infarcts and help in the differential diagnosis of bone and joint complaints in patients with sickle cell disorders. When acute symptoms are present, scintigraphic studies should be more revealing than conventional radiographic examination.

In patients with hemolytic anemia, the marrow is expanded symmetrically and uniformly throughout the axial skeleton and extremities (Fig. 28.13A). It is more extensive in patients with sickle cell anemia (Hb S/S) than in those with S/C hemoglobin disease (Hb S/C) or sickle thalassemia (Hb S-Thal) (Fig. 28.13B). When BMS are obtained in patients with Hb S/S, the long bones are clearly outlined in their entirety. A distinct triangular pattern of increased marrow activity can be identified in the distal femora, proximal tibiae, and distal tibiae. Histologic examination of marrow indicates that the expansion involves all three elements (erythrocytic, granulocytic, and megakaryocytic); however, the red cell precursors predominate. In sickle cell pa-

tients, bone scan may show generally increased uptake in the skeleton, especially in the lower extremities (Fig 28.14). This is most likely due to increased blood flow to both bone and bone marrow caused by significant bone marrow expansion.

BMS is specifically useful in monitoring the course of events during and after sickle cell crises. Immediately after a painful crisis with skeletal involvement, areas of marrow infarct appear devoid of activity surrounded by active marrow (Fig. 28.15). The site of the infarct seen on the BMS usually corresponds to the region of tenderness. There may be slight swelling and warmth over the area of infarction as well. The extent of involvement is best seen in the first week after an occlusive crisis. Marrow infarct has been seen most often in the lower extremities; followed by the upper extremities; and, less often, the axial skeleton. A focal or extensive area of infarct can occur in any part

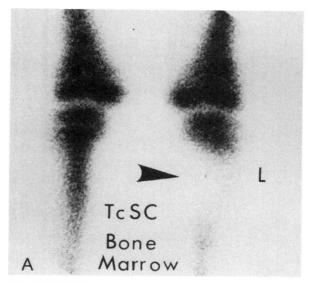

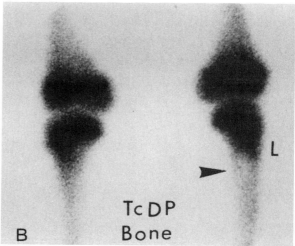

FIGURE 28.15. Active marrow and bone infarcts of the tibia. This 8-year-old patient with sickle cell anemia complained of pain in an area below the knee. **A:** The marrow scans performed 4 days after the onset of symptoms shows a larger and more distinct defect in the same location. This combination is diagnostic of an infarct. **B:** The bone scan obtained 1 day following the onset of pain revealed a subtle negative defect in the upper tibia.

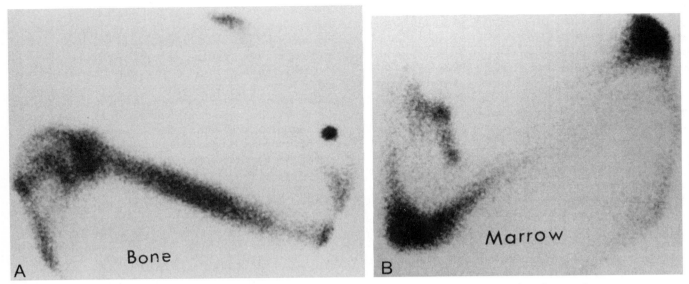

FIGURE 28.16. Subacute bone and marrow infarcts. This patient was seen because of persistent pain in the right arm for more than 2 weeks. **A:** The bone scan shows the diffuse uptake of the bone-seeking agent in the humerus. **B:** The marrow scan demonstrates decreased marrow activity in most of the humerus corresponding to the bone abnormality. This combination is consistent with infarct older than a few days, although long-standing osteomyelitis with extension to the bone can cause similar findings.

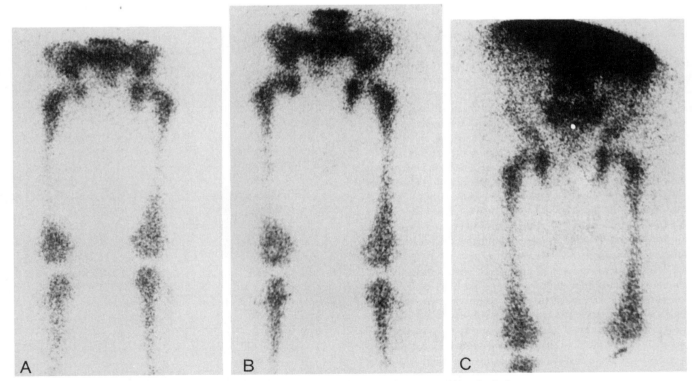

FIGURE 28.17. Marrow regeneration following infarction. This 2-year-old boy had a bone marrow scan because of bone pain. Several abnormalities are found including a defect in the left femur and left ischium **(A)**. Repeat scans after 2 weeks **(B)** and 6.5 months **(C)** show the gradual repopulation of these areas.

of a long bone. Generally, not more than a few separate areas are involved; however, extensive infarcts involving multiple sites can also occur (109). Demonstration of infarcts in the midportion of the spine, lower ribs, and lower sternum is impossible using radiocolloid scans because of intense tracer uptake in the liver and spleen (110). This limitation can be overcome by using Tc-NSAb (35). Initially, bone scans either appear normal or show decreased activity in the area of the infarct (a negative defect) (100) (Fig. 28.15). The extent of the infarct on bone scan is less impressive than that on BMS. Because of the collaterals between the nutrient and periosteal arteries, the damage in the bone is usually less than that in the bone marrow. Bone scans after 10 to 14 days show a rim of increased activity around the area of infarct resulting from reactive bone formation (Fig. 28.16). As reactive bone formation continues, several weeks later the area of infarct shows an abnormal density on x-ray film. The area of abnormality may then stay positive for increased activity on the bone scan for several months, whereas radiographic change can be permanent. Follow-up BMS in asymptomatic patients with old marrow infarcts may show normalization of the defects, indicating repopulation of active bone marrow (110). Younger patients appear to repopulate their infarcted marrow more often than older subjects (Fig. 28.17). Marrow fibrosis after infarcts is more commonly seen in adult patients (111). Fifty percent of the patients studied with BMS in the asymptomatic state showed areas of decreased activity that very likely represent fibrosis resulting from previous infarct (109).

Necrotic tissue in the marrow may serve as a nidus for infection and subsequent osteomyelitis. BMS in conjunction with bone and/or gallium scan has been useful to differentiate infarct from osteomyelitis in sickle cell patients (112). Concordant negative defects on both marrow and bone scans appear to be a useful indicator of marrow infarcts. When the BMS reveals a large photopenic defect and the uptake on the bone scan is normal or mildly decreased, infarct is a very likely diagnosis regardless of the duration of the symptoms. Increased uptake on a bone scan up to 3 days from the onset of symptom is indicative of an infection causing hyperemia in the bones or joints, especially in the presence of either a normal or minimally abnormal BMS. A marrow defect by infection is appreciated only when the disease is relatively advanced. Increased uptake on a bone scan after 4 or more days from the onset of symptoms, however, does not reliably separate osteomyelitis from infarct (113). When differentiation of osteomyelitis from infarct is of clinical concern, bone scan should be performed as soon as possible, preferably within 72 hours of the onset of pain (113). It has been reported that in most patients with infarcts, the affected sites do not show increased gallium uptake compared with marrow activity (112). This observation may suggest that a gallium scan could be more useful than a bone scan after several days from the onset of symptoms. However, it should be noted that, in the series reported, only four patients with infarction were imaged 7 or more days after the onset of symptoms (16 days being the maximum time interval). Combined WBC and marrow imaging has been used for the same purpose and has been found to be useful (114).

The incidence of AVN of the femoral head is low in younger children. In adolescent and adult patients with sickle cell anemia,

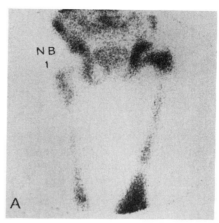

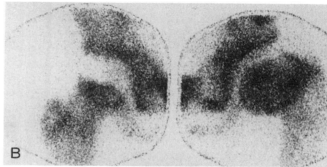

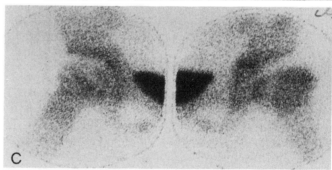

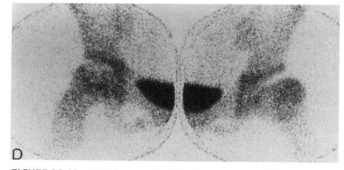

FIGURE 28.18. Aseptic necrosis of the femoral head with subsequent repair. This is an example of avascular necrosis of the femoral head in an 8-year-old girl with sickle cell anemia. **A:** The marrow scan was performed because of right hip pain. It shows the right femoral head and neck to be devoid of activity. **B:** A bone scan performed 2 weeks later confirmed the vascular necrosis of right femoral head. Note that the involvement is less extensive than indicated by the marrow scan. The changes in the left femoral head are due to a previous osteotomy following avascular necrosis on that side. Repeat bone scans show the gradual return of activity to the right femoral head 2 months **(C)** and 7 months **(D)** later.

AVN of the femoral head is the most disabling of bone lesions. Therefore, early diagnosis is of great importance in the management of the patients. BMS may not be useful to detect early AVN in patients with absent or minimal bone marrow in the femoral heads (in patients with normal hematologic states). However, in sickle cell patients, BMS may give the first evidence of AVN in the head of the femur (Fig. 28.18), humerus, or the knee (115). Reactive bone formation occurs around the necrotic marrow and bone very soon after the onset of the infarct (116). Based on this pathologic finding, bone scan has been used to detect early AVN. Both bone and bone marrow scans are very efficient in early detection of AVN in patients with sickle cell anemia (100). X-ray film may not show any abnormality early after the onset of AVN. Later, however, changes consistent with AVN will appear along with subsequent bony destruction.

Combined bone and marrow scans are helpful in differentiating arthropathies other than those related to vasoocclusive crises (115). Patients with septic arthritis, synovitis, and a variety of arthritides with no osseous destruction have a normal marrow scan and the bone scan shows diffuse increased activity on both sides of the joint space, indicating only hyperemia. In patients with a fracture or extraosseous causes of joint involvement, the marrow scan appears normal and can rule out infarct as a contributing factor. An old infarct can cause bony sclerosis adjacent to the sacroiliac joint and x-ray film may erroneously suggest ankylosing spondylitis. A negative defect on BMS may suggest an old infarct with subsequent fibrosis, and the bone scan will appear within normal limits (117). Noninflammatory joint effusions often occur during painful crises. Microvascular thrombi are thought to be the cause of effusions by synovial biopsies (118). When BMS was done, evidence of marrow infarct adjacent to the involved joints was found (115). Excellent correlation between the effused joints and the scan findings of marrow infarct suggested that these joint effusions may be due to marrow infarct in the adjacent bone.

The liver and spleen can be evaluated as part of BMS in patients with sickle cell disorders. The liver appears larger than normal, and the spleen may appear devoid of activity, indicating functional asplenia (119) (Fig. 28.19A). In patients with Hb S/C or Hb S-Thal, the spleen may appear larger than normal. Of interest is the uptake of the bone-seeking agent in the area of the spleen in patients with functional asplenia. This finding may reflect calcification in the spleen (Fig. 28.19**B**).

Infarct involving the yellow marrow results in loss of signal from the tissue on MRI and, therefore, is readily seen as decreased intensity on T1WI. In hematopoietic marrow, infarcts are isointense or minimally hyperintense on T1WI. These findings are difficult to detect on T1WI. On T2WI, the infarcts show very high signal. However, the time required for signal alteration in acute infarct can take several days. Acute osteomyelitis results in infiltration of normal marrow by inflammatory cells. As a result of increased cellularity and water content, the infected region is manifested as an ill-defined area of decreased SI on T1WI and increased SI on T2WI. The areas of involvement in chronic osteomyelitis are better demarcated (120).

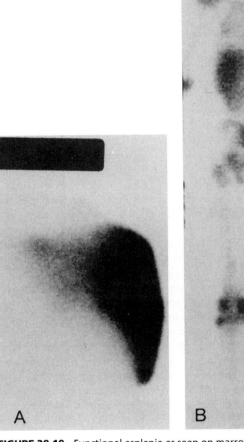

FIGURE 28.19. Functional asplenia as seen on marrow and bone scan. **A:** A liver-spleen scan of a patient with sickle cell anemia hemoglobinopathy shows function asplenia. **B:** A bone scan performed a few days earlier reveals significant deposition of the bone-seeking agent in an area corresponding to the location of the spleen. This combination (functional asplenia with the uptake bone agent) was commonly noted in our patient population.

SUMMARY

Bone marrow imaging has played a limited role in the day-to-day practice of nuclear medicine over the past 3 decades. This is mainly due to the lack of an optimal agent that addresses important clinical questions. In many of the hematologic disorders in which the state of the marrow function is of importance for appropriate management decisions, BMS is of limited value. BMS is of interest in the evaluation of patients with cancer and infection in which bone marrow abnormalities are focal in nature and can be detected by scintigraphic techniques. The role of BMS techniques that visualize these abnormalities as negative defects is limited in such circumstances and, therefore, is of minimal value. FDG PET and MRI are the two emerging techniques that may become the two modalities of choice for this purpose. Particularly, FDG PET, because of its ability to image the entire body to determine the state of disease activity, has the promise of becoming an important examination of the bone marrow in a variety of disorders including cancer and infection.

REFERENCES

1. Datz F, Taylor AJ. The clinical use of radionuclide bone marrow imaging. *Semin Nucl Med* 1985;15:239–259.
2. Engstedt L et al. In vivo localization of colloidal Au198 intravenously injected in polycythemia vera. *Acta Radiol* 1958;49:66–71.
3. Aburano T et al. 99mTc HMPAO-labeled leukocytes for hematopoietic marrow imaging. Comparison with 111In chloride. *Clin Nucl Med* 1992;17:938–944.
4. Greenberg M, Atkins H, Schiffer L. Erythropoietic and reticuloendothelial function in bone marrow in dogs. *Science* 1966;152:526–528.
5. Van Dyke D, Shkurkin C, Price D et al. Differences in distribution of erythropoietic and reticuloendothelial marrow in hematological disease. *Blood* 1967;30:364–374.
6. Munz D, Sandrock D, Rilinger N. Comparison of immunoscintigraphy and colloid scintigraphy of bone marrow. *Lancet* 1990;336:258–259.
7. Kniseley R, Andrews G, Edwards C et al. Bone marrow and skeletal scanning. *Radiol Clin North Am* 1969;8:265–290.
8. Nelp W, Larson S, Lewis R. Distribution of erythron and the RES in the bone marrow organ. *J Nucl Med* 1967;8:430–436.
9. Desai A, Thakur M. Radiopharmaceuticals for spleen and bone marrow studies. *Semin Nucl Med* 1985;15:229–238.
10. Hotze A et al. Kombinierte Knochenmark- und Skelettszintigraphie bei ossaeren und myelogenen Erkrankungen. *Fortschr Roentgenstr* 1984;140:717.
11. Blend M, Pavel D. Bone marrow imaging: a comparison study using a 99Tcm-sulphur colloid versus a new 99Tcm-microaggregated albumin. *Nucl Med Commun* 1986;7:787–789.
12. Kalin B, Kimiaei S, Jacobsson H. A better target-to-background activity ratio using a large-sized colloid compared to a nano-sized colloid for scintigraphy of the peripheral bone marrow. A study in mice and humans. *Nucl Med Commun* 1993;14:219–224.
13. Munz D. Bone marrow imaging: basic concepts and clinical results. *Der Nuklearmed* 1984;4:251–268.
14. Hotze A, Mahlstedt F, Wolf F. *Bone marrow imaging. Techniques, findings, interpretation* Darmstadt: GIT Verlag Ernst Giebeler, 1984.
15. Lentle B et al. Detecting bone marrow metastases at the time of examining the liver with radiocolloid. *J Nucl Med* 1987;28:184–187.
16. Padhy A et al. Marrow uptake index (MUI): a quantitative scintigraphic study of bone marrow in aplastic anemia. *Thymus* 1987;10:137–146.
17. Ferrant A, Rodhain J, Leners N et al. Quantitative assessment of erythropoiesis in bone marrow expansion areas using 52Fe. *Br J Haematol* 1986;62:247–255.
18. Anger H, Van Dyke D. Human bone marrow distribution shown in vivo by iron-52 and the positron scintillation camera. *Science* 1964;144:1587–1589.
19. Fordham E, Ali A. Radionuclide imaging of bone marrow. *Semin Hematol* 1981;18:222–239.
20. Goodwin D, Goode R, Brown L et al. 111In-labeled transferrin for the detection of tumors. *Radiology* 1971;100:175–179.
21. Farrer P, Saha G, Katz M. Further observations of the use of 111In-transferrin for the visualization of bone marrow in man. *J Nucl Med* 1973;14:384–395.
22. Arrago J et al. Diagnostic value of BMS with 111indium-transferrin and 99m technetium-colloids in myelofibrosis. *Am J Hematol* 1985;18:275–282.
23. Beamish M, Brown E. The metabolism of transferrin bound 111In and Fe-59 in the rat. *Blood* 1974;43:693–701.
24. McNeil B, Holman B, Button L et al. Use of indium chloride scintigraphy in patients with myelofibrosis. *J Nucl Med* 1974;15:647–651.
25. Sayle B, Fawcett H, Gardner F. Indium-111 chloride bone marrow imaging in chronic renal disease. *Clin Nucl Med* 1985;10:498–500.
26. Chipping P, Klonizakis I, Lewis S. Indium chloride scanning: a comparison with iron as a tracer for erythropoiesis. *Clin Lab Haematol* 1980;2:255–263.
27. McNeil B, Rappaport J, Nathan D. Indium chloride scintigraphy: an index of severity in patients with aplastic anemia. *Br J Haematol* 1976;34:599–604.
28. Reske S. Recent advances in bone marrow scanning. *Eur J Nucl Med* 1991;18:203–221.
29. Reske S et al. 99mTc labelled NCA-95/CEA-antibodies (TcNCAA) for immunoscintigraphy of hematopoietic bone marrow in man. I. Antibody distribution in normal bone marrow. In Höfer A, Bergmann H, eds. *Radioactive isotope in Klinik und forschung.* Stuttgart: Schattauer, 1990.
30. Becker W, Borst U, Fischback W et al. Kinetic data on in-vivo labeled granulocytes in humans with a murine 99mTc labeled monoclonal antibody. *Eur J Nucl Med* 1989;15:361–366.
31. Mojiminiyi S, Shepstone B. Bone marrow immunoscintigraphy [Letter]. *Lancet* 1989;1:725–726.
32. Altehoefer C, Blum U, Bathmann J et al. Comparative diagnostic accuracy of magnetic resonance imaging and immunoscintigraphy for detection of bone marrow involvement in patients with malignant lymphoma. *J Clin Oncol* 1997;15:1754–1760.
33. Metz S, Kolthoff B, Siegel E et al. Multi-compartment model for the monoclonal 99mTc anti-granulocyte antibody BW 250/183. *Eur J Nucl Med* 1990;19:632.
34. Tavassoli M, Yoffey J. *Bone marrow. Structure and function.* New York: Alan Riss, 1983.
35. Reske S, Buell U. Reduced Technetium-99m labelled NCA-95/CEA-antibody uptake in the liver due to gentle antibody reconstitution. Technical note. *Eur J Nucl Med* 1990;17:38.
36. Steinstraesser A et al. A novel 99mTc labelled antibody for in vivo targeting of granulocytes. *J Nucl Med* 1988;29:925.
37. Axelsson B, Kalin B. Comparison of 111In granulocytes and 99mTc albumin colloid for bone marrow scintigraphy by the use of quantitative SPECT imaging. *Clin Nucl Med* 1990;15:473–479.
38. Kim C et al. Significance of diffusely decreased marrow uptake on 111In labeled white blood cells. *Radiology* 1990;177:161.
39. Gallagher B, Fowler J, Gutterson N et al. Metabolic trapping as a principle of radiopharmaceutical design: some factors responsible for the biodistribution of [18F] 2-deoxy-2-fluoro-D-glucose. *J Nucl Med* 1978;19:1154–1161.
40. Warburg O, Wind F, Negleis E. On the metabolism of tumors in the body. In: Warburg O, ed. *The metabolism of tumors.* London: Constable, 1930:254–270.
41. Monakhov N, Neistadt E, Shavlovskii M et al. Physicochemical properties and isoenzyme composition of hexokinase from normal and malignant human tissues. *J Natl Cancer Inst* 1978;61:27–34.
42. Shreve P, Anzai Y, Wahl R. Pitfalls in oncologic diagnosis with FDG PET imaging: physiologic and benign variants. *Radiographics* 1999;19:61–77.
43. Hashimoto M. Pathology of bone marrow. *Acta Haematol* 1962;27:193–216.
44. Bonner H. The blood and the lymphoid organs. In: Rubin E, Farber JL, eds. *Pathology.* Philadelphia: Lippincott, 1988.
45. Bourgeois P et al. Bone marrow scintigraphy in breast cancer. *Nucl Med Commun* 1989;10:389–400.
46. Rudberg U, Uden R, Ahlback S. Colloid scintigraphy showing red bone marrow extension in patients with prostatic carcinoma. *Acta Radiol* 1992;33:97–102.
47. Kim C, Reske S, Alavi A. Bone marrow scintigraphy. In: Boles MA, Henkin RE, eds. *Nuclear Medicine: principles and practice.* St. Louis: Mosby, 1995.
48. Bourgeois P, Malarme M, Van Franck R et al. Bone marrow scintigraphy in prostatic carcinomas. *Nucl Med Commun* 1991;12:35–45.
49. Haubold-Reuter B, Duewell S, Schilcher B et al. The value of bone

scintigraphy, bone marrow scintigraphy and fast spin-echo magnetic resonance imaging in staging of patients with malignant solid tumours: a prospective study. *Eur J Nucl Med* 1993;20:1063–1069.

50. Fritz P, Adolph J, Bubeck B et al. Knochenmarkszintigraphie mit Radiokolloiden bei Skelettmetastasen. *Fortschr Röntgenstr* 1986;144:689.

51. Gosfield Er, Alavi A, Kneeland B. Comparison of radionuclide bone scans and magnetic resonance imaging in detecting spinal metastases. *J Nucl Med* 1993;34:2191–2198.

52. Kosuda S, Kaji T, Yokoyama H et al. Does bone SPECT actually have lower sensitivity for detecting vertebral metastasis than MRI? *J Nucl Med* 1996;37:975–978.

53. Hanna S, Fletcher B, Fairclough D et al. Magnetic resonance imaging of disseminated bone marrow disease in patients treated for malignancy. *Skeletal Radiol* 1991;20:79–84.

54. Lien H, Taksdal I, Scheistroen M et al. Focal regeneration of irradiated bone marrow: a pitfall in MR imaging. *AJR* 1995;165:742–743.

55. Perrin-Resche I, Bizais Y, Buhe T et al. How does iliac crest bone marrow biopsy compare with imaging in the detection of bone metastases in small cell lung cancer? *Eur J Nucl Med* 1993;20:420–425.

56. Nishimura R, Nagao K, Miyayama H et al. Diagnostic problems of evaluating vertebral metastasis from breast carcinoma with a higher degree of malignancy. *Cancer* 1999;85:1782–1788.

57. Walker R, Kessar P, Blanchard R et al. Turbo STIR magnetic resonance imaging as a whole-body screening tool for metastases in patients with breast carcinoma: preliminary clinical experience. *J Magn Reson Imaging* 2000;11:343–350.

58. Chung J, Kim Y, Yoon J et al. Diagnostic usefulness of F-18 FDG whole body PET in detection of bony metastases compared to 99mTc MDP bone scan. *J Nucl Med* 1999;40:96.

59. Bury T, Barreto A, Daenen F et al. Fluorine-18 deoxyglucose positron emission tomography for the detection of bone metastases in patients with non-small cell lung cancer. *Eur J Nucl Med* 1998;25:1244–1247.

60. Durski J, Srinivas S, Segall G. Comparison of FDG-PET and bone scans for detecting skeletal metastases in patients with non-small cell lung cancer. *Clin Positron Imaging* 2000;3:97–105.

61. Cook G, Fogelman I. The role of positron emission tomography in the management of bone metastases. *Cancer* 2000;88:2927–2933.

62. Minn H, Soini I. [18F]fluorodeoxyglucose scintigraphy in diagnosis and follow up of treatment in advanced breast cancer. *Eur J Nucl Med* 1989;15:61–66.

63. Shreve P, Grossman H, Gross M et al. Metastatic prostate cancer: initial findings of PET with 2-deoxy-2-[F-18]fluoro-D-glucose. *Radiology* 1996;199:751–756.

64. Cook G, Fogelman I. The role of positron emission tomography in skeletal disease. *Semin Nucl Med* 2001;31:50–61.

65. Franzius C, Sciuk J, Daldrup-Link H et al. FDG-PET for detection of osseous metastases from malignant primary bone tumours: comparison with bone scintigraphy. *Eur J Nucl Med* 2000;27:1305–1311.

66. Papac R. Bone marrow metastases: a review. *Cancer* 1994;74:2403–2413.

67. McKenna R. The bone marrow manifestations of Hodgkin's disease, the non-Hodgkin's lymphomas, and lymphoma-like disorders. In: Knowles DM, ed. *Neoplastic hematopathology*. Baltimore: Williams & Wilkins, 1992.

68. Hoane B, Shields A, Porter B et al. Detection of lymphomatous bone marrow involvement with magnetic resonance imaging. *Blood* 1991;78:728–738.

69. Moog F, Bangerter M, Kotzerke J et al. 18-F-fluorodeoxyglucose-positron emission tomography as a new approach to detect lymphomatous bone marrow. *J Clin Oncol* 1998;16:603–609.

70. Linden A, Zankovich R, Theissen P et al. Malignant lymphoma: bone marrow imaging versus biopsy. *Radiology* 1989;173:335–339.

71. Moog F, Kotzerke J, Reske S. FDG PET can replace bone scintigraphy in primary staging of malignant lymphoma. *J Nucl Med* 1999;40:1407–1413.

72. Reske S, Karstens J, Glockner W et al. Radioimmunoimaging for diagnosis of bone marrow involvement in breast cancer and malignant lymphoma. *Lancet* 1989;335:299–301.

73. Bizzi A, Movsas B, Tedeschi G et al. Response of Non-Hodgkin's lymphoma to radiation therapy: early and long-term assessment with H-1 MR spectroscopic imaging. *Radiology* 1995;194:271–276.

74. Carr R, Barrington S, Madan B et al. Detection of lymphoma in bone marrow by whole-body positron emission tomography. *Blood* 1998;91:3340–3346.

75. Hollinger E, Alibazoglu H, Ali A et al. Hematopoietic cytokine-mediated FDG uptake simulates the appearance of diffuse metastatic disease on whole-body PET imaging. *Clin Nucl Med* 1998;23:93–98.

76. Kostakoglu L, Goldsmith S. Fluorine-18 fluorodeoxyglucose positron emission tomography in the staging and follow-up of lymphoma: is it time to shift gears? *Eur J Nucl Med* 2000;27:1564–1578.

77. DeSchrijver M et al Scintigraphy of inflammation with nanometer-sized colloidal tracers. *Nucl Med Commun* 1987;8:895.

78. Reske S et al. Localisation of subacute and chronic inflammatory lesions by means of 99mTc labelled murine monoclonal anti-NCA-antibodies. *J Nucl Med* 1989;30:797.

79. Brandhorst I et al. *Scintigraphic bone marrow status in acquired immunodeficiency syndromes* (AIDS): first results in 22 patients. In: Nuklearmedizin N, Schmidt HAE, Ell PJ, et al., eds. Stuttgart: Schattauer, 1986.

80. Lind P et al. Immunoscintigraphy of inflammatory processes with a Technetium-99m-labeled monoclonal antigranulocyte antibody (MAB BW 250/183). *J Nucl Med* 1990;31:417.

81. King A et al. Imaging of bone infection with labelled white blood cells: role of contemporaneous bone marrow imaging. *Eur J Nucl Med* 1990;17:148.

82. Feigin D, Strauss H, James A. The bone marrow scan in experimental osteomyelitis. *Skeletal Radiol* 1976;1:103.

83. Morrison W, Schweitzer M, Bock G et al. Diagnosis of osteomyelitis: utility of fat-suppressed contrast-enhanced MR imaging. *Radiology* 1993;189:251–257.

84. Deely D, Schweitzer M. MR imaging of bone marrow disorders. *Radiol Clin North Am* 1997;35:193–212.

85. Golde D, Gulati S. The myeloproliferative diseases. In: Isselbacher KJ, Braunwald E, Wilson JD, et al., eds. Harrison's principles of internal medicine. McGraw-Hill, 1994, 1757–1764.

86. Widding A, Stilbo I, Hansen S et al. Scintigraphy with nanocolloid Tc 99m in patients with small cell lung cancer, with special reference to bone marrow and hepatic metastasis. *Eur J Nucl Med* 1990;16:717–719.

87. Reske S et al. Immunoscintigraphy of bone marrow with 99mTc labelled NCA-95/CEA antibodies (TcNCAA). Comparison with bone scanning, plane radiographs and HAMA-response. *J Nucl Med* 1990;31:751.

88. Holl G, Wudel E, Koppenhagen K et al. False positive granulocyte scintigraphy in a patient with acute leukemia. Case report. *Eur J Nucl Med* 1988;14:628.

89. Wahren B et al. Clinical evaluation of NCA in patients with chronic myelocytic leukemia. *Int J Cancer* 1982;29:133.

90. Dibos P, Judisch J, Spaulding M et al. Scanning and reticuloendothelial system in hematological disease. *Johns Hopkins Med J* 1972;130:68–81.

91. Jamar F, Field C, Leners N et al. Scintigraphic evaluation of the haemopoietic bone marrow using a 99mTc-anti-granulocyte antibody: a validation study with 52Fe. *Br J Haematol* 1995;90:22–30.

92. Hotta T, Murate T, Inoue C et al. Patchy haemopoiesis in long-term remission of idiopathic aplastic anaemia. *Eur J Haematol* 1990;45:73–77.

93. Merrick M, Gordon-Smith E, Lavender J et al. A comparison of 111In with 52Fe and 99mTc-sulfur colloid for bone marrow scanning. *J Nucl Med* 1975;16:66–68.

94. Abdel-Dayem H, Sanchez J, al-Mohannadi S et al. Diffuse thallium-201-chloride uptake in hypermetabolic bone marrow following treatment with granulocyte stimulating factor. *J Nucl Med* 1992;33:2014–2016.

95. Palestro C, Roumanas P, Kim C et al. Early and late skeletal effects of radiation therapy on 111In labeled leukocyte imaging. *Clin Nucl Med* 1992;17:269–273.

96. Alavi A, McCloskey J, Steinberg M. Early detection of avascular necrosis of the femoral head by technetium-99m diphosphonate bone scan: a preliminary report. *Clin Orthop* 1977;127:137–141.

97. Munz D, Hör G. Symmetric visualization of femoral heads in reticulo-endothelial bone marrow scanning in adults: correlation with peripheral expansion of the bone marrow organ. *Eur J Nucl Med* 1983;8: 109.

98. Sarikaya I, Sarikaya A, Holder L. The role of single photon emission computed tomography in bone imaging. *Semin Nucl Med* 2001;31: 3–16.

99. Beltran J, Herman L, Burk J et al. Femoral head avascular necrosis: MR imaging with clinical-pathologic and radionuclide correlation. *Radiology* 1988;166:215–220.

100. Lutzker L, Alavi A. Bone and marrow imaging in sickle cell disease: diagnosis of infarction. *Semin Nucl Med* 1976;6:83–93.

101. Ficat R. Vascular pathology of femoral-head necrosis. *Orthopade* 1980; 9(4):238–244.

102. Mitchell D, Kressel H, Arger P et al. Avascular necrosis of the femoral head: morphologic assessment by MR imaging, with CT correlation. *Radiology* 1986;161:739–742.

103. Mitchell D, Burk DJ, Vinitski S et al. The biophysical basis of tissue contrast in extracranial MR imaging. *AJR* 1987;149:831–837.

104. Mitchell M, Kundel H, Steinberg M et al. Avascular necrosis of the hip: comparison of MR, CT, and scintigraphy. *AJR* 1986;147:67–71.

105. Mitchell M, Kundel H, Steinberg M et al. Avascular necrosis of the hip: comparison of MR, CT, and scintigraphy. *AJR* 1986;147:67–71.

106. Borgies P et al. Diagnosis of heterotopic bone marrow in the mediastinum using 52Fe and positron emission tomography. *Eur J Nucl Med* 1989;15:761–763.

107. Sweet D, Madewell J. Pathogenesis of osteonecrosis. In: Resnick DK, Niwayama G, eds. *Diagnosis of bone and joint disorder*. Philadelphia: W.B. Saunders, 1981:2780–2831.

108. Ballas S. Treatment of pain in adults with sickle cell disease. *Ant J Hematol* 1990;34:49–54.

109. Alavi A, Bond J, Kuhl D et al. Scan detection of bone marrow infarct in sickle cell disorders. *J Nucl Med* 1974;15:1003–1007.

110. Alavi A, Heyman S, Kim H. Scintigraphic examination of bone and marrow infarcts in sickle cell disorders. *Semin Roentgenol* 1987; 22: 213–224.

111. Diggs L. Bone and joint lesions in sickle cell disease. *Clin Orthop* 1967;52:119–143.

112. Kahn CJ et al. Combined bone marrow and gallium imaging. Differentiation of osteomyelitis and infarction in sickle hemoglobinopathy. *Clin Nucl Med* 1988;13:443–449.

113. Kim H et al. Differentiation of bone and bone marrow infarcts from osteomyelitis in sickle cell disorders. *Clin Nucl Med* 1989;14: 249–254.

114. Palestro C et al. Diagnosis of musculoskeletal infection using combined 111In labeled leukocyte and 99mTc SC marrow imaging. *Clin Nucl Med* 1992;17:128–129.

115. Alavi A, Schumacher H, Dorwart B et al. Bone marrow scans in evaluating arthropathy in sickle cell disorders. *Arch Intern Med* 1976; 136:436–440.

116. D'Aubigne R, Postel M, Mazabraud A et al. Idiopathic necrosis of the femoral head in adults. *J Bone Joint Surg* 1965;47B:612–633.

117. Alavi A. Scintigraphic detection of bone and marrow infarction in sickle cell disorders. In: Bohrer SF, ed. *Bone ischemia and infarction in sickle cell disease*. St. Louis: Warren H. Green, 1981:274–304.

118. Schumacher H, Andrews R, McLaughlin G. Arthropathy in sickle cell disease. *Am Intern Med* 1973;78:201–211.

119. Pearson H, Spencer R, Cornelius E. Functional asplenia in sickle cell anemia. *N Engl J Med* 1969;281:923–926.

120. Vogler JI, Murphy W. Bone marrow imaging. *Radiology* 1988;168: 679–693.

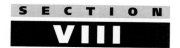

ENDOCRINOLOGY

29

LABORATORY (*IN VITRO*) ASSESSMENT OF THYROID FUNCTION

JOHN E. FREITAS
MILTON D. GROSS
SALIL D. SARKAR

Thyroid disease is commonly encountered in clinical practice and its diagnosis has been facilitated by the continued development of sensitive and specific *in vitro* tests for assessment of thyroid function. With the introduction of the third-generation serum measurement of thyroid-stimulating hormone (TSH), the clinician now has an almost ideal screening tool for the initial evaluation of thyroid dysfunction, as well as a very useful monitor for long-term fine-tuning of thyroid hormone replacement or suppression therapy (1). However, the TSH assay does have limitations in the daily evaluation of patients with suspected or known thyroid disease that still render the more traditional *in vitro* tests of thyroid function of value. The plethora of *in vitro* thyroid function tests still offered by some laboratories leads to redundant testing at increased cost, but more and more laboratories are streamlining their requisitions to direct the referring physician to a more appropriate ordering sequence. Direct measurements of serum free thyroxine (FT_4), the physiologically active hormone, have replaced the more traditional total thyroxine (TT_4) and indirect FT_4 determinations in many laboratories, but have not eliminated disparate or misleading values in certain patients or patient populations [e.g., nonthyroidal illness (NTI) and/or altered thyroid-binding proteins].

THYROID PHYSIOLOGY

Normal thyroid hormone secretion is maintained by the classic negative feedback interaction between the hypothalamus, anterior pituitary, and the thyroid. The tripeptide thyrotropin-releasing hormone (TRH), synthesized in the median basal hypothalamus and secreted into the hypophyseal-portal system, interacts with anterior pituitary thyrotroph receptors to stimulate biosynthesis and release of TSH. Once released, TSH stimulates thyroxine (T_4) and triiodothyronine (T_3) synthesis (10:1 ratio) and release from the thyroid gland. Circulating T_4 binds to the thyrotroph membrane receptors and is metabolized to T_3 intracellularly. It is the latter hormone's intranuclear occupancy that exerts its well-recognized negative feedback control of pituitary TSH secretion. Circulating total T_3 is primarily derived (80%) from peripheral monodeiodination (5'-deiodinase) of T_4 by liver, kidney, and other tissues.

Thyroid hormone (T_4 and T_3) is present in blood reversibly complexed to thyroid-binding globulin (TBG—high affinity, low capacity), transthyretin (TTR—intermediate affinity and capacity), and albumin (ALB—low affinity but high capacity). Bound and free thyroid hormone are in equilibrium and changes in TBG affinity and/or capacity have profound effects on total (bound + free) T_4 and to a lesser extent total T_3 measured concentrations, but FT_4 and free T_3 (FT_3) are maintained in the reference range (Table 29.1). Less commonly, inherited TTR and ALB variants with increased T_4 affinity can also give rise to TT_4 elevations. Only a small percentage of circulating T_4 (0.03%) and T_3 (0.3%) exist in the free physiologically active state, but it is the free thyroid hormone that exerts its tissue effects through intracellular nuclear receptor binding with the subsequent formation of a thyroid hormone-receptor complex. This complex is felt to activate or suppress thyroid hormone regulated genes that modulate cellular function.

The alterations in the regulation of thyroid hormone production that occur in normal physiologic states such as pregnancy are instructive. During the early to mid first trimester, maternal TBG levels rapidly increase two- to threefold in response to rising estrogen concentrations with a slight reduction in maternal FT_4 and FT_3. This reduction leads to feedback stimulation of the pituitary-thyroid axis with reestablishment of basal serum TSH concentrations at a slightly higher set point in the second trimester, which persists to term (2). Also occurring late in the first trimester is the direct stimulation of maternal thyroid hormone production by rising human chorionic gonadotropin (hCG). There appears to be partial inhibition of the pituitary-thyroid axis with a transient reduction in serum TSH associated

J.E. Freitas: Radiology Department, University of Michigan Medical School, Ann Arbor, MI, and Radiology Department, St. Joseph Mercy Hospital, Ypsilanti, MI.

M.D. Gross: Departments of Radiology and Internal Medicine, Division of Nuclear Medicine, University of Michigan and Department of Veterans Affairs Health Systems, Ann Arbor, MI.

S.D. Sarkar: Department of Nuclear Medicine, Albert Einstein College of Medicine of Yeshiva University, and Department of Nuclear Medicine, Jacobi Medical Center, Bronx, NY.

Table 29.1. *Conditions Associated with Changes in Thyroid Binding Globulin Capacity or Affinity*

1. Decreased serum thyroid-binding globulin
   A. Genetic — X-linked familial trait
   B. Acquired
      1. Diseases — Severe nonthyroidal illness, protein-calorie malnutrition. Nephrotic syndrome. Chronic renal failure, protein-losing enteropathy, cirrhosis, acromegaly, hyperthyroidism, diabetic ketoacidosis, Cushing's syndrome, lymphosarcoma
      2. Drugs — Glucocorticoids, danazol, L-asparaginase
      3. Hormonal — Androgen excess due to virilizing tumors, testosterone, and anabolic steroids
2. Increased serum thyroid-binding globulin
   A. Genetic — X-linked familial trait
   B. Acquired
      1. Diseases — Chronic active hepatitis, myeloma, acute intermittent porphyria, infectious hepatitis, AIDS, hypothyroidism, oat cell carcinoma, angioneurotic edema
      2. Drugs — Methadone, heroin, perphenazine, clofibrate
      3. Hormonal — Estrogen therapy, hyperestrogenic states (pregnancy, molar pregnancy, estrogen-producing tumor, newborn)
3. Inhibited T4 and T3 binding to thyroid-binding globulin
   A. Acquired
      1. Drugs — Salicylates, phenylbutazone, fenoclofenac, mitotane, phenytoin, halofenate, 5-fluorouracii

with peak hCG concentrations. In less than 25% of normal pregnancies, basal serum TSH is noted to be abnormally low transiently at 10 to 14 weeks gestation secondary to this hCG effect.

Fetal TSH and T_4 production begins at approximately 14 weeks but remains at quite low levels to 20 weeks and then gradually rises to term. Fetal T_3 concentrations show a similar pattern during the second and third trimesters, but most T_4 production is inactivated by monodeiodination (5-deiodinase) to reverse T_3 (RT_3). The degree of transplacental T_4 transfer from the maternal to the fetal circulation remains controversial, but current consensus is that a small but significant T_4 transfer does occur that is essential to fetal neural growth and organization (3). At delivery with abrupt cooling of the term newborn in the extrauterine environment, there is a rapid rise in TSH, which peaks at 30 minutes and gradually returns to neonatal basal concentrations by 48 hours. In response to the TSH rise, there is a prolonged rise in thyroid hormones characterized by a marked increase in T_3 (three- to sixfold) within 4 to 6 hours (TSH-stimulated thyroidal secretion) and a gradual further increase (T_4 to T_3 conversion) to a peak at 24 to 30 hours. There is a more gradual rise in serum TT_4 and FT_4 concentrations, which peak at 24 to 36 hours and slowly decline over 2 to 3 weeks. TT_4, FT_4, T_3, and TSH concentrations are highest in the neonate and decline progressively over 15 years to adult concentrations. In preterm infants, the hypothalamic-pituitary-thyroid system has not fully matured and the TSH, TT_4, FT_4, and T_3 responses to delivery are blunted and TT_4 and FT_4 concentrations are lower than in term infants throughout the

neonatal period. The more premature the infant is at delivery, the greater the decrement in TT_4, FT_4, and T_3 concentrations seen.

IN VITRO TESTS OF THYROID FUNCTION

In vitro thyroid function tests are immunoassays initially based on the principle of competitive protein binding. In traditional radioimmunoassay (RIA), a radioactive-labeled antigen competes with the unlabeled antigen (analyte or ligand) for a limited number of binding sites on the specific antibody (Fig. 29.1). The RIA approach allows measurement of many different hormones and other biologic molecules because antibodies can be raised to a wide spectrum of both naturally occurring and synthetic substances. RIA sensitivity, the minimal detectable antigen concentration, is dependent on the antibody's affinity constant, the labeled antigen's specific activity, nonspecific binding, and assay experimental error. Nonisotopic immunoassay systems that use enzyme (IEMA) and fluorescent (IFMA) labels are widely available for measuring T_4 and T_3 and have supplanted isotopic techniques in most laboratories.

To improve immunoassay sensitivity especially for low molecular weight analytes, immunoradiometric assays (IRMAs) were introduced using a radiolabeled antibody with a high affinity constant, high specific activity, and low nonspecific binding. In an IRMA system, the sample analyte or ligand binds to a labeled antibody present in excess (Fig. 29.2) (4). The unbound labeled antibody is then bound to a solid phase (immobilized) antigen inversely proportional to the sample analyte concentration. If the count emitted by the labeled antibody bound to the solid phase antigen is measured, this remains a competitive immunoassay. However, if the labeled antibody bound to the analyte is counted directly, this is a noncompetitive immunoassay. An improvement in the original IRMA system has been the sandwich technique using two antibodies, each one directed against a different epitope (antigenic site) on the analyte (Fig. 29.3) (5). The sandwich or two-site immunoassay is a noncompetitive assay. The analyte or ligand acts as a bridge between the

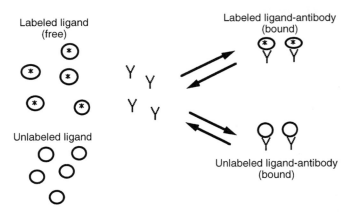

FIGURE 29.1. Radioimmunoassay diagram. The radioactive-labeled ligand (antigen) competes with unlabeled ligand present in the patient's serum for a limited number of binding sites on the specific antibody.

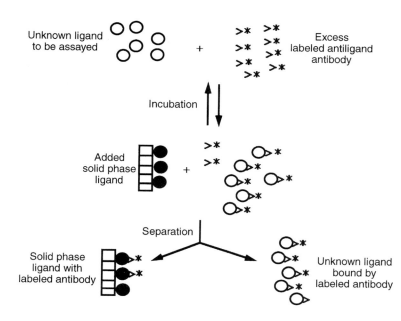

FIGURE 29.2. Immunoradiometric diagram. The labeled antibody in excess binds the ligand in step 1. Solid phase ligand is then added to remove remaining excess labeled antibody in step 2. After separation in step 3, either the liquid or solid phase-bound labeled antibody can be counted. The liquid phase counts are directly proportional to the unknown ligand concentration.

solid phase and liquid-phase (labeled) antibodies. In this highly sensitive technique, the amount of solid-phase bound radioactivity directly reflects the sample analyte concentration. Nonisotopic labels (enzymatic, fluorescent, and chemiluminescent) have been coupled with spectrophotometric, fluorometric, and chemiluminometric signal detection systems to further enhance the sensitivity of the sandwich-type immunometric assays (IMAs)

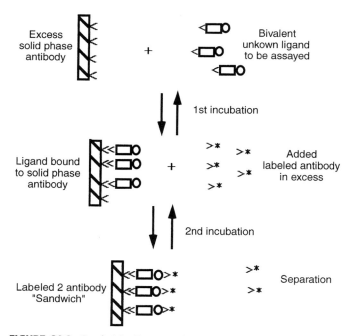

FIGURE 29.3. Sandwich diagram. The ligand binds to excess solid phase antibody directed against one of the ligand's epitopes. The complex is then exposed to a second labeled antibody in excess. This second antibody is directed to the other epitope on the ligand. After separation, the solid phase bound counts are directly proportional to the unknown ligand concentration.

(Fig. 29.4) (6). Nonisotopic labels can have much higher specific activity than isotopic labels allowing shorter incubation times. When used in conjunction with a noncompetitive two-site assay system, incubation times can be measured in minutes, ideally suited to fully automated immunoanalyzers readily available in most laboratories.

T_4 and T_3 Measurements

The TT_4 measurement has outlived its usefulness in most clinical situations but is still offered as a thyroid function test in many laboratories. TT_4 can be measured cost effectively by RIA or fluorescence polarization. Although commonly used in the past to screen patients with suspected thyroid dysfunction, the TT_4 value alone (reference range: 4.8 to 12.4 µg/dL) is a measurement of biologically inactive, protein-bound hormone that may not accurately reflect the patient's thyroid status because of alterations in carrier protein binding. Abnormal TT_4 values are more often caused by alterations in T_4 binding than by hyperthyroidism or hypothyroidism. Serum total T_3 (TT_3) measured by similar methodology to TT_4 may be used to confirm the diagnosis of hyperthyroidism especially in the 5% of hyperthyroid patients with normal TT_4 values, so-called T_3 thyrotoxicosis. Although TT_3 values are affected to a lesser extent than are TT_4 values by alterations in carrier protein binding, TT_3 values often correlate poorly with thyroid status because they can be influenced dramatically by drugs or disease processes that alter T_4 metabolism (Fig. 29.5). It is not well recognized that TT_4 and TT_3 concentrations are age-dependent with highest concentrations seen in the first year of life and declining gradually to adult values by age 16 to 18. TT_3 values exhibit the highest reference interval (90 to 221 ng/dL) at 1 to 11 months with a gradual decline to adult values (60 to 180 ng/dL) by age 16 to 18. Approximately 10% to 15% of normal children demonstrate elevated TT_3 values when compared inappropriately to the adult reference range,

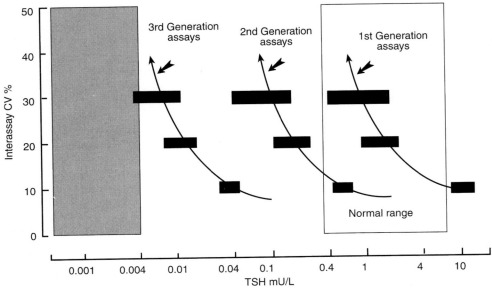

FIGURE 29.4. First- to third-generation thyroid-stimulating hormone (TSH) diagram. A comparison of interassay precision expressed as percent coefficient of variation for first-generation radioimmunoassays and second- and third-generation immunoradiometric assays for TSH measurement. The solid bars represent 95% confidence limits for varying TSH levels for each TSH assay generation. (From Spencer CA. Thyroid profiling for the 1990's: free T_4 estimate or sensitive TSH measurement. *J Clin Immunoassay* 1989;112:82, with permission.)

a point often overlooked in pediatric referrals for suspected hyperthyroidism (7).

Free Thyroxine Index

Because FT_4 and FT_3 values correlate more closely with thyroid clinical status than do TT_4 and TT_3 values, FT_4 (and less often FT_3) values are determined either indirectly as a FT_4 index (FT_4I or T_7) or by direct measurement. To estimate FT_4 concentration, the T_3 resin uptake (T_3RU) test or thyroid hormone binding ratio (THBR) test is often used to assess T_4-binding proteins. The T_3RU reflects the relative saturation of an individual patient's TBG binding sites by T_4. The less the number of available binding sites present on the patient's TBG, the greater will be the T_3RU value and vice versa (Table 29.2). The T_3RU value (expressed as a percentage) is obtained by dividing the resin-bound counts by the residual serum counts after separation. The THBR value can then be obtained by dividing the T_3RU value by a pooled serum reference. The FT_4I is calculated by multiplying the TT_4 by the T_3RU test (or THBR). However, marked TBG alterations (e.g., pregnancy or genetic variant) may not be fully corrected by the T_3RU value, generating an elevated FT_4I. The utility of the FT_4I in patients with known or suspected thyroid disease is shown in Fig. 29.6.

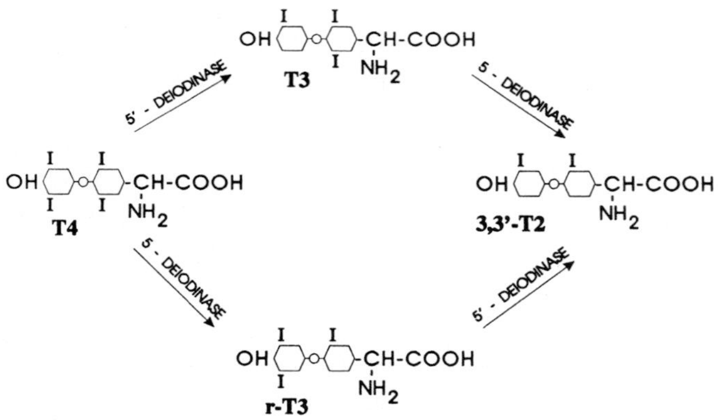

Free Thyroxine

Direct measurements of FT_4 by direct or tracer equilibrium dialysis, analog T_4, or direct solid-phase anti-T_4 RIA methodologies has supplanted FT_4I measurements in many laboratories

FIGURE 29.5. Thyroxine (T_4) metabolism and its metabolites. T_4 is metabolized to triiodothyronine (T_3) and reverse triiodothyronine (rT_3). In the presence of 5'-deiodinase deficiency, T_4 is metabolized preferentially to rT_3. (From Troncone L, Shapiro B, Satta MA et al., eds. *Thyroid diseases: basic science, pathology, clinical and laboratory diagnoses.* Boca Raton, FL: CRC Press, 1994:206, with permission.)

Table 29.2. *Effect of Altered Thyroid-Binding Proteins on TT_4, T_3RU, FT_4I, and FT_4*

TT_4	T_3RU	FT_4I	FT_4	Clinical diagnosis
I	I	I	I	Hyperthyroidism
D	D	D	D	Hypothyroidism
I	D	N	N	TBG excess
D	I	N	N	TBG deficiency
I	N	I	N	Dysalbuminemia
D	I	N	N	Hypoalbuminemia
I	I	I	N	Thyroid autoantibody
D	I	D	N - I	Low T_4 nonthyroidal illness
I	D	N - I	N - I	High T_4 nonthyroidal illness

I, increased; D, decreased; N, normal figures correlation chart.
TBG, thyroid-binding globulin.

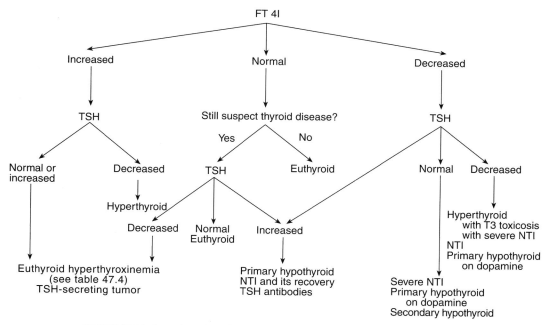

FIGURE 29.6. Free thyroxine algorithm for adults with suspected thyroid disease.

(8). Direct equilibrium dialysis is the "gold standard" but is not suited to high patient volume operations. Analog T_4 assays use the failure of the analog to bind to serum proteins while maintaining an affinity for an antibody to T_4. However, many T_4 analogs do bind to some extent to serum proteins, predominantly serum albumin, generating spurious results in situations such as severe NTI or familial dysalbuminemic hyperthyroxinemia (FDH) in which albumin levels are altered. A commonly used alternative FT_4 assay uses a two-step incubation procedure with initial serum equilibration of a solid-phase (paramagnetic microparticle) anti-T_4 antibody and separation of serum from the antibody, followed by the addition of acridinium ester-labeled T_3 to the solid-phase antibody. Using chemiluminescent technology to determine the number of unoccupied binding sites, the signal intensity is inversely proportional to the amount of FT_4 in the patient sample (9). This immunoassay (reference range: 0.70 to 1.48 ng/dL) and others demonstrate excellent correlation with the gold standard, direct equilibrium dialysis, in the assessment of patients with thyroid dysfunction and NTI but are not entirely free of interference (e.g., heterophile antibodies, nonspecific immunoglobulins) (Table 29.2). When suspected, adding nonimmune globulin as a "blocker" can minimize immunoglobulin-mediated interference. The utility of the FT_4I in patients with known or suspected thyroid disease is shown in Fig. 29.6.

FT_3 concentrations can be determined using similar methodologies described for FT_4, and such measurements (reference range: 1.71 to 3.71 pg/mL) have clinical usefulness in confirming a suspected diagnosis of T_3 thyrotoxicosis and in evaluating some patients with euthyroid hyperthyroxinemia. RT_3, a T_4 metabolite produced by 5-deiodinase action on the inner ring of T_4, has no significant biologic activity, but its excessive production may serve a protective mechanism in NTI. In differentiating

patients with NTI from sick hypothyroid patients, RT_3 measurement may provide important management information because it is high in the former and low in the latter patients.

TSH Measurement

The usefulness of the serum TSH assay has expanded as its sensitivity has increased from first- to third-generation immunoassays (Fig. 29.4). The serum TSH concentration drives T_4 and T_3 secretion with FT_4 and FT_3 exerting negative feedback inhibition at the pituitary on TSH secretion. Minute changes in FT_4 concentration produce an amplified serum TSH response as a result of the log-linear serum TSH-FT_4 relationship (10). A twofold change in FT_4 concentration induces a 160-fold change in serum TSH concentration. In the presence of an intact pituitary-thyroid axis, the serum TSH concentration is the most sensitive indicator and the single best test to diagnose thyroid dysfunction. This has led to the use of the serum TSH immunoassay as a screening tool in patients with a low pretest likelihood of disease, and the American Thyroid Association now recommends that adults be screened by serum TSH measurement beginning at age 35 and every 5 years thereafter (11,12). A typical chemiluminescent (ICMA) third-generation assay uses the two-antibody sandwich technique with solid phase antibody specific for the TSH β-subunit and a second acridinium ester-labeled antibody directed to the nonspecific TSH α-subunit. The third-generation TSH assays differentiate suppressed hyperthyroid from low but euthyroid values (assay sensitivity to 0.01 mIU/L) but demonstrate no significant differences for patients whose second-generation values are 0.1 mIU/L or greater (Fig. 29.7).

However, such low-end sensitivity may vary as much as one order of magnitude (coefficient of variation above 30%) depend-

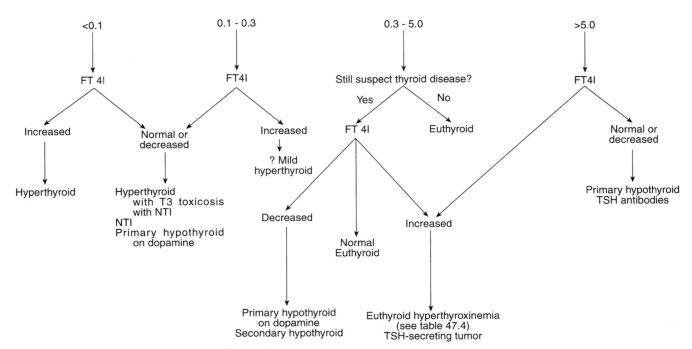

FIGURE 29.7. Serum thyroid-stimulating hormone algorithm for adults with suspected thyroid disease.

ing on the skill and ability of laboratory personnel (13). To ensure reasonable reproducibility of the current in-house TSH immunoassay, each laboratory must address functional detection limit, percent cross-reactivity, linearity of response, recovery, accuracy, precision, matrix effects, interference, "hook effect," and percent overlap between hyperthyroid and euthyroid serum. The specificity of the third-generation assays is excellent, but some patient samples with endogenous heterophile antibodies, especially human anti-mouse antibodies and rheumatoid factors, give factitiously elevated concentrations, although the frequency of such interference can be reduced by adding nonimmune immunoglobulins to the test reagents (14,15). The presence of measurable TSH values in a clinically hyperthyroid patient is more likely to be secondary to assay technical error than the presence of heterophile antibodies.

Using a third-generation assay, hyperthyroid patients can usually be distinguished from patients with NTI or hypothalamic-pituitary dysfunction (10). However, some overlap of TSH values does exist requiring correlation with FT_4 concentrations, additional clinical information, and, perhaps, a period of observation in some patients. With the demonstration that many patients receiving thyroid hormone replacement were being overtreated despite FT_4I values in the reference range, there has been considerable emphasis placed on the use of TSH to closely monitor such replacement therapy (16). Serum TSH reflects the patient's long-term thyroid status more accurately than the more immediate changes that occur in T_4 concentrations following ingestion of thyroxine tablets. Serum TSH values in the reference range are desired in thyroid hormone replacement of primary

hypothyroidism but not necessarily in congenital hypothyroidism (CH). Noncompliant patients on thyroxine replacement therapy may demonstrate serum TSH elevation despite normal FT_4 concentrations. The patient's compliance should be ascertained before increasing thyroxine dosage to correct TSH elevation. Similarly, serum TSH is used to ensure that thyroid cancer patients receive appropriate but not excessive suppression of TSH, a thyroid growth-stimulating factor. Unfortunately, there is no consensus concerning the optimal TSH value for monitoring such patients using third-generation assays. Using a second-generation assay, many thyroidologists administered T_4 doses that suppressed serum TSH to ≤0.1 mIU/L. Reassay of serum samples with values less than 0.1 mIU/L (second-generation assay) with a third-generation assay demonstrated that 24% of samples had values less than 0.01 mIU/L. Serum TSH suppression to less than 0.01 mIU/L is probably excessive and most thyroidologists are satisfied with third-generation TSH values of less than 0.1 mIU/L for their thyroid cancer patients at high risk for recurrence or mortality. For low-risk patients, serum TSH suppression less than 0.3 mIU/L is probably reasonable, although some thyroidologists choose to maintain such patients in the euthyroid range especially after several years of uneventful observation.

Patients with primary hypothyroidism demonstrate elevated TSH values, but not all patients with elevated TSH concentrations are hypothyroid. Transient TSH elevations (usually <20 mIU/L) can be seen in hospitalized patients recovering from serious illnesses or injuries, and further evaluation should be delayed until the medical condition has stabilized unless impending myxedema coma (very rare) is present. Normal or increased TSH values can be seen with hyperthyroidism secondary to TSH-secreting pituitary tumors or selective pituitary resistance to thyroid hormone (17,18). Differentiation can be difficult but a TSH-secreting adenoma is likely to be present if the thyrotropin releasing hormone-induced TSH response is blunted or suppressed, the TSH fails to decrease to T_3 administration, or the α-subunit/whole TSH molar ratio is high (19).

CH is detected in 1 in 4,000 infants by neonatal hypothyroidism screening programs with an incidence of 2,500 infants yearly worldwide. Screening programs in the United States and Canada usually use a two-tiered procedure of T_4, followed by TSH in those infants with T_4 values approximately ≤ 7 µg/dL or 2.1 standard deviations below the mean daily value (20,21). These programs use 72- to 120-hour postdelivery filter paper blood spot specimens. Earlier sampling at 24 to 48 hours can be misleading because of the normal physiologic TSH surge of the newborn. Unfortunately, such sampling is encouraged by the recent trend of 1- to 2-day postdelivery discharges of mother and newborn (40% of newborns in some areas). Simultaneous T_4/TSH determination on the same specimen would be the ideal approach for rapid diagnosis. With the T_4, then TSH if needed, approach, newborns with TBG deficiency (incidence 1 in 5,000 to 10,000) or with hypothalamic-pituitary hypothyroidism (incidence 1 in 50,000) are also identified. Using the TSH first approach, these newborns are not identified. No matter which screening approach is adopted, it is estimated that 5% to 10% of newborns with CH are missed because they have normal screening T_4 and TSH concentrations (21). The serum TSH remains elevated in some infants with CH despite adequate T_4 replacement (10 to 15 µg/kg/day for the first year), perhaps resulting from a disordered pituitary set point for TSH secretion (22). Adequate replacement should be monitored by TT_4 measurements (not TSH) at 3, 6, and 12 months of age, with the goal to maintain TT_4 greater than 10 µg/dL.

Thyroglobulin Measurements

Serum thyroglobulin (TG) is released normally from the thyroid gland as part of T_4 and T_3 secretion and can be measured by a variety of commercial methodologies with varying sensitivities and specificities. Sandwich IRMA, IEMA, ICMA, and IFMA techniques provide highly sensitive (assay sensitivity to 0.2 ng/mL) and specific TG assays. However, 4% to 15% of patients with well-differentiated thyroid cancer and the majority of patients with Hashimoto's thyroiditis (HT) demonstrate serum TG autoantibodies that can interfere with the assays, generating spurious low or high (IRMA) or falsely low results (IEMA, IFMA) (23). Most laboratories screen TG samples for the presence of autoantibodies by adding TG to samples and assessing TG recovery, which is decreased if autoantibodies are present. Fortunately, certain assays promise some relief from endogenous anti-TG autoantibody interference by using monoclonal antibodies directed against different TG epitopes (24).

Serum TG can be used to differentiate factitious hyperthyroidism from thyrotoxicosis or destructive thyroiditis, but its more common application is in the long-term monitoring of well-differentiated thyroid cancer. Serum TG is not useful in

monitoring patients with well-differentiated thyroid cancer treated only by lobectomy without radioiodine ablation. The better the low-end sensitivity and specificity of the assay, the better the clinical usefulness of the assay in detecting circulating serum TG released from residual normal or neoplastic tissue following thyroid cancer surgery. Commercial assays with known improved specificity and freedom from interference from endogenous anti-TG antibodies should be selected in patients with known autoimmune thyroid disease and well-differentiated thyroid cancer to preclude the likelihood of the obtained TG values being reported as spurious, falsely low, or nondiagnostic. IMAs with sensitivity limits of 0.2 to 5.0 ng/mL have proved a useful thyroid cancer management tool. It is important to know, when interpreting serum TG values, whether the specimen was obtained during thyroid hormone suppression or not. Measurements obtained while the patient is on suppressive doses of thyroid hormone are usually significantly lower than measurements obtained after thyroid hormone is withdrawn. When engaged in long-term monitoring of thyroid cancer patients, it is important to compare sequential results with the same assay and under the same conditions (e.g., on or off T_4). Interassay comparisons are likely to provide misleading information and are not recommended because the TG assay has not been standardized and each laboratory must determine its own reference range.

In 86 patients with well-differentiated thyroid cancer treated with near-total thyroidectomy and radioiodine ablation, follow-up TG (assay sensitivity to 1.0 ng/mL) monitoring at 1-year demonstrated TG values that were undetectable in 94% (on T_4) and in 68% (off T_4) of patients, respectively, without evidence of residual ^{131}I-concentrating thyroid tissue (successful ablation). In patients with residual ^{131}I-concentrating thyroid tissue (unsuccessful ablation) but no evidence of metastatic disease, TG values were undetectable in 74% on T_4 but in only 2% off T_4. The results described may vary considerably depending on the particular TG assay used even if the assay sensitivity limits are similar. Patients with detectable TG values on T_4 who demonstrate only small increases in their TG value off T_4 usually do not have significant disease, but occasionally metastatic disease is present. In patients with regional or distant metastases, TG values are almost invariably detectable or high on T_4 although some patients with lymph node metastases have TG values less than 1 ng/mL. Patients with bone and/or lung metastases exhibit higher TG values than do patients with lymph node metastases, but there is only a rough correlation of TG values with tumor burden. Similar results have been reported by others (14,25–28). Serum TG is more sensitive than ^{131}I scintigraphy in detection of metastatic thyroid carcinoma and periodic serum TG sampling is essential in any long-term thyroid cancer monitoring program (28,29). In many programs, TG values are obtained on and off T_4 at periodic intervals whereas, in other programs, TG values are obtained on T_4 only as long as TG values stay below a predetermined threshold value (e.g., <10 ng/mL) and there is no evidence of cancer recurrence. The advent of recombinant human TSH (rTSH, Thyrogen) enables an alternative approach in patients unable or unwilling to undergo T_4 withdrawal. (30). In patients taking T_4, measuring TG following rTSH intramuscular administration has been shown to be quite effective in detecting thyroid cancer recurrence using stimulated TG cut-off values in the 3 to 5 ng/mL range.

In patients with hyperthyroidism but with a low radioactive iodine uptake, differentiation between factitious hyperthyroidism and destructive thyroiditis (subacute or silent thyroiditis) can be made on the basis of serum TG values. In patients taking thyroid hormone surreptitiously, TG secretion is suppressed and serum TG values are low or undetectable, but patients with destructive thyroiditis leak preformed TG and demonstrate markedly elevated serum TG values (31,32). Patients with destructive thyroiditis treated early in their course with glucocorticoids (but not salicylates) can demonstrate a marked drop in TG values, and this should be borne in mind when interpreting TG values of referred patients (33). Because patients with factitious hyperthyroidism often have a history of prior thyroid disease, the possibility of TG antibody interference in the assay should be excluded.

Neonates with congenital primary hypothyroidism may be athyreotic (30%), dyshormonogenic (10%), or have ectopic thyroid tissue (60%) (22,34). Athyreotic infants have low or undetectable TG values, but TG values overlap between ectopic (normal or elevated TG values) and dyshormonogenic (markedly elevated TG values) subgroups (35).

Calcitonin Measurements

The secretion of serum calcitonin (CT), a single-chain 32-amino acid peptide, mainly by the parafollicular thyroid C-cells is modulated by extracellular calcium levels primarily, but pentagastrin, β-adrenergic agonists, growth hormone releasing hormone, and various gastrointestinal peptides stimulate CT secretion (36). The definitive role of CT in calcium homeostasis remains unknown, but CT exerts its metabolic effects by binding to cell membrane receptors of osteoclasts to inhibit osteoclastic bone resorption. CT also acts on the kidneys to enhance calcium, phosphate, magnesium, and sodium excretion. CT is also produced at extrathyroidal sites (lungs, thymus, gastrointestinal tract, central nervous system, and bladder) and thyroidectomized patients have detectable CT values (37). CT is now commonly measured by ICMA using two mouse monoclonal antibodies to human CT (reference range: < 4.1 pg/mL).

Serum CT is most commonly used as a tumor marker for the presence of C-cell hyperplasia or sporadic or familial medullary thyroid carcinoma (MTC). In patients with palpable or metastatic MTC, baseline CT values are usually diagnostic, but pentagastrin or pentagastrin-calcium provocative testing of stored intrathyroidal CT has been standard practice for screening for familial MTC disease. However, the identification of mutations of the RET proto-oncogene located on chromosome 10 as the causative gene in familial MTC, multiple endocrine neoplasia type 2 (MEN 2) A and B families, has revolutionized the screening approach to these syndromes (38). Using five different molecular techniques, 95% of familial MTC or MEN 2 families show characteristic germline mutations in genomic DNA extracted from peripheral white blood cells. In such affected families, genetic testing can be used as the sole determinant for management decisions in family members, but each individual should be studied with independent samples sent to two separate

laboratories to reduce false-positive and negative results. Such a DNA-based screening approach is highly cost-effective when compared with repetitive provocative testing. In families with proven germline transmission of MTC but no identifiable RET mutation, provocative testing of CT is indicated. Both pentagastrin (0.5 μg/kg 5-second intravenous bolus) and calcium (2 to 3 mg/kg of elemental calcium as 1-minute infusion), alone or as a combination infusion, stimulate CT secretion with CT values obtained at −5, 0, 2, 5, and 10 minutes. CT values peak early (2 to 5 minutes) after stimulus injection and usually rise to greater than 50 pg/mL in patients with subclinical MTC or C-cell hyperplasia. A single normal stimulation test does not exclude the presence of occult disease in family members of a MEN IIA kindred, and sequential studies at regular intervals are required. Such sequential studies in family members should begin early (age 1 in some programs) and continue at 2-year intervals until age 35. Because 95% of family members at risk for MTC will be detected by this age, screening at 5-year intervals thereafter appears reasonable (39,40). Peak CT levels less than 100 pg/mL can be seen as affected family members transit from normal to abnormal CT responses with sequential provocative testing. Total thyroidectomy at age 5 to 7 is recommended for affected individuals detected by DNA-based screening and at the time of provocative test conversion in others. Persistent or recurrent CT concentrations postthyroidectomy are seen in 5% to 15% of affected individuals screened by provocative testing suggesting that metastatic disease was already present when sequential provocative testing first became abnormal. Following total thyroidectomy, stimulatory testing should be performed on at least two occasions. Patients with normal stimulatory testing on both occasions can be considered cured (41).

Thyroid Autoantibodies

Patients with autoimmune thyroid disease demonstrate circulating thyroid antibodies directed against the autoantigens, thyroid peroxidase (TPO), TG, TSH receptor (TSHR), sodium iodide symporter, TSH, T_4, and T_3. TPO (present in 90% of HT patients) and TG autoantibodies (50% of patients) are most commonly measured to support or confirm the diagnosis of HT and are detectable by hemagglutination, RIA, IRMA, and immunosorbent techniques (42,43). However, high anti-TPO and, to a lesser extent, anti-TG titers can be seen in patients with primary thyroid lymphoma, and this should be considered in the appropriate clinical setting (44). Significant titers of anti-TPO are also present in many patients with Graves' disease and are found in lesser titers in nonthyroid autoimmune diseases such as rheumatoid arthritis, systemic lupus erythematosus, pernicious anemia, Sjögren's syndrome, Addison's disease, and type I diabetes mellitus.

Thyroid-stimulating antibodies (TSab) are antibodies directed against TSHR that exert a stimulatory effect on thyroidal secretion of T_4 and T_3. Such TSHR antibodies are detected by two different assays: a bioassay, in which cyclic adenosine monophosphate (cAMP) generation is measured, and a radioreceptor assay, in which the inhibition of labeled TSH binding, is measured. Most patients with active Graves' disease demonstrate thyroid-stimulating immunoglobulin (TSI) activity (cAMP generation assay) and up to 85% of these patients demonstrate TSH binding inhibition (TBII) activity (45). TSI and TBII activity is less commonly detected in patients with euthyroid Graves' disease (approximately half of such patients). TSab values are usually superfluous in the diagnosis of Graves' disease but can be helpful in certain clinical situations. The presence of significantly elevated titers of TSab activity in the serum of a third-trimester expectant mother with active or previously treated Graves' disease can be useful in predicting the likelihood (2% to 10% risk) of the development of neonatal Graves' disease and its attendant 16% mortality rate (46,47).

The prevalence of antibodies to TSH, T_4, and T_3 is variable but should be considered especially in patients with autoimmune thyroid disease when the patient's clinical status does not correlate with measurements of serum TSH, T_4, T_3, or FT_4 (15). Most laboratories can readily detect the presence of interfering antibodies when this possibility is raised.

DRUG EFFECTS ON THYROID HORMONE LEVELS AND FUNCTION

Numerous drugs can change TT_4 and TT_3 values by altering TBG capacity or affinity as shown in Table 29.3. Drugs can also change FT_4 and TSH values, in addition to TT_4 and TT_3 values, by various mechanisms altering thyroid hormone metabolism, gastrointestinal absorption, thyroid hormone secretion and/or release, and the hypothalamic-pituitary-thyroid axis (Table 29.3).

Thionamides

Propylthiouracil and methimazole, the two principal antithyroid drugs, are often used for the control of hyperthyroidism before

^{131}I or surgery or the definitive treatment of Graves' disease and toxic nodular goiter. Thionamides decrease hormone synthesis by inhibiting oxidation and organic binding of iodide, as well as coupling of iodotyrosines. They may alter thyroglobulin function and decrease thyroid growth response to thyroid-stimulating antibodies (TSAb) in Graves' disease (48–51). The levels of TSAb, which are responsible for the hyperthyroidism of Graves' disease, are also decreased during thionamide therapy, and permanent remission may occur after 6 to 12 months. Presumably, removal of the thyroid-stimulating factors allows the underlying autoimmune thyroiditis, the etiologic basis of Graves' disease, to pursue its natural course toward eventual hypothyroidism. Finally, propylthiouracil is known to inhibit the peripheral monodeiodination of T_4 with the result that smaller amounts of the more potent T_3 are formed.

β-Blockers

β-Adrenergic blocking agents are routinely used to decrease the end-organ responses to excess thyroid hormone and help provide relief from the symptoms of hyperthyroidism: palpitations, nervousness, heat intolerance, and insomnia. Propranolol, the most commonly used β-blocker, also inhibits the peripheral conversion of T_4 to T_3. Other β-blockers, sucfsh as atenolol and metoprolol, are predominantly cardioselective in their effects.

Corticosteroids

Large amounts of glucocorticoids acutely decrease TSH secretion and the conversion of T_4 to T_3 and are used in the treatment of thyroid storm. Steroids have an antiinflammatory effect, which may be used in the treatment of selected patients with subacute thyroiditis and in the management of Graves' ophthalmopathy, especially after radioiodine therapy. Chronic hypercortisolism, as in Cushing's syndrome, may lead to decreased TSH response to TRH and may mask some autoimmune symptoms in some patients with HT (51).

Iodide and Lithium

Iodides in large doses inhibit the synthesis of thyroid hormones (52–54). This includes iodine-containing organic compounds used for therapy, i.e., expectorants, mucolytics, antiasthmatics, and topical antiseptics. Because of their additional rapid effects on thyroid hormone release in hyperthyroidism, iodides (saturated solution of potassium iodide or Lugol's solution) can also be used for the acute control of severe thyrotoxicosis and thyroid storm. However, escape from the effects of iodide may occur, and therapy for hyperthyroidism should be combined with thionamides.

The iodinated contrast agents, e.g., iopanoic acid, affect the conversion of T_4 to T_3 by inhibition of 5′-deiodinase activity and may decrease intrathyroidal thyroid hormone levels. These drugs also may be used for short-term control of severe thyrotoxicosis (53).

Lithium interferes with thyroid hormone synthesis and decreases the secretion of thyroid hormone. Chronic therapy may

Table 29.3. *Drug Effects on Thyroid Function*

Site of action and drug	TT_4	FT_4	T_3	TSH
1. Thyroid hormone metabolism				
Amiodarone, iopanoic acid, ipodate	I/D	I/D	D	N
Phentoin, phenobarbital, rifampin	D	D	N	N,I
Glucocorticoids, propylthiouracil, β-adrenergic antagonists	N	N	D	N
2. Gastrointestinal absorption				
Colestipol, cholestyramine, (inhibit oral L-thyroxine absorption)	D	D	D	I
3. Hypothalamic-pituitary-thyroid axis				
Amphetamines	I	I	N,I	I
Dopamine	D	D	D	D
Glucocorticoids, octreotide	N	N	N	D
4. Thyroid hormone synthesis/release				
Iodides (Hashimoto's thyroiditis, nodular goiter)	D	D	D	I
Ketoconazole	I	I	I	D
Lithium (Hashimoto's thyroiditis)	D	D	D	I
Methimazole, propylthiouracil	D	D	D	I
Sulfonamides, sulfonylureas	D	D	D	I
Aminogluthemide	D	D	D	I

I, increased; D, decreased; N, normal.
TSH, thyroid-stimulating hormone.

result in goiter and hypothyroidism, especially in patients with antithyroid antibodies and preexisting autoimmune thyroiditis. (55). This drug is not routinely used in the treatment of hyperthyroidism but may provide an alternative to iodides in patients with iodide allergy (56).

Other Drugs

Amiodarone

Amiodarone, a cardiac antiarrhythmic agent, is used for the control of tachyarrhythmias and coronary artery disease and is often associated with thyroid dysfunction. Iodine excess (75 mg of iodide per 200 mg of active drug) accounts for the principal effects on thyroid function that can be very prolonged as a result of the slow tissue clearance of amiodarone metabolites (57). Although most patients treated with amiodarone remain euthyroid, TT_4, FT_4, and rT_3 levels increase and TT_3 levels decrease as a result of 5'-deiodinase inhibition. TSH remains normal or slightly elevated during the first few months of therapy in patients without thyroid disease. Thyroid dysfunction occurs in about 15% of patients that can manifest as either hypothyroidism or the abrupt development of hyperthyroidism. Hypothyroidism as a result of amiodarone can occur in normal thyroid glands, although the presence of autoimmune thyroiditis (HT) is an important risk factor. The release of excessive iodide and an intrinsic failure of escape from iodide (the Wolff Chaikoff effect) is considered to be the etiology for the development of amiodarone-induced hypothyroidism. Amiodarone-induced hyperthyroidism is a more complex process that has two more or less distinct subtypes. Type I amiodarone-induced hyperthyroidism in areas of iodine deficiency occurs as a result of an acute iodine load (Jod-Basedow phenomenon) whereas type II amiodarone-induced hyperthyroidism is a destructive thyroiditis apparently induced by amiodarone itself (57). Further complicating the issue of amiodarone-induced hyperthyroidism is the presence of mixed types with characteristics of both types I and II. (57)

Hepatic Enzyme-Inducing Drugs

Hepatic glucuronidation and to some extent sulfation, with subsequent excretion via bile into feces, plays an important role in thyroid hormone metabolism. Drugs that induce hepatic enzymes, including phenobarbital, phenytoin, carbamazepine, nicardipine, rifampin, and imidazole antibiotics, enhance the metabolism of thyroid hormone (55) (Table 29.3). As a result of lowered thyroid hormone levels, there is a compensatory increase in TSH leading to goiter formation. Dilantin and carbamazepine have other minor effects including competitive inhibition of T_4 binding to TBG and suppression of TSH response to TRH (55, 58). The net clinical effect of these two drugs, however, is usually a euthyroid status.

Altered TBG Levels or TBG-Binding

Drugs affecting thyroid-binding proteins do not alter thyroid physiology per se, but do influence the results of thyroid function

tests (58,59) (Table 29.1). The measured levels of TT_4 and T_3 may be increased or decreased without altering free hormone levels (58,60). Increased TBG often results from high estrogen levels and is often seen in women taking oral contraceptives, in pregnancy, and in newborn infants. Decreased TBG may be secondary to androgenic and anabolic steroids and L-asparaginase. Both increased and decreased TBG may occur as familial disorders (Table 29.3). Aspirin, phenylbutazone, heparin, and furosemide interfere with protein binding of thyroid hormone and may lead to decreased TT_4 with normal or increased free hormone concentrations (55) (Table 29.1).

Miscellaneous Drugs

Cytokine therapy is associated with a significant incidence of hypothyroidism (61,62). These therapeutic agents may exacerbate underlying autoimmune thyroid disease and cause transient hyperthyroidism (63). Iron salts, known to decrease blood levels of certain drugs, have been shown to reduce the efficacy of thyroxine replacements in patients with hypothyroidism (64). It has been suggested that binding of iron to thyroxine decreases its intestinal absorption. Both dopamine and octreotide have been shown to decrease TSH. Aminogluthemide, tolbutamide, and sulfonamides have also been observed to increase TSH levels in some patients (55).

INTERPRETATIVE PITFALLS OF *IN VITRO* THYROID FUNCTION TESTS

Interpretation of serum TT_4 and TT_3 values would be simple if thyroid hormone elevation meant either hyperthyroidism or TBG excess, and low thyroid hormone values indicated hypothyroidism or TBG deficiency. However, the meaning of an elevated TT_4, a normal serum TSH, or a low serum TT3 is dependent on the individual patient's clinical situation, and any interpretation of thyroid function tests requires an understanding of potential modifying factors such as genetic variants, drug interactions, intercurrent illnesses, and assay limitations.

Euthyroid Hyperthyroxinemia

Elevated TT_4 values in patients without a previous history of thyroid disease may indicate hyperthyroidism, but such elevations occur more often in the absence of demonstrable thyroid disease. TT_4 elevation from TBG excess and L-thyroxine therapy have already been discussed, but there is a less well-recognized transient TT_4 and FT_4 elevation that commonly persists for up to 9 hours following oral L-thyroxine ingestion. Blood sampling for TT_4 and FT_4 should be performed before L-thyroxine ingestion (65). Causes of hyperthyroidism and so-called euthyroid hyperthyroxinemia are shown in Table 29.4. T_4-binding protein abnormalities such as the autosomal dominant FDH syndrome in which an albumin variant has increased avidity for T4, but not T3, are not infrequent (66) (Table 29.3). The T_3RU, TT_3, and TSH values are normal, but the TT_4 and FTI are elevated in FDH. The FT_4 may or may not be falsely elevated depending

Table 29.4. *Differential Diagnosis of Hyperthyroxinemia*

Euthyroid	Hyperthyroid
Dependent upon T_4 binding proteins	Graves' disease
Genetic	
Increased TBG (see Table 29.2)	Plummer's disease
	Destructive thyroiditis
Increased albumin or transthyreitin avidity	Subacute thyroiditis
Acquired	Silent thyroiditis
Liver disease	Iatrogenic or factitious hyperthyroidism
Multiple diseases	Jod-Basedow disease
Drugs (see Table 3)	Pituitary tumor
Independent of T_4 binding proteins	Nontumorous hyperplasia
Acute psychiatric illness	
Acute nonthyroidal illness	Struma ovarii
Drugs (see Table 29.4)	Functioning metastatic thyroid carcinoma
Generalized resistance to thyroid hormone (GRTH)	Molar TSH-induced hyperthyroidism
Endogenous T_4 antibodies	
Familial 5'-deiodinase defect	

TBG, thyroid-binding globulin; TSH, thyroid-stimulating hormone.

on the limitations of the particular FT_4 assay employed. A similar familial syndrome is also seen with a TTR variant that exhibits increased T_4 avidity (67).

Drug-induced hyperthyroxinemia is seen with iopanoic acid and sodium ipodate (oral cholecystographic agents), amiodarone, and amphetamines. These agents decrease TT_3 leading to increased TT_4 (by 25% to 30%) and TSH (for a few weeks for cholecystographic agents, months for amiodarone) by their pharmacologic block of peripheral and pituitary deiodination of T_4 to T_3 (55). Although other well-known drugs such as propylthiouracil, propranolol (at doses >320 mg/day), and glucocorticoids block peripheral T_4 to T_3 conversion, hyperthyroxinemia does not ensue because of their failure to sufficiently block pituitary T_4 to T_3 deiodination (68). The TT_4 and TT_3 elevation seen in amphetamine abusers appears to be due to a central stimulation of TSH secretion and disappears with drug withdrawal (69).

As many as 33% of acute psychiatric admissions demonstrate elevated TT_4 or FT_4 values (18%) but normal TT_3 values (70). The initial TT_4 or FT_4 elevation is transient with gradual return to normal over 7 to 14 days without thyroid-directed therapy. The TT_3 and FT_3 values are not increased and serum TSH remains in the normal range. Although some patients demonstrate a blunted TSH response to a TRH challenge, this does not correlate with FT_4 elevation. Differentiation from mild T_4 thyrotoxicosis is possible by measuring serum TSH and FT_3, and observation is recommended until the clinical situation clarifies with time.

Slight elevation of TT_4, but low normal to low TT_3, is seen with aging alone probably as a result of impaired monodeiodination of T_4 to T_3. The TT_4, FT_4 (more commonly), and FT_4I are occasionally elevated in patients with NTI, but the TT_3 is low or low normal and rT_3 is markedly elevated as a result of

5'-deiodinase deficiency (71). Fortunately, contemporary serum TSH values are normal in both of these clinical situations. As the acute illness resolves, FT_4 and TT_4 values return to the normal range as T3 rises. Hyperthyroxinemia resulting from increased serum TBG level is seen in chronic active hepatitis, primary biliary cirrhosis, the acute phase of viral hepatitis, and in acute intermittent porphyria (72). FT_4 is usually normal unless concomitant hypothyroidism is present. Occasionally, patients with acute alcoholic hepatitis demonstrate transient TT_4 and FT_4 elevations of unknown mechanism. A normal serum TSH helps to exclude hyperthyroidism in this setting. Lastly, the TT_4, FT_4, and TT_3 are elevated in the syndromes of thyroid hormone resistance in which resistance to thyroid hormone may involve both peripheral and pituitary tissues (over 300 cases), peripheral tissues only (52 cases), or pituitary only (1 case) (19). Familial generalized resistance (GRTH), the most common syndrome, is manifested by goiter and excess thyroid hormone production despite clinical euthyroidism. In such patients, the serum TSH is inappropriately normal or elevated from failure of the negative feedback inhibition resulting from pituitary resistance. The mechanism of the peripheral and pituitary resistance is probably variable, but mutations in thyroid hormone receptors have been confirmed in families with generalized and peripheral resistance. Although rare, GRTH should be considered in any patient with markedly elevated thyroid hormone values but absent or minimal signs and/or symptoms of thyrotoxicosis.

Euthyroid Hypothyroxinemia

Low TT_3 levels are commonly seen in older adults and in patients with severe NTI because of impaired monodeiodination of T_4 to T_3. T_3 production is markedly reduced, the T_3 metabolic clearance rate is increased, and decreased T_3 binding to serum proteins is present. T_3 values resulting from these additive effects are usually less than 30 ng/dL, if they are detectable. In the absence of renal failure, rT_3 values are markedly elevated because metabolic clearance is reduced (73). With increasing illness severity, TT_4 falls as T_4 binding to serum proteins decreases and/or TBG concentration falls. The TT_4 concentration is low more often than that of FT_4. The FT_4 may be normal or low (depending on patient and assay) and the TT_3 is low, but the serum TSH should be detectable. This physiologic adaptation to severe illness (euthyroid sick syndrome) is seen in 30% to 50% of patients in a medical intensive care unit. Yet, the prevalence of true hypothyroidism or hyperthyroidism in patients with NTI is less than 1% (72). The severity of the TT_4 changes correlates with subsequent mortality, with greater than 80% mortality seen for patients with TT_4 less than 3.0 µg/dL as compared with a 15% mortality in patients with TT_4 levels greater than 5.0 µg/dL (74,75). However, T_4 administration in replacement doses does not improve survival (76). FT_4 values by direct equilibrium dialysis are variable, with low (2.3%) and high values (26%) seen (77). Serum TSH is probably the best indicator of thyroid status, although it is recognized that TSH suppression in hypothyroid patients with concomitant severe illness does occur especially in conjunction with dopamine and glucocorticoid therapy (8). In patients with NTI, both the FT_4 and TSH should be routinely ordered if thyroid disease is suspected.

Drug-induced hypothyroxinemia is infrequent (see Table 29.2). Phenytoin interferes with T_4 protein binding and accelerates T_4 metabolism leading to low TT_4, FT_4, and FT_4I despite normal TT_3 and TSH, whereas large doses of aspirin, fenclofenac, and phenylbutazone induce low TT_4, FT_4I, and TT_3 but normal FT_4 and TSH. Dopamine can lower TT_4, FT_4, TT_3, and TSH values, especially in the NTI setting (55).

ROLE OF *IN VITRO* TESTS IN EVALUATION OF THYROID DISORDERS

A detailed discussion of this topic is beyond the scope of this chapter. The underlying pathophysiologic mechanisms for the common thyroid diseases causing hyperthyroidism and hypothyroidism, however, are briefly discussed.

Nodular Goiter

The classic description of the evolution of thyroid nodules by Taylor (78), and subsequent studies has helped to clarify this subject, although controversies remain (79–82). There is considerable heterogeneity in thyroid cell function in response to TSH and in growth (replication) rates. These individual cell characteristics are transferred probably for the first few generations, and there may be a tendency in some cells, over decades, to form nodules consisting of clone(s) with increased function. The higher incidence of nodular thyroid disease often with subclinical hyperthyroidism in the older adult population supports this hypothesis. Although growth is influenced by TSH stimulation and by the availability of iodine, the cells are capable of inheriting acquired changes in (TSH-induced) growth capacities and may not require TSH stimulation after a certain point. Thus, some cell clusters eventually acquire new and stable growth rates that cannot be slowed significantly by TSH suppression. This mechanism may explain why suppressive thyroid hormone therapy may fail to decrease nodule size (83). Recent studies suggest an additional mechanism for nodular growth constitutively activating gain-of-function mutations of the TSH receptor (84,85). The extranodular thyroid tissue may well possess clones of cells with the same function as those in the toxic nodule, but because of their smaller numbers and lower overall function, such tissue accumulates less radiotracer and may appear to be suppressed.

Heterogeneity in cell function suggests that cold adenomas may originate from cells that have relatively decreased function to begin with, or, alternatively, a hot adenoma may subsequently become cold because cell function and heterogeneity are dynamic processes that change over time (79,80). Lastly, hemorrhage and necrosis in a hot adenoma is an alternative explanation for cold lesion on thyroid scanning (78).

Graves' Disease

Given the complexities of the immune system, the pathophysiologic mechanisms responsible for Graves' disease are not entirely understood and continue to be the subject of considerable debate. Regardless of the underlying mechanisms, the immediate cause of Graves' hyperthyroidism seems clearer. Patients have TSH receptor autoantibodies (TRAb), produced by lymphocytes within the thyroid that are either stimulatory or inhibitory (49). (See the section on thyroid autoantibodies.) Successful treatment with radioiodine or thionamides has been associated with a decrease in stimulating antibodies and increase in blocking antibodies (86,87).

Although the underlying immunopathologic mechanisms remain unclear, environmental factors influencing immunoregulation have been implicated as precipitating factors for excess TSAb production. A number of infectious agents, including *Yersinia enterocolitica,* have been linked to Graves' disease. Such a hypothesis is attractive, particularly in light of the occasional occurrence of Graves' disease in unrelated couples (88,89). Mental stress often precedes the onset of Graves' disease and could perhaps be a precipitating factor by virtue of its inhibitory effect on immune suppression (90). It is also known that a genetic predisposition exists for Graves' disease and that the underlying abnormalities for Graves' disease and Hashimoto's disease are closely related. The occurrence of each of these disorders in different members of the same family, as well as reports of monozygotic twins, one with Graves' disease, the other with HT, support a common basis for these two disorders (91).

The possible relationship between sustained thyroid stimulation with TSAb or TSH and neoplastic change is an important consideration. Graves' disease is associated with a somewhat higher incidence of thyroid cancer and probably a more aggressive tumor behavior (92).

Subacute Thyroiditis

Subacute thyroiditis, also called de Quervain's or granulomatous thyroiditis, is an inflammatory thyroid disorder believed to be the result of a viral infection. The disorder may occur in clusters and has a seasonal prevalence (88). Although earlier attempts were directed at isolating a single virus as the causative agent for subacute thyroiditis, it now appears that a large number of viruses may be associated with the disorder.

Typically, the entire gland is involved; however, the condition may begin in only a part of the thyroid with subsequent involvement of other areas. The clinical symptoms may last from a few weeks to a few months. The patient may be hyperthyroid initially as a result of release of thyroid hormone from the damaged gland. At this stage, it is usually impossible to image the thyroid with ^{99m}Tc-pertechnetate or radioiodine and the 24-hour uptake is very low and is an important clue in diagnosis (93). Subsequently, as intrathyroidal stores of hormone are depleted, the patient becomes hypothyroid. Eventually, thyroid function returns to normal. Over an extended period of a few years, however, some patients may become hypothyroid (94).

The possibility of autoimmune sequelae of subacute thyroiditis has been entertained in light of the findings of antithyroid antibodies including TRAb in this disorder and reports of the sequential occurrence of subacute thyroiditis and Graves' disease (88). In the vast majority of cases, however, no permanent immune-related condition is found, and the thyroid autoantibodies may represent a nonspecific response to released thyroid antigens.

Postpartum Thyroiditis and Silent Thyroiditis

The term *postpartum thyroiditis* refers to a clinical syndrome characterized by hyperthyroidism that resolves spontaneously, and the hyperthyroid or destructive phase is associated with the inability to image the thyroid gland. In this respect, postpartum thyroiditis resembles subacute thyroiditis. As with subacute thyroiditis, there are three stages in the disease course—hyperthyroidism, hypothyroidism, and, finally, euthyroidism, although not all stages are clinically recognizable. Although similarities exist, these conditions are not necessarily identical pathologic entities.

Thyroiditis is a common manifestation of postpartum thyroid dysfunction caused by exacerbation of an underlying autoimmune process, presumably as a result of immune "rebound" after pregnancy. Increase in thyroid autoantibody levels in the first trimester or at delivery is associated with a higher incidence of postpartum thyroid dysfunction, and the condition may recur in subsequent pregnancies (95–99). The reported exacerbation of autoimmune thyroid disease by cytokine therapy with resultant transient hyperthyroidism may represent an analogous condition (61–63).

The term *silent* or *painless* thyroiditis has been used loosely to describe any syndrome of transient hyperthyroidism. Histopathologic confirmation is sparse, and although these cases may represent a mixed bag of different entities, most are probably autoimmune (98,100). It is also conceivable that occasional outbreaks of silent thyroiditis in the past actually represented thyrotoxicosis factitia resulting from the ingestion of beef products containing bovine thyroid gland rich in hormone and iodine (101).

Jod-Basedow Phenomenon

Excess intake of iodide can lead to either hypothyroidism or hyperthyroidism, although, in most instances, a euthyroid status is maintained by autoregulatory mechanisms (55,102). Iodide-induced hyperthyroidism, also known as the Jod-Basedow phenomenon, occurs more often in areas of iodine deficiency where, presumably, the thyroid gland is more hyperplastic as a result of TSH stimulation. For the same reason, a higher incidence of iodide-induced hyperthyroidism is also seen in patients with nodular thyroid glands. A number of sources of excess iodide have been identified, including foods such as seaweed and milk (in certain areas), drugs such as amiodarone and topical iodine, and radiographic contrast dyes. The use of therapeutic potassium iodide in areas of endemic iodine deficiency also may be a predisposing factor.

Hyperthyrotropin States

Trophoblastic tumors, including hydatidiform mole and choriocarcinoma, are another potential cause of hyperthyroidism. hCG has TSH-like effects on the thyroid and is believed to have a role in the regulation of thyroid function in normal pregnancy (103). Although high levels of hCG could theoretically cause the hyperthyroidism of trophoblastic disease, some investigators have implicated a variant and more potent form of hCG (103, 104).

Hyperthyroidism resulting from pituitary-TSH excess is an uncommon condition (105). Hyperthyroidism generally results from selective, or relatively greater, resistance to the action of thyroid hormone at the pituitary level compared with that in peripheral tissues. The pituitary, unable to "sense" increasing levels of thyroid hormone, continues to respond to TRH stimulation with increased TSH secretion that, in turn, increases T_4 and T_3 levels. Thyrotoxic manifestations ensue because peripheral tissue response to thyroid hormone is preserved. Some patients with TSH excess hyperthyroidism may have a pituitary defect in converting T_4 to T_3, i.e., abnormality in the pituitary (type II) 5'-deiodinase, with the result that intrapituitary T_3 levels are decreased and TSH production is increased. Pituitary hyperplasia and microadenomas have been found in some patients with TSH-excess hyperthyroidism, possibly resulting, at least in some instances, from chronic TRH stimulation resulting from the absence of negative feedback at the pituitary level.

Thyrotropin levels that are high relative to circulating thyroid hormone levels, as in the disorder described earlier, fall under the category of inappropriate TSH secretion (106). However, not all instances of inappropriate TSH secretion are associated with hyperthyroidism. Thus, generalized (i.e., pituitary and peripheral tissue) resistance to thyroid hormone is not associated with hyperthyroidism. Similarly, drugs such as iopanoic acid and amiodarone, which decrease the conversion of T_4 to T_3 in pituitary as well as in peripheral tissues, may cause relative increase in T_4 levels in the absence of TSH suppression.

Autoimmune Thyroid Disease

Autoimmune thyroiditis is the most common cause of hypothyroidism. The terms *autoimmune thyroiditis* and *HT* are often used interchangeably, although Hashimoto's disease originally was described as the goitrous variety of autoimmune thyroiditis characterized by diffuse lymphocytic infiltration, fibrosis, atrophy of follicular cells, and eosinophilic changes in some follicular cells (Hürthle cells). Variations in histologic characteristics may occur, particularly in childhood, adolescence, and the postpartum period, and atrophic and fibrous forms also occur. Despite varying histology, these entities share a common pathogenetic mechanism, namely a T-cell mediated organ-specific autoimmune process. A genetic predisposition for this disorder is present, although environmental factors, such as excess iodides and infection, also may play a role (88,107,108). HT is associated with increased levels of autoantibodies to TPO (antimicrosomal) and thyroglobulin. Levels of anti-TPO antibodies generally correlate with the degree of thyroid dysfunction. These antibodies also inhibit peroxidase enzyme, which is responsible for organification of trapped iodine. Autoimmune thyroiditis or HT is not a specific clinical entity. Patients with this disorder usually present with goiter with or without hypothyroidism. Occasionally, they may present with transient hyperthyroidism followed, over time, by hypothyroidism. Such a course is typical in the postpartum period. (See the section on postpartum thyroiditis.)

Iodine-Deficiency Thyroid Disease

Iodine deficiency continues to be a cause of thyroid disorders in certain parts of the world (107). Endemic goiter with or without hypothyroidism and endemic cretinism with or without neurologic deficits are the hallmarks of iodine deficiency. As mentioned earlier, the severity of the neurologic deficits in endemic cretinism probably is related to both fetal and maternal thyroid function (109).

Endemic goiter today is probably related to a combination of factors including iodine deficiency; deficiency of another trace element, selenium; and presence of environmental goitrogens (110,111). Among the latter, the role of industrial chemicals, which promote metabolic disposal of thyroid hormone and lead to TSH-mediated thyroid growth, was discussed earlier. (See the section on hepatic enzyme-inducing drugs.) In addition, a number of foods, particularly cassava, release thiocyanate after ingestion. The goitrogenic effect of thiocyanate is related primarily to its inhibitory effect on iodide trapping by the thyroid gland.

Iodine Excess Thyroid Disease

Iodine excess occasionally may lead to goiter formation with or without hypothyroidism. Large amounts of iodine may decrease synthesis and release of thyroid hormone (Wolff Chaikoff effect), and a dose-dependent increase in the incidence of hypothyroidism has been found in areas of high dietary iodine uptake (112). The development of iodide goiter in the past from the use of therapeutic iodides for pulmonary conditions is in accord with this mechanism. Although foods such as seaweed are a frequent source of excess iodine in certain populations, other sources include drugs such as amiodarone and ipodate.

Excess iodine intake probably can lead to goiter formation and hypothyroidism in the absence of underlying thyroid disease. However, it is also well known that autoimmune thyroid disease is highly sensitive to the hypothyroid effects of exogenous iodides, a phenomenon used for the control of hyperthyroidism following radioiodine therapy or thyroidectomy. Perhaps the most intriguing aspect of iodide-induced goitrogenesis is the possibility that iodides may initiate or promote autoimmune thyroiditis (107,108). Epidemiologic findings appear to support this view (111). A change from iodine-deficiency to iodine-sufficiency in some regions has been associated with an increase in the incidence of autoimmune thyroid disease and no decrease in goiter prevalence.

Other Conditions

Central hypothyroidism is an uncommon disorder arising from the failure of TSH or TRH secretion. The condition usually results from tumors, surgery, or radiation therapy involving the pituitary or hypothalamus and from ischemic necrosis of the pituitary (Sheehan's syndrome). A subtler and intriguing form of hypothyroidism may occur in psychiatric illness. A subgroup of patients with refractory depression appears to respond to treatment when thyroid hormone is added to the antidepressant drug regimen (113). Although these patients are thought to have CNS-mediated hypothyroidism, the exact mechanism is unclear. Decrease in CNS β-adrenergic receptor function has been implicated, although abnormalities in other neurotransmitter systems cannot be excluded.

REFERENCES

1. Kaplan MM. Clinical perspectives in the diagnosis of thyroid disease. *Clin Chem* 1999;45:1377–1383.
2. Glinoer D. The regulation of thyroid function in pregnancy: pathways of endocrine adaptation from physiology to pathology. *Endocr Rev* 1997;18:404–433.
3. Glinoer D, Delange F. The potential repercussions of maternal, fetal, and neonatal hypothyroxinemia on the progeny. *Thyroid* 2000; 10: 871–887.
4. Martino E, Bambini G, Bartalena L et al. Human serum thyrotropin measurements by ultrasensitive immunoradiometric assay as a first line test in the evaluation of thyroid function. *Clin Endocrinol* 1986; 24:141–148.
5. Garcia EJ, Fiori A. Radioimmunoassay and competitive binding analysis. In: Rocha A, Harbert J, eds. *Textbook of nuclear medicine: basic science.* Philadelphia: Lea & Febiger, 1978:341.
6. Chan DW. Automation of thyroid function testing. *Clin Lab Med* 1993;13:631–644.
7. Zurakowski D, DiCanzio J, Majzoub JA. Pediatric reference intervals for serum thyroxine, triiodothyronine, thyrotropin, and free thyroxine. *Clin Chem* 1999;45:1087–1090.
8. Kaptein EM. Clinical application of free thyroxine determinations. *Clin Lab Med* 1993;13:653–672.
9. Liewendahl K, Melamies L, Helenius T et al. Automated and manual serum free thyroxine assays evaluated with equilibrium dialysis. *Scand J Clin Lab Invest* 1994;54:347–351.
10. Spencer CA, LoPresti JS, Patel A et al. Applications of a new chemiluminometric thyrotropin assay to subnormal measurement. *J Clin Endocrinol Metab* 1990;70:452–460.
11. Ladenson PW, Singer PA, Ain KB et al. American Thyroid Association guidelines for detection of thyroid dysfunction. *Arch Inter Med* 2000;160:1573–1575.
12. Helfand M, Redfern CC. Screening for thyroid disease: an update. *Ann Intern Med* 1998;129:144–158.
13. Thonnart B, Messian O, Linhart NC et al. Ten highly sensitive thyrotropin assays compared by receiver-operating characteristic curves analysis. Results of a prospective multicenter study. *Clin Chem* 1988; 34:691–695.
14. Bayer MF. Effective laboratory evaluation of thyroid status. *Med Clin North Am* 1991;75:1–26.
15. Despres N, Grant AM. Antibody interference in thyroid assays: a potential for clinical misinformation. *Clin Chem* 1998;44: 2557–2559.
16. Klee GG, Hay ID. Assessment of sensitive thyrotropin assays for an expanded role in thyroid function testing: proposed criteria for analytic performance and clinical utility. *J Clin Endocrinol Metab* 1987; 64:461–471.
17. Weintraub BD, Gershengorn MC, Kourides IA et al. Inappropriate secretion of thyroid stimulating hormone. *Ann Intern Med* 1981;95: 339–351.
18. Beckers A, Abs R, Mahler C et al. Thyrotropin-secreting pituitary adenomas: report of seven cases. *Clin Endocrinol Metab* 1991;72: 477–483.
19. Refetoff S. Resistance to thyroid hormone. *Clin Lab Med* 1993;13: 563–581.
20. Fisher DA, Dussault JH, Foley TP et al. Screening for congenital hypothyroidism: results of screening one million North American infants. *J Pediatr* 1979;94:700–705.
21. Dussault JH. Neonatal screening for congenital hypothyroidism. *Clin Lab Med* 1993;13:645–652.
22. Fisher, DA. Clinical review 19. Management of congenital hypothyroidism. *J Clin Endocrinol Metab* 1991;72:523–529.

23. Seesko HG, Wells SA. Thyroid tumors. In: Mercer DW, Herberman RB, eds. *Immunodiagnosis of cancer,* 2nd ed. New York: Dekker, Marcel, 1990:431–452.
24. Piechaczyk M, Baldet L, Pau B et al. Novel immunoradiometric assay of thyroglobulin in serum with use of monoclonal antibodies selected for lack of cross-reactivity with autoantibodies. *Clin Chem* 1989;35:422–424.
25. Pacini F, Lari R, Mazzeo S et al. Diagnostic value of a single serum thyroglobulin determination on and off thyroid suppressive therapy in the follow-up of patients with differentiated thyroid cancer. *Clin Endocrinol* 1985;23:405–411.
26. Black EG, Sheppard MC, Hoffenberg R. Serial thyroglobulin measurements in the management of differentiated thyroid carcinoma. *Clin Endocrinol* 1987;27:115–120.
27. Schlumberger M, Tubiana M. Serum Tg measurements and total body I-131 scans in the follow-up of thyroid cancer patients. In: Hamburger JI, ed. *Diagnostic methods in clinical thyroidology.* New York: Springler-Verlag, 1989:147–157.
28. Mazzaferri EL, Kloos RT. Is diagnostic iodine-131 scanning with recombinant human TSH useful in the follow-up of differentiated thyroid cancer after thyroid ablation? *J Clin Endocrinol Metab* 2000; 87:1490–1498.
29. Lubin E, Mechlis-Frish S, Zatz S et al. Serum thyroglobulin and iodine-131 whole body scan in the diagnosis and assessment of treatment for metastatic differentiated thyroid carcinoma. *J Nucl Med* 1994;35:257–262.
30. Mazzaferri EL. Recombinant human thyrotropin symposium: An overview of the management of papillary and follicular thyroid carcinoma. *Thyroid* 1999;9:421–427.
31. Madeddu G, Casu AR, Constanza C et al. Serum thyroglobulin levels in the diagnosis and follow-up of subacute "painful" thyroiditis. *Arch Intern Med* 1985;145:243–247.
32. Mariotti S, Martino E, Cupini C et al. Low serum thyroglobulin as a clue to the diagnosis of thyrotoxicosis factitia. *N Engl J Med* 1982; 307:410–412.
33. Yamamoto M, Saito S, Sakurada T et al. Effect of prednisolone and salicylate on serum thyroglobulin level in patients with subacute thyroiditis. *Clin Endocrinol* 1987;27:339–344.
34. Klein RZ. Infantile hypothyroidism: then and now. Results of neonatal screening. *Curr Prob Pediatr* 1985;15:1–58.
35. Heinze HJ, Shulman DI, Diamond FB et al. Spectrum of serum thyroglobulin elevation in congenital thyroid disorders. *Thyroid* 1993; 3:37–40.
36. Austin LA, Heath H III. Calcitonin: physiology and pathology. *N Engl J Med* 1981;304:269–278.
37. Becker KL, Snider RH, Moore CF et al. Calcitonin in extrathyroidal tissues of man. *Acta Endocrinol (Copenh)* 1979;92:746–751.
38. Wohllk N, Cote GJ, Evans DB et al. Application of genetic screening information to the management of medullary thyroid carcinoma and multiple endocrine neoplasia type 2. *Endocrinol Metab Clin North Am* 1996;25:1–25.
39. Ponder BA, Ponder MA, Coffey R et al. Risk estimation and screening in families of patients with medullary thyroid carcinoma. *Lancet* 1988; 1:397–401.
40. Gagel RF, Jackson CE, Block MA et al. Age-related probability of development of hereditary medullary thyroid carcinoma. *J Pediatr* 1982;101:941–946.
41. Gagel RF, Tashjian AH Jr, Cummings T et al. The clinical outcome of prospective screening for multiple endocrine neoplasia type 2a. An 18-year experience. *N Engl J Med* 1988;318:478–484.
42. Brown J, Solomon DH, Beall GN et al. Autoimmune thyroid disease—Graves' and Hashimoto's. *Ann Intern Med* 1978;88:379–391.
43. Volpe R. The role of autoimmunity in hypoendocrine and hyperendocrine function with special emphasis on autoimmune thyroid disease. *Ann Intern Med* 1977;87:86–99.
44. Hamburger JI, Miller JM, Kini SR. Lymphoma of the thyroid. *Ann Intern Med* 1983;99:685–693.
45. Orgiazzi J. Anti-TSH receptor antibodies in clinical practice. *Endocrinol Metab Clin North Am* 2000;29:339–355.
46. Matsuura N, Konishi J, Fujieda K et al. TSH-receptor antibodies in mothers with Graves' disease and outcome in their offspring. *Lancet* 1988;1:14–17.
47. Tamaki H, Amino N, Aozasa M et al. Universal predictive criteria for neonatal overt thyrotoxicosis requiring treatment. *Am J Perinatol* 1988;5:152–158.
48. Cooper DS. Antithyroid drugs. *N Engl J Med* 1984;311:1353.
49. Tamai H, Kasagi K, Takaichi Y et al. Development of spontaneous hypothyroidism in patients with Graves' disease treated with antithyroidal drugs: clinical, immunological, and histological findings in 26 patients. *J Clin Endocrinol Metab* 1989;69:49.
50. Rees Smith B, McLachlan SM, Furmariak J. Autoantibodies to the thyrotropin receptor. *Endocr Rev* 1988;9:106–121.
51. Rubello D, Sonino N, Casara D et al. Acute and chronic effects of high glucocorticoid levels on hypothalamic-pituitary-thyroid axis in man. *J Endocr Invest* 1992;15:437–441.
52. Klein I, Levey GS. Iodide excess and thyroid function. *Ann Intern Med* 1983;98:406–409.
53. Brown RS, Cohen JH, Braverman LE. Successful treatment of massive acute thyroid hormone poisoning with iopanoic acid. *J Pediatr* 1998; 132:903–905.
54. Konno N, Makita H, Yuri K et al. Association between dietary iodine intake and prevalence of subclinical hypothyroidism in the coastal regions of Japan. *J Clin Endocrinol Metab* 1994;78:393–397.
55. Surks, M, Sievert R. Drug therapy: drugs and thyroid function. *N Engl J Med* 1998;333:1688–1694.
56. Perrild H, Hegedus L, Baastrup PC et al. Thyroid function and ultrasonically determined thyroid size in patients receiving long-term lithium treatment. *Am J Psychiatry* 1990;147:1518–1521.
57. Martino E, Bartalena L, Bogazzi F et al. The effects of amiodarone on the thyroid. *Endocr Rev* 2001;22:240–254.
58. Wenzel KW. Pharmacologic interference with *in vitro* tests of thyroid function. *Metabolism* 1981;30:717–721.
59. Bartalena L. Recent achievements in studies on thyroid hormone-binding proteins. *Endocr Rev* 1990;11:47–64.
60. Yabu Y, Amir SM, Ruiz M et al. Heterogeneity of thyroxine binding by serum albumins in normal subjects and patients with familial dysalbuminemic hyperthyroxinemia. *J Clin Endocrinol Metab* 1985;60:451–459.
61. Atkins MB, Mier JW, Parkinson DR et al. Hypothyroidism after treatment with interleukin-2 and lymphokine-activated killer cells. *N Engl J Med* 1988;318:1557–1563.
62. Kung AW, Jones BM, Lai CL. Effects of interferon-γ therapy on thyroid function, T-lymphocyte subpopulations and induction of autoantibodies. *J Clin Endocr Metab* 1990;71:1230–1234.
63. Sauter NP, Atkins MB, Mier JW. Transient thyrotoxicosis and persistent hypothyroidism due to acute autoimmune thyroiditis after interleukin-2 and interferon-α therapy for metastatic carcinoma: a case report. *Am J Med* 1992;92:441–444.
64. Campbell NRC, Hasinoff BB, Stalts H et al. Ferrous sulfate reduces thyroxine efficacy in patients with hypothyroidism. *Ann Int Med* 1992;117:1010–1013.
65. Ain KB, Pucino F, Shiver TM et al. Thyroid hormone levels affected by time of blood sampling in thyroxine-treated patients. *Thyroid* 1993;3:81–85.
66. Lee WNP, Golden MP, Van Herle AJ et al. Inherited abnormal thyroid-binding protein causing selective increase of total serum thyroxine. *J Clin Endocrinol Metab* 1979;49:292–299.
67. Moses AC, Lawlor J, Haddow J et al. Familial euthyroid hyperthyroxinemia resulting from increased thyroxine binding to thyroxine-binding pre-albumin. *N Engl J Med* 1982;306:966–969.
68. Borst GC, Eil C, Burman KD. Euthyroid hyperthyroxinemia. *Ann Intern Med* 1983;98:366–377.
69. Morley JE, Shafer RB. Thyroid function screening in new psychiatric admissions. *Arch Intern Med* 1982;142:591–593.
70. Spratt DI, Pont A, Miller MB et al. Hyperthyroxinemia in patients with acute psychiatric disorders. *Am J Med* 1982;73:41–48.
71. Gavin LA, Rosenthal M, Cavalieri RR. The diagnostic dilemma of hyperthyroxinemia in acute illness. *JAMA* 1979;242:251–253.
72. Cavalieri RR. The effects of nonthyroid disease and drugs on thyroid function tests. *Med Clin North Am* 1991;75:27–39.

73. Kaptein EM, Robinson WJ, Grieb DA et al. Peripheral serum thyroxine, triiodothyronine and reverse triiodothyronine kinetics in the low thyroxine state of acute non-thyroidal illness: a non-compartmental analysis. *J Clin Invest* 1982;69:526–535.

74. Kaptein EM, Weiner JM, Robinson WJ et al. Relationship of altered thyroid hormone indices to survival in nonthyroidal illnesses. *Clin Endocrinol* 1982;16:565–574.

75. Slag MF, Morley JE, Elson MK et al. Hypothyroxinemia in critically ill patients as a predictor of high mortality. *JAMA* 1981;245:43–49.

76. Brent G, Hershman JM. Thyroxine therapy in patients with severe nonthyroidal illnesses and low serum thyroxine concentration. *J Clin Endocrinol Metab* 1986;63:1–8.

77. Nelson JC, Tomei RT, Wilcox RB. Altered T4 binding, disordered pituitary-thyroid regulation and thyroid diagnosis in nonthyroidal illnesses (NTI). *Thyroid* 1992;2:S–26.

78. Taylor S. The evolution of nodular goiter. *J Clin Endocrinol Metab* 1953;54:1232–1237.

79. Studer H, Peter HJ, Gerber H. Natural heterogeneity of thyroid cells: the basis for understanding thyroid function and nodular goiter growth. *Endocr Rev* 1989;10:125–135.

80. Studer H, Gerber H, Zbaeren J et al. Histomorphological and immunohistochemical evidence that the human nodular goiters grow by episodic replication of multiple clusters of thyroid follicular cells. *J Clin Endocrinol Metab* 1992;75:1151–1158.

81. Rieu M, Bekka S, Sambor B et al. Prevalence of subclinical hyperthyroidism and relationship between thyroid hormonal status and thyroid ultrasonographic parameters in patients with non-toxic nodular goiter. *Clin Endocrinol* 1993;39:67–71.

82. Sawin CT, Geller A, Wolf PA et al. Low serum thyrotropin concentrations as a risk factor for atrial fibrillation in older persons. *N Engl J Med* 331;1249:1949–1952.

83. Gharib H, Mazaferri EL. Thyroxine suppressive therapy in patients with nodular thyroid disease. *Ann Int Med* 1998;128:386–394.

84. Tonacchera M, Chiovato L, Pinchera A et al. Hyperfunctioning thyroid nodules in toxic multinodular goiter share activating thyrotropin receptor mutations with solitary toxic adenoma. *J Clin Endocrinol Metab* 1998;88:492–498.

85. Paschke A, Ludgate M. The thyrotropin receptor in thyroid diseases. *N Engl J Med* 1997;337:1675–1681.

86. Rees Smith B, McLachla SM, Furmariak J. Autoantibodies to the thyrotropin receptor. *Endocr Rev* 1988;9:106–121.

87. Woeber K. The year in review: the thyroid. *Ann Int Med* 1999;131:959–962.

88. Tomer Y, Davies TF. Infection, thyroid disease and autoimmunity. *Endocr Rev* 1993;14:107–120.

89. McIver B, Morris JC. The pathogenesis of Graves' disease. *Endocrinol Metab Clin North Am* 1998;27:73–89.

90. Locke S, Ader R, Besedovsky H et al. *Foundations of psychoneuroimmunology.* New York: Aldine, 1985.

91. Chertow BS, Fidler WJ, Farriss BL. Graves' disease and Hashimoto's thyroiditis in monozygous twins. *Acta Endocrinol* 1973;72:18–24.

92. Mazzaferri EL. Thyroid cancer and Graves' disease. *J Clin Endocrinol Metab* 1990;70:826–829.

93. Smallridge RC, DeKeyser FM, van Herle AJ et al. Thyroid iodine content and serum thyroglobulin; clues to the natural history of destruction-induced thyroiditis. *J Clin Endocrinol Metab* 1986;62:1213–1219.

94. Benker G, Olbricht TH, Windeck R et al. the sonographical and function sequelae of de Quervain's subacute thyroiditis; long-term follow-up. *Acta Endocrinol* 1988;117:435–441.

95. Parker RH, Beierwaltes WH. Thyroid antibodies during pregnancy and in the newborn. *J Clin Endocrinol Metab* 1961;21:792–801.

96. Stegnaro-Green A, Roman SH, Cobin RH et al. A prospective study of lymphocyte-initiated immunosuppression in normal pregnancy: evidence of a T-cell etiology for postpartum thyroid dysfunction. *J Clin Endocr Metab* 1992;74:645–653.

97. Amino N, Tada H, Hidaka Y et al. Screening for postpartum thyroiditis. *J Clin Endocrinol Metab* 1999;84:1813–1821.

98. LaVolsi VA. Postpartum thyroiditis: the pathology slowly unravels. *Am J Clin Pathol* 1993;100:193–195.

99. Mizukami Y, Michigishi T, Nonomura A et al. Postpartum thyroiditis: a clinical, histologic, and immunopathologic study of 15 cases. *Am J Clin Pathol* 1993;100:200–205.

100. Morrison J, Caplan RH. Typical and atypical ("silent") subacute thyroiditis in a wife and husband. *Arch Int Med* 1978;138:45–48.

101. Kinney JS, Hurwitz EB, Fishbein DB et al. Community outbreak of thyrotoxicosis: epidemiology, immunogenetic characteristics, and long-term outcome. *Am J Med* 1988;84:10–18.

102. Woeber, K. Update on management of hyperthyroidism and hypothyroidism. *Arch Fam Med* 2000;9:743–747.

103. Kennedy RL, Darne J. The role of hCG in regulation of the thyroid gland in normal and abnormal pregnancy. *Obstet Gynecol* 1991;78:298–307.

104. Mann K, Hoermann R. Thyroid stimulation by placental factors. *J Endocrinol Invest* 1993;16:378–384.

105. Bodenner D, Lash R. Thyroid disease mediated by molecular defects in cell surface and nuclear receptors. *Am J Med* 1998;105:524–538.

106. Jackson JA, Verdonk CA, Spiekerman AM. Euthyroid hyperthyroxinemia and inappropriate secretion of thyrotropin. Recognition and diagnosis. *Arch Int Med* 1987;147:1311–1313.

107. Boyages SC. Iodine deficiency disorders. *J Clin Endocrinol Metab* 1993;77:587–591.

108. Sundick RS, Herdegen DM, Brown TR et al. The incorporation of dietary iodine into thyroglobulin increases its immunogenicity. *Endocrinology* 1987;120:2078–2084.

109. Porterfield SP, Hendrich CE. The role of thyroid hormones in prenatal and neonatal neurological development—current perspectives. *Endocr Rev* 1993;14:94–106.

110. Curran PG, DeGroot LJ. The effect of hepatic enzyme-inducing drugs on thyroid hormones and the thyroid gland. *Endocr Rev* 1991;12:135–150.

111. Beierwaltes WH. Endocrine imaging in the management of goiter and thyroid nodules: Part I. *J Nucl Med* 1991;32:1455–1461.

112. Konno N, Makita H, Yuri K et al. Association between dietary iodine intake and prevalence of subclinical hypothyroidism in the costal regions of Japan. *J Clin Endocrinol Metab* 1994;78:393–397.

113. Howland RH. Thyroid dysfunction in refractory depression: implications for pathophysiology and treatment. *J Clin Psychiatry* 1993;54:47–54.

30

THYROID IMAGING

WILLIAM H. MARTIN
MARTIN P. SANDLER

Several imaging modalities, including nuclear medicine, sonography, x-ray fluorescent scanning, single photon emission computed tomography (SPECT), positron emission tomography (PET), x-ray transmission computed tomography (CT), and magnetic resonance imaging (MRI), have been used in an attempt to provide a noninvasive diagnosis in the care of patients with diseases of the thyroid gland. In this chapter, we discuss the imaging modalities used in the diagnosis of thyroid disorders.

EMBRYOLOGY

The thyroid gland can be recognized in the human embryo by the end of the first month after conception when the embryo is 3.5 to 4 mm long. The gland evolves from a medial primordium arising from two lateral primordia derived from the fourth and fifth branchial pouch complex. Toward the end of the fourth week of embryonic development, the thyroid is a bilobed structure. The lobes are joined together by the thyroglossal duct, which is attached to the ventral floor of the pharynx. The duct becomes a solid stalk and begins to atrophy by the sixth week, maintaining its pharyngeal connection in the form of a permanent pit (foramen caecum) situated at the apex of the V-shaped sulcus terminalis on the dorsum of the tongue. Toward the end of the seventh week, the gland assumes a new position at the level of the developing trachea while the pharynx grows forward. At this stage a narrow isthmus of developing thyroid tissue joins the two lobes located on either side of the trachea. Cells of the lower portion of the duct differentiate into thyroid tissue to form the pyramidal lobe. Thyroid tissue can be found anywhere between the base of the tongue and the retrosternal anterior mediastinum (Fig. 30.1). Part of the lateral lobe of the thyroid is derived from the ventral portion of the last branchial pouch, which remains as a separate gland known as the *ultimobranchial body* (1). This tissue is the source of origin of the parafollicular, or C, cells that secrete calcitonin (2), a 32-amino-acid polypeptide regulated by the same calcium sensor expressed in parathyroid cells. Although calcitonin affects renal handling of calcium and inhibits osteoclast-mediated bone resorption, the physiologic role of calcitonin in humans remains uncertain (2). Thyroid follicles begin developing by the eighth week of gestation and acquire colloid material by the third month (1). By approximately 10.5 weeks, the human fetal thyroid gland concentrates iodine and synthesizes the entire spectrum of organically bound iodinated hormones, including thyroxine (T_4) (3). Congenital abnormalities of the thyroid gland can be related to its embryologic development, including numerous hereditary enzyme deficiencies involved in the biosynthesis of T_4 (4) as well as agenesis and hemiagenesis.

ANATOMY

The thyroid gland is normally located in the lower part of the neck and consists of two lobes joined by an isthmus that crosses the second and third tracheal rings anteriorly (5). The thyroid is one of the largest endocrine organs, weighing approximately 15 to 25 g, and is enveloped by the pretracheal fascia. The isthmus measures approximately 2 cm $\times$ 2 cm $\times$ 0.5 cm. The individual lobes have an ellipsoid configuration—a pointed superior pole and poorly defined inferior pole merging medially toward the isthmus. Each lobe is approximately 2.0 to 2.5 cm in both thickness and width at its largest diameter and is approximately 4 to 4.5 cm long. A pyramidal lobe is present in 30% to 50% of patients. This lobe projects upward from the isthmus most often from the left lobe; it is only rarely active, however, except when there is diffuse thyroidal hyperplasia (6).

The thyroid gland is closely fixed to the anterior and lateral aspects of the trachea by loose connective tissue. A fibrous capsule, which invests the gland, is connected to the pretracheal fascia and causes the thyroid to move upward with deglutition. In most cases, the upper margin of the isthmus lies just below the cricoid cartilage, which provides an excellent landmark for locating the thyroid gland. The carotid arteries, jugular veins, and sternocleidomastoid muscles are lateral to the gland.

Two pairs of parathyroid glands are located superiorly and inferiorly along the posterior aspect of the thyroid lobes (see Chapter 32). The blood supply to the thyroid gland is from the superior thyroidal artery arising from the external carotid artery and from the inferior thyroidal artery, which emanates from the

W.H. Martin: Department of Radiology and Radiological Sciences, Vanderbilt University Medical Center, Nashville, TN.
M.P. Sandler: Department of Radiology and Radiological Sciences, Vanderbilt University Medical Center, Nashville, TN.

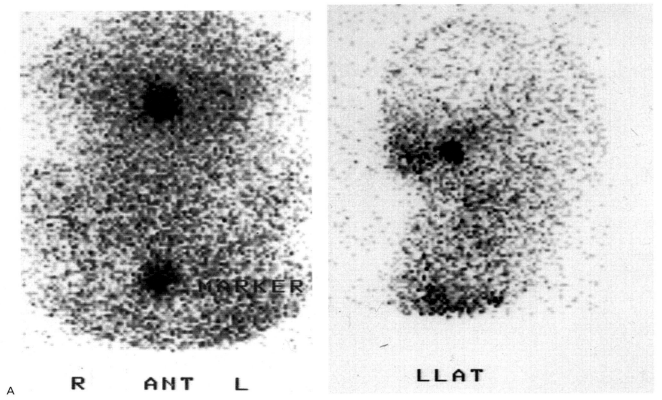

A R ANT L

LLAT B

FIGURE 30.1. Anterior **(A)** and lateral **(B)** ^{99m}Tc pertechnetate images show lingual thyroid at the base of the tongue. Increased background activity is suggestive of the coexistent hypothyroidism typical of ectopia.

thyrocervical trunk off the subclavian artery. The right lobe of the thyroid is frequently more vascular and slightly larger than the left. It also tends to enlarge more in disorders associated with a diffuse increase in gland size. A wide capillary network surrounds each follicle, and veins are derived from a perifollicular plexus. The veins accompany the arteries and drain into the jugular veins. Copious lymphatic vessels drain to locoregional nodes, including the deep cervical nodes in the tracheoesophageal groove and along the internal jugular veins as well as to the superior mediastinal nodes. The recurrent laryngeal nerve is adjacent to the posterior aspect of each thyroid lobe.

PHYSIOLOGY

See Chapter 29.

MEASUREMENT OF RADIOIODINE UPTAKE IN THE THYROID

Radioiodine uptake (RAIU) in the thyroid is a kinetic, nonimaging measurement of the percentage of an administered radioiodine dose incorporated by the thyroid over a standard time period, an individual measurement representing a single point in a dynamic process (7,8). This is illustrated with a continuous

plot of radioiodine uptake versus time (Fig. 30.2) that shows uptake increases gradually over 18 to 24 hours after oral administration. Although most patients with thyrotoxicosis have a similar pattern of uptake with an elevated percentage accumulation at 24 hours, an occasional patient with a high intrathyroidal turnover of iodine is incorrectly classified as having normal thyroid function on the basis of a normal 24-hour value. An early measurement, 4 to 6 hours after administration of the radioiodine, is useful to avoid this error.

Method

RAIU studies usually are performed with oral or intravenous administration of the radiotracer. ^{131}I sodium iodide is most frequently used, at a dose of 5 to 15 μCi, because orally administered iodine is rapidly and fairly completely absorbed in the fasting state (9). The rate of absorption, however, can vary from patient to patient and even from time to time for the same patient, so early uptake measurements (30 minutes to 4 hours after administration of the radionuclide) may be unreliable (10). Therefore, 24-hour RAIU measurements are used most often clinically. Measurements obtained within 30 minutes after intravenous injection or 2 to 6 hours after oral administration reflect thyroid trapping, whereas those obtained more than 6 hours after administration reflect organification (11). ^{131}I is available in liquid or capsule form, and reliable measurements can be

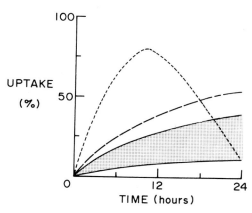

FIGURE 30.2. Radioiodine uptake versus time. Euthyroid range is represented by the *stippled area* and the typical hyperthyroid range by the *broken line*. In thyrotoxicosis, iodine uptake and turnover can be so rapid that the radioiodine is incorporated into thyroid hormone and discharged before the 24-hour measurement (*short broken line*) can be obtained. (From Powers TA. Radioiodine thyroid uptake measurement. In Sandler MP, Patton JA, Partain CL, eds. *Thyroid and parathyroid imaging.* Norwalk, CT: Appleton-Century-Crofts, 1986:181, with permission).

obtained with either (12–14). Capsules are easier to handle and allow less airborne exposure to workers. Artifactual depression in RAIU due to delayed or decreased absorption of commercially provided radioiodine capsules was reported in the 1970s but is no longer a problem (12–14).

Patient preparation for an uptake study is straightforward, although certain precautions must be taken. Because food present within the stomach can impair absorption, the patient should fast for 4 hours before administration of radioiodine to enhance absorption. The examiner should ascertain whether any iodine-containing agents or drugs known to affect thyroid function have been administered (Table 30.1). It also is important to know whether any isotopic studies have been recently performed. Because patients can be unaware of the radioactive na-

Table 30.1. *Factors Interfering in Thyroid Imaging*

Factor	Period
Iodide	
Lugol. SSKI	1–3 wk
Radiographic contrast agents	
Intravenous pyelogram angiogram	1–3 wk
Gallbladder agents	2–3 wk
Bronchogram	1 mo
Myelogram	Year
Antithyroid drugs (propylthiouracil, methimazole, perchlorate)	
Thyroid hormones	1 wk
Levo thyroxine (Synthroid[a])	4–6 wk
Triiodothyronine (Cytomel[a])	2 wk
Thyroid disease	
Thyroiditis acute phase	Transient
Hypothyroidism (primary, secondary, tertiary)	Permanent
Congenital and migrational problems of the thyroid	Permanent

[a]Brand names.
From Ashkar FS. Thyroid imaging and function studies. *Clin Nucl Med* 1981;6:P77–86.

ture of the examination, it is useful to make a preliminary background count over the thyroid to check for residual activity. If ^{131}I is used for the uptake measurements, administration of ^{99m}Tc pertechnetate (^{99m}Tc) as for a thyroid scan, should be delayed until after completion of the RAIU study to avoid errors due to coincidence counts from the ^{99m}Tc. If ^{131}I is present, background counts must be measured before administration of the uptake dose so that they can be accounted for in the uptake calculation.

A thyroid detector probe usually is used to perform thyroid uptake measurements. This consists of an open collimated sodium iodide crystal coupled to a single photomultiplier tube with accompanying electronics. Room background counts are obtained to detect isotope contamination or gross equipment malfunction (15). A scintillation camera with a pinhole collimator can be used to obtain uptake measurements identical to those obtained with a conventional uptake probe (16).

With the probe, uptake measurement is performed by means of counting both the patient dose (capsule) and a standard capsule of similar activity in a neck phantom. The phantom is an acrylic container machined to the size of the average neck with a small hole into which the capsule can be inserted. Each capsule is counted for at least 10,000 counts (standard deviation, 1%), and the result is expressed in counts per minute (cpm). The counts are obtained at a standard distance of 25 to 35 cm from the phantom (this varies from system to system), which is also used for counting patient activity. After a background count is obtained over the thyroid, the dose capsule is administered to the patient. The patient is instructed to return in 4 and in 24 hours, at which time measurements are again obtained of the standard capsule, the patient thyroid, and the thigh. The latter measurement is used to correct for nonthyroid blood-pool activity and is taken at a point equal to the diameter of the neck (17). Percentage uptake can than be calculated as follows:

$$\% \ Uptake = \frac{Thyroid \ cmp\left(t\right) - Thigh \ cpm\left(t\right)}{Standard \ cmp\left(t\right)}$$
$$\times \frac{Standard \ cpm\left(0\right)}{Patient \ capsule \ cpm\left(0\right)} \times 100$$

where *cmp(0)* is counts per minute at the time of administration and *cpm(t)* is counts per minute at time *t*.

The second term in the equation is necessary because capsules, even of the same lot number, can contain different activities. Use of one capsule as a standard without normalizing it to the patient dose capsule can cause large errors in the uptake measurement (18). Each laboratory should establish a normal range of values because the uptake measurements are influenced by dietary iodine (19) and vary with geographic location (20). Normal values are expressed as the mean of the uptake in the population ± 2 standard deviations, but usually are written as a range, such as 10% to 25% at 24 hours. RAIU can be as high as 70% from birth to 3 days of age but declines to adult levels by 1 year of age (21).

Other methods used to estimate background contribution include measuring the neck activity with a lead shield covering the thyroid and quantifying the proportion of total body radioiodine in the neck of a patient with thyroid disease. This value averages 2.5% from 2 to 120 minutes after the dose is administered. Because nonthyroid activity usually is insignificant after the first several hours, these techniques are important only in early uptake measurements, plasma clearance measurements, and the perchlorate discharge test (22). To circumvent the problems of background estimation and the use of standards, the ratio of neck count rate at 15 minutes to that at 5 minutes after intravenous injection of radioiodine was proposed (23). This value was found as sensitive as that obtained with 24-hour RAIU suppression and stimulation testing.

Other Techniques

To circumvent the problem of a high radiation burden from ^{131}I (approximately 5 to 15 rad to the thyroid), several other methods have been used to measure RAIU. When ^{123}I (1.55 μCi) is substituted for ^{131}I with a counting time of 4 minutes for a fractional standard deviation of 5%, the radiation dose is reduced to 55 mrad (24). However, a variety of technical problems can adversely affect the accuracy of RAIU determinations if ^{123}I is used; these have been reviewed by Chervu et al. (25). Whereas it is preferable to not use calculated decay-corrected counts for the standard when ^{131}I is used, it is even more important to count a standard ^{123}I capsule at each time period because of the increased error that occurs with fluctuation in high line voltage and resultant drift in the pulse-height analyzer. Because of the lower energy of ^{123}I (159 keV), there is significant photon absorption by the neck. Error is introduced by the variations in thyroid depth, size, and shape, and this error is less of a problem with the higher energy photons of ^{131}I. Use of the usual neck phantoms leads to underestimation of gland depth and can cause uptake errors as high as 25% owing to the higher tissue attenuation—15% per centimeter for ^{123}I, and 11% per centimeter for ^{131}I (26). To overcome this limitation, advantage is taken of the simultaneous emission of a 28-keV x-ray with a technique called *coincidence counting*. This allows quantitation of the absolute amount of ^{123}I independently of the geometric configuration, volume, and depth of the gland. ^{124}I contamination of ^{123}I also contributes to the error, which increases with time because of the longer physical half-life of ^{124}I (25). Furthermore, most uptake probes are unable to handle the high count rates of scanning doses when ^{123}I (200 to 300 μCi) is used for uptake measurements. The result is severe dead-time losses as high as 60% when the capsule standard is counted. This results in artifactual elevation of RAIU determinations (27). For this reason, ^{123}I uptake measurements are more accurate when a camera rather than an uptake probe is used if scanning doses of ^{123}I are administered (28).

^{132}I, which has a half-life of 2.33 hours, has been used for uptake measurements in an attempt to decrease the radiation dosage, especially in examinations of pediatric patients. Estimates of 50- to 100-fold reduction in exposure have been reported (29). Levy and Ashburn (30) developed the following formula for uptake measurements with this isotope:

$$\% \text{ Uptake} = \frac{\text{Neck cpm} - 2.4(\text{thigh cpm})}{\text{Standard cpm}} \times 100$$

The factor 2.4 was derived by blocking thyroid uptake with super-saturated potassium iodide for 2 days before administration of a 10-μCi dose of ^{132}I and measuring neck to thigh ratios.

^{99m}Tc is trapped but not organified by the thyroid. Maximum uptake occurs 10 to 20 minutes after intravenous injection. The following crude but relatively accurate estimates of thyroid uptake can be obtained by means of comparing thyroid to salivary gland activity 20 minutes after injection:

- Normal: thyroid $\geq$ salivary with background activity present
- Low: thyroid $<$ salivary with increased background activity
- High: thyroid $>>$ salivary with no background activity

The overall accuracy of this method compared with that of RAIU is 94% (31).

Normal thyroid uptake of ^{99m}Tc pertechnetate (^{99m}Tc) is only 0.3% to 3.75% of the injected dose. Although high and constantly varying levels of neck background activity represent a source of error (32), high degrees of correlation between ^{99m}Tc and ^{131}I uptake have been reported by many investigators (33–35). A standard scintillation camera equipped with a parallel hole collimator can be used. A normalized background is subtracted from the thyroid region of interest (32,35).

In an attempt to obviate neck background measurements, quantitation of ^{99m}Tc uptake has been measured by means of counting over the thyroid and the thigh. Use of the 10-minute to 2-minute thyroid ratio and the 15-minute neck-to-thigh ratio resulted in correct identification of more than 90% of cases of hypothyroidism and hyperthyroidism, whereas 84% of cases of normal thyroid function were correctly classified (36). In another technique, the gamma camera is used without a collimator. Counts are obtained 45 minutes after injection with the patient seated 6 feet (1.8 m) from the crystal with and without a lead shield over the thyroid. The uptake measurement is calculated as follows:

$$\% \text{ Uptake} = \frac{\text{Unshielded cpm} - \text{Shielded cpm} \times 100}{\text{Unshielded cpm}}$$

A correlation of 0.99 was obtained in a series of 19 patients who also had standard RAIU measurements obtained. The use of ^{99m}Tc pertechnetate has several advantages over the use of radioiodine. It is quicker, requires only a single visit to the nuclear medicine suite, is less expensive, is readily available in most departments, and has a more favorable dosimetry profile (37). Conversion of the ^{99m}Tc uptake value to a more conventional 24-hour ^{131}I uptake value can be accomplished with a simple formula (34).

Thyroid Diseases Affecting Uptake

In general, any disorder associated with increased iodine turnover causes elevation in RAIU. The elevated RAIU of hyperthyroid Graves' disease is typical. However, not all patients with elevated RAIU have thyrotoxicosis. Patients with iodine deficiency, dyshormonogenesis, and chronic autoimmune thyroiditis typically have elevated RAIU despite euthyroidism or mild hypothyroidism (38,39). Conversely, hypothyroidism with low iodine turnover is associated with decreased RAIU. Other thyroid disorders with low RAIU include subacute (de Quervain's) thyroiditis, thyrotoxicosis factitia, silent thyroiditis, struma ovarii, and functional metastatic thyroid cancer. In these cases of atypical hyperthyroidism, low RAIU indicates passive discharge of preformed thyroid hormone (thyroiditis) or an extrathyroidal source of the hormone (40).

Nonthyroidal Factors Affecting Uptake

Factors other than thyroid disease can adversely affect the measurement of RAIU (Table 30.1). Expansion of the iodine pool by means of ingestion or parenteral administration of iodine-containing agents is the greatest problem in this regard. As little as 1 mg of iodine can significantly reduce RAIU, and a single oral dose of iodine greater than 10 mg can decrease the 24-hour RAIU 98%, to a value less than 1.5% (41). Medications containing potassium iodide, such as expectorants, have many times this amount of iodine. Intravenous radiographic contrast agents contain several grams of iodine and can suppress uptake measurements for 4 to 6 weeks, whereas non–water-soluble myelographic agents left in the subarachnoid space can suppress uptake indefinitely (42).

This problem is illustrated by the fact that a progressive decrease in RAIU values among persons with normal thyroid function occurred during the 1960s. Pittman et al. (43) in 1968 reported a significant decline in normal 24-hour RAIU from 28.7% ± 6.5% in 1959 to 15.4% ± 6.8% related to euthyroid expansion of the iodine pool by excessive dietary iodine intake largely attributable to consumption of iodized bread (150 μg per slice). Other authors also have found a similar decrease in normal ranges attributable to a variety of iodide sources, including dairy products, cake mixes, cereals, medications, iodized water supplies, and even goitrogens, such as rapeseed and peanut oils (44–47). One milligram of iodine per liter of drinking water is reported to depress 24-hour uptake from 17% to 6%. The widespread use of iodized salt has played a pivotal role in the reduction of RAIU values in the western population with normal thyroid function. The high levels of iodide used in processed foods and restaurant offerings may represent another cause of depressed RAIU in the U.S. population.

Other nonthyroid factors affecting RAIU include use of thiouracil drugs, steroids, and goitrogenic agents, such as cabbage, turnips, kale, and rutabaga. These materials decrease uptake by inhibiting hormonal output (48). Chronic renal failure depresses uptake by impairing iodide clearance and expanding the body pool (49). Multihormonal contraceptives also diminish RAIU, possibly by a similar mechanism (50). Increased uptake can be caused by iodine depletion in patients with inflammatory bowel disease, chronic diarrhea, or nephrotic syndrome and in those consuming sodium-restricted diets or taking diuretics (42,51).

Perchlorate Discharge Test

The perchlorate ion is trapped but not organified, as is the pertechnetate ion. Consequently, when administered in milligram quantities, perchlorate ion competes with iodine for thyroid uptake, and because of its higher affinity for the symporter, it is able to displace thyroidal radioiodine that has not been organified. Because of the high intrathyroidal iodide pool in patients with iodine organification defects, perchlorate has been used to detect

organification defects occurring in Hashimoto chronic thyroiditis and congenital enzyme deficiencies (52). After a baseline RAIU measurement is obtained, the patient ingests 1 g of potassium perchlorate. In examinations of children, an intravenous dose of 3 mg/kg body weight has been used (53). RAIU is measured 60 to 90 minutes after administration of perchlorate. Healthy persons have no change in thyroid counts before or after administration of perchlorate. A positive test result is characterized by at least a 10% to 15% decline in count rate (54). Although the sensitivity of the perchlorate discharge test is proportional to the severity of the organification defect, the sensitivity can be greatly enhanced with simultaneous administration of 500 μg of stable sodium iodide with the perchlorate dose (55). The iodine-perchlorate discharge test can be used to detect not only congenital organification defects but also relatively subtle defects in patients with a variety of thyroid disorders, including chronic autoimmune thyroiditis, controlled Graves' disease, and previous thyroidectomy for benign disease. These are the patients who are susceptible to iodine-induced hypothyroidism (56). Because pertechnetate is not organified, it cannot be used for the discharge test (11).

Thyroid Stimulation and Suppression Test

In the past, thyroid reserve after inflammatory disease, ^{131}I therapy, or surgery, was used to differentiate primary from secondary hypothyroidism. It was evaluated by means of measurement of the response of the gland to exogenous thyroid-stimulating hormone (TSH). This study was performed by means of measuring RAIU before and immediately after 3 days of injections of bovine TSH. RAIU doubled or increased at least 15% in healthy persons (15). However, bovine TSH is allergenic, and many patients with hypothyroidism have a normal response. The test consequently has been replaced with the highly sensitive assay of serum TSH (57). Thyroid function and RAIU increase with administration of recombinant human TSH (rhTSH), but this test is used only in the evaluation (and sometimes treatment) of patients with differentiated thyroid cancer (58).

The most sensitive indicator of hyperthyroidism is the loss of thyroid control by TSH. This was previously studied by means of examining the RAIU response to exogenous thyroid hormone. The triiodothyronine (T_3 [Cytomel]) suppression test is performed by means of administering 100 μg of T_3 daily for 7 days. RAIU decreases normally at least 50% (15). Failure of suppression indicates thyroid autonomy (17). An easier and more convenient yet as effective variation of the T_3 suppression test has been described in which 10 days of T_4 and ^{99m}Tc pertechnetate uptake and imaging are used (59). With the availability of a highly sensitive TSH assay, however, this test has been abandoned for the diagnosis of hyperthyroidism (57). The T_3 suppression test is still occasionally used in the determination of thyroid nodule autonomy.

Although measurement of RAIU played an important role early in the laboratory investigation of thyroid disease, it has largely been supplanted by newer *in vitro* tests (see Chapter 29). The diagnosis of hyperthyroidism and hypothyroidism is now made by means of measurement of circulating levels of TSH, T_4, and T_3. Nevertheless, there are several situations in which

RAIU determination remains useful. The most common of these is the estimation of ^{131}I dosage for the management of hyperthyroidism associated with Graves' disease (see Chapter 31) and autonomously functioning nodules (60). In cases of atypical hyperthyroidism, such as thyroiditis and thyrotoxicosis factitia, RAIU is frequently the only means of determining the passive release or exogenous source of hormone (37,40,61,62).

After discontinuance of antithyroid drug therapy for Graves' disease, approximately 50% to 80% of patients have a relapse and recurrent hyperthyroidism within 1 year. Early uptake measurements performed with either ^{131}I or ^{99m}Tc have been reported to be useful in following the cases of patients undergoing antithyroid drug therapy. Although patients taking methimazole or propylthiouracil can appear clinically and biochemically to have normal thyroid function, the critical question is whether to withdraw or continue the drug. Because these agents do not affect the trapping mechanism, early uptake measurements can be used to determine whether relapse will occur after discontinuance (37,61,63). The best predictor of recurrence of hyperthyroidism after withdrawal of drug treatment is reported to be the disappearance of circulating thyrotropin receptor–stimulating immunoglobulins (TSIg), but the relapse rate is still 20% to 50% even in this population (64). In summary, no single test or combination of tests is accurate for ascertaining which patients with Graves' disease will or will not have a relapse after discontinuance of antithyroid medications.

CLINICAL APPLICATIONS

Normal and Abnormal Thyroid Gland

Several modalities are available to image a normal or an abnormal thyroid gland. Functional imaging of the thyroid gland is performed by means of scintigraphy with a variety of radioisotopes. Imaging to define anatomic features and determine the blood flow of the thyroid gland is accomplished by means of duplex and color flow Doppler sonography, CT, and MRI.

The objectives of imaging the thyroid gland are as follows:

1. Assessment of anterior neck masses in neonates and of neonatal hypothyroidism
2. Detection of a space-occupying lesion when clinical suspicion is high
3. Detection of additional space-occupying lesion (multinodular goiter)
4. Characterization of the lesion (solid, cyst, calcification, cystic degeneration)
5. Evaluation of the trapping and organification activity of a space-occupying lesion relative to the thyroid parenchyma (hyperfunctioning, hypofunctioning, or autonomous)
6. Definition of cervical lymph node involvement
7. Determination of extrathyroidal extension into adjacent tissues (aerodigestive tract)
8. Determination of the vascularity of a lesion
9. Detection of local recurrence or persistent residual tissue after thyroid excision
10. Evaluation of a substernal mass
11. Identification of thyroid tissue in ectopic locations (thyroglossal duct, struma ovarii) with functional imaging

Plain Radiography

On plain radiographs, the incidental finding of irregular calcific foci or dense calcifications in the thyroid region may help identify a previously unsuspected space-occupying lesion. A plain radiograph also may show the soft-tissue density of lobar or diffuse thyromegaly with or without displacement or compression of the trachea.

Scintigraphy

With the development of fine-needle aspiration biopsy (FNA) for the evaluation of nodular disease combined with the exquisite anatomic detail provided by sonography, CT, and MRI, the use of thyroid scintigraphy has decreased appropriately. However, it will continue to play an important role in the functional evaluation of a variety of thyroid disorders as well as the detection of metastatic thyroid cancer. ^{99m}Tc pertechnetate is the most readily available radionuclide for thyroid imaging. Like iodine, pertechnetate ions (TcO_4^-) are trapped by the thyroid in the same manner as iodine through an active transport mechanism, but pertechnetate ions are not organified (33,65–68). ^{123}I is both trapped and organified by the thyroid gland, so overall assessment of thyroid function is possible. Because ^{123}I is cyclotron-produced, it is expensive and has a relatively short half-life of 13.6 hours. Therefore long-term storage is a problem, and notice is necessary for imaging. Because of the high thyroid and total-body radiation dose from β emission (Table 30.2) and its inferior image quality, ^{131}I is rarely used for thyroid imaging other than for assessment of metastatic thyroid cancer.

The choice of radionuclide for routine imaging of the thyroid gland is between ^{99m}Tc and ^{123}I. A disadvantage of imaging with pertechnetate is that it is only trapped and not organified in the follicles. Early imaging after intravenous administration is associated with relatively high background activity. Imaging with ^{99m}Tc, however, provides diagnostic information equivalent to that obtained with ^{123}I imaging in most cases (67,68). When it is essential to assess both organification and trapping, ^{123}I scintigraphy can be performed later.

Planar imaging is similar for both radiopharmaceuticals. Anterior and anterior oblique images are acquired with a high-resolution pinhole collimator with a 3- to 6-mm insert. This allows detection of nodules as small as 5 mm. The oblique views

Table 30.2. *Patient Dose from Various Thyroid Scanning Agents*

Agent	Activity administered (mCi)	Whole-body dose (mrad)	Thyroid dose (rad)
^{131}I	0.05	23	65.0
^{125}I	0.05	20	41.0
^{123}I	0.20	6	2.6
^{99m}Tc	5–15.00	70	0.6[a]
Fluorescent	None	None	0.015–0.06

1 mCi = 37 MBq; 1 rad = 0.01 Gy.
[a]Critical organ—stomach, 1.25 rad.
From Sandler MP, Rao BK, Patton JA, et al. Thyroid imaging. In: Sandler MP, Patton JA, Cross M, et al., eds. Endocrine imaging. Norwalk, CT: Appleton & Lange, 1992:197, with permission.

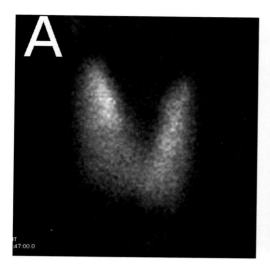 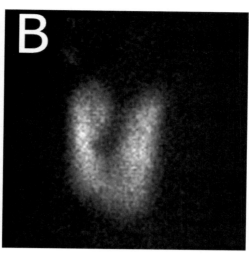

FIGURE 30.3. A small posteromedial cold nodule in the right lobe is depicted only on the oblique **(B)** ^{99m}Tc image. The anterior image **(A)** is normal.

allow detection of small nodules obscured by overlying or underlying physiologic activity (Fig 30.3). A radioactive ^{57}Co marker is placed on the sternal notch and often on the chin to provide anatomic landmarks. Some institutions also place a 5-cm line marker in the field of view to aid in estimating the size of the gland or nodule. An additional anterior view usually is acquired with the collimator pulled back several centimeters so that the salivary glands and mediastinum are included in the field of view.

For ^{99m}Tc pertechnetate imaging, 200,000-count images are acquired 20 minutes after intravenous injection of 5 to 10 mCi (for adults). For ^{123}I imaging, 50,000-count images are acquired 6 and 24 hours after oral administration of 200 to 300 μCi. Because there is less background activity with ^{123}I than with

^{99m}Tc pertechnetate, these count rates provide comparable image quality. Palpable nodules can be localized on the scintigram with lead "cold" markers or ^{57}Co "hot" markers. Marking extrathyroidal palpable nodules is especially important. SPECT with both ^{99m}Tc and ^{123}I has been reported.

On scintigrams the thyroid gland appears as two ellipsoid structures slightly angled toward each other inferiorly and connected by a thin isthmus. The degree of activity in the isthmus is highly variable. The gland shows uniform peripheral activity, with an occasional increase in the central part of the lobes owing to their ellipsoid configuration and the increased central thickness of the gland. With pertechnetate imaging, salivary gland, buccal mucosa, esophageal, and blood-pool background activity are seen with the thyroid gland (Figs. 30.4 and 30.5). Salivary

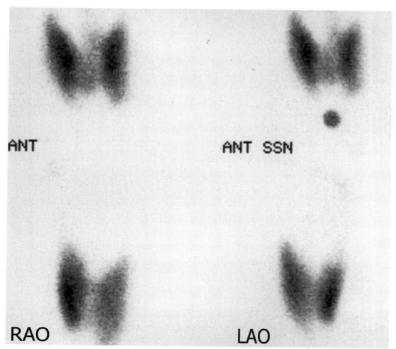

FIGURE 30.4. ^{99m}Tc thyroid scan shows normal thyroid-to-salivary and thyroid-to-background ratios in the usual four views.

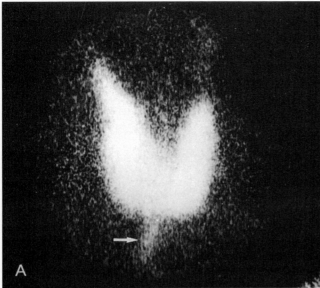

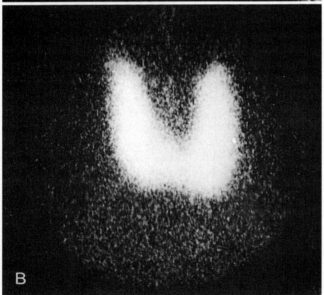

FIGURE 30.5. Midline esophageal ⁹⁹ᵐTc activity (*arrow*) **(A)** disappears **(B)** when the patient swallows water. (Reproduced by permission from Sandler MP, Patton JA, Sacks GA, et al. Scintigraphic thyroid imaging. In: Sandler MP, Patton JA, Partain CL, eds. *Thyroid and parathyroid imaging.* Norwalk, CT: Appleton-Century-Crofts, 1986:112).

gland activity often is absent during the delayed phase of ¹²³I imaging.

The lateral border of a normal thyroid lobe usually is slightly concave to straight but can be mildly convex. Marked concavity suggests the presence of a cold nodule, and exaggerated convexity often is associated with diffuse goiter. Although the lobes are generally symmetric in size, the right lobe sometimes is somewhat larger than the left. The lobes can be angulated toward each other in a U- or V-shaped configuration. The pyramidal lobe, a remnant of the distal thyroglossal duct, is identified in fewer than 10% of patients with normal thyroid function but is visualized in as many as 40% of patients with Graves' disease

(6). Extrathyroidal linear activity near the midline frequently is caused by radioactivity excreted into the esophagus from the salivary glands. Esophageal activity is most often inferior to the gland and slightly to the left of midline. It should disappear or change in location or intensity after water is swallowed (Fig. 30.5).

Sonography

Sonography of the thyroid gland is performed in the transverse, sagittal, and oblique coronal planes with phased linear-array high-frequency transducers (7.5 to 10 MHz). The thyroid gland is medial to the common carotid artery and jugular vein, which are useful landmarks. A normal thyroid gland has a homogenous echogenicity greater than that of the adjacent strap muscles. The thyroid lobes joined by the isthmus are anterolateral to the air-containing trachea. The homogeneously echogenic pattern of the thyroid gland probably is caused by the numerous follicles, which range from 0.02 mm to 0.9 mm in diameter. Because the axial resolution of real-time scanners is approximately 0.5 mm, diffuse echogenicity of the thyroid gland is most likely due to the microscopic structures within the follicles. Anterior and lateral to the thyroid, the sternocleidomastoid muscle is an easily identifiable landmark. Posterior to the thyroid gland on the left, a round structure measuring approximately 1.5 cm in diameter with higher central echogenicity is the nondistended esophagus.

Sonography is the modality of choice for screening patients at high risk of thyroid cancer to detect clinically nonpalpable nodules as small as 2 mm (69). These high-risk groups of patients are those with a history of the following:

1. Familial thyroid carcinoma, particularly the medullary variant
2. Multiple endocrine neoplasia, type 2
3. Previous exposure to ionizing radiation (therapeutic irradiation to scalp, face, mediastinum)
4. Previous exposure to atomic fallout
5. Inhabitation at uranium- and thorium-rich regions

Other indications for sonography (69) include the following:

1. Differentiation of a solitary nodule from multinodular disease
2. Follow-up evaluation of the size of a solitary nodule during suppressive therapy or over time
3. Characterization of the nodule before biopsy (degeneration is common in nodules larger than 1 cm in diameter, and biopsy yields a suboptimal cytologic sample)
4. Detection of thyroidal calcifications
5. Detection of cervical lymph node metastases, including postsurgical recurrences
6. Definition of any extrathyroidal extension of a neoplasm
7. Detection of thyroglossal duct cyst
8. Differentiation of a thyroid nodule from a nonthyroid mass (parathyroid, lymph node)
9. Guidance for needle biopsy

Color flow Doppler imaging of thyroid nodules has depicted perinodular and intranodular flow, but the finding is nonspecific (70). Arteriovenous shunting, high flow rates, and hypervascularity occur in large tumors and in hyperplastic glands of patients with Graves' disease (71).

Computed Tomography

The iodinated contrast material needed for optimal neck imaging with CT interferes with functional evaluation of a thyroid nodule with radiotracers (Table 30.1). Therefore CT is not routinely used as a primary imaging modality in the evaluation of a thyroid lesion. CT is useful to detect extrathyroidal (tracheal, laryngeal, and esophageal) extension of a malignant lesion of the thyroid, to detect lymph node metastases, and to differentiate a thyroid nodule from a nonthyroid mass. Because of the relative expense and the need for administration of contrast medium, CT often is reserved for selected cases with complex anatomic features and for assessment of the mediastinum if necessary.

The thyroid gland is seen as a homogeneous structure with higher attenuation values than those of the adjacent soft tissues anterior to the trachea (40 to 60 Hounsfield units [HU]; normal soft tissue, 20 to 30 HU; water 0 to 15 HU). This difference is accentuated considerably after the administration of intravenous contrast medium. CT provides precise definition of the borders of the thyroid gland and the relation of the gland to neighboring soft tissue, vascular, and aerodigestive structures. Ultrasonography, CT, and MRI are not accurate in differentiation of benign and malignant thyroid nodules (72).

Magnetic Resonance Imaging

MRI provides excellent anatomic detail of the thyroid gland with proton-density and surface coil imaging. CT and MRI have been used for accurate assessment of the size of enlarged glands, but palpation is probably sufficient for most clinical purposes.

X-Ray Fluorescent Scanning

X-ray fluorescent (XRF) scanning of the thyroid with an external source of ^{241}Am provides unique and valuable information for clinical diagnosis and defines the distribution of stable iodine within the gland and thus the past functional status of the gland. The characteristic fluorescent x-ray emitted from stable intrathyroidal ^{127}I through its interaction with the ^{241}Am photons produces an emission image that gives direct information about the size and shape of the thyroid (73), This is achieved with a low dose of radiation to the thyroid and a negligible dose of extrathyroidal radiation (Table 30.2) (74). Thus it allows physiologic measurements of thyroid function in groups with normal and high radiation risk, including children and pregnant women. XRF scanning also can be used to evaluate thyroid disorders in the presence of a flooded iodine pool (73).

Developmental Thyroid Abnormalities

Hemiagenesis of the thyroid probably occurs in no more than 1 per 2,000 persons; there is a female preponderance of 3:1. Agenesis occurs less frequently. The left lobe is absent in 80% and the isthmus in 50% of persons with this abnormality. Hemiagenesis with an isthmus (Fig. 30.6) resembles a hockey stick (75). A full spectrum of disorders can occur in the remaining lobe, including Graves' disease, multinodular goiter, thyroiditis, and adenocarcinoma. Differentiation of hemiagenesis from autonomous toxic nodule with suppression of extranodular tissue usually can be achieved scintigraphically by means of raising the intensity of the data on the monitor screen or with ^{201}Tl or ^{99m}Tc sestamibi imaging (76). Sonography and CT also can be used.

Thyroid tissue can be present anywhere along the embryologic descent from the base of the tongue to the superior mediastinum (77). Ectopic thyroid tissue usually is hypofunctioning,

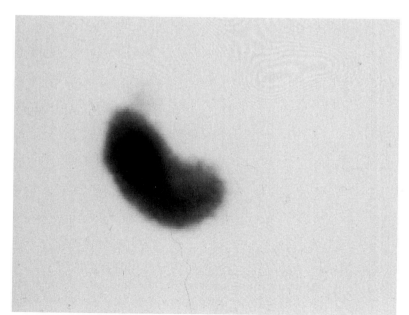

FIGURE 30.6. Diffuse toxic goiter with hemiagenesis. ^{99m}Tc scan shows absence of the left lobe and the typical hockeystick pattern of hemiagenesis. The absence of salivary gland and background activity suggests hyperthyroidism. Surgical absence of the left lobe would have a similar appearance. (From Sandler MP, Martin WH, Moody EB. Endocrine imaging. In Habibian MR, Delbeke D, Martin WH, et al., eds. *Nuclear medicine imaging: a teaching file.* Philadelphia: Lippincott Williams & Wilkins, 1999:36, with permission.)

incapable of maintaining euthyroidism in the absence of eutopic thyroid tissue. Lingual or upper cervical thyroid tissue (Fig. 30.1) can be present in the neonate or child as a midline mass with or without obstructive symptoms; it usually is accompanied by hypothyroidism. Scintigraphic visualization with ^{99m}Tc pertechnetate or ^{123}I establishes the diagnosis and obviates biopsy or surgical resection. The mass regresses with initiation of T$_4$ therapy. Lateral thyroid rests rarely occur, but they, too, usually are hypofunctioning. Thyroglossal duct cysts, which at physical examination rise with protrusion of the tongue, often contain ectopic follicular thyroid cells but not usually enough to be detectable with scintigraphy. In rare instances, detached mediastinal remnants, ovarian thyroid rests, struma ovarii, and struma cordis occur. All of these developmental and abnormal rests can function, can hyperfunction, and can be involved with adenocarcinoma of the thyroid. In the presence of a eutopic functioning thyroid gland, all functioning ectopic thyroid tissue should be considered metastatic until found otherwise (Fig. 30.7).

Multinodular Goiter

The importance of identifying a multinodular goiter relates to the lower incidence of malignant growth (1% to 6%) than in patients with a single cold nodule (10% to 20%) (78,79), although patients with multinodular goiter may have a higher incidence of thyroid cancer than do persons without goiter. A dominant cold nodule out of proportion in size to other cold foci should be subjected to biopsy, because the incidence of

carcinoma is similar to that for solitary cold nodule (79). Although patients with multinodular goiter do not have hypothyroidism (Hashimoto thyroiditis is likely if the patient has hypothyroidism), many eventually have hyperthyroidism that necessitates treatment.

Pathophysiology

See Chapter 29.

Scintigraphy

The scintigraphic appearance of a multinodular goiter is generalized inhomogeneity with multiple cold (hypofunctioning) areas interspersed between focal areas of normal and increased activity in an asymmetrically enlarged thyroid gland (Fig. 30.8). The differential diagnosis includes Hashimoto's thyroiditis, multiple adenoma, and multifocal carcinoma. If the gland is hyperfunctioning, the diagnosis of toxic multinodular goiter is assured.

Ultrasonography

When only a solitary thyroid nodule is identified with palpation, ultrasonography easily depicts nodules 2 to 3 mm in diameter, increasing the rate of detection of multinodular goiter when only a solitary thyroid nodule is detected by means of clinical palpation (Fig. 30.9) (69). Because available data on the incidence of malignant growth in a multinodular goiter are related to

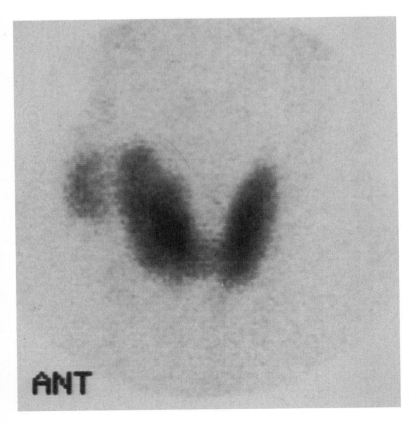

FIGURE 30.7. Papillary carcinoma of the thyroid was found at surgery in this patient with a solitary hypofunctioning nodule in the upper pole of the right lobe. The extrathyroidal ^{99m}Tc activity lateral to the right lobe represents metastatic lymphadenopathy.

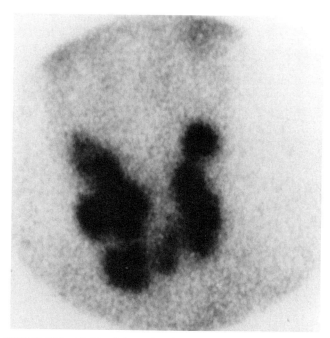

FIGURE 30.8. Multinodular goiter is manifested by asymmetric goitrous enlargement accompanied by multiple bilateral foci of both decreased and increased ^{99m}Tc activity.

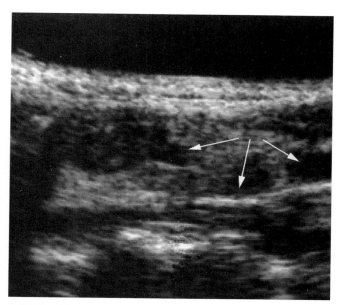

FIGURE 30.9. Longitudinal sonogram shows multinodular goiter, which is recognized by the presence of multiple hypoechoic nodules (*arrows*).

clinically palpable goiters, the significance of small nonpalpable nodules detected with ultrasonography remains uncertain. The presence of an ultrasonographically detected incidental subcentimeter nodularity does not obviate biopsy of a dominant palpable nodule (80).

Computed Tomography and Magnetic Resonance Imaging

Multinodular goiters can be easily identified with CT and MRI because of their anatomic appearance (Fig. 30.10). CT typically shows a goitrous thyroid as heterogeneous and displays nodular enlargement of one or both lobes with cysts and often calcification. Hemorrhage occurs in 60% of cases (81). On MR images, multinodular goiter is typically heterogeneous, with an isointense signal or increased signal intensity on T1-weighted images and mixed signal intensity on T2-weighted images (81). Contrast enhancement is typically diffuse and mottled on CT scans and MR images. In some instances, all imaging modalities show a uniform parenchymal appearance in an enlarged thyroid gland.

X-ray Fluorescent Scanning

In a series of 83 patients with multinodular goiter, the mean total iodine content of 10.3 ± 6.9 mg was not significantly different from that of normal thyroid glands, indicating a reduction in iodine content per milligram of thyroid tissue (73).

Solitary Thyroid Nodule

The treatment of patients with a solitary thyroid nodule remains controversial and relates to the high incidence of nodules, the

relative infrequency of cancer, and the relatively low morbidity and mortality associated with malignant tumors of the thyroid. Thyroid nodules can contain normal thyroid tissue, benign inactive tissue (which can be solid, cystic, or mixed solid and cystic), hyperplastic or autonomously functioning benign tissue, or malignant tissue (Table 30.3).

Table 30.3. *Causes of Solitary Palpable Nodule*

Benign	Malignant	
	Primary	Secondary
Adenoma	Carcinoma	Kidney, pancreas,
Adenomatous	Papillary	esophagus,
hyperplasia in a	adenocarcinoma	rectum,
goiter	Follicular carcinoma	melanoma,
Adenomatous nodule	Clear cell carcinoma	lung,
Cyst	Oxyphil carcinoma	lymphoma
Colloid nodules	Medullary carcinoma	
Chronic thyroiditis	Undifferentiated	
Subacute thyroiditis	carcinoma	
Miscellaneous	Small cell carcinoma	
Amyloid	Giant cell carcinoma	
Hemochromatosis	Epidermoid carcinoma	
Malignant Nodules	Other malignant	
	tumors	
	Lymphoma	
	Sarcoma	
	Malignant	
	teratoma	
	Osteogenic sarcoma	

From Sandler MP, Patton JA, Sacks GA, et al. Scintigraphy thyroid imaging. In: Sandler MP, Patton JA, Partain Cl, eds. *Thyroid and parathyroid imaging.* Norwalk, CT: Appleton & Lange, 1986:125, with permission.

Classification of the Causes of Solitary Thyroid Nodule

Nodular thyroid disease is more common among women than among men, and the incidence increases with age. Series of autopsy examinations of the thyroid have documented a 50% incidence of nodules. In 75% of these cases, there are multiple nod- ules, and 4% contain primary occult carcinoma (82). In the Framingham study a 4% incidence of nodular goiters were found with palpation (5% uninodular, 1% multinodular) in an unselected series of 5,000 healthy persons 30 to 59 years of age (83). Miller (84) reported an 11% incidence of nodular goiter in the adult female population; 4% of the lesions were found malignant at surgery (84).

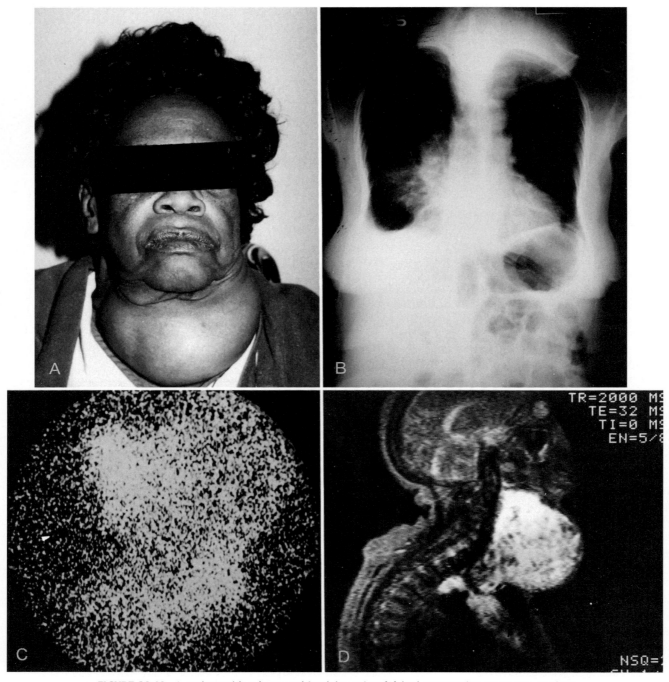

FIGURE 30.10. A patient with a large multinodular goiter **(A)** had compressive symptoms. **B:** Chest radiograph shows a large, right-sided mass. **C:** ^{131}I scintigraphic image shows a large diffuse multinodular goiter with retrosternal extension. **D:** Sagittal T2-weighted magnetic resonance image shows involvement of both the anterior and posterior mediastinum. (From Sandler MP, Patton JA. Multimodality imaging of the thyroid and parathyroid glands. *J Nucl Med* 1987;28:125, with permission.)

Evaluation of Patients with Solitary Thyroid Nodule

The investigation of a solitary thyroid nodule is directed at differentiating benign lesions of many causes from a malignant nodule to prevent indiscriminate surgical intervention. The evaluation of patients with solitary nodules consists of a history and physical examination, thyroid function tests, thyroid imaging, and thyroid biopsy.

Clinical Examination

The incidence of thyroid cancer is threefold to fourfold higher among patients exposed to radiation than it is in the general population (85,86), and there is a higher incidence of benign nodularity in this population. From 1940 through 1960, young persons often underwent radiation therapy for acne, thymic enlargement, or benign conditions of the tonsils or adenoid tissue. It is estimated that more than 1 million such persons are living in the United States. Internal exposure to radioiodine during childhood as occurred with the Chernobyl accident (87) and with nuclear weapons testing in Nevada (88) increases the risk of thyroid carcinoma as much as 62-fold (89). The latency period for malignant tumors of the thyroid among these patients is approximately 5 years or less, but the period can continue into adult life. The incidence is linearly related to the radiation dose up to 1,500 rad (3 to 5 cancers/106 persons per rad per year). High doses of radiation used for the management of hyperthyroidism and malignant tumors of organs other than the thyroid are more likely to cause late hypothyroidism, but patients with lymphoma receiving therapeutic radiation to the neck have an increased incidence of thyroid nodularity and thyroid cancer (90). A family history of thyroid carcinoma should be sought. Medullary carcinoma of the thyroid (MTC) can occur in a familial autosomal dominant pattern with or without features of multiple endocrine neoplasia (91,92), and familial occurrence of papillary carcinoma has been reported (93). The presence of MTC can be established by means of measuring its secretory product, calcitonin. The genetic mutation for multiple endocrine neoplasia, type 2, has been isolated to the *ret* proto-oncogene, so genetic screening of family members of an affected individual is appropriate (94). Prophylactic thyroidectomy, usually before 6 years of age, is recommended for all children in whom a *ret* mutation is identified.

Attention to the patient's age is important, because the prevalence of thyroid nodules among children is fivefold to tenfold lower than it is among adults (<1.5%), but 17% to 25% of thyroid nodules in children are malignant, making thyroid cancer the third most common solid tumor in childhood and adolescence (95,96). Because thyroid cancer is only twice as common among women as it is among men, a solitary thyroid nodule is more likely to be malignant in a man because of the frequent occurrence of thyroid nodules among women (97).

Physical findings that suggest a malignant lesion in the thyroid include size of the nodule and the presence of fixation to adjacent structures, tracheal deviation, and enlarged cervical lymph nodes (98). Rapid increase in the size of a nodule, although suggestive of malignant growth, often is caused by benign hemorrhage or cystic degeneration. The differential diagnosis of a solitary thyroid nodule includes parathyroid enlargement (adenoma, carcinoma, or cyst), lymphadenopathy, branchial cyst, and thyroglossal duct cyst. Some patients with agenesis of a thyroid lobe have a palpable nodule caused by compensatory hypertrophy of the remaining lobe (Fig. 30.6).

Laboratory assessment can be useful in that only rare patients with hyperthyroidism or hypothyroidism have coexistent thyroid cancer. In a patient with an elevated level of thyroid autoantibodies, a thyroid nodule most likely represents chronic Hashimoto thyroiditis, although thyroid cancer can occur among patients with autoimmune thyroiditis (80). Some investigators have recommended screening patients who have thyroid nodules by means of serum thyroglobulin (99) and serum calcitonin (100) determinations to increase the accuracy of FNA and clinical assessment.

Hypofunctioning Thyroid Nodules

Scintigraphy. A hypofunctioning, or cold, nodule on a thyroid scintigram is a focal region that takes up less radioisotope than the rest of the thyroid gland—85% to 90% of solitary nodules are hypofunctioning (Fig. 30.11). Although malignant tumors of the thyroid do not effectively concentrate radioisotopes, taking up only 1% to 10% of the activity accumulated by normal thyroid tissue, only 10% to 20% of cold nodules are malignant. The other 80% to 90% of cold nodules are degenerative nodules, hemorrhagic benign nodules, cysts, inflammatory nodules (e.g., Hashimoto's thyroiditis or de Quervain's thyroiditis), infiltrative disorders (e.g., amyloid or hemochromatosis), or nonthyroid neoplasms (101). An indeterminate nodule (4% to 7% of solitary nodules) is a palpable nodule larger than 1 cm in diameter that cannot be detected with scintigraphy. It has the same significance as a cold, hypofunctioning nodule, emphasizing the importance of correlating the scintigraphic findings with the findings of the physical examination. When indeterminate nodules are combined with cold nodules, the sensitivity for detection of thyroid carcinoma is 97%, but the specificity and positive predictive value are only 15% to 20%. Extrathyroidal activity on the thyroid scan of a patient with palpable lymph nodes and a solitary thyroid nodule, although rare, in most instances represents metastatic cancer of the thyroid (Fig. 30.7).

Ultrasonography. Ultrasonography is not especially useful for differentiating benign from malignant thyroid nodules (69). The presence of peripheral eggshell calcification on ultrasound or CT scans suggests a benign process, but multiple, small, highly echogenic foci on ultrasound scans are strongly suggestive of the microcalcifications present within malignant tumors (Fig. 30.12). The traditional role of ultrasonography to separate cystic from solid lesions is outdated. True thyroid cysts are rare, and small, solid colloid-rich nodules can appear anechoic with through-transmission. Predominantly cystic lesions usually have at least a small solid component and generally are a benign nodule with cystic degeneration. Cystic adenocarcinoma is rare but cannot be reliably differentiated from benign lesions by means of ultrasonography. Although most thyroid cancers are hypoechoic, as many as 10% are isoechoic, and follicular adenomas often are hypoechoic. Hyperechoic nodules almost always are benign, but they are uncommon. A hypoechoic halo surround-

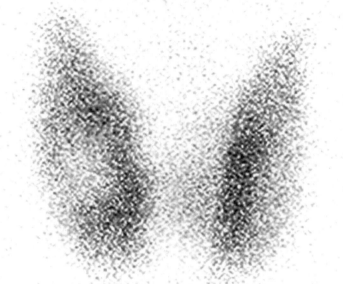

A

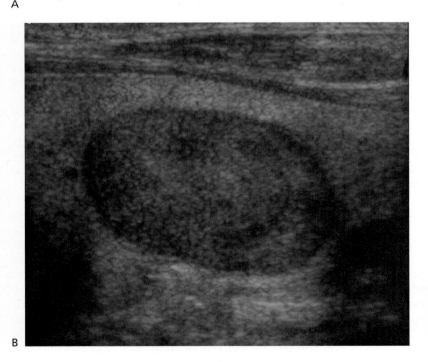

B

FIGURE 30.11. **A:** ^{123}I scintigram shows a large, hypofunctioning right thyroid nodule. **B:** The nodule is hypoechoic with a surrounding halo suggestive of benignity. Because of a history of radiation exposure, the nodule was resected. Histologic examination showed the lesion was malignant.

ing an isoechoic or hypoechoic nodule usually is an indicator of benignity, but some papillary carcinomas (20%) may have a halo (Fig. 30.11). Carcinoma of the thyroid sometimes have marked intranodular blood flow at color flow Doppler imaging, but the finding is not specific (70,102). Ultrasonography can reliably depict additional small nodules in patients with a solitary palpable thyroid nodule (69,103). Approximately 50% of patients with clinical evidence of a solitary nodule have multiple nodules at ultrasonography. Among those with multiple nodules, one third have three or more nodules. Approximately 90%

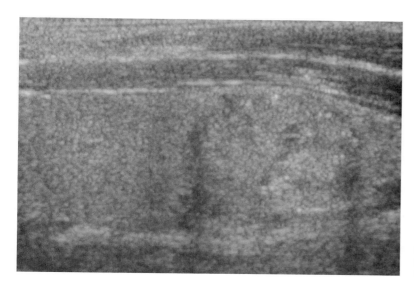

FIGURE 30.12. Ultrasound image shows a palpable thyroid nodule with numerous punctate echogenic foci representing calcifications typical of papillary carcinoma.

of clinically palpable nodules are at least 1 cm in diameter, whereas more than 70% of the other nodules not identified clinically are smaller than 1 cm in diameter. Therefore a palpable solitary nodule represents a multinodular gland in approximately 50% of patients. Multinodular goiter is considered a benign process with a risk of malignant growth in the range of 1% to 5% (78). Small, occult (nonpalpable) thyroid nodules detected at ultrasonography almost never are malignant and should be considered clinically unimportant unless they have other features of malignant growth or the nodule grows (104,105). For instance, in a patient with a dominant cold nodule associated with multinodular goiter, further assessment is warranted (80). In a series of 95 patients with multinodular goiter, 14% of dominant nodules were malignant at biopsy, a risk similar to that of solitary cold nodule in patients without concurrent multinodular goiter (106). Similarly, for a patient with a history of radiation exposure, detection of a clinically inapparent nodule at ultrasonography necessitates further evaluation (85,86,107). Ultrasonography is accurate in the assessment of nodule size (69,108), but the rate of growth of a nodule and response to T_4 suppressive therapy are not reliable in differentiating benign from malignant disease (108).

Computed Tomography and Magnetic Resonance Imaging. Neither CT nor MRI is helpful for differentiating benign from malignant thyroid nodules in the absence of local invasion of normal anatomic structures, extension into the mediastinum, or cervical lymphadenopathy. *In vitro* MRI of thyroid biopsy specimens have revealed abnormal values on T1- and T2-weighted images of both benign and malignant lesions without clear differentiation (109). The metastatic nodes in papillary carcinoma can become markedly enhanced (hypervascular), show increased signal intensity on T1-weighted images (increased thyroglobulin content or hemorrhage), and reveal punctate calcifications (72). Any anterior neck mass with a cystic component accompanied by a mural nodule or calcification is

suspected to be carcinoma within a thyroglossal duct cyst (Fig. 30.13) (110).

Differentiation between benign and malignant thyroid nodules is not possible on the basis of T1- and T2-weighted measurements alone (Figs. 30.10 and 30.13). Colloid cysts have prolonged T2-weighted values characteristic of simple fluids, and hemorrhagic cysts have relatively lower T2-weighted values. Adenoma has a wide range of T1-weighted values, although they are generally prolonged, overlapping those of thyroid carcinoma. Findings at MRI may suggest malignant disease of the thyroid on the basis of distorted anatomic features of the thyroid and invasion of surrounding structures. High-field surface-coil MRI can depict characteristic pathologic features of the pseudocapsule

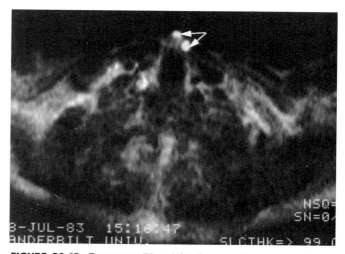

FIGURE 30.13. Transverse T2-weighted magnetic resonance image shows a thyroglossal duct cyst. Two discreet foci of high signal intensity in the midline and in the left lobe of the thyroid were found at surgery to be papillary carcinoma. (From Smith FW, Runge VM, Sandler MP, et al. Magnetic resonance imaging in thyroid disease. In: Sandler MP, Patton JA, Partain CL, eds. *Thyroid and parathyroid imaging.* Norwalk CT: Appleton-Century-Crofts, 1986:344, with permission.)

and hemorrhagic degeneration and contribute to the noninvasive differential diagnosis of thyroid masses (81).

X-Ray Fluorescent Scanning. Quantitative XRF imaging has been proposed for the evaluation of solitary cold thyroid nodules (73). With this technique, the *in vivo* iodine content of a solitary nodule and that of a corresponding region of normal tissue in the contralateral lobe are measured. The iodine content ratio of the nodule versus normal tissue is calculated and used as a predictor of benignity (Fig. 30.14). XRF scanning is useful only for investigation of a solitary cold nodule (Fig. 30.15). The spatial resolution of a rectilinear scanner limits the size of a solitary nodule in which the amount of iodine can be quantitated with XRF to approximately 1 cm. XRF imaging is not useful to differentiate the pathologic types of malignant tumors of the thyroid. This technique, in conjunction with careful clinical judgment, can be used to ascertain which patients are at low risk of malignant disease and can probably undergo conservative treatment.

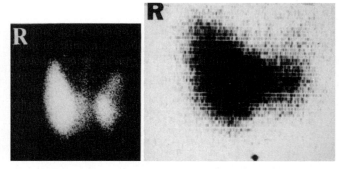

FIGURE 30.15. ^{99m}Tc pertechnetate scan (*left*) and x-ray fluorescent scan (*right*) of a patient with a solitary palpable nodule at the superior pole of the left lobe. The hypofunctioning nodule in the left upper lobe had an iodine content ratio of 0.29 (< 0.6) and was found at surgery to be malignant.

Because it is a nonradioisotopic technique, XRF scanning can be used to evaluate a solitary thyroid nodule in pediatric and pregnant patients without exposing extrathyroidal tissue to radiation.

Other Nuclear Medicine Techniques. Because of the poor specificity of ^{99m}Tc and ^{123}I scintigraphy and of ultrasonography, CT, and MRI for the differentiation of benign and malignant thyroid nodules tumor-avid agents have been investigated. Although combining FNA and ^{99m}Tc or ^{123}I scintigraphy for the preoperative assessment of thyroid nodules is sufficient in most cases, the cytologic findings often do not provide enough information to establish a diagnosis, especially of follicular neoplasm. Both ^{201}Tl and ^{99m}Tc sestamibi are nonspecific tumor imaging agents that have been used in the evaluation of thyroid nodules and in the localization of metastatic disease after surgery for thyroid cancer (111). After injection of 3 mCi ^{201}Tl, planar anterior images are acquired with a pinhole collimator 20 minutes and 3 hours after injection. Thyroid scans are performed 20 minutes and 2 to 3 hours after administration of 15 to 20 mCi ^{99m}Tc sestamibi. Whereas benign lesions tend either to not take up these agents or to not retain them at delayed imaging, malignant nodules usually are hot or "warm" on initial images and retain a greater degree of the radiopharmaceutical than does normal or benign tissue on delayed images. The sensitivity is relatively high, but the specificity is somewhat disappointing owing to radiopharmaceutical uptake and retention by follicular adenoma.

In one study, ^{201}Tl was used for imaging of 246 patients with thyroid nodule, 101 of whom had carcinoma. The sensitivity for detection of palpable carcinoma was 87%, but the specificity was only 58% owing to uptake by benign neoplasms (112). The sensitivity was poor for detection of tumors less than 1.5 cm in diameter and for partially necrotic tumors. In a more recent prospective study with 78 patients with solitary hypofunctioning thyroid nodules undergoing preoperatively ^{201}Tl scintigraphy (113), 86% of the 65 benign lesions were less than or equal in uptake to normal thyroid tissue 3 hours after administration of the radionuclide, and 85% of the malignant lesions were hot on delayed images, but 14% of the benign lesions also showed increased activity on the delayed images.

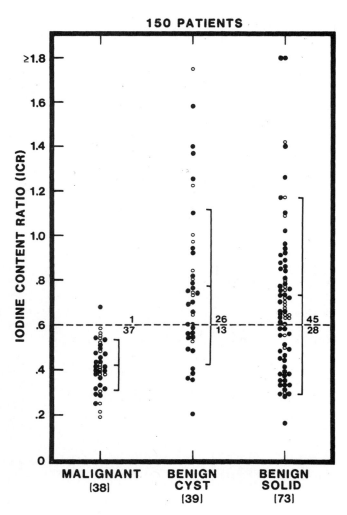

FIGURE 30.14. Iodine content ratios determined before surgery for 150 patients with solitary cold nodules show that almost no carcinomas had ratios greater than 0.6. (From Patton JA, Sandler MP, Partain CL. Prediction of benignity of the solitary (cold) thyroid nodule by fluorescent scanning. *J Nucl Med* 1985;26:463, with permission.)

In a report of 71 patients undergoing preoperative ^{99m}Tc sestamibi scintigraphy, 91% of the 23 carcinomas were detected with ^{99m}Tc sestamibi, and only 11% of the benign lesions were detected (114). In another report describing 52 patients with cold nodules undergoing sestamibi imaging, increased ^{99m}Tc sestamibi uptake increased eightfold the likelihood of detection of malignant growth; the presence of a cold ^{99m}Tc sestamibi defect (in contradistinction to an isointense, or warm, lesion) excluded malignancy (115). Therefore both ^{99m}Tc sestamibi and ^{201}Tl imaging are useful adjuncts to FNA with cytologic examination in the evaluation of solitary thyroid nodules, especially when results of the latter are inconclusive. Increased uptake of the radiopharmaceutical within the nodule, particularly on delayed images, increases the likelihood of the presence of malignant growth, whereas decreased uptake in the nodule almost excludes malignant disease. Isointense, or warm, nodular uptake is nonspecific. Because ^{201}Tl and ^{99m}Tc sestamibi uptake within thyroid tissue is independent of circulating TSH and iodine concentrations (76,116), ^{201}Tl and ^{99m}Tc sestamibi scintigraphy can be used to determine the anatomic features and functionality of the thyroid when ^{99m}Tc pertechnetate or ^{123}I scans are not useful, such as in evaluation of patients taking thyroid hormone, with subacute thyroiditis, or with an expanded iodine pool. ^{99m}Tc tetrofosmin behaves similarly to ^{99m}Tc sestamibi in the evaluation of thyroid disorders (117).

^{18}F-fluorodeoxyglucose (^{18}F-FDG), a positron-emitting analog of D-glucose, accumulates in tissues with high glycolytic demand. *In vitro* studies have shown that both benign and malignant thyroid tumors accumulate ^{18}F-FDG (118). Preliminary clinical studies of PET in the preoperative diagnosis of suspected thyroid carcinoma have shown increased ^{18}F-FDG uptake in most malignant lesions (differentiated, Hürthle cell, anaplastic, and medullary carcinoma) with little overlap with the degree of uptake in benign lesions (119–121). One study, however, showed overlap of ^{18}F-FDG uptake between benign (nodular goiter and follicular adenoma) and malignant lesions (122), and increased ^{18}F-FDG uptake in autoimmune thyroiditis has been reported (123). Focal uptake within the thyroid should, however, always be interpreted as suggestive of neoplasm, even if found incidentally (124). In summary, because of limited specificity and sparse clinical data, ^{18}F-FDG PET is not currently recommended in the initial diagnostic evaluation of patients with suspected thyroid carcinoma.

Needle Biopsy of the Thyroid

FNA of the thyroid gland had been adopted at most institutions in the western world by the early 1980s and is now universally accepted as the most accurate technique, other than thyroidectomy, for differentiating benign from malignant thyroid nodules in both adults and children (125,126). This procedure is benign and simple, and it yields important diagnostic information about the thyroid nodule. In a series of FNA involving 18,183 patients, 4% of nodules were malignant, and 27% had findings suggestive of malignant growth or did not provide enough information to establish a diagnosis (126). Physicians must be aware that a biopsy that does not lead to a diagnosis is of no value in the prediction of benignity of the solitary thyroid nodule; 10% to 30% of nodules with cytologic findings suggestive of malignant growth or that do not provide enough information for a diagnosis are malignant (126). An experienced cytopathologist is critical to the accuracy of the biopsy. The cytopathologist must take care to avoid making a diagnosis when a sample is of insufficient cellularity. If this precaution is followed, the false-negative rate is generally only 1% to 2%, and the specificity is in the range of 85% to 95%. Ultrasound guidance for FNA of 1- to 2-cm nodules and of complex nodules may enhance diagnostic accuracy (127). Aspiration and cytologic analysis of the cyst fluid are unsatisfactory in most cases. Ultrasound-guided FNA of the solid component of a complex or cystic mass is accurate in 94% of cases (128). Some investigators have recommended that FNA be the initial investigative procedure in the evaluation of patients with solitary thyroid nodules and that scintigraphy be reserved for "follicular" neoplasms. This strategy can delay the diagnosis of a functioning autonomous thyroid nodule (AFTN). Biopsy is generally not recommended for AFTN.

Functioning Thyroid Nodules

A hot or warm nodule concentrates the radioisotope to a greater degree than does a normal thyroid gland. A hot thyroid nodule in most cases is benign, because malignant tissue rarely has normal scintigraphic activity (129–131). The incidence of hot nodules among patients with discrete thyroid nodules varies from 7% to 25% (132). A functioning thyroid nodule in a patient with normal thyroid function can be classified as either a hypertrophic nodule or autonomous adenoma (AFTN). If the person has hyperthyroidism, however, the hot thyroid nodule is an AFTN.

Hypertrophic Nodule. Hypertrophic nodules are TSH-dependent and are thought to develop as a result of either inflammatory or degenerative insult to the gland. Those areas of the thyroid that survive the insult respond to elevated levels of TSH and become hypertrophied to compensate for defective hormone synthesis in the gland. The net effect is the appearance of a hot or warm nodule, as often occurs with multinodular goiter.

Autonomous Adenoma. AFTNs arise independently of TSH stimulation and are clonal neoplasms probably resulting from somatic mutations (133). They are clinically discrete, usually solitary, and can occur at any age. Before modern-day sensitive TSH assays became available, only 20% of cases of hyperthyroidism were diagnosed when patients with AFTN came to medical attention. Most of the patients were older than 40 years, and the nodules were larger than 2.5 to 3.0 cm in diameter. Only 10% of cases of normal thyroid with an AFTN were thought to progress to thyrotoxicosis over several years of follow-up study (134). A more recent review of 49 patients with AFTN revealed that biochemical hyperthyroidism, often subclinical, was present in 74% of patients when they came to medical attention. During a mean of follow-up period of 31 months, nodules enlarged in 33% of patients not receiving definitive therapy, and 24% of patients with normal thyroids eventually had hyperthyroidism (135).

Cystic degeneration of an AFTN is common (frequency, 27% or more) and appears as an area of central photopenia surrounded by normal or increased activity on scintigraphic images (owl's-eye appearance). A similar scintigraphic finding is present after ^{131}I therapy for AFTN. Degeneration only rarely results in resolution of subclinical hyperthyroidism (135). The occurrence of carcinoma is exceedingly rare, and changes of necrosis should not be confused with malignant growth.

The introduction of sensitive TSH assays has simplified the evaluation of AFTN and has revealed a high prevalence of subclinical hyperthyroidism (135). In view of the current increased awareness of adverse consequences associated with subclinical hyperthyroidism and the rarity of spontaneous resolution of hyperthyroidism in patients with AFTN (despite a propensity for spontaneous hemorrhage and degeneration), definitive therapy is recommended. Both radioiodine therapy and hemithyroidectomy have high cure rates and a low posttreatment incidence of hypothyroidism (25%) (see Chapter 31) (136,137). Administration of iodine, as in the form of radiographic contrast media, can induce transient hyperthyroidism in patients with a nontoxic AFTN (Jod-Basedow phenomenon). If clinically indicated, especially in the care of elderly patients with coexistent cardiac disease, the administration of β-blockers before radiographic studies should be considered.

Hypertrophic versus Autonomous Functioning Thyroid Nodules. The T_3 suppression test allows differentiation of autonomous versus hypertrophic nodules. In this test, a ^{99m}Tc scan is performed after the patient is given 100 μg T_3 daily for 7 days. This is followed by a second ^{99m}Tc scan. The autonomous nodule, being functionally independent of TSH, continues to appear hot (Fig. 30.16). Hypertrophic nodules do not show increased trapping because the hypothalamic-pituitary-thyroid axis has been suppressed by the exogenous T_3. An easier and more convenient yet as effective variation of the T_3 suppression test has been described in which 10 days of T_4 administration and ^{99m}Tc pertechnetate uptake and imaging are used (59). In patients with hyperplastic nodularity, the TSH level is normal or elevated. A suppressed TSH level is typical of AFTN. The separation of these two entities is important, because treatment of patients with a hypertrophic nodule should be suppression with long-term T_4 administration. However, with the advent of the sensitive TSH assay, the T_3 suppression test is only rarely used clinically (60).

Disparate Thyroid Imaging. Disparate thyroid imaging is dissociation between trapping and organification, measured with ^{99m}Tc and ^{123}I imaging, respectively (Fig. 30.17). It occurs in 2% to 8% of thyroid nodules and is not specific for malignant disease. It has been observed in patients with adenomatous goiter and follicular adenoma when the nodule retains its ability to concentrate monovalent anions (pertechnetate and iodine) but no longer has the ability to organify iodine (67,68,138). A common subcellular defect has been postulated to account for the nonspecificity of this finding, multinodular goiter having the highest frequency of discrepancy (68,139).

In their study of 316 patients with nodular thyroid disease, Kusic et al. (68) found six different patterns of disparate imaging

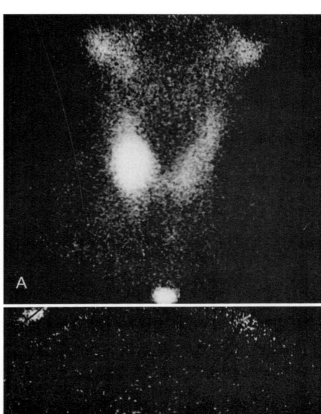

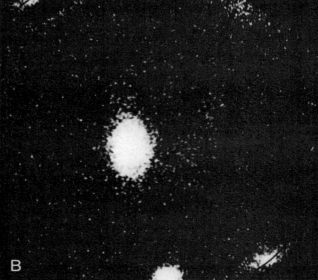

FIGURE 30.16. Effect of liothyronine suppression on an autonomous thyroid nodule. **A:** Baseline scan shows a hot nodule in the right lobe without suppression of extranodular ^{99m}Tc activity. **B:** After administration of liothyronine, suppression of all extranodular thyroid activity is consistent with autonomously functioning adenoma. (From Sandler MP, Patton JA, Sacks GA, et al. Scintigraphic thyroid imaging. In: Sandler MP, Patton JA, Partain CL, eds. *Thyroid and parathyroid imaging.* Norwalk, CT: Appleton-Century-Crofts 1986:129, with permission.)

and an incidence of 5% to 8% (Table 30.4). Twelve carcinomas were found (4%), but none in nodules showing discrepancies. Ryo et al. (67) found incongruence between ^{99m}Tc and ^{123}I scans of 40 of 122 patients (33%). Many of the nodules were hot or warm ^{99m}Tc abnormalities that were cold at ^{123}I imaging. If it is assumed that 8% of hot nodules on ^{99m}Tc images are cold on ^{123}I images and that 10% of those nodules are malignant, fewer than 1% of hot nodules are malignant. Routine re-imaging of hot nodules by means of scanning with radioiodine therefore

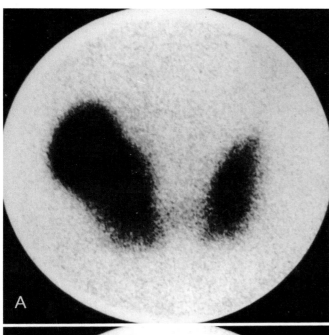

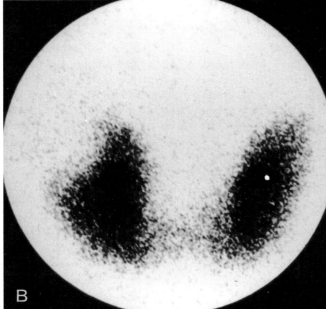

FIGURE 30.17. Discrepancy between ⁹⁹ᵐTc and ¹²³I scans. **A:** ⁹⁹ᵐTc scan shows a hot nodule in the upper pole of the right lobe. **B:** ¹²³I scintigram shows the nodule is hypofunctioning and poses a 10% to 20% risk of malignant disease. (From Sandler MP, Rao BK, Patton JA, et al. *Thyroid imaging.* In: Sandler MP, Patton JA, Gross M, et al., eds. *Endocrine imaging.* Norwalk, CT: Appleton & Lange 1992:197, with permission.)

is probably not necessary because discrepancies are far more likely to be caused by benign thyroid disorders than by malignant lesions (68). Initial thyroid imaging with ¹²³I should be reserved for (a) patients at increased risk of malignancy, that is, prepubertal patients, men, and patients with a childhood history of head and neck irradiation or a family history of malignant disease of the thyroid and for (b) patients in whom a substernal pathologic condition is a consideration (see later, Retrosternal Goiter).

Table 30.4. *Types of Discrepancy*

⁹⁹ᵐTc hot/¹²³I normal
⁹⁹ᵐTc hot/¹²³I cold
⁹⁹ᵐTc normal/¹²³I cold
⁹⁹ᵐTc normal/¹²³I hot
⁹⁹ᵐTc cold/¹²³I normal
⁹⁹ᵐTc cold/¹²³I hot

Modified from Kusic Z, Becker DV, Saenger EL, et al. Comparison of technetium-99m and iodine-123 imaging of thyroid nodules: correlation with pathologic findings. *J Nucl Med* 1990;31:393–399, with permission.

Malignant Disease and Functioning Thyroid Nodules. Focal hot nodules on iodine thyroid scintigrams are associated with an exceedingly low incidence of malignant growth (130). Autonomously functioning thyroid nodules that are differentiated carcinoma are extremely rare; only 18 such cases have been reported in the literature (131). Most reported cases of "hot" carcinoma represent the coexistence of a small malignant tumor adjacent to a benign hot lesion (140). Only a small number of well-documented cases of hot carcinoma have been reported in the literature (141,142). The case described by Ghose et al. (141) showed a high radioiodine content in the carcinoma at autoradiography. That described by Sandler et al. (142) (Fig. 30.18) showed a low in vitro iodine content measured with XRF. A cold area within a hot nodule is suggestive of carcinoma within a hyperfunctioning adenoma, although hemorrhage into a functioning adenoma is more likely. Tumor-avid imaging with ⁹⁹ᵐTc sestamibi or possibly ¹⁸F-FDG may play a role in the assessment of such a situation because malignant neoplasms usually cause intense and persistent tracer uptake, whereas a benign AFTN does not (143).

When a palpable nodule corresponds in position to a uniformly hot area on an iodine scintigram, a malignant lesion is unlikely but not completely excluded. Some follicular adenomas undergo malignant degeneration (144). Thus hyperfunctioning nodules clinically suggestive of the presence of malignant growth or in patients at high risk of carcinoma should not always be presumed benign according to scintigraphic criteria.

Hyperthyroidism

Hyperthyroidism is a clinical syndrome that results from the presence of supraphysiologic circulating levels of thyroid hormones and can occur as a consequence of numerous disease processes (Table 30.5). Most cases of hyperthyroidism are caused by increased endogenous synthesis and secretion of thyroid hormones from the thyroid, but destruction-induced thyrotoxicosis, iodide-induced hyperthyroidism (Jod-Basedow phenomenon), and other less common etiologic factors must be considered. Clinical history and physical examination combined with measurement of circulating hormones and thyroid autoantibodies, thyroid scintigraphy, and RAIU tests usually lead to identification and differentiation of the various diseases.

Graves' Disease

Clinical Examination

When hyperthyroidism and diffuse goiter are accompanied by exophthalmus or pretibial myxedema, the diagnosis of Graves'

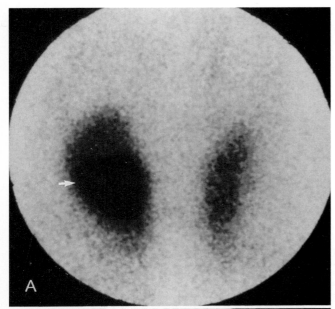

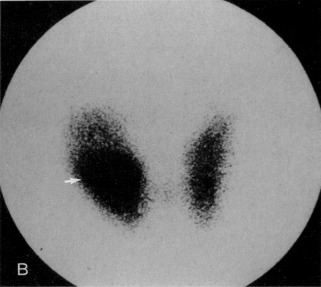

FIGURE 30.18. Thyroid carcinoma. **A:** ^{99m}Tc image shows a hot nodule in the lower pole of the right lobe (*arrow*). **B:** ^{123}I scintigram shows a hyperfunctioning nodule found at surgery to be a malignant functioning nodule (*arrow*). (From Sandler MP, Fellmeth B, Salhany KE, et al. Thyroid carcinoma masquerading as a solitary benign hyperfunctioning nodule. *Clin Nucl Med* 1988;13:411, with permission.)

Table 30.5. *Classification of Hyperthyroidism*

A Thyroid gland (≈95%)
  Diffuse toxic goiter (Graves' disease)
  Toxic nodular goiter
    Multinodular (Plummer's disease)
    Solitary nodule
  Thyroiditis (subacute)
B Exogenous thyroid hormone/iodine (≈4%)
  Iatrogenic
  Factitious
  Iodine-induced (Jod-Basedow)
C Rarely encountered causes (≈1%)
  Hypothalamic-pituitary neoplasms
  Struma ovarii
  Excessive production of human chorionic gonadotropin by trophoblastic tissue
  Metastatic thyroid carcinoma

From Sandler MP, Patton JA, Sacks GA, et al. Scintigraphy thyroid imaging. In: Sandler MP, Patton JA, Partain C, eds. *Thyroid and parathyroid imaging.* Norwalk, CT: Appleton & Lange, 1986:113, with permission.

Scintigraphy

The presence of TSIg in patients with Graves' disease results in both increased trapping and increased organification of iodide by the thyroid gland. Scintigraphic imaging of patients with Graves' disease with ^{99m}Tc reveals diffusely increased thyroidal activity with minimal blood-pool background and salivary gland activity that resembles, in many respects, normal scintiscan findings in the thyroid gland (Fig. 30.19). The gland frequently but not always appears enlarged, usually symmetrically. A pyramidal lobe can be visualized in as many as 43% (6) of patients with Graves' disease.

Patients with diffuse toxic goiter in most cases have increased ^{131}I uptake 4 and 24 hours after administration of the radionuclide. Some patients with Graves' disease have normal 24-hour RAIU because of very rapid ^{131}I turnover, that is, early uptake and rapid turnover of the radioisotope, so that the thyroid is depleted of the tracer within 24 hours, but early (4- to 6-hour) uptake is elevated in these instances. The low RAIU (usually 5% or less) among hyperthyroid patients with subacute thyroiditis, postpartum thyroiditis, silent thyroiditis, or surreptitious administration of thyroid hormone is easily differentiated from the normal RAIU that occurs in an occasional patient with Graves' disease.

In a series of 178 patients with hyperthyroidism and no suspicion of thyroid nodularity, 152 patients (85%) had typical Graves' disease, but 9% had Graves' disease with functioning or nonfunctioning nodules, 3% had unexpected subacute thyroiditis, and 3% had an AFTN (145). Scintigraphy therefore is important in the treatment of patients with Graves' disease, because 15% of those patients may have associated nodularity or another diagnosis such as AFTN or subacute thyroiditis.

A cold nodule in toxic diffuse goiter can be a functioning but TSH-dependent benign adenoma (Marine-Lenhart syndrome), another benign process, or thyroid carcinoma (Fig. 30.20) (146, 147). Marine-Lenhart syndrome occurs with a frequency of 3% to 4% among patients with Graves' disease. In Marine-Lenhart

disease can be made confidently. Other symptoms and signs of hyperthyroidism are nonspecific, as are the conventional laboratory findings of increased serum levels of T_4 and T_3 and suppressed serum levels of TSH. Because of the autoimmune causation of Graves' disease (see Chapter 29), elevated levels of circulating thyroid autoantibodies (microsomal and thyroglobulin) are present in 90% of patients. These also can occur, however, in patients with silent thyroiditis, postpartum thyroiditis, iodide-induced hyperthyroidism, and occasionally even in patients with subacute thyroiditis. Increased titers of TSIg can be measured if clinically warranted.

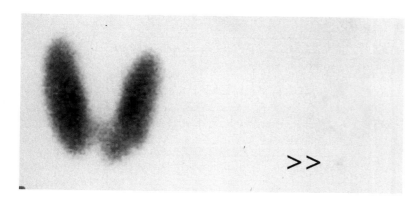

FIGURE 30.19. Graves' disease. Homogenous symmetric increased ^{99m}Tc uptake with absent background and salivary gland activity is consistent with the presence of diffuse toxic goiter. Uptake is so intense that the ^{57}Co sternal notch marker (*arrows*) is barely visible.

syndrome, a thyroid scan shows an enlarged gland with one or two poorly functioning cold nodules. The nodule is TSH-dependent, but the paranodular tissue is TSH-independent (the adenomatous cells have receptors for TSH but not for TSIg). After endogenous (posttreatment) or exogenous stimulation with rhTSH, function in the nodule returns (146,147). The nodule therefore appears cold during thyrotoxic Graves' disease, but it becomes functional after a radioiodine-induced period of euthyroidism and appears hot. At scintigraphy, however, malignant growth cannot be excluded if a cold nodule is not TSH-dependent (administration of rhTSH and ^{99m}Tc should allow visualization of the nodule in the hyperthyroid state.). Although the coexistence of thyroid carcinoma with Graves' disease is not common, it may be more common than in the general population. In one study, 16 of 886 patients undergoing thyroidectomy for Graves' disease (2%) were found to have thyroid carcinoma, 38% of which were 1 cm in diameter or larger (148). Among

315 consecutively enrolled, untreated patients with Graves' disease, 49 (16%) had thyroid nodules larger than 8 mm and an additional 57 (18%) had nodularity that developed during a routine follow-up period. Only one nodule was malignant (149). Thus nodularity is relatively common, a frequency of approximately 15% when the patient comes to medical attention and an additional 18% during the follow-up period. Malignant growth (0.3% of patients; 1% of nodules) is relatively rare. Palpable or cold nodules in patients with Graves' disease usually should be subjected to biopsy, with or without ultrasound guidance, before ^{131}I therapy, because FNA cytologic findings are difficult to interpret after radiation therapy (150). An alternative is thyroidectomy for hyperthyroidism and hypofunctioning nodule (151).

Ultrasonography

In Graves' disease, the thyroid gland is diffusely and homogeneously hypoechoic because of the abundance of colloid and the numerous dilated vessels throughout the gland. A pulsatile pattern of multiple small areas of intrathyroidal flow seen diffusely throughout the gland in both systole and diastole on color flow Doppler images is called *thyroid inferno* (71).

Magnetic Resonance Imaging

Patients with Graves' disease have prolonged values on T1-weighted images (152). MRI of patients with Graves' disease, however, is of limited value compared with the numerous modalities currently available for diagnosing this disorder and differentiating it from other causes of hyperthyroidism.

X-Ray Fluorescent Scanning

XRF imaging can be used to differentiate uncontrolled Graves' disease from diffuse multinodular goiter. The images are similar, however, to those obtained with radioisotope scintigraphy. In the evaluation of patients with Graves' disease, an increase in gland size and iodine content is seen. In the evaluation of patients with diffuse multinodular goiter, an increase in gland size, but with a patchy iodine distribution, is seen (73).

Toxic Nodular Goiter

Clinical Examination

Toxic nodular goiter can be caused by multiple adenomatous nodules or a solitary hyperfunctioning adenoma (see Chapter

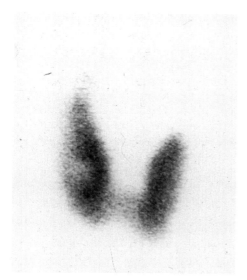

FIGURE 30.20. In this patient with thyrotoxic diffuse goiter, a solitary hypofunctioning nodule is present in the right lobe. Radioactive iodine uptake was 46%. This nodule could represent coexistent thyroid carcinoma, a benign nodule or Marine-Lenhart syndrome. (From Sandler MP, Martin WH, Moody EB. Endocrine imaging. In: Habibian MR, Delbeke D, Martin WH, et al., eds. *Nuclear medicine imaging: a teaching file.* Philadelphia: Lippincott Williams & Wilkins, 1999:49, with permission.)

29). Patients with toxic nodular goiter usually are older than those with diffuse toxic goiter (Graves' disease) and are more likely to have cardiac complications. Patients with solitary toxic nodules often are younger, varying in age from adolescence to adulthood. Solitary toxic nodules are slightly more common among men, whereas the sex incidence is roughly equal among patients with toxic multinodular goiter.

Physical examination of patients with a solitary nodule or multinodular goiter in association with hyperthyroidism is not specific for toxic multinodular goiter (Plummer's disease), because this combination can occur in patients with subacute thyroiditis, iodide-induced thyrotoxicosis, or iatrogenic hyperthyroidism (suppression of TSH with exogenous thyroid hormone in a patient with a euthyroid multinodular goiter). Clinical examination reveals classic features of hyperthyroidism, but exophthalmus and pretibial myxedema are absent. Thyroid autoantibodies and TSIg typically are absent.

Scintigraphy

At scintigraphy, toxic multinodular goiter is seen as asymmetric irregular enlargement of the gland with heterogeneous distribution of the radiopharmaceutical throughout the gland. Focal areas of increased activity represent islands of autonomously hyperfunctioning tissue, whereas the areas of decreased activity represent relatively normal thyroid tissue suppressed by excessive thyroid activity or are degenerated nodules. There is also decreased background and salivary gland activity (Fig. 30.21). The 24-hour radioiodine uptake in toxic nodular goiter can be elevated but more frequently is within the high normal range. Malignant growth in a toxic nodule or goiter is rare (<1%).

The differential diagnosis of a solitary toxic nodule with suppression of all extranodular tissue (Fig. 30.22) (due to TSH suppression by the high thyroid hormone levels) includes hemiagenesis, previous hemithyroidectomy, and lobar involvement by thyroiditis or neoplasm. Ultrasonography and CT can be used to identify suppressed thyroid tissue in the contralateral aspect

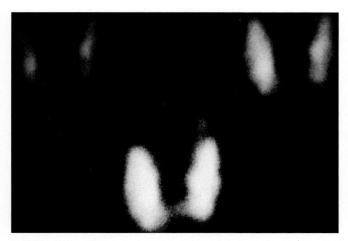

FIGURE 30.21. ^{99m}Tc scintigram shows multiple hyperfunctioning foci interspersed throughout both lobes with diminished background and salivary gland activity due to toxic multinodular goiter. (From Sandler MP, Patton JA, Sacks GA. Thyroid imaging. In: Sandler MP, Patton JA, Shaff MI, et al., eds. *Correlative imaging.* Baltimore: Williams & Wilkins; 89:230, with permission.)

of the neck, but frequently some contralateral thyroid tissue can be identified on the ^{99m}Tc or ^{123}I scintiscan if the intensity is increased on the computer monitor. Because TSH is not a major factor in the thyroid uptake of ^{201}Tl and ^{99m}Tc sestamibi (76), either can be used in the visualization of suppressed thyroid tissue in patients with AFTN, but ^{201}Tl is somewhat superior to ^{99m}Tc sestamibi for visualization of suppressed thyroid tissue.

Management of solitary hyperfunctioning adenoma can be accomplished by means of surgery, radioactive iodine therapy (136,137) (see Chapter 31), or percutaneous intranodular injection of ethanol (153). Thiouracil therapy is not a rational long-term alternative. Surgery usually is the treatment of choice of younger patients. Higher doses of ^{131}I, 15 to 25 mCi, are required for successful management of toxic AFTN because this lesion is relatively radioresistant (136). Treatment with percutaneous ethanol can be considered a useful alternative to surgery and radioiodine administration, but repeated instillation frequently is necessary (153,154).

Thyroiditis

Thyroiditis can be classified as acute, subacute, chronic, and other rare forms (Table 30.6).

Acute Thyroiditis

Acute suppurative or infectious thyroiditis is rare and usually is caused by hematogenous infection by bacteria, fungi, or parasites. Immunosuppressed patients may be particularly susceptible. In general, nuclear imaging plays a minor role in diagnosis and management. A variety of causative organisms have been isolated from aspirates. These include *Staphylococcus aureus, Streptococcus* and *Salmonella* organisms, *Escherichia coli, Mycobacterium tuberculosis,* and *Actinomyces* organisms (155). Infection is by means of local spread from adjacent structures, such as a persistent thyroglossal duct, or from distant sites through the lymphatic or blood vessels. The thyroid gland may have focal or diffuse areas of necrosis, hemorrhage, and suppuration. Abscess formation is not infrequent.

Patients with suppurative thyroiditis have acute onset of localized pain over the thyroid gland accompanied by systemic manifestations of infection. The gland is erythematous and tender. Cervical lymphadenopathy and leukocytosis are present. Patients have normal thyroid function, and RAIU is normal. Scintigraphy usually is not requested, but it may reveal areas of hypofunction corresponding to sites of tenderness. CT or ultrasonography often is used to define the extent of disease and the presence of abscess formation.

Subacute Thyroiditis

Subacute thyroiditis, also known as de Quervain's thyroiditis or granulomatous thyroiditis, is a benign, self-limited inflammatory disease of the thyroid gland most likely of viral causation (156). Epstein-Barr virus, cytomegalovirus, coxsackievirus, mumps virus, influenza virus, human immunodeficiency virus, and adenovirus all have been incriminated. The thyroid gland can be affected either diffusely or focally. Extensive cellular destruction occurs with leukocyte and subsequent lymphocyte infiltration accompanied by destruction-induced release of preformed thy-

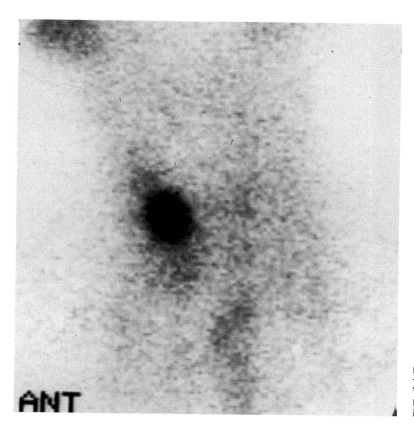

FIGURE 30.22. A patient with thyrotoxicosis and a palpable thyroid mass was found to have a solitary focus of increased ^{99m}Tc activity in the right neck with no extranodular activity. Image shows diminished background and salivary gland activity that suggest toxic autonomously functioning adenoma.

roid hormones. After a variable interval of weeks to months, the inflammatory process subsides with regeneration of the thyroid follicles and eventual attainment of euthyroidism.

The spectrum of clinical manifestations of subacute thyroiditis varies considerably. This disorder probably is more common than is typically thought and affects women five times more

Table 30.6. *Classification of Thyroiditis*

A Acute suppurative or nonsuppurative
    Bacterial: *Staphylococcus aureus*
    Streptococcus hemoliticus, or *Streptococcus pneumoniae*
    Fungal: actinomycosis
    Other organisms excluding viruses
Synonyms:
B Subacute thyroiditis (de Quervain's thyroiditis, giant cell thyroiditis, pseudotuberculous thyroiditis, silent thyroiditis)
    Viral: coxsackie, mumps, influenza, adenovirus
C Chronic thyroiditis (autoimmune)
    Lymphocytic thyroiditis (Hashimoto's struma)
    Chronic fibrous variant
    Lymphocytic thyroiditis of childhood and adolescence
    Asymptomatic atrophic thyroiditis
    Idiopathic myxedema
D Fibrous (Riedels') thyroiditis
E Radiation thyroiditis
F Traumatic thyroiditis
G Miscellaneous (e.g., amyloidosis, sarcoidosis)

From Sandler MP, Patton JA, Sacks GA, et al. Scintigraphy thyroid imaging. In: Sandler MP, Patton JA, Partain CL, eds. *Thyroid and parathyroid imaging.* Norwalk, CT: Appleton & Lange, 1986:116, with permission.

frequently than it does men. Patients may have a prodromal illness, but in most cases, there is a sudden onset of diffuse or localized pain over the gland, which can radiate to the jaw or the ear. The thyroid gland may be exquisitely tender to palpation and frequently is mildly to moderately enlarged. Symptomatic hyperthyroidism is present in 50% of patients when they seek medical attention and persists for several weeks to months. Serum thyroglobulin, T_4, and T_3 levels are increased owing to release of preformed thyroid hormones from the gland. Autoantibodies and TSIg usually are not present at significant titers. During the hyperthyroid phase, there is appropriate suppression of TSH. Injury to the follicular cells impairs the normal cellular trapping mechanism. Scintigraphy may show diffusely decreased radionuclide uptake (Fig. 30.23) or isolated areas of impaired uptake within the gland. Thyroidal RAIU is markedly decreased to less than 5%. During the recovery phase, RAIU may be elevated before returning to normal. Ultrasonography during the acute thyrotoxic phase shows diffuse hypoechogenicity similar to that of Graves' disease, but color flow Doppler imaging shows no increased vascularity, thus differentiating it from Graves' disease (157). Intense ^{67}Ga uptake is seen with subacute thyroiditis, but it also occurs with neoplastic involvement, acute suppurative thyroiditis, autoimmune thyroiditis, silent thyroiditis, amiodarone-induced hyperthyroidism, Graves' disease, and even benign adenomatous goiter (158–164). Differentiation from Graves' disease is easy because of the association of elevated thyroid hormone levels with increased RAIU in patients with Graves' disease. Although patients with chronic thyroiditis rarely have

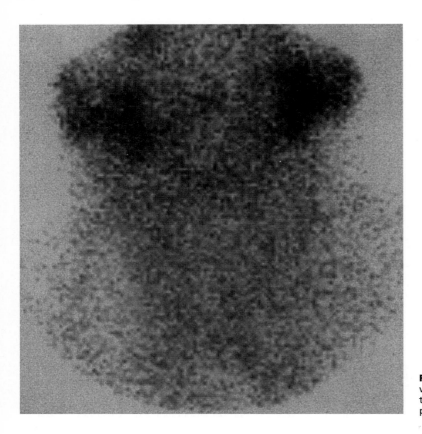

FIGURE 30.23. Markedly decreased ^{99m}Tc thyroidal activity with increased background activity in this patient with thyrotoxicosis is most consistent with subacute thyroiditis. Silent or postpartum thyroiditis would have a similar appearance.

a tender goiter, reminiscent of subacute thyroiditis, RAIU usually is normal or elevated, and the level of thyroid antibodies is invariably elevated.

A second variety of thyrotoxic subacute thyroiditis is called *silent lymphocytic thyroiditis* and is similar in manifestation to subacute granulomatous thyroiditis except for the absence of pain, tenderness, and prodromal systemic symptoms (156). No giant cells are present at histologic examination, and the cause is thought to be exacerbation of underlying autoimmune thyroid disease. Thyroid autoantibodies are present in high titers but often diminish as the thyrotoxic phase resolves. As in subacute granulomatous thyroiditis, destruction-induced hyperthyroidism is accompanied by markedly suppressed RAIU and mild thyromegaly (Fig. 30.23), all of which resolve over months. This entity occurs more frequently among women in the postpartum period (*postpartum thyroiditis*) and tends to recur with subsequent pregnancies. Many of these women eventually have long-term permanent hypothyroidism (165).

Chronic Thyroiditis

Hashimoto (166) first described lymphocytic thyroiditis in 1912. The spectrum of autoimmune thyroid disease encompasses Graves' disease and the various types of autoimmune lymphocytic thyroiditis (AIT). The most important types of AIT are chronic goitrous (Hashimoto's) thyroiditis and chronic atrophic thyroiditis, both of which are characterized by lymphocytic infiltration, fibrosis, and loss of follicular epithelium. Other overlapping variants include postpartum, silent, juvenile, and focal thyroiditis (167). Although there is a proliferation of B-cell thyroid autoantibodies, destruction of follicular cells and impairment of iodide organification are a T cell–mediated phenomenon affected by elaboration of a variety of toxic cytokines. There is a polygenetic susceptibility, *HLA* (DR3 and DR5) being one of the involved genes. The mean annual incidence of clinical AIT is approximately 3.5 per 1,000 women and 1 per 1,000 men, but results of epidemiologic studies indicate an increasing incidence (168). Almost all patients with lymphocytic thyroiditis have detectable antithyroglobulin and antiperoxidase (antimicrosomal) antibodies (167). Further evidence of an autoimmune causation is supported by a high association with other autoimmune diseases such as Graves' disease, pernicious anemia, diabetes mellitus, Addison's disease, autoimmune polyglandular syndromes, and a variety of rheumatologic diseases. The true prevalence of the disease is difficult to define. As many as 40% of U.S. white women older than 20 years have evidence of focal AIT at autopsy; this prevalence increases to 55% by the age of 80 years (169). High concentrations of thyroid autoantibodies can be detected in 30% of women and 10% of men older than 55 years and are present in 43% of female relatives of patients with clinical AIT (170). Therefore there is biochemical and autopsy evidence that AIT is extremely common in the white female population. Six percent to 8% of women have subclinical hypothyroidism that manifests as normal serum T_4 and increased serum TSH levels usually in association with high serum antithyroid antibodies. These cases of subclinical disease progress to overt hypothyroidism at a rate of 5% per year (167).

The most common initial clinical manifestation is the development of diffuse thyroid enlargement, with hypothyroidism in 50% of cases. Atrophic AIT can be associated with TSH receptor–blocking antibodies. Some patients have pain over the thyroid gland or rapid thyroid enlargement with marked discomfort. Hyperthyroidism with increased ^{131}I uptake is an infrequent manifestation of Hashimoto disease (3% to 5%) and is called *Hashitoxicosis*.

Elevated antiperoxidase or antithyroglobulin antibody titers are the most specific laboratory findings to establish the diagnosis of AIT, typically making biopsy unnecessary. RAIU can be normal, elevated, or suppressed in patients with chronic lymphocytic thyroiditis, depending on the stage of the disease. Scintigraphy reveals inhomogeneous activity throughout the gland in 50% and a pattern suggestive of either hot or cold nodules or a combination of both in 30% of patients (52). Twenty percent of patients with lymphocytic thyroiditis have normal findings at scintigraphic imaging. Ultrasonography shows reduced echogenicity in most patients with Hashimoto thyroiditis, but the ultrasonographic findings can be normal or appear similar to those of multinodular goiter (171). In summary, the scintigraphic and sonographic findings are so varied that Hashimoto's thyroiditis is in the differential diagnosis of nearly every thyroid scan.

The differential diagnosis includes euthyroid colloid goiter that can be readily differentiated because of the marked elevation of thyroid antibody titer in patients with AIT. Because both conditions are managed similarly, identification of AIT is most helpful to stimulate a search for other autoimmune disorders. Hyperthyroidism or hypothyroidism in association with AIT is helpful to differentiate it from malignant disease of the thyroid, but thyroid cancer can coexist with autoimmune thyroiditis (80). The presence of a dominant hypofunctioning nodule or cervical lymphadenopathy suggests a malignant tumor of the thyroid, and FNA is indicated. Therapy with T_4 corrects for hypothyroidism, suppresses TSH release, and can result in involution of TSH-dependent areas within the goiter.

Amiodarone-induced Thyrotoxicosis

Amiodarone is a highly lipophilic antiarrhythmic pharmaceutical containing 75 mg iodine per tablet with a half-life of more than 3 months. As expected, RAIU decreases to less than 4% in patients with normal thyroid function after amiodarone therapy is initiated. Approximately 6% of treated patients have iodine-induced hypothyroidism, perhaps related to coexistent Hashimoto's thyroiditis. However, 3% of amiodarone-treated patients eventually have thyrotoxicosis. Two varieties of amiodarone-induced thyrotoxicosis have been described (172). Type I is caused by iodide-induced hyperthyroidism (Jod-Basedow phenomenon) in patients with preexisting nodular goiter or subclinical Graves' disease. Because of the prolonged half-life of amiodarone, the hyperthyroidism can be refractory to medical therapy. Type II is amiodarone-induced destructive thyroiditis. This more common variety occurs among patients without preexisting thyroid disease, is not associated with thyroid antibodies, and does not have histologic features of subacute or autoimmune thyroiditis. The thyrotoxicosis persists for 1 to 3 months but resolves more rapidly with glucocorticoid administration. The RAIU of type II amiodarone-induced thyrotoxicosis

is near zero but RAIU also can be very low in type I disease. If RAIU is more than 5%, the presence of type I disease is likely (172). Of more use in the differentiation of these two types is color flow Doppler sonography. Type I amiodarone-induced thyrotoxicosis has normal or increased flow, whereas type II has decreased flow and patchy echogenicity. Type I disease usually responds to antithyroid drug administration in combination with perchlorate, but thyroidectomy may be necessary. The role of ^{131}I therapy in the management of type I amiodarone-induced thyrotoxicosis is controversial. Type II disease responds promptly to steroid treatment and is ameliorated by means of administration of propylthiouracil and oral cholecystographic agents such as ipodate (Oragrafin).

Exogenous Thyroid Hormone

Iatrogenic and factitious (or surreptitious) hyperthyroidism (62) are caused by administration of excessive doses of thyroid hormone and are clinically, biochemically, and scintigraphically indistinguishable. In both instances, patients have clinical and biochemical thyrotoxicosis. Elevated circulating thyroid hormones suppress TSH release by the pituitary gland and decrease thyroidal RAIU to near zero. Scintigraphy reveals impaired thyroid trapping and poor or absent uptake by the thyroid gland in association with an increase in background and salivary gland activity (Fig. 30.24). Factitious hyperthyroidism can be extremely difficult to diagnose because of the accompanying psychiatric disturbance. Clinically, patients with this disorder can be differentiated from those with endogenous hyperthyroidism because the former have suppressed thyroglobulin levels and low

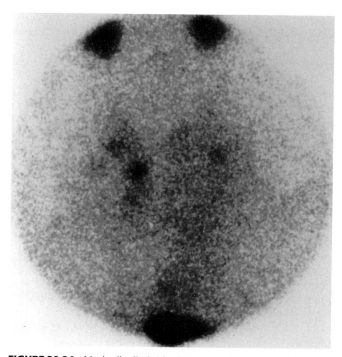

FIGURE 30.24. Markedly diminished thyroid uptake with relatively increased salivary gland and background activity in a patient with multinodular goiter who is taking thyroxine suppression therapy. Anatomic detail cannot be discerned.

RAIU. The differential diagnosis includes all causes of hyperthyroidism associated with a decrease in RAIU, all of which are associated with elevated levels of circulating thyroglobulin rather than the suppressed serum thyroglobulin level that occurs with factitious hyperthyroidism.

Iodine-induced Thyrotoxicosis

For healthy persons, ingestion of excess iodine does not cause thyrotoxicosis. Jod-Basedow disease is an unusual condition of thyrotoxicosis induced in susceptible persons by consumption of exogenous iodine (supplemented bread and dairy products, iodine-containing radiographic contrast media, and various antiarrhythmic cardiac drugs) (56). The disorder occurs most frequently among older patients with underlying thyroid disease, such as nontoxic multinodular goiter, euthyroid AFTN, or previously managed (euthyroid) Graves' disease, but it is actually quite rare in iodide-replete areas. RAIU is near zero because of flooding of the extrathyroidal iodine pool. The pathophysiologic mechanism is not well understood (see Chapter 29).

Central Hyperthyroidism

In all forms of conventional hyperthyroidism, serum TSH is undetectable (<0.05 μU/mL), because the pituitary thyrotroph is extremely sensitive to even minimal elevations of serum free T_4 or T_3. Central hyperthyroidism is a rare syndrome in which hyperthyroidism is caused by hypersecretion of TSH by the pituitary gland with resultant diffuse toxic goiter and elevated RAIU in the face of an inappropriately elevated, that is, detectable, serum level of TSH (62). The two causes of this entity are (a) TSH-producing pituitary adenoma and (b) the syndrome of partial resistance to thyroid hormone in which the pituitary gland is resistant to the feedback inhibitory effects of high circulating levels of thyroid hormones while the peripheral tissues remain sensitive and allow the patient to experience the consequences of hyperthyroidism. This subject has been reviewed (173). It is critical to differentiate these patients from those with the more common causes of hyperthyroidism that manifest as suppressed TSH levels to avoid inappropriate thyroidectomy or radioiodine therapy. These thyrotroph adenomas are usually, but not always, larger than 1 cm in diameter and often are invasive. They are differentiated from partial hormone resistance by their inability to mount a TSH response to thyrotropin-releasing hormone and by excessive secretion of α subunit. Thyrotroph adenomas usually are somatostatin receptor positive, can be visualized with ^{111}In octreotide scintigraphy, and respond to somatostatin therapy with a reduction in size and relief of hyperthyroidism (174). These large, invasive pituitary neoplasms sometimes do not resolve with hypophysectomy, even when this operation is combined with external radiation therapy (175). If the hyperthyroidism cannot be controlled postoperatively with systemic somatostatin therapy, thyroid ablation with radioiodine is appropriate.

Thyrotoxicosis of Hydatidiform Mole, Choriocarcinoma, and Hyperemesis Gravidarum

There is abundant evidence that human chorionic gonadotropin (hCG) is a weak TSH agonist. Trophoblastic tumors, hydatidiform mole, and choriocarcinoma often cause hyperthyroidism because they secrete large amounts of hCG, especially the asialo molecular variant with its enhanced thyrotropic potency. When the serum level of hCG exceeds approximately 200 IU/mL, hyperthyroidism is likely present. There is a correlation between the biochemical severity of hyperthyroidism and the serum level of hCG in these patients. Removal of the mole or effective chemotherapy for choriocarcinoma cures the hyperthyroidism (176).

In normal pregnancy, when hCG levels are highest at 10 to 12 weeks of gestation, serum TSH levels are suppressed, presumably because of slight increases in free T_4 concentration. Hyperemesis gravidarum, defined as severe vomiting in early pregnancy that causes weight loss and ketonuria, usually is associated with hCG concentrations higher than those normally occurring in pregnancy. Approximately one third to two thirds of patients with hyperemesis gravidarum have evidence of increased thyroid function. Only a small proportion of these patients have clinical hyperthyroidism, called *gestational thyrotoxicosis*. These patients probably secrete asialo variants of hCG with increased thyroid-stimulating activity, similar to that among patients with trophoblastic tumors (176).

Struma Ovarii

In approximately 1% to 2% of benign ovarian teratomas, functioning thyroid tissue is a major component and is called *struma ovarii*. Most of these patients have normal thyroid function, but in rare instances the tumor produces sufficient thyroid hormone to cause hyperthyroidism. Woodruff et al. (177) found only 13 cases among 2,000 ovarian tumors, and Kempers et al. (178) reported eight cases of struma ovarii with hyperthyroidism. The diagnosis of struma ovarii should be suspected when a patient with thyrotoxicosis has a pelvic mass. The eutopic cervical thyroid is suppressed, as evidenced by low RAIU over the neck with nonvisualization of thyroid tissue in the neck. The ectopic thyroid tissue can be visualized in the pelvis with ^{99m}Tc pertechnetate or radioiodine, and the hyperthyroidism resolves with resection of the tumor (179).

Metastatic Thyroid Carcinoma

Over the past several years, a great deal of attention has been directed at the simultaneous occurrence of hyperthyroidism and thyroid cancer. Fifteen percent to 33% of patients with Graves' disease may have associated nodularity or another diagnosis, such as AFTN or subacute thyroiditis (145,149). Two percent of patients undergoing thyroidectomy for Graves' disease and fewer than 1% of patients who undergo ultrasonography and FNA are reported to have thyroid carcinoma (148,149). The evaluation and treatment of these patients remains controversial, as recently reviewed by Mazzaferri (180).

Hyperthyroidism due to overproduction of thyroid hormone by differentiated metastatic lesions of thyroid cancer is quite rare; only 56 cases have been documented (181–185). Most but not all of the reported cases were follicular carcinoma, and the demographic features of the patients were no different from those of patients follicular carcinoma without hyperthyroidism. The overall survival rate also is similar. Approximately 60% of cases are diagnosed as thyrotoxicosis at initial presentation; the other cases occur months to years later, at the time of disease progression. The hyperthyroidism is caused by autonomous function of numerous, bulky ^{131}I-avid metastatic lesions and responds well to ^{131}I therapy.

Retrosternal Goiter

The most common neoplasms of the anterior mediastinum are thymoma, lymphoma, and germ-cell tumor. Although substernal aberrant thyroid accounts for only 7% to 10% of all mediastinal masses, the noninvasive demonstration of radioiodine uptake within a mediastinal mass is important because definitive tissue diagnosis is otherwise considered imperative before initiation of treatment, be it surgery, radiation therapy, or chemotherapy (186,187). FNA can be used effectively to obtain an accurate tissue diagnosis in 86% of cases of mediastinal masses (188).

Most goiters in the superior mediastinum arise from the cervical gland (189). Although clear continuity between the cervical and intrathoracic components usually is present in cases of extension of mediastinal goiter, the connection may be only a narrow fibrous band. In such cases, as well as in the presence of a primary intrathoracic goiter, lack of continuity between the cervical gland and the thoracic mass does not exclude the diagnosis of mediastinal goiter (Fig. 30.25). The clinical presentation of symptoms of mediastinal compression associated with a palpable goiter and mediastinal mass on a chest radiograph suggests but is not specific for the diagnosis of substernal goiter (Fig. 30.10) (186,187, 189). The preoperative diagnosis of thyroid mediastinal mass frequently requires the use of radioiodine scintigraphy, CT, or MRI (186,188,189). Contrast-enhanced spiral CT is the study of choice for evaluating an anterior mediastinal mass and often leads to an accurate diagnosis solely on the basis of the characteristic CT appearance of the various disease processes (187). CT findings of intrathoracic goiter include continuity with the cervical gland, focal calcification, high attenuation values (>70 HU), and marked enhancement after intravenous administration of contrast medium (186,187,189). These features, although suggestive of intrathoracic goiter, are not specific for the diagnosis of mediastinal thyroid mass. MRI is indicated when CT findings are equivocal and as the first-line method in particular situations, such as suspected involvement of the posterior mediastinum.

Scintigraphy

Radionuclide scanning has been the standard method for determining whether a mediastinal mass is functioning thyroid tissue. Because of high background activity related to surrounding blood-pool activity, ^{99m}Tc images are suboptimal and difficult to interpret. [123]I is the radionuclide of choice for imaging retrosternal thyroid masses. [131]I is no longer used because of the high radiation dose to the thyroid (Table 30.1). Because of delayed imaging and a high degree of specificity, ^{123}I yields high-quality images of thoracic goiters, even when uptake is relatively decreased (Fig. 30.26). The most common cause of false-negative

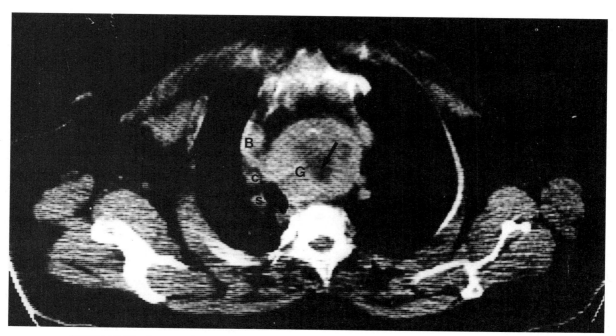

FIGURE 30.25. Computed tomographic scan shows a complete intrathoracic goiter (G) with areas of low attenuation consistent with necrosis (arrow). The brachiocephalic veins (B), carotid artery (c), and subclavian artery (s) surround the mass. (From Shaff MI, Price AC, Sandler MP, et al. Computed tomography and thyroid disease. In: Sandler MP, Patton JA, Partain CL, eds. *Thyroid and parathyroid imaging.* Norwalk, CT: Appleton-Century-Crofts, 1986:329, with permission.)

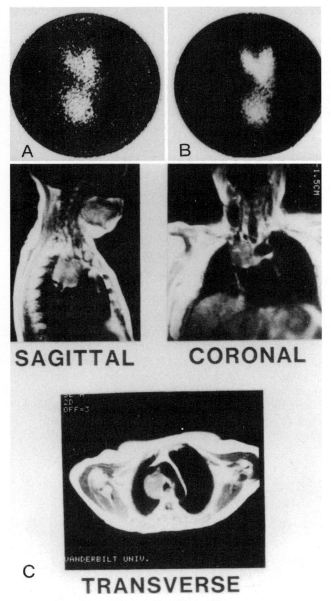

FIGURE 30.26. ^{131}I scintigraphic image **(A)**, ^{123}I scintigraphic image **(B)**, and magnetic resonance images **(C)** show functioning substernal goiter that extends into the mediastinum. (From Sandler MP, Patton JA, Sacks GA, et al. Evaluation of intrathoracic goiter with I-123 scintigraphy and nuclear magnetic imaging. *J Nucl Med* 1984;25:874, with permission.)

findings on thyroid scans in the evaluation for mediastinal goiter is recent exposure of the patient to exogenous iodine, usually from preceding contrast-enhanced CT. Rare false-positive findings on thyroid scans caused by mediastinal teratoma, as by ovarian struma, have been reported (190), as has RAIU within thymic tissue (191). ^{123}I SPECT has been successfully performed on patients with multinodular goiter to assess thyroid function and extension of the goiter in relation to the airways (192). Although occult carcinoma of the thyroid is found in as many as 17% of thoracic goiters, the incidence of "clinically significant" cancer was less than 4% in an analysis of 15 reports comprising

1,267 patients (193). ^{201}Tl, ^{99m}Tc sestamibi, and FDG PET also can be used to investigate mediastinal goiter, but all are nonspecific and can accumulate in other neoplasms that occur within the mediastinum, including lymphoma, invasive thymoma, and germ-cell tumors (194,195).

The management of mediastinal goiter is surgical resection. These large masses do not regress with T_4 suppressive therapy but can occasionally be managed successfully with 30 to 125 mCi doses of ^{131}I (196). The management of other anterior mediastinal masses varies with the histologic findings.

Neonatal Hypothyroidism

Congenital hypothyroidism (CHT) has an incidence of 1 case per 2,500 to 5,000 births, and most infants do not have signs or symptoms of hypothyroidism at birth (197). Therefore newborns in most developed countries are screened for CHT by means of measurement of serum TSH or T_4 level. Infants with CHT lose 3 or 4 IQ points each month that diagnosis and adequate T_4 replacement therapy are delayed, so a delay beyond 6 to 8 weeks of life is likely to be associated with impairment of intellectual function (198,199).

Because of the institution of newborn screening programs in the 1970s, the mental retardation of CHT has been eradicated (197). Although iodine deficiency is a common cause of CHT in some parts of the world, thyroid dysgenesis (agenesis, hypoplasia, ectopia) is the most common cause in the industrialized world and United States (197). There are several causes of transient CHT, so hormone replacement therapy is stopped for most children when they are 3 to 4 years of age so that the diagnosis and the need for lifelong treatment can be confirmed.

Thyroid scintigraphy is performed immediately after CHT is confirmed by means of repeated serum T_4 and TSH determinations. Although ^{123}I scintigraphy can be used to assess CHT, it is complicated by the necessity for oral administration and delayed acquisitions. ^{99m}Tc pertechnetate typically is used because of its ease of administration, ready availability, and its ability for easy detection of eutopic and ectopic thyroid tissue as well as for assessment of the degree of thyroidal uptake (Table 30.7). With a pinhole collimator, a close-up and a more distant view (to include the face and chest) in the anterior projection as well as a lateral view are acquired 20 to 30 minutes after intravenous injection of 500 μCi ^{99m}Tc pertechnetate. The image is normal when screening results are falsely positive (200). A small focus of usually relatively faint uptake cephalic to the thyroid cartilage is consistent with ectopia and indicates the need for lifelong T_4 therapy. A eutopic enlarged gland with increased uptake, usually marked, is most consistent with dyshormonogenesis. A small proportion of these cases of enlargement are caused by transient immaturity of the iodine organification mechanism, and the gland is normal at reassessment after 3 years of age (201). Nonvisualization of the thyroid at scintigraphy is caused by agenesis in more than 90% of cases. In the other cases, the presence of maternal transmission of TSH-receptor blocking antibodies causes nonvisualization. The latter patients have normal thyroid function at reassessment when these maternal antibodies have cleared the child's system. Patients with a nonvi-

Table 30.7. *Causes, Laboratory Findings, and Scintigraphic Findings in Congenital Hypothyroidism*

Diagnosis	Serum thyroxine level (μg/dL)	Serum thyrotropin level (mU/L)	$^{99m}TcO_4$ Scan
Primary (all cases)	<4–6	>20	Variable
Agenesis			Nonvisualization
Maternal antibodies			Nonvisualization
Ectopic-rudimentary			Small ectopic
Dyshormonogenesis			Large, hyperactive
Maternal ^{131}I therapy			Nonvisualization, hypoactive
Endemic goiter			Large, hypoactive
Pendred syndrome			Large, hypoactive
Miscellaneous			Variable
Secondary (all cases)	<4	<0.01	Nonvisualization, hypoactive
End organ (all cases)	Normal	Normal	Normal

Modified from Sfakianakis GN, Ezuddin SH, Sanchez JE, et al. Pertechnetate scintigraphy in primary congenital hypothyroidism. *J Nucl Med* 1999;40:799–804, with permission of the Society of Nuclear Medicine.

sualized gland or patients with images suggesting dyshormonogenesis undergo reevaluation at 3 to 4 years of age to exclude transient CHT. Patients with ectopia do not need reassessment.

Thyroid scintigraphic examination of neonates is indispensable in the proper diagnostic evaluation of congenital hypothyroidism, because it (a) allows a more specific diagnosis, (b) is cost-effective for selecting patients for subsequent reassessment to uncover transient CHT and discontinue thyroid hormone replacement therapy (200), and (c) defines the presence of dyshormonogenesis, which is familial and necessitates genetic counseling.

Detection of Thyroid Carcinoma and Metastatic Thyroid Disease

Thyroid carcinoma accounts for 90% of all endocrine malignant tumors and 1.5% of all malignant tumors. Approximately 19,000 new cases occur annually in the United States; 75% of these occur among women. Thyroid cancer causes only 0.4% of all cancer deaths, or approximately 1,200 per year (202). These statistics show a significant increase over the past decade. However, because differentiated thyroid cancer (DTC), which constitutes 80% of cases of thyroid carcinoma, grows slowly, occurs in young persons, and frequently is responsive to therapy (15-year survival rate, 90%), annual evaluation of every patient must continue for decades. Almost 200,000 patients living in the United States have undergone thyroidectomy for thyroid cancer and need regular assessment. In recent years, the number of radiopharmaceuticals used in the detection and ongoing evaluation of thyroid carcinoma has expanded to include not only ^{131}I but also ^{123}I, ^{201}Tl, ^{99m}Tc sestamibi, ^{99m}Tc tetrofosmin, ^{99m}Tc furifosmin, pentavalent ^{99m}Tc dimercaptosuccinic acid [^{99m}Tc-(V)-DMSA],^{123}I/^{131}I metaiodobenzylguanidine (MIBG), somatostatin receptor analogs, ^{18}F-FDG, and radiolabeled monoclonal antibodies (111). The utility of the various radio-

pharmaceuticals depends on the histologic type of thyroid cancer present. Although 80% of malignant tumors of the thyroid are DTC (papillary and follicular), MTC (7%), lymphoma (5%), and undifferentiated anaplastic carcinoma (<5%) present specific challenges in imaging. Carcinoma metastatic to the thyroid is a not an uncommon finding at autopsy. Clinically, however, it typically is an incidental finding at ultrasonography, CT, or MRI in the evaluation of a patient who has been treated for a nonthyroid malignant tumor or who has a malignant tumor in a contiguous structure; cervical lymphadenopathy often is present (203).

Differentiated Thyroid Carcinoma

Seventy percent to 80% of cases of DTC are of the papillary or mixed papillary-follicular histologic type; the others are follicular. The behavior of the two tumor types differs. Papillary carcinoma typically metastasizes to locoregional lymph nodes and the lungs, and follicular carcinoma disseminates hematogenously to the bones. DTC usually maintains the capacity to trap and organify iodine and to synthesize and release thyroglobulin. These characteristics of DTC allow postthyroidectomy management of iodine-avid disease with high-dose ^{131}I and the monitoring of therapy with radioiodine scintigraphy and measurement of thyroglobulin in the serum. However, dedifferentiation occurs to a variable extent with both types of DTC with loss of the iodide symporter or loss of thyroglobulin expression, thus presenting challenges for imaging and follow-up evaluation of these patients. Other, less differentiated malignant tumors of the thyroid have characteristics such as calcitonin expression or increased metabolism that allow specific imaging and posttherapy monitoring as well. A thorough discussion of therapy is presented in Chapter 31.

The traditional methods of follow-up evaluation of patients with DTC are whole-body radioiodine scintigraphy and monitoring of serum level of thyroglobulin. ^{131}I uptake by functioning thyroid carcinoma and metastatic lesions usually is less than 10% that of normal thyroid tissue (204). Therefore distant and nodal metastases may not be visualized at radioiodine scintigraphy before ablation of the postsurgical thyroid remnant. Optimal ^{131}I uptake by neoplastic tissue also depends on TSH stimulation. Adequate endogenous TSH levels of greater than 30 μU/mL can be attained 2 weeks after discontinuance of exogenous T$_3$ (liothyronine) therapy or 4 to 6 weeks after discontinuance of T$_4$ therapy (204).

The symptoms of hypothyroidism accompanying withdrawal of thyroid hormone can be quite bothersome to many patients (58,205), even to the extent that compliance with follow-up evaluation is compromised (206). Parenteral administration of exogenous bovine TSH used in the past is now obsolete (207). Administration of rhTSH to stimulate radioiodine uptake (and thyroglobulin release) can be used in patients maintained on thyroid hormone therapy (58,208,209). Parenteral administration of 0.9 mg rhTSH on 2 successive days results in a peak TSH level of 124 μU/mL versus 71 μU/mL after withdrawal of thyroid hormone. In a multicenter trial with 226 patients, findings on 4-mCi ^{131}I scans acquired during T$_4$ therapy after administration of rhTSH were congruent with or superior to findings on thyroid hormone–withdrawal scans in 93% of patients. There was no significant difference in detection rate for metastases. When this imaging modality was coupled with rhTSH-stimulated thyroglobulin measurement, the detection rate of disease or tissue limited to the thyroid bed was 93% and for metastatic disease was 100% (208). These results were confirmed in a report of 289 patients, 128 of whom underwent rhTSH-stimulated ^{131}I imaging and the others T_4-withdrawal imaging; there was no difference in diagnostic accuracy (209). The rapid clearance of background activity in these patients with normal thyroid function (as opposed to those with hypothyroidism) does not affect radioiodine retention by the tumor (210). Therefore radioiodine scintigraphy is performed under conditions of TSH stimulation—either endogenous stimulation through thyroid hormone withdrawal or exogenous stimulation through administration of rhTSH.

Thyroglobulin is a complex iodinated glycoprotein synthesized and released by both benign and malignant thyroid cells but by no other tissues. The level of circulating thyroglobulin is normally 1 to 25 ng/dL, but thyroglobulin should be undetectable in the absence of functioning thyroid tissue. This measurement is of little use in the differential diagnosis of thyroid nodules (99,211) but is quite useful as a tumor marker in the postoperative follow-up evaluation of patients with DTC after ^{131}I ablation of the normal remnant. An elevated serum thyroglobulin level (>2 ng/mL) in such patients is a highly sensitive and specific indicator of the presence of residual or metastatic thyroid carcinoma (212,213). Even patients with "false-positive" thyroglobulin elevations frequently are found to have metastatic disease at follow-up examinations (204,208,209,214). Thyroglobulin release is TSH-dependent, even from malignant tissue (215). Thyroglobulin determinations made after withdrawal of thyroid hormone are, in most reports, more sensitive for the detection of metastases than are levels measured in patients undergoing suppressive therapy (216,217). It is generally reported that 90% of patients with metastases have an elevated thyroglobulin level during thyroid hormone therapy (213). In a large, multicenter trial, however, that included 30 patients with ^{131}I uptake outside the thyroid bed, an elevated thyroglobulin level (>2 ng/mL) was detected in only 80% of patients taking thyroid hormone but in 100% of patients given rhTSH or who had experienced withdrawal of thyroid hormone (208). Some authors have recommended radioiodine scintigraphy only in the evaluation of patients with elevation in serum thyroglobulin level (218). Other experts, however, including the National Cancer Center Network, have advocated radioiodine scintigraphy in combination with TSH-stimulated measurements of serum thyroglobulin, because of the occurrence of recurrent disease in the absence of TSH-stimulated elevation in thyroglobulin level (209,219,220). The assay for thyroglobulin is inaccurate in the presence of antithyroglobulin antibodies, so all serum should be screened for such antibodies (221). Preliminary evidence suggests that measurement of circulating thyroglobulin mRNA by means of reverse transcription polymerase chain reaction technology is more sensitive than is serum thyroglobulin measurement and is unaffected by the presence of thyroglobulin antibodies (222).

Whole-body radioiodine scintigraphy is first performed 6 to 10 weeks after thyroidectomy and 2 weeks after discontinuance of exogenous T_3 therapy. Because mCi doses of ^{131}I can have adverse effects on a fetus, pregnancy should be excluded before administration. Static whole-body images are acquired 48 to 72 hours after oral administration of 2 to 5 mCi of ^{131}I. Images acquired at 96 hours can be useful in equivocal or suspicious cases (223). Serum TSH levels greater than 30 μU/mL should be confirmed before scanning to assure adequate stimulation (205,224). The usual protocol for rhTSH-stimulated imaging is as follows: (a) intramuscular administration of 0.9 mg rhTSH on Monday and Tuesday, (b) oral administration of 4 mCi ^{131}I on Wednesday, (c) withdrawal of serum for thyroglobulin measurement and acquisition of whole-body images on Friday. ^{99m}Tc pertechnetate scanning is not a sensitive method of following patients for metastatic disease (225), and routine serial bone scans are not generally useful (226). Consumption of a low-iodine diet can significantly increase RAIU into metastatic lesions (227). Although the specificity of ^{131}I scanning is 95%, one must not confuse normal physiologic activity in the salivary glands, nose, gastric mucosa, urinary bladder, intestines, and lactating breast with metastatic disease (Fig. 30.27). Because of hepatic catabolism of iodothyronines, diffuse liver uptake is physiologic if benign or malignant functioning thyroid tissue is present. Furthermore, rare false-positive scan results have been caused by the presence of body secretions (urine, saliva, lactation, and perspiration), pathologic transudates, Zenker's diverticulum, Meckel's diverticulum, Warthin's tumor, scrotal hydrocele, bronchogenic tumor, gastric tumor, and other nonthyroid pathologic conditions (228). More accurate localization of metastatic lesions can be attained with CT radioiodine fusion imaging, the results of which often contribute to patient care (Fig. 30.28) (229,230). In rare instances, ^{131}I uptake has been seen in Hürthle cell, medullary, and anaplastic tumors.

The sensitivity of ^{131}I scintigraphy for the detection of persistent or metastatic thyroid carcinoma is 50% to 70%, depending in part on the diagnostic dose of ^{131}I used (213,216,231). The radiation burden from ^{131}I administration is moderate, so an optimal scanning dosage is difficult to determine. If the patient receives a therapeutic dose of 100 to 200 mCi (3.7 to 5.4 GBq) of ^{131}I, a posttherapy scan 3 to 7 days later can increase the rate of detection of metastatic lesions as much as 45% (232,233). The combination of ^{131}I imaging and serum thyroglobulin determination augments the detection of metastatic disease to 85% to 100% (212,213,217,234). A schedule of follow-up examinations every 6 to 12 months is recommended until serum thyroglobulin is undetectable and radioiodine scintigraphy shows no uptake (219). Scanning every 2 to 3 years can then be instituted considering that 50% of recurrences of DTC manifest more than 5 years after initial treatment.

Stunning is the phenomenon in which the initial diagnostic dose of ^{131}I (3 to 5 mCi) reduces trapping of the subsequently administered therapeutic dose (Fig. 30.29). The frequency of this effect and its clinical significance are controversial (235), but the few quantitative uptake studies performed seem to confirm a 30% to 50% reduction of therapeutic RAIU compared with the diagnostic dose (236,237). The most elegant study prospectively demonstrated a highly significant reduction in uptake after a

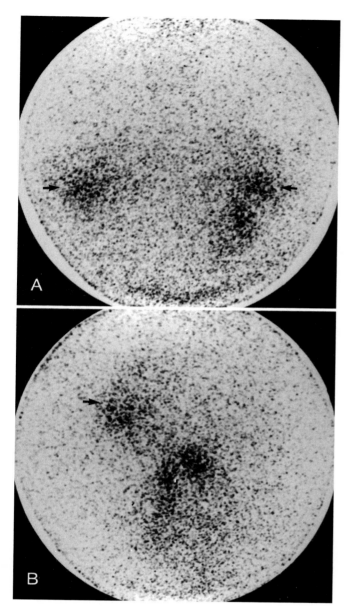

FIGURE 30.27. Whole-body ¹³¹I anterior **(A)** and confirming lateral **(B)** scintigraphic images show bilateral physiologic ¹³¹I activity in lactating breasts There is no evidence of radioiodine-avid metastatic disease.

phy with 1.0 to 1.5 mCi for the initial postsurgical examination in the hope of avoiding the damaging effects of ¹³¹I β radiation (241). Although there is little if any difference in the sensitivity for detection of thyroid remnant and cervical metastases with ¹²³I as opposed to ¹³¹I imaging, the sensitivity for detection of distant metastases may be somewhat lower with ¹²³I (242–244).

Because of the limited sensitivity of radioiodine scintigraphy for the detection of DTC metastases, and because radioiodine scintigraphy is inconvenient for patients owing to the necessity for thyroid hormone withdrawal (or rhTSH administration) and several visits to the nuclear medicine facility, other DTC-avid radiopharmaceuticals have been sought. These include ²⁰¹Tl, ⁹⁹ᵐTc sestamibi, ⁹⁹ᵐTc tetrofosmin, ⁹⁹ᵐTc furifosmin, somatostatin receptor analogs, and ¹⁸F FDG (111). The advantages of these substances include (a) the ability to detect tumor deposits that are not iodine-avid, including somewhat less differentiated varieties such as Hürthle cell (245), tall cell, and insular carcinoma, (b) the ability to image euthyroid patients who are taking T₄ for replacement, and (c) the ability to image patients who have an expanded iodine pool related to administration of iodinated contrast material. These agents have all been found to yield false negative findings in a sizable minority of patients with iodine-avid DTC, so they are most importantly used in the patient population that is ¹³¹I scan-negative but thyroglobulin positive. This constitutes approximately 10% to 15% of patients with negative results of diagnostic radioiodine scintigraphy and is indicative of the presence of persistent or recurrent tumor. These alternative radiopharmaceuticals should not be used instead of ¹³¹I scintigraphy unless the patient is known from earlier studies to be ¹³¹I-negative. Although skeletal metastases of DTC are mostly osteolytic, results of ⁹⁹ᵐTc diphosphonate scintigraphy often are positive among patients with bone metastases (64% to 85%) but may not accurately demonstrate the extent of disease (226,246,247).

Although imaging for DTC with ²⁰¹Tl, ⁹⁹ᵐTc agents, and ¹⁸F FDG is more convenient for patients because withdrawal from thyroid hormone is not necessary (not TSH-dependent) and imaging is not dependent on iodine trapping, these agents do not accumulate well in normal thyroid tissue. Hence imaging is not as sensitive as is imaging with ¹³¹I or ¹²³I in detecting the presence of a postoperative thyroid remnant (248). ²⁰¹Tl whole-body scintigraphy does, however, have a sensitivity of 60% to 90% for the detection of metastatic DTC, including ¹³¹I-negative, thyroglobulin-positive metastatic lesions (Fig. 30.30) (195, 248–253). False-positive findings can be caused by nonthyroid tumors, vascular structures, and salivary glands. Use of ²⁰¹Tl SPECT can increase the sensitivity for detection of small metastatic foci, especially in patients with disseminated micronodular pulmonary metastases (250). ⁹⁹ᵐTc sestamibi has compared favorably with thallium in the detection of thyroid metastases and may be preferable because of its near-ideal imaging characteristics (254). ⁹⁹ᵐTc sestamibi is highly sensitive for the detection of cervical and mediastinal lymphadenopathy but is less useful for detection of pulmonary metastases and is no better than conventional radiographic imaging for detection of distant metastases. In a large multicenter trial with 222 patients, the sensitivity of imaging with ²⁰¹Tl and ⁹⁹ᵐTc sestamibi was significantly less than of ¹⁸F-FDG PET (195). Other investigators have

first dose of ¹³¹I to 171 consecutively enrolled patients with benign thyrotoxic disease. This finding correlated strongly with the absorbed energy dose from the initial dose (238). This result seems to establish that stunning does exist and that it is purely a radiobiologic inhibitory phenomenon related to absorbed dose, but the effects on outcome of ¹³¹I therapy are as yet unsettled. There are qualitative data that show stunning is more prominent among patients with thyroid cancer receiving higher diagnostic doses. These data have prompted many investigators to recommend scanning doses of 3 mCi or less (239). In a report on 255 patients who underwent scanning with only 2 mCi of ¹³¹I, clinically evident stunning occurred in only 5 (2%) patients (240). As an alternative, some institutions perform ¹²³I scintigra-

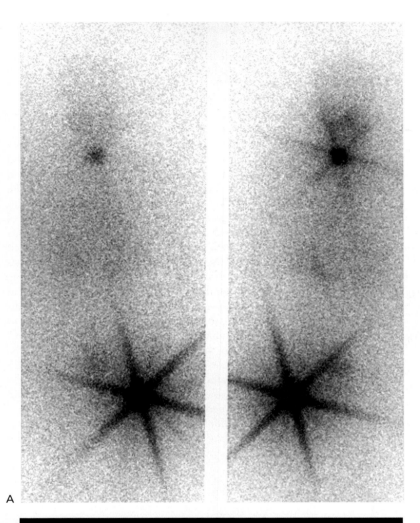

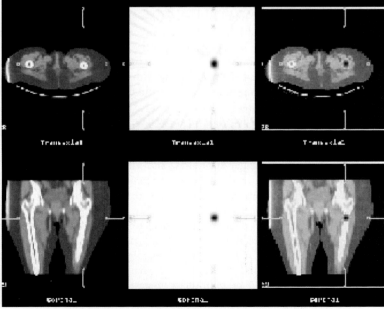

FIGURE 30.28. A: Whole-body posttherapy image shows markedly increased activity in the thyroid bed most compatible with physiologic activity in the postoperative remnant. However, a large focus of intense activity in the pelvis or at the groin would suggest the presence of distant metastasis. **B:** Fusion of CT and SPECT images allows accurate localization of the metastatic lesion to the proximal left femur.

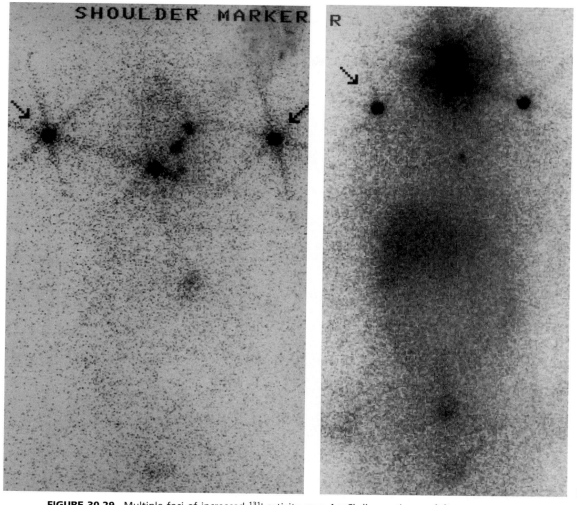

FIGURE 30.29. Multiple foci of increased ^{131}I activity on a 4-mCi diagnostic scan **(A)** are not present on the images **(B)** acquired 1 week after administration of a 150-mCi therapeutic dose. These findings are consistent with stunning.

found ^{18}F-FDG and ^{201}Tl to have similar sensitivity for the detection of metastases; congruency was present for 94% of lesions (251). ^{99m}Tc tetrofosmin and ^{99m}Tc furifosmin have sensitivities similar to that of ^{99m}Tc sestamibi for detection of DTC metastases (241,252,253,255–258). CT and MRI are more useful for detection of intrathoracic and intraabdominal disease.

Somatostatin receptor scintigraphy is more commonly used in the assessment of MTC and other neuroendocrine tumors, but nonmedullary carcinoma of the thyroid also expresses somatostatin receptors. In 95% of Hürthle cell carcinoma patients having serum Tg levels greater than 10 mg/ml, but results have been disappointing in patients with non-Hürthle cell DTC (259, 260).

Metastatic lesions of thyroid carcinoma that are poorly visualized with ^{131}I have been imaged with ^{18}F-FDG PET while patients continued thyroid hormone suppressive therapy (Fig. 30.31). The first systematic investigation comparing radioiodine scintigraphy and ^{18}F-FDG PET showed that 19 of 26 patients (73%) with negative results of ^{131}I scans had positive results

of ^{18}F-FDG PET scans; four of the lesions were Hürthle cell carcinoma (261). Their findings have been confirmed by numerous investigators (195,251,262–268). The conclusion is that ^{18}F-FDG imaging is particularly helpful in the evaluation of patients with elevated thyroglobulin levels but negative findings at radioiodine scintigraphy (269). Dietlein et al. (266,267) compared the value of radioiodine, ^{99m}Tc sestamibi, and ^{18}F-FDG imaging in the follow-up evaluation of patients with DTC. The sensitivity was 50% for ^{18}F-FDG or ^{99m}Tc sestamibi imaging alone, 61% for radioiodine imaging alone, and 86% for FDG and radioiodine imaging combined. The sensitivity of ^{18}F-FDG PET in a more selected population of patients with elevated thyroglobulin levels and negative results of posttherapy radioiodine scans was 82% (266,267). Similar conclusions were reached in a large multicenter trial with 222 patients. The sensitivity of ^{18}F-FDG PET was 85% for the patients with negative results of radioiodine scintigraphy and was significantly higher for ^{18}F-FDG than for ^{201}Tl or ^{99m}Tc sestamibi imaging (195). In a cohort of 18 patients with elevated thyroglobulin levels but nega-

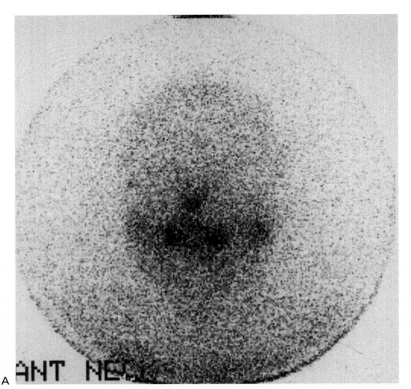
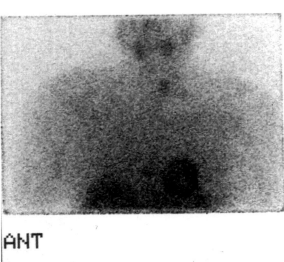
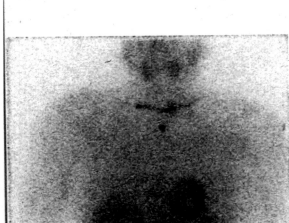

FIGURE 30.30. Metastatic thyroid carcinoma. In a patient with an elevated serum thyroglobulin level but a negative ^{131}I scan **(A)**, ^{201}Tl imaging **(B)** reveals a focus of increased activity in the left neck related to tracheoesophageal metastatic lymphadenopathy found at surgery.

tive results of diagnostic ^{131}I scans, Wang et al. (262) found that ^{18}F-FDG PET had a positive predictive value of 92%. The authors concluded that ^{18}F-FDG PET in this selected population changed the treatment of 50% of the patients (262). Management was reportedly altered in 55% of a similar cohort in another report (268). In a review of 14 studies, ^{18}F-FDG PET had a consistently high sensitivity for detection of recurrent neoplasm in patients with elevated serum thyroglobulin levels and negative results of radioiodine scintigraphy (269). ^{18}F-FDG PET does appear to be more sensitive for detection of tumor deposits in direct proportion to the degree of elevation in serum thyroglobulin level (50% for thyroglobulin 10 to 20 ng/mL and 93% for thyroglobulin >100 ng/mL). This finding is probably representative of tumor volume, but it has been reported to identify (265), 70% of cervical nodes less than 1 cm in diameter (264). There is preliminary evidence that ^{18}F-FDG PET may have prognostic importance. In a series of 125 patients undergoing annual follow-up radioiodine scintigraphy, serum thyroglobulin determination, and ^{18}F-FDG PET, the 3-year survival rate was only 18% among patients with a high volume of ^{18}F-FDG–avid

disease versus 96% among those with less bulky disease. No patient with ^{18}F-FDG-negative distant metastases died (263). Although almost all PET performed on patients with DTC has been performed with the patient in the euthyroid state, preliminary data suggest that TSH stimulation increases sensitivity for detection of metastatic disease as much as 30% with a 63% increase in tumor-to-background ratio (270). The discordance between ^{131}I and ^{18}F-FDG uptake is controversial but is theoretically related to increased glucose transport in less differentiated tumors that have lost their ability to trap iodine. Metaanalysis of seven reports indicated that 75% of patients with recurrent DTC have positive results of ^{131}I scans (271). Many of the others can be successfully treated with high-dose ^{131}I therapy subsequently demonstrating positive findings on posttherapy scans (272). However, the long-term success of ^{131}I therapy in the care of patients with negative results of radioiodine scintigraphy and elevated thyroglobulin levels continues to be controversial in regard to outcome (273). Over a 12-year follow-up period, 89% of patients with negative results of diagnostic radioiodine scintigraphy but elevated serum thyroglobulin levels

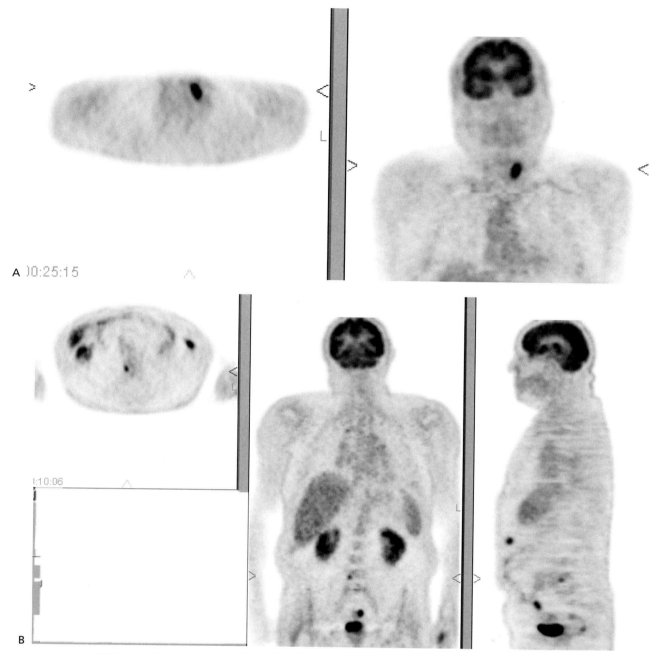

FIGURE 30.31. In a patient with Hürthle cell carcinoma and a rising serum thyroglobulin level, ultrasonography revealed a left hypervascular mass suggestive of metastatic adenopathy. Results of ^{131}I scintigraphy were negative, but ^{18}F-FDG imaging **(A)** shows not only the left cervical metastatic lesion but also a small hypermetabolic focus in the lumbar spine **(B)**.

and no radiographic evidence of tumor had a significant reduction in serum thyroglobulin level, 68% down to undetectable levels, without ^{131}I or any other treatment. Therefore the extent of disease and advisability of surgical treatment of some of these patients with positive results of posttherapy scans and elevated thyroglobulin levels may be better demonstrated with ^{18}F-FDG PET combined with conventional cross-sectional imaging. Patients with elevated serum thyroglobulin levels and negative re-

sults of ^{131}I scans after ^{131}I therapy are best evaluated with ^{18}F-FDG PET. The results lead to a change in management in more than 50% of cases.

Ultrasonography, CT, and MRI are adjunctive imaging modalities in defining the extent of metastatic disease. At ultrasonography, metastatic adenopathy tends to be round rather than ellipsoid with a replaced hilum and low-resistance flow rates during Doppler spectral analysis. The sensitivity for detection of

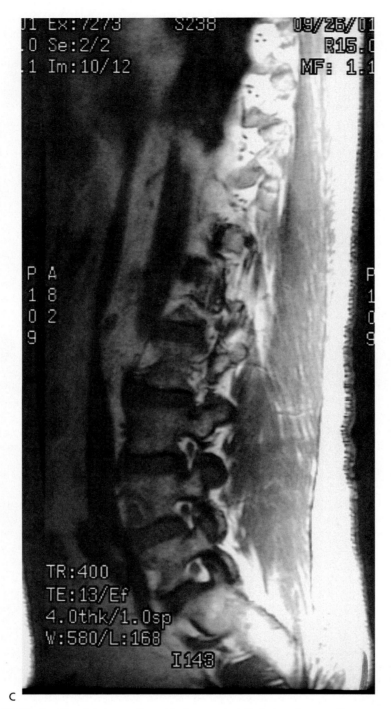

FIGURE 30.31. *Continued.* Later confirmed to be a metastatic lesion at magnetic resonance imaging (C).

cervical adenopathy is greater than 90% when ultrasonography is used (256,257,274). CT and MRI are more useful for detection of intrathoracic and intraabdominal disease.

In summary, most patients who have negative (results of) radioiodine scintigraphy but elevated serum thyroglobulin levels undergo ^{131}I scanning after receiving a therapeutic dose of [131]I.

If no metastatic lesions are identified at posttherapy radioiodine scintigraphy, the patient is observed with a combination of conventional imaging, including chest radiographs, ultrasonography of the neck, and cross-sectional imaging with or without the use of alternative radiopharmaceuticals. ^{18}F-FDG seems to be the radiopharmaceutical of choice, and imaging with this agent would be expected to be more sensitive than would imaging with ^{99m}Tc sestamibi or ^{201}Tl for small-volume disease (252, 253,257,258).

Medullary Carcinoma of the Thyroid

Approximately 3% to 5% of all cases of thyroid cancer are MTC. MTC is an intermediate-grade malignant lesion that occurs in both a sporadic (80%) and a familial (20%) form (275). There is autosomal dominant inheritance in families with multiple endocrine neoplasia, type 2A and type 2B, as well as in the syndrome of familial MTC associated with germline mutations of the *ret* proto-oncogene located on chromosome 10. Because there is a 4% to 10% prevalence of "cryptic" heritable disease in the absence of a definite family history, all patients with MTC should undergo *ret* gene testing. Nearly 50% of patients have metastatic cervical adenopathy when they initially seek medical attention. When the lesion is clinically palpable, surgical cure is rarely achieved despite performance of regional lymphadenectomy, but the 10-year survival rate is 86% even with persistent postoperative hypercalcitoninemia (276). The 5-year survival rate is 94% among patients with metastatic lymphadenopathy but only 41% among those with extranodal disease (277). Only in the occasional patient with MTC is the tumor radioiodine-avid, but clinical response does occur among such patients (278). Typically, however, MTC does not concentrate iodine, so ^{131}I scintigraphy is not useful, and ^{131}I treatment results in no improvement in survival or recurrence rate (279). The "bystander" effect is probably not of clinical importance.

Recurrent or persistent disease is easily detected through the presence of elevated serum levels of calcitonin and carcinoembryonic antigen (CEA) (275), but the optimal modality for localization of metastases continues to evolve. The long-term utility of procedures for localization of metastatic MTC is controversial. Some reports suggest that as many as 40% of cases of persistent postoperative hypercalcitoninemia can be resolved with repeated microdissection of residual metastatic nodes in the neck with an accompanying improved prognosis (280–282). Other authors report postoperative normalization of calcitonin levels in only 6% to 15% of patients at reoperation (283,284). However, most investigators report relief of symptoms and a decrease in the occurrence of distant metastases in patients who respond to repeated surgery with a 50% or more reduction in serum calcitonin level (283,284). Therefore many surgeons reoperate on a patient with MTC and significantly elevated calcitonin levels, particularly if there is no extranodal disease, in the hope of relieving symptoms, decreasing the rate of progression, and prolonging survival.

Selective venous catheterization for serum calcitonin determination is a sensitive and specific localization method (281,282, 285,286), but it is invasive and technically demanding. CT and MRI provide a high degree of spatial resolution for the purposes of surgical planning and are similar to or slightly inferior to radionuclide scanning for the detection and localization of recurrent of MTC (284,287-289). As with other thyroid tumors, both ^{201}Tl and ^{99m}Tc sestamibi have proved highly sensitive and specific in the diagnosis of MTC, but only if basal calcitonin

levels are greater than 1,000 pg/mL (248,290–292). In a similar manner, ^{18}F-FDG PET is evolving into a primary modality for detection of MTC (293). The sensitivity was 73% among 20 consecutively evaluated patients with MTC and elevated calcitonin levels (294,295) and 94% in a cohort of 36 patients with MTC (Fig. 30.32) (296). ^{99m}Tc-(V)-DMSA localizes in a high percentage of MTC tumors (283,289,297–299). Pentavalent DMSA resembles the phosphate ion and is taken up by tumors, such as MTC and osteosarcoma, in which calcification is a well-recognized phenomenon (300). However, ^{99m}Tc-(V)-DMSA uptake also occurs in thyroid amyloidosis (301), and amyloid deposition within MTC is characteristic (275). False-negative results on ^{201}Tl and ^{99m}Tc-(V)-DMSA scans are most frequent among patients with only mildly elevated serum calcitonin levels, a finding probably indicative of low tumor volume (297).

Somatostatin receptors and CEA are present on the cell surface of many medullary carcinomas (302). Most metastatic lesions of MTC can be visualized with ^{111}In-labeled somatostatin receptor scintigraphy. A few false-positive foci are seen owing to the presence of chronic inflammation and somatostatin receptor–positive tumors other than MTC, but sensitivity was reported initially to be approximately 90% (287,302,303). More recently, in examinations of 25 patients with recurrent MTC, ^{111}In octreotide imaging depicted 65% of lesions, whereas ^{99m}Tc-(V)-DMSA imaging depicted only 34% (283). In a study with 14 patients with recurrent MTC, ^{111}In octreotide identified 78% of patients with recurrent disease but detected only 44% of metastatic lesions; ^{99m}Tc-(V)-DMSA identified only 57% of patients and 30% of lesions (289). Somatostatin-receptor scintigraphy is insensitive for detecting hepatic tumor owing to the presence of physiologic hepatic uptake. Several studies have shown a relatively high incidence of cases of hepatic metastases not shown on CT scans but confirmed at staging laparoscopy. Among 36 patients with recurrent MTC, multiple, subcentimeter, hypervascular metastatic lesions of the liver were found preoperatively in 89% of patients only by means of hepatic angiography (296). There is preliminary evidence to support the utility of radiolabeled anti-CEA antibodies in the detection of recurrence of MTC (304). This modality offers hope for therapy as well.

Like other neuroectodermal tumors, 40% to 50% of MTC take up ^{123}I/^{131}I MIBG (305,306). Although less sensitive than ^{201}Tl, ^{99m}Tc-(V)-DMSA, and ^{99m}Tc MIBI imaging, ^{131}I MIBG imaging is highly specific and may thus be useful in conjunction with other localization modalities (285). Furthermore, the therapeutic efficacy of high-dose (100 to 300 mCi) ^{131}I MIBG imaging of patients with significant uptake appears promising (307–309). Although a complete response is uncommon, a partial response with considerable palliation of symptoms and hormonal improvement has occurred in most patients. Therapy for this otherwise difficult malignant disease should improve over the next several years.

In summary, early detection of recurrent MTC and localization of metastases is important because microdissection offers the chance for long-term remission or cure for some patients (6% to 40%), relief of symptoms, reduction in the occurrence of distant metastases, and possibly prolongation of survival. No

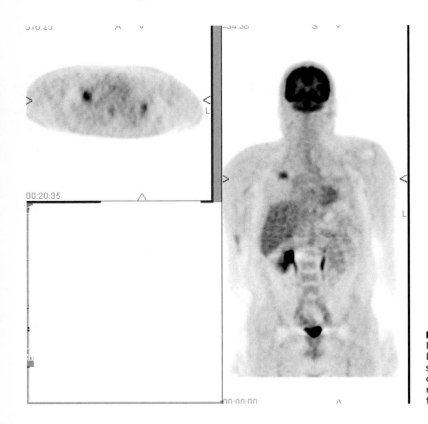

FIGURE 30.32. Young man with previously resected medullary thyroid carcinoma and an increasing serum calcitonin level. ^{18}F-FDG image shows increased pulmonary activity that suggests the presence of metastatic disease. A computed tomographic scan obtained several months earlier and a concurrent ^{111}In octreotide scan both were interpreted as negative for metastatic disease.

single diagnostic modality can reliably demonstrate the full extent of disease in these patients, but the combination of cross-sectional radiography (ultrasonography, CT, MRI) with scintigraphy using ^{111}In octreotide or ^{18}F-FDG PET is proving helpful. Radioguided surgery with radiolabeled anti-CEA antibodies or other radiopharmaceuticals offers perhaps the best hope for the detection and resection of very small metastatic lesions (283), but there is a growing consensus that most patients with evidence of recurrent or persistent MTC may need laparoscopy or hepatic angiography before embarking on repeated surgery for cure (296).

Thyroid Lymphoma and Anaplastic Carcinoma

Lymphoma of the thyroid constitutes less than 5% of all malignant tumors of the thyroid and only 2% of all cases of extranodal lymphoma. It usually manifests as a rapidly enlarging painless goiter in an elderly patient with preexisting AIT (310) with or without accompanying hypothyroidism. [99m]Tc and ^{131}I scintigraphy are of little utility in differentiating lymphomatous involvement from thyroiditis. At ultrasonography, thyroid lymphoma usually can be differentiated from unaffected tissue as an extremely hypoechoic masses intermingled with echogenic structures. Ultrasonography, CT, and MRI are comparable in the detection of the primary tumor and nodal metastases (311, 312). Preliminary data suggest that ^{201}Tl and ^{99m}Tc sestamibi imaging can be useful in the detection of thyroid lymphoma and in assessment of response to therapy (313). [67]Ga scanning is not helpful, usually showing uptake similar to that of Hashimoto thyroiditis and anaplastic carcinoma (314). FDG activity is increased in lymphoma, and PET can be useful in defining extrathyroidal disease, but biopsy is required. Treatment consists of external radiation therapy and combination chemotherapy. The survival rate is nearly 100% at 8 years in the absence of distant disease (310).

Undifferentiated or anaplastic carcinoma of the thyroid accounts for fewer than 5% of malignant tumors of the thyroid. It manifests most frequently as a rapidly enlarging goiter in an elderly person. The survival rate is extremely poor (315). [99m]Tc and ^{123}I scintigraphy show nonspecific areas of diminished activity. Although results of ^{67}Ga scintigraphy usually are positive, this modality contributes little to preoperative diagnosis or postoperative follow-up evaluation (316). Preliminary reports indicate that imaging with ^{201}Tl or ^{99m}Tc sestamibi can be useful in the evaluation of recurrent anaplastic carcinoma, especially if findings at CT or ultrasonography are equivocal (249,317). Ultrasonography and CT often reveal calcification and necrosis extending into surrounding tissue and regional or mediastinal adenopathy (318). Although the median survival period is less than 6 months, aggressive multimodality radiation therapy and chemotherapy among patients without distant metastases can result in a few enduring responses of more than 2 years (319).

ACKNOWLEDGMENT

The authors thank Thomas A. Powers, MD, and Bhaskara K. Rao, MD, for their previous contributions to this chapter.

REFERENCES

1. Pintar JE. Normal development of the hypothalamic-pituitary-thyroid axis. In: Utiger RO, ed. *Werner and Ingbar's the thyroid: a fundamental and clinical text,* 8th ed. Philadelphia: Lippincott Williams & Wilkins, 2000:7–19.
2. Martin TJ, Moseley JM, Sexton PM. Calcitonin. In: DeGroot LJ, Jameson JL, eds. *Endocrinology,* 4th ed. Philadelphia: WB Saunders, 2001:999–1008.
3. Villee DB. Development of endocrine function in the human placenta and fetus (second of two parts). *N Engl J Med* 1969;281:533–541.
4. Villee DB. *Human endocrinology: a developmental approach.* Philadelphia: WB Saunders, 1975.
5. Clark OH. Surgical anatomy. In: Braverman LE, Utiger RD, eds. *Werner & Ingbar's the thyroid: a fundamental and clinical text,* 8th ed. Philadelphia: Lippincott Williams & Wilkins, 2000:455–461.
6. Levy HA, Sziklas JJ, Rosenberg RJ, et al. Incidence of a pyramidal lobe on thyroid scans. *Clin Nucl Med* 1982;7:560–561.
7. Ashkar FS. Thyroid imaging and function studies. *Clin Nucl Med* 1981;6:P77–86.
8. Goolden AW. Tests of thyroid function in vivo. *J Clin Pathol* 1975;28:244–247.
9. Cavalieri RR. Trace elements. In: Goodhard RS, Shils ME, eds. *Modern nutrition in health and disease,* 6th ed. Philadelphia: Lea & Febiger, 1980:396.
10. Ficken VJ, Adams GD, Allen EW, et al. Absorption of iodide following oral administration. *Clin Nucl Med* 1983;8:9(abst).
11. Thyroid radionuclide uptake measurements. *Int J Appl Radiat Isotl* 1972;23:305–313.
12. Green JP, Wilcox JR, Marriott JD, et al. Thyroid uptake of 131-I: further comparisons of capsules and liquid preparations. *J Nucl Med* 1976;17:310–312.
13. Robertson JS, Verhasselt M, Wahner HW. Use of 123-I for thyroid uptake measurements and depression of 131-I thyroid uptakes by incomplete dissolution of capsule filler. *J Nucl Med* 1974;15:770–774.
14. Halpern S, Alazraki N, Littenerg R, et al. I-131 thyroid uptakes: capsule versus liquid. *J Nucl Med* 1973;14:507–510.
15. Hamburger JI. Application of the radioiodine uptake to the clinical evaluation of thyroid disease. *Semin Nucl Med* 1971;1:287–300.
16. Prince JR, Dukstein WG, White WE, et al. An evaluation of the 24-hour RAIU test performed with an Auger camera and a pinhole collimator. *Clin Nucl Med* 1979;4:471–475.
17. Rosenberg IN. Evaluation of thyroid function. *N Engl J Med* 1972;286:924–927.
18. Lawrence CA, Russell ME, Davis RP, et al. The effect of capsule content variations on thyroid uptake results. *J Nucl Med* 1970;11:561–563.
19. Hooper PL, Turner JR, Conway MJ, et al. Thyroid uptake of I-123 in a normal population. *Arch Intern Med* 1980;140:757–758.
20. Oddie TH, Pirnique FG, Fisher DA, et al. Geographic variation of radioiodine uptake in euthyroid subjects. *J Clin Endocrinol Metab* 1968;28:761–765.
21. Hayek A, Stanbury JB. The diagnostic use of radionuclides in the thyroid disorders of childhood. *Semin Nucl Med* 1971;1:334–344.
22. Steward RD, Murray IP. The estimation of extra-thyroidal neck tissue radioactivity during thyroidal radioiodine uptake measurements. *J Nucl Med* 1967;8:678–685.
23. Rosenthall L. A quantitative analysis of the effect of thyroid suppression and stimulation on 131-I thyroid trapping. *Radiology* 1973;108:353–357.
24. Herman MW, Spiegler P, Koontz R, et al. Coincidence counting of 123-I in pediatric thyroid studies. *Radiology* 1974;113:455–458.
25. Chervu S, Chervu LR, Goodwin PN, et al. Thyroid uptake measurements with I-123: problems and pitfalls [Concise Communication]. *J Nucl Med* 1982;23:667–670.
26. Martin PM, Rollo FD. Estimation of thyroid depth and correction for I-123 uptake measurements. *J Nucl Med* 1977;18:919–924.
27. Lee KH, Siegel ME, Fernandez OA. Discrepancies in thyroid uptake

28. Benjamin RS, Amro A, El-Desouki MI. Measurement of iodine-123 thyroid uptake using a gamma camera with LEAP collimator. *J Nucl Med Technol* 1999;27:215–219.
29. Hardy-Young S, Blackburn G. Congenital thyrotoxicosis: case report and results of 132-iodine uptake studies. *J Endocrinol* 1968;41:299–300.
30. Levy BS, Ashburn W. Thyroid-uptake studies using 132-I. *J Nucl Med* 1969;10:286–289.
31. Sostre S, Parikh S. A visual index of thyroid function. *Clin Nucl Med* 1979;4:59–63.
32. Hayes MT, Wesselossky B. Simultaneous measurement of thyroid trapping (Tc-99m) and binding (I-131): clinical and experimental studies in man. *J Nucl Med* 1973;14:785–792.
33. Burke GA, Halko A, Silverstein GE, et al. Comparative thyroid uptake studies with I-131 and 99m-Tc. *J Clin Endocrinol Metab* 1972;34:630–637.
34. Smith JJ, Croft BY, Brookeman VA, et al. Estimation of 24-hour thyroid uptake of I-131 sodium iodide using a 5-minute uptake of technetium-99m pertechnetate. *Clin Nucl Med* 1990;50:80–83.
35. Higgins HP, Ball D, Eastham S. 20-min 99m Tc thyroid uptake: a simplified method using the gamma camera. *J Nucl Med* 1973;14;907–911.
36. Schneider PB. Simple, rapid thyroid function testing with 99mTc-pertechnetate thyroid uptake ratio and neck/thigh ratio. *Am J Roentgenol* 1979;132:249–253.
37. Kirkegaard C, Friis T, Molholm Hansen JE, et al. The diagnostic and prognostic value of the 20-minute 99mTc-uptake in the thyroid gland. *Acta Endocrinol* 1973;74:659–665.
38. Wing J, Kalk WJ, Ganda C. High radioisotope uptakes in patients with hypothyroidism. *S Afr Med J* 1982;62:892–893.
39. Ramtoole S, Maisey MN, Clarke SE, et al. The thyroid scan in Hashimoto's thyroiditis: the great mimic. *Nucl Med Commun* 1988;9:639–645.
40. Hamburger JI. Pitfalls in the laboratory diagnosis of atypical hyperthyroidism. *Arch Intern Med* 1979;139:96–98.
41. Sternthal E, Lipworth L, Stanley B, et al. Suppression of thyroid radioiodine uptake by various doses of stable iodine. *N Engl J Med* 1980;303:1083–1088.
42. McDougall IR, Cavalieri RR. In vivo radionuclide tests and imaging. In: Braverman LE, Utiger RD, eds. *Werner & Ingbar's the thyroid: a fundamental and clinical text,* 8th ed. Philadelphia: Lippincott Williams & Wilkins, 2000:355–375.
43. Pittman JA Jr, Dailey GE III, Beschi RJ. Changing normal values for thyroidal radioiodine uptake. *N Engl J Med* 1969;280:1431–1434.
44. Alazraki NP, Halpern SE, Ashburn WL. A re-evaluation of 131-I thyroid uptakes. *Radiology* 1972;105:611–614.
45. Wong ET, Schultz AL. Changing values for the normal thyroid radioactive iodine uptake test. *JAMA* 1977;238:1741–1743.
46. Ericsson UB, Thorel JI. Decreased radioiodine uptake values without increase in urinary iodine excretion. *Acta Med Scand* 1981;209:293–297.
47. Freund G, Thomas WC Jr, Bird ED, et al. Effect of iodinated water supplied on thyroid function. *J Clin Endocrinol Metab* 1966;26:619–624.
48. Grayson RR. Factors which influence the radioactive iodine thyroidal uptake test. *Am J Med* 1960;28:397.
49. Beckers C, van Ypersele de Strihou, Coche E, et al. Iodine metabolism in severe renal insufficiency. *J Clin Endocrinol Metab* 1969;29:93–96.
50. Barsivala V, Virkar K. Thyroid functions of women taking oral contraceptives. *Contraception* 1974;9:305–314.
51. Jarnerot G. The thyroid in ulcerative colitis and Crohn's disease, I: thyroid radioiodide uptake and urinary iodine excretion. *Acta Med Scand* 1975;197:77–81.
52. Fisher DA, Oddie TH, Johnson DE, et al. The diagnosis of Hashimoto's thyroiditis. *J Clin Endocrinol Metab* 1975;40:795–801.
53. Greig WR. Radionuclide evaluation of thyroid disease in children. *Semin Nucl Med* 1973;3:3–25.
54. Baschieri L, Benditti A, Deluca F, et al. Evaluation and limitations

of the perchlorate test in the study of thyroid function. *J Clin Endocrinol Metab* 1963;23:786.

55. Takeuchi K, Suzuki H, Horiuchi Y, et al. Significance of iodide-perchlorate discharge test for detection of iodine organification defect of the thyroid. *J Clin Endocrinol Metab* 1970;31:144–146.

56. Roti E, Vagenakis AG. Effect of excess iodide: clinical aspects. In: Braverman LE, Utiger RD, eds. *Werner & Ingbar's the thyroid: a fundamental and clinical text,* 8th ed. Philadelphia: Lippincott Williams & Wilkins, 2000:721–732.

57. Toft AD. Clinical practice. Subclinical hyperthyroidism. *N Engl J Med* 2001;345:512–516.

58. Ladenson PW, Braverman LE, Mazzaferri EL, et al. Comparison of administration of recombinant human thyrotropin with withdrawal of thyroid hormone for radioactive iodine scanning in patients with thyroid carcinoma. *N Engl J Med* 1997;337:888–896.

59. Ramos CD, Zantut-Wittmann DE, Tambascia MA, et al. Thyroid suppression test with L-thyroxine and [^{99m}Tc] pertechnetate. *Clin Endocrinol (Oxf)* 2000;52:471–477.

60. Burch HB, Shakir F, Fitzsimmons TR, et al. Diagnosis and management of the autonomously functioning thyroid nodule: the Walter Reed Army Medical Center experience, 1975–1996. *Thyroid* 1998; 8:871–880.

61. Myhill J. Thyroid testing during drug administration. *Med J Aust* 1969;1:422–424.

62. Cooper DS, Ridgway EC, Maloof F. Unusual types of hyperthyroidism. *J Clin Endocrinol Metab* 1978;7:199–220.

63. Schleusener H, Schwander J, Fischer C, et al. Prospective multicenter study on the prediction of relapse after antithyroid drug treatment in patients with Graves' disease. *Acta Endocrinol (Copenh)* 1989;120: 689–701.

64. Talbot JN, Duron F, Feron R, et al. Thyroglobulin, thyrotropin, and thyrotropin binding inhibiting immunoglobulins assayed at the withdrawal of antithyroid drug therapy as predictors of relapse of Graves' disease within one year. *J Endocrinol Invest* 1989;12:589–595.

65. Atkins HL, Richards P. Assessment of thyroid function and anatomy with technetium-99m pertechnetate. *J Nucl Med* 1968;9:7–15.

66. dos Remedios LV, Weber PM, Jasko IA. Thyroid scintiphotography in 1000 patients; rational use of 99m-Tc and I-131 compounds. *J Nucl Med* 1971;12:673–677.

67. Ryo UY, Vaidya PV, Schneider AB, et al. Thyroid imaging agents: a comparison of I-123 and Tc-99m pertechnetate. *Radiology* 1983; 148:819–822.

68. Kusic Z, Becker DV, Saenger EL, et al. Comparison of technetium-99m and iodine-123 imaging of thyroid nodules: correlation with pathologic findings. *J Nucl Med* 1990;31:393–399.

69. Simeone JR, Daniels GH, Mueller RP, et al. High-resolution real-time sonography of the thyroid. *Radiology* 1982;145:431–435.

70. Lupi A, Cerisara D, Orsolon P, et al. Thyroid nodules and Doppler ultrasonography: a new element for an old puzzle? *Minerva Endocrinol* 1999;24:7–10.

71. Ralls PW, Mayekawa DS, Lee KP, et al. Color-flow Doppler sonography in Graves' disease: "thyroid inferno." *Am J Roentgenol* 1988;150: 781–784.

72. Weber AL, Randolph G, Aksoy FG. The thyroid and parathyroid glands: CT and MR imaging and correlation with pathology and clinical findings. *Radiol Clin North Am* 2000;1105–1129.

73. Patton JA, Sandler MP. X-ray fluorescent scanning. In: Sandler MP, Patton JA, Partain CL, eds. *Thyroid and parathyroid imaging.* Norwalk, CT: Appleton-Century-Crofts, 1986:247–274.

74. Esser PD, McAfee JG, Subramanian G. Estimated absorbed radiation doses to adults. In: Freeman LM, ed. *Freeman and Johnson's clinical radionuclide imaging,* 3rd ed. Orlando, FL: Grune & Stratton, 1984: 1521.

75. Melnick JC, Stemkowski PE. Thyroid hemiagenesis (hockey stick sign): a review of the world literature and a report of four cases. *J Clin Endocrinol Metab* 1981;52:247–251.

76. Erdil TY, Onsel C, Kanmaz B, et al. Comparison of 99mTc-methoxyisobutyl isonitrile and ^{201}T1 scintigraphy in visualization of suppressed thyroid tissue. *J Nucl Med* 2000;41:1163–1167.

77. Okstad S, Mair Ilos, Sundsfiord JA, et al. Ectopic thyroid tissue in the head and neck. *J Otolaryngol* 1986;115:52–55.

78. Brown CI. Pathology of the cold nodule. *Clin Endocrinol Metab* 1981; 10:235–245.

79. Ashcraft MW, Van Herle AJ. Management of thyroid nodules, II: scanning techniques, thyroid suppressive therapy, and fine needle aspiration. *Head Neck Surg* 1981;3:297–322.

80. Ridgway EC. Clinical review 30: Clinician's evaluation of a solitary thyroid nodule. *J Clin Endocrinol Metab* 1992;74:231–235.

81. Noma S, Kanaoka M, Minami S et al: Thyroid masses: MR imaging and pathologic correlation. *Radiology* 1988;168:759–764.

82. Mortensen JD, Woolner LB, Bennett WA. Gross and microscopic findings in clinically normal thyroid glands. *J Clin Endocrinol Metab* 1955;15:1270–1280.

83. Vander JB, Gaston EA, Dawber TR. Significance of solitary nontoxic thyroid nodules: preliminary report. *N Engl J Med* 1954;251: 970–973.

84. Miller JM. Carcinoma and thyroid nodules: the problem in an endemic goiter area. *N Engl J Med* 1955;252:247–251.

85. Refetoff S, Harrison J, Karanfilski BT, et al. Continuing occurrence of thyroid carcinoma after irradiation to the neck in infancy and childhood. *N Engl J Med* 1975;292:171–175.

86. Schneider AB, Favus MJ, Stachura ME, et al. Incidence, prevalence, and characteristics of radiation-induced thyroid tumors. *Am J Med* 1978;64:243–252.

87. Astakhova LN, Anspaugh LR, Beebe GW, et al. Chernobyl-related thyroid cancer in children of Belarus: a case-control study. *Radiat Res* 1998;150:349–356.

88. National Cancer Institute. *Estimated exposures and thyroid doses received by the American people from I-131 in fallout following Nevada atmospheric nuclear bomb test.* Bethesda, MD: National Institutes of Health, 1977.

89. Nikiforov Y, Gnepp DR, Fagin JA. Thyroid lesions in children and adolescents after the Chernobyl disaster: implications for the study of radiation tumorigenesis. *J Clin Endocrinol Metab* 1996;81:9–14.

90. Hancock SL, Cox RS, McDougall IR. Thyroid disease after treatment of Hodgkin's disease. *N Engl J Med* 1991;325:599–605.

91. Hill CS Jr, Ibanez ML, Samaan NA, et al. Medullary (solid) carcinoma of the thyroid gland: an analysis of the M.D. Anderson Hospital experience with patients with the tumor, its special features, and its histogenesis. *Medicine (Baltimore)* 1973;52:141–171.

92. Keiser R, Beaven MA, Doppman J, et al. Sipple's syndrome: medullary thyroid carcinoma, pheochromocytoma, and parathyroid disease. *Ann Intern Med* 1973;78:561–579.

93. Rios A, Rodrigues JM, Illana J, et al. Familial papillary carcinoma of the thyroid: report of three families. *Eur J Surg* 2001;167:339–343.

94. Wells SA, Franz C. Medullary carcinoma of the thyroid. *World J Surg* 2000;24:952–956.

95. Scott MD, Crawford JD. Solitary thyroid nodules in childhood: is the incidence of thyroid carcinoma declining? *Pediatrics* 1975;58: 521–525.

96. Khurana KK, Labrador E, Izquierdo R, et al. The role of fine-needle aspiration biopsy in the management of thyroid nodules in children, adolescents, and young adults: a multi-institutional study. *Thyroid* 1999;9:383–386.

97. Schottenfeld D, Gershman ST. Epidemiology of thyroid cancer. *Clin Bull* 1977;7:98–101.

98. Shimaoka K, Badillo J, Sokal JE, et al. Clinical differentiation between thyroid cancer and benign goiter: an evaluation. *JAMA* 1962;181: 179–185.

99. Ongphiphadhanakul B, Rajatanavin R, Chiemchanya S, et al. Systematic inclusion of clinical and laboratory data improves diagnostic accuracy of fine-needle aspiration biopsy in solitary thyroid nodules. *Acta Endocrinol (Copenh)* 1992;126:233–237.

100. Rieu M, Lame MC, Richard A, et al. Prevalence of sporadic medullary thyroid carcinoma: the importance of routine measurement of serum calcitonin in the diagnostic evaluation of thyroid nodules. *Clin Endocrinol (Oxf)* 1995;42:453–460.

101. Psarra RA, Papadopoulos SN, Livada D, et al. The single thyroid nodule. *Br J Surg* 1974;59:545–548.

102. Rago T, Vitti P, Chiovato L, et al. Role of conventional ultrasonography and color flow-Doppler sonography in predicting malignancy in 'cold' thyroid nodules. *Eur J Endocrinol* 1998;138:41–46.

103. Tan GH, Gharib H, Reading CC. Solitary thyroid nodule: comparison between palpation and ultrasonography. *Arch Intern Med* 1995;155:2418–2423.

104. Brander AE, Vikinkoski VP, Nickels JI, et al. Importance of thyroid abnormalities detected at US screening: a 5-year follow-up. *Radiology* 2000;215:801–806.

105. Burguera B, Gharib H. Thyroid incidentalomas: prevalence, diagnosis, significance, and management. *Endocrinol Metab Clin North Am* 2000;29:187–203.

106. Sachmechi I, Miller E, Varatharajah R, et al. Thyroid carcinoma in single cold nodules and in cold nodules of multinodular goiter. *Endocr Pract* 2000;6:5–7.

107. Bucci A, Shore-Freedman E, Gierlowski T, et al. Behavior of small thyroid cancers found by screening radiation-exposed individuals. *J Clin Endocrinol Metab* 2001;86:3711–3716.

108. Cooper DS. Thyroid suppression therapy for benign nodular disease. *J Clin Endocrinol Metab* 1995;80:331–334.

109. de Certaines J, Herry JY, Lancien G, et al. Evaluation of human thyroid tumors by proton nuclear magnetic resonance. *J Nucl Med* 1982;23:48–51.

110. Branstetter BF, Weissman JL, Kennedy TL, et al. The CT appearance of thyroglossal duct carcinoma. *Am J Neuroradiol* 2000;21:1547–1550.

111. Casara D, Rubello D, Saladini G. Role of scintigraphy with tumor-seeking agents in the diagnosis and preoperative staging of malignant thyroid nodules. *Biomed Pharmacother* 2000;54:334–336.

112. Koizumi M, Taguchi H, Goto M, et al. Thallium-201 scintigraphy in the evaluation of thyroid nodules: a retrospective study of 246 cases. *Ann Nucl Med* 1993;7:147–152.

113. Sinha PS, Beeby DI, Ryan P. An evaluation of thallium imaging for detection of carcinoma in clinically palpable solitary, nonfunctioning thyroid nodules. *Thyroid* 2001;11:85–89.

114. Sathekge MM, Mageza RB, Muthuphei MN, et al. Evaluation of thyroid nodules with technetium-99m MIBI and technetium-99m pertechnetate. *Head Neck* 2001;23:305–310.

115. Mezosi E, Bajnok L, Gyory F, et al. The role of technetium-99m methoxyisobutylisonitrile scintigraphy in the differential diagnosis of cold thyroid nodules. *Eur J Nucl Med* 1999;26:798–803.

116. Alonso O, Mut F, Lago G, et al. 99Tc(m)-MIBI scanning of the thyroid gland in patients with markedly decreased pertechnetate uptake. *Nucl Med Commun* 1998;19:257–261.

117. Klain M, Maurea S, Cuocolo A, et al. Technetium-99m tetrofosmin imaging in thyroid diseases: comparison with Tc-99m-pertechnetate, thallium-201 and Tc-99m-methoxyisobutylisonitrile scans. *Eur J Nucl Med* 1996;23:1568–1574.

118. Joensuu H, Ahonen A, Klemi PJ. 18F-fluorodeoxyglucose imaging in preoperative diagnosis of thyroid malignancy. *Eur J Nucl Med* 1988;13:502–506.

119. Bloom AD, Adler LP, Shuck JM. Determination of malignancy of thyroid nodules positron emission tomography. *Surgery* 1993;114:728–735.

120. Sasaki M, Ichiya Y, Kuwabara Y, et al. An evaluation of FDG-PET in the detection and differentiation of thyroid tumors. *Nucl Med Commun* 1997;18:957–963.

121. Uematsu H, Sadato N, Ohtsubo T, et al. Fluorine-18-fluorodeoxyglucose PET versus thallium-201 scintigraphy evaluation of thyroid tumors. *J Nucl Med* 1998;39:453–459.

122. Uchida Y, Matsuno N, Minoshima S, et al. Diagnostic value of 18F-FDG PET in primary and metastatic thyroid cancer. *J Nucl Med* 1995;36:196P.

123. Yasuda S, Shohtsu A, Ide M, et al. Chronic thyroiditis: diffuse uptake of FDG at PET. *Radiology* 1998;207:775–778.

124. Ramos CD, Chisin R, Yeung HW, et al. Incidental focal thyroid uptake on FDG positron emission tomographic scans may represent a second primary tumor. *Clin Nucl Med* 2001;26:193–197.

125. Hamburger JI. Diagnosis of thyroid nodules by fine needle biopsy: use and abuse. *J Clin Endocrinol Metab* 1994;79:335–339.

126. Gharib H, Goellner JR. Fine-needle aspiration biopsy of the thyroid: an appraisal. *Ann Intern Med* 1993;118:282–289.

127. Leenhardt L, Hejblum G, Franc B, et al. Indications and limits of ultrasound-guided cytology in the management of nonpalpable thyroid nodules. *J Clin Endocrinol Metab* 1999;84:24–28.

128. Braga M, Cavalcanti C, Collaco LM, et al. Efficacy of ultrasound-guided fine-needle aspiration biopsy in the diagnosis of complex thyroid nodules. *J Clin Endocrinol Metab* 2001;86:4089–4091.

129. Jackson IMD, Thomson JA. The relationship of carcinoma to the solitary thyroid nodule. *Br J Surg* 1967;54:1007–1010.

130. Freitas JE, Gross MD, Ripley S, et al. Radionuclide diagnosis and therapy of thyroid cancer: current status report. *Semin Nucl Med* 1985;15:106–131.

131. Appetecchia M, Ducci M. Hyperfunctioning differentiated thyroid carcinoma. *J Endocrinol Invest* 1998;21:189–192.

132. Sisson JC, Bartold SP, Bartold SL. The dilemma of a solitary thyroid nodule: resolution through decision analysis. *Semin Nucl Med* 1978;8:59–71.

133. Namba H, Matsuo K, Fagin JA. Clonal composition of benign and malignant human thyroid tumors. *J Clin Invest* 1990;86:120–125.

134. Hamburger JI. Evolution of toxicity in solitary nontoxic autonomously functioning thyroid nodules. *J Clin Endocrinol Metab* 1980;50:1089–1093.

135. Shakir F, Fitzsimmons TR, Jaques DP, et al. Diagnosis and management of the autonomously functioning thyroid nodule: the Walter Reed Army Medical Center experience, 1975–1996. *Thyroid* 1998;8:871–880.

136. Huysmans DA, Corstens FH, Kloppenborg PW. Long-term follow-up in toxic solitary autonomous thyroid nodules treated with radioactive iodine. *J Nucl Med* 1991;32:27–30.

137. Meier DA, Dworkin HJ. The autonomously functioning thyroid nodule. *J Nucl Med* 1991;32:30–32.

138. Shambaugh GE 3d, Quinn JL, Oyasu R, et al. Disparate thyroid imaging: combined studies with sodium pertechnetate Tc-99m and radioactive iodine. *JAMA* 1974;228:866–869.

139. Cavalieri RR. Impaired peripheral conversion of thyroxine to triiodothyronine. *Annu Rev Med* 1977;28:57–65.

140. Khan O, Ell PJ, Maclennan KA, et al. Thyroid carcinoma in a autonomously hyperfunctioning thyroid nodule. *Postgrad Med J* 1981;57:172–175.

141. Ghose MK, Genuth SM, Abellera RM, et al. Functioning primary thyroid carcinoma and metastases producing hyperthyroidism. *J Clin Endocrinol Metab* 1971;33:639–646.

142. Sandler MP, Fellmeth B, Salhany KE, et al. Thyroid carcinoma masquerading as a solitary benign hyperfunctioning nodule. *Clin Nucl Med* 1988;13:410–415.

143. Vattimo A, Bertelli P, Cintorino M, et al. Hürthle cell tumor dwelling in hot thyroid nodules: preoperative detection with technetium-99m-MIBI dual-phase scintigraphy. *J Nucl Med* 1998;39:822–825.

144. Murray D. The thyroid gland. In Kovacs K, Asa SL, eds. *Functional endocrine pathology*. Cambridge, UK: Blackwell Scientific, 1991:293–374.

145. Lacey NA, Jones A, Clarke SE. Role of radionuclide imaging in hyperthyroid patients with no clinical suspicion of nodules. *Br J Radiol* 2001;74:486–489.

146. Park HM, Zieverink S, Ransburg RC, et al. Marine-Lenhart syndrome: Graves' disease with poorly functioning nodules. In: *Proceedings of VII International Thyroid Congress*. Canberra, Australia: Academy of Science, 1980:641.

147. Charkes ND. Graves' disease with functioning nodules (Marine-Lenhart syndrome). *J Nucl Med* 1972;13:885–892.

148. Hales IB, McElduff, Crummer P, et al. Does Graves' disease or thyrotoxicosis affect the prognosis of thyroid cancer. *J Clin Endocrinol Metab* 1992;75:886–889.

149. Cantalamessa L, Baldini M, Orsatti A, et al. Thyroid nodules in Graves' disease and the risk of thyroid carcinoma. *Arch Intern Med* 1999;159:1705–1708.

150. Centeno BA, Szyfelbein WM, Daniels GH, et al. Fine needle aspiration biopsy of the thyroid gland in patients with prior Graves' disease

treated with radioactive iodine: morphologic findings and potential pitfalls. *Acta Cytol* 1996;40:1189–1197.

151. Wang CY, Chang TJ, Chang TC, et al. Thyroidectomy or radioiodine? The value of ultrasonography and cytology in the assessment of nodular lesions in Graves' hyperthyroidism. *Am Surg* 2001;67:721–726.

152. Sandler MP, Patton JA. Multimodality imaging of the thyroid and parathyroid glands. *J Nucl Med* 1987;28:122–129.

153. Martino E, Murtas ML, Loviselli A, et al. Percutaneous intranodular ethanol injection for treatment of autonomously functioning thyroid nodules. *Surgery* 1992;112:1164–1165.

154. Livraghi T, Paracchi A, Ferrari C, et al. Treatment of autonomous thyroid nodules with percutaneous ethanol injection: 4-year experience. *Radiology* 1994;190:529–533.

155. Farwell AP. Infectious thyroiditis. In: Braverman LE, Utiger RD, eds. *Werner & Ingbar's the thyroid: a fundamental and clinical text,* 8th ed. Philadelphia: Lippincott Williams & Wilkins, 2000:1044–1050.

156. Emerson CH, Farwell AP. Sporadic silent thyroiditis, postpartum thyroiditis, and subacute thyroiditis. In: Braverman LE, Utiger RD, eds. *Werner & Ingbar's the thyroid: a fundamental and clinical text,* 8th ed. Philadelphia: Lippincott Williams & Wilkins, 2000:578–589.

157. Hiromatsu Y, Ishibashi M, Miyake I, et al. Color Doppler ultrasonography in patients with subacute thyroiditis. *Thyroid* 1999;9:1189–1193.

158. Templ A, Berna L, Camacho V, et al. 67 Ga-citrate scintigraphy as a determiner in the diagnosis of a subacute thyroiditis. *Rev Esp Med Nucl* 2001;20:36–39.

159. Bando Y, Ushiogi Y, Toya D, et al. Painless thyroiditis associated with severe inflammatory reactions in amyloid goiter: a case report. *Endocr J* 2001;48:323–329.

160. Achong DM, Snow KJ. Gallium-avid painless thyroiditis in a patient with AIDS. *Clin Nucl Med* 1994;19:413–415.

161. Miyamoto S, Kasagi K, Takeuchi R, et al. Ga-67 citrate accumulation in adenomatous goiter. *Clin Nucl Med* 1992;17:803–805.

162. Castellucci RP, Gardner DF, Haden HT, et al. Autoimmune thyroiditis manifested as a systemic febrile illness: diagnosis by gallium scan and fine needle aspiration biopsy. *South Med J* 1989;82:647–649.

163. Allard JC, Lee VW, Franklin P. Thyroid uptake of gallium in Graves' disease. *Clin Nucl Med* 1988;13:663–666.

164. Ling MC, Dake MD, Okerlung MD. Gallium uptake in the thyroid gland in amiodarone-induced hyperthyroidism. *Clin Nucl Med* 1988;13:258–259.

165. Premawardhana LDKE, Parkes AB, Ammari F, et al. Postpartum thyroiditis and long-term thyroid status: prognostic influence of thyroid peroxidase antibodies and ultrasound echogenicity. *J Clin Endocrinol Metab* 2000;85:71–75.

166. Hashimoto H. Zur kenntnis der lymphomatösen veränderung der schiddruse (struma lymphomatosa). *Langenbecks Arch Klin Chir* 1912;97:219–248.

167. Weetman, AP. Chronic autoimmune thyroiditis. In: Braverman LE, Utiger RD, eds. *Werner & Ingbar's the thyroid: a fundamental and clinical text,* 8th ed. Philadelphia: Lippincott Williams & Wilkins, 2000:721–732.

168. Vanderpump MPJ, Tunbridge WMG. The epidemiology of thyroid diseases. In: Braverman LE, Utiger RD, eds. *Werner & Ingbar's the thyroid: a fundamental and clinical text,* 8th ed. Philadelphia: Lippincott Williams & Wilkins, 2000:467–473.

169. Okayasu I, Hara Y, Nakamura K, et al. Racial and age-related differences in incidence and severity of focal autoimmune thyroiditis. *Am J Clin Pathol* 1994;101:698–702.

170. Prentice LM, Phillips DI, Sarsero D, et al. Geographical distribution of subclinical autoimmune thyroid disease in Britain: a study using highly sensitive direct assays for autoantibodies to thyroglobulin and thyroid peroxidase. *Acta Endocrinol (Copenh)* 1990;123:493–498.

171. Pederson OM, Aardal NP, Larssen TB, et al. The value of ultrasonography in predicting autoimmune thyroid disease. *Thyroid* 2000;10:251–259.

172. Daniels GH. Amiodarone-induced thyrotoxicosis. *J Clin Endocrinol Metab* 2001;86:3–8.

173. McDermott MT, Ridgway EC. Central hyperthyroidism. *Endocrinol Metab Clin North Am* 1998;27:187–203.

174. Caron P, Arlot S, Bauters C, et al. Efficacy of the long-acting octreotide formulation (octreotide-LAR) in patients with thyrotropin-secreting pituitary adenomas. *J Clin Endocrinol Metab* 2001;86:2849–2853.

175. Brucker-Davis F, Oldfield EH, Skarulis MC, et al. Thyrotropin-secreting pituitary tumors: diagnostic criteria, thyroid hormone sensitivity, and treatment outcome in 25 patients followed at the National Institutes of Health. *J Clin Endocrinol Metab* 1999;84:476–486.

176. Hershman JM. Human chorionic gonadotropin and the thyroid: hyperemesis gravidarum and trophoblastic tumors. *Thyroid* 1999;9:653–657.

177. Woodruff JD, Rauh JT, Markley RL. Ovarian struma. *Obstet Gynecol* 1966;27:194–201.

178. Kempers RD, Dockerty MB, Hoffman DL, et al. Struma ovarii ascites, hyperthyroid, and asymptomatic syndromes. *Ann Intern Med* 1970;72:883–893.

179. Grandet PJ, Remi MH, Struma ovarii with hyperthyroidism. *Clin Nucl Med* 2000;25:763–765.

180. Mazzaferri EL.Thyroid cancer and Graves' disease: the controversy ten years later. *Endocr Pract* 2000;6:221–225.

181. Paul SJ, Sisson JC. Thyrotoxicosis caused by thyroid cancer. *Endocrinol Metab Clin North Am* 1990;19:593–612.

182. Guglielmi R, Pacella CM, Dottorini ME, et al. Severe thyrotoxicosis due to hyperfunctioning liver metastases from follicular carcinoma: treatment with (131)I and interstitial laser ablation. *Thyroid* 1999;9:173–177.

183. Salvatori M, Saletnich I, Rufini V, et al. Severe thyrotoxicosis due to functioning pulmonary metastases of well-differentiated thyroid cancer. *J Nucl Med* 1998;39:1202–1207.

184. Sisson JC, Carey JE. Thyroid carcinoma with high levels of function: treatment with (131)I. *J Nucl Med* 2001;42:975–983.

185. Kasagi K, Takeuchi R, Miyamoto S, et al. Metastatic thyroid cancer presenting as thyrotoxicosis: report of three cases. *Clin Endocrinol (Oxf)* 1994;40:429–434.

186. Mark JB. Management of anterior mediastinal tumors. *Semin Surg Oncol* 1990;6:286–290.

187. Tecce PM, Fishman EK, Kuhlman JE. CT evaluation of the anterior mediastinum: spectrum of disease. *Radiographics* 1994;14:973–990.

188. Shabb NS, Fahl M, Shabb B, et al. Fine-needle aspiration of the mediastinum: a clinical, radiologic, cytologic, and histologic study of 42 cases. *Diagn Cytopathol* 1998;19:428–436.

189. Bashist B, Ellis K, Gold RP. Computed tomography of intrathoracic goiters. *Am J Roentgenol* 1983;140:455–460.

190. Fernandez-Ulloa M, Maxon HR, Mehta S, et al. Iodine-131 uptake by primary lung adenocarcinoma: misinterpretation of 131I scan. *JAMA* 1976;236:857–858.

191. Davidson J, McDougall IR. How frequently is the thymus seen on whole-body iodine-131 diagnostic and post-treatment scans? *Eur J Nucl Med* 2000;27:425–430.

192. Chen JJS, LaFrance ND, Rippin R, et al. Iodine-123 SPECT of the thyroid in multinodular goiter. *J Nucl Med* 1988;29:110–113.

193. Humphrey ML, Burman KD. Retrosternal and intrathoracic goiter. *Endocrinologist* 1992;2:195–201.

194. Huang TS, Chieng PU, Chang CC, et al. Positron emission tomography for detecting iodine-131 nonvisualized metastases of well-differentiated thyroid carcinoma: two case reports. *J Endocrinol Invest* 1998;21:392–398.

195. Grunwald F, Kalicke T, Feine U, et al. Fluorine-18 fluorodeoxyglucose positron emission tomography in thyroid cancer: results of a multicentre study. *Eur J Nucl Med* 1999;26:1547–1552.

196. Bonnema SJ, Bertelsen H, Mortenson J, et al. The feasibility of high dose iodine 131 treatment as an alternative to surgery in patients with a very large goiter: effect on thyroid function and size and pulmonary function. *J Clin Endocrinol Metab* 1999;84:3636–3641.

197. Fisher DA, Sussault JH, Foley TP. Screening for congenital hypothyroidism: results of screening one million North American infants. *J Pediatr* 1979;94:700–705.

198. Fisher DA. Management of congenital hypothyroidism. *J Clin Endocrinol Metab* 1991;72:523–529.

199. Klein AH, Meltzer S, Kenny FM. Improved prognosis in congenital hypothyroidism treated before age three months. *J Pediatr* 1972;81: 912–915.

200. Sfakianakis GN, Ezuddin SH, Sanchez JE, et al. Pertechnetate scintigraphy in primary congenital hypothyroidism. *J Nucl Med* 1999;40: 799–804.

201. Nose O, Harada T, Miyai K, et al. Transient neonatal hypothyroidism probably related to immaturity of thyroidal iodine organification. *J Pediatr* 1986;108:573–576.

202. *Cancer facts and figures, 2000.* New York: American Cancer Society, 2000.

203. Takashima S, Takayama F, Wang JC, et al. Radiologic assessment of metastases to the thyroid gland. *J Comput Assist Tomogr* 2000;24: 539–545.

204. Mazzaferri EL. Radioiodine and other treatments and outcomes. In: Braverman LE, Utiger RD, eds. *Werner & Ingbar's the thyroid: a fundamental and clinical text,* 8th ed. Philadelphia: Lippincott Williams & Wilkins, 2000:904–929.

205. Goldman JM, Line BR, Aamodt RL, et al. Influence of triiodothyronine withdrawal time on I-131 uptake post-thyroidectomy for thyroid cancer. *J Clin Endocrinol Metab* 1980;50:734–739.

206. Comtois R, Theriault C, Del Vecchio P. Assessment of the efficacy of iodine-131 for thyroid ablation. *J Nucl Med* 1993;34:1927–1930.

207. Krishnamurthy GT. Human reaction to bovine TSH [Concise Communication]. *J Nucl Med* 1978;19:284–286.

208. Haugen BR, Pacini F, Reiners C, et al. A comparison of recombinant human thyrotropin and thyroid hormone withdrawal for the detection of thyroid remnant or cancer. *J Clin Endocrinol Metab* 1999;84: 3877–3885.

209. Robbins RJ, Tuttle RM, Sharaf RN, et al. Preparation by recombinant human thyrotropin or thyroid hormone withdrawal are comparable for the detection of residual differentiated thyroid carcinoma. *J Clin Endocrinol Metab* 2001;86:619–625.

210. Sarkar SD, Afriyie MO, Palestro CJ. Recombinant human thyroid-stimulating hormone-aided scintigraphy: comparison of imaging at multiple times after I-131 administration. *Clin Nucl Med* 2001;26: 392–395.

211. DeGroot LJ, Hoye K, Refetoff S, et al. Serum antigens and antibodies in the diagnosis of thyroid cancer. *J Clin Endocrinol Metab* 1977;45: 1220–1223.

212. van Sorge-van Botel RA, van Eck-Smit BL, Goslings BM. Comparison of serum thyroglobulin, 131-I and 201-Tl scintigraphy in the postoperative follow-up of differentiated thyroid cancer. *Nucl Med Commun* 1993;14:365–372.

213. Lupin E, Mechlis-Frish S, Zatz S. Serum thyroglobulin and iodine-131 whole-body scan in the diagnosis and assessment of treatment for metastatic differentiated thyroid carcinoma. *J Nucl Med* 1994;35: 257–262.

214. Black EG, Sheppard MC. Serum thyroglobulin measurements in thyroid cancer: evaluation of "false" positive results. *Clin Endocrinol* 1991;35:519–520.

215. Schlumberger M, Charbord P, Fragu P, et al. Circulating thyroglobulin and thyroid hormones in patients with metastases of differentiated thyroid carcinoma: relationship to serum thyrotropin levels. *J Clin Endocrinol Metab* 1980;51:513–519.

216. Ashcraft MW, Van Herle AJ. The comparative value of serum thyroglobulin measurements and iodine-131 total body scans in the follow-up study of patients with treated differentiated thyroid cancer. *Am J Med* 1981;71:806–814.

217. Schneider AB, Line BR, Goldman JM, et al. Sequential serum thyroglobulin determinations, I-131 scans, I-131 uptakes after triiodothyronine withdrawal in patients with thyroid cancer. *J Clin Endocrinol Metab* 1981;53:1199–1206.

218. Cailleux AF, Baudin E, Travagli JP, et al. Is diagnostic iodine-131 scanning useful after total thyroid ablation for differentiated thyroid cancer? *J Clin Endocrinol Metab* 2000;85:175–178.

219. Mazzaferri EL, Kloos RT. Using recombinant human TSH in the management of well-differentiated thyroid cancer: current strategies and future directions. *Thyroid* 2000;10:767–778.

220. Westbury C, Vini L, Fisher C, et al. Recurrent differentiated thyroid cancer without elevation of serum thyroglobulin. *Thyroid* 2000;10: 171–176.

221. Spencer CA, Takeuchi M, Kazarosyan M, et al. Serum thyroglobulin autoantibodies: prevalence, influence on serum thyroglobulin measurement, and prognostic significance in patients with differentiated thyroid carcinoma. *J Clin Endocrinol Metab* 1998;83:1121–1127.

222. Ringel MD, Balducci-Silano PL, Anderson JS, et al. Quantitative reverse transcription-polymerase chain reaction of circulating thyroglobulin messenger ribonucleic acid for monitoring patients with thyroid carcinoma. *J Clin Endocrinol Metab* 1999;94:4037–4042.

223. Briele B, Hotze A, Grunwald F, et al. Increased sensitivity of whole-body scintigraphy with I-131 for the detection of iodine-accumulating metastases by means of delayed imaging. *Nuklearmedizin* 1990;29: 264–268.

224. Nutting C, Hyer S, Vini L, et al. Failure of TSH rise prior to radioiodine therapy for thyroid cancer: implications for treatment. *Clin Oncol (R Coll Radiol)* 1999;11:269–271.

225. Campbell CM, Khafagi FA. Insensitivity of 99mTc pertechnetate for detecting metastases of differentiated thyroid carcinoma. *Clin Nucl Med* 1990;15:1–4.

226. DeGroot LJ, Reilly M. Use of isotope bone scans and skeletal survey x-rays in the follow-up of patients with thyroid carcinoma. *J Endocrinol Invest* 1984;7:175–179.

227. Lakshmanan M et al. A simplified low iodine diet in I-131 scanning and therapy of thyroid cancer. *Clin Nucl Med* 1988;12:866–868.

228. Shapiro B, Rufini V, Jarwan A, et al. Artifacts, anatomical and physiological variants, and unrelated disease that might cause false-positive whole-body 131-I scans in patients with thyroid cancer. *Semin Nucl Med* 2000;30:115–132.

229. Martin WH, Patton JA, Delbeke D, et al. Improved localization of endocrine sites using an integrated CT-SPECT fused imaging system. *J Nucl Med* 2000;41:49P.

230. Even-Sapir E, Keidar Z, Sachs J, et al. The new technology of combined transmission and emission tomography in evaluation of endocrine neoplasms. *J Nucl Med* 2001;42:998–1004.

231. Waxman A, Ramanna L, Chapman N. The significance of I-131 scan dose in patients with thyroid cancer: determination of ablation [Concise Communication]. *J Nucl Med* 1981;22:861–864.

232. Spies WG, Wojtowizc CH, Spies SM, et al. Value of post-therapy whole-body I-131 imaging in the evaluation of patients with thyroid carcinoma having undergone high-dose I-131 therapy. *Clin Nucl Med* 1989;14:793–800.

233. Pacini FL, Lippi F, Formica N, et al. Therapeutic doses of iodine-131 revealed undiagnosed metastases in thyroid cancer patients with detectable serum thyroglobulin levels. *J Nucl Med* 1987;28: 1888–1891.

234. Ikekubo K, Hino M, Ito H, et al. The early detection of metastatic differentiated thyroid cancer using 131-I total body scan and treatment with 131-I. *Jpn J Nucl Med* 1991;28:247–259.

235. Morris LF, Waxman AD, Braunstein GD. The nonimpact of thyroid stunning: remnant ablation rates in ^{131}I-scanned and nonscanned individuals. *J Clin Endocrinol Metab* 2001;86:3501–3511.

236. Leger FA, Izembart M, Dagousset F, et al. Decreased uptake of therapeutic doses of iodine-131 after 185-MBq iodine-131 diagnostic imaging for thyroid remnants in differentiated thyroid carcinoma. *Eur J Nucl Med* 1998;25:242–246.

237. Huie D, Medvedec M, Dodig D, et al. Radioiodine uptake in thyroid cancer patients after diagnostic application of low-dose [131]I. *Nucl Med Commun* 1996;17:839–842.

238. Sabri O, Zimny M, Schreckenberger M, et al. Does thyroid stunning exist? A model with benign thyroid disease. *Eur J Nucl Med* 2000; 27:1591–1597s.

239. Muratet JP, Daver A, Minier JF, et al. Influence of scanning doses of iodine-131 on subsequent first ablative treatment outcome in patients operated on for differentiated thyroid carcinoma. *J Nucl Med* 1998; 39:1546–1550.

240. McDougall IR. Does stunning occur after 74 MBq ^{131}I in patients with differentiated thyroid cancer? *J Nucl Med* 2001;42:158P.

241. Haugen BR, Lin EC. Isotope imaging for metastatic thyroid cancer. *Endocrinol Metab Clin North Am* 2001;30:469–492.

242. Mandel SJ, Shankar LK, Benard F, et al. Superiority of iodine-123 compared with iodine-131 scanning for thyroid remnants in patients with differentiated thyroid cancer. *Clin Nucl Med* 2001;26:6–9.

243. Park HM, Park YH, Zhou XH. Detection of thyroid remnant/metastases without stunning: an ongoing dilemma. *Thyroid* 1997;7:277–280.

244. Yaakob W, Gordon L, Spicer KM, et al. The usefulness of iodine-123 whole-body scans in evaluating thyroid carcinoma and metastases. *J Nucl Med Technol* 1999;27:279–281.

245. Balon HR, Fink-Bennet TD, Stoffer SS. Technetium-99m-sestamibi uptake by recurrent Hürthle cell carcinoma of the thyroid. *J Nucl Med* 1992;33:1393–1395.

246. Alam MS, Takeuchi L, Kasage K, et al. Value of combined technetium-99m hydroxymethylene diphosphate and thallium-201 imaging in detecting bone metastases from thyroid carcinoma. *Thyroid* 1997;7:705–712.

247. Schirrmeister H, Buck A, Guhlmann A, et al. Anatomical distribution and sclerotic activity of bone metastases from thyroid cancer assessed with F-18 sodium fluoride positron emission tomography. *Thyroid* 2001;11:677–683.

248. Ramanna L, Waxman A, Braunstein G. Thallium-201 scintigraphy in differentiated thyroid cancer: comparison with radioiodine scintigraphy and serum thyroglobulin determinations. *J Nucl Med* 1991;32:441–445.

249. Iida Y, Hidaka A, Hatabu H, et al. Follow-up study of postoperative patients with thyroid cancer by thallium-201 scintigraphy and serum thyroglobulin measurement. *J Nucl Med* 1991;32:2098–2100.

250. Charkes ND, Vitti RA, Brooks K. Thallium-201 SPECT increases detectability of thyroid cancer metastases. *J Nucl Med* 1990;31:147–153.

251. Shiga T, Tsukamoto E, Nakada K, et al. Comparison of (18)F-FDG, (131)I-Na, and (201)T1 in diagnosis of recurrent or metastatic thyroid carcinoma. *J Nucl Med* 2001;42:414–419.

252. Seabold JE, Gurll N, Schurrer ME, et al. Comparison of 99mTc-methoxyisobutyl isonitrile and [201]T1 scintigraphy for detection of residual thyroid cancer after ^{131}I ablative therapy. *J Nucl Med* 1999;40:1434–1440.

253. Nishiyama Y, Yamamoto Y, Ono Y, et al. Comparison of 99Tcm-tetrofosmin with [201]T1 and ^{131}I in the detection of differentiated thyroid cancer metastases. *Nucl Med Commun* 2000;21:917–923.

254. Briele B, Hotze AL, Kropp J, et al. Comparison of 99mTc-MIBI and Tl-201-chloride in the follow-up of patients with differentiated thyroid carcinoma. *J Nucl Med* 1992;33:844.

255. Alam MS, Kasagi K, Misaki T, et al. Diagnostic value of technetium-99m methoxyisobutyl isonitrile (99mTc-MIBI) scintigraphy in detecting thyroid cancer metastases: a critical evaluation. *Thyroid* 1998;8:1091–100.

256. Casara D, Rubello D, Saladini G, et al. Clinical approach in patients with metastatic differentiated thyroid carcinoma and negative ^{131}I whole body scintigraphy: importance of 99mTc MIBI scan combined with high resolution neck ultrasonography. *Tumori* 1999;85:122–127.

257. Rubello D, Mazzarotto R, Casara D. The role of technetium-99m methoxyisobutylisonitrile scintigraphy in the planning of therapy and follow-up of patients with differentiated thyroid carcinoma after surgery. *Eur J Nucl Med* 2000;27:431–440.

258. Ng DC, Sundram FX, Sin AE. 99mTc-sestamibi and ^{131}I whole-body scintigraphy and initial serum thyroglobulin in the management of differentiated thyroid carcinoma. *J Nucl Med* 2000;41:631–635.

259. Gorges R, Kahaly G, Muller-Brand J, et al. Radionuclide-labeled somatostatin analogues for diagnostic and therapeutic purposes in nonmedullary thyroid cancer. *Thyroid* 2001;11:647–659.

260. Valli N, Catargi B, Ronci N, et al. Evaluation of indium-111 pentetreotide somatostatin receptor scintigraphy to detect recurrent thyroid carcinoma in patients with negative radioiodine scintigraphy. *Thyroid* 1999;9:583–589.

261. Joensuu H, Ahonen A. Imaging of metastases of thyroid carcinoma with fluorine-18 fluorodeoxyglucose. *J Nucl Med* 1987:28:910–914.

262. Wang W, Macapinlac H, Larson SM, et al. [18F]-2-fluoro-2-deoxy-D-glucose positron emission tomography localizes residual thyroid cancer in patients with negative diagnostic ^{131}I whole body scans and elevated serum thyroglobulin levels. *J Clin Endocrinol Metab* 1999;84:2291–2302.

263. Wang W, Larson SM, Fazzari M, et al. Prognostic value of [18F]fluorodeoxyglucose positron emission tomographic scanning in patients with thyroid cancer. *J Clin Endocrinol Metab* 2000;85:1107–1113.

264. Yeo JS, Chung JK, So Y, et al. F-18-fluorodeoxyglucose positron emission tomography as a presurgical evaluation modality for I-131 scan–negative thyroid carcinoma patients with local recurrence in cervical lymph nodes. *Head Neck* 2001;23:94–103.

265. Schulter B, Bohuslavizki KH, Beyer W, et al. Impact of FDG PET on patients with differentiated thyroid cancer who present with elevated thyroglobulin and negative ^{131}I scan. *J Nucl Med* 2001;42:71–76.

266. Dietlein M, Scheidhauer K, Voth E, et al. Fluorine-18 fluorodeoxyglucose positron emission tomography and iodine-131 whole body scintigraphy in the follow-up of differentiated thyroid cancer. *Eur J Nucl Med* 1997;24:1342–1348.

267. Dietlein M, Scheidhauer K, Voth E, et al. Follow-up of differentiated thyroid cancer: what is the value of FDG and sestamibi in the diagnostic algorithm? *Nuklearmedizin* 1998;37:6–11.

268. Alnafisi NS, Driedger AA, Coates G, et al. FDG PET of recurrent or metastatic ^{131}I-negative papillary thyroid carcinoma. *J Nucl Med* 2000;41:1010–1015.

269. Hooft L, Hoekstra OS, Deville W, et al. Diagnostic accuracy of 18F-fluorodeoxyglucose positron emission tomography in the follow-up of papillary or follicular thyroid cancer. *J Clin Endocrinol Metab* 2001;86:3779–3786.

270. Moog F, Linke R, Manthey N, et al. Influence of thyroid-stimulating hormone levels on uptake of FDG in recurrent and metastatic differentiated thyroid carcinoma. *J Nucl Med* 2000;41:1989–1995.

271. Maxon HR, Smith HS. Radioiodine-131 in the diagnosis and treatment of metastatic well-differentiate thyroid cancer. *Endocrinol Metab Clin North Am* 1990;19:958–718.

272. Pineda JD, Lee T, Ain K, et al. Iodine-131 therapy for thyroid cancer patients with elevated thyroglobulin and negative diagnostic scan. *J Clin Endocrinol Metab* 1995;80:1488–1492.

273. Pacini F, Agate L, Elisei R, et al. Outcome of differentiated thyroid cancer with detectable serum Tg and negative diagnostic ^{131}I whole body scan: comparison of patients treated with high ^{131}I activities versus untreated patients. *J Clin Endocrinol Metab* 2001;86:4092–7097.

274. Frilling A, Gorges R, Tecklenborg K, et al. Value of preoperative diagnostic modalities in patients with recurrent thyroid carcinoma. *Surgery* 2000;128:1067–1074.

275. Ball DW, Baylin SB, de Bustros AC. Medullary thyroid carcinoma. In: Braverman LE, Utiger RD, eds. *Werner & Ingbar's the thyroid: a fundamental and clinical text,* 8th ed. Philadelphia: Lippincott Williams & Wilkins, 2000:930–943.

276. van Heerden JA, Grant CS, Gharib H, et al. Long term course of patients with persistent hypercalcitoninemia after apparent curative primary surgery for medullary thyroid carcinoma. *Ann Surg* 1990;212:395–400.

277. Ellenhorn JDI, Shah JP, Brennan MF. Impact of therapeutic regional lymph node dissection for medullary carcinoma of the thyroid gland. *Surgery* 1993;114:1078–1081.

278. Hellman DE, Kartchner M, Van Antwerp JD, et al. Radioiodine in the treatment of medullary carcinoma of the thyroid. *J Clin Endocrinol Metab* 1979;48:451–455.

279. Saad MF, Guido JJ, Samaan NA. Radioactive iodine in the treatment of medullary carcinoma of the thyroid. *J Clin Endocrinol Metab* 1983;57:124–128.

280. Gagel RF, Robinson MF, Donovan DT, et al. Medullary thyroid carcinoma: recent progress. *J Clin Endocrinol Metab* 1993;76:809–814.

281. Norton JA, Doppman JL, Brennan MF. Localization and resection

of clinically inapparent carcinoma of the thyroid. *Surgery* 1980;87:616–622.

282. Medina-Franco H, Herrera MF, Lopez G, et al. Persistent hypercalcitoninemia in patients with medullary thyroid cancer: a therapeutic approach based on selective venous sampling for calcitonin. *Rev Invest Clin* 2001;53:212–217.

283. Adams S, Acker P, Lorenz M, et al. Radioisotope-guided surgery in patients with pheochromocytoma and recurrent medullary thyroid carcinoma: a comparison of preoperative and intraoperative tumor localization with histopathologic findings. *Cancer* 2001;92:263–270.

284. Kebebew E, Kikuchi S, Duh QY, et al. Long-term results of reoperation and localizing studies in patients with persistent or recurrent medullary thyroid cancer. *Arch Surg* 2000;135:895–901.

285. Lupoli G, Lombardi G, Panza N, et al. (131-I-meta-iodobenzylguanidine scintigraphy and selective venous catheterization after thyroidectomy for medullary thyroid carcinoma. *Med Oncol Tumor Pharmacother* 1991;8:7–13.

286. Frank-Raue K, Raue F, Buhr HJ, et al. Localization of occult persisting medullary thyroid carcinoma before microsurgical reoperation: high sensitivity of selective venous catheterization. *Thyroid* 1992;2:113–117.

287. Dorr U, Wurstlin S, Frank-Raue K, et al. Somatostatin receptor scintigraphy and magnetic resonance imaging in recurrent medullary thyroid carcinoma: a comparative study. *Horm Metab Res* 1993;27[Suppl]:48–55.

288. Wang Q, Takashima S, Fukuda H, et al. Detection of medullary thyroid carcinoma and regional lymph node metastases by magnetic resonance imaging. *Arch Otolaryngol Head Neck Surg* 1999;125:842–848.

289. Arslan N, Ilgan S, Yuksel D, et al. Comparison of In-111 octreotide and Tc-99m (V) DMSA scintigraphy in the detection of medullary thyroid tumor foci in patients with elevated levels of tumor markers after surgery. *Clin Nucl Med* 2001;26:683–688.

290. Hoefnagel CA, Delprat CC, Marcuse HR, et al. Role of thallium-201 total-body scintigraphy in follow-up of thyroid carcinoma. *J Nucl Med* 1986;27:1854–1857.

291. Talpos GB, Jackson CE, Froelich JW, et al. Localization of residual medullary thyroid cancer by thallium/technetium scintigraphy. *Surgery* 1985;98:1189–1196.

292. O'Driscoll CM, Baker F, Casey MJ, et al. Localization of recurrent medullary thyroid carcinoma with technetium-99m-methoxyisobutylnitrile scintigraphy: a case report. *J Nucl Med* 1991;32:2281–2283.

293. Conti FS, Durski JM, Bacqai F, et al. Imaging of locally recurrent and metastatic thyroid cancer with positron emission tomography. *Thyroid* 1999;9:797–804.

294. Gasparoni P, Rubello D, Ferlin G. Potential role of fluorine-18-deoxyglucose (FDG) positron emission tomography (PET) in the staging of primitive and recurrent medullary thyroid carcinoma. *J Endocrinol Invest* 1997;20:527–530.

295. Brandt-Mainz K, Muller SP, Gorges R, et al. The value of fluorine-18 fluorodeoxyglucose PET in patients with medullary thyroid cancer. *Eur J Nucl Med* 2000;27:490–496.

296. Esik O, Szavcsur P, Szakall S Jr, et al. Angiography effectively supports the diagnosis of hepatic metastases in medullary thyroid carcinoma. *Cancer* 2001;91:2084–2095.

297. Udelsman R, Mojiminiyi OA, Soper ND, et al. Medullary carcinoma of the thyroid: management of persistent hypercalcitonaemia utilizing [99mTc](V) dimercaptosuccinic acid scintigraphy. *Br J Surg* 1989;76:1278–1782.

298. Mojiminiyi OA, Udelsman R, Soper ND, et al. Pentavalent 99mTc DMSA scintigraphy: prospective evaluation of its role in the manage-ment of patients with medullary carcinoma of the thyroid. *Clin Nucl Med* 1991;16:259–262.

299. Bigsby RJ, Lepp EK, Litwin DEM, et al. Technetium-99m pentavalent dimercaptosuccinic acid and thallium-201 in detecting recurrent medullary carcinoma of the thyroid. *Can J Surg* 1992;35:388–392.

300. Ohta H, Yamamoto K, Endo K, et al. A new imaging agent for medullary carcinoma of the thyroid. *J Nucl Med* 1984;25:323–325.

301. Ohta H, Hatabu H, Endo K, et al. 99mTc(V)-DMSA accumulation in thyroid amyloidosis. *Clin Nucl Med* 1991;16:778–779.

302. Kwekkeboom DJ, Reubi JC, Lamberts SW, et al. The potential value of somatostatin receptor scintigraphy in medullary thyroid carcinoma. *J Clin Endocrinol Metab* 1993;76:1413–1417.

303. Dorr U, Frank-Raue K, Raue F. The potential value of somatostatin receptor scintigraphy in medullary thyroid carcinoma. *Nucl Med Commun* 1993;14:439–445.

304. Peltier P, Curtet C, Chatal JF, et al. Radioimmunodetection of medullary thyroid cancer using a bispecific anti-CEA/anti-indium-DTPA antibody and an indium-111-labeled DTPA dimer. *J Nucl Med* 1993;34:1267–1273.

305. Troncone L, Rufini V, Montemaggi P, et al. The diagnostic and therapeutic utility of radioiodinated metaiodobenzylguanidine (MIBG): 5 years of experience. *Eur J Nucl Med* 1990;16:325–335.

306. Skowsky WR, Wilf LH. Iodine-131 metaiodobenzylguanidine scintigraphy of medullary carcinoma of the thyroid. *South Med J* 1991;84:636–641.

307. Troncone L, Rufini V, Maussier ML, et al. The role of [131I] metaiodobenzylguanidine in the treatment of medullary thyroid carcinoma: results in five cases. *J Nucl Biol Med* 1991;35:327–332.

308. Clarke SE. [131I]metaiodobenzylguanidine therapy in medullary thyroid cancer: Guy's hospital experience. *J Nucl Biol Med* 1991;35:323–326.

309. Hoefnagel CA, Delprat CC, Valdes Olmos RA. Role of [131I]metaiodobenzylguanidine therapy in medullary thyroid carcinoma. *J Nucl Biol Med* 1991;35:334–336.

310. Matsuzuka F, Miyauchi A, Katayama S, et al. Clinical aspects of primary thyroid lymphoma: diagnosis and treatment based on our experience of 119 cases. *Thyroid* 1993;3:93–99.

311. Shibata T, Noma S, Nakano Y, et al. Primary thyroid lymphoma: MR appearance. *J Comput Assist Tomogr* 1991;15:629–633.

312. Takashima S, Morimoto S, Ikezoe J, et al. Primary thyroid lymphoma: comparison of CT and US assessment. *Radiology* 1989;171:439–443.

313. Scott AM, Kostakoglu L, O'Brien JP, et al. Comparison of technetium-99m-MIBI and thallium-201-chloride uptake in primary thyroid lymphoma. *J Nucl Med* 1992;33:1396–1398.

314. Kasagi K, Hatabu H, Tokuda Y, et al. Lymphoproliferative disorders of the thyroid gland: radiological appearances. *Br J Radiol* 1991;64:569–575.

315. Nel CJC, van Heerden JA, Goellner JR, et al. Anaplastic carcinoma of the thyroid: a clinicopathologic study of 82 cases. *Mayo Clin Proc* 1985;60:51–58.

316. Senga O, Miyakawa M, Shirota H, et al. Comparison of Tl-201 and Ga-67-citrate scintigraphy in the diagnosis of thyroid tumor [Concise Communication]. *J Nucl Med* 1982;23:225–228.

317. Montes TC, Munoz C, Rivero JI, et al. Uptake of Tc-99m sestamibi and Tc-99m MDP in anaplastic carcinoma of the thyroid (nondiagnostic CT and ultrasound scans). *Clin Nucl Med* 1999;24:355–356.

318. Takashima S, Morimoto S, Ikezoe J, et al. CT evaluation of anaplastic thyroid carcinoma. *Am J Roentgenol* 1990;154:1079–1085.

319. Nilsson O, Lideberg J, Zedenius J, et al. Anaplastic giant cell carcinoma of the thyroid gland: treatment and survival over a 25-year period. *World J Surg* 1998;22:725–730.

31

RADIOIODINE TREATMENT OF THYROID DISEASE

R. MICHAEL TUTTLE
DAVID V. BECKER
JAMES R. HURLEY

RADIOIODINE TREATMENT OF HYPERTHYROIDISM

Introduction

Thyrotoxicosis is a clinical symptom complex caused by elevated thyroid hormone levels. The term hyperthyroidism is limited to those causes of thyrotoxicosis associated with abnormal, autonomous hyperfunction of the thyroid gland. The most common cause of hyperthyroidism is antibody mediated stimulation of the thyroid gland known as Graves' disease whereas hyperfunctioning autonomous nodules (Plummer's disease) are a less common cause more often seen in older patients. Other forms of thyrotoxicosis are those due to increased release of thyroid hormone from the gland by an inflammatory process, as in subacute thyroiditis and, rarely, by increased secretion of thyroid hormone by stimulation of the thyroid by excess pituitary thyroid-stimulating hormone (TSH).

In Graves' disease and toxic nodular goiter, the absence of treatment methods that can correct the etiologic abnormality directs treatment to manipulations that reduce the level of circulating thyroid hormone. This can be accomplished with antithyroid drugs, surgery, or radioactive iodine therapy. Each of these methods is effective, but they all are reported, in an extensive medical literature, to have widely varying cure and relapse rates, frequencies of side effects, and differences in cost and convenience. As a result, although hyperthyroidism can be treated effectively, the outcome of any specific treatment cannot be predicted in any individual patient.

Establishing the Diagnosis

Before instituting definitive treatment, the diagnosis of hyperthyroidism must be confirmed and its etiology established. Clini-

cal examination usually reveals the generally recognized and widely known symptoms of thyrotoxicosis, reflecting the elevated levels of thyroid hormones.

The diagnosis of thyrotoxicosis is supported by tests that demonstrate elevated levels of serum thyroxine (T_4) and/or triiodothyronine (T_3) with an associated suppressed serum TSH. An elevated thyroidal radioiodine uptake confirms that active secretion by the thyroid gland is the source of the elevated serum hormone levels. The thyroid scan will show whether the process is diffuse, involving the entire thyroid gland as in Graves' disease, or is localized to one or more autonomous areas (with suppression of the function of the remaining thyroid tissue), indicating the presence of toxic nodular goiter. Conversely, a very low radioactive iodine (RAI) uptake with essentially no visible uptake on the RAI scan is consistent with a transient thyroiditis, excess iodine intake, or surreptitious use of thyroid hormone.

Therapeutic Options

Antithyroidal Drug Therapy

Antithyroid drugs have been widely used since their introduction in the early 1940s and are often used for the initial management of hyperthyroidism in selected patients (1–4). Although symptomatic control can be achieved in almost all patients with these agents with adequate dosage and frequent administration, the incidence of permanent remission varies from 10% to 40%.

Induction of permanent remission after antithyroid drugs occurs most often in younger individuals with mild disease of short duration and with relatively small goiters. A trial of 12 months or so under close observation is usually sufficient to determine whether a permanent remission is likely to occur. Failure to induce permanent remission after an adequate trial of antithyroid drugs and a desire to avoid the potential morbidity and cost of surgical thyroidectomy often lead to the selection of radioiodine therapy.

Toxic reactions to antithyroid drugs are relatively infrequent, occurring in about 5% to 7% of adults (1). They are most likely to occur within a few months of the initiation of therapy and are usually minor, including skin rash and drug fever. Less common

R.M. Tuttle: Assistant Professor of Medicine, Cornell School of Medicine, Memorial Sloan Kettering Cancer Center, New York, NY.

D.V. Becker: Professor, Department of Radiology and Medicine, Cornell University Medical Center, and Director, Division of Nuclear Medicine, The New York Hospital-Cornell Medical Center, New York, NY.

J.R. Hurley: Associate Professor, Department of Medicine and Radiology, Cornell University Medical College, and Associate Director, Division of Nuclear Medicine, The New York Hospital-Cornell Medical Center, New York, NY.

reactions include leukopenia, hepatitis, agranulocytosis, and migratory polyarthrits.

Thyroidectomy

Surgical thyroidectomy has been in use since the early 1900s, and wide experience has established its effectiveness and benefits in producing a permanent cure of hyperthyroidism in up to 85% of patients (5). A relapse rate of 5% to 20% has been reported. As with radioiodine, the frequency of relapse can be decreased by removing more tissue but only at the cost of a higher incidence of early hypothyroidism.

Surgery has the disadvantage of a significant morbidity and occasional mortality, depending to a major degree on the skill of the surgeon. As the use of radioiodine has increased, surgical experience with this disease has diminished with the result that surgical morbidity has increased, although it remains a viable and effective option for many patients.

Radioactive Iodine

Radioiodine (cyclotron-produced ^{130}I) was first used for the treatment of hyperthyroidism in 1941 by Hertz and Roberts at Massachusetts General Hospital (6). However, it was not until after World War II, in the early 1950s, that ^{131}I became widely available to clinicians as a byproduct of atomic bomb production. Extensive experience established it as an effective, practical, and inexpensive agent to permanently control hyperthyroidism. In contrast to surgery, it avoids the potential of serious operative complications and has the advantages of permitting outpatient treatment with eventual, if not immediate, control of almost all clinical hyperthyroidism.

In the United States, of the three major modalities used in the treatment of hyperthyroidism, ^{131}I appears to be generally preferred for the majority of adult patients. Its efficacy is unquestioned and sufficient data have accumulated in the 40 years of its use to provide convincing evidence of its safety (4).

Clinical Aspects of Treatment with Radioactive Iodine

Graves' Disease

With few exceptions, Graves' disease can be cured with radioiodine treatment. How rapidly this occurs depends, to a significant degree, on the amount of radioiodine administered. The majority of patients are cured by the initial administration of radioiodine, and those not cured usually have amelioration of their symptoms. Persistent disease requires repeat treatment, and a second administration of ^{131}I usually cures the 10% to 40% of Graves' disease patients requiring additional treatment.

A wide variety of approaches and radioiodine dose strategies have been used, all with a high degree of success. However, the different methods of treatment appear only to alter the proportion of early to late hypothyroidism and the rate at which a response is achieved. Nevertheless, there are significant arguments to be made for and against the different approach. These issues are discussed in detail in the technical aspects section that follows.

Toxic Nodular Goiter: Autonomously Functioning Thyroid Nodule(s)

Hyperthyroidism resulting from autonomous hyperfunctioning nodules that suppress the function of the nonnodular thyroid tissue theoretically represents an ideal situation for radioiodine treatment. In these patients, radioiodine is selectively accumulated by the autonomous nodule(s) while the uptake of RAI by the rest of the gland is suppressed because of greatly decreased pituitary TSH secretion (7). The administered radioiodine exerts its maximum effect within the hyperfunctioning tissue and affects the remaining thyroid tissue to a much lesser degree, if at all. After adequate treatment, function in the autonomous nodule diminishes and, as thyroid hormone levels decrease, TSH secretion is normalized. The extranodular tissue previously suppressed is then stimulated by TSH and usually regains normal function. A relatively large nodule (usually more than 3 cm in diameter) usually predominates in toxic nodular goiter, but other small localized areas of autonomy within the gland are usually present and multiple clinically evident nodules are not uncommon. Toxic nodular goiter must be differentiated from Graves' disease (toxic diffuse goiter) with incidental nodules. In the latter, the nodules on scanning usually contain less radioiodine than the diffusely hyperfunctioning surrounding nonnodular thyroid tissue.

Although radioiodine is generally considered the treatment of choice for most patients with toxic nodules, surgery is sometimes preferred in children or in the presence of large nodules, particularly those with symptomatic tracheal compression (7). Surgery is often more efficient management because it more rapidly produces euthyroidism, particularly because repeat radioiodine administration may be required more often than in Graves' disease. Antithyroid drugs do not induce permanent remissions in patients with toxic nodules, although they can be helpful in controlling the symptoms of hyperthyroidism.

Relatively large amounts of radioiodine are usually required for adequate treatment of toxic nodular goiter, probably because of the inhomogeneity of distribution of radioiodine. If adequate amounts of ^{131}I are given, often two to five times as much as for Graves' disease, such patients can almost always be cured. Because of the amount of radioiodine required and its irregular distribution, there is a possibility of localized acute radiation damage with discharge of hormone and exacerbation of hyperthyroidism. Although it is infrequent, this may be a potential problem in older people and those with complicating illness. In such patients, preparation with antithyroid drugs before ^{131}I will deplete hormone stores and decrease the possibility of aggravation of disease.

Although hyperthyroidism can be controlled and shrinkage of the nodule is frequent, complete disappearance of large toxic nodules is uncommon. Postradioiodine hypothyroidism after treatment of toxic nodules with ^{131}I is uncommon.

Radioactive Iodine and Pregnancy

Because iodide readily crosses the placental barrier, radioiodine is absolutely contraindicated in pregnancy. Because the fetal thyroid begins to accumulate iodine between the tenth to twelfth week of gestation, ^{131}I could affect the fetal thyroid if given at or after that time. It is also inappropriate earlier in pregnancy because of exposure of the fetus to unnecessary radiation from maternal ^{131}I as well as from ^{131}I crossing the placenta.

Because a patient may be unaware that she is pregnant, it is advisable to obtain a reliable pregnancy test before the administration of radioiodine therapy to women in whom this possibility exists. A history of regular menses, absence of exposure, or use of adequate birth control measures has sometimes proven unreliable evidence that the patient is not pregnant.

Treatment of Children

The medical management of hyperthyroid children is often difficult and complicated (8). In adults, the overall complication rate of antithyroid drugs is about 5% to 7%; in children however, 10% to 25% is more common and an incidence as high as 40% has been reported. In addition, permanent remission following drug therapy appears to be even less frequent than in adults, and problems in compliance with drug schedules are common.

Although thyroidectomy is often recommended as definitive therapy in children, the incidence of surgical complications in this age group is significantly higher than in adults, presumably because of the smaller size of the neck structures.

Because surgery and antithyroid drugs can have expected and significant immediate morbidity in children, the argument has been made that the remote potential of an as yet unsubstantiated hazard of radioactive iodine is preferable and that RAI should be the treatment of choice in hyperthyroid children.

Technical Aspects of Treatment with Radioactive Iodine

Biologic Basis of Radioiodine Use

The use of radioiodine for treatment of hyperthyroidism is based on the radiation-induced cell changes resulting from the highly energetic β-rays emitted by [131]I. The accumulation of the isotope at the cell-colloid interface results in inhibition of thyroid follicular cell function and damage to cell mechanisms of reproduction. The magnitude of such effect appears directly proportional to the radiation dose. However, determination in advance of the precise radiation dose required for specific physiologic effects is difficult, if not impossible.

The absorbed radiation dose (measured in rad or Gray), is determined by the total amount of radiation energy deposited in the tissue and the tissue mass. The effect of radiation on the thyroid depends on the absorbed radiation dose, the tissue response (radiosensitivity), and the quality (i.e., the linear energy transfer) of the radiation.

It is important to differentiate between the number of millicuries administered to the patient and the radiation dose received by the thyroid gland. The radiation dose (rad) to the thyroid is related not only to the amount of radioiodine administered (millicuries), but also to the fraction deposited in the gland (the thyroid uptake) and the duration of its retention by the thyroid (the biologic half-life). These parameters can be measured following a pretherapy tracer and used to estimate the amount of administered radioiodine required to deliver a desired radiation dose. The uptake of the treatment administration by the thyroid can similarly be measured to provide a direct estimate of the amount of radiation actually received by the thyroid. Factors that cannot be measured readily but that may influence radiation effects include the shape or geometry of the gland and the microscopic distribution of radionuclide.

These parameters, whether measured or assumed, represent the basis for all methods of therapeutic radioiodine administration. It appears that no particular strategy for determination of the number of millicuries to be administered for therapy has any particular advantage in minimizing subsequent hypothyroidism, although there are practical, theoretic, and investigational differences among them. As a result, the tendency has been to use the simplest, least expensive, and least cumbersome method.

Dose Strategies

Fixed Millicurie Administration

The simplest method of radioiodine administration is to give an identical number of millicuries to all patients in a particular clinical category. Many clinics use a standard 3 to 7 mCi (111 to 259 MBq) of ^{131}I given orally. About 60% of the patients so treated develop a remission within 3 to 4 months. Many of the rest show improvement, and, when necessary, a second treatment is given following which only about 10% to 15% remain hyperthyroid and require further treatment. A number of modifications of the fixed dose method have been proposed, including increasing the number of millicuries given to patients with larger glands, to those with severe disease, and for a variety of other less well-specified factors.

The strategy of fixed millicurie administration has the limitation that there is little correlation between the millicuries administered to the patient and the rad dose delivered to the thyroid gland. This is due in part to the wide range of radioiodine uptake of hyperthyroid patients, which varies greatly (from 30% to 100%) and does not correlate with either the severity of symptoms or the mass of the gland. To provide some uniformity for evaluation, any method used should, at the very least, use the measured uptake by the thyroid. Because radiation dose is related to the amount of radioactivity deposited in each gram of thyroid, some estimate of gland weight should also enter into the determination of the amount of radioiodine to be administered.

Delivered Microcuries Per Gram

The most widely used method attempts to deposit a specified number of microcuries of ^{131}I in each gram of thyroid tissue. This method requires that both thyroid uptake be measured and gland weight be estimated. It assumes an average biologic half-life that is considered to be essentially constant for all patients, although it is known to vary widely. Estimates of thyroid size, although most commonly based on physical examination estimates, can also be reliably determined using ultrasonography. Many practitioners today use 100–120 μCi per gram for the usual patient with the diffusely enlarged thyroid of hyperthyroid Graves' disease (approximately 10,000 rads).

If it is desirable to accelerate the process of therapy to minimize the duration of symptoms in a severely hyperthyroid patient, administration of a larger amount of radioiodine (up to 160 to 200 μCi/g, 5,920 to 7,400 kBq/g) will produce a more rapid and more certain response. The associated higher incidence of hypothyroidism may be an acceptable consequence in such situations. Because larger glands are thought to be inherently more resistant to radioiodine, a larger amount of radioiodine (i.e., more microcuries per gram) may also be given to individuals with large goiters.

To calculate the amount of radioiodine to be administered on the basis of delivered microcuries per gram, the following formula may be used.

$$\text{Administered } \mu\text{Ci} = \frac{\mu\text{Ci/g desired} \times \text{gland wt (g)} \times 100}{\% \text{ uptake (24 hr)}} \quad [1]$$

Modifications of this formula have been proposed to compensate directly for variations in thyroidal turnover rate and indirectly by including a factor in the dose formula that is based on the level of the protein-bound ^{131}I in the serum.

Delivered Rad (Dosimetry)

Attempts to deliver precise amounts of radiation to the thyroid appear to have no significant clinical advantage over simpler and easier methods of estimating administered amounts of ^{131}I. Nevertheless, the use of a method based on a universally accepted radiologic unit, the rad or Gray, has significant advantages, not the least of which is providing a basis for intercomparison of results. Much of the large experience with radioiodine treatment available reports only millicuries administered, a largely meaningless figure. Although it is clear that radiation sensitivity may vary considerably from one individual to the next, the contributing factors characterizing such sensitivity cannot be analyzed and understood until some scientifically consistent dosimetry formulation is applied. Until radioiodine treatment is reported in terms of delivered radiation dose and conceptualized in terms of estimated units of absorbed radiation, we can expect little improvement in our approach to therapy.

It is possible to convert microcuries per gram to rad by simplifying the dosimetry formulas, because many factors are relatively constant and others necessarily vary only within a limited range and often can be assumed. Because most of the effective radiation dose from ^{131}I comes from the relatively high-energy β-rays, the Quimby-Marinelli (9) formulation produces almost identical results (within about 3%) as that from the medium internal radiation dose (MIRD) absorbed dose calculations. The following formula relates thyroidal radiation dose (rad) to thyroid uptake and gland weight.

$$\text{Administered } \mu\text{Ci} = \frac{\text{rad desired} \times \text{gland wt (g)} \times 100}{\% \text{ uptake (24 hr)} \times 93} \quad [2]$$

This formula assumes a biologic half-life of 24 days (equiva-

lent to an effective half-life of 6 days) and the appropriate physical constants.

If biologic half-life is measured, it can be used to calculate the effective half-life (all in units of days), as follows.

$$t_{1/2\text{eff}} = \frac{t_{1/2\text{biol}} \times t_{1/2\text{phys}}}{t_{1/2\text{biol}} + t_{1/2\text{phys}}} \quad [3]$$

By changing the constant in Eq. 2, it can be rewritten to include the effective half-life and to allow calculation of the amount of administered radioiodine required to provide a desired number of rad delivered to the thyroid.

$$\text{Administered } \mu\text{Ci} = \frac{\text{rad desired} \times \text{gland wt (g)} \times 6.67}{t_{1/2\text{eff}} \times \% \text{ uptake (24 hr)}} \quad [4]$$

The philosophy of the therapist with regard to the relative desirability of rapid cure (which may be achieved only at the expense of a higher early and total incidence of hypothyroidism) weighs strongly in selecting radiation dose. One is left to decide dose on the basis of individual experience, which is, of course, only gained after use of a particular dose schedule and careful follow-up and analysis. In this context, 10,000 rads appears to be a reasonable starting point.

Rapid Thyroid Turnover of Radioiodine ("Small Pool")

About 10% to 15% of hyperthyroid patients have been found to have a very rapid thyroidal turnover of iodine and, therefore, a very short biologic half-life of radioiodine in the thyroid (10, 11). These patients are believed to have a relatively small thyroidal iodine pool. This situation often follows antithyroid drug administration that is known to deplete thyroidal iodine. It may also occur following prior thyroid surgery or ^{131}I treatment of Graves' disease or in patients with Hashimoto's thyroiditis.

Rapid thyroidal turnover of radioiodine decreases the delivered thyroidal radiation dose from each millicurie of ^{131}I initially deposited in the thyroid. Because of the smaller thyroidal iodine pool, the specific activity of ^{131}I-labeled thyroid hormone secreted by the gland is greatly increased. Serum levels of protein-bound ^{131}I (PB^{131}I), which are usually less than 0.5% of administered activity per liter at 24 hours, may be strikingly elevated (up to 4% of the administered activity per liter and higher). This is important because extrathyroidal radiation dose, including, most notably, the bone marrow dose, in hyperthyroid patients is largely dependent on blood radioactivity. Because the PB^{131}I remains in the blood longer than ^{131}I (iodide), it contributes the greatest proportion of the whole-body and marrow radiation dose delivered from radioiodine administration.

In patients with a small thyroidal iodine pool, radioiodine therapy given in any standard dose strategy is likely to be unsuccessful. Patients with small pool syndrome can be identified when the 4 hour uptake is significantly higher than the 24 hour uptake, the calculated biological half life is short of the PB^{131}I is elevated. Because a considerable proportion of hyperthyroid patients may receive antithyroid drugs as initial therapy, this may be a frequent occurrence and suggests the usefulness of pretherapy studies of iodine metabolism. Under these circumstances it is advisable to increase the amount of radioiodine administered because of antithyroid drug-associated radioresistance.

Clinical Management Issues

Before Radioiodine Treatment

For the majority of patients with uncomplicated mild hyperthyroidism, preparation for ^{131}I therapy with antithyroid drugs is unnecessary (1,2,12). However, in high-risk patients with severe hyperthyroidism, with complicating diseases (particularly cardiovascular), and in the older age groups, it is reasonable and appropriate to bring these patients to a euthyroid state with antithyroid drugs (thioamides) before they receive radioactive iodine. In such circumstances, this medication can be discontinued as little as 48 to 72 hours before administration of ^{131}I or continued at a reduced dose during therapy. If necessary, the drugs can be reinstituted at a full blocking dose within a few days, although it is preferable to wait a week if clinically feasible. There may be significant hazard, however, in the sudden withdrawal or interruption of long-term antithyroid drug therapy in severely hyperthyroid patients because an exacerbation of disease may occur associated with an abrupt increase in serum thyroid hormone levels within 24 to 48 hours (13).

Use of antithyroid drugs routinely as initial therapy in all hyperthyroid patients will often delay the institution of definitive therapy because in many of these patients a permanent remission is unlikely. Antithyroid drugs may increase radioresistance and unless an increase (usually arbitrary) is made in the amount of administered radioiodine, treatment failure may occur (2). Radioresistance appears to be clinically more significant in patients pretreated with propylthiouracil than in those pretreated with methimazole (14).

β-Adrenergic blocking agents (e.g., propranolol, metoprolol), although not affecting thyroid hormone synthesis or secretion, ameliorate some of the peripheral manifestations of hyperthyroidism through action on β-adrenergic receptors. Radioiodine uptake and serum T_4 levels are not altered. However, inhibition of peripheral conversion of T_4 to T_3 by propranolol does occur and will reduce serum T_3 levels. However, longer acting β-blockers have the advantage of once a day dosing and probably increased patient compliance. The major clinical effects of these drugs include reduction in heart rate and relief of palpitations. They may also improve such distressing symptoms as anxiety, restlessness, tremor, and sweating, although symptomatic relief is rarely complete. β-Blocking agents are particularly useful because they make the patient more comfortable but do not interfere with most diagnostic tests or with radioiodine therapy.

Immediate Posttreatment Period

The major impact of radioiodine therapy occurs within 3 months of treatment. Hyperthyroid symptoms are unlikely to be affected until 4 to 6 weeks have elapsed, although the enlarged thyroid may decrease in size earlier. During this period, supplemental β-adrenergic blocking agents are useful to ameliorate symptoms. Thioamides may be used to control hyperthyroidism following radioiodine treatment. However, such medications should not generally be instituted immediately because their use within 1 week of treatment will increase thyroidal iodine turnover rate and reduce the anticipated radiation dose to the gland.

Marked decrease in the size of the thyroid suggests that a significant response to treatment has occurred. If at 3 months the patient has improved clinically but is still hyperthyroid, further supplemental drug therapy should be considered. Antithyroid drugs or iodine could be administered if symptoms are disturbing because further response to the radioiodine may only appear slowly over the subsequent 3 to 9 months.

If at 3 months the symptoms of hyperthyroidism are still significant, serum thyroid hormones remain elevated, and the thyroid has not decreased in size, repeat treatment with ^{131}I should be considered. Retreatment is rarely undertaken before 3 months after therapy. However, if there is no sign of improvement in clinical status at 8 weeks in a seriously ill patient, additional ^{131}I might be given at that time. Patients should be monitored closely following ^{131}I therapy and seen as often as their clinical situation requires. Transient hypothyroidism (as well as transient euthyroidism) is sometimes seen in the months immediately following radioiodine treatment.

Retreatment with Radioactive Iodine

There are as many approaches to retreatment as to initial therapy. Following radioiodine therapy, the residual thyroid tissue usually shows a more rapid thyroidal ^{131}I turnover than was seen previously. This shorter biologic half-life implies that to deliver the same amount of radiation as in the initial treatment, a larger amount of ^{131}I must be given. If the biologic half-life is measured and included in the calculations (Eq. 4), it is reasonable to deliver the same number of rads as for the initial treatment. If other methods are used to determine the amount of ^{131}I to be given, 20% to 30% more radioiodine should be deposited in the thyroid than for initial therapy.

Posttherapy Hypothyroidism

It was not realized until more than 10 years after radioiodine therapy was introduced that the posttreatment incidence of hypothyroidism was substantial. Later studies showed not only a high early incidence (from 26% to 43% in the first year after treatment) but also a subsequent regular annual increment of hypothyroidism.

At present, it is not possible to predict outcome in any individual patient, and because the incidence of hypothyroidism is considerable regardless of dose, it has been suggested that large amounts of ^{131}I should be given routinely to produce earlier and more certain control. Some therapists are willing to accept, and sometimes prefer, the consequent high early (and late) incidence of hypothyroidism. With such a strategy, permanent supplementation with thyroid hormone is started at the earliest possible moment.

Hypothyroidism following radioiodine treatment is probably due, at least in part, to the effect of radiation in impairing the reproductive capacity of follicular cells and a resultant gradually shrinking functional follicular cell population. There is evidence, however, that hypothyroidism is a natural consequence of the autoimmune pathophysiologic processes of Graves' disease. Malone and Cullen (15) have suggested that the linear relationship between radiation dose and hypothyroidism accounts for the early incidence. Late hypothyroidism, which occurs at a relatively fixed rate, appears independent of dose and may be more related to the natural history of the disease. This regular incremental late appearance also occurs after surgery, and there were a number of reports of late hypothyroidism and impaired thyroid reserve following remission of hyperthyroidism induced by antithyroid drugs (16,17).

Because it is not possible to predict which patients will develop hypothyroidism and when hypothyroidism will develop, the need for careful long-term follow-up seems obvious. This problem is made more difficult because in many areas radioiodine therapy is administered by specialists in nuclear medicine and radiology who are often hospital based and are rarely in a position to provide long-term care for the patients they treat. Long-term follow-up should be made an integral part of the treatment regimen.

Complications of Radioiodine Treatment

When radioiodine was first introduced widely in the late 1950s and the 1960s there was considerable concern about the possible hazards of the use of radiation for the treatment of a nonmalignant disease. Almost 50 years of experience with ^{131}I in about 1 million patients worldwide has demonstrated what must really be considered an impressive lack of complications. It is the demonstrated safety as well as the effectiveness of ^{131}I compared with the known frequency of side effects of antithyroid drugs and surgery that make ^{131}I such an important therapeutic agent for the treatment of hyperthyroidism.

Early Complications

Exacerbation of Hyperthyroidism
There have been a number of case reports of exacerbation of hyperthyroidism following radioiodine therapy and a few instances (in the 1950s and 1960s) of thyroid crisis or death following treatment. In several reports of thyroid storm following radioiodine therapy, however, the data suggest that withdrawal of antithyroid drugs may be as important a contributing factor as the radioiodine. Clinical exacerbation of hyperthyroidism after ^{131}I treatment does occur, but it appears to be rare.

The possibility of exacerbation of hyperthyroidism suggests that patients with existing cardiac disease and at risk of such complications should receive careful management of their heart disease, as well as antithyroid drugs to deplete thyroidal hormone content before receiving ^{131}I therapy.

New or Worsening Orbitopathy
Retrospective reports over many years have not demonstrated that any particular therapy of Graves disease was more likely than any other to be associated with an increased incidence of thyroid eye disease. However, a recent study reported a signifi-

cantly increased risk (33%) of new or worsening orbitopathy in patients treated with radioiodine compared with those treated with surgery or antithyroid drugs (18). In this study, patients treated with ^{131}I were allowed to become hypothyroid before replacement therapy with thyroid hormone was started, but those treated with surgery or antithyroid drugs were not. In a subsequent study by the same investigators, routine administration of T_4 replacement within 2 weeks of radioiodine therapy reduced the incidence of orbitopathy to only 11% (19). This data confirms an older clinical observation suggesting that hypothyroidism appearing in Graves' disease patients after radioiodine (and other forms of treatment) may be associated with worsening thyroid eye disease.

Patients without clinically detectable orbitopathy are apparently unlikely to develop significant eye disease after radioiodine treatment, although patients who do have significant eye involvement before treatment have an increased risk of an exacerbation of eye disease after radioiodine. The use of oral prednisone in doses of 0.3 to 0.4 mg/kg/day started at the time of radioiodine has been reported to prevent worsening of orbitopathy after treatment.

Late Complications

Leukemia
External ionizing radiation (usually more than 50 rad) has been reported to lead to an increased occurrence of leukemia with a peak incidence about 6 years after exposure. A single treatment of ^{131}I, in the process of delivering between 5,000 and 12,000 rads to the thyroid, delivers about 8 to 16 rads to the blood. The possibility that radioiodine treatment might lead to an increase in leukemia was a matter of early concern. In 1961, the Cooperative Thyrotoxicosis Follow-Up Study was established to test for an increase in the incidence of leukemia (20). In a comparison of 18,000 radioiodine-treated patients with 10,000 surgically treated patients, with each group followed for a total of about 115,000 patient years, no difference between these groups was seen in the adjusted incidence rate of leukemia for age, sex, or type of leukemia.

Induction of Neoplasms
External radiation and that from radioisotopes of iodine deposited in the thyroid gland can induce thyroid neoplasms in animals. External x-ray therapy (ranging from 16 to 1,200 rads) to the head and neck of infants and children is associated with the appearance of a significant number of thyroid neoplasms following a latent period of 5 to 35 years. The relevance of late effects of external x-ray therapy of children to the possible sequelae of ^{131}I therapy of hyperthyroid adults is uncertain. Significant differences in the biologic effectiveness of external x-ray, as compared with internally deposited ^{131}I, have been reported, with differences in the rate of induction of neoplasms varying by a factor of 3 to 20.

It is generally believed that children are more radiosensitive than adults, particularly with regard to the development of thyroid neoplasia. Experience with the induction of thyroid nodules and cancer 7 to 35 years after x-ray therapy to the head and neck of children cannot be applied to the different situation of internal radiation from ^{131}I because of differences in the rate of delivery of the radiation and its distribution. Although there is relatively little experience with long-term follow-up of radioiodine-treated children, a number of studies have not found deleterious effects in more than 700 children treated with radioiodine. The long life expectancy during which malignant changes might appear and the apparent increased radiosensitivity in children suggest that it would be prudent to withhold radioiodine treatment from children unless other alternatives have failed.

Genetic Consequences

A variety of genetic abnormalities have been shown to occur in some animals after exposure to radiation. There is little evidence of such effects in humans. Radioiodine dosimetry studies suggest that the average woman in the course of receiving a single radioiodine treatment receives about 2 rads to the ovaries (21). This gonadal dose is of the same magnitude as that delivered from such radiologic diagnostic procedures as barium enemas, intravenous pyelograms, and pelvic computed tomography (CT) scans.

To detect genetic abnormalities that might occur following radioiodine treatment would require very large populations carefully followed over several generations, and such studies are unlikely to be undertaken. Limited data are available from examination of the reproductive history of young people treated with large amounts of ^{131}I for thyroid cancer, and these have shown no detectable effect on birth history or fertility.

The administration of radioiodine as treatment for hyperthyroidism is not considered to be a contraindication to subsequent pregnancy on the basis of existing data. However, it does seem wise to avoid pregnancy for at least 6 months following RAI therapy. Nevertheless, a number of clinicians prefer not to use radioactive iodine as the initial form of therapy in young women who anticipate having children in the immediate future.

RADIOACTIVE IODINE TREATMENT OF THYROID CANCER

Introduction

A large body of evidence indicates that radioiodine (^{131}I) is of value in the management of papillary and follicular thyroid cancers (22,23). Papillary and follicular thyroid cancers, which are collectively referred to as differentiated thyroid cancer, originate from thyroid follicular cells. Although they usually appear as an area of decreased activity (cold nodule) on preoperative radionuclide images obtained when TSH levels are normal, about 75% will concentrate radioiodine under intense TSH stimulation. Because the cells that comprise anaplastic thyroid cancer, thyroid lymphoma, and medullary thyroid cancer do not have the capability to concentrate iodine, radioactive iodine therapy is very unlikely to be of any value in the treatment of these types of thyroid cancer.

Metastases capable of collecting radioiodine (functioning metastases) can often be treated effectively by giving the patient a large amount of radioiodine. Uptake in cervical lymph node metastases is usually completely eliminated. However, in most patients with unresected locally invasive thyroid cancer or distant metastases, radioiodine treatment is only palliative. Life may be prolonged and symptoms relieved, but almost all patients with bone metastases, and over half of those with lung metastases, eventually die of their disease.

Perhaps more importantly, administration of therapeutic amounts of radioiodine to patients without any evidence of residual thyroid cancer following surgery significantly decreases the risk of recurrence of thyroid cancer and the risk of death resulting from thyroid cancer. This type of treatment, called ablation, presumably has its effect through the destruction of microscopic foci of residual or metastatic thyroid cancer.

Surgical Management

There is a wide range of opinion regarding optimal surgery for differentiated thyroid cancer (24,25). In addition to decreasing recurrence rates in moderate to high risk patients, a total or near total thyroidectomy has several advantages over lobectomy alone, including:

1. Sufficient thyroid tissue is removed to result in TSH elevation, which increases the chance of detecting functioning residual cancer on postoperative whole-body imaging. TSH elevation also increases the effectiveness of radioiodine ablation in destroying microscopic metastases.
2. A smaller mass of residual normal thyroid results in more successful RAI ablation of the normal thyroid remnant.
3. The smaller amount of residual thyroid tissue provides less competition for radioiodine given for treatment of functioning metastases and permits use of a smaller amount of radioiodine for ablation.

Stratification of Risk

The first and most important step in postoperative management of patients with differentiated thyroid cancer is to analyze the factors that affect the risks of recurrence and death. Patients at high risk of dying from thyroid cancer should be treated aggressively, whereas patients with a low risk of disease specific mortality should not be overtreated.

Papillary thyroid cancer is an uncommon cause of death. The cancer specific mortality at 20 years is only 5.5%. However, through careful analysis of risk factors patients can be subdivided into high- and low-risk groups (Table 31.1). The high-risk group, about 15% of the total, has a 40% risk of dying of papillary cancer by 20 years. The low-risk group, almost 85% of the total, has a 1% risk of dying of papillary cancer by 20 years (26, 27).

Postoperative Management

Patients who have cancers less than 1.5 cm in size and without lymph node metastases, extrathyroidal extension, vascular invasion, or distant metastases; who have undergone only a lobectomy; and who have low levels of serum thyroglobulin (Tg) are placed on levothyroxine (T$_4$) and followed clinically. All other moderate- to high-risk patients undergo whole-body imaging with radioiodine to look for functioning metastases. We prefer to wait 4 to 6 weeks following thyroidectomy before performing

Table 31.1. *Risk Stratification for Papillary and Follicular Thyroid Cancers*

Parameter	Low risk	High risk
Age at diagnosis	<45 yrs	>45 yrs
Size	<1.5 cm	>4 cm
Local invasion	Absent	Present
Vascular invasion	Absent	Present
Pathologic grade	Well differentiated	Poorly differentiated
Gross multifocal disease	Absent	Present
DNA ploidy	Diploid	Aneuploid
Cervical metastasis	Absent	Controversial*
Distant metastasis	Absent	Present
Time from nodule detection to initial therapy	<1 yr	>1 yr

*Lymph node metastases are often associated with increased risk of local recurrence but not disease specific mortality.

radioiodine studies. This allows time for the patient to recover from surgery, for reestablishment of blood supply to the operative site, for circulating T4 to fall to undetectable levels, and for any stable iodine used in the setting of surgery to be excreted.

During this period the patient is maintained on T_3, which is begun about a week after surgery. The usual dose is 25 μg twice daily. However, some patients, especially older individuals, develop hyperthyroid symptoms on this dose. If this occurs, the dose can be reduced to 12.5 μg 2 or 3 times per day. Two weeks before whole-body imaging, T_3 is discontinued to permit TSH to rise to maximum levels, and 1 week before, the patient begins a low iodine diet.

Patients with evidence of functioning metastatic thyroid cancer on whole-body images are treated with radioiodine. Patients with known residual cancer or metastases that do not collect radioiodine when whole-body imaging is performed in the setting of a significantly elevated TSH (greater than 30 μU/mL) are placed on T_4 and considered for other forms of treatment, such as external radiation therapy combined with adjuvant doxorubicin.

Patients with negative whole-body scans and no evidence of residual cancer are evaluated for ablation. Radioiodine ablation is the administration of a therapeutic amount of radioiodine to patients without any evidence of functioning residual thyroid cancer following surgery. It has been found empirically to decrease the risk of recurrence and death resulting from thyroid cancer in patients with more than low risk for development of recurrence or death, presumably through the destruction of microscopic foci of residual cancer capable of concentrating radioiodine. The decision whether to ablate and how much radioiodine to use is based on risk factor analysis as described previously.

Patient Preparation for Whole-Body Imaging, Ablation, and Treatment

Before radioiodine is administered for whole-body imaging, ablation, or treatment of thyroid cancer, conditions should be optimized so that uptake of radioiodine is as high as possible. This

will increase both the sensitivity of whole-body imaging and the effectiveness of treatment, because doubling the uptake is equivalent to giving twice as much radioiodine. A number of factors affect uptake, but only serum TSH and inorganic iodine can be easily manipulated.

Thyroid Stimulating Hormone

Differentiated thyroid cancer cells have receptors for TSH but are much less sensitive to stimulation of uptake than normal thyroid follicular cells (28,29). High TSH levels (greater than 30 (μU/mL) are required to insure detection of all thyroid cancers that are capable of function. To achieve high TSH concentrations required for RAI ablation or therapy, it is necessary to induce hypothyroidism by first surgically removing or ablating most of the normal thyroid and then withdrawing thyroid hormone for a prolonged period.

When replacement thyroid hormone is not given after total thyroidectomy, TSH elevation may be detectable within 2 weeks. However, maximum TSH concentration is usually not reached for 4 to 6 weeks, and patients with more than a few grams of normal thyroid tissue may remain euthyroid indefinitely with a normal or only slightly elevated TSH.

Except for brief periods of evaluation and treatment, patients with well-differentiated thyroid cancer should be maintained on sufficient thyroid hormone to suppress TSH. Before whole-body imaging, ablation, or treatment, thyroid hormone must be discontinued to induce temporary hypothyroidism and TSH elevation. If only T_3 has been given, TSH is almost always significantly elevated within 2 weeks.

T_4 disappears from the serum much more slowly than T3 and TSH may remain suppressed for as long as 4 weeks after it has been stopped. To avoid a prolonged period of symptomatic hypothyroidism, patients taking T_4 may be switched to T_3 6 weeks before the planned procedure. T_3 is then discontinued a minimum of 2 weeks before administration of radioiodine.

Serum TSH should be determined before administration of radioiodine for whole-body imaging, ablation, or therapy to be sure that it is sufficiently elevated. In an occasional patient, TSH will fail to rise because of an abnormality of the hypothalamus or pituitary. Some patients, usually older, whose TSH has been completely suppressed by high doses of thyroid hormone for prolonged periods of time, may require more than 2 weeks without T_3 before TSH rises above 30 μU/mL. In these patients, an additional week or two without T_3 usually results in further TSH elevation. If not, consideration should be given to injection of recombinant human TSH (30).

Serum Inorganic Iodine Concentration

The second major determinant of radioiodine uptake is the serum inorganic iodine concentration. Because stable and radioactive iodine atoms compete to enter thyroid follicular cells at the level of the iodine trap, an increase in the number of inorganic iodine atoms in the blood decreases the uptake of radioiodine, whereas a decrease in the inorganic iodine concentration results in a higher uptake of radioiodine.

Avoiding Excess Iodine

Unfortunately, iodine is ubiquitous in the medical environment. Very large amounts are often given for diagnostic radiographic procedures in the form of iodinated radiographic contrast. Following these procedures, substantial amounts of iodine may remain in the body for prolonged periods. This is especially true in patients who are hypothyroid or who have poor renal function. Administration of iodinated radiographic contrast should be avoided in patients with differentiated thyroid cancer who may require whole-body imaging and/or treatment in the near future. It must be pointed out that the older contrast agents and the new nonionic contrast agents *both* contain large amounts of iodine. If contrast has been given or must be given, the following minimum time intervals should elapse before radioiodine studies are initiated: (a) water soluble contrast given intravenously: 2 months; (b) gallbladder agents: 4 months; (c) water soluble contrast given for myelography, cisternography, or bronchography: 3 months; (d) iodinated oil given for myelography, cisternography, bronchography, or lymphangiography: unknown.

Another major but subtler source of iodine contamination is antiseptics containing iodine, which are increasingly used on all hospitalized patients. The iodine is readily absorbed through the skin, raises the concentration of inorganic iodine in the blood, and lowers the radioiodine uptake. These should be avoided for at least 2 weeks before radioiodine studies.

Low Iodine Diets

The total iodine content of the American diet is almost 1,000 μg/day, far in excess of the recommended daily allowance. However, recent studies emphasize a trend toward lower iodine excretion rates over the last 20 to 30 years. Low iodine diets can be effective in lowering iodine excretion and increasing uptake. We ask our patients to follow a low iodine diet beginning 1 week before radioiodine administration and continuing until at least 24 hours after ablation or treatment with radioiodine. The instructions we give are shown in Table 31.2. In our experience, following the diet doubles the uptake of radioiodine in most patients. If a formal low iodine diet is not used, patients should at least be asked to avoid vitamins, food supplements, and medications containing iodine and foods that are particularly high in iodine, including fish, shellfish, and foods that may contain seaweed. Seaweed, often in the form of kelp, may also be present in some nutritional supplements.

Ancillary Techniques for Stimulating Uptake

Injection of Thyroid Stimulating Hormone

Intramuscular injection of bovine TSH has been shown to stimulate radioiodine uptake by both normal thyroid and functioning thyroid cancer. However, injection of bovine TSH has several drawbacks. Blood levels are only transiently elevated, allergic reactions may occur, and neutralizing antibodies may be formed against both bovine and human TSH, causing TSH resistance. For this reason, the prolonged high levels of endogenous TSH that can be achieved following removal or ablation of normal thyroid tissue are preferred. Recently, recombinant human TSH has been approved for radioactive iodine scanning in thyroid cancer patients (31,32). Preliminary studies indicated that recombinant human TSH may also be effectively used for ablation and therapy of known metastases (30). However, the proper dosage of both recombinant TSH and radioactive iodine are yet to be clearly defined.

Diuretic Administration

Both acute and chronic diuresis has been used in combination with low iodine diets to lower serum inorganic iodine concentrations and increase uptake of radioiodine by thyroid cancer. We have not found diuretics to have any advantage over a well-maintained low iodine diet alone. However, a combination of diuresis and intravenous saline can be used to increase the clearance of radioiodine from the body following high-dose radioiodine treatment of metastatic disease.

Whole-Body Imaging with Radioiodine

Whole-body imaging is performed after administration of a tracer of ^{131}I to detect functioning metastatic thyroid cancer and/or residual normal thyroid. In addition to imaging, quantitative studies should be performed to determine the percent uptake of radioiodine by any functioning tissue. This information permits estimation of radiation dose and can be used to calculate the amount of radioiodine required for ablation or to predict the response of metastases to treatment. If high dose radioiodine treatment of distant metastases is a possibility, serial determinations of whole-body and whole-blood activity should be performed to permit calculation of the maximum amount of radioiodine that can be safely administered to the patient.

Patients should be prepared for whole-body imaging by initiating a low iodine diet a week before the tracer as described in the section on patient preparation. The required elevation in TSH is then achieved following either discontinuation of thyroid hormone for a sufficient length of time to maximize TSH or injection of recombinant human TSH. Recent studies have demonstrated that disease detection based on radioactive iodine scan-

Table 31.2. *Low Iodine Diet*

Foods and medications that contain iodine may interfere with the procedure that is planned for you. We would like you to stop taking any iodine containing medications and any of the foods listed below until the procedure has been completed.

Vitamins and food supplements—Check the label. If iodine is present, do not take.

Kelp or seaweed—Very high in iodine. Common in Asian food, especially Japanese. Unless you are an expert, avoid Asian foods.

Ocean fish and shellfish—These are particularly high in iodine.

Iodized salt—Check the label. If your salt contains iodine, buy non-iodized salt.

Milk, ice cream, and yogurt—You may have a small amount of milk in coffee or on cereal—hard cheese *may* be eaten.

Cured or spicy meats—Bacon, ham, sausage, salami, etc. Fresh meat is OK.

Very salty foods—Potato chips, pretzels, salted nuts, etc.

Commercial white bread and rolls—Homemade or local bakery bread, whole wheat, rye, cracked wheat, etc. are OK.

Commercial pizza and chili—Homemade is OK.

Canned fruits and vegetables—Fresh and frozen are OK.

Instant coffee—Drip or percolator coffee is OK.

Tea, including herbal tea and commercial lemonade.

Bright red foods, pills or capsules—Some red food dyes contain iodine.

Sensitivity For Disease Detection

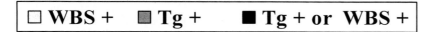

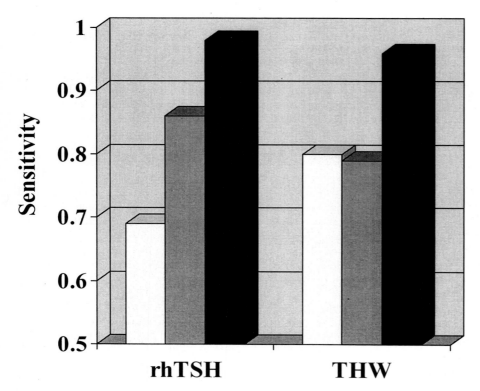

FIGURE 31.1. The sensitivity for detection of metastatic disease is given for whole-body radioactive iodine scanning and stimulated thyroglobulin (greater than or equal to 2 ng/mL) when used as single, isolated tests and when used in combination. The maximal sensitivity for detection of metastatic disease with both hypothyroid withdrawal (THW, *right side*) and recombinant human TSH stimulation (rhTSH, *left side*) is achieved when the results of both the stimulated thyroglobulin and the whole-body diagnostic radioactive iodine scan are taken together. Furthermore, when both tests are considered in an individual patient, there is no significant difference in the sensitivity for disease detection between traditional hypothyroid withdrawal and recombinant human TSH stimulation (33).

ning and serum Tg stimulation is essentially identical using either method of preparation (Fig. 31.1) (33). Blood is drawn for TSH and Tg just before administration of an oral tracer of ^{131}I. When using the recombinant TSH stimulation approach, it is critical that a serum Tg be obtained 72 hours following the second TSH injection. It is the combination of this stimulated Tg value with the interpretation of the radioactive iodine scan that provides maximal sensitivity for detection of residual or recurrent disease.

Size of Tracer

There is wide variability in the amount of ^{131}I recommended for whole-body imaging. It has been well-established that a progressive increase in millicuries (mCi) administered results in a progressive increase in the number of foci of either residual normal thyroid or thyroid cancer that are detected on whole-body images. In the past, this led to the routine use of 10 mCi tracers in many nuclear medicine departments. Recently, it has also been shown that use of large tracers results in decreased uptake of subsequent therapeutic radioiodine (stunning), decreasing the effectiveness of ablation or treatment. We, and others, recommend use of a 2.0 mCi ^{131}I tracer for whole-body imaging with

some exceptions. For example, when performing follow-up whole-body imaging in patients who have been treated with radioiodine for metastases but who are currently thought to be free of disease, higher scanning doses of 5 mCi seem reasonable.

Timing of Imaging

Imaging of the anterior neck and chest and areas of known or suspected metastases is performed at 24 hours. Because radioiodine is excreted slowly in hypothyroid patients, especially if they have been on a low iodine diet, considerable background activity is usually present at 24 hours. Full whole-body imaging is, therefore, delayed for 48 or 72 hours, resulting in a considerably improved target-to-background ratio. In some patients, especially those with diffuse pulmonary metastases that have already been treated with radioiodine, very faint uptake may be detectable only 5 to 7 days after administration of the tracer.

Technical Details

The best images are anterior and lateral neck images performed on a scintillation camera with a collimator designed specifically for use with ^{131}I. If a medium-energy collimator is used, septal penetration will significantly degrade the images. If there is a choice, the camera with the thickest crystal should be used as this will improve counting efficiency. Additional spot images of the neck are useful in identifying and localizing cervical lymph node metastases. Accurate anatomic marking of the images is essential for accurate interpretation, especially the neck images.

If there is substantial activity in residual normal thyroid, septal penetration by the higher energy γ-rays from ^{131}I may significantly degrade the image. Reimaging with a lead shield over the "hot spot" may improve image quality. The problem of septal penetration can also be eliminated by using a pinhole collimator. For patients with focal neck activity, neck palpation with placement of markers at appropriate anatomical sites is the best way to determine whether foci of uptake are in the thyroid bed, thyroglossal duct, or lymph nodes.

Interpretation

When nonphysiologic foci of radioiodine concentration are present outside the neck on whole-body images, especially when correlated with radiographic abnormalities, the presence of metastatic well-differentiated thyroid cancer can be assumed. However, most foci of uptake on whole-body images are due to physiologic sites of radioiodine accumulation. Contamination of skin, hair, or clothing with radioactive urine or saliva also occurs commonly.

Sites of Physiologic Radioiodine Concentration

Interpretation of whole-body images requires knowledge of the physiologic extrathyroidal sites where ^{131}I normally accumulates in the body. Activity is commonly present in the nose, presumably resulting from persistence of radioiodine that leaks out of nasal capillaries when blood levels are high shortly after administration of the tracer. The salivary glands and stomach trap radioiodine from the blood and secrete it into the mouth and stomach. As long as inorganic radioiodine is present in the blood these structures will be visualized. Radioactive saliva is usually detected in the mouth and may also be present in the esophagus. Any patient with central chest activity should be reimaged standing after drinking a glass of water. Saliva may also contaminate the beard or, in patients who drool onto their pillow at night, the hair. Radioiodine binds permanently to hair and cannot be removed by washing.

The majority of the radioiodine will be excreted in the urine, and the bladder will be visualized as long as inorganic radioiodine is present in the blood. Patients should be asked to void immediately before imaging the pelvis. Radioiodine may also be present in bladder diverticula or in the ureter or renal pelvis in patients with obstructive uropathy. Radioiodine is excreted via the colon, and the large intestine is almost always visualized. The liver normally contains a large fraction of the body's thyroid hormone stores. If residual normal thyroid or thyroid cancer capable of synthesizing radioactive thyroid hormone is present, the liver may show diffuse radioactivity on whole-body images. When hepatic metastases occur, they are virtually always focal. Radioiodine is rarely concentrated by the gallbladder, and we have observed a case of appendiceal retention of radioiodine.

Sites of Artifactual Radioiodine Concentration

Artifactual areas of radioiodine concentration are also common. These are most often caused by contamination of clothes or skin with urine, less often with saliva. In one instance a handkerchief contaminated with radioactive nasal mucus was present in the pocket of the patient's gown. Areas of inflammation, usually of the skin, may result in transudation of radioiodine into adjacent soft tissue with slow clearance resulting in a hot spot on scan. Any area of abnormal uptake on whole-body imaging that does not appear to be physiologic should be investigated by examining the region and if necessary removing clothes, scrubbing the area, and reimaging the patient. Imaging the clothes (without the patient) may reveal the location of artifactual uptake.

Interpretation of Neck Images

Interpretation of the neck images is often difficult. Foci of uptake well away from the thyroid bed laterally or inferiorly are almost always due to functioning thyroid cancer in cervical lymph nodes. Foci of uptake at the level of the sternal notch are usually due to metastatic foci in paratracheal lymph nodes, which are one of the earliest sites of metastasis. Foci of uptake in or near the midline above the thyroid bed are almost always due to normal thyroid cells in pyramidal lobe or thyroglossal duct. This uptake often, but not always, has a linear component. Small foci of uptake just at or above the upper pole regions may be due to unrecognized thin extensions of the lobes that have been transected at surgery. If uptake is present above a lobe that did not contain thyroid cancer, it can be presumed to be in normal thyroid cells. However, if it is above a lobe that did contain thyroid cancer, it is safer to presume that it represents a metastasis in a cervical lymph node.

Interpretation of residual uptake in the thyroid bed is based on the extent of the primary cancer. If there was no evidence of extrathyroidal extension or incomplete surgical resection, uptake in either thyroid bed can be assumed to be due to residual normal thyroid cells. However, if tumor did penetrate the thyroid capsule or extend to within 2 mm of the surgical margin of resection, uptake in the ipsilateral thyroid bed must be presumed to be residual thyroid cancer.

Ablation

To avoid confusion the term *ablation* will be used when radioiodine is administered to destroy residual normal thyroid and/or microscopic metastases in the absence of detectable functioning thyroid cancer. The term *treatment* will be used when radioiodine is used to destroy functioning thyroid cancer whether or not normal thyroid tissue is present.

Indications for Ablation

There is evidence that radioiodine given to patients who appear to be free of disease after surgical treatment for the purpose of destroying residual normal thyroid decreases the risk of recurrence and death (23,34). Wong et al. (35), using decision analysis, estimated that radioiodine ablation reduced the risk of recurrence by 54%. However, there is no significant decrease in risk for patients with primary cancers less than 1.5 cm in size who have no evidence of extrathyroidal invasion, multifocal cancer, extensive vascular invasion, or lymph node metastases. Radioiodine ablation probably decreases the risk of recurrence by destruction of microscopic metastases that are known to be present in both the opposite thyroid lobe and the ipsilateral lymph nodes in 90% of patients with papillary thyroid cancer.

Ancillary Benefits from Ablation

Elimination of residual normal thyroid with its relatively high uptake of radioiodine should increase uptake in metastases by making more radioiodine available to them.

Patients with residual normal thyroid tissue often have detectable Tg even when TSH is totally suppressed, whereas those who have undergone ablation usually have low or undetectable Tg. Tg is more sensitive in detecting recurrences in the latter group (36).

Quantity of Radioiodine Administered for Ablation

Fixed Millicurie Amount

Most laboratories use a standard amount of radioiodine for ablation regardless of the size of the thyroid remnant or the uptake of radioiodine. For many years this was between 75 and 150 mCi, and most of the published data on the effectiveness of ablation in reducing the risk of recurrence and death was obtained from patients given 50 mCi or more. Such large amounts of radioiodine eliminate detectable uptake in residual thyroid tissue in most patients. Previously, hospitalization was required for administration of 30 mCi or more of radioactive iodine. Recent changes in the federal guidelines allow much larger doses to be given as outpatient provided appropriate safety guidelines are followed.

At the present, a lively debate persists between advocates of low-dose ablation and those who believe that high-dose ablation is more effective. The data are difficult to sort out because of differences in patient preparation (low iodine diets can double uptake and thus double the effectiveness of a given amount of radioiodine) and in scanning doses (larger doses are more likely to reveal residual uptake).

It appears paradoxical that 30 mCi of radioiodine will completely destroy the thyroid remnant in some patients, whereas 150 mCi may not be sufficient in others. The explanation lies in the *radiation dose* delivered to the remnant. This depends not only on the number of mCi administered but also on the size of the remnant, the percent uptake, and the effective half-life ($t_{1/2eff}$) of ^{131}I in the remnant.

$$\text{Rads delivered} = \frac{\text{mCi } ^{131}I \times t_{1/2eff} \times \% \text{ uptake} \times 1500}{\text{remnant weight (g)}} \quad [5]$$

Patients with small remnants and high uptakes may receive a large radiation dose from 30 mCi whereas those with large remnants and low uptakes may receive a small and inadequate dose from 150 mCi.

Recommendations

For patients with no evidence of residual thyroid cancer following surgery and a negative radioiodine whole-body scan, the decisions whether to ablate or not and how much radioiodine to use are based on risk factor analysis. Many staging systems have been proposed for well-differentiated thyroid cancer but most are relatively cumbersome. We also dislike numerical systems that obscure specific risk factors. We use a modification of the staging system proposed by Mazzaferri and Jhiang (37), which appears to be the simplest and most directly applicable to postoperative management. The recommendations regarding ablation are ours. They assume that radioiodine whole-body imaging shows no functioning metastases.

Stage 1 patients have a primary cancer less than 1.5 cm in size and no high-risk factors. They have an 8% risk of recurrence and virtually no risk of death. They do not benefit from radioiodine ablation.

Stage 2 patients have one or more of these risk factors: a primary cancer between 1.5 and 4.5 cm in size, cervical lymph node metastases, and/or more than three gross foci of cancer within the thyroid. Those with extrathyroidal extension, marked vascular invasion, or distant metastases are excluded. We recommend low-dose ablation using 30 to 100 mCi for stage 2 patients. If only a lobectomy has been performed, we do not recommend completion thyroidectomy. However, patients with multifocal disease undergo ultrasound imaging of the remaining lobe with completion thyroidectomy if this shows one or more discrete nodules.

Stage 3 patients have one or more of these risk factors: primary cancer greater than 4.5 cm in size, extrathyroidal invasion, and/or extensive vascular invasion. Those with distant metastases are excluded. We recommend high-dose (150 mCi) ablation for stage 3 patients. In this group, we also recommend completion thyroidectomy before ablation for patients who have undergone only a lobectomy, because we do not believe that ablation is effective in decreasing the risk of recurrence unless radioiodine is given when TSH is significantly elevated.

Repeat whole-body imaging is performed 5 to 10 days after ablation because this may occasionally show uptake in metastatic thyroid cancer not appreciated on preablation whole-body images performed after a smaller radioiodine tracer. T_4 is administered to suppress TSH, and the patients are followed clinically. In the absence of any evidence of recurrence, routine follow-up whole-body imaging is performed 1 year after ablation. The usual criteria for successful ablation are absence of any focal uptake on neck images, a neck uptake of less than 1%, and a stimulated serum thyroglobulin <2 ng/mL. If these scans are negative, the patients enter long-term follow-up.

If the initial ablation dose is not successful, most laboratories will give a second dose of radioactive iodine, often giving a larger amount of radioiodine for the second ablation. Repeat ablation is less likely to succeed than the initial ablation.

Complications of Ablation

Ablation with up to 150 mCi of ^{131}I is not associated with life-threatening complications (a single case of leukemia has been reported in a patient receiving 100 mCi of ^{131}I) (38). However, transient headache or nausea, sialadenitis with temporary loss of taste, and/or a transient drop in the sperm count may occur. These are more common when more than 100 mCi of ^{131}I are given.

Radiation thyroiditis commonly occurs when an entire thyroid lobe is ablated. Symptoms may begin 1 to 10 days after ablation and consist of pain and tenderness in the remnant. Discomfort or pain on swallowing is frequent, and pain may radiate into the ear or chest. There may be slight swelling over the remnant. Less often there is severe and/or persistent pain and rarely the swelling may be intense enough to cause partial airway obstruction. Radiation thyroiditis is usually associated with transient elevation of thyroid hormone levels resulting from release of thyroid hormones from the remnant.

Mild discomfort can be treated with routine analgesics, but severe pain or swelling requires administration of corticosteroids. Prednisone 30 mg daily is usually effective and can be tapered rapidly over 7 days. It may be necessary to repeat the course of prednisone once or twice before symptoms totally resolve. Because radiation thyroiditis with transient elevation of T_3 and T_4 is so common after ablation of an entire lobe, we do not start replacement thyroid hormone immediately but check thyroid function tests at 2- to 4-week intervals. Thyroid hormone is started once serum T_4 begins to fall.

Treatment of Thyroid Cancer with Radioiodine (^{131}I)

Effectiveness of Treatment

Radioiodine is the most effective treatment for metastatic or residual thyroid cancers that have the ability to concentrate it. Unfortunately, not all thyroid cancer does. In a review of the literature, Maxon and Smith (39) concluded that about three fourths of recurrences and metastases from well-differentiated thyroid cancer were capable of concentrating radioiodine. There was no difference between papillary and follicular cancers.

Radioiodine has a number of advantages when compared with external radiation therapy. Most importantly, the delivered radiation dose is often greater. The maximum dose that can safely be delivered using external radiation therapy is on the order of 6,000 rads and is limited by radiation to surrounding structures. The β-rays from ^{131}I have an average tissue penetration of only 0.45 mm and a maximum penetration of 1.8 mm. Because there is little radiation to surrounding structures, the radiation dose to the cancer from treatment with radioiodine is limited only by the incidental whole-body radiation. External radiation is delivered to discrete areas, and any thyroid cancer cells outside those areas are not affected. Radioiodine seeks out all functioning thyroid cancer cells in the body regardless of whether their presence has been detected, and, therefore, all are irradiated. Furthermore, radioiodine treatment can be repeated whereas external radiation can be delivered only once.

The effectiveness of radioactive iodine in the treatment of metastatic disease varies depending on the location of the metastases. In a review of literature, Maxon and Smith (39) found complete resolution by scan in 68% of patients treated for lymph

node metastases and in 46% of those treated for pulmonary metastases but only in 7% of those treated for bone metastases. Treatment had no apparent effect in 12% of lymph node metastases, 24% of lung metastases, and 54% of bone metastases. These differences in response to treatment may reflect the mass of cancer present. Among patients with lung metastases, those with negative chest x-ray films but diffuse lung uptake on whole-body imaging with radioiodine are most likely to have a complete response to radioiodine treatment. Those who have multiple small metastases detectable on chest x-ray film are less likely to have a complete response, whereas those with nodular metastases greater than 1 cm in diameter have the poorest response.

Although it is rarely possible to eliminate uptake from bony metastases, radioiodine treatment relieves pain in about one third of instances. For patients with large bony metastases, a combination of radioiodine treatment and external radiation may yield a better response than either treatment alone.

Evaluation for Treatment

Radiation treatment of well-differentiated thyroid cancer consists of administering a large amount of ^{131}I in hopes of destroying the cancer cells. Because significant complications may result, radioiodine treatment should be carried out only when there is a reasonable expectation that it will benefit the patient. Candidates for radioiodine treatment should meet the following five criteria:

1. The patient has biopsy proven differentiated thyroid cancer.
2. Residual thyroid cancer is present.
3. Adequate surgery has been performed.
4. The residual thyroid cancer concentrates radioiodine.
5. Treatment with radioiodine will deliver an effective radiation dose to the cancer without risk of major complications.

Estimating Radiation Dose to Metastases

Although most laboratories document the presence of uptake in thyroid cancer before treatment with radioiodine, few attempt to estimate the radiation dose that will be delivered. The lack of enthusiasm for pretreatment estimation of radiation dose is probably due in part to the time-consuming nature of the measurements required and, in part, to the relative paucity of information on methodology in the clinical literature. However, such estimates can be made and used to predict the outcome of treatment. Maxon et al. (40) performed lesional dosimetry and calculated an estimated radiation dose in 26 patients with 67 foci of metastatic thyroid cancer, primarily in cervical lymph nodes. Response to treatment was evaluated by follow-up whole-body imaging with 2 mCi of ^{131}I, and only metastases with no detectable uptake were classified as responding. Of 48 metastases with a predicted radiation dose of over 8,000 rads, 47 responded. Twelve of 19 metastases with a predicted radiation dose with less than 8,000 rads also responded, but none of those with the predicted radiation dose of less than 3,500 rads responded. In a subsequent report, 26 of 29 (90%) of lymph node metastases responded to a radiation dose of over 8,500 rads (41).

Estimation of the radiation dose to a focus of metastatic thyroid cancer is the same as estimating the radiation dose to a thyroid remnant before radiation using Eq. 1, discussed earlier. For convenience, this equation is rearranged here to yield results in rads/mCi administered, which allows rapid calculation of the radiation dose for different amounts of administered radioiodine.

$$\text{rads/mCi} = \frac{t_{1/2\text{eff}} \times \% \text{ uptake} \times 150}{\text{mass of lesion (g)}} \quad [6]$$

Practical Application of Estimated Radiation Dose

The importance of radiation dose estimations in making treatment decisions has yet to be established. As previously noted, Maxon et al. (41), were able to eliminate uptake in lymph node metastases in 74% of patients by delivering more than 8,500 rads. However, lymph node metastases generally respond very well to treatment with radioiodine, and little data is available on the response of lesions in bone, lung, liver, or brain. A dose of 8,000 rads would seem to be low for a cancerocidal dose, because radiation from ^{131}I appears to have less biologic effect on a rad-per-rad basis than that from external radiation therapy, and 30,000 rads is needed to ablate normal thyroid tissue with radioiodine. Clearly, more work is required in this area. On the other hand, even though treatment of patients with an estimated radiation dose between 5,000 and 30,000 rads may not cure the cancer, it often results in regression, relief of symptoms, and prolongation of life. It is also possible to retreat many patients who have persistent uptake resulting in a greater cumulative radiation dose.

Quantity of Radioiodine Administered for Treatment

The usual practice in treating metastatic thyroid cancer is to give a standard amount of radioiodine to all patients. Most laboratories use between 100 and 150 mCi, and the administration of up to 200 mCi has generally been without serious complications. A common variation is to adjust the amount of radioiodine based on the location of the metastases. Patients with presumed residual cancer in the thyroid bed are given 100 mCi, those with metastases in cervical lymph nodes 150 to 175 mCi, those with metastases in the lungs 175 to 200 mCi, and those with bony metastases 200 mCi.

A different approach was advocated by Benua et al. (42) and Leeper (43). Rather than setting a fixed mCi limit, they individualized treatment so that each patient with life-threatening disease received the maximum "safe" amount of radioiodine—that is, the largest amount that would not result in significant complications. On the basis of extensive experience in the use of large amounts of radioiodine, they set an empirical upper limit of 200 rads for the radiation dose to the blood and 120 mCi for whole body retention of radioiodine 48 hours after treatment. Patients with diffuse pulmonary metastases were further limited to no more than 80 mCi whole body retention at 48 hours. Using this protocol, Leeper reported treating 70 patients with an average of 309 mCi of [131]I (range 70 to 659 mCi) without permanent bone marrow suppression, leukemia, or pulmonary fibrosis. The limiting factor for most patients was the radiation dose to the

blood. Ten patients received less than 200 mCi because a larger amount would have delivered more than 200 rads to the blood. In one patient, 200 mCi would have delivered 560 rads to the blood (43). Using the same protocol since 1980, we have had equally satisfactory results.

The dosimetry calculations require determination of whole-blood radioiodine concentration and whole-body radioiodine retention 4 hours after administration of a tracer of ^{131}I and then daily for 4 days as described in the section on whole-body imaging. A simple computer program for performing the necessary calculations is available from Dr. Pat Zanzonico of Memorial Sloan Kettering Cancer Center in New York.

It is clear from data previously reviewed that treatment with 100 to 200 mCi of radioiodine usually eradicates uptake in iodine-concentrating tissue in the thyroid bed or cervical lymph nodes. However, in patients with lung or bone metastases, uptake of radioiodine often persists. If uptake in metastatic thyroid cancer is not eliminated by one or two treatments with radioiodine, it is very unlikely it will be eradicated by subsequent treatment. Failure to eradicate uptake generally indicates a poor prognosis.

Recommendations

We recommend administration of 150 mCi of radioiodine for minimal residual cancer in the thyroid bed and/or metastases to cervical lymph nodes and 200 mCi for mediastinal lymph node metastases. We prefer to treat patients with life-threatening disease (gross residual thyroid cancer in the neck following surgery or distant metastases) with a maximum safe amount of radioiodine based on the Memorial Hospital dosimetry protocol as described earlier. If they are treated with a fixed dose schedule, such patients should be given 200 mCi of radioiodine. Fixed dose schedules should be adjusted downwards for children and small adults.

We wish to stress the importance of giving an adequate amount of radioiodine for initial treatment. It is unwise to try to minimize whole-body radiation by using a small amount with the intention of retreating with a larger amount if uptake persists. Functioning metastases treated with small amounts of radioiodine may lose their ability to concentrate radioiodine while retaining their ability to grow. However, in no case should the amount of radioiodine administered exceed the capacity of the treating facility to safely handle large amounts of radioiodine. Small laboratories and hospitals that are not adequately equipped and do not have trained nursing personnel available may find it preferable to refer patients with life-threatening disease to institutions that have the capability of administering larger amounts of radioiodine.

Maximizing the Radiation Dose

The radiation dose delivered to functioning thyroid cancer is determined in part by the percentage uptake of radioiodine and in part by its biologic half-life. An increase in uptake or a prolongation of the biologic half-life results in a larger radiation dose and increases the probability of a successful outcome. Standard techniques used to increase uptake are discussed in the section on whole-body imaging and include ablation of residual normal thyroid tissue, prolonged withdrawal of thyroid hormone to increase TSH, avoidance of iodine containing medications and x-ray contrast material, and low iodine diets. Less often employed manipulations include injection of exogenous TSH and administration of diuretics before treatment.

Lithium

The use of lithium to prolong the biologic half-life of radioiodine in thyroid cancer is currently under investigation (44). Movius et al. (45), reported on the use of lithium in seven patients with metastatic, well-differentiated thyroid cancer. After initial radioiodine kinetics, they were placed on lithium carbonate 900 mg per day, which resulted in blood levels of 0.8 to 1.2 mg/dL. The radioiodine kinetics were then repeated. In 10 of the 12 cancers, the biologic half-life was prolonged with a median increase of 52%. This resulted in an increase in the mean radiation dose to the lesions of 30%. All of the metastases whose radiation dose was augmented by at least 25% had initial biologic half-lives of less than 6 days. Lithium has significant toxicity, and the margin for safety between therapeutic and toxic blood levels is small. Furthermore, renal excretion is slowed by hypothyroidism. If lithium is administered, daily determination of serum of lithium levels is necessary.

Decreasing TSH After Treatment

High levels of TSH may shorten the biologic half-life of radioiodine in some thyroid cancers. Resumption of full replacement doses of T_3 24 hours after treatment with radioiodine causes a rapid decrease in TSH and may prolong the biologic half-life of radioiodine in the cancer.

Practical Management

Informed consent is obtained from all patients before treatment following a thorough discussion of the risks and benefits. A pregnancy test is performed on all women who are less than 5-years postmenopause. The details of hospitalization, isolation, treatment, and so forth should be discussed thoroughly in advance. Patients should also be instructed on precautions to be followed after discharge to minimize radiation exposure to other family members. The hospital staff should have detailed written instructions on the care of patients treated with radioiodine and the procedures to be followed. Ideally, all radioiodine treatment is carried out in the same unit so that the staff become familiar with the procedure. The patient is admitted to a single room with a private bathroom and is confined to that room until cleared by the radiation safety officer. Unless they are seriously ill and require prolonged close attention, radiation exposure of the staff will be low (46,47).

If more than 150 to 200 mCi of radioiodine is given, an intravenous infusion of 5% dextrose and water at a rate of 125 mL/hour can be given to insure adequate hydration. No solid food is permitted from 4 hours before treatment until 1 hour after to promote rapid absorption of radioiodine and minimize stomach radiation. Advance orders are written for oral and intravenous antiemetics in case of nausea. In our experience, vomiting within the first few hours after treatment with radioiodine is rare and usually due to anxiety.

After administration of radioiodine, the patient is encouraged to drink freely and to urinate once an hour to minimize radiation to the bladder and pelvic area. Frequent use of lemon wedges or sour hard candy has been recommended to stimulate salivary flow and decrease the risk of radiation-induced sialoadenitis. However, some patients have difficulty tolerating frequent use of these acidic preparations. Any type of long-lasting candy or cough drop should stimulate adequate salivary flow and, in our experience, is more likely to be used consistently. If vomiting does occur shortly after treatment, the vomitus may contain significant amounts of radioiodine. An attempt should be made to assay it to determine the quantity present.

Because prolonged retention of ^{131}I in the gut increases whole-body radiation dose, patients should be encouraged to use milk of magnesia and/or bisacodyl suppositories to have daily bowel movements throughout the period of whole-body imaging and treatment.

In most instances only a small percentage of the radioiodine given for treatment is taken up by the cancer. In the first 24 hours, 40% to 60% is usually excreted in the urine and an additional 20% to 30% is excreted in the second 24 hours. Regulations regarding disposal of this highly radioactive urine vary and should be checked with the hospital radiation safety officer and/or the office of radiation control. Small amounts of radioiodine are also present in saliva, nasal mucus, and sweat. Items that may be contaminated with these substances should be handled with gloves, stored in secure plastic bags, and monitored for residual radioactivity before disposal. The sharps container in the room should also be monitored for radioactivity before disposal. After the patient has been discharged, the room, and especially the bathroom, should be wipe-tested and decontaminated. In our experience, the telephone mouthpiece is often the most highly contaminated object.

The radiation dose delivered to the cancer in the first 24 hours after treatment usually causes sufficient damage to inhibit further uptake of radioiodine. We therefore begin treatment with thyroid hormone at 24 hours to induce a rapid return to euthyroidism. The purpose is to decrease whole-body radiation by accelerating the excretion of radioiodine. Rapid lowering of TSH may also slow release of radioiodine from the cancer and thus increase the delivered radiation dose. If only a daily replacement dose of T_4 is given to profoundly hypothyroid patients, it may require several weeks for serum T_4 to rise into the normal range and even longer before symptoms of hypothyroidism disappear and TSH is suppressed. We therefore start our patients on T_4 plus T_3 25 µg, two or three times daily. This is safe in acutely hypothyroid patients who are otherwise normal but should be used with caution in patients with cardiovascular disease. An alternative to the addition of T_3 is to administer loading doses of T_4, giving two to three times the normal daily replacement for a period of 3 to 5 days. When T_3 is given, it is stopped after 7 to 10 days. The low iodine diet is discontinued 24 hours after treatment.

In patients treated with over 200 mCi of radioiodine, whole-body retention should be monitored to be sure that the predicted radiation dose to the blood is not exceeded. This can be accomplished by counting the patient daily with a radiation detector in a fixed geometry. In patients with highly functional tumors and high uptakes, radiolabeled proteins may be released into the blood if the cancer receives a high radiation dose. This may result in whole-blood activity that is higher following therapy than after the pretherapy tracer. If this occurs, the radiation dose to the blood may be greater than predicted. It is possible to follow whole-blood radioactivity after therapy in such patients by drawing 10 mL of blood into a syringe and counting it in a dose calibrator.

If urinary excretion is slower than predicted, it can be accelerated by inducing a diuresis with intravenous saline and oral furosemide. If blood radioactivity is significantly higher than predicted and likely to result in excessive bone marrow radiation it should be possible to reduce it by plasmapheresis. Because persistent blood activity is due to protein bound radioactive T_4 and T_3, it cannot be removed by dialysis.

We also attempt to determine uptake and biologic half-life of radioiodine in metastases after treatment. After therapy it is also possible to use single photon emission computed tomography (SPECT) to determine uptake in metastases because more photons are available following treatment. Uptake is almost always lower and the biologic half-life often shorter than before treatment, probably because of early radiation damage to the cancer. About 1 week after treatment complete whole-body imaging is performed on a scintillation camera. These images provide better definition of the extent of disease than the pretherapy images and may show unexpected sites of involvement, especially in patients with bony metastases.

A complete blood count (CBC) and platelet count is always performed before treatment and several weeks after treatment. The nadir for the white count and platelet count usually occurs about 6 weeks after therapy. If the 4-week values are low, counts are checked weekly until they rise again. T_4 and TSH are checked at 4 weeks. If TSH is not within the normal range, the dose of T_4 is increased. T_4, TSH, and Tg are all checked at 8 weeks and the dose of T_4 adjusted to insure complete suppression of TSH. For patients who have significant metastatic disease (e.g.,

bone, lung, liver, brain) TSH is maintained undetectable in a third-generation TSH assay.

Follow-Up and Retreatment

The interval between treatments for patients with metastatic thyroid cancer depends on the response to the previous treatment and also on the extent and location of the metastatic disease. The size of the metastases can be assessed with ultrasound for cervical lymph nodes and with CT or magnetic resonance imaging (MRI) for bone and lung lesions. Determination of serum Tg provides an overall indication of the mass of functioning cancer.

It is preferable to wait 1 year between treatments because this is felt to reduce the risk of leukemia. However, if there is convincing evidence of disease progression (an increase in Tg or an increase in the size of the metastases) the patient should be retreated even if the interval from the previous treatment is as short as 3 months.

Most authorities recommend that patients who have been treated with radioiodine for functioning thyroid cancer undergo whole-body imaging at regular intervals, most commonly yearly, until there is no detectable uptake for 2 consecutive years and then every 2 to 5 years. Most would retreat with a large amount of radioiodine if there were any detectable uptake on whole-body imaging performed following a large radioiodine tracer. Some investigators have administered multiple therapeutic doses as high as 300 mCi to patients who have negative diagnostic whole-body scans but persistently elevated Tg following total thyroidectomy and ablation of residual normal thyroid. Most of these patients have specific radioiodine uptake in either residual normal thyroid or thyroid cancer when imaged following a large therapeutic dose of ^{131}I, and Tg declines in the majority. However, Tg remains elevated in about half.

In many cases with wide spread metastatic disease, it is very unlikely that radioactive iodine will eliminate all thyroid cancer

Table 31.3. *Complications from Treatment of Thyroid Cancer with* [131]I

	Complication	Comments
Early complications	Nausea, headache	Common
	Sialoadenitis	10–15% incidence over first 6 months after therapy
	Pain, swelling in metastatic lesions	Uncommon, but can be lead to serious complications with brain metastases or spinal column metastases
	Bone marrow suppression	Transient, nadir 6 weeks after therapy
Long-term complications	Leukemia	Slight increased risk with very high cumulative doses (more than 500–800 mCi)
	Permanent bone marrow suppression	Rarely seen with cumulative doses less than 1 Ci
	Unusual, and rare complications	Hypoparathyroidism, recurrent laryngeal nerve injury
	Radiation pneumonitis, pulmonary fibrosis	Possible in patients with diffuse pulmonary metastases that concentrate RAI well
	Anaplastic transformation	Probably unrelated to RAI, more likely an uncommon event in the natural history of some thyroid cancers
	Risk of second malignancy	Unlikely, never proven
	Infertility	Transient gonadal dysfunction, perhaps slightly premature menopause, no effect on subsequent fertility
	Genetic effects	No adverse effects on fetal outcome following RAI treatments

RAI, radioactive iodine.

cells from the body. If after one or more treatments with radioiodine, whole-body imaging shows very low uptake, the size of the metastases is stable or declining on radiographic imaging, and Tg is stable or declining, we do not retreat. We continue follow-up of such patients with serum Tg and radiographic imaging at gradually increasing intervals. We also keep TSH suppressed by third-generation assay. However, we do not perform routine whole-body imaging with radioiodine, wishing to avoid TSH stimulation of the residual cancer cells. Whole-body imaging with radioiodine is performed only if we decide to retreat the metastases because of increasing size and/or Tg. On the other hand, we do not have a fixed upper limit for the cumulative amount of radioiodine used to treat aggressive metastatic disease and have given several patients over 2 Ci of ^{131}I. This is generally tolerated well, especially if the interval between treatments is a year or more. These patients usually develop a mild chronic anemia and slightly low platelet count.

Complications

Serious complications are rare after an initial treatment with 200 mCi of radioiodine or less, but the risk increases with larger initial treatments or following the administration of large cumulative amounts (43). This subject is summarized in Table 31.3.

REFERENCES

1. Cooper DS. Antithyroid drugs for the treatment of hyperthyroidism caused by Graves' disease. *Endocrinol Metab Clin North Am* 1998;27:225–247.
2. Tuttle RM. Effect of pretreatment with antithyroid drugs on the failure rate of radioiodine therapy in Graves' disease. *Endocrinologist* 2000;10:356–360.
3. Becker DV. Choice of therapy for Graves' hyperthyroidism. *N Engl J Med* 1984;311:464–466.
4. Wartofsky L, Glinoer D, Solomon B et al. Differences and similarities in the diagnosis and treatment of Graves' disease in Europe, Japan and the United States. *Thyroid* 1991;1:129–135.
5. Werga-Kjellman P, Zedenius J, Tallstedt L et al. Surgical treatment of hyperthyroidism: a ten-year experience. *Thyroid* 2001;11:187–192.
6. Hertz S, Roberts A. Application of radioactive iodine in therapy of Graves' disease. *J Clin Invest* 1942;21:624.
7. Erickson D, Gharib H, Li H et al. Treatment of patients with toxic multinodular goiter. *Thyroid* 1998;8:277–282.
8. Kraiem Z, Newfield RS. Graves' disease in childhood. *J Pediatr Endocrinol Metab* 2001;14:229–243.
9. Quimby EH, Feitelberg S. Radioactive isotopes in medicine and biology. In: Quimby EH, Feitelberg S, eds. *Basic physics and instrumentation.* Philadelphia: Lea & Febiger, 1961.
10. Barandes M, Hurley JR, Becker DV. Implications of rapid intrathyroidal iodine turnover for 131-I therapy: the small pool syndrome. *J Nucl Med* 1973;14:379.
11. Jackson GL. Calculated low dose radioiodine therapy of thyrotoxicosis. *Int J Nucl Med* Biol 1975;2:80–81.
12. Kaplan MM, Meier DA, Dworkin HJ. Treatment of hyperthyroidism with radioactive iodine. *Endocrinol Metab Clin North Am* 1998;27:205–223.
13. Burch HB, Solomon BL, Cooper DS et al. The effect of antithyroid drug pretreatment on acute changes in thyroid hormone levels after (131)I ablation for Graves' disease. *J Clin Endocrinol Metab* 2001;86:3016–3021.
14. Imseis RE, Vanmiddlesworth L, Massie JD et al. Pretreatment with propylthiouracil but not methimazole reduces the therapeutic efficacy

of iodine-131 in hyperthyroidism. *J Clin Endocrinol Metab* 1998;83:685–687.
15. Malone JF, Cullen MJ. Two mechanisms for hypothyroidism after 131-I therapy. *Lancet* 1976;2:73.
16. Irvine WJ, Toft AD, Lidgard GP et al. Occasional survey: spectrum of thyroid function in patients remaining in remission after antithyroid drug therapy for thyrotoxicosis. *Lancet* 1977;2:179.
17. Wood LC, Ingbar SH. Hypothyroidism as a late sequela in patients with Graves' disease treated with antithyroid agents. *J Clin Invest* 1979;64:1429.
18. Tallstedt L, Lundell G, Blomgren H et al. Does early administration of thyroxine reduce the development of Graves' ophthalmopathy after radioiodine treatment? *Eur J Endocrinol* 1994;130:494.
19. Kung AW, Yau CC, Cheng A. The incidence of ophthalmopathy after radioiodine therapy for Graves' disease: prognostic factors and the role of methimazole. *J Clin Endocrinol Metab* 1994;79:542–546.
20. Saenger EL, Thoma GE, Tompkins EA. Incidence of leukemia following treatment of hyperthyroidism. Preliminary report of the Cooperative Thyrotoxicosis Therapy Follow-Up Study. *JAMA* 1968;205:855.
21. Robertson JS, Gorman CA. Gonadal radiation dose and its genetic significance in radioiodine therapy of hyperthyroidism. *J Nucl Med* 1976;17:826–835.
22. Daniels GH. Radioiodine and thyroid cancer: some questions, controversies, and considerations. *Endocr Pract* 2001;7:320–323.
23. Mazzaferri EL, Kloos RT. Clinical review 128: current approaches to primary therapy for papillary and follicular thyroid cancer. *J Clin Endocrinol Metab* 2001;86:1447–1463.
24. Kebebew E, Clark OH. Differentiated thyroid cancer: "complete" rational approach. *World J Surg* 2000;24:942–951.
25. Shaha AR. Thyroid cancer: extent of thyroidectomy. *Cancer Control* 2000;7:240–245.
26. Hay ID. Papillary thyroid carcinoma. *Endocrinol Metab Clin North Am* 1990;19:545–576.
27. Shaha AR, Shah JP, Loree TR. Risk group stratification and prognostic factors in papillary carcinoma of thyroid. *Ann Surg Oncol* 1996;3:534–538.
28. Clark OH. TSH suppression in the management of thyroid nodules and thyroid cancer. *World J Surg* 1981;5:39–47.
29. Bronnegard M, Torring O, Boos J et al. Expression of thyrotropin receptor and thyroid hormone receptor messenger ribonucleic acid in normal, hyperplastic, and neoplastic human thyroid tissue. *J Clin Endocrinol Metab* 1994;79:384–389.
30. Robbins RJ, Tuttle RM, Sonenberg M et al. Radioiodine ablation of thyroid remnants after preparation with recombinant human thyrotropin. *Thyroid* 2001;11:865–869.
31. Ladenson PW, Braverman LE, Mazzaferri EL et al. Comparison of administration of recombinant human thyrotropin with withdrawal of thyroid hormone for radioactive iodine scanning in patients with thyroid carcinoma. *N Engl J Med* 1997;337:888–896.
32. Haugen BR, Pacini F, Reiners C et al. A comparison of recombinant human thyrotropin and thyroid hormone withdrawal for the detection of thyroid remnant or cancer. *J Clin Endocrinol Metab* 1999;84:3877–3885.
33. Robbins RJ, Tuttle RM, Sharaf RN et al. Preparation by recombinant human thyrotropin or thyroid hormone withdrawal are comparable for the detect of residual differentiated thyroid carcinoma. *J Clin Endocrinol Metab* 2001;86:619–625.
34. Hurley JR. Management of thyroid cancer: radioiodine ablation, "stunning," and treatment of thyroglobulin-positive, (131)I scan-negative patients. *Endocr Pract* 2000;6:401–406.
35. Wong JB, Kaplan MM, Meyer KB et al. Ablative radioactive iodine therapy for apparently localized thyroid carcinoma: a decision analytic perspective. *Endocrinol Metab Clin North Am* 1990;19:741–760.
36. Torrens JI, Burch HB. Serum thyroglobulin measurement. Utility in clinical practice. *Endocrinol Metab Clin North Am* 2001;30:429–467.
37. Mazzaferri EL. Long-term outcome of patients with differentiated thyroid carcinoma: effect of therapy. *Endocr Pract* 2000;6:469–476.
38. Beierwaltes WH. The treatment of thyroid carcinoma with radioactive iodine. *Semin Nucl Med* 1978;8:79–94.

39. Maxon HR III, Smith HD. Radioiodine-131 in the diagnosis and treatment of metastatic well-differentiated thyroid cancer. *Endocrinol Metab Clin North Am* 1990;19:685–718.

40. Maxon HR, Thomas SR, Hertzberg VS et al. Relation between effective radiation dose and outcome of radioiodine therapy for thyroid cancer. *N Engl J Med* 1983;309:937–941.

41. Maxon HR III, Englaro EE, Thomas SR et al. Radioiodine-131 therapy for well-differentiated thyroid cancer—a quantitative radiation dosimetric approach: outcome and validation in 85 patients. *J Nucl Med* 1992;33:1132–1136.

42. Benua RS, Cicale NR, Sonenberg M et al. The relation of radioiodine dosimetry to results and complications in the treatment of metastatic thyroid cancer. *Am J Roentgenol* 1962;87:171–182.

43. Leeper R. Controversies in the treatment of thyroid cancer: the New York Memorial Hospital approach. *Thyroid Today* 1982;5:1–4.

44. Koong SS, Reynolds JC, Movius EG et al. Lithium as a potential adjuvant to 131I therapy of metastatic, well differentiated thyroid carcinoma. *J Clin Endocrinol Metab* 1999;84:912–916.

45. Movius EG, Robbins J, Pierce LR et al. The value of lithium in radioiodine therapy of thyroid carcinoma. In: Medeiros-Neto G, Gaitan E, eds. *Frontiers in thyroidology,* vol 2. New York: Plenum, 1986: 1269–1272.

46. Castronovo FP Jr, Beh RA, Veilleux NM. Dosimetric considerations while attending hospitalized I-131 therapy patients. *J Nucl Med Technol* 1982;10:157–160.

47. Ibis E, Wilson CR, Collier BD et al. Iodine-131 contamination from thyroid cancer patients. *J Nucl Med* 1992;33:2110–2115.

32

PARATHYROID GLANDS

WILLIAM H. MARTIN
MARTIN P. SANDLER

Primary hyperparathyroidism is a common endocrinopathy, especially in older women, with an estimated 100,000 new cases diagnosed annually in the United States (1–3). Its diagnosis has been simplified by ubiquitous automated biochemical screening of the general population for serum calcium and by improvements in the accuracy of the assay for serum parathyroid hormone (PTH). Its therapy, however, is controversial. Because many patients are asymptomatic and only a minority will subsequently develop symptoms and/or complications of hyperparathyroidism, many authorities recommend only annual follow-up, reserving definitive surgical therapy only for those who progress (4–7). Because many patients may be lost to follow-up and because predicting which uncomplicated patients will progress over subsequent years is impossible (4,5), some advocate surgical resection of the offending parathyroid gland(s) in most patients, even if symptoms are difficult to define (8,9). Once the diagnosis has been made and the decision to proceed with surgery has been reached, controversy surrounds the use of preoperative localization studies. Because bilateral neck exploration with identification of all four parathyroid glands and resection of the pathologic gland(s) by an experienced surgeon results in cure of the hyperparathyroidism in approximately 90% to 97% of patients (10–14), many still follow the dictum, "The best way of locating the parathyroid glands is to localize an experienced parathyroid surgeon" (15). However, despite the controversy regarding the cost-effectiveness of routine preoperative imaging, many surgeons are at present inclined to request localization before embarking on neck exploration. The high sensitivity and specificity provided by ^{99m}Tc-sestamibi (^{99m}Tc-MIBI) scintigraphy have rewarded the clinicians with a highly accurate modality, leading to a resurgence of parathyroid scintigraphy over the past several years. In part because of the accuracy of modern-day parathyroid scintigraphy, the therapy of hyperparathyroidism is evolving rapidly.

ANATOMY AND PHYSIOLOGY

The parathyroid glands are oval, reddish brown structures situated along the posterior aspect of the thyroid lobes. In 85% of individuals, there are four parathyroid glands, two upper and two lower, each weighing approximately 35 to 40 mg with dimensions of 6 × 3 mm. A supernumerary fifth gland occurs in approximately 10% to 13% of people, the most common site being the thymus, and as few as two and as many as eight glands have been reported. Three percent of individuals have only three glands (16). The superior parathyroid glands arise from the fourth branchial pouch and migrate in close association with the thyroid lobes, so only 1% of the superior parathyroid glands are located ectopically. Aberrant superior glands may be found between the thyroid and the esophagus, within the carotid sheath, behind the innominate vein, or even in the posterior mediastinum (17). The inferior parathyroid glands arise from the third branchial cleft and migrate caudally with the thymus gland. Normally the inferior parathyroid glands migrate only as far as the inferior poles of the thyroid gland but may descend with the thymus into the mediastinum. The close embryologic relationship between the inferior parathyroid glands and the thymus is reflected by the fact that the position of the inferior parathyroid glands is more variable than that of the superior glands, with only 60% of them located in the immediate vicinity of the lower pole of the thyroid gland (17). The remaining ectopic glands are located within the superior pole of the thymus (39%), the mediastinum (2%), within the thyroid gland (up to 3.5%) (18,19), and other miscellaneous positions from the angle of the jaw to the arch of the aorta (Fig. 32.1).

The arterial supply of the parathyroids is variable, depending on the location of the gland, the presence of vascular variants, and previous neck surgery. The venous drainage is also variable, although the effluent of all four glands is usually through the inferior thyroid vein. Venous drainage may vary with ectopic locations, previous surgery, and vascular variants such as a lateral accessory vein. Knowledge of the venous drainage is a prerequisite for successful venous sampling (20). The predominant epithelial cell of the parathyroid gland is the chief cell, which is responsible for the synthesis and secretion of PTH. The oxyphil cell, making up less than 5% of normal adult glands, is of uncertain significance.

W.H. Martin: Department of Radiology and Radiological Sciences, Vanderbilt University Medical Center, Nashville, TN.
M.P. Sandler: Department of Radiology and Radiological Sciences, Vanderbilt University Medical Center, Nashville, TN.

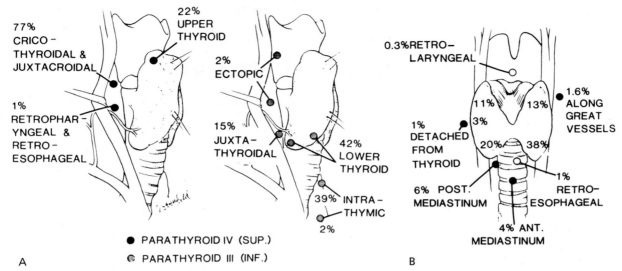

● PARATHYROID IV (SUP.)

⊕ PARATHYROID III (INF.)

A

B

FIGURE 32.1. Normal and aberrant distribution of parathyroid glands. **A:** The inferior parathyroid glands may lie within the fascial sheath of the thyroid gland or behind and outside the fascial sheath. Glands that occupy the first position tend to descend in front of the trachea into the superior mediastinum, whereas if the gland occupies the lateral position, the tumor tends to extend posteroinferiorly behind the esophagus into the posterior mediastinum. (From Sacks GA, Eisenberg H, Pallotta J. Parathyroid adenomas: cinearteriography. *AJR* 1980;135:535, with permission.) **B:** Localizations of adenomas include posterior to the superior or inferior pole of the thyroid gland, thymus, posterosuperior mediastinum (in the tracheoesophageal groove at the level of the cervicothoracic junction), behind the sternohyoid muscle at the level of the thoracic inlet, anterior or lateral to the aortic arch or brachiocephalic vessels, intrathyroidal, at the carotid bifurcation, retrolaryngeal, in the phrenic nerve, in the pharynx or esophageal wall, and in the heart. (From Wang CA. The anatomic basis of parathyroid surgery. *Ann Surg* 1976;183:271, with permission.)

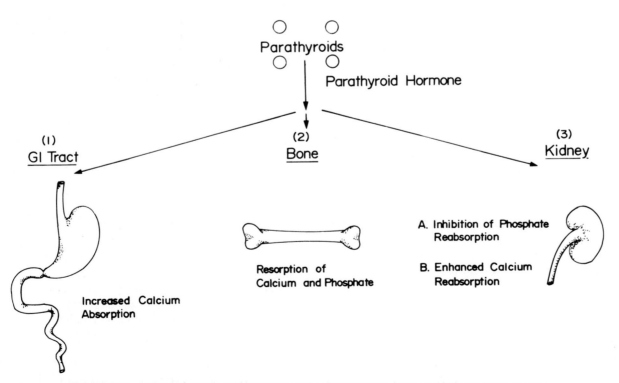

FIGURE 32.2. Actions of parathyroid hormone on the digestive tract, bone, and kidneys. (From Sandler MP, Patton JA, Fleischer AC et al. Parathyroid imaging. In: Sandler MP, Patton JA, Groce MD et al., eds. *Thyroid and parathyroid imaging.* Norwalk, CT: Appleton & Lang, 1992:353, with permission.)

PTH is an 84-amino acid polypeptide with a molecular weight of 9,500 Daltons that is synthesized, stored, and secreted by the parathyroid glands. Parathormone is largely responsible for the regulation and maintenance of calcium and phosphorus homeostasis by its action on bone, small intestine, and the kidneys. PTH has four principle actions (Fig. 32.2): (a) increased calcium absorption from the gastrointestinal tract, (b) osteoclastic stimulation with resultant resorption of calcium and phosphorus from bone, (c) inhibition of phosphate reabsorption by the proximal renal tubules resulting in phosphaturia, and (d) enhancement of renal tubular calcium reabsorption. The secretion of PTH is modulated by the circulating serum calcium level in a classical feedback loop mechanism (21).

PATHOPHYSIOLOGY

Hypoparathyroidism

Hypofunction of the parathyroid glands most commonly results from inadvertent damage or removal of several parathyroid glands at the time of thyroidectomy or parathyroidectomy or from total parathyroidectomy performed for parathyroid hyperplasia or carcinoma. Less common causes of hypofunction include idiopathic or autoimmune disease, secretion of a structurally abnormal PTH, or functional such as in patients with hypomagnesemia. Symptomatology resulting from the hypocalcemia of hypoparathyroidism is manifested by neuromuscular irritability resulting in paresthesias, tetany, and convulsions. Chronic hypoparathyroidism may result in dense bones, cataracts, and intracerebral calcifications (21). The diagnosis of hypoparathyroidism is clinical and biochemical; imaging does not play an important role in its diagnosis or management.

Hyperparathyroidism

The diagnosis of hyperparathyroidism is usually made by a finding of elevated circulating levels of calcium accompanied by elevated serum PTH levels. Other causes of hypercalcemia related to parathyroid disease include familial hypocalciuric hypercalcemia, in which there is a mutation of the calcium-sensor gene resulting in a shift in the parathyroid cells' set point for calcium, and lithium-induced hypercalcemia resulting from the interference by lithium with the parathyroid calcium sensor, eventually resulting in parathyroid hyperplasia (21). There are numerous causes of non-PTH-dependent hypercalcemia such as vitamin D intoxication, thiazide diuretics, and sarcoidosis or other granulomatous inflammatory processes. However, the most important and common parathyroid-independent cause of hypercalcemia is humoral hypercalcemia of malignancy. This is caused by the overproduction of PTH-related protein (PTHrP). Elevated circulating levels of PTHrP occur in a majority of patients with malignancy and hypercalcemia. PTHrP binds to the PTH receptor and mimics all the actions of PTH (21). A wide variety of tumors overproduce PTHrP. The differentiation of hyperparathyroidism from other etiologies of hypercalcemia is based on elevated circulating levels of PTH. Imaging studies are used for localization rather than diagnosis.

In primary hyperparathyroidism, an abnormal parathyroid gland or glands secrete an excessive amount of PTH. In contrast, increased secretion of PTH that is an appropriate response to hypocalcemia is termed *secondary hyperparathyroidism*, most commonly seen in patients with chronic renal insufficiency. Tertiary hyperparathyroidism occurs when one or more hyperplastic glands in a patient with secondary hyperparathyroidism become autonomously functioning resulting in hypercalcemia. In primary hyperparathyroidism, the excessive secretion of PTH leads secondarily to hypercalcemia, hypophosphatemia, relative hypocalciuria, and resorption of bone.

In the past, up to 70% of patients presented with nephrolithiasis and up to 25% of patients presented with osteitis fibrosa cystica manifested by osteoporosis, pathologic fractures, and brown tumors (Fig. 32.3) (2,5,22,23). Many patients also presented with gastrointestinal (GI) symptoms including peptic ulcer disease and pancreatitis, neuropsychiatric symptoms, hypertension, and fatigue.

However, with the advent of multichannel analyzer determination of serum calcium levels in routine screening, over 80% of patients now are either asymptomatic or have only nonspecific symptoms with or without osteoporosis; and only 17% now exhibit nephrolithiasis (8). The syndrome of primary hyperparathyroidism results from a single adenoma in 80% to 85% of cases, with multiple adenomas, multigland hyperplasia, and parathyroid carcinoma accounting for the remainder (Table 32.1) (23–25). The disease is more frequent in women (3:1) and increases with age but may occasionally be seen in young people. As a result of routine screening, the prevalence of primary hyperparathyroidism has risen from 0.05% to 0.5 % with an incidence in older women of almost 200 cases per 100,000 persons for a prevalence of 1.8% (3).

Parathyroid adenomas are caused by somatic mutations and subsequent clonal expansion of the mutant cells, probably related to deletion of tumor suppressor genes (21). The cause of sporadic primary hyperplasia is unknown but appears to be due to a polyclonal proliferation. Patients with familial hyperparathyroidism usually exhibit multigland hyperplasia. In patients with multiple endocrine neoplasia type 1 (MEN 1), hyperparathyroidism occurs in 95%, often accompanied by pituitary and/or islet cell tumors. Hyperparathyroidism occurs less often in patients with multiple endocrine neoplasia type 2A (MEN 2A) (5% to 20%) in concert with pheochromocytoma and medullary carcinoma of the thyroid. These are autosomal dominant syn-

Table 32.1. *Pathologic Classification of Parathyroid Lesions in Patients with Primary Hyperparathyroidism*

Class	Type	Percent
Adenomas	Single	80
Hyperplasia	Chief cell	15
	Clear cell	1
Carcinoma		4

From Sandler MP, Patton JA, Sacks GA, Gordon L. Parathyroid imaging. In: Sandler MP, Patton JA, Shaff MI, et al., eds. *Correlative imaging.* Baltimore: Williams & Wilkins, 1989;255, with permission.

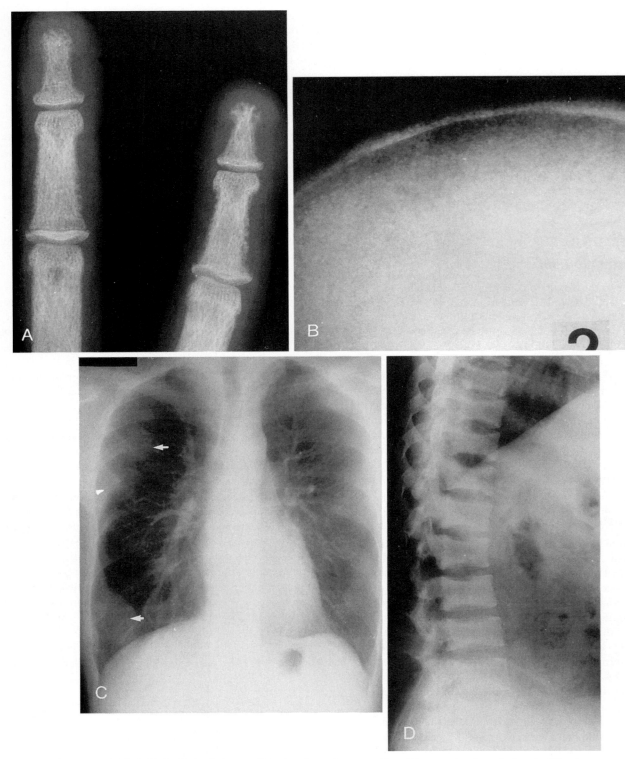

FIGURE 32.3. Skeletal abnormalities in primary hyperparathyroidism may be characterized by **(A)** sub-periosteal resorption at the radial aspect of the phalanges of the hand, **(B)** trabecular resorption in the diploe of the cranium, **(C)** generalized osteopenia with brown tumors (*arrows*), **(D)** dense vertebral endplates, and **(E)** ^{201}Tl (or ^{99m}Tc-MIBI) scintigraphy may reveal brown tumors or increased mandibular activity and periarticular and soft tissue calcifications. (From Falke THM, Schipper J, Patton JA et al. Parathyroid glands. In: Sandler MP, Patton JA, Groce MD et al., eds. *Endocrine imaging.* Norwalk, CT: Appleton & Lang, 1992;154, with permission.)

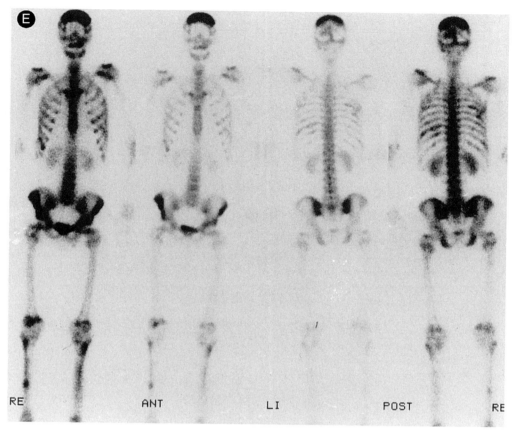

RE   ANT   LI   POST   RE

FIGURE 32.3. *Continued.*

dromes related to specific gene mutations on chromosome 11 for MEN 1 and on chromosome 10 for MEN 2. There are two additional autosomal dominant forms of primary hyperparathyroidism that are not associated with multiple endocrine neoplasia.

The distinction between adenoma and hyperplasia is important, because hypercalcemia resulting from adenoma can be cured by resection of the offending gland or glands, whereas that resulting from hyperplasia is more difficult to treat surgically and requires total or near-total parathyroidectomy.

Parathyroid carcinoma is a rare entity that accounts for less than 1% of patients with primary hyperparathyroidism (26), although it may be more common in Japan and in Italy than previously recognized (27). In contrast to the mild hypercalcemia of benign hyperparathyroidism, patients with carcinoma often present with calcium levels greater than 14 mg/dL (normal 8.5 to 10.6 mg/dL) and marked elevations in PTH levels, usually accompanied by symptoms of hypercalcemia, bone pain, fractures, renal colic, and even a palpable neck mass. It is an indolent tumor with a relatively low malignant potential with functioning metastases occurring in the local regional nodes (30%) and lungs (40%) (26).

Parathyroid cysts are rare, are usually not associated with hypercalcemia, and are discovered incidentally. Although most are small and asymptomatic, they may occasionally be large enough to cause hoarseness or odynophagia and may extend into the mediastinum. Ultrasound (US)-guided fine needle aspiration may produce a clear fluid rich in PTH and devoid of thyroglobulin, virtually pathognomonic of parathyroid cyst (28).

Imaging of Hyperparathyroidism

Although patients with mild hyperparathyroidism may be followed clinically without definitive therapy, the only effective therapy available is surgical resection of the offending gland or glands. The traditional operative procedure is a bilateral exploration of the neck under general endotracheal anesthesia with adenomectomy, usually with multigland biopsy. Using the standard approach, experienced surgeons have reported a cure rate of over 90% (10–14). For hyperplasia, subtotal parathyroidectomy (3.5 glands) or total parathyroidectomy plus autotransplantation are recommended (29). If there are relative contraindications to neck surgery, arteriographic ablation or percutaneous ethanol injection under US guidance may be effective (30,31). With the increasing prevalence of the disease, less experienced surgeons are being called on to care for these patients with failure rates perhaps as high as 20% (32). Furthermore, the degree of hypercalcemia is directly proportional in general to the size of the adenoma (16), so more patients with smaller adenomas are

Table 32.2. *Etiology of Failed Parathyroid Surgery*[a]

Class	Number of patients
Multiple abnormal glands	50
Localization in ectopic position	40
Supernumerary parathyroid glands	17
Surgeon inexperience	12
Metastatic parathyroid cancer	4
Errors on frozen section examination	4

[a]One or a combination of reasons based on 89 reoperations.
From Levin KE, Clark OH. The reasons for failure in parathyroid operation. *Arch Surg* 1989;124:911–915, with permission.

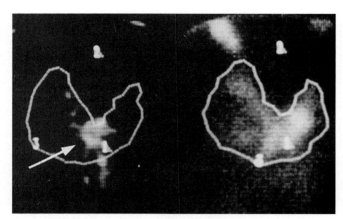

FIGURE 32.4. A 65-year-old woman with primary hyperparathyroidism. The final summed radioiodinated toluidine blue (RTB) image (*left panel*) demonstrates a parathyroid adenoma located in the isthmus and the adjacent left thyroid lobe (*arrow*). The location of the adenoma is defined by the thyroid region-of-interest superimposed on the RTB image from the ^{99m}Tc thyroid image (*right panel*) and by markers at the sternal notch and thyroid cartilage. The ^{99m}Tc thyroid scan (*right panel*) demonstrates an asymmetrically enlarged right lobe with a large cold nodule. (Courtesy of CWASTS, C. Sheba Medical Center Tel-Hashomer/Ramat GAM, Israel.)

undergoing surgical treatment for mild hyperparathyroidism. In fact, a 5% to 10% recurrence rate usually related to aberrant or ectopically located glands or recurrent hyperplasia (Table 32.2) occurs (32–34). Reexploration is technically more difficult and is accompanied by a higher morbidity and poorer success rate (60%) than the initial operative procedure (14,34,35). Diseased parathyroid glands are often aberrantly located, and the availability of accurate, noninvasive imaging can be of great assistance to the surgeon (34). Before 1992, preoperative parathyroid localization using noninvasive imaging demonstrated poor sensitivity with a high rate of false-positive findings. With the development of ^{99m}Tc-MIBI parathyroid scintigraphy in 1989 (36), the high sensitivity and specificity of this modality (25,37–45) has permitted highly effective preoperative localization of parathyroid disease.

HISTORICAL PERSPECTIVES

In 1965 the use of ^{75}Selenium-labeled amino acid analog of methionine (selenomethionine), was introduced as a scintigraphic agent for parathyroid scanning (46). Because of its suboptimal imaging characteristics and the associated low sensitivity (40%) and specificity (51%) for detecting parathyroid adenomas, ^{75}selenomethionine scintigraphy was abandoned by the mid-1980s (47).

Toluidine blue is a vital stain similar to methylene blue that stains pathologic parathyroid glands when injected intravenously because of binding to nucleic acids and mucopolysaccharides (48,49); surrounding tissues are stained only lightly and wash out rapidly (50). In the mid-1970s, ^{131}I-labeled toluidine blue scintigraphy yielded only a slight improvement over ^{75}selenomethionine scintigraphy (51,52). However, when computerized scintigraphic and superimposition capabilities became available in the 1980s, the use of dual-isotope radioiodinated toluidine blue (RTB) and ^{99m}Tc-pertechnetate scintigraphy resulted in sensitivities of 87% to 93%, a specificity of 94%, and an accuracy of 92% (Fig. 32.4) (53,54). The technique suffers from the requirement for the patient to remain motionless during the 45- to 60-minute acquisition. In Europe and Asia, the identification of parathyroid pathology is aided by the intraoperative infusion of nonradiolabeled methylene blue with sensitivities reported to be greater than 95% (55–57). However, the use of ^{123}I-labeled methylene blue has proved unsatisfactory for preoperative imaging of parathyroid adenomas with a sensitivity of only 20% (58).

In 1983, the use of combined ^{99m}Tc-pertechnetate and ^{201}Tl subtraction imaging for the localization of parathyroid adenomas was described (59,60). This technique is based on the principal that thyroid and parathyroid tissue will both take up ^{201}Tl, whereas only thyroid tissue will trap ^{99m}Tc-pertechnetate. The accumulation of ^{201}Tl in a parathyroid adenoma is nonspecific, most likely related to the high cellularity and/or vascularity of the tumor. ^{201}Tl is a nonspecific tumor imaging agent, and false-positive findings may be seen in both benign and malignant thyroid neoplasms, as well as in Hashimoto's thyroiditis, inflammatory cervical nodes, sarcoidosis, brown tumors, metastatic carcinoma, and lymphoma (60–67). ^{201}Tl imaging is a useful modality for the detection of parathyroid carcinoma (Fig. 32.5).

Although a variety of protocols have been used, most commonly the ^{201}Tl planar images are acquired first using a pinhole collimator after the injection of 2 mCi because of the lower energy of ^{201}Tl and the desire to avoid downscatter of ^{99m}Tc photons into the ^{201}Tl window. Immediately after completion of the ^{201}Tl acquisition, 2 mCi of ^{99m}Tc-pertechnetate are injected, and the thyroid images are acquired 10 to 15 minutes later. The patient must remain motionless during the entire acquisition if the images are to be coregistered and subtracted. Any remaining foci of ^{201}Tl activity after subtraction of the ^{99m}Tc counts theoretically represent pathologic parathyroid activity (Fig. 32.6). The advantages of subtraction scintigraphy include a relatively high sensitivity and specificity as well as the potential to identify both aberrant and ectopic glands (46, 59–64,68–75). In a review of 14 reports encompassing 317 patients with primary hyperparathyroidism, the sensitivity of dual-isotope ^{99m}Tc/^{201}Tl scintigraphy was 82% with 5% false-positive findings and an accuracy of 78% (76). The detection of hyperplasia and of adenomas smaller than 300 mg was relatively low (approximately 50%), and patient motion during the acquisition of the two sets of images may result in both false-

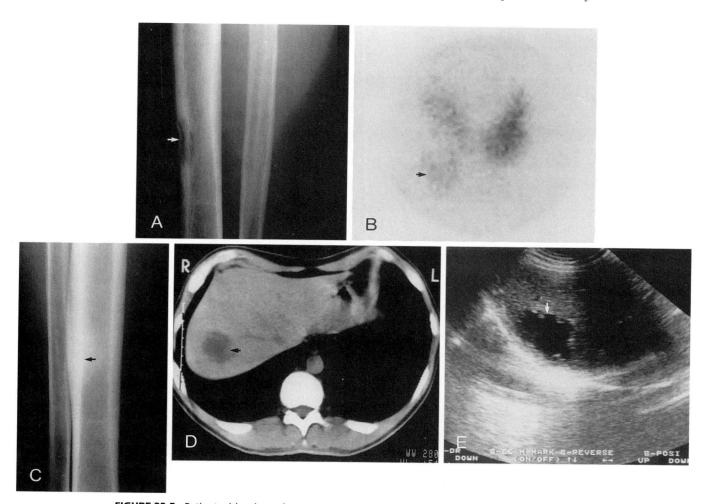

FIGURE 32.5. Patient with primary hyperparathyroidism presented with a tumor of the tibia **(A)**. ^{201}Tl imaging **(B)** revealed an abnormal right lower parathyroid adenoma *(arrow)*. After surgery, the brown tumors gradually recalcified **(C)**. Severe hypercalcemia recurred 1 year later. CT **(D)**, ultrasound **(E)**, and MRI **(F)** revealed a solitary cystic mass within the right lobe of the liver. *(Figure continues.)*

positive and false-negative interpretations because of misregistration of the data sets (65). Other technical factors such as image distortion caused by pinhole collimation and normalization artifacts may also contribute to interpretive errors (61,64,65). The low count rate of ^{201}Tl may contribute to false-negative findings for lesions deep in the neck or mediastinum, but sensitivity in these regions remains respectable (Fig. 32.7); rapid washout of ^{201}Tl from a parathyroid adenoma has been reported as a false negative (77).

In an attempt to increase sensitivity for the detection of smaller adenomas, ^{123}I/^{201}Tl dual-isotope subtraction imaging was reported to detect adenomas smaller than 300 mg (69) (Fig. 32.8). However, because of the simplicity and reliability of ^{99m}Tc-MIBI scintigraphy, ^{99m}Tc/^{201}Tl or ^{123}I/^{201}Tl subtraction imaging is only rarely used in current clinical practice.

^{99m}TC-MIBI PARATHYROID IMAGING

^{99m}Tc-MIBI is a radiopharmaceutical with lipophilic cationic properties used for both myocardial perfusion and tumor imaging (36,45,78–84). Distribution of ^{99m}Tc-MIBI is proportional to blood flow, and once intracellular it is sequestered primarily within the mitochondria (85–87). The accumulation of ^{99m}Tc-MIBI within the mitochondria and cytoplasm of cells is in response to the electrical potentials generated across the membrane bilayers of both the cell and mitochondria. The large number of mitochondria present in the cells of parathyroid adenomas (and other tumors) may be responsible for the avid uptake and slow release of ^{99m}Tc-MIBI in parathyroid adenomas compared with surrounding thyroid tissue (88). A number of studies have shown that ^{99m}Tc-MIBI is maintained within mitochondria with a concentration of up to 1,000 times greater than the extracellular concentration and that these concentrations are maintained longer than ^{201}Tl (45,86,87). There is also developing evidence that ^{99m}Tc-MIBI is preferentially taken up and retained in mitochondria-rich oxyphil parathyroid cells to the extent that parathyroid lesions with an oxyphil cell content above 25% usually retain ^{99m}Tc-MIBI whereas those with lower oxyphil cell content may not and those with no oxyphil cells do not (88, 89). It is therefore thought that one explanation for false-nega-

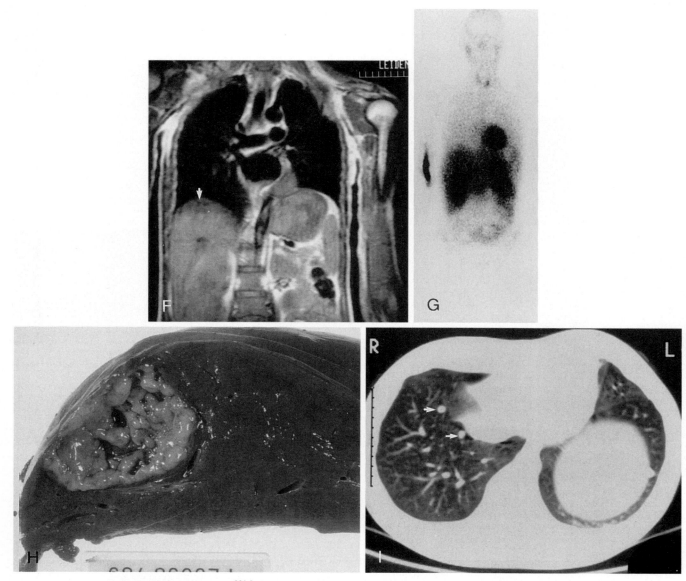

FIGURE 32.5. *Continued.* ^{201}Tl scintigraphy **(G)** failed to identify the liver or any other lesions. During surgery, a large encapsulated cystic tumor was resected **(H)** that consisted of parathyroid hormone producing parathyroid tissue at histopathology, consistent with parathyroid carcinoma metastasis. One year later, multiple pulmonary metastases were identified at the time of recurrent hypercalcemia **(I)**. (From Falke THM, Schipper J, Patton JA et al. Parathyroid glands. In: Sandler MP, Patton JA, Groce MD et al., eds. *Endocrine imaging.* Norwalk, CT: Appleton & Lang, 1992:156–158, with permission.)

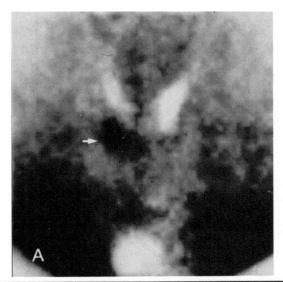

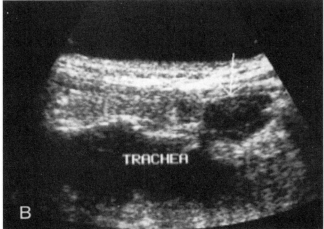

FIGURE 32.6. ^{99m}Tc/^{201}Tl subtraction image in the anterior projection using a conversion collimator from a patient with a suspected parathyroid adenoma **(A)**. A parathyroid adenoma is identified at the inferior pole of the right lobe of the thyroid **(B)**. Longitudinal sonogram shows a hypoechoic parathyroid adenoma inferior to the right thyroid lobe. (From Sandler MP, Patton JA, Sacks GA et al. Parathyroid imaging. In: Sandler MP, Patton JA, Shaff MI et al., eds. *Correlative imaging: nuclear medicine, magnetic resonance, computed tomography, ultrasound.* Baltimore: Williams & Wilkins 1989:253–264, with permission.)

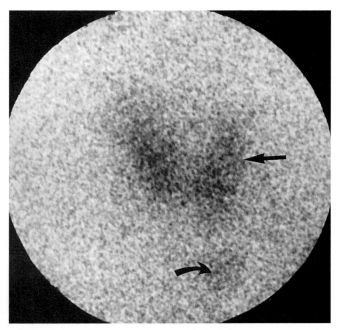

FIGURE 32.7. ^{201}Tl scintigram identifies the thyroid gland (*straight arrow*) and a left anterior mediastinal parathyroid adenoma (*curved arrow*).

is a nonspecific tumor-imaging agent that can be taken up by both benign and malignant thyroid lesions including adenoma, differentiated thyroid cancer, Hürthle cell carcinoma, medullary thyroid carcinoma, and primary thyroid lymphoma, as well as inflammatory and metastatic nodes (36,82–84,96–99), potentially adversely affecting the specificity of parathyroid scintigraphy (Fig. 32.9).

Most commonly, ^{99m}Tc-MIBI parathyroid scintigraphy is

tive findings with ^{99m}Tc-MIBI may be rapid washout in adenomas containing few oxyphil cells (90,91).

Similar to ^{201}Tl, ^{99m}Tc-MIBI is rapidly taken up by normal thyroid tissue with peak accumulation at 3 to 5 minutes and a rapid half-time clearance of approximately 60 minutes (36,92). This uptake is not affected by exogenous thyroid hormone or iodine administration (93–95). The uptake of ^{99m}Tc-MIBI within parathyroid tissue is higher than the uptake by thyroid tissue, and the activity remains relatively stable over 2 hours. ^{201}Tl uptake by parathyroid tissue, on the other hand, is similar to that of thyroid tissue, and ^{201}Tl activity declines with time (88). This explains the better visualization of parathyroid adenomas at 2 to 3 hours after ^{99m}Tc-MIBI injection, allowing for physiologic thyroid washout. However, like ^{201}Tl, ^{99m}Tc-MIBI

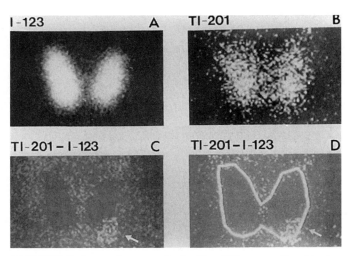

FIGURE 32.8. Images from a patient with a 700-mg parathyroid adenoma (*small arrow*). Images obtained by subtracting the ^{123}I data **(A)** from the ^{201}Tl data **(B)** reveal a solitary focus of ^{201}Tl activity near the inferior pole of the left lobe of the thyroid. (From Pacard D, D-Armour P, Carrier L et al. Localization of abnormal parathyroid(s) using thallium-201/iodine-123 subtraction scintigraphy in patients with primary hyperparathyroidism. *Clin Nucl Med* 1987;12:1, with permission.)

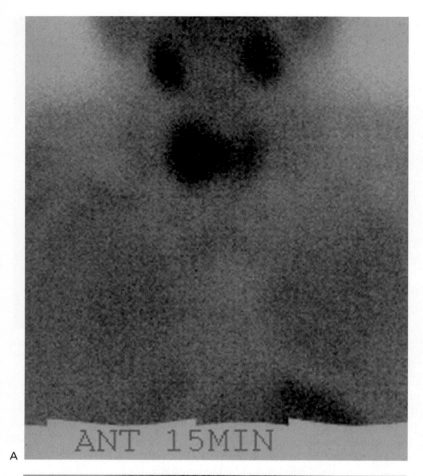

A

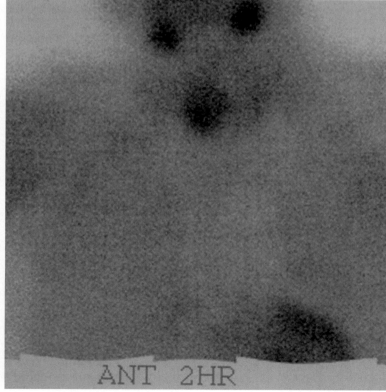

B

FIGURE 32.9. Early 99mTc-MIBI imaging **(A)** demonstrates a large focus of increased activity at the midportion of the right lobe of the thyroid with a normal appearing left lobe. The delayed image **(B)** reveals washout of the left lobar activity but persistence of the right lobe focus. *(Figure continues.)*

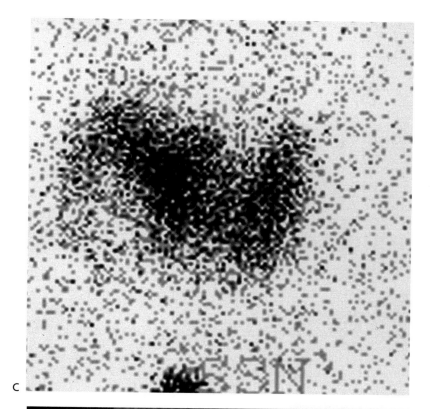

C

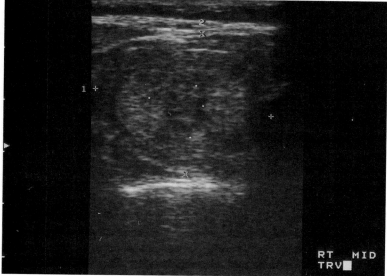

D

FIGURE 32.9. *Continued.* A ^{123}I scan **(C)** reveals a large cold nodule in the right lobe, congruent with the abnormality seen on 99mTc-MIBI image. Sonography **(D)** shows a solid right thyroid nodule but no parathyroid adenoma. Benign or malignant thyroid pathology may result in false-positive 99mTc-MIBI (or 201Tl) findings.

performed as a double-phase study based on the differential washout of 99mTc-MIBI from the thyroid versus parathyroid adenoma. With this approach, planar images of the neck and mediastinum are obtained with a preset 10-minute time for each image using a large field of view camera with a low energy, high-resolution parallel-hole collimator. The initial set is obtained at 10 to 15 minutes and the second set at 2 to 3 hours after the injection of 20 to 25 mCi of 99mTc-MIBI. Ideally, myocardial activity is excluded from the field of view.

A focus of increased activity in the neck or mediastinum that

either progressively increases over the duration of the study or persists on delayed imaging in contrast to the decreased thyroidal activity on the delayed imaging is interpreted as differential washout and therefore consistent with parathyroid pathology (Fig. 32.10). Semiquantitative analysis with regions of interest drawn around normal thyroid tissue and the focal "parathyroid" abnormality have been reported with parathyroid/thyroid ratios of 1.24 ± 0.23 for early images and 1.46 ± 0.20 on delayed images as consistent with parathyroid pathology (100), but visual analysis is sufficient for clinical purposes. An analysis of 32 re-

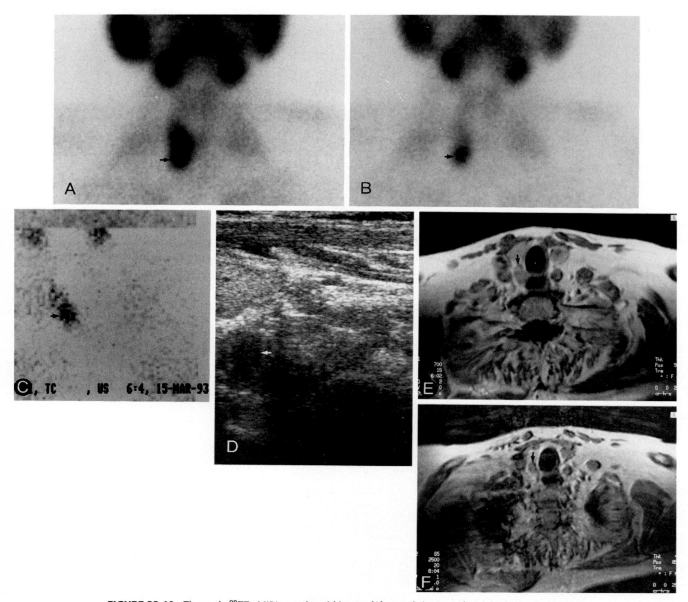

FIGURE 32.10. The early ^{99m}Tc-MIBI parathyroid image **(A)** reveals increased activity in the lower pole of the right thyroid lobe; left lobar activity is absent because of prior lobectomy. The delayed image **(B)** reveals only a small focus of increased activity at the inferior pole of the right lobe consistent with parathyroid adenoma. ^{99m}Tc/^{201}Tl subtraction imaging **(C)** identifies a parathyroid adenoma at the inferior pole of the right thyroid lobe (*arrow*). Longitudinal sonogram **(D)** shows a hypoechoic parathyroid adenoma inferior to the right thyroid lobe (*arrow*). Transverse MRI T1-weighted image **(E)** identifies a parathyroid adenoma inferior to the right thyroid lobe (*arrow*). Proton density weighted MRI **(F)** reveals slightly increased signal intensity in the parathyroid adenoma (*arrow*).

ports using this double-phase technique for the detection of abnormal parathyroid glands was reported to be successful in 671 of 803 (84%) patients who had adenomas and was successful in 59 of 93 (63%) patients with multiglandular disease or hyperplasia (37) (Fig. 32.11). In a recent metaanalysis of 6,331 patients undergoing initial surgery for primary hyperparathyroidism over a 10-year period, the mean sensitivity and specificity of preoperative ^{99m}Tc-MIBI imaging for the detection of a solitary adenoma was reported to be 91% and 99%, respectively (25). This analysis, unlike the prior one, excluded patients with famil-

ial hyperparathyroidism and multiple endocrine neoplasia who often have multiglandular disease. This accounts for the higher (87%) than unusual incidence of solitary adenoma in this analysis. Although sensitivity has been reported to decrease for adenomas smaller than 300 mg, many investigators at present report the ability to reliably detect adenomas larger than 100 mg (38).

Contrary to the findings of initial investigators, rapid clearance of ^{99m}Tc-MIBI from adenomas does occasionally occur, resulting in false-negative interpretations of delayed images (90, 91) (Fig. 32.12). This is particularly true for some large adeno-

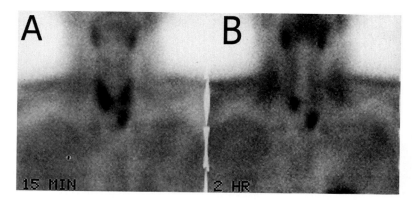

FIGURE 32.11. Immediate **(A)** and delayed **(B)** ^{99m}Tc-MIBI imaging reveals a focus of increased activity at the inferior tip of the right lobe of the thyroid and a focus of increased activity at the base of the left neck, consistent with dual parathyroid adenomas. Hyperplasia may appear similarly.

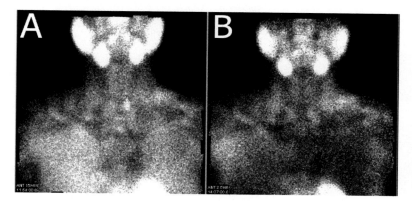

FIGURE 32.12. In this woman with primary hyperparathyroidism and prior thyroidectomy, a solitary focus of increased activity in the left neck on the immediate image **(A)** is suggestive of parathyroid adenoma, despite the washout on the delayed image **(B)**. At surgery, a 99-mg left parathyroid adenoma was found deep in the tracheoesophageal groove. Although atypical, parathyroid adenomas may be visualized on immediate images and washout on delayed views.

mas, although early imaging results are usually positive with large adenomas. Despite the presence of US-detectable thyroid abnormalities in a large minority of patients with hyperparathyroidism (101), the incidence of false-positive findings (resulting from thyroid disease) when using this double-phase technique is quite small, as evidenced by the high reported specificities, generally greater than 95%. Correlation with US images when appropriate or occasionally obtaining delayed images at 4 to 6 hours may be helpful. Single photon emission computed tomography (SPECT) imaging is useful for accurate localization, especially in the mediastinum, and may improve sensitivity when planar images are negative (39–42). This is particularly true

for smaller tumors in the tracheoesophageal groove and ectopic lesions; fusion imaging may also aid in accurate localization, particularly within the mediastinum (Fig. 32.13). There is some concern, though poorly documented, that false-positive findings may be seen more often using SPECT. Visualization of physiologic activity in the myocardial wall of the right atrial appendage should not be mistaken for a mediastinal adenoma (102) (Fig. 32.14).

Dual-isotope imaging using either ^{99m}Tc-pertechnetate or ^{123}I subtraction imaging for thyroid counts has also been reported (38,39). Sensitivity may be slightly higher than with the single isotope technique, and specificity is improved in the face

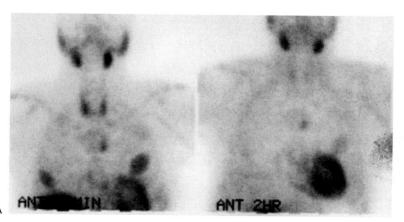

FIGURE 32.13. In this man with prior parathyroidectomy for tertiary hyperparathyroidism and recurrent hypercalcemia, immediate (*left panel*) and delayed (*right panel*) ^{99m}Tc-MIBI imaging **(A)** reveals an ectopic parathyroid adenoma in the mediastinum. The large foci of increased activity in the thorax represent brown tumors of the ribs. (*Figure continues.*)

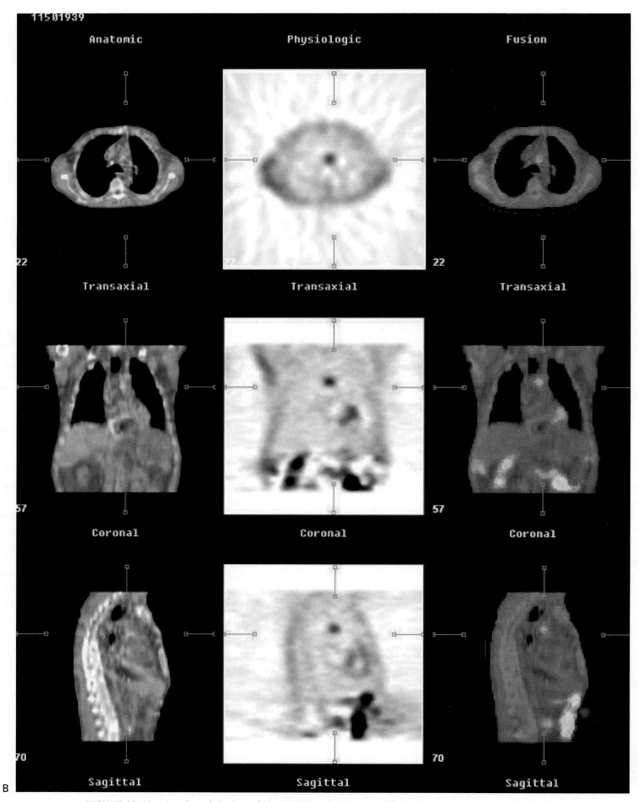

FIGURE 32.13. *Continued.* Fusion of the SPECT and CT images **(B)** localized the adenoma, facilitating successful resection.

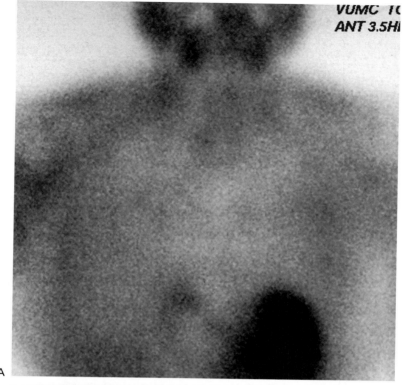

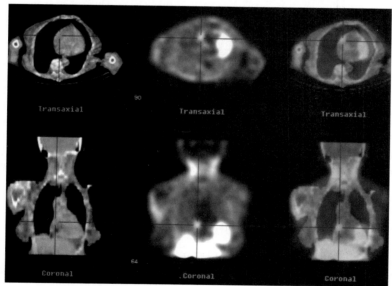

FIGURE 32.14. Immediate (not shown) and delayed 99mTc-MIBI imaging **(A)** in a woman with persistent primary hyperparathyroidism; the only focus of activity identified is in the region of the right atrial appendage, and was not consistent with a parathyroid adenoma. SPECT images **(B)** are confirmatory for physiologic right atrial appendage activity.

of thyroid disease. Similar disadvantages as with 201Tl/99mTc subtraction imaging persist. A variety of protocols have been used by different investigators, but most often 123I is administered orally 6 hours before imaging followed by an intravenous injection of 10 to 20 mCi of 99mTc-MIBI and immediate image acquisition with the patient still on the table. Because of its simplicity, accompanied by less cost and similar accuracy, the

dual-phase 99mTc-MIBI protocol is used for routine clinical purposes in most centers. In specific patients, a dual-isotope technique may be useful.

When 99mTc-MIBI scintigraphy is directly compared with 99mTc/201Tl subtraction imaging, sensitivity is consistently higher with 99mTc-MIBI (44,45). 99mTc-MIBI also performs well in comparison to other modalities such as US, computed tomography (CT), and magnetic resonance imaging (MRI) in patients undergoing initial surgery and in those undergoing reoperation (43,103–106).

The high sensitivity and specificity of parathyroid imaging for parathyroid localization using ^{99m}Tc-MIBI scintigraphy has stimulated interest in the preoperative assessment of patients initially undergoing evaluation for hyperparathyroidism, as well as in patients undergoing reoperation for recurrent or persistent disease. Furthermore, there has been interest in the use of this technique for rapid differentiation of primary hyperparathyroidism versus the humoral hypercalcemia malignancy in patients with severe hypercalcemia, as well as in the evaluation of patients with chronic renal failure and tertiary hyperparathyroidism. The evaluation of patients with parathyroid autotransplantation and recurrent hypercalcemia has also been advanced by the use of ^{99m}Tc-MIBI scintigraphy.

Although controversy exists regarding the optimal imaging necessary for the evaluation of these patients, there is no doubt that ^{99m}Tc-MIBI is the radiopharmaceutical of choice for parathyroid scintigraphy.

PREOPERATIVE IMAGING

Because an experienced surgeon successfully localizes parathyroid adenomas on at least 90% of initial surgeries (10–14) and because a highly accurate imaging modality has not in the past been available, the general consensus has been that preoperative imaging is not necessary and/or is not cost effective for patients undergoing initial neck exploration (6,13,14). In fact, many still follow the dictum, "The best way of locating the parathyroid glands is to localize an experienced parathyroid surgeon." (15). Proponents of imaging before the first surgery cite the use of directed surgery (as opposed to bilateral neck exploration), reduction in operative time, and virtual elimination of reoperations as reasons to obtain ^{99m}Tc-MIBI imaging preoperatively. (14,25,107–109) Furthermore, it must be realized that in only approximately 50% of patients can all four parathyroid glands be visualized during surgery (10). In the 5% to 10% of cases in which surgical failure occurs, it is due to abnormal location of the tumor within the neck or mediastinum, failure to recognize hyperplasia, or an undiscovered fifth gland. (12,14,32,34,35, 110–113).

Because the success of reoperation is lower than that of initial surgery (60%) and morbidity is higher (14,34,35,103, 114–116), a concerted effort must be directed toward avoiding reoperation. Over the past decade, three developments have led surgeons to alter the traditional surgical approach to patients with hyperparathyroidism: (a) the ^{99m}Tc-MIBI imaging technique has provided surgeons with a highly accurate preoperative localization modality (25,37–45), (b) the "quick" intraoperative PTH assay has provided an accurate assessment of the hormonal response to the gland(s) excision with a turnaround time of 15 minutes (117–119), and (c) the development of miniaturized handheld gamma probes has proven useful for localization intraoperatively and for confirmation of successful excision (120–124). The intraoperative probe is a collimated device that detects gamma photons and relays them through a preamplifier and a signal processor producing an audio signal and a digital display of the count rate. At present, the commercially available probes have either NaI(Tl) scintillating crystals or a semiconductor detector, CdZnTe or CdTe. The CdZnTe and CdTe detectors do not require photomultiplier tubes, thus permitting miniaturization. Although the available probes vary in shielding and collimation with resultant different performance characteristics, they all perform adequately in the clinical setting.

Because surgical excision of a single gland is performed in more than 80% of parathyroidectomy cases (10,25,37) (Table 32.3), preoperative localization with ^{99m}Tc-MIBI permits unilateral exploration of the neck when imaging provides unequivocal findings of a single adenoma. If the intraoperative 20-minute postexcision quick PTH levels fall to less than 70% of the preoperative level, the procedure is deemed successful and contralateral exploration is avoided (34,119,125,126). Unilateral exploration of the neck reduces morbidity and surgical complications such as recurrent laryngeal nerve paresis, postoperative hemorrhage, infection, and hypoparathyroidism (118,127). It has been demonstrated that, in cases in which correct preoperative localization permitted unilateral parathyroidectomy, the time for surgery and anesthesia was significantly reduced (109,118,128).

The technique of minimally invasive radioguided parathyroidectomy (MIRP) was developed in the late 1990s, and a number of investigators have reported success using this technique (120–122,124,127,129,130). The subject has recently been reviewed (131). After unequivocal unilateral detection of a solitary adenoma with ^{99m}Tc-MIBI in 80% of unselected or 87% of selected patients (25), the patient is taken to the operating room either the same morning or on a different day and undergoes a 2.5- to 4-cm incision often under local anesthesia. The surgeon is directed to the offending gland using a handheld gamma probe. In the case of intrathyroidal adenoma, intrathymic adenoma, or adenoma located deep in the tracheoesophageal groove, the use of preoperative imaging and an intraoperative probe can greatly enhance the surgeon's ability to identify the pathologic adenoma (Figs. 32.12 and 32.15). Intraoperative success can be confirmed by counting the *ex vivo* adenoma and comparing those counts to the *in vivo* parathyroid plus thyroid counts or by using a quick PTH assay. In this manner, multiglandular disease should be easily recognized (119,132,133). Numerous investigators have now reported surgical success rates of 90% to 100% using the MIRP technique (119,120,123,124,131,134).

The management and imaging costs of patients with multigland and ectopic disease who fail initial surgical exploration

Table 32.3. *Surgical Procedure in 109 Patients with Primary Hyperparathyroidism*

Procedure	Number of patients
Extirpation of one gland	89 (82%)
Extirpation of two glands	4 (4%)
Subtotal parathyroidectomy	13 (12%)
Biopsy	3 (3%)

From Heslinga JM. Enige heelkundige aspecten van hyperparathyreoidie (Thesis). Leiden: Pasmans JH, 1987:(English summary) 115–119, with permission.

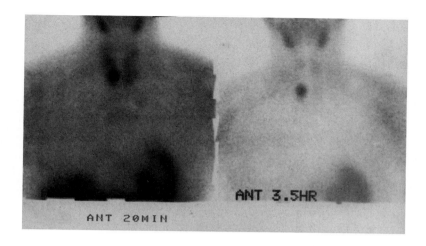

FIGURE 32.15. Anterior immediate (*left panel*) and 3.5-hour delayed (*right panel*) ^{99m}Tc-MIBI images reveal a focus of increased activity at the inferior right thyroid pole. On the delayed images, there is virtually complete washout of physiologic thyroid activity. At surgery an intrathyroidal non-palpable parathyroid adenoma was identified only with the aid of radioguidance and with knowledge of the preoperative scintigraphic findings.

(7%) might justify the cost of routine preoperative localization with ^{99m}Tc-MIBI even without taking into consideration the lower costs associated with unilateral explorations (135). However, many of the advantages of preoperative localization will not be evident unless the surgeon limits the surgical procedure to a unilateral approach and unless the gamma probe or quick PTH assay is used for intraoperative confirmation of successful excision (107,127,136,137). A number of investigators have documented shortened length of hospital stay, fewer operative failures, and less morbidity associated with MIRP (118,127, 134). Denham and Norman (25) estimated a savings of 37% per patient, whereas Goldstein et al. (134) estimated a 47% reduction in hospital costs, primarily related to the use of local anesthesia and discharge within 5 hours of surgery. In the United States $282 million was spent on parathyroidectomies in 1997 (138); if a 37% to 47% savings can be realized, this would translate to a $104 to $133 million savings annually.

The use of MIRP is precluded in patients at high risk of having multigland disease, such as those with familial hyperparathyroidism, MEN, and secondary or tertiary hyperparathyroidism. In a recent metaanalysis of 6,331 patients with nonfamilial, non-MEN sporadic hyperparathyroidism, only 12% of patients had multiglandular disease (9% hyperplasia and 3% multiple adenomas) (25). With a ^{99m}Tc-MIBI sensitivity of 90% and a specificity of 99%, the risk of missing multigland disease is estimated to be less than 1% (Fig. 32.16). Intraoperative confirmation of successful excision using a gamma probe or quick PTH assay should limit failures even further (119). In support of this is the low incidence for persistent and recurrent hyperparathyroidism reported by investigators performing MIRP, no higher than that reported with conventional bilateral exploration (120–122,124,127,129–131). The technique of MIRP using ^{99m}Tc-MIBI scintigraphy is significantly changing the management of primary hyperparathyroidism (120,130,131,139–141).

REOPERATION FOR PERSISTENT OR RECURRENT HYPERPARATHYROIDISM

There is universal agreement in the need for accurate preoperative imaging for localization in patients with primary or tertiary

hyperparathyroidism undergoing reoperative parathyroid exploration (142,143), in patients undergoing parathyroid surgery after previous thyroidectomy (144) (Fig. 32.12), and in patients in whom nonsurgical treatment of primary hyperparathyroidism is contemplated (30,145). Thirty percent of patients with persistent or recurrent hyperparathyroidism eventually undergo two or more additional surgeries before cure is attained (35,146).

Due in part to anatomic distortion related to scarring, the complication rate in patients undergoing repeat neck exploration after an initial failed surgery may be tenfold higher than after initial neck exploration with permanent hypoparathyroidism occurring in 3% to 16% (116) and a fivefold increase in vocal cord paralysis (115). The success rate may be as low as 60% (14,103,114), but improves to almost 90% (with a similar reduction in morbidity) if preoperative localization is successful (34, 116,147).

The usual cause of initial surgical failure (persistent disease) is the presence of either unrecognized parathyroid hyperplasia (Fig. 32.17) or ectopic parathyroid tissue either in the neck or mediastinum (34,35,113) (Figs. 32.13 and 32.18). Whereas 4% to 8% of glands are located ectopically in patients undergoing successful initial parathyroidectomy, ectopia accounts for 24% to 39% of missed lesions (111,112), and multiglandular disease is over twice as common at reoperation as compared with initial surgery (34,35). Recurrent hyperparathyroidism or that occurring after an interval of 6 to 12 months of normocalcemia usually is due to unresected hyperplastic glands, but occasionally it may be related to a second adenoma or parathyroid carcinoma.

If the initial surgery was performed by an experienced parathyroid surgeon, the offending "missed" gland(s) is usually located within the mediastinum or in another ectopic location, whereas 90% of missed glands in patients operated on by less experienced surgeons occur in the neck (32). A variety of imaging modalities has been used for the localization of disease in patients with recurrent or persistent hyperparathyroidism. US is less sensitive in patients with previously operated necks and is less sensitive in detecting ectopic glands and mediastinal glands (103, 105,148). CT imaging may be compromised by artifact from metallic clips in the neck. Most investigators have recommended a combination of ^{99m}Tc-MIBI scintigraphy and MRI. The re-

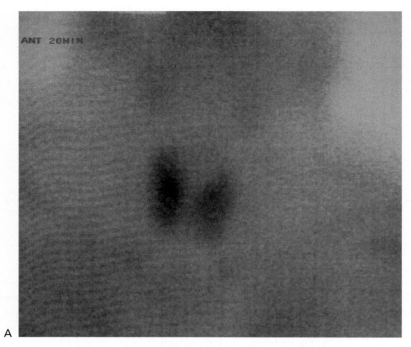

A

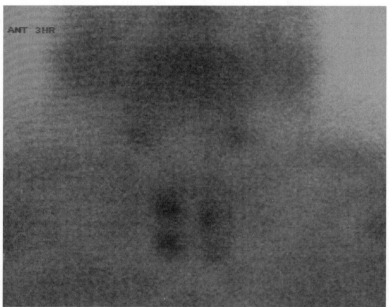

B

FIGURE 32.16. Anterior immediate **(A)** and delayed **(B)** ^{99m}Tc-MIBI imaging demonstrates four-gland hyperplasia in this patient with chronic renal failure. Although four glands may not always be identified, more than one gland is usually demonstrated in patients with multiglandular disease.

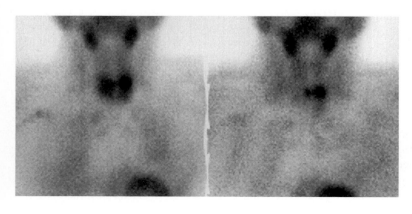

FIGURE 32.17. In this patient with multiple endocrine neoplasia (MEN 1) and prior bilateral parathyroidectomy, persistent hyperparathyroidism is explained by the identification of bilateral superior hyperplastic parathyroid glands, the left being larger than the right on immediate (*left panel*) and delayed (*right panel*) ^{99m}Tc-MIBI imaging.

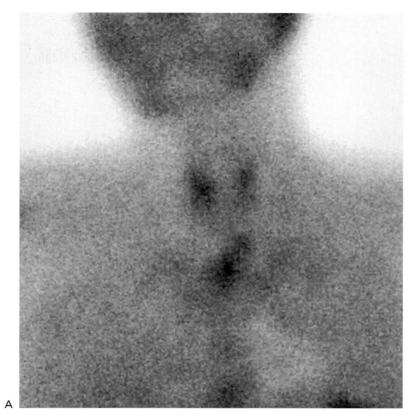

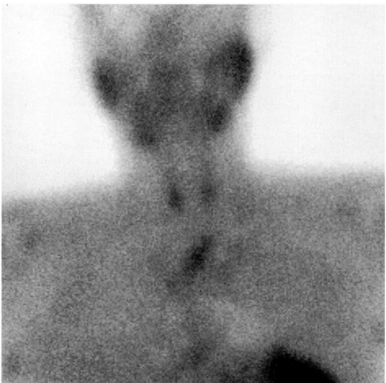

FIGURE 32.18. In this patient with chronic renal failure and tertiary hyperparathyroidism, parathyroid-ectomy may have been unsuccessful if preoperative ^{99m}Tc-MIBI imaging had not been performed. Two superior hyperplastic parathyroid glands are identified on the immediate and delayed ^{99m}Tc-MIBI images in a eutopic location, but the inferior hyperplastic glands are located within the superior mediastinum, the right gland being more inferior than the left.

sults of both of these modalities have improved in more recent reports as compared with initial studies (43,44,103–106). MRI provides excellent anatomic detail with high resolution and contrast, as well as the absence of significant artifact from surgical clips in the neck. Recent reports indicate that MRI is approximately 82% to 88% sensitive and ^{99m}Tc-MIBI scintigraphy is approximately 79% to 85% sensitive for the accurate localization of parathyroid pathology in patients with recurrent or persistent hyperparathyroidism (43,103–106) (Figs. 32.13 and 32.17). The combination of these two modalities in most reports has provided a substantial increase in sensitivity and positive predictive value in the range of 89% to 94%.

Evidence is accumulating that reoperation may be successfully performed using the MIRP technique if unequivocal cervical or upper mediastinal localization can be demonstrated (120, 130,131,141). Bonjer et al. (120) found that MIRP was successful in 89% of patients reoperated on for recurrent/persistent hyperparathyroidism.

SECONDARY AND TERTIARY HYPERPARATHYROIDISM AND AUTOTRANSPLANTATION

Despite advances in dialysis technique and pharmacologic therapy for secondary hyperparathyroidism in chronic renal failure patients, parathyroidectomy with or without autotransplantation of parathyroid tissue into the muscles of the neck or forearm is still performed in approximately 2% of patients annually, and up to 4% per year of renal transplant patients require parathyroidectomy for tertiary hyperparathyroidism (149). Parathyroid autotransplantation is also often performed at the time of total parathyroidectomy for primary parathyroid hyperplasia (29).

Although some investigators have reported that ^{99m}Tc-MIBI imaging can identify over 80% of hyperplastic glands in renal failure patients, others have found it to be less useful (150) (Fig. 32.17). Five percent to 8% of patients undergoing successful surgery for secondary or tertiary hyperparathyroidism experience a recurrence, regardless of whether autotransplantation is used, and 14% of patients with primary parathyroid hyperplasia experience a recurrence after total parathyroidectomy with autotransplantation (151). As in other patients with recurrent or persistent disease, these patients require localization procedures before re-exploration. Scintigraphy is an ideal method to determine whether such recurrences are graft-dependent, because either ^{201}Tl or ^{99m}Tc-MIBI can localize and functionally characterize the reimplanted parathyroid tissue (141,152). ^{99m}Tc-MIBI may be more effective than US or MRI for this application.

OTHER RADIONUCLIDE IMAGING TECHNIQUES

^{99m}Tc-tetrofosmin is a radiopharmaceutical similar to ^{99m}Tc-MIBI and is used primarily for myocardial perfusion scintigraphy. Like ^{99m}Tc-MIBI, it too demonstrates mitochondrial uptake and has been shown to be effective in the detection of a variety of neoplasms. Reports to date regarding the utility of ^{99m}Tc-tetrofosmin imaging for parathyroid pathology in patients with hyperparathyroidism encompass over 220 patients

(121,153–167). The sensitivity for detection of both parathyroid adenomas and hyperplasia with tetrofosmin is similar to that of ^{99m}Tc-MIBI. However, ^{99m}Tc-tetrofosmin does not clear from normal thyroid tissue in the same manner as ^{99m}Tc-MIBI, so dual-phase scintigraphy is less useful with tetrofosmin than with ^{99m}Tc-MIBI (156,159,163). As with ^{99m}Tc-MIBI, detection rate is higher with larger tumors and in patients with higher PTH levels (155). In view of the poor washout of thyroidal ^{99m}Tc-tetrofosmin, subtraction imaging using ^{99m}Tc-pertechnetate (154,159,160,166) or SPECT (121,154,162) may heighten sensitivity. Unlike ^{99m}Tc-MIBI, the uptake and retention of ^{99m}Tc-tetrofosmin does not appear to be proportional to the number of mitochondria-rich oxyphil cells within parathyroid adenomas (164). As with ^{99m}Tc-MIBI, false-positive findings with benign and malignant thyroid lesions occur (162). In a single report of the use of ^{99m}Tc-furifosmin in 10 patients with parathyroid adenomas, ^{99m}Tc-furifosmin detected 100% of the adenomas and demonstrated thyroidal clearance similar to what is seen with ^{99m}Tc-MIBI (168).

^{18}F-fluorodeoxyglucose (^{18}F-FDG) is a positron-emitting glucose analog used most commonly to identify malignant neoplasms characterized by high ^{18}F-FDG accumulation, although some low-grade tumors, such as pituitary adenoma and thyroid adenoma, may also demonstrate ^{18}F-FDG avidity (169). ^{18}F-FDG positron emission tomography (PET) has been reported to have sensitivity for the detection of parathyroid adenomas ranging from 22% to 94% (170–172). Specificity has been as low as 64%, related primarily to inflammatory lymphadenopathy but also to benign thyroid neoplasms. As with other nuclear medicine imaging modalities, the detection of hyperplastic glands is lower, in the range of 29% to 50%. A single case report indicates that ^{18}F-FDG PET may be superior to ^{99m}Tc-MIBI for detection of recurrent parathyroid carcinoma (173). In view of the frequency (78%) of persistent or recurrent hyperparathyroidism after initial surgery for parathyroid carcinoma and the relatively limited sensitivity of various imaging modalities for localization (^{99m}Tc-MIBI 79%, MR 93%, CT 67%, and US 69%), ^{18}F-FDG or ^{11}C-methionine PET may assume a major role in the detection of recurrent parathyroid carcinoma (174).

^{11}C-methionine is another positron-emitting radiopharmaceutical used for tumor imaging with the advantage that it is less prone to accumulate in inflammatory lesions. There is preliminary evidence that ^{11}C-methionine PET may be of great utility in patients with recurrent or persistent hyperparathyroidism who have negative, equivocal, or misleading anatomic imaging or ^{99m}Tc-MIBI scintigraphy (175–179). There appear to be fewer false positives, with an incidental thymoma being the only false-positive finding reported to date (180). ^{11}C-methionine PET appears to be of particular use in patients with difficult clinical situations, such as persistent hyperparathyroidism including MEN-1 patients, and in patients having undergone autotransplantation. ^{11}C-methionine PET may be a good alternative before attempting invasive localization using arteriography and venous sampling.

ALTERNATIVE IMAGING MODALITIES

In addition to scintigraphy, US, CT, MRI, angiography, and venous sampling are used to localize parathyroid pathology. All of these techniques depend to a varying degree on the size of the abnormal gland, with the exception of venous sampling.

Ultrasonography

US evaluation of the parathyroid gland employs a 7- to 10-MHz transducer and is capable of detecting enlarged parathyroid glands when they are in a eutopic cervical location. Normal parathyroid glands are usually not detectable because of their small (2 to 3 mm) size. Ectopic glands are more difficult to detect, and US cannot be used to identify mediastinal parathyroid adenomas. Thyroid nodules (particularly posteriorly located) and cervical lymph nodes (especially within the tracheo-esophageal groove) may mimic parathyroid pathology (181), but thyroid nodules generally appear less vascular than parathyroid adenomas. US identification of parathyroid adenomas has a sensitivity of 64% with a specificity of 94% (181), although the sensitivity is highly dependent on size and somewhat dependent on location (182). Parathyroid adenomas are typically homogeneously hypoechoic with a hyperechoic capsule and are uniformly hypervascular (181) (Figs. 32.6 and 32.10). The sensitivity for detection of parathyroid hyperplasia is 30% to 69%, and only occasionally are all four hyperplastic glands identified as abnormal (183). Although US is often used in the preoperative evaluation of patients undergoing initial surgery (184), it plays a limited role in the evaluation of patients with persistent or recurrent hyperparathyroidism following initial neck exploration. Initial enthusiasm for intraoperative US for localization has given way to radioguidance with ^{99m}Tc-MIBI. As for thyroid lesions, sonography can be used for guided percutaneous biopsy of neck masses to aid in differentiating parathyroid versus thyroid or nodal origin (185). Cytology, immunocytochemistry, and radioimmunoassay for PTH or thyroglobulin may be conducted to evaluate the aspirated material.

Computed Tomography

The accuracy of CT for the detection of parathyroid adenomas is dependent on tumor size. It has a sensitivity of approximately 70% with a specificity of 90% for adenomas (186). The use of intravenous contrast is necessary to distinguish vessels from adjacent soft tissue structures and parathyroid masses. Contrast enhancement occurs in only 25% of parathyroid tumors, generally the larger ones (186). Advantages of CT include the ability to image the entire neck and mediastinum, but disadvantages include the requirement for contrast enhancement, as well as anatomic distortion from scarring and streak artifacts resulting from metal clips from prior thyroid or parathyroid surgery (103). CT is sensitive for detection of parathyroid tumors situated in the retroesophageal or retrosternal location. The sensitivity for detection of hyperplasia using CT varies from 45% to 88% (183).

Magnetic Resonance Imaging

MRI is widely used in evaluating neck pathology because it offers excellent soft tissue contrast without the need for intravenous

iodinated contrast material, and metal surgical clips produce fewer artifacts than with CT. Standard T1, T2, and postcontrast T1-weighted imaging is employed. Normal parathyroid glands are not visualized using MRI (187), but parathyroid adenomas and hyperplastic glands are typically bright on T2-weighted images and enhance on postcontrast T1-weighted images (Fig. 32.10). However, approximately 40% of abnormal glands have atypical MR signal characteristics resulting from fibrosis, hemorrhage, or fat (187–189). The MRI characteristics of parathyroid adenomas, however, are nonspecific and may be seen with other neck masses and with lymphadenopathy (190). Although sensitivity is reported to be 74% to 92% for identification of parathyroid adenomas, the more recent series report sensitivities of 85% to 92% (103–106). As with other imaging modalities, MRI is less sensitive for detection of hyperplasia (40% to 74%) (104, 114,190). Most recently, MRI has been reported to be highly sensitive for detection of parathyroid pathology in patients with recurrent or persistent hyperparathyroidism with sensitivities in the range of 85% to 90% (43,103–106).

Invasive Techniques

Selective parathyroid arteriography produces a blush or stain of abnormal parathyroid glands because of their high degree of vascularity. It is expensive and technically challenging, morbidity is significant, and sensitivity is not particularly high (20,191, 192). Bilateral venous sampling for PTH may be slightly more sensitive than arteriography (20) but, at present, is only rarely necessary in confusing cases of persistent or recurrent hyperparathyroidism. Interestingly, some investigators have reported successful use of the quick PTH assay with intraoperative sampling of the bilateral jugular veins for localization of an ectopic adenoma when cervical exploration has been otherwise unsuccessful (193,194).

SUMMARY

Because of the large number of patients with relatively mild hyperparathyroidism and small adenomas or hyperplasia, preoperative imaging is now often performed before initial surgery. Although US is a sensitive modality for the identification of eutopic cervical enlarged parathyroid glands, ^{99m}Tc-MIBI scintigraphy using a dual-phase technique is the preferred modality in these patients. In patients without a family history or known MEN, lateralization with preoperative ^{99m}Tc-MIBI scintigraphy allows a less invasive, less expensive, and safer unilateral neck exploration with the aid of a handheld gamma probe (MIRP). No imaging modality is highly sensitive for differentiating hyperplasia from adenoma(s). In patients with persistent or recurrent primary hyperparathyroidism the combination of ^{99m}Tc-MIBI scintigraphy and MRI is recommended with a combined sensitivity of 92% to 94% (43,103–106,195). Invasive techniques are only rarely necessary.

ACKNOWLEDGEMENTS

The authors would like to thank Theo M. Falke, MD, and Jaap Schipper, MD, for their previous contributions to this chapter.

REFERENCES

1. Palmer M, Jakobsson S, Akerstrom G et al. Prevalence of hypercalcemia in a health survey: a 14-year follow-up study of serum calcium values. *Eur J Clin Invest* 1988;18:39–46.
2. Heath H III, Hodgson SF, Kennedy MA. Primary hyperparathyroidism. Incidence, morbidity, and potential economic impact in a community. *N Engl J Med* 1980;302:189–193.
3. Christensson T, Hellström K, Wengle B. Clinical and laboratory findings in subjects with hypercalcaemia. A study including cases with primary hyperparathyroidism detected in a health screening. *Acta Med Scand* 1976;200:355–360.
4. Lafferty FW, Hubay CA. Primary hyperparathyroidism. A review of the long-term surgical and nonsurgical morbidities as a basis for a rational approach to treatment. *Arch Intern Med* 1989;149:789–796.
5. Scholz DA, Purnell DC. Asymptomatic primary hyperparathyroidism. 10-year prospective study. *Mayo Clin Proc* 1981;56:473–478.
6. Consensus development conference statement. Diagnosis and management of asymptomatic hyperparathyroidism. *J Bone Miner Res* 1991;6:S9–S13.
7. Weigel RJ. Nonoperative management of hyperparathyroidism: present and future. *Curr Opin Oncol* 2001;13:33–38.
8. Silverberg SJ et al. Therapeutic controversies in primary hyperparathyroidism. *J Clin Endocrinol Metab* 1999;84:2275–2285.
9. Talpos GB, Bone HG, Kleerekoper M et al. Randomized trial of parathyroidectomy in mild asymptomatic primary hyperparathyroidism: patient description and effects of the SF-36 health survey. *Surgery* 2000;128:1013–1020.
10. van Heerden JA, Grant CS. Surgical treatment of primary hyperparathyroidism: an institutional perspective. *World J Surg* 1991;15:688–692.
11. Auguste, L-J, Attie JN, Schnaap D. Initial failure of surgical exploration in patients with primary hyperparathyroidism. *Am J Surg* 1990;160:333–336.
12. Edis AJ, Sheedy PF, Beahrs OH et al. Results of reoperation for hyperparathyroidism, with evaluation of preoperative localization studies. *Surgery* 1978;84:384–393.
13. Roe SM, Burns RP, Graham LD et al. Cost-effectiveness of preoperative localization studies in primary hyperparathyroid disease. *Ann Surg* 1994;219:582–586.
14. Satava RM, Beahrs OH, Scholz DA. Success rate of cervical exploration for hyperparathyroidism. *Arch Surg* 1975;110:625–628.
15. Broadie TA. Location, location, location. *Am Surg* 1997;63:567–572.
16. Castleman B, Roth SI. *Tumors of the parathyroid glands.* Atlas of tumor pathology AFIP second series, fasicle 14. Washington DC:, 1978.
17. Wang C. The anatomic basis of parathyroid surgery. *Ann Surg* 1976;183:271–275.
18. Al-suhaili AR, Lynn J, Lavender JP. Intrathyroidal parathyroid adenoma: preoperative identification and localization by parathyroid imaging. *Clin Nucl Med* 1988;13:512–514.
19. Kang EH, Schiebler ML, Gefter WB et al. MR demonstration of bilateral intrathyroidal parathyroid glands. *J Comput Assist Tomogr* 1988;12:349–350.
20. Miller Dl, Doppman JL, Krudy AG et al. Localization of parathyroid adenomas in patients who have undergone surgery: Part II. Invasive procedures. *Radiology* 1987;162:138–141.
21. Bringhurst FR, Demay MB, Kronenberg HM. Hormones and disorders of mineral metabolism. In: Wilson JD, Foster DW, Kronenberg HM et al., eds. *Williams textbook of endocrinology,* 9th ed. Philadelphia: WB Saunders, 1998:1155–1210.
22. Mundy GR, Cove DH, Fisken R. Primary hyperparathyroidism: changes in the pattern of clinical presentation. *Lancet* 1980;1:1317–1320.
23. Trigonis C, Hamberger B, Farnebo LO et al. Primary hyperparathyroidism—changing trends over fifty years. *Acta Chir Scand* 1983;149:675–679.
24. Thompson NW, Eckhauser FE, Harness JK: The anatomy of primary hyperparathyroidism. *Surgery* 1982;92:814–821.
25. Denham DW, Norman J. Cost-effectiveness of preoperative sestamibi scan for primary hyperparathyroidism is dependent solely upon the surgeon's choice of operative procedure. *J Am Coll Surg* 1998;186:293–304.
26. Shane E. Parathyroid carcinoma. *J Clin Endocrinol Metab* 2001;86:485–493.
27. Favia G, Lumachi G, Polistina F et al. Parathyroid carcinoma: sixteen new cases and suggestions for correct management. *World J Surg* 1998;22:1225–1230.
28. Rangnekar N, Bailer WJ, Ghani A et al. Parathyroid cysts. Report of four cases and review of the literature. *Int Surg* 1996;81:412–414.
29. Wells SA, Ellis GJ, Gunnells JC et al. Parathyroid autotransplantation in primary parathyroid hyperplasia. *N Engl J Med* 1976;295:57–62.
30. Verges BL, Cercueil JP, Vaillant G et al. Results of ultrasonically guided percutaneous ethanol injection into parathyroid adenomas in primary hyperparathyroidism. *Acta Endocrinol* 1993;129:381–387.
31. Pallotta JA, Sacks BA, Moller DE et al. Arteriographic ablation of cervical parathyroid adenomas. *J Clin Endocrin Metab* 1989;69:1249–1255.
32. Weber CJ, Sewell CW, McGarity WC. Persistent and recurrent sporadic primary hyperparathyroidism: histopathology, complications, and results of reoperation. *Surgery* 1994;116:991–998.
33. Levin KE, Clark OH. The reasons for failure in parathyroid operation. *Arch Surg* 1989;124:911–914.
34. Thompson GB, Grant CS, Perrier ND et al. Reoperative parathyroid surgery in the era of sestamibi scanning and intraoperative parathyroid hormone monitoring. *Arch Surg* 1999;84:699–704.
35. Brennan MF, Nortan JA. Reoperation for persistent and recurrent hyperparathyroidism. *Ann Surg* 1985;201:40–44.
36. Coakley AJ, Kettle AG, Wells CP et al. Tc-99m-sestamibi: a new agent for parathyroid imaging. *Nucl Med Commun* 1989;10:791–794.
37. Taillefer R. Parathyroid scintigraphy. In: Khalkhali J, Maublant JC, Goldsmith J, eds. *Nuclear oncology: diagnosis and therapy.* Philadelphia: Lippincott Williams & Wilkins, 2001:221–244.
38. Hindie E, Melliere D, Perlemuter L et al. Primary hyperparathyroidism: higher success rate of first surgery after preoperative Tc-99m sestamibi-I-123 subtraction scanning. *Radiology* 1997;204:221–228.
39. Neumann DR, Esselstyn CB, Go RT et al, Comparison of double-phase Tc-99m-sestamibi subtraction SPECT in hyperparathyroidism. *AJR* 1997;169:1671–1674.
40. Moka D, Voth E, Dietlein M et al. Technetium 99m-MIBI SPECT: A highly sensitive diagnostic tool for localization of parathyroid adenomas. *Surgery* 2000;128:29–35.
41. Schurrer ME, Seabold JE, Gurll NJ et al. Sestamibi SPECT scintigraphy for detection of postoperative hyperfunctional parathyroid glands. *AJR* 1996;166:1465–1470.
42. Billotey C, Sarfati E, Aurengo A et al. Advantages of SPECT in technetium 99m-sestamibi parathyroid scintigraphy. *J Nucl Med* 1996;37:1773–1778.
43. Gotway MB, Reddy GP, Webb WR et al. Comparison between MR imaging and 99m-Tc MIBI scintigraphy in the evaluation of recurrent or persistent hyperparathyroidism. *Radiology* 2001;218:783–790.
44. Peeler BB, Martin WH, Sandler MP et al. Sestamibi parathyroid scanning and preoperative localization studies for patients with recurrent/persistent hyperparathyroidism or significant comorbid conditions: development of an optimal localization strategy. *Am Surg* 1997;63:37–46.
45. O'Doherty M, Kettle A, Collins R et al. Parathyroid imaging with technetium-99m-sestamibi: preoperative localization and tissue uptake studies. *J Nucl Med* 1992;33:313–318.
46. Potchen EJ, Adelstein SJ, Dealy JB. Radioisotopic localization of the overactive human parathyroid. *AJR* 1965;93:955–961.
47. Waldorf JC, van Heerden JA, Gorman CA et al. (^{75}Se) Selenomethionine scanning for parathyroid localization should be abandoned. *Mayo Clin Proc* 1984;59:534–537.
48. Kang GS, DiGiulio W. Potential value of toluidine blue analogs as parathyroid scanning agents. *J Nucl Med* 1968;9:643–644.
49. Archer EG, Potchen EJ, Studer R et al. Tissue distribution of I-125-toluidine blue in the rat. *J Nucl Med* 1972;13:85–91.
50. Hurvitz RJ, Hurvitz S, Morgenstern L. *In-vivo* staining of the parathyroid glands and pancreas. *Arch Surg* 1967;95:274–277.

51. Yeager RM, Krementz ET. Toluidine blue in identification of parathyroid glands at operation. *Ann Surg* 1969;169:829–838.

52. Krementz ET, Yeager R, Howley W et al. The first 100 cases of parathyroid tumor from Charity Hospital of Louisiana. *Ann Surg* 1971;173:872–873.

53. Zwas ST, Czerniak A, Boruchowsky S et al. Preoperative parathyroid localization by superimposed iodine-131 toluidine blue and technetium-99m pertechnetate imaging. *J Nucl Med* 1987;28:298–307.

54. Czernick A, Zwas ST, Shustik O et al. The use of radioiodinated toluidine blue for preoperative localization of parathyroid pathology. *Surgery* 1991;110:832–838.

55. Takei H, Iino Y, Endo K et al. The efficacy of technetium-99m-MIBI scan and intraoperative methylene blue staining for the localization of abnormal parathyroid glands. *Surg Today* 1999;29:307–312.

56. Muslumanoglu M, Terzioglu T, Ozarmagan S et al. Comparison of preoperative imaging techniques (thallium technetium scan and ultrasonography) and intraoperative staining (with methylene blue) in localizing the parathyroid glands. *Radiol Med (Torino)* 1995;90:444–447.

57. Derom A, Wallaert P, Janzing H et al. Intraoperative identification of parathyroids by means of methylene blue. *Acta Chir Belg* 1994;94:97–100.

58. Blower PJ, Kettle AG, O'Doherty MJ et al. ^{123}I-methylene blue: an unsatisfactory parathyroid imaging agent. *Nucl Med Commun* 1992;13:522–527.

59. Ferlin G, Borsato N, Camerani M et al. New perspectives in localizing enlarged parathyroids by technetium-thallium subtraction scan. *J Nucl Med* 1983;24:438–441.

60. Young AE, Gaunt JI, Croft DN et al. Localization of parathyroid adenomas by thallium-201 and technetium-99m subtraction scanning. *Br Med J (Clin Res Ed)* 1983;286:1384–1386.

61. Basarab RM, Manni A, Harrison TS. Dual isotope subtraction parathyroid scintigraphy in the preoperative evaluation of suspected hyperparathyroidism. *Clin Nucl Med* 1985;10:300–314.62.

62. Punt CJ, DeHooge P, Hoekstra JB. False-positive subtraction scintigram of the parathyroid glands due to metastatic tumor. *J Nucl Med* 1985;26:155–156.

63. Fukuchi M, Hyodo K, Tachibana K et al. Marked thyroid uptake of thallium-201 in patients with goiter: case report. *J Nucl Med* 1977;18:1199–1201.

64. Borsato N, Zanco P, Camerani N et al. Scintigraphy of the parathyroid glands with 201Tl: experience with 250 operated patients. *Nucl Med* 1989;28:26–28.

65. Blue PW, Crawford G, Dydek GJ. Parathyroid subtraction imaging—pitfalls in diagnosis. *Clin Nucl Med* 1989;14:47–57.

66. Shimaoka K, Parthasarethy KL, Friedman M et al. Disparity of radioiodine and radiothallium concentrations in chronic thyroiditis. *J Med* 1980;11:401–412.

67. Yang CJC, Seabold JE, Gurll NJ. Brown tumor of bone: a potential source of false-positive thallium 201 localization. *J Nucl Med* 1989;30:1264–1267.

68. Gooding GAW, Okerlund MD, Stark DD et al. Parathyroid imaging: comparison of double-tracer (T1-201, Tc-99m) scintigraphy and high resolution US. *Radiology* 1986;161:57–64.

69. Picard D, D'Amour P, Carrier L et al. Localization of abnormal parathyroid gland(s) using thallium-201/iodine-123 subtraction scintigraphy in patients with primary hyperparathyroidism. *Clin Nucl Med* 1987;12:60–64.

70. Macfarlane SD, Hanelin LG, Taft DA et al. Localization of abnormal parathyroid glands using thallium-201. *Am J Surg* 1984;148:7–12.

71. Fogelman I, McKillop JH, Bessent RG et al. Successful localization of parathyroid adenoma by thallium-201 and technetium-99m subtraction scintigraphy: description of an improved technique. *Eur J Nucl Med* 1984;9:545–547.

72. Okerlund MD, Sheldon K, Corpuz S et al. A new method with high sensitivity and specificity for localization of abnormal parathyroid glands. *Ann Surg* 1984;381–387.

73. Percival RC, Blake GM, Urwin GH et al. Assessment of thallium pertechnetate subtraction scintigraphy in hyperparathyroidism. *Br J Radiol* 1985;58:131–135.

74. Winzelberg GG, Hydovitz JD, O'Hara KR et al. Prospective comparison of 201Tl/Tc 99m pertechnetate parathyroid subtraction scintigraphy and high-resolution parathyroid ultrasonography in patients with suspected parathyroid adenomas. *Radiology* 1985;155:231–235.

75. Park CH, Intenzo C, Cohen HE. Dual tracer imaging for localization of parathyroid lesions. *Clin Nucl Med* 1986;11:237–241.

76. Hauty M, Swartz K, McClung M et al. Technetium thallium scintiscaning for localization of parathyroid adenomas and hyperplasia: a reappraisal. *Am J Surg* 1987;153:479–486.

77. Greenberg SB, Park CH, Intenzo C. Dynamic or early imaging in dual tracer parathyroid scintigraphy. *Clin Nucl Med* 1986;11:627–628.

78. Jones AG, Abrams MJ, Davison A et al. Biological studies of a new class of technetium complexes: the hexakis (alkylisonitrile) technetium (I) cations. *Int J Nucl Med Biol* 1984;11:225–234.

79. Piwnica-Worms D, Kronauge JF, Holman BL et al. Comparative myocardial uptake characteristics of hexakis (alkylisonitrile) technetium (I) complexes: effect of lipophilicity. *Invest Rad* 1989;24:25–29.

80. Holman BL, Jones AG, Lister-James J et al. A new Tc-99m-labeled myocardial imaging agent, hexakis (t-butylisonitrile) technetium (I) [Tc-99m TBI]: initial experience in the human. *J Nucl Med* 1984;25:1350–1355.

81. Wackers FJTh, Berman DS, Maddahi J et al. Technetium-99m hexakis 2-methoxyisobutyl isonitrile: human biodistribution, dosimetry, safety, and preliminary comparison to thallium-201 for myocardial perfusion imaging. *J Nucl Med* 1989;30:301–311.

82. Maffioli L, Steens J, Pauwels E et al. Applications of 99mTc-sestamibi in oncology. *Tumori* 1996;82:12–21.

83. Hassan IM, Sahweil A, Constantinides C et al. Uptake and kinetics of Tc-99m hexakis 2-methoxy isobutyl isonitrile in benign and malignant lesions in the lungs. *Clin Nucl Med* 1989;14:333–340.

84. Yamamoto Y, Nishiyama Y, Satoh K et al. Comparative evaluation of Tc-99m MIBI and Tl-201 chloride SPECT in non-small-cell lung cancer mediastinal lymph node metastases. *Clin Nucl Med* 2000;25:29–32.

85. Chiu ML, Kronange JF, Piwnica-Worms D. Effect of mitochondrial and plasma-membrane potentials on accumulation of hexakis (2-methoxyisobutylisonitrile) technetium in cultured mouse fibroblasts. *J Nucl Med* 1990;31:1646–1653.

86. Crane P, Laliberte R, Heminway S et al. Effect of mitochondrial viability and metabolism on technetium-99m-sestamibi myocardial retention. *Eur J Nucl Med* 1993;20:20–25.

87. Backus M, Piwnica-Worms D, Hockett D et al. Microprobe analysis of Tc-MIBI in heart cells: calculation of mitochondrial membrane potential. *Am J Physiol* 1993;265:178–187.

88. Sandrock D, Merino MJ, Norton JA et al. Ultrastructural histology correlates with results of thallium 201/technetium 99m parathyroid subtraction scintigraphy. *J Nucl Med* 1993;34:24–29.

89. Carpentier A, Jeannotte S, Verreault J et al. Preoperative localization of parathyroid lesions in hyperparathyroidism: relationship between technetium-99m-MIBI uptake and oxyphil cell content. *J Nucl Med* 1998;39:1441–1444.

90. Staudenherz A, Telfeyan D, Steiner F et al. Scintigraphic pitfalls in giant parathyroid glands. *J Nucl Med* 1995;36:467–469.

91. Benard F, LeFebre B, Beuvon F et al. Parathyroid scintigraphy: rapid washout of technetium 99m MIBI from a large parathyroid adenoma. *J Nucl Med* 1995;34:241–243.

92. Mitchell BK, Cornelius EA, Zoghbi S et al. Mechanisms of technetium-99m-sestamibi parathyroid imaging and the possible role of p-glycoprotein. *Surgery* 1996;120:1039–1045.

93. Erdil TY, Onsel C, Kanmaz B et al. Comparison of 99mTc-methoxyisobutyl isonitrile and 201T1 scintigraphy in visualization of suppressed thyroid tissue. *J Nucl Med* 2000;4:1163–1167.

94. Osmanagaoglu K, Schelstraete K, Lippens M et al. Visualization of parathyroid adenoma with Tc-99m MIBI in a case with iodine saturation and impaired thallium uptake. *Clin Nucl Med* 1993;18:214–216.

95. Alonso O, Mut F, Lago G et al. 99Tc(m)-MIBI scanning of the thyroid gland in patients with markedly decreased pertechnetate uptake. *Nucl Med Commun* 1998;19:257–261.

96. Scott AM, Kostakoglu L, O'Brien JP et al. Comparison of technetium

99m MIBI and thallium 201 chloride uptake in primary thyroid lymphoma. *J Nucl Med* 1992;33:1396–1398.

97. Ng DC, Sundram FX, Sin AE. 99mTc-sestamibi and 131I whole-body scintigraphy and initial serum thyroglobulin in the management of differentiated thyroid carcinoma. *J Nucl Med* 2000;41:631–635.

98. Dadparvar S, Chevres A, Tulchinsky M et al. Clinical utility of technetium-99m methoxisobutylisonitrile imaging in differentiated thyroid carcinoma: comparison with thallium-201 and iodine-131 Na scintigraphy, and serum thyroglobulin quantitation. *Eur J Nucl Med* 1995; 22:1330–1338.

99. Klieger P, O'Mara R. A case of active sarcoid mimicking a mediastinal parathyroid adenoma on Tc-99m sestamibi imaging. *Clin Nucl Med* 1998;23:534–535.

100. Taillefer R, Boucher YV, Potvin C et al. Detection and localization of parathyroid adenomas in patients with hyperparathyroidism using a single radionuclide imaging procedure with technetium-99m-sestamibi (double-phase study). *J Nucl Med* 1992;33:1801–1807.

101. Laing VO, Frame B, Block MA. Associated primary hyperparathyroidism and thyroid lesions. *Arch Surg* 1969;98:709–712.

102. Mlikotic A, Mishkin FS. Visualization of the right atrial appendage during sestamibi scintigraphy. *Clin Nucl Med* 2000;25:848–849.

103. Numerow LM, Morita ET, Clark OH et al. Persistent/recurrent hyperparathyroidism: a comparison of sestamibi scintigraphy, MRI, and ultrasonography. *J Magn Reson Imaging* 1995;5:702–708.

104. Lee VS, Spritzer CE, Coleman RE et al. The complementary roles of fast spin-echo MR imaging and double-phase 99m Tc-sestamibi scintigraphy for localization of hyperfunctioning parathyroid glands. *AJR* 1996;167:1555–1562.

105. Giron J, Ouhayoun E, Dahan M et al. Imaging of hyperparathyroidism: US, CT, MRI and MIBI scintigraphy. *Eur J Radiol* 1996;21: 167–173.

106. Fayet P, Hoeffel C, Fulla Y et al. Technetium-99m sestamibi scintigraphy, magnetic resonance imaging and venous blood sampling in persistent and recurrent hyperparathyroidism. *Br J Radiol* 1997;70: 459–464.

107. Casas AT, Burke GJ, Mansberger AR Jr et al. Impact of technetium-99m-sestamibi localization on operative time and success of operations for primary hyperparathyroidism. *Am Surg* 1994;60:12–16.

108. Carter WB, Sarfati MR, Fox KA et al. Preoperative detection of sporadic parathyroid adenomas using technetium-99m-sestamibi: what role in clinical practice? *Am Surg* 1997;63:317–321.

109. Chheda H, Farrell C. Minimally invasive parathyroidectomy for primary hyperparathyroidism: decreasing operative time and potential complications while improving cosmetic results. *Ann Surg* 1998;64: 391–396.

110. Levin KE, Clark OH. The reasons for failure in parathyroid operation. *Arch Surg* 1989;124:911–914.

111. Brennan MF, Marx SJ, Doppman J et al. Results of reoperation for persistent and recurrent hyperparathyroidism. *Ann Surg* 1981;194: 671–676.

112. Gaz RD, Doubler PB, Wang CA. The management of 50 unusual hyperfunctioning parathyroid glands. *Surgery* 1987;102:949–957.

113. Carty, SE, Norton JA.. Management of patients with persistent or recurrent primary hyperparathyroidism. *World J Surg* 1991;15: 716–723.

114. Peck WW, Higgins CB, Fisher MR et al. Hyperparathyroidism: comparison of MR imaging with radionuclide scanning. *Radiology* 1987; 163:415–420.

115. Patow CA, Norton JA, Brennan MF. Vocal cord paralysis and reoperative parathyroidectomy. A prospective study. *Ann Surg* 1986;203: 282–285.

116. Jaskowiak N, Norton JA, Alexander HR et al. A prospective trial evaluating a standard approach to reoperation for missed parathyroid adenomas. *Ann Surg* 1996;224:308–322.

117. Irvin GL, Prudhomme DL, Deriso GT et al. A new approach to parathyroidectomy. *Ann Surg* 1994;219:574–581.

118. Carty SE, Worsey J, Virji MA et al. Concise parathyroidectomy: The impact of preoperative SPECT 99mTc sestamibi scanning and intraoperative quick parathormone assay. *Surgery* 1997;122:1107–1114.

119. Wilkinson RH Jr, Leight GS Jr, Garner SC et al. Complementary

120. Bonjer HJ, Bruining HA, Pols HA et al. Intraoperative nuclear guidance in benign hyperparathyroidism and parathyroid cancer. *Eur J Nucl Med* 1997;24:246–251.

121. Gallowitsch HJ, Fellinger J, Kresnik E et al. Preoperative scintigraphic and intraoperative scintimetric localization of parathyroid adenoma with cationic Tc-99m complexes and a hand-held gamma-probe. *Nuklearmedizin* 1997;36:13–18.

122. Haigh PI, Glass EC, Singer FR et al. The role of preoperative Tc-99m-sestamibi scanning and intraoperative gamma probe localization for minimally invasive parathyroidectomy. *J Nucl Med* 1999;40:50P.

123. Kotz D. Advancing medical care: the role of nuclear medicine in radioguided surgery. *J Nucl Med* 1998;39:13N,15N,21N.

124. Singer JA, Sardi A, Conaway G et al. Minimally invasive parathyroidectomy utilizing a gamma detecting probe intraoperatively. *Md Med J* 1999;48:55–58.

125. Sfakianakis GN, Irvin GL III, Foss J et al. Efficient parathyroidectomy guided by SPECT-MIBI and hormonal measurements. *J Nucl Med* 1996;37:798–804.

126. Sofferman RA, Standage J, Tang ME. Minimal-access parathyroid surgery using intraoperative parathyroid hormone assay. *Laryngoscope* 1998;108:1497–1503.

127. Norman J, Chheda H, Farrell C. Minimally invasive parathyroidectomy for primary hyperparathyroidism: decreasing operative time and potential complications while improving cosmetic results. *Am Surg* 1998;64:391–396.

128. Bergman JA, Pallant R. Thallium/technetium subtraction scanning for primary hyperparathyroidism: scan sensitivity and effect on operative time. *Ear Nose Throat J* 1998;77:404–407.

129. Norman J, Chheda H. Minimally invasive parathyroidectomy facilitated by intraoperative nuclear mapping. *Surgery* 1997;122: 998–1003.

130. Norman J, Denham D. Minimally invasive radioguided parathyroidectomy in the reoperative neck. *Surgery* 1998;124:1088–1092.

131. Howe JR. Minimally invasive parathyroid surgery. *Surg Clin North Am* 2000;80:1399–1426.

132. Berger AC, Libutti SK, Bartlett DL et al. Heterogeneous gland size in sporadic multiple gland parathyroid hyperplasia. *J Am Coll Surg* 1999;188:382–389.

133. Shen W, Sabanci U, Morita ET et al. Sestamibi scanning is inadequate for directing unilateral neck exploration for first-time parathyroidectomy. *Arch Surg* 1997;132:969–974.

134. Goldstein RE, Blevins L, Delbeke D et al. Effect of minimally invasive radioguided parathyroidectomy on efficacy, length of stay, and costs in the management of primary hyperparathyroidism. *Ann Surg* 2000; 231:732–742.

135. Sofferman RA, Nathan MH. The ectopic parathyroid adenoma: a cost justification for routine preoperative localization with technetium Tc-99m sestamibi scan. *Arch Otolaryngol Head Neck Surg* 1998;124: 649–654.

136. Wei JP, Burke GJ. Cost utility of routine imaging with Tc-sestamibi in primary hyperparathyroidism before initial surgery. *Am Surg* 1997; 63:1097–1100.

137. Roe SM, Brown PW, Pate LM et al. Initial cervical exploration for parathyroidectomy is not benefited by preoperative localization studies. *Am Surg* 1998;64:503–507.

138. Sosa JA, Powe NR, Levine MA et al. Cost implications of different surgical management strategies for primary hyperparathyroidism. *Surgery* 1998;124:1028–1035.

139. Robertson GS, Johnson PR, Bolia A et al. Long-term results of unilateral neck exploration for preoperatively localized nonfamilial parathyroid adenomas. *Am J Surg* 1996;172:311–314.

140. Sofferman RA, Nathan MH, Fairbank JT et al. Perioperative technetium Tc-99m sestamibi imaging: paving the way to minimal access parathyroid surgery. *Arch Otolaryngol Head Neck Surg* 1998;124: 649–654.

141. Hung GU, Wu HS, Tsai SC et al. Recurrent hyperfunctioning para-

thyroid gland demonstrated on radionuclide imaging and an intraoperative gamma probe. *Clin Nucl Med* 2000;25:348–350.

142. Grant CS, Charboneau JW, James EM et al. Reoperative parathyroid surgery. *Wien Klin Wochenschr* 1988;100:360–363.

143. Clark OH, Way LW, Hunt TK. Recurrent hyperparathyroidism. *Ann Surg* 1976;184:391–402.

144. Kadowaki MH, Fulton N, Scark C et al. Difficulties of parathyroidectomy after previous thyroidectomy. *Surgery* 1989;106:1018–1023.

145. Solbiati L, Giangrande A, De Pra L et al. Percutaneous ethanol injection of parathyroid tumors under ultrasound guidance: treatment for secondary hyperparathyroidism. *Radiology* 1985;155:607–610.

146. Wang CA. Parathyroid reexploration: a clinical and pathological study of 112 cases. *Ann Surg* 1977;186:140–145.

147. Shen W, Duren M, Morita E et al. Reoperation for persistent or recurrent primary hyperparathyroidism. *Arch Surg* 1996;131:861–869.

148. Kang YS, Rosen K, Clark OH et al. Localization of abnormal parathyroid glands of the mediastinum with MR imaging. *Radiology* 1993;189:137–141.

149. Decker PA, Cohen EP, Doffek KM et al. Subtotal parathyroidectomy in renal failure: still needed after all these years. *World J Surg* 2001;25:708–712.

150. Chesser Am, Carroll MC, Lightowler C et al. Technetium-99m methoxy isobutyl isonitrile (MIBI) imaging of the parathyroid glands in patients with renal failure. *Nephrol Dial Transplant* 1997;12:97–100.

151. Gasparri G, Camandona M, Abbona GC et al. Secondary and tertiary hyperparathyroidism: causes of recurrent disease after 446 parathyroidectomies. *Ann Surg* 2001;233:65–69.

152. McCall AR, Calandra D, Lawrence AM et al. Parathyroid autotransplantation in forty-four patients with primary hyperparathyroidism: the role of thallium scanning. *Surgery* 1986;4:614–620.

153. Garcia Vicente A, Soriano Castrejon A, Rodado Marina S et al. Minimally invasive parathyroid surgery with 99mTc-sestamibi scintigraphy and probe-radioguided surgery: preliminary results. *Rev Esp Med Nucl* 2000;19:403–408.

154. Gallowitsch HJ, Mikosch P, Kresnik E et al. Comparison between 99mTc-tetrofosmin/pertechnetate subtraction scintigraphy and 99mTc-tetrofosmin SPECT for preoperative localization of parathyroid adenoma in an endemic goiter area. *Invest Radiol* 2000;35:453–459.

155. Hiromatsu Y, Ishibashi M, Nishida H et al. Technetium-99m tetrofosmin parathyroid imaging in patients with primary hyperparathyroidism. *Intern Med* 2000;39:101–106.

156. Vallejos V, Martin-Comin J, Gonzalez MT et al. The usefulness of Tc-99m tetrofosmin scintigraphy in the diagnosis and localization of hyperfunctioning parathyroid glands. *Clin Nucl Med* 1999;24:959–964.

157. Giordano A, Marozzi P, Meduri G et al. Quantitative comparison of technetium-99m tetrofosmin and thallium-201 images of the thyroid and abnormal parathyroid glands. *Eur J Nucl Med* 1999;26:907–911.

158. Martinez-Lazaro R, Cortes A. Hyperplasia of all four parathyroid glands in renal failure visualized by Tc-99m tetrofosmin scintigraphy. *Nephrol Dial Transplant* 1999;14:1795–1796.

159. Apostolopoulos DJ, Houstoulaki E, Giannakenas C et al. Technetium-99m-tetrofosmin for parathyroid scintigraphy: comparison to thallium-technetium scanning. *J Nucl Med* 1998;39:1433–1441.

160. Vallejos V, Martin-Comin J, Mora J et al. Use of 99mTc-tetrofosmin scintigraphy in the diagnosis of patients with hyperparathyroidism. *Rev Esp Med Nucl* 1998;17:94–101.

161. Ishibashi M, Nishida H, Hiromatsu Y et al. Comparison of technetium-99m-MIBI, technetium-99m-tetrofosmin, ultrasound and MRI for localization of abnormal parathyroid glands. *J Nucl Med* 1998;39:320–324.

162. Gallowitsch HJ, Mikosch P, Kresnik E et al. Technetium 99m tetrofosmin parathyroid imaging. Results with double-phase study and SPECT in primary and secondary hyperparathyroidism. *Invest Radiol* 1997;32:459–465.

163. Fjeld JG, Erichsen K, Pfeffer PF et al. Technetium-99m-tetrofosmin for parathyroid scintigraphy: a comparison with sestamibi. *J Nucl Med* 1997;38:831–834.

164. Ishibashi M, Nishida H, Strauss HW et al. Localization of parathyroid glands using technetium-99m-tetrofosmin imaging. *J Nucl Med* 1997;38:706–711.

165. Giordano A, Meduri G. Differences between technetium-99m tetrofosmin and technetium-99m sestamibi in parathyroid scintigraphy. *Eur J Nucl Med* 1997;24:347.

166. Giordano A, Meduri G, Marozzi P. Parathyroid imaging with 99Tcm-tetrofosmin. *Nucl Med Commun* 1996;17:706–710.

167. Aigner RM, Fueger GF, Nicoletti R Parathyroid scintigraphy: comparison of technetium-99m methoxyisobutylisonitrile and technetium-99m tetrofosmin studies. *Eur J Nucl Med* 1996;23:693–696.

168. Aigner RM, Fueger GF, Wolf G. Parathyroid scintigraphy: first experiences with technetium (III)-99m-Q12. *Eur J Nucl Med* 1997;24:326–329.

169. Martin WH, Delbeke D, Habibian RH. Oncologic imaging. In: Habibian MR, Delbeke D, Martin WH et al., eds. *Nuclear medicine imaging: a teaching file.* Philadelphia: Lippincott Williams & Wilkins, 1999:619–722.

170. Neumann DR, Esselstyn CB Jr, MacIntyre WJ et al. Regional body FDG-PET in postoperative recurrent hyperparathyroidism. *J Comput Assist Tomogr* 1997;21:25–28.

171. Neumann DR, Esselstyn CB, MacIntyre WJ et al. Comparison of FDG-PET and sestamibi-SPECT in primary hyperparathyroidism. *J Nucl Med* 1996;37:1809–1815.

172. Neumann DR, Esselstyn CB Jr, MacIntyre WJ et al. Primary hyperparathyroidism: preoperative parathyroid imaging with regional body FDG PET. *Radiology* 1994;192:509–512.

173. Neumann DR, Esselstyn CB, Kim EY. Recurrent postoperative parathyroid carcinoma: FDG-PET and sestamibi-SPECT findings. *J Nucl Med* 1996;37:2000–2001.

174. Kebebew E, Arici C, Duh QY et al. Localization and reoperation results for persistent and recurrent parathyroid carcinoma. *Arch Surg* 2001;136:878–885.

175. Lawson MA, Targovnik JH, Chen K et al. Three cases of primary hyperparathyroidism (PHP) with prior failed surgery where culprit lesions were identified by 11C-Methionine positron emission tomography (PET) and accurately localized with PET-MRI coregistration. *Clin Positron Imaging* 2000;3:31–36.

176. Hellman P, Skogseid B, Oberg K et al. Primary and reoperative parathyroid operations in hyperparathyroidism of multiple endocrine neoplasia type 1. *Surgery* 1998;124:993–999.

177. Cook GJ, Wong JC, Smellie WJ et al. [11C]Methionine positron emission tomography for patients with persistent or recurrent hyperparathyroidism after surgery. *Eur J Endocrinol* 1998;139:195–197.

178. Sundin A, Johansson C, Hellman P et al. PET and parathyroid L-[carbon-11]methionine accumulation in hyperparathyroidism. *J Nucl Med* 1996;37:1766–1770.

179. Hellman P, Ahlstrom H, Bergstrom M et al. Positron emission tomography with 11C-methionine in hyperparathyroidism. *Surgery* 1994;116:974–981.

180. Adler LP, Akhrass R, Ma D et al. False-positive parathyroid scan leading to sternotomy: incidental detection of a thymoma by C-11 methionine positron emission tomography. *Surgery* 1997;122:116–119.

181. Mazzeo S, Caramella D, Lencioni R et al: Usefulness of echo-color Doppler in differentiating parathyroid lesions from other cervical masses. *Eur Radiol* 1997;7:90–95.

182. Reading CC, Charboneau JW, James EM. High resolution parathyroid sonography. *AJR* 1982;139:539–546.

183. Stark DD, Gooding, GA, Moss AA et al. Parathyroid imaging: comparison of high-resolution CT and high-resolution sonography. *AJR* 1983;141:633–638.

184. Clark OH, Duy QY. Primary hyperparathyroidism: a surgical perspective. *Endocrinol Metab Clin North Am* 1989;18:701–714.

185. Solbiati L, Montali G, Croce F et al. Parathyroid tumors detected by fine-needle aspiration biopsy under ultrasonic guidance. *Radiology* 1983;148:793–797.

186. Stark DD, Gooding GAW, Moss AA et al. Parathyroid imaging: comparison of high-resolution CT and high-resolution sonography. *AJR* 1983;141:633–638.

187. Lee VS, Spritzer CE. MR imaging of abnormal parathyroid glands. *AJR* 1998;170:1097–1103.
188. Seelos KC, DeMarco R, Clark OH et al. Persistent and recurrent hyperparathyroidism: assessment with gadopentelate dimeglumine-enhanced MR imaging. *Radiology* 1990;177:373–378.
189. Nakahara H, Noguchi S, Murakami N et al. Gadolinium-enhanced MR imaging of thyroid and parathyroid masses. *Radiology* 1997;202:765–772.
190. Stevens SK, Chang JM, Clark OH et al. Detection of abnormal parathyroid glands in postoperative patients with recurrent hyperparathyroidism: sensitivity of MR imaging. *AJR* 1993;160:607–612.
191. McIntyre RJ, Kumpe DA, Liechty RD. Reexploration and angiographic ablation for hyperparathyroidism. *Arch Surg* 1994;129:499–503.
192. Mitchell BK, Merrell RC, Kinder BK. Localization studies in patients with hyperparathyroidism. *Surg Clin North Am* 1995;75:483–498.
193. Bergenfelz A, Algotsson L, Roth B et al. Side localization of parathyroid adenomas by simplified intraoperative venous sampling for parathyroid hormone. *World J Surg* 1996;20:358–360.
194. Yamashita H, Noguchi S, Futata T et al. Usefulness of quick intraoperative measurements of intact parathyroid hormone in the surgical management of hyperparathyroidism. *Biomed Pharmacother* 2000;54(Suppl 1):108s–111s.
195. Erdman WA, Breslau NA, Weinreb JC et al. Noninvasive localization of parathyroid adenomas: comparison of X-ray computerized tomography, ultrasound, scintigraphy and MRI. *Magn Reson Imaging* 1989;7:187–194.

33

BONE DENSITOMETRY AND THE DIAGNOSIS OF OSTEOPOROSIS

GLEN M. BLAKE
IGNAC FOGELMAN

Over the past decade, osteoporotic fractures have come to be recognized as one of the most serious problems in public health. For a 50-year-old white woman, the lifetime risk of suffering a fragility fracture is estimated to be 30% to 40%, which compares with the figures for breast cancer and cardiovascular disease of 9% to 12% and 30% to 40%, respectively (1). For men, the risks of an osteoporotic fracture are about one third of those in women. Fractures of the spine, hip, or wrist are the sites most often associated with osteoporosis, although epidemiologic studies show that fractures at most other sites in the skeleton are also implicated (2). In the United States in 1995 the total health care costs attributable to osteoporotic fractures exceeded $13 billion (3), a figure that is expected to rise to between $30 and $40 billion by the year 2020 (4). Of these costs, about two thirds are attributable to hip fractures. As well as incurring greater costs, hip fractures cause greater morbidity and mortality than other types of fracture. One in five people die in the first year after a hip fracture, and one in four older patients require a higher level of long-term care (5). Also, it should not be forgotten that fractures at other sites may also cause substantial pain and disability.

The increased recognition of the scale of morbidity and mortality attributable to osteoporosis has led to a major effort by the pharmaceutical industry to develop new treatments for the prevention of fractures (6–13). Estrogen deficiency following the menopause is one of the best-documented causes of postmenopausal bone loss and can be prevented by hormone replacement therapy (HRT) (14,15). Although estrogen is effective in preventing osteoporosis and in relieving menopausal symptoms, many women do not continue with HRT because of side effects such as bleeding, weight gain, and breast tenderness (16), as well as concerns about the risk of breast and other hormone-related cancers (17,18). Consequently, much effort has been devoted to developing alternative treatments for osteoporosis. Among these, the bisphosphonates (BPs) are becoming increasingly recognized as the treatment of choice at the present (19–21). An-

other new class of therapeutic agents is the selective estrogen receptor modulators (SERMs), compounds that mimic the beneficial effects of estrogen on osteoporosis while antagonizing the effects on the breast and uterus (22,23). The use of parathyroid hormone (PTH) is also being investigated and is likely to have a major impact on the treatment of osteoporosis in the next few years (24–26). Although PTH requires administration by daily self-injection, unlike estrogen, BPs, and SERMs it acts by stimulating bone formation rather than inhibiting bone resorption. It therefore leads to larger increases in bone density than these other treatments (25) and has been shown to dramatically reduce the incidence of vertebral and other fractures (26). It is important not to forget that nonpharmacologic approaches such as programs to reduce the number of falls in older adults (27–29) and the use of hip protectors (30) might also make an important contribution to the prevention of osteoporotic fractures.

Associated with the growing awareness of the significance of osteoporosis for public health and the development of new approaches to its prevention, the past decade has seen a rapid evolution of new radiologic techniques for the noninvasive assessment of skeletal integrity (31,32) (Table 33.1). The technique most associated with the recent growth in bone densitometry is dual-energy x-ray absorptiometry (DXA) (33). DXA was developed in the mid-1980s from the earlier technique of dual photon absorptiometry (DPA) by replacing the ^{153}Gd radionuclide source with an x-ray tube. With its advantages of high precision, short scan times, low radiation dose, and stable calibration, DXA has proved well suited to meet the need for scanning equipment to assist in the diagnosis of osteoporosis and to aid decisions about treatment.

THE DEFINITION OF OSTEOPOROSIS

In the early 1990s, a consensus meeting defined osteoporosis as "a systemic skeletal disease characterized by low bone mass and microarchitectural deterioration of bone tissue, with a consequent increase in bone fragility and susceptibility to fracture" (34). It should be noted that this definition does not require an individual to have sustained a fracture before a diagnosis of osteoporosis is made but introduces the concept of low bone

G.M. Blake: Department of Nuclear Medicine, Guy's Hospital, London, UK.

I. Fogelman: Nuclear Medicine, Division of Radiological Sciences, Guy's, King's and St. Thomas' Medical School, London, UK.

TABLE 33.1. *Characteristics of Different Bone Densitometry Techniques*

Technique	Regions of interest	Units reported	Precision (%CV)	Effective dose (μSv)
DXA	PA spine	BMD (g/cm^2)	1%	1–10
	Proximal femur		1–2%	1–10
	Total body		1%	3
QCT	Spine	BMD (g/cm^3)	3%	50–500
pDXA	Forearm	BMD (g/cm^2)	1–2%	0.1
	Calcaneus		1–2%	0.1
pQCT	Forearm	BMD (g/cm^3)	1–2%	0.3
RA	Phalanx	BMD (g/cm^2)	1–2%	0.01–10
QUS	Calcaneus	BUA (dB/MHz)	2–5%	None
	Calcaneus	SOS (m/s)	0.1–1%	None
	Tibia	SOS (m/s)	1–2%	None
	Multi-site	SOS (m/s)	1–2%	None

DXA, dual energy x-ray absorptiometry; QCT, quantitative computed tomography; pDXA, peripheral DXA; pQCT, peripheral QCT; RA, radiographic absorptiometry; QUS, quantitative ultrasound; BMD, bone mineral density; BUA, broadband ultrasonic attenuation; SOS, speed of sound.

mass and its relationship to increased fracture risk. Although it could be argued that it is wrong to define a disease on the basis of what is essentially a risk factor, i.e., low bone density, there is nevertheless some logic to this because fractures tend to occur late in the disease process when skeletal integrity is already severely compromised. It is therefore desirable to identify those individuals at high risk with a view to instituting appropriate treatment.

Today, there is general agreement that measurements of bone mineral density (BMD) are the most effective way of identifying those patients most at risk of fracture. Indeed, the widespread availability of bone densitometry systems has led to working definitions of osteoporosis that are increasingly based on measurements of BMD. In 1994, a World Health Organization (WHO) study group recommended a clinical definition of osteoporosis based on a BMD measurement of the spine, hip, or forearm expressed in standard deviation (SD) units called T-scores (35,36). The T-score is calculated by taking the difference between a patient's measured BMD and the mean BMD of healthy young adults matched for gender and ethnic group and expressing the difference relative to the young adult population SD.

$$\text{T-score} = \frac{\text{Measured BMD} - \text{Young adult mean BMD}}{\text{Young adult standard deviation}}$$

A T-score indicates the difference between the patient's measured BMD and the ideal peak bone mass achieved by a young adult (37). A negative T-score therefore indicates either a failure to achieve the optimal peak bone mass or the subsequent effects of aging or disease on BMD. In the WHO report, a patient is classified as having osteoporosis if her T-score ≤2.5 at the spine, hip, or forearm (Table 33.2). The WHO study group also proposed an intermediate state referred to as osteopenia that was defined by a T-score between −2.5 and −1. A T-score ≥−1 was regarded as normal. A fourth state of "established osteoporosis" was also proposed, denoting osteoporosis as defined previously but in the presence of one or more documented fragility fractures.

The WHO study group definitions of osteoporosis, osteopenia, and normal are intended to identify patients with high, intermediate, and low risk of fracture, respectively. However, an important limitation of these definitions is that they apply only to DXA measurements of the spine, hip, or forearm. As will be discussed later, they cannot automatically be applied to other BMD measurement sites or to other technologies such as quantitative computed tomography (QCT) or quantitative ultrasound (QUS) (Table 33.1).

The rationale for the WHO definition of osteoporosis is that it captures around 30% of all white postmenopausal women (1). As explained previously, this figure approximates to the lifetime risk of fracture for a 50-year-old woman. In comparison, it can be argued that the WHO definition of osteopenia captures too high a percentage of women to be clinically useful, and nowadays this term is being used less often, particularly in the context of therapeutic decision making. In contrast, the WHO definition of osteoporosis has had a major influence on clinical practice, to the extent that if the question is "Does this patient have osteoporosis, yes or no?," this is now regarded as a T-score issue.

Alongside the T-score, another useful way of expressing BMD measurements is by using Z-scores (38). Like the T-score, the Z-score is expressed in units of the population SD. However, instead of comparing the patient's BMD with the young adult mean, it is compared with the mean BMD expected for the patient's peers, e.g., for a healthy normal subject matched for age, gender, and ethnic origin.

$$\text{Z-score} = \frac{\text{Measured BMD} - \text{Age matched mean BMD}}{\text{Age matched standard deviation}}$$

Table 33.2. *The WHO Study Group Recommendations for the Definitions of Osteoporosis and Osteopenia*

Terminology	T-score definition
Normal	T ≥ −1.0
Osteopenia	−2.5 < T < −1.0
Osteoporosis	T ≤ −2.5
Established osteoporosis	T ≤ −2.5 in the presence of one or more fragility fractures

From 35,36.

Although Z-scores cannot be used to diagnose osteoporosis, they nevertheless remain a useful concept because they express the patient's risk of sustaining an osteoporotic fracture relative to his or her peers. Every reduction of 1 SD in BMD equates to an approximately twofold increase in the likelihood of fracture (39). It follows that patients with a Z-score less than −1 are at a substantially increased risk of fracture compared with their peers.

TECHNIQUES AVAILABLE FOR BONE DENSITOMETRY

Table 33.1 lists the methods currently available for the noninvasive assessment of the skeleton for the diagnosis of osteoporosis and/or the evaluation of an increased risk of fracture. These include DXA, spinal QCT, peripheral dual-energy x-ray absorptiometry (pDXA), peripheral quantitative computed tomography (pQCT), radiographic absorptiometry (RA), and QUS. These techniques differ substantially in fundamental methodology, in clinical discrimination and utility, and in general availability and cost. Each is reviewed briefly in the following discussion. The reader can find further information about these techniques in several comprehensive reviews (31,32,40,41).

Dual X-Ray Absorptiometry

Over the past decade, DXA has established itself as the most widely used method of measuring BMD because of its advantages of high precision, short scan times, and reasonable cost. DXA equipment (Fig. 33.1) allows scanning of the spine and hip (Fig. 33.2**A** and **B**), usually regarded as the most important measurement sites because they are frequent sites of fractures that cause the greatest impairment to quality of life and the greatest morbidity and mortality. A measurement of hip BMD has been shown to be the most reliable way of evaluating the risk of hip fracture (39,42–44). Also, because of the metabolically active trabecular bone in the vertebral bodies, the spine is

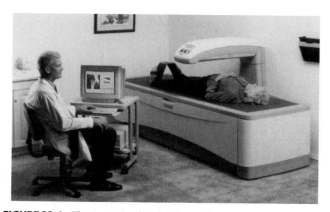

FIGURE 33.1. The Lunar Prodigy fan-beam dual-energy x-ray absorptiometry scanner (GE Lunar, Madison, WI). Densitometers such as this are most often used for measuring spine and hip bone mineral density but can also be used for total body, forearm, and lateral projection studies of the spine.

regarded as the optimal site for monitoring response to treatment (45).

The fundamental principle behind DXA is the measurement of the attenuation profiles through the body using x-ray photons of two different energies (33) (Fig. 33.3). Because the x-ray attenuation coefficient depends on atomic number and photon energy, separate measurement of the high- and low-energy x-ray profiles enables the soft tissue contribution to be subtracted from the low-energy attenuation profile. This leaves a bone attenuation profile that reflects the "areal" density (i.e., the mass per unit projected area) of bone mineral (hydroxyapatite). Because an image with high spatial resolution is not a prerequisite for a satisfactory measurement, radiation dose to the patient as measured by the effective dose is very low (1 to 10 μSv) (46) and is comparable to the average daily dose from natural background radiation.

It is widely recognized that the accuracy of DXA scans is limited by the variable composition of soft tissue. Because of its higher hydrogen content, the attenuation coefficient of fat is different from that of lean tissue. Differences in the soft tissue composition in the path of the x-ray beam through bone compared with the adjacent soft tissue reference area will cause errors in the BMD measurements, which have been examined in a number of studies (47,48). Svendsen et al. (48) reported a cadaver study in which the effect of fat inhomogeneity on the random component of the accuracy errors for BMD measurements in the spine, hip, and forearm were examined. The root mean square accuracy errors were reported to be 3% for forearm, 5% for spine, and 6% for femoral neck and total hip BMD.

The first generation of DXA scanners used a pinhole collimator, producing a pencil beam coupled to a single scintillation detector in the scanning arm. Since then the most significant development has been the introduction of new systems that use a slit collimator to generate a fan beam coupled to a linear array of solid state detectors. As a result, image resolution has improved, and scan times have shortened from around 5 to 10 minutes for the early pencil beam models to 10 to 30 seconds for the latest fan-beam systems. Radiation dose to patients is somewhat higher for fan-beam systems compared with pencil beam, and for centers with a larger patient workload it might be necessary to limit the resulting scatter dose to technologists by ensuring that the operator's console is at least 2 or 3 m from the patient (49).

Quantitative Computed Tomography

QCT has the advantage that it determines the true three-dimensional ("volumetric") bone density (units: mg/cm^3) compared with the two-dimensional areal density measured by DXA. QCT is usually applied to measure the trabecular bone in the vertebral bodies (50) (Fig. 33.4). The measurement can be performed on any clinical computed tomography (CT) scanner, if the patient is scanned with an external reference phantom to calibrate the CT numbers to bone equivalent values. Most CT manufacturers provide a software package to automate the placement of the regions-of-interest (ROIs) within the vertebral bodies. Patient dose is much lower than for standard CT scans, if the examination is performed correctly (51). QCT studies are generally per-

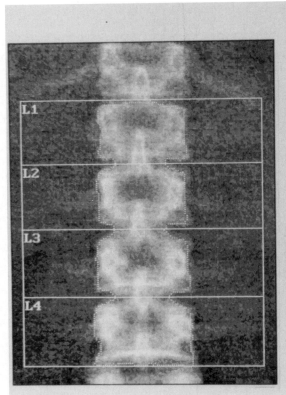

BMD(L1-L4) = 0.797 g/cm^2

Region	BMD	T(30.0)		Z	
L1	0.702	-2.02	76%	-1.68	79%
L2	0.764	-2.40	74%	-2.01	78%
L3	0.825	-2.35	76%	-1.95	79%
L4	0.873	-2.21	78%	-1.79	82%
L1-L4	0.797	-2.27	76%	-1.88	79%

A

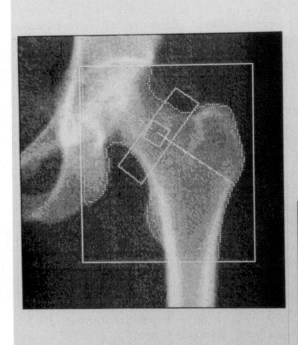

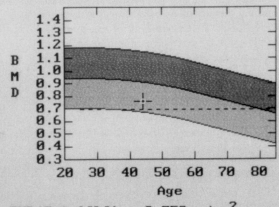

BMD(Total[L]) = 0.752 g/cm^2

Region	BMD	T		Z	
Neck	0.571	-2.51 (25.0)	67%	-2.11	71%
Troch	0.577	-1.25 (25.0)	82%	-1.05	84%
Inter	0.905	-1.26 (35.0)	82%	-1.12	84%
TOTAL	0.752	-1.56 (25.0)	80%	-1.30	83%
Ward's	0.495	-2.04 (25.0)	67%	-1.23	77%

B

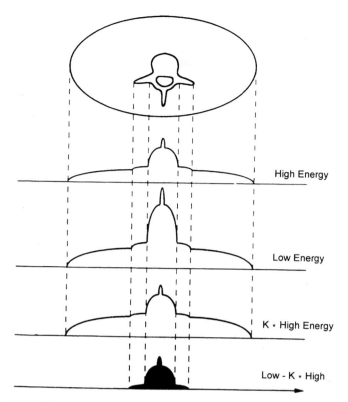

FIGURE 33.3. The principles of operation of a dual-energy x-ray absorptiometry scanner. The top two profiles show the attenuation curves for the high-energy and the low-energy photons in the x-ray beam. The high-energy profile is then multiplied by a factor *k* so that the soft tissue attenuation matches that in the low-energy profile. When the modified high-energy profile is subtracted from the low-energy profile the distribution of bone mineral density is left.

High Energy

Low Energy

K * High Energy

Low - K * High

formed using a single kV setting (single energy QCT), when the principal source of error is the variable composition of the bone marrow. However, a dual-kV scan (dual-energy QCT) is also possible. This reduces the accuracy errors but at the price of poorer precision and higher radiation dose. The advantage of spinal QCT is the high responsiveness of the vertebral trabecular bone to aging and disease (32,50). The principal disadvantage is the cost of the equipment.

Peripheral DXA, Peripheral QCT, and Radiographic Absorptiometry

Despite the widespread popularity of spine and hip DXA, there is continuing interest in the development of new devices for

assessing the peripheral skeleton (52). The first bone densitometers were forearm scanners that used the technique of single photon absorptiometry (SPA) based on a ^{125}I radionuclide source (53). Follow-up of patients after SPA studies has shown that forearm bone density measurements can predict fracture risk over 25 years (54). In recent years the technology has been updated by replacing the radionuclide source with a low voltage x-ray tube (40 to 60 kV_p) and by using the principles of DXA to perform BMD scans of the distal forearm (Fig. 33.5**A** and **B**) and the calcaneus. The advantages of pDXA systems include the small footprint of the devices, relatively low cost, and extremely low effective dose [0.1 μSv (55)].

Just as pDXA devices were developed as an alternative to DXA scanning of the central skeleton, small dedicated pQCT systems are also available for measuring the forearm (52). These devices have the advantage of separating the trabecular and cortical bone of the ultradistal radius and of reporting volumetric density. In addition to the use of pQCT measurements of trabecular bone (56) for the investigation of osteoporosis, the detailed geometrical measurements of the cortical shell also allow the calculation of structural parameters of bone strength that can be related to the fracture load at different skeletal sites (57).

RA is a technique developed many years ago for assessing bone density in the hand that has attracted renewed interest (52). It has the advantage of using conventional x-ray equipment with the addition of a small aluminum wedge in the image field for calibration. The radiographic film image is scanned into a personal computer (PC) and then processed automatically using a specially developed software application to measure BMD in the phalanges. Recently the technique has been further updated by the introduction of small tabletop units that incorporate direct digital acquisition of the x-ray image of the hand (Fig. 33.6). Another old technique that has been reintroduced with improvements derived from modern image processing is radiogrammetry in which bone mass in the forearm and phalanges is estimated from measurements of the outer periosteal diameter and the diameter of the inner medullary space made on a good quality radiograph. One advantage of RA and radiogrammetry is their potential for general use based on the widespread availability of conventional film radiography.

Peripheral x-ray absorptiometry methods such as those described previously have obvious advantages when selecting bone densitometry methodologies suitable for use in physicians' offices or in primary care clinics in the community. However, epidemiologic studies show that the discriminatory ability of peripheral BMD measurements to predict hip fractures is somewhat poorer than when hip BMD measurements are used (39,

FIGURE 33.2. **A:** Part of a computer printout from a dual-energy x-ray absorptiometry (DXA) scan of the spine. The printout shows (clockwise from left) *(1)* scan image of lumbar spine, *(2)* patient's age and bone mineral density (BMD) plotted with respect to the reference range, and *(3)* BMD figures for individual vertebrae and total spine (L1 to L4) together with interpretation in terms of T-scores and Z-scores. **B:** Part of a computer printout from a DXA scan of the hip. The printout shows (clockwise from left) *(1)* scan image of proximal femur, *(2)* patient's age and BMD for the total femur region-of-interest (ROI) plotted with respect to the NHANES III reference range (76), *(3)* BMD figures for five different ROIs in the hip (femoral neck, greater trochanter, intertrochanteric, total femur, and Ward's triangle) together with interpretation in terms of T-scores and Z-scores using the NHANES III reference range. (From Fogelman I, Blake GM. Different approaches to bone densitometry. *J Nucl Med* 2000;41:2015–2025, with permission.)

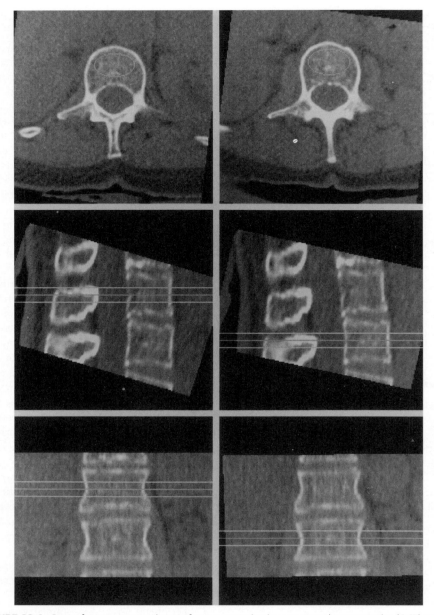

FIGURE 33.4. Part of a computer printout from a quantitative computed tomography (QCT) scan of the spine showing transverse, sagittal, and coronal images of two lumbar vertebrae. The study was analyzed using a commercially available QCT software package (Mindways Software Inc, San Francisco, CA).

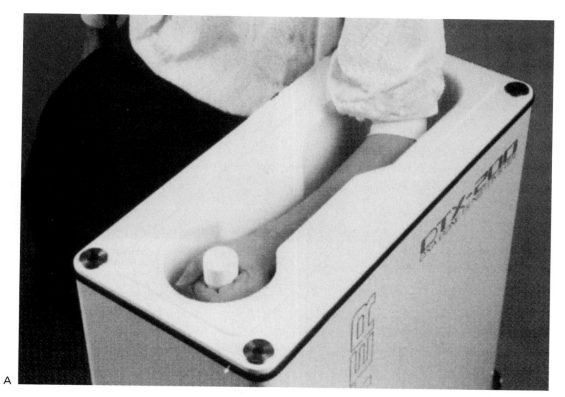

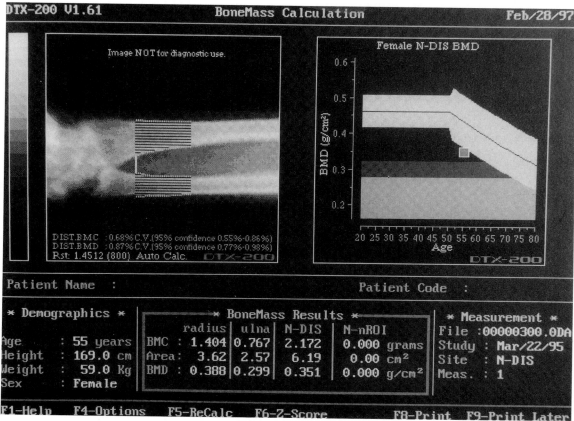

FIGURE 33.5. A: The Osteometer DTX-200 peripheral dual-energy x-ray absorptiometry (pDXA) scanner (Osteometer Meditech, Hawthorne, CA). Densitometers such as this are usually used for measuring forearm. Some pDXA systems can also make measurements of the heel. **B:** Computer printout from a pDXA scan of the distal forearm. The scan was performed on the DTX-200 system shown in **(A).**

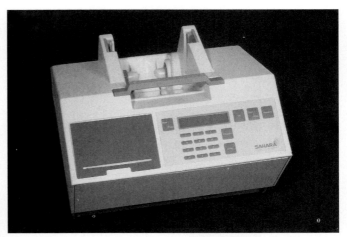

FIGURE 33.7. The Hologic Sahara system for performing quantitative ultrasound measurements in the heel (Hologic Inc., Bedford, MA). Devices such as this measure broadband ultrasonic attenuation and speed of sound in the calcaneus. In the Sahara system the two measurements are combined to provide an estimate of heel bone mineral density.

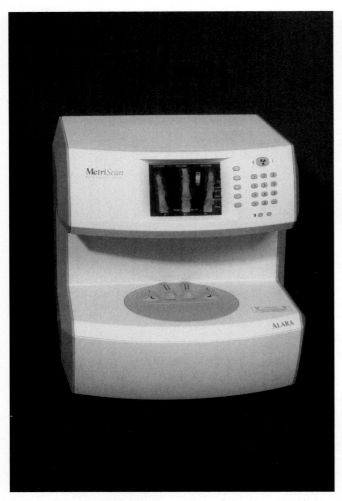

FIGURE 33.6. The Alara MetriScan digital radiography system for performing radiographic absorptiometry scans of the hand. Note the small calibration wedge is visible between the fingers on the scan image (Alara Inc., Hayward, CA).

42–44). Also, the changes in forearm BMD in response to HRT, BPs, and SERMs are relatively small, making such measurements less suitable than spine BMD for monitoring response to treatment (58,59). Finally, despite the fact that the radiation dose is extremely low, peripheral x-ray devices are subject to government regulatory requirements that control the use of radiography equipment, including the training of technologists and physicians in the principles of radiation safety.

Quantitative Ultrasound

QUS is a technique for measuring the peripheral skeleton that has raised considerable interest in recent years (41,52,60,61). There is a wide variety of equipment available, with most devices using the heel as the measurement site (Fig. 33.7). The calcaneus is chosen because it encompasses a large volume of trabecular bone between relatively flat faces and is readily accessible for transmission measurements. The physical principles of QUS measurements are outlined in Fig. 33.8**A–C.** An ultrasound

pulse passing through bone is strongly attenuated as the signal is scattered and absorbed by trabeculae. Attenuation (measured in decibels) increases linearly with frequency, and the slope of the relationship is referred to as the broadband ultrasonic attenuation (BUA) (Fig. 33.8**C**). BUA is reduced in patients with osteoporosis, because there are fewer trabeculae in the calcaneus to attenuate the signal. As well as BUA, most QUS systems also measure the speed of sound (SOS) in the heel by dividing the distance between the ultrasound transducers by the propagation time (Fig. 33.8**A**). SOS values are reduced in patients with osteoporosis because the loss of mineralized bone leads to a reduction in the elastic modulus. Some manufacturers combine the BUA and SOS values into a single parameter referred to as "stiffness" or the "quantitative ultrasound index" (QUI). These combinations have no particular physical meaning but may improve precision and discrimination by averaging out errors such as those caused by temperature variations (62). With early generation QUS devices the patient's foot was placed in a water bath to couple the ultrasound signal to the heel. However, most later devices are dry contact systems in which transducer pads covered with ultrasound gel are pressed against the patient's heel.

A major attraction of bone ultrasound devices is that they do not use ionizing radiation and therefore avoid the regulatory requirements for x-ray systems. Also, the instrumentation is relatively inexpensive and several devices, especially among the dry systems, are designed to be portable. Therefore, ultrasound could be more widely used than conventional DXA scanners, which are largely restricted to hospital-based osteoporosis clinics. Moreover, evidence from several large prospective studies of incident fractures confirms that QUS measurements are as predictive of hip fracture risk as other types of peripheral measurement (63–65).

However, there are a number of limitations to QUS measurements. In general, the fracture studies mentioned previously were conducted in older populations aged ≥70 years, examined only hip fracture risk, and used the earlier generation of water-based

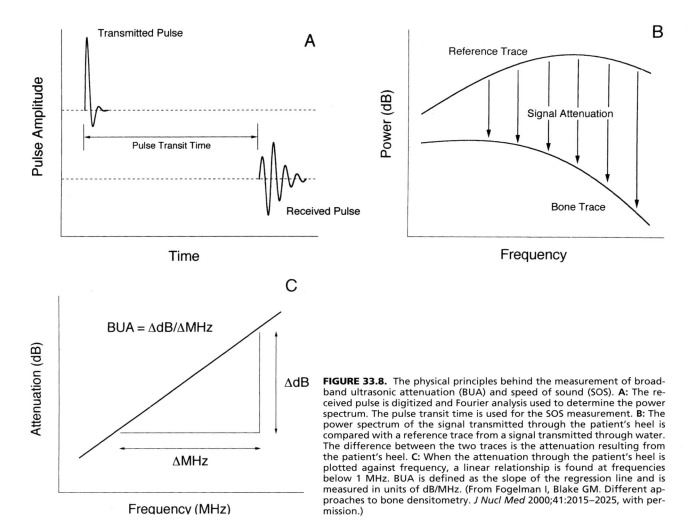

FIGURE 33.8. The physical principles behind the measurement of broadband ultrasonic attenuation (BUA) and speed of sound (SOS). **A:** The received pulse is digitized and Fourier analysis used to determine the power spectrum. The pulse transit time is used for the SOS measurement. **B:** The power spectrum of the signal transmitted through the patient's heel is compared with a reference trace from a signal transmitted through water. The difference between the two traces is the attenuation resulting from the patient's heel. **C:** When the attenuation through the patient's heel is plotted against frequency, a linear relationship is found at frequencies below 1 MHz. BUA is defined as the slope of the regression line and is measured in units of dB/MHz. (From Fogelman I, Blake GM. Different approaches to bone densitometry. *J Nucl Med* 2000;41:2015–2025, with permission.)

calcaneal QUS systems. Thus, the success of QUS in predicting fracture risk in younger patients remains uncertain. Another difficulty with QUS studies is that they are not readily encompassed within the WHO definitions of osteoporosis and osteopenia that, as emphasized previously, should be applied only to DXA scans of the spine, hip, or forearm. The difficulty with generalizing the WHO definition of osteoporosis to other types of measurement is that, although spine and femur T-scores measured by DXA decline with age in a generally similar manner, the relationship can be markedly different for other techniques such as QCT and at least some QUS devices (66) (Fig. 33.9).It is clear that a more inclusive paradigm than a T-score threshold of −2.5 applied to every technique is required if most types of peripheral measurement are to be properly incorporated. Recently, Kanis and Glüer (67) proposed that a measurement of hip BMD should be regarded as the gold standard for the definition of osteoporosis. For the other techniques, such as QUS intervention, thresholds would be developed so that measurements could be interpreted in terms of a 5-year hip fracture risk equivalent to that defined by a femur BMD T-score of −2.5. At the time of writing this review, these proposals to set up device specific equivalent T-scores are still under discussion (68).

There are also a number of technical limitations to QUS. Many devices use a foot support that positions the patient's heel between fixed transducers. Thus, the measurement site is not readily adapted to different sizes and shapes of the calcaneus, and the exact anatomic site of the measurement varies from patient to patient. However, this problem is avoided by imaging QUS systems that perform a raster scan of the heel and ensure a more consistent placement of the measurement site (69). Finally, it is generally agreed that the relatively poor precision of QUS measurements makes many devices unsuitable for monitoring patients' response to treatment (70).

RELATIONSHIP BETWEEN BONE MEASUREMENT SITES

The spine and hip are generally regarded as the most important BMD measurement sites because they are the sites of the osteoporotic fractures that cause the greatest impairment of quality of life and the greatest morbidity and mortality. Many would still consider spine BMD the optimal measurement because of its sensitivity to the changes associated with aging, disease, and

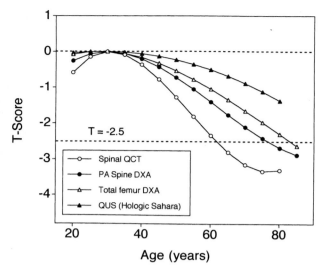

FIGURE 33.9. Age-related decline in mean T-score for white female subjects for *(1)* spine dual-energy x-ray absorptiometry (DXA) (Hologic manufacturer's reference range), *(2)* femoral neck DXA [NHANES III reference range (76)], *(3)* spinal quantitative computed tomography [data from Cann et al. (84)], and *(4)* quantitative ultrasound of the calcaneus [data from Frost, Blake and Fogelman (85)]. (From Blake GM, Fogelman I. Bone densitometry and the diagnosis of osteoporosis. *Semin Nucl Med* 2001;31:69–81, with permission.)

therapy. However, it has the disadvantage that in older adults the measurements are often affected by the presence of degenerative changes that lead to the artificial elevation of BMD values. This becomes an increasing problem after the age of 70 but can occur earlier. Others would argue that hip BMD is the most useful measurement because it is the most predictive of hip fracture risk (39,42–44), which is clinically the most important fracture. For this reason a consensus is developing that the femur should be the gold standard for bone densitometry measurements (67, 68). In practice, when DXA measurements are carried out, spine and hip BMD are usually both available for evaluation.

Because osteoporosis is common and is a primary care disease, there is a need for a simpler and more accessible evaluation than DXA of the central skeleton, which is generally found only in large hospitals. There is therefore considerable interest in pDXA and QUS devices because such systems are smaller and cheaper than DXA. Because osteoporosis is a systemic disease, bone loss is not limited to the axial skeleton. However, correlation coefficients between BMD measurements at different skeletal sites are typically around $r \approx 0.6$ to 0.7, and thus a measurement at one site is far from being a perfect predictor of that at any other. Correlations between QUS and BMD measurements are even poorer, with coefficients of around $r \approx 0.4$ to 0.5. Thus, whatever intervention threshold is chosen as the basis for recommending treatment, different groups of patients will be selected depending on the measurement site and technology in use. This raises the important questions of how well the different types of densitometry measurements perform at identifying the patients most at risk of fracture and how the advantage of one technique compared with another may be quantified.

WHICH MEASUREMENT IS BEST?

The most rigorous and convincing method of comparing the ability of different technologies and measurement sites to predict osteoporotic fractures is through prospective studies of incident fractures. One of the largest and most ambitious of these studies is the Study of Osteoporotic Fractures (SOF) that involved more than 9,000 women aged 65 years and older recruited in four regions of the United States (71). A commonly used descriptive approach to presenting data from such studies is to divide subjects into four quartiles based on their baseline BMD values and to plot the fracture risk for the patients in each quartile. Figure 33.10 shows SOF data for hip fracture risk (42) plotted in this way. The data show that patients in the lowest quartile of hip BMD have approximately ten times the risk of hip fracture of patients in the highest quartile. Statistical analyses of epidemiologic studies are performed using a "gradient of risk" model in which fracture risk increases exponentially with decreasing BMD (Fig. 33.10, inset). Mathematically, this is done using a proportional hazard model for prospective studies or logistic regression for cross-sectional studies (72). The results are expressed in terms of the relative risk (RR), which is defined as the increased risk factor for each 1 SD decrease in BMD.

The distribution of BMD values for the general population of healthy subjects of a given age approximates to a Gaussian curve. If the BMD values are expressed in Z-score units, the distribution curve has a mean of zero and a SD of 1.0 (Fig. 33.11**A**). When the Gaussian curve describing the general population is combined with the exponential equation describing the dependence of fracture risk on BMD to infer the BMD distribution of the future fracture population, this latter is predicted to be a second Gaussian curve with the same SD as the general population but with its peak offset to lower BMD values by a Z-score difference of $\beta = \ln(RR)$ (73) (Fig. 33.11**A**). By integrating the two Gaussian curves from $-\infty$ to any chosen BMD treatment threshold (say, the Z-score equivalent to a T-score of -2.5), the percentage of subjects in the fracture population and the general population with BMD values below the chosen threshold can be estimated and used to draw a receiver operating characteristic (ROC) curve that shows the true-positive fraction (those patients who later sustain a fracture and were correctly identified to be at risk) plotted against the false-positive fraction (those patients identified as being a risk but who never actually sustain a fracture) (73) (Fig. 33.11**B**). Fig. 33.11**B** shows that if treatment is recommended for patients with the lowest 30% of BMD values for devices with RR values of 1.5, 2.0, 2.5, or 3.0, the measurements will identify 45%, 57%, 65%, and 72%, respectively, of patients who later sustain a fracture. It is clear that the best technique in terms of providing the optimal discrimination of future fracture cases is the one with the largest RR value.

Fig. 33.12 shows SOF data presented by Black et al. (43) for the RR values for hip fracture risk for different BMD sites. With around 250 fracture cases included in this analysis, the study presents compelling evidence that hip fracture risk is best predicted by a measurement of femur BMD. For a wider view of the merits of measurement sites other than the hip, a meta-

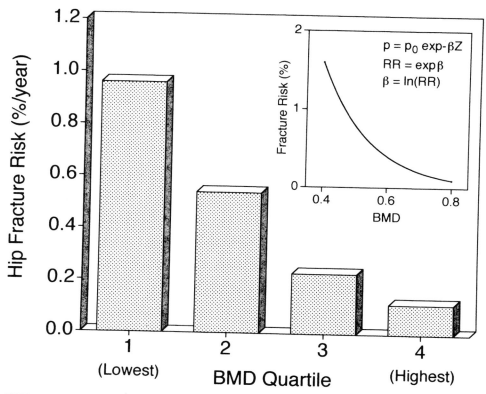

FIGURE 33.10. Incidence of hip fracture by bone mineral density (BMD) quartile for femoral neck BMD [data from Cummings et al. (42)]. The inset figure illustrates the gradient of risk model in which data from prospective studies of incident fractures are modeled by an exponential increase in fracture risk with decreasing BMD.

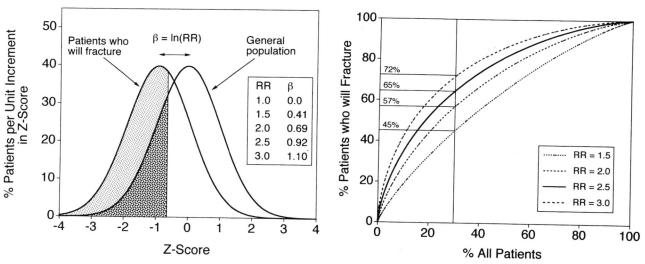

FIGURE 33.11. **A:** Gaussian curves representing the distribution of bone mineral density (BMD) values in a fracture population compared with the age-matched general population. The curve representing the fracture population has the same standard deviation as the curve representing the general population but is offset to lower BMD values by a Z-score difference of β = ln(RR). **B:** By integrating the two Gaussian curves in **(A)**, the percentage of subjects in each group who fall below any chosen BMD threshold can be estimated and used to draw receiver operating characteristic (ROC) curves that show the true-positive fraction (those patients who sustain a fracture and were correctly identified to be at risk) plotted against the false-positive fraction (those patients identified as being at risk but who never actually have a fracture). The ROC curves are drawn for relative risk (RR) values of 1.5, 2.0, 2.5, and 3.0. If a decision were made to treat patients with the lowest 30% of BMD values then devices with these RR values would identify, respectively, 45%, 57%, 65%, and 72% of patients who will later sustain a fracture.

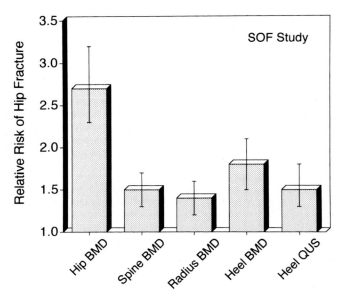

FIGURE 33.12. Relative risk values for 5-year hip fracture incidence for bone mineral density measurements of the femoral neck, lumbar spine, forearm, and heel and quantitative ultrasound measurements of the heel. The figure is drawn from data reported by Black, Palmero, and Bauer (43).

analysis of fracture studies is required. Such an analysis was published by Marshall et al. (39), and their collated data for the prediction of different types of fracture from BMD measurements at different skeletal sites are shown in Fig. 33.13. Although these results are consistent with the earlier conclusion that hip BMD is best for predicting hip fracture risk, the degree to which spine BMD best predicts vertebral fractures or radius BMD forearm fractures is less conclusive. Interestingly, when assessed by the ability to predict fractures occurring at any site, RR figures for different measurement sites are closely comparable.

REFERENCE RANGES

If the WHO criterion of a hip or spine DXA T-score ≤ -2.5 (or alternatively a device specific equivalent T-score for other types of measurement) is used to make treatment decisions, then it is apparent that any errors in the mean BMD or population SD of the reference group could have a significant influence on clinical decision making. The great majority of centers providing a scanning service use reference ranges provided by the equipment manufacturers, and issues over the accuracy of these ranges have caused controversy in the past (74). This continues to be a problematic area in view of the large number of new devices that are being introduced for the assessment of the skeleton. However, for femur DXA the problem is now largely resolved

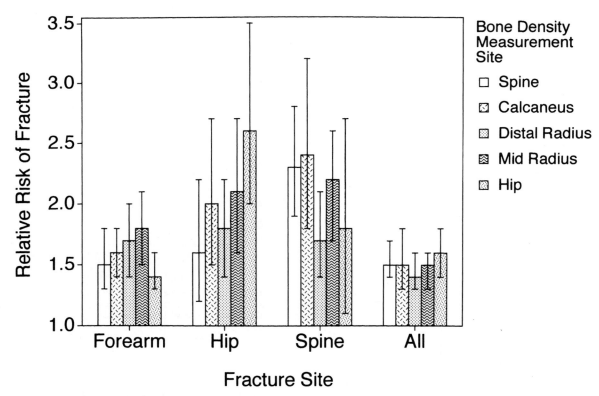

FIGURE 33.13. Relative risk values for fractures at different skeletal sites for bone density measurements in the spine, heel, distal radius, midradius, and hip. Data are taken from the meta-analysis of prospective studies collated by Marshall, Johnell, and Wedel (39).

after a report by the International Committee for Standards in Bone Measurement (ICSBM) (75), which recommended that hip BMD measurements should be interpreted using the total femur ROI and the hip BMD reference ranges derived from the U.S. NHANES III study (76). The NHANES III project studied a nationally representative sample of over 14,000 men and women with approximately equal numbers of non-Hispanic white, non-Hispanic black, and Mexican Americans. Data were gathered using densitometers operated from trailers so that subjects from all regions of the United States could be included. The ICSBM report recommends use of the total femur ROI instead of the previously widely used femoral neck site because of its improved precision and because it is the hip region that is most readily implemented on all manufacturers' systems.

Many centers have already acted on these recommendations, and they are increasingly being used for scan interpretation. It is important to note that these changes affect the percentage of patients who are diagnosed as having osteoporosis at the hip. Using the total femur ROI and the NHANES III reference range, fewer patients will be diagnosed as having osteoporosis, as compared with using the femoral neck ROI and the manufacturer's reference range (77). There is no definite right or wrong answer in this situation. What is more important is to have a consistent approach, and it is certainly highly desirable to have universally accepted DXA BMD criteria for the diagnosis of osteoporosis.

One advantage of presenting bone densitometry results in terms of T-scores is that they avoid the confusion caused by the raw BMD figures that differ for different manufacturers' equipment (78). The ICSBM Committee has addressed this latter issue by publishing equations that allow each manufacturer to express their BMD values on a consistent scale in standardized units (sBMD: units mg/cm^2) (75,79). Their report also included figures for the NHANES III total femur reference data converted into sBMD values.

CLINICAL DECISION MAKING

With the development of new treatments for preventing osteoporosis and the wider availability of bone densitometry equipment, much debate has centered on the issues of the clinical indications for the diagnostic use of bone densitometry and recommendations for the initiation of treatment based on the findings. In the United States, an influential report was published by the National Osteoporosis Foundation (NOF) (80). In Europe similar reports have been issued by the European Foundation for Osteoporosis (EFFO) (1), and in the United Kingdom by the Royal College of Physicians (RCP) (81).

The NOF report (80) included a sophisticated set of guidelines for therapeutic intervention. Various nomograms were developed that incorporate age, BMD, and four other risk factors for osteoporosis (Table 33.3). An interesting aspect of the NOF approach is that the calculations for therapeutic intervention are based on the concept of a quality adjusted life year (QALY) costed at $30,000. This is a relatively high value and one that would not be considered appropriate for application in Europe. This implies that there may have to be different BMD criteria

Table 33.3. *Risk Factors for Osteoporosis Additional to Age and BMD Incorporated in the NOF Guidelines for Therapeutic Intervention^a*

History of fracture after age 40
History of hip, wrist or vertebral fracture in a first-degree relative
Being in lowest quartile for body weight [≤57.8 kg (127 lb)]
Current cigarette smoking habit

BMD, bone mineral density.
^{a}Reproduced from National Osteoporosis Foundation guidelines (80,82).

for therapeutic intervention in different countries throughout the world. It also follows from the NOF approach that there will be different thresholds for intervention depending on the cost of treatment. Although the NOF report is an extremely important document with an extensive review of the relevant background information, it is nevertheless complex, and it is unlikely that primary care physicians will instigate treatment based on such a scheme. The NOF subsequently published a physicians' handbook with simplified recommendations that included the availability of BMD measurements for all women older than the age of 65 years and in all postmenopausal women younger than the age of 65 in whom clinical risk factors are present (82). Even if desirable, such a recommendation is simply not feasible in Europe at the present time.

Clinical guidelines for the prevention and treatment of osteoporosis in the United Kingdom were recently published by the RCP (81). These concluded that at present there is no consensus for a policy of population screening using BMD scans. Instead a case finding strategy is recommended for referring patients for bone densitometry based on a list of widely accepted clinical risk factors (Table 33.4). The list is identical to that previously published in the EFFO report (1). The RCP report also recom-

Table 33.4. *Risk Factors Providing Indications for the Diagnostic Use of Bone Densitometry^a*

1. Presence of strong risk factors
   - Estrogen deficiency
       Premature menopause (age <45 years)
       Prolonged secondary amenorrhoea (>1 year)
       Primary hypogonadism
   - Corticosteroid therapy
       Prednisolone >7.5 mg/day for 1 year or more
   - Maternal family history of hip fracture
   - Low body mass index (<19 kg/m^2)
   - Other disorders associated with osteoporosis
       Anorexia nervosa
       Malabsorption syndrome
       Primary hyperparathyroidism
       Posttransplantation
       Chronic renal failure
       Hyperthyroidism
       Prolonged immobilization
       Cushing's syndrome
2. Radiographic evidence of osteopenia and/or vertebral deformity
3. Previous fragility fracture, especially of the hip, spine, or wrist
4. Loss of height, thoracic kyphosis (after radiographic confirmation of vertebral deformities)

^{a}Table reproduced from the Royal College of Physicians guidelines (81).

mended a DXA T-score of ≤ -2.5 as the basis for instigating therapy.

It is important to emphasize that the WHO definition of osteopenia ($-2.5 < T < -1$) is not useful in isolation with regard to decisions about treatment, because it captures too high a percentage of postmenopausal women and, in fairness, was never intended to be used in this way. The evidence available from clinical trials indicates that it is the patients with the most severe disease who benefit most from antiresorptive therapies such as BPs (8,13). Thus there seems to be a consensus supporting the use of a T-score of ≤ -2.5 as the appropriate intervention threshold for instigating treatment in white women. However, it is important to take all the other relevant clinical factors into account such as those listed in Tables 33.3 and 33.4. In particular, the age of the patient and whether there is a history of previous fragility fractures are important independent predictors of future fracture risk.

No consensus has yet emerged on what intervention thresholds are appropriate in men and other ethnic groups. However, the revised guidelines recently published by Kanis and Glüer (67) recommended that the same absolute BMD thresholds applied to white women should also apply to these other groups.

WHAT IF DIFFERENT TYPES OF MEASUREMENT DISAGREE?

Given the wide range of different types of bone densitometry measurement now available, there is clearly cause for concern about the potential for conflicting findings between different techniques. If two types of measurement were to correlate perfectly ($r = 1.0$), they would identify exactly the same patients in the high-risk group. However, in practice different types of measurement often correlate poorly, with $r \approx 0.6$ to 0.7 between BMD results from different sites, and $r \approx 0.4$ to 0.5 between QUS and BMD measurements. This raises the issue of how concerned clinicians should be that, because of the imperfect correlations, different patients are selected for treatment on the basis of different sites and techniques.

To understand this problem, it should be borne in mind that there is no such thing as an absolute fracture threshold. As demonstrated by the normal distribution curves for fracture and nonfracture patients (Fig. 33.11**A**), there will always be a substantial overlap between measurements from these two populations. This situation is to be expected given that most osteoporotic fractures are multifactorial and, in addition to low BMD, will depend on other issues such as accidents and the propensity to fall. It is therefore clear that, depending on the rules agreed for the clinical interpretation of BMD measurements, only a certain percentage of those patients scanned who later go on to sustain a fracture will be identified as being in the high-risk group. Depending on the correlation coefficient between them, different types of measurement are identifying different individuals from this fracture group.

This situation is illustrated in Fig. 33.14, which compares the treatment decisions based on two different types of bone densitometry measurement referred to as BMD1 and BMD2 for 100 future fracture patients. For the purposes of Fig. 33.14

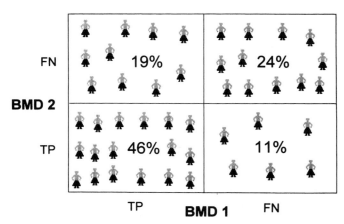

FIGURE 33.14. Comparative agreement of the interpretation of two different types of bone densitometry measurement for 100 future fracture patients. It is assumed that the two measurements have relative risk (RR) values of 2.5 for BMD1 and 2.0 for BMD2, that the correlation coefficient between the measurements is $r = 0.6$, and that patients are recommended for treatment if they are in the lowest 30% of bone mineral density (BMD) values. A total of 65% of patients would have true-positive (TP) scans based on a measurement of BMD1 compared with 57% based on BMD2. The figure shows that 46% of patients would have TP scans by both BMDs, and 24% of cases would have false-negative (FN) scans by both BMDs. The BMD1 measurement would identify 19% of patients in the high-risk group who were missed by BMD2, whereas the BMD2 measurement would identify 11% of patients missed by BMD1. The figure emphasizes that different types of BMD measurements select different groups of individuals from the total pool of patients that will eventually sustain a fracture and that the most effective technique is the one with the highest RR value.

it is assumed that the two types of measurements have RR values of 2.5 and 2.0, respectively; that the correlation coefficient between the measurements is $r = 0.6$; and that patients are recommended for treatment if they are in the lowest 30% of BMD values. A total of 65% of patients would have true positive scans based on a measurement of BMD1 compared with 57% based on BMD2. However, the BMD1 measurement would identify 19% of patients as at risk who were missed by BMD2, whereas the BMD2 measurement would identify 11% of patients missed by BMD1. Fig. 33.14 emphasizes that different types of BMD measurements select different groups of individuals from the total pool of patients who will eventually sustain a fracture and that the most effective technique is the one with the largest RR value.

It is clear that bone densitometry studies provide a measure of fracture risk that is analogous to assessment of blood pressure with regard to the risk of stroke or to measurement of cholesterol with regard to the risk of developing ischemic heart disease (39). BMD measurements are well suited to the study of populations, in which they are effective in identifying patients who have a higher than average risk of fracture but are less good at identifying those specific individuals who will later sustain a fracture.

SUMMARY AND CONCLUSION

The past decade saw the proving (in large clinical trials) of several types of new treatment for the prevention of osteoporosis such as BPs, SERMs, and PTH. Alongside these developments, the pace of technologic innovation was rapid, with the introduction of new radiologic methods for the noninvasive assessment of patients' bone density status. DXA scanning of the hip and spine remains the gold standard, although there is now a wider appreciation of the need for smaller, cheaper devices for scanning the peripheral skeleton if the many millions of women most at risk of a fragility fracture are to be identified and treated. Several sets of guidelines for the clinical use of bone densitometry have been published and most have included recommendations for intervention thresholds for initiating treatment in white women. The WHO criterion of a T-score ≤ -2.5 has been especially influential, although it cannot automatically be applied to the techniques other than DXA of the spine and hip or in men or patients from other ethnic groups.

At present, most experts do not advocate mass screening of the population for osteoporosis, and instead the guidelines recommend a case-finding strategy based on identifying patients with generally accepted clinical risk factors. However, with the widespread availability of QUS systems, this view may change. The advantages of QUS outlined previously mean that it may have a role in many specialist departments and primary care facilities. However, in view of the large number of commercial devices available, there are concerns about whether all the reference ranges are accurate and appropriate. As emphasized previously, the WHO definition of a T-score of ≤ -2.5 cannot automatically be applied to QUS, and there is a consensus emerging towards defining intervention thresholds for peripheral devices based on estimates of absolute fracture risk. It seems premature to advocate the routine use of QUS until these issues have been resolved and appropriate clinical strategies have been agreed. Nevertheless, it is probable that ultrasound will be widely used for the assessment of the skeleton within the next 5 to 10 years, and at that point there would effectively be screening for osteoporosis.

ACKNOWLEDGMENTS

Sections of this review article were adapted and modified with permission of the Society of Nuclear Medicine (83).

REFERENCES

1. Kanis JA, Delmas P, Burckhardt P et al., on behalf of the European Foundation for Osteoporosis and Bone Disease. Guidelines for diagnosis and treatment of osteoporosis. *Osteoporos Int* 1997;7:390–406.
2. Seeley DG, Browner WS, Nevitt MC et al. Which fractures are associated with low appendicular bone mass in elderly women? *Ann Intern Med* 1991;115:837–842.
3. Ray NF, Chan JK, Thamer M et al. Medical expenditures for the treatment of osteoporotic fractures in the United States in 1995: report from the National Osteoporosis Foundation. *J Bone Miner Res* 1997; 12:24–35.
4. Chrischilles E, Shireman T, Wallace R. Costs and health effects of osteoporotic fractures. *Bone* 1994;15:377–386.
5. Schurch M-A, Rizzoli R, Mermillod B et al. A prospective study on socio-economic aspects of fracture of the proximal femur. *J Bone Miner Res* 1996;11:1935–1942.
6. Chapuy MC, Arlot ME, Duboeuf F et al. Vitamin-D3 and calcium to prevent fractures in elderly women. *N Engl J Med* 1992;327: 1637–1642.
7. Black DM, Cummings SR, Karpf DB et al. Randomised trial of the effect of alendronate on risk of fracture in women with existing vertebral fractures. *Lancet* 1996;348:1535–1541.
8. Cummings SR, Black DM, Thompson DE et al. Effect of alendronate on risk of fracture in women with low bone density but without vertebral fracture: results from the Fracture Intervention Trial. *JAMA* 1998; 280:2077–2082.
9. Ettinger B, Black DM, Mitlak BH et al. Reduction of vertebral fracture risk in postmenopausal women with osteoporosis treated with raloxifene: results from a 3-year randomized clinical trial. *JAMA* 1999;282: 637–645.
10. Harris ST, Watts NB, Genant HK et al. Effects of risedronate treatment on vertebral and nonvertebral fractures in women with postmenopausal osteoporosis. *JAMA* 1999;282:1344–1352.
11. Reginster J-Y, Minne HW, Sorensen OH et al. Randomised trial of the effects of risedronate on vertebral fractures in women with established postmenopausal osteoporosis. *Osteoporos Int* 2000;11:83–91.
12. Chesnut CH, Silverman S, Andriano K et al. A randomized trial of nasal spray salmon calcitonin in postmenopausal women with established osteoporosis: the prevent recurrence of osteoporotic fractures study. *Am J Med* 2000;109:267–276.
13. McClung MR, Geusens P, Miller PD et al. Effect of risedronate treatment on hip fracture risk in elderly women. *N Engl J Med* 2001;344: 333–340.
14. Lufkin EG, Wahner HW, O'Fallon WM et al. Treatment of postmenopausal osteoporosis with transdermal oestrogen. *Ann Intern Med* 1992; 117:1–9.
15. Grady D, Rubin SM, Petitti DB et al. Hormone therapy to prevent disease and prolong life in postmenopausal women. *Ann Intern Med* 1992;117:1016–1037.
16. Ryan PJ, Harrison R, Blake GM et al. Compliance with hormone replacement therapy (HRT) after screening for postmenopausal osteoporosis. *Br J Obstet Gynaecol* 1992;99:325–328.
17. Collaborative group on hormonal factors in breast cancer. Breast cancer and hormone replacement therapy: collaborative reanalysis of data from 51 epidemiological studies of 52,705 women with breast cancer and 108,411 women without breast cancer. *Lancet* 1997;350:1047–1059.
18. Rodriguez C, Patel AV, Calle EE et al. Estrogen replacement therapy and ovarian cancer mortality in a large prospective study of US women. *JAMA* 2001;285:1460–1465.
19. Liberman UA, Weiss SR, Bröll J et al. Effect of oral alendronate on bone mineral density and the incidence of fractures in postmenopausal osteoporosis. *N Engl J Med* 1995;333:1437–1443.
20. Mortensen L, Charles P, Bekker PJ et al. Risedronate increases bone mass in an early postmenopausal population: two years of treatment plus one year of follow-up. *J Clin Endocrinol Metab* 1998;83:396–402.
21. Tonino RP, Meunier PJ, Emkey R et al. Skeletal benefits of alendronate: 7-year treatment of postmenopausal osteoporotic women. *J Clin Endocrinol Metab* 2000;85:3109–3115.
22. Delmas PD, Bjarnason NH, Mitlak BH et al. Effects of raloxifene on bone mineral density, serum cholesterol concentrations, and uterine endometrium in postmenopausal women. *N Engl J Med* 1997;337: 1641–1647.
23. Cummings SR, Eckert S, Krueger KA et al. The effect of raloxifene on risk of breast cancer in postmenopausal women: results from the MORE randomised trial. *JAMA* 1999;281:2189–2197.
24. Cosman F, Lindsay R. Is parathyroid hormone a therapeutic option for osteoporosis? A review of the clinical evidence. *Calcif Tissue Int* 1998;62:475–480.
25. Lindsay R, Nieves J, Formica C et al. Randomised controlled study of effect of parathyroid hormone on vertebral-bone mass and fracture incidence among postmenopausal women on oestrogen with osteoporosis. *Lancet* 1997;350:550–555.
26. Neer RM, Arnaud CD, Zanchetta JR et al. Effect of recombinant human parathyroid hormone (1-34) fragment on spine and non-spine fractures and bone mineral density in postmenopausal osteoporosis. *N Engl J Med* 2001;344:1434–1441.

27. Close J, Ellis M, Hooper R et al. Prevention of falls in the elderly trial (PROFET): a randomised controlled trial. *Lancet* 1999;353:93–97.

28. Robertson MC, Devlin N, Gardner MM et al. Effectiveness and economic evaluation of a nurse delivered home exercise programme to prevent falls. I: randomised controlled trial. *BMJ* 2001;322:697–701.

29. Robertson MC, Devlin N, Gardner MM et al. Effectiveness and economic evaluation of a nurse delivered home exercise programme to prevent falls. 2: controlled trial in multiple centres. *BMJ* 2001;322:701–704.

30. Kannus P, Parkkari J, Niemi S et al. Prevention of hip fracture in elderly people with use of a hip protector. *N Engl J Med* 2000;343:1506–1513.

31. Genant HK, Engelke K, Fuerst T et al. Noninvasive assessment of bone mineral and structure: state of the art. *J Bone Miner Res* 1996;11:707–730.

32. Grampp S, Genant HK, Mathur A et al. Comparisons of non-invasive bone mineral measurements in assessing age-related loss, fracture discrimination and diagnostic classification. *J Bone Miner Res* 1997;12:697–711.

33. Blake GM, Fogelman I. Technical principles of dual energy x-ray absorptiometry. *Semin Nucl Med* 1997;27:210–228.

34. Consensus Development Conference. Diagnosis, prophylaxis and treatment of osteoporosis. *Am J Med* 1993;94:646–650.

35. WHO Technical Report Series 843. *Assessment of fracture risk and its application to screening for postmenopausal osteoporosis.* Geneva: World Health Organization, 1994.

36. Kanis JA, Melton LJ, Christiansen C et al. The diagnosis of osteoporosis. *J Bone Miner Res* 1994;9:1137–1141.

37. Heaney RP, Abrams S, Dawson-Hughes B et al. Peak bone mass. *Osteoporos Int* 2000;11:985–1009.

38. Blake GM, Fogelman I. Interpretation of bone densitometry studies. *Semin Nucl Med* 1997;27:248–260.

39. Marshall D, Johnell O, Wedel H. Meta-analysis of how well measures of bone mineral density predict occurrence of osteoporotic fractures. *BMJ* 1996;312:1254–1259.

40. Blake GM, Wahner HW, Fogelman I. *The evaluation of osteoporosis: dual energy x-ray absorptiometry and ultrasound in clinical practice,* 2nd ed. London: Martin Dunitz, 1999.

41. Njeh CF, Hans D, Fuerst T et al. *Quantitative ultrasound: assessment of osteoporosis and bone status.* London: Martin Dunitz, 1999.

42. Cummings SR, Black DM, Nevitt MC et al. Bone density at various sites for prediction of hip fractures. *Lancet* 1993;341:72–75.

43. Black DM, Palermo L, Bauer D. How well does bone mass predict long-term risk of hip fracture? *Osteoporos Int* 2000;11(Suppl 2):S59 (abst).

44. Woodhouse A, Black DM. BMD at various sites for the prediction of hip fracture: a meta-analysis. *J Bone Miner Res* 2000;15(Suppl 1):S145(abst).

45. Eastell R. Treatment of postmenopausal osteoporosis. *N Engl J Med* 1998;338:736–746.

46. Njeh CF, Fuerst T, Hans D et al. Radiation exposure in bone mineral assessment. *Appl Rad Isotope* 1999;50:215–236.

47. Tothill P, Pye DW. Errors due to non-uniform distribution of fat in dual x-ray absorptiometry of the lumbar spine. *Br J Radiol* 1992;65:807–813.

48. Svendsen OL, Hassager C, Skodt V et al. Impact of soft tissue on invivo accuracy of bone mineral measurements in the spine, hip, and forearm: a human cadaver study. *J Bone Miner Res* 1995;10:868–873.

49. Patel R, Blake GM, Batchelor S et al. Occupational dose to the radiographer in dual X-ray absorptiometry: a comparison of pencil-beam and fan-beam systems. *Br J Radiol* 1996;69:539–543.

50. Cann CE. Quantitative CT for determination of bone mineral density: a review. *Radiology* 1988;166:509–522.

51. Kalender WA. Effective dose values in bone mineral measurements by photon absorptiometry and computed tomography. *Osteoporos Int* 1992;2:82–87.

52. Glüer C-C, Jergas M, Hans D. Peripheral measurement techniques for the assessment of osteoporosis. *Semin Nucl Med* 1997;27:229–247.

53. Cameron JR, Sorensen JA. Measurement of bone mineral *in vivo*: an improved method. *Science* 1963;142:230–232.

54. Düppe H, Gärdsell P, Nilsson B et al. A single bone density measurement can predict fractures over 25 years. *Calcif Tissue Int* 1997;60:171–174.

55. Patel R, Blake GM, Fogelman I. Radiation dose to the patient and operator from a peripheral dual x-ray absorptiometry system. *J Clin Densitom* 1999;2:397–401.

56. Schneider PF, Fischer M, Allolio B et al. Alendronate increases bone density and bone strength at the distal radius in postmenopausal women. *J Bone Miner Res* 1999;14:1387–1393.

57. Augat P, Reeb H, Claes LE. Prediction of fracture load at different skeletal sites by geometric properties of the cortical shell. *J Bone Miner Res* 1996;11:1356–1363.

58. Faulkner KG. Bone densitometry: choosing the proper skeletal site to measure. *J Clin Densitom* 1998;1:279–285.

59. Hoskings D, Chilvers CE, Christiansen C et al. Prevention of bone loss in postmenopausal women under 60 years of age. Early postmenopausal intervention cohort study group. *N Engl J Med* 1998;338:485–492.

60. Njeh CF, Boivin CM, Langton CM. The role of ultrasound in the assessment of osteoporosis: a review. *Osteoporos Int* 1997;7:7–22.

61. Njeh CF, Fuerst T, Diessel E et al. Is quantitative ultrasound dependent on bone structure? A reflection. *Osteoporos Int* 2001;12:1–15.

62. Nicholson PH, Bouxsein ML. Influence of temperature on ultrasonic properties of the calcaneus in situ. *J Bone Miner Res* 1999;14(Suppl 1):S498(abst).

63. Hans D, Dargent-Molina P, Schott AM et al. Ultrasonographic heel measurements to predict hip fracture in elderly women: the EPIDOS prospective study. *Lancet* 1996;348:511–514.

64. Bauer DC, Glüer C-C, Cauley JA et al. Broadband ultrasonic attenuation predicts fractures strongly and independently of densitometry in older women. *Arch Intern Med* 1997;157:629–634.

65. Pluijm SMF, Graafmans WC, Bouter LM et al. Ultrasound measurements for the prediction of osteoporotic fractures in elderly people. *Osteoporos Int* 1999;9:550–556.

66. Faulkner KG, VonStetton E, Miller P. Discordance in patient classification using T-scores. *J Clin Densitom* 1999;2:343–350.

67. Kanis JA, Glüer C-C. An update on the diagnosis and assessment of osteoporosis with densitometry. *Osteoporos Int* 2000;11:192–202.

68. Black DM. Revision of T-score BMD diagnostic thresholds. *Osteoporos Int* 2000;11(Suppl 2):S58(abst).

69. Fournier B, Chappard C, Roux C et al. Quantitative ultrasound imaging at the calcaneus using an automatic region of interest.*Osteoporos Int* 1997;7:363–369.

70. Glüer C-C. Quantitative ultrasound techniques for the assessment of osteoporosis—expert agreement on current status. *J Bone Miner Res* 1997;12:1280–1288.

71. Cummings SR, Black DM, Nevitt MC et al. Appendicular bone density and age predict hip fracture in women. The Study of Osteoporotic Fractures Research Group. *JAMA* 1990;263:665–668.

72. Hui SL, Slemenda CW, Carey MA et al. Choosing between predictors of fractures. *J Bone Miner Res* 1995;10:1816–1822.

73. Blake GM, Fogelman I. Peripheral or central densitometry: does it matter which technique we use? *J Clin Densitom* 2001;4:83–96.

74. Faulkner KG, Roberts LA, McClung MR. Discrepancies in normative data between Lunar and Hologic DXA systems. *Osteoporos Int* 1996;6:432–436.

75. Hanson J. Standardization of femur BMD [Letter]. *J Bone Miner Res* 1997;12:1316–1317.

76. Looker AC, Wahner HW, Dunn WL et al. Updated data on proximal femur bone mineral levels of US adults. *Osteoporos Int* 1998;8:468–489.

77. Chen Z, Maricic M, Lund P et al. How the new Hologic hip reference values affect the densitometric diagnosis of osteoporosis. *Osteoporos Int* 1998;8:423–427.

78. Genant HK, Grampp S, Glüer C-C et al. Universal standardization for dual x-ray absorptiometry: patient and phantom cross-calibration results. *J Bone Miner Res* 1994;9:1503–1514.

79. Steiger P. Standardization of spine BMD measurements [Letter]. *J Bone Miner Res* 1995;10:1602–1603.

80. National Osteoporosis Foundation. Osteoporosis: review of the evidence for prevention, diagnosis, and treatment and cost-effectiveness analysis. *Osteoporos Int* 1998;8(Suppl 4):S7–S80.

81. Royal College of Physicians. *Osteoporosis: clinical guidelines for prevention and treatment.* London, England: Royal College of Physicians, 1999.

82. National Osteoporosis Foundation. *Physicans guide to prevention and treatment of osteoporosis.* Washington DC: National Osteoporosis Foundation, 1998.

83. Fogelman I, Blake GM. Different approaches to bone densitometry. *J Nucl Med* 2000;41:2015–2025.

84. Cann CE, Genant HK, Kolb FO et al. Quantitative computed tomography for prediction of vertebral fracture risk. *Bone* 1985;6:1–7.

85. Frost ML, Blake GM, Fogelman I. Contact quantitative ultrasound: an evaluation of precision, fracture discrimination, age-related bone loss and applicability of the WHO criteria. *Osteoporos Int* 1999;10: 441–449.

Diagnostic Nuclear Medicine, Fourth Edition. Edited by M.P. Sandler, R.E. Coleman, J.A. Patton, F.J.Th. Wackers, A. Gottschalk. Lippincott Williams & Wilkins, Philadelphia 2003.

34

ADRENAL SCINTIGRAPHY AND METAIODOBENZYLGUANIDINE THERAPY OF NEUROENDOCRINE TUMORS

MILTON D. GROSS
BRAHM SHAPIRO
CHUONG BUI
BARRY L. SHULKIN
JAMES C. SISSON

The unique feature of the evaluation of adrenal disorders with radionuclides is the functional nature of the imaging information as contrasted with the principal anatomy-based imaging modalities of computed tomography (CT) and magnetic resonance (MR) (1). The radiotracers used to image the adrenal cortex and medulla are metabolic probes of adrenal and neuroendocrine physiology and provide information regarding individual gland function and anatomy (Table 34.1). In disorders of sympathomedulla tissues, scintigraphy provides whole-body screening for extraadrenal disease and possible radionuclide therapy of malignant pheochromocytomas and other neuroendocrine tumors. Adrenal gland imaging by any modality, however, is not indicated until the clinical and biochemical diagnosis of an adrenal cortical or sympathomedulla disorder is firmly established so that subsequent imaging procedures can be tailored to the best clinical and scintigraphic advantage.

ADRENAL CORTEX

Radiopharmaceuticals

Attempts at developing suitable radiopharmaceuticals for adrenocortical imaging have spanned the last four decades (2). In

M.D. Gross: Departments of Radiology (Division of Nuclear Medicine) and Internal Medicine, University of Michigan Medical Center, Ann Arbor, MI, and Department of Veterans Affairs Health System, Nuclear Medicine Service, Ann Arbor, MI.

B. Shapiro: Division of Nuclear Medicine, Department of Radiology, University of Michigan, and Department of Veterans Affairs Health Systems, Ann Arbor, MI.

C. Bui: Division of Nuclear Medicine, Department of Radiology, University of Michigan, and Department of Veterans Affairs Health Systems, Ann Arbor, MI.

B.L. Shulkin: Division of Nuclear Medicine, Department of Radiology, University of Michigan, Department of Veterans Affairs Health Systems, Ann Arbor, MI.

J.C. Sisson: Division of Nuclear Medicine, Department of Radiology, University of Michigan, Department of Veterans Affairs Health Systems, Ann Arbor, MI.

the 1960s, the biodistribution of ^{14}C-labeled cholesterol and other compounds important in adrenocortical metabolism were studied extensively. The rationale for evaluating cholesterol derives from the knowledge that it is a principal precursor in the synthesis of adrenocortical steroids.

In 1969, Counsell et al. (3) synthesized [131]I 19-iodocholesterol, a novel radiopharmaceutical, which provided adrenal-to-liver ratios as high as 168:1 and adrenal-to-kidney ratios on the order of 300:1. In 1970 the adrenal glands of a patient with Cushing's disease were successfully visualized using this agent (4,5).

A second radiopharmaceutical for adrenocortical imaging, ^{131}I-6-iodomethyl-19-norcholesterol (NP-59), first recognized as a contaminant formed in the synthesis of [131]I 19-iodocholesterol with significantly greater avidity for the adrenal cortex than its predecessor, was subsequently developed (6). NP-59 has greater *in vivo* stability and less deiodination with diminished thyroidal uptake of free ^{131}I activity than [131]I 19-iodocholesterol and, as a result of these attributes, is the radiopharmaceutical of choice for adrenocortical imaging (7,8). [75]Se has been used to label various cholesterol derivatives with imaging results that are similar to those obtained with NP-59. A ^{75}Se-labeled 6β derivative has been marketed outside of the United States as Scintadren (9).

Low-density lipoproteins (LDLs), the principal carriers of cholesterol, can also be labeled either with radioiodine ^{111}In or ^{99m}Tc metal chelates and show specific LDL-receptor mediated adrenocortical uptake (10). More recently reversible and irreversible inhibitors of enzymes of adrenal hormone biosynthesis have been used to image the adrenal cortex (11). Successful adrenocortical imaging in animals has been demonstrated with ^{11}C-etiomidate and ^{11}C-metiomidate, whereas an intermediate of aerobic metabolism, ^{11}C-acetate, has been used to image benign adrenal masses (12).

Factors affecting localization and metabolism of the radio-

Table 34.1. *Radiopharmaceuticals for Adrenal Gland Imaging*

Mechanism(s) of uptake	Radiopharmaceutical	Metabolic activity	Target
Receptor-mediated			
	[131]I-19-iodocholesterol	Mediated by LDL receptor[a]	Adrenal cortex
	^{131}I-6-iodocholesterol	"	"
	[131]I-6β-iodomethylnorcholesterol	"	"
	^{75}Se-selenomethylnorcholesterol	"	"
	[131]I, ^{123}I, ^{111}In, ^{99m}Tc-low density lipoproteins	"	"
Active transport into neurosecretory granules			
	^{123}I-metaiodobenzylguanidine (^{123}I-MIBG)	Neuronal blocker	Neuroendocrine
	^{131}I-metaiodobenzylguanidine (^{131}I-MIBG)[c]	"	"
	^{125}I-metaiodobenzylguanidine (^{125}I-MIBG)[c]	"	"
	^{131}I-aminoiodobenzylguanidine (^{131}I-AIBG)[c]	"	"
	[211]At-astatobenzylguanidine ([211]At-MABG)[c]	"	"
	^{11}C-epinephrine	Catecholamine	"
	^{11}C-hydroxyephedrine (^{11}C-HED)	Catecholamine analog	"
	^{11}C-phenylephrine	Catecholamine analog	"
	^{18}F-dopamine	Catecholamine	"
Metabolic intermediate			
	^{18}F-fluorodeoxyglucose (^{18}F-FDG)	Glucose analog	Neoplasms
	^{11}C-acetate	TCA intermediate[b]	Adrenal adenoma
	^{11}C-etiomidate/^{11}C-metiomate	Enzyme inhibitor	"

[a]LDL, low density lipoprotein
[b]TCA, tricarboxylic acid cycle
[c]therapeutic or potential therapeutic radiopharmaceutical.

cholesterols have been studied extensively by Gross et al. (13) (Table 34.2). The radiocholesterols are conveyed in plasma associated with specific transport LDLs. The effects of cholesterol on adrenal gland radiocholesterol uptake are multifactorial and may be a result of adrenal lipoprotein receptor, down-regulation, and pool dilution effects (14,15). Furthermore, uptake is positively influenced by corticotropin-releasing hormone (CRH) and adrenocorticotropic hormone (ACTH) and negatively influenced by dexamethasone (or other exogenous or endogenously secreted glucocorticoids) suppression of hypothalamic CRH and pituitary ACTH secretion (4,16).

Once located within the adrenal cortex, the radiocholesterol derivatives are esterified like native cholesterol but are not further metabolized. Thus, significant iodinated steroids or metabolites are not found following the administration of NP-59 (17). There is, however, an enterohepatic circulation of the radiocholesterol derivatives that may, at times (especially in studies using dexamethasone), interfere with adrenal imaging studies (18). The lack of mobilization of the radiocholesterol derivatives into the metabolic pathways of steroid hormone biosynthesis and the relatively large size of the intraadrenal cholesterol pool helps to explain the prolonged retention of these agents within the adrenal cortex, with discernible imaging of the adrenals for as long as 2 to 3 weeks after radiotracer administration (9).

Dosimetry

The dosimetry of NP-59 is shown in Table 34.3. Radiation exposures are not trivial and demand a confirmed clinical and biochemical diagnosis before imaging. The combination of dexamethasone will decrease adrenal cortical exposure by about 50% (19).

Table 34.2. *Drugs that Interfere with NP-59 and MIBG Uptake*

Mechanisms	Drugs
Radiocholesterol	
Inhibit aldosterone action on the distal nephron	Spironolactone
Suppress cortisol biosynthesis/secretion	Ketoconazole
Stimulate renin/angiotensin secretion	Diuretics
	Oral contraceptives
Suppress ACTH/cortisol biosynthesis/secretion	Glucocorticoids (i.e., dexamethasone)
Decrease cholesterol/stimulate LDL receptor	Cholesterol lowering agents
Decrease LDL receptor activity	Hypercholesterolemia/genetic
Metaiodobenzylguanidine	
Inhibition of type I uptake	Tricyclic antidepressants
	Cocaine
	Labetalol
Inhibition of uptake in neurosecretory granules	Reserpine
Granule uptake competition	Norepinephrine
	Serotonin
	Guanethidine
Granule content depletion	Reserpine
	Guanethidine
	Labetalol
	Sympathomimetic amines
Calcium mediated	Calcium antagonists

ACTH, adrenocorticotropic hormone; LDL, low-density lipoprotein.

Table 34.3. *Agents, Methods, and Dosimetry of Radiopharmaceuticals for Adrenal Scintigraphy*

Radiopharmaceuticals	NP-59[a]	SMC[b]	131I-MIBG	123I-MIBG[c]
Thyroid blockade[d] (SSKI 1 drop or Lugol's 2 drops in beverage tid)	Start 2 days before injection and continue for 14 days	Not required	Start 2 days before injection and continue for 6 days	Start 2 days before injection and continue for 4 days
Adult dose (i.v.)	37 MBq	9.25 MBq	18.5 MBq–37 MBq	370 MBq
Shelf-life	2 weeks; frozen	6–8 wks; room temp.	2 weeks; 4°C	24 h; 4°C
% Uptake/adrenal	0.07%–0.26%	0.07%–0.30%	0.01%–0.22%	0.01%–0.22%
Dosimetry (cGy/dose)	–	–	From package insert	From package insert
Adrenal	28–88	6.1	0.38–0.75	8–28
Ovaries	8.0	1.9	0.14–0.27	0.35
Liver	2.4	3.5	1.45–2.90	0.32
Kidneys	2.2	–	0.16–0.32	–
Spleen	2.7	–	1.10–2.20	–
Urinary bladder	–	–	1.40–2.80	–
Thyroid	150[e]	0.43[e]	0.17[e]–0.33[e]	17.7[e]
Whole body	1.2	1.4	–	0.29
Effective dose equivalent	–	–	0.35–0.70	–
Beta emission	Yes	No	Yes	No
Laxative (e.g., bisacodyl 5–10 mg p.o. bid)	Begin 2 days before & continue during imaging	No	Begin postinjection	Begin postinjection
Imaging interval postradiotracer administration (optional additional imaging times)	*Non-DS:* 1 or more days 5, 6, or 7 postinjection	7 (14) days postinjection	24, 48 (72) hours postinjection	2–6, 24 (48) hours postinjection
	DS: 1 or more early: (3), 4 & one or more late: 5, 6, or 7 days postinjection	(no large published experience with DS scans)		
Collimator	High-energy, parallel hole	Medium energy, parallel hole	High-energy, parallel hole	Low energy, parallel hole
Principal photopeak (abundance)	364 keV (81%)	137 keV (61%), 265 keV (59%), 280 keV (25%)	364 keV	159 keV
Window	20% window	20% window	20% window	20% window
Imaging time/counts (per view)	20 min/100K	20 min/200K (±SPECT)	20 min/100K	10 min (at 3 hours); 20 min/1M (±SPECT)

[a]131I-iodomethylnorcholesterol.
[b]75Se-selenomethylnorcholesterol.
[c]0%–1.4% 125I contamination.
[d]Patients allergic to iodine may be given potassium perchlorate 200 mg every 8 hours after meals or triiodothyronine 20 mg every 8 hours.
[e]No thyroid blockade (can be reduced to 1%–2% by iodide administration).
DS, dexamethasone suppression; K, thousand counts; M, million counts.
From Kloos RT, Khafali F, Gross MD, Shapiro B. Adrenal (Section 10). In: Maisey MN, Britton KE, Collier BD, eds. *Clinical nuclear medicine,* 3rd ed. London: Chapman and Hall Medical, 1998:359, with permission.

Technique

Patient Preparation

Patients are pretreated for 1 to 2 days before and for 10 to 14 days after radiopharmaceutical injection with saturated potassium iodide solution (SSKI), 3 drops twice daily, to block thyroidal uptake of free radioiodine. The thyroid may also be blocked with potassium perchlorate, 200 mg orally, at least 30 to 60 minutes before radiopharmaceutical injection and four times daily thereafter for 7 to 10 days after injection (8) (Table 34.3).

Dose and Route of Radiopharmaceutical Administration

The routine imaging dose of NP-59 is 1 mCi (37MBq)/1.7 m² of body surface area administered intravenously. The specific

activity ranges from 1 to 5 mCi (37 to 185 MBq)/mg of cholesterol base. The injection is given slowly over a 1- to 2-minute interval. The only adverse reaction encountered has been a tingling sensation in the arms and legs when a rapid injection technique has been used (8).

Imaging Sequence and Views Obtained

For standard or baseline scans without hormonal manipulation, imaging is performed beginning 4 to 5 days after radiopharmaceutical administration (Table 34.3). This allows for clearance of background activity. If at the time of initial imaging background activity is excessive, further delays of 24 to 48 hours usually yield more favorable target-to-background radioactivity ratios (8). 131I activity in the liver, colon, and gallbladder may interfere with visualization of the adrenal, and a mild laxative administered the day before imaging may be useful in an attempt to reduce colonic activity (20). Administration of a fatty meal or a cholecystagogue can be used to reduce gallbladder activity (21).

The posterior view affords the best single projection for adrenal imaging. In this view, the adrenals are nearest to the gamma-camera, and the patient may be studied prone, supine, or sitting. The preferred imaging device is a wide-field-of-view gamma-camera equipped with a high-energy, parallel-hole collimator. An 80-keV window is centered around 364 keV (8). Routine images are collected for a duration of 20 minutes or for a minimum of 50,000 counts/image. Lateral and anterior views are often necessary to fully interpret the findings on the posterior view. Single photon emission computed tomography (SPECT) imaging may be of utility in adrenal cortical imaging, despite the problems posed by low relative counts and the high-energy photon of ^{131}I (22) (Table 34.3).

Suppression Scans

Adrenal imaging in patients with non-cortisol-producing lesions often requires hormonal manipulation with suppression of pituitary ACTH secretion by dexamethasone. The current recommended dose is 4 mg of dexamethasone in divided doses every 6 hours for 7 days before NP-59 administration and for a 5-day postinjection interval or until the imaging sequence is completed (13,16) (Table 34.3). Coadministration of diuretics or spironolactone may also result in spurious, early adrenocortical imaging and misinterpretation of dexamethasone suppression studies (23). During suppression imaging, it is often helpful to localize the kidneys with a small amount of ^{99m}Tc-DTPA (9). This facilitates proper patient positioning before initiation of data acquisition and anatomic aids in the identification of adrenocortical activity.

ACTH-Stimulated Scans

ACTH can be used to stimulate the uptake of precursor LDL-derived cholesterol and radiocholesterol into the adrenal cortex. Given intravenously ACTH can be used to augment uptake in hypoadrenal states and to document function of otherwise suppressed glands in patients with Cushing's adenoma and in asymmetrically functioning adrenals in patients with incidentally discovered adrenal masses (24).

In more recent studies the absence of iodocholesterol uptake in a hyperfunctioning adrenal mass has been used to predict the success of catheter directed adrenocortical ablation therapy in patients with primary aldosteronism (25).

Interpretation of the Normal Adrenal Scintiscan

Following radiotracer injection, the concentration of radioactivity in the adrenal cortex rises rapidly and plateaus within the first 48 hours. However, the background activity remains high, and imaging is ordinarily delayed until 4 to 5 days after injection to achieve more favorable target-to-background ratios (8).

Gallbladder radioactivity can be confused with the right adrenal. In the posterior view, the gallbladder is inferolateral to the right adrenal, whereas on the lateral projection it can be readily recognized by its anterior location. When both adrenals are visualized, misinterpretation of gallbladder activity is rarely a problem. However, confusion can arise during dexamethasone suppression scintigraphy, especially with delayed or lateralizing patterns of adrenal visualization (21). Occasionally, colonic activity interferes with visualization of the adrenals. Laxatives should be administered and the imaging procedures repeated (20).

Clinical Applications

The clinical spectrum of adrenocortical neoplasms that can be approached with scintigraphy are outlined in Table 34.4.

Cushing's Syndrome

The initial application of adrenal imaging was in Cushing's syndrome in which diagnostic accuracy is greater than 95% in depicting hyperplasia, carcinoma, or adenoma as a cause(s) for glucocorticoid excess (8,9). However, anatomic imaging and selective intracranial venous sampling has been especially useful in depicting the central etiologies of ACTH-dependent Cushing's syndrome. The patterns of iodocholesterol imaging in hypercortisolism reflect the pathophysiology involved and are outlined in Table 34.5.

Excessive ACTH secretion from either pituitary or ectopic source(s) is the most common cause of Cushing's syndrome. Symmetric visualization of the adrenals in patients with bio-

Table 34.4. *Adrenal Gland and Related Neuroendocrine Tumors*

Cortex	Medulla/Sympathetic paraganglia
Adenoma	Pheochromocytoma[a] (benign and
Aldosteronoma	malignant)
Cushing's adenoma	Neuroblastoma
Androgen-secreting	Ganglioneuroma
Incidentally discovered[b]	Ganglioblastoma
(nonhypersecreting)	Paraganglioma
	Carotid body tumors
Hyperplasia[c]	Other neuroendocrine tumors[f]
(symmetric/asymmetric)	Carcinoid
	Medullary thyroid cancer
Adrenocortical carcinoma[d]	Islet cell tumors
Metastasis to adrenal	Insulinoma
	Glucagonoma
Gonadal neoplasms[e]	Somatostatinoma
	VIPoma
	Merkel cell

[a]familial (MEN IIA/MEN IIB), bilateral, extra-adrenal.
[b]can include cyst, myelolipoma, etc.
[c]non-adenomatous hyperfunction.
[d]hypersecretory malignancy.
[e]arrhenoblastoma.
[f]>imaging sensitivity with somatostatin analogs.
VIPoma, vasoactive intestinal peptide-secreting neoplasm.

Table 34.5. *Imaging Patterns in Cushing's Syndrome (Without Dexamethasone Suppression)*

Scintigraphic pattern	Type of Cushing's syndrome
Bilateral symmetrical imaging	ACTH dependent; hypothalamic; pituitary Cushing's disease; ectopic ACTH syndrome; ectopic CRF syndrome
Bilateral asymmetrical imaging	ACTH independent nodular hyperplasia[a] (However all causes listed above may rarely cause asymmetrical hyperplasia)
Unilateral imaging	Adrenal adenoma[b]; adrenal remnants[b,e]; ectopic adenocortical tissue[c]
Bilateral nonvisualization	Adrenal carcinoma[b,e]; severe hypercholesterolemia[d]

[a]Almost always asymmetrical.
[b]Cortisol secreting lesions suppress tracer uptake into contralateral gland.
[c]Usually only one focus present, occasionally more than one focus may be present in ectopic locations or metastatic sites.
[d]A potential cause for interference with the effectiveness of study.
[e]Very rarely tumors (and metastases) may accumulate sufficient tracer to image.
ACTH, adrenocorticotropic hormone; CRF, corticotrophin-releasing factor.

chemically confirmed glucocorticoid excess is invariably due to adrenal hyperplasia, and adrenal scintigraphy is rarely indicated as the cause(s) of glucocorticoid excess is elsewhere.

Asymmetric, but bilateral, NP-59 uptake (>50%) suggests ACTH-independent hyperplasia (8,26) (Fig. 34.1). It is important to recognize this imaging pattern because conventional medical or surgical treatment for ACTH-independent hyperplasia is not effective. Moreover, if nodular, marked asymmetric adrenal anatomy is demonstrated by CT or magnetic resonance imaging (MRI) a mistaken diagnosis of unilateral adrenal disease can be made, unilateral adrenalectomy would not be curative

because of unrecognized hyperplasia of the contralateral adrenal. Although an infrequent occurrence, this clinical dilemma illustrates the need for correlation of both anatomic and functional imaging information (8,27). In a review by Fig et al. (28), NP-59 scintigraphy correctly identified all cases of cortical nodular hyperplasia, whereas in the same series CT was less successful.

Nonvisualization of one adrenal gland with increased uptake in the other gland is characteristic of adrenal adenoma in patients with hypercortisolism (8,26) (Fig. 34.2). ACTH is suppressed by the excessive secretion of glucocorticoids and accounts for the nonvisualization of the normal gland. Adenomas as small as 0.5 cm in diameter have been identified as the etiology of this scan pattern (8). The scintiscan identifies both the abnormal physiology and the site of excessive glucocorticoid secretion with high sensitivity and accuracy (28). Bilateral nonvisualization in patients with Cushing's syndrome usually indicates the presence of a hyperfunctioning adrenocortical carcinoma (8). The accumulation of radiocholesterol by the tumor is typically inadequate for visualization, but excessive glucocorticoid secretion suppresses hypothalamic/pituitary trophic hormones (CRF and ACTH) and radiotracer uptake into the contralateral gland (29). There are, however, scattered reports of some functioning adrenocortical carcinomas and their metastases imaging with radiocholesterol. The degree of cellular differentiation may play a role in the ability to accumulate radiocholesterol in the visualization of these malignant adrenocortical neoplasms (28).

Primary Aldosteronism

The diagnosis of primary aldosteronism is established by finding elevated plasma and/or urinary aldosterone levels associated with low or suppressed renin activity (30). Primary aldosteronism can

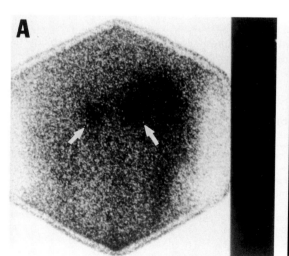 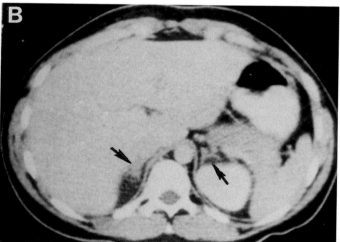

FIGURE 34.1. A posterior ^{131}I-6-iodomethyl-19-norcholesterol scan **(A)** in a patient with adrenocorticotropic hormone independent Cushing's syndrome. There is bilateral adrenal accumulation of iodocholesterol (*arrows*). The corresponding computed tomography scan **(B)** depicts an abnormal right and normal left adrenal. (From Fig LM, Ehrmann D, Gross MD et al. The localization of abnormal adrenal function in the ACTH-dependent Cushing syndrome. *Ann Intern Med* 1988;109:547–553, with permission.)

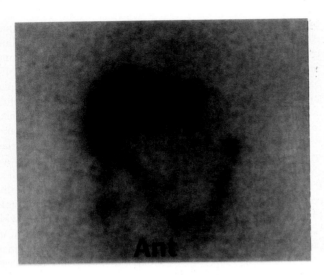 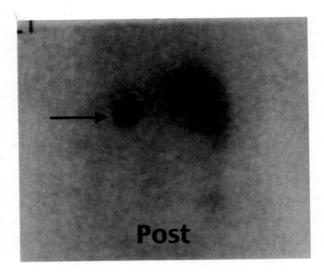

Day 4
(No Dex. suppression)

FIGURE 34.2. Anterior (*Ant*) and posterior (*Post*) ^{131}I-6-iodomethyl-19-norcholesterol scans in a patient with adrenocorticotropic hormone independent Cushing's syndrome with unilateral left adrenal accumulation (*arrow*) confirming the presence of hyperfunction of the left adrenal with suppression of the right adrenal gland.

be due to adrenal adenoma or to bilateral adrenal hyperplasia, and correct management is dependent on distinguishing these two diagnostic possibilities. Because aldosteronomas are small (usually less than 2 cm in diameter) and often associated with macronodules, it is difficult to unequivocally state that a "nodular" abnormality detected by CT or MRI is solely responsible for the hormone excess. Adrenal vein hormone sampling may be definitive but is invasive and has associated morbidity (30).

Dexamethasone Suppression Scans

To increase the specificity of adrenal scintigraphy, the dexamethasone suppression scan was introduced (31). The dose of dexamethasone used for scintigraphy has been empirically established to take advantage of the "window" of suppressibility of the normal adrenal cortex (suppression interval) and imaging to distinguish normal adrenal function from that of adenoma and bilateral adrenal hyperplasia (13,16).

Interpretation of the dexamethasone suppression scan depends on the time sequence after radiocholesterol injection during which the adrenal gland(s) visualize. Initial images are obtained on the second or third day following injection, and, if necessary, imaging continues daily until the fifth postinjection day. In normal subjects on dexamethasone suppression (4 mg daily for 7 days before iodocholesterol injection), the adrenals are either not visualized at all or are seen at the end of the imaging sequence (day 5). Early unilateral adrenal visualization (<5 days) suggests adrenal adenoma, whereas bilateral early adrenal visualization (<5 days) suggests hyperplasia (13,16) (Fig. 34.3) (Table 34.6). Using the suppression regimen outlined ear-

lier and these criteria, the accuracy of the dexamethasone suppression scan exceeds 90% (25,32). More recently, SPECT has been used to identify adrenal adenomas responsible for primary aldosteronism (33).

Adrenal Hyperandrogenism

Excessive androgen production can be due to hypersecretion from the ovaries or the adrenals or due to the peripheral conversion of precursor steroids to androgens (34). Although a nonadrenal source of the excess hormone production can be established in the majority of patients, those with an adrenal component

Table 34.6. *Scintigraphic Imaging in Aldosteronism (With Dexamethasone Suppression)*

Scintigraphic pattern	Type of aldosteronism
Symmetrical bilateral early imaging (before day 5)	Bilateral autonomous hyperplasia; secondary aldosteronism[a]
Unilateral early imaging (before day 5)	Unilateral adenoma (Conn's tumor); unilateral malignant aldosterone secreting tumor (rare)
Symmetrical late imaging (on or after day 5); nondiagnostic pattern	Normal adrenals; dexamethasone suppressible aldosteronism (rare)

[a]Should be excluded by measurement of renin and aldosterone levels and should not require imaging.

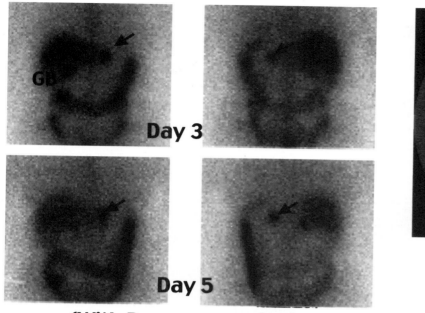

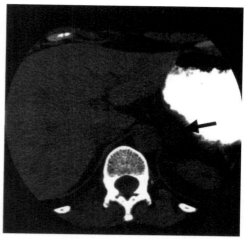

Day 3

Day 5

(With Dex. suppression)

A

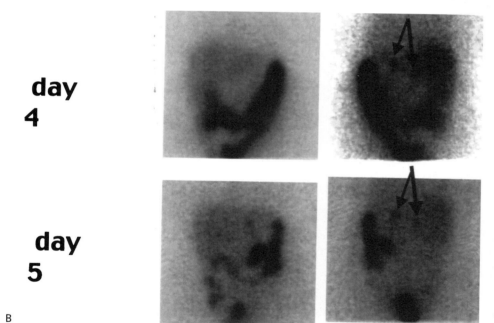

day
4

day
5

B

FIGURE 34.3. A: Dexamethasone suppression ^{131}I-6-iodomethyl-19-norcholesterol imaging in primary aldosteronism resulting from a left adrenal adenoma (*arrow*) at 3- and 5-days postinjection. Note the appearance of the right adrenal on the day 5 images. The computed tomography scan demonstrates an enlarged left adrenal (*arrow*). **B:** Bilateral adrenal hyperplasia (*arrows*) is depicted on dexamethasone suppression ^{131}I-6-iodomethyl-19-norcholesterol imaging as bilateral radiotracer accumulation on day 4 postinjection.

are probably greater than previously estimated (35,36). Dexamethasone suppression scintigraphy has been used to evaluate patients in whom an adrenal source of androgen hypersecretion is suspected (37).

Gonadal Hyperfunction

The excessive secretion of gonadal steroids has been depicted by the accumulation of iodocholesterol into abnormal glands. Because cholesterol is a precursor compound in the biosynthesis

of gonadal steroids, hyperfunction has been localized by scintigraphic techniques. Success has been reported in the identification of both ovarian (arrhenoblastoma) and testicular neoplasms (38–40). Incidental reports of nonneoplastic processes that have been imaged with iodocholesterol are rare. Localization of functional ovarian disease, such as hyperthecosis, stromal hyperplasia, or polycystic ovaries, has been demonstrated (41). Testicular imaging with iodocholesterol has been reported in normal subjects and patients with functioning neoplasms (42,43). Adrenal rest tissues have been identified within the testes of children with congenital adrenocortical enzyme deficiencies (44).

Incidentally Discovered Adrenal Mass (Incidentaloma)

A growing body of evidence suggests that adrenal gland asymmetry and nodularity found on CT examinations may be a normal finding (45). In the absence of clinical manifestations of adrenal gland dysfunction, these "lesions" have been referred to as "inci-

dentalomas" (45). Over the past few years a significant effort has been directed toward the noninvasive evaluation of these masses that include novel adaptations to imaging with CT or MRI as a means to distinguish nonhypersecretory, benign, adrenal masses from adrenal metastases and adrenocortical carcinoma (46). Gross and others have shown in euadrenal patients that the presence of radiocholesterol uptake by an adrenal mass identified on CT that exceeds the anatomically normal adrenal is most characteristic of a benign nonhypersecretory neoplasm (e.g., adenomas). Alternatively, diminished or absent radiocho-

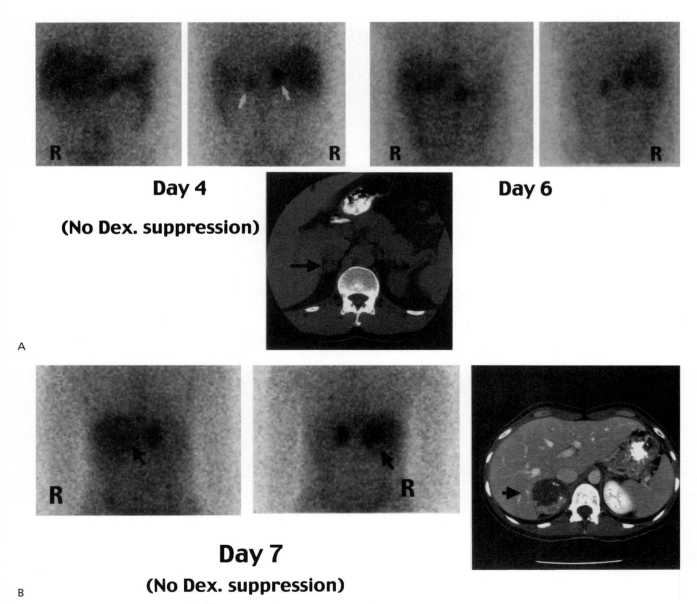

FIGURE 34.4. A: ^{131}I-6-iodomethyl-19-norcholesterol (NP-59) imaging in a patient with an incidentally discovered right adrenal mass. The uptake of iodocholesterol in the abnormal adrenal is greater that the contralateral anatomically normal gland (concordant imaging) and is compatible with a nonhypersecretory adrenal adenoma. **B:** NP-59 imaging in a patient with an incidentally discovered right adrenal mass (arrow). The uptake of iodocholesterol in the abnormal adrenal is less than the contralateral anatomically normal gland (discordant imaging) and is compatible with a space-occupying adrenal lesion.

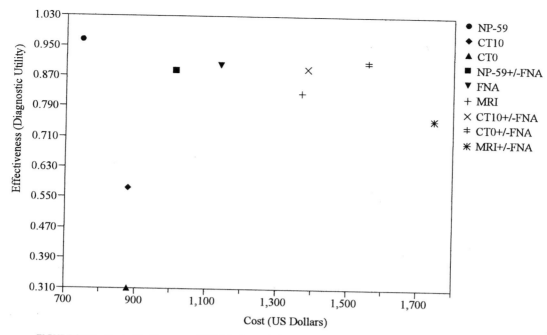

FIGURE 34.5. Cost effectiveness of ^{131}I-6-iodomethyl-19-norcholesterol in the evaluation of incidentally discovered adrenal masses in comparison to other diagnostic modalities. Effectiveness (diagnostic utility) is a probability-weighted utility of the four diagnostic test outcomes: true positive, true negative, false positive, and false negative. The assigned utility values range from −1 (worst possible or least desirable) to +1 (best possible or most desirable outcome) with intermediate values between −1 to +1. CT10, computed tomography (CT) cutoff for adenoma at 10 HU; CT0, CT cutoff for adenoma at 0 HU. (From Dwamena B, Kloos RT, Fendrick AM et al. Diagnostic evaluation of the adrenal incidentaloma: decision and cost-effectiveness analysis. *J Nucl Med* 1998;39:707–712, with permission.)

lesterol uptake by an adrenal mass is compatible with a space-occupying or malignant process (47) (Fig. 34.4) (Table 34.7). The scintiscan is thus useful in identifying those adrenal masses that would benefit from further diagnostic studies (i.e., adrenal biopsy) and is the most cost-effective means of evaluation when

compared with other routine, diagnostic modalities (48) (Fig. 34.5).

ADRENAL MEDULLARY IMAGING

Radiopharmaceuticals

Radiolabeled catecholamines and their analogs were among the first compounds evaluated as potential agents for imaging the adrenal medulla. ^{14}C-labeled dopamine demonstrated significant localization in the normal human adrenal medulla, as well as in neuroblastoma and pheochromocytoma (49,50). Iodination of dopamine was readily accomplished but provided an agent with insufficient adrenal medulla uptake for imaging (51). Other approaches have been attempted but were without success until attention was turned toward the neuronal blocking agents as potential compounds for adrenomedullary imaging (52). The original agent evaluated was bretylium, which demonstrated good adrenal medulla uptake in the dog but insufficient accumulation in man (52). Along these lines, Wieland et al. (53) evaluated a number of guanethidine analogs and among these, the iodobenzylguanidines radioiodinated in both the *para* and *meta* positions demonstrated avid concentration in the adrenal medullas of several experimental animal species. The *meta* isomer, metaiodobenzylguanidine (MIBG) demonstrated significantly earlier uptake with lower background activity and less *in vivo*

Table 34.7. *Scintigraphic Imaging in Incidentally Discovered Adrenal Masses*

Scintigraphic pattern	Etiology
Symmetrical	Normal adrenal (mass not in adrenal) adenoma <2 cm diameter Nonhypersecretory benign adenoma
Asymmetrical (concordant)[a] Asymmetrical (discordant)[b]	Space-occupying lesions; adrenal cyst, myelolipoma, pheochromocytoma; adrenal carcinoma, metastasis
Unilateral	Hyperfunctioning adrenal mass; Cushing adenoma (aldosteronism-rare), nonhypersecretory adenoma (see asymmetrical-concordant) space-occupying lesion (see asymmetrical discordant)

[a]Concordant, uptake increased on side of CT/MRI localized adrenal mass.
[b]Discordant, uptake decreased on side of CT/MRI localized mass.

deiodination (54). MIBG has subsequently been shown to localize in diagnostically useful concentrations in adrenal medullary tumors (55) and in adrenal medullary hyperplasia (56), with much less uptake in the normal adrenal medulla (57). Variations on the benzylguanidine theme have been used to image adrenergic tissues with various radioisotopes and modifications of the parent compound (i.e., aminobenzylguanidine) (1) (Table 34.1).

The localization of MIBG and analogs is thought to be through the norepinephrine reuptake mechanisms, with entry of the agent into catecholamine storage vesicles of adrenergic nerve endings and the cells of the adrenal medulla (58). Supporting this concept are a series of experiments indicating that uptake can be prevented or reduced with pretreatment with reserpine and tricyclic antidepressants and other commonly used drugs that must be excluded before MIBG scintigraphy (53,54,58,59) (Table 34.2). More importantly, however, was the finding that α- and β-adrenergic blockade does not interfere with the uptake of MIBG, and, with the exception of labetalol which has an inhibitory action on amine uptake, clinical studies can be safely performed during treatment for hypercatecholaminemia (55,58, 59).

Hydroxyephedrine (HED), an analog of norepinephrine that may be labeled with ^{11}C for use in positron emission tomography (PET), is concentrated into adrenergic nerve terminals by the norepinephrine uptake mechanism (60,61). This was the first positron-emitting tracer of the adrenergic nervous system suitable for human studies (62). More recently, high specific activity ^{11}C-epinephrine has been useful for quantitative imaging studies of the sympathetic nervous system (63). Fluorine-18-fluorodeoxyglucose (^{18}F FDG) has also been used to image neuroendocrine neoplasms (64).

Radiation Dosimetry

Clearance of radioiodinated MIBG from the blood is rapid, with approximately two thirds of the dose excreted into the urine in the first 24 hours after administration. The radiation dosimetry for ^{123}I and ^{131}I-MIBG is summarized in Table 34.3. The thyroid dosimetry is presented with and without iodide administration, and most of the absorbed dose is due to the uptake of radioiodine released by *in vivo* deiodination (65).

Technique

Patients are pretreated with a stable iodine preparation beginning 1 day before and continuing for 1 week after the administration of MIBG. No other pretreatment is required (55,66). The preferred imaging device is a large-field-of-view gamma-camera with a ½-inch thick crystal. For studies with ^{131}I, a high-energy, parallel-hole collimator should be employed. For studies with ^{123}I, a low-energy, high-resolution collimator should be used (Table 34.3). In suspected pheochromocytoma, the entire body is imaged with multiple overlapping anterior and posterior composite views from the skull to the infra pelvic region. Although most pheochromocytomas will be visualized at 48 hours, there is some variability that necessitates imaging at 24, 48, and 72

hours following injection with ^{131}I-MIBG. Each image should contain between 50,000 and 100,000 counts. ^{123}I-MIBG provides excellent images as early as 6-hours postinjection and with late 24-hour images. Radioactive surface markers can be used for anatomic orientation, and, in selected cases, one or more additional radiopharmaceuticals can be administered for more specific anatomic localization. It is often useful to outline the kidneys, liver, spleen, skeleton, cardiac blood pool, and/or left ventricular myocardium to aid interpretation of the MIBG scan (57,58,66,67). Studies with ^{11}C-HED, ^{11}C-epinephrine, and ^{18}F FDG afford much earlier imaging of pheochromocytomas and other neuroendocrine tumors within minutes postinjection (68).

Interpretation of the Normal Sympathomedulla Scan

In the normal subject, radioactivity is routinely seen in the salivary glands, liver, spleen, and bladder. Kidney uptake is early and may be transient. Variable amounts of radioactivity are seen in the myocardium and lungs. Free radioiodine will localize in the thyroid and stomach and on later images may be seen in the colon. The normal adrenal medulla is infrequently visualized with ^{131}I-MIBG (less than 20% of cases at 48 hours) and is never seen with more than faint activity (57). The normal adrenal medulla is seen on ^{123}I-MIBG studies but is not imaged on PET studies with ^{11}C-HED, ^{11}C-epinephrine, or ^{18}F FDG, but salivary gland, heart, liver, kidney, and bladder activity are seen in normal subjects undergoing PET scans with these agents (62, 68).

Clinical Application

The clinical spectrum of neuroendocrine neoplasms that can be approached with scintigraphy is outlined in Table 34.4.

Pheochromocytoma Localization

The majority of pheochromocytomas are sporadic and are localized within the adrenal gland (66). When these tumors are greater than 1.5 cm in diameter, they are readily visualized by CT (69). As a "hot spot" imaging technique, MIBG scintigraphy detects both large and small lesions and has the additional advantage that in up to 10% of cases there can be multifocal and/or metastatic disease present at virtually any site(s) within the body. These lesions have been detected by the total body screening examination outlined earlier (55,57,66) (Fig. 34.6). MIBG scintigraphy is of particular value in the localization of extraadrenal pheochromocytomas. These lesions occur at many locations from the base of the skull to the pelvis and often are not detected by CT because of their size and close relationship to other structures (70,71) (Fig. 34.7). Venous catecholamine sampling may indicate the level of a given lesion, but this is not a practical means of surveying the entire body. This screening ability is also of particular value when recurrent pheochromocytomas are suspected. Recurrence can be due to the development of a new

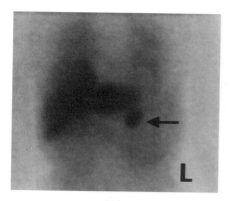
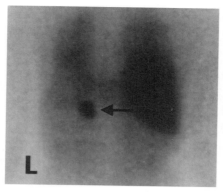
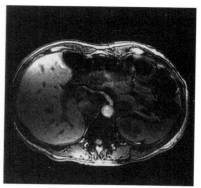

FIGURE 34.6. An intraadrenal pheochromocytoma (*arrow*) is depicted on a ^{123}I-metaiodobenzylguanidine scan and on magnetic resonance imaging of the abdomen.

primary tumor, distant metastases, or local areas of recurrent tumor(s). Conventional imaging procedures often fail because of distorted anatomy and, in the case of CT, the presence of metal clips in the operative field(s). The MIBG scan is unaffected by these factors (55). Shapiro et al. (72) have reported their experience in 30 cases of malignant pheochromocytoma studied with MIBG. The most common sites of metastatic disease are the skeleton, lymph nodes, lung, and peritoneum. MIBG scintigraphy is the single most sensitive technique for evaluating all of these sites as compared with other radionuclide studies such as bone and liver scanning and CT (58) (Fig. 34.8).

Other Clinical Applications

MIBG imaging has proven useful in several other conditions. Patients with multiple endocrine neoplasia type 2 (MEN 2) have been studied. This disorder is transmitted by an autosomal dominant pattern and is characterized by parathyroid hyperplasia, medullary thyroid carcinoma (MTC), and adrenal medullary hyperplasia or pheochromocytoma in the case of MEN 2A and by medullary carcinoma of thyroid, mucosal ganglioneuromata, and adrenal medullary hyperplasia or pheochromocytoma in

MEN 2B. MIBG uptake has been suggested as a potential means of following the course of the development of adrenal medullary disease in this disorder and may depict the transition from medullary hyperplasia to pheochromocytoma (Fig. 34.9). Serial scintigraphy may assist in the proper timing of surgical intervention to diminish the risk of sudden death in patients with potential catecholamine excess and delay as long as possible the consequences of bilateral adrenalectomy, the only available treatment for these patients with adrenal medulla dysfunction in MEN 2 (56).

Patients with neurofibromatosis have also been studied with MIBG scintigraphy. These patients have a somewhat increased incidence of pheochromocytoma, and because of the difficulty of differentiation of pheochromocytoma from retroperitoneal neurofibromata, functional imaging with MIBG has distinct utility and efficacy in these patients (73). Further, the role of MIBG imaging in the management of neuroblastoma is well established (74,75). Scintigraphy has been shown useful for the detection, staging, and monitoring responses to therapy and in the distinction of residual tumor from scar. Higher quality images are provided with ^{123}I-MIBG rather than ^{131}I-MIBG and thus demonstrates higher sensitivity and specificity than ^{131}I-

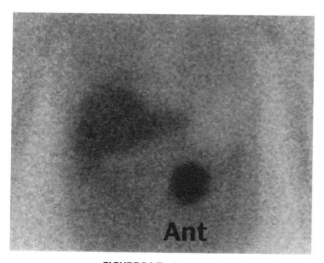
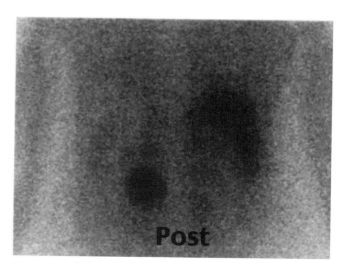

FIGURE 34.7. An extraadrenal pheochromocytoma is depicted on a ^{123}I-metaiodobenzylguanidine scan.

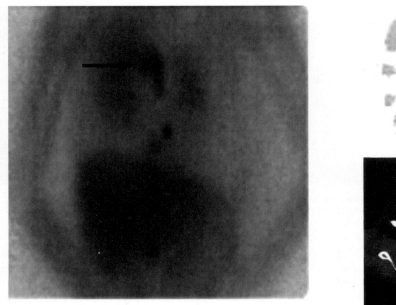

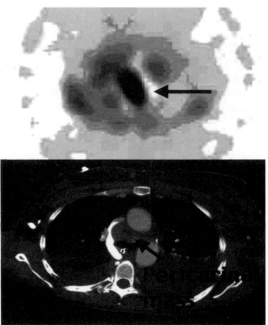

FIGURE 34.8. A metastatic pheochromocytoma on ^{123}I-metaiodobenzylguanidine scintigraphy. Para-aortic metastatic disease and a pericardial metastasis (*arrow*) are identified.

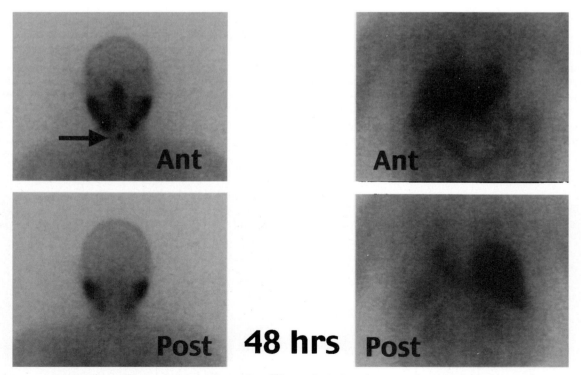

FIGURE 34.9. ^{123}I-metaiodobenzylguanidine (^{123}I-MIBG) scintigraphy in a patient with multiple endocrine neoplasia type 2 and medullary thyroid carcinoma after thyroidectomy, depicted as a solitary focus of MIBG uptake in the thyroid bed (*arrow*).

MIBG. There is some concern, however, that bone metastases may be missed using ^{123}I-MIBG (76). However, others have demonstrated both ^{131}I and ^{123}I-MIBG scintigraphy superior to bone scintigraphy for the detection of skeletal involvement in neuroblastoma, in which false-positive findings are uncommon and usually the result of gastrointestinal or renal visualization (77). In addition, carcinoid, MTC, and a wide variety of other neuroendocrine tumors have been imaged with ^{131}I and ^{123}I-MIBG with varying degrees of success (78–80).

^{11}C-labeled HED, ^{11}C-epinephrine, and ^{18}F FDG have been used to localize pheochromocytoma and neuroblastoma (66,81). High-quality PET images of these tumors are obtained as early as 10 minutes following injection and are comparable to SPECT

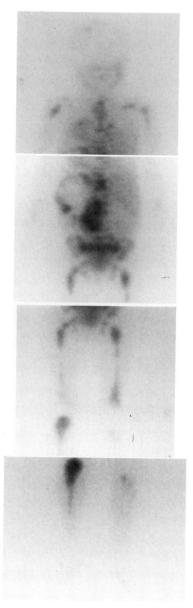

FIGURE 34.10. Widespread ^{131}I-metaiodobenzylguanidine uptake to include bone marrow metastases is seen in metastatic neuroblastoma.

images obtained 24 hours following ^{123}I-MIBG (82) (Figs. 34.10 and 34.11).

THERAPY OF NEUROENDOCRINE TUMORS WITH RADIOIODINATED METAIODOBENZYLGUANIDINE

The strikingly intense uptake and prolonged retention of tracer doses of ^{131}I-MIBG observed in metastatic pheochromocytoma deposits raised the possibility of therapy with this and other related radiopharmaceuticals (82–88). Furthermore, other neuroendocrine tumors of the amine precursor uptake and decarboxylation (APUD) type such as neuroblastoma, carcinoid, and MTC accumulate MIBG have been candidates for experimental radionuclide therapy (89–91).

Therapy of Pheochromocytoma With MIBG

^{131}I-MIBG has been administered in large doses for the experimental therapy of malignant pheochromocytoma and other neuroendocrine neoplasms that demonstrated avid accumulation of the radiopharmaceutical (92). ^{131}I-MIBG has been given in multiple doses (cumulative maximum ~35 GBq) spread over 12 months with dosimetry estimates of beta radiation that range from 1,000 cGy to 40,000 cGy (92–95). In a recent review of 116 patients treated with varying doses of ^{131}I-MIBG [~3.7 GBq (100 mCi) to 11.1 GBq (300 mCi)] multiple investigators report partial responses (≥50% decline in catecholamine and metabolite levels and/or ≥50% or greater decrease in tumor volume) in 18% to 88% of patients (92–95) (Table 34.8). Sustained, partial remissions with marked improvement in symptoms have been noted to extend in some patients over 2 to 3 years or more (95–97) (Table 34.8). Objective improvements have been noted in pain from bone and retroperitoneal metastases, a decline in blood pressure in concert with falling catecholamine levels, and an improved overall sense of well-being (92–95). Decreases in tumor volume, catecholamine excretion, and the number of metastases were noted only after multiple doses of ^{131}I-MIBG (92). Modest bone marrow depression with mild transient thrombocytopenia and leukopenia were often observed. Bone marrow failure associated with MIBG therapy was observed in two patients with diffuse bony metastases after second and third dose of ^{131}I-MIBG to each, respectively (96). Nausea and vomiting have been associated with whole-body doses of greater than 80 cGy and despite continuous, stable iodide administration, two patients developed late hypothyroidism (96,97).

In an attempt to optimize the therapeutic approach to malignant pheochromocytoma ^{131}I-MIBG therapy has been combined with multiple drug chemotherapy. Combination chemotherapy (cyclophosphamide 750 mg/m^2, dacarbazine 600 mg/m^2, and vincristine 1.4 mg/m^2) in two patients who also received ^{131}I-MIBG (three doses each of 85 to 90 cGy, with a cumulative dose/patient of 31.5 and 22.5 GBq, respectively) were reported to have further reductions of tumor volume (to undetectable in one patient), whereas in another patient there was normalization in vanillylmandelic acid (VMA) excretion (98). These data sug-

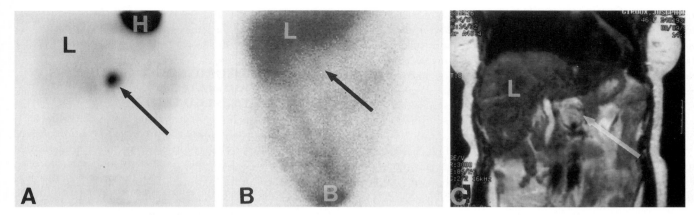

FIGURE 34.11. Malignant pheochromocytoma in a patient 14 years after left adrenalectomy and nephrectomy. A transverse ^{11}C-hydroxyephedrine (^{11}C-HED) positron emission tomography (PET) **(A)** and a ^{123}I-metaiodobenzylguanidine (^{123}I-MIBG) single photon emission computed tomography (SPECT) **(B)** scans of the midabdomen demonstrating intense accumulation of both tracers (*arrows*) in a recurrent, malignant pheochromocytoma. C: A magnetic resonance scan of the abdomen depicts the left perirenal mass (*arrow*) and correlates with the site of uptake on the ^{11}C-HED PET and ^{123}I-MIBG SPECT scans. B, bladder; H, heart; L, liver.

Table 34.8. ^{131}I-MIBG Therapy Results in Malignant Pheochromocytoma[a]

	Range	No or %	Mean[d] ± SD	Median
Number of doses administered	1–11	—	3.3[d] ± 2.2	[b]
Age at MIBG therapy (yrs)	12–76[d]	—	—	—
Site of primary (%): Adrenal	—	77	—	—
Extra adrenal	—	21	—	—
Both sites	—	2	—	—
Sites of metastases (%)				
Soft tissue	—	39	—	—
Bone	—	13	—	—
Both sites	—	48	—	—
Specific activity of dose (mCi/M mol)	10–15	—	—	—
Radiation dose to tumor (when calculated[e]) (rads)	100–19790	—	—	—
Individual dose activity (mCi)	—	—	158	—
Cumulative dose activity (mCi)	98–2322	—	490[d] ± 350	—
Initial response rate (%)				
-Symptomatic	—	78	—	—
-Hormonal	—	45[b]	—	—
-Tumor volume	—	30[b,c]	—	—
-Complete response	—	4.3	—	—
Adverse Effects (no of cases) total[c] (radiation sickness)				
-Marrow	—	47	—	[b]
-Liver	—	25	—	—
-Hypertensive	—	4	—	—
Crisis	—	1	—	—
Duration of follow-up (months)	13–108	—	30.9[d] ± 23.1	[b]
Fraction of responders	—	45	—	—
Relapsing or progressing (%) in study period				
Interval from response to relapse or progression (months)	—	—	29.3[d] ± 31.1	19
Fraction of responders				
eventually dying (%) in study period	—	33	—	—
Interval from response to deaths (months)	—	—	23.2[d] ± 8.1	22
Fraction of nonresponders				
eventually dying (%) in study period	—	45	—	—
Interval from therapy to death in nonresponders (month)	—	14.3[d] ± 8.3	13	

[a]Data (24 centers in 10 countries from 1983 10 1996) derived from Lohk-L et al. *Endocrinol Invest* 1997;20:648–858, with permission
[b]There were five complete, durable hormonal and tumor responders (4.3%).
[c]Soft tissue lesions were more responsive than those in bone.
[d]17 of 116 patients were ≤18 years of age.
[e]Available in only 35 of 116 cases.

gest that ^{131}I-MIBG and chemotherapy can be combined with an additive therapeutic effect. In more recent studies in a transplantable pheochromocytoma animal model, ^{76}Br-metabromobenzylguanidine has shown promise as a potential diagnostic (positron emitting) and therapeutic (beta emitting) radiopharmaceutical (97,99).

Therapy of Neuroblastoma with Radioiodinated-MIBG

Neuroblastoma is the second most common solid tumor of childhood that often presents at an advanced stage with a bleak prognosis (<25% long-term remission in stage IV disease) (74, 75). For patients with stage IV and III tumors that fail to respond or in those that relapse after standard therapy, the outlook is worse, prompting the use of aggressive and experimental salvage therapies including high dose multidrug chemotherapy, autologous or allogenic bone marrow transplant, and antineuroblastoma monoclonal antibodies (both as unlabeled immunotherapy and as ^{131}I-labeled radioimmunotherapy) (100). Because most neuroblastoma deposits show intense and prolonged uptake of diagnostic tracer doses of ^{131}I or ^{123}I-MIBG, large doses of radioiodinated-MIBG have been used to treat metastatic neuroblastoma (74,75,101–106) (Table 34.9).

The experience to date with ^{131}I-MIBG has demonstrated that moribund patients with very large tumor burdens do not show a significant benefit. Very widespread marrow infiltration by neuroblastoma is associated with increased radiation myelotoxicity (resulting primarily from high marrow radiation dose from the ^{131}I-MIBG taken up by tumor in the marrow space) (104–107,110). Some patients who show no objective evidence of tumor response may demonstrate striking, but temporary, subjective palliation (e.g., decrease in pain, decrease in narcotic use, and resolution of tumor fever). Objective tumor responses are achieved in a minority of patients (102,103,105–109). These are only rarely complete, and relapse is not infrequent (Table 34.9). Nevertheless, some prolonged survivals have been achieved at 50 and 60 months (102,103).

Alternative protocols using ^{131}I-MIBG given early in the course of the disease (in some cases before chemotherapy) have shown some success (90,110–112). ^{131}I-MIBG therapy has been used to render otherwise inoperable stage III tumors suitable for resection, and ^{131}I-MIBG has been administered as a prelude to bone marrow transplant (either in place of or in addition to whole-body external irradiation). Therapy with ^{131}I-MIBG provides a differential specific delivery of radiation to tumor that is not achieved by unselective external irradiation.

The dose-limiting factor for ^{131}I-MIBG therapy is irreversible bone marrow depression. Doses of ^{131}I-MIBG below 2.5 Gy have been shown to achieve tumor doses of 50 Gy with only transient thrombocytopenia and leukopenia (113). MIBG has been combined, either before or after, with chemotherapy and radiation therapy in the treatment of neuroblastoma (101). Cisplatin has been combined with ^{131}I-MIBG therapy with some success (114). Hyperbaric oxygen has been used to overcome tumor hypoxia and combined with ^{131}I-MIBG has increased survival in high-risk patients from 12% to 32% at 28-months posttherapy (115).

Because one of the patterns of neuroblastoma metastases is microscopic tumor foci scattered throughout the bone marrow (single cells or small cell clusters) and because some patients who initially respond to ^{131}I-MIBG relapse with diffuse marrow tumor infiltration, ^{125}I-MIBG has been used as an alternative therapeutic radiopharmaceutical (116–118). The β-particles from ^{131}I may escape small tumor deposits resulting in a low radiation dose to the tumor (108). In contrast, the low-energy Auger electrons from ^{125}I are far less penetrating and deliver most of their energy within a few millimeters (116–118). The ^{125}I-MIBG would be expected to be taken up into the cytoplasm of neuroblastoma cells from where the nucleus would be significantly irradiated (109,117,118). An alternative alpha-emitting labeled benzylguanidine analog, ^{211}Astatine-labeled meta-astatobenzyl guanidine (^{211}AT-MABG) and an ^{211}astatine-labeled fluorobenzylguanidine analog have had some therapeutic success in *in vitro* studies (119,120).

Table 34.9. *^{131}I-MIBG Therapy of Neuroblastoma*

Center	Patients	Complete remission	Partial remission	Stable	Progressive disease	Not evaluable	Objective response
Amsterdam	66	7	29	18	9	3	57%
Univ Frankfort	15		9	1	5		60%
Univ Tubingen	25	4	6	6		9	63%
Other German ctrs	20	1	3	8		8	33%
Multicenter France	26			10	16		0%
Genova/Brescia	43	2	5	23	12	1	17%
Royal Marsden	5	1	1			3	100%
Multicenter UKCCSG	25		8	9	7	1	33%
Gemelli, Rome	14	2	3	5	2	2	42%
Univ Michigan	14		1	3	10		7%
INT, Milan	7		2	2	3		29%
UCSF, San Francisco	11		2	2	7		18%
Univ Turin	5		1	1	3		20%
Total	276	17	70	88	74	27	35%

From Tepmongkol S, Heyman S. *Medical and pediatric oncology.* 1999;32:427–431, with permission.

Table 34.10. *¹³¹I-MIBG Therapy of Other Neuroendocrine Tumors*

Responses	Carcinoid	Medullary thyroid cancer
Complete response	0	1
Partial response	10	5
Stable disease	28	8
Progressive disease	11	4
Nonevaluable	2	0
Total	51	18

From Shapiro B et al. *Q J Nucl Med* 1995;39(Suppl 1):55–57, with permission.

Therapy of Other Neuroendocrine Tumors with Radioiodinated-MIBG

In addition to pheochromocytoma and neuroblastoma, a wide range of neuroendocrine tumors of the APUD series show MIBG uptake sufficient for diagnostic scintigraphy. In principle, any tumor demonstrating intense and prolonged uptake of tracer doses of ¹³¹I or ¹²³I-MIBG might be treated with large doses of ¹³¹I-MIBG (87,90,91,104). The reported experience in these cases is smaller than for pheochromocytoma and neuroblastoma, but both carcinoid tumors and MTC have been treated with ¹³¹I-MIBG (90,104,121–123) (Table 34.10).

SUMMARY

The challenge of radionuclide adrenal and neuroendocrine scintigraphy lies in understanding the unique functional interplay of these imaging agents with adrenal physiology and pathophysiology so that studies of functional localization are properly performed and interpreted. These studies must be modified and tailored for each case to obtain the greatest diagnostic return. When conducted in the proper clinical setting (reasonable suspicion based on clinical features and biochemical studies), both adrenal cortical and neuroendocrine imaging have significant clinical utility and demonstrable efficacy. The therapeutic use of radiolabeled-MIBG and analogs for pheochromocytoma, neuroblastoma, and other APUDomas offers a promising approach for the future.

ACKNOWLEDGMENTS

This work is supported by NCI (CA-90015), NIAMDD (RO1-AM-21477-02 RAD), HEW 3M01-RR-0042-21 S1 CLR, and the Department of Veterans Affairs Health System. We acknowledge the Phoenix Memorial Laboratory for the use of the radiochemical facilities.

REFERENCES

1. Kloos RT, Khafagi F, Gross MD et al. Adrenal (Section 10). In: Maisey MN, Britton KE, Collier BD, eds. *Clinical nuclear medicine,* 3rd ed. London: Chapman and Hall Medical, 1998:357–380.
2. Shapiro B, Gross MD, Shulkin BL. Radioisotope diagnosis and ther-
apy of malignant pheochromocytoma. *Trends Endocrinol Metab* 2001; 12:469–475.
3. Counsell RE, Ranade VV, Blair RJ et al. Tumor localizing agents. IX. Radioiodinated cholesterol. *Steroids* 1970;16:317–328.
4. Blair RJ, Beierwaltes WH, Lieberman LM et al. Radiolabeled cholesterol as an adrenal scanning agent. *J Nucl Med* 1971;12:176–182.
5. Beierwaltes WH, Lieberman LM, Ansari AA et al. Visualization of human adrenal glands by *in vivo* scintillation scanning. *JAMA* 1971; 216:275–277.
6. Basmadjian GP, Hetzel KR, Ice RD et al. Synthesis of a new adrenal cortex imaging agent 6-¹³¹I-iodomethyl-19-norcholest-5(10)-en-3-ol (NP-59). *J Labeled Compd* 1975;11:427–432.
7. Sarkar SD, Beierwaltes WH, Ice RD et al. A new and superior adrenal scanning agent, NP-59. *J Nucl Med* 1975;16:1038–1042.
8. Thrall JH, Freitas JE, Beierwaltes WH. Adrenal scintigraphy. *J Nucl Med* 1978;18:23–41.
9. Shapiro B, Britton KE, Hawkins LA et al. Clinical experience with ⁷⁵Se-selenomethylnorcholesterol adrenal imaging. *Clin Endocrinol* 1981;15:19.
10. Beierwaltes WH, Wieland DM, Mosley ST et al. Imaging of the adrenal glands with radiolabeled inhibitors of enzymes. *J Nucl Med* 1978;19:20–23.
11. Isaacsohn JL, Lees AM, Lees RS et al. Adrenal imaging with technetium-99m-labelled low density lipoproteins. *Metabolism* 1986;35: 364–366.
12. Bergström M, Bonasma TA, Bergström E et al. *In vitro* and *in vivo* primate evaluation of carbon-11 etiomidate and carbon-11 metiomidate as potential tracers for PET imaging of the adrenal cortex and its tumors. *J Nucl Med* 1998;39:982–987.
13. Gross MD, Valk TW, Swanson DP et al. The role of pharmacologic manipulation in adrenal cortical scintigraphy. *Semin Nucl Med* 1981; 11:128–148.
14. Gordon L, Mayfield RK, Levine JH et al. Failure to visualize adrenal glands in a patient with bilateral adrenal hyperplasia. *J Nucl Med* 1980;21:49–51.
15. Valk T, Gross M, Swanson D et al. The relationship of serum lipids to adrenal gland uptake of 6-¹³¹I-iodomethyl-19-norcholesterol in Cushing's syndrome. *J Nucl Med* 1980;21:1069–1072.
16. Gross MD, Freitas JE, Swanson DP et al. The normal dexamethasone suppression adrenal scintiscan. *J Nucl Med* 1979;20:1131–1135.
17. Fukushi S, Nakajima K, Miura T et al. Comparative study of adrenal scanning agents, 6-iodomethyl-19-norcholest-5(10)-en-3-ol-¹³¹I (NCh-6-¹³¹I) and 131-I-19-iodocholesterol (CL-19-¹³¹I). *Jpn J Nucl Med* 1976;13:775–779.
18. Lynn MD, Gross MD, Shapiro B. Enterohepatic circulation and distribution of I-131-6B-iodomethyl-19-norcholesterol (NP-59). *Nucl Med Res Commun* 1986;7:625–630.
19. Carey JE, Thrall JH, Freitas JE et al. Absorbed dose to the human adrenals from iodomethyl-norcholesterol (I-131) "NP-59." *J Nucl Med* 1979;20:60–62.
20. Shapiro B, Nakajo M, Gross MD et al. Value of bowel preparation in adrenocortical scintigraphy with NP-59. *J Nucl Med* 1983;24: 732–734.
21. Juni JE, Gross MD. Bilateral visualization on adrenal cortical scintigraphy. *Semin Nucl Med* 1983;13:168–170.
22. Ishimura J, Kawanaka M, Fukuchi M. Clinical application of SPECT in adrenal imaging with I-131-6B-iodomethyl-19-norcholesterol. *Clin Nucl Med* 1989;14:278–281.
23. Fischer M, Vetter W, Winterg B et al. Adrenal scintigraphy in primary aldosteronism. Spironolactone as a cause of incorrect classification between adenoma and hyperplasia. *Eur J Nucl Med* 1982;7:222–224.
24. Nakajo M, Sakata H, Shirona K et al. Application of ACTH stimulation to adrenal imaging with radiocholesterol. *Clin Nucl Med* 1983; 8:112–120.
25. Nakajo M, Nakabeppu Y, Tsuchimochi S. Scintigraphic assessment of therapeutic success in aldosteronomas treated by transcatheter arterial embolization using absolute ethanol. *J Nucl Med* 1997;38:237–241.
26. Gross MD, Valk TW, Freitas JE et al. The relationship of adrenal iodomethylnorcholesterol uptake to indices of adrenal cortical func-

tion in Cushing's syndrome. *J Clin Endocrinol Metab* 1981;52:1062–1066.

27. Smals AGH, Pieters G, Van Haelst V et al. Macronodular adrenocortical hyperplasia in long-standing Cushing's disease. *J Clin Endocrinol Metab* 1984;58:25–31.

28. Fig LM, Ehrmann D, Gross MD et al. The localization of abnormal adrenal function in the ACTH-dependent Cushing syndrome. *Ann Intern Med* 1988;109:547–553.

29. Schteingart DE, Seabold JE, Gross MD et al. Iodocholesterol adrenal tissue uptake and imaging in adrenal neoplasms. *J Clin Endocrinol Metab* 1981;52:1156–1161.

30. Ganguly A. Primary aldosteronism. *N Engl J Med* 1998;339:1828–1834.

31. Conn JW, Cohen EL, Herwing KR. The dexamethasone-modified adrenal scintiscan in hyporeninemic aldosteronism (tumor vs. hyperplasia). A comparison with adrenal venography and adrenal venous aldosterone. *J Lab Clin Med* 1976;88:841–855.

32. Freitas JE, Grekin RJ, Thrall JH et al. Adrenal imaging with iodomethylnorcholesterol (I-131) in primary aldosteronism. *J Nucl Med* 1979;20:7–12.

33. Ishimura J, Fukuchi M. High diagnostic accuracy of qualitative adrenal SPECT imaging without dexamethasone suppression in primary aldosteronism. *J Nucl Med* 1992;33:384.

34. Givens JR. Hirsutism and hyperandrogenism. *Adv Intern Med* 1976;21:221–247.

35. Kirschner MA, Bardin CW. Androgen production and metabolism in normal and virilized women. *Metabolism* 1972;21:667–688.

36. Leventhal ML, Scommegna A. Multiglandular aspects of Stein-Leventhal syndrome. *Am J Obstet Gynecol* 1963;87:445–451.

37. Gross MD, Freitas JE, Swanson DP et al. Dexamethasone suppression adrenal scintigraphy in hyperandrogenism. *J Nucl Med* 1981;22:12–17.

38. Nakajo M, Sakata H, Shinohara S. Positive imaging of arrhenoblastoma of the ovary with 131-I-aldosterol: case report. *Jpn J Nucl Med* 1979;16:472.

39. Barkan AL, Cassorla F, Loriaux DL et al. Steroid and gonadotrophin secretion in a patient with a 30-year history of virilization due to a lipoid-cell ovarian tumor. *Obstet Gynecol* 1984;64:287.

40. Carpenter DC, Wahner HW, Salassa RM et al. Demonstration of steroid producing gonadal tumors by external scanning with the use of NP-59. *Mayo Clin Proc* 1979;54:332–334.

41. Mountz JM, Gross MD, Shapiro B et al. Scintigraphic localization of ovarian dysfunction. *J Nucl Med* 1988;29:1644–1650.

42. Leonard JM, Rudd TG, Burgess EC et al. Concentration of radiolabeled cholesterol in a feminizing adenoma of the testis. *J Nucl Med* 1979;20:307–309.

43. Gross MD, Thrall JH, Beierwaltes WH. The adrenal scan: a current status report on radiotracers, dosimetry and clinical utility. In: Freeman LM, Weissman HS, eds. *Nuclear medicine annual.* New York: Raven Press, 1980:127–175.

44. Stakianakis GN, Sotos J, Vasquez S. Adrenal gland and ectopic adrenal tissue imaging in children with congenital adrenal hyperplasia. *J Nucl Med* 1979;20:622(abst).

45. Kloos RT, Gross MD, Francis IR et al. Incidentally discovered adrenal masses. *Endocr Rev* 1995;16:460–484.

46. Barzon L, Boscaro M. Diagnosis and management of adrenal incidentalomas. *J Urol* 2000;163:398–407.

47. Gross MD, Shapiro B, Francis IR et al. Scintigraphic evaluation of clinically silent adrenal masses. *J Nucl Med* 1994;35:1145–1152.

48. Dwamena B, Kloos RT, Fendrick AM et al. Diagnostic evaluation of the adrenal incidentaloma: decision and cost-effectiveness analysis. *J Nucl Med* 1998;39:707–712.

49. Lieberman LM, Beierwaltes WH, Varma VM et al. Labeled dopamine concentration in human adrenal medulla and in neuroblastoma. *J Nucl Med* 1969;10:93–97.

50. Anderson BG, Beierwaltes WH, Harrison TS et al. Labeled dopamine concentration in pheochromocytomas. *J Nucl Med* 1973;14:781–784.

51. Fowler JS, MacGregor RR, Wolf AP. Radiopharmaceuticals. Halogenated dopamine analogs: synthesis and radiolabeling of 6-iododopamine and tissue distribution studies in animals. *J Med Chem* 1976;19:356–360.

52. Korn N, Buswink A, Yu T et al. A radioiodinated bretylium analog as a potential agent for scanning the adrenal medulla. *J Nucl Med* 1977;18:87–89.

53. Wieland DM, Wu JL, Brown LE et al. Radiolabeled adrenergic neuron blocking agents: adrenal medulla imaging with (131I) iodobenzylguanidine. *J Nucl Med* 1980;21:349–353.

54. Wieland DM, Brown LE, Tobes MC et al. Imaging the primate adrenal medulla with (123I) and (131I) metaiodobenzylguanidine [Concise communication]. *J Nucl Med* 1981;22:358–364.

55. Sisson JC, Frager MS, Valk TW et al. Scintigraphic localization of pheochromocytoma. *N Engl J Med* 1981;305:12–17.

56. Valk TW, Frager MS, Gross MD et al. Spectrum of pheochromocytoma in multiple endocrine neoplasia: a scintigraphic portrayal using 131-I-metaiodobenzylguanidine. *Ann Intern Med* 1981;94:762–767.

57. Nakajo M, Shapiro B, Copp J et al. The normal and abnormal distribution of the adrenomedullary imaging agent I-131-metaiodobenzylguanidine (I-MIBG) in man: evaluation by scintigraphy. *J Nucl Med* 1983;24:672–682.

58. Shapiro B, Wieland DM, Brown LE et al. 131I-meta-iodobenzylguanidine (MIBG) adrenal medullary scintigraphy: interventional studies. In: Spencer RP, ed. *Interventional nuclear medicine.* New York: Grune & Stratton, 1983:451–481.

59. Khafagi FA, Shapiro B, Fig LM et al. Labetalol reduces iodine-131 MIBG uptake by pheochromocytoma and normal tissues. *J Nucl Med* 1989;30:481–489.

60. Rosenspire KC, Haka MS, Jewett DM et al. Synthesis and preliminary evaluation of (11C) metahydroxyephedrine: a false neurotransmitter agent for heart neuronal imaging. *J Nucl Med* 1990;31:1328–1334.

61. Schwaiger M, Kalff V, Rosenspire KC et al. The noninvasive evaluation of the sympathetic nervous system in the human heart by PET. *Circulation* 1990;82:457–464.

62. Shulkin BL, Wieland DM, Schwaiger M et al. PET scanning with hydroxyepinephrine: an approach to the localization of pheochromocytoma. *J Nucl Med* 1992;33:1125–1131.

63. Chakraborty PK, Gildersleeve DL, Jewett DM et al. High yield synthesis of high specific activity R-(-) epinephrine for routine PET studies in humans. *Nucl Med Biol* 1993;20:939–944.

64. Shulkin BL, Koeppe RA, Francis IR et al. Pheochromocytomas that do not accumulate metaiodobenzylguanidine: localization with PET and administration of FDG. *Radiology* 1993;186:711–715.

65. Swanson DP, Carey JE, Brown LE et al. *Human absorbed dose calculations for iodine 131 and iodine 123 labeled metaiodobenzylguanidine (MIBG): a potential myocardial and adrenal medulla imaging agent.* Proceedings of the 2nd International Symposium on Radiopharmaceutical Dosimetry, Oak Ridge, TN, 1980.

66. Shapiro B, Sisson JC, Beierwaltes WH. Experience with the use of 131-I-metaiodobenzylguanidine for locating pheochromocytomas. In: Raynaud C, ed. *Nuclear medicine and biology.* Vol. II. Paris: Pergamon Press, 1982:1265.

67. Lynn MD, Shapiro B, Sisson JC et al. Portrayal of pheochromocytoma and normal human adrenal medulla by 123I-metaiodobenzylguanidine (123I-MIBG). *J Nucl Med* 1984;25:436.

68. Shulkin BL. PET epinephrine studies of pheochromocytoma. *J Nucl Med* 1995;36:22–23P.

69. Witteles RM, Kaplan EL, Roizen MF. Sensitivity of diagnostic and localization tests for pheochromocytoma in clinical practice. *Arch Int Med* 2000;160:2521–2524.

70. Laursen K, Damgaard-Pedersen K. CT for pheochromocytoma diagnosis. *AJR* 1980;134:277–280.

71. Shapiro B, Sisson JC, Kalff V et al. The location of middle mediastinal pheochromocytomas. *J Thorac Cardiovasc Surg* 1984;87:814–820.

72. Shapiro B, Sisson JC, Lloyd R et al. Malignant pheochromocytoma: clinical, biochemical and scintigraphic characterization. *Clin Endocrinol* 1984;20:189–203.

73. Kalff V, Shapiro B, Lloyd R et al. The spectrum of pheochromocytoma in hypertensive patients with neurofibromatosis. *Arch Intern Med* 1982;142:2092–2097.

74. Shulkin BL, Shapiro B. Radioiodinated meta-iodobenzylguanidine in

the management of neuroblastoma. In: Pochedly C, ed. *Neuroblastoma.* Boca Raton, FL: CRC Press, 1990:171–198.

75. Gelfand MJ. Metaiodobenzylguanidine in children. *Semin Nucl Med* 1993;23:231–242.

76. Gordon I, Peters AM, Gutman A et al. Tc-99m bone scans are more sensitive than I-123 MIBG scans for bone imaging in neuroblastoma. *J Nucl Med* 1990;31:129–134.

77. Shulkin BL, Shapiro B, Hutchinson RJ. ^{131}I-MIBG and bone scintigraphy for the detection of neuroblastoma. *J Nucl Med* 1992;33:1735–1740.

78. Von Moll L, McEwan AJ, Shapiro B et al. ^{131}I-MIBG scintigraphy of neuroendocrine tumors other than pheochromocytoma and neuroblastoma. *J Nucl Med* 1987;28:979–988.

79. Van Gils APG, Wander Mey AGL, Moogma RPLM et al. Iodine-123-metaiodobenzylguanidine scintigraphy in patients with chemodectomas of the head and neck region. *J Nucl Med* 1990;31:1147–1155.

80. Bomanji J, Levison DA, Zuzarte J et al. Imaging of carcinoid tumors with iodine-123 metaiodobenzylguanidine. *J Nucl Med* 1987;28:1907–1910.

81. Shulkin BL, Wieland DM, Baro ME et al. PET studies of neuroblastoma with carbon 11-hydroxyephedrine. *J Nucl Med* 1993;33:220.

82. Sisson JC, Shapiro B, Beierwaltes WH et al. Radiopharmaceutical treatment of malignant pheochromocytoma. *J Nucl Med* 1984;25:197–206.

83. Shapiro B, Sisson JC, Lloyd RV et al. Malignant pheochromocytoma: clinical, biochemical and scintigraphic characterization. *Clin Endocrinol (Oxf)* 1984;20:189–203.

84. Shapiro B, Copp JE, Sisson JC et al. 131-I-metaiodobenzylguanidine for the locating of suspected pheochromocytoma: experience in 400 cases (441 studies). *J Nucl Med* 1985;26:576–585.

85. Sisson JC, Shapiro B, Beierwaltes WH et al. Treatment of malignant pheochromocytomas with a new radiopharmaceutical. *Trans Assoc Am Physicians* 1983;96:209–217.

86. Shapiro B, Fig LM, Gross MD et al. Radiochemical diagnosis of adrenal disease. *Crit Rev Clin Lab Sci* 1989;27:265–298.

87. Shapiro B, Fig LM. General principles and perspectives of cancer therapy with radiopharmaceuticals. *J Nucl Med Allied Sci* 1990;34:260–264.

88. Shapiro B, Fig LM. Medical therapy of pheochromocytoma. In: Barkan A, ed. Medical therapy of endocrine tumors. *Endocrinol Metab Clin North Am* 1989;18:443–481.

89. McEwan AJ, Shapiro B, Sisson JC et al. Radioiodobenzylguanidine for the scintigraphic location and therapy of adrenergic tumors. *Semin Nucl Med* 1985;15:132–153.

90. Shapiro B. Summary, conclusions, and future directions of 131-I-metaiodobenzylguanidine therapy in the treatment of neural crest tumors. *J Nucl Biol Med* 1991;35:357–363.

91. Von Moll L, McEwan AJ, Shapiro B et al. 131-I-MIBG scintigraphy of neuroendocrine tumors other than pheochromocytoma and neuroblastoma. *J Nucl Med* 1987;28:979–988.

92. Shapiro B, Sisson JC, Wieland DM et al. Radiopharmaceutical therapy of malignant pheochromocytoma with 131-I-metaiodobenzylguanidine: results from 10 years of experience. *J Nucl Biol Med* 1991;35:269–276.

93. Sisson JC, Shapiro B. Neural crest tumors, treatment. In: Wagner HN Jr, Szabo Z, Buchanan JW, eds. *Principles of nuclear medicine,* 2nd ed. Philadelphia: WB Saunders, 1995:680–686.

94. Hoefnagel CA, Lewington VJ. MIBG therapy. In: Murray IPC, Ell PJ, eds. *Nuclear medicine in clinical diagnosis and treatment.* Edinburgh: Churchill Livingstone, 1998:1067–1082.

95. Loh K-C, Fitzgerald PA, Matthay KK et al. The treatment of malignant pheochromocytoma with iodine-131 metaiodobenzylguanidine (131I-MIBG): a comprehensive review of 116 reported patients. *J Endocrinol Invest* 1997;20:648–658.

96. Lewington VJ, Zivanovic MA, Tristam M et al. Radiolabeled metaiodobenzylguanidine targeted radiotherapy for malignant pheochromocytoma. *J Nucl Biol Med* 1991;35:280–283.

97. Shapiro B, Sisson JC, Wieland DM et al. Radiopharmaceutical therapy of malignant pheochromocytoma with ^{131}I] metaiodobenzylguanidine: results from 10 years of experience. *J Nucl Biol Med* 1991;35:269–276.

98. Sisson JC, Shapiro B, Shulkin BL et al. Treatment of malignant pheochromocytoma with 131-I metaiodobenzylguanidine and chemotherapy. *Am J Clin Oncol* 1999;22:364–370.

99. Clerc J, Mardon K, Galons H et al. Assessing intratumor distribution and uptake with MBBG versus MIBG imaging and targeting xenografted PC-12 pheochromocytoma cell line. *J Nucl Med* 1995;36:859–866.

100. Niethammer D, Handgretinger R. Clinical strategies for the treatment of neuroblastoma. *Eur J Cancer* 1995;31A:568–571.

101. Tepmongkol S, Heyman S. [131]I MIBG therapy in neuroblastoma: mechanisms, rationale, and current status. *Med Pediatr Oncol* 1999;32:427–431.

102. Moyes JSE, McCready VR, Fullbrook AC. *Neuroblastoma: MIBG in its diagnosis and management.* Berlin/Heidelberg: Springer-Verlag, 1989:1–168.

103. International workshop on the role of [131-I]meta-iodobenzylguanidine in the treatment of neural crest tumors. Rome, Italy, September 6–7, 1991. Conference proceedings (49 contributions). *J Nucl Biol Med* 1991;35:177–357.

104. Sisson JC, Hutchinson R, Carey J et al. Toxicity from treatment of neuroblastoma with 131-I-meta-iodobenzylguanidine. *Eur J Nucl Med* 1988;14:337–340.

105. Troncone L, Rufini V, Montemoggi P et al. The diagnostic and therapeutic utility of radio-iodinated meta-iodobenzylguanidine (MIBG): 5 years of experience. *Eur J Nucl Med* 1990;16:325–335.

106. Troncone L, Rufini V, Daidone MS et al. 131-I-MIBG in the radiometabolic treatment of tumors originating from the neural crest. *Acta Med Romana* 1993;31:470–475.

107. Hutchinson RJ, Sisson JC, Shapiro B et al. 131-I-metaiodobenzylguanidine treatment in patients with refractory advanced neuroblastoma. *Am J Clin Oncol* 1992;15:226–232.

108. Cunningham SH, Mairs RJ, Wheldon TE et al. Toxicity to neuroblastoma cells and spheroids of benzylguanidine conjugated to radionuclides with short range emissions. *Br J Cancer* 1998;77:2061–2068.

109. Sisson JC, Shapiro B, Hutchinson RJ et al. Treatment of neuroblastoma with 125-I-MIBG: the Michigan experience. Proceedings of the international meeting "Ten years of experience in neuroblastoma: quo vadis MIBG." German Societies of Nuclear Medicine and Pediatric Oncology. Sylt Germany, April 25–26, 1994.

110. Sisson JC, Hutchinson R, Carey J et al. Toxicity from treatment of neuroblastoma with 131-I-meta-iodobenzylguanidine. *Eur J Nucl Med* 1988;14:337–340.

111. Mastrangelo R, Tornesello A, Mastrangelo S. Role of ^{131}I-Metaiodobenzylguanidine in the treatment of neuroblastoma. *Med Pediatr Oncol* 1998;31:22–26.

112. de Kraker J, Hoefnagel CA, Caron H et al. First line targeted radiotherapy, a new concept in the treatment of advanced stage neuroblastoma. *Eur J Cancer* 1995;31:600–602.

113. Sisson JC, Shapiro B, Hutchinson RJ et al. Predictors of toxicity in treating patients with neuroblastoma by radiolabeled metaiodobenzylguanidine. *Eur J Nucl Med* 1994;21:46–52.

114. Mastrangelo R, Tornesello A, Lasorella A et al. Optimal use of the 131-I-meta-iodobenzylguanidine and cisplatin combination in advanced neuroblastoma. *J Neuro Oncol* 1997;31:153–158.

115. Voute PA, van de Kleij AJ, de Kraker J et al. Clinical experience with radiation enhancement by hyperbaric oxygen in children with recurrent neuroblastoma stage IV. *Eur J Cancer* 1995;31A:596–560.

116. Sisson JC, Kwok CS, Hutchinson RJ et al. Radiation effects of I-131-MIBG and I-125-MIBG. In: DeNardo GL, Lewis JP, Raventos A et al., eds. *ACNP/SNM joint symposium on biology of radionuclide therapy.* Washington, DC: American College of Nuclear Physicians, 1989:243–251.

117. Sisson JC, Hutchinson RJ, Shapiro B et al. Iodine 125-I-MIBG to treat neuroblastoma: preliminary report. *J Nucl Med* 1990;31:1479–1485.

118. Sisson JC, Shapiro B, Hutchinson RJ. Treatment of neuroblastoma with 125-I-metaiodobenzylguanidine. *J Nucl Biol Med* 1991;35: 255–259.
119. Vaidyanathan G, Harrison C, Walsh P et al. *In vivo* cytotoxicity of m-[At-211] astatobenzylguanidine (MABG). *J Nucl Med* 1993;34: 218P.
120. Vaidyanathan G, Zhao X-G, Larsen RH et al. 3-[^{211}At]-astato-4-fluorobenzyl-guanidine: a potential therapeutic agent with prolonged retention by neuroblastoma cells. *Br J Cancer* 1997;76:226–233.

121. Bestagno M, Pizzocaro C, Pagliaini R et al. Results of 131-I-metaiodobenzylguanidine treatment in metastatic carcinoid. *J Nucl Biol Med* 1991;35:343–345.
122. Bomanji J, Britton KE, Ur E et al. Treatment of malignant phaeochromocytoma, paraganglioma and carcinoid tumours with 131-I-metaiodobenzylguanidine. *Nucl Med Comm* 1993;14:856–861.
123. Shapiro B, Sisson JC, Shulkin B et al. The current status of radioiodinated metaiodobenzylguanidine therapy of neuro-endocrine tumors. *Q J Nucl Med* 1995;39(Suppl 1):55–57.

Diagnostic Nuclear Medicine, Fourth Edition. Edited by M.P. Sandler, R.E. Coleman, J.A. Patton, F.J.Th. Wackers, A. Gottschalk. Lippincott Williams & Wilkins, Philadelphia 2003.

35

SOMATOSTATIN RECEPTOR SCINTIGRAPHY

DIK J. KWEKKEBOOM
MARION DE JONG
ERIC P. KRENNING

SOMATOSTATIN AND SOMATOSTATIN RECEPTORS

Somatostatin is a peptide hormone consisting of 14 amino acids (SS-14). It is present in the hypothalamus, the cerebral cortex, the brainstem, the gastrointestinal tract, and the pancreas. Somatostatin receptors have been identified on many cells of neuroendocrine origin, comprising, among others, the somatotroph cells of the anterior pituitary, the thyroid C-cells, and the pancreatic islet cells (1,2). Also, cells not known as classically neuroendocrine, such as lymphocytes (3), may possess these receptors (Fig. 35.1).

Somatostatin receptors are structurally related integral membrane glycoproteins. At the moment, five subtypes of human somatostatin receptors have been cloned (4–7). The somatostatin analogue octreotide inhibits somatostatin binding to the receptor subtype 2 in the low nanomolar range (0.1 to 1 nM), in contrast to higher values (lower affinity) for types 3 and 5 (10 to 100 nM) and 1 and 4 (>1,000 nM). All subtypes mediate their effects via inhibition of adenylate cyclase activity (8). Especially subtype 2 can be visualized *in vitro* with $[^{125}I\text{-}Tyr^3]$-octreotide autoradiography and *in vivo* during scintigraphy with radiolabeled octreotide derivatives. In general, the distribution of the high affinity binding of SS-14 to human tissues is similar to that of the cloned somatostatin receptor subtype 2 (octreotide-receptor). Insulinomas form one of the exceptions to this rule, because SS-14 binding to this tumor may go hand in hand with the presence of other somatostatin receptor subtypes that do not bind octreotide with high affinity.

SOMATOSTATIN EFFECTS *IN VITRO* AND *IN VIVO*

In the central nervous system (CNS), somatostatin acts as a neurotransmitter, whereas its hormonal activities include the in-

hibition of the physiologic and tumorous release of growth hormone (GH), insulin, glucagon, gastrin, serotonin, and calcitonin (9). Other actions are (a) an antiproliferative effect on tumors, as has been found in cultured breast cancer cell lines, cultured small cell lung carcinoma (SCLC) cell lines, numerous animal tumor models, and in neuroendocrine tumors in man, and (b) specific regulation of immune responses (10). The antiproliferative effect is ascribed to (a) inhibition of growth via induction of somatostatin receptors; (b) inhibition of the release of hormones and growth factors such as GH, bombesin, and insulin-like growth factor I (IGF-I); (c) inhibition of angiogenesis; and (d) modulation of immunologic activity (10).

DISTRIBUTION OF SOMATOSTATIN RECEPTORS IN DISEASE STATES

Besides on normal tissue (11), somatostatin receptors were demonstrated in neuroendocrine tumors, many of which are derived from cells belonging to the amine precursor uptake and decarboxylation (APUD) system (12,13). These neuroendocrine tumors may contain secretory granules (14). Also, somatostatin receptors were identified in tumors of the CNS (15,16), breast (17), lung (18), lymphoid tissue (19,20), and tissues affected by activated leukocytes.

The affinity of somatostatin for its receptor on tumors and lymphomas is in the low nanomolar range. In general, neuroendocrine tumors, lymphomas, and activated leukocytes have an increased density of somatostatin receptors, which enables their *in vitro* and *in vivo* visualization with radiolabeled somatostatin analogues. Furthermore, studies with autoradiography showed that veins in surrounding tissue of various human cancers, and possibly also in tissues affected by certain inflammatory diseases, may express a high density of somatostatin receptors (21). The importance of this finding with regard to the *in vivo* visualization is yet to be established.

[^{111}IN-DTPA^0]OCTREOTIDE, A SOMATOSTATIN ANALOGUE FOR SOMATOSTATIN RECEPTOR SCINTIGRAPHY

In vitro receptor binding studies using $[^{123}I\text{-}Tyr^3]$-octreotide and $[^{111}In\text{-}DTPA^0]$octreotide show affinities for the rat brain cortex

D.J. Kwekkeboom: Department of Nuclear Medicine, University Hospital of Rotterdam, Rotterdam, The Netherlands.

M. De Jong: Department of Nuclear Medicine, University Hospital of Rotterdam, Rotterdam, The Netherlands.

E.P. Krenning: Department of Nuclear Medicine, University Hospital of Rotterdam, Rotterdam, The Netherlands.

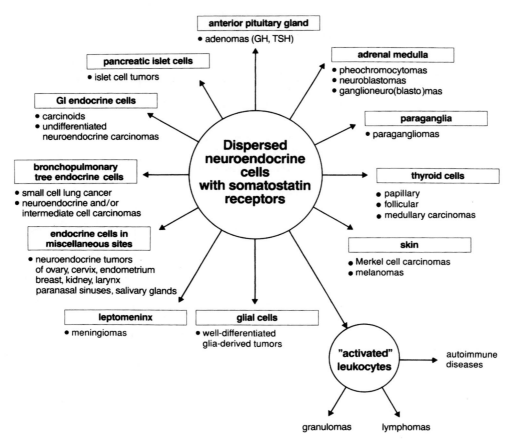

FIGURE 35.1. Tumors and diseases with neuroendocrine cells and/or activated leukocytes with increased density of somatostatin receptors, which can be visualized with [^{111}In-DTPA-D-Phe^1]-octreotide scintigraphy. (Modified from Lamberts SWJ, Krenning EP, Reubi JC. The role of somatostatin and its analogs in the diagnosis and treatment of tumors. *Endocr Rev* 1991;12:450–482, with permission.)

in the low nanomolar range with the highest affinity for the first radioligand (22).

The molecular weights of SS-14 and its chelated analogue [DTPA^0]octreotide are 1.6 and 1.4 kDa, respectively. Thus, the maximal peak blood level after intravenous injection of 10 μg [DTPA^0]octreotide in man is 0.5 nM, assuming an instant passage into the interstitium and a complete distribution in an extracellular volume of 14 L. The simultaneous renal clearance of this analogue might prevent [DTPA^0]octreotide from reaching a concentration at the membrane receptor that equals the receptor affinity. In rats bearing implanted somatostatin receptor positive tumors, pretreatment with a high dose of unlabeled octreotide blocks the binding of injected radiolabeled octreotide, pointing to *in vivo* saturation of the receptor (23). The metabolic properties of [^{111}In-DTPA^0]octreotide turn out to be similar in rat and man.

SCINTIGRAPHY: TECHNIQUE AND NORMAL FINDINGS

Scanning Protocol

The preferred dose of [^{111}In-DTPA^0]octreotide (with at least 10 μg of the peptide) is about 200 MBq. With such a dose it is possible to perform single photon emission computed tomography (SPECT), which may increase the sensitivity to detect somatostatin receptor-positive tissues and gives a better anatomic delineation than planar views. The acquisition of sufficient counts per view and also obtaining spot images with a sufficient counting time instead of performing whole-body scanning with a too low count density are other important points that may make the difference between a successful localizing study and a disappointing one.

Planar images are obtained with a double head or large field-of-view gamma-camera, equipped with medium-energy parallel-hole collimators. The pulse height analyzer windows are centered over both ^{111}In photon peaks (172 keV and 245 keV) with a window width of 20%. The acquisition parameters for planar images (preferably spot views) are 300,000 preset counts or 15 minutes per view for the head and neck, and 500,000 counts or 15 minutes for the remainder of the body. If whole-body acquisition is used, scan speed should not exceed 3 cm/minute. Using higher scan speeds, like 8 cm/minute, will result in failure to recognize small somatostatin receptor-positive lesions and lesions with a low density of these receptors (24). For SPECT images with a triple-head camera the acquisition parameters are 40 steps of 3 degrees each, 128 × 128 matrix, and at least 30 seconds per step (45 seconds for SPECT of the head). SPECT analysis is performed with a Wiener or Metz filter on original data. The filtered data are reconstructed with a Ramp filter.

Because of its relatively long effective half-life, [^{111}In-DTPA^0]octreotide is a radiolabeled somatostatin analogue that can be used to visualize somatostatin receptor-bearing tumors efficiently after 24 and 48 hours, when interfering background radioactivity is minimized by renal clearance. Planar and SPECT studies are therefore preferably performed 24 hours after injection of the radiopharmaceutical. A higher lesion detection rate of 24 hours planar imaging over 4 hours acquisition was reported by Jamar et al. (25), as well as the additional value of SPECT imaging. Planar studies after 24 and 48 hours can be carried out with the same protocol. Repeat scintigraphy after 48 hours is especially indicated when 24 hours scintigraphy shows accumulation in the abdomen, which may also represent radioactive bowel content.

Normal Scintigraphic Findings and Artifacts

Normal scintigraphic features include visualization of the thyroid, spleen, liver, and kidneys and, in some patients, visualization of the pituitary. Also, the urinary bladder and the bowel (to a variable degree) are usually visualized (Fig. 35.2). The visualization of the pituitary, thyroid, and spleen is due to receptor binding. Uptake in the kidneys is for the most part due to reabsorption of the radiolabeled peptide in the renal tubular cells

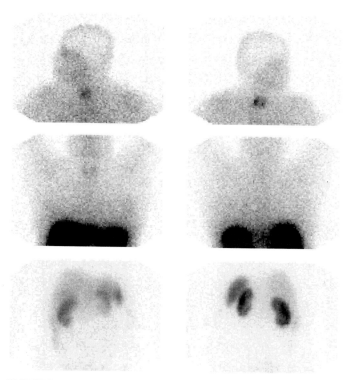

FIGURE 35.2. Normal scintigraphy with visualization of the pituitary and thyroid (*upper images,* lateral views of the head); fainter visualization of the thyroid because of scaling (*middle images*); anterior (*left*) and posterior (*right*) views of the chest; uptake in the liver, spleen, and the kidneys and also some bowel activity (*lower images*); anterior (*left*) and posterior (*right*) views of the abdomen.

after glomerular filtration, although somatostatin receptors have been demonstrated in human renal tubular cells and vasa recta (26). There is a predominant renal clearance of the somatostatin analogue, although hepatobiliary clearance into the bowel also occurs, necessitating the use of laxatives to facilitate the interpretation of abdominal images.

False-positive results of somatostatin receptor imaging (SRI) have been reported. In virtually all cases the term *false positive* is a misnomer because somatostatin receptor-positive lesions (not related to the pathology for which the investigation is performed) are present. Examples are the visualization of the gallbladder, thyroid abnormalities, accessory spleens, recent cerebrovascular accidents (CVAs), activity at the site of a recent surgical incision, and so forth. Many of these have been reviewed by Gibril et al. (27). Also, chest uptake after irradiation and diffuse breast uptake in female patients can be mistaken for other pathology. In some patients, the coexistence of two different somatostatin receptor-positive diseases should be considered. Diminished uptake in the spleen resulting from ongoing treatment with (unlabeled) octreotide may occur, which may be accompanied by a lower liver uptake. In case of hepatic metastases, this phenomenon may be misinterpreted as a better uptake in the liver metastases.

During octreotide treatment, the uptake of [^{111}In-DTPA^0] octreotide in somatostatin receptor-positive tumors and the spleen is diminished. This represents the analogy of blocking the receptor binding of iodinated octreotide with excess unlabeled octreotide in *in vitro* autoradiography. Yet, in our experience and that of others, neuroendocrine tumors may remain visible during treatment with octreotide, although the tumor uptake of [^{111}In-DTPA^0]octreotide may be less (up to 50%) than without octreotide treatment. In this respect, it should be taken into account that many of these tumors contain high numbers of somatostatin receptors, and that even high doses of octreotide (1, 500 μg/day or more subcutaneously) may not result in complete occupancy of the somatostatin receptors. It should also be considered that the expression of receptors on a tumor is not a steady state but a process in which recycling of receptors may occur.

DOSIMETRY

The effective dose equivalent of 3 to 6 mCi [^{111}In-DTPA^0]octreotide (8 to 16 mSv) is comparable to values for other ^{111}In-labeled radiopharmaceuticals (28) and is acceptable in view of the clinical indications. Furthermore, these radiation doses have to be compared with the values of commonly used imaging techniques for these clinical indications, e.g., computed tomography (CT) (chest: 7 to 11 mSv) and angiography (5 to 25 mSv).

IMAGING RESULTS IN NEUROENDOCRINE AND OTHER TUMORS

Pituitary Tumors

On virtually all GH-producing pituitary adenomas, somatostatin receptors are present (Fig. 35.3). Also, *in vivo* SRI is posi-

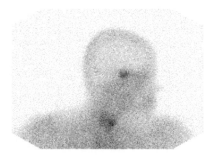

FIGURE 35.3. Moderate uptake at the site of a pituitary adenoma.

tive in most cases (29,30), but other pituitary tumors as well as pituitary metastases from somatostatin receptor-positive neoplasms, parasellar meningiomas, lymphomas, or granulomatous diseases of the pituitary may be positive. Therefore the diagnostic value of SRI in pituitary tumors is limited (31).

Controversy exists as to the relationship between the calculated tumor to background ratios in pituitary acromegaly using SRI with [¹¹¹In-DTPA⁰]octreotide and the extent of suppressibility of GH levels during octreotide treatment. Most investigators find no or only a weak correlation, however (30,32). SRI, therefore, does not seem to have a role in deciding whether or not to treat an acromegalic patient with octreotide.

Because of the limited effect of octreotide on hormone secretion by clinically nonfunctioning pituitary tumors, both *in vivo* and *in vitro,* and because of the absence of tumor shrinkage in the majority of patients studied, octreotide treatment in patients with a clinically nonfunctioning pituitary tumor does not seem promising (33,34). Therefore, there is no role for SRI in treatment selection (31).

Endocrine Pancreatic Tumors

The majority of the endocrine pancreatic tumors can be visualized using SRI (Fig. 35.4). Therefore, SRI can be of great value in localizing tumor sites in this type of patients and also in those cases in which surgery is indicated but no tumor localization can be found with conventional imaging modalities, which is often the case. Reported data on the sensitivity of SRI in patients with gastrinomas vary from about 60% to 90% (35–38), and part of the discrepancy in results is likely due to insufficient scanning technique (especially short acquisition time), not per-

forming SPECT studies, or injection of relatively low doses of [¹¹¹In-DTPA⁰]octreotide, all of which lead to a poorer performance of SRI.

Using ultrasound, CT, magnetic resonance imaging (MRI), and/or angiography, endocrine pancreatic tumors can be localized in about 50% of cases (39). Endoscopic ultrasound has been reported to be very sensitive in detecting endocrine pancreatic tumors, also when CT or transabdominal ultrasound fail to demonstrate the tumor (40). Studies comparing the value of endoscopic ultrasonography with SRI in the same patients point to more favorable results for SRI (36,38). Gibril et al. (37) published the results of a prospective study in 80 patients with Zollinger-Ellison syndrome, comparing SRI with a variety of other imaging techniques, as well as angiography. They found that SRI was as sensitive as all of the other imaging studies combined and advocated its use as the first imaging method to be used in these patients because of its sensitivity, simplicity, and cost effectiveness. Lebtahi et al. (41) reported that the results of SRI in 160 patients with gastroenteropancreatic (GEP) tumors modified patient classification and surgical therapeutic strategy in 25% of patients. Also, Termanini et al. (42) reported that SRI altered patient management in 47% of 122 patients with gastrinomas. However, results in patients with insulinomas are disappointing, possibly because part of these tumors may either be somatostatin receptor-negative or contain somatostatin receptors that do not bind octreotide.

Carcinoids

Reported values for the detection of known carcinoid tumor localizations vary from 80% to nearly 100% (43–45) (Fig. 35.5).

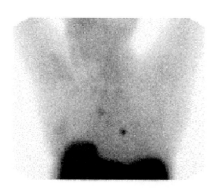

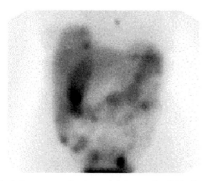

FIGURE 35.5. Intense uptake in multiple carcinoid lesions. Metastases in the chest *(upper image)* and in the abdomen and liver *(lower image).*

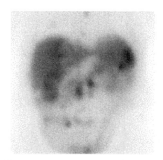

FIGURE 35.4. Intense uptake at multiple sites of a neuroendocrine tumor, with metastases in the abdomen, liver, and spine.

Also, the detection of unexpected tumor sites, not suspected with conventional imaging, is reported by several investigators (43,45,46).

Treatment with octreotide may cause a relief of symptoms and a decrease of urinary 5-HIAA levels in patients with the carcinoid syndrome (47). In patients with the carcinoid syndrome, SRI, because of its ability to demonstrate somatostatin receptor-positive tumors, could therefore be used to select those patients who are likely to respond favorably to octreotide treatment. On the other hand, only for those patients who have somatostatin receptor-negative tumors is chemotherapy effective (48).

The impact on patient management is fourfold: SRI may detect resectable tumors that would be unrecognized with conventional imaging techniques, it may prevent surgery in patients whose tumors have metastasized to a greater extent than can be detected with conventional imaging, it may direct the choice of therapy in patients with inoperable tumors, and it may be used to select patients for peptide receptor radionuclide therapy (PRRT, see later).

Paragangliomas

In virtually all patients with paragangliomas, tumors are readily visualized (49) (Fig. 35.6). Unexpected additional paraganglioma sites are often found. Multicentricity and distant metastases are each reported to occur in 10% of patients; in our study with SRI, we found multiple sites of pathology in 9 of 25 patients (36%) with a known paraganglioma (49). One of the major advantages of SRI is that it provides information on potential tumor sites in the whole body in patients with paraganglioma. It could thus be used as a screening test, to be followed by CT scanning, MRI, or ultrasound of the sites at which abnormalities are found.

Medullary Thyroid Carcinoma and Other Thyroid Cancers

In patients with medullary thyroid carcinoma (MTC) the sensitivity of SRI to detect tumor localizations is 50% to 70% (50, 51). In a series of 17 patients with MTC whom we studied (50), the ratio of CT over carcinoembryonic antigen (CEA) levels was

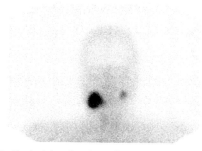

FIGURE 35.6. Typical localization of abnormal accumulation during somatostatin receptor imaging in a patient with bilateral carotid body paragangliomas. Single photon emission computed tomography is mandatory in these patients because the intense uptake in one lesion may mask other sites of pathology.

significantly higher in patients in whom SRI was successfully applied. This may imply that somatostatin receptors can be detected *in vivo* on the more differentiated forms of MTC. Also, SRI is more often positive in patients with high serum tumor markers and large tumors (51) and seems therefore less suitable to demonstrate microscopic disease (51,52).

Although papillary, follicular, and anaplastic thyroid cancers and also Hürthle-cell carcinomas do not belong to the group of classical neuroendocrine tumors, the majority of patients with these cancers show uptake of radiolabeled octreotide during SRI (53,54). Also, it is not necessary to withdraw patients from L-thyroxine suppression therapy to perform SRI (55). Interestingly, differentiated thyroid cancers that do not take up radioactive iodine may show radiolabeled octreotide accumulation (53). In some patients, this could open new therapeutic options: operation, if the number of observed lesions is limited, or, alternatively, PRRT if the uptake is sufficient.

Merkel Cell Tumors

Trabecular carcinomas of the skin, or Merkel cell tumors, are aggressive neoplasms that tend to occur in the sun-exposed skin. Often these tumors metastasize and, despite therapy, disease-related death is high. Ultrastructurally and immunocytochemically, the majority of these tumors have neuroendocrine characteristics.

In four out of the five patients studied with SRI in whom tumor had also been detected by CT and/or ultrasound, these sites were recognized on the scintigrams. In two patients, SRI demonstrated more metastatic tumor localizations than previously recognized (56).

If SRI were performed in patients with Merkel cell tumors, the sites of abnormal accumulation of radioactivity could thereafter be visualized using CT scanning or ultrasound and biopsies could be taken. Establishing the extent of the disease in this way may ensure an optimal choice of treatment for these tumors.

Small Cell Lung Carcinoma (SCLC)

With SRI the primary tumors can be demonstrated in virtually all patients with SCLC (57–59). Some of the known metastases may be missed, however; especially, several authors report the unexpected finding of brain metastases (57,58). Others however, have reported the lack of any additional information with SRI (60).

Of special interest are two groups of patients in whom the additional information provided by SRI may have therapeutic consequences: those in whom unexpected cerebral metastases are found and those in whom the additional information leads to upstaging from limited disease (LD) to extensive disease (ED). Adding SRI to the staging protocol in patients with SCLC would lead to an upstaging in 5 of 14 patients (36%) out of a group of 26 untreated patients who we studied (58) (who seemingly had LD with conventional imaging only). With conventional imaging, cerebral metastases were detected in two patients. SRI suggested cerebral metastases in these two and in another five patients as well. In four of them, cerebral metastases became manifest within 1 year.

Inclusion of SRI in the staging protocol of patients with SCLC may lead to upstaging in some of the patients with LD. The cost increase as compared with a conventional workup only must be weighed against an unnecessary treatment in part of patients with LD (i.e., local chest radiotherapy if a complete remission is achieved) (61). Applying SRI in the workup of patients with SCLC would demonstrate otherwise undetected brain metastases. From a radiotherapeutic point of view, it would be preferable to irradiate brain metastases when they are small. Therefore, the cost increase compared with the conventional workup is justified by the therapeutic consequences: irradiation of the brain at an early stage, which may lead to a postponement of neurologic symptoms and a better quality of life.

Breast Cancer

SRI localized 39 of 52 primary breast cancers (75%) (62). Imaging of the axillae showed nonpalpable cancer-containing lymph nodes in 4 of 13 patients with subsequently histologically proven metastases (Fig. 35.7). A special remark has to be made with respect to the observation of bilateral and diffuse physiologic breast uptake in normal females. This faint uptake is present in about 15% of patients 24 hours postinjection and is clearly different from the more localized accumulation at the site of breast cancer. At the moment the basis for this finding is unknown. In the follow-up after a mean of 2.5 years, SRI in 28 of the 37 patients with an originally somatostatin receptor-positive cancer was positive in 2 patients with clinically recognized metastases, as well as in 6 of the remaining 26 patients who were symptom free. SRI may be of value in selecting patients for clinical trials with somatostatin analogues or other medical treatments. Furthermore, SRI is sensitive for detecting recurrences of somatostatin receptor-positive breast cancer.

Malignant Lymphomas

Although in many patients with non-Hodgkin's lymphoma (NHL) one or more lesions may be somatostatin receptor-positive, receptor-negative lesions also occur in a substantial number of patients (63). Also, uptake of [^{111}In-DTPA^0]octreotide in lymphomas is lower as compared with the uptake in neuroendocrine tumors (64). In a prospective study in 50 untreated patients

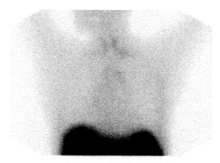

FIGURE 35.7. Faint uptake in a presumed lymph node just below and left of the thyroid in a patient with metastatic breast carcinoma. Computed tomography revealed no abnormalities in this region. The patient had Horner's syndrome.

with low-grade NHL, SRI was positive 84% (42/50) of patients (65). In 20% of patients, SRI revealed lesions that had not been demonstrated by conventional staging procedures. However, in 19 patients (38%), SRI missed lesions. Because of the limited sensitivity, SRI is recommended only in selected cases of NHL.

In 126 consecutive untreated patients with histologically proven Hodgkin's disease the results of SRI were compared with physical and radiologic examinations (66). SRI was positive in all patients. The lesion-related sensitivity was 94% and varied from 98% for supradiaphragmatic lesions to 67% for infradiaphragmatic lesions. In comparison with CT scanning and ultrasonography, SRI provided superior results for the detection of Hodgkin's disease localizations above the diaphragm. In stages I and II supradiaphragmatic patients, SRI detected more advanced disease in 18% (15/83) of patients, resulting in an upstaging to stage III or IV, thus directly influencing patient management. These data support the validity of SRI as a powerful imaging technique for the staging of patients with Hodgkin's disease.

Melanoma

Positive results of SRI have been reported in 16 out of 19 patients with melanoma (67). The exact impact of SRI on staging and patient management remains to be determined.

Neuroblastomas and Pheochromocytomas

In about 90% of patients with neuroblastoma, SRI visualized tumor deposits (68). Patients with neuroblastomas that are somatostatin receptor-positive *in vitro* have a longer survival compared with the receptor-negative ones (69). A drawback of the use of SRI for localization of this tumor in the adrenal gland is the relatively high radioligand accumulation in the kidneys. Metaiodobenzylguanidine (MIBG) scintigraphy is preferred for its localization in this region.

In a large retrospective study in patients operated for pheochromocytoma, the overall preoperative detection rate for tumors larger than 1 cm in diameter was 90% for ^{123}I-MIBG and only 25% for SRI (70). Most of the patients had primary benign pheochromocytomas. In patients with metastases, SRI detected lesions in seven of eight patients, including ^{123}I-MIBG negative cases. Therefore, it can be concluded that SRI should be tried in suspicious metastatic pheochromocytomas, especially if ^{123}I-MIBG is negative.

Cushing's Syndrome

In a study of 19 patients with Cushing's syndrome, none of the pituitary adenomas of 8 patients with Cushing's disease (or the adrenal adenoma of another patient) could be visualized with SRI (71). In 8 of the other 10 patients, the primary ectopic corticotropin or corticotropin-releasing hormone (CRH) secreting tumors were successfully identified with SRI. Phlipponneau et al. (72) and Weiss et al. (73) have reported their successful localizations of a 6-mm diameter corticotropin-secreting bronchial carcinoid and a 10-mm diameter corticotropin-secreting-

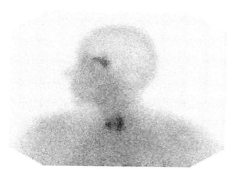

FIGURE 35.8. Moderate uptake in a parasellar meningioma.

bronchial carcinoid with one lymph node metastasis, respectively. Therefore, SRI can be included as a diagnostic step in the workup of Cushing's syndrome with a suspected ectopic corticotropin or CRH-secreting tumor. Others, however, conclude that although SRI may be helpful in selected cases, it is not a significant advance over conventional imaging (74).

Brain Tumors

SRI localizes meningiomas in virtually all patients (75,76) (Fig. 35.8). The majority of well-differentiated astrocytomas (grade I and II) are somatostatin receptor-positive, whereas the undifferentiated glioblastomas (grade IV) are receptor-negative. An inverse relationship between the presence of somatostatin and epidermal growth factor (EGF) receptors has been observed. In grade III astrocytomas both receptors can be found (77). Astrocytomas have been visualized with SRI (76). A prerequisite for the localization with this radioligand is a locally open blood-brain barrier. Especially in the lower graded astrocytomas this barrier may be unperturbed. Therefore, the grading of glia-derived brain tumors with SRI is at this moment not promising.

IMAGING RESULTS IN OTHER DISEASES

In vivo SRI is also positive in a number of granulomatous and autoimmune diseases, such as sarcoidosis, tuberculosis, Wegen-

er's granulomatosis, de Quervain's thyroiditis, aspergillosis, Graves' hyperthyroidism, and Graves' ophthalmopathy (78–80). It is expected that SRI may contribute to a more precise staging and a better evaluation of several of these diseases.

Sarcoidosis

In a cross-sectional study in 46 patients with sarcoidosis, known mediastinal, hilar, and interstitial disease was recognized in 36 of 37 patients (81) (Fig. 35.9). Also, such pathology was found in 7 other patients who had normal chest x-rays. In 5 of these, SRI pointed to interstitial disease. SRI was repeated in 13 patients. In 5 of 6 patients who had a chest x-ray film monitored improvement of disease activity, SRI also showed a decrease of pathologic uptake. In 2 of 5 patients in whom the chest x-ray film was unchanged, but serum angiotensin-converting enzyme (ACE) concentrations decreased and lung function improved, a normalization was found with SRI. To determine the value of SRI in the follow-up of patients with sarcoidosis, a prospective longitudinal study will have to be performed.

Uveitis may be the presenting symptom of sarcoidosis. In our experience, in patients with uveitis, SRI is often helpful because of the typical pattern of uptake in the mediastinum, lung hila, and parotid glands that can be seen in patients who eventually appear to have sarcoidosis, even when the chest x-ray film or CT are normal. Thus, SRI can be used to reach a diagnosis and also influence the decision of how to treat this type of patient.

Graves' Disease

In Graves' hyperthyroidism, accumulation of radiolabeled octreotide in the thyroid gland is markedly increased and correlates with serum levels of free thyroxine and thyrotropin binding inhibiting immunoglobulins. *In vitro* studies showed that the follicular cells express somatostatin receptors in Graves' disease (82). In clinically active Graves' ophthalmopathy, the orbits show accumulation of radioactivity 4 hours and 24 hours after injection of [^{111}In-DTPA^0]octreotide (79). SPECT is required for a proper interpretation of orbital scintigraphy. There is also a correlation between orbital [^{111}In-DTPA^0]octreotide uptake

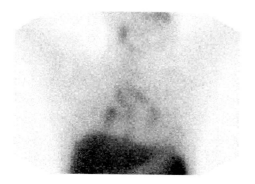
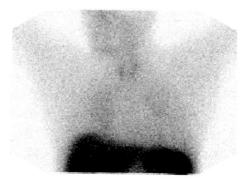

FIGURE 35.9. The typical pattern of bihilar and mediastinal uptake in a patient with sarcoidosis *(left image)*. Often, the parotid glands are also involved. The right image shows diffuse uptake in the lungs in a patient with interstitial sarcoidosis.

and Clinical Activity Score and Total Eye Score (79,83). Also, uptake is high in clinically active disease, but low if ophthalmopathy is inactive (80). The clinical value of SRI in Graves' disease has yet to be established. Possibly this technique could select those patients with Graves' ophthalmopathy who might benefit from treatment with octreotide (80,83).

SCINTIGRAPHY: SUMMARY

[^{111}In-DTPA^0]octreotide is a radiopharmaceutical with a great potential for the visualization of somatostatin receptor-positive tumors. The overall sensitivity of SRI to localize neuroendocrine tumors is high. In a number of neuroendocrine tumor types, as well as in Hodgkin's disease, inclusion of SRI in the localization or staging procedure may be very rewarding, either in terms of cost effectiveness, patient management, or quality of life. The value of SRI in patients with other tumors, like breast cancer, or in patients with granulomatous diseases has to be established.

SURGICAL PROBE

The application of radiolabeled peptides may be clinically useful in another way: After the injection of [^{111}In-DTPA^0]octreotide, tumor localizations can be detected by the surgeon by means of a handheld probe that is used during the operation (84,85). This may especially be of value if small tumors with a high receptor density are present, for instance gastrinomas.

PEPTIDE RECEPTOR RADIONUCLIDE THERAPY

In patients with somatostatin receptor-positive pathology, SRI is useful if it can localize otherwise undetectable disease or if it can be used for treatment selection (usually the choice between symptomatic treatment with somatostatin analogues or other medical treatment). In patients with known metastatic disease, however, in whom little or no treatment alternatives are available, SRI has a limited role. This situation changes if imaging has a sequel in treatment. The request for iodine scans of the thyroid would be a fraction of what it is if radioiodine treatment were not available. In analogy, the option of treatment with radiolabeled somatostatin analogues may become the impetus to SRI.

As soon as the success of peptide receptor scintigraphy for tumor visualization became clear, the next logical step was to try to label these peptides with radionuclides emitting α- or β-particles, or Auger or conversion electrons, and to perform radiotherapy with these radiolabeled peptides.

[^{111}In-DTPA^0]Octreotide Therapy

Radionuclide therapy with high doses of [^{111}In-DTPA^0]octreotide has been performed in a clinical phase 1 study. In 30 end-stage patients with mostly neuroendocrine tumors who received up to a cumulative dose of 74 GBq, the only side effects were

a transient decline in platelet counts and lymphocyte subsets (86).

The typical dose per administration was 6,000 to 7,000 MBq ^{111}In incorporated in 40 to 50 μg [DTPA^0]octreotide. Doses were given with at least 2-week intervals between administrations, and a total of 8 administrations were aimed for, increasing in a few patients to about 20 administrations. Patients were scanned 3 and 7 days after each administration of the radiotherapeutic dose. Uptakes decreased slowly or remained the same if the interval between the successive administrations was less than 1 month. In patients who had 6 or more administrations of 6,000 to 7,000 MBq of [^{111}In-DTPA^0]octreotide with intervals of maximally 1 month between administrations, uptake in the tumor was still clearly visible after the last administration. Of the 21 patients who received a cumulative dose of more than 20 GBq, some reduction in tumor size was found in 6 and stable disease in 8. There was a tendency towards better results in patients with a high tumor uptake (86). The observed responses to this radionuclide therapy are in agreement with internalization of [^{111}In-DTPA^0]octreotide into tumor cells and with an antiproliferative effect also shown in other studies (87,88).

[^{90}Y-DOTA^0,Tyr^3]Octreotide Therapy

^{111}In-coupled peptides, because of the small particle range of the Auger electrons and therefore short tissue penetration, are not ideal for radionuclide therapy. Recently, another somatostatin analogue, [DOTA^0, Tyr^3]octreotide (DOTATOC) was developed, to which the high-energy β-emitter ^{90}Y can be linked in a very stable manner (89,90). In studies in patients and rats, the uptake of radioactivity in known somatostatin receptor-positive organs and tumors was higher after ^{111}In-DOTATOC than after [^{111}In-DTPA^0]octreotide (91,92). Patient studies showed favorable results of ^{90}Y-DOTATOC treatment (89,93). Also, a study comparing both the uptake of ^{111}In-DOTATOC and ^{86}Y-DOTATOC, as well as the effects of treatment with ^{90}Y-DOTATOC in the same patients has started (94). The absorbed radiation dose to the kidneys may pose a problem in PRRT. In rats it was shown that the renal uptake of [^{111}In-DTPA^0]octreotide could be reduced by positively charged amino acids, e.g., with about 50 % by single intravenous administration of 400 mg/kg L-lysine or D-lysine (95). Therefore, during PRRT with ^{90}Y-DOTATOC, an infusion containing the positively charged amino acids L-lysine and L-arginine is given during and after the infusion of the radiopharmaceutical, to reduce the kidney uptake. A recent analysis of the results of ^{90}Y-DOTATOC treatment in a phase 1 trial in 22 end-stage patients with progressive disease shows a partial tumor response in 2, a minor response in 3, and stable disease in 10 patients (94). A phase 2 trial of ^{90}Y-DOTATOC treatment in patients with SCLC and breast cancer is expected to start soon.

[^{177}Lu-DOTA^0,Tyr^3]Octreotate Therapy

The somatostatin analogue [DOTA^0,Tyr^3]octreotate has a nine-fold higher affinity for the somatostatin receptor subtype 2 if compared with [DOTA^0,Tyr^3]octreotide. Also, labeled with the beta and gamma emitting radionuclide ^{177}Lu, this compound

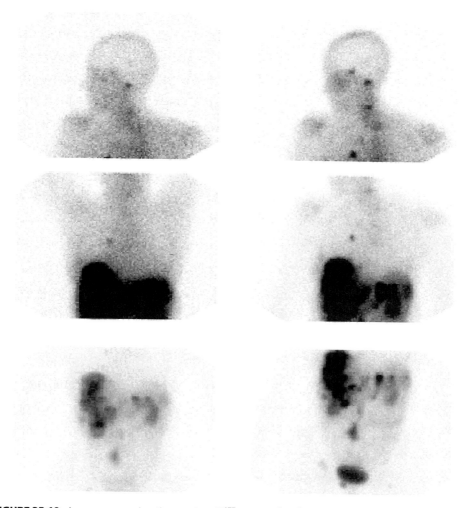

FIGURE 35.10. Images comparing the uptake of [^{177}Lu-DOTA^0,Tyr^3]octreotate and [^{111}In-DTPA^0]octreotide 24-hours postinjection in a patient with a metastasized neuroendocrine tumor. *Left column:* [^{111}In-DTPA^0]octreotide; *right column:* [^{177}Lu-DOTA^0,Tyr^3]octreotate. Note that the biodistribution in liver, spleen, and kidneys is similar for both radiopharmaceuticals and that the uptake in the tumors is higher with [^{177}Lu-DOTA^0,Tyr^3]octreotate.

was shown very successful in terms of tumor regression and animal survival in a rat model (91,96,97).

In a study in patients, the uptake after 24 hours, expressed as percentage of the injected dose of [^{177}Lu-DOTA^0,Tyr^3]octreotate (^{177}Lu-octreotate), was comparable to that after [^{111}In-DTPA^0]octreotide for kidneys, spleen, and liver, but was three- to fourfold higher for four of five tumors (98) (Fig. 35.10). From this study, it was concluded that in comparison with the radionuclide coupled somatostatin analogues that are currently available for somatostatin receptor-mediated radiotherapy, ^{177}Lu-octreotate potentially represents an important improvement because of the higher absorbed doses that can be achieved to most tumors with about equal doses to potentially dose-limiting organs and because of the lower tissue penetration range of ^{177}Lu if compared with ^{90}Y, which may be especially important for small tumors. In a very recent preliminary evaluation of the antitumor effects of this new radiopharmaceutical in 21 patients with neuroendocrine tumors who received their maximal cumu-

lative dose of 600 to 800 mCi, a partial remission (i.e., a tumor volume reduction of more than 50%) was found in 6/21 (29%) patients, at the first follow-up 6 to 8 weeks after the last treatment. Because ^{177}Lu emits β-radiation of an energy comparable to that of ^{131}I, which in thyroid disease exerts its maximal effect 3 to 6 months after administration, these results of PRRT with ^{177}Lu-octreotate may be expected to even improve with longer follow-up.

OUTLOOK

The basis of somatostatin receptor scintigraphy and its reported possibilities, especially in nuclear oncology, are promising for the future usefulness of other small radiolabeled peptides, especially as complementary radioligands for octreotide. Tumor localization, differentiation and staging of tumor types by *in vivo* mapping of tumorous peptide receptors, localization of metastases expressing different peptide receptors by administration of a "cocktail" of radioligands, and impact on the choice of drugs for cancer treatment are all possible features to be addressed by nuclear medicine in the future. Also, PRRT using radionuclides with appropriate particle ranges may become a new treatment modality. One might consider the use of radiolabeled somatostatin analogues first in an adjuvant setting after surgery of somatostatin receptor-positive tumors to eradicate occult metastases and second for treatment of cancer recurrence at a later stage.

REFERENCES

1. Reubi JC, Maurer R. Autoradiographic mapping of somatostatin receptors in the rat CNS and pituitary. *Neuroscience* 1985;15:1183–1193.
2. Patel YC, Amherdt M, Orci L. Quantitative electron microscopic autoradiography of insulin, glucagon and somatostatin binding sites on islets. *Science* 1982;217:1155–1156.
3. Sreedharan SP, Kodama KT, Peterson KE et al. Distinct subsets of somatostatin receptors on cultured human lymphocytes. *J Biol Chem* 1989;264:949–953.
4. Yamada Y, Post SR, Wang K et al. Cloning and functional characterization of a family of human and mouse somatostatin receptors expressed in brain, gastrointestinal tract, and kidney. *Proc Natl Acad Sci U S A* 1992;89:251–255.
5. Yamada Y, Reisine T, Law SF et al. Somatostatin receptors; an expanding gene family: cloning and functional characterization of human SSTR 3, a protein coupled to adenylyl cyclase. *Mol Endocrinol* 1992; 6:2136–2142.
6. Rohrer L, Raulf F, Bruns C et al. Cloning and characterization of a fourth human somatostatin receptor. *Proc Natl Acad Sci U S A* 1993; 90:4196–4200.
7. Yamada Y, Kagimoto S, Kubota A et al. Cloning, functional expression and pharmacological characterization of a fourth (hSSTR4) and a fifth (hSSTR5) human somatostatin receptor subtype. *Biochem Biophys Res Comm* 1993;195:844–852.
8. Patel YC, Greenwood MT, Warszynska A et al. All five cloned somatostatin receptors (hSSTR1-5) are functionally coupled to adenylyl cyclase. *Biochem Biophys Res Comm* 1994;198:605–612.
9. Brazeau P. Somatostatin: a peptide with unexpected physiologic activities. *Am J Med* 1986;81(Suppl 6B):8–13.
10. Lamberts SWJ, Krenning EP, Reubi JC. The role of somatostatin and its analogs in the diagnosis and treatment of tumors. *Endocr Rev* 1991; 12:450–482.
11. Reubi JC, Kvols L, Krenning EP et al. Distribution of somatostatin receptors in normal and tumor tissue. *Metabolism* 1990;39:78–81.
12. Reubi JC, Krenning EP, Lamberts SWJ et al. *In vitro* detection of somatostatin receptors in human tumors. *Metabolism* 1992;41: 104–110.
13. Reubi JC, Laissue J, Krenning EP et al. Somatostatin receptors in human cancer: incidence, characteristics, functional correlates and clinical implication. *J Steroid Biochem Mol Biol* 1992;43:27–35.
14. Pearse AGE, Polak JM, Heath CM. Polypeptide hormone production by "carcinoid" APUDomas and their relevant cytochemistry. *Virchows Arch [B]* 1974;16:95–109.
15. Reubi JC, Maurer R, Klijn JGM et al. High incidence of somatostatin receptors in human meningiomas: biochemical characterization. *J Clin Endocrinol Metab* 1986;63:433–438.
16. Reubi JC, Lang W, Maurer R et al. Distribution and biochemical characterization of somatostatin receptors in tumors of the human central nervous system. *Cancer Res* 1987;47:5758–5765.
17. Reubi JC, Waser B, Foekens JA et al. Somatostatin receptor incidence and distribution in breast cancer using receptor autoradiography: relationship to EGF-receptors. *Int J Cancer* 1990;46:416–420.
18. Reubi JC, Waser B, Sheppard M et al. Somatostatin receptors are present in small-cell but not in non-small-cell primary lung carcinomas: relationship to EGF receptors. *Int J Cancer* 1990;45:269–274.
19. Reubi JC, Waser B, Vanhagen M et al. *In vitro* and *in vivo* detection

20. of somatostatin receptors in human malignant lymphomas. *Int J Cancer* 1992;50:895–900.
21. Reubi JC, Horisberger U, Waser B et al. Preferential location of somatostatin receptors in germinal centers of human gut lymphoid tissue. *Gastroenterology* 1992;103:1207–1214.
22. Reubi JC, Horisberger U, Laissue J. High density of somatostatin receptors in veins surrounding human cancer tissue: role in tumor-host interaction? *Int J Cancer* 1994;56:681–688.
23. Bakker WH, Alberts R, Bruns C et al. [¹¹¹In-DTPA-D-Phe¹]-octreotide, a potential radiopharmaceutical for imaging of somatostatin receptor-positive tumors: synthesis, radiolabeling and *in vitro* validation. *Life Sci* 1991;49:1583–1591.
24. Bakker WH, Krenning EP, Reubi JC et al. *In vivo* application of [¹¹¹In-DTPA-D-Phe¹]-octreotide for detection of somatostatin receptor-positive tumors in rats. *Life Sci* 1991;49:1593–1601.
25. Van Uden A, Steinmeijer MVJ, De Swart J et al. Imaging with octreoscan: haste makes waste. *Eur J Nucl Med* 1999;26:1022P.
26. Jamar F, Fiasse R, Leners N et al. Somatostatin receptor imaging with indium-111-pentetreotide in gastroenteropancreatic neuroendocrine tumors: safety, efficacy and impact on patient management. *J Nucl Med* 1995;36:542–549.
27. Reubi JC, Horisberger U, Studer UE et al. Human kidney as target for somatostatin: high affinity receptors in tubules and vasa recta. *J Clin Endocrinol Metab* 1993;77:1323–1328.
28. Gibril F, Reynolds JC, Chen CC et al. Specificity of somatostatin receptor scintigraphy: a prospective study and effects of false-positive localizations on management in patients with gastrinomas. *J Nucl Med* 1999;40:539–553.
29. Krenning EP, Bakker WH, Kooij PPM et al. Somatostatin receptor scintigraphy with [¹¹¹In-DTPA-D-Phe¹]-octreotide in man: metabolism, dosimetry and comparison with [¹²³I-Tyr³]-octreotide. *J Nucl Med* 1992;33:652–658.
30. Ur E, Mather SJ, Bomanji J et al. Pituitary imaging using a labelled somatostatin analogue in acromegaly. *Clin Endocrinol* 1992;36: 147–150.
31. Legovini P, De Menis E, Billeci D et al. ¹¹¹Indium-pentetreotide pituitary scintigraphy and hormonal responses to octreotide in acromegalic patients. *J Endocrinol Invest* 1997;20:424–428.
32. Kwekkeboom DJ, de Herder WW, Krenning EP. Receptor imaging in the diagnosis and treatment of pituitary tumors. *J Endocrinol Invest* 1999;22:80–88.
33. Duet M, Ajzenberg C, Benelhadj S et al. Somatostatin receptor scintigraphy in pituitary adenomas: a somatostatin receptor density index can predict hormonal and tumoral efficacy of octreotide *in vivo*. *J Nucl Med* 1999;40:1252–1256.
34. De Bruin TWA, Kwekkeboom DJ, Van 't Verlaat JW et al. Clinically nonfunctioning pituitary adenoma and octreotide response to long term high dose treatment, and studies *in vitro*. *J Clin Endocrinol Metab* 1992;75:1310–1317.
35. Merola B, Colao A, Ferone D et al. Effects of a chronic treatment with octreotide in patients with functionless pituitary adenomas. *Horm Res* 1993;40:149–155.
36. Kwekkeboom DJ, Krenning EP, Oei HY et al. Use of radiolabeled somatostatin to localize islet cell tumors. In: Mignon M, Jensen RT, eds. *Frontiers of gastro-intestinal research*, vol 23. Endocrine tumors of the pancreas. New York: Karger, 1995:298–308.
37. De Kerviler E, Cadiot G, Lebtahi R et al. Somatostatin receptor scintigraphy in forty-eight patients with the Zollinger-Ellison syndrome. *Eur J Nucl Med* 1994;21:1191–1197.
38. Gibril F, Reynolds JC, Doppman JL et al. Somatostatin receptor scintigraphy: its sensitivity compared with that of other imaging methods in detecting primary and metastatic gastrinomas. A prospective study. *Ann Intern Med* 1996;125:26–34.
39. Zimmer T, Stolzel U, Bader M et al. Endoscopic ultrasonography and somatostatin receptor scintigraphy in the preoperative localisation of insulinomas and gastrinomas. *Gut* 1996;39:562–568.
40. Lunderquist A. Radiologic diagnosis of neuroendocrine tumors. *Acta Oncol* 1989;28:371–372.
41. Rösch T, Lightdale CJ, Botet JF et al. Localization of pancreatic endo-

crine tumors by endoscopic ultrasonography. *N Engl J Med* 1992;326:1721–1726.

41. Lebtahi R, Cadiot G, Sarda L et al. Clinical impact of somatostatin receptor scintigraphy in the management of patients with neuroendocrine gastroenteropancreatic tumors. *J Nucl Med* 1997;38:853–858.

42. Termanini B, Gibril F, Reynolds JC et al. Value of somatostatin receptor scintigraphy: a prospective study in gastrinoma of its effect on clinical management. *Gastroenterology* 1997;112:335–347.

43. Kwekkeboom DJ, Krenning EP, Bakker WH et al. Somatostatin analogue scintigraphy in carcinoid tumors. *Eur J Nucl Med* 1993;20:283–292.

44. Kalkner KM, Janson ET, Nilsson S et al. Somatostatin receptor scintigraphy in patients with carcinoid tumors: comparison between radioligand uptake and tumor markers. *Cancer Res* 1995;55(Suppl 23):5801–5804.

45. Westlin JE, Janson ET, Arnberg H et al. Somatostatin receptor scintigraphy of carcinoid tumours using the [111In-DTPA-D-Phe1]-octreotide. *Acta Oncol* 1993;32:783–786.

46. Ahlman H, Wängberg B, Tisell LE. Clinical efficacy of octreotide scintigraphy in patients with midgut carcinoid tumours and evaluation of intraoperative scintillation detection. *Br J Surg* 1994;81:1144–1149.

47. Kvols LK, Moertel CG, O'Connell MJ et al. Treatment of the malignant carcinoid syndrome. *N Eng J Med* 1986;315:663–666.

48. Kvols LK. Medical oncology considerations in patients with metastatic neuroendocrine carcinomas. *Semin Oncol* 1994;21(Suppl 13):56–60.

49. Kwekkeboom DJ, Van Urk H, Pauw KH et al. Octreotide scintigraphy for the detection of paragangliomas. *J Nucl Med* 1993;34:873–878.

50. Kwekkeboom DJ, Reubi JC, Lamberts SWJ et al. *In vivo* somatostatin receptor imaging in medullary thyroid carcinoma. *J Clin Endocrinol Metab* 1993;76:1413–1417.

51. Tisell LE, Ahlman H, Wängberg B et al. Somatostatin receptor scintigraphy in medullary thyroid carcinoma. *Br J Surg* 1997;84:543–547.

52. Adams S, Baum RP, Hertel A. Comparison of metabolic and receptor imaging in recurrent medullary thyroid carcinoma with histopathological findings. *Eur J Nucl Med* 1998;25:1277–1283.

53. Postema PTE, De Herder WW, Reubi JC et al. Somatostatin receptor scintigraphy in non-medullary thyroid cancer. *Digestion* 1996;1(Suppl):36–37.

54. Gulec SA, Serafini AN, Sridhar KS et al. Somatostatin receptor expression in Hurthle cell cancer of the thyroid. *J Nucl Med* 1998;39:243–245.

55. Haslinghuis LM, Krenning EP, de Herder WW et al. Somatostatin receptor scintigraphy in the follow-up of patients with differentiated thyroid cancer. *J Endocrinol Invest* 2001;24:415–422.

56. Kwekkeboom DJ, Hoff AM, Lamberts SWJ et al. Somatostatin analogue scintigraphy: a simple and sensitive method for the *in vivo* visualization of Merkel cell tumors and their metastases. *Arch Dermatol* 1992;128:818–821.

57. Kwekkeboom DJ, Kho GS, Lamberts SW et al. The value of octreotide scintigraphy in patients with lung cancer. *Eur J Nucl Med* 1994;21:1106–1113.

58. Bombardieri E, Crippa F, Cataldo I et al. Somatostatin receptor imaging of small cell lung cancer (SCLC) by means of 111In-DTPA octreotide scintigraphy. *Eur J Cancer* 1995;31A:184–188.

59. Reisinger I, Bohuslavitzki KH, Brenner W et al. Somatostatin receptor scintigraphy in small-cell lung cancer: results of a multicenter study. *J Nucl Med* 1998;39:224–227.

60. Kirsch CM, von Pawel J, Grau I et al. Indium-111 pentetreotide in the diagnostic work-up of patients with bronchogenic carcinoma. *Eur J Nucl Med* 1994;21:1318–1325.

61. Kwekkeboom DJ, Lamberts SWJ, Habbema JD et al. Cost-effectiveness analysis of somatostatin receptor scintigraphy. *J Nucl Med* 1996;37:886–892.

62. Van Eijck CH, Krenning EP, Bootsma A et al. Somatostatin-receptor scintigraphy in primary breast cancer. *Lancet* 1994;343:640–643.

63. Van Hagen PM, Krenning EP, Reubi JC et al. Somatostatin analogue scintigraphy of malignant lymphomas. *Br J Haematol* 1993;83:75–79.

64. Leners N, Jamar F, Fiasse R et al. Indium-111-pentetreotide uptake in endocrine tumors and lymphoma. *J Nucl Med* 1996;37:916–922.

65. Lugtenburg PJ, Lowenberg B, Valkema R et al. Somatostatin receptor scintigraphy in the initial staging of low-grade non-Hodgkin's lymphomas. *J Nucl Med* 2001;42:222–229.

66. Lugtenburg PJ, Krenning EP, Valkema R et al. Somatostatin receptor scintigraphy useful in stage I-II Hodgkin's disease: more extended disease identified. *Br J Haematol* 2001;112:936–944.

67. Hoefnagel CA, Rankin EM, Valdés Olmos RA et al. Sensitivity versus specificity in melanoma imaging using iodine-123 iodobenzamide and indium-111 pentetreotide. *Eur J Nucl Med* 1994;21:587–588.

68. Krenning EP, Kwekkeboom DJ, Bakker WH et al. Somatostatin receptor scintigraphy with [111In-DTPA-D-Phe1]- and [123I-Tyr3]-octreotide: the Rotterdam experience with more than 1000 patients. *Eur J Nucl Med* 1993;20:716–731.

69. Moertel CL, Reubi JC, Scheithauer BS et al. Expression of somatostatin receptors in childhood neuroblastoma. *Am J Clin Pathol* 1994;102:752–756.

70. Van der Harst E, de Herder WW, Bruining HA et al. [(123)I]metaiodobenzylguanidine and [(111)In]octreotide uptake in benign and malignant pheochromocytomas. *J Clin Endocrinol Metab* 2001;86:685–693.

71. De Herder WW, Krenning EP, Malchoff CD et al. Somatostatin receptor scintigraphy: its value in tumor localization in patients with the Cushing syndrome caused by ectopic corticotropin and/or CRH secretion. *Am J Med* 1994;96:305–312.

72. Philipponneau M, Nocaudie M, Epelbaum J et al. Somatostatin analogs for the localization and preoperative treatment of an ACTH-secreting bronchial carcinoid tumor. *J Clin Endocrinol Metab* 1994;78:20–24.

73. Weiss M, Yellin A, Husza'r M et al. Localization of adrenocorticotropic hormone-secreting bronchial carcinoid tumor by somatostatin-receptor scintigraphy. *Ann Intern Med* 1994;121:198–199.

74. Torpy DJ, Chen CC, Mullen N et al. Lack of utility of (111)In-pentetreotide scintigraphy in localizing ectopic ACTH producing tumors: follow-up of 18 patients. *J Clin Endocrinol Metab* 1999;84:1186–1192.

75. Haldemann AR, Rosler H, Barth A et al. Somatostatin receptor scintigraphy in central nervous system tumors: role of blood-brain barrier permeability. *J Nucl Med* 1995;36:403–410.

76. Schmidt M, Scheidhauer K, Luyken C et al. Somatostatin receptor imaging in intracranial tumours. *Eur J Nucl Med* 1998;25:675–686.

77. Reubi JC, Horisberger U, Lang W et al. Coincidence of EGF receptors and somatostatin receptors in meningiomas but inverse, differentiation-dependent relationship in glial tumors. *Am J Pathol* 1989;134:337–344.

78. Vanhagen PM, Krenning EP, Reubi JC et al. Somatostatin analogue scintigraphy in granulomatous diseases. *Eur J Nucl Med* 1994;21:497–502.

79. Postema PTE, Krenning EP, Wijngaarde R et al. [111In-DTPA-D-Phe1]-octreotide scintigraphy in thyroidal and orbital Graves' disease: a parameter for disease activity? *J Clin Endocrinol Metab* 1994;79:1845–1851.

80. Krassas GE, Dumas A, Pontikides N et al. Somatostatin receptor scintigraphy and octreotide treatment in patients with thyroid eye disease. *Clin Endocrinol (Oxf)* 1995;42:571–580.

81. Kwekkeboom DJ, Krenning EP, Kho GS et al. Octreotide scintigraphy in patients with sarcoidosis. *Eur J Nucl Med* 1998;25:1284–1292.

82. Reubi JC, Waser B, Friess H et al. Regulatory peptide receptors in goiters of the human thyroid. *J Nucl Med* 1997;38(Suppl):266P.

83. Gerding MN, van der Zant FM, van Royen EA et al. Octreotide-scintigraphy is a disease-activity parameter in Graves' ophthalmopathy. *Clin Endocrinol (Oxf)* 1999;50:373–379.

84. Modlin IM, Cornelius E, Lawton GP. Use of an isotopic somatostatin receptor probe to image gut endocrine tumors. *Arch Surg* 1995;130:367–373.

85. Wangberg B, Forssell-Aronsson E, Tisell LE et al. Intraoperative detection of somatostatin-receptor-positive neuroendocrine tumours using indium-111-labelled DTPA-D-Phe1-octreotide. *Br J Cancer* 1996;73:770–775.

86. Krenning EP, De Jong M, Kooij PPM et al. Radiolabelled somatostatin analogue(s) for peptide receptor scintigraphy and radionuclide therapy. *Ann Oncol* 1999;10(Suppl 2):23–29.

87. Fjalling M, Andersson P, Forssell-Aronsson E et al. Systemic radionu-

clide therapy using indium-111-DTPA-D-Phe1-octreotide in midgut carcinoid syndrome. *J Nucl Med* 1996;37:1519–1521.

88. McCarthy KE, Woltering EA, Espenan GD et al. *In situ* radiotherapy with 111In-pentetreotide: initial observations and future directions. *Cancer J Sci Am* 1998;4:94–102.

89. Otte A, Jermann E, Behe M et al. DOTATOC: a powerful new tool for receptor-mediated radionuclide therapy. *Eur J Nucl Med* 1997;24:792–795.

90. De Jong M, Bakker WH, Krenning EP et al. Yttrium-90 and indium-111 labelling, receptor binding and biodistribution of [DOTA^0,d-Phe^1,Tyr^3]octreotide, a promising somatostatin analogue for radionuclide therapy. *Eur J Nucl Med* 1997;24:368–371.

91. De Jong M, Breeman WAP, Bakker WH et al. Comparison of ^{111}In-labeled somatostatin analogues for tumor scintigraphy and radionuclide therapy. *Cancer Res* 1998;58:437–441.

92. Kwekkeboom DJ, Kooij PPM, Bakker WH et al. Comparison of indium-111-DOTATOC and indium-111-DTPA-octreotide in the same patients: biodistribution, kinetics, organ and tumor uptake. *J Nucl Med* 1999;40:762–767.

93. Paganelli G, Zoboli S, Cremonesi M et al. Receptor-mediated radionuclide therapy with 90Y-DOTA-D-Phe1-Tyr3-Octreotide: preliminary report in cancer patients. *Cancer Biother Radiopharm* 1999;14:477–483.

94. Valkema R, Jamar F, Jonard P et al. Targeted radiotherapy with ^{90}Y-SMT487 (OctreoTher™): a phase I study. *J Nucl Med* 2000;41:111P.

95. Bernard BF, Krenning EP, Breeman WA et al. D-lysine reduction of indium-111 octreotide and yttrium-90 octreotide renal uptake. *J Nucl Med* 1997;38:1929–1933.

96. Erion JL, Bugaj JE, Schmidt MA et al. High radiotherapeutic efficacy of [Lu-177]-DOTA-Y(3)-octreotate in a rat tumor model. *J Nucl Med* 1999;40:223P.

97. De Jong M, Breeman WA, Bernard BF et al. [177Lu-DOTA(0),Tyr3]octreotate for somatostatin receptor-targeted radionuclide therapy. *Int J Cancer* 2001;92:628–633.

98. Kwekkeboom DJ, Bakker WH, Kooij PPM et al. [^{177}Lu-DOTA^0,Tyr^3]octreotate: comparison with [^{111}In-DTPA^0]octreotide in patients. *Eur J Nucl Med* 2001;28:1319–1325.

36

PET FOR CLINICAL DIAGNOSIS AND RESEARCH IN NEUROENDOCRINE TUMORS

BARBRO ERIKSSON
MATS BERGSTRÖM
HÅKAN ÖRLEFORS
ANDERS SUNDIN
KJELL ÖBERG
BENGT LÅNGSTRÖM

PET IN ONCOLOGY

A revolutionary development in synthetic chemistry has supplied a range of new potential tracers for positron emission tomography (PET). Some of these tracers have been tested in clinical research to define their possible role in clinical diagnosis (1), whereas others are still used in research projects. Depending on the tracer employed, one can selectively measure the function of different metabolic pathways of interest or expression of receptors and enzymes. This approach may also offer an opportunity to measure metabolic changes in tumors after treatment. At present, the routine evaluation of tumor response to treatment has relied on anatomic changes [computed tomography (CT) and magnetic resonance imaging (MRI)] demonstrating alterations in growth as reflected by tumor size. However, changes in tumor size may take weeks to months to develop before the success or failure of therapy is evident, and there is a definite value to search for methods in which response is revealed early in the treatment. It has been suggested that PET with its potential for characterization of physiology could serve this purpose.

^{18}F-deoxyglucose (^{18}F-FDG) is the most widely used agent for imaging tumors with PET. As a means of staging cancer disease, PET with ^{18}F-FDG has proven to be a most valuable method and a method that should be used as a primary investigation in several tumor types. In addition to numerous studies using ^{18}F-FDG to stage and diagnose cancer, investigators have also demonstrated that the uptake of this tracer often declines after successful treatment (2). ^{18}F-FDG is, however, not mechanistically directly coupled to tumor metabolism but rather indicates the expression of glucose transporters and could therefore be expected to fail sometimes in assessment of tumor response, especially early after treatment. Furthermore, it is not a selective tracer for tumor imaging because many cell types express the glucose transporter. For example, macrophages, which invade tumors and are found in inflammatory lesions, demonstrate increased uptake of ^{18}F-FDG.

NEUROENDOCRINE TUMORS

Neuroendocrine tumors derive from endocrine cells, usually contain secretory granules, and have the capacity to produce biogenic amines and polypeptide hormones. Twenty years ago, Pearse presented the so-called *a*mine *p*recursor *u*ptake and *de*carboxylation (APUD) concept based on the observation that certain cells have the capacity to take up and decarboxylate amine precursors such as 5-hydroxytryptophan (5-HTP) and L-dihydroxyphenylalanine (L-DOPA). Tumors derived from these cells were consequently called APUDoma (3).

Carcinoids are usually classified according to embryonic origin into foregut, midgut, and hindgut carcinoids, a classification that is clinically relevant because these different tumors have different tendencies to metastasize and have different symptomatology (4).

The midgut carcinoid, usually originating from cells in the small intestine, has a relatively high tendency to metastasize via local lymph nodes to the liver, and most patients have liver metastases at diagnosis. At this stage most patients present with the carcinoid syndrome, including symptoms of flush, diarrhea, bronchoconstriction, and right-sided heart failure, caused by overproduction of substances such as serotonin and tachykinins

B. Eriksson: Department of Medical Sciences, University Hospital, Uppsala, Sweden

M. Bergström: Uppsala University PET-Centre, University Hospital, Uppsala, Sweden

H. Örlefors: Department of Medical Sciences, University Hospital, Uppsala, Sweden

A. Sundin: Department of Radiology, University Hospital, Uppsala, Sweden

K. Öberg: Department of Medical Sciences, University Hospital, Uppsala, Sweden

B. Långström: Uppsala University PET-Centre, University Hospital, Uppsala, Sweden

(5). Serotonin is produced by the carcinoid tumor cells via two enzymatic steps: first, tryptophan is 5-hydoxylated to 5-HTP, which in turn is decarboxylated to serotonin [5-hydroxytryptamine (5-HT)] by aromatic amino acid decarboxylase (AADC). Serotonin circulating in the blood is predominantly bound to platelets. Unbound serotonin is oxidatively amidated to 5-hydroxyindoleacetic acid (5-HIAA). 5-HIAA is excreted in the urine and has until now been one of the most important tumor markers for diagnosis and treatment follow-up in carcinoid patients (6).

Carcinoids of foregut origin, such as bronchial and gastric carcinoids have a lower tendency to metastasize to the liver, and they infrequently produce serotonin because of a lack of AADC. Instead other substances are produced, such as pancreatic polypeptide (PP), human chorionic gonadotropin (hCG)-alpha, adrenocorticotropic hormone (ACTH), and histamine. Hindgut carcinoids metastasize in about 20% of cases and rarely present hormonal symptoms or elevation of U-5-HIAA despite the content of peptides and hormones in the tumors.

Endocrine pancreatic tumors (EPTs) are classified according to hormone production and associated symptoms into the following clinical syndromes: insulinomas, gastrinomas, watery diarrhea hypokalemia achlorhydria (WDHA) syndrome, glucagonomas, and somatostatinomas. In malignant tumors, mixed syndromes are common as a result of production of multiple hormones from the tumors. About one third of EPTs are hormonally silent despite their content and production of hormones and these tumors are called nonfunctioning tumors. EPTs can also be part of the multiple endocrine neoplasia (MEN) 1 syndrome, in which multiple pancreatic tumors are almost always found.

Diagnostic Methods in Neuroendocrine Tumors

The diagnostic methods that are currently available, including CT, ultrasonography, and MRI, often fail to localize small primary tumors, e.g., insulinomas and gastrinomas. Selective angiography has often been used to localize small tumors, but this procedure is invasive and often falsely positive. Endoscopic ultrasonography is a new technique, which is relatively sensitive but not available in all centers. Ultrasonography performed intraoperatively has shown the greatest sensitivity, but it is always of advantage to the surgeon to know the localization of the tumor preoperatively.

Today, octreotide scintigraphy (OctreoScan), based on the presence of somatostatin receptors (SSTR 1 to 5) in 80% to 90% of neuroendocrine tumors, is a routine investigation in all newly diagnosed patients with neuroendocrine gastrointestinal tumors (7). Diagnostically, it has meant a great improvement, because it is a whole-body examination and the patient's disease can be staged. Furthermore, it is a predictive test for sensitivity to somatostatin analog treatment (8). The method may have problems in localizing small tumors and tumors that lack somatostatin receptor 2 (SSTR2), e.g., 50% of insulinomas.

Medical Treatment

Carcinoids and EPTs grow slowly but have a malignant potential and the majority of patients have multiple liver metastases at diagnosis, which means that they are beyond surgical cure. Medical treatment is warranted, and during the past 10 to 20 years several therapeutic options have been developed. Alpha-interferon (IFN) and somatostatin analogs and combinations of them are established therapies in both carcinoids and EPTs and can control hormonal symptoms by reducing circulating hormone levels for extended periods (9,10). In a small group of patients (10% to 15%), a significant reduction in tumor size (>50%) can be noted, but in the majority of patients tumor size remains unchanged on CT or MRI. However, during IFN treatment the number of tumor cells was reduced and replaced by fibrosis (11). Furthermore, high-dose somatostatin analog treatment induces apoptosis in the tumors of responding patients (12). These phenomena cannot be detected by conventional radiologic methods. Specific chemotherapy with streptozocin in combination with 5-fluorouracil and doxorubicin can be effective in malignant EPT and produces biochemical and/or radiologic responses in 50% of patients with a median duration of 2 years (9). In contrast, midgut carcinoids have been rather resistant to various combinations of chemotherapeutic drugs (10). However, in a subset of carcinoid tumors, particularly foregut carcinoids (lung, thymus), the combination of cisplatin plus etoposide has produced remarkable remissions. That is also true for anaplastic EPT.

PET EXAMINATIONS WITH ¹¹C-LALBELED 5-HTP

For visualization of tumors in general, the primary PET tracers have been and still are ^{18}F-FDG and ^{11}C-labeled methionine (13). In a small pilot study, we showed that the uptake of methionine was low in neuroendocrine tumors compared with the normally high uptake in liver and pancreas. Also PET with FDG in a small number of patients failed to show enhanced accumulation of this tracer. Similar observations were made comparing the value of ^{18}F-FDG PET to octreotide scintigraphy in the imaging of neuroendocrine tumors (14). Increased uptake of ^{18}F-FDG (reflecting increased glucose metabolism) could only be seen in a small number of less-differentiated neuroendocrine tumors with high proliferative activity and without somatostatin receptors (negative octreotide scintigraphy).

Neuroendocrine tumors have previously been classified as APUDomas, based of Pearse's old characterization of amine precursor uptake and decarboxylation. Because increased serotonin synthesis is one of the diagnostic criteria of the carcinoid syndrome, it appeared rational to use a labeled precursor for serotonin as a tracer. In a pilot trial, tryptophan labeled with ^{11}C was used but did not show high uptake in carcinoid liver metastases as compared with normal liver. Tryptophan uptake is predominantly related to amino acid transport and protein synthesis, and therefore the liver uptake is dominating. However, 5-HTP ^{11}C-labeled in the β position showed a very high uptake in the tumors as compared with normal organs, including the liver (Figs. 36.1 and 36.2). Kinetic analysis of the tracer uptake indicated irreversible trapping of the tracer in the tumors (15).

In further PET studies using specific positioning labeling of 5-HTP in the β and carboxyl positions, the process of uptake

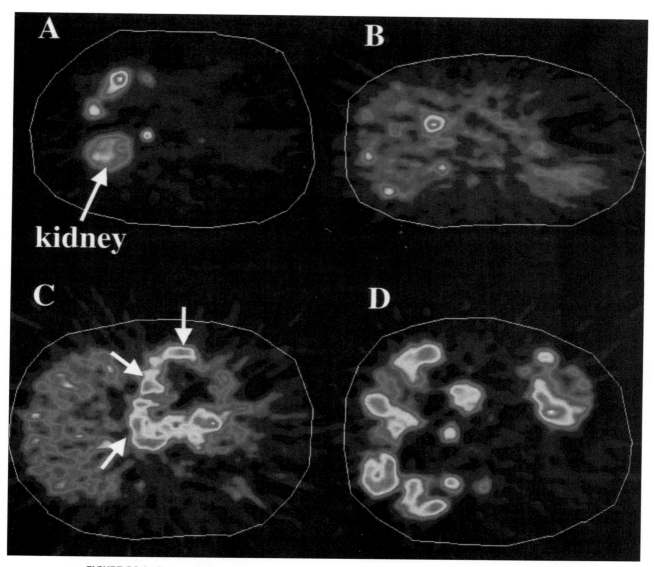

FIGURE 36.1. Four patients with carcinoid metastases in the liver, examined with positron emission tomography after the administration of ^{11}C-labeled 5-hydroxytryptophan. Patients **(A)** and **(B)** have four to five metastases observed in the sections. Patient **(C)** has one very large and necrotic metastasis, whereas patient **(D)** has practically the whole liver full of tumors.

and rapid decarboxylation of the tracer to serotonin was demonstrated (16). The basis of the latter study is that, when the tracer is labeled in the β position, the radioactivity (after decarboxylation) will be contained in ^{11}C-serotonin, which is stored in secretory granules. With the label in the carboxy position, decarboxylation will remove ^{11}C-CO_2, which leaves the tissue, whereas the formed serotonin is unlabeled (Fig. 36.3).

Visualization of Tumors

In a first study, eighteen consecutive patients with neuroendocrine gastrointestinal tumors (midgut 14, foregut 1, hindgut 1, and EPTs 2) were examined with ^{11}C-5-HTP (15). All patients except two (1 EPT and the hindgut carcinoid) had elevations of U-5-HIAA. All patients showed significantly increased uptake

of the tracer in tumorous tissue including those with normal U-5-HIAA. Metastases in the liver, lymph nodes, pleura, and the skeleton showed accumulation of the tracer. More lesions could be detected with PET in comparison with CT. The selective and high uptake in tumor tissue compared with surrounding normal tissue (high tumor-to-background ratio) produced a very good tumor visibility. These initial optimistic results have now been confirmed in more than 200 PET studies in patients with neuroendocrine tumors. PET-HTP is now a routine method in our hospital for the staging of neuroendocrine tumor disease.

Pharmacologic Modulation of Tracer Uptake

In most patients, a high concentration of radioactivity was observed in the renal pelvis resulting from the excretion of the

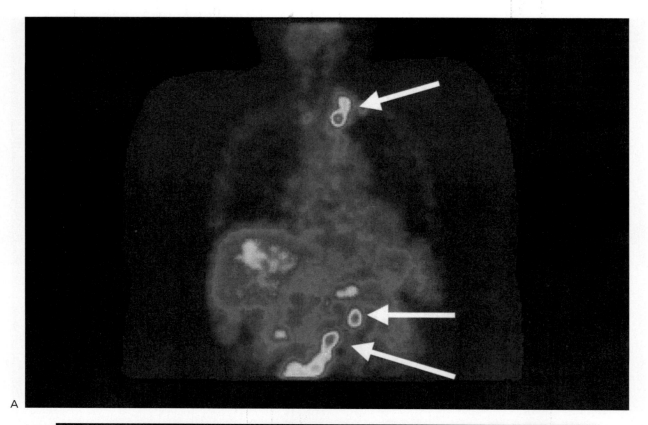

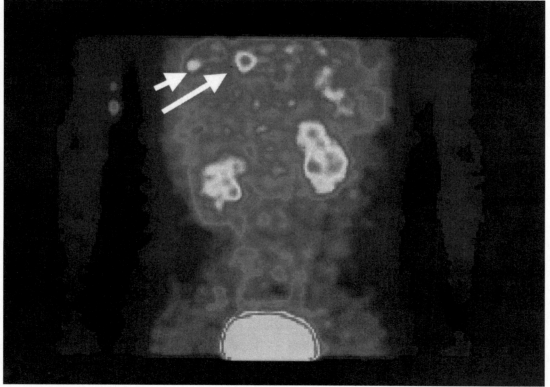

FIGURE 36.2. Whole-body positron emission tomography examinations with ^{11}C-labeled 5-hydroxy-tryptophan, demonstrating in **(A)** an ectopic adrenocorticotropic hormone-producing bronchial carcinoid and in **(B)** lung metastases in another patient.

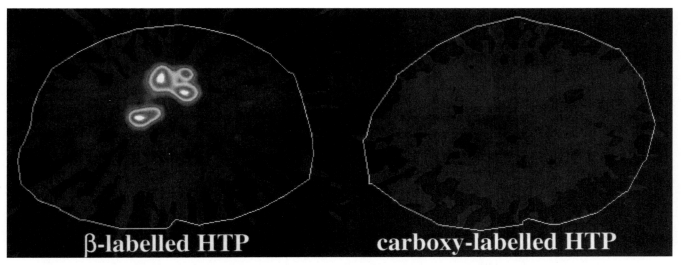

FIGURE 36.3. Positron emission tomography with ^{11}C-5-hydroxytryptophan (5-HTP) in a patient with carcinoid metastases in the abdomen. A very high uptake is noted with HTP-labeled in the β position (*left image*), in which (after carboxylation) the label is converted to serotonin. When the same section is examined with HTP in the carboxy position (*right image*), in which decarboxylation releases the label as CO_2, no increased uptake is noted.

tracer in the urine. Often this very high radioactivity produced streaky artifacts in the area of interest, which made the interpretation of images difficult. The mechanism behind this phenomenon is that ^{11}C-HTP is decarboxylated to ^{11}C-serotonin in the vascular system and in some well-perfused organs, and the formed ^{11}C-serotonin is effectively removed by the kidneys. Studies were done in rats using different drugs (decarboxylase inhibitors, monoamine oxidase inhibitors, inhibitors of tubular transport) to modulate the relative uptake in different organs, and it was found that decarboxylase inhibitors that block the peripheral amino acid decarboxylase could decrease the renal excretion significantly (17). In a human trial, the radioactivity uptake in the renal pelvis decreased sixfold and the tumoral uptake increased threefold if the patient was pretreated with the decarboxylase inhibitor carbidopa (18). Peroral premedication with carbidopa is therefore routinely used in association with PET studies with HTP.

Therapy Monitoring

PET with 5-HTP can also be used to study metabolic effects of treatment in the tumors (15). Ten patients receiving different types of treatment (IFN $n = 4$, IFN plus somatostatin analog $n = 2$, and somatostatin analogs $n = 4$) were followed before and at different time intervals after start of treatment (4 days and 3, 6, and 12 months). When changes in the transport rate constant for the uptake of 5-HTP were compared with changes in U-5-HIAA during treatment, there was a greater than 95% correlation using regression analysis. Thus, PET with HTP might be a valuable complement for therapy monitoring especially in tumors lacking tumor markers such as enhanced 5-HIAA or chromogranin A.

PET WITH ^{11}C-LABELED L-DIHYDROXYPHENYLALANINE (L-DOPA)

It is uncommon for patients with EPT to have elevation of U-5-HIAA as a sign of perturbed serotonin synthesis. It was therefore suggested that another amine precursor, L-DOPA would be a valid tracer for these tumors.

L-DOPA is an amino acid that is converted to the catecholamine dopamine by AADC. In addition to its role as a precursor of adrenaline and noradrenaline, dopamine is a transmitter substance in the central and peripheral nervous system. In this context ^{11}C-labeled L-DOPA was used as a tracer for dopamine synthesis.

Visualization of Tumors

Twenty-two consecutive patients with biochemically verified EPTs were examined with ^{11}C-labeled L-DOPA (19). Six patients had clinical symptoms of gastrinoma, four had glucagonomas, three had insulinomas, six had nonfunctioning tumors, one had WDHA syndrome, and two had mixed functioning tumors. Six patients had the MEN 1 syndrome. Increased uptake of the tracer in the primary tumor and metastases could be seen in 10 patients, mainly functioning tumors (gastrinomas, glucagonomas) (Fig. 36.4). With L-DOPA as a tracer, nonfunctioning tumors were not detected. Also small insulinomas (not detected by any other preoperative radiologic technique but by intraoperative ultrasonography) were difficult to visualize.

Therapeutic Monitoring

Two patients (one gastrinoma and one glucagonoma) treated with high-dose somatostatin analogs (lanreotide, 12 mg/day)

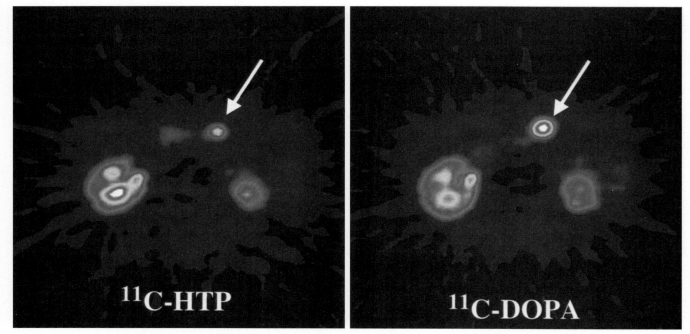

FIGURE 36.4. Patient with endocrine pancreas tumor, examined both with 5-hydroxytryptophan (*left image*) and with L-dihydroxyphenylalanine (*right image*).

were examined with PET and L-DOPA before treatment and after 6 months of treatment (20). At 6 months, both patients had improved symptomatically and biochemically with reduction in hormone levels. Paradoxically, PET after 6 months showed a threefold increase in the uptake of L-DOPA compared with PET before treatment. The explanation for this finding is not obvious, but we suggest that it indicates that high-dose somatostatin analog treatment inhibits exocytosis of peptides and amines (more than synthesis). Before treatment, high amounts of ^{11}C-dopamine are formed and stored in granules but are rapidly released from the tumor cells via exocytosis. After somatostatin treatment, the ^{11}C-dopamine formed remains in the granules inside the cells, thereby giving a high signal in the images. In the same study (20), we validated that the tracer was decarboxylated by comparison of the kinetics of ^{11}C-L-DOPA labeled in either the carboxyl or β position.

Pharmacologic Modulation

To optimize the *in vivo* examination of patients, the effect of different agents on the uptake of L-DOPA was investigated in different organs in rats (21,22). The effect of decarboxylase inhibitors indicated a decreased renal excretion of L-DOPA, whereas COMT inhibitors increased the uptake in the normal pancreas.

[18]F-Labeled L-Fluoro-DOPA

Although we do not have experience in the use of ^{18}F-labeled L-fluoro-DOPA, we have suggested that this tracer should be almost equivalent to ^{11}C-L-DOPA. Small differences do exist with respect to affinity to different enzymes. In line with our

observations on modulation by enzyme inhibitors, decarboxylase and COMT inhibition in association with the PET study should increase the tumor uptake and contrast to the surrounding tissues. In other centers a few studies have been performed with positive results. The advantage of ^{18}F-L-fluoro-DOPA is its better availability within the PET field and the longer half-life of the radionuclide, but our own experience suggests that ^{11}C-HTP has superior biologic characteristics.

[11]C-5-HTP AS A UNIVERSAL TRACER IN WHOLE-BODY PET

The observation in our previous study that several patients without elevation of U-5-HIAA had high uptake of 5-HTP in the tumors encouraged further exploration of this tracer as a valuable tracer for the diagnosis of neuroendocrine tumors. Furthermore, the possibility of modulating the uptake of 5-HTP with carbidopa has facilitated the performance of whole-body PET, i.e., examination of both the abdomen and thorax in the same investigation despite the short half-life of [11]C (Fig. 36.2). In a first study, eight patients with biochemically verified neuroendocrine tumors [five with suspect ACTH-producing tumors and three with EPT (nonfunctioning $n = 2$ and insulinoma $n = 1$)] underwent whole-body PET with 5-HTP in addition to CT/MRI and octreotide scintigraphy. Conventional radiology (CT/MRI) was initially considered negative in all eight patients. Octreotide scintigraphy could demonstrate tumors in two cases, whereas PET could visualize tumors in six cases (three ACTH-producing lung/thymic carcinoids and all three EPTs). With the PET images at hand, the tumors could be identified on MRI and CT images in five cases. All six patients with positive PET examinations were operated on, and the PET findings could be verified.

We now recommend that patients with neuroendocrine tumors be investigated with PET-HTP as reduced whole-body studies. The patient should be pretreated with carbidopa. Scanning commences 10 minutes after administration of the tracer, starting in the lower pelvic region. The studies are made in three-dimensional (3D) mode to increase the sensitivity. Typically three to four fields are sufficient to cover the important aspects of the body, and the acquisition times are slightly adjusted to compensate for radioactive decay.

FDG-PET IN NEUROENDOCRINE CANCERS

There is a subgroup of patients who have poorly differentiated tumors, which, for example, lack somatostatin receptors and the expression of chromogranin A. The tumors may show the content of another marker for neuroendocrine differentiation—synaptophysin. The proliferation capacity, as evaluated using the proliferation marker Ki-67, is usually high in these tumors as compared with the more common well-differentiated neuroendocrine tumors. In this patient category, we have found that PET with 5-HTP might be negative, whereas ^{18}F-FDG PET usually is positive and can be used for staging (Fig. 36.5) and therapeutic monitoring, which is in agreement with the findings of Adams et al. (14).

PET SOMATOSTATIN SCINTIGRAPHY

The possibility of using ^{68}Ga coupled to somatostatin analogs has been proposed by Hoffman et al. (23). This group has shown that ^{68}Ga-octreotide can be produced on a routine basis, using ^{68}Ga obtained from a generator and thus obviating the need for a cyclotron. Furthermore, they showed that ^{68}Ga-octreotide has a better tumor-to-background ratio than ^{111}In-octreotide and that scanning can be performed within an hour after tracer administration. Finally, this method takes advantage of the superior resolution and sensitivity of the PET camera compared with

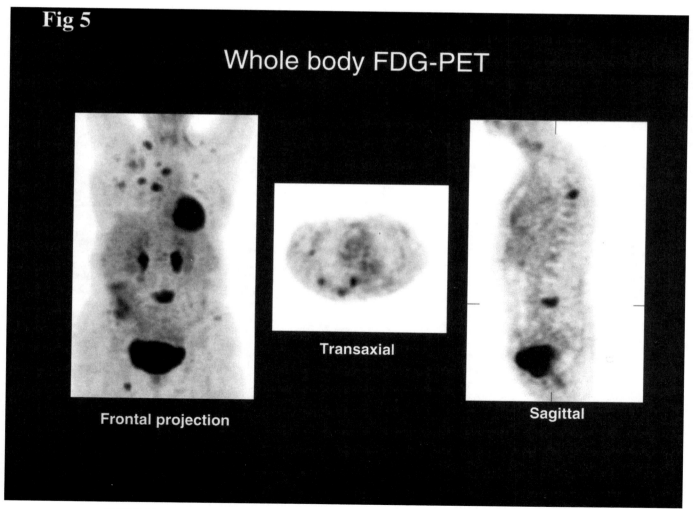

FIGURE 36.5. Patient with a primary neuroendocrine tumor in the colon (resected), multiple liver metastases, and bone metastases that were discovered with ^{18}F-FDG PET.

a gamma-camera. In a small pilot group, we have confirmed the experience of Hoffman et al.

It is too early to say whether ^{68}Ga-octreotide-PET will replace PET-HTP as a diagnostic tool. We have previously documented that some metastatic lesions might be somatostatin receptor negative and hence not appear in octreotide scintigraphy images, although they would be positive with PET-HTP. The opposite is also true. This might suggest a complementary role of octreotide scintigraphy and HTP for diagnosis, whereas octreotide scintigraphy is the method of choice for decisions regarding somatostatin treatment.

CURRENT STATUS

At present, greater than 90% of neuroendocrine tumors can be visualized with PET using the tracers now available, notably HTP. PET with 5-HTP can be used to screen the thorax and abdomen (whole-body PET) for small primary tumors that cannot be detected by other methods including octreotide scintigraphy. In several preoperative evaluations, PET has provided crucial information to the surgeon, thanks to the excellent tumor visibility, which in turn depends on the high tumor-to-background ratio and good spatial resolution. It is clear that PET with HTP is the most sensitive method for detecting extent of metastases, superior to octreotide scintigraphy, CT, and MRI in this respect. However, lack of availability and high cost affect its extensive use. It is therefore reasonable to use PET-HTP adequately in the investigation route for neuroendocrine tumors, especially to exclude metastases in cases in which a clinical diagnosis of neuroendocrine tumor is made when CT is negative or when tumor burden is so limited that surgery is an option.

PET can also be used to monitor functional parameters reflecting effects of treatment in the tumors, which other methods can not.

For neuroendocrine cancers with a high proliferation index, PET with ^{18}F-FDG can be used.

ACKNOWLEDGMENTS

This work was supported by the Swedish Cancer Foundation, Söderberg's Foundation and Lions Cancer Foundation.

REFERENCES

1. Shields AF, Graham MM, Spence AM. The role of PET imaging in clinical oncology; a current status report. *Nucl Med Annu* 1995: 129–168.
2. Findlay M, Young H, Cunningham D et al. Noninvasive monitoring of tumor metabolism using fluorodeoxyglucose and positron emission tomography in colorectal cancer liver metastases: correlation with tumor response to fluorouracil. *J Clin Oncol* 1996;14:700–708.
3. Pearse AGE. The APUD concept and hormone production. *Clin Endocrinol Metab* 1980;17:211–222.
4. Williams ED, Sandler M. The classification of carcinoid tumors. *Lancet* 1963;1:238–239.
5. Thorson A, Björck G, Björkman G et al. Malignant carcinoid of the small intestine with metastases to the liver, valvular disease of the right side of the heart (pulmonary stenosis and tricuspid regurgitation with septal defects), peripheral vasomotor symptoms, bronchoconstriction and an unusual type of cyanosis, a clinical and pathological syndrome. *Ann Heart J* 1954;47:795–817.
6. Norheim I, Öberg K, Theodorsson-Norheim E et al. Malignant carcinoid tumors: an analysis of 103 patients with regard to tumor localization, hormone production and survival. *Ann Surg* 1987;206:115–125.
7. Krenning EP, Kweekeboom DJ, Bakker WH et al. Somatostatin receptor scintigraphy with [^{111}I-DTPA-D-Phe^1]- and [^{123}Tyr^3]-octreotide: the Rotterdam experience with more than 1.000 patients. *Eur J Nucl Med* 1993;20:716–731.
8. Tiensuu Janson E, Westlin JE, Eriksson B et al. [^{111}In-DTPA-D-Phe^1]-octreotide scintigraphy in patients with carcinoid tumors—the predictive value for somatostatin analogue treatment. *Eur J Endocrinol* 1994; 131:575–576.
9. Eriksson B, Öberg K. An update of the medical treatment of malignant endocrine pancreatic tumors. *Acta Oncol* 1993;32:203–208.
10. Öberg K, Eriksson B. The role of interferons in the management of carcinoid tumors. *Acta Oncol* 1991;30:519–522.
11. Andersson T, Eriksson B, Lindgren PG et al. Effects of interferon on tumor tissue content in liver metastases during interferon treatment. *Cancer Res* 1990;50:3413–3415.
12. Imam H, Eriksson B, Lukinius A et al. Induction of apoptosis in neuroendocrine tumors of the digestive system during treatment with somatostatin analogs. *Acta Oncol* 1997;36:607–614.
13. Bergström M, Muhr C, Lundberg PO. *In vivo* study of amino acid distribution and metabolism in pituitary adenomas using positron emission tomography with 11-C-D-methionine and 11-C-L-methionine. *J Compat Assist Tomogr* 1987;11:384–389.
14. Adams S, Baum R, Rink T et al. Limited value of fluorine-18 fluorodeoxyglucose positron emission tomography for the imaging of neuroendocrine tumours. *Eur J Nucl Med* 1998;25:79–83.
15. Örlefors H, Sundin A, Lilja A et al. Positron emission tomography (PET) with 5-hydroxytryptophan (5-HTP) in the diagnosis and treatment follow-up of carcinoid tumors. *J Clin Oncol* 1998;7:2534–2541.
16. Sundin A, Eriksson B, Bergström M et al. Demonstration of [^{11}C]-5-hydroxy-L-tryptophan accumulation and decarboxylation in carcinoid tumors by specific positioning labeling in positron emission tomography. *Nucl Med Biol* 2000;27:33–41.
17. Bergström M, Lu L, Eriksson B et al. Modulation of organ uptake of ^{11}C-labeled 5-hydroxytryptophan. *Biogenic Amines* 1996;12:477–485.
18. Örlefors H, Sundin A, Bergström M et al. *In vivo* modulation of 11C-5-HTP uptake in neuroendocrine gut tumors using PET (*manuscript*).
19. Ahlström H, Eriksson B, Bergström M et al. Pancreatic neuroendocrine tumors: diagnosis with PET. *Radiology* 1995;195:333–337.
20. Bergström M, Eriksson B, Öberg K et al. *In vivo* demonstration of enzyme activity in endocrine pancreatic tumors—decarboxylation of ^{11}C-dopamine. *J Nucl Med* 1996;36:32–37.
21. Bergström M, Lu L, Marquez M et al. Modulation of organ uptake of ^{11}C-labelled L-DOPA. *Nucl Med Biol* 1997;24;15–19.
22. Bergström M, Marquez M, Eriksson B et al. COMT inhibition increases the pancreas uptake of ^{11}C-L-DOPA. *Scand J Gastroenterol* 1996;31:1216–1222.
23. Henze M, Schumacher J, Hipp P et al. PET imaging of somatostatin receptors using (68Ga)DOTA-D-Phe-Tyr-Octreotide: first result in patients with meningiomas. *J Nucl Med* 2001;42:1053–1056.

Diagnostic Nuclear Medicine, Fourth Edition. Edited by M.P. Sandler, R.E. Coleman, J.A. Patton, F.J.Th. Wackers, A. Gottschalk. Lippincott Williams & Wilkins, Philadelphia 2003.

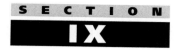

NEUROLOGY

37

SPECT BRAIN IMAGING

FREDERICK J. BONTE
MICHAEL D. DEVOUS, SR.

Roy and Sherrington (1) identified the relationship between brain physiologic activity and brain blood flow in 1890. Measurements of whole brain blood flow were made by Kety and Schmidt (2) using nitrous oxide as their tracer. Their method was soon adapted to the use of radionuclide tracers principally [133]Xe (3), which was either inhaled by the patient or injected in solution, permitting measurements to be made with scintillation detectors placed on the scalp. It could yield quantitative regional brain blood flow data (4). The development of scintillation multiprobe units soon followed, enabling investigators to quantify regional cerebral blood flow (RCBF), or perfusion, simultaneously within individual regions of the cortex. However, multiprobe systems with their poor spatial resolution and capability of measuring only surface blood flow, led to the rapid development of scanning devices. This development was led by Kuhl and his associates (5) and provided three-dimensional imaging capabilities. Single photon emission computed tomography (SPECT) soon became the method of choice for RCBF studies. Stokely et al. (6) devised a rotating four-detector SPECT scanner, which optimized the use of inhaled ^{133}Xe as a tracer. SPECT imaging systems next took the form of an Anger camera (7) mounted on a gantry that enabled it to be rotated around the patient's head, and soon rotating camera systems were developed using multiple cameras, which provided improved resolution and sensitivity.

Meanwhile, SPECT RCBF radiopharmaceuticals appropriate to the new imaging systems made their appearance in rapid succession: ^{123}I-iodoamphetamine (IMP) (8), and the [99mTc]-labeled compounds hexamethyl propyleneamine oxime (HMPAO, exametazime, Ceretec, Nycomed Amersham Inc.) (9), and ethyl cysteinate dimer (ECD, Neurolite, Merck du Pont Inc.) (10). Although these three agents enabled greatly improved resolution, none of them provided the quantitative data available with the use of [133]Xe. Furthermore, although it is used in many countries outside the United States, [123]IMP is at present not commercially available in this country.

With tracers other than ^{133}Xe, obtaining quantitative data from SPECT has presented a problem. Investigators have used several methods based on establishing regions-of-interest (ROIs) and comparing counts within these ROI with some standard such as the cerebellar cortex, the occipital cortex, and a given section of the brain that contains the ROIs that are being evaluated. Several years ago Devous et al. (11) compared visual interpretation of brain blood flow SPECT images with results derived from various semiquantitative methods in which ROI methods were used. They found no significant difference in the accuracy in interpretation between the two methods. Furthermore, the cerebellar cortex is subject to diaschises, even in the dementias, and the occipital cortex perfusion has been found to be quite variable in some of the affective disorders.

The theory and practice of SPECT image acquisition, processing and display are considered at length in Chapter 4. An approach to quantitation has been made with the development of voxel comparison methods, for example, the statistical parametric mapping of Friston et al. (12) performed with image data placed in a three-dimensional stereotactic system such as that of Talairach and Tournoux (13).

Further advances in imaging devices include the development of ring SPECT detectors, such as the CERASPECT imager (14), as well as development of techniques for fusing RCBF images with anatomic studies, such as those made with computed tomography (CT) or magnetic resonance imaging (MRI). Imaging devices with multiple simultaneous capabilities have been developed, some of which promise resolution on par with positron emission tomography (PET).

BRAIN SPECT IN CEREBROVASCULAR DISEASE

The measurement of RCBF in patients with cerebrovascular diseases was the earliest application of brain SPECT. There are numerous reports concerning the role of SPECT RCBF imaging in stroke, transient ischemic attacks (TIAs), subarachnoid hemorrhage (SAH), arteriovenous malformation (AVM), and other derangements of cerebral hemodynamics. Several valuable reviews are available (15–17). Many of these reports promote both diagnostic and prognostic roles for SPECT RCBF imaging of cerebrovascular disease, although some criticisms have been

F.J. Bonte: Nuclear Medicine Center, Department of Radiology, The University of Texas Southwestern Medical Center at Dallas, and Parkland Memorial Hospital, Dallas, TX

M.D. Devous, Sr.: Department of Radiology and Nuclear Medicine and Nuclear Medicine Center, Department of Radiology. The University of Texas Southwestern, Medical Center, Dallas, TX

raised that investigations to date have not directly addressed the questions of greatest importance to the referring physician (18).

Stroke

Reduced RCBF following stroke occurs instantly; thus, SPECT is useful in the detection of acute cerebral ischemia (15,19). In contrast, CT or MRI is typically normal for the first hours to days after the ictus. The difference in sensitivity between structural and functional imaging modalities disappears within about 72 hours. In addition, the sensitivity of SPECT is significantly reduced for lacunar infarctions. Sensitivity for lesion detection is also affected by the phenomenon of luxury perfusion (17,19) whereby perfusion and metabolism become decoupled beginning approximately 5 days after the ictus and continuing for as much as 20 days, possibly producing false-negative scans. Thus, acute RCBF imaging is effective, whereas imaging during the subacute phase is less sensitive.

SPECT imaging may also be useful in delineation of stroke subtypes. Because evolving therapies are subtype-specific, it becomes increasingly important to rapidly provide accurate subtyping. In acute infarctions, distinguishing between the appropriateness of anticoagulation or thrombolytic therapy may depend on the demonstration of the physiologic significance of an angiographically demonstrable lesion.

Early SPECT and Prognosis

Estimation of clinical outcome early in the course of infarction is important for both clinical investigations and patient management. Clinical measures (20) are often used but with limited success (21). Anatomic imaging has limited prognostic capability (22). Since the original writing of this chapter, there has been a substantial expansion of the literature regarding the relationship between SPECT RCBF abnormalities and outcome. In the early literature a direct relationship between RCBF and clinical outcome was both supported (20–35) and refuted (36–39). Improved correlation between RCBF and outcome has been achieved with measurement of the volume of the RCBF defect relative to the volume of structural defect (31). Mountz et al. (31) compared CT lesions to those on SPECT in chronic stroke patients. The ratio between SPECT and CT volume defect sizes strongly correlated with outcome, with larger ratios associated with better outcomes. The volume of the flow lesion alone may also enhance prognostication (16,40,41).

Most recent literature indicates that SPECT predicts improvement following stroke with an accuracy similar to the Canadian Neurologic Scale (CNS). Also, the initial perfusion defect on SPECT correlates with stroke severity and outcome as assessed by the National Institutes of Health (NIH) stroke scale and the Barthel Index, which demonstrates the feasibility of SPECT for selecting or stratifying patients in clinical trials during the first hours of stroke. In some studies SPECT seems superior, whereas in others it does not perform quite as well as the CNS or NIH scales. This depends on how early after stroke the RCBF data are obtained, earlier data having stronger predictive value. For example, Giubilei et al. (42) examined SPECT and clinical scores in a probabilistic model, finding that although

neurologic scores did have the highest predictive power, SPECT conducted within 6 hours of onset had a significant added value, providing a 92% predictive power for poor neurologic outcome.

Several recent studies illustrate the prognostic value of early SPECT RCBF imaging. Alexandrov et al. (43) performed SPECT scans an average of 5 days after onset in 458 stroke patients. They showed that a simple visual interpretation scheme (RCBF normal, increased, mixed, low, or absent) correlated with stroke lesion volume and short-term (2 week) outcome as measured by the CNS. Specifically, 97% of patients with normal and increased HMPAO uptake had good recovery, whereas 62% with absent perfusion had poor outcome. Multiple logistic regression identified the CNS score as the strongest outcome predictor, but the SPECT rating had additional prognostic value independent of the CNS score and improved the predictive power of the CNS score. This improvement was primarily due to distinguishing patients with a moderate focal RCBF decrease from those with complete absence of brain perfusion when studied *within the first 72 hours of stroke.* Thus, SPECT does have a prognostic role *if* performed early after stroke.

Lees et al. (44) studied 63 patients by CT, SPECT, and mean transit time for a median of 1, 3, or 2 days, respectively, from symptom onset and correlated results with the 3-month poststroke Barthel Index. Stepwise logistic regression identified the lesion volume on SPECT as the only significant predictor of good functional outcome (Barthel score greater than 70) with an overall predictive accuracy of 73%. Similarly, Laloux et al. (45) examined correlations between early SPECT and outcome in 55 patients. (SPECT was obtained within the first 24 hours in 82% of the patients.) Multivariate analysis demonstrated that only the size of hypoperfusion functioned as an independent predictor for the functional state at 1-month poststroke ($p = 0.004$), whereas the CNS was a predictor for mortality ($p = 0.009$).

Experimental evidence in animals suggests that severely ischemic tissue in which ionic disruption has occurred may be viable for less than 1 to 2 hours. However, mildly to moderately ischemic tissue, in which electrical function is disturbed without loss of ionic homeostasis (the ischemic penumbra), is viable for up to 3 hours in a rat model of middle cerebral artery occlusion and for 6 to 8 hours in baboons and squirrel monkeys (46). Thus, early reperfusion should be of critical importance to tissue salvage and clinical recovery. Reperfusion in the first 24 to 48 hours of cerebral ischemia has been found in a limited number of SPECT and PET studies. In some of these reports, reperfusion was associated with a beneficial clinical outcome, whereas one paper each reported a variable association and no clinical benefit with reperfusion. In two early studies, Baird et al. (47) found regions of increased HMPAO uptake in SPECT scans obtained within 48 hours of symptom onset in 11 patients with normal CT 7 to 14 days poststroke, and Sperling and Lassen (48) observed increased HMPAO uptake within 48 hours of stroke onset in regions without infarction on chronic CT.

Perhaps the clearest study of SPECT data truly early after onset is that of Shimosegawa et al. (49) who studied 31 patients within 6 hours after stroke onset, comparing RCBF to follow-up CT at 5 days postinfarct. The authors noted that hyperperfusion was present in some stroke patients even within 6 hours of onset and that *no areas of hyperperfusion resulted in infarcted tissue* (defined by CT). The lesion to contralateral hemisphere ratio at 6 hours poststroke differed significantly between infarcted tissue (0.48 ± 0.14), and peri-infarct tissue (0.75 ± 0.10, $p < 0.02$). The authors concluded that brain destined for infarction can be distinguished from viable surviving tissue if the lesion to contralateral ratio is less than 0.6 for SPECT images obtained within 6 hours of stroke onset. Baird et al. (47) recently studied 53 patients with serial ^{99m}Tc-HMPAO SPECT in the first 48 hours following ischemic stroke. In a multiple linear regression analysis they found that only age ($p < 0.01$) and the percentage change in volume of reperfused cerebral tissue between the 24- and 48-hour scans ($p < 0.01$) provided independent prognostic information, concluding that an early reperfusion window does indeed exist in humans. They also found a correlation between the SPECT defect size in the first 24 hours and outcome in *post-hoc* univariate analyses. However, this was not observed in the multiple linear regression analysis, suggesting that a close relation between the neurologic score at admission and the size of the perfusion defect occurred and that the neurologic score is a stronger predictor (a common finding, see earlier discussion). Finally, the authors concluded that because serial changes in cerebral perfusion within the first 24 to 48 hours are of independent prognostic value, whereas perfusion defect size in the first 24 hours was not, hemodynamic changes occurring after 24 hours may significantly affect outcome and possibly account for the disparate results between studies described in the literature.

Future studies may incorporate location and mechanism of the ischemia in prognostic models. For example, motor deficits resulting from cortical ischemia are better correlated with SPECT RCBF than those of subcortical or small vessel origin (50,51). Also, even in subcortical infarcts, aphasia, neglect, and sensory abnormalities are better correlated with cortical hypoperfusion (39,52). Although further work on prognosis and outcome is needed, most data to date suggest that SPECT scanning early after stroke is a useful tool for estimating outcome after cerebral infarction.

SPECT and Thrombolytic Therapy in Acute Stroke

RCBF studies in the early hours after stroke onset suggest that perfusion abnormalities fall into three broad categories: (a) acute focal absence of RCBF implies failure of collateral flow distal to obstruction and poor prognosis, suggesting that benefit from acute treatment is unlikely for patients with this type of hemodynamic insult; (b) acutely decreased but not absent RCBF indicates some collateral flow and better opportunity for recovery—such patients may be the best target group for therapeutic intervention; and (c) normal RCBF during the first hours of ischemia identifies patients with reversible deficits, for whom thrombolytic therapy is unnecessary. These categorizations and their relationship to thrombolytic therapy choices and likely outcome are schematically illustrated in Fig. 37.1. Increased HMPAO uptake (hyperfixation) is also observed after reperfusion and is normally also associated with improved outcome.

Baird et al. (47,53) were among the first to examine SPECT in thrombolytic therapy. They compared the extent of reperfusion between patients who had received thrombolytic therapy

Stroke, SPECT and Thrombolysis

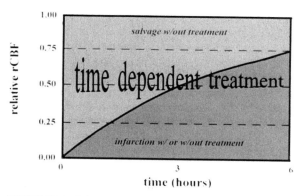

FIGURE 37.1. Schematic representation of acute stroke regional cerebral blood flow (RCBF) categorizations and their relationship to thrombolytic therapy and likely outcome. Normal or only modestly reduced RCBF during the first hours of ischemia identifies patients with reversible deficits for whom thrombolytic therapy may not be needed (*top of diagram*). Acutely decreased but not absent RCBF indicates some collateral flow and better opportunity for recovery; such patients may be the best target group for thrombolytic therapy (*middle of diagram*). Acute focal absence of RCBF implies failure of collateral flow distal to obstruction and poor prognosis, suggesting an unlikely benefit from acute treatment for patients with this type of hemodynamic insult (*bottom of drawing*).

and a control group studied during the same period (who were ineligible to receive such therapy) to determine if, among all patients, reperfusion led to improved outcome. They studied 57 patients (22 treated with streptokinase) each of whom had SPECT studies performed before streptokinase administration and 24 hours later. On the second study, there was only a trend for patients who received streptokinase to be more likely to develop at least partial reperfusion. However, when they considered all patients, including those with no SPECT abnormality on the initial study, those who did not reperfuse had higher mortality rates ($p < 0.008$), less neurologic improvement ($p = 0.016$), and more functional disability ($p < 0.001$) than patients who had reperfusion or had initially normal perfusion.

Ezura et al. (54) studied 17 patients with an abnormal initial RCBF and a normal initial CT treated with tPA within 6 hours from onset. They found a tendency toward an inverse time-dependent relationship between cortical infarction and residual relative (to the contralateral normal hemisphere) RCBF. Furthermore, in 10 patients whose occluded arteries did not recanalize within 6 hours, cortical areas with residual relative RCBF of more than 70% did not develop infarction. They observed a single case with hemorrhagic transformation in which the relative RCBF was below 35%. The authors concluded that patients with RCBF between 35% and 70% (moderate ischemia involving the cortex) are the best candidates for fibrinolytic therapy.

In an intriguing study, Hanson et al. (55) prospectively studied 14 patients by HMPAO SPECT within 6 hours of symptom onset (mean time of 3.2 hours from symptom onset to SPECT); scans were repeated at 24 hours. The severity of the SPECT abnormality on the admission scan (a semiquantitative asymmetry index) correlated with the severity of the admission NIH stroke scale ($p < 0.05$), with poor long-term outcome based on the Barthel Index ($p < 0.001$) and with complications of cerebral hemorrhage and massive cerebral edema ($p < 0.005$). Seven of the 14 patients were randomized to tPA treatment and 7 to a glutamate antagonist trial. Both trials remain blinded at the time of this report; thus, the relationship between RCBF and treatment is unknown. Patients fell into three patterns: (a) patients with mild asymmetry (both of whom demonstrated good long-term recovery); (b) intermediate asymmetry with variable outcome (although 8/9 showed clinical improvement on the NIH stroke scale with relatively good long-term outcome and only one had hemorrhagic conversion); and (c) those with severe asymmetry, all of whom had very poor long-term outcome. One patient in this latter group showed 24-hour hyperperfusion with no clinical benefit. Although the initial scan related to outcome and to the NIH stroke scale, there was no correlation between the change in RCBF between initial and 24-hour scans and the change in clinical assessment on the NIH stroke scale over that same time. In fact 5 patients showed improvement in SPECT at 24 hours without any corresponding clinical improvement, suggesting that 24-hour restoration of blood flow is not early enough to provide clinical benefit. There was also a relationship between the SPECT graded score and the Barthel Index, such that asymmetry greater than 40% routinely led to poor Barthel Index at 3 months (≤ 60). Similarly, admission SPECT scan scores with greater than 50% asymmetry were routinely associated with cerebral edema or hemorrhage. The authors concluded that early SPECT imaging may be useful for selecting or stratifying patients in clinical therapeutic trials.

Cerebrovascular Reserve

It is important to determine the degree to which underlying disease has exhausted the normal RCBF reserve capacity and the degree to which collateral supplies have been recruited as a countermeasure. Measurements of cerebrovascular reserve may be particularly effective in assessing the need for acute interventions following stroke or the risk status for secondary strokes. Although CO_2 is an effective vasodilator in the cerebrovascular system, often administered by inhalation to challenge cerebral vasoreactivity, the administration of acetazolamide, a carbonic anhydrase inhibitor and potent cerebral vasodilator, is a more convenient and effective alternative (15,56–58). Intravenous administration of 1-g acetazolamide leads to a uniform increase in RCBF throughout the normal brain that peaks at 20 minutes and lasts for about 1 hour, gradually returning to normal over a 2- to 3-hour span. Diseased or at-risk areas show little or no response. Side effects are minimal, including mild paresthesias and diuresis.

Acetazolamide stress testing has been used to assess cerebrovascular reserve in patients with TIA, stroke, arteriovenous malformation, epilepsy, and dementia (15,56–58). In the latter two instances the purpose of the test is to determine whether alterations in resting RCBF are of neuronal or vascular origin. Primary neuronal dysfunction (such as in Alzheimer's disease) produces RCBF abnormalities only as an epiphenomenon, through autoregulation. Such areas have a normal acetazolamide response.

Transient Ischemic Attacks (TIA)

Determining the cause of a TIA (thrombotic, embolic, or hemodynamic origin) has substantial impact on patient management. RCBF SPECT imaging in TIA patients may be of value in assessing both the severity of the existing ischemia and the response of an ischemic area to medical or surgical intervention and may clarify the mechanism of ischemia (59) or identify patients at the highest risk for subsequent infarction in the first week following TIA. However, it is important to note that the sensitivity of RCBF imaging in TIA declines with time, from 60% in the first 24 hours to a level below 40% at 1 week after the event (15,19). This sensitivity may be enhanced both early and late after the ischemic event by examination of cerebrovascular reserve with acetazolamide (59).

Sample Images in Cerebrovascular Disease

Under the most common setting for imaging RCBF (eyes and ears open in a dimly lit environment with minimal auditory "white noise"), the normal RCBF distribution shows symmetric flow distribution between homologous regions, with little anterior/posterior variance (Fig. 37.2). In some instances there is greater activity in the cerebellum than in the cerebrum (more common with HMPAO than with ECD). When RCBF is interrupted, these patterns change dramatically. We herein provide three such examples. In acute stroke, RCBF is the first characteristic of the CNS to change, and substantial image alterations can result (Fig. 37.3), usually without concomitant structural changes unless hemorrhage occurs. Over time, the RCBF deficit can resolve because of luxury perfusion (Fig. 37.4, *top row*), a process that takes place some time between day 5 and day 30 posticus. However, if crossed cerebellar diaschisis is present (Fig. 37.4, *bottom row*), it will persist even during the luxury perfusion phase. When exhaustion of cerebrovascular reserve is the primary finding (typically in TIA, but also seen in completed stroke), a baseline study can be normal (Fig. 37.5, *top*). Administration of a cerebral vasodilator (such as acetazolamide) can then be used to demonstrate the presence, extent, and severity of cerebrovascular reserve failure (Fig. 37.5, *bottom*). This information is very valuable in presurgical management of patients in whom surgical intervention is considered and in assessment of the risk of a future stroke in all patients with underlying cerebrovascular disease.

In summary, SPECT RCBF images provide a sensitive early measure of cerebral ischemia and may provide both diagnostic and prognostic information in stroke patients. However, little change in the referral pattern from neurologists that would include frequent SPECT scans has been observed. The opportunities for productive focused studies with SPECT RCBF imaging to significantly impact the management of patients with cerebrovascular disease are abundant. With increasing opportunities for acute treatment, more sophisticated algorithms for patient management in recovery, and new opportunities for treatment of the penumbra in subacute and chronic stroke, SPECT brain imaging in cerebrovascular disease should be an important component of patient care.

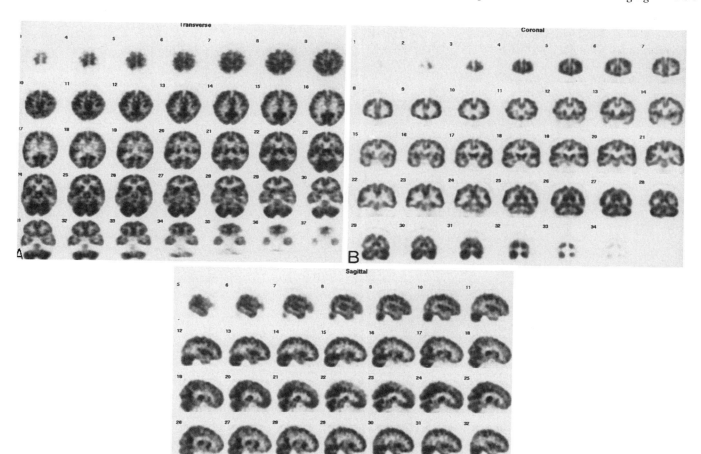

FIGURE 37.2. This is a normal regional cerebral blood flow single photon emission computed tomography scan made with ^{99m}Tc-hexamethyl propyleneamine oxime and a triple-camera scanner. **A:** Contiguous set of transaxial sections providing optimal views of cerebral and cerebellar cortex, pons, basal ganglia, and thalami. Note the slight separation of hemispheres in a mature individual with mild cerebral atrophy. **B:** Contiguous coronal sections provide especially good visualization of the inferior temporal lobes and cross sections of basal ganglia and lobes of the thalamus. **C:** Contiguous sagittal sections from subject's left (*upper*) to right (*lower*) provide useful views of frontal sensory motor and parietal cortex superiorly and inferior temporal lobe cortex. (Courtesy S. Petras, Toshiba America Inc.)

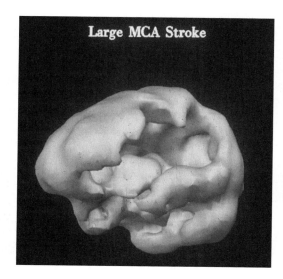

FIGURE 37.3. Three-dimensional surface-rendered single photon emission computed tomography (SPECT) regional cerebral blood flow (RCBF) images obtained 9-hours postictus in a 58-year-old woman suffering from stroke. Computed tomography images were normal at this time, whereas SPECT RCBF images portray both the distribution and severity of altered perfusion.

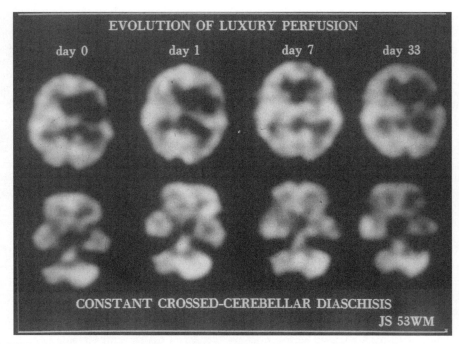

FIGURE 37.4. Transverse images from a midcortical (*upper row*) and cerebellar (*lower row*) level in a 53-year-old male stroke patient. Note the presence of a cortical defect and crossed cerebellar diaschisis at day zero. Cortical perfusion normalizes via the process of luxury perfusion by day seven. However, crossed-cerebellar diaschisis persists even during the luxury perfusion stage.

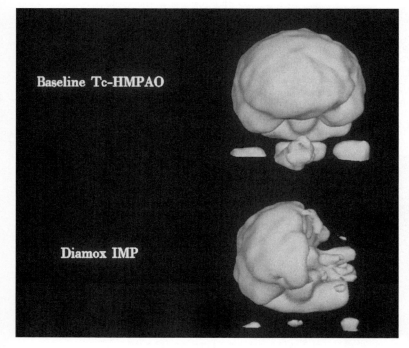

FIGURE 37.5. Dual-isotope baseline and vasodilated regional cerebral blood flow (RCBF) images in a patient with transient ischemic attacks (TIAs). Upper image shows normal surface rendered three-dimensional RCBF image at rest, whereas bottom image demonstrates significant left hemispheric failed vasodilator reserve. Such images illustrate the degree of failed reserve that can be present in TIA patients without evidence of substantial resting RCBF alterations.

ADEQUACY OF COLLATERAL RCBF WITH PROJECTED LARGE VESSEL SACRIFICE

In the course of dealing with certain head and neck neoplasms or lesions such as aneurysms affecting large cerebral vessels, the neurologic surgeon may be obliged to contemplate sacrificing a major vessel, such as the internal carotid or middle cerebral artery. The clinical state of the patient will depend on the adequacy of collateral circulation that may be established after the vessel is sacrificed. In 1911, Matas tested the adequacy of cerebral circulation by applying pressure to the great vessels in the neck. Interventional neuroradiologists now approach this problem by means of an intraarterial balloon catheter, incorporating RCBF SPECT into the procedure to provide needed information about the adequacy of collateral blood flow (60).

In the present version of this test, a balloon catheter is advanced to the level at which projected ligation will occur and the catheter balloon is expanded, occluding the vessel. The neuroradiologist then observes the patient for signs and symptoms of ischemia for a period of 30 to 45 minutes. If symptoms occur, the balloon is rapidly deflated, and the patient's symptoms usually subside. However, some patients who tolerate such an occlusion without the development of symptoms have been found subsequently to develop neurologic deficits when the major artery is sacrificed. The balloon test has been expanded to include the intravenous injection of a radiopharmaceutical such as ^{99m}Tc-HMPAO or ECD at the end of the equilibration. Because the distribution of the agent is stable for some time after administration, the neuroradiologist may conclude the examination in a timely manner. The patient is then taken to the nuclear medicine facility where a scan is performed. If the scan shows positive findings in the form of regionally decreased RCBF, it is necessary to secure a baseline study to determine whether the perfusion deficit resulted from balloon occlusion or was a preexisting lesion. The baseline study is often done on the following day. If the baseline RCBF returns to normal, it can be assumed that the deficit resulted from balloon occlusion. However, if the SPECT scan made following occlusion is normal in appearance, the patient is judged able to tolerate vessel sacrifice, and no baseline scan is required (61).

The appearance of an abnormal study is seen in Fig. 37.6. The patient was a woman who was known to have an intracerebral aneurysm. Fig. 37.6A–C are transverse sections from a study made with ^{99m}Tc-HMPAO, which was injected approximately 30 minutes after the inflation of a balloon near the origin of the left middle cerebral artery. Arrows indicate areas of perfusion deficit on the patient's left side extending from the base to the supraventricular portion of the left hemisphere. The perfusion

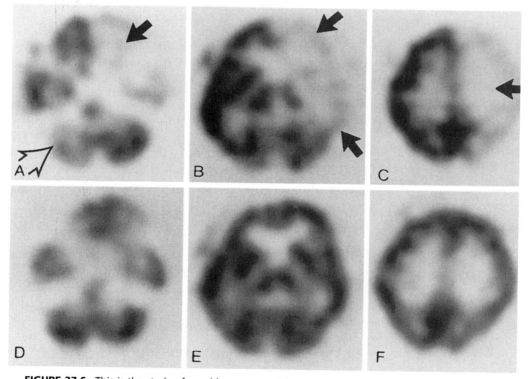

FIGURE 37.6. This is the study of an older woman with a known intracerebral aneurysm who was a candidate for vessel ligation. These studies were performed with ^{99m}Tc-hexamethyl propyleneamine oxime (HMPAO) and a triple-camera scanner. **A–C:** Selected frames from a study in which ^{99m}Tc-HMPAO was injected approximately 30 minutes after the inflation of a balloon near the origin of the middle cerebral artery. There are extensive regional cerebral blood flow (RCBF) defects throughout the left middle cerebral distribution (*solid arrows*). There is also a right crossed cerebellar diaschisis (*open arrow*). **D–F:** ^{99m}Tc-HMPAO baseline study performed 7 days later, showing a complete return of normal RCBF pattern on the patient's left and disappearance of the diaschisis. The study suggests that the patient would not tolerate ligation at the projected level.

on the right side is normal except for a reduction in RCBF within the right cerebellar hemisphere. The large deficit on the left side is consistent in volume with occlusion of anterior and middle cerebral arteries, with the maintenance of flow in the posterior circulation. Fig. 37.6**D–F** show the baseline study that was performed on the following day. Perfusion on the left side is normal at all levels and has also returned to a normal level in the right cerebellum, indicating that an immediate crossed diaschisis had occurred following occlusion of the left internal carotid artery, with the cessation of signals through the fronto-ponto-cerebellar fibers. This test remains a useful addition to the neuroradiologist's armamentarium.

NEUROLOGIC DISEASES

Migraine

Friberg (62) has reviewed RCBF studies made in patients undergoing migraine attacks. During the aura that may precede an attack, there is often a temporary reduction in whole-brain flow, followed by a rise to values above normal during the headache phase of the migraine attack. However, blood flow increases of 30% or more are not capable of causing headache, because values of this magnitude are often encountered in an acetazolamide (ACZ) challenge test (56) during which no headache occurs. The cause of migraine symptoms, therefore, cannot be explained on the basis of SPECT findings.

Huntington's Disease

Although several SPECT RCBF studies have found reduced flow to caudate and putamen, the findings tend to occur when the disease is established. It has been shown that PET may identify abnormalities in ^{18}F-deoxyglucose (^{18}F-FDG) imaging in individuals with an appropriate genetic background who are at risk for the disease. PET would seem to be the modality of choice in this disorder.

Chronic Fatigue Syndrome

The status of this entity has been debated for many years, but recent work suggests that it is a real disease of unknown origin. Costa et al. (63), using SPECT and ^{99m}Tc-HMPAO studied 24 patients with chronic fatigue syndrome, comparing the scans of these patients with the scans of 24 normal volunteers. The principal finding was hypoperfusion of the brainstem, which they found to be significant to the level of $p < 0.0001$. They also studied many groups of patients with other neurologic diseases without identifying a similar finding. Ichise et al. (64), using a similar SPECT technique, also identified occasional areas of reduced RCBF in frontal and parietal cortex. Joyce et al. (65) reviewed the current literature and found that children with the diagnosis of chronic fatigue syndrome seem to have a much higher recovery rate than do adults, and they point out that the older the patient, the less likely that recovery becomes.

Parkinson's Disease

Parkinson's disease (PD) is one of the major disabling diseases of older adults, with distressing motor symptoms and a high incidence of dementia. Brain blood flow SPECT has not been found to be useful in detecting the disease, but Seibyl et al. (66) have developed radiopharmaceuticals labeled with ^{123}I (Fig. 37.7) that are capable of labeling the dopamine transporter, a decline in which occurs with clinical PD. ^{123}I-β-CIT, a member of the tropane family, has been found to be an effective dopamine transporter label, yielding striatal SPECT scans capable of identifying PD. They have also studied ^{123}I-FP-CIT (67), which appears to have much faster washout than does ^{123}I-β-CIT. The latter may be the preferred radiopharmaceutical. Maraganore et al. (68) have used this compound to identify not only patients with clinical PD but also relatives at risk for the development of PD by reduced striatal uptake. Kung et al. (69) have succeeded in labeling a tropane with ^{99m}Tc (TRODAT-1), which will also label dopamine transporters and represents a promising development in a field that remains experimental.

Prion Disease

Within the past several years, neurodegenerative disease resulting from a deformed protein molecule, the prion, has been identified as the probable cause of entities such as scrapie in sheep (70) and bovine encephalopathy in cattle (reaching epidemic proportions in the United Kingdom), as well as human diseases such as kuru, Creutzfeldt-Jakob disease (CJD), and familial insomnia. Imaging findings have been confusing, with no single pattern emerging as yet. CJD is reported to have caused diminished flow in the left hemisphere on ^{99m}Tc-HMPAO scan (71), whereas familial and sporadic fatal insomnia (71) has been shown on ^{18}FDG PET, which has demonstrated markedly reduced metabolic activity in the thalamus. We have observed a single proven case of CJD, in which there was markedly diminished SPECT RCBF in both posterior parietal regions and the entire occipital region, including the visual cortex, in a patient who was blind when studied. Seemingly, bovine encephalopathy has crossed over to humans, appearing as new variant CJD in a number of people in Britain (72) and most recently in France (72). de Silva et al. (71) have reported the use of HMPAO SPECT in two histopathologically confirmed cases of "mad cow" disease, which showed diminished perfusion of the cerebral cortex. More case reports are required to establish the various patterns assumed by central nervous system prion disease.

Substance Abuse

Disseminated cortical lesions have been observed by Holman et al. (73) in patients with a history of cocaine, crack cocaine, and heroin use. Because there is considerable overlap in drugs used within groups of patients with AIDS, it is difficult to be certain of the cause of these defects, because AIDS has been shown to produce similar lesions (74). Lesions resulting from substance abuse in the absence of AIDS have been shown to resolve in patients who have terminated intravenous narcotic use (73).

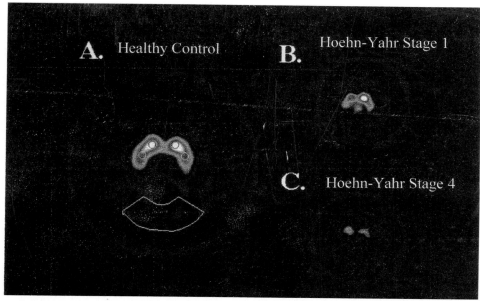

FIGURE 37.7. Transaxial single photon emission computed tomography (SPECT) images at the level of striatum in healthy control (7A) and idiopathic Parkinson's disease (PD) patient Hoehn-Yahr Stage 1-mild (7B) and Stage 4-severe (7C) obtained 24 hours following the injection of ^{123}I β-CIT. The patient in 7B has unilateral right-side symptoms. SPECT demonstrates bilateral reductions of striatal uptake, more pronounced on the side contralateral to motor symptoms. The patient in 7C has severe manifestations of PD. (Courtesy of John B. Seibyl M.D.)

Cortical RCBF defects resembling those seen in patients indulging in intravenous drug abuse have also been identified in patients with a history of inhalation of industrial solvents, including substances such as glue, cleaning solutions, and paint (74), and they have been seen in certain patients with chronic fatigue syndrome (74).

There are other underlying differences in response to cocaine use, as shown by Levin et al. (75). These authors studied a group of cocaine users who did not have AIDS and who were ostensibly otherwise healthy. Twelve of 13 men had abnormal scans, whereas only 5 of 13 female users showed the distinctive abnormalities, which, in this group, were found in the frontal and temporal lobes and in the striatum. Several of the subjects in each group abused other substances in addition to cocaine. When they were excluded, 8 of 9 male users had hypoperfusion lesions, which were seen in only 1 of the 9 women. The remainder of the female cocaine users had normal scans. The reason for this gender difference is not known, but this finding may assume importance in assessing RCBF SPECT scans in drug abusers.

Neurotoxicity

Many classes of chemical agents will damage the central nervous system. These include simple compounds such as CO and illuminating gas and other compounds such as methanol, hexane, and the various organophosphate compounds (76). The latter may be in the form of insecticides or even toxic nerve gases such as sarin, tabun, and several others. All of these agents may destroy one or another portion of the striatum. Occasionally these lesions may be so severe as to cause reduced RCBF deficits visible on

SPECT scans (76), but probably these lesions are imaged to best advantage with MRI. Cell death has been shown with magnetic resonance spectroscopy as well (77). This subject is covered in greater detail by Spencer and Butterfield (78).

Head Trauma

Brain injury resulting from head trauma has been studied with RCBF SPECT by a number of groups, notably Abdel-Dayem et al. (79), Ichise et al.(80), Jacobs et al. (81), and others. Repeated head injury, such as sustained by boxers, is well known to result in frontal brain atrophy and traumatic parkinsonism, and severe head injury can lead to permanent coma, dementia, or mental retardation. SPECT findings may be striking in these individuals, but the study will not contribute to the management of such patients. Of greater recent interest has been the study of relatively mild trauma and its late consequences (82) (Fig. 37.8). Both direct and contrecoup injuries, manifested by reduced RCBF, have been described. To some extent, neuropsychologic deficits can be traced to SPECT findings, such as loss of short-term memory with demonstrable temporal lobe injury.

Of special interest are the findings of Jacobs et al. (81) that SPECT alterations correlate well with the severity of trauma and that a negative initial SPECT study is a reliable predictor of a favorable clinical outcome. They add that in cases with initial positive SPECT findings, a follow-up SPECT and clinical data are necessary, to which an MRI is often added.

The previous comments relate principally to closed head injuries. SPECT plays a lesser role in open head injuries but may be useful in evaluating such residuals as posttraumatic epilepsy.

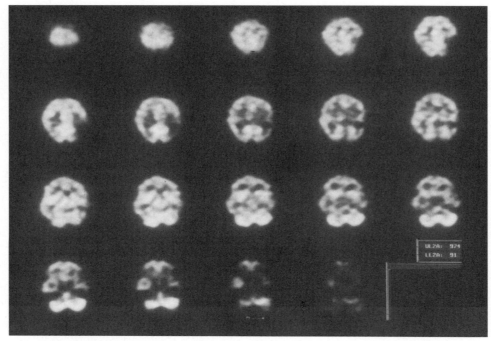

FIGURE 37.8. The patient was a 26-year-old woman with recent onset of headache and possible seizures. She had suffered a moderate head injury in an auto accident at the age of 8 with loss of consciousness of short duration. She had apparently made a complete clinical recovery and had no sequential signs or symptoms until recently. Transaxial sections made with ^{99m}Tc-hexamethyl propyleneamine oxime and a triple-camera single photon emission computed tomography show left posterior parietal hypoperfusion extending inferiorly into the left temporal lobe. Magnetic resonance imaging is said to have shown findings suggestive of remote injury, and the patient denied any significant trauma subsequent to her original injury.

Epilepsy

Epilepsy, the commonest cause of seizures, has been classified as generalized (grand mal, absence) or partial epilepsy. SPECT imaging has contributed little to the diagnosis and management of generalized epilepsy and is seldom employed for the study of this disorder. However, considerable attention has been paid to the partial epilepsies, most of which are medically treatable. There is, unfortunately, an appreciable fraction of all patients with partial epilepsy who are or who become refractory to medical treatment. Under these circumstances it is now common practice to search for a seizure focus that can be surgically removed with as little damage to fluent tissue as possible. A considerable literature has developed on refractory epilepsy; a meta-analysis was performed by Devous et al. (83), who identified 30 publications dealing with the use of SPECT RCBF imaging to localize a potentially surgically treatable seizure focus. It must be borne in mind that SPECT is one of a number of pieces of evidence, which may include CT, MRI, EEG, and the placement of intracranial electrodes for optimal localization.

It has been shown, both experimentally and in patients, that during the seizure or ictal episode, there will often be detectable hyperperfusion in the immediate vicinity of the seizure focus site (84–87). Also, it is not uncommon for the hyperperfusion to persist for a short period following the end of the seizure, in what is called the postictal period (84,88). Between seizures, in what is termed the interictal period, it is common for the seizure

focus site to be hypoperfused, thus aiding in its localization. The appearance of these findings in a patient with a temporal lobe seizure focus site is seen in Fig. 37.9. In Figure 37.9**A,** a coronal view from a scan performed with a triple-camera scanner with fan-beam collimators and stabilized and with ^{99m}Tc-HMPAO,

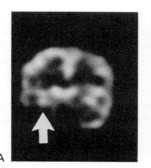 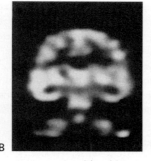

A   B

FIGURE 37.9. This is the study of a young woman with a history of seizures for many years. She had increasing numbers of both simple and complex partial seizures that had recently become difficult to control with medication. Studies were done with ^{99m}Tc-hexamethyl propyleneamine oxime (HMPAO) and a triple-camera scanner. **A:** Anterior coronal section shows markedly diminished flow in the inferior right temporal lobe with the patient in an interictal state. **B:** Anterior coronal section with injection made during a complex partial seizure. An experimental stabilized form of ^{99m}Tc-HMPAO was used. Note the marked increase in flow in the inferior portion of the right temporal lobe where regional cerebral blood flow is now higher than on the normal left side.

there is markedly reduced RCBF in the inferior right temporal lobe, compared with the normal left side. The patient had been placed in an epilepsy observation facility (84,87). When EEG and video evidence showed him to be having a seizure, a qualified attendant went to his bedside and injected 740 MBq of the radiopharmaceutical from a syringe that had been kept at his bedside for this purpose. Because stabilized ^{99m}Tc-HMPAO has a relatively long washout period, it was possible to wait until the following morning to obtain the scan; the coronal view is seen in Fig. 37.9**B**, in which there is now evidence of marked hyperperfusion in the inferior right temporal lobe. This combination of findings is the optimal SPECT scan evidence of the presence of a seizure focus in the temporal lobe. Devous et al. (84) found that in patients with temporal lobe seizures, interictal scans had a sensitivity of 44% and ictal scans a 97% sensitivity. If a postictal scan was substituted for an ictal procedure, sensitivity fell to 75%. In general, ictal scans have been found to match most closely the results of intracranial EEG electrodes in identifying seizure focus sites.

Obsessive-Compulsive Disorder

RCBF SPECT imaging studies (89–91) seem to show that there is a circuit involved in the production of obsessive-compulsive responses. The cingulate and orbitofrontal cortical regions seem to be involved, together with the right caudate nucleus. Regional blood flow values may depend on whether the patient is at rest or undergoing a stimulus that will produce an obsessive-compulsive response, as in the study of Rauch et al. (92), although the reverse findings were observed by Busatto et al. (89), employing statistical parametric mapping (see Chapter 4) These investigators showed significantly reduced flow in the right lateral orbitofrontal cortex and in the left anterior cingulate. The study of Hoehn-Saric et al. (93) is interesting in that elevated RCBF in the frontal cortex declined when the patients were restudied after the administration of fluoxetine. Thus, it would appear that a number of the previously mentioned structures are involved in a circuit that may be activated in some manner to produce an obsessive-compulsive response. Perhaps flow is at a normal level between such responses. At any rate, additional work seems to be required on this subject.

The Dementias

With an aging population, the American public has become aware of these diseases, which will pose severe social and financial problems for many families in the years to come. Several of the dementing diseases can be identified in the initial screening: These include hypothyroidism and apathetic hyperthyroidism, which may be treated for cure; certain vitamin deficiencies that respond to a reinforced diet; and neurosyphilis and several infectious diseases, which also respond to appropriate therapy. These diseases, together with multiinfarct dementia, when identified in initial screening, are referred to appropriate physicians for further treatment. However, the most common of the dementias is Alzheimer's disease (AD), which appears to be a family of diseases associated with abnormalities on at least four chromosomes (94). It may be familial or sporadic, but its incidence

begins to grow steadily as the population reaches its sixties. It has been estimated that the chance of developing AD by age 65 varies between 5% and 15%. Thereafter, the incidence increases steadily, and one's chances of developing the disease by age 85 have been estimated to be as high as 45%. It is possible that the incidence declines slightly in the very old. Family physicians, internists, and geriatricians, in addition to neurologists and psychiatrists, have become very familiar with the early signs and symptoms of AD and have become adept in the diagnosis of typical AD, with its complaints of short-term memory loss and visuospatial difficulties (95).

There is a good deal of literature about the use of RCBF SPECT in the diagnosis of AD (95–102), and several series with prospective diagnoses and histopathologic confirmation have been started. Our own study, (95) sponsored by the National Institute on Aging of the National Institutes of Health, has now reached 87 patients and 29 normal controls with the following results: for the diagnosis of AD: sensitivity = 55/64 = 85.9% [74.5% to 93.0%, 95% confidence limits (CL)]; specificity = 18/23 = 78.3% (55.8% to 91.7% CL); positive predictive value = 55/61 = 90.2% (79.1% to 95.9% CL); negative predictive value = 18/26 = 69.2% (48.1% to 84.9% CL).

In recent years, the RCBF SPECT scans in the foregoing series were performed with ^{99m}Tc-HMPAO and a triple-camera scanner with fan-beam collimation. The diagnostic success rate is satisfactory, but errors in diagnosis are encountered, in part because of the long survival of patients following the initial SPECT study, which is not repeated. The interval between SPECT and histopathologic confirmation averages approximately 5 years and may be as long as 12 years. Long survival occurs often in patients with AD.

With RCBF SPECT, the initial finding in early AD is usually reduced RCBF in the inferior portions of one or both temporal lobes (left more often than right) (Fig. 37.10) along the medial and inferior cortical surfaces. With MRI the earliest sign of AD is shrinkage of one or both hippocampi, as seen on coronal sections (103). With SPECT, as the disease progresses, extensive hypoperfusion develops in the superior temporal lobes, as well as the mid and superior portions of the parietal cortical areas. Frontal hypoperfusion may also be noted in the prefrontal, lateral frontal, and supraorbital cortex (Fig. 37.11). Recently, Minoshima et al. (102) have shown that hypoperfusion of the posterior cingulate cortex is an early and frequent sign of AD, which is confirmed in our material (95). Rarely, AD may occur with an almost exclusively frontal RCBF reduction, rendering the SPECT diagnosis quite difficult (105). In the late stages of AD, parietal temporal and frontal hypoperfusion is seen, but the sensory/motor and occipital cortical areas are relatively spared, together with the striatum (Fig. 37.11**B**).

Occasionally, AD may coexist with PD. The latter is characterized histopathologically by the presence of cellular inclusions of α-synuclein, the Lewy bodies (LBs). However, an increasingly common discovered cause of dementia is a combination of AD with a primarily cortical distribution of LBs (106–109). Histopathologically, the amyloid plaques and neurofibrillary tangles of AD have their usual distribution, but there may be many LBs in the frontal, temporal, and parietal cortical areas. Few, if any, LBs are to be found in the visual association cortex [Brodmann

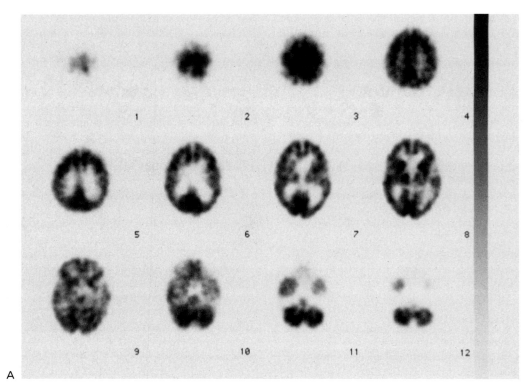

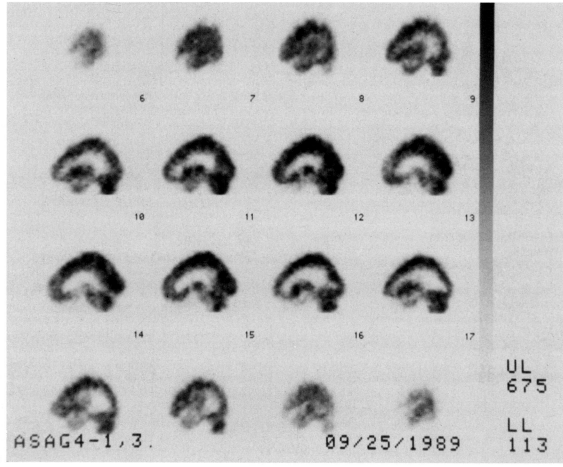

FIGURE 37.10A & B.

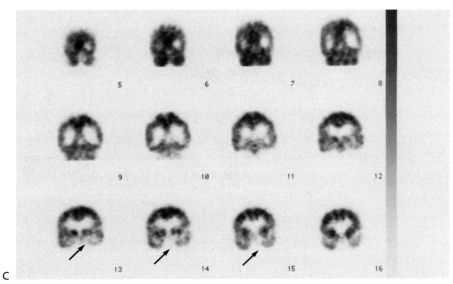

FIGURE 37.10. The patient was a 74-year-old man with possible recent onset of short-term memory loss. He was otherwise healthy and his psychologic test scores were within normal limits. ^{99m}Tc-hexamethyl propyleneamine oxime regional cerebral blood flow single photon emission computed tomography scan, made with a triple-camera scanner, was obtained, and the coronal views from this study are shown. The only positive finding was hypoperfusion of the medial and inferior cortex of the inferior left temporal lobe (*arrows*). This patient died 26 months later. Autopsy showed mild Alzheimer's disease principally confined to the inferior left temporal lobe.

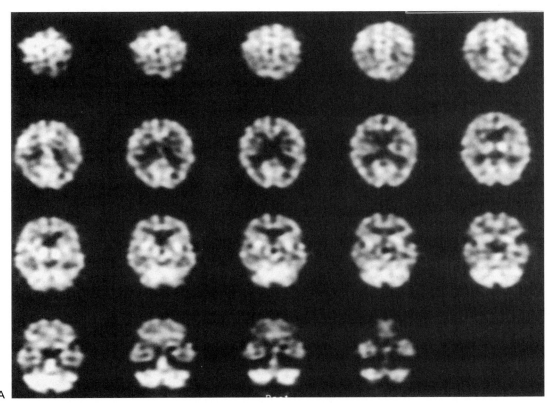

FIGURE 37.11. A set of transaxial views from a ^{99m}Tc-hexamethyl propyleneamine oxime regional cerebral blood flow single photon emission computed tomography study made with a triple-camera scan and fan-beam collimation. The patient was a 71-year-old man with evidence of advanced dementia with short-term memory loss and visuospatial difficulties. **A:** A set of transaxial views shows mild atrophy with separation of the hemispheres and moderate reduction of cortical flow except for the superior frontal region. Cerebellum and striatum appear normally perfused, as does the visual cortex. *(Figure continues.)*

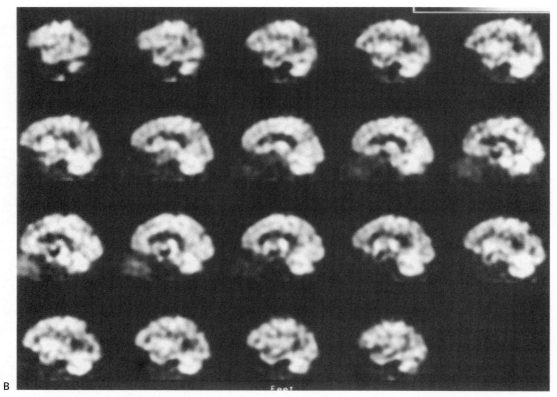

FIGURE 37.11. *Continued.* **B:** A set of sagittal views shows reduced flow in frontal, temporal, and sagittal regions, sparing the sensory/motor cortex, which is characteristic of Alzheimer's disease (AD). Also spared is the perfusion of the occipital cortex. At autopsy, this patient was found to have severe AD by all histopathologic rating systems.

areas (B) 18 & 19]. It is interesting to note that there is a higher incidence of depression and of visual hallucinations in patients with AD plus LB (108). In the final stages of AD plus LB disease, AD predominates. A higher proportion of patients with this disorder are men, as opposed to AD alone. Figure 37.12 shows views from the SPECT study of a patient with proven AD plus LB. Note the marked hypoperfusion of the occipital cortex (*arrow*). This finding has been identified on both SPECT (110) and PET (111), and it is a useful differential finding on scan interpretation.

In some cases of AD plus LB, the cortical hypoperfusion extends superiorly from the occipital cortex into the parietal region. Even in the absence of other signs of AD, this may prove to be a useful diagnostic finding.

The second most numerous group of dementias in many clinics comprises from 10% to 20% of all patients with dementias. They are referred to as a group as the frontotemporal dementias. The best known of these is probably Pick's disease (112), which, on SPECT, often shows general cortical hypoperfusion with especially severe changes in the frontal cortex extending posteriorly into the temporal lobes. Patients often exhibit a rigid, and sometimes abusive, personality, but this is shared by a number of other diseases of the frontotemporal group. The diagnosis is made histopathologically with identification of the cellular inclusions (Pick bodies). Pick's disease, itself, may behave atypically. One case in our series showed an entirely posterior presentation, causing us to misdiagnose this patient's disease as

AD. A typical case of Pick's disease is seen in Fig. 37.13. There is marked frontal atrophy with separation of the hemispheres and severe inferior frontal hypoperfusion involving prefrontal, cingulate, and lateral frontal cortical regions. The superior frontal cortex seems less involved. Changes are slightly more marked on the right than on the left, and there is slight disparity in the perfusion of the cerebellar hemispheres, with a possible left crossed diaschisis. The patient was a 62-year-old man, whose disease ran a rapid course. He died 16 months after the examination shown in the Fig. 37.13, and the histopathologic diagnosis was Pick's disease. The striatum and thalamus are often said to be involved. Although the striatum appears to be normally perfused in Fig. 37.13, there may be moderate hypoperfusion of the thalamus. Other dementing diseases may present in a primarily frontal manner including frontotemporal dementia, progressive supranuclear palsy, and multisystem degeneration, as well as some of the dysphonias (113–117). The occasional case of chronic alcohol abuse, neurosyphilis, or AIDS may also be accompanied by hypoperfusion in the frontal area.

As mentioned previously, patients suffering from true multiinfarct dementia (95) are identified early in the screening process and referred to the vascular disease service, because dementia is usually secondary to brain infarction. However, occasionally multiinfarct dementia does not progress in the typical "stair-step" fashion thought to be typical of this form of dementia, but instead progresses rather smoothly, and is referred for a SPECT scan to obtain further information about what usually

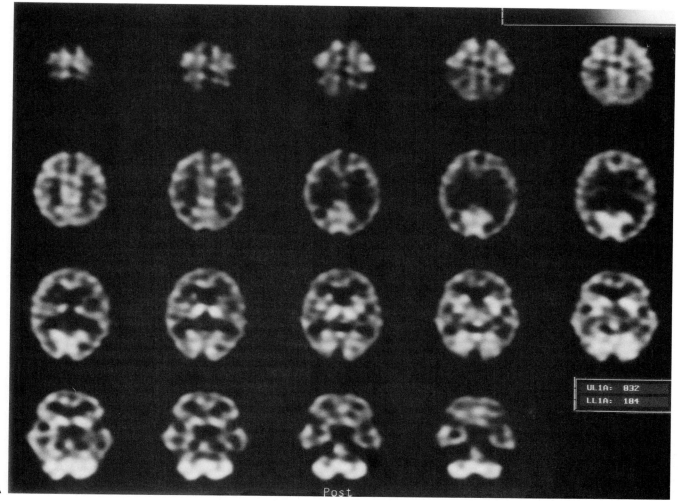

FIGURE 37.12. ⁹⁹ᵐTc-hexamethyl propyleneamine oxime regional cerebral blood flow single photon emission computed tomography made with triple-camera scanner and fan-beam collimation. The patient was a 71-year-old man with a 3-year history of progressive loss of short-term memory and recent onset of tremor and rigidity, the latter suggesting Parkinson's disease, in addition to his early history that was more consistent with Alzheimer's disease (AD). **A:** Rather marked reduction in cortical blood flow, with the usual sparing of the superior frontal cortex, the visual cortex, the striatum, and the cerebellum. A certain amount of atrophy is present with separation of the hemispheres. There may be slight diminution in perfusion of the right caudate and putamen with respect to the left, but the finding is marginal. *(Figure continues.)*

appears to be a non-AD dementia. Figure 37.14 shows a typical case involving a 68-year-old woman whose SPECT scan shows separate areas of infarction in the right frontal, right posterior temporal, and left frontoparietal regions. On further investigation, it was found that the cause of her multiple infarcts was periodic showers of emboli from a defective heart valve prosthesis. When the defective valve was replaced and anticoagulation therapy was started, her embolic episodes ceased and, with healing, her dementia improved. In patients who are noted to have opacities in the white matter, termed leukoaraiosis, there appears to be no relationship with dementia. Heiss et al. (118) have found little value in RCBF SPECT for the differential diagnosis between AD and vascular dementia.

The differential diagnosis of the dementias may assume considerable importance in the near future, because possible treatments for AD are now under development. Schenk et al. (119),

using an appropriate strain of mice, have shown that these animals may be immunized against the development of amyloid plaques and that older animals who have developed numerous plaques tend to lose them when treated immunologically. Wolozin et al. (120) have described decreased prevalence of AD associated with treatment by HMG-CoA reductase inhibitors (statins). It may therefore soon be important to identify those patients with true AD so that they may enter a treatment protocol (121).

PSYCHIATRIC DISEASES

Affective Disorders

Unipolar and bipolar depression are serious illnesses that greatly influence the lives of patients who contract them. However,

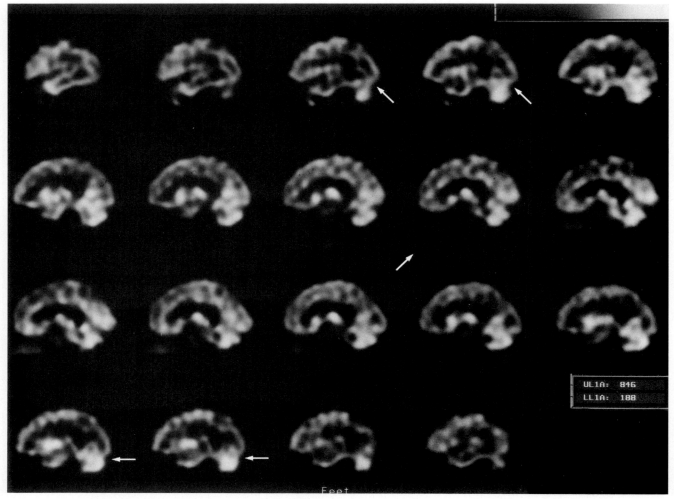

FIGURE 37.12. *Continued.* **B:** A set of sagittal views once again shows relative sparing of frontal flow and the sensory/motor cortex. However, there is markedly reduced flow in the posterior cortex, including the occipital region (*arrows*). This area of markedly reduced flow seems to extend superiorly into the posterior parietal region. At autopsy, this patient had evidence of AD, but also had a profusion of cortical Lewy bodies. The perfusion pattern is characteristic of a small group of patients with this combined disorder in our autopsy series.

severe depression and manic-depressive disease are accompanied by few anatomic findings, unless they follow an episode such as brain injury, treatment of a brain neoplasm, or the development of the fatal disease, which may trigger episodes of an affective nature. There is a voluminous body of research, much of it conducted with the aid of various imaging modalities. Much of what has been learned suggests that these diseases arise in and around the limbic system and its various connections (122–126, 128–131). The several brain structures that may play roles in the affective disorders include prefrontal and frontal cortex, temporal cortex, the hippocampus, and amygdala. The entorhinal cortex, the insula, both anterior and posterior aspects of the cingulate cortex, and the parietal cortex have also been implicated. Dopamine, serotonin, and norepinephrine systems all communicate with various portions of the structures named previously, and their receptors and transporters may play major roles in these diseases. There may be a genetic background, but

twin studies have shown disparity in incidence in monozygotic, as well as fraternal, twins, indicating the presence of other factors or a very complex genetic background (127).

Findings in imaging studies have been confusing; Kuhl et al. (122) found decreased glucose metabolism in the lateral prefrontal cortex, whereas Drevets et al. (124), studying RCBF with a PET technique, found increased RCBF in left prefrontal cortex and in the left amygdala. Indeed, Drevets et al. found increased RCBF in the left amygdala in patients who were ill or in remission, suggesting a basic role for this structure. A consensus seems to have arisen, however, favoring flow and metabolic reduction in the prefrontal cortex (125). Mayberg (126) has suggested a model of depression in which blood flow and metabolic rate in dorsal cortical regions such as the dorsal prefrontal, inferior parietal, and cingulate is reduced, whereas ventral paralimbic areas such as the orbitofrontal cortex, insula, hippocampus, and a portion of the cingulate are increased in depressed patients

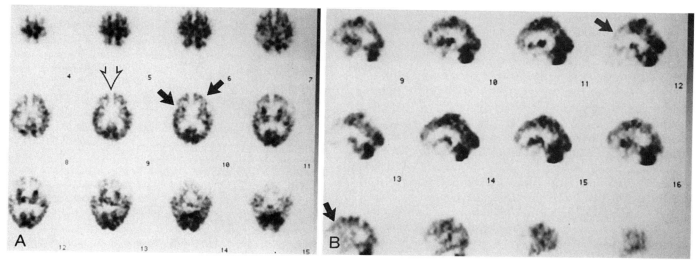

FIGURE 37.13. This is the study of an older man who had autopsy-proven Pick's disease. The study was performed with ^{99m} Tc-hexamethyl propyleneamine oxime and a triple-camera scanner. **A:** Transaxial sections show reduced frontal flow bilaterally (*solid arrows*) and frontal atrophy with separation of the hemisphere in the frontal region (*open arrow*). **B:** Sagittal sections show reduced flow in the anterior and inferior portions of both frontal lobes. Note sparing of the motor-sensory cortex and the posterior superior parietal area. (From Bonte FJ, Horn J, Tinter R et al. Single photon tomography in Alzheimer's disease and the dementias. *Semin Nucl Med* 1990;20:342–352, with permission.)

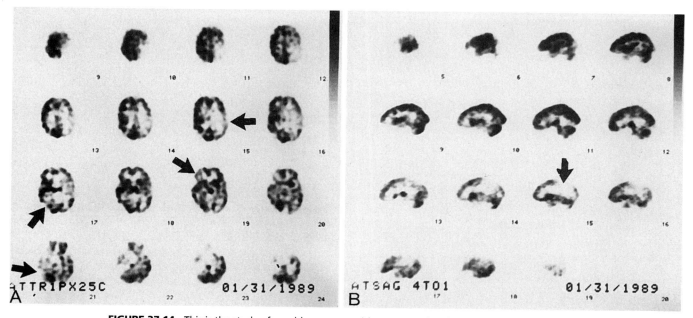

FIGURE 37.14. This is the study of an older woman with proven multiinfarct dementia. The study was performed with ^{99m}Tc-hexamethyl propyleneamine oxime and a triple-camera scanner. **A:** Transaxial sections show areas of reduced flow (*arrows*) resulting from infarctions in inferior right temporal and frontal regions and in the left parietal region. **B:** Sagittal sections show reduced regional cerebral blood flow in the anterior superior parietal region impinging on the sensory-motor cortex not usually seen in Alzheimer's disease.

and in normal controls with self-induced sadness. A balance between these two sets of structures is thought to represent the normal state, and Mayberg believes that the behavior of the rostral component of the anterior cingulate cortex is predictive of treatment responders, with abnormal decreases in patients who will not respond to treatment. At any rate, the rostral cingulate may play a mediating role between the various components involved.

An additional finding has been identified in RCBF SPECT studies of patients with unipolar depression and a few patients with bipolar disease who were depressed at the time of study: reduced RCBF in the visual association cortex, Brodmann (B) areas 18 and 19. These were initially identified in older patients referred for dementia study, who were depressed but not demented. Over the years, the finding of reduced RCBF in B 18 and 19 was identified occasionally in depressed patients who were mature but not elderly and finally in young adults. During that time, Kowatch et al. (132) were authorized to perform baseline ^{99m}Tc-HMPAO RCBF SPECT studies on a group of children with clinical evidence of depression, plus a group of normal controls, within the age range of 11 to 18 years. The study, which had been approved by the National Institutes of Health

in addition to the Southwestern Institutional Review Board, was intended as a baseline study before the administration of an experimental drug. The latter phase of the study was canceled, but during examination of the available material, it was found that of 21 depressed patients, 8 had reduced RCBF in B18 and 19, but 13 patients did not. None of the 18 control subjects showed scan abnormality. Initially, it was thought advisable to publish this novel finding, to bring it to the attention of other investigators (135), and the results are seen in Fig. 37.15.

We next decided to appraise the areas of reduced RCBF in both adolescent patient groups, comparing them with the normal controls (135). All groups had a mean age of 14.5 years. The method selected was statistical parametric mapping, as described by Friston et al. (136). Images of individual patients and controls were registered in Talairach space (137) and processed for uncorrected k and uncorrected Z. Fig. 37.16**A** and **B** show statistical parametric mapping (SPM) maps in transaxial, sagittal, and coronal projections in which all findings, representing voxel groups with significantly reduced RCBF, are projected to the midplane in each projection. There are two different sets of patterns. The larger group of 13 patients have anterior findings of the general sort described previously, whereas the 8 patients with reduced B18 and 19 RCBF have a significantly different

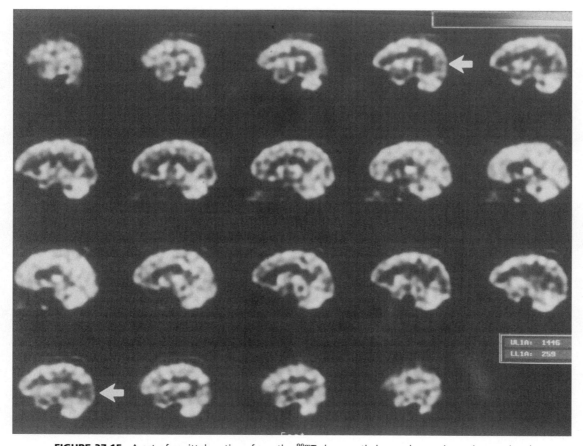

FIGURE 37.15. A set of sagittal sections from the ^{99m}Tc-hexamethyl propyleneamine oxime regional cerebral blood flow single photon emission computed tomography study of a 26-year-old man with a history of intermittent depression, who was presently having an acute episode for which he was not receiving medication. Arrows indicate areas of hypoperfusion in the visual association cortex (B18 and 19). As far as is known, the patient had no visual abnormalities.

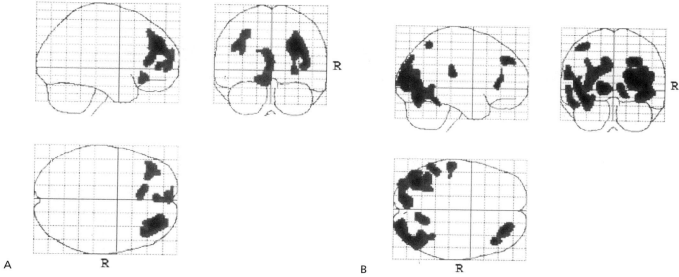

FIGURE 37.16. **A:** Derived from the study of 13 patients, ages 11 to 18, whose ^{99m}Tc-hexamethyl propyleneamine oxime regional cerebral blood flow (RCBF) single photon emission computed tomography studies were compared with those of 18 normal control children, ages 11 to 18, by the process of statistical parametric mapping (136). Areas of reduced flow in each of the three views are projected to a plane in the midline. The pattern of reduced RCBF is statistically significant. Voxel groups seem to represent the commonly accepted anterior pattern involving a number of limbic system. **B:** The result of the comparison of the scan data of eight patients, ages 11 to 18 years, whose individual scans showed posterior B18 and 19 hypoperfusion, using the process of statistical parametric mapping. Note that a primarily posterior pattern is obtained in this group. The clinical difference and possible implications of the pattern differences is unknown at this time. Similar findings have been noted in a group of patients and controls in the 20- to 50-year-old age group.

pattern of voxel groups with principal findings seen in the posterior cortex (Fig. 37.16**B**). A review of the literature shows that other investigators, such as Upadhyaya et al. (123) and Drevets et al. (124), had also identified reduced occipital flow in depressed patients but had not commented on the finding. The reason for selective posterior localization of low-flow areas in the smaller group is not known, but it has been found in groups of adults as well. Thus far there does not appear to be any unique clinical distinction between the patient groups with different sets of findings, and further investigation is required. Among possibilities considered were abnormalities in the dopamine system, originating with the dopaminergic neurons of the retina, or even some biochemical factor that altered the distribution of ^{99m}Tc-HMPAO (135).

Schizophrenia

The role of brain blood flow SPECT in schizophrenia remains problematic. Most positive findings have involved the frontal cortex, usually on the patient's left side (138). In addition, Verhoeff et al. (139) have identified abnormalities in the distribution of benzodiazepine receptor imaging (using the tracer ^{123}I-Iomazenil) with findings localized in the left precentral gyrus. Temporal lobe abnormalities have been identified with both MRI and magnetic resonance (MR) spectroscopy (140,141), whereas additional abnormalities in the thalamus in schizophrenia patients has been reported by Omori et al. (140) using the same modalities. However, Falke et al. (142) have noted no histopath-

ologic evidence of degeneration in the thalamus and caudate in schizophrenic patients. Challenge tests, such as the Wisconsin Card Sorting test, have elicited interesting findings by several groups. Steinberg et al. (143) have found ^{133}Xe to be especially useful for obtaining both baseline and challenge tests on the same day, because of the rapid clearance of radioxenon. Positive findings have been identified in the form of reduction of frontal flow as the result of the changing strategy of the Wisconsin Card Sorting test. Min et al. (144), using ^{99m}Tc-ECD, concluded that positive and negative symptoms of schizophrenia are related to dysfunctions in different regions of the brain, with varying patterns. Thus, the usefulness of SPECT imaging in schizophrenia has not been clearly established.

An interesting observation was made by Matsuda et al. (145), who demonstrated a significant increase in left superior temporal uptake of ^{123}I-IMP in a patient who was having an auditory hallucination. These authors also noted that the localization disappeared when the patient was asymptomatic. Thus, at least in some patients there is a physiologic basis for this and perhaps other hallucinatory symptoms.

DIFFERENTIAL DIAGNOSIS OF BRAIN LESIONS IN PATIENTS WITH AIDS

A frequent complication of AIDS is the development of brain lesions. These often present as ring lesions on MRI studies, which do not permit further diagnosis between the possibilities

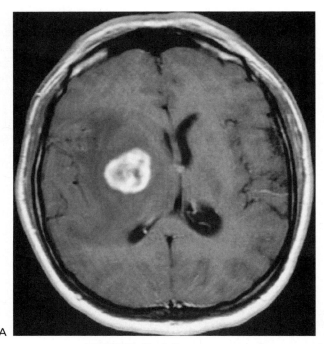

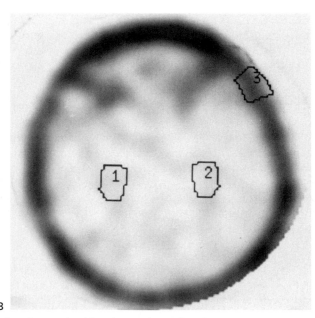

FIGURE 37.17. A: Transverse magnetic resonance imaging view made with unknown factors but showing a ring lesion in the right cerebrum in a patient known to have AIDS. **B:** A ^{201}Tl scan that shows the presence of three regions-of-interest (ROIs). No concentration appears within ROI 1, and the lesion was shown to be a granuloma resulting from toxoplasmosis. (Courtesy of W.A. Erdman M.D.)

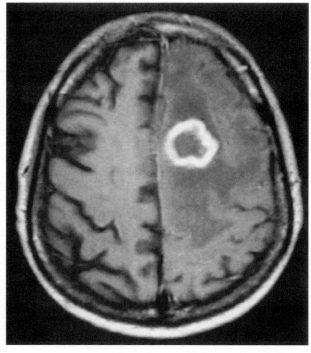

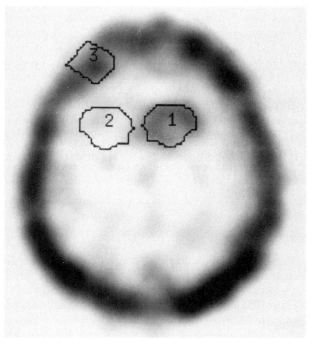

FIGURE 37.18. A: Transverse magnetic resonance imaging scan made with unknown factors, showing a ring lesion in the anterior superior white matter of the left cerebrum. **B:** Three regions-of-interest (ROIs) constructed as before. Note that the concentration of ^{201}Tl in ROI 1 is greater than that in ROI 2 and is equal to that in ROI 3 in the scalp. The diagnosis was lymphoma, which was confirmed in this patient who is known to have AIDS. (Courtesy of W.A. Erdman M.D.)

of lymphoma and one of the granulomatous diseases. Among the latter, toxoplasmosis is probably the most common, but tuberculomas may also occur in this fashion. Brain SPECT presents an opportunity for an almost immediate differential diagnosis. A dose of 185 MBq (5 mCi) of ^{201}Tl as thallous chloride is administered intravenously, and SPECT imaging can begin as early as 5 minutes later. The principle of the test is that the tracer should accumulate in lymphoma and not in one of the granulomas. Ruiz et al. (146) apparently looked for localization of uptake in the suspect lesions, but Erdman et al. (147) point out that faint uptakes may represent false-positive localization. Erdman et al. require concentration in the rim of the ring lesion that is greater than or equal to the concentration in the scalp. This method has a very high sensitivity in a small group of patients. An additional point made by Ruiz et al. is that thin rings most often accompany granulomatous lesions, whereas thick rings are almost exclusively seen with lymphoma.

Figure 37.17**A** is a transverse MRI view showing a ring lesion indenting and displacing the midportion of the right lateral ventricle; Fig. 37.17**B** is a ^{201}Tl scan that shows the presence of three ROIs. ROI 1 is placed over the lesion, R0I 2 is in the identical contralateral location, and ROI 3 is in the scalp. Note that there is no concentration within ROI 1. The lesion was shown to be a granuloma resulting from toxoplasmosis.

Figure 37.18**A** is a transverse MRI scan showing a ring lesion in the anterior superior white matter of the left cerebral hemisphere. In Figure 37.18**B,** three ROIs have been constructed as before. Note that the concentration of ^{201}Tl in ROI 1 is greater than that in ROI 2 and is equal to that in ROI 3 that is placed in the scalp. The diagnosis was lymphoma, which was shown to be correct. Both of the patients shown also suffered from AIDS.

Because of the rapidity with which results can be obtained, this test is often used in the differential diagnosis of MRI-demonstrable brain lesions in patients suffering from AIDS.

BRAIN TUMOR IMAGING

High-grade gliomas, certain metastases, and several other types of poorly differentiated brain neoplasms are treated with various combinations of surgery, radiation therapy, and chemotherapy. Changes that follow treatment may include edema and radiation necrosis. In a patient who develops symptoms following treatment, a decision must be made as to whether symptoms are caused by edema and necrosis or recurrence of the primary neoplasm. Because of physical changes that occur within the treated volume, CT and MRI are often not helpful in evaluating tumor viability. ^{201}Tl, administered intravenously as thallous chloride, has been found to localize in malignant residuals in a series of patients who had been treated for malignant gliomas (148).

Kim et al. (149) proposed establishing an ROI around the lesion in question and its mirror ROI on the opposite side of the brain, a technique described previously for differentiating malignant from inflammatory and granulomatous lesions. Kim et al. found that a ratio of maximum counts per pixel in the tumor ROI over matching counts in the homologous ROI gave

a ratio of approximately 3.5:1, which was statistically significant. Others have used the method of Erdman et al. (147), described previously, in which localization within a nodule that equaled or exceeded that of the scalp was thought to be abnormal. Figure 37.19**A** and **B** illustrate the accumulation of densities secondary to treatment of a glioma, within which ^{201}Tl could not identify a residual. Figure 37.20**A** and **B** shows a large area of suspected necrosis, but there is a sharp localization of ^{201}Tl within it (in an area later shown to be residual malignant tumor). This remains a

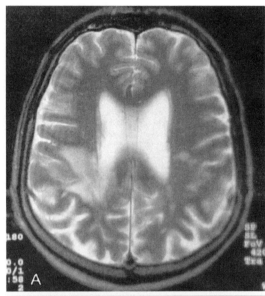

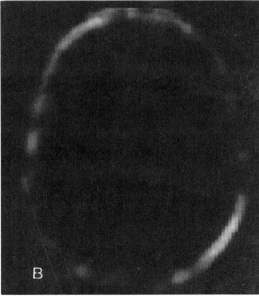

FIGURE 37.19. This is the study of a young man with a long history of seizures and recent discovery of a high right posterior frontal mass which was found to be a composite astrocytoma and oligodendroglioma. Resection was ruled out and the patient received radiation therapy. **A.** Follow-up transaxial MRI shows ill-defined lesion along the posterior aspect of the right lateral ventricle. **B.** Transaxial section from ^{201}Tl SPECT study shows no evidence of tracer localization, and no evidence of recurrent tumor. (Case courtesy of H. Chehabi and D. Lilien.)

preparation of the figures, and the support of grants NIH NIA
2 P30 12300 and Nycomed-Amersham, Inc.

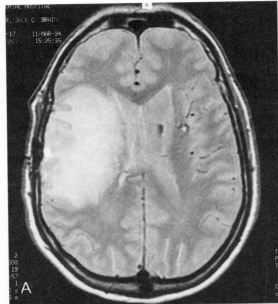
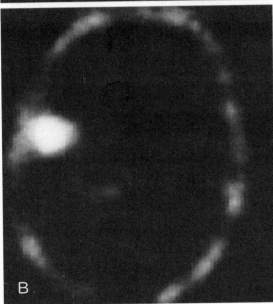

FIGURE 37.20. This is the study of an elderly man who was found to have a right inferior frontoparietal glioma. The lesion was treated with partial resection and postoperative stereotactic radiosurgery. There has been a recent onset of symptoms. **A.** Follow-up transaxial MRI shows a large right frontoparietal mass representing edema and necrosis. Recurrent tumor cannot be definitely identified. **B.** Transaxial 201Tl SPECT shows evidence of conspicuous localization within the region of the mass, indicating recurrent or persistent neoplasm. (Case courtesy of H. Chehabi and D. Lilien.)

useful procedure, because the amount of thallium used is small, and SPECT imaging can begin within 5 minutes of administration of the tracer dose.

ACKNOWLEDGMENTS

The authors wish to acknowledge the help of Ms. Carol Gibson in preparation of the manuscript, Ms. Dorothy Smith in the

REFERENCES

1. Roy CS, Sherrington CS. On the regulation of the blood supply of the brain. *J Physiol (London)* 1890;11:85–108.
2. Kety SS, Schmidt CF. The nitrous oxide method for quantitative determination of cerebral blood flow in man: theory, procedure and normal values. *J Clin Invest* 1948;27:476–483.
3. Lassen NA, Munck O. The cerebral blood flow in man determined by the use of radioactive krypton. *Acta Physiol Scand* 1955;33:30–49.
4. Obrist WD, Thompson HK Jr, King HC. Determination of regional cerebral blood flow by inhalation of 133–xenon. *Circ Res* 1967;20:124–135.
5. Kuhl DE, Edwards RQ, Ricci AR et al. Quantitative section scanning using orthogonal tangent correction. *J Nucl Med* 1972;13:447–448(abst).
6. Stokely EM Sveinsdottir, Lassen NA et al. A single photon dynamic computer assisted tomograph (DCAT) for imaging brain function in multiple cross-sections. *J Comput Assist Tomogr* 1980;4:230–240.
7. Anger HO. Scintillation camera with multichannel collimators. *J Nucl Med* 1964;5:515–531.
8. Winchell HS, Baldwin RM, Lin JH. Development of I-123 labeled amines for brain studies: localization of (I-123) iodophenylalkylamines in rat brain. *J Nucl Med* 1980;21:940–946.
9. Neirinckx RD, Burke JF, Harrison RC et al. The retention mechanism of technetium-99m-HMPAO: intracellular reaction with glutathione. *J Cereb Blood Flow Metab* 1988;8:S4–S12.
10. Walovitch RC, Hill TC, Garrity ST et al. Characterization of technetium-99m-L, L-ECD for brain perfusion imaging. 1: Pharmacology of technitum-99m ECD in non human primates *J Nucl Med* 1989;30:1892–1901.
11. Devous MD Sr, Thisted RA, Jagust WJ et al. Meta-analysis of SPECT brain imaging in dementia. *J Nucl Med* 1995;36:107P(abst).
12. Friston J, Holmes AP, Worsley KJ et al. Statistical parametric maps in functional imaging: a general linear approach. *J Human Brain Map* 1995;2:189–210.
13. Talairach J, Tournoux P. *Co-planar stereotaxic atlas of the human brain.* New York: Thieme Medical Publishers, 1988.
14. Smith AP, Genna S. Imaging characteristics of ASPECT, a single-crystal ring camera for dedicated brain SPECT. *J Nucl Med* 1989;30:796.
15. Devous MD Sr, Brass LM. SPECT imaging in cerebrovascular disease. In: Murray IPC, Ell PJ, eds. *Nuclear medicine in clinical diagnosis and treatment.* London: Churchill-Livingstone, 1995:559–574.
16. Fayad PB, Brass LM. Single photon emission computed tomography in cerebrovascular disease. *Stroke* 1991;22:950–954.
17. Hellman RS, Tikofsky RS. An overview of the contributions of regional cerebral blood flow studies in cerebrovascular disease. Is there a role for single photon emission computed tomography? *Sem Nucl Med* 1990;20:303–324.
18. Brass LM, Rattner Z. Single photon emission computed tomography in cerebral vascular disease. In: Weber DA, Devous MD, Tikofsky RS, eds. *Workshop on brain SPECT perfusion imaging: optimizing imaging acquisition and processing.* DOE CONF-9110368. 1992;77–88.
19. De Roo M, Mortelmans L, Devos P et al. Clinical experience with Tc-99m HM-PAO high resolution SPECT of the brain in patients with cerebrovascular accidents. *Eur J Nucl Med* 1989;15:9–15.
20. Allen CMC. Predicting the outcome of acute stroke: a prognostic score. *J Neurol Neurosurg Psychiatry* 1984;47:475–480.
21. Oxbury JM, Greenhall RCD, Grainger KMR. Predicting the outcome of stroke: acute stage after cerebral infarction. *BMJ* 1975;3:125–127.
22. Levy DE, Caronna JJ, Lapinski RH et al. Clinical predictors of recovery from ischemic stroke. In: Reivich M, Hurtig HI, eds. *Cerebrovascular diseases.* New York: Raven Press, 1983;121–128.
23. Costa DC, Ell PJ. 99mTc-HMPAO washout in prognosis of stroke. *Lancet* 1989;1:213–214.
24. Defer G, Moretti JL, Cesaro P et al. Early and delayed SPECT using

N-isopropyl p-iodoamphetamine iodine 123 in cerebral ischemia. A prognostic index for clinical recovery. *Arch Neurol* 1987;44:715–718.

25. Feeney DM, Baron JC. Diaschisis. *Stroke* 1986;17:817–830.
26. Heiss W, Zeiler K, Havelec L et al. Long-term prognosis in stroke related to cerebral blood flow. *Arch Neurol* 1977;34:671–676.
27. Kushner M, Alavi A, Reivich M et al. Contralateral cerebellar hypometabolism following cerebral insult: a positron emission tomographic study. *Ann Neurol* 1984;15:425–434.
28. Kushner M, Reivich M, Fieschi C et al. Metabolic and clinical correlates of acute ischemic infarction. *Neurology* 1987;37:1103–1110.
29. Lassen NA, Sperling B. ^{99m}Tc-bicisate reliably images CBF in chronic brain diseases but fails to show reflow hyperemia in subacute stroke: report of a multicenter trial of 105 cases comparing ^{133}Xe and ^{99m}Tc-bicisate (ECD, Neurolite) measured by SPECT on same day. *J Cereb Blood Flow Metab* 1994;14:S44–S48.
30. Moretti JL, Cinotti L, Cesaro P et al. Amines for brain tomoscintigraphy. *Nucl Med Comm* 1978;8:581–595.
31. Mountz JM, Modell JG, Foster NL et al. Prognostication of recovery following stroke using the comparison of CT and technetium-99m HM-PAO SPECT. *J Nucl Med* 1990;31:61–66.
32. Nakagawara J, Nakamura J, Takeda R et al. Assessment of post ischemic reperfusion and diamox activation test in stroke using ^{99m}TC-ECD SPECT. *J Cereb Blood Flow Metab* 1994;14:S49–S57.
33. Nagata K, Yunoki K, Sumie K et al. Regional cerebral blood flow correlates of aphasia outcome in cerebral hemorrhage and cerebral infarction. *Stroke* 1986;17:417–423.
34. Pantano P, Veron JC, Samson Y et al. Crossed cerebellar diaschisis. Further studies. *Brain* 1986;109:677–694.
35. Yoon BW, Roh JK, Myung HJ et al. Assessment of regional cerebral blood flow (rCBF) in ischemic stroke using Tc-99m HMPAO SPECT—comparison with CT and MR findings. *J Korean Med Sci* 1991;6:21–29.
36. Demeurisse G, Verhas M, Capon A et al. Lack of evolution of the cerebral blood flow during clinical recovery of a stroke. *Stroke* 1983;14:77–81.
37. Hayman LA, Taber KH, Jhingran SG et al. Cerebral infarction. Diagnosis and assessment of prognosis by using ^{123}IMP-SPECT and CT. *AJNR* 1989;10:557–562.
38. Lee RGL, Hill TC, Holman BL et al. Predictive value of perfusion defect size using N-isopropyl-(I-123)-p-iodoamphetamine emission tomography in acute stroke. *J Neurosurg* 1984;61:449–452.
39. Vallar G, Perani D, Cappa SF et al. Recovery from aphasia and neglect after subcortical stroke: neuropsychological and cerebral perfusion study. *J Neurol Neurosurg Psychiatry* 1988;51:1269–1276.
40. Bushnell DL, Gupta S, Micoch AG et al. Prediction of language and neurological recovery after cerebral infarction with SPECT imaging using N-isopropyl-(I-123)-p-iodoamphetamine. *Arch Neurol* 1989;46:665–669.
41. Limburg M, van Royen EA, Hijdra A et al. rCBF-SPECT in brain infarction: when does it predict outcome? *J Nucl Med* 1991;32:383–387.
42. Giubilei F, Lenzi GL, Di Piero V et al. Predictive value of brain perfusion single-photon emission computed tomography in acute cerebral ischemia. *Stroke* 1990;21:895–900.
43. Alexandrov AV, Black SE, Ehrlich LE et al. Simple visual analysis of brain perfusion on HMPAO SPECT predicts early outcome in acute stroke. *Stroke* 1996;27:1537–1542.
44. Lees KR, Weir CJ, Gillen GJ et al. Comparison of mean cerebral transit time and single-photon emission tomography for estimation of stroke outcome. *Eur J Nucl Med* 1995;22:1261–1267.
45. Laloux P, Rachelle F, Jamart J et al. Comparative correlations of HMPAO SPECT indices, neurologic score, and stroke subtypes with clinical outcome in acute carotid infarcts. *Stroke* 1995;26:816–821.
46. Baird AE, Austin MC, McKay WJ et al. Changes in cerebral tissue perfusion in the first 48 hours of ischemic stroke: Relation to clinical outcome. *J Neurol Neurosurg Psychiatry* 1996;61:26–29.
47. Baird AE, Donnan GA. Increased 99mTc-HMPAO uptake in ischemic stroke. *Stroke* 1993;24:1261–1262.
48. Sperling B, Lassen NA. Increased ^{99m}Tc-HMPAO uptake in ischemic stroke [Letter]. *Stroke* 1993;24:1262.
49. Shimosegawa E, Hatazawa J, Inugami A et al. Cerebral infarction

within six hours of onset: prediction of completed infarction with Technetium-99m-HMPAO SPECT. *J Nucl Med* 1994;35:1097–1103.
50. Foster NL, Mountz JM, Bluelein LA et al. Blood flow imaging of a posterior circulation stroke. Use of technetium Tc 99m hexamethyl-propyleneamine oxime and single photon emission computed tomography. *Arch Neurol* 1988;45:687–690.
51. Seiderer M, Krappel W, Moser E et al. Detection and quantification of chronic cerebrovascular disease: comparison of MR imaging, SPECT, and CT. *Radiology* 1989;170:545–548.
52. Bogousslavsky J, Delaloye-Bischof A, Regli F et al. Prolonged hypoperfusion and early stroke after transient ischemic attack. *Stroke* 1990;21:40–46.
53. Baird AE, Donnan GA, Austin MC et al. Reperfusion after thrombolytic therapy in a ischemic stroke measured by single-photon emission computed tomography. *Stroke* 1994;25:79–85.
54. Ezura M, Takahashi A, Yoshimoto T. Evaluation of regional cerebral blood flow using single-photon emission tomography for the selection of patients for local fibrinolytic therapy of acute cerebral embolism. *Neurosurg Rev* 1996;19:231–236.
55. Hanson FK, Grotta JC, Rhoades H et al. Value of single-photon emission-computed tomography in acute therapeutic trials. *Stroke* 1993;24:1322–1329.
56. Bonte FJ, Devous MD Sr, Reisch JS. The effect of acetazolamide on regional cerebral blood flow in normal human subjects as measured by single photon emission computed tomography. *Invest Radiol* 1988;23:564–568.
57. Chollet F, Celsis P, Clanet M et al. SPECT study of cerebral blood flow reactivity after acetazolamide in patients with transient ischemic attacks. *Stroke* 1989;20:458–464.
58. Vorstrup S. Tomographic cerebral blood flow measurements in patients with ischemic cerebrovascular disease and evaluation of the vasodilatory capacity by the acetazolamide test. *Acta Neurol Scan* 1988;114(Suppl):1–48.
59. Bogousslavsky J, Miklossy J, Regli F et al. Subcortical neglect: neuropsychological, SPECT, and neuropathological correlations with anterior choroidal artery territory infarction. *Ann Neurol* 1988;23:448–452.
60. Eckard DA, Purdy PD, Bonte FJ. Crossed cerebellar diaschisis and loss of consciousness during balloon occlusion of the internal carotid artery. *AJNR* 1992;13.
61. Mathews D, Walker BS, Purdy P et al. Brain blood flow SPECT in temporary balloon occlusion of carotid and intracerebral arteries. *J Nucl Med* 1993;34:1239–1243.
62. Friberg L. Cerebral blood flow changes in migraine: methods, observations and hypotheses. *J Neurol* 1991;238:S12–S17.
63. Costa DC, Tannock C, Brostoff J. Brainstem perfusion is impaired in chronic fatigue syndrome. *QJM* 1995;88:767–773.
64. Ichise M, Salit IE, Abbey SE et al. Assessment of regional cerebral perfusion by Tc-99m HMPAO RCBF SPECT in chronic fatigue syndrome. *Nucl Med Commun* 1992;13:767–772.
65. Joyce J, Hotopf M, Wessely S. The prognosis of chronic fatigue and chronic fatigue syndrome: A systematic review. *QJM* 1997;90:223–233.
66. Seibyl JP, Marek K, Sheff K et al. Iodine-123-β-CIT and Iodine-123-FPCIT SPECT measurement of dopamine transporters in healthy subjects and Parkinson's patients. *J Nucl Med* 1998;39:1500–1508.
67. Booij J, Tissing HG, Boer GJ et al. (123I) FP-CIT SPECT shows a pronounced decline striatal dopamine transporter labeling in early and advanced Parkinson's disease. *J Neurol Neurosurg Psychiatry* 1997;62:133–140.
68. Maraganore DM, O'Connor MK, Bower JH et al. Detection of preclinical Parkinson's disease in at-risk family members with the use of ^{123}I-β-CIT SPECT: an exploratory study. *Mayo Clinic Proc* 1999;74:681–685.
69. Kung HF, Kim H-J, Kung M-P et al. Imaging of dopamine transporters in humans with Technetium 99m TRODAT-1. *Eur J Nucl Med* 1996;23:1527–1530.
70. Prusiner SB. Novel proteinaceous infectious particles cause scrapie. *Science* 1982;216:136–144.
71. de Silva R, Patterson J, Hadley D et al. Single photon emission com-

puted tomography in the identification of new variant Creutzfeldt-Jacob disease: case reports. *BMJ* 1998;316:593–594.

72. World Health Organization. *New variant Creutzfeldt-Jakob disease in France.* Geneva: WHO Publications, 1999.

73. Holman BL, Mendelson J, Garada B et al. Regional cerebral blood flow improves with treatment in chronic cocaine polydrug users. *J Nucl Med* 1993;34:723–727.

74. Bonte FJ, Devous MD Sr, Holman BL. Single photon emission computed tomographic imaging of the brain. In: Sandler MP, Coleman RE, Wackers FJT, et al., eds. *Diagnostic nuclear medicine,* 3rd ed. Baltimore: Williams & Wilkins, 1996:1087.

75. Levin JM, Holman BL, Mendelson JH et al. Gender differences in cerebral perfusion in cocaine abuse: ^{99m}TC-HMPAO SPECT study of drug abusing women. *J Nucl Med* 1994;35:1902–1909.

76. Haley RW, Kurt TM. Self-reported exposure to neurotoxic chemical combinations in the Gulf War: a cross-sectional epidemiologic study. *JAMA* 1997;277:231–237.

77. Hantson P, Duprez T, Mahieu P. Neurotoxicity to the basal ganglia shown by magnetic resonance imaging (MRI) following poisoning by methanol and other substances. *Clinical Toxicol* 1997;35:151–161.

78. Spencer PS, Butterfield PG. Environmental agents and Parkinson's disease. In: Ellenberg JH, Koller WC, Langston JW, eds. *Etiology of Parkinson's disease.* New York: Marcel Dekker, 1995:319–364.

79. Abdel-Dayem HM, Sadek SA, Kouris K et al. Changes in cerebral perfusion after acute head injury: comparison of CT with Tc-99m HMPAO RCBF SPECT. *Radiology* 1987;165:221–226.

80. Ichise M, Chung D-G, Wang P et al. Technetium-99m HMPAO SPECT, CT and MRI in the evaluation of patients with chronic traumatic brain injury: a correlation with neuro-psychological performance. *J Nucl Med* 1994;35:217–226.

81. Jacobs A, Put E, Ingels M et al. Prospective evaluation of technetium 99m-HMPAO SPECT in mild and moderate traumatic brain injury. *J Nucl Med* 1994;35:942–947.

82. Hofman PAM, Stapart SZ, Van Kroonenburgh MJPG et al. MR imaging single-photon emission CT, and neural cognitive performance after mild traumatic brain injury. *AJNR* 2001;22:441–449.

83. Devous MD Sr, Thisted RA, Morgan GF et al. SPECT brain imaging in epilepsy: a meta-analysis. *J Nucl Med* 1998;39:285–293.

84. Devous MD Sr, Leroy RF, Homan RW. Single-photon emission tomography in epilepsy. *Semin Nucl Med* 1990;20:325–341.

85. Oliveira AJ, da Costa JC, Hilario LN et al. Localization of the epileptogenic zone by ictal and interictal SPECT with ^{99m}Tc ECD in patients with medically refractory epilepsy. *Epilepsia* 1999;40:693–702.

86. Vera P, Kaminska A, Cieuta C et al. Use of subtraction ictal SPECT co-registered to MRI for optimizing the localization seizure foci in children. *J Nucl Med* 1999;40:786–792.

87. Smith BJ, Karvellis KC, Cronan S et al. Developing an effective program to complete ictal SPECT in the epilepsy monitoring unit. *Epilepsy Res* 1999;33:189–197.

88. O'Brien TJ, Brinkmann BH, Mullan BP. Comparative study of ^{99m}Tc ECD and ^{99m}Tc HMPAO for peri-ictal SPECT: qualitative and quantitative analysis. *J Neurol Neurosurg Psychiatry* 1999;66:331–339.

89. Busatto GF, Zamignani DR, Buchpiguel CA et al. A voxel-based investigation of regional cerebral blood flow abnormalities in obsessive-compulsive disorder using single photon emission tomography (SPECT). *Psychiatry Res Neuroimaging* 2000;99:15–27.

90. Saxena S, Brody AL, Schwartz JM et al. Neuroimaging in frontal-subcortical circuitry in obsessive-compulsive disorder. *Br J Psychiatry* 1998;173(Suppl 35):26–38.

91. Rubin RT, Villanueva-Meyer J, Ananth J et al. *Arch Gen Psychiatry* 1992;49:695–702.

92. Rauch SL, Jenike MA, Alpert NM et al. Regional cerebral blood flow measured during symptom provocation in obsessive-compulsive disorder using oxygen-labeled carbon dioxide and positron emission tomography. *Arch Gen Psychiatry* 1994;57:62–70.

93. Hoehn-Saric R, Pearlson GD, Harris GJ et al. Effects of fluoxetine on regional cerebral blood flow in obsessive-compulsive patients. *Am J Psychiatry* 1991;148:1243–1245.

94. Rosenberg RN. The molecular and genetic basis of AD: the end of the beginning. *Neurology* 2000;54:2045–2054.

95. Bonte FJ, Weiner MF, Bigio EH et al. Brain blood flow in the demen-

tias: SPECT with histopathologic correlation in 54 patients. *Radiology* 1997;202:793–797.

96. Claus JJ, Van Harskamp F, Breteler M et al. The diagnostic value of SPECT with Tc 99m HMPAO and Alzheimer's disease: a popular-based study. *Neurology* 1994;44:454–561.

97. Neary D, Snowden JS, Shields RA et al. Single photon emission tomography using 99mT HM-PAO in the investigation in dementia. *J Neurol Neurosurg Psychiatry* 1987;50:1101–1109.

98. Di Patre PL, Read SL, Cummings JL et al. Progression of clinical deterioration and pathological changes in patients with Alzheimer disease evaluated at biopsy and autopsy. *Arch Neurol* 1999;56:1254–1261.

99. Osimani A, Ichise M, Chung D et al. SPECT for differential diagnosis for dementia and correlation of RCBF with cognitive impairment. *Can J Neurol Sci* 1994;21:104–111.

100. Imran MB, Kawashima R, Awata S et al. Tc-99m HMPAO SPECT in the evaluation of Alzheimer's disease: correlation between neuropsychiatric evaluation and CBF images. *J Neurol Neurosurg Psychiatry* 1999;66:228–232.

101. Parvezi JP, Van Hoesen GW, Damasio A. The selective vulnerability of brainstem nuclei to Alzheimer's disease. *Ann Neurol* 2001;49:53–66.

102. Minoshima S, Foster NL, Kuhl DE. Posterior cingulate cortex in Alzheimer's disease. *Lancet* 1994;344:895.

103. Jack CR, Petersen RC, O'Brien PC et al. MR-based hippocampal volumetry in the diagnosis of Alzheimer's disease. *Neurology* 1992;42:183–188.

104. Galynker H, Dutta E, Vilks N et al. Hypofrontality and negative symptoms in patients with dementia of the Alzheimer type. *Neuropsychiatry Neuropsychol Behav Neurol* 2000;13:53–59.

105. Johnson JK, Head E, Kim R et al. Clinical and pathological evidence for a frontal variant of Alzheimer's disease. *Arch Neurol* 1999;56:1233–1239.

106. Defebvre L, Leduc V, Duhamel A et al. Technetium HMPAO SPECT in dementia with Lewy bodies, Alzheimer's disease and idiopathic Parkinson's disease. *J Nucl Med* 1999;40:956–962.

107. Ishii K, Yamaji S, Kitagaki H et al. Regional cerebral blood flow difference between dementia with Lewy bodies and AD. *Neurology* 1999;53:413–416.

108. Lopez OL, Wisniewski S, Hamilton RL et al. Predictors of progression in patients with AD and Lewy bodies. *Neurology* 2000;54:1774–1779.

109. Mori E, Shimomura T, Fujimori M et al. Visuoperceptual impairment in dementia with Lewy bodies. *Arch Neurol* 2000;57:483–489.

110. Donnemiller J, Heilmann J, Wenning GK et al. Brain perfusion scintigraphy with 99mTc-HMPAO or 99mTc-ECD and 123I β-CIT-photon emission tomography in dementia of the Alzheimer type and diffuse Lewy body disease. *Eur J Nucl Med* 1997;24:320–325.

111. Albin RL, Minoshima S, D'Amato CJ et al. Fluoro-deoxyglucose positron emission tomography in diffuse Lewy body disease. *Neurology* 1996;47:462–466.

112. Binetti G, Locascio JJ, Corkin S et al. Differences between Pick disease and Alzheimer disease in clinical appearance and rate of cognitive decline. *Arch Neurol* 2000;57:225–232.

113. Bugiani O, Murrell JR, Giaccone G et al. Fronto-temporal dementia and corticobasal degeneration in a family with a P301S mutation in tau. *J Neuropathol Exp Neurol* 1999;58:667–677.

114. Willert C, Spitzer C, Herzer R et al. Early manifestation of fronto-temporal dementia. *Nervenarzt* 2000;71:44–49.

115. Chow TW, Miller BL, Hayashi VN et al. Inheritance of fronto-temporal dementia. *Arch Neurol* 1999;56:817–822.

116. Chapman SB, Rosenberg RN, Weiner MF et al. Autosomal dominant progressive syndrome of motor-speech loss with dementia. *Neurology* 1997;49:1298–1306.

117. Mesulam MM. Primary progressive aphasia. *Ann Neurol* 2001;49:425–432.

118. Heiss W, Mielke R, Kessler J et al. *Joint science world wide—ageing in dementia.* 2001.

119. Schenk D, Barbour R, Dunn W et al. Immunization with amyloid-β accentuates Alzheimer's disease like pathology in the PDAPP mouse. *Nature* 1999;400:173–177.

120. Wolozin B, Kellman W, Celesia GG et al. Decreased prevalence of

Alzheimer's disease associated with HMG-CoA reductase inhibitors. *Soc Neurosci* 1999;25:13.9(abst).

121. Janus C, Pearson J, McLaurin J et al. A β peptide immunization reduces behavioural impairment and plaques in a model of Alzheimer's disease. *Nature* 2000;408:21–28.

122. Kuhl DE, Metter EJ, Riege WH. Patterns of cerebral glucose utilization in depression, multiple infarct dementia, and Alzheimer's disease. In: Sokoloff L ed. *Brain imaging and brain function.* New York: Raven Press, 1985:211–225.

123. Upadhyaya AK, Abouy-Saleh MT, Wilson K et al. A study of depression in old age using single-photon emission computerized tomography. *Br J Psychiatry* 1990;157(Suppl 9):76–81.

124. Drevets, WC, Videen TO, Price JL et al. A functional anatomical study of unipolar depression. *J Neuroscience* 1992;12:3628–3641.

125. Bonne O, Krausz Y, Gorfine M et al. Cerebral hypoperfusion in medication resistant depressed patients assessed by Tc99m HMPAO SPECT. *J Affective Disorder* 1996;41:163–171.

126. Mayberg HS. Limbic-cortical dysregulation: a proposed model of depression. *Neuropsych* 1997;9:471–481.122.

127. Nemeroff CB. The neurobiology of depression. *Sci Am* 1998;278: 42–57.

128. Abou-Saleh MT, Suhaili A, Karim L et al. Single photon emission tomography with 99mTC-HMPAO in patients with depression. *J Affect Disord* 1999;55:115–123.

129. Grasby PM. Imaging strategies in depression. *J Psychopharmacology* 1999;13:346–351.

130. Rampello L, Nicoletti F, Nicoletti F. Dopamine in depression: therapeutic implications. *CNS Drugs* 2000;13:35–45.

131. Kumar A, Bilker W, Lavretsky H et al. Volumetric asymmetries in late-onset mood disorders. An attenuation of frontal asymmetry with depression severity. *Psychiatry Res Neuroimaging* 2000;100:41–47.

132. Kowatch RA, Devous MD, Sr, Harvey DC et al. A SPECT HMPAO study of regional cerebral blood flow in depressed adolescents and normal controls. *Prog Neuropsychopharmacol Biol Psychiatry* 1999;23: 643–656.

133. Bonte FJ. Brain blood flow SPECT: posterior deficits in young patients with depression. *Clin Nucl Med* 1999;24:696–697.

134. Bonte FJ, Devous MD Sr, Harris TS et al. Occipital brain perfusion deficits in children with major depressive disorders. *J Nucl Med* 2000; 41:200P(abst).

135. Bonte FJ, Trivedi MH, Devous MD Sr et al. Occipital brain perfusion deficits in children with major depressive disorder. *J Nucl Med* (in press).

136. Friston KJ, Holmes AP, Worsley KJ et al. Statistical parametric maps in functional imaging: a general linear approach. *Hum Brain Mapp* 1995;2:189–210.

137. Talairach J, Tournoux P. *Co-planar stereotaxic atlas of the human brain.* New York: Thieme Medical Publishers, 1988.

138. Rains GD, Sauer K, Kant C. Cognitive impairment consistent with left fronto-temporal abnormality in schizophrenia patients. *J Neurotherapy* 2001;6:1–4.

139. Verhoeff NP, Soares JC, D'Souza CD et al. (123 I) Iomazenil SPECT benzodiazepine receptor imaging in schizophrenia. *Psychiatry Res* 1999;91:163–173.

140. Omori M, Murata T, Kimura H et al. Thalamic abnormalities in patients with schizophrenia revealed by proton magnetic resonance spectroscopy. *Psychiatry Res* 2000;98:155–162.

141. Kegeles LS, Shungu DC, Angilvel S et al. Hippocampal pathology in schizophrenia: Magnetic resonance imaging and spectroscopy studies. *Psychiatry Res* 2000;98:163–175.

142. Falke E, Han LY, Arnold SE. Absence of neurodegeneration in the thalamus and caudate of patients with schizophrenia. *Psychiatry Res* 2000;93:103–110.

143. Steinberg JL, Devous MD Sr, Paulman RG. Wisconsin card sorting activated regional cerebral blood flow in first break and chronic schizophrenic patients and normal controls. *Schizophrenia Research* 1996; 19:177–187.

144. Min SK, An SK, Jon DI et al. Positive and negative symptoms and regional cerebral perfusion in antipsychotic-naïve schizophrenic patients: a high-resolution SPECT study. *Psychiatry Res* 1999;90: 159–168.

145. Matsuda H, Gyobu T, Ii M et al. Increased accumulation of N-isopropyl-(I-123) t-iodoamphetamine in the left auditory area in a schizophrenic patient with auditory hallucinations. *Clin Nucl Med* 1988;13:53–55.

146. Ruiz A, Ganz WI, Donovan PMJ et al. Use of thallium-201 brain SPECT to differentiate cerebral lymphoma from toxoplasma encephalitis in AIDS patients. *AJNR* 1994;15:1885–1894.

147. Erdman WA, Skiest D, Chang W et al. CNS lymphoma vs. toxoplasma: are subjective thallium SPECT interpretations worthwhile? *J Nucl Med* 1999;40:200P.

148. Kaplan WD, Takronan T, Morris A et al. Thallium-201 brain tumor imaging: a comparative study with pathologic correlation. *J Nucl Med* 1987;28:47–52.

149. Kim KT, Black KL, Marciano D et al. Thallium SPECT imaging of brain tumors: methods and results. *J Nucl Med* 1990;32:965–969.

38

ROLE OF POSITRON EMISSION TOMOGRAPHY IN THE INVESTIGATION OF NEUROPSYCHIATRIC DISORDERS

ANDREW B. NEWBERG
ABASS ALAVI

In the 1960s, Kuhl and Edwards (1) developed emission tomography to image the biodistribution of radionuclides and used it to obtain scans of the brain. This technique was later named single photon emission computed tomography (SPECT) and was used to study a number of neurologic disorders, as well as to accurately demonstrate the regional distribution of various tracers in the central nervous system (CNS) (2). SPECT studies employ single photon emitting radionuclides such as iodine or technetium that are labeled to a specific compound. The initial SPECT radiopharmaceuticals were designed to demonstrate breakdowns in the blood–brain barrier. With the introduction of contrast-enhanced computed x-ray tomography, the need for SPECT to reveal blood–brain barrier abnormalities was significantly reduced. Concurrent with these developments, it was realized that positron-emitting radionuclides allow the synthesis of biologically important radiotracers because the elements used for labeling are identical or close to those that are naturally contained in such compounds. Thus, radionuclides such as ^{11}C, ^{18}F, and ^{13}N appear useful in producing a vast number of tracers that are usable for studying body chemistry and function (3). The emitted positron travels a short distance before meeting an electron and annihilating to produce two 511-keV γ-rays that travel in opposite directions, approximately 180 degrees from each other. Modern positron emission tomography (PET) instruments have a resolution in the range of 4 to 6 mm compared with that of a SPECT machine, which has a range of approximately 8 to 10 mm. Today, the resolution of PET has approached the theoretical limit of a few millimeters, resulting in considerable improvement of image quality (4).

One major development, which revealed the ability of PET to elucidate regional brain metabolism and function, was the synthesis of ^{18}F-fluorodeoxyglucose (^{18}F-FDG). This was achieved by close collaboration between investigators from Brookhaven National Laboratory and from the University of Pennsylvania (5). At the same time, significant progress was made in designing and manufacturing PET instruments, allowing for the generation of transaxial images of various structures in the body (6,7).

PET, along with a variety of radiotracers, has been used to study many physiologic and pathologic states throughout the body. However, its applications in studying the brain, as a research and as a diagnostic clinical tool, have revealed some extraordinary findings. PET studies may influence the management of the patient in neuropsychiatric disorders including seizures, brain tumors, movement disorders (8,9), dementia (10), schizophrenia, and obsessive compulsive disorder (11).

The two most commonly used radiopharmaceuticals for PET imaging (Table 38.1) are ^{18}F-FDG, which measures the cerebral metabolic rate for glucose (CMRGlc), and ^{15}O H$_2$O (12), which measures regional cerebral blood flow (RCBF). These tracers have been used to investigate a wide variety of neurologic disorders such as dementia and psychiatric illnesses but have also been used to study the effects of various physiologic stimuli on the human CNS. In addition to these two radiopharmaceuticals, many other positron emitting compounds, including neurotransmitter analogues, have been synthesized over the past two decades (Table 38.1) for measuring receptor and other chemical activities (13–20). The following includes a review of the literature that deals with the applications of PET to CNS function in both physiologic and pathologic states.

NORMAL AGING

^{18}F-FDG PET findings in normally aging brain (Fig. 38.1) as reported in the literature have been inconsistent. A number of investigators described diminished regional glucose metabolism in the temporal, parietal, somatosensory, and especially the frontal regions (21–26). Our group has shown that cortical metabolic rates measured by ^{18}F-FDG PET were reduced in older control subjects in comparison to young controls with more

A.B. Newberg: Division of Nuclear Medicine, University of Pennsylvania Medical Center, Philadelphia, PA.

A. Alavi: Division of Nuclear Medicine, University of Pennsylvania Medical Center, Philadelphia, PA.

Table 38.1. *Radioligands Commonly Used in Neurologic PET Imaging*

Compound	Application
^{15}O H$_2$O	Blood flow
^{18}F fluorodeoxyglucose	Glucose metabolism
^{15}O O$_2$	Oxygen metabolism
^{11}C L-methionine	Amino acid metabolism
^{11}C raclopride, ^{11}C methylspiperone	Dopamine receptor activity
^{18}F fluoroethylspiperone, ^{18}F spiperone	
^{11}C carfentanil, ^{11}C etorphine	Opiate receptor activity
^{11}C flunitrazepam	Benzodiazepine receptor activity
^{11}C scopolamine, ^{11}C quinuclidinyl benzilate	Muscarinic cholinergic receptors
6-^{18}F fluoro-L-DOPA, 4-^{18}F fluoro-m-tyrosine	Presynaptic dopaminergic system
^{11}C ephedrine, ^{18}F fluorometaraminol, 6-^{18}F fluorodopamine	Adrenergic terminals

Based on Diksic M, Reba RC, eds. Radiopharmaceuticals and brain pathology studied with PET and SPECT. Boca Raton: CRC Press, 1991; and Phelps ME. PET: a biological imaging techniques. *Neurochemical Research* 1991;16:929–940.

prominent decreases in the frontal and somatosensory cortices (27). Minor health problems appeared to have no significant effects on regional or whole brain CMRGlc. Another study also suggested that there is an age-related decrease in temporal lobe activity (28). These metabolic changes appear to be asymmetric and also affect men and women differently (29). For example, the left parietal lobe showed a greater decrease with age compared with the right, whereas the right frontal lobe showed a greater decrease than the left. Women were found to have greater age-related decreases than men do in the thalamus and hippocampus. On the other hand, men experienced a greater decline in left hemispheric metabolism compared with women who typically had either symmetric decreases or greater decreases in the right hemisphere.

PET imaging has also demonstrated not only that there are focal abnormalities attributable to the aging process but also that there may be modifications of large-scale network operations that are used for various cognitive and memory related tasks (30–33). PET imaging has demonstrated similar decrements during fine motor tasks, suggesting possible neurologic mechanisms for the decline in such tasks with age (34). Also, visual processing appears to be associated with different brain areas in older as compared with younger individuals. One study demonstrated that younger subjects tended to activate the temporo-occipital areas, whereas older subjects activated the fronto-occipital pathways during certain types of visual perception (35). Another study also demonstrated increased frontal lobe, as well as medial temporal lobe, activity in older subjects performing visual memory tasks (36). Similar findings have been reported for visual face recognition tasks (37). Verbal memory tasks are similarly associated with a larger recruitment of brain structures with increased activity in both prefrontal cortices (38), as well as the occipital regions (39).

Yoshii et al. (40) used a large number of healthy volunteers to determine the effects of gender, age, brain volume, and cerebrovascular risk factors on CMRGlc values as determined with ^{18}F-FDG PET. When brain atrophy was not considered, mean CMRGlc values were lower in older patients, particularly in the frontal, parietal, and temporal regions. Also, women had significantly higher mean CMRGlc than men. When covariate analysis was used to account for brain atrophy, the effects of age and gender on CMRGlc were no longer significant. Therefore, age-related brain atrophy can influence the analysis of PET studies and should to be taken into consideration in such studies (41–43).

Recent studies have also suggested that there are significant age-related declines in the activity of specific neurotransmitter systems. In the dopaminergic system, there appears to be an age-related decline not only in the striatum but also in a number of cortical areas as well (44). The cortical areas particularly involved include the frontal, temporal, and parietal lobes. This decline in dopaminergic activity has also been shown to be significantly correlated with the age-related decline in cognitive function (45, 46), as well as with the expression of extrapyramidal disorders (47). Although there appears to be similar decreases in dopamine receptors in both men and women, women appear to have increased endogenous striatal dopamine concentration (48). It may be the case that dopamine changes associated with age are also closely correlated with decreases in cerebral metabolism (49). That such correlations remained significant even after correcting for age effects suggests that dopamine may influence frontal, cingulate, and temporal metabolism regardless of age. Other studies have demonstrated age-related declines in muscarinic acetylcholinergic receptors, which occurred more rapidly in women compared with men (50), although the clinical relevance of such a decline is uncertain (51). Similar decreases with aging have been observed in serotonin receptors (52,53). PET imaging has even been useful in detecting chemical and other molecular changes associated with aging. For example, one study showed increasing levels of monoamine oxidase B activity with aging (54).

ALZHEIMER'S DISEASE AND RELATED DISORDERS

Dementia is usually defined as a chronic, cognitive impairment. Dementia has a number of possible causes including Alzheimer's disease (AD), Parkinson's disease (PD), Huntington's disease (HD), Wilson's disease, multiinfarct dementia (MID), human immunodeficiency virus, multiple sclerosis, and Jakob-Creutzfeldt disease. AD is the most prevalent cause of dementia with an estimated 2 million individuals in the United States incapacitated by AD.

Alzheimer's Disease

The criteria for the diagnosis of AD were defined by the Working Group of the National Institute of Neurological and Communicative Disorders and Stroke and the Alzheimer's Disease and Related Disorders Association (NINCDS-ADRDA) in 1984 (55). The criteria for the diagnosis of AD require evidence of

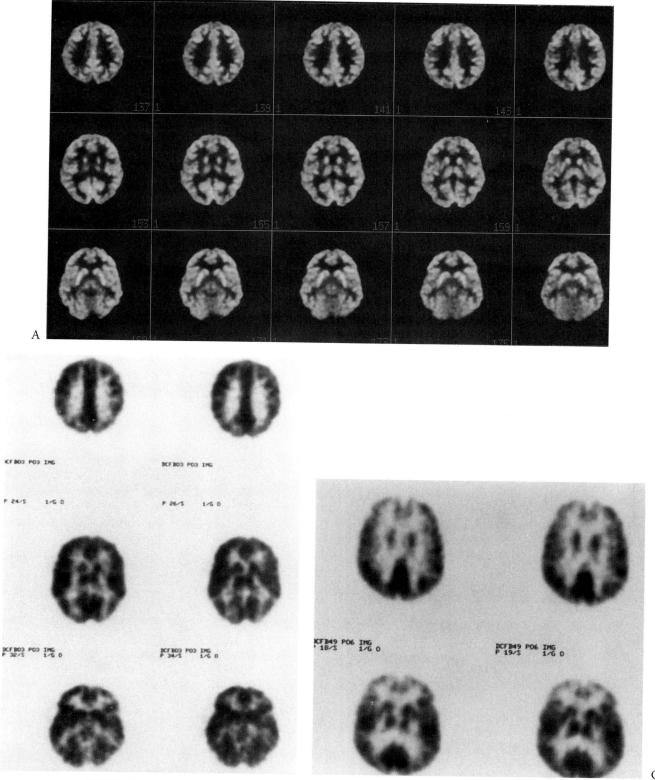

FIGURE 38.1. A: PET image of normal subject using a high-resolution gadolinium oxyorthosilicate PET camera. The resolution of 2.5 to 3 mm is superior to prior PET cameras and demonstrates significant cortical and subcortical detail. PET images of a normal subject **(B)** shows symmetrical tracer uptake throughout the cortex and striatum in comparison to the PET images of a healthy elderly subject **(C)** showing mild hypometabolism in the frontal lobes bilaterally.

progressive, chronic cognitive deficits in the middle-aged and older patients with no identifiable underlying cause. Unfortunately, although it is possible to make an accurate diagnosis of dementia in most patients with severe disease, it is very difficult to differentiate between AD and other dementing disorders in patients with mild disease (56,57). It is believed that functional imaging studies such as PET might help in making the diagnosis of AD and in elucidating the mechanisms underlying the disorder.

Since 1980, a large number of studies have used PET in the assessment of patients with AD (58–66). Initial ^{18}F-FDG PET studies, comparing CMRGlc in patients with AD to age-matched, healthy controls, showed that there is a 20% to 30% decrease in whole brain CMRGlc values in patients with AD when compared with healthy age-matched controls (67). Other studies showed that patients with AD have decreased whole brain glucose metabolism (CMRGlc), and the bilateral parietal and temporal lobes are particularly affected (68–72). This parietal hypometabolism (Fig. 38.2) is often referred to as representing the "typical" pattern of AD and may be particularly pronounced in patients younger than 65 years (73). In fact, in a study of 26 patients with cognitive dysfunction, bilateral parietal hypometabolism was successful in predicting AD as much as 13 months before the clinical diagnosis of AD by NINCDS-ADRDA criteria (74). However, it should be noted that although the bilateral parietal pattern is highly predictive of AD (75,76), the pattern is not pathognomic for AD and may be seen in patients with

PD, bilateral parietal subdural hematomas, bilateral parietal stroke, and bilateral parietal radiation therapy ports (77). One particularly disturbing feature in some AD patients is concomitant delusional misidentification syndrome (DMS). When compared with AD patients without DMS, the DMS group had significant hypometabolism in the orbitofrontal and cingulate areas bilaterally and left medial temporal areas (78). These findings were believed to be associated with the delusional formation and were also associated with significant bilateral hypermetabolism in the sensory association cortices.

Several more recent studies have attempted to distinguish AD from controls and other types of dementia based on different metabolic measures, as well as genetic and physiologic measures (79). One study compared the difference between mesocortical temporal hypometabolism and the neocortical temporal lobe and found that a mesocortical/neocortical ratio of 1 as a cutoff print was highly sensitive and specific in the diagnosis of AD (80). Parietotemporal hypometabolism is associated with familial AD in individuals from both amyloid precursor protein mutation and chromosome 14 linked families (81).

However, it has proven much more difficult to distinguish AD patients from non-Alzheimer's dementia (NAD) patients (Fig. 38.2) based on qualitative and quantitative analysis of cerebral metabolism (82). Both AD and NAD are associated with similar degrees of global dysfunction as reflected in significantly decreased whole brain CMRGlc values and often have similar types of regional metabolic changes (83).

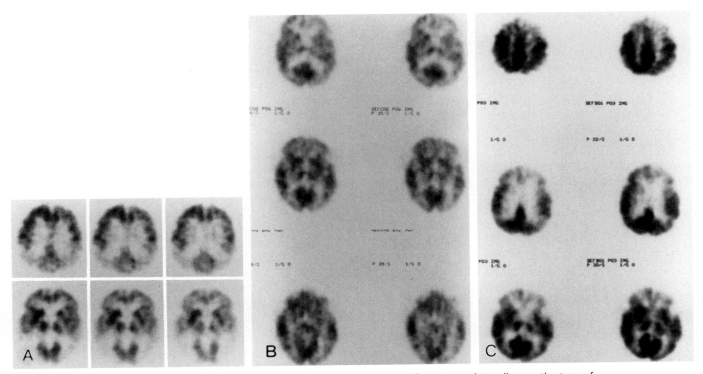

FIGURE 38.2. A ^{18}F-FDG PET imaging in dementia shows specific patterns depending on the type of dementia. A patient with Alzheimer's disease (**A**) shows marked bilateral temporoparietal hypometabolism. A PET study of a subject with atypical dementia (**B**) shows a diffuse hypometabolism throughout the cortex. The PET image of a patient with frontal lobe dementia (**C**) shows marked hypometabolism in both frontal lobes compared with the metabolism in the parieto-occipital area.

Postmortem histopathologic studies of the brains of AD patients have revealed senile plaques and neurofibrillary tangles (84–86), particularly in the areas observed to be involved on PET images. However, this is not always the case. Neuronal degeneration is most pronounced in the hippocampus and amygdaloid nucleus followed by the inferior temporal lobe and posterior central parietal region (87,88). One striking finding is clear-cut involvement of the hippocampus and the amygdaloid nucleus in the early stages of AD with only subtle abnormalities in other sites (89–91). Van Housen et al. (92) showed that only certain subfields of the hippocampal formation were affected by cell loss, neurofibrillary tangles, and neuritic plaques in patients with AD.

In patients with AD of varying severity, the magnitude and extent of hypometabolism appear to correlate with the severity of the dementia symptoms. Moderately affected patients show significantly decreased metabolism in the left midfrontal lobes, bilateral parietal lobes, and the superior temporal regions. In patients with severe AD, the same regions are affected, but the hypometabolism is much more pronounced. In all patients, the parietal lobes show the greatest changes, with a 38% decrease in patients with moderate AD and a 53% decrease in patients with severe AD. The premotor cortex has similar decreases in moderately and severely demented patients. Furthermore, the metabolic ratio between the parietal and premotor and the parietal and prefrontal cortices correlates significantly with the degree of cognitive impairment in patients with moderate dementia. Longitudinal studies have shown that CMRGlc values decrease more rapidly over time in patients with AD than in age-matched control subjects. There was also a more severe decrement in the parietal lobe metabolism compared with the frontal lobes over time.

Other areas (sensorimotor and visual cortices, subcortical nuclei, brainstem, and cerebellum) have relatively preserved CMRGlc (93) except in patients with specific neuropsychologic deficits (94–97). For example, patients with abnormalities in their visuospatial skills have hypometabolism in the right hemisphere as compared with the left. It has been suggested that certain asymmetric changes may be due to the focal onset and progression of AD, although these asymmetries may also be due to patient selection. There was no correlation between the age of AD patients and the type of asymmetric changes (98). Studies correlating CMRGlc to mini-mental status examination scores and other neuropsychologic testing have more consistently shown a relationship between these measures in patients with AD, which has been particularly true when parietal and temporal lobe metabolic rates have been compared with neuropsychologic deficits.

Several studies have compared AD patients to controls while performing cerebral activation studies. For example, a study by Duara et al. (99) showed that AD patients had relative increases in cerebral activation during a reading memory test that were similar to those in controls. Another study of AD patients demonstrated relative asymmetric activation (right greater than left) more so in men than in women during a verbal memory task (100). The authors concluded that these findings suggest differential effects in men and women with AD. The results of these activation studies do not yet show a clear distinction between the change in glucose metabolism during various activation tasks in AD patients, and further research will be necessary to better elucidate the effects of AD on resting and activation-related cerebral metabolism.

In the past decade, investigators have suggested that measured values of various functional parameters might require correction for brain atrophy because PET scans do not have adequate resolution to separate metabolically inactive ventricular and sulcal CSF spaces from the rest of the brain (101,102). Magnetic resonance imaging (MRI) volumetric determinations have been used to correct the CMRGlc values obtained by PET. AD patients, with more atrophy when compared with controls, show a greater increase in corrected CMRGlc values than normal subjects. One study demonstrated that AD patients showed significant decreases in mean whole brain CMRGlc compared with controls before atrophy correction, with no difference after correction (103). These results indicated that the brain tissue in AD patients may utilize glucose at levels similar to that of normal tissue. However, AD patients have considerably less brain tissue. This notion also further enhances the conclusion reached in the aforementioned activation studies, which showed appropriate activation and, hence, viability of the brain tissue in AD patients compared with controls.

The most important potential role for PET is in the evaluation of therapeutic interventions for AD. The relatively recent development of several pharmaceuticals for AD provides an important area for PET imaging. Patients can be imaged before therapy to determine who might be the best candidates for therapy. Patients can also be followed longitudinally to determine the effectiveness of the pharmaceutical intervention. Also, PET imaging can be useful in the physiologic evaluation of various pharmacologic interventions. One PET study explored how donepezil affected acetylcholinesterase activity (104). Donepezil hydrochloride reportedly provides nearly complete inhibition of cerebral cortical acetylcholinesterase activity in patients with AD. However, this study demonstrated an average of only 27% inhibition of acetylcholinesterase activity. This finding suggests that the clinical trials of donepezil are not reflecting the actual degree of pharmacologic activity and suggests that further investigation of the effects of this drug is warranted.

A PET study of the use of tacrine in patients with AD demonstrated improvement of nicotinic receptors (measured as ^{11}C-nicotine binding), cerebral blood flow, and cognitive tests (trail making test and block design test) that preceded improvements in glucose metabolism (105). These improvements were observed in both short- and long-term treatment regimens. Propentofylline (PPF) has been explored as a potential pharmacologic intervention in patients with both vascular dementia, as well as AD, because of the elaboration of inflammatory cytokines and neurotoxic free radicals, decreased secretion of nerve growth factor by astrocytes, excess release of glutamate with associated neurotoxicity, and loss of cholinergic neurons in these two types of dementia. A phase II study using PET showed significant improvements in cerebral glucose metabolism in patients with both vascular dementia and AD after treatment with PPF. Patients treated with a placebo had significant decreases in cerebral metabolism during the same period (106).

Thus, PET continues to play a major role in the study and

diagnosis of AD. It can aid in the diagnosis and the determination of the course and severity of the disease. Furthermore, with improved methods for quantitative analysis of specific regions such as the hippocampus, PET may help further unravel the pathophysiologic changes in AD. The role of PET imaging will be significantly enhanced as successful therapeutic interventions evolve in the treatment of AD. This will be of particularly great importance in the management of patients with early AD.

Multiinfarct Dementia

A number of ^{18}F-FDG PET reports described changes that are seen in MID and how they differ from those in patients with AD. MID is characterized by multiple infarcts throughout the brain (both white and gray matter) and is associated with a stepwise progression of dementia symptoms. In patients with MID, PET images show scattered focal areas of hypometabolism (107) corresponding to the multiple sites of abnormalities seen on MRI. Thus, qualitative PET can be used to distinguish MID from AD. Pawlik et al. (108) showed that PET was the most sensitive test for distinguishing dementias of vascular origin from other disorders. PET has also been used to quantitatively measure glucose metabolic rates in patients with MID and to compare the results to patients with AD (109). In this study, patients with MID were found to have whole brain CMRGlc values comparable to those in patients with AD and markedly decreased compared with controls. Thus, quantitative PET may not be as useful in distinguishing MID from AD. In this study, which corrected CMRGlc values for brain atrophy, it was found that although patients with AD do not have significantly different corrected metabolic values compared with controls, MID patients showed significantly reduced glucose metabolism even after atrophy correction. This finding may suggest that hypometabolism in MID is disproportionate to the degree of atrophy. This implies that in MID patients, in contrast to AD, there is decreased metabolism in the remaining adjacent brain tissue in addition to a loss of brain volume secondary to infarction. There is also reduced RCBF and regional cerebral metabolism rate of oxygen (rCMRO$_2$) without an increase in the regional oxygen extraction fraction (rOEF) in patients with AD and MID. The oxygen extraction fraction refers to the amount of oxygen extracted from the blood by a quantity of brain tissue. However, in two studies, increased rOEFs were observed in the periphery of chronic ischemic infarcts in such patients (110,111). A more recent study showed decreased mean RCBF and rCMRO$_2$ with comparable rOER values in all cerebral regions except in the cerebellum in MID patients compared with multiinfarct patients without dementia (112). In patients with lacunes and leukoaraiosis with dementia, mean RCBF and rCMRO$_2$ were decreased with increased rOER in all cerebral regions except in the cerebellum compared with those patients without dementia. Thus, the PET findings in demented patients with multiple large infarcts are in agreement with the concept of MID, and in demented patients with lacunes and leukoaraiosis, the PET pattern suggests a state of misery perfusion not only in the deep structures but also in the whole cerebral cortex.

Primary Progressive Aphasia

Primary progressive aphasia (PPA) was first described by Mesulam (113) as a disorder without signs of a generalized dementia. The age at onset is generally in the presenium with initial symptoms of an anomic aphasia. However, impairments in reading, writing, and verbal comprehension are experienced. Most patients have specific deficits with running speech, auditory repetition, confrontation naming, reading comprehension, and writing. Patients with this type of language impairment also have had deficits in closely associated abilities such as praxis and calculation (114,115). One of the critical issues is whether PPA is a separate entity or merely one of several possible presentations of AD. In Mesulam's study, some of the patients did progress to AD. Furthermore, AD is often associated with marked language difficulties, including anomia with significant deficits in confrontational naming (116).

Several reports describe ^{18}F-FDG PET imaging findings in patients with PPA. Chawluk et al. (117) showed that PPA patients had a markedly decreased glucose metabolism in the left parietal and left temporal lobes. However, it was noted that PPA patients had no contralateral or global abnormalities on PET as are usually seen in AD. Tyrrell et al. (118) reported six cases of PPA in which PET studies revealed hypometabolism localized to the left hemisphere, specifically the left temporal lobe. A similar finding of hypometabolism in the left supramarginal gyrus and its surrounding areas was reported in a patient with a conduction aphasia with no other signs of dementia (119). Only one of the six patients had hypometabolism on the right side as well. Kempler et al. (120) analyzed PET and computed tomography (CT) in three patients with the presentation of PPA. They concluded that PPA does not have a uniform syndrome complex, that there was only mild atrophy in the left temporal lobe, and that left temporal lobe metabolism was markedly reduced.

Our laboratory used ^{18}F-FDG PET in PPA patients and found a markedly decreased glucose metabolism in the left temporal lobe compared with controls and glucose metabolism similar to those in AD patients (121). The left/right ratio of glucose metabolic rates was markedly lower not only in the temporal lobes but in all other lobes as well, compared with controls and AD patients. This finding suggests that PPA is a hemispheric process and that the metabolic derangements extend beyond the focus of the language center. However, PPA was well distinguished from AD patients and the typical AD pattern.

Pick's Disease

Pick's disease is a neurodegenerative dementia with a predilection for the frontal and temporal lobes where Pick bodies are noted on histopathologic examination. The disease is associated with cognitive and language dysfunction, as well as behavioral changes. The most common finding in PET images (Fig. 38.2) is hypometabolism in the frontal and anterior temporal lobes bilaterally (122–125). This pattern of anterior hypometabolism is consistent with the findings on histopathologic examination, as well as frontal and temporal lobe atrophy on CT and magnetic resonance (MR) images (126,127). The small number of studies reported in the literature may not allow determination of the accuracy of ^{18}F-FDG PET imaging in the diagnosis of Pick's disease. Furthermore, there are disorders, such as other frontal lobe dementias (Fig. 38.2) and schizophrenia, that also may have a pattern of frontal lobe hypometabolism, and these should be considered in the differential diagnosis. However, clinical findings are significantly different.

BRAIN TUMORS

Primary intracranial tumors comprise approximately 5% to 9% of all cancers and carry a median survival of approximately 1 year. Furthermore, gliomas represent 50% of all intracranial tumors. PET can play an important role in the evaluation and management of patients with brain tumors, including the grading of tumors, determination of prognosis, and the differentiation of recurrent tumor from radiation necrosis (128,129).

Many of the studies of brain tumors with PET were done using ^{18}F-FDG, although studies have been reported in which [11]C L-methionine (reflecting neutral amino acid transport) and ^{11}C putrescine (130–133) have been used. Most ^{18}F-FDG studies have concluded that high-grade tumors are hypermetabolic (Fig. 38.3), whereas low-grade tumors are hypometabolic. In a study of 72 patients by DiChiro et al. (130), the mean CMRGlc (measured with ^{18}F-FDG) was 4.0 ± 1.8 mg glucose/100 g/minute for low-grade tumors, whereas high-grade tumors had a CMRGlc of 7.4 ± 3.5 mg glucose/100 g/minute. Other groups (134–136) have corroborated the finding of hypermetabolism in high-grade tumors and hypometabolism in low-grade tumors. One distinction from this typology is juvenile pilocytic astrocytoma, which typically has a high glucose metabolism despite its benign nature (137,138). Other studies have shown increased metabolism in mixed neuronal-glial tumors such as gangliogliomas, which must be considered in making a diagnosis, especially in young patients with brain tumors in the presence of uncharacteristic morphologic features (139). An interesting study comparing ^{18}F-FDG uptake with microvascular blood volume using functional magnetic resonance imaging (fMRI) showed that the two measures correlated significantly and were also matched to the degree of angiogenesis as determined by histopathologic means (140). It should be mentioned that quantitative analysis of metabolism in which the tumor site is compared with the contralateral normal brain tissue appears to be the most successful means for making the diagnosis of brain tumor, whereas standardized uptake values do not appear to be as reliable (141). It should be noted that PET cannot differentiate between primary lymphomas of the CNS, brain secondaries, or malignant gliomas, because all of these may be hypermetabolic (142). In fact, a PET study of brain metastases from small cell lung cancer indicated increased rCMRGlc, RCBF, and rCBV in tumor tissue even though there was a high degree of variability in these measures (143). However, no correlation between survival and metabolic or hemodynamic parameters could be demonstrated. After radiotherapy, the mean tumor rCMRglu decreased, whereas RCBF and rCBV remained unchanged.

There are studies that have examined the metabolic parameters related to various types of tumors. For example, in a comparison of low-grade astrocytomas and oligodendrogliomas, both tumor types exhibited a glucose hypometabolism, whereas me-

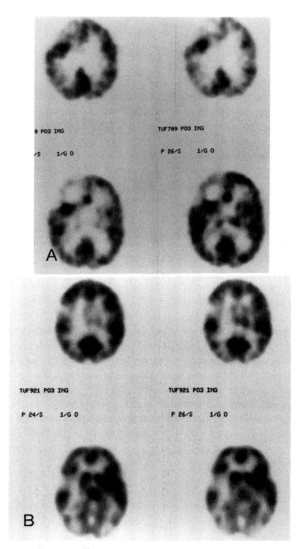

FIGURE 38.3. A: A ^{18}F-FDG PET image of a high-grade glioma in the frontotemporal area showing the tumor as an area of increased glucose metabolism with central necrosis. **B:** In contrast, a low-grade brain tumor in the frontoparietal area reveals reduced metabolic activity at the site of abnormality seen on magnetic resonance image.

thionine uptake was high in all oligodendrogliomas and was either decreased, normal, or moderately increased in astrocytomas (144). This study suggested that despite similar radiologic and clinical presentations, these different types of low-grade gliomas are metabolically different. Hypometabolism has also associated with local edema, cystic changes, necrosis near the tumor, and areas neuronally connected to the tumor (145,146). There have also been distant metabolic abnormalities, such as in the contralateral cerebellar hemisphere, associated with brain tumors called crossed cerebellar diaschisis (147). There can also be crossed cortical diaschisis associated with cerebellar tumors (148).

Newer studies have explored the use of PET for surgical planning of the extent of the tumor that requires resection, as well as for determining eloquent areas of cortical function to be avoided during surgery (149,150). ^{18}F-FDG PET has also been successful in determining the prognosis of patients with brain tumors (151,152). PET can more accurately predict the degree of malignancy of a tumor than CT or MRI, and PET has also been shown to predict survival in patients with gliomas more accurately than either CT or MRI (147,148,151–153). ^{18}F-FDG uptake in gliomas is regionally related to the presence of anaplasia (153). Alavi et al. (135) found that the median survival of patients with hypermetabolic gliomas was 7 to 11 months from the time of diagnosis, whereas the median survival of patients with low-grade gliomas was 33 months with a range of 1 to more than 7 years. Similar findings with regard to the ability of ^{18}F-FDG PET to determine prognosis were reported by several other groups (154,155).

Interestingly, ^{18}F-FDG PET images do not always correlate with CT scans. Although most of the hypermetabolic tumors show enhancement on CT, only 50% of the low-grade tumors show enhancement, a sign often attributed to a high degree of malignancy. Furthermore, ^{18}F-FDG PET is more accurate than CT in predicting the degree of malignancy when the two do not correlate. A more recent study demonstrated that hypermetabolism on PET imaging that extended beyond the area of contrast enhancement on MRI may be of value in predicting rapid progression of high-grade glioma (156).

Although ^{18}F-FDG PET appears to be useful in grading brain tumors and determining their prognosis, PET also has another advantage over anatomic imaging. Unlike CT or MRI, PET can distinguish radiation necrosis from tumor recurrence (157–160). The sensitivity for making this determination may be as high as 86% with a specificity as high as 56% (161). However, others have questioned how useful this approach may be in distinguishing necrosis from active tumor (162). In general, areas of radiation necrosis are hypometabolic (Figs. 38.4, 38.5, and 38.6), whereas tumor recurrence appears hypermetabolic on ^{18}F-FDG PET. Radiation necrosis has been associated with hypometabolism in the white matter only, whereas necrosis re-

sulting from chemotherapy was associated with gray matter changes in addition to white matter abnormalities. These investigators were also able to distinguish an area of tumor recurrence among necrotic changes. Furthermore, they found no false-positive or false-negative results in this study.

^{18}F-FDG PET has also been used to determine tumor response to radiation and/or chemotherapy and eventual patient survival. Phillips et al. (163) found a marked decrease in rCMRGlc in a patient with medulloblastoma 1 day after the administration of methotrexate. Twenty-four hours after a cycle of an eight-drug chemotherapy regimen, Rozental et al. (164, 165) found that glioblastomas had an increase of 20% to 100% in glucose uptake compared with before chemotherapy. Furthermore, the patient's survival was found to be inversely related to the amount of increase in CMRGlc. Ogawa et al. (166) used PET to measure blood volume and glucose metabolism in tumor tissue in response to radiation therapy. One month after therapy, there were significant reductions of 30% to 65% in glucose metabolism in the tumor tissue, but the surrounding brain tissue showed no significant changes. Furthermore, the patients whose tumors had decreased glucose metabolism after radiation therapy tended to have a better prognosis than those who did not show such a response.

Tumors have been studied using ^{11}C-methionine (MET) and PET, which has been useful for outlining tumor activity and developing treatment plans, as well as for determining prognosis with the less active tumors having a better overall prognosis (167,168). ^{11}C-MET PET has also been shown to be useful in the differentiation of tumor recurrence from radiation necrosis and delineation of the extent of the tumor (169). PET has also been used to study nucleic acid metabolism in brain tumors using ^{18}F-fluorodeoxyuridine (FUDR). In general, FUDR offers high contrast in the study of brain tumors because of the low uptake by normal brain tissue and is capable of differentiating between high-grade and low-grade tumors (170).

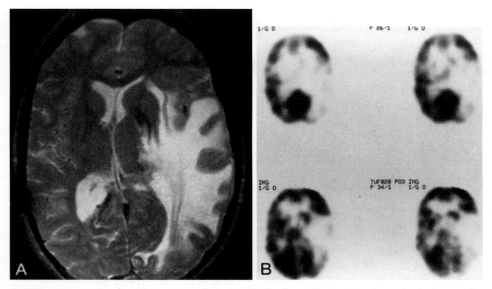

FIGURE 38.4. A: A magnetic resonance imaging (MRI) of a patient with primary brain tumor after radiation therapy shows high-intensity signal and surrounding edema. This MRI is not able to distinguish recurrent tumor from radiation necrosis. **B:** The corresponding ^{18}F-FDG PET image shows the same area as a hypometabolic region suggesting that this is all related to radiation effects.

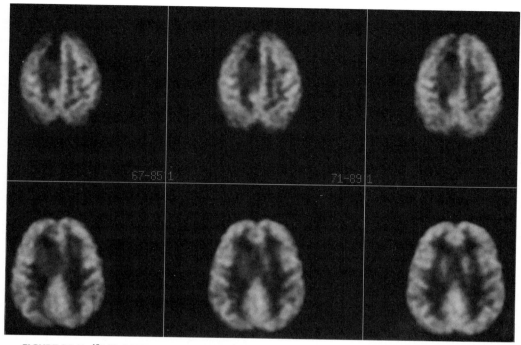

FIGURE 38.5. ^{18}F-FDG PET using high-resolution gadolinium oxyorthosilicate scanner in a patient with prior astrocytoma in the right frontal lobe after surgery and radiation therapy. The patient presented with worsening symptoms, and the scan demonstrated hypometabolism in the prior tumor region consistent with radiation necrosis.

MOVEMENT DISORDERS

Parkinson's Disease

PD is caused by loss of the pigmented neurons in the substantia nigra and the locus ceruleus and is characterized by the triad of bradykinesia, tremor, and rigidity. The loss of pigmented neurons is associated with decreased production of dopamine, de-

creased storage of dopamine, and nigrostriatal system dysfunction. It is believed that initially there is an upregulation of dopamine receptors (171,172) followed by a downregulation that occurs as the disease progresses. Eventually, PD can lead to dementia in 20% to 30% of the patients.

The decrease in size of the substantia nigra, resulting from degeneration of the neurons or from iron deposition, can be

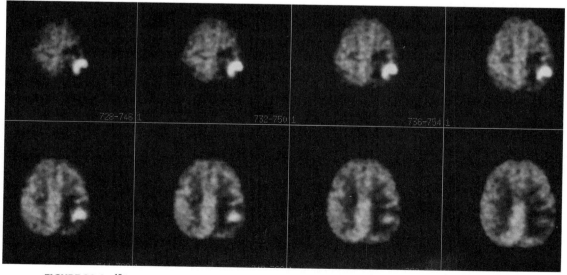

FIGURE 38.6. ^{18}F-FDG PET using high-resolution gadolinium oxyorthosilicate scanner in a patient with prior glioma in the right parietal region after radiation therapy. The patient presented with worsening symptoms, and the scan demonstrated intense activity within an area of hypometabolism consistent with recurrent tumor.

observed on MR images (173). However, CT and MRI are primarily used to rule out other intracranial disorders. Furthermore, Huber et al. (174) showed that MRI was not useful in differentiating dementia of PD from that of AD. PET offers the ability to study not only cerebral metabolism but also the dopamine transmitter receptor system, which may prove extremely useful in the diagnosis of PD, as well as in the determination of the pathophysiology of this disease (175–178).

Several groups have reported hypermetabolism in the basal ganglia in early, untreated PD (179,180). Similarly, hemiparkinsonism is associated with hypermetabolism in the contralateral basal ganglia (181,182). However, one group found no significant striatal changes in patients with PD (183,184). Another group (185) reported decreases in glucose metabolism in the basal ganglia contralateral to the side of the symptoms in patients with hemiparkinsonism-hemiatrophy syndrome. PD patients have been shown to have mild diffuse cortical hypometabolism compared with controls. Furthermore, this hypometabolism correlates with the severity of bradykinesia but is unrelated to the duration of the disease.

Regarding therapy, one study demonstrated that hypometabolism in the striatum and inferior thalamus in the side contralateral to the predominant parkinsonian signs was associated with L-DOPA unresponsiveness, whereas hypermetabolism in the striatum and inferior thalamus contralateral to the predominant side were found in L-DOPA-responsive patients (186). Several groups have indicated that L-DOPA therapy does not correct or change the local or global metabolic rates. However, Blesa et al. (187) reported a reversal of pallidal hypermetabolism with L-DOPA therapy. Another study by Jenkins et al. (188) indicated that PD patients had improved activation in the supplementary motor cortex during a motor function task when akinesia was reversed with apomorphine infusion (a dopamine agonist).

Dementia associated with PD appears to be associated with a uniform cerebral hypometabolism. However, severe dementia in PD may be indistinguishable from AD on PET images (Fig. 38.7), because both show significant bilateral parietal hypometabolism (189). Peppard et al. (190) showed that PD patients with dementia differed from PD patients without dementia in that the former had hypometabolic perirolandic and angular gyrus regions. However, PD patients with dementia did not have significantly different CMRGlc values than AD patients (191). Furthermore, the parietal cortex/caudate-thalamus ratio negatively correlated with the severity and duration of the disease in PD patients, as well as in AD patients. The results from these studies indicate that PD patients with dementia may suffer from an underlying Alzheimer-type process or may have a dementia specifically associated with the PD that affects the frontal lobes. The dopaminergic system may also play a role in the dementia symptoms of PD because reduced presynaptic dopamine activity in the caudate is associated with impairment in neuropsychologic tests measuring verbal fluency, working memory, attentional functioning, and somatosensory discrimination (192–194). In PD without dementia, iodobenzovesamicol (an *in vivo* marker of the vesicular acetylcholine transporter binding) was reduced only in the parietal and occipital cortex, but demented PD subjects had extensive cortical binding decreases similar to early-onset AD.

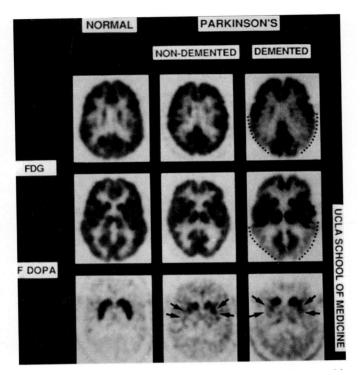

FIGURE 38.7. Two patients with Parkinson's disease (PD), one with associated dementia and one without dementia, are compared with a healthy control subject. The first two rows show glucose metabolism in these subjects. The PD patient without dementia shows essentially a normal pattern of metabolism, whereas the PD patient with dementia shows biparietotemporal hypometabolism that is similar to the pattern seen in patients with Alzheimer's disease. The bottom row are 18F-fluorodopa positron emission tomography studies that show decreased tracer uptake in the putamen of the PD patients. (From Mazziotta JC. Movement disorders. In: Mazzlotta JC, Gilman S, eds. *Clinical brain imaging: principles and applications.* Philadelphia: Davis, 1992:244–293, with permission.)

PET imaging in PD has also been performed with [18F] fluorodopa (FDOPA) to evaluate presynaptic dopaminergic function and has shown abnormalities in the nigrostriatal dopaminergic projection (195,196), as well as reduced basal ganglia activity (Fig. 38.8), especially in patients with the "on/off" phenomena (197,198). Others have argued that the limited spatial resolution of PET with FDOPA may result in substantial underestimation of the true rate of FDOPA uptake and metabolism *in vivo* and

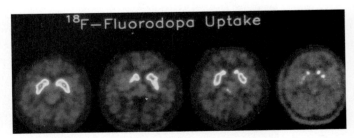

FIGURE 38.8. 18F-fluorodopa images of the brain from left to right include, a normal subject, a patient with Parkinson's disease, a patient with DOPA-responsive dystonia, and a patient with juvenile parkinsonism. All three patients show reduced uptake of this radiopharmaceutical in the basal ganglia region.

may also obscure regional heterogeneity in the neurochemical pathology of PD (199). Garnett et al. (200) showed that, in hemiparkinsonism, there is a marked decrease in activity in the contralateral basal ganglia. However, there is also decreased activity, although to a lesser extent, in the ipsilateral basal ganglia. More recent studies have also shown that tracers measuring the dopamine transporter system may also have a role in the study of patients with PD because they show significant declines in dopamine transporter activity (201–204).

FDOPA studies have been used to investigate clinical course and the effects of therapy in patients with PD. Patients with PD have been followed longitudinally and were found to have a mean decrease in the accumulation of FDOPA by 1.7% per year over 3 years. Furthermore, there have been reports that the decrease in activity correlates with the worsening of bradykinesia scores. L-DOPA therapy appears to have differential biologic effects depending on the type of patient treated. For example, in patients with mild PD, L-DOPA infusion decreased DOPA influx in the putamen, whereas in patients with advanced PD, L-DOPA induced significant upregulation of DOPA influx (205). This study might explain the less graded clinical response to L-DOPA in advanced PD and potentially explain the pathogenesis underlying motor fluctuations. More recent PET studies have demonstrated that although loss of putamen dopamine storage predisposes PD patients to motor complications, it cannot be the only factor determining when such motor symptoms arise clinically (206). Additional PET studies suggest that loss of striatal dopamine storage capacity along with pulsatile exposure to exogenous L-DOPA results in pathologically raised synaptic dopamine levels and deranged basal ganglia opioid transmission. This, rather than altered dopamine receptor binding, may be the cause of inappropriate overactivity of basal ganglia-frontal projections, resulting in breakthrough involuntary movements (207).

A number of new surgical techniques have been developed for the treatment of PD, and their effect has been observed with PET. For example, pallidotomy has been associated with increased activation of premotor areas and reduced hyperactivity of the lentiform nucleus (208–210). Pallidal (GPi) and subthalamic (STN) stimulation also increase activation of premotor areas but decrease activation in the primary motor area (211, 212). Suppression of unilateral tremor with thalamic stimulation has been shown to be associated with a reduction in cerebellar blood flow. These findings corroborate the general notion that increased activity in the subthalamic-pallidal projection is directly implicated in the pathophysiology of PD and that surgical techniques that block these output nuclei leads to partial restoration of cortical physiology.

Another PET technique involves the use of ^{11}C-nomifensine, which is a potent inhibitor of presynaptic dopamine and norepinephrine reuptake sites. The greatest uptake in normal subjects occurs in the striatal dopaminergic nerve terminals and the norepinephrine uptake sites in the thalamus, and there is a decline in uptake with age (213). Several groups (201,211) showed that in PD patients younger than 65 years, there is a marked reduction in striatal uptake of ^{11}C-nomifensine, most pronounced in the putamen with the caudate slightly less affected. However, in older PD patients, there is similar binding activity to age-

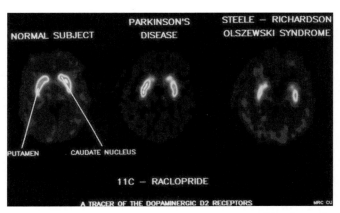

FIGURE 38.9. Positron emission tomographic scans of basal ganglia ^{11}C-raclopride uptake integrated over the 60 minutes after the intravenous tracer administration in a normal control subject, an untreated patient with Parkinson's disease (PD), and a patient with progressive supranuclear palsy (PSP). The patient with PD has normal striatal tracer uptake, but there is reduced uptake in the patient with PSP, particularly in the caudate nucleus.

matched controls. Furthermore, in hemiparkinsonism, there is decreased striatal uptake of ^{11}C-nomifensine bilaterally, with a greater decrease on the contralateral side. It should also be noted that studies have compared ^{11}C-nomifensine to FDOPA PET in PD patients and have found similar decreases, both qualitatively and quantitatively (201,214).

Imaging with [11]C N-methylspiperone (NMSP, a postsynaptic D2 receptor antagonist) has shown variable results in activity early in the disease and decreased tracer binding in advanced PD (215–218). It should also be noted that PET imaging with NMSP in hemiparkinsonism patients has shown bilateral variability in striatal uptake (219). [11]C NMSP has also been useful in the study of the effects of dopaminergic medication on PD patients. The use of dopaminergic medication is expected to show decreased NMSP uptake in the basal ganglia because of downregulation of the receptor system. However, Wijnand et al. (219) found a bilateral increase in receptor binding following therapy. It was suggested that this unexpected increase might be the result of persistent postsynaptic D2 receptor hypersensitivity or a change in the local pharmacokinetics of the tracer.

[11]C-raclopride has also been used to investigate D2 receptors in PD patients (Fig. 38.9). An increase in ^{11}C-raclopride activity (receptor upregulation) has been observed in the striatum contralateral to hemiparkinsonian symptoms in early disease. This corroborates the theory of initial upregulation of dopamine receptors followed by subsequent downregulation as the disease progresses (220). Brooks et al. (218) found that PD patients did not differ significantly in ^{11}C-raclopride uptake in the striatum compared with controls, although two of the six patients did have marked increases in putamen tracer uptake.

Huntington's Disease

HD is an autosomal dominant disorder that usually presents in middle age. HD is characterized by progressive motor abnormalities such as involuntary choreiform movements and akinetic rigidity, as well as behavioral disturbances and progressive cognitive deterioration (221). Furthermore, HD is commonly associated with dementia symptoms. Neuropathologic studies have shown neuronal degeneration in the striatum with the caudate more involved than the putamen (222). Although the mechanism that causes HD is unknown, it is believed to be the result of excitatory amino acid toxicity (perhaps caused by the low levels of inhibitory neurotransmitters), which destroys the neurons (223).

PET studies of HD patients have consistently found hypometabolism in the caudate and putamen nuclei (224–227) (Fig. 38.10), which often precedes the atrophy as determined by CT (224,228–230). These changes have also been shown to be reversible when HD patients were treated with fetal striatal tissue transplantation (231).

Most studies do not report cortical changes in glucose metabolism. However, Kuwert et al. (232) reported cortical hypometabolism in 23 HD patients compared with controls. The duration of the chorea correlated significantly with the decline in rCMRGlc in the frontoparietal and temporo-occipital areas. Furthermore, the frontoparietal and temporo-occipital

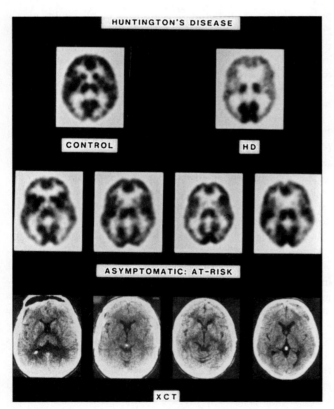

FIGURE 38.10. Comparison of patient with Huntington's disease (HD) and a patient at risk for developing HD compared with a normal control subject. The HD patient shown at the upper right shows decreased metabolism in the caudate nuclei compared with the healthy control patient shown at the *upper left*. The bottom two rows are ¹⁸F-FDG PET and computed tomography (CT) images from four patients who were asymptomatic but at risk for HD. The four CT scans (*bottom row*) are all normal. However, the metabolic activity in the caudate nuclei of these patients at risk for HD range from a normal appearance (*far left*) to one similar to that of the symptomatic HD patient (*far right*). (From Mazziotta JC, Phelps ME, Pahl JJ et al. Reduced cerebral glucose metabolism in asymptomatic patients at risk or Huntington's disease. *N Engl J Med* 1987;316:357–362, with permission.)

rCMRGlc correlated with the severity of dementia in the HD patients. These results suggest that involvement of the cerebral cortex of HD, especially in patients with cognitive impairment, may be of importance in explaining clinical findings.

Young et al. (233) showed that HD patients have caudate hypometabolism in all stages of the disease, whereas hypometabolism of the putamen is normal in the early stages. This might reflect the greater involvement of the caudate over the putamen in the neuropathologic studies. Furthermore, they found that the degree of caudate hypometabolism correlated with the patient's overall functional capacity, whereas putamen hypometabolism correlated with the severity of motor disturbances. Other groups found similar correlations between caudate hypometabolism and neuropsychologic deficits in verbal learning and memory (234, 235).

Several studies have been performed to determine whether the diagnosis of HD can be established in asymptomatic patients who are at risk for developing the disease. The results from these studies have been mixed. Mazziotta et al. (227) found hypometabolism in the caudate of 31% of 58 at-risk patients. When the caudate hypometabolism was compared with DNA polymorphism studies that identified the HD gene in at-risk patients, there was a concordance rate of 91%. Although other investigators (236,237) have corroborated this success, Young et al. (238) did not find any significant difference in caudate metabolism between patients at risk for developing HD and control subjects. A PET study of dopamine receptors suggested that this method might demonstrate receptor loss in asymptomatic carriers, although it was not clear that this technique would be able to predict progression to disease (239). Thus, it remains controversial whether PET can be used to help determine which at-risk patients will progress to symptomatic HD. Therefore, PET might be most useful as a complement to DNA testing in evaluating at-risk patients.

PET has also been used to study the changes in the dopaminergic pathways in HD patients. Leenders et al. (240) used ¹⁸F-fluorodopa and found normal striatal uptake but a decreased D2 receptor density. This finding is believed to be consistent with the neuropathology of HD, which consists of neuronal loss in the neostriatum while the nigrostriatal pathway remains intact. Other investigators (217,241) have found similar decreases in dopamine receptor densities in the basal ganglia of HD patients. Thus, these types of receptor studies with PET might be very useful in elucidating the neuropathologic mechanism underlying HD. Studies have also demonstrated decreased opioid activity in the striatum of HD patients (242). Conversely, a PET study with ¹¹C Flumazenil demonstrated an upregulation of γ-aminobutyric acid (GABA) receptors in the striatum of HD patients (243). However, an earlier study showed that caudate benzodiazepine receptor density is already severely impaired when other subcortical structures reveal only minor abnormalities (244).

Dystonia

Idiopathic torsional dystonia (ITD) is a dominantly inherited disorder with features including frequently repetitive, sustained muscle contractions. Chase et al. (245) found that patients with ITD have significantly increased glucose metabolism in the lenticular nuclei contralateral to the affected limbs. Two of the six patients studied also had increased metabolism in the contralateral caudate. However, another group (246) found increased metabolism in the striatum in only one of five patients. Stoessl et al. (247) studied 14 patients with idiopathic torticollis and found no significant changes in glucose metabolism compared with controls, but there was an abnormal covariance between thalamic function and the striatum.

Dopa-responsive dystonia represents a minority of patients with dystonia who have dramatic responses to L-DOPA therapy. It is believed that these patients have a defect in the dopamine synthetic pathway (at the tyrosine hydroxylase step) that is bypassed with the administration of L-DOPA. Sawle et al. (248) studied six of these patients with ^{18}F-fluorodopa PET. The results indicated that these patients had significant decreases in FDOPA uptake in the caudate and putamen, suggesting that this disorder is not related to defective synthesis of dopamine but to a defect in the decarboxylation, vesicular uptake, and storage of dopamine (as reflected by the decreased FDOPA uptake). Several other groups have reported similar decreases in dopamine uptake in dystonic patients (249,250). More recent studies have demonstrated an elevated ^{11}C-raclopride binding index in the putamen and caudate nucleus of these patients compared with controls and PD patients. The increase of ^{11}C-raclopride binding may be interpreted either as reduced tracer displacement by endogenous dopamine or as an alteration of the receptor features resulting from chronic dopamine deficiency (251).

Progressive Supranuclear Palsy

Progressive supranuclear palsy (PSP) is a disease that causes a paralyzed gaze, dystonia, axial rigidity, and, eventually, dementia. PSP is associated with hypometabolism of the basal ganglia, thalamus, pons, and cerebral cortex but not the cerebellum (252, 253). Foster et al. (252) found that the superior frontal cortex has the most significant involvement. D'Antona et al. (254) also reported frontal hypometabolism in patients with PSP. It also appears, based on MRI analysis, that corpus callosum atrophy is present in PSP and is associated with cognitive impairment and cerebral cortical hypometabolism, especially in the frontal cortical region (255). Goffinet et al. (253) used ^{18}F-FDG PET to show that the motor and premotor areas were severely hypometabolic (Fig. 38.11). The authors suggested that this pattern could be due to disconnection from the subcortical structures. Other studies have demonstrated more globally decreased cerebral metabolism in PSP with or without a predilection for the frontal lobes (256,257). Leenders et al. (250) also found significantly decreased dopamine formation and storage in the striatum in PSP patients. This decrease also correlated with the degree of reduced frontal blood flow.

Wilson's Disease

Wilson's disease is an autosomal recessive disorder of copper metabolism that can eventually result in movement disorders (including spasticity, rigidity, and chorea) and psychiatric disorders resulting from a buildup of copper in the brain. ^{18}F-FDG PET studies have shown that patients with Wilson's disease have

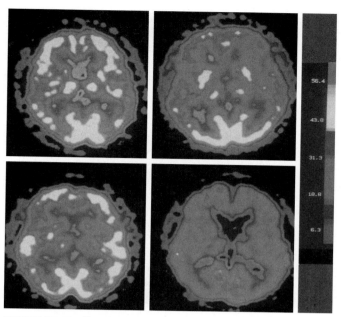

FIGURE 38.11. ^{18}F-FDG PET images at the level of the basal ganglia of an age-matched control (*left upper*) and three patients with progressive supranuclear palsy (PSP) are shown. Compared with the control subject, the most frequent pattern in patients with PSP is decreased metabolism in frontal lobes bilaterally, which also selectively affects the motor cortex (*right upper*). However, a normal pattern (*right lower*) may be seen. Diffuse hypometabolism (*right lower*) is marked in some patients. (From Gaffinet AM, DeVolder AG, Gillain C et al. Positron tomography demonstrates frontal lobe hypometabolism in progressive supranuclear palsy. *Ann Neurol* 1989;25:131–139, with permission.)

significantly decreased glucose metabolism in the cerebellum and striatum compared with controls (258–260). Cortical and thalamic glucose metabolism was also significantly decreased but to a lesser degree. In addition, decreases in the cerebellum, thalamus, and cortex correlated with the degree of pyramidal signs. With therapy, the observed reductions of metabolism are observed to normalize (261), and patients recently started on decoppering therapy had significantly reduced rCMRGlc values compared with patients on therapy for a longer duration. Hawkins et al. (260) found reduced cortical gray and central white matter glucose metabolism (particularly in the frontal region) and decreases in the lenticular nuclei in patients with neurologic symptoms from Wilson's disease (Fig. 38.12). Pappata et al. (262), however, did not find significant decrements in cortical metabolism in patients with Wilson's disease despite marked cognitive impairment. The dopaminergic system may also be affected in Wilson's disease, but early studies suggest that the striatal degeneration comprises a complex pathology involving both afferent and efferent projections (263). However, there do appear to be improvements in dopaminergic function with therapy (264).

CEREBROVASCULAR DISORDERS

Cerebrovascular disease is the third leading cause of death in the United States and affects approximately half a million people.

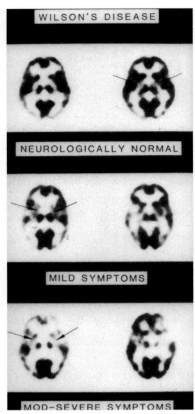

FIGURE 38.12. ^{18}F-FDG PET images of three patients diagnosed with Wilson's disease. The *top row* images of a neurologically asymptomatic patient show only a mild decrease in metabolism in the lenticular nuclei. The *middle row* images are of a patient with mild neurologic impairment and show a moderate decrease in metabolism in the lenticular nuclei. The patient with moderate-to-severe neurologic dysfunction not only shows a markedly decreased metabolism in the lenticular nuclei, but also shows hypometabolic areas in the temporal and frontal cortices and the right thalamus. (From Hawkins RA, Mazziotta JC, Phelps ME. Wilson's disease studied with FDG and positron emission tomography. *Neurology* 1987;37:1707–1711, with permission.)

However, stroke is often associated with a poor outcome in part because of the lack of understanding of the mechanisms that underlie stroke and the process by which recovery may take place. PET imaging has been of great benefit in advancing the understanding of the pathophysiology of cerebrovascular disorders (265–268). PET (as well as SPECT) imaging allows for the detection of stroke earlier and with higher sensitivity than anatomic imaging with either MRI or CT. Furthermore, PET imaging has been useful in evaluating the extent of the functional damage, because areas not immediately affected by the infarct may show hypometabolism or decreased blood flow. Initial stroke severity has been shown to correlate with the "initially affected" volume as determined by PET, whereas neurologic deterioration during the first week after stroke correlates with the proportion of the initially affected volume that infarcted, and functional outcome correlates with the final infarct volume (269).

In patients who have suffered a stroke, there is a characteristic uncoupling between CBF and metabolism in the infarcted area (270–274). Several studies using ^{15}O H$_2$O have described "mis-

ery perfusion" in and near areas of infarct within the first hours to days after a stroke (Fig. 38.13). This misery perfusion is described as a relative decrease in RCBF compared with the regional glucose metabolism (rCMRGlc) or oxygen metabolism (rCMRO$_2$). Further studies have shown that there is a marked increase in the rOEF in response to the diminished blood flow (275,276). However, a recent study has shown no correlation between the degree of misery perfusion and angiographic findings in patients with carotid artery occlusion (277).

A recent study demonstrated that the oxygen consumption significantly decreased between the acute and chronic phases of stroke, but that acute-stage mesial-prefrontal metabolism was significantly correlated with neurologic recovery (278). This study also showed that there was a delayed intrahemispheric remote hypometabolism that developed while the patient was clinically recovering and appears to be related to infarct size. Neurologic recovery was not a function of thalamic hypometabolism but appeared to be influenced by mesial-prefrontal metabolism, possibly because this region is part of a network that has an important compensatory role in motor recovery.

Approximately 1 week after infarct, "luxury perfusion" occurs, which is a relative increase of RCBF compared with cerebral metabolism (279). Wise et al. (276) found that RCBF increased compared with rCMRO$_2$ over several days postinfarct. Furthermore, there was a subsequent decrease in the rOEF in the infarcted area 18 hours to 7 days after the infarct. This is believed to reflect mitochondrial dysfunction and energy failure of the damaged tissue.

In addition to the infarcted area, there exists a "penumbral"

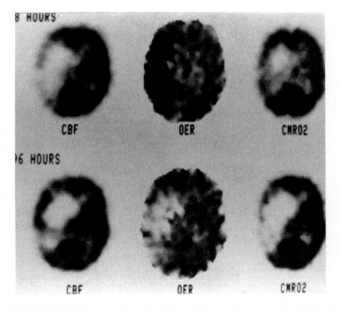

FIGURE 38.13. Images showing the relation between cerebral blood flow oxygen extraction and oxygen metabolism after a right middle cerebral artery stroke. Shortly after stroke (8 hours), there is misery perfusion with decreased blood flow, increased oxygen extraction, and increased metabolism. Ninety-six hours later, there is luxury perfusion with increased blood flow, decreased oxygen extraction, and decreased oxygen metabolism. (From Frackowiak R, Wise R. Positron tomography in ischemia cerebrovascular disease. *Neurol Clin* 1983;1:183–201, with permission.)

zone, a hypometabolic and presumably ischemic area that surrounds the infarct core (280). This area also has increased rOEF suggesting that this area has decreased perfusion relative to the necessary oxygen requirements. If blood flow to this ischemic area is restored before irreversible damage occurs, then the tissue will likely recover and resume normal function (281).

Distant from the ischemic and the stroke sites, there are regions that also show alterations in metabolism despite being normal on anatomic imaging studies such as CT or MRI (282–286). However, it is not completely certain what are the clinical consequences of these distant hypometabolic regions (287). The most distinctive and characteristic example of such remote effects is crossed cerebellar diaschisis, first described by Baron et al. (288). Crossed cerebellar diaschisis refers to hypometabolism and hypoperfusion in the cerebellar cortex contralateral to the site of the infarct in the cortex and usually occurs during the first 2 months after infarction (289). It is believed that this is due to an interruption of the cerebro-ponto-cerebellar pathways as a result of the stroke. Interestingly, patients with persistent cerebellar diaschisis have a decrease in oxygen consumption that is less than the decrease in glucose utilization (290). This uncoupling of oxygen consumption and glucose utilization may reflect a change in brain metabolism caused by deafferentation. Another study did demonstrate that the degree of neurologic improvement was worse in the patients with cerebellar diaschisis, which may be simply be reflective of more severe and widespread ischemia resulting in the diaschisis (291). There are also other areas that are hypometabolic after a cortical infarct (292). These areas include the ipsilateral thalamus, the ipsilateral caudate nucleus, and the ipsilateral primary visual cortex (if the infarct is in the anterior visual pathways). A recent study also demonstrated a decline in oxygen metabolism in the unaffected hemisphere from the acute to the subacute stage, which suggests a delayed effect from transcallosal fiber degeneration (293).

PET studies have not been shown to be as successful in assessing risk of stroke or the potential outcome of surgical intervention in patients with carotid artery disease (294–296). Count-based PET measurement of OEF without arterial sampling has been shown to accurately predict the risk of stroke in patients with carotid artery occlusion (297). This is corroborated somewhat by another study that demonstrated a lower frequency of hemodynamic abnormalities in asymptomatic patients (298). However, in an earlier study of patients with carotid artery disease being treated with antithrombotic medication, there was no difference in the incidence of stroke in patients with normal and those with abnormal hemodynamics. The same group found no correlation between the degree of carotid artery stenosis and the hemodynamic measures of the cerebral circulation in 19 patients with significant carotid artery occlusion. However, in patients before and after extracranial-intracranial bypass surgery, decreases in rCBV and normalization of the RCBF/rCBV ratio were found after surgery (299). Despite this finding, only 3 of 21 patients who underwent bypass surgery suffered ipsilateral stroke within 1 year. Furthermore, none of the 23 patients who did not have surgery, but had PET findings similar to those in the surgical group, had a stroke. The conclusion from this study was that the PET results of the hemodynamic status of patients

with carotid artery disease could not adequately predict which patients would benefit from bypass surgery.

There have been several studies that have correlated the functional recovery in patients with stroke with functional changes on their PET scans (300,301). For example, rCMRGlc measured early after stroke have shown that receptive language disorders best correlate with metabolism in the left superior temporal cortex, and word fluency best correlate with metabolism in the left prefrontal cortex (302). A PET study of patients with left inferior frontal gyrus strokes and resulting aphasia demonstrated a stronger-than-normal response in the homologous right inferior frontal gyrus (303). Although the level of activation in the right inferior frontal gyrus did not correlate with verbal performance, increased activity in the perilesional area occurred in the two patients who gave the best performance in certain verbal tasks and who also showed the most complete recovery from aphasia. Similar results were described in several other studies of patients with aphasia secondary to stroke that demonstrated increased right temporal lobe activity as a mechanism to compensate for the impaired left hemispheric function (304,305). However, the best degree of speech restoration has been found in those patients with at least some preservation of activity in the left temporal lobe that can ultimately be incorporated into the functional language network (306,307). Another study measuring CBF associated with passive elbow movement showed that hemiplegic stroke initially activated the bilateral inferior parietal cortex, contralateral sensorimotor cortex, ipsilateral dorsolateral prefrontal cortex, supplementary motor area, and cingulate cortex but later included activation of the ipsilateral premotor area (308). These results suggested that recovery from hemiplegia is accompanied by changes of brain activation in sensory and motor systems.

PET studies have also been used to monitor the success of various treatment regimens. PET has been used to evaluate the effects of thrombolytic therapy in acute stroke and has found that critically hypoperfused tissue can be preserved by early reperfusion and that large infarcts can be prevented by early reperfusion to misery perfused but viable tissue (309). Imaging of benzodiazepine receptors by flumazenil PET distinguishes between irreversibly damaged and viable penumbra tissue early after acute stroke (310,311). In the future, functional imaging modalities that could eventually include tracers for neuronal integrity might be used to help in the selection of patients for thrombolytic therapy possibly permitting the extension of the critical time period for inclusion of patients to aggressive stroke management strategies (312). Hakim et al. (313) found that stroke patients treated with nimodipine had a greater increase in the RCBF in the ischemia core (7 days after the infarct) than did patients receiving placebo. There was also an increase in RCBF in the penumbral zone in the nimodipine group compared with the placebo group (but these results were not statistically significant). Another study using ^{18}F-FDG PET found that patients on nimodipine had greater increases in glucose metabolism in the affected areas compared with controls (314).

HEAD TRAUMA

There have been a limited number of studies using PET in the evaluation of patients with head trauma. One of the problems with the use of PET in these cases is that PET cannot distinguish between structural damage and cerebral dysfunction because these may all result in areas of decreased metabolism (315). Thus, it is helpful to compare PET to anatomic images such as those obtained by MRI or CT, especially because cerebral dysfunction can extend beyond the boundary of anatomic lesions (316) and may even appear in remote locations from the trauma.

Lesions such as cortical contusions, intracranial hematoma, and resultant encephalomalacia have metabolic effects that are confined primarily to the site of injury. However, subdural and epidural hematomas often cause widespread hypometabolism and may even affect the contralateral hemisphere (317). Another entity, diffuse axonal injury, has been found to cause diffuse cortical hypometabolism (Figs. 38.14 and 38.15), but there is a particularly marked decrease in metabolism in the parieto-occipital cortex (318). Furthermore, crossed cerebellar diaschisis, as well as ipsilateral cerebellar hypometabolism, has been found in head injury patients with supratentorial lesions (319).

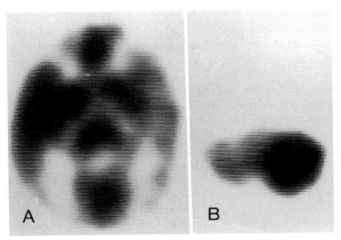

FIGURE 38.15. **A:** Positron emission tomography image of a head injury patient shows the effects of a left epidural hematoma with subsequent decreased metabolism in the entire left hemisphere. **B:** In the cerebellum of this patient, there is cerebellar diaschisis shown as a decreased metabolism in the contralateral cerebellum.

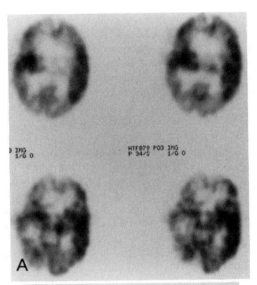

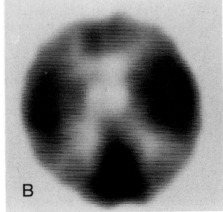

FIGURE 38.14. Two positron emission tomography images of patients suffering from head injury. **A:** One patient developed diffuse axonal injury characterized by globally decreased metabolism. This finding is in comparison to a patient **(B)** with normal metabolism in most of the cortical areas except the frontal lobe that was the area involved in the injury.

There has generally been a good correlation between the severity of head trauma as measured by the Glasgow Coma Scale (GCS) and the extent of whole brain hypometabolism. Patients with persistent symptoms in minor head injury may have associated corresponding deficits in neuropsychologic testing, as well as in cerebral metabolism (320). Global and regional metabolic rates have been found to improve as patients recover from head trauma. Another study demonstrated that regionally decreased glucose metabolism was observed in 88% of patients (321). The prevalence of global cortical CMRGlc reduction was higher in severely head-injured patients (86% vs. 67% mild-moderate), although the absolute values were similar across the injury severity spectrum. The level of consciousness, as measured by the GCS, correlated poorly with the global cortical CMRGlc value, although the correlation was better for mildly head injured patients. As many as half of patients with head injury may also have increased glucose metabolism as early as 1 week after injury (322). This hyperglycolysis may occur either regionally or globally and also suggests that the metabolic state of the traumatically injured brain should be defined differentially in terms of glucose and oxygen metabolism. However, PET imaging may not be as helpful in determining overall prognosis in head injury patients, particularly children and adolescents, with respect to rehabilitation (323).

Also, after head injury, even though a patient may be in a persistent vegetative state, the brain actually responds to the emotional attributes of sound or speech. This was determined using PET to measure CBF changes when a story was told by a patient's mother (324). During auditory presentation, there was increased activity in the rostral anterior cingulate, right middle temporal, and right premotor cortices.

AIDS DEMENTIA

Patients with HIV infection may have very subtle metabolic changes, such as mildly increased activity in the basal ganglia and parietal lobes, even though they have no changes in neuropsychologic function (325). However, other groups have demonstrated that changes in basal ganglia, thalamus, and temporal lobes are correlated with cognitive decline (326). AIDS dementia complex (ADC) is a frequent complication of AIDS. Unfortunately, it is often difficult to attribute this finding to the direct effects of the virus on the brain because these patients can acquire opportunistic infections or lymphoma that can mimic the symptoms of ADC (327). ^{18}F-FDG PET can therefore be of value in differentiating superimposed lymphoma from opportunistic infections, which typically appear less active compared with tumor (328–330). PET and SPECT have been useful in showing abnormalities in the subcortical gray matter and the cerebral cortex in these patients (331). However, a SPECT study by Holman et al. (332) found that similar abnormalities were found in ADC patients and in chronic cocaine and polydrug abusers. Therefore, the diagnosis of ADC must be made with caution because the dementia symptoms may also be related to the polydrug abuse in these patients.

ALCOHOLISM

Studies of alcoholic patients with PET have generally found decreased whole brain metabolic activity (333–335). One study by Wik et al. (335) used CT and ^{18}F-FDG PET to examine patients with alcoholism. They found that alcoholic patients had reductions of 20% to 30% in both cortical and subcortical brain regional metabolism compared with controls. Although the hypometabolism was diffusely distributed, the parietal areas were found to be disproportionately affected. Other studies have reported frontal lobe hypometabolism. Also, studies have reported metabolic deficits in the left hemisphere more often than in the right (336). A recent study also suggests that there may be differences in the cerebral metabolism in women with alcoholism compared with men, because women had less of a decrease in metabolism compared with men (337). Patients with chronic alcoholism and cerebellar degeneration have been found to have significantly reduced rCMRGlc in the superior vermis compared with controls (338). Volkow et al. (339) reported that the decrease in metabolism in chronic alcoholics correlated with the time since they last consumed alcohol. There were decreases in frontal and parietal metabolism that did not follow this pattern, suggesting that these changes might be a long-term component of the effects of chronic alcoholism. However, patients who remained abstinent or who had minimal alcohol during longitudinal follow-up showed partial recovery of glucose metabolism in two of three divisions of the frontal lobes and improvement on neuropsychologic tests of general cognitive and executive functioning, whereas the patients who relapsed had further declines in these areas (340). Examining the metabolic changes associated with detoxification showed a significant increase in global and regional (primarily frontal lobe) measures predominantly within 16 to 30 days (341). Further follow-up did not demonstrate additional changes, suggesting that the effects of detoxification occur in the first 30 days.

Studies have also begun to explore the effects of alcohol on various neurotransmitter systems within the brain. GABA-ben-zodiazepine receptor function is altered in alcoholics as demonstrated by decreased sensitivity to lorazepam administration in the thalamus, basal ganglia, orbitofrontal cortex, and cerebellum and may account for the decreased sensitivity to the effects of alcohol and benzodiazepines in these subjects (342,343). For example, studies have shown low dopamine D2 receptor densities and less conclusive changes in the dopamine transporter densities among late-onset alcoholics, and low presynaptic DA function was observed in the left caudate of two patients, suggesting that this stage of alcoholism may be a heterogeneous disorder (344,345). One study reported reduced binding in the striatal monoaminergic presynaptic terminals in severe chronic alcoholic patients, suggesting that the damaging effects of severe chronic alcoholism on the CNS are more extensive than previously considered (346). A comparison of alcoholics with controls with a serotoninergic challenge demonstrated activation of the basal ganglia circuits involving the orbital and prefrontal areas in controls but a blunted response among alcoholics (347). In a related study of alcoholic patients on disulfiram, there was decreased cerebral glucose metabolism and decreased flumazenil influx and distribution volume in patients receiving disulfiram, suggesting that this drug may be an important factor in the functional imaging studies of alcoholic patients (348).

COCAINE ABUSE

The use of cocaine has steadily increased over the past few decades and has reached an almost epidemic proportion. Cocaine is one of the most addictive and toxic abused drugs (349). PET studies have the potential of elucidating the mechanisms of the effects and the addictive properties of cocaine (350). Initial studies with [^{11}C] cocaine showed maximal uptake in the basal ganglia (351). This uptake was very rapid, reaching peak concentration in 4 to 8 minutes after injection and a clearance half-life of 20 minutes. Preadministration of nomifensine, which blocks the presynaptic reuptake of dopamine and norepinephrine, was shown to block the uptake of cocaine in the basal ganglia in this study. Another study has shown that the euphoric effects of cocaine correspond directly to the concentration of the drug in the basal ganglia (352,353), corroborating the findings of the PET scan results.

Brain metabolism studies have shown that acute administration of cocaine in chronic cocaine abusers results in decreased metabolism in the cortical and subcortical structures. Furthermore, the extent of metabolic decrease correlated with the subjective evidence of the euphoria. In patients with chronic cocaine abuse, the duration since detoxification affects the cerebral glucose metabolism. Volkow et al. (354) showed decreased frontal activity 8 days to 2 months after last cocaine use (more extensive decrement in the left compared with the right hemisphere) in chronic abusers compared with controls. Another study of the acute changes after withdrawal of the drug showed that 1 week after last cocaine use, these patients had hypermetabolism in the orbitofrontal cortex and the basal ganglia compared with normal controls and those studied 1 month after last cocaine use (355). Furthermore, hypermetabolism in these regions correlated with the subjective craving for cocaine. A follow-up study also showed similar findings, particularly affecting the right hemisphere, but this study indicated that dopamine enhancement is not sufficient to increase metabolism in the frontal regions (356). The predominant correlation of craving within the right but not the left brain regions suggests laterality of the addiction response. Interestingly, a similar pattern has been reported in patients with obsessive-compulsive disorder (OCD) (357), although it is not clear whether the ritualistic behavior in OCD is comparable to the addictive behavior of cocaine abusers. However, it is known that the orbitofrontal cortex and basal ganglia, areas involved in cocaine abuse, are also involved in a circuit regulating repetitive behavior (358). In terms of the actual craving for cocaine, one PET study showed a pattern of increased activity in limbic (amygdala and anterior cingulate) CBF and decreases in the basal ganglia while watching a video designed to induce craving (359), whereas another study showed activation of the temporal insula (involved with autonomic control) and the orbitofrontal cortex (involved with expectancy and reinforcement) during a craving stimulus (360).

PET receptor studies have attempted to determine the relationship between cocaine and dopamine receptors in the basal ganglia. Furthermore, it has been shown that increased dopamine plays an important role in cocaine's euphoric properties and that a decrease in dopamine presynaptic activity plays a role in withdrawal and possibly addictive properties (361,362). Another study suggested that the thalamic dopamine pathways are also important in cocaine addiction (363). Cocaine has been shown to significantly block dopamine transporters (364). The levels of blockade were comparable across several different routes of administration including intravenous, intranasal, and smoked cocaine. Interestingly, smoked cocaine induced significantly greater self-reports of a "high" than the other routes, likely resulting from the speed in which the cocaine is delivered to the brain because there was no difference in the overall dopamine transporter blockade. Another study demonstrated that cocaine abusers have an enhanced sensitivity to lorazepam, suggesting that there is a disruption of GABA pathways that may reflect, in part, cocaine withdrawal (365). This same study noted that cocaine abusers also have intense sleepiness induced by lorazepam, suggesting potential clinical consequences of prescribing such medications to cocaine abusers.

SCHIZOPHRENIA

PET has been widely used in the study of the functional abnormalities in schizophrenia (366–368). It has been hypothesized that schizophrenia is most commonly associated with frontal lobe dysfunction (369,370), although some early studies did not report such a finding (371–373). One study showed that the degree of frontal hypometabolism correlated with negative symptoms, as opposed to positive symptoms (374), although other studies have found an association between positive symptoms and decreased frontal activity (375). A refinement of the proposed hypothesis for the underlying cause of dysfunction in schizophrenia ascribes the hypofrontal pattern to those schizophrenic patients with a predominance of negative symptoms (376,377). These patients tend to be older and have a long

history of neuroleptic therapy. On the other hand, younger patients with predominantly positive symptoms usually do not have a hypofrontal pattern. Also, the frontal lobe activity may change during the course of the disorder and may be more prominent in the acute setting (378), or frontal lobe changes may vary with specific symptoms in an individual patient (379). There are other areas that may also be affected including the anterior cingulate (380) and the thalamus and striatum (381–383) (Fig. 38.16). Liddle et al. (384,385) proposed three syndromes of symptoms in schizophrenics with corresponding PET patterns of RCBF: (a) patients with psychomotor poverty syndrome and diminished word generating ability have decreased perfusion of the dorsolateral prefrontal cortex, (b) patients with the disorganization syndrome have impaired inhibition of inappropriate responses and have increased RCBF of the right anterior cingulate gyrus, and (c) patients with the reality distortion syndrome have increased perfusion in the medial temporal lobe at a locus that is activated in normal subjects during the internal monitoring of eye movements.

More recent work has tried to establish specific networks of structures related to the clinical manifestations of schizophrenia. For example, there is a correlation between the anterior thalamus and the frontal cortex, a key element in the thalamo-cortical-striatal circuit suggested to be abnormal in some models of schizophrenia (386,387). The findings from this study also showed that schizophrenics have lower correlations between frontal lobe activity and activity in other structures consistent with frontal cortical dysfunction.

A number of PET studies have been performed to determine whether left hemispheric dysfunction can be detected in schizophrenics. Several studies have found that, at rest, patients with schizophrenia have increased perfusion and metabolism in the left hemispheric cerebral cortex relative to the right (388–390). They also found that the severity of the symptoms of schizophrenia correlated with the degree of hyperactivation of the left hemisphere and not with the degree of hypofrontality. A more recent study has shown that patients lack asymmetry in caudate dopamine transporter binding, which conforms with the concept of disrupted brain lateralization in schizophrenia (391).

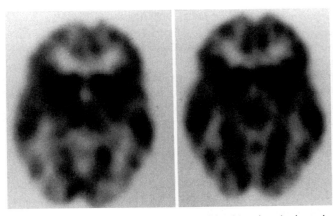

FIGURE 38.16. ^{18}F-FDG PET of a patient with schizophrenia shows increased metabolism in the caudate nuclei bilaterally compared with the cortical metabolism. All changes in metabolism are symmetric.

Cerebral activation studies have improved the understanding of the deficits associated with schizophrenia. ^{18}F-FDG PET studies in which a subject underwent specific frontal lobe activation tests of sustained attention by continuous performance tasks found decreased activation of the frontal lobes in schizophrenic patients compared with controls (392,393). DeLisi et al. (394) found that schizophrenic patients had higher left temporal lobe metabolic rates compared with controls when there was sensory stimulation of the right arm. Another study (395) compared PET and electroencephalogram (EEG) findings in schizophrenic and control subjects performing various simple and complex motor tasks. Although no changes were observed in the schizophrenic or control group during simple motor tasks, the schizophrenic group had decreased activation in the supplementary motor and the contralateral sensorimotor cortices during complex motor tasks compared with controls. During a continuous performance task, schizophrenics showed negative correlations of task performance with anterior cingulate activity, suggesting that overactivity of that region, which is involved in mental effort and whose metabolic rate is typically lower in schizophrenic patients, may also result in the impairment of task performance in these patients (396). Patients with schizophrenia also fail to activate the anterior cingulate gyrus during selective attention performance (397). Schizophrenia patients with negative symptoms have been found to have a lesser activation in the left hemisphere during word generation with compensatory changes in the right hemisphere (398). Schizophrenia is also associated with attenuated right thalamic and right prefrontal activation during the recognition of novel visual stimuli and with increased left prefrontal cortical activation during impaired episodic recognition of previously seen visual stimuli (399). Similarly, patients with schizophrenia fail to activate cortical-cerebellar-thalamic-cortical circuitry during recall of both well-learned and novel word lists (400). Frontal cortex function during memory retrieval is more impaired in schizophrenic patients (401, 402). Volkow et al. (403) found that with eye-tracking tasks, schizophrenic patients had lower correlations between anterior and posterior cortical areas and between the thalamus and neocortical areas compared with controls. Furthermore, these results indicate a marked derangement in the pattern of interactions among various brain regions in schizophrenics. The results of most of these activation studies provide evidence for abnormal thalamic and prefrontal cortex function in schizophrenia (404), although another study showed a cingulated gyrus/parietal lobe dysfunction underlying impairment of working memory processes during a random number generation task in schizophrenia (405). There has also been evidence of hippocampal dysfunction during episodic memory retrieval in schizophrenia (406). Interestingly, schizophrenic patients have also failed to show graded memory task-related decreases in activity in the left superior temporal and inferior parietal gyrus, which is typically seen in control subjects (407,408).

In addition to the metabolic and blood flow studies, PET offers imaging of dopamine receptors in schizophrenic patients (409,410). This is particularly useful because the dopaminergic system has been implicated in the pathophysiology of this disorder, as well as the site of action for neuroleptic drugs, the primary therapeutic modality considered effective in these patients. Most

investigators have reported no differences in dopamine receptor density or affinity in the basal striatum between schizophrenics and controls (411–413). However, several reports have found an increased density of dopamine receptors in both neuroleptic naïve and previously treated but drug-free schizophrenic patients (414,415). Another group (416) found increases in dopamine activity in patients with manic depressive psychosis, suggesting that increased dopamine activity might be a feature of psychotic illness in general and may not be specific to schizophrenia. A more recent study detected decreased FDOPA uptake in neuroleptic naïve schizophrenics (417). Another study demonstrated that depressive symptoms in neuroleptic-naïve first-admission schizophrenia patients have low presynaptic dopamine function (418). There has been no evidence of a change in serotonin receptors in patients with schizophrenia (419,420), although some investigators have reported a decrease in the frontal lobes in neuroleptic naïve patients (421).

PET studies have also evaluated the effects of therapeutic interventions in patients with schizophrenia. Early studies reported a general increase in glucose metabolism, particularly in the left temporal lobe, following neuroleptic treatment, but there was no change in the anteroposterior gradient (422,423). Schizophrenic patients that responded to haloperidol treatment typically had a "normalizing" effect on metabolic activity in the striatum; the metabolic rate while they were receiving haloperidol was higher than that while they were receiving placebo (424). Nonresponders were more likely to show a worsening of hypofrontality and an absence of change in the striatum during the treatment condition. Another study corroborated this finding such that a haloperidol challenge caused widespread decreases in absolute metabolism in nonresponsive patients but not in the responsive patients (425). Studies have shown that that there is a high dopamine D2 receptor occupancy, particularly in the basal ganglia, in early treatment with neuroleptics and that this occupancy was dose dependent and associated not only with the therapeutic effect but also with side effects such as hyperprolactinemia and extrapyramidal signs (426–428). Upregulation of dopamine D2 receptors has also been shown to be associated with a regional increase of blood flow and metabolism in the basal ganglia (429). Furthermore, the D2 receptor occupancy has been shown to decrease as the drug levels decreased on withdrawal of treatment (409, 410). Interestingly, patients who are resistant to neuroleptic therapy have similar D2 receptor blockade compared with patients who do respond clinically to therapy (430,431).

The data suggest that both traditional and novel antipsychotics with high affinity for dopamine D2 receptors are associated with a substantial increase in D2 receptor binding. The present data in humans agree well with animal data that implicate D2 receptor-mediated mechanisms in motor hyperactivity. Interestingly, a new atypical antipsychotic, quetiapine, shows a transiently high D2 occupancy that decreases to very low levels by the end of the dosing interval, which may account for its lower incidence of extrapyramidal side effects (432). PET has also been used to evaluate other new drugs such as amoxapine and olanzapine, which have a profile similar to that of other atypical antipsychotics with a higher occupancy of serotonin receptors compared with D2 receptors (433,434). PET imaging has demonstrated sex differences related to the effects with antipsychotic medications (clozapine and fluphenazine) with women having a reduction in cingulated gyrus metabolism compared with men (435). In men, fluphenazine was associated with a much greater elevation in basal ganglia metabolic rates than was clozapine, whereas women demonstrated nearly equal increases on both fluphenazine and clozapine.

MOOD DISORDERS

The most common finding on PET imaging in depressed patients is a global dysfunction as demonstrated by decreased cerebral blood flow (436) and decreased cerebral metabolism (437). Furthermore, some studies have indicated that decreased cerebral blood flow might correlate with the degree of depression. One group (438,439) found that patients with depression had whole brain decreases in blood flow, with the left anterior cingulate gyrus and the left dorsolateral prefrontal cortex particularly affected. Furthermore, depressed patients who also had cognitive impairment were found to have decreased RCBF in the left medial frontal gyrus and increased RCBF in the cerebellar vermis compared with depressed patients without cognitive dysfunction. Decreased activity in a localized area in the prefrontal cortex ventral to the genu of the corpus callosum has been demonstrated in both familial bipolar depressives and familial unipolar depressives (440). Even during non-rapid eye movement (non-REM) sleep, depressed patients have decreased frontal and limbic metabolic activity in association with posterior cortical increases (441). There are typically decreases in serotonergic system including both 1A and 2A receptors in the limbic and neocortical areas (442–444).

A ^{18}F-FDG PET study by Kumar et al. (445) showed that patients with late-age onset of depression have decreased metabolism throughout the cortex and even in many subcortical structures (Fig. 38.17 and 38.18). Furthermore, these decreases were of the same or greater magnitude compared with patients with AD. However, AD patients more likely had the typical temporoparietal hypometabolism pattern on PET images, whereas the depression patients tended to have more global hypometabolism. The serotonin type 2A receptor does not appear to be affected in late-life onset depression, although there is a decrease in binding to this receptor type in patients with AD (446). Depressed patients with concomitant anxiety symptoms demonstrated specific metabolic changes with increased activity in the right parahippocampal and left anterior cingulate regions and decreased activity in the cerebellum, left fusiform gyrus, left superior temporal, left angular gyrus, and left insula (447). The authors concluded that anxiety symptoms are associated with changes in specific brain regions that partially overlap with those in primary anxiety disorders and differ from those associated with depression.

Recent studies have also explored treatment-related effects in patients with depression. On pretreatment scans, lower metabolism in the left ventral anterior cingulate gyrus, ventrolateral prefrontal cortex, and orbitofrontal cortex has been associated with a better treatment response to paroxetine (448). Furthermore, there is decreased activity in limbic and striatal areas and increased activity in the dorsal cortical areas (including the prefrontal, parietal, anterior, and posterior cingulated areas) associated with improvements in clinical symptoms (449). The clinical improvement in depressed patients treated with paroxetine is also associated with an increase in the density of serotonin type 2A receptors in the frontal cortex (450,451). However, the reduction in 5-hydroxytryptamine 1A (5-HT1A) receptor binding in depressed patients was not changed by selective serotonin reuptake inhibitor treatment (452). Also, depressed patients showed a significant reduction in available serotonin type 2A

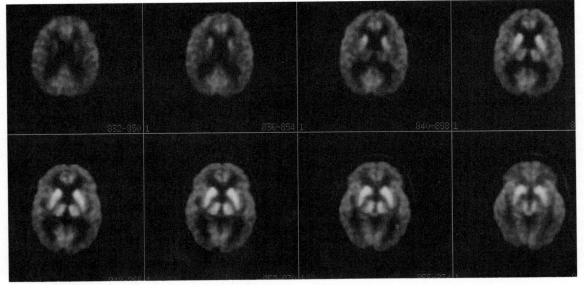

FIGURE 38.17. ^{18}F-FDG PET using high-resolution gadolinium oxyorthosilicate scanner in a patient with symptoms of a major depressive episode demonstrates markedly decreased metabolism throughout the cortex with relative sparing of the basal ganglia and thalami.

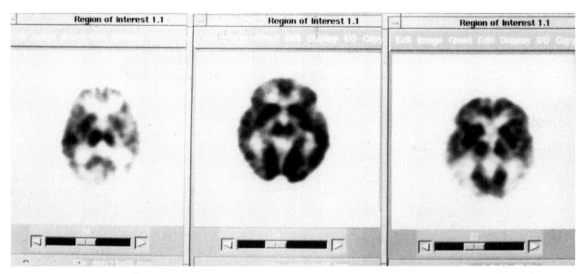

FIGURE 38.18. ^{18}F-FDG PET images of a subject with depression (*right*) compared with a normal control (*center*) and a patient with Alzheimer's disease (AD) (*left*). The patient with depression has decreased metabolism throughout the cortical and even the subcortical structures compared with the control subject. Note that the depressed patient shows a marked decrease in metabolism diffusely, whereas the patient with AD has hypometabolism primarily in the parietal areas bilaterally.

receptors in the brain following desipramine treatment (453). In a study of sleep deprivation, high pretreatment metabolic rates and overall posttreatment decreases in metabolic rates in the medial prefrontal cortex and anterior cingulated gyrus (particularly on the right) were associated with those depression patients who responded well to sleep deprivation therapy (454, 455).

Another group used PET to study cerebral glucose metabolism in bipolar patients (456,457). They found that bipolar patients who are actively depressed have decreased global metabolism. As their depression improves, they have increases in their cerebral metabolism. In contrast, unipolar patients were found to have normal global metabolic rates that did not correlate with clinical symptoms. These investigators also found a decreased caudate/hemispheric metabolic ratio in depressed unipolar patients. Furthermore, this ratio increased as symptoms of depression improved. Buchsbaum et al. (458) found a decreased anteroposterior gradient in bipolar depressed patients but not in unipolar patients. More recent work has demonstrated that bipolar depression is associated with a pattern of prefrontal hypometabolism, whereas a cerebello-posterior cortical hypermetabolism may be observed in bipolar patients. Thus, in depressed patients, PET might be useful in distinguishing unipolar from bipolar patients, a distinction that would have significant implications for the patient's treatment and prognosis (459). Some bipolar patients also have psychotic symptoms and have been found to have elevations in D2 dopamine receptor density likely associated with the psychotic symptoms and not the mood disorder (460).

Other receptor types have been studied in patients with mood disorders. FDOPA uptake in the left caudate was significantly lower in depressed patients with psychomotor retardation than in patients with high impulsivity and in comparison subjects (461).

OBSESSIVE-COMPULSIVE DISORDER

Several studies have used ^{18}F-FDG PET to investigate patients with OCD. Early results have generally shown that OCD patients have increased cerebral metabolism in the orbital region of the frontal cortex and the caudate nuclei compared with controls (462–465). However, there has not been a consistent observation of increased activity in the caudate. One study also found increased metabolism in the cingulate gyrus of OCD patients compared with controls (438). PET has been used to explore the effects of different types of therapy in OCD. One study demonstrated that higher glucose metabolism in the orbitofrontal cortex (OFC) was associated with greater improvement with behavioral therapy and a worse outcome with fluoxetine treatment (466). Behavior therapy responders also had significant bilateral decreases in caudate metabolism (467). Furthermore, patients who responded to paroxetine had significantly lower metabolic rates in the right anterolateral OFC and right caudate nucleus, and lower pretreatment metabolism in both the left and right OFC predicted greater improvement with treatment (468). These results suggest that subjects with differing patterns of metabolism preferentially respond to behavioral therapy versus medication. In patients with OCD, behavioral therapy responders have been shown to have significant bilateral decreases in caudate glucose metabolic rates compared with poor responders (469). This study, as well as others, also suggested that there is a prefrontal cortico-striato-thalamic network that mediates the symptoms of OCD (470).

ANXIETY DISORDERS

PET has been employed to attempt to gain a better understanding of the neurophysiologic mechanisms underlying anxiety disorders. Rieman et al. (471–473) studied patients with panic disorders using H_2O PET and found that these patients have increased rCBF in the right parahippocampal gyrus in lactate-vulnerable patients (patients in whom intravenous infusion of sodium lactate can induce a panic attack) in a resting, nonpanic state, compared with controls. During a lactate-induced panic attack, the patients had increased rCBF bilaterally in the temporal poles, the claustrum, and the lateral putamen. In patients with generalized anxiety disorder, there was a decrease in the glucose metabolism in the right occipital and frontal cortex after benzodiazepine administration, suggesting that the anxiety response might be related more to overactivity in the right hemisphere. Furthermore, this overactivity can be corrected with benzodiazepine therapy. Patients with simple phobias might also be expected to have changes in cerebral metabolism or blood flow. However, Mountz et al. (474) did not find any changes in these patients in either the resting state or when exposed to a phobic stimuli compared with controls. This finding conflicts with the reports of anxiety response in normal patients mentioned previously. Further elucidation of the mechanisms underlying anxiety are needed.

EPILEPSY AND OTHER SEIZURE DISORDERS

Epilepsy affects 0.5% to 1.0% of the population, can cause focal or generalized seizures, and usually begins in childhood. In general, during an epileptic seizure, cerebral metabolism and blood flow are markedly increased. The focus of partial seizures can be identified using ^{18}F-FDG PET because these areas have increased metabolism during the seizure and decreased metabolism in the interictal period (475–479). It has been shown that single hypometabolic regions can be identified in 55% to 80% of patients with focal EEG abnormalities (480–482). However, performing ictal PET studies is somewhat impractical because of the short half-life of the positron emitters and other logistic reasons. One of the most effective treatments for partial epilepsy, refractory to medical intervention, is surgical removal of the involved area. Using high-resolution PET images, accurate localization of seizure foci can be achieved to aid in selecting the appropriate surgical intervention (483). It also appears that certain clinical features affect the metabolic and cerebral blood flow findings (484). The degree of asymmetry in the region of the seizure focus appears greater with increasing duration of the seizure disorder. However, another study did not find any association between complex partial seizure frequency or lifetime number of secondarily caused generalized seizures and hippocampal volume or metabolism (485). Cerebral glucose metabolism appears to have a greater rate of increase in asymmetry than does cerebral blood flow. These results indicate an uncoupling of cerebral metabolism and blood flow that is progressive and results from the differential response of glucose metabolism and blood flow to chronic seizure activity. The type of seizure preceding the PET study may also affect the metabolic landscape such that hypometabolism is limited to the epileptogenic zone if the preceding seizure is focal limbic, whereas patients with widespread limbic seizures have hypometabolism that included one or several additional areas of the limbic cortex (486).

Another important aspect of seizure studies is how to distinguish those patients who will do well postoperatively from those who will be less likely to benefit from temporal lobectomy. Several PET studies did not find any correlation between the severity of abnormal temporal lobe activity and the frequency of postoperative seizures (487,488). However, these studies had a limited number of patients and may not have been able to detect statistical differences. Other studies have shown that in those patients with hypometabolism only in the affected temporal lobe, there is a higher likelihood of a successful postsurgical outcome (489–491). It has also been shown that patients with a greater degree of hypometabolism in the temporal lobe (i.e., a more distinct asymmetry) tended to have a better outcome than those with a lesser degree of asymmetry (492,493). It may be that those patients without significant hypometabolism of the affected temporal lobe (i.e., minimal asymmetry between the temporal lobes) might have extratemporal or bitemporal seizure foci. These patients may therefore be less amenable to surgical resection. This is corroborated by other studies that have shown that patients with hypometabolism detected in the opposite hemisphere to the epileptic focus on EEG may be more likely to have postoperative seizures (494) and those patients with extratemporal hypometabolism tend to have a higher likelihood of postoperative seizures (495). We have recently reported that the ^{18}F-FDG PET finding of thalamic hypometabolism may be an important added measure in the evaluation of patients with temporal lobe epilepsy (TLE) with regard to postoperative seizure outcome (496). Compared with patients with no thalamic asymmetry, patients with ipsilateral thalamic hypometabolism had a slightly higher risk and those with contralateral hypometabolism had a markedly increased risk for having postoperative seizures.

The temporal lobe is the most common focus of partial epilepsy (Figs. 38.19 and 38.20). Studies show that the sensitivity

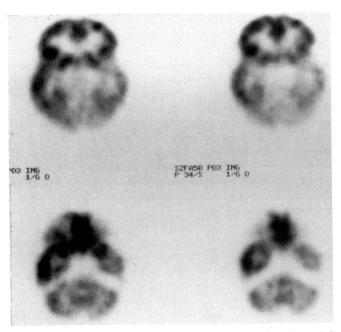

FIGURE 38.19. ^{18}F-FDG PET of a patient with a seizure focus in the left temporal lobe shown as hypometabolism in that area during postictal imaging.

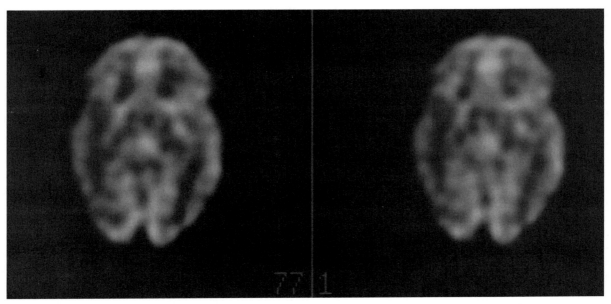

FIGURE 38.20. ^{18}F-FDG PET scan in a patient with medically refractory seizures that demonstrates hypometabolism in the right temporal region consistent with a seizure focus.

of PET in detecting TLE foci is greater than 70% in patients with partial complex seizures using ^{18}F-FDG (497–501) or ^{15}O CO$_2$ (502–504). However, a study by Sperling et al. (505) has shown a positive finding on PET in 44% of patients with TLE who had normal CT scans. One FDG PET study showed ipsilateral hypometabolism of the seizure focus in the temporal pole but relatively increased metabolism in the ipsilateral mesiobasal region (506). Contralateral to the seizure focus, metabolism was increased in the lateral temporal cortex and mesiobasal regions. A study using statistical parametric mapping (SPM) compared hemispheric asymmetry on ^{18}F-FDG PET images in patients with mesial TLE with controls (507). When the SPM program was used to detect temporal interhemispheric asymmetry, hypometabolism was identified on the side chosen for resection in most cases (sensitivity, 71%; specificity, 100%) and was predictive of favorable postsurgical outcome in 90% of the patients.

The other major site of seizure focus in partial epilepsy is the frontal lobe. Because many of these seizures begin in the medial or inferior aspects of the frontal lobe, scalp EEG readings do not provide adequate localization of foci (508,509). Franck et al. (510) used ^{18}F-FDG PET to study 13 patients with presumed frontal lobe epilepsy (FLE) and found PET to be the best modality for localizing seizure foci in this location. In addition, the authors suggested that PET might help in determining the site of surgical excision or suggest a contraindication to surgical intervention in patients with multiple or bilateral foci. One study of 180 surgical specimens from patients with FLE found a high correlation between hypometabolic regions on PET images and structural, histopathologic changes in the surgical specimens, again demonstrating the value of PET in detecting seizure foci (511).

Performing ictal PET studies is somewhat impractical because of the relatively short half-life of positron emitting isotopes such

as ^{18}F and other logistic reasons (512). However, several ictal PET studies have been reported in the literature that have been successful in detecting seizure foci in patients with partial seizures as hypermetabolic areas (513). Complex partial seizures are associated with bilaterally increased cerebral blood flow in a number of cortical areas, particularly the temporal and frontal lobes (514). In addition, these patients also had increased blood flow to the subcortical nuclei, which are activated during ictus.

PET imaging to measure various neurotransmitter systems has been employed to study patients with seizures. Initial studies of benzodiazepine receptor activity in TLE showed decreased benzodiazepine receptor activity in the medial temporal lobe (515). This reduction in benzodiazepine receptor activity may correlate with the frequency of seizures (516). A more recent study compared the results obtained from ^{18}F-FDG and ^{11}C-flumazenil (517). ^{18}F-FDG PET images showed a large area of hypometabolism in the epileptogenic temporal lobe (as determined by other diagnostic studies including scalp EEG and MRI). Both ^{18}F-FDG PET and ^{11}C-flumazenil PET reliably revealed the epileptogenic temporal lobe and neither agent proved superior to the other. Another study compared changes in benzodiazepine receptors in the thalami of patients with TLE (518). The dorsal medial nuclei showed significantly lower glucose metabolism and ^{11}C-flumazenil binding on the side of the epileptic focus. Interestingly, the lateral thalami showed bilateral hypermetabolism and increased ^{11}C-flumazenil binding.

FLE is associated with significantly reduced benzodiazepine receptor density in the anterior cerebellum contralateral to the seizure focus (519). On the other hand, mesial temporal lobe seizures were associated with reductions in the ipsilateral cerebellum. Another study reported that frontal lobe seizure foci were correctly identified by ^{11}C-flumazenil PET as an area of decreased benzodiazepine receptor density in all patients studied

(520). Several other studies of benzodiazepine receptors showed that the areas of abnormal benzodiazepine receptor binding was more extensive than anatomic abnormalities observed on MRI or even than the hypometabolic areas observed on interictal FDG PET (521,522).

CEREBRAL ACTIVATION STUDIES

One of the most intriguing uses of PET is to measure cerebral activation during various physiologic stimulation paradigms. The results from such studies may help define specific areas of the brain that are responsible for various aspects of thought, speech, sensation, movement, emotion, and other complicated functions. In the past decade, there have probably been several thousand brain activation studies using PET imaging, as well as the more recent development of functional MRI. This section considers some of the basic targets and elements of these experiments but obviously will not provide an exhaustive analysis of such studies. Usually the subjects who undergo an activation study serve as their own control group because they are scanned at rest and during stimulation. However, there have been conflicting reports regarding how a resting state should be identified. Greenberg et al. (523) found that when subjects are imaged with both eyes and ears closed, there is no significant difference between the metabolism in the right and left hemispheres. However, Mazziotta et al. (524) did find significantly decreased metabolism in some right hemispheric structures under these same conditions. Subjects imaged with both eyes and ears opened with low level ambient light and noise have been found to have no asymmetries in hemispheric metabolism (525), although Finkelstein et al. (526) did find left hemispheric activation in some subjects.

Kushner et al. (527) used ^{18}F-FDG PET to study the retinotopic organization in the primary visual cortex. The results from this study showed that visual stimulation of either hemifield resulted in increased metabolism in the contralateral striate cortex. Furthermore, there was slightly increased metabolism in the right frontal and parietal cortices compared with the left, suggesting that the right hemisphere might be more specialized to visual processing than the left. Phelps et al. (528) found that metabolic activation of the striate and peristriate areas correlated with increasing the complexity of visual stimulation. Subjects had increases in metabolism of 45% in the striate and 59% in the peristriate areas when observing a complex outdoors scene compared with the subject at rest with eyes closed. The determination of visual forms and position may occur in slightly different parts of the brain with form determination activating the occipitotemporal area and position determination activating the occipitoparietal area (529). The parietofrontal network, as well as the right hippocampus, may also play an important role in the ability to generate topographic maps of the environment (530).

A number of studies have investigated the neurophysiologic response to various word tasks, including listening to words, identifying words, and speaking words. Petersen et al. (531) used ^{15}O H$_2$O to measure changes in blood flow in subjects who were given several different types of visual and auditory tests.

They found that specific areas of the brain were responsible for different functions. These were identified as the primary receptive area for visual or auditory perception of single words, the articulation-association area used for producing verbal output when an identified word is spoken, and the semantic processing area that is activated when a subject is asked to determine a use for a particular identified word. Using ^{18}F-FDG PET, Greenberg et al. (523) found that when subjects listened monaurally to a meaningful English story, the contralateral superior temporal lobe was activated more than the ipsilateral temporal cortex. However, Mazziotta et al. (532) found that subjects hearing the story had activation of the left temporal lobe regardless of which ear was stimulated. In addition, if the subject was stimulated by musical chords, the right inferior frontal, parietal, and superior temporal lobes were activated. Interestingly, if subjects were asked to discriminate between sequences of tones, those who used analytic schemes for discrimination had increased metabolism in the left hemisphere, whereas nonanalytic subjects had increased metabolism in the right hemisphere. There have been other reports describing studies in which more specific paradigms have been administered to determine the precise location of functional sites (533).

Studies have also explored the brain areas involved in quantitation and have found that during calculation there was activation in the medial frontal/cingulate gyri, left dorsolateral prefrontal cortex, left anterior insular cortex and right anterior insular cortex/putamen, left lateral parietal cortex, and the medial thalamus (534). Another study examined more specific areas involved in handling numbers; the processing of arabic digits produced activation of the occipitoparietal areas, as well as a the right anterior insula (535).

Heiss et al. (536) and other groups have used PET in measuring cerebral activity with memory challenges. In general, memory function is associated with activation of limbic structures and the temporal, parietal, and occipital association areas (537, 538). Friston et al. (537) indicated that the particular areas involved with word memory function are the prefrontal cortex, the superior parietal cortex, and the left parahippocampal region. Decreases in the physiologic activation of these areas is often associated with memory deficit states such as AD and transient global amnesia. (The latter has been found to be associated with a decreased metabolism bilaterally in the mesial temporal lobe.) There also appear to be subtle differences between males and females in brain activation during memory tasks that may account for why women usually perform better on such tasks (539). PET studies of how the brain retrieves complex memories has shown that information about the auditory components of multisensory events is stored in the auditory responsive cortex but interestingly is reactivated at retrieval, suggesting that part of an encoded stimulus complex can evoke the whole experience on retrieval (540). A study of visual memory of faces showed that recent memory for faces is primarily a frontal-lobe task, whereas well-learned recognition memory for faces uses a more distributed neural circuit that includes the visual areas, which appear to serve as memory-storage sites (541). Finally, autobiographic memory retrieval results in significantly increased activity in the left frontal cortex with concomitant activation in the inferior temporal and occipital lobes in the left hemisphere (542).

These PET activation studies have helped to elucidate our understanding of cerebral function and its relation to mental activities and behavior (543–545). For example, investigators (546–548) have found that when subjects performed purposely willed tasks or tasks that required sustained attention, there was activation of the prefrontal cortex. The medial prefrontal cortex, temporoparietal junction, basal temporal regions, and extrastriate cortex may actually form a network for processing information about intentions and make inferences about other people's mental states, based on the ability to make inferences about other creatures' actions (549). PET imaging may even help determine how human beings perceive reality and keep a running story of events that happen via activation of the orbitofrontal cortex, which may sort out mental associations that pertain to ongoing reality (550). PET offers the ability to study how the brain works and may eventually determine more specifically the interrelationships between various neural structures and how these structures correlate with specific mental tasks.

Emotions are another important facet of brain function that have been evaluated with PET. It appears that the anterior paralimbic regions of the brain mediate negative emotional states such as guilt in healthy individuals (551). The amygdala also appears involved in arousing stimuli, and not just emotionally aversive stimuli (552). Similarly, anger has been associated with activation of the left orbitofrontal cortex, right anterior cingulate cortex affective division, and bilateral anterior temporal poles (553).

CONCLUSION

Overall, PET imaging will continue to play a major role in the evaluation of patients with a variety of neurologic and psychiatric disorders. PET will be useful in the clinical setting to assist with diagnosis, follow clinical course, evaluate patients for therapy, and assess the effects of therapeutic interventions. PET imaging will also continue to help unlock the mysteries of the human brain by establishing how various structures function independently and as a complex network to provide human beings with the extensive set of sensory, experiential, behavioral, and cognitive abilities.

REFERENCES

1. Kuhl DE, Edwards RQ. Image separation of radioisotope scanning. *Radiology* 1963;80:653–662.
2. Kuhl DE, Edwards RQ, Ricci AR et al. The MARK IV system for radionuclide computed tomography of the brain. *Radiology* 1976;121:405–413.
3. Alavi A, Hirsch LJ. Studies of central nervous system disorders with single photon emission computed tomography and positron emission tomography. Evolution over the past 2 decades. *Semin Nucl Med* 1991;21:58–81.
4. Budinger TF. Future developments in positron-emission tomography for incorporation into the clinical sphere. *Invest Radiol* 1993;28(Suppl 3):S142–143.
5. Ido T, Wan CN, Casella V et al. Labeled 2-deoxyglucose analogs. 18F-labeled 2-deoxyglucose-2-fluoro-D-glucose, 2-deoxy-2-fluoro-D-manose and 14C-2-deoxy-2-fluoro-D-glucose. *J Label Comp Radiopharm* 1978;14:175–183.
6. Ter-Pogossian MM, Phelps ME, Hoffman EJ et al. A positron emission transaxial tomography for nuclear medicine imaging (PET). *Radiology* 1975;114:89–98.
7. Phelps ME, Hoffman EJ, Mullani NA et al. Design considerations for a positron emission transaxial tomograph (PET-III). *IEEE Trans Nucl Sci NS* 1976;23:516–522.
8. Therapeutic and Technology Assessment Subcommittee of the American Academy of Neurological Assessment. Positron emission tomography. *Neurology* 1991;41:163–167.
9. Shtern F. Positron emission tomography as a diagnostic tool: a reassessment based on literature review. *Invest Radiol* 1992;27:165–168.
10. The Workshop Panel. Advances in clinical imaging using positron emission tomography. National Cancer Institute workshop statement. *Arch Intern Med* 1990;150:735–739.
11. Fu CHY, McGuire PK. Functional neuroimaging in psychiatry. *Phil Trans R Soc Lond B* 1999;354:1359–1370.
12. Diksic M, Reba RC, eds. *Radiopharmaceuticals and brain pathology studied with PET and SPECT*. Boca Raton: CRC Press, 1991.
13. Kung HF. Overview of radiopharmaceuticals for diagnosis of central nervous disorders. *Crit Rev Clin Lab Sci* 1991;28:269–286.
14. Maziere B, Maziere M. Positron emission tomography studies of brain receptors. *Fundam Clin Pharmacol* 1991;5:61–91.
15. Gatley SJ, DeGrado TR, Kornguth ML et al. Radiopharmaceuticals for positron emission tomography: development of new, innovative tracers for measuring the rates of physiologic and biochemical processes. *Acta Radiol (Stockh)* 1990;374(Suppl):7–11.
16. Kopin TJ. In-vivo quantitative imaging of catecholaminergic nerve terminals in brain and peripheral organs using positron emission tomography (PET). *J Neural Transm* 1990;32(Suppl):19–27.
17. Sadzot B, Mayberg HS, Frost JJ. Detection and quantification of opiate receptors in man by positron emission tomography. Potential applications to the study of pain. *Neurophysiol Clin* 1990;20:323–334.
18. Frost JJ. Receptor imaging by positron emission tomography and single-photon emission computed tomography. *Invest Radiol* 1992;27(Suppl 2):S54–S58.
19. Abadie P, Baron JC, Bisserbe JG et al. Central benzodiazepine receptors in human brain: estimation of regional Bmax and KD values with positron emission tomography. *Eur J Pharmacol* 1992;213:107–115.
20. Varastet M, Brouillet E, Chavoix C et al. In vivo visualization of central muscarinic receptors using [11C] quinuclidinyl benzilate and positron emission tomography in baboons. *Eur J Pharmacol* 1992;213:275–284.
21. Mielke R, Kessler J, Szelies B et al. Normal and pathological aging—findings of positron-emission-tomography. *J Neural Trans* 1998;105:821–837.
22. Moeller JR, Ishikawa T, Dhawan V et al. The metabolic topography of normal aging. *J Cerebr Blood Flow Metab* 1996;16:385–398.
23. Chawluk JB, Alavi A, Dann R et al. Positron emission tomography in aging and dementia: effect of cerebral atrophy. *J Nucl Med* 1987;28:431–437.
24. Kuhl DE, Metter EJ, Rieger WH et al. Effects of human aging on patterns of local cerebral glucose utilization determined by the 18-F fluorodeoxyglucose method. *J Cerebr Blood Flow Metab* 1987;7:S411.
25. deLeon M, George A, Tomanelli J et al. Positron emission tomography studies of normal aging, a replication of PET III and 18-FDG using PET IV and II-CDG. *Neurobiol Aging* 1987;8:319–323.
26. Weiss D, Souder E, Alavi A et al. Effects of normal aging on whole brain and regional glucose metabolism as assessed by F-18 positron emission tomography. *J Nucl Med* 1990;31:771.
27. Loessner A, Alavi A, Lewadnrowski KU et al. Regional cerebral function determined by FDG-PET in healthy volunteers: normal patterns and changes with age. 1995;36:1141–1149.
28. Eberling JL, Nordahl TE, Kusubov N et al. Reduced temporal lobe glucose metabolism in aging. *J Neuroimaging* 1995;5:178–182.
29. Murphy DGM, DeCarli C, McIntosh AR et al. Sex differences in human brain morphometry and metabolism: an in vivo quantitative

magnetic resonance imaging and positron emission tomography study on the effect of aging. *Arch Gen Psychiatry* 1996;53:585–594.

30. Cabeza R, Anderson ND, Houle S et al. Age-related differences in neural activity during item and temporal-order memory retrieval: a positron emission tomography study. *J Cog Neurosci* 2000;12: 197–206.

31. Reuter-Lorenz PA, Jonides J, Smith EE et al. Age differences in the frontal lateralization of verbal and spatial working memory revealed by PET. *J Cog Neurosci* 2000;12:174–187.

32. Cabeza R, Grady CL, Nyberg L et al. Age-related differences in neural activity during memory encoding and retrieval: a positron emission tomography study. *J Cog Neurosci* 1997;17:391–400.

33. Della-Maggiore V, Sekuler A, Grady CL et al. Corticolimbic interactions associated with performance on a short-term memory task are modified by age. *J Neurosci* 2000;20:8410–8416(Online).

34. Calautti C, Serrati C, Baron JC. Effects of age on brain activation during auditory-cued thumb-to-index opposition: A positron emission tomography study. *Stroke* 2001;32:139–146(Online).

35. Levine BK, Beason-Held LL, Purpura KP. Age-related differences in visual perception: a PET study. *Neurobiol Aging* 2000;21:577–584.

36. McIntosh AR, Sekuler AB, Penpeci C et al. Recruitment of unique neural systems to support visual memory in normal aging. *Curr Biol* 1999;9:1275–1278.

37. Grady CL, McIntosh AR, Bookstein F. Age-related changes in regional cerebral blood flow during working memory for faces. *Neuroimage* 1998;8:409–425.

38. Madden DJ, Turkington TG, Provenzale JM et al. Adult age differences in the functional neuroanatomy of verbal recognition memory. *Human Brain Mapping* 1999;7:115–135.

39. Hazlett EA, Buchsbaum MS, Mohs RC et al. Age-related shift in brain region activity during successful memory performance. *Neurobiol Aging* 1998;19:437–445.

40. Yoshii F, Barker WW, Chang JY et al. Sensitivity of cerebral glucose metabolism to age, gender, brain volume, brain atrophy, and cerebrovascular risk factors. *J Cerebr Blood Flow Metab* 1988;8:654–661.

41. Clark C, Hayden M, Hollenberg S et al. Controlling for cerebral atrophy in positron emission tomography data. *J Cerebr Blood Flow Metab* 1987;7:510–512.

42. Alavi A, Newberg A, Souder E et al. Quantitative analysis of PET and MRI data in normal aging and Alzheimer's disease: atrophy weighted total brain metabolism and absolute whole brain metabolism as reliable discriminators. *J Nucl Med* 1993;34:1681–1687.

43. Schlageter NL, Horwitz B, Creasey H et al. Relation of measured brain glucose utilization and cerebral atrophy in man. *J Neurol Neurosurg Psychiatry* 1987;50:779–785.

44. Kaasinen V, Vilkman H, Hietala J et al. Age-related dopamine D2/D3 receptor loss in extrastriatal regions of the human brain. *Neurobiol Aging* 2000;21:683–688.

45. Volkow ND, Gur RC, Wang GJ et al. Association between decline in brain dopamine activity with age and cognitive and motor impairment in healthy individuals. *Am J Psychiatry* 1998;155:344–349.

46. Backman L, Ginovart N, Dixon RA et al. Age-related cognitive deficits mediated by changes in the striatal dopamine system. *Am J Psychiatry* 2000;157:635–637.

47. Wang Y, Chan GL, Holden JE et al. Age-dependent decline of dopamine D1 receptors in human brain: a PET study. *Synapse* 1998;30: 56–61.

48. Pohjalainen T, Rinne JO, Nagren K et al. Sex differences in the striatal dopamine D2 receptor binding characteristics in vivo. *Am J Psychiatry* 1998;155:768–773.

49. Volkow ND, Logan J, Fowler JS et al. Association between age-related decline in brain dopamine activity and impairment in frontal and cingulate metabolism. *Am J Psychiatry* 2000;157:75–80.

50. Yoshida T, Kuwabara Y, Sasaki M et al. Sex-related differences in the muscarinic acetylcholinergic receptor in the healthy human brain—a positron emission tomography study. *Ann Nucl Med* 2000;14: 97–101.

51. Lee KS, Frey KA, Koeppe RA et al. In vivo quantification of cerebral muscarinic receptors in normal human aging using positron emission tomography and [11C]tropanyl benzilate. *J Cereb Blood Flow Metab* 1996;16:303–310.

52. Rosier A, Dupont P, Peuskens J et al. Visualisation of loss of 5-HT2A receptors with age in healthy volunteers using [18F]altanserin and positron emission tomographic imaging. *Psychiatr Res* 1996;68: 11–22.

53. Meltzer CC, Smith G, Price JC et al. Reduced binding of [18F]altanserin to serotonin type 2A receptors in aging: persistence of effect after partial volume correction. *Brain Res* 1998;813:167–171.

54. Fowler JS, Volkow ND, Wang GJ et al. Age-related increases in brain monoamine oxidase B in living healthy human subjects. *Neurobiol Aging* 1997;18:431–435.

55. McKhann G, Drachman D, Folstein M et al. Clinical diagnosis of Alzheimer's disease: report of the NINCDS-ADRDA Work Group under the auspices of Department of Health and Human Services Task Force on Alzheimer's Disease. *Neurology* 1984;34:939–944.

56. Tierney MC, Gisher RH, Lewis AJ et al. The NINCDS-ADRDA Workgroup criteria for the clinical diagnosis of probable Alzheimer's disease. A clinical pathological study of 57 cases. *Neurology* 1988;38: 359–364.

57. Joachim CL, Morris JH, Selkow DJ. Clinical diagnosed Alzheimer's disease. Autopsy results in 150 cases. *Ann Neurol* 1988;24:50–56.

58. Friedland RP, Budinger TF, Brant-Zawadzki M et al. The diagnosis of Alzheimer-type dementia. A preliminary comparison of positron emission tomography and proton magnetic resonance. *JAMA* 1984; 252:2750–2752.

59. Friedland RP, Jagust WJ; Huesman RH et al. Regional cerebral glucose transport and utilization in Alzheimer's disease. *Neurology* 1989; 39:1427–1434.

60. Foster NL, Chase TN, Mansi L et al. Cortical abnormalities in Alzheimer's disease. *Ann Neurol* 1984;16:649–654.

61. Cutler NR, Haxby J, Duara R et al. Clinical history, brain metabolism, and neurophysiological function in Alzheimer's disease. *Ann Neurol* 1985;18:298–309.

62. Foster NL, Chase TN, Patronas NJ et al. Cerebral mapping of apraxia in Alzheimer's disease by positron emission tomography. *Ann Neurol* 1986;19:139–143.

63. Loewenstein DA, Barker WW, Chang JY et al. Predominant left hemisphere metabolic dysfunction in dementia. *Arch Neurol* 1989;46: 146–152.

64. Jagust WJ, Friedland RP, Budinger TF et al. Longitudinal studies of regional cerebral metabolism in Alzheimer's disease. *Neurology* 1988; 38:909–912.

65. Haxby JC, Grady CL, Koss E et al. Heterogeneous anterior-posterior metabolic patterns in dementia of the Alzheimer type. *Neurology* 1988; 38:1853–1863.

66. Sheridan PH, Sato S, Foster N et al. Relations of EEG alpha background to parietal lobe function in Alzheimer's disease as measured by positron emission tomography and psychometry. *Neurology* 1988; 38:747–750.

67. Alavi A, Reivich M, Ferris S et al. Regional cerebral glucose metabolism in aging and senile dementia as determined by 18F-deoxyglucose and positron emission tomography. In: Hoyer S, ed. *The aging brain—physiological and pathophysiological aspects.* Berlin: Springer-Verlag, 1982:87–195.

68. Heiss WD, Kessler J, Szelies B et al. Positron emission tomography in the differential diagnosis of organic dementias. *J Neural Transm* 1991;33(Suppl):13–19.

69. Jamieson DG, Chawluck JB, Alavi A et al. The effect of disease severity on local cerebral glucose metabolism in Alzheimer's disease. *J Cerebr Blood Flow Metab* 1987;7:S410.

70. Kumar A, Schapiro MB, Grady C et al. High-resolution PET studies in Alzheimer's disease. *Neuropsychopharmacology* 1991;4:35–46.

71. Bonte FJ, Hom J, Tinter R et al. Single photon tomography in Alzheimer's disease and the dementias. *Semin Nucl Med* 1990;20:342–352.

72. Rapoport SI, Horowitz B, Grady CL et al. Abnormal brain glucose metabolism in Alzheimer's disease as measured by positron emission tomography. *Adv Exp Med Biol* 1991;291:231–248.

73. Ichimiya A, Herholz K, Mielke R et al. Difference of regional cerebral

metabolic pattern between presenile and senile dementia of the Alzheimer type: a factor analytic study. *J Neurol Sci* 1994;123:11–17.

74. Kuhl DE, Small GW, Riege WH et al. Cerebral metabolic patterns before the diagnosis of probable Alzheimer's disease. *J Cereb Flood Flow Metab* 1987;7:406(abst).

75. Frackowiak R, Pozilli C, Legg N et al. Regional cerebral oxygen supply and utilization in dementia. A clinical and physiological study with oxygen-15 and positron emission tomography. *Brain* 1981;104: 753–788.

76. Foster NL, Mann U, Mohr E et al. Focal cerebral glucose hypometabolism in definite Alzheimer's disease. *Ann Neurol* 1989;26:132–133.

77. Mazziotta JC, Frackowiak RSJ, Phelps ME. The use of positron emission tomography in the clinical assessment of dementia. *Semin Nucl Med* 1992;22:232–246.

78. Mentis MJ, Weinstein EA, Horwitz B. Abnormal brain glucose metabolism in the delusional misidentification syndromes: a positron emission tomography study in Alzheimer disease. *Biol Psychiatry* 1995; 38:438–449.

79. Jelic V, Nordberg A. Early diagnosis of Alzheimer disease with positron emission tomography. *Alzheimer Dis Assoc Disord* 2000;14(Suppl 1):S109–113.

80. Cohen, RM, Andreason PJ, Sunderland T. The ratio of mesial to neocortical temporal lobe blood flow as a predictor of dementia. *J Am Geriatr Soc* 1997;45:329–333.

81. Kennedy AM, Rossor MN, Frackowiak RS. Positron emission tomography in familial Alzheimer disease. *Alzheimer Dis Assoc Disord* 1995; 9:17–20.

82. Newberg A, Alavi A, Souder E et al. A comparison of FDG-PET and MRI data from patients with atypical dementias and Alzheimer's disease (AD). *J Nucl Med* 1992;33:965(abst).

83. Newberg A, Alavi A, Clark C. Comparison of FDG-PET and levels of tau protein in the diagnosis of patients with dementia. *J Nucl Med* 2000;41:64P.

84. Brun A, Gustafson L. Distribution of cerebral degeneration in Alzheimer's disease: a clinicopathological study. *Arch Psychiatr Nervenkr* 1976;223:15–33.

85. Perry EK, Tomlinson BE, Blessed G et al. Neuropathologic and biochemical observations on the noradrenergic system in Alzheimer's disease. *J Neurol Sci* 1981;51:279–287.

86. Terry RD, Katzman R. Senile dementia of the Alzheimer type. *Ann Neurol* 1983;14:497–506.

87. Brun A, Englund E. Regional pattern of degeneration in Alzheimer's disease: neuronal loss and histopathological grading. *Histopathology* 1981;5:549–564.

88. Mitzutani T, Amano N, Sasaki H et al. Senile dementia of Alzheimer type characterized by laminar neuronal loss exclusively in the hippocampus, parahippocampus and medial occipitotemporal cortex. *Acta Neuropathol* 1990;80:575–580.

89. Brun A, Gustafson L. Limbic lobe involvement in presenile dementia. *Arch Psychiatr Nervenkr* 1978;226:79–93.

90. Hubbard BM, Fenton GW, Anderson JM. A quantitative histological study of early clinical and preclinical Alzheimer's disease. *Neuropathol Appl Neurobiol* 1990;16:111–121.

91. Katzman R, Saitoh T. Advances in Alzheimer's disease. *FASEB J* 1991; 5:278–286.

92. Van Housen GW, Hyman BT. Hippocampal formation: anatomy and the pattern of pathology in Alzheimer's disease. *Prog Brain Res* 1990;83:445–457.

93. Kushner M, Tobin M, Alavi A et al. Cerebellar glucose consumption in normal and pathologic states using fluorine-FDG and PET. *J Nucl Med* 1987;28:1667–1670.

94. Chase TN, Foster NL, Fedio P et al. Regional cortical dysfunction in Alzheimer's disease as determined by positron emission tomography. *Ann Neurol* 1984;15:S170–174.

95. Haxby JC, Duara R, Grady CL et al. Relationship between neuropsychological and cerebral metabolic asymmetries in early Alzheimer's disease. *J Cereb Blood Flow Metab* 1985;5:193–200.

96. McGeer EG, Peppard RP, McGeer PL et al. 18-Fluorodeoxyglucose positron emission tomography studies in presumed Alzheimer cases. *Can J Neurol Sci* 1990;17:1–11.

97. Grady CL, Haxby JV, Schlageter NL et al. Stability of metabolic and neuropsychological asymmetries in dementia of the Alzheimer type. *Neurology* 1986;36:1390–1392.

98. Koss E, Friedland RP, Ober BA. Differences in lateral hemispheric asymmetries of glucose utilization between early- and late-onset Alzheimer type dementia. *Am J Psychiatry* 1985;142:638–640.

99. Duara R, Barker WW, Chang J et al. Viability of neocortical function shown in behavioral activation state PET studies in Alzheimer's disease. *J Cerebr Blood Flow Metab* 1992;12:927–934.

100. Siegel BV Jr, Shihabuddin L, Buchsbaum MS et al. Gender differences in cortical glucose metabolism in Alzheimer's disease and normal aging. *J Neuropsychiatry Clin Neurosci* 1996;8:211–214.

101. Chawluk JB, Dann R, Alavi A et al. The effect of focal cerebral atrophy in positron emission tomographic studies of aging and dementia. *Nucl Med Biol* 1990;17:797–804.

102. Labbe C, Froment JC, Kennedy A et al. Positron emission tomography metabolic data corrected for cortical atrophy using magnetic resonance imaging. *Alzheimer Dis Assoc Disord* 1996;10:141–170.

103. Alavi A, Newberg A, Souder E et al. Is absolute whole brain glucose metabolism a sensitive marker for Alzheimer's disease? *J Nucl Med* 1992;33:940(abst).

104. Kuhl DE, Minoshima S, Frey KA et al. Limited donepezil inhibition of acetylcholinesterase measured with positron emission tomography in living Alzheimer cerebral cortex. *Ann Neurol* 2000;48:391–395.

105. Nordberg A, Amberla K, Shigeta M et al. Long-term tacrine treatment in three mild Alzheimer patients: effects on nicotinic receptors, cerebral blood flow, glucose metabolism, EEG, and cognitive abilities. *Alzheimer Dis Assoc Disord* 1998;12:228–237.

106. Mielke R, Moller HJ, Erkinjuntti T et al. Propentofylline in the treatment of vascular dementia and Alzheimer-type dementia: overview of phase I and phase II clinical trials. *Alzheimer Dis Assoc Disord* 1998; 12(Suppl 2):S29–S35.

107. Duara R. Utilization of positron emission tomography in research and clinical applications. In: Duara R, ed. *Frontiers of clinical neuroscience*, vol 10. New York: Wiley Liss, 1990:1–12.

108. Pawlik G, Holthoff V, Rudolf J et al. Vasculitic dementia. Characteristic changes of regional brain function demonstrated by PET. *J Cerebr Blood Flow Metab* 1989;9(Suppl 1):S534.

109. Alavi A, Newberg A, Souder E et al. Comparison of quantitative MRI and PET between patients with dementia of the Alzheimer type and multi-infarct dementia. *J Stroke Cerebrovasc Dis* 1992;2:218–221.

110. Gibbs J, Frackowiak R, Legg N. Regional cerebral blood flow and oxygen metabolism in dementia due to vascular disease. *Gerontology* 1986;32(Suppl 1):84–89.

111. Pozilli C, Itoh M, Matsuzawa T et al. Positron emission tomography in minor ischemic stroke using oxygen-15-steady state technique. *J Cerebr Blood Flow Metab* 1987;7:137–144.

112. De Reuck J, Decoo D, Marchau M et al. Positron emission tomography in vascular dementia. *J Neurol Sci* 1998;154:55–61.

113. Mesulam MM. Slowly progressive aphasia without generalized dementia, *Ann Neurol* 1982;11:592–598.

114. Gordon B, Selnes O. Progressive aphasia "without dementia:" evidence of more widespread involvement. *Neurology* 1984;34:102.

115. Luzzatti C, Poeck K. An early description of slowly progressive aphasia. *Arch Neurol* 1991;48:228–229.

116. Shuttleworth EC, Huber SJ. The naming disorder of dementia of Alzheimer type. *Brain Lang* 1988;34:222–234.

117. Chawluk JB, Mesulam MM, Hurtig H et al. Slowly progressive aphasia without generalized dementia: studies with positron emission tomography. *Ann Neurol* 1986;19:68–74.

118. Tyrrell PJ, Warrington EK, Frackowiak RSJ, et al. Heterogeneity in progressive aphasia due to focal cortical atrophy. *Brain* 1990;113: 1321–1336.

119. Hachisuka K, Uchida M, Nozaki Y et al. Primary progressive aphasia presenting as conduction aphasia. *J Neurol Sci* 1999;167:137–141.

120. Kempler D, Metter EJ, Riege WH et al. Slowly progressive aphasia: three cases with language, memory, CT and PET data. *J Neurol Neurosurg Psychiatry* 1990;53:987–993.

121. Newberg A, Alavi A, Souder E et al. Quantitative PET and MRI analysis in patients with primary progressive aphasia (PPA). *J Nucl Med* 1992;33:857(abst).

122. Kamo H, McGeer PL, Harrop R et al. Positron emission tomography and histopathology in Pick's disease. *Neurology* 1988;38:228(abst).

123. Kamo H, McGeer R, Harrop R et al. Positron emission tomography and histopathology in Pick's disease. *Neurology* 1987;37:439.

124. Salmon E, Maquet P, Sadzot B et al. Positron emission tomography in Alzheimer's and Pick's disease. *J Neurol* 1988;235:S1.

125. Lieberman AP, Trojanowski JQ, Lee VM et al. Cog, neuroimaging, and pathological studies in a patient with Pick's disease. *Ann Neurol* 1998;43:259–265.

126. Groen JJ, Hekster REM. Computed tomography in Pick's disease. Findings in a family affected in three consecutive generations. *J Comput Assist Tomogr* 1982;6:907–911.

127. Wechsler AF, Verity MA, Rosenchein S et al. Pick's disease. A clinical computed tomographic, and histologic study with Golgi impregnation observations. *Arch Neurol* 1982;39:287–290.

128. Wilson CB. Metabolic imaging of human brain tumors. *Semin Neurol* 1989;9:388–393.

129. DiChiro G. Positron emission tomography using (18F) fluorodeoxyglucose in brain tumors. A powerful diagnostic and prognostic tool. *Invest Radiol* 1986;22:360–371.

130. DiChiro G, DeLaPaz RL, Brooks RA et al. Glucose utilization of cerebral gliomas measured by 18F fluorodeoxy-glucose and positron emission tomography. *Neurology* 1982;32:1323–1329.

131. O'Tuama LA. Methionine transport in brain tumors. *J Neuropsychiatry* 1989;1(Suppl 1):S37–S44.

132. Hiesiger E, Logan J, Wolf AP et al. Serial PET studies of human cerebral malignancy with (1-11C) putrescine (11C-PUT) and (1-11C)2-deoxy-D-glucose (11C-2DG). *J Nucl Med* 1986;27:889(abst).

133. Patronas NJ, Brooks RA, DeLaPaz RL et al. Glycolytic rate (PET) and contrast enhancement (CT) in human cerebral gliomas. *AJNR* 1983;4:533–535.

134. Alavi J, Alavi A, Dann R et al. Metabolic brain imaging correlated with clinical features and brain tumors. *J Nucl Med* 1985;18:P64(abst).

135. Alavi JB, Alavi A, Chawluk J et al. Positron emission tomography in patients with glioma. A predictor of prognosis. *Cancer* 1988;62:1074–1078.

136. Delbeke D, Meyerowitz C, Lapidus RL et al. Optimal cutoff levels of F-18 fluorodeoxyglucose uptake in the differentiation of low-grade from high-grade brain tumors with PET. *Radiology* 1995;195:47–52.

137. Katschten B, Stevenaert A, Sadzot B et al. Preoperative evaluation of 54 gliomas by PET with fluorine-18-fluorodexyglucose and/or carbon-11-methionine. *J Nucl Med* 1998;39:778–785.

138. Fulham MJ, Melisi JW, Nishimiya J et al. Neuroimaging of juvenile pilocytic astrocytomas: an enigma. *Radiology* 1993;189:221–225.

139. Meyer PT, Spetzger U, Mueller HD et al. High F-18 FDG uptake in a low-grade supratentorial ganglioma: a positron emission tomography case report. *Clin Nucl Med* 2000;25:694–697.

140. Aronen HJ, Pardo FS, Kennedy DN et al. High microvascular blood volume is associated with high glucose uptake and tumor angiogenesis in human gliomas. *Clin Cancer Res* 2000;6:2189–2200.

141. Hustinx R, Smith RJ, Benard F et al. Can the standardized uptake value characterize primary brain tumors on FDG-PET? *Eur J Nucl Med* 1999;26:1501–1509.

142. Roelcke U, Leenders KL. Positron emission tomography in patients with primary CNS lymphoma. *J Neuro-Oncol* 1999;43:231–236.

143. Lassen U, Andersen P, Daugaard G et al. Metabolic and hemodynamic evaluation of brain metastases from small cell lung cancer with positron emission tomography. *Clin Cancer Res* 1998;4:2591–2597.

144. Derlon JM, Petit-Taboue MC, Chapon F et al. The in vivo metabolic pattern of low-grade brain gliomas: a positron emission tomographic study using 18F-fluorodeoxyglucose and 11C-L-methylmethionine. *Neurosurgery* 1997;40:276–287.

145. DeLaPaz RL, Patronias NJ, Brooks RA et al. Positron emission tomographic study of suppression of gray matter glucose utilization by brain tumors. *AJNR* 1983;4:826–829.

146. Patronas NJ, DiChiro G, Smith BH et al. Depressed cerebellar glucose metabolism in supratentorial tumors. *Brain Res* 1984;291:93–101.

147. Otte A, Roelcke U, von Ammon K et al. Crossed cerebellar diaschisis and brain tumor biochemistry studied with positron emission tomography, [18F]fluorodeoxyglucose and [11C]methionine. *J Neurol Sci* 1998;156:73–77.

148. Newberg AB, Alavi A, Alavi J. Contralateral cortical diaschisis in a patient with cerebellar astrocytoma after radiation therapy. *Clin Nucl Med* 2000;25:431–433.

149. Gross MW, Weber WA, Feldmann HJ et al. The value of F-18-fluorodeoxyglucose PET for the 3-D radiation treatment planning of malignant gliomas. *Int J Radiat Oncol Biol Phys* 1998;41:989–995.

150. Kaplan AM, Lawson MA, Spataro J et al. Positron emission tomography using [18F] fluorodeoxyglucose and [11C] l-methionine to metabolically characterize dysembryoplastic neuroepithelial tumors. *J Child Neurol* 1999;14:673–677.

151. Coleman RE, Hoffman JM, Hanson MW et al. Clinical application of PET for the evaluation of brain tumors. *J Nucl Med* 1991;32:616–622.

152. Deshmukh A, Scott JA, Palmer EL et al. Impact of fluorodeoxyglucose positron emission tomography on the clinical management of patients with glioma. *Clin Nucl Med* 1996;21:720–725.

153. Goldman S, Levivier M, Pirotte B et al. Regional glucose metabolism and histopathology of gliomas. A study on positron emission tomography-guided stereotactic biopsy. *Cancer* 1996;78:1098–1106.

154. Patronas NJ, DiChiro G, Kufta C et al. Prediction of survival in glioma patients by means of positron emission tomography. *J Nucl Med* 1985;18:P64(abst).

155. Herholz K, Ziffling P, Staffen W et al. Uncoupling of hexose transport and phosphorylation in human gliomas demonstrated by PET. *Eur J Cancer Clin Oncol* 1988;24:1139–1150.

156. Vlassenko AG, Thiessen B, Beattie BJ et al. Evaluation of early response to SU101 target-based therapy in patients with recurrent supratentorial malignant gliomas using FDG PET and Gd-DTPA MRI. *J Neuro-Oncol* 2000;46:249–259.

157. De Witte O, Levivier M, Violon P et al. Prognostic value positron emission tomography with [18F]fluoro-2-deoxy-D-glucose in the low-grade glioma. *Neurosurgery* 1996;39:470–476.

158. DiChiro G, Oldfield E, Wright DC et al. Cerebral necrosis after radiotherapy and/or intraarterial chemotherapy for brain tumors. PET and neuropathologic studies. *AJR* 1988;150:189–198.

159. Rozental JM, Levine RL, Nickles RJ et al. Changes in glucose uptake by malignant gliomas: preliminary study of prognostic significance. *J Neurooncol* 1991;10:75–83.

160. Patronas NJ, DiChiro G, Brooks RA et al. Work in progress: (18F) fluorodeoxyglucose and positron emission tomography in the evaluation of radiation necrosis of the brain. *Radiology* 1982;144:885–889.

161. Ricci PE, Karis JP, Heiserman JE et al. Differentiating recurrent tumor from radiation necrosis: Time for reevaluation of positron emission tomography? *AJNR* 1998;19:407–413.

162. Olivero WC, Dulebohn SC, Lister JR. The use of PET in evaluating patients with primary brain tumors: Is it useful? *J Neurol Neurosurg Psychiatry* 1995;58:250–252.

163. Phillips PC, Dhawan V, Stother SC et al. Reduced cerebral glucose metabolism and increased brain capillary permeability following high-dose methotrexate chemotherapy: a positron emission tomography study. *Ann Neurol* 1979;6:371–388.

164. Rozental JM, Robbins HI, Finlay J et al. "Eight-drugs-in-one-day" chemotherapy administered before and after radiotherapy to adult patients with malignant glioma. *Cancer* 1989;63:2475–2481.

165. Rozental JM, Robbins HI, Finlay J et al. Eight-drugs-in-one-day chemotherapy in postirradiated adult patients with malignant gliomas. *Med Pediatr Oncol* 1989;17:471–476.

166. Ogawa T, Uemura K, Shishido F et al. Changes of cerebral blood flow and oxygen and glucose metabolism following radiochemotherapy of gliomas. A PET study. *J Comput Assist Tomogr* 1988;12:290–297.

167. Ogawa T, Inugami A, Hatazawa J et al. Clinical positron emission tomography for brain tumors: comparison of fluorodeoxyglucose F 18 and L-methyl-11C-methionine. *AJNR* 1996;17:345–353.

168. Nuutinen J, Sonninen P, Lehikoinen P et al. Radiotherapy treatment planning and long-term follow-up with [(11)C]methionine PET in patients with low-grade astrocytoma. *Int J Radiat Oncol Biol Phys* 2000;48:43–52.

169. Sonoda Y, Kumabe T, Takahashi T et al. Clinical usefulness of 11C-

MET PET and 201T1 SPECT for differentiation of recurrent glioma from radiation necrosis. *Neurol Medico-Chir* 1998;38:342–347.

170. Kameyama M, Tsurumi Y, Shirane R et al. Multiparametric analysis of brain tumors with PET. *J Cerebr Blood Flow Metab* 1987;7(Suppl 1):S466.

171. Mardsen CD. Basal ganglia disease. *Lancet* 1982;2:1141–1147.

172. Marsden CD. The mysterious motor function of the basal ganglia. *Neurology* 1982;32:514–539.

173. Braffman BH, Grossman RI, Goldberg HI et al. MR imaging of Parkinson's disease with spin-echo and gradient sequences. *AJR* 1989;152:159–165.

174. Huber SJ, Shuttleworth EC, Christy JA et al. Magnetic resonance imaging in dementia of Parkinson's disease. *J Neurol Neurosurg Psychiatry* 1989;52:1221–1227.

175. Aquilonius S-M. What has PET told us about Parkinson's disease. *Acta Neurol Scand* 1991;136:37–39.

176. Calne DB, Snow BJ. PET imaging in Parkinsonism. *Adv Neurol* 1993;60:484–487.

177. Eidelberg D. Positron emission tomography studies in parkinsonism. *Neurol Clin* 1992;10:421–433.

178. Guttman M. Dopamine receptors in Parkinson's disease. *Neurol Clin* 1992;10:377–386.

179. Rougemont D, Baron JC, Collard P et al. Local cerebral glucose utilization in treated and untreated patients with Parkinson's disease. *J Neurol Neurosurg Psychiatry* 1984;47:824–830.

180. Eidelberg D, Moeller JR, Dhawan V et al. The metabolic anatomy of Parkinson's disease. Complementary (18F) fluorodeoxyglucose and (18F) fluorodopa positron emission tomographic studies. *Move Dis* 1990;5:203–213.

181. Martin WRW, Beckman JH, Calne DB et al. Cerebral glucose metabolism in Parkinson's disease. *Can J Neurol Sci* 1984;11:169–173.

182. Martin WRW, Stoessel A et al. Positron emission tomography in Parkinson's disease. Glucose and dopa metabolism. *Adv Neurol* 1986;45:95–98.

183. Kuhl DE, Metter EJ, Riege WH. Patterns of local cerebral glucose utilization determined in Parkinson's disease by the (18F) fluorodeoxyglucose method. *Ann Neurol* 1984;15:419–424.

184. Kuhl DE, Metter EJ, Riege WH et al. Patterns of cerebral glucose utilization in Parkinson's disease and Huntington's disease. *Ann Neurol* 1984;15(Suppl):S119–S125.

185. Przedborski S, Goldman S, Giladi N et al. Positron emission tomography in hemiparkinsonism-hemiatrophy syndrome. *Adv Neurol* 1993;60:501–505.

186. Dethy S, Van Blercom N, Damhaut P et al. Asymmetry of basal ganglia glucose metabolism and dopa responsiveness in parkinsonism. *Move Dis* 1998;13:275–280.

187. Blesa R, Blin J et al. Levodopa-reduced glucose metabolism in striato-pallidothalamocortico circuit in Parkinson's disease. *Neurology* 1991;41:359.

188. Jenkins IH, Fernandez W, Playford ED et al. Impaired activation of the supplementary motor area in Parkinson's disease is reversed when akinesia is treated with apomorphine. *Ann Neurol* 1992;32:749–757.

189. Mazziotta JC. Movement disorders. In: Maziotta JC, Gilman S, eds. *Clinical brain imaging: principles and applications.* Philadelphia: Davis, 1992:244–293.

190. Peppard RF, Martin WR, Clark CM et al. Cortical glucose metabolism in Parkinson's and Alzheimer's disease. *J Neurosci Res* 1990;27:561–568.

191. Kuhl DE, Metter EJ, Benson DF et al. Similarities of cerebral glucose metabolism in Alzheimer's and parkinsonian dementia. *J Nucl Med* 1985;26:P69(abst).

192. Rinne JO, Portin R, Ruottinen H et al. Cog impairment and the brain dopaminergic system in Parkinson disease: [18F]fluorodopa positron emission tomographic study. *Arch Neurol* 2000;57:470–475.

193. Weder BJ, Leenders KL, Vontobel P et al. Impaired somatosensory discrimination of shape in Parkinson's disease: association with caudate nucleus dopaminergic function. *Human Brain Mapping* 1999;8:1–12.

194. Holthoff-Detto VA, Kessler J, Herholz K et al. Functional effects of striatal dysfunction in Parkinson disease. *Arch Neurol* 1997;54:145–150.

195. Martin WR. Parkinson's disease: positron emission tomographic studies. *Semin Neurol* 1989;9:345–350.

196. Nahmias C, Garnett ES, Firnau G et al. Striatal dopamine distribution in parkinsonian patients during life. *J Neurol Sci* 1985;69:223–230.

197. Leenders KL, Palmer AJ, Quinn N et al. Brain dopamine metabolism in patients with Parkinson's disease measured with positron emission tomography. *J Neurol Neurosurg Psychiatry* 1986;49:853–860.

198. Leenders KL, Salmon EP, Tyrrell P et al. The nigrostriatal dopaminergic system assessed in vivo by positron emission tomography in healthy volunteer subjects and patients with Parkinson's disease. *Arch Neurol* 1990;47:1290–1298.

199. Rousset OG, Deep P, Kuwabara H et al. Effect of partial volume correction on estimates of the influx and cerebral metabolism of 6-[(18)F]fluoro-L-dopa studied with PET in normal control and Parkinson's disease subjects. *Synapse* 2000;37:81–89.

200. Garnett ES, Nahmias C, Firnau G. Central dopaminergic pathways in hemiparkinsonism examined by positron emission tomography. *Can J Neurol Sci* 1984;11:174–179.

201. Nurmi E, Ruottinen HM, Kaasinen V et al. Progression in Parkinson's disease: a positron emission tomography study with a dopamine transporter ligand [18F]CFT. *Ann Neurol* 2000;47:804–808.

202. Lee CS, Samii A, Sossi V et al. In vivo positron emission tomographic evidence for compensatory changes in presynaptic dopaminergic nerve terminals in Parkinson's disease. *Ann Neurol* 2000;47:493–503.

203. Ouchi Y, Kanno T, Okada H et al. Presynaptic and postsynaptic dopaminergic binding densities in the nigrostriatal and mesocortical systems in early Parkinson's disease: a double-tracer positron emission tomography study. *Ann Neurol* 1999;46:723–731.

204. Ouchi Y, Yoshikawa E, Okada H et al. Alterations in binding site density of dopamine transporter in the striatum, orbitofrontal cortex, and amygdala in early Parkinson's disease: compartment analysis for beta-CFT binding with positron emission tomography. *Ann Neurol* 1999;45:601–610.

205. Torstenson R, Hartvig P, Langstrom B et al. Differential effects of levodopa on dopaminergic function in early and advanced Parkinson's disease. *Ann Neurol* 1997;41:334–340.

206. Brooks DJ. PET studies and motor complications in Parkinson's disease. *Trends Neurosci* 2000;23(Suppl):S101–108.

207. Brooks DJ, Piccini P, Turjanski N et al. Neuroimaging of dyskinesia. *Ann Neurol* 2000;47(Suppl 1):S154–158.

208. Brooks DJ, Samuel M. The effects of surgical treatment of Parkinson's disease on brain function: PET findings. *Neurology* 2000;55(Suppl 6):S52–59.

209. Henselmans JM, de Jong BM, Pruim J et al. Acute effects of thalamotomy and pallidotomy on regional cerebral metabolism, evaluated by PET. *Clin Neurol Neurosurg* 2000;102:84–90.

210. Eidelberg D, Moeller JR, Ishikawa T et al. Regional metabolic correlates of surgical outcome following unilateral pallidotomy for Parkinson's disease. *Ann Neurol* 1996;39:450–459.

211. Limousin P, Greene J, Pollak P et al. Changes in cerebral activity pattern due to subthalamic nucleus or internal pallidum stimulation in Parkinson's disease. *Ann Neurol* 1997;42:283–291.

212. Davis KD, Taub E, Houle S et al. Globus pallidus stimulation activates the cortical motor system during alleviation of parkinsonian symptoms. *Nature Med* 1997;3:671–674.

213. Tedroff J, Aquilonius S-M, Hartvig P et al. Monoamine re-uptake sites in the human brain evaluated by means of 11C-nomifensine and positron emission tomography. The effects of age and Parkinson's disease. *Acta Neurol Scand* 1988;77:192–201.

214. Tedroff J, Aquilonius S-M, Hartvig P et al. Striatal kinetics of (11C)-(+)-nomifensine and 6-(18F) fluoro-L-dopa in Parkinson's disease measured with positron emission tomography. *Acta Neurol Scand* 1990;81:24–30.

215. Shinotoh H, Hirayama K, Tateno Y. Dopamine D1 and D2 receptors in Parkinson's disease and striatonigral degeneration determined by PET. *Adv Neurol* 1993;60:488–493.

216. Rinne JO, Laihinen K, Nagren J et al. PET demonstrates different

behavior of striatal dopamine D-1 and D-2 receptors in early Parkinson's disease. *J Neurosci Res* 1990;27:494–499.

217. Sawle GV, Brooks DJ, Ibanez V et al. Striatal D2 receptor density is inversely proportional to dopa uptake in untreated hemi-Parkinson's disease. *J Neurol Neurosurg Psychiatry* 1990;53:177.

218. Brooks DJ, Ibanez V, Sawle GV et al. Striatal D2 receptor status in patients with Parkinson's disease, striatonigral degeneration, and progressive supranuclear palsy, measured with 11C raclopride and positron emission tomography. *Ann Neurol* 1992;31:184–192.

219. Wijnand A, Rutgers F, Lakke JPW et al. Tracing of dopamine receptors in hemiparkinsonism with positron emission tomography (PET). *J Neurol Sci* 1987;80:237–248.

220. Antonini A, Schwarz J, Oertel WH et al. Long-term changes of striatal dopamine D2 receptors in patients with Parkinson's disease: a study with positron emission tomography and [11C]raclopride. *Move Dis* 1997;12:33–38.

221. Mazziotta JC. Huntington's disease: studies with structural imaging techniques and positron emission tomography. *Semin Neurol* 1989; 9:360–369.

222. Vonsattel JP, Myers RH, Stevens TJ et al. Neuropathological classification of Huntington's disease. *J Neuropathol Exp Neurol* 1985;44: 559–577.

223. Koh JY, Peters S, Choi DW. Neurons containing NADPH-diaphorase are selectively resistant to quinolate toxicity. *Science* 1985;230: 561–563.

224. Phelps ME, Mazziota JC, Wapenski J et al. Cerebral glucose utilization and blood flow in Huntington's disease. *J Nucl Med* 1985;26: 47.

225. Kuwert T, Lange HW, Langin KJ et al. Cerebral glucose consumption measured by PET in patients with and without psychiatric symptoms of Huntington's disease. *Psychiatr Res* 1989;29:361–362.

226. Pahl JJ. Cerebral metabolic decline. A biochemical marker of genetic expression in Huntington's disease. *Adv Funct Neuroimaging* 1989; 2:3–8.

227. Mazziotta JC, Phelps ME, Pahl JJ et al. Reduced cerebral glucose metabolism in asymptomatic patients at risk for Huntington's disease. *N Engl J Med* 1987;316:357–362.

228. Brooks DJ, Frackowiak RSJ. PET and movement disorders. *J Neurol Neurosurg Psychiatry* 1989;52(Suppl):S68–S77.

229. Kuhl DE, Phelps ME, Markham CH et al. Cerebral metabolism and atrophy in Huntington's disease determined by 18-F-FDG and computed tomographic scan. *Ann Neurol* 1982;12:425–434.

230. Hayden MR, Martin WRW, Stoessl AJ et al. Positron emission tomography in the early diagnosis of Huntington's disease. *Neurology* 1986;36:888–894.

231. Bachoud-Levi AC, Remy P, Nguyen JP et al. Motor and cognitive improvements in patients with Huntington's disease after neural transplantation. *Lancet* 2000;356:1975–1979.

232. Kuwert T, Lange HW, Langen KJ et al. Cortical and subcortical glucose consumption measured by PET in patients with Huntington's disease. *Brain* 1990;113:1405–1423.

233. Young AV, Penney JB, Starosta-Rubinstein S et al. PET scan investigations of Huntington's disease. Cerebral metabolic correlates of neurological features and functional decline. *Ann Neurol* 1986;29: 296–303.

234. Berent S, Goerdani B, Lehtinen S et al. Positron emission tomographic scan investigations of Huntington's disease. Cerebral metabolic correlates of cognitive function. *Ann Neurol* 1988;23:541–546.

235. Kuwert T, Sures T, Herzog H et al. On the influence of spatial resolution and of the size and form of regions of interest on the measurement of regional cerebral metabolic rates by positron emission tomography. *J Neural Transm* 1992;37(Suppl):53–66.

236. Hayden MR, Hewitt J, Martin WRW et al. Studies in persons at risk for Huntington's disease. *N Engl J Med* 1987;317:382–383.

237. Hayden MR, Hewitt J, Stoessl AJ et al. The combined use of positron emission tomography and DNA polymorphisms for preclinical detection of Huntington's disease. *Neurology* 1987;37:1441–1447.

238. Young AB, Penney JB, Starosta-Rubinstein S et al. Normal caudate glucose metabolism in persons at risk for Huntington's disease. *Arch Neurol* 1987;44:254–257.

239. Weeks RA, Piccini P, Harding AE et al. Striatal D1 and D2 dopamine receptor loss in asymptomatic mutation carriers of Huntington's disease. *Ann Neurol* 1996;40:49–54.

240. Leenders KL, Frackowiak RSJ, Quinn N et al. Brain energy metabolism and dopaminergic function in Huntington's disease measured in vivo using positron emission tomography. *Mov Disord* 1986;1: 69–77.

241. Wong DF, Links JM, Wagner HN et al. Dopamine and serotonin receptors measured in vivo in Huntington's disease with C-11-N-methylspiperone PET imaging. *J Nucl Med* 1985;26:P107(abst).

242. Weeks RA, Cunningham VJ, Piccini P et al. 11C-diprenorphine binding in Huntington's disease: a comparison of region of interest analysis with statistical parametric mapping. *J Cerebr Blood Flow Metab* 1997; 17:943–949.

243. Kunig G, Leenders KL, Sanchez-Pernaute R et al. Benzodiazepine receptor binding in Huntington's disease: [11C]flumazenil uptake measured using positron emission tomography. *Ann Neurol* 2000;47: 644–648.

244. Holthoff VA, Koeppe RA, Frey KA et al. Positron emission tomography measures of benzodiazepine receptors in Huntington's disease. *Ann Neurol* 1993;34:76–81.

245. Chase TN, Tamminga CA, Burrows H. Positron emission tomographic studies of regional cerebral glucose metabolism in idiopathic dystonia. *Adv Neurol* 1988;50:237–241.

246. Gilman S, Junck L, Young AB et al. Cerebral metabolic activity in idiopathic dystonia studied with positron emission tomography. *Adv Neurol* 1988;50:231–236.

247. Stoessl AJ, Martin WRW, Clark C et al. PET studies of cerebral glucose metabolism in idiopathic torticollis. *Neurology* 1986;36: 653–657.

248. Sawle GV, Leenders KL, Brooks DJ et al. Dopa-responsive dystonia: [18F] dopa positron emission tomography. *Ann Neurol* 1991;30: 24–30.

249. Martin WRW, Stoessl AJ, Palmer M et al. PET scanning in dystonia. *Adv Neurol* 1988;50:223–228.

250. Leenders KL, Quinn N, Frackowiak RSJ et al. Brain dopaminergic system studied in patients with dystonia using positron emission tomography. *Adv Neurol* 1988;50:243–247.

251. Kunig G, Leenders KL, Antonini A et al. D2 receptor binding in dopa-responsive dystonia. *Ann Neurol* 1998;44:758–762.

252. Foster NL, Gilman S, Berent S et al. Cerebral hypometabolism in progressive supranuclear palsy studied with positron emission tomography. *Ann Neurol* 1988;24:399–406.

253. Goffinet AM, De Volder AG, Gillain C et al. Positron tomography demonstrates frontal lobe hypometabolism in progressive supranuclear palsy. *Ann Neurol* 1989;25:131–139.

254. D'Antona R, Baron JC et al. Subcortical dementia. Frontal cortex hypometabolism detected by positron tomography in patients with progressive supranuclear palsy. *Brain* 1985;108:785–799.

255. Yamauchi H, Fukuyama H, Nagahama Y et al. Atrophy of the corpus callosum, cognitive impairment, and cortical hypometabolism in progressive supranuclear palsy. *Ann Neurol* 1997;41:606–614.

256. Santens P, De Reuck J, Crevits L et al. Cerebral oxygen metabolism in patients with progressive supranuclear palsy: a positron emission tomography study. *Eur Neurol* 1997;37:18–22.

257. Leenders KL, Frackowiak RSJ, Lees AJ. Steel-Richardson-Olszewski syndrome. Brain energy metabolism, blood flow, and fluorodopa uptake measured by positron emission tomography. *Brain* 1988;111: 615–630.

258. Schlaug G, Hefter H, Engelbrecht V et al. Neurol impairment and recovery in Wilson's disease: evidence from PET and MRI. *J Neurol Sci* 1996;136:129–139.

259. Kuwert T, Hefter H, Scholz D et al. Regional cerebral glucose consumption measured by positron emission tomography in patients with Wilson's disease. *Eur J Nucl Med* 1992;19:96–101.

260. Hawkins RA, Mazziotta JC, Phelps ME. Wilson's disease studied with FDG and positron emission tomography. *Neurology* 1987;37: 1707–1711.

261. Cordato DJ, Fulham MJ, Yiannikas C. Pretreatment and posttreat-

ment positron emission tomographic scan imaging in a 20-year-old patient with Wilson's disease. *Move Dis* 1998;13:162–166.

262. Pappata S, Levasseur M, Tran-Dinh S et al. PET study of cerebral glucose utilization in 10 patients with Wilson's disease. *J Cerebr Blood Flow Metab* 1989;9:S23.

263. Westermark K, Tedroff J, Thuomas KA. Neurological Wilson's disease studied with magnetic resonance imaging and with positron emission tomography using dopaminergic markers. *Move Dis* 1995;10:596–603.

264. Schlaug G, Hefter H, Nebeling B et al. Dopamine D2 receptor binding and cerebral glucose metabolism recover after D-penicillamine-therapy in Wilson's disease. *J Neurol* 1994;241:577–584.

265. Baron J, Frackowiak R, Herholz K et al. Use of PET methods for measurement of cerebral energy metabolism and hemodynamics in cerebrovascular disease. *J Cerebr Blood Flow Metab* 1989;9:723–742.

266. Baron J, Lebiun-Granolie P, Collar P et al. Noninvasive measurement of blood flow, oxygen consumption and glucose utilization in the same brain regions in man by positron emission tomography. Concise communication. *J Nucl Med* 1982;23:391–399.

267. Brooks DJ. The clinical role of PET in cerebrovascular disease. *Neurosurg Rev* 1991;14:91–96.

268. Kushner M, Reivich M, Fieschi C et al. Metabolic and clinical correlates of acute ischemic infarction. *Neurology* 1987;37:1103–1110.

269. Read SJ, Hirano T, Abbott DF et al. The fate of hypoxic tissue on 18F-fluoromisonidazole positron emission tomography after ischemic stroke. *Ann Neurol* 2000;48:228–235.

270. Ackerman R, Correia J, Alpert N et al. Positron imaging in ischemic stroke disease using compound labeled with oxygen-15. *Arch Neurol* 1981;38:537–543.

271. Baron J, Bousser M, Comar D et al. Noninvasive tomograph study of cerebral blood flow and oxygen metabolism in vivo. *Eur Neurol* 1981;20:273–284.

272. Baron J, Rougemont D, Bousser M et al. Local CBF, oxygen extraction fraction (OEF) and CMRO2. Prognostic value in recent supratentorial infarction in humans. *J Cerebr Blood Flow Metab* 1983;3:A–2(abst).

273. Lenzi G, Frackowiak R, Jonres T. Cerebral oxygen metabolism and blood flow in human cerebral ischemic infarction. *J Cerebr Blood Flow Metab* 1982;2:321–335.

274. Kuhl DE, Phelps M, Kowell A et al. Effects of stroke on local cerebral metabolism and perfusion. Mapping by emission tomography of 18FDG and 12NH3. *Ann Neurol* 1980;8:47–69.

275. Baron J, Rougemont D, Bousser M et al. Local interrelationships of cerebral oxygen consumption and glucose utilization in normal subjects and in ischemic stroke patients. *J Cerebr Blood Flow Metab* 1984;4:140–149.

276. Wise R, Bernardi S, Frackowiak R et al. Serial observations on the pathophysiology of acute stroke. The transition from ischemia to infarction as reflected in regional oxygen extraction. *Brain* 1983;106:197–222.

277. Derdeyn CP, Shaibani A, Moran CJ et al. Lack of correlation between pattern of collateralization and misery perfusion in patients with carotid occlusion. *Stroke* 1999;30:1025–1032.

278. Iglesias S, Marchal G, Viader F et al. Delayed intrahemispheric remote hypometabolism. Correlations with early recovery after stroke. *Cerebrovasc Dis* 2000;10:391–402.

279. Lassen N. The luxury perfusion syndrome and its possible relation to acute metabolic acidosis localized within the brain. *Lancet* 1966;2:1113–1115.

280. Marchal G, Evans A, Dagher A et al. The evolution of cerebral infarction with time. A PET study of the ischemia penumbra. *J Cerebr Blood Flow Metab* 1987;7(Suppl 1):S99.

281. Baron J, Bousser M, Rey A et al. Reversal of focal "misery-perfusion syndrome" by extra-intracranial arterial bypass in hemodynamic cerebral ischemia. *Stroke* 1981;12:454–459.

282. Feeney D, Baron J. Diaschisis. *Stroke* 1986;17:817–830.

283. Kushner M, Alavi A, Reivich M et al. Contralateral cerebellar hypometabolism following cerebral insult. A positron emission tomographics study. *Ann Neurol* 1984;15:425–434.

284. Pantano P, Baron J, Samson Y et al. Crossed cerebellar diaschisis. Further studies. *Brain* 1986;109:634–677.

285. Herholz K, Heindel W, Rackl A et al. Regional cerebral blood flow in leukoaraiosis and atherosclerotic carotid disease. *Arch Neurol* 1990;47:392–397.

286. Powers J, Grubb R, Raichle M. Physiological response to focal cerebral ischemia in humans. *Ann Neurol* 1984;16:546–552.

287. Iglesias S, Marchal G, Viader F et al. Delayed intrahemispheric remote hypometabolism. Correlations with early recovery after stroke. *Cerebrovasc Dis* 2000;10:391–402.

288. Baron J, Bousser M, Comar D et al. Crossed cerebellar diaschisis in human supratentorial brain infarction. *Trans Am Neurol Assoc* 1980;105:459–461.

289. Baron J, Bousser MG, Comar D. Crossed cerebellar diaschisis. A remote functional depression secondary to supratentorial infarction in man. *J Cerebr Blood Flow Metab* 1981;1:S500–S501.

290. Yamauchi H, Fukuyama H, Nagahama Y et al. Uncoupling of oxygen and glucose metabolism in persistent crossed cerebellar diaschisis. *Stroke* 1999;30:1424–1428.

291. De Reuck J, Decoo D, Lemahieu I et al. Crossed cerebellar diaschisis after middle cerebral artery infarction. *Clin Neurol Neurosurg* 1997;99:11–16.

292. Broich K, Alavi A, Kushner M. Positron emission tomography in cerebrovascular disorders. *Semin Nucl Med* 1992;22:224–232.

293. Iglesias S, Marchal G, Rioux P et al. Do changes in oxygen metabolism in the unaffected cerebral hemisphere underlie early neurological recovery after stroke? A positron emission tomography study. *Stroke* 1996;27:1192–1199.

294. Powers W, Tempel L, Grubb R. Influence of cerebral hemodynamics on stroke risk. One-year follow-up of 38 medically treated patients. *Ann Neurol* 1989;25:325–330.

295. Powers W, Grubb R, Raichle M. Clinical results of extracranial-intracranial bypass-surgery in patients with hemodynamic cerebrovascular disease. *J Neurosurg* 1989;70:61–67.

296. Leblanc R. Physiologic studies of cerebral ischemia. *Clin Neurosurg* 1991;37:289–311.

297. Derdeyn CP, Videen TO, Simmons NR et al. Count-based PET method for predicting ischemic stroke in patients with symptomatic carotid arterial occlusion. *Radiology* 1999;212:499–506.

298. Derdeyn CP, Yundt KD, Videen TO et al. Increased oxygen extraction fraction is associated with prior ischemic events in patients with carotid occlusion. *Stroke* 1998;29:754–758.

299. Samson Y, Baron J, Bousser M. Effects of extra-intracranial arterial bypass on cerebral blood flow and oxygen metabolism in humans. *Stroke* 1985;16:609–616.

300. Heiss WD, Kessler J, Karbe H et al. Cerebral glucose metabolism as a predictor of recovery from aphasia in ischemic stroke. *Arch Neurol* 1993;50:958–964.

301. Powers W, Fox P. Positron emission tomography measurements of cerebral blood flow and metabolism. How can they be used to study functional recovery from stroke? (An American perspective). In: Ginsberg M, Dietrich W, eds. *Cerebrovascular diseases* (16th research Princeton conference). New York: Raven Press, 1989.

302. Karbe H, Kessler J, Herholz K et al. Long-term prognosis of poststroke aphasia studied with positron emission tomography. *Arch Neurol* 1995;52:186–190.

303. Rosen HJ, Petersen SE, Linenweber MR et al. Neural correlates of recovery from aphasia after damage to left inferior frontal cortex. *Neurology* 2000;55:1883–1894.

304. Ohyama M, Senda M, Kitamura S et al. Role of the nondominant hemisphere and undamaged area during word repetition in poststroke aphasics. A PET activation study. *Stroke* 1996;27:897–903.

305. Karbe H, Thiel A, Weber-Luxenburger G et al. Brain plasticity in poststroke aphasia: what is the contribution of the right hemisphere? *Brain Lang* 1998;64:215–230.

306. Heiss WD, Kessler J, Thiel A et al. Differential capacity of left and right hemispheric areas for compensation of poststroke aphasia. *Ann Neurol* 1999;45:430–438.

307. Warburton E, Price CJ, Swinburn K et al. Mechanisms of recovery

from aphasia: evidence from positron emission tomography studies. *J Neurol Neurosurg Psychiatry* 1999;66:155–161.

308. Nelles G, Spiekramann G, Jueptner M et al. Evolution of functional reorganization in hemiplegic stroke: a serial positron emission tomographic activation study. *Ann Neurol* 1999;46:901–909.

309. Heiss WD, Grond M, Thiel A et al. Tissue at risk of infarction rescued by early reperfusion: a positron emission tomography study in systemic recombinant tissue plasminogen activator thrombolysis of acute stroke. *J Cerebr Blood Flow Metab* 1998;18:1298–1307.

310. Heiss WD, Grond M, Thiel A et al. Permanent cortical damage detected by flumazenil positron emission tomography in acute stroke. *Stroke* 1998;29:454–461.

311. Heiss WD, Kracht L, Grond M et al. Early [(11)C]Flumazenil/H(2)O positron emission tomography predicts irreversible ischemic cortical damage in stroke patients receiving acute thrombolytic therapy. *Stroke* 2000;31:366–369.

312. Heiss WD, Graf R, Grond M et al. Quantitative neuroimaging for the evaluation of the effect of stroke treatment. *Cerebrovasc Dis* 1998; 2(Suppl):23–29.

313. Hakim A, Evans A, Berger L et al. The effect of nimodipine on the evolution of human cerebral infarction studies by PET. *J Cerebr Blood Flow Metab* 1989;9:523–534.

314. Heiss W, Holthoff V, Pawlik G et al. Effect of nimodipine on regional cerebral glucose metabolism in patients with acute ischemic stroke as measured by positron emission tomography. *J Cerebr Blood Flow Metab* 1990;10:127–132.

315. Langfitt TW, Obrist WD, Alavi A et al. Computerized tomography, magnetic resonance imaging, and positron emission tomography in the study of brain trauma. Preliminary observations. *J Neurosurg* 1986; 64:760–767.

316. Alavi A, Fazekas T, Alves W et al. Positron emission tomography in the evaluation of head injury. *J Cerebr Blood Flow Metab* 1987;7: S646(abst).

317. George JK, Alavi A, Zimmerman RA et al. Metabolic (PET) correlates of anatomic lesions (CT/MRI) produced by head trauma. *J Nucl Med* 1989;30:802(abst).

318. Alavi A. Functional and anatomic studies of head injury. *J Neuropsychiatry* 1989;1:S45–S50.

319. Alavi A, Mirot A, Newberg A et al. F-18 PET evaluation of crossed cerebellar diaschisis in head injury. *J Nucl Med* 1997;38:1717–1720.

320. Ruff RM, Crouch JA, Troster AI et al. Selected cases of poor outcome following minor brain trauma: Comparing neuropsychological and positron emission tomography assessment. *Brain Injury* 1994;8: 297–308.

321. Bergsneider M, Hovda DA, Lee SM et al. Dissociation of cerebral glucose metabolism and level of consciousness during the period of metabolic depression following human traumatic brain injury. *J Neurotrauma* 2000;17:389–401.

322. Bergsneider M, Hovda DA, Shalmon E et al. Cerebral hyperglycolysis following severe traumatic brain injury in humans: a positron emission tomography study. *J Neurosurg* 1997;86:241–251.

323. Worley G, Hoffman JM, Paine SS et al. 18-Fluorodeoxyglucose positron emission tomography in children and adolescents with traumatic brain injury. *Dev Med Child Neurol* 1995;37:213–220.

324. de Jong BM, Willemsen AT, Paans AM. Regional cerebral blood flow changes related to affective speech presentation in persistent vegetative state. *Clin Neurol Neurosurg* 1997;99:213–216.

325. Hinkin CH, van Gorp WG, Mandelkern MA et al. Cerebral metabolic change in patients with AIDS: report of a six-month follow-up using positron-emission tomography. *J Neuropsychiatry Clin Neurosci* 1995;7:180–187.

326. van Gorp WG, Mandelkern MA, Gee M et al. Cerebral metabolic dysfunction in AIDS: findings in a sample with and without dementia. *J Neuropsychiatry Clin Neurosci* 1992;4:280–287.

327. Heald AE, Hoffman JM, Bartlett JA et al. Differentiation of central nervous system lesions in AIDS patients using positron emission tomography (PET). *Int J STD AIDS* 1996;7:337–346.

328. Hoffman JM, Waskin HA, Schifter T et al. FDG-PET in differentiating lymphoma from nonmalignant central nervous system lesions in patients with AIDS. *J Nucl Med* 1993;34:567–575.

329. Villringer K, Jager H, Dichgans M et al. Differential diagnosis of CNS lesions in AIDS patients by FDG-PET. *J Comp Assist Tomogr* 1995;19:532–536.

330. O'Doherty MJ, Barrington SF, Campbell M et al. PET scanning and the human immunodeficiency virus-positive patient. *J Nucl Med* 1997;38:1575–1583.

331. Kramer EL, Sanger JJ. Brain imaging in acquired immunodeficiency syndrome dementia complex. *Semin Nucl Med* 1990;20:353–363.

332. Holman BL, Garada B, Johnson KA et al. A comparison of brain perfusion SPECT in cocaine abuse and AIDS dementia complex. *J Nucl Med* 1992;33:1312–1315.

333. Samson Y, Baron JC, Feline A et al. Local cerebral glucose utilization in chronic alcoholics, a positron tomography study. *J Neurol Neurosurg Psychiatry* 1986;49:1165–1170.

334. Sach H, Russel JAG, Christman DR et al. Alterations in regional cerebral glucose metabolic rate in non-Korsakoff chronic alcoholism. *Arch Neurol* 1987;44:1242–1251.

335. Wik G, Borg S, Sjogren I et al. Positron emission tomography determination of regional cerebral glucose metabolism in alcohol-dependent men and healthy controls using 11C-glucose. *Acta Psychiatr Scand* 1988;78:234–241.

336. Volkow ND, Fowler JS. Neuropsychiatric disorders. Investigation of schizophrenia and substance abuse. *Semin Nucl Med* 1992;22: 254–267.

337. Wang GJ, Volkow ND, Fowler JS et al. Regional cerebral metabolism in female alcoholics of moderate severity does not differ from that of controls. *Alcohol Clin Exp Res* 1998;22:1850–1854.

338. Gilman S, Adams K, Koeppe RA et al. Cerebellar hypometabolism in alcoholic cerebellar degeneration studied with FDG and PET. *Neurology* 1988;38:365.

339. Volkow ND, Wang G-J, Hitzemann R et al. Decreased cerebral response to inhibitory neurotransmission in alcoholics. *Am J Psychiatry* 1993;150:417–422.

340. Johnson-Greene D, Adams KM, Gilman S et al. Effects of abstinence and relapse upon neuropsychological function and cerebral glucose metabolism in severe chronic alcoholism. *J Clin Exp Neuropsychol* 1997;19:378–385.

341. Volkow ND, Wang GJ, Hitzemann R et al. Recovery of brain glucose metabolism in detoxified alcoholics. *Am J Psychiatry* 1994;151: 178–183.

342. Volkow ND, Wang GJ, Begleiter H et al. Regional brain metabolic response to lorazepam in subjects at risk for alcoholism. *Alcohol Clin Exp Res* 1995;19:510–516.

343. Volkow ND, Wang GJ, Hitzemann R et al. Decreased cerebral response to inhibitory neurotransmission in alcoholics. *Am J Psychiatry* 1993;150:417–422.

344. Volkow ND, Wang GJ, Fowler JS et al. Decreases in dopamine receptors but not in dopamine transporters in alcoholics. *Alcohol Clin Exp Res* 1996;20:1594–1598.

345. Tiihonen J, Vilkman H, Rasanen P et al. Striatal presynaptic dopamine function in type 1 alcoholics measured with positron emission tomography. *Mol Psychiatry* 1998;3:156–161.

346. Gilman S, Koeppe RA, Adams KM et al. Decreased striatal monoaminergic terminals in severe chronic alcoholism demonstrated with (+)[11C]dihydrotetrabenazine and positron emission tomography. *Ann Neurol* 1998;44:326–333.

347. Hommer D, Andreasen P, Rio D et al. Effects of m-chlorophenylpiperazine on regional brain glucose utilization: a positron emission tomographic comparison of alcoholic and control subjects. *J Neurosci* 1997;17:2796–2806.

348. Gilman S, Adams KM, Johnson-Greene D et al. Effects of disulfiram on positron emission tomography and neuropsychological studies in severe chronic alcoholism. *Alcohol Clin Exp Res* 1996;20:1456–1461.

349. Johanson CE, Fishman MW. The pharmacology of cocaine related to its abuse. *Pharmacol Rev* 1989;41:3–52.

350. Strickland TL, Miller BL, Kowell A et al. Neurobiology of cocaine-induced organic brain impairment: contributions from functional neuroimaging. *Neuropsychol Rev* 1998;8:1–9.

351. Fowler JS, Volkow ND, Wolf AP et al. Mapping cocaine binding sites in human and baboon brain in vivo. *Synapse* 1989;4:371–377.

352. Cook CE, Jeffcoat AR, Perez-Reys M. Pharmacokinetic studies of cocaine and phencyclidine in man. In: Barnett G, Chiang CN, eds. *Pharmacokinetics and pharmacodynamics of psychoactive drugs.* Foster City, CA: Biomedical Publications, 1985:48–74.

353. London ED, Cascella NG, Wong DF et al. Cocaine-induced reduction of glucose utilization in human brain. A study using positron emission tomography and (Fluorine-18)-fluorodeoxyglucose. *Arch Gen Psychiatry* 1990;47:567–574.

354. Volkow ND, Hitzemann R, Wang GJ et al. Long-term frontal brain metabolic changes in cocaine abusers. *Synapse* 1992;11:184–190.

355. Volkow ND, Fowler JS, Wolf AP et al. Changes in brain glucose metabolism in cocaine dependence and withdrawal. *Am J Psychiatry* 1991;148:621–626.

356. Volkow ND, Wang GJ, Fowler JS et al. Association of methylphenidate-induced craving with changes in right striato-orbitofrontal metabolism in cocaine abusers: implications in addiction. *Am J Psychiatry* 1999;156:19–26.

357. Baxter L, Phelps M, Mazziotta J et al. Local cerebral glucose metabolic rates in obsessive-compulsive disorder. A comparison with rates in unipolar depression and normal controls. *Arch Gen Psychiatry* 1987; 44:211–218.

358. Modell JG, Mountz JM, Curtis G et al. Neurophysiologic dysfunctions in basal ganglia limbic striatal and thalamocortical circuit as a pathogenetic mechanism of obsessive compulsive disorder. *J Neuropsychiatry* 1989;1:27–36.

359. Childress AR, Mozley PD, McElgin W et al. Limbic activation during cue-induced cocaine craving. *Am J Psychiatry* 1999;156:11–18.

360. Wang GJ, Volkow ND, Fowler JS et al. Regional brain metabolic activation during craving elicited by recall of previous drug experiences. *Life Sci* 1999;64:775–784.

361. Schlaepfer TE, Pearlson GD, Wong DF et al. PET study of competition between intravenous cocaine and [11C]raclopride at dopamine receptors in human subjects. *Am J Psychiatry* 1997;154:1209–1213.

362. Wu JC, Bell K, Najafi A et al. Decreasing striatal 6-FDOPA uptake with increasing duration of cocaine withdrawal. *Neuropsychopharmacology* 1997;17:402–409.

363. Volkow ND, Wang GJ, Fowler JS et al. Decreased striatal dopaminergic responsiveness in detoxified cocaine-dependent subjects. *Nature* 1997;386:830–833.

364. Volkow ND, Wang GJ, Fischman MW et al. Effects of route of administration on cocaine induced dopamine transporter blockade in the human brain. *Life Sci* 2000;67:1507–1515.

365. Volkow ND, Wang GJ, Fowler JS et al. Enhanced sensitivity to benzodiazepines in active cocaine-abusing subjects: a PET study. *Am J Psychiatry* 1998;155:200–206.

366. Liddle PF. PET scanning and schizophrenia—what progress? *Psychiatrol Med* 1992;22:557–560.

367. Sedvall G. The current status of PET scanning with respect to schizophrenia. *Neuropsychopharmacology* 1992;7:41–54.

368. Cleghorn JM, Zipursky RB, List SJ. Structural and functional brain imaging in schizophrenia. *J Psychiatry Neurosci* 1991;16:53–74.

369. Kim JJ, Mohamed S, Andreasen NC et al. Regional neural dysfunctions in chronic schizophrenia studied with positron emission tomography. *Am J Psychiatry* 2000;157:542–548.

370. Andreasen NC, O'Leary DS, Flaum M et al. Hypofrontality in schizophrenia: distributed dysfunctional circuits in neuroleptic-naive patients. *Lancet* 1997;349:1730–1734.

371. Gur RE, Resnick SM, Alavi A et al. Regional brain function in schizophrenia I. A positron emission tomography study. *Arch Gen Psychiatry* 1987;44:119–125.

372. Sheppard G, Gruzelier J, Manchanda R et al. Positron emission tomographic scanning in predominantly never-treated acute schizophrenic patients. *Lancet* 1983;2:1448–1452.

373. Wiesel FA, Wik G, Sjogren I et al. Regional brain glucose metabolism in drug-free schizophrenic patients and clinical correlates. *Acta Psychiatr Scand* 1987;76:628–641.

374. Volkow ND, Wolf AP, Van Gelder P et al. Phenomenological correlates of metabolic activity in 18 patients with chronic schizophrenia. *Am J Psychiatry* 1987;144:151–158.

375. McGuire PK, Quested DJ, Spence SA et al. Pathophysiology of 'positive' thought disorder in schizophrenia. *Br J Psychiatry*1998;173:231–235.

376. Buchanan RW, Breier A, Kirkpatrick B et al. The deficit syndrome. Functional and structural characteristics. *Schizophr Res* 1991;4:400–401.

377. Schroder J, Buchsbaum MS, Siegel BV et al. Cerebral metabolic activity correlates of subsyndromes in chronic schizophrenia. *Schizophr Res* 1996;19:41–53.

378. Spence SA, Hirsch SR, Brooks DJ et al. Prefrontal cortex activity in people with schizophrenia and control subjects. Evidence from positron emission tomography for remission of 'hypofrontality' with recovery from acute schizophrenia. *Br J Psychiatry* 1998;172:316–323.

379. Sabri O, Erkwoh R, Schreckenberger M et al. Correlation of positive symptoms exclusively to hyperperfusion or hypoperfusion of cerebral cortex in never-treated schizophrenics. *Lancet* 1997; 349:1735–1739.

380. Haznedar MM, Buchsbaum MS, Luu C et al. Decreased anterior cingulate gyrus metabolic rate in schizophrenia. *Am J Psychiatry* 1997; 154:682–684.

381. Early TS, Reiman EM, Raichle ME et al. Left globus pallidus abnormality in never-medicated patients with schizophrenia. *Proc Natl Acad Sci U S A* 1987;84:561–563.

382. Hazlett EA, Buchsbaum MS, Byne W et al. Three-dimensional analysis with MRI and PET of the size, shape, and function of the thalamus in the schizophrenia spectrum. *Am J Psychiatry* 1999;156:1190–1199.

383. Buchsbaum MS, Someya T, Teng CY et al. PET and MRI of the thalamus in never-medicated patients with schizophrenia. *Am J Psychiatry* 1996;153:191–199.

384. Liddle PF, Friston KJ, Frith CD et al. Cerebral blood flow and mental processes in schizophrenia. *J R Soc Med* 1992;85:224–227.

385. Liddle PF, Friston KJ, Frith CD et al. Patterns of cerebral blood flow in schizophrenia. *Br J Psychiatry* 1992;160:179–186.

386. Katz M, Buchsbaum MS, Siegel BV Jr et al. Correlational patterns of cerebral glucose metabolism in never-medicated schizophrenics. *Neuropsychobiology* 1996;33:1–11.

387. Siegel BV Jr, Buchsbaum MS, Bunney WE Jr et al. Cortical-striatal-thalamic circuits and brain glucose metabolic activity in 70 unmedicated male schizophrenic patients. *Am J Psychiatry* 1993;150:1325–1336.

388. Gur RE, Chin S. Laterality in functional brain imaging studies of schizophrenia. *Schizophr Bull* 1999;25:141–156.

389. Gur RE, Resnick SM, Gur RC et al. Regional brain function in schizophrenia. II. Repeated evaluation with positron emission tomography. *Arch Gen Psychiatry* 1987;44:126–129.

390. Gur RE, Resnick SM, Gur RC. Laterality and frontality of cerebral blood flow and metabolism in schizophrenia. Relationship to symptom specificity. *Psychiatr Res* 1989;27:325–334.

391. Laakso A, Vilkman H, Alakare B et al. Striatal dopamine transporter binding in neuroleptic-naive patients with schizophrenia studied with positron emission tomography. *Am J Psychiatry* 2000;157:269–271.

392. Cohen RM, Semple WE, Gross M et al. From syndrome to illness. Delineating the pathophysiology of schizophrenia with PET. *Schizophr Bull* 1988;14:169–176.

393. Cohen RM, Semple WE, Gross M et al. Dysfunction in a prefrontal substrate of sustained attention in schizophrenia. *Life Sci* 1987;43:2031–2039.

394. DeLisi LE, Buchsbaum MS, Holcomb HH et al. Increased temporal lobe glucose use in chronic schizophrenic patients. *Biol Psychiatry* 1989;25:835–851.

395. Gunther W. MRI-SPECT and PET-EEG findings on brain dysfunction in schizophrenia. *Prog Neuro-Psychiatropharmacol Biol Psychiatry* 1992;16:445–462.

396. Siegel BV Jr, Nuechterlein KH, Abel L et al. Glucose metabolic correlates of continuous performance test performance in adults with a history of infantile autism, schizophrenics, and controls. *Schizophr Res* 1995;17:85–94.

397. Carter CS, Mintun M, Nichols T et al. Anterior cingulate gyrus dysfunction and selective attention deficits in schizophrenia: [15O]H2O PET study during single-trial Stroop task performance. *Am J Psychiatry* 1997;154:1670–1675.

398. Artiges E, Martinot JL, Verdys M et al. Altered hemispheric functional

dominance during word generation in negative schizophrenia. *Schizophr Bull* 2000;26:709–721.

399. Heckers S, Curran T, Goff D et al. Abnormalities in the thalamus and prefrontal cortex during episodic object recognition in schizophrenia. *Biol Psychiatry* 2000;48:651–657.

400. Crespo-Facorro B, Paradiso S, Andreasen NC et al. Recalling word lists reveals "cognitive dysmetria" in schizophrenia: a positron emission tomography study. *Am J Psychiatry* 1999;156:386–392.

401. Heckers S, Goff D, Schacter DL et al. Functional imaging of memory retrieval in deficit vs nondeficit schizophrenia. *Arch Gen Psychiatry* 1999;56:1117–1123.

402. Carter CS, Perlstein W, Ganguli R et al. Functional hypofrontality and working memory dysfunction in schizophrenia. *Am J Psychiatry* 1998;155:1285–1287.

403. Volkow ND, Wolf AP, Brodie JD et al. Brain interactions in chronic schizophrenics under resting and activation conditions. *Schizophr Res* 1988;1:47–53.

404. Andreasen NC, O'Leary DS, Cizadlo T et al. Schizophrenia and cognitive dysmetria: a positron-emission tomography study of dysfunctional prefrontal-thalamic-cerebellar circuitry. *Proc N Acad Sci* 1996;93:9985–9990.

405. Artiges E, Salame P, Recasens C et al. Working memory control in patients with schizophrenia: a PET study during a random number generation task. *Am J Psychiatry* 2000;157:1517–1519.

406. Heckers S, Rauch SL, Goff D et al. Impaired recruitment of the hippocampus during conscious recollection in schizophrenia. *Nature Neurosci* 1998;1:318–323.

407. Fletcher PC, McKenna PJ, Frith CD et al. Brain activations in schizophrenia during a graded memory task studied with functional neuroimaging. *Arch Gen Psychiatry* 1998;55:1001–1008.

408. Ragland JD, Gur RC, Glahn DC et al. Frontotemporal cerebral blood flow change during executive and declarative memory tasks in schizophrenia: a positron emission tomography study. *Neuropsychology* 1998;12:399–413.

409. Hyde TM, Weinberger DR. The brain in schizophrenia. *Semin Neurol* 1990;10:275–285.

410. Sedvall G. Monoamines and schizophrenia. *Acta Psychiatr Scand* 1990;358(Suppl):7–13.

411. Okubo Y, Suhara T, Suzuki K et al. Decreased prefrontal dopamine D1 receptors in schizophrenia revealed by PET. *Nature* 1997;385:634–636.

412. Sedvall G, Farde L, Hall H et al. PET scanning—a new tool in clinical psychopharmacology. *Psychiatropharmacol Ser* 1988;5:27–33.

413. Farde L, Nordstrom A-L, Eriksson L et al. Comparison of methods used with (11C)NMSP for the PET-determination of central D2 dopamine receptors. *Clin Neuropharmacol* 1990;13:87–88.

414. Wong DF, Wagner HN Jr, Tune LE et al. Positron emission tomography reveals elevated D2 dopamine receptors in drug-naive schizophrenics. *Science* 1986;234:1558–1563.

415. Tune L, Barta P, Wong D et al. Striatal dopamine D2 receptor quantification and superior temporal gyrus: volume determination in 14 chronic schizophrenic subjects. *Psychiatr Res* 1996;67:155–158.

416. Seeman P, Guan HC, Niznik HB. Endogenous dopamine lowers the dopamine D2 receptor density as measured by (3H)raclopride: implications for positron emission tomography of the human brain. *Synapse* 1989;3:96–97.

417. Elkashef AM, Doudet D, Bryant T et al. 6-(18)F-DOPA PET study in patients with schizophrenia. Positron emission tomography. *Psychiatr Res* 2000;100:1–11.

418. Hietala J, Syvalahti E, Vilkman H et al. Depressive symptoms and presynaptic dopamine function in neuroleptic-naive schizophrenia. *Schizophr Res* 1999;35:41–50.

419. Verhoeff NP, Meyer JH, Kecojevic A et al. A voxel-by-voxel analysis of [18F]setoperone PET data shows no substantial serotonin 5-HT(2A) receptor changes in schizophrenia. *Psychiatr Res* 2000;99:123–135.

420. Okubo Y, Suhara T, Suzuki K et al. Serotonin 5-HT2 receptors in schizophrenic patients studied by positron emission tomography. *Life Sci* 2000;66:2455–2464.

421. Ngan ET, Yatham LN, Ruth TJ et al. Decreased serotonin 2A receptor

densities in neuroleptic-naive patients with schizophrenia: a PET study using [(18)F]setoperone. *Am J Psychiatry* 2000;157:1016–1018.

422. Volkow ND, Brodie JD, Wolf AP et al. Brain metabolism in patients with schizophrenia before and after acute neuroleptic administration. *J Neurol Neurosurg Psychiatry* 1986;49:1199–1202.

423. Resnick SM, Gur RE, Alavi A et al. Positron emission tomography and subcortical glucose metabolism in schizophrenia. *Psychiatr Res* 1988;24:1–11.

424. Buchsbaum MS, Potkin SG, Siegel BV Jr et al. Striatal metabolic rate and clinical response to neuroleptics in schizophrenia. *Arch Gen Psychiatry* 1992;49:966–974.

425. Bartlett EJ, Brodie JD, Simkowitz P et al. Effect of a haloperidol challenge on regional brain metabolism in neuroleptic-responsive and nonresponsive schizophrenic patients. *Am J Psychiatry* 1998;155:337–343.

426. Kapur S, Zipursky R, Jones C et al. Relationship between dopamine D(2) occupancy, clinical response, and side effects: a double-blind PET study of first-episode schizophrenia. *Am J Psychiatry* 2000;157:514–520.

427. Farde L, Wiesel FA, Halldin C et al. Central D2-dopamine receptor occupancy in schizophrenic patients treated with antipsychotic drugs. *Arch Gen Psychiatry* 1988;45:71–76.

428. Kapur S, Remington G, Jones C et al. High levels of dopamine D2 receptor occupancy with low-dose haloperidol treatment: a PET study. *Am J Psychiatry* 1996;153:948–950.

429. Miller DD, Andreasen NC, O'Leary DS et al. Effect of antipsychotics on regional cerebral blood flow measured with positron emission tomography. *Neuropsychopharmacology* 1997;17:230–240.

430. Wolkin A, Barouche F, Wolf AP et al. Dopamine blockade and clinical response. Evidence for two biological subgroups of schizophrenia. *Am J Psychiatry* 1989;146:905–908.

431. Martinot JL, Pailliere-Martinot ML, Loc HC et al. Central D2 receptor blockade and antipsychotic effects of neuroleptics. Preliminary study with positron emission tomography. *Psychiatr Psychiatrobiol* 1990;5:231–240.

432. Kapur S, Zipursky R, Jones C et al. A positron emission tomography study of quetiapine in schizophrenia: a preliminary finding of an antipsychotic effect with only transiently high dopamine D2 receptor occupancy. *Arch Gen Psychiatry* 2000;57:553–559.

433. Kapur S, Cho R, Jones C et al. Is amoxapine an atypical antipsychotic? Positron-emission tomography investigation of its dopamine2 and serotonin2 occupancy. *Biol Psychiatry* 1999;45:1217–1220.

434. Kapur S, Zipursky RB, Remington G et al. 5-HT2 and D2 receptor occupancy of olanzapine in schizophrenia: a PET investigation. *Am J Psychiatry* 1998;155:921–928.

435. Cohen RM, Nordahl TE, Semple WE et al. The brain metabolic patterns of clozapine- and fluphenazine-treated female patients with schizophrenia: evidence of a sex effect. *Neuropsychopharmacology* 1999;21:632–640.

436. O'Connell RA, Van Heertum RL, Holt AR et al. Single photon emission computed tomography in psychiatry. *Clin Nucl Med* 1987;12(Suppl 9):13.

437. Phelps ME, Mazziotta JC, Baxter L et al. Positron emission tomographic study of affective disorders. Problems and strategies. *Ann Neurol* 1984;15(Suppl):S149–S156.

438. Bench CJ, Friston KJ, Brown RG et al. The anatomy of melancholia—focal abnormalities of cerebral blood flow in major depression. *Psychiatrol Med* 1992;22:607–615.

439. Dolan RJ, Bench CJ, Brown RG et al. Regional cerebral blood flow abnormalities in depressed patients with cognitive impairment. *J Neurol Neurosurg Psychiatry* 1992;55:768–773.

440. Drevets WC, Price JL, Simpson JR Jr et al. Subgenual prefrontal cortex abnormalities in mood disorders. *Nature* 1997; 386:824–827.

441. Ho AP, Gillin JC, Buchsbaum MS et al. Brain glucose metabolism during non-rapid eye movement sleep in major depression. A positron emission tomography study. *Arch Gen Psychiatry* 1996;53:645–652.

442. Yatham LN, Liddle PF, Shiah IS et al. Brain serotonin receptors in major depression: a positron emission tomography study. *Arch Gen Psychiatry* 2000;57:850–858.

443. Drevets WC, Frank E, Price JC et al. Serotonin type-1A receptor imaging in depression. *Nucl Med Biol* 2000;27:499–507.
444. Biver F, Wikler D, Lotstra F et al. Serotonin 5-HT2 receptor imaging in major depression: focal changes in orbito-insular cortex. *Br J Psychiatry* 1997;171:444–448.
445. Kumar A, Newberg A, Alavi A et al. Regional cerebral glucose metabolism in late life depression and Alzheimer's disease: a preliminary positron emission tomography study. *Proc Natl Acad Sci U S A* 1993; 90:7019–7023.
446. Meltzer CC, Price JC, Mathis CA et al. PET imaging of serotonin type 2A receptors in late-life neuropsychiatric disorders. *Am J Psychiatry* 1999;156:1871–1878.
447. Osuch EA, Ketter TA, Kimbrell TA et al. Regional cerebral metabolism associated with anxiety symptoms in affective disorder patients. *Biol Psychiatry* 2000;48:1020–1023.
448. Brody AL, Saxena S, Silverman DH et al. Brain metabolic changes in major depressive disorder from pre- to post-treatment with paroxetine. *Psychiatr Res* 1999;91:127–139.
449. Mayberg HS, Brannan SK, Tekell JL et al. Regional metabolic effects of fluoxetine in major depression: serial changes and relationship to clinical response. *Biol Psychiatry* 2000;48:830–843.
450. Zanardi R, Artigas F, Moresco R et al. Increased 5-hydroxytryptamine-2 receptor binding in the frontal cortex of depressed patients responding to paroxetine treatment: a positron emission tomography scan study. *J Clin Psychiatropharmacol* 2001;21:53–58.
451. Meyer JH, Kapur S, Eisfeld B et al. The effect of paroxetine on 5-HT(2A) receptors in depression: an [(18)F]setoperone PET imaging study. *Am J Psychiatry* 2001;158:78–85.
452. Sargent PA, Kjaer KH, Bench CJ et al. Brain serotonin1A receptor binding measured by positron emission tomography with [11C]WAY-100635: effects of depression and antidepressant treatment. *Arch Gen Psychiatry* 2000;57:174–180.
453. Yatham LN, Liddle PF, Dennie J et al. Decrease in brain serotonin 2 receptor binding in patients with major depression following desipramine treatment: a positron emission tomography study with fluorine-18-labeled setoperone. *Arch Gen Psychiatry* 1999;56:705–711.
454. Wu J, Buchsbaum MS, Gillin JC et al. Prediction of antidepressant effects of sleep deprivation by metabolic rates in the ventral anterior cingulate and medial prefrontal cortex. *Am J Psychiatry* 1999;156:1149–1158.
455. Smith GS, Reynolds CF 3rd, Pollock B et al. Cerebral glucose metabolic response to combined total sleep deprivation and antidepressant treatment in geriatric depression. *Am J Psychiatry* 1999;156:683–689.
456. Baxter LR, Phelps ME, Mazziotta JC et al. Cerebral metabolic rates for glucose in mood disorders. *Arch Gen Psychiatry* 1985;42:441–447.
457. Schwartz JM, Baxter LR, Mazziotta JC et al. The differential diagnosis of depression. Relevance of positron emission tomography studies of cerebral glucose metabolism to the bipolar-unipolar dichotomy. *JAMA* 1987;258:1368–1374.
458. Buchsbaum M, Wu J, Haier R et al. Positron emission tomography assessment of effects of benzodiazepines on regional glucose metabolic rate in patients with anxiety disorder. *Life Sci* 1986;40:2393–2400.
459. Morris P, Rapoport GI. Neuroimaging and affective disorder in late life: a review. *Can J Psychiatry* 1990;35:347–354.
460. Pearlson GD, Wong DF, Tune LE et al. In vivo D2 dopamine receptor density in psychotic and nonpsychotic patients with bipolar disorder. *Arch Gen Psychiatry* 1995;52:471–477.
461. Martinot M, Bragulat V, Artiges E et al. Decreased presynaptic dopamine function in the left caudate of depressed patients with affective flattening and psychomotor retardation. *Am J Psychiatry* 2001;158: 314–316.
462. Baxter L, Schwartz J, Mazziotta J et al. Cerebral glucose metabolic rates in nondepressed patients with obsessive-compulsive disorder. *Am J Psychiatry* 1988;145:1560–1563.
463. Nordahl TE, Benkelfat C, Semple W et al. Cerebral glucose metabolic rates in obsessive compulsive disorder. *Neuropsychopharmacology* 1989;2:23–28.
464. Swedo SE, Schapiro MB, Grady CL et al. Cerebral glucose metabolism in childhood-onset obsessive-compulsive disorder. *Arch Gen Psychiatry* 1989;46:518–523.
465. Insel TR, Winslow JT. Neurobiology of obsessive-compulsive disorder. *Psychiatr Clin North Am* 1992;15:813–824.
466. Brody AL, Saxena S, Schwartz JM et al. FDG-PET predictors of response to behavioral therapy and pharmacotherapy in obsessive compulsive disorder. *Psychiatr Res* 1998;84:1–6.
467. Schwartz JM, Stoessel PW, Baxter LR et al. Systematic changes in cerebral glucose metabolic rate after successful behavior modification treatment of obsessive-compulsive disorder. *Arch Gen Psychiatry* 1996; 53:109–113.
468. Saxena S, Brody AL, Maidment KM et al. Localized orbitofrontal and subcortical metabolic changes and predictors of response to paroxetine treatment in obsessive-compulsive disorder. *Neuropsychopharmacology* 1999;21:683–693.
469. Schwartz JM, Stoessel PW, Baxter LR Jr et al. Systematic changes in cerebral glucose metabolic rate after successful behavior modification treatment of obsessive-compulsive disorder. *Arch Gen Psychiatry* 1996; 53:109–113.
470. Rauch SL, Jenike MA, Alpert NM et al. Regional cerebral blood flow measured during symptom provocation in obsessive-compulsive disorder using oxygen 15-labeled carbon dioxide and positron emission tomography. *Arch Gen Psychiatry* 1994;51:62–70.
471. Reiman E, Rachle M, Butler F et al. A focal brain abnormality in panic disorder: a severe form of anxiety. *Nature* 1984;310:683–685.
472. Reiman E, Rachle M, Robbins E et al. Neuroanatomical correlates of a lactate-induced anxiety attack. *Arch Gen Psychiatry* 1989;46: 493–500.
473. Reiman E, Rachle M, Robbins E et al. The application of positron emission tomography to the study of panic disorder. *Am J Psychiatry* 1986;143:469–477.
474. Mountz J, Modell J, Wilson M et al. PET evaluation of cerebral blood flow during anxiety state in simple phobia. *Arch Gen Psychiatry* 1989; 46:501–504.
475. Abou-Khalil BW, Siegel GJ, Sackellares JC et al. Positron emission tomography studies of cerebral glucose metabolism in chronic partial epilepsy. *Ann Neurol* 1987;22:480–486.
476. Engel J Jr, Brown WJ, Kuhl DE et al. Pathologic findings underlying focal temporal lobe hypometabolism in partial epilepsy. *Ann Neurol* 1982;12:518–528.
477. Engel J Jr, Kuhl DE, Phelps ME et al. Comparative localization of the epileptic foci in partial epilepsy by PCT and EEG. *Ann Neurol* 1982;12:529–537.
478. Theodore WH, Brooks R, Sato S et al. The role of positron emission tomography in the evaluation of seizure disorders. *Ann Neurol* 1984; 15(Suppl):S1176–S1179.
479. Theodore WH, Newmark ME, Sato S et al. 18F-fluorodeoxyglucose positron emission tomography in refractory complex partial seizures. *Ann Neurol* 1983;13:537.
480. Henry TR, Sutherling WW, Engel J Jr et al. Interictal cerebral metabolism in partial epilepsies of neocortical origin. *Epilepsy Res* 1991;10: 174–182.
481. Engel J Jr. PET scanning in partial epilepsy. *Can J Neurol Sci* 1991; 18(Suppl):588–592.
482. Duncan R. Epilepsy, cerebral blood flow, and cerebral metabolic rate. *Cerebrovasc Brain Metab Rev* 1992;4:105–121.
483. Utsubo H, Chuang SH, Hwang PA et al. Neuroimaging for investigation of seizures in children. *Pediatr Neurosurg* 1992;18:105–116.
484. Breier JI, Mullani NA, Thomas AB et al. Effects of duration of epilepsy on the uncoupling of metabolism and blood flow in complex partial seizures. *Neurology* 1997;48:1047–1053.
485. Spanaki MV, Kopylev L, Liow K et al. Relationship of seizure frequency to hippocampus volume and metabolism in temporal lobe epilepsy. *Epilepsia* 2000;41:1227–1229.
486. Savic I, Altshuler L, Baxter L et al. Pattern of interictal hypometabolism in PET scans with fludeoxyglucose F 18 reflects prior seizure types in patients with mesial temporal lobe seizures. *Arch Neurol* 1997; 54:129–136.
487. Theodore WH, Katz D, Kufta C et al. Pathology of temporal lobe foci: correlation with CT, MRI and PET. *Neurology* 1990;40:797–803.
488. Theodore WH, Gaillard WD, Sato S et al. Positron emission tomo-

graphic measurement of cerebral blood flow and temporal lobectomy. *Ann Neurol* 1994;36:241–244.

489. Manno EM, Sperling MR, Ding X et al. Predictors of outcome after anterior temporal lobectomy: positron emission tomography. *Neurology* 1994;44:2331–2336.

490. Radtke RA, Hanson MW, Hoffman JM et al. Temporal lobe hypometabolism on PET: predictor of seizure control after temporal lobectomy. *Neurology* 1993;43:1088–1092.

491. Wong C-Y, Geller EB, Chen EQ et al. Outcome of temporal lobe epilepsy surgery predicted by statistical parametric PET imaging. *J Nucl Med* 1996;37:1094–1100.

492. Theodore WH, Sato S, Kufta C et al. Temporal lobectomy for uncontrolled seizures: The role of positron emission tomography. *Ann Neurol* 1992;32:789–794.

493. Delbeke D, Lawrence SK, Abou-Khalil BW et al. Postsurgical outcome of patients with uncontrolled complex partial seizures and temporal lobe hypometabolism on 18FDG-positron emission tomography. *Invest Radiol* 1996;31:261–266.

494. Benbadis SR, So NK, Antar MA et al. The value of PET scan (and MRI and Wada test) in patients with bitemporal epileptiform abnormalities. *Arch Neurol* 1995;52:1062–1068.

495. Swartz BE, Tomiyasu U, Delgado-Escueta AV et al. Neuroimaging in temporal lobe epilepsy: test sensitivity and relationships to pathology and postoperative outcome. *Epilepsia* 1992;33:624–634.

496. Newberg A, Alavi A, Sperling M et al. Thalamic metabolic asymmetry on FDG-PET scans as a determinant of seizure outcome after temporal lobectomy. *J Nucl Med* 1997;38:92P.

497. Engel J Jr, Kuhl DE, Phelps ME. Patterns of human local cerebral glucose metabolism during epileptic seizures. *Science* 1982;218:64–66.

498. Theodore WH, Fishbein D, Dubinsky R. Patterns of cerebral glucose metabolism in patients with partial seizures. *Neurology* 1988;38:1201–1206.

499. Markand ON, Salanova V, Worth R et al. Comparative study of interictal PET and ictal SPECT in complex partial seizures. *Acta Neurol Scand* 1997;95:129–136.

500. Salanova V, Markand O, Worth R et al. FDG-PET and MRI in temporal lobe epilepsy: relationship to febrile seizures, hippocampal sclerosis and outcome. *Acta Neurol Scand* 1998;97:146–153.

501. Knowlton RC, Laxer KD, Ende G et al. Presurgical multimodality neuroimaging in electroencephalographic lateralized temporal lobe epilepsy. *Ann Neurol* 1997;42:829–837.

502. Bernardi S, Trimble MR, Frackowiak RSJ et al. An interictal study of partial epilepsy using positron emission tomography and oxygen-15 inhalation method. *J Neurol Neurosurg Psychiatry* 1983;46:473–477.

503. Franck G, Maquet P, Sadzot B et al. Contribution of positron emission tomography to the investigation of epilepsies of frontal lobe origin. *Adv Neurol* 1992;57:471–485.

504. Och RF, Yamamoto Y, Gloor P. Correlations between the positron emission tomography measurement of glucose metabolism and oxygen utilization in focal epilepsy. *Neurology* 1984;34(Suppl 1):125.

505. Sperling M, Wilson G, Engel J Jr et al. Magnetic resonance imaging in intractable partial epilepsy: correlative studies. *Ann Neurol* 1986;20:57–62.

506. Rubin E, Dhawan V, Moeller JR et al. Cerebral metabolic topography in unilateral temporal lobe epilepsy. *Neurology* 1995;45:2212–2223.

507. Van Bogaert P, Massager N, Tugendhaft P et al. Statistical parametric mapping of regional glucose metabolism in mesial temporal lobe epilepsy. *Neuroimage* 2000;12:129–138.

508. Quesney LF, Olivier A, Andermann F et al. Preoperative EEG investigation in patients with frontal lobe epilepsy: trends, results and pathophysiological considerations. *J Clin Neurophysiol* 1987;4:208–209.

509. Rasmussen T. Surgery of frontal lobe epilepsy. In: Purpura DP, Penry JK, Walter RD, eds. *Advances in neurology*, vol 8. New York: Raven Press, 1975.

510. Franck G, Maquet P, Sadzot B et al. Contribution of positron emission tomography to the investigation of epilepsies of frontal lobe origin. *Adv Neurol* 1992;57:471–485.

511. Robitaille Y, Rasmussen T, Dubeau F et al. Histopathology of non-neoplastic lesions in frontal lobe epilepsy: review of 180 cases with recent MRI and PET correlations. *Adv Neurol* 1992;57:499–511.

512. Alavi A, Hirsch LJ. Studies of central nervous system disorders with single photon emission computed tomography and positron emission tomography. Evolution over the past 2 decades. *Semin Nucl Med* 1991;21:58–81.

513. Chugani HT, Rintahaka PJ, Shewmon DA. Ictal patterns of cerebral glucose utilization in children with epilepsy. *Epilepsia* 1994;35:813–822.

514. Theodore WH, Balish M, Leiderman D et al. Effect of seizures on cerebral blood flow measured with 15O-H2O and positron emission tomography. *Epilepsia* 1996;37:796–802.

515. Savic I, Persson A, Roland P et al. In-vivo demonstration of reduced benzodiazepine receptor binding in human epileptic foci. *Lancet* 1988;2:863–866.

516. Savic I, Svanborg E, Thorell JO. Cortical benzodiazepine receptor changes are related to frequency of partial seizures: a positron emission tomography study. *Epilepsia* 1996;37:236–244.

517. Debets RM, Sadzot B, van Isselt JW et al. Is 11C-flumazenil PET superior to 18FDG PET and 123I-iomazenil SPECT in presurgical evaluation of temporal lobe epilepsy? *J Neurol Neurosurg Psychiatry* 1997;62:141–150.

518. Juhasz C, Nagy F, Watson C et al. Glucose and [11C]flumazenil positron emission tomography abnormalities of thalamic nuclei in temporal lobe epilepsy. *Neurology* 1999;53:2037–2045.

519. Savic I, Thorell JO. Localized cerebellar reductions in benzodiazepine receptor density in human partial epilepsy. *Arch Neurol* 1996;53:656–662.

520. Savic I, Thorell JO, Roland P. [11C]flumazenil positron emission tomography visualizes frontal epileptogenic regions. *Epilepsia* 1995;36:1225–1232.

521. Arnold S, Berthele A, Drzezga A et al. Reduction of benzodiazepine receptor binding is related to the seizure onset zone in extratemporal focal cortical dysplasia. *Epilepsia* 2000;41:818–824.

522. Richardson MP, Koepp MJ, Brooks DJ et al. Benzodiazepine receptors in focal epilepsy with cortical dysgenesis: an 11C-flumazenil PET study. *Ann Neurol* 1996;40:188–198.

523. Greenberg JH, Reivich M, Alavi A et al. Metabolic mapping of functional activity in man with 18F-fluoro-deoxyglucose technique. *Science* 1981;212:678–680.

524. Mazziotta JC, Phelps ME, Carson RE et al. Tomographic mapping of human cerebral metabolism: sensory deprivation. *Ann Neurol* 1982;12:435–444.

525. Mazziotta JC, Phelps ME, Carson RE et al. Tomographic mapping of human cerebral metabolism. Normal unstimulated state. *Neurology* 1981;31:503–516.

526. Finkelstein S, Alpert NM, Ackerman RH et al. Positron brain, imaging—normal patterns and asymmetries. *Brain Cogn* 1982;1:286–293.

527. Kushner MJ, Rosenquist A, Alavi A et al. Cerebral metabolism and patterned visual stimulation. A positron emission tomographic study of the human visual cortex. *Neurology* 1988;38:89–95.

528. Phelps ME, Huhl DE, Mazziotta JC. Metabolic mapping of the brain's response to visual stimulation. Studies in man. *Science* 1981;211:1445–1448.

529. Vidryanszky Z, Gulyas B, Roland PE. Visual exploration of form and position with identical stimuli: functional anatomy with PET. *Human Brain Mapping* 2000;11:104–116.

530. Mellet E, Briscogne S, Tzourio-Mazoyer N et al. Neural correlates of topographic mental exploration: the impact of route versus survey perspective learning. *Neuroimage* 2000;12:588–600.

531. Petersen SE, Fox BT, Posner MI et al. Positron emission tomographic studies of the cortical anatomy of single-word processing. *Nature* 1988;331:585–589.

532. Mazziotta JC, Phelps ME, Carson RE. Tomographic mapping of human cerebral metabolism. Auditory stimulation. *Neurology* 1982;32:921–928.

533. Wise R, Hadar U, Howard D et al. Language activation studies with positron emission tomography. *Ciba Found Symp* 1991;153:218–228.

534. Cowell SF, Egan GF, Code C et al. The functional neuroanatomy of simple calculation and number repetition: A parametric PET activation study. *Neuroimage* 2000;12:565–573.

535. Pesenti M, Thioux M, Seron X et al. Neuroanatomical substrates of arabic number processing, numerical comparison, and simple addition: a PET study. *J Cog Neurosci* 2000;12:461–479.

536. Heiss WD, Pawlik G, Holthoff V et al. PET correlates of normal and impaired memory functions. *Cerebrovasc Brain Metab Rev* 1992; 4:1–27.

537. Friston KJ, Grasby PM, Frith CD et al. The neurotransmitter basis of cognition: psychopharmacological activation studies using positron emission tomography. *Ciba Found Symp* 1991;163:76–87.

538. Raichle ME. Memory mechanisms in the processing of words and word-like symbols. *Ciba Found Symp* 1991;163:198–204.

539. Nyberg L, Habib R, Herlitz A. Brain activation during episodic memory retrieval: sex differences. *Acta Psychiatrol* 2000;105:181–194.

540. Nyberg L, Habib R, McIntosh AR et al. Reactivation of encoding-related brain activity during memory retrieval. *Proc Natl Acad Sci U S A* 2000;97:11120–11124.

541. Wiser AK, Andreasen N, O'Leary DS et al. Novel vs. well-learned memory for faces: a positron emission tomography study. *J Cog Neurosci* 2000;12:255–266.

542. Conway MA, Turk DJ, Miller SL et al. A positron emission tomography (PET) study of autobiographical memory retrieval. *Memory* 1999; 7:679–702.

543. Volkow ND, Tancredi LR. Biol correlates of mental activity studied with PET. *Am J Psychiatry* 1991;148:439–443.

544. Haxby JV, Grady CL, Ungerleider LG et al. Mapping the functional neuroanatomy of the intact human brain with brain work imaging. *Neuropsychologia* 1991;29:539–555.

545. Baron J. Testing cerebral function: will it help the understanding or diagnosis of central nervous system disease? *Ciba Found Symp* 1991; 163:250–261.

546. Corbetta M, Miezin FM, Shulman GL et al. Selective attention modulates extrastriate visual regions in humans during visual feature discrimination and recognition. *Ciba Found Symp* 1991;163:165–175.

547. Frith CD, Friston K, Liddle PF et al. Willed action and the prefrontal cortex in man: a study with PET. *Proc R Soc Lond* 1991;244:241–246.

548. Pardo JV, Fox PT, Raichle ME. Localization of a human system for sustained attention by positron emission tomography. *Nature* 1991; 349:61–64.

549. Castelli F, Happe F, Frith U et al. Movement and mind: a functional imaging study of perception and interpretation of complex intentional movement patterns. *Neuroimage* 2000;12:314–325.

550. Schnider A, Treyer V, Buck A. Selection of currently relevant memories by the human posterior medial orbitofrontal cortex. *J Neurosci* 2000;20:5880–5884.

551. Shin LM, Dougherty DD, Orr SP et al. Activation of anterior paralimbic structures during guilt-related script-driven imagery. *Biol Psychiatry* 2000;48:43–50.

552. Taylor SF, Liberzon I, Koeppe RA. The effect of graded aversive stimuli on limbic and visual activation. *Neuropsychologia* 2000;38: 1415–1425.

553. Dougherty DD, Shin LM, Alpert NM et al. Anger in healthy men: a PET study using script-driven imagery. *Biol Psychiatry* 1999;46: 466–472.

Diagnostic Nuclear Medicine, Fourth Edition. Edited by M.P. Sandler, R.E. Coleman, J.A. Patton, F.J.Th. Wackers, A. Gottschalk. Lippincott Williams & Wilkins, Philadelphia 2003.

39

SPECT IMAGING OF CEREBRAL NEUROTRANSMISSION

ANA M. CATAFAU

Electric impulses were thought to be the main mechanism responsible for signal transmission between neurons. Now it is recognized that the events responsible for the generation of these electric impulses are of a chemical nature. These events take place in the synapse, that is, the interface between the axonal terminal of the presynaptic neurons and the dendrites of the postsynaptic neurons. During cerebral neurotransmission, chemical compounds (neurotransmitters) are released from the presynaptic neuron to the synaptic cleft, where they reach proteins (receptors) located in the membrane of the postsynaptic neuron. The neurotransmitter-receptor interaction leads to changes in ion channels of the postsynaptic membrane, thus generating the electric impulse or action potential, which is responsible for the release of neurotransmitters from the axonal terminal. After the interaction with receptors, neurotransmitters are cleared from the synapse via enzymatic metabolism or reuptake by proteins called transporters that are located on the membrane of the presynaptic terminal.

Study of neurotransmission is important because dysfunction of specific neurotransmission systems has been implicated in most neurologic and psychiatric diseases. In most cases, drugs used for treatment of neuropsychiatric diseases or for the symptoms of these diseases have been designed to counteract involved neurotransmission abnormalities. Examples are given in Table 39.1. A method for the study of cerebral neurotransmission *in vivo* such as single photon emission computed tomography (SPECT) allows investigation of the pathophysiology of neuropsychiatric diseases and will contribute to the design of new drugs and therapeutic strategies and consequently to advances in psychopharmacology.

Before the development of SPECT and positron emission tomography (PET), the study of cerebral neurotransmission in humans was carried out only *in vitro* on postmortem brain homogenates or by means of autoradiography of brain slices previously incubated with ^{3}H- or ^{125}I-labeled ligands, which provided elegant images on the distribution of several synaptic elements. However, dynamic interactions that occur in the live brain, such

as modulation between systems or competition with endogenous neurotransmitters, are not usually considered in postmortem studies of neurotransmission.

Several ligands for receptors and transporters have been successfully labeled for SPECT imaging with gamma-emitter isotopes such as ^{123}I and ^{99m}Tc. The relatively long half-life of these isotopes, the relative simplicity of the methods that can be applied for neurotransmission assessment, and the availability of the equipment make the study of cerebral neurotransmission with SPECT cost effective. SPECT of the dopaminergic system has already been added to the arsenal of nuclear medicine tools in the clinical setting. For this system, receptors, transporters, and endogenous dopamine release can be imaged using SPECT. This chapter focuses on how to perform and interpret neurotransmission SPECT imaging in a practical manner for routine clinical use. Information about ligand-target interaction, radioligands, methodology, and interpretation of this technique, as well as the main clinical applications and research findings, are provided.

CONCEPTS FOR PRACTICAL PERFORMANCE OF NEUROTRANSMISSION SPECT IMAGING

A knowledge of the interaction between the ligand and the receptor or transporter (ligand-target interaction) is needed to understand the kinetic properties of the radioligands for SPECT imaging of cerebral neurotransmission. Particular technical aspects of this procedure, as well as the assessment of the images, are also based on the special nature of the ligand-target interaction and the radioligand's kinetics.

In the live brain, the target-ligand interaction is a dynamic process. Classically, a three-compartmental model is used to represent SPECT radioligand kinetics. The universally used law of mass action is used to explain the bimolecular reaction of drug-receptor. Specific binding to the receptor occurs while free ligand is in excess. When the amount of free ligand equals the amount of bound ligand, equilibrium is achieved (1). The compartmental model proposed for neurotransmission SPECT is shown in Fig. 39.1. In this model, $C_{\#}$ represents compartments, $k_{\#}$ are the transfer rate constants (sec^{-1}) that measure transit of the radioligand between compartments, and $V_{\#}$ is the quantity of

A.M. Catafau: Clinical Pharmacology Discovery Medicine, Centre of Excellence for Drug Discovery, Psychiatry, Barcelona, Spain.

Table 39.1. *Neurotransmission Systems Involved in Neuropsychiatric Diseases and Corresponding Drugs Used for their Treatment*

Neurotrans-mission system	Receptor	Disease	Medication
Dopaminergic	$D_{1,2,3,4}$	Parkinson's	L-Dopa
		Schizophrenia	Typical antipsychotics
Serotoninergic	$5HT_{1A, 1B, 1C}$	Depression	SSRIs
	$5HT_{2A, 2B}$	OCD	SSRIs
		Schizophrenia	Atypical antipsychotics
GABAergic	$GABA_{A, B}$	Anxiety	
		Epilepsy	Benzodiazepines
Cholinergic	$M_{1,2,3}$	Huntington's	Tacrine,
	Nicotinic	Alzheimer's	Donepezile

OCD, obsessive compulsive disorder; SSRIs, selective serotonin reuptake inhibitors.

radioligand distributed in each compartment. After intravenous administration of the radioligand, the first compartment in which it is located is the plasma (C_1 or vascular compartment). The ligand crosses the intact blood–brain barrier and enters the brain (k_1). The initial distribution of the tracer in the brain is proportional to cerebral blood flow, and images acquired during this time are quite similar to cerebral perfusion SPECT images (2,3). At this stage, most of the radioligand is found in the cerebral tissue both in free and nonspecifically bound fractions (C_2 or nondisplaceable compartment) and is progressively bound to the specific target (k_3) (C_3, specific binding fraction or target compartment). The radioligand can also be displaced from the target to the nondisplaceable compartment (k_4) and can come back to the blood (k_2). The radioligand is progressively bound to the target until equilibrium is reached. At equilibrium, there is no net transfer of radioligand between compartments.

The terms *affinity, dissociation,* and *density* are crucial to understand the ligand-target interaction, the desirable requirements for radioligands (4,5), and the outcome quantification parameter obtained from SPECT imaging—the binding potential (BP). Affinity refers to the ability of the ligand to recognize and be bound to a specific target and relates to molecular specificity. This concept is the inverse of dissociation, which refers to the ability of the ligand to unbind from the target. If the dissociation

constant is expressed as k_d, then affinity is $1/k_d$. The term density refers to the number or concentration of the target (e.g., receptors or transporters). Saturability is related to target density. Receptors are present in the brain in very low concentration (approximately 10^{-12} mol/g), and if a ligand is delivered in excess, the receptors will be saturated. If all the targets were bound by the ligand, then the maximum binding of the ligand would be a measure of the target density. Therefore, density is expressed as B_{max} (maximum binding). However, in the live brain, a certain number of targets are occupied by endogenous neurotransmitter. Thus, B'_{max} is used to represent the density of *free* target, that is, the number of targets that are available for the ligand because they are not already occupied. The outcome measurement of SPECT imaging reflects the density of the target or synaptic element of interest. This measurement is the BP, defined as B_{max}/Kd (6). However, quantification of BP with SPECT requires dynamic acquisitions over time and serial blood samples, which makes the method difficult and the procedure impractical for routine clinical use. Therefore, the measurement that can be obtained in the more simple and widely used SPECT approach (see Methodology section) can be defined as $BP^* = V''_3 = BP/V_2$, V_2 is the quantity of radioligand distributed in the nondisplaceable compartment at equilibrium (7,8).

RADIOLIGANDS FOR SPECT IMAGING OF CEREBRAL NEUROTRANSMISSION

To be suitable for cerebral neurotransmission SPECT imaging, the main requirements of a ligand are (a) to freely diffuse across the intact blood–brain barrier, (b) to have a low nonspecific tissular absorption, (c) to have a high affinity for the target (e.g., receptor or transporter), (d) to have a slow dissociation rate from the target, and (e) to have low or polar metabolites that do not cross the blood–brain barrier (1,5). To avoid saturability of the targets, very low concentrations of ligands must be injected, which implies the preparation of radioligands with very high specific activities (in the Curies per nanomole range).

High binding affinity and slow dissociation rate are needed for SPECT detection of the specific binding sites after clearance of the radioligand from the blood and from the nonspecifically bound tissues. A slow metabolism of the tracer compared with the SPECT timing is also desirable. Typically, radioligands for SPECT have slow metabolism and slow dissociation rates. Hence, after a bolus injection of the radioligand, the uptake ratio of the region rich in target to the region free of target increases until a steady-state condition is achieved. This steady-state condition, in which the uptake ratio remains constant, can be maintained long enough to perform single static SPECT imaging, that is, for 30 to 45 minutes. Washout of the ligand from the brain occurs afterwards (Fig. 39.2).

Neurotransmission SPECT imaging in humans is already possible using radioligands for the dopaminergic, serotoninergic, γ-aminobutyric acid (GABA)ergic, and muscarinic cholinergic systems (Table 39.2). For the dopaminergic and serotoninergic systems, it is possible to image receptors and transporters (9–20). For the GABAergic and muscarinic systems, radioligands for human use have been developed only for receptors (21–25).

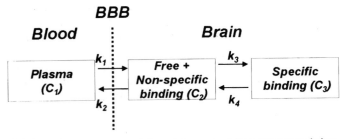

FIGURE 39.1. Compartmental model proposed for neurotransmission single photon emission computed tomography.

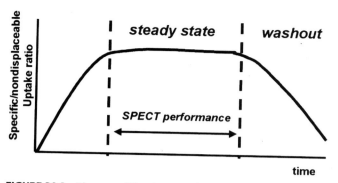

FIGURE 39.2. Diagram of the changes of the specific/nondisplaceable uptake ratios expected over time after a bolus injection of a radioligand for single photon emission computed tomography (SPECT). The single SPECT acquisition has to be performed during steady state.

Table 39.3. *Radioligands in Study for Cerebral Neurotransmission SPECT Imaging*

Target	Radioligand	Reference
Serotonin 5HT$_{1A}$ R	^{123}I-p-MPPI	26
Nicotinic acetylcholine R	^{123}I-A-85380	27
Vesicular acetylcholine transporter	^{123}I-DRC140	28
Opioid R	[125]I-7alpha-O-IA-DPN	29

R, receptor.

SPECT of the dopaminergic system can be performed on a routine clinical basis, because the receptor ligand ^{123}I-IBZM and the dopamine transporter (DAT) ligand ^{123}I-FP-CIT are already registered and commercially available in Europe. Radioligands for other synaptic elements such as serotonin 5-hydroxytryptamine 1A (5-HT$_{1A}$) receptors, nicotinic acetylcholine receptors, and opioid receptors, as well as for the vesicular acetylcholine transporter, have been proven suitable for SPECT in animals and are promising future ligands if human studies are successful (26–29) (Table 39.3). All radioligands for neurotransmission SPECT are labeled with ^{123}I, except for the DAT ligand TRO-DAT, which has been successfully labeled with [99m]Tc (18). Obviously, future development of technetium-labeled ligands will further expand the availability of neurotransmission SPECT imaging.

Table 39.2. *Radioligands for Neurotransmission SPECT Imaging in Humans*

Target	Radioligand	Reference
Dopaminergic D$_2$R (postsynaptic)	^{123}I-IBZM	9
	^{123}I-Epipride	10
	^{123}I-BF	11
	^{123}I-Iodospiperone	12
	^{123}I-Iodolisuride	13
DA transporter (presynaptic)	^{123}I-β-CIT	14
	^{123}I-FP-CIT	15
	^{123}I-IPT	16
	^{123}I-PE2I	17
	^{99m}Tc-TRODAT-1	18
Benzodiazepinic R	^{123}I-Iomazenil	21
	^{123}I-NNC-13-8241	22
Serotoninergic 5HT$_{2A}$ R	^{123}I-R91150	19
5HT transporter	^{123}I-β-CIT	14
	^{123}I-ADAM	20
Muscarinic acetylcholine R	^{123}I-IDEX	23
	^{123}I-IQNP	24
NMDA glutamate R	^{123}I-MK-00801	25

R, receptor; DA, dopamine; 5HT, serotonine; NMDA, N-methyl-D-aspartate.

METHODOLOGY OF NEUROTRANSMISSION SPECT

Several methodologic approaches have been proposed for neurotransmission SPECT imaging. The radioligand can be injected as a bolus (generally over a 10-second period, flushed with saline) or as a bolus plus constant infusion of variable duration and rates of infusion that depend on the radioligand and the purpose of the study (30,31). With regard to acquisition protocols, dynamic studies can be performed that acquire several sets of SPECT images from the time of injection to the end of the study, or a conventional single static SPECT acquisition can be performed during the steady-state condition.

Study Designs

Protocols including constant infusion and dynamic acquisition are appropriate for research, allowing more accurate quantification and overcoming the problem of lipophilic metabolites when present (32). These protocols are also appropriate for imaging intrasynaptic release of endogenous neurotransmitters, as demonstrated for dopamine (31). However, dynamic SPECT acquisition needs adequate temporal resolution in case short acquisition times are required. In addition, these studies are long lasting, requiring acquisition of SPECT images for several hours. Constant infusions from 7 to 9 hours have been reported, using several ligands for dopamine receptor imaging (31–33). Furthermore, a larger radiation exposure to the subjects is entailed. In addition, serial blood samples (arterial and or venous) have to be drawn to correct for metabolites of the radioligand, and data must also be decay-corrected. Hence, these protocols are impractical for neurotransmission SPECT performance in a routine clinical setting.

On the other hand, the bolus injection followed by a conventional single SPECT acquisition during steady state is a simpler approach that allows quantification of BP from a single-point measurement of tracer uptake in target-rich and target-poor cerebral regions. Factors that may interfere with the accuracy of the results, such as plasma clearance of the radioligand, can be integrated in the assessment, thus improving the reliability of the results (34). This is the protocol used in clinical practice for diagnosis purposes, because it improves patient compliance and makes the study more feasible and cost effective. Extensive research has also been reported using this simpler approach, which is the focus of this chapter.

Using the bolus injection and single SPECT acquisition protocol, the SPECT acquisition must be performed during the steady-state condition described previously. Fig. 39.2 outlines the sequence of uptake ratio changes measured by SPECT from the time of injection. Specific/nonspecific uptake ratio (defined later) progressively increases from the time of injection until equilibrium is achieved. Then, a steady-state condition, in which the specific/nonspecific uptake ratio remains constant, is maintained long enough to enable a conventional SPECT acquisition (2). SPECT imaging must be performed at this time, before washout begins. Recommended acquisition timing lots depend on the radioligand. For ^{123}I-IBZM, the steady-state condition has been reported between 60- and 180-minutes postinjection (35) and for ^{123}I-FP-CIT between 3- and 6-hours postinjection (15). General rules to define SPECT acquisition parameters and reconstruction do not differ from those already described for cerebral perfusion SPECT imaging, although some special issues have been reported (36).

Data Analysis

For data analysis, the region-of-interest (ROI) method is used. ROIs are placed on cerebral regions rich in the target element and on a cerebral region free of the target element (Fig. 39.3). Uptake of the radioligand in the target-rich regions (e.g., the striatum for dopamine receptor or transporters or the cerebral cortex for serotonin receptors) reflects the specific binding fraction. Counts obtained from the target-free regions (e.g., cerebellum or a cerebral cortex region, such as the frontal or the occipital

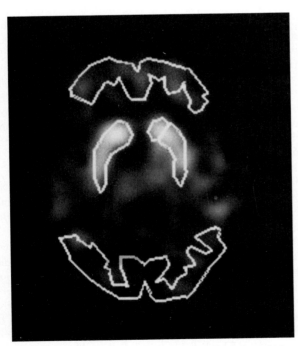

FIGURE 39.3. Example of regions-of interest (ROIs) that can be used for data analysis. On a dopamine transporter (DAT) SPECT slice at the basal ganglia level, specific uptake is obtained from the ROIs placed on caudate, putamen, and/or the whole striatum. The nondisplaceable activity is obtained from a ROI placed in a DAT-free region, such as the occipital cortex or the frontal cortex.

lobes for dopamine receptors or transporters, or the cerebellum for serotonin receptors) reflect the free and nonspecifically bound fraction. BP* (or V_3'') is expressed as the ratio of specific/nonspecific uptake, or more accurately as the ratio of [specific − (free + nonspecific)]/(free + nonspecific) uptake.

ROIs can be drawn directly on SPECT images or can be drawn on the magnetic resonance imaging (MRI) of the subject if coregistration with SPECT is used (Fig. 39.4). First, tridimensional realignment of the SPECT and MRI images is performed, then the ROIs are drawn on the MRI and copied to the corresponding SPECT slices. However, because of the low spatial resolution of SPECT images, fiducial markers that can be identified in both the SPECT and MRI scans should be placed in the same location on the head of the patient during both procedures. Plastic masks and laser beams for positioning can also help. Automated registration methods of brain receptor SPECT images through intermediary transmission CT have been reported (37), although they are not implemented yet. Nevertheless, for routine clinical purposes, even visual assessment has been reported to be suitable for neurotransmission SPECT images. The normal pattern depends on the radioligand used. At steady state, the maximum uptake is seen in the cerebral regions rich in the target, and poor activity is seen in the remaining cerebral regions. Dopamine receptors and transporters show the same normal SPECT patterns, because both elements are equally distributed throughout the brain. Because dopaminergic D2 receptors (D2Rs) and DAT are concentrated in the striatum, only this structure shows high tracer uptake (Fig. 39.5). In cases of asymmetric uptake between hemispheres or between structures (e.g., caudate vs. putamen), visual assessment is feasible (3,38,39) (Fig. 39.6). However, in cases of symmetrical abnormalities the relationship between target and background is more difficult to assess only with visual inspection, and quantification is recommended.

Interpretation

Neurotransmission SPECT provides information on the distribution, density, and degree of occupancy of the synaptic element that is studied. For imaging interpretation, the law of mass action and the compartmental model described previously must be kept in mind. Influence of interfering medications in the radioligand uptake has to be taken into account, because competition between the drug and the radioligand for the target synaptic site leads to a decreased binding of the radioligand. Therefore, history of medication has to be carefully done before the SPECT procedure, and a complete washout of drugs that may interfere with the study is required. Under these conditions, a decreased uptake of the radioligand can reflect: (a) decreased density or affinity (as assessed by the BP*) of the target element or (b) increased occupancy by the endogenous neurotransmitter (if no interfering drugs are present). Inversely, an increased uptake of the radioligand may reflect: (a) increased density or affinity of the target element or (b) a deficit of the endogenous neurotransmitter in the synaptic cleft.

In addition to the effects from medication, up-regulation and down-regulation phenomena, as well as neuronal loss, are factors to consider when interpreting neurotransmission SPECT images. Recently, agonist-mediated receptor internalization has

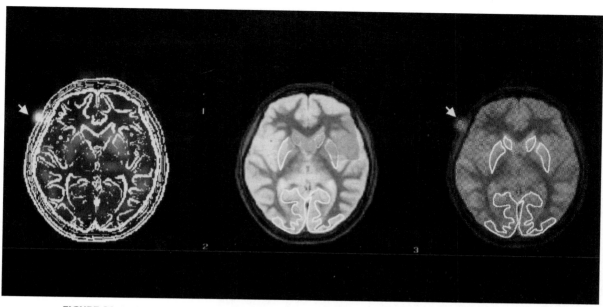

FIGURE 39.4. Coregistration method. After single photon emission computed tomography-magnetic resonance imaging (SPECT-MRI) realignment, regions-of-interest (ROIs) are drawn on the MRI and copied to the corresponding SPECT slice for analysis. Arrows point to fiducials used for realignment.

been proposed to play an important role in characterizing receptor-ligand interactions with *in vivo* neurotransmission imaging techniques (40).

CLINICAL APPLICATIONS OF NEUROTRANSMISSION SPECT

Most of the reported experience with neurotransmission SPECT has been with the dopaminergic system (for a review, see reference 41). This system is involved in important neurologic and psychiatric diseases, such as Parkinson's disease and other movement disorders, schizophrenia, and substance abuse. Also, there has been successful development of radioligands for dopamine receptors and transporters. Consequently, the only established clinical indication for neurotransmission SPECT is the assessment of the dopaminergic system in parkinsonisms. Dementias and cerebrovascular disease are other potential clinical applications of neurotransmission SPECT with radioligands for dopaminergic and other systems. Finally, extensive and interesting research work has been done in schizophrenia and other psychiatric diseases, providing insight into the pathophysiology and contributing to drug development. In this section of the chapter, established and potential clinical applications, as well as the main research findings of neurotransmission SPECT, are described.

Parkinsonism

DATs are located in the membrane of the presynaptic nigrostriatal dopaminergic neurons. Therefore, DAT ligands (Table 39.2) are useful in detecting the loss of functional dopaminergic presynaptic neuron terminals in the striatum. Degeneration of these nigrostriatal neurons is present in parkinsonian syndromes such

as Parkinson's disease (PD) and the Parkinson-plus syndromes, such as multiple system atrophy (MSA) and progressive supranuclear palsy (PSP) (42). All these diseases present with parkinsonism as a common feature. Symptoms of parkinsonism are tremor, rigidity, and bradykinesia, and the diagnosis of parkinsonism can be made if two of these three symptoms are present in any combination. However, there are other diseases that may present with parkinsonism and do not involve degeneration of the nigrostriatal neurons. This is the case in essential tremor and parkinsonian syndromes secondary to medication, toxins, encephalitis, vascular disease, and others. Treatment and prognosis in terms of disease progression are different for each clinical entity (42). For example, L-DOPA is ineffective in patients with essential tremor, a disease known as "benign parkinsonism" because of its smooth progression. Parkinsonian syndromes entail more awkward progression, especially MSA and PSP. Within parkinsonian syndromes, PD presents the best response to L-DOPA; PSP and MSA require higher doses or other therapeutic strategies (Table 39.4). The diagnosis of these diseases is based on clinical criteria, because the formal diagnosis can only be made postmortem. Clinical criteria can be specific in advanced stages of these diseases, but misleading diagnoses have been reported to be as frequent as 25% (43). SPECT of DAT is helpful in the diagnosis of patients with clinically uncertain parkinsonian syndromes (44, 45) (Figs. 39.6 and 39.7). The expected patterns of DAT uptake, which depend on the neuropathology of each disease, are summarized in Table 39.4.

DAT ligands are unable to discriminate between PD and Parkinson-plus syndromes (e.g., MSA and PSP), because degeneration of the presynaptic dopaminergic neuron is present in all these diseases. However, MSA and PSP may also exhibit degeneration of the postsynaptic neurons where the dopaminergic D2Rs are located and therefore may show decreased stria-

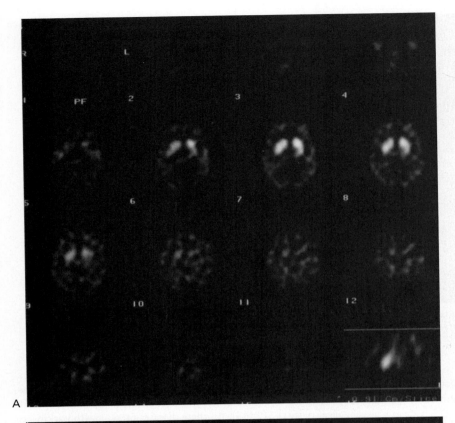

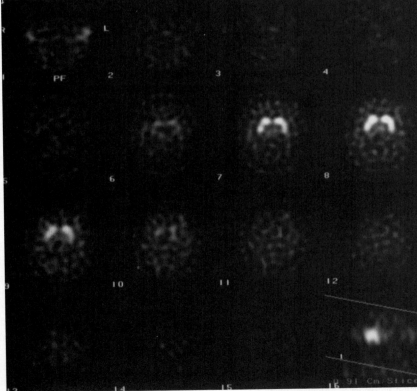

FIGURE 39.5. Normal single photon emission computed tomography images of (**A**) dopaminergic D2 receptor using ^{123}I-IBZM and (**B**) dopamine transporter with ^{123}I-FP-CIT. Intense uptake in the striatum and mild uptake in the remaining cerebral regions is seen.

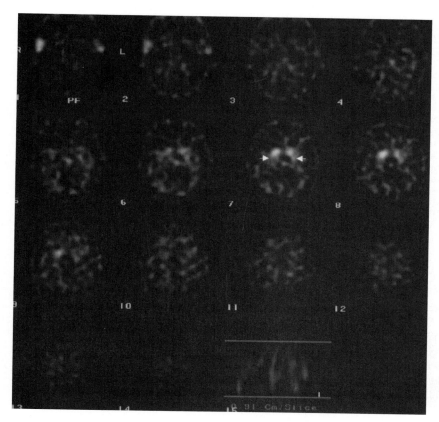

FIGURE 39.6. Abnormal pattern of dopamine transporter uptake, corresponding to a patient with Parkinson's disease. Note the decreased uptake in both putamen, which is more marked in the right hemisphere (*arrows*). Compare to the normal ^{123}I-FP-CIT uptake pattern of Fig. 39.5**B**. Right hemisphere is on the left-hand side.

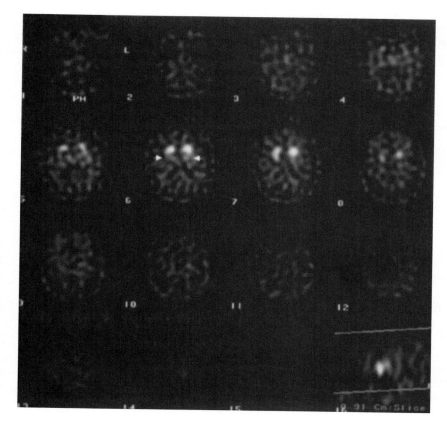

FIGURE 39.7. Bilateral dopamine transporter uptake decrease in both putamen in a patient with parkinsonian syndrome. Compare to the normal ^{123}I-FP-CIT uptake pattern of Fig. 39.5**B**.

Table 39.4. *Striatal DAT Uptake in Striatum in the Most Frequent Misdiagnosis of Patients with Parkinsonism*

Disease	Degeneration of presynaptic dopaminergic neurons	Responsiveness to L-DOPA	DAT uptake
PD	Yes	Yes	Decreased
PSP	Yes	Yes[a]	Decreased
MSA	Yes	Yes[a]	Decreased
CBD	Yes	Yes[a]	Decreased
Secondary PS	No	No	Normal
ET	No	No	Normal

PD, Parkinson's disease; PSP, progressive supranuclear palsy; MSA, multisystem atrophy; CBD, corticobasal degeneration; PS, parkinsonian syndrome; ET, essential tremor; DAT, dopamine transporter.
[a]At higher doses than PD.

tal uptake of D2R ligands (Table 39.2) on the SPECT, whereas striatal D2Rs are preserved or may be increased in PD because of up-regulation (46,47). Therefore, once the diagnosis of parkinsonian syndrome has been suggested by a DAT SPECT, differential diagnosis of PD versus MSA or PSP may be carried out with D2R SPECT. Fig. 39.8 shows a flow chart for the use of SPECT of the dopaminergic system in the diagnosis of parkinsonism. With the introduction of technetium-labeled DAT ligands, such as ^{99m}Tc-TRODAT, the possibility of scanning DAT and D2R simultaneously in the same patient might prove feasible, as well as time and cost effective (48).

Confirmation of the clinical diagnosis may be helpful before surgical interventions such as pallidotomy or subthalamic stimulation. Apart from confirming or ruling out a parkinsonian syndrome, SPECT of DAT can be useful in monitoring disease progression and in the early diagnosis, which would become critical indications for future neuroprotective therapies (45).

Epilepsy

Two neurotransmission systems have been imaged with SPECT in epileptic patients, the GABAergic and the muscarinic cholin-

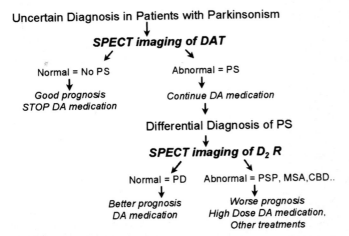

FIGURE 39.8. Flow chart for the diagnosis of parkinsonism using single photon emission computed tomography of the dopaminergic system.

ergic systems. There is evidence of loss of GABA$_A$ and muscarine cholinergic receptors in pathology studies of temporal lobectomy specimens. Decreases in ^{123}I-Iomazenil and ^{123}I-IDEX have consequently been reported in epileptic patients with temporal lobe epilepsy. Reduced regional cerebral blood flow (rCBF) in the epileptic focus has also been described with cerebral perfusion SPECT, and this may influence the uptake of the neuroreceptor radioligands, because of reduced tracer delivery to the focus. However, comparison of neuroreceptor SPECT with cerebral perfusion SPECT imaging in the interictal situation has demonstrated higher sensitivity and accuracy of the former for seizure focus localization (3,49,50). Decreased BP has been reported in patients with normal interictal rCBF SPECT and normal MRI. This is a promising area not only for clinical diagnosis but for contribution to medication effect assessment and drug development.

Dementias

Most work with neurotransmission SPECT has been focused on Alzheimer's disease (AD). Initial studies were carried out with dopaminergic and GABAergic radioligands. SPECT may be helpful in the differential diagnosis between AD and Lewy body dementia, because the latter exhibits decreased D2R and DAT uptake (51,52). The potential usefulness of SPECT imaging of the dopaminergic neurotransmission in the differentiation of these two diseases deserves further investigation. Furthermore, ^{123}I-Iomazenil SPECT has been tested as a marker of neuronal loss in AD patients. The same pattern described with cerebral perfusion SPECT imaging, that is, decreased uptake in temporoparietal areas have been found using ^{123}I-Iomazenil. However, mismatches reported when comparing both procedures include a wider, clearer, and broader area of decreased uptake with ^{123}I-Iomazenil (39), as well as preserved benzodiazepine receptors in areas with impaired CBF (53). These findings suggest a greater sensitivity and accuracy of benzodiazepine receptor SPECT in the detection of neuronal damage in AD, because the neuronal density is a more specific parameter than neuronal function. Uptake of muscarinic acetylcholine receptors using ^{123}I-IDEX (54) and ^{123}I-IQNB (55) is decreased in specific cerebral areas involved in AD (i.e., temporoparietal regions) and also in Pick's disease. These uptake decreases can be seen in mismatch with ^{18}F-D-glucose (FDG) PET patterns, that is, there are greater deficits in muscarinic receptors than in cerebral metabolism or, on the contrary, better preservation of muscarinic receptors than metabolism in specific cerebral regions (55). The glutamate (NMDA) receptor ligand ^{123}I-MK-801 (56) has also been used in AD patients. However, further evidence of the clinical usefulness of these radioligands in the diagnosis and/or clinical management of AD patients is needed. More recently, nicotinic acetylcholine receptor ligands are being tested as potential candidates for SPECT imaging in humans with application in dementias (57).

Cerebrovascular Disease

As a marker of neuronal damage and viability, SPECT imaging of benzodiazepine receptors has been used in cerebrovascular disease. No uptake in the necrotic core of the cerebral infarct, slightly decreased uptake in the peri-infarct region, and preserved uptake of ^{123}I-iomazenil in the misery perfusion region and in remote deafferentiated areas has been reported (58,59). Moreover, decreased iomazenil uptake has been found in reperfused and structurally preserved cerebral cortex as evidence of mild injury or incomplete infarction (60). Benzodiazepine receptor SPECT has also been suggested as a prognostic marker of aphasia in patients with cerebral infarction (61).

NEUROTRANSMISSION SPECT IN RESEARCH

Most research using neurotransmission SPECT imaging has been focused on psychiatry. Many of the advances in the pathophysiologic and neuropharmacologic aspects of psychiatric diseases achieved during the last decade can be attributed to neurotransmission SPECT and PET studies. Schizophrenia is the most extensively investigated disease, followed by alcoholism and depression.

Schizophrenia

In schizophrenia, neurotransmission SPECT has been used to investigate the pathophysiology and the mechanism of action of antipsychotics. Most studies have been performed using SPECT of D2Rs with ^{123}I-IBZM (for a review, see reference 41), although other receptors, such as serotoninergic, GABAergic, and muscarinic, have also been investigated in schizophrenic patients. More recently, this technique is being used to study possible associations between genetic traits and cerebral receptor expression (62).

SPECT in Pathophysiology Research

SPECT of the dopaminergic system is an enticing tool to use in the research of schizophrenia, in which a dopaminergic hypothesis is involved. Because dopaminergic hyperactivity has been implicated in schizophrenia, initial studies searched for a higher D2R density in schizophrenics than in normal controls and reported inconsistent results. A meta-analysis has revealed that, although about 70% of patients show increased D2R density, this parameter cannot be considered as a specific or consistent marker for schizophrenia (63). Subgroups of patients based on psychopathologic scores or symptomatology (i.e., positive vs. negative symptom predominance), as well a prognostic factors (64) have been investigated in an attempt to elucidate the reason for the inconsistency in the increased D2R density finding, but no conclusion has been reached. Extrastriatal D2R density in the mesial temporal cortex can also be studied by using SPECT with ligands such as ^{123}I-epidepride, but experience in this field is still scarce (65). Initial research is being done with transporters. A SPECT study has not found alterations of either DAT in the striatum or serotonin transporter in the brainstem of schizophrenic patients (66).

Amphetamine challenge has been used to indirectly measure endogenous dopamine release in the synaptic cleft using ^{123}I-IBZM SPECT. The basis of such studies is the competition between endogenous dopamine and the radioligand for the D2R. Using the paradigm of bolus plus constant infusion, amphetamine can be injected at equilibrium, and the displacement of the radioligand from the D2R induced by the released dopamine causes a decrease in the IBZM uptake that can be measured by SPECT (31). These studies have revealed a larger amphetamine-induced striatal ^{123}I-IBZM displacement in schizophrenic patients than in controls and in acutely psychotic than in chronically stable patients (67). Neurotransmission imaging is supporting the involvement of the glutamatergic system in schizophrenia (68). This increased amphetamine-induced response may result from a disruption of glutamatergic systems regulating dopaminergic cell activity, as recently demonstrated in a ^{123}I-IBZM SPECT study in normal subjects (69).

Finally, the implication of the GABAergic system in the pathophysiology of schizophrenia is being investigated with SPECT and benzodiazepine receptor ligands such as ^{123}I-Iomazenil (70, 71). However, so far results are conflicting, and most of them have failed to find abnormalities.

SPECT and Mechanism of Action of Antipsychotics

Antipsychotic action is mediated by the blockade of D2R. Competition between the antipsychotic drug and the SPECT radioligand allows the SPECT measurement of drug-induced occupancy, which can be expressed as a percentage of baseline (Figs. 39.9 and 39.10) (1). Since, the PET study of Farde et al. (72) in which a therapeutic window of D2R occupancy between 60% to 80% was reported to provide optimal antipsychotic response with minimal extrapyramidal side effects, many SPECT studies have been carried out to measure the D2R and 5-HT$_{2A}$ (73) and even muscarinic acetylcholine (74) receptor occupancy induced by several typical and atypical antipsychotics at different dosage regimens (41). In general, higher D2R occupancy has been reported for typical antipsychotics such as haloperidol than for atypical antipsychotics, which show in addition 5-HT$_{2A}$ occupancy. However, degrees of receptor occupancy induced by atypical antipsychotics vary among studies. Most studies are performed at a single time under stable doses of antipsychotic. Recently, the time after the last dose has been suggested to be a crucial parameter to consider when investigating the D2R occupancy of atypical antipsychotics. For atypical antipsychotics such as clozapine, different occupancies have been found at 2 hours (70%) and at 12 hours (50%) after the last dose (75). The recently proposed hypothesis by Kapur and Seeman (76) claims that differences in affinity for the D2R rather than the degree of D2R occupancy account for the differences between typical and atypical antipsychotics.

Alcoholism

Neurotransmission SPECT is contributing to the investigation of dysfunction of the dopaminergic, GABAergic, and serotoninergic systems in alcoholism. SPECT findings support a decreased GABA-benzodiazepine (77) and extrastriatal D2/D3 receptor density (78), as well as a decreased DAT density (79) in alcoholism. The D2R density has been suggested to be a potential

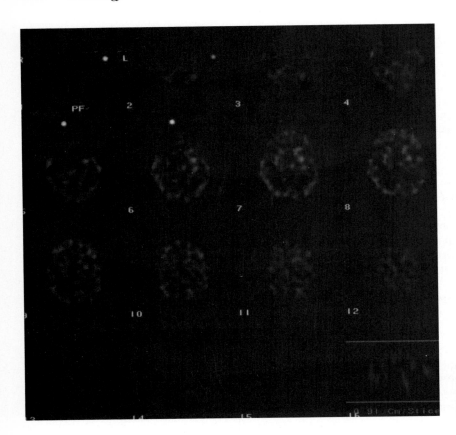

FIGURE 39.9. ^{123}I-IBZM single photon emission computed tomography of a schizophrenic patient on haloperidol. Absence of striatal uptake, corresponding to a dopaminergic D2 receptor occupancy of 89%. Compare to the normal ^{123}I-IBZM uptake pattern of Fig. 39.5A.

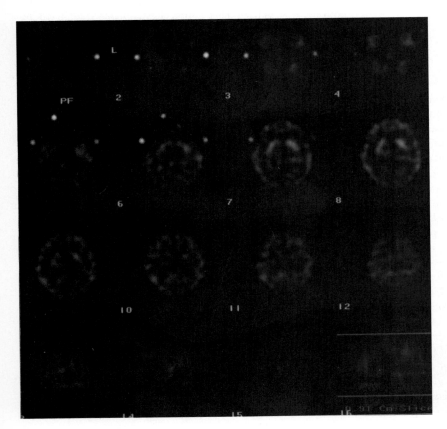

FIGURE 39.10. ^{123}I-IBZM single photon emission computed tomography of a schizophrenic patient on ziprasidone. Bilateral decreased uptake in the striatum, corresponding to a dopaminergic D2 receptor occupancy of 57%. Compare to the normal ^{123}I-IBZM uptake pattern of Fig. 39.5A.

marker for predicting relapse in alcoholic patients (80). Moreover, SPECT seems to be useful in measuring the serotonin transporter genotype (81).

Depression

Although serotonin has been the main neurotransmitter involved in depression, most SPECT studies have been focused on the dopaminergic system, probably because of the wider availability of radioligands for the latter system. Decreased levels of serotonin transporters in the midbrain region of subjects with major depression have been reported in a SPECT study (for a review see reference 82). A decreased binding of IBZM to D2R has been suggested in depressed patients who respond to either medical (83–85) or sleep deprivation (86) therapies. Amphetamine-induced dopamine release studies seem to support a role of the dopaminergic system in depression (87), but further experience will be needed before conclusions can be made.

SUMMARY

SPECT is a feasible tool for the study of cerebral neurotransmission *in vivo*. The wide availability of SPECT equipment and the relative simplicity of the methods that can be applied for neurotransmission assessment support its growing use for routine clinical purposes. Involvement of the dopaminergic system in the pathophysiology of important neuropsychiatric diseases, together with the availability of radioligands for dopamine receptors and transporters, have lead to extensive SPECT research of this system. Main results of this experience have been the clinical application of the SPECT of the dopaminergic system in parkinsonism and advances in the pathophysiology and neuropharmacology of schizophrenia. There is increasing evidence of the potential clinical use of SPECT radioligands for other neurotransmission systems, particularly the GABAergic in epilepsy, dementias, and cerebrovascular disease. The development of other radioligands for SPECT is an active area of research. The possibility of studying genotype expressions with this technique supports the future use of SPECT imaging of cerebral neurotransmission in genetics.

REFERENCES

1. Kerwin RW, Pilowsky LS. Traditional receptor theory and its application to neuroreceptor measurements in functional imaging. *Eur J Nucl Med* 1995;22:699–710.
2. Verhoeff NPLG. Imaging neurotransmission and neuroreceptors—physiological and pharmacological basis. In: Costa DC, Morgan GF, Lassen NA, eds. *New trends in nuclear neurology and psychiatry.* John Libbey & Co Ltd, 1993:25–36.
3. Boundy KL, Rowe CC, Black AB et al. Localization of temporal lobe epileptic foci with iodine-123 iododexetimide cholinergic neuroreceptor single-photon emission computed tomography. *Neurology* 1996;47:1015–1020.
4. Maziere B, Maziere M. Where have we got to with neuroreceptor mapping of the human brain? *Eur J Nucl Med* 1990;16:817–835.
5. Kegeles LS, Mann JJ. In vivo imaging of neurotransmitter systems using radiolabeled receptor ligands. *Neuropsychopharmacology* 1997;17:293–307.
6. Mintun MA, Raichle ME, Kilbourn MR et al. A quantitative model for the in vivo assessment of drug binding sites with positron emission tomography. *Ann Neurol* 1984;15:217–227.
7. Ichise M, Meyer JH, Yonekura Y. An introduction to PET and SPECT neuroreceptor quantification models. *J Nucl Med* 2001;42:755–763.
8. Innis RB. Single photon emission computed tomography imaging of dopaminergic function: presynaptic transporter, postsynaptic receptor, and "intrasynaptic" transmitter. *Adv Pharmacol* 1998;42:215–219.
9. Kung HF, Pan S, Kung MP et al. In vitro and in vivo evaluation of [123I]IBZM: a potential CNS D-2 dopamine receptor imaging agent. *J Nucl Med* 1989;30:88–92.
10. Kessler RM, Ansari MS, Schmidt DE et al. High affinity dopamine D2 receptor radioligands. 2. [125I]epidepride, a potent and specific radioligand for the characterization of striatal and extrastriatal dopamine D2 receptors. *Life Sci* 1991;49:617–628.
11. Kung MP, Kung HF, Billings J et al. The characterization of IBF as a new selective dopamine D-2 receptor imaging agent. *J Nucl Med* 1990;31:648–654.
12. Saji H, Iida Y, Magata Y et al. Preparation of 123I-labeled 2′-iodospiperone and imaging of D2 dopamine receptors in the human brain using SPECT. *Int J Rad Appl Instrum B* 1992;19:523–529.
13. Chabriat H, Levasseur M, Vidailhet M et al. *In-vivo* SPECT imaging of D2 receptor with iodine-iodolisuride: results in supranuclear palsy. *J Nucl Med* 1992;33:1481–1485.
14. Neumeyer JL, Wang S, Gao Y et al. N-omega-fluoroalkyl analogs of (1R)-2 beta-carbomethoxy-3 beta-(4-iodophenyl)-tropane (beta-CIT): radiotracers for positron emission tomography and single photon emission computed tomography imaging of dopamine transporters. *J Med Chem* 1994;37:558–561.
15. Booij J, Andringa G, Rijks LJ et al. 123I-FP-CIT binds to the dopamine transporter as assessed by biodistribution studies in rats and SPECT studies in MPTP-lesioned monkeys. *Synapse* 1997;27:183–190.
16. Kung MP, Essman WD, Frederick D et al. IPT: a novel iodinated ligand for the CNS dopamine transporter. *Synapse* 1995;20:316–324.
17. Guilloteau D, Emond P, Baulieu JL et al. Exploration of the dopamine transporter: in vitro and in vivo characterization of a high-affinity and high-specificity iodinated tropane derivative (E)-N-(3-iodoprop-2-enyl)-2beta-carbomethoxy-3beta-(4′-methylphenyl)nortropane (PE2I). *Nucl Med Biol* 1998;25:331–337.
18. Kung MP, Stevenson DA, Plössl K et al. [99mTc] TRODAT-1: a novel technetium-99m complex as a dopamine transporter imaging agent. *Eur J Nucl Med* 1997;24:372–380.
19. Mertens J, Terriere D, Sipido V et al. Radiosynthesis of a new radioiodinated ligand for serotonin-5HT2-receptors, a promising tracer for gamma-emission tomography. *J Labelled Comp Radiopharm* 1994;34:795–806.
20. Choi SR, Hou C, Oya S et al. Selective in vitro and in vivo binding of [(125)I]ADAM to serotonin transporters in rat brain. *Synapse* 2000;38:403–412.
21. Abi-Dargham A, Krystal JH, Anjivel S et al. SPECT measurement of benzodiazepine receptors in human brain with 123I-Iomazenil: kinetic and equilibrium paradigms. *J Nucl Med* 1994;35:228–238.
22. Kuikka JT, Hiltunen J, Foged C et al. Initial human studies with single-photon emission tomography using iodine-123 labelled 3-(5-cyclopropyl-1,2,4-oxadioazo-3-yl)-7-yodo-5,6-dihidro-5-methyl-6-oxo-4H-imidazol[1,5-a][1,4]-benzodiazepine (NNC-13-8241). *Eur J Nucl Med* 1996;16:273–280.
23. Mueller-Gartner HW, Wilson AA, Dannals RF et al. Imaging muscarinic cholinergic receptors in human brain in vivo with SPECT, I-123-4-iododexetimide. *J Cereb Blood Flow Metab* 1992;12:562–570.
24. Nobuhara K, Farde L, Halldin C et al. SPET imaging of central muscarinic acetylcholine receptors with iodine-123labelled E-IQNP and Z-IQNP. *Eur J Nucl Med* 2001;28:13–24.
25. Brown DR, Wyper DJ, Owens J et al. 123Iodo-MK-801: a SPECT agent for imaging the pattern and extent of glutamate (NMDA) receptor activation in Alzheimer's disease. *J Psychiatr Res* 1997;31:605–619.
26. Passchier J, van Waarde A. Visualization of serotonin-1A (5-HT1A) receptors in the central nervous system. *Eur J Nucl Med* 2001;28:113–129.
27. Zoghbi SS, Tamagnan G, Baldwin MF et al. Measurement of plasma

metabolites of (S)-5-[(123)I]iodo-3-(2-azetidinylmethoxy)pyridine of A-85380. *Nucl Med Biol* 2001;28:91–96.

28. Bando K, Naganuma T, Taguchi K et al. Piperazine analog of vesamicol: in vitro and in vivo characterization for vesicular acetylcholine transporter. *Synapse* 2000;38:27–37.

29. Wang RF, Tafani JA, Zajac JM et al. A radioiodinated 7alpha-O-iodoallyl diprenorphine for mapping opioid receptors. *Neuropeptides* 1999;33:498–502.

30. Seibyl JP, Woods SW, Zoghibi SS et al. Dynamic SPECT imaging of dopamine D2 receptors in human subjects with iodine-123-IBZM. *J Nucl Med* 1992;33:1964–1971.

31. Laruelle M, Abi-Dargham A, van Dyck CH et al. SPECT imaging of striatal dopamine release after amphetamine challenge. *J Nucl Med* 1995;36:1182–1190.

32. Varrone A, Fujita M, Verhoeff NPLG et al. Test-retest reproducibility of extrastriatal dopamine D2 receptor imaging with [123I] epidepride SPECT in humans. *J Nucl Med* 2000;41:1343–1351.

33. Ichise M, Ballinger J, Golan H et al. Noninvasive quantification of dopamine D2 receptors with iodine-123-IBF SPECT. *J Nucl Med* 1996;37:513–520.

34. Laruelle M. The role of model-based methods in the development of single scan techniques. *Nucl Med Biol* 2000;27: 637–642.

35. Verhoeff NPLG, Brüke T, Podreka I et al. Dynamic SPECT in two healthy volunteers to determine the optimal time for in vivo D2 dopamine receptor imaging with ^{123}I-IBZM using the rotating gamma camera. *Nucl Med Com* 1991;12:687–697.

36. Links JM. Special issues in quantitation of brain receptors and related markers by emission computed tomography. *Q J Nucl Med* 1998;42: 158–165.

37. Van Laere K, Koole M, D'Asseler Y et al. Automated stereotactic standardization of brain SPECT receptor data using single-photon transmission images. *J Nucl Med* 2001;42:361–375.

38. Benamer TS, Patterson J, Grosset DG et al. Accurate differentiation of parkinsonism and essential tremor using visual assessment of [123I]-FP-CIT SPECT imaging: the [123I]-FP-CIT study group. *Mov Disord* 2000;15:503–510.

39. Fukuchi K, Hashikawa K, Seike Y et al. Comparison of iodine-123-iomazenil SPECT and technetium-99m-HMPAO-SPECT in Alzheimer's disease. *J Nucl Med* 1997;38:467–470.

40. Laruelle M. Imaging synaptic neurotransmission with in vivo binding competition techniques: a critical review. *J Cereb Blood Flow Metab* 2000;20:423–451.

41. Verhoeff NPLG. Radiotracer imaging of dopaminergic transmission in neuropsychiatric disorders. *Psychopharmacology* 1999;147:217–249.

42. Oertel WH, Quinn NP. Movement disorders parkinsonism. In: *Neurological disorders: course and treatment*. American Academy Press, 1996: 715–772.

43. Meara J, Bhowmick BK, Hobson P. Accuracy of diagnosis in patients with presumed Parkinson's Disease. *Age Ageing* 1999;28:99–102.

44. Booij J, Speelman JD, Horstink MWIM et al. The clinical benefit of imaging striatal dopamine transporters with 123I-FP-CIT SPET in differentiating patients with presynaptic parkinsonism from those with other forms of parkinsonism. *Eur J Nucl Med* 2001;28:266–272.

45. Tatsch K. Imaging of the dopaminergic system in parkinsonism with SPET. *Nucl Med Commun* 2001;22:819–827.

46. Hierholzer J, Cordes M, Venz S et al. Loss of dopamine-D2 receptor binding sites in Parkinsonian plus syndromes. *J Nucl Med* 1998;39: 954–960.

47. van Royen EA, Verhoeff NPLG, Speelman JD et al. Multiple system atrophy and progressive supranuclear palsy. Diminished striatal D2 dopamine receptor activity demonstrated by 123I-IBZM single photon emission computed tomography. *Arch Neurol* 1993;50:513–516.

48. Dresel SH, Kung MP, Huang XF et al. Simultaneous SPECT studies of pre- and postsynaptic dopamine binding sites in baboons. *J Nucl Med* 1999;40:660–666.

49. Kuji I, Sumiya H, Tsuji S et al. Asymmetries of benzodiazepine receptor binding potential in the inferior medial temporal lobe and cerebellum detected with 123I-iomazenil SPECT in comparison with 99mTc-HMPAO SPECT in patients with partial epilepsy. *Ann Nucl Med* 1998; 12:185–190.

50. Tanaka F, Yonekura Y, Ikeda A et al. Presurgical identification of epileptic foci with iodine-123 iomazenil SPET: comparison with brain perfusion SPET and FDG PET. *Eur J Nucl Med* 1997;24:27–34.

51. Walker Z, Costa DC, Janssen AG et al. Dementia with Lewy bodies: a study of post-synaptic dopaminergic receptors with iodine-123 iodobenzamide single-photon emission tomography. *Eur J Nucl Med* 1997; 24:609–614.

52. Donnemiller E, Heilmann J, Wenning GK et al. Brain perfusion scintigraphy with ^{99m}Tc-HMPAO or ^{99m}Tc-ECD and ^{123}I-B-CIT single-photon emission tomography in dementia of the Alzheimer-type and diffuse Lewy body disease. *Eur J Nucl Med* 1997;24:320–325.

53. Ohyama M, Senda M, Ishiwata K et al. Preserved benzodiazepine receptors in Alzheimer's disease measured with C-11 flumazenil PET and I-123 iomazenil SPECT in comparison with CBF. *Ann Nucl Med* 1999; 13:309–315.

54. Claus JJ, Dubois EA, Booij J et al. Demonstration of a reduction in muscarinic receptor binding in early Alzheimer's disease using iodine-123 dexetimide single-photon emission tomography. *Eur J Nucl Med* 1997;24:602–608.

55. Heinz A, Jones DW, Raedler T et al. Neuropharmacological studies with SPECT in neuropsychiatric disorders. *Nucl Med Biol* 2000;27: 677–682.

56. Brown DR, Wyper DJ, Owens J et al. 123Iodo-MK-801: a SPECT agent for imaging the pattern and extent of glutamate (NMDA) receptor activation in Alzheimer's disease. *J Psychiatr Res* 1997;31:605–619.

57. Fujita M, Tamagnan G, Zoghbi SS et al. Measurement of alpha4beta2 nicotinic acetylcholine receptors with [123I*5-I-A-85380 SPECT. *J Nucl Med* 2000;41:1552–1560.

58. Sasaki M, Ichiya Y, Kuwabara Y et al. Benzodiazepine receptors in chronic cerebrovascular disease: comparison with blood flow and metabolism. *J Nucl Med* 1997;38:1693–1698.

59. Hatazawa J, Satoh T, Shimosegawa E et al. Evaluation of cerebral infarction with iodine 123-iomazenil SPECT. *J Nucl Med* 1995;36: 2154–2161.

60. Nakagawara J, Sperling B, Lassen NA. Incomplete brain infarction of reperfused cortex may be quantitated with iomazenil. *Stroke* 1997;28: 124–132.

61. Koshi Y, Kitamura S, Ohyama M et al. Benzodiazepine receptor imaging with iomazenil SPECT in aphasic patients with cerebral infarction. *Ann Nucl Med* 1999;13:223–229.

62. Martinez D, Gelernter J, Abi-Dargham A et al. The variable number of tandem repeats polymorphism of the dopamine transporter gene is not associated with significant change in dopamine transporter phenotype in humans. *Neuropsychopharmacology* 2001;24:553–560.

63. Zakzanis KK, Hansen KT. Dopamine D2 densities and the schizophrenic brain. *Schizophr Res* 1998;32:201–206.

64. Catafau AM, Pérez V, Corripio I et al. Striatal dopaminergic D2 receptor density: a prognostic marker in schizophrenia? *Eur J Nucl Med* 2001;28:1034.

65. Hall H, Halldin C, Jerning E et al. Autoradiographic comparison of [125I]epidepride and [125I]NCQ 298 binding to human brain extrastriated dopamine receptors. *Nucl Med Biol* 1997;24:389–393.

66. Laruelle M, Abi-Dargham A, van Dyck C et al. Dopamine and serotonin transporters in patients with schizophrenia: an imaging study with [(123)I]beta-CIT. *Biol Psychiatry* 2000;47:371–379.

67. Abi-Dargham A, Gil R, Krystal J et al. Increased striatal dopamine transmission in schizophrenia: confirmation in a second cohort. *Am J Psychiatry* 1998;155:761–767.

68. Bressan RA, Pilowsky L. Imaging the glutamatergic system in vivo-relevance to schizophrenia. *Eur J Nucl Med* 2000;1723–1731.

69. Kegeles LS, Abi-Dargham A, Zea-Ponce Y et al. Modulation of amphetamine-induced striatal dopamine release by ketamine in humans: implications for schizophrenia. *Biol Psychiatry* 2000;48:627–640.

70. Verhoeff NP, Soares JC, D'Souza CD et al. [123I]Iomazenil SPECT benzodiazepine receptor imaging in schizophrenia. *Psychiatry Res* 1999; 91:163–173.

71. Busatto GF, Pilowsky LS, Costa DC et al. Correlation between reduced in vivo benzodiazepine receptor binding and severity of psychotic symptoms in schizophrenia. *Am J Psychiatry* 1997;154:56–63.

72. Farde L, Wiesel FA, Halldin C et al. Central D2-dopamine receptor

occupancy in schizophrenic patients treated with antipsychotic drugs. *Arch Gen Psychiatry* 1988;45:71–76.

73. Travis MJ, Busatto GF, Pilowsky LS et al. 5-HT2A receptor blockade in patients with schizophrenia treated with risperidone or clozapine. A SPET study using the novel 5-HT2A ligand 123I-5-I-R-91150. *Br J Psychiatry* 1998;173:236–241.

74. Raedler TJ, Knable MB, Jones DW et al. In vivo olanzapine occupancy of muscarinic acetylcholine receptors in patients with schizophrenia. *Neuropsychopharmacology* 2000;23:56–68.

75. Jones C, Kapur S, Remington G et al. Transient dopamine D2 occupancy in low EPS-incidence drugs: PET evidence. *Biol Psychiatry* 2000; 47:112.

76. Kapur S, Seeman P. Does fast dissociation from the dopamine d(2) receptor explain the action of atypical antipsychotics?: A new hypothesis. *Am J Psychiatry* 2001;158:360–369.

77. Abi-Dargham A, Krystal JH, Anjilvel S et al. Alterations of benzodiazepine receptors in type II alcoholic subjects measured with SPECT and [123I]iomazenil. *Am J Psychiatry* 1998;155:1550–1555.

78. Kuikka JT, Repo E, Bergstrom KA et al. Specific binding and laterality of human extrastriatal dopamine D2/D3 receptors in late onset type 1 alcoholic patients. *Neurosci Lett* 2000;292:57–59.

79. Repo E, Kuikka JT, Bergstrom KA et al. Dopamine transporter and D2-receptor density in late-onset alcoholism. *Psychopharmacology (Berl)* 1999;147:314–318.

80. Guardia J, Catafau AM, Batlle F et al. Striatal dopaminergic D(2) receptor density measured by [(123)I]iodobenzamide SPECT in the prediction of treatment outcome of alcohol-dependent patients. *Am J Psychiatry* 2000;157:127–129.

81. Heinz A, Jones DW, Mazzanti C et al. A relationship between serotonin transporter genotype and in vivo protein expression and alcohol neurotoxicity. *Biol Psychiatry* 2000;47:643–649.

82. Staley JK, Malison RT, Innis RB. Imaging of the serotonergic system: interactions of neuroanatomical and functional abnormalities of depression. *Biol Psychiatry* 1998;44:534–549.

83. Klimke A, Larisch R, Janz A et al. Dopamine D2 receptor binding before and after treatment of major depression measured by [123I]IBZM SPECT. *Psychiatry Res* 1999;90:91–101.

84. Larisch R, Klimke A, Vosberg H et al. In vivo evidence for the involvement of dopamine-D2 receptors in striatum and anterior cingulate gyrus in major depression. *Neuroimage* 1997;5:251–260.

85. Ebert D, Feistel H, Loew T et al. Dopamine and depression—striatal dopamine D2 receptor SPECT before and after antidepressant therapy. *Psychopharmacology (Berl)* 1996;126:91–94.

86. Ebert D, Feistel H, Kaschka W et al. Single photon emission computerized tomography assessment of cerebral dopamine D2 receptor blockade in depression before and after sleep deprivation—preliminary results. *Biol Psychiatry* 1994;35:880–885.

87. Anand A, Verhoeff P, Seneca N et al. Brain SPECT imaging of amphetamine-induced dopamine release in euthymic bipolar disorder patients. *Am J Psychiatry* 2000;157:1108–1114.

40

CEREBROSPINAL FLUID IMAGING

SANDRA K. LAWRENCE
DOMINIQUE DELBEKE
C. LEON PARTAIN
MARTIN P. SANDLER

Cerebrospinal fluid (CSF) flow and dynamics have been extensively studied. The first description of CSF was made by Cotugno (1) in 1774. Fifty years later Magendie (2,3) began outlining the architecture of the ventricular system and subarachnoid spaces. CSF production was localized in the choroid plexus by Faivre (4) in 1854. Key and Retzius (5), later supported by Weed (6,7), proposed that CSF is reabsorbed by the arachnoid granulations of Pacchioni. Later authors suggested that there were additional areas of CSF production (8–13) and CSF reabsorption (12,14–18).

The combination of choroid plexus CSF production with arachnoid granulation resorption of CSF implied the concept of flow of CSF from lateral ventricles to subarachnoid spaces. In 1943, based on the Monroe-Kellie doctrine (7) (the sum of the intracranial volumes of brain, blood, and CSF must be constant), O'Connell (19) postulated that the CSF circulation driving force could be secondary to net volume expansion of pulsatile intracranial arteries. Beering (20) alternatively suggested the driving force behind CSF motion was the pulsatile expansion and contraction of the choroid plexus.

The combination of Welch's (21) published findings on the mechanical function of CSF values and Di Chiro's (22) studies using radionuclide cisternography (RC) to access CSF flow further supported the active circulation theories. Subsequent animal experiments only partially supported the hypothesis, but in 1966 Di Chiro proposed the two-way theory of bulk transport. In bulk transport, CSF flows from the ventricles caudally into the third ventricle, out into the posterior compartment of the spinal cord from the foramina of Luschka and Magendie, with a caudal flow in the posterior compartment of the spinal canal. There is a cephalad direction of CSF flow in the anterior compartment of the spinal canal ascending to the vertex and the arachnoid granulations.

Although controversies persisted, current standard texts and teaching have been that CSF is produced and absorbed everywhere in the subarachnoid spaces, but primary CSF production is in the choroid plexus, transport is by bulk flow into the subarachnoid spaces with a two-way spinal canal circulation, and primary reabsorption is in the arachnoid granulations (23–25).

Further work with RC established the "normal" CSF flow patterns. James et al. (26) noted that radiopharmaceuticals injected intrathecally into the lumbar subarachnoid spaces normally reached the basal cisterns by 1 hour, the frontal poles and Sylvian fissure area in 2 to 6 hours (Fig. 40.1), the cerebral convexities by 12 hours, and the arachnoid villi in the sagittal sinus area by 24 hours (Fig. 40.2). Movement of radioactivity within the CSF compartment did not appear to be influenced by patient posture or activity nor by barbotage at the time of injection (27). Additional investigations by Milhorat (28) and James et al. (29) established that the flow of the CSF, as reflected by radionuclide movement, has both central and superficial routes to the parasagittal region. Radioactivity was not normally detected in the ventricular system, presumably because CSF flow was from the ventricles into the remainder of the CSF space (28,29). When radioactivity was introduced directly into the ventricular system, it normally appeared in the basal cisterns within minutes. From the basal cisterns, movement of the radioactivity was similar to the movement observed after lumbar intrathecal injections. CSF flow to the area of arachnoid villi was mainly through the lateral and anterior or superficial and central communicating pathways (30).

With a lumbar subarachnoid injection, the central (anterior) pathway had two principal routes. The superior one leads from the suprasellar cistern through the cisterna lamina terminalis and callosal cistern, passing medially into the interhemispheric cistern and then upward to the parasagittal area (26,31). The inferior route was from the basal cisterns to the quadrigeminal plate cistern, passing through the posterior portion of the callosal cistern into the interhemispheric cistern and then upward to the parasagittal region (32).

The superficial (lateral) route of CSF flow was through the Sylvian cistern, between the posterior surface of the frontal lobes and the anterior surface of the temporal lobes, and over the cerebral convexity to the parasagittal region (30). This estab-

S.K. Lawrence: Department of Radiology and Radiological Sciences, Vanderbilt University Medical Center, Nashville, TN.

D. Delbeke: Department of Radiology and Radiological Sciences, Vanderbilt University Medical Center, Nashville, TN.

C.L. Partain: Department of Radiology and Radiological Sciences, Vanderbilt University Medical Center, Nashville, TN.

M.P. Sandler: Department of Radiology and Radiological Sciences, Vanderbilt University Medical Center, Nashville, TN.

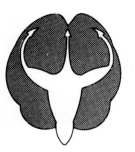
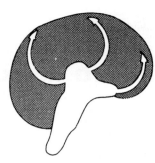

FIGURE 40.1. Expected radiopharmaceutical 2 hours after lumbar subarachnoid injection (arrows indicate radiopharmaceutical movement). No ventricular radioactivity is present on either anterior (*left*) or lateral (*right*) views. (From James AE, Deland FH, Hodges EJ III et al. Cerebrospinal fluid (CSF) scanning cisternography. *AJR* 1970;110:74–79, with permission.)

lished CSF model is currently being challenged by new findings with magnetic resonance imaging (MRI) and RC.

More recent studies are providing new information that is reshaping our understanding of normal physiology and CSF dynamics. Newer investigations describe the arrival of an arterial systolic pulse wave that causes internal regions of the brain to move caudally and to extend a compressive force on the three

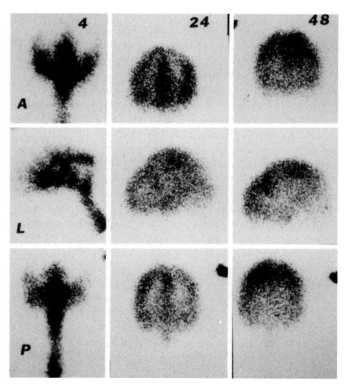

FIGURE 40.2. Radionuclide cisternography of cerebrospinal fluid (CSF) flow. Typical nuclear medicine CSF study at 4 hours (*left*), 24 hours (*center*), and 48 hours (*right*) after injection. Anterior (*A*), left lateral (*L*), and posterior (*P*) views are shown. Anterior view at 4 hours (*top left*) shows central radioactivity between the hemispheres and in the basal cisterns inferiorly. Lateral activity is present in Sylvian fissure areas. Left lateral view at 4 hours (*middle left*) shows radioactivity inferiorly in the basal cisterns and more superiorly in the quadrigeminal plate cisterns, as well as some radioactivity in the Sylvian area.

ventricles, initiating CSF antegrade injection with retrograde CSF flow during phases of the cardiac cycle (33–35). The outflow from the cranial cavity into the subarachnoid space is, therefore, dependent on size and timing of the intracranial arterial expansion during systole and indirectly by a fronto-occipital "volume wave" (25). The instantaneous blood flow increase in the superior sagittal sinus at the beginning of systole is considered to reflect a direct pressure transmission via the subarachnoid spaces and may be an important prerequisite for maintaining normal intracranial pressure (ICP) and cerebral blood flow (CBF) (25).

Contrary to traditional views of unidirectional flow proposed by Di Chiro, MRI velocity imaging studies have shown large oscillatory bidirectional CSF flow that permits rapid mixing between chambers (25,33–35), with the spinal flow channel described as a "meandering river" (25). In an RC study with MRI correlation, Grietz concluded that bulk flow is not necessary to explain transport of radionuclide tracers in the subarachnoid spaces because the main absorption of CSF is not necessarily through the arachnoid granulations (35–37). In addition, a major part of the CSF transportation to the vascular compartment is likely to occur via the perivascular and extracellular spaces of the central nervous system (25). Transventricular absorption of CSF represents a major compensatory mechanism for stabilizing volume and increased interventricular pressure, with the elimination of periventricular edematous fluid via the blood–brain barrier and vascular compartment (38). Normal velocity patterns of CSF have been verified by independent studies (39–47). Recent studies suggest increased aqueductal flow velocity (48) and increased lateral brain motion (49) in patients with normal pressure hydrocephalus (NPH). Circadian variations of CSF production were recently documented and may play a role in disease (50). Slow movement of CSF may contribute to the elevation of CSF protein and albumin content in neurologic diseases other than spinal obstruction (51). Further investigations into the CSF circulation and associated intracranial dynamics are warranted.

CEREBROSPINAL FLUID LEAKAGE

The first CSF leak was described by Tillaux in 1877 (52). Galen later proposed that CSF rhinorrhea occurred when CSF was purged into the nose through the infundibulum and ethmoid bone (32). For CSF to extravasate or leak there must be a compromise in both the dura and the bone. In CSF rhinorrhea, the region of interest is the skull base from the frontal sinuses to the temporal bone. Pneumatization of the paranasal sinuses and mastoids results in bone that is less dense and, therefore, more susceptible to thinning from age or increased ICP and to trauma (53). This thinning is particularly evident lateral to the cribriform plate, where the floor of the anterior fossa turns upward to join the orbital plate of the frontal bone and forms the roof of the ethmoid (Fig. 40.3). This point is further weakened as a result of dural attachment. It is here that most "cribriform plate" fractures actually occur (Fig. 40.4), because the cribriform plate is a relatively sturdy structure despite being traversed by the olfactory channels (53). Occasionally, rhinorrhea is secondary

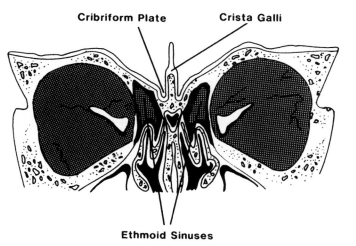

FIGURE 40.3. Frontal view at level of crista galli and ethmoid sinuses. Note the sharp upward turn of the floor of the anterior fossa toward the downward sloping orbital roof. This point is weak because of the dural attachment.

Table 40.1. *Classification of Cerebrospinal Fluid Rhinorrhea*[a]

Traumatic
    Postoperative (iatrogenic)
    Other trauma (accidental)
Nontraumatic
    High pressure leaks
        Tumors
        Hydrocephalus
            Communicating
            Obstructive
    Normal pressure leaks
        Congenital anomalies
        Focal bone atrophy or thinning with acquired meningocele or meningoencephalocele
        Erosions
            Tumor
            Osteomyelitis

[a]Modified from Ommaya AK, Di Chiro G, Baldwin M, Pennybacker JB. Non-traumatic cerebrospinal fluid rhinorrhea. *J Neurol Neurosurg Psychiatry* 1968;31:214–255.

to leakage into a mastoid cell with communication via the middle ear cavity and eustachian tube to the nasopharynx. Otorrhea usually occurs via a temporal bone defect but may not be clinically evident without a concomitant tympanic membrane tear or after myringotomy (54).

A classification of CSF leaks was given by Ommaya (Table 40.1), with an addition to the table proposed by Kaufman et al. (55). About 80% of CSF rhinorrhea cases are the result of direct head trauma, 16% are iatrogenic trauma from surgery, and 4% are spontaneous or nontraumatic (56).

Most direct head trauma occurs as a result of traffic accidents (57,58). CSF rhinorrhea occurs in 2% to 6% of unselected head injuries and 11% of skull fractures (56,59–61). Fractures resulting in CSF leakage primarily involve the ethmoid sinus and cribriform plate but can involve the frontal sinus, the facial bones (particularly LeFort II fractures that extend into the nasal cavity), the petrous bone (fluid enters the nasal cavity via the eustachian tube), and the middle cranial fossa floor [via the pterygoid recess of the sphenoid sinus (59,60,62–64)]. On computed tomography (CT) a distinct bony fracture may not be apparent without very thin slices, but pneumocephalus or air/fluid levels in the sinuses may be evident (65).

Depending on the location of the traumatic defect, patients can present with rhinorrhea, otorrhea, otorhinorrhea, periorbital edema, or neurologic deficit (52–66). Although anosmia has been reported in 78% of posttraumatic patients with CSF rhinorrhea (67), a more recent study by Hubbard et al. (68) noted normal olfaction in 77% of posttraumatic patients with cribri-

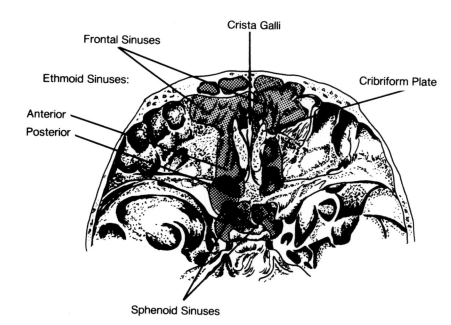

FIGURE 40.4. Anterior skull base viewed from above. Fractures are the most common pathology involving the paranasal sinuses and cribriform plate that leads to cerebrospinal fluid rhinorrhea.

form plate defects. Interestingly, in the same study, 20% of the cases had the CSF leakage site contralateral to the nasal fluid drip (68). This was probably secondary to dislocation of the vomer from the crista galli, which allowed fluid leaking from one cribriform plate to cross to the opposite nostril (56). Thus, clinical lateralization is not reliable in posttraumatic CSF leaks (68). Traumatic CSF leaks are usually apparent immediately or during the first 48 hours after injury, but sometimes the presentation is delayed for years (59–61,69). The fistula tract may become occluded by a plug of brain herniating through the fracture line, preventing complete healing of the dura. However, in 50% to 70% of traumatic CSF leaks, there is spontaneous resolution within 1 week, with up to 90% to 95% resolution in 6 months (59,70–73).

Iatrogenic postoperative CSF leaks usually occur following nasal and transphenoidal surgery. In a series of 57 patients with CSF leaks reported by Lantz et al. (53) nearly 33% were following pituitary surgery.

Spontaneous or nontraumatic CSF leaks characteristically persist intermittently for years and are categorized as either high- or normal-pressure leaks. High-pressure leak etiologies include noncommunicating hydrocephalus or rarely communicating hydrocephalus, benign intracranial hypertension, or direct erosion from a benign or malignant neoplastic process (52,74). Normal-pressure leaks have been associated with osteomyelitis; with the empty sella syndrome (75); and with various congenital anomalies including meningocele, encephalocele, and focal olfactory atrophy or cribriform plate defect. Spontaneous temporal bone CSF leaks are very rare, with only 42 total reported cases, most of which presented in the seventh decade (54). Spontaneous temporal bone CSF leaks are primarily secondary to herniation of aberrant arachnoid granulations along the dural plate, with the bone dura dehiscence distant to the otic capsule (76). Ninety-four percent involve the middle fossa (tegmen) and 6% involved the posterior fossa (54). Clinical symptoms include hearing loss (61%), ear fullness (35%), otorrhea (30%), rhinorrhea (21%), and meningitis (19%) (54). Although there are various rare causes of congenital temporal CSF leaks, the primary etiology is Mondini dysplasia of the osseous and membranous labyrinth (77). Complete spontaneous closure of any nontraumatic CSF leak occurs in less than 33% of cases (72); usually the leak requires surgical repair (56).

Spontaneous intracranial hypotension is also known to occur under other conditions such as lumbar puncture, spinal surgery, fracture of the thoracic spine, inadvertent puncture during epidural anesthesia, or the Valsalva maneuver during some sporting activities such as weight-lifting. These patients present with postural headache associated with low CSF pressure (78).

Pyrogenic meningitis is the most serious complication of CSF leakage. Meningitis is the major complication of traumatic rhinorrhea, occurring in 25% to 50% of untreated fistula (67,68, 73), in 10% of cases during the first 7 days of trauma (56), and in 10% of cases several years after the spontaneous cessation of leakage (56). Although there is a higher percentage of patients that develop meningitis with traumatic CSF leaks, meningitis remains a serious risk in spontaneous cases as well (52). Consequently, early surgery is appropriate in patients with substantial posttraumatic leak, delayed presentation of a posttraumatic leak, or a spontaneous leak, because these patients have a significantly higher risk of meningitis and a lower rate of spontaneous resolution.

Diagnosis of Cerebrospinal Fluid Leak

Accurate demonstration of a CSF leak is essential for effective surgical repair but has proven to be a difficult diagnostic challenge. This is clearly illustrated by the number of available diagnostic examinations, both clinical and radiographic.

Clinically, the majority of CSF leaks produce only a small volume of fluid and are often only intermittently active. CSF has a higher glucose content than nasal secretions, and glucose measurement has served as a confirmation of a CSF leak. An old laboratory method of glucose evaluation involved placing a drop of suspected fluid onto filter paper; a yellow rim around the drop indicated CSF. Alternatively, a glucose oxidase strip only requires a drop of fluid for glucose determination. Unfortunately, both lacrimal and nasal secretions contain glucose with subsequent false-positive findings as high as 52% reported (79, 80,81). However, absence of glucose essentially eliminates CSF rhinorrhea. If an adequate sample is obtainable, a protein concentration less than 200 mg/dL, or a glucose value that is 60% of a concomitant serum glucose value, suggests that the fluid is CSF (82). The most specific laboratory test is immunoelectrophoresis identification of CSF B-2 transferrin bands, because it is definitive even when the specimen is contaminated by blood, saliva, or nasal secretions (83).

Radiographic procedures used to diagnose a CSF leak include plain skull films (53), complex motion tomography (53), intralumbar injection of dyes (indigo carmine, methylene blue, or fluorescein) (84), RC alone (85,86), digital subtraction cisternography/fluoroscopy (87), and MRI (88). Because high resolution computed tomography (HRCT) with iopamidol or iohexol contrast is now widely available, is required for preoperative delineation of surgical anatomy, and has relatively high sensitivity of 81% to 87% for CSF leak localization (52, 74), it is currently the first-line radiographic evaluation study (Fig. 40.5). In 1987, Flynn et al. (89) established RC combined with intranasal pledgets, which offered a higher sensitivity and specificity for the diagnosis of a CSF leak compared with contrasted CT study; however, definitive anatomic localization of the CSF leak remains a limiting factor for considering this as a first-line study. However, the nuclear medicine study is advantageous for symptomatic patients with small intermittent CSF leaks because it is performed over a longer time (up to 48 hours), thus increasing the chance of CSF leak detection (71,90,91). In addition, RC allows for detection of CSF spinal leaks that would require extensive time and cost using contrast HRCT (92,93). Single photon emission computed tomography (SPECT) cisternography after intralumbar injection of ^{123}I-labeled albumin was recently proposed as a valuable diagnostic tool for evaluation of small intermittent leaks in the difficult area of the cribriform plate (94). Because there was no controlled comparison with ^{111}In diethylenetriaminepentaacetic acid (DTPA) planar scintigraphy with pledget/plasma ratios on the eight patients studied (94), the increased cost and time required for SPECT may not be justified as the first-line nuclear medicine study unless there

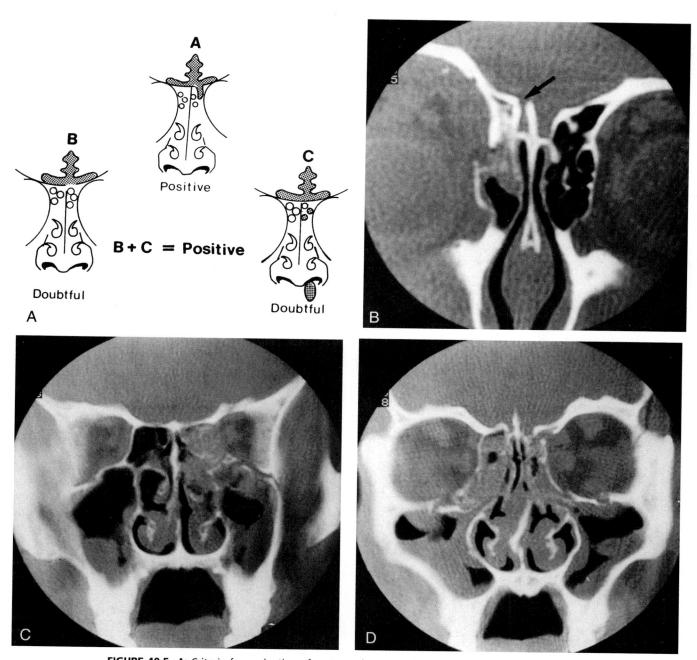

FIGURE 40.5. **A:** Criteria for evaluation of contrasted computed tomography (CT) cisternography in cerebrospinal fluid (CSF) rhinorrhea. **A:** Contrast passes through a bony defect. **B:** Site of fracture of bony defect alone is doubtful. **C:** Contrast visualized in paranasal sinus nasal cavity or on cotton pledget alone also doubtful, but positive in combination with **B**. **B:** Medial orbital roof fracture. Direct prone coronal CT scan showing a fracture (*arrow*) and ethmoid density in this patient with an acute CSF leak. **C and D:** Medial roof fracture. Two prone CT scans in the same patient as in **B** at slightly different levels. **C:** A large oblique fracture extends across the left maxilla. **C and D:** Comminution in the ethmoid region. Such fractures could result in CSF leaks.

is a substantially higher detection rate of CSF leak. In the most difficult cases, intraoperative intrathecal injection using fluorescein dye diluted with 10 mL of autologous CSF into the subarachnoid spaces may localize the CSF leak (54). However, there is a risk of seizures or temporary paralysis with this study (95).

Radionuclide studies have proven to be a sensitive and accurate method of examination for CSF leaks. RC with intranasal pledget placement was first performed with ^{24}Natrium by Crow et al. (96) in 1956. Evaluation has been performed with a variety of radiopharmaceutical tracers including ^{131}I human serum albumin (22), ^{99m}Tc-transferrin (97), ^{169}Yb-DTPA (98), ^{111}In-DTPA (90), and ^{99m}Tc-DTPA (89). The sensitivity detection of a CSF leak has ranged from 50% to 100% depending on the technique (61,89,99), with a specificity that approaches 100% (89). The image quality of ^{99m}Tc and ^{111}In are preferred. ^{111}In-DTPA is an excellent radiopharmaceutical for CSF scintigraphy because it is hydrophilic (100), does not accumulate in brain tissue (101), and with the DTPA ligand has a plasma $T_{1/2}$ less than 2 hours providing minimal background activity (101). Although ^{99m}Tc offers the advantage of a lower radiation dose, easy availability, and better imaging resolution, for small intermittent leaks ^{111}In-DTPA (500 μCi dose) can provide valuable 24-hour, 48-hour, and even 72-hour images if needed.

Maintaining the patient in a supine position until the actual scan time of imaging is advocated to pool the radiopharmaceutical in the basal cisterns. CSF leakage can often be increased by compression of the internal jugular vein or by performance of a Valsalva maneuver (54). These maneuvers can help decrease the number of false-negative studies in patients with intermittent CSF leakage.

Various administrative techniques and protocols have been used. Although the suboccipital puncture method had difficulty detecting cribriform plate leaks (102), other invasive techniques, such as cisternal puncture (103), direct injection via burr holes (85), and overpressure cisternography (104), reported high detection rates. However, they also reported higher morbidity than with lumbar injection. Most institutions use an intrathecal lumbar injection route.

After an intrathecal lumbar injection, patients are scanned with a scintillation camera for a single lumbar spine image to ensure proper placement of the tracer into the subarachnoid spaces. Because most CSF leaks occur near the basilar cisterns, head imaging should occur between 1 to 3 hours after a lumbar injected dose. Optimally, head images should coincide with the radioactive bolus at the CSF leak; therefore, scanning or obtaining a single image at half-hour intervals would allow more precise determination. However, most institutions acquire their head images in the anterior, posterior, and both lateral projections at standard protocol times of 2-hour, 6-hour, and 24-hour postinjection. If needed 48-hour, and even 72-hour, images can be obtained. When spontaneous intracranial hypotension is suspected, there is slow CSF circulation to the convexity and rapid appearance of renal and urinary bladder activity. Often the CSF leak is not detected on the images, but occasionally an image of a "Christmas tree" or "railroad pattern" can be identified along the spinal canal. Therefore, images of the entire spinal canal and of the bladder should be obtained (105,106).

Note that with posterior nasopharyngeal leaks, the CSF may be swallowed with subsequent false-negative images and pledget evaluation. To increase detection of posterior nasopharyngeal leaks an evaluation of a gastric secretion activity/serum activity ratio has been advocated (98). A less invasive technique involves acquiring an anterior abdominal view at 24 hours, and at 48 hours if needed (74,91). Note that a long exposure time can be required for abdominal-view acquisitions.

For suspected otorrhea, a single pledget can be placed in each external auditory meatus. For patients with rhinorrhea, knowledge of the anatomic pathway of sinus drainage aids in both physical and diagnostic examination of leaks via pledget activity. The frontal and ethmoid sinuses open into the middle meatus,

the frontal opens anterior to the ethmoid, and the sphenoid sinus opens anteriorly into the sphenoethmoidal recess of the nasal cavity. In a small percent of posttraumatic CSF leaks, lateralization will not be reliable (68), but usually the pledget with the highest abnormal count rate is assumed to have been closest to the CSF leak site. Protocols differ as to the total number and placement timing of the 0.5-mL volume intranasal pledgets.

Because CSF is absorbed into the blood stream via arachnoid villi, some radioactivity is distributed into normal nasal secretions. Therefore, most institutions presently use the protocol that compares the activity in the nasal pledgets to plasma activity for which normal values have been established in a study of 16 patients without known abnormalities (107). In this protocol, two pledgets with an absorptive capacity of 0.5 mL are placed in each nostril. The pledgets are inserted 2 hours after intrathecal injection of 0.5 mCi of ^{111}In-DTPA and remain in place for 4 hours. Five milliliters of anticoagulated venous blood is withdrawn at the time of placement and removal of the pledgets. The activity in the cotton pledgets and 0.5-mL aliquots of plasma are counted separately for 10 minutes in a scintillation well counter with a window setting at 150 to 250 keV. Sample counts can be expressed in terms of counts per gram to normalize for differences in pledget size and amounts of absorbed fluid. A ratio of the nasal secretion to the blood value can thus be used to detect the presence of a CSF leak. The results are expressed as the ratio of pledget activity to the average of the two plasma samples. The normal intranasal pledget/plasma ratio is 1.3 (107). In patients with active CSF leak the ratio is usually between 2 and 10 (74), but a pledget/plasma ratio of more than 1.5 is interpreted as positive evidence of a CSF leak. Marked pledget count asymmetry is suspicious, even if not greater than the 1.3 ratio; a new set of pledgets for a longer time should be considered. Nearly 100% of CSF leaks can be diagnosed by a combination of the various isotopic techniques previously described, and a high percentage can be localized (71,89–91,99, 108) (Fig. 40.6).

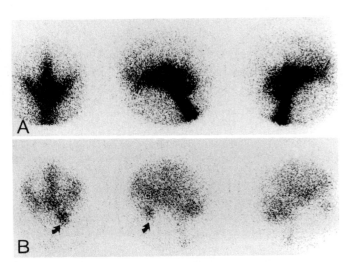

FIGURE 40.6. After intrathecal injection of ^{111}In-DTPA, questionable cerebrospinal fluid (CSF) leak activity is seen on the 4-hour images **(A)**, but obvious activity at 24 hours indicates CSF leak (**B**, *arrows*).

Injection Problems

Although examination of CSF leaks by radionuclide studies is relatively easy to perform and has a high degree of accuracy, there are minor injection problems that should be noted. Extra-arachnoid (subdural or epidural) injection of radiopharmaceuticals results in delayed progression to the cranial area. This can be detected by the rapid transfer of activity into blood and urine or by the characteristic Christmas tree or railroad track spinal image. There may be a lack of anatomic specificity with this appearance, and active leakage is often necessary for detection. Finally, there is a possibility of aseptic meningitis secondary to an endotoxin-contaminated tracer; however, with the sterile high purity commercial test kits currently available the incidence is very low (74).

HYDROCEPHALUS

With the introduction of CT and MRI, a quick, noninvasive radiographic study became available to accurately assess ventricular size and often to establish the presence of an underlying abnormality. Pneumoencephalography and nuclear medicine examinations became less important both in diagnosis and management of hydrocephalus, whether on an obstructive or communicating basis.

Both hydrocephalus and atrophy are characterized by ventricular dilatation (the term *hydrocephalus ex-vacuo* is inappropriate and should be discontinued in favor of atrophy (109). Hydrocephalus is differentiated from cortical atrophy with compensatory dilatation of the ventricles and cisterns by evaluation of CT and MRI images, which demonstrated marked ventricular enlargement out of proportion to sulcal enlargement (Fig. 40.7). Questionable cases in the past were evaluated with radionuclide cisternogram.

RC is performed using a lumbar intrathecal injection of ^{111}In-DTPA. Obtaining a posterior image of the lower spine 15 to 30 minutes after injection documents advancement of the injected radiopharmaceutical. In adults, head imaging is performed at 4, 24, and 48 hours in the anterior, left lateral, and posterior projections (Fig. 40.2). In pediatric patients, 2-, 12-, and 24-hour images may be required because of a more rapid CSF flow (105,110). In normal adults, tracer activity enters the basal cisterns and extends into the interhemispheric and sylvian fissures by 3 to 4 hours forming Neptune's triumvirate, with subsequent activity over the convexities by 24 hours. Normally, there is no reflux of activity into the lateral ventricles. Occasionally, however, a transient reflux into the lateral ventricles is seen before 24 hours, but this has not been considered significant (105). Use of ^{111}In-DTPA for cisternography delivers approximately 0.1 rad/mCi total body, 2.3 rad/mCi to the brain, and 1.3 rad/mCi to the spinal cord (105).

Possible mechanisms that account for the development of hydrocephalus include (a) obstructive hydrocephalus (communicating or noncommunicating), (b) decreased CSF absorption, (c) NPH, and (d) overproduction of CSF (choroid plexus tumors).

The communicating obstructive hydrocephalus or extraventricular obstructive hydrocephalus (EVOH) occurs within the subarachnoid spaces or cisterns and usually follows subarachnoid hemorrhage (SAH) or an inflammatory process. It is felt to secondarily diminish absorption as a result of a dysfunctional arachnoid villi/venous sinus interface or lack of ventricular clearing as a result of cell damage to the ependymal lining (107,110).

Noncommunicating obstructive hydrocephalus or intraventricular obstructive hydrocephalus (IVOH) occurs within the ventricular system down to and including the fourth ventricle outlet foramina. CT or MRI findings vary with the site and duration of the blockage, with the ventricle system enlarging proximal to the obstruction. Of the congenital etiologies, aqueductal stenosis is the most common, followed by Arnold-Chiari malformation and Dandy-Walker cyst (107). Any type of neoplasm adjacent to or within the ventricle can result in obstruction. Brainstem gliomas, intraventricular ependymomas, and colloid cysts of the third ventricle are most common (107).

Although there are case reports of inborn normotensive hydrocephalus without intellectual sequelae (111), NPH is characteristically associated with the triad of dementia, incontinence, and ataxia in conjunction with enlarged ventricles and normal CSF pressure (112,113). The etiology of NPH continues to be investigated; some investigators report a high incidence of hyperdynamic CSF flow in the cerebral aqueduct (48,92,114). In 1993, Xiong et al. (115) proposed that the NPH symptoms were not secondary to ventricular dilatation and damage to adjacent brain parenchyma but rather to the corpus callosum impingement by the falx cerebri. This finding is indirectly supported by Larsson et al. (116) who reported that the reversibility of the symptoms in NPH are independent of the total CSF

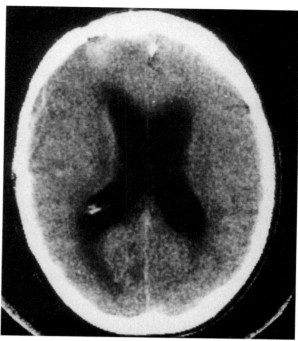

FIGURE 40.7. Hydrocephalus several months following subarachnoid hemorrhage. Note lack of convexity sulci definition in addition to the ventricular enlargement. There are several areas of infarcts, which are complications of the subarachnoid hemorrhage.

clearance and that factors other than quantitative CSF dynamics alone accounts for the pathophysiology of NPH.

RC has become a less important diagnostic tool for diagnosis of NPH. The early investigations of RC in NPH patients described classic diagnostic findings of early entry of the radiopharmaceutical into the lateral ventricles that persists at 24 and 48 hours with impairment of flow over the convexities of the brain demonstrated by delayed or absent activity. (117,118) (Fig. 40.8). These findings suggested the NPH patient would benefit from diversionary ventriculoperitoneal (VP) shunt surgery (119, 120). Later investigations have proven that this pattern is not specific and that there are false positives with no improved outcome from VP shunting (121–125).

Although 40% to 87% of NPH patients will improve after VP shunting (116,126), the relatively high complication rate (up to 31%) (113), which includes death (126), has prompted continued investigations for a preoperative positive predictor of VP shunt outcome. Unfortunately, past predictive value of anticipating the clinical outcome of VP shunting has been difficult and far from consistent (127,128). In 1984, Sano et al. (129) emphasized that CSF shunting was not beneficial for idiopathic NPH cases with multilacunar infarction by tomographic measurement of CBF. Vanneste et al. (124) retrospectively evaluated 75 NPH patients using presurgical clinical data, CT scans, nonquantitative radionuclide scintigraphy, and postsurgical outcome with these conclusions: (a) the predictive value of nonquantitative RC is low and (b) nonquantitative RC offers no advantage in selection of patients for a shunt versus comparison to combined clinical and CT data alone. However, Larsson et al. (116) investigated quantitative cisternography using ^{99m}Tc-DTPA and reported that the radioactivity ratio of ventricular activity to total intracranial activity (V/T) positively correlated with the degree of VP shunt improvement. All patients with a V/T ratio greater than 32% had good improvement, although ratios less than 32% did not exclude good outcome. In 1991, Kamiya et al. (130) evaluated N-isopropyl-p-iodine-123-iodoamphetamine (^{123}I-IMP) SPECT before and after CSF removal. They reported that frontal blood flow increased compared with temporal flow after CSF removal in all patients with SAH who improved after VP shunt procedure. Another study compared ^{99m}Tc hexamethylpropyleneamine oxime (HMPAO) SPECT to intrathecal injection of ^{111}In-DTPA RC and CT scan for predictive outcome of VP shunting (126). Although there was no correlation between cisternography pattern and clinical shunt outcome, there was a statistically significant poor shunt outcome; NPH patients had concurrent Alzheimer-type dementia (126). In a ^{123}I-IMP SPECT study in childhood hydrocephalus, the authors counted radioactivity in region-of-interest (ROI), calculated a reabsorption ratio (RR), and reported all negative-RR cases had poor VP shunt outcome, whereas all positive-RR cases had good VP shunt outcome (131). These recent nuclear medicine studies are promising, but whether nuclear medicine plays a role in prognostic information for hydrocephalus treatment remains to be determined; further evaluation of quantitative CSF flow assessment with MRI (132) and measurement of periventricular water proton relaxation times (133) may prove to be better prognostic indicators for VP shunt procedures.

CEREBROSPINAL FLUID SHUNTS

The widespread use of diversionary shunts in treating various forms of hydrocephalus has created the need for a simple method to analyze changes in CSF flow, to determine shunt patency, and to determine the cause of complications. Initial diagnosis of shunt patency and adequacy of CSF flow in many cases is made by examination of the patient and inspection of the subcutaneous CSF reservoir. If the reservoir in an alert patient readily resumes its shape after compression, it is reasonably clear that the shunt is adequately functioning. If the pumping chamber compresses but does not refill and return to its original shape, proximal occlusion is likely. When there is undue resistance to compression, there may be obstruction at the valve or distal catheter. Suspected shunt dysfunction evaluation often includes CT and puncture of the shunt system for measurement of CSF pressure, bacterial culture, and hematology and chemistry laboratory analysis.

Proximal and distal flow can be evaluated by tapping the reservoir percutaneously. If CSF is obtained with the unidirectional valve distal to the port, patency of the proximal portion of the shunt is assumed. In addition, when using a manometer, a rapid descent to closing pressure of the valve suggests shunt patency. If no CSF is obtained initially, the pumping chamber is depressed. If the manometer column falls only after pumping,

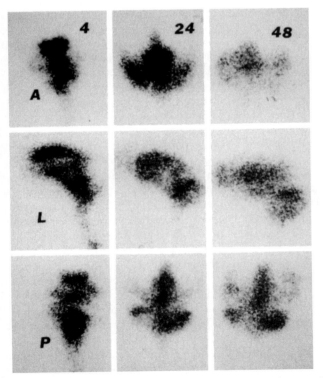

FIGURE 40.8. Normal pressure hydrocephalus. Typical nuclear medicine cerebrospinal fluid scan at 4 hours (*left*), 24 hours (*center*), and 48 hours (*right*) after injection. Anterior (*A*), left lateral (*L*), and posterior (*P*) views are shown. Notice the marked ventricular penetration by the radiopharmaceutical.

there is a presumed distal obstruction. If the column fails to drop even with pumping, then the valve is probably obstructed.

Clarification of the shunt dysfunction may require the evaluation of CSF shunt dynamics by radionuclide shuntography (Fig. 40.9). Radionuclide studies using ^{111}In-DTPA (134), ^{99m}Tc-DTPA (135), or ^{99m}Tc provide diagnostic information that is minimally invasive but accurate in the determination of shunt patency. With the imaging characteristics of 140 keV, short $T_{1/2}$, low cost, low radiation dose, and easy availability, ^{99m}Tc agents are preferred for CSF shunt imaging. Use of ^{99m}Tc-DTPA allows for decreased background activity secondary to increased renal extraction and excretion. A delayed image demonstrating activity within the kidneys suggests some degree of distal limb patency. The effective dose equivalent for a normally functioning shunt with a technetium agent is 0.07 mSv, and only 0.1 mSv with distal obstruction (136).

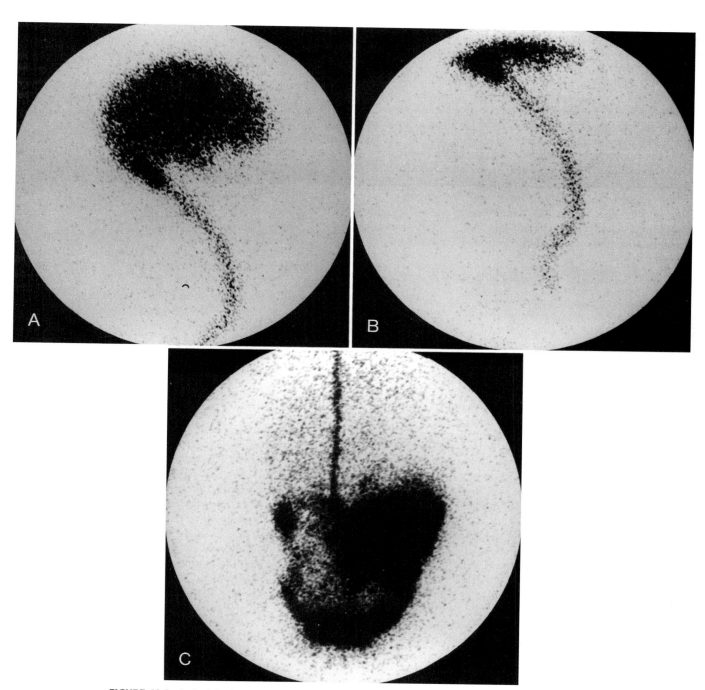

FIGURE 40.9. A: Activity is visualized superior to the shunt reservoir with good dispersement demonstrating patency of the proximal limb. **B:** Activity is only seen in the path of the shunt tubing at 30 minutes. No free activity is seen in the abdomen (versus expected normal tree flow in **C**). This represents occlusion to the distal limb of the shunt.

Familiarity with the exact type and configuration of shunt system is essential before performing a CSF shunt study (137). Shunt types include VP, ventriculojugular, ventriculoatrial, and lumboperitoneal. Patients with ventriculoatrial shunts have a higher complication rate (107).

Common complications of CSF shunt surgery secondary to excessive negative ICP from overdrainage of CSF include ventricular blockage, subdural hematoma, craniosynostosis, chronic headache, and slit ventricle syndrome (120,138–141). Other commonly recognized complications are infection and thromboembolism (107). Superior vena cava obstruction and immune complex glomerulonephritis are seen particularly with ventriculoatrial shunts (107). Disconnection of the shunt catheter or distal catheter knotting or kinking are more common in children (142). Distal limb VP complications include tip occlusion from fibrous adhesion or encasement, pseudocyst formation, tip perforation (bowel wall, abdominal wall, scrotal wall, pelvic organs, gallbladder), and shunt tip migration (143–147).

A patent shunt is not necessarily equivalent to adequate flow (138). Functional obstruction of the antisiphon device (ASD) can cause symptomatic ventriculomegaly despite radionuclide evidence of shunt patency (148). Chronic irritation of the peritoneum or subclinical peritonitis can secondarily prevent good CSF resorption through the peritoneum (138). When intraabdominal pressure exceeds the CSF pressure there can be resistance to CSF outflow into the peritoneal cavity (149). Interestingly, this has been reported from use of a corset or during periods of constipation (149).

A shunt injection is performed under strictly aseptic conditions; the radiopharmaceutical is injected via a 25-gauge needle into the shunt reservoir. The distal catheter is manually occluded during the procedure so that the radiopharmaceutical will reflux into the ventricular system. If the one-way valve is located proximal to the port, no reflux of activity would be expected in the ventricle system. Serial postinjection gamma-camera images are obtained to monitor the ventricles and flow of the CSF into the distal shunt catheter. The distal shunt tubing is visualized as a linear band of radioactivity. In VP shunts, there should be free flow of radioactivity at the distal tip of a functioning shunt. Signs of inadequate shunt function include

1. A reservoir that requires pumping to initiate flow or in which resistance is encountered when injecting tracer into the chamber
2. Lack of free intraperitoneal flow or a loculated collection of activity at the peritoneal tip represents distal obstruction
3. Extravasation of injected radiopharmaceutical or pooling at the reservoir site, which suggests a break in the shunt tubing secondary to mechanical stress or discontinuity of connections
4. Absence of reflux into the ventricular system and rapid filling of the distal shunt or failure of the radiopharmaceutical to clear from the ventricles after several hours, which represents proximal limb obstruction
5. Nonvisualization of the parotid glands after 30 minutes, which represents distal obstruction of a ventriculovascular shunt (normal parotid gland activity appears in 5 to 30 minutes)
6. Absence of lung activity using ^{99m}Tc-MAA with a ventriculoatrial shunt, which represents distal shunt obstruction

Patients occasionally have progressive hydrocephalus or intermittent symptoms of ICP despite the presence of an apparently functioning CSF diversionary shunt. Even though radionuclide studies are capable of demonstrating shunt patency, this is reflected only at the time of the study and no indication is given of the functional adequacy of the shunt. Several quantitative radionuclide methods for determining shunt patency and flow have been described but have met with variable success (119, 150–152). Attempts can be made to quantify shunt function as a percentage disappearance of the radioactivity from the lateral ventricles for various time intervals (153). This is feasible if the volume of the valve and reservoir and disappearance rate of the tracer are known (152,154). For example, with a Rickham reservoir and Hakim valve, the normal half-disappearance time of ^{99m}Tc-DTPA from the valve is 0.5 to 6 minutes (149,155).

In addition to accurately assessing the clearance characteristics of an individual shunt, Chervu et al. (156) have shown the necessity of first developing a calibration curve for the whole shunt mechanism. Fortunately, most institutions limit themselves to the use of one or two shunt systems making it possible for only one or two calibration curves to suffice. Sources of error that have been shown to distort clearance values include radioactive contamination of the overlying tissue at the injection site, introduction of an air bubble into the system, and failure to consider the entire configuration of the shunt apparatus, including the type of reservoir and valve (153).

CEREBROSPINAL AND MONOCLONAL ANTIBODIES

In 1957, Pressman (157) proposed the use of paired labeling in the determination of tumor-localizing antibodies. Extensive investigations of monoclonal antibodies for imaging tumors resulted (158–160). In 1992, the first commercially available monoclonal antibodies for imaging received Food and Drug Administration (FDA) approval. The concept of a "magic bullet" monoclonal antibody that would selectively localize and destroy tumor tissue continues to be investigated. Although there has been little success with large-bulk tumors (161,162), there is a therapeutic advantage when the tumor is confined to a single compartment (163).

Even with advances in chemotherapy and radiotherapy, malignant meningitis is devastating with mean survival of 2 to 3 months (164,165). Several studies showed that many tumors that metastasize to the leptomeninges are radiosensitive (166–168). Early investigations used a heavy molecular weight complex of ^{198}Au colloid-labeled antibodies, but there was concern over a high radiation dose to the cauda equina (170–173). More recent studies with monoclonal antibodies labeled with the short-range β-emitter ^{131}I successfully irradiated disseminated meningeal tumor yet spared the spinal cord and brain from excessive radiation (168). The direct intrathecal administration of radiolabeled monoclonal antibodies not only provides tumor imaging capabilities but also, at treatment dose levels, has resulted in clinical remission, neurologic improvement, and prolonged patient survival (167,168,173).

ACKNOWLEDGMENTS

The authors would like to thank Ann C. Price M.D., Val M. Runge M.D., and A. Everette James, Jr. for their previous contributions to this chapter.

REFERENCES

1. Cotugno D. The first description of the spinal fluid. By Domenico Cotugno, 1775. *Clin Orthop* 1998;227:6–9.
2. Magendie F. Memoire sur le liquide qui se trouve dans le crène et l'épine de l'homme et des animaux. *J Physiol Exp Pathol* 1825;5: 27–32.
3. Magendie F. *Recherchés sur le liquide céphalo-rachidien ou cérébrospinal.* Academie des Sciences Paris: France, 1842.
4. Faivre E. *Compt rend de l'Acad des Sciences* Academie des Sciences, Paris, France, 1854;34:424.
5. Key A, Retzius G. Studien in der anatomie des nervensystems und des bindegewebes. Royal Academy of Sciences, Stockholm: Sweden, 1875.
6. Weed LH. Studies on the cerebrospinal fluid III. The pathways of escape from the subarachnoid spaces with particular reference to the arachnoid villi. *J Med Res* 1914;26:51–60.
7. Weed LH. Some limitation of the Monro-Kellie hypothesis. *Arch Surg* 1929;18:1049–1053.
8. Beering EA. Water exchange of central nervous system and cerebrospinal fluid. *J Neurosurg* 1952;9:275–280.
9. Cestan, Laborde, Riser M. La perméabilité méninge n'est qu'un des modes la permeabilité vasculaire. *Presse Méd* 1925;33:1330–1332.
10. Greenberg DM, Aird RB, Boelter MDD et al. A study with radioactive isotopes of the permeability of the blood-cerebrospinal fluid barrier to ions. *Am J Physiol* 1943;140:47–52.
11. Sweet WH, Selverstone B, Soloway S et al. Studies of formation, flow and absorption of cerebrospinal fluid. II. Studies with heavy water in normal man. In: *Surgical forum. Clinical Congress of American College of Surgeons.* Philadelphia: WB Saunders, 1951.
12. Sweet WH, Brownell GL, Scholl JA et al. The formation, flow and absorption of CSF; newer concepts based on studies with isotopes. *Res Publ Ass Nerv Ment Dis* 1954;34:101–105.
13. Wallace GB, Brodie BB. On the source of cerebrospinal fluid. The distribution of bromide and iodide throughout the central nervous system. *J Pharmacol Exp Ther* 1940;70:418–421.
14. Dandy WE, Blackfan KD. Internal hydrocephalus. An experimental, clinical and pathological study. *Am J Dis Child* 1914;8:406–408.
15. Dandy WE. Where is cerebrospinal fluid absorbed? *JAMA* 1929;92: 2012–2015.
16. Howart F, Cooper ERA. The fate of certain foreign colloids and cristalloids after subarachnoid injection. *Acta Anat* 1955;25:112–117.
17. Mott FW. The Oliver-Sharpey lectures on cerebrospinal fluid. Lecture I: The physiology of cerebrospinal fluid. *Lancet* 1910;2:1–12.
18. Kiss F, Sattler J. Struktur und Funktion der Pacchionischen Granulationen. *Anat Anz* 1956;103:273–276.
19. O'Connell JEA. The vascular factor in intracranial pressure and the maintenance of the cerebrospinal fluid circulation. *Brain* 1943;66: 204–207.
20. Beering EA Jr. Circulation of the cerebrospinal fluid: demonstration of the choroid plexus as the generator of the force for flow of fluid and ventricular enlargement. *J Neurosurg* 1962;19:405–413.
21. Welch K, Friedman V. The cerebrospinal fluid valves. *Brain* 1960; 83:454–458.
22. Di Chiro G. Movement of cerebrospinal fluid in human beings. *Nature* 1964;204:290–293.
23. McComb JG. Recent research into the nature of the cerebrospinal fluid formation and absorption. *J Neurosurg* 1983;59:369–374.
24. Go KG. Cerebral pathophysiology. *An integral approach with some emphasis on clinical implications.* Amsterdam: Elsevier Science Publishers, 1991.
25. Greitz D. Cerebrospinal fluid circulation and associated intracranial dynamics: a radiologic investigation using MR imaging and radionuclide cisternography. *Acta Radiol* 1993;386(Suppl):1–23.
26. James AE, DeLand FH, Hodges FJ III et al. Cerebrospinal fluid (CSF) scanning: cisternography. *Am J Roentgenol Rad Ther* 1970;110:74–79.
27. Di Chiro G. Observation on the circulation of the cerebrospinal fluid. *Acta Radiol Diagn* 1966;5:988–991.
28. Milhorat TH. Choroid plexus and cerebrospinal fluid production. *Science* 1969;166:1514–1518.
29. James AE, Strecker EP, Kouigsmark B et al. Alterations in CSF absorption in experimental communicating hydrocephalus. In: *Proceedings of the Society of Neurological Surgeons.* Los Angeles: 1973.
30. James AE. Cerebrospinal fluid imaging (cisternography). In: Gottschalk A, Potchen EJ, eds. *Diagnostic nuclear medicine,* 1st ed. Baltimore: Williams & Wilkins, 1976:303–323.
31. James AE, DeLand FH, Hodges FJ III et al. Cisternography: its role in normal pressure hydrocephalus. *JAMA* 1970;213:1615–1620.
32. Thomason St C. *The cerebrospinal fluid: its spontaneous escape from the nose.* London: Cassell, 1899.
33. Feinberg DA. Modern concepts of brain motion and cerebrospinal fluid flow. *Radiology* 1992;185:630–635.
34. Feinberg DA, Mark AS. Cerebrospinal fluid flow evaluated by inner volume magnetic resonance velocity imaging. *Acta Radiol (Stockh)* 1986;369(Suppl):766–770.
35. Feinberg DA, Mark AS. Human brain motion and cerebrospinal fluid circulation demonstrated with MR velocity imaging. *Radiology* 1987; 163:793–799.
36. Ahmadi J, Gomez DG, Pavese AM et al. Evidence for transventricle absorption in the hydrocephalic dog. *Invest Radiol* 1979;14:432–437.
37. Takei F, Shapiro K, Kohn I. Influence of the rate of ventricular enlargement on the white matter water content in progressive feline hydrocephalus. *J Neurosurg* 1987;66:577–583.
38. Deo-Narine V, Gomez DG, Vullo T et al. Direct in vivo observation of transventricular absorption in the hydrocephalic dog using magnetic resonance imaging. *Invest Radiol* 1994;29:287–293.
39. Enzmann DF, Pelc NJ. Normal flow patterns of intracranial and spinal cerebrospinal fluid defined with phase-contrast cine MR imaging. *Radiology* 1991;178:467–474.
40. Enzmann DR, Pelc NJ. Phase-contrast MR imaging in measurement of brain motion. *Radiology* 1992;185:653–660.
41. Nitz WR, Bradley WG, Watanabe AS et al. Flow dynamics of cerebrospinal fluid: assessment with phase-contrast velocity MR imaging performed with retrospective cardiac gating. *Radiology* 1992;183: 395–405.
42. Quencer RM, Donavan-Post MJ, Hinks RS. Cine MR in the evaluation of normal and abnormal CSF flow. Intracranial and intraspinal studies. *Neuroradiology* 1990;32:371–377.
43. Kahn T, Müller E, Lewin JS et al. MR measurement of spinal CSF flow with the RACE technique. *J Comput Assist Tomogr* 1992;16: 54–57.
44. Thomsen C, Stahlberg F, Stubgaard M et al., The Scandinavian Flow Group. Fourier analysis of cerebrospinal fluid flow velocities. MR imaging study. *Radiology* 1990;177:659–663.
45. Poncelet BP, Wedeen VJ, Weisskoff RM et al. Brain parenchyma motion: measurement with cine echo-planar MR imaging. *Radiology* 1992;185:645–651.
46. Berstrand G, Gerströ M, Nordell B et al. Cardiac gated MR imaging of cerebrospinal fluid flow. *J Comput Assist Tomogr* 1985;9:1003–1008.
47. Levy LM, DiChiro G. MR phase imaging and cerebrospinal fluid flow in the head and spine. *Neuroradiology* 1990;32:399–404.
48. Bradley WG Jr, Whittemore AR, Kortman KE et al. Marked cerebrospinal fluid void: indicator of successful shunt in patients with suspected normal-pressure hydrocephalus. *Radiology* 1991;178: 459–466.
49. Wahkloo AK, Jungling F, Hennig J. Pulsatile brain motion in normals and patients with NPH. In: *Book of abstracts: Society of Magnetic Reso-*

nance in Medicine 1992. Berkeley, CA: Society of Magnetic Resonance in Medicine, 1992:627(abst).

50. Nilsson C, Stahlberg F, Thomsen C et al. Circadian variation in human cerebrospinal fluid production measured by magnetic resonance imaging. *Am J Physiol* 1992;262:R20–R24.

51. Nau R, Emrich D, Prange HW. Inverse correlation between disappearance of intrathecally injected ^{111}In-DTPA from CSF with CSF protein content and CSF-to-serum albumin ratio. *J Neurol Sci* 1993;115:102–104.

52. Colquhoun IR. CT cisternography in the investigation of cerebrospinal fluid rhinorrhea. *Clin Radiol* 1993;47:403–408.

53. Lantz EJ, Forbes GS, Brown ML et al. Radiology of cerebrospinal fluid rhinorrhea. *Am J Roentgenol* 1980;135:1023–1030.

54. Pappas DG Jr, Hoffman RA, Cohen NL et al. Spontaneous temporal bone cerebrospinal fluid leak. *Am J Otol* 1992;6:534–539.

55. Kaufman B, Nulsen FE, Weiss MH et al. Acquired spontaneous non-traumatic normal-pressure cerebrospinal fluid fistulas originating from the middle fossa. *Radiology* 1977;122:379–387.

56. Loew F, Pertuiset B, Chaumier EE et al. Traumatic, spontaneous and postoperative CSF rhinorrhoeae. In: Symon L, ed. *Advances and technical standards in neurosurgery.* Vienna: Springer-Verlag, 1984:11:169–207.

57. Leech P. Cerebrospinal fluid leakage, dural fistulae and meningitis after basal skull fracture. *Injury* 1974;6:141–149.

58. Robinson RG. Cerebrospinal fluid rhinorrhea, meningitis and pneumonocephalus due to non-missile injuries. *Aust NZ J Surg* 1970;39:328–334.

59. Brisman R, Hughes JEO, Mount L. Cerebrospinal fluid rhinorrhea and the empta sella. *J Neurosurg* 1969;31:538–543.

60. Brisman R, Hughes JEO, Mount LA. Cerebrospinal fluid rhinorrhea. *Arch Neurol* 1970;22:245–252.

61. Park JI, Strelzow VV, Friedman WH. Current management of cerebrospinal fluid rhinorrhea. *Laryngoscope* 1983;93:1294–1300.

62. Yeates AE, Blumenkopf B, Drayer BP et al. Spontaneous CSF rhinorrhea arising from the middle cranial fossa CT demonstration. *Am J Neuroradiol* 1984;5:820–821.

63. Lewin W, Cairns H. Fractures of the sphenoid sinus with cerebrospinal rhinorrhoea. *Br Med J* 1951;1:1–6.

64. Lewin W. Cerebrospinal fluid rhinorrhea in closed head injury. *Br J Surg* 1954;42:1–18.

65. Odrezin GT, Royal SA, Young DW et al. High resolution computed tomography of the temporal bone in infants and children: a review. *Int J Pediatr Otorhinolaryngol* 1990;19:15–31.

66. Wetmore SJ, Herrmann P, Fisch U. Spontaneous cerebrospinal fluid otorrhea. *Am J Otol* 1987;8:96–102.

67. Manelfe C, Cellerier P, Sobel D et al. Cerebrospinal fluid rhinorrhea: evaluation of metrizamide cisternography. *AJR* 1982;132:471–476.

68. Hubbard JL, McDonald TJ, Pearson BW et al. Spontaneous cerebrospinal fluid rhinorrhea: evolving concepts in diagnosis and surgical management based on the Mayo Clinic experience from 1970 through 1982. *Neurosurgery* 1985;16:314–320.

69. Russell T, Cummins BH. Cerebrospinal fluid rhinorrhea 34 years after trauma: a case report and review of the literature. *Neurosurgery* 1984;15:705–706.

70. Guo-Xaun B. Diagnosis and treatment of cerebrospinal rhinorrhea on a rhinological basis. *Chin Med J (Engl)* 1983;96:877–880.

71. McKusick KA. The diagnosis of traumatic cerebrospinal fluid rhinorrhea. *J Nucl Med* 1977;18:1234–1235.

72. Naidich TP, Moran CJ. Precise anatomic localization of atraumatic sphenoethmoidal cerebrospinal fluid rhinorrhea by metrizamide CT cisternography. *J Neurosurg* 1980;53:222–228.

73. Prere J, Puech JL, Deroover N et al. Rhinorrhea and meningitis due to post-traumatic osteo-meningeal defects in the anterior cranial fossa. Diagnosis with water-soluble CT cisternography. *Neuroradiology* 1986;13:278–285.

74. Jeffrey PJ, Sostre S, Scherer LR et al. Bowel visualization during indium-111 labeled diethylene triamine penta-acetic acid cisternography due to massive cerebrospinal fluid leak. *Eur J Nucl* 1990;17:365–369.

75. Gallardo E, Schacter D, Caceres E et al. The empty sella: results of treatment in 76 successive cases and high frequency of endocrine and neurological disturbances. *Clin Endocrinol* 1992;37:529–533.

76. Gracek RR, Leipzig B. Congenital cerebrospinal otorrhea. *Ann Otol Rhinol Laryngol* 1979;88:358–365.

77. Schuknecht HG. Mondini dysplasia: a clinical and pathological study. *Ann Otol Rhinol Laryngol* 1980;89(Suppl):1–23.

78. Ommaya AK, DiChiro G, Baldwin M et al. Non-traumatic cerebrospinal fluid rhinorrhea. *J Neurol Neurosurg Psychiatry* 1968;31:214–255.

79. Gadeholt H. The reaction of glucose oxidase test paper in normal nasal secretion. *Acta Otolaryngol (Stockh)* 1964;58:271–272.

80. Kogoy J, Trieff NM, Winkelmann P et al. Glucose in nasal secretions: diagnostic significance. *Arch Otolaryngol* 1972;95:225–227.

81. Hull HF, Morrow G. Glucorrhoea revisited. *JAMA* 1975;234:1052–1055.

82. Myer CM, Miller GW, Ball JB. Spontaneous cerebrospinal fluid otorrhea. *Ann Otol Rhinol Laryngol* 1985;94:96–97.

83. Irjala K, Suonpaa J, Laurent B. Identification of CSF leakage by immunofixation. *Arch Otolaryngol Head Neck Surg* 1979;105:447–454.

84. Calcaterra TC. Diagnosis and management of ethmoid cerebrospinal rhinorrhea. *Otolaryngol Clin North Am* 1985;18:99–105.

85. Mamo L, Cophigon J, Rey A et al. A new radionuclide method for the diagnosis of post traumatic cerebrospinal fistulae. *J Neurosurg* 1982;57:92–98.

86. Front D, Penning L. Occult spontaneous cerebrospinal fluid rhinorrhoea diagnosed by isotope cisternography. *Neuroradiology* 1971;2:167–169.

87. Byrne JV. Ingram CE, MacVicar D et al. Digital subtraction cisternography: a new approach to fistula localization in cerebrospinal fluid rhinorrhea. *J Neurol Neurosurg Psychiatry* 1990;53:1072–1075.

88. Nickalas P, Dutcher PO, Kido DK et al. New imaging techniques in diagnosis of cerebrospinal fluid fistula. *Laryngoscope* 1988;98:1065–1068.

89. Flynn BM, Butler SP, Quinn RJ et al. Radionuclide cisternography in the diagnosis and management of cerebrospinal leaks: the test of choice. *Med J Aust* 1987;146:82–84.

90. Glaubitt D, Haubrich J, Cordini-Voutsas M. Detection and quantitation of intermittent CSF rhinorrhea during prolonged cisternography with ^{111}In-DPTA. *AJNM* 1983;1:391–398.

91. Zu'bi SM, Kirkwood R, Abbasy M et al. Intestinal activity visualized on radionuclide cisternography in patients with cerebrospinal fluid leak. *J Nucl Med* 1991;32:151–153.

92. Maeda T, Ishida H, Matsuda H et al. The utility of radionuclide myelography and cisternography in the progress of cerebrospinal fluid leaks. *Eur J Nucl Med* 1984;9:416–418.

93. Primean M, Carrier L, Milette P et al. Spinal cerebrospinal fluid leak demonstrated by radioisotopic cisternography. *Clin Nucl Med* 1988;13:701–703.

94. Nielsen JT, Anderson K, Nielsen BV et al. Detection of rhinorrhea by cisternography in combination with single photon emission tomography, following lumbar injection of iodine-123-labeled albumin. *Eur J Nucl Med* 1992;19:966–970.

95. Mahaley MS Jr, Odom GL. Complication following intrathecal injection of fluorescein. *J Neurosurg* 1966;25:298–299.

96. Crow HJ, Keogh C, Northfield DWC. The location of cerebrospinal fluid fistulae. *Lancet* 1956;2:325–327.

97. Matin P, Goodwin DA. Cerebrospinal fluid scanning with 111-In. *J Nucl Med* 1971;12:668–672.

98. Doge H, Johannsen BA. Radioactivity in gastric juice—a simple adjunct to the Yb-169 DPTA cisternographic diagnosis of CSF rhinorrhea: concise communication. *J Nucl Med* 1977;18:1202–1204.

99. Oberson R. Radioisotopic diagnosis of rhinorrhea. *Radiol Clin Biol* 1972;41:28–35.

100. Thyrrel DA. The kinetics of ^{111}In-DTPA for cisternography. In: Cox PH, ed. *Progress in radiopharmacology,* vol 3. The Hague: Martinus Nijhoff, 1982:213–222.

101. McAfee JG, Gagne G, Atkins HL et al. Biological distribution and excretion of DTPA labeled with Tc-99m and In-111. *J Nucl Med* 1979;20:1273–1278.

102. Otto HJ, Koch RD. Indikation und aussagewert der szintigraphie der

intrakraniellen liquorräume. *Psychiatry Neurol Med Psychol* 1980;32: 658–662.

103. Di Chiro G, Ommaya AK, Ashburn WL et al. Isotope cisternography in the diagnosis and follow-up of cerebrospinal fluid rhinorrhea. *J Neurosurg* 1967;28:522–524.

104. Curnes JT, Vincent LM, Kowalsky RJ et al. CSF rhinorrhea: detection and localization using overpressure cisternography with Tc-99m-DPTA. *Radiology* 1985;154:795–799.

105. Benamor M, Tainturier C, Graveleau P et al. Radionuclide cisternography in spontaneous intracranial hypotension. *Clin Nucl Med* 1998; 23:150–151.

106. Ali SA, Cesani F, Zuckermann JA et al. Spinal-cerebrospinal fluid leak demonstrated by radiopharmaceutical cisternography. *Clin Nucl Med* 1998;23:152–155.

107. McKusick KA, Malmud LS, Kardella PA et al. Radionuclide cisternography: normal values for nasal secretions of intrathecally injected ^{111}In DTPA. *J Nucl Med* 1973;14:933–934.

108. Ashburn WL, Harbert JC, Briner WH et al. Cerebrospinal fluid rhinorrhea studies with gamma scintillation camera. *J Nucl Med* 1968; 9:523–529.

109. Osborn AG, ed. *Diagnostic neuroradiology,* 1st ed. St. Louis: Mosby-Year Book, 1994:752–754.

110. Henriksson L, Voigt K. Age-dependent differences of distribution and clearance pattern in normal RIHSA cisternograms. Neuroradiology 1976;12:103–107.

111. Gruwald F, Schlnus R. Isotope cisternography with indium-111 DTPA in a patient with nearly no intellectual deficits and extensive hydrocephalus. *Clin Nucl Med* 1989;5:352–353.

112. Hakim S. Some observations on CSF pressure. *Hydrocephalic syndrome in adults with "normal" CSF pressure (recognition of a new syndrome)* [Thesis No. 957]. Bogotà Columbia: Javeriana University School of Medicine, 1964.

113. Peterson RC, Modri B, Laws E. Surgical treatment of idiopathic hydrocephalus in elderly patients. *Neurology* 1985;35:307–311.

114. Schroth G, Klose U. Cerebrospinal fluid flow, III. Pathological cerebrospinal fluid pulsations. *Neuroradiology* 1992;35:16–19.

115. Xiong G, Rauch RA, Hagino N et al. An animal model of corpus callosum impingement as seen in patients with normal pressure hydrocephalus. *Invest Radiol* 1993;28:46–50.

116. Larsson A, Moonen M, Bergh AC et al. Predictive value of quantitative cisternography in normal pressure hydrocephalus. *Acta Neurol Scand* 1990;81:327–332.

117. Bannister R, Gilford E, Kocen R. Isotope encephalography in the diagnosis of dementia due to communicating hydrocephalus. *Lancet* 1967;1014–1017.

118. Patten DH, Benson DF. Diagnosis of normal-pressure hydrocephalus by RISA cisternography. *J Nucl Med* 1968;9:457–461.

119. James AE Jr, DeBlanc HJ Jr, DeLand FH et al. Refinements in cerebrospinal fluid diversionary shunt evaluation by cisternography. *AJR* 1972;115:766–773.

120. McCullough DC, Harbert JC, Di Chiro G et al. Prognostic criteria for cerebrospinal fluid shunting from isotope cisternography in communicating hydrocephalus. *Neurology* 1970;20:594–598.

121. Black PM. The normal pressure hydrocephalus syndrome. In: Scott RM, ed. *Concepts in neurosurgery: hydrocephalus.* Baltimore: Williams & Wilkins, 1990;3:102–114.

122. Greenberg JO, Shenkin HA, Adam R. Idiopathic normal pressure hydrocephalus—a report of 73 patients. *J Neurol Neurosurg Psychiatry* 1977;40:336–341.

123. Benzel EC, Pelletier AL, Levy PG. Communicating hydrocephalus in adults: prediction of outcome after ventricular shunting procedures. *Neurosurgery* 1990;26:655–660.

124. Vanneste J, Augustijn P, Davies GA et al. Normal pressure hydrocephalus: is cisternography still useful in selecting patients for a shunt? *Arch Neurol* 1992;49:366–370.

125. Vanneste J, van Acker R. Normal pressure hydrocephalus: did literature alter management? *J Neurol Neurosurg Psychiatry* 1990;53: 564–568.

126. Granado JM, Diaz F, Alday R. Evaluation of brain SPECT in the diagnosis and prognosis of the normal pressure hydrocephalus syndrome. *Acta Neurochir* 1991;112:88–91.

127. Mathew NT, Meyer JS, Hertmann A et al. Abnormal cerebrospinal fluid-blood flow dynamics. Implications in diagnosis, treatment and prognosis in normal pressure hydrocephalus. *Arch Neurol* 1975;32: 657–664.

128. Symon L, Hinzpeter T. The enigma of normal pressure hydrocephalus: tests to select patients for surgery and to predict shunt function. *Clin Neurosurg* 1977;24:285–333.

129. Sano K, Tamura A, Segawa H et al. Cerebral circulation in NPH: tomographic measurement of CBF. In: *Annual report of the Ministry of Health and Welfare, "Normal pressure hydrocephalus."* Tokyo: Ministry of Health and Welfare, 1984;49–53.

130. Kamiya K, Yamashita N, Nagai H et al. Investigation of normal pressure hydrocephalus by 123-I IMP SPECT. *Neurol Med Chiro* 1991; 31:503–507.

131. Shinoda M, Yamaguchi T, Tanaka Y et al. Single photon emission computerized tomography in childhood hydrocephalus. *Child's Nerv Syst* 1992;8:219–221.

132. Jack CR, Mokri B, Laws ER et al. MR findings in normal-pressure hydrocephalus: significance and comparison with other forms of dementia. *J Comput Assist Tomogr* 1987;11:923–931.

133. Tamaki N, Shirakuni T, Ehara K et al. Characterization of periventricular edema in normal-pressure hydrocephalus by measurement of water proton relaxation times. *J Neurosurg* 1990;73:864–870.

134. Graff-Radford NR, Rezai K, Godersky JC et al. Regional cerebral blood flow in normal pressure hydrocephalus. *J Neurol Neurosurg Psychiatry* 1987;50:1589–1596.

135. Gilday D, Kellam J. In-DTPA evaluation of CSF diversionary shunts in children. *J Nucl Med* 1973;14:920–925.

136. Sty JR, D'Souza BJ, Daniels D. Nuclear anatomy of diversionary central nervous system shunts in children. *Clin Nucl Med* 1978;3: 271–273.

137. Johnson R, Ahlberg J, Mattsson S et al. Patient exposure when using ^{99}Tc-DTPA for evolution of cerebrospinal fluid shunt patency. *Acta Radiol* 1988;29:378–380.

138. Altman J, James AE Jr. Ventriculo-venous cerebrospinal fluid shunts: roentgenologic analysis. *AJR* 1971;112:237–250.

139. Tokoro K, Chiba Y. Optimum position for an antisiphon device in a cerebrospinal fluid shunt system. *Neurosurgery* 1991;29;4:519–525.

140. Becker DP, Nelsen FE. Control of hydrocephalus by valve regulated venous shunt maintenance. *J Neurosurg* 1968;28:215–218.

141. Harwood-Nash DC. Radiology of shunt complications. In: Harwood-Nash DC, Ritz CR, eds. *Neuroradiology in infants and children,* vol 2. St. Louis: CV Mosby, 1976:651–667.

142. Fox JL, McCullough DC, Green RC. Effect of cerebrospinal fluid shunts on intracranial pressure and on cerebrospinal fluid dynamics. 2. A new technique of pressure measurements: results and concepts. 3. A concept of hydrocephalus. *J Neurol Neurosurg Psychiatry* 1973; 36:302–312.

143. Eschelman DJ, Lee VW. Lesser sac cerebrospinal fluid collection. An unusual complication of a ventriculoperitoneal shunt. *Clin Nucl Med* 1990;6:415–417.

144. Agha FP, Amendola MA, Shirazi KK et al. Unusual complications of ventriculoperitoneal shunts. *Radiology* 1982;146: 323–326.

145. Goldfine SF, Turetz F, Beck AR et al. Cerebrospinal fluid intraperitoneal cyst: an unusual abdominal mass. *AJR* 1978;130:568–572.

146. Grosfeld JL, Cooney DR, Smith J et al. Intra-abdominal complications following ventriculoperitoneal shunt procedures. *Pediatrics* 1974;54:791–796.

147. Fischer EG, Shillito J Jr. Large abdominal cyst: a complication of peritoneal shunts. Report of three cases. *J Neurosurg* 1969;31: 441–444.

148. Mai DT, Vasinrapee P, Cook RE. Diagnosis of abdominal cerebrospinal fluid pseudocyst by scintigraphy. *Clin Nucl Med* 1993;18: 237–238.

149. Dreake JM, de Silva MC, Rutka JT. Functional obstruction of an antisiphon devise by raised tissue capsule pressure. *Neurosurgery* 1993; 32:137–139.

150. Uvebrant P, Sixt R, Bjure J et al. Evaluation of cerebrospinal fluid

shunt function in hydrocephalic children using ^{99m}Tc-DTPA. *Child's Nerv Syst* 1992;8:76–80.

151. DiChiro G, Grove AS Jr. Evaluation of surgical and spontaneous cerebrospinal fluid shunts by isotope scanning. *J Neurosurg* 1966;24:743–748.

152. Matin P, Goodwin DA, DeNardo GL. Cerebrospinal fluid scanning and ventricular shunts. *Radiology* 1970;94:435–438.

153. Harbert J, Haddad D, McCullough D. Quantitation of cerebrospinal fluid shunt flow. *Radiology* 1974;112:379–387.

154. Ackerman M, de Tover G, Quist G. Radioisotope ventriculography and cisternography in noncommunicating hydrocephalus. In: *Proceedings of the symposium on cisternography and hydrocephalus.* Springfield: IL, Charles C. Thomas, 1973.

155. Rudd TG, Shurtleff DB, Loeser JD et al. Radionuclide assessment of cerebrospinal fluid shunt function in children. *J Nucl Med* 1973;14:683–686.

156. Chervu S, Chervu LR, Vallabhajosyula DM et al. Quantitative evaluation of cerebrospinal fluid shunt flow. *J Nucl Med* 1984;25:91–95.

157. Pressman D, Day ED, Blau M. The use of paired labelling in the determination of tumour-localising antibodies. *Cancer Res* 1957;17:845–850.

158. Coakham HB, Garson J, Brownell B et al. Monoclonal antibodies as reagents for brain tumour diagnosis: a review. *J R Soc Med* 1984;77:780–787.

159. Carrel S, Acciolla RS, Carmagnola AL et al. A common melanoma associated antigen detected by monoclonal antibody. *Cancer Res* 1980;40:2523–2528.

160. Bourdon MA, Coleman RE, Blasberg RG et al. Monoclonal antibody localisation in subcutaneous and intracranial human glioma xenografts. *Anticancer Res* 1984;4:133–140.

161. Mach JP, Forni M, Ritschard J. Use of radiolabelled monoclonal anti CEA antibodies for the detection of human carcinomas by external photoscanning and immunoscintigraphy. *Immunol Today* 1981;2:283–249.

162. Davies AG, Richardson RB, Bourne SP et al. Immunolocalisation of human brain tumours. In: Bleehan NM, ed. *Tumors of the brain.* New York: Springer-Verlag, 1986:99–112.

163. The Hammersmith Oncology Group and the Imperial Cancer Research Fund. Antibody-guided irradiation of malignant lesions: three cases illustrating a new method of treatment. *Lancet* 1984;1:1441–1443.

164. Madelyn OE, Chernik NL, Posner JB. Infiltration of the leptomeninges by systemic cancer: a clinical and pathological study. *Arch Neurol* 1974;30:122–137.

165. Ongerboer de Visser BW, Somers R, Nooyen WH et al. Intraventricular methotrexate therapy of leptomeningeal metastasis from breast carcinoma. *Neurology* 1983;33:1565–1572.

166. Hustu HO, Aur RJA, Verzosa MS et al. Prevention of central nervous system leukaemia by irradiation. *Cancer* 1973;32:585–597.

167. Lashford LS, Davies AG, Richardson RB et al. A pilot study of ^{131}I monoclonal antibodies in the therapy of leptomeningeal tumour. *Cancer* 1988;61:857–868.

168. Richardson RB, Kemshead JT, Davies AG. Dosimetry of intrathecal iodine-131 monoclonal antibody in cases of neoplastic meningitis. *Eur J Nucl Med* 1990;17:42–48.

169. Gold LH, Kieffer SA, D'Angio GJ et al. Current status of intrathecal radiogold in treatment of medulloblastoma. *Acta Radiol* 1972;11:329–340.

170. Metz O, Stoll W, Plenert W. Meningosis prophylaxis with intrathecal ^{198}Au-colloid and methotrexate in childhood acute lymphocytic leukaemia. *Cancer* 1982;49:224–228.

171. Doge H, Hliscs R. Intrathecal therapy with ^{198}Au-colloid for meningosis prophylaxis. *Eur J Nucl Med* 1984;9:125–128.

172. D'Angio GJ, French LA, Stadlan EM et al. Intrathecal radioisotopes for the treatment of brain tumours. *Clin Neurosurg* 1968;15:288–300.

173. Coakham HB, Richardson RB, Davies AG et al. Neoplastic meningitis from a pineal tumour treated by antibody guided irradiation via the intrathecal route. *Br J Neurosurg* 1988;2:199–209.

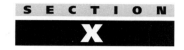

SECTION
X

NEPHROLOGY

41

RENAL RADIONUCLIDES AND IN VITRO QUANTITATION

MICHELLE G. CAMPBELL
THOMAS A. POWERS

RENAL PHYSIOLOGY

The kidney integrates three major functions—the regulatory, the endocrine, and the excretory—to maintain a homeostatic internal environment.

The regulatory role of the kidney involves the maintenance of acid base balance, pH, blood volume, and electrolytes. Secretion and activation of hormones accounts for the endocrine role of the kidney.

The excretory function of the kidney relies on passive glomerular filtration, active tubular secretion, and reabsorption. The functioning unit of the kidney is the nephron. Each of the body's two kidneys contains about 1 million nephrons, which are composed of a glomerulus, a proximal tubule, a loop of Henle, a distal tubule, and a collecting tubule. The primary function of the nephron is to clear the blood of unnecessary or foreign substances. The kidneys receive approximately 20% of the cardiac output, and the glomerulus filters about 20% of this 600 mL/minute of plasma to produce 180 L/day of essentially protein-free fluid. Renal blood flow, filtrate characteristics, and number of functioning nephrons all affect glomerular filtration rate (GFR). A mean glomerular pressure gradient of 40 mm Hg is required for glomerular filtration. This is accomplished by controlling renal plasma flow and resistance via the angiotensin system. The efferent arteriole constricting effects of angiotensin II provide the added resistance needed to drive the filtrate through the glomerulus when the arterial plasma pressure is inadequate. Through these regulatory mechanisms GFR is maintained when the arterial blood pressure is between 70 and 120 mm Hg. Substance size, charge, and shape also determine whether a particular substance will be filtered in the glomerulus. Compounds that have a molecular weight below 300 dalton and are polar in charge are preferentially filtered. The average GFR is 120 mL/minute and decreases as nephrons are lost as a result of advancing age.

In the proximal tubule, water, sodium, bicarbonate, amino acids, and glucose are reabsorbed leaving 30% to 40% of the original glomerular filtrate to pass into the loop of Henle. By means of a countercurrent exchange mechanism, the loop of Henle further alters the urine by selective transport of electrolytes and varying permeability to water. The distal convoluted tubules alter the osmolality according to the presence or absence of antidiuretic hormone (ADH) to produce either a concentrated (ADH present) or dilute urine (ADH absent) (1,2).

RADIONUCLIDES

Many factors play a role in the choice of a renal radiopharmaceutical. Agents are now available to measure perfusion, functional morphology, and excretion. The development of the scintillation scanner in 1950, prompted investigators to begin imaging the kidneys after injection of iodine-labeled agents. Initially, the transit time of radiolabeled Diodrast was too rapid to complete the 30-minute renal scan available at that time. Using individual scintillation probes, the first renogram was performed in the late 1950s to measure the transit time through each kidney of radiolabeled ^{131}I-orthoiodohippurate (^{131}I-OIH). Successful static images with ^{131}I-OIH were soon to follow.

[99m]Tc-labeled glucoheptonate (GHA), 2,3-dimercaptosuccinic acid (DMSA), and diethylenetriaminepentaacetic acid (DTPA) were developed in the 1970s to supplement ^{131}I-OIH. ^{99m}Tc-mercaptoacetyltriglycine (MAG3) is an even more recent agent. Perfusion agents such as ^{99m}Tc-DTPA, ^{99m}Tc-MAG3, and ^{99m}Tc-GHA allow bolus administration with visualization of the abdominal aorta and iliac vessels within 30 seconds of administration. In addition, excretion can be evaluated when using ^{99m}Tc-MAG3 and ^{99m}Tc-DTPA. GHA can evaluate the renal morphology. ^{99m}Tc-DMSA is also a functional morphologic agent similar to ^{99m}Tc-GHA; however, it provides a higher radiation dose per mCi. The primary radiopharmaceuticals for evaluation of excretion are ^{131}I-OIH, ^{99m}Tc-DTPA, and ^{99m}Tc-MAG3 (3–7) (see Tables 41.1 and 41.2).

[99m]Tc-Glucoheptonate

The chemical structure of both GHA and ^{99m}Tc-GHA is shown in Fig. 41.1.

M.G. Campbell: Department of Radiology and Radiological Sciences, Vanderbilt University Medical Center, Nashville, TN.

T.A. Powers: Department of Radiology, Vanderbilt University Medical Center, Nashville, TN.

Table 41.1. *Radionuclides*

Characteristic	[131]I	[99m]Tc hours
$t_{1/2}$ physical	8 days	6
Photon energy (keV)	364	140
Dose (mCi)	0.25–0.3	2–15

Renal Handling

^{99m}Tc-GHA is handled by the kidney through glomerular filtration and tubular cell fixation. Of the injected dose, 80% to 90% is eliminated by glomerular filtration and the other 10% to 20% by tubular secretion. A portion of that eliminated by tubular secretion is fixated by the proximal convoluted tubules and provides the cortical detail on delayed images. Maximal renal concentration of ^{99m}Tc-GHA occurs at 15 minutes and decreases rapidly. The protein-bound ^{99m}Tc-GHA is cleared by tubular secretion, but the protein-free portion is excreted by glomerular filtration. Approximately 6.9% of an injected dose of ^{99m}Tc-GHA is protein bound at 10 minutes, but this drops to 2.4% at 20 minutes. Also, ^{99m}Tc-GHA has minimal hepatic uptake resulting in a high kidney to liver ratio (8).

At one time, the same method of excretion was thought to be used by both ^{99m}Tc-DMSA and ^{99m}Tc-GHA. Lee and Blaufox (8) suggested that ^{99m}Tc-GHA is accumulated in the proximal tubule by the same active transport enzyme mechanism of para-aminohippuric acid (PAH) and hippuran. They demonstrated a blockade of ^{99m}Tc-GHA uptake by PAH and probenecid that was not found by Yee et al. (9) when they examined the effect of PAH and probenecid on ^{99m}Tc-DMSA.

Dosimetry

Arnold et al. (6) characterized many of the technetium-labeled agents used for renal imaging. They determined that 14.6% of the injected dose localized in the kidneys. Radiation dose esti-

Table 41.2. *Dosimetry*

Radiopharmaceutical	Organ	Dose (rem/mCi)
[99m]Tc-Mag3	Bladder wall	.44
	Kidneys	.015
	Ovaries	.022
	Uterus	.048
^{131}I-OIH	Bladder	4.8
	Kidneys	.056
	Ovaries	.077
	Uterus	.177
^{99m}Tc-GHA	Kidneys	.170
	Bladder	.80
	Gonads	.020
^{99m}Tc-DTPA	Bladder	.35
	Kidneys	.014
	Ovaries	.020
	Uterus	.041
^{99m}Tc-DMSA	Kidneys	.62
	Bladder	.28
	Gonads	.022

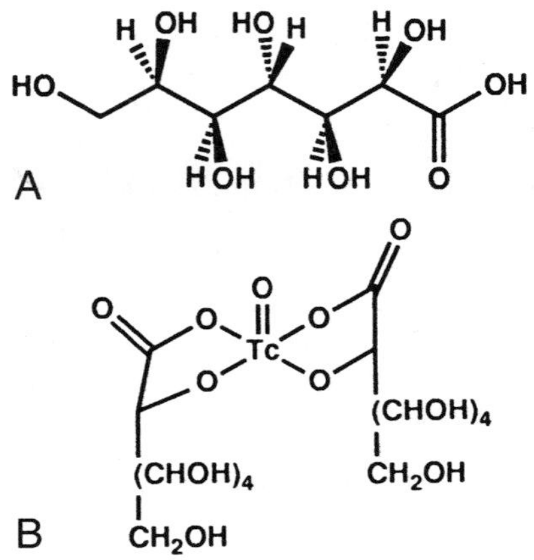

FIGURE 41.1. The chemical structure of **(A)** glucoheptonate (GHA) and of **(B)** ^{99m}Tc-GHA.

mates were made assuming a urine flow rate of 60 cc/hour, and assuming three daytime voids and one overnight void. Also, the bladder was assumed to be empty at the time of injection. Using the Medical Internal Radiation Dose (MIRD) committee methods, the radiation dose to the kidneys was determined to be 0.170 rem per mCi and for the bladder, 0.80 rem per mCi. The large percentage of ^{99m}Tc-GHA that is rapidly eliminated in the urine is responsible for the larger radiation dose to the bladder mucosa. Consequently, the radiation dose to the kidneys is much less (see Table 41.2). The administered adult dose range for ^{99m}Tc-GHA is 10 to 15 mCi. Adjustments must be made for pediatric patients.

Imaging Characteristics

All of the technetium-labeled pharmaceuticals capitalize on technetium's ideal 140 keV energy for imaging. Because approximately 80% to 90% of the injected dose is cleared by glomerular filtration, the cortex, collecting system, and ureters are visualized on early images. This provides information on glomerular function. The other 10% to 20% of the injected dose is fixated by the tubular cells and is responsible for the cortical morphology on the delayed images. This aids in the detection of renal scarring and other morphologic characteristics (10). This dual method of ^{99m}Tc-GHA excretion displays the cortex, collecting system, and ureters (11) (Fig. 41.2).

There have been reports of biliary excretion of ^{99m}Tc-GHA, especially in fasting patients and in patients with renal insufficiency (12,13). Penicillin, penicillamine, acetaminophen, and trimethoprim-sulfamethoxazole also may increase biliary excretion (14).

Specific Uses

^{99m}Tc-GHA has several uses in renal imaging. The primary use has been detailed evaluation of the cortex. Because ^{99m}Tc-GHA delivers a lower dose to the kidneys than the other main cortical agent, ^{99m}Tc-DMSA, it may be used when both perfusion and cortical morphology must be evaluated. There are a few potential

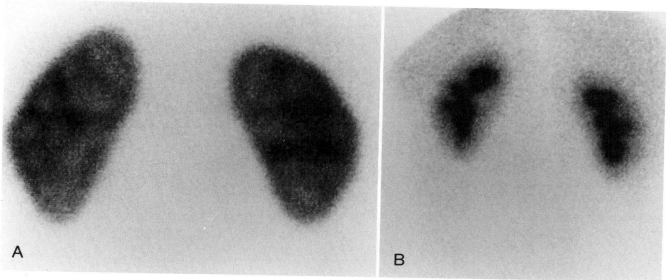

FIGURE 41.2. A: Early glucoheptonate images displaying the cortex and collecting system. **B:** Late gluco-heptonate images demonstrating the cortical morphology.

disadvantages to using ^{99m}Tc-GHA. Activity occasionally seen in the gallbladder and small bowel may overlay the right kidney and obscure interpretation. In the setting of obstruction, accumulation of activity within the renal pelvis may also make interpretation difficult (15). On delayed static images, the reduced activity in the renal pelvis gives better cortical detail in the hilar region. The use of ^{99m}Tc-GHA in detecting renal mass lesions such as tumor, cyst, abscess, and infarct has been well documented (16). In addition, ^{99m}Tc-GHA renal scanning has been shown to have a greater accuracy than intravenous urogram (IVU) in detecting renal mass lesions (17).

^{99m}Tc-DMSA

The chemical structure of DMSA and Tc-DMSA is shown in Fig. 41.3.

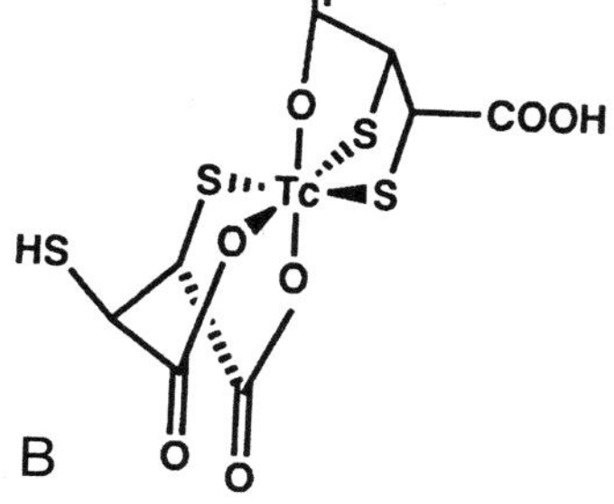

FIGURE 41.3. The chemical structure of **(A)** 2,3-dimercaptosuccinic acid (DMSA), and of **(B)** ^{99m}Tc-DMSA.

Renal Handling

^{99m}Tc-DMSA is excreted in the urine by glomerular filtration and tubular secretion. ^{99m}Tc-DMSA is cleared within 10 minutes of injection. Twelve percent of the injected dose is retained 1-hour postinjection (6).

De Lange et al. (18) found that ^{99m}Tc-DMSA is 90% protein bound and that peritubular uptake accounted for 65% of excretion and glomerular filtration is 35%. The free fraction in plasma is 24%, with 3% of the injected dose seen as a free fraction within 15 minutes and 27% within 70 minutes (19).

Poor ^{99m}Tc-DMSA uptake in the presence of normal ^{99m}Tc-DTPA uptake has been reported in patients with tubulointerstitial renal disease, demonstrating that ^{99m}Tc-DMSA is an indicator of functioning tubular renal mass and not renal function. The precise mechanism of tubular uptake remains unclear (20). Provoost et al. (21) induced a generalized proximal tubular dysfunction in rats by administering sodium maleate and found a 31.5% decrease in the amount of ^{99m}Tc-DMSA retained in the kidney with a 23.3% increase in the amount found in the bladder. They speculated that this enhanced excretion was caused by either an inhibition of tubular reabsorption or a rapid cellular release.

Dosimetry

^{99m}Tc-DMSA delivers the highest radiation dose per mCi to the kidney, approximately 0.62 rems per mCi, and 0.28 rems per mCi to the bladder (6). There is a concern of a high radiation dose with ^{99m}Tc-DMSA. The radiation dose of ^{99m}Tc-DMSA per mCi is three times higher than that of ^{99m}Tc-GHA. However, the dose of ^{99m}Tc-DMSA is about one third that of ^{99m}Tc-GHA. The higher percentage of cortical fixation with DMSA allows a smaller injected dose. The radiation dose to the kidneys, therefore, is equal in ^{99m}Tc-GHA and ^{99m}Tc-DMSA. Furthermore, the lower accumulation of ^{99m}Tc-DMSA in the bladder

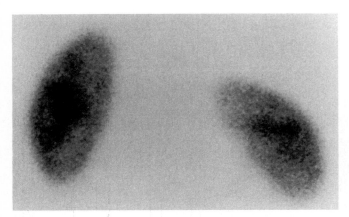

FIGURE 41.4. ^{99m}Tc-2,3-dimercaptosuccinic acid images providing detailed cortical resolution.

gives a lower radiation dose to the gonads than ^{99m}Tc-GHA (10). The administration dose range for adults is 2 to 5 mCi.

Imaging Characteristics

^{99m}Tc-DMSA is a cortical scanning agent that localizes in the proximal tubule. It is only minimally excreted and produces images of functioning renal mass (22). It provides good resolution of the cortical outline and avoids the difficulty in interpretation that is often encountered with ^{99m}Tc-GHA when activity accumulates in the collecting system (Fig. 41.4) (23).

Specific Uses

^{99m}Tc-DMSA is one of the two cortical imaging agents in renal imaging. It produces more detailed cortical images than ^{99m}Tc-GHA. ^{99m}Tc-DMSA, however, should not be used as a perfusion agent because it delivers a significant radiation dose when a bolus injection is required (15). Rossleigh et al. (24), as well as many other investigators, demonstrated the superior sensitivity of ^{99m}Tc-DMSA to intravenous urography for the evaluation of renal scarring in infants.

According to Gordon (25), ^{99m}Tc-DMSA is indicated in children for evaluation and/or detection of renal scars, small kidneys, duplicated collecting systems, renal masses, and systemic hypertension. Shanon et al. (26) found that ^{99m}Tc-DMSA renal scanning was more sensitive (94%) than either intravenous pyelography (IVP) (76%) or ultrasonography (65%) in detection of renal scars in children. In addition to agreeing with Shanon, Elison et al. (23) found a correlation between cortical defects and severity of reflux on voiding cystourethrogram. Goldraich et al. (27) prospectively evaluated 299 refluxing kidneys; although they found an 88% concordance between IVP and DMSA scanning, they also had a 12% discordance. Thirty-four of 37 kidneys showed evidence of scarring with DMSA and had normal IVP. Repeat IVP 1 to 3 years later demonstrated scarring in 30 of 34 kidneys. This indicates that defects on ^{99m}Tc-DMSA scanning may become apparent before changes are noted on IVP. Six children in the study had an acute urinary tract infection (UTI) at the time of their follow-up scan. The images demonstrated

new scars that subsequently disappeared on repeat ^{99m}Tc-DMSA imaging 4 weeks later. Although many more children would need to be studied in this clinical situation, these findings suggest that ^{99m}Tc-DMSA scanning may identify kidneys at risk for scarring. ^{99m}Tc-DMSA scanning has many advantages over IVP. It offers a lower radiation dose, is not affected by overlying bowel gas or bones, and avoids possible allergic reactions (26).

^{99m}Tc-DMSA has also been used to evaluate renal function by single photon emission computed tomography (SPECT) quantitation. ^{99m}Tc-DMSA uptake was compared with creatine clearance and serum creatinine in 20 patients with varying renal disease. SPECT quantitation of ^{99m}Tc-DMSA was found to correlate with the serum creatinine ($r = 0.89$) and creatinine clearance ($r = 0.76$) (28).

^{99m}Tc-DTPA

The chemical structure of DTPA and the technetium-labeled form of DTPA is shown in Fig. 41.5.

Renal Handling

^{99m}Tc-DTPA is used to measure renal perfusion and both global and differential glomerular filtration. It is excreted solely by glomerular filtration. Ninety percent of the injected dose is excreted at 24 hours, and only 5% to 10% is bound to plasma proteins at 1 hour. ^{99m}Tc-DTPA has a rapid clearance with a half-time of 70 minutes and a biologic half-life of 1 to 2 hours (6).

Dosimetry

Stabin et al. (7) found that the radiation dose to the kidneys of ^{99m}Tc-DTPA was equivalent to that of ^{99m}Tc-MAG3. ^{99m}Tc-DTPA delivered 0.014 rems per mCi to the kidneys and 0.35 rems per mCi to the bladder. The administrated dose range for adults is 10 to 15 mCi.

Imaging Characteristics

The technetium label and the method of excretion make ^{99m}Tc-DTPA a good agent for measurement of GFR and perfusion.

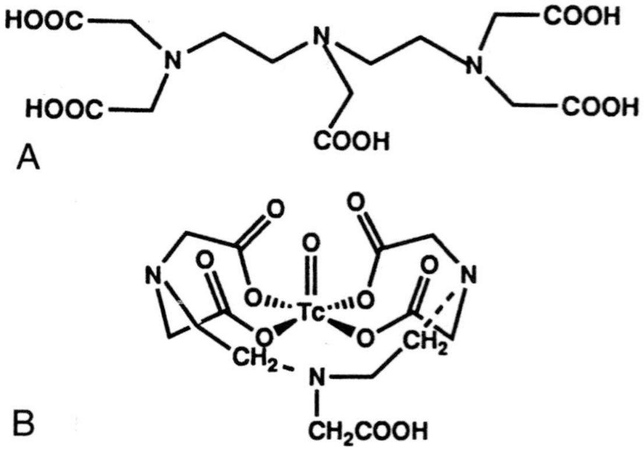

FIGURE 41.5. The chemical structure of **(A)** diethylenetriaminepentaacetic acid (DTPA), and of the **(B)** ^{99m}Tc-labeled form of DTPA.

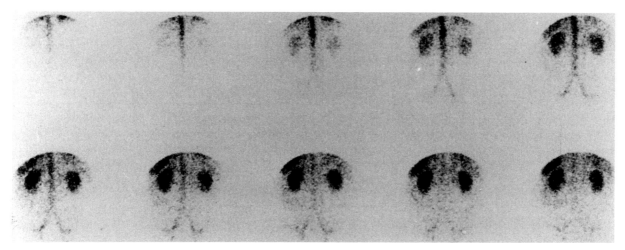

FIGURE 41.6. Perfusion images following bolus administration of ^{99m}Tc-diethylenetriaminepentaacetic acid.

It is not useful in evaluating cortical detail because the low extraction efficiency (20%) results in a low target-to-background ratio, especially in patients with poor renal function, and often makes image interpretation difficult (29).

Specific Uses

Because ^{99m}Tc-DTPA is excreted solely by glomerular filtration, it may be used to quantitate GFR. ^{99m}Tc-DTPA has a clearance that is 5% less than that of inulin, the gold standard, resulting in an acceptable clinical measure of the global and differential GFR. Its low cost, low radiation dose, and availability make ^{99m}Tc-DTPA the ideal radiopharmaceutical for GFR measurements (15).

Perfusion studies are important in the evaluation of the renal transplant patients. Deteriorating renal function in this population may be attributed to either rejection or acute tubular necrosis. The diminished perfusion seen in rejection is differentiated from the normal perfusion seen in acute tubular necrosis. Rapid frame acquisition following bolus injection permit comparison of iliac artery perfusion to renal artery perfusion (Fig. 41.6) (15). ^{99m}Tc-MAG3 is used more frequently and provides the additional information of excretory and morphologic function. ^{99m}Tc-MAG3 also provides more accurate measure of perfusion in the patients with significant renal impairment (29).

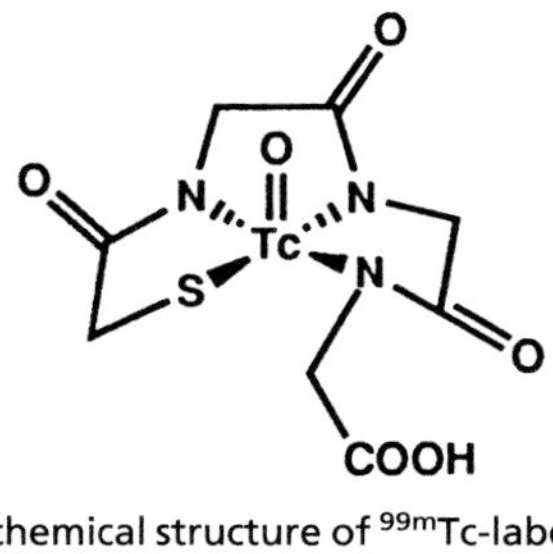

Hippuran/Mercaptoacetyltriglycine

Chemical Structure

^{99m}Tc-MAG3 was introduced by Fritzberg et al. (30) in 1986 and is a triamide monomercaptide (Fig. 41.7). Fig. 41.8 shows the structure of ^{131}I-OIH.

Renal Handling

Eighty percent of ^{131}I-OIH is secreted by the tubules, and 20% is filtered by the glomerulus. The extraction fraction of hippuran is approximately 65% with a rapid clearance half-time of 30 minutes. Maximum concentration in the kidney occurs at 3 to 5 minutes, and by 7 to 10 minutes only 50% remains (31). ^{99m}Tc-MAG3 excretion is similar to ^{131}I-OIH, but only about 2% is excreted by glomerular filtration. Some have suggested that the excretion of ^{99m}Tc-MAG3 is comparable to the secretory rate of the proximal convoluted tubule and that ^{99m}Tc-MAG3 excretion should be referred to as the tubular extraction rate or TER (32).

Taylor et al. (31) compared image quality, excretion, clearance, and time activity or renogram curves of ^{131}I-OIH and ^{99m}Tc-MAG3 in normal volunteers. The clearance of ^{99m}Tc-MAG3 was more rapid than that of ^{131}I-OIH, 1.30 L/minute and 0.88 L/minute, respectively. In addition, the 30-minute excretion and renogram curves for both radiopharmaceuticals were almost identical. The image quality, however, was superior

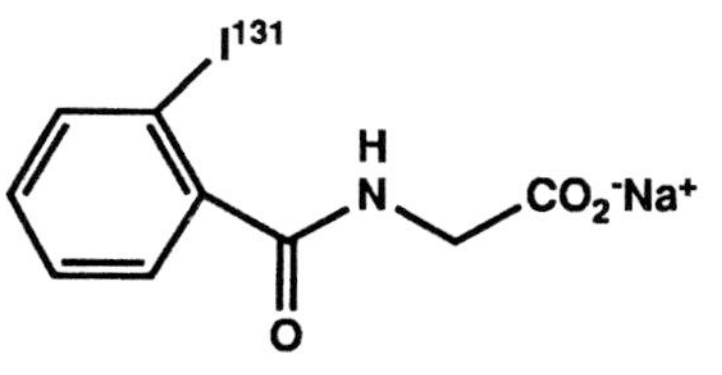

FIGURE 41.7. The chemical structure of ^{99m}Tc-labeled mercaptoacetyltriglycine.

FIGURE 41.8. The chemical structure of ^{131}I-orthoiodohippurate.

with ^{99m}Tc-MAG3 in all 10 normal volunteers (30). In patients with varying degrees of renal impairment, the ^{99m}Tc-MAG3 images were again superior to those obtained with ^{131}I-OIH. Also, the 30-minute excretion was not significantly different, but the time to peak was more rapid for ^{99m}Tc-MAG3 (32). Bubeck et al. (33) compared ^{99m}Tc-Mag 3 and ^{131}I-OIH protein binding, volume of distribution, red blood cell (RBC) binding, and biologic half-lives. They reported that the plasma protein binding of ^{99m}MAG3 was 90%, compared with 70% for ^{131}I-OIH. The volume of distribution as a percent of body weight was 16.6% for ^{99m}Tc-MAG3 and 10% for ^{131}I-OIH. They found that ^{99m}Tc-MAG3 was bound to RBCs to a lesser extent, 5.1% compared with 15.3%. The higher intravascular concentration and subsequent lower volume of distribution of ^{99m}Tc-MAG3 was attributed to the higher plasma protein binding of ^{99m}Tc-MAG3 as compared with ^{131}I-OIH. About 70% of the administered dose of both radiopharmaceuticals was excreted by 30 minutes. ^{99m}Tc-MAG3 was also found to have a lower affinity for tubular transport proteins than ^{131}I-OIH. The greater effect of PAH on ^{99m}Tc-MAG3 clearance demonstrated in their study supported this premise.

There have been reports of hepatobiliary activity following administration of kit-prepared ^{99m}Tc-MAG3. Initially, this hepatobiliary activity was attributed to the impurities in the kit formulations. However, there have been several other reports of hepatobiliary activity using the same kit-prepared ^{99m}Tc-MAG3 in patients with normal to poor renal function (29,34–36). In one study using kit-formulated ^{99m}Tc-MAG3 in normal volunteers and in patients with renal failure, the investigators found that gallbladder activity at 30 to 60 minutes and intestinal activity at 3 hours was 0.5% and 1%, respectively. In the renal failure patients, the gallbladder activity and intestinal activity at the same time points were 1% and 5%, respectively (37).

Dosimetry

Stabin et al. studied the radiation dosimetry for ^{99m}Tc-MAG3, ^{99m}Tc-DTPA, and ^{131}I-OIH in humans by standard MIRD techniques. They calculated the radiation dose estimates assuming clinical doses of 370 mBq (10 mCi) of ^{99m}Tc-DTPA and ^{99m}Tc-MAG$_3$ and 11.1 mBq (30 µCi) of ^{131}I-OIH and a rapid urinary voiding schedule. Patients were expected to void within 30 minutes of the study and every 4 hours thereafter. In addition, radiation doses were calculated per injected unit, on a slow voiding schedule and assuming no renal clearance. They found that the technetium-labeled compounds ^{99m}Tc-DTPA and ^{99m}Tc-MAG3 had similar radiation doses per unit injected activity. Although the radiation dose delivered by ^{131}I-OIH was 3 to 10 times higher, the actual patient radiation burden was essentially the same because of the lesser quantity administered. The rapid voiding schedule reduced the radiation dose to the bladder and gonads by a factor of two to three and to the kidneys by 10%. When Stabin et al. (7) estimated the radiation dose assuming no renal clearance, they calculated the doses to the kidneys to be 13 rads for ^{99m}Tc-DTPA, 15 rads for ^{99m}Tc-MAG3, and 150 rads for ^{131}I-OIH. This supports the concern for elevated radiation doses delivered by ^{131}I-OIH to patients with renal

obstruction and suggests using a different radionuclide in this clinical setting.

In normal renal function, the higher intravascular concentration of ^{99m}Tc-MAG3 accounts for the slightly larger radiation dose to the kidneys in the face of similar elimination curves. However, in patients with renal impairment, the longer physical half-life of ^{131}I-OIH delivers a significantly higher radiation dose (33).

The normal adult dose range is 250 to 300 µCi for ^{131}I-OIH and 5 to 10 mCi for ^{99m}Tc-MAG3.

Imaging Characteristics

^{131}I-OIH has an extraction efficiency of 70% to 90% in normal volunteers and thus a high target-to-background ratio (38). However, ^{131}I-OIH emits 364-keV γ-rays and β-particles, resulting in poor resolution and high radiation dose (39) (Fig. 41.9). Currently, thin crystals and low-energy collimators are routinely used. It is difficult to find the high-energy collimators and thicker crystals required to obtain high-quality images with the high-energy ^{131}I analogs (40). ^{123}I-OIH produces better resolution because of the 159-keV γ-photon and absence of β emission. However, because ^{123}I has a 13-hour half-life and requires cyclotron synthesis, it is expensive and not readily available.

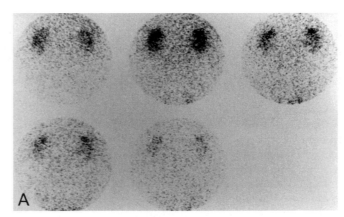

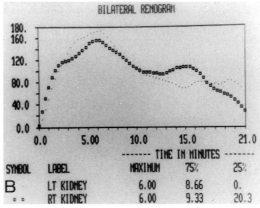

FIGURE 41.9. Renogram performed with ^{131}I-orthoiodohippurate. **A:** The posterior static images. **B:** The corresponding renogram time activity curves.

The discovery of a technetium tubular agent has used technetium's ideal imaging properties with 140-keV photon production, technetium's lack of β emission, and half-life of 6 hours to produce lower radiation dose, higher counting efficiency, and better resolution (39).

Specific Use

^{99m}Tc-MAG3 is the most widely used renal radionuclide. This agent is useful for evaluating renal morphology, perfusion, and function in one study (Fig. 41.10) (39).

^{131}I-OIH has been the agent of choice for the measurement of effective renal plasma flow (ERPF) (15). Russell et al. (41) measured ERPF with both ^{131}I-OIH and ^{99m}Tc-MAG3 by a single injection and single plasma clearance method in 50 patients. A proportional relationship was found between the ERPF measured by both agents. They determined a correction constant of 0.563 to correct the ERPF value obtained with ^{99m}Tc-MAG3 to that obtained with ^{131}I-OIH. The corrected ^{99m}Tc-MAG3 value had a correlation coefficient of 0.96 with the ^{131}I-OIH values.

Most investigators recommend ^{99m}Tc-DMSA or even ^{99m}Tc-GHA to evaluate the renal parenchyma. Gordon et al. (42) compared ^{99m}Tc-DMSA and ^{99m}Tc-MAG3 in detecting focal renal defects and predicting differential renal function. These investigators found that ^{99m}Tc-MAG3 had a sensitivity and a specificity of 88% in detecting focal renal abnormalities. In addition, differential function between the two radiopharmaceuticals had a high correlation ($r^2 = 0.97$). They felt that ^{99m}Tc-MAG3, in children with UTIs, had a high likelihood of detecting focal renal defects and providing accurate assessment of differential renal function. Perfusion, as with any of the technetium-labeled agents, can be evaluated with ^{99m}Tc-MAG3 by rapidly acquiring the frames after bolus administration.

Many have suggested that ^{99m}Tc-MAG3 replace ^{99m}Tc-DTPA and ^{131}I-OIH in the evaluation of renal transplants. ^{99m}Tc-MAG3 images were shown to be of better quality than those produced with ^{131}I-OIH. Also, the higher radiation dose with the iodine-labeled pharmaceuticals is avoided with the technetium-labeled analog. Dubovsky et al. (43) also felt that the higher percentage of ^{99m}Tc-MAG3 retained in the parenchyma provided better detection of renal lesions than ^{99m}Tc-DTPA.

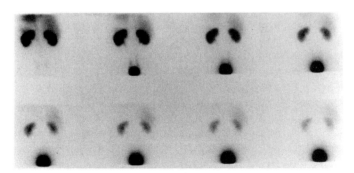

FIGURE 41.10. ^{99m}Tc-mercaptoacetyltriglycine renogram images obtained in the posterior projection.

MEASUREMENT OF FUNCTION

Glomerular Filtration Rates

The introduction of radionuclides and their use in monitoring renal function has made serial measurements of GFRs and ERPF less time consuming and less demanding to both the patient and the technologist. GFR is the clearance rate of a substance that is excreted from the body by glomerular filtration and is not secreted or reabsorbed by the tubules. Ideally, this substance is not protein bound, does not enter RBCs, and is not changed in the process (44). Assuming the substance is cleared solely by glomerular filtration, this rate can be inferred by observing the rate of disappearance of the substance from the blood, the rate of appearance of the substance in the urine, or the amount of uptake of the substance in the kidneys. The methods in the nuclear medicine department capitalize on either measuring the activity in the urine, in the blood, or, by using the gamma-camera, in the kidneys. Although gamma-camera or external probe techniques provide differential function and avoid urine and blood sampling, correction for attenuation by overlying liver and spleen must be addressed (45).

Classically, GFR is the urinary clearance of inulin after a steady state is achieved by a continuous intravenous infusion. GFR is then calculated according to the following formula.

$$\text{Clearance} = \frac{UV}{P}$$

where U is the urine inulin concentration in milligrams per milliliters and V is the urinary flow rate in milliliters per minute. P represents the plasma inulin concentration also in milligrams per milliliter. This method requires both continuous infusion and urine sampling (44).

To measure GFR an agent must be excreted entirely by glomerular filtration and not be protein bound. The prototype is inulin. The clearance of 5'CN ethylenediaminetetraacetic acid (EDTA) is equivalent to inulin and has been reported to be the most accurate radio-labeled measure of GFR, but it is not commercially available in the United States (46). ^{131}I-labeled iothalamate has been used instead of ^{51}Cr-EDTA in the United States but has the disadvantage of high radiation doses. More recently, ^{99m}Tc-DTPA has been employed to measure GFR. Because the clearance of ^{99m}Tc-DTPA is 5% less than that of inulin, ^{99m}Tc-DTPA underestimates the true GFR (47). This is acceptable clinically because creatinine clearance has an error of 10% to 15%. The low radiation dose, low expense, and opportunity for renal imaging make ^{99m}Tc-DTPA the agent of choice for the measurement of GFR (15).

The inconvenience of urine collection can be circumvented when the renal clearance can be extrapolated to infinite time. This can be accomplished only when the agent is excreted solely by glomerular filtration, the renal function is not too low, and the patient is not too edematous. When these criteria are met, the plasma clearance can be estimated from one or two plasma samples and the complete clearance curve need not be obtained. This avoids the obvious pitfall of urine collection errors and the need for multiple blood samples. In some instances, blood samples are avoided by using the gamma-camera detectors. The gamma-camera techniques do not require urine or blood samples and are faster than creatinine clearance. An additional advantage to the gamma-camera technique over the standard plasma methods is that differential function can be calculated (46).

The two methods of radionuclide administration for GFR measurements are continuous infusion and single bolus injection. Clinically, the single injection technique has been routinely used. The principle of the continuous infusion method is that once equilibrium is established, the rate of disappearance of the tracer via glomerular filtration is equivalent to the rate of infusion. The rate of infusion can then be substituted for *UV* in the clearance equation. One potential source of error in the continuous infusion method is the buildup of ^{99m}Tc-DTPA metabolites that are cleared at a slower rate than ^{99m}Tc-DTPA. This may artificially overestimate the plasma concentration of tracer and therefore underestimate clearance (44).

The most convenient, least demanding method of measuring GFR is by measuring the plasma clearance after single bolus injection. Clearance can be calculated according to

$$clearance = \frac{injected\ dose}{area\ under\ plasma\ concentration\ curve}$$
$$= \frac{D}{\int P(t) \cdot dt}$$

The most accurate model of excretion of a GFR tracer is a dual-compartment model that follows a biexponential curve. The initial phase of the curve is rapid and represents the redistribution of tracer into the extracellular space. The second portion of the curve is much slower and represents elimination of the tracer by glomerular filtration once distribution in the extracellular space is complete (Fig. 41.11).

The area under the plasma concentration curve is the sum of these two components.

$$P(t) = Ae^{-a1t} + Be^{-a2t}$$

To accurately represent activity in the two compartments, a complete plasma clearance curve must be obtained. This requires

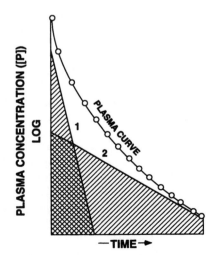

FIGURE 41.11. The dual-compartment elimination curve of a glomerular filtration rate agent. 1 represents the rapid distribution into the extracellular or intravascular space. 2 represents the elimination of the tracer via glomerular filtration.

blood samples from 5 minutes up to 5 hours. If plasma samples are obtained before distribution in the extracellular fluid, the area under the curve will be underestimated and the clearance subsequently overestimated (44).

A simplified method of measuring GFR by the single injection technique is to obtain plasma samples 2, 3, and 4 hours after injection. At this time, equilibration with the extracellular fluid (ECF) will be complete. By using this method, often referred to as the slope intercept method, the initial fast component of the plasma concentration curve will be disregarded and will, therefore, provide GFR values greater than the true GFR. The amount of this error is greatly reduced in patients with poor renal function (44).

Waller et al. (48) used a reference GFR by obtaining half-hour blood samples and corrected the GFR for the single compartment model and for body surface area. This group found the closest correlation to the reference GFR when two blood samples at 2 hours and 4 hours were obtained. The standard error of GFR estimate was 2.8 mL/minute. The least accurate measure was the external detector method where the standard error was greater than 10 mL/minute.

There has been an alternate method of GFR measurement reported that accounts for the volume of distribution. GFR can be calculated from the product of the rate constant of the exponential clearance and the volume of distribution of activity. The volume of distribution of activity is calculated from the estimated activity per unit volume assuming dilution had occurred instantaneously. A correction factor is applied to account for the activity already cleared by the kidneys during the distribution phase. Without this factor, the volume of distribution would be overestimated (48). Fawdry and Gruenewald (49) studied 800 GFR studies obtained by the standard two-sample slope intercept method and compared these to a 3-hour volume of distribution method. They found that the accuracy of the volume of distribution method was greatest when the GFR was between 60 to 100 mL/minute.

Mulligan et al. (50) examined several methods of measuring GFR with ^{99m}Tc-DTPA. As stated previously, GFR can be calculated from the activity in single or multiple blood samples, from the accumulation of radioactivity in the urine, or from counts obtained solely from the gamma-camera. Mulligan et al. found that the two plasma sample technique of Russell and the urinary sample technique developed by Jackson were the most accurate methods over a large range of renal function. The Russell method involves obtaining blood samples at either 30 and 180 minutes or at 60 and 180 minutes and applying this data to the linear dual-compartment model of Sapirstein that follows.

$$GFR \cong \frac{Qo}{\int_o^\infty Pdt} = \frac{Qo}{\dfrac{C1_0}{\lambda_1} + \dfrac{C2_0}{\lambda_2}}$$

where Qo is the injected dose; $\int_o^\infty Pdt$ = is dual-exponential integration of six-point plasma disappearance curve by curve stripping; $C1_0$, $C2_0$ = the value of the monoexponential compartment curves of the dual-exponential disappearance curve at time 0, and λ_1, λ_2 = rate constants of the two monoexponential compartment curves.

For the 30- and 180-minute Russell sample method, the GFR was calculated thus

$$\text{GFR} = \left[\frac{Qo \ln(P_{30}/P_{180})}{150} \times \exp \frac{30 \ln P_{180} - 180 \ln P_{30}}{150} \right]^{0.979}$$

where Qo is the injected dose and P_{time} is the activity of plasma samples drawn.

In the Jackson urinary method, the GFR is calculated from the terminal slope of a plasma disappearance curve. The initial portion of this curve was obtained by externally measuring the blood pool activity in the heart and extrapolating this data to the postvoid bladder image. The total urinary activity was corrected for unexcreted residual bladder activity and the GFR calculated thus:

$$\text{GFR} \cong \frac{TUA}{\int_0^T P dt} = \frac{TUA}{\overset{...}{P}(T)}$$

TUA is the total urinary activity corrected for residual volume; $\int_0^T P dt$ = portion of $\int_0^\infty P dt$ from 0 to T; T is the time of postvoid bladder image; and $\overset{...}{P}$ = mean plasma activity.

This method was found to be as accurate as the two-sample plasma method discussed earlier. However, as stated previously, urinary methods are inconvenient and prone to collection errors (50).

More recently, the optimal sample time following a single injection was evaluated for GFR measurements assuming the two-compartment model. Russell found that for the most accurate values, sample times must begin by 10 minutes and continue for at least 240 minutes. Although he felt that the long time interval evaluated was more important than the number of samples, six blood samples were recommended. The duration of sampling needed to be at least 3 hours because the slow component of excretion accounted for most of the clearance. The accuracy obtained by these methods, although essential in research, is seldom required clinically (51).

The gamma-camera method of GFR and ERPF measurements is seldom used for global measurements and is discussed more extensively in regard to differential measurements. However, it is discussed briefly here. Chachati et al. (52) reviewed Gates' technique of global and differential GFR measurements following injection of ^{99m}Tc-DTPA. Using a scintillation camera, the fraction of the injected dose in the kidneys was determined 1 to 3 minutes after injection and compared with the GFR obtained by simultaneous infusion of inulin. The renal function of the study group varied from normal to anuric and included nine patients with either one kidney or a nephrostomy tube. The GFR was calculated according to Gates' (53) equation.

$$\% \text{ Uptake} = \frac{\dfrac{\text{kidney count} - \text{background}}{e^{-uy}}}{\text{injected dose}} \times 100$$

where Y is the renal depth and μ is the attenuation coefficient for ^{99m}Tc.

This group found a good correlation between Gates' method of GFR measurements and inulin clearance in global measurements ($r = 0.86$, $n = 24$, $p < 0.001$) and in the unilateral group ($r = 0.91$, $n = 9$, $p < 0.001$). Subsequent investigators, however, have demonstrated a poor correlation between the gamma-camera method of Gates and a complete plasma dual-compartment reference method (50).

There have been reports of impurities in the commercial preparations of ^{99m}Tc-DTPA that have resulted in GFR errors. This has been attributed to protein binding. Ultrafiltration before use has diminished the amount of impurities and thus the error in GFR (54).

The spectrum of accuracy varies widely based on the method chosen to calculate GFR. The complete plasma clearance curve is the most accurate but requires multiple blood samples. The two-plasma blood sample is only slightly more accurate than the one-plasma sample method, whereas the gamma-camera techniques are less accurate than all of the plasma methods. However, the gamma-camera technique has been shown to be more accurate than creatinine clearance and, furthermore, does not require either plasma or urine samples.

Effective Renal Plasma Flow

ERPF is another parameter of renal function. As inulin clearance is the gold standard in glomerular filtration, PAH is the gold standard for ERPF measurements. Although the measurements of PAH clearance are very accurate, this method requires constant infusion, is inconvenient, and lacks precision. For these reasons, PAH clearance is now rarely used to measure renal function (46).

As with GFR measurements, many methods of ERPF measurements have been reported in the literature. Most of the variety is between the number of plasma samples and the timing of these blood samples (up to six plasma samples). The model of ^{131}I-OIH distribution and secretion follows biexponential decay according to the same dual-compartmental model that the GFR agent ^{99m}Tc-DTPA follows. The first portion of the decay curve represents the distribution of ^{131}I-OIH in the extracellular fluid (the first compartment) and dominates the initial 10 to 15 minutes after ^{131}I-OIH administration. The second portion of the curve represents the intravascular (second compartment) clearance of ^{131}I-OIH by the kidney and begins about 15 to 20 minutes after ^{131}I-OIH injection. The complete plasma concentration curve can be plotted when multiple blood samples are obtained over approximately 60 minutes, although the minimal gain in accuracy of the additional samples and the inconvenience to both the technologist and patient make this technique unfeasible clinically. The most common technique of ERPF measurement is a single bolus administration of ^{131}I-OIH followed by either one or two plasma samples (55).

For an agent to measure renal plasma flow, it must have an extraction efficiency of 100%. PAH is the nearest to the ideal agent with an extraction efficiency of 90% and with tubular excretion. Because PAH is not completely extracted, the term *effective renal plasma flow* is used when this agent quantitates renal plasma flow. The two radionuclides that most closely resemble the incomplete extraction and tubular excretion of PAH are ^{131}I-OIH and ^{99m}Tc-MAG3 (44). ^{131}I-OIH clearance is slightly less than that of PAH. When using a single injection technique, however, the measurements obtained with ^{131}I-OIH correlate well with those obtained from constant infusion of PAH. The correlation is felt to be secondary to the competing effects of ^{131}I-OIH's lower clearance and the inability of the single injection technique to accurately quantitate the first few minutes of the plasma time activity curve. These errors tend to cancel (46).

Since 1982, the single injection, single-sample method for ERPF measurements has been an established method according to Dubovsky and Russell. The single sample is drawn about 44 minutes after ^{131}I-OIH is administered and, therefore, discounts the extracellular distribution phase by assuming equilibrium has been obtained. This method is the simplest and least time consuming of the plasma techniques (55).

The two-plasma sample technique has been reported to be more accurate. Russell et al. (56) compared the one- and two-plasma sample techniques to a complete reference curve. The reference data was obtained from six to nine plasma samples drawn between 10 and 90 minutes. The single-sample ERPF measurement was obtained from a 44-minute postinjection sample. The two-sample method ERPF was obtained by calculating the ERPF from two samples in the reference curve. Russell et al. found that the residual standard deviation of the two-plasma sample method (20 mL/minute) was approximately half that obtained from a single sample (48 mL/minute). In addition, the optimal time interval for the two samples was 8.7 minutes and 92 minutes postbolus injection. This group recommended the single injection, two-plasma sample method of ERPF calculation only when accuracy is critical (research) and further advised obtaining the samples at 10 to 15 minutes and at 60 to 90 minutes postinjection.

The slope intercept method also uses two plasma samples after a single bolus injection of ^{131}I-OIH. However, the two samples are drawn between 30 and 60 minutes. These samples can be used only to estimate the clearance portion of the decay curve and, like the single-sample method, it disregards the extracellular equilibration. Consequently, the volume of distribution and the ERPF is overestimated. This method offers little advantage over the single-sample method and furthermore requires an additional plasma sample.

Lear et al. proposed a new two-compartment, two-sample technique and compared this technique to the single 44-minute sample technique and to the slope intercept technique. This group based their new technique on the volume of distribution and on the exchange between the intravascular and extravascular space observed in healthy and unhealthy patients. The volume of distribution is the sum of the intravascular and extravascular volumes. They noted that the intravascular (V1) and extravascular (V2) components had a stable rate of exchange (k/V1, k/V2) over a wide spectrum of renal function. The fraction of the volume of distribution contained in V1 ranged from 0.5 to 0.6 with the V1 = 0.6 × Vd in healthy individuals and V1 = 0.6 × Vd in patients with severe renal disease. In this model, V1 was assumed to equal to V2, and the sum was equal to the volume of distribution (Vd). Following is the biexponential decay curve of the two-compartment model.

$$\frac{dC_1}{dt} = -\left[\text{ERPF} \cdot \left(\frac{C_1}{V_1}\right)\right] - \left[\left(\frac{k}{V_1}\right) \cdot C_1\right] + \left[\left(\frac{k}{V_1}\right) \cdot C_2\right]$$

$$\frac{dC_2}{dt} = \left(\frac{k}{V_2}\right) \cdot \left(C_1 - C_2\right)$$

where C_1 is the ^{131}I-OIH concentration in compartment 1; C_2 is the ^{131}I-OIH concentration in compartment 2; k is the rate constant of intercompartmental exchange; and *ERPF* is the effective renal plasma flow.

When assuming that V1 = V2, and V1 = 0.5 Vd, and k/V1 = 0.5, the equation is simplified to

$$\frac{dC_1}{dt} = -\left[\text{ERPF} \cdot \left(\frac{C_1}{V_1}\right)\right] - \left[0.05 \cdot \left(C_1 - C_2\right)\right]$$

$$\frac{dC_2}{dt} = 0.05 \cdot \left(C_1 - C_2\right)$$

A personal computer then set certain conditions and generated a time concentration curve that best fit the data obtained at 40 and 60 minutes. The ERPF and volume of distribution was then calculated. With this method there were certain assumptions that do not always hold true. V1 will not always equal 0.5 × Vd and k will not be constant in all patients. This group reported, however, that resulting errors in ERPF values were smaller than errors found in other techniques. In addition, adjustments to V1 and Vd were suggested in different clinical settings and the computer program was provided to accomplish the corresponding calculations. The advantage of this technique over the slope intercept method is that this method accounts for the extravascular distribution time (55).

ERPF has been measured by a gamma-camera method both globally and differentially. Chachati et al. (52) examined a gamma-camera method of ERPF calculations following ^{131}I-OIH injection and compared this to the PAH infusion method. The basis of the gamma-camera method was to determine the fraction of the injected dose of ^{131}I-OIH 1-2 minutes after administration according to Schlegel's equation.

$$\text{Relative uptake} = \frac{\text{kidney count} - \text{background} \times Y^2}{\text{1 minute count of injected dose}} \times 100$$

where Y is the renal depth calculated thus; *left kidney:* 13.2 (weight/height) + 0.7; and *right kidney:* 13.3 (weight/height) + 0.7.

The renal depth calculation was developed by Tonnesen and cited by Schlegel and Hamway (57). Chachati and his group (52) found a good correlation between PAH clearance and ERPF ($r = 0.84$, $n = 22$, $p < 0.001$). The gamma-camera methods are infrequently used to measure global function and are discussed more fully during the review of differential renal function.

^{99m}Tc-MAG3 has a clearance that is nearly half that of ^{131}I-OIH. However, ERPF measurements reported with ^{99m}Tc-MAG3 have correlated with those of ^{131}I-OIH (58). Using a dual-channel technique, ERPF was calculated following simultaneous administration of ^{131}I-OIH and ^{99m}Tc-MAG3 and after obtaining a 44-minute plasma sample. The proportionality constant between ^{131}I-OIH and ^{99m}Tc-MAG3 was 0.563. By taking the product of the ^{99m}Tc-MAG3 activity and 0.563 and substituting this value for ^{131}I-OIH activity, the ERPF values in 50

patients agreed with those obtained with ^{131}I-OIH ($r = 0.96$) (59).

One- and two-plasma sample methods for evaluating ERPF with ^{99m}Tc-MAG3 were compared by Russell et al (60). The single plasma sample was drawn at 43 minutes and resulted in an error of 19 mL/minute (residual standard deviation). The 43-minute sample time was the optimum over a large range of renal function. Longer sample times in poor renal function and shorter sample times in patients with good renal function can be used when renal function is known in advance. The 43-minute sample time is preferred by these investigators in cases of unknown renal function. The two-plasma sample technique resulted in an error of 7 mL/minute (standard residual deviation) when the samples were obtained at 12 and 94 minutes. Note that the suggested sample times for ^{99m}Tc-MAG3 are almost identical to those recommended for ^{131}I-OIH. Finally, these investigators felt that the accuracy needed for clinical decision making was provided by the single-sample technique and that the two-sample method should be reserved for research purposes when accuracy is essential.

Muller-Suur et al. (61) found that a single sampling time of 60 minutes provided a smaller error of 15 mL/minute as compared with the 19 mL/minute found by Russell et al. at 43 minutes. Furthermore, this group reported a regression equation to convert the ERPF values obtained with ^{99m}Tc-MAG3 to the more familiar corresponding ^{131}I-OIH values. Muller-Suur et al. used the equation

$$ERPF = 1.86 \times C\ (MAG3) + 4.6$$

The obvious advantage of the superior dosimetry of ^{99m}Tc-MAG3 over ^{131}I-OIH makes ^{99m}Tc-MAG3 the ideal agent for ERPF measurements. The normal ERPF value obtained with ^{131}I-OIH is 600 mL/minute, and the normal clearance of ^{99m}Tc-MAG3 is 370 mL/minute.

Renogram

Following bolus injection of a tubular agent (^{131}I-OIH or ^{99m}Tc-MAG3), serial images of the kidney are obtained every 2 to 3 minutes. To minimize tissue attenuation, these images are anterior images in the transplant patient and posterior images in native kidneys. Regions-of-interest (ROIs) are then drawn around the kidneys and a time activity curve, the renogram curve, is generated from the activity in the kidney. This curve represents several different components of radionuclide distribution, the vascular phase, the concentration phase, and the excretory phase. Because the kidneys receive approximately 20% of the cardiac output, the initial phase of the curve is rapidly upsloping and represents renal perfusion. This begins about 15 to 20 seconds after injection and reaches an inflection point at 20 to 40 seconds. Renal tubular function and background activity also affect the slope. The second portion of the renogram curve has milder increase in activity reaching a peak within 3 to 5 minutes. This portion of the curve represents tubular accumulation. By about 3 to 5 minutes, the activity in the kidney begins to accumulate in the bladder via the collecting system. This is

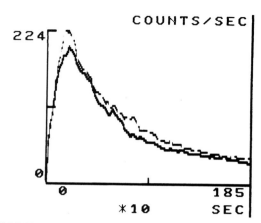

FIGURE 41.12. A normal time activity renogram curve with activity in counts on the vertical axis and time in tens of seconds on the horizontal axis.

represented by a rapidly falling curve (Fig. 41.12). In addition, a curve can be generated that represents the perfusion only. Rapidly acquired frames immediately following the bolus of either ^{99m}Tc-MAG3 or ^{99m}Tc-DTPA delineate the aorta and the kidneys. Normally, activity is seen in the kidneys within 3.5 seconds of being seen in the aorta.

The shape of the renogram curve is affected by many factors. Prerenal insults will affect the perfusion portion of the curve. Renal diseases such as glomerulonephritis will affect the tubular function portion of the curve, whereas postrenal diseases such as obstruction will prevent activity from reaching the bladder and affect the excretory portion of the curve (62).

Differential Function

The disadvantage of the foregoing techniques for the measurement of GFR and ERPF is that the measurements are global measurements and individual kidney function is not addressed. Gamma-camera techniques have been developed to measure both global and differential GFR and ERPF. Most do not require urine samples, and, although most do not require plasma samples, several do use one plasma sample. The obvious advantage to gamma-camera techniques is that they are not invasive. However, this comes at a price. The accuracy of these techniques is not always comparable to the plasma clearance methods but is usually superior to creatinine clearance.

Global and differential GFR measurements use the gamma-camera to produce a renogram after ^{99m}Tc-DTPA bolus injection and apply this data to the following equation to obtain the individual kidney glomerular filtration rate (IKGFR).

$$\frac{dR(t)}{dt} = \alpha \cdot P(t)$$

where dR is the rate of renal uptake; P is the plasma concentration; and α is the constant of proportionality and represents IKGFR.

Once correction has been made for background, the IKGFR should be constant for up to 2.5 minutes after injection. This is the minimum time it takes for the radionuclide to transit the renal ROI (63). Many variations on this equation were reported separately by Rutland (64) and Rehling et al. (65) in 1985.

One of the problems of accurate gamma-camera imaging of ^{99m}Tc-DTPA is the low extraction efficiency and subsequent low target-to-background ratio. The background correction is the main source of error in this method. The liver, spleen, adrenals, renal hilar vessels, intestine, and soft tissue all contribute to background. These organs vary in their ratio of intravascular to extravascular activity, and no single area accurately represents the intravascular and extravascular components of background. Perirenal, subrenal, suprarenal, and heart activity have all been used in an attempt to approximate the background correctly. Bell and Peters (66) reported that extravascular chest wall activity contributed to an error in background cardiac blood pool estimation and resulted in overestimation of IKGFR by a factor of 1.17.

Piepsz et al. (67) addressed the problem of background correction. This group reported a double background correction method that combines the area ratio method and the linear fit method. The area ratio method is stated as

$$Rb(t) = Rc(t) + T(t) + aP(t)$$

where $T(t)$ represents the extravascular component and $aP(t)$ is the fraction of blood pool activity included in the background ROI. $Rb(t)$ is the noncorrected renal activity and $Rc(t)$ is the background corrected renal activity. Thus, the background can be corrected by the area ratio as

$$\text{Background activity} = T'(t) + a'P(t)$$

where $T'(t)$ is the extravascular component in the perirenal space. Assuming that the activity in the perirenal space is an approximate of the extravascular component in the renal space, $T = T'$. By subtracting the previous two equations and dividing them by $P(t)$ one finds

$$\frac{Rc(t)}{P(t)'} = \frac{C \cdot \int P(t)dt}{P(t)} + (a - a')$$

where $a - a'$ is the fraction of the intravascular component not corrected for by the area ratio method. This is an equation for a straight line. The slope of this line is the clearance that has been corrected for both intravascular and extravascular activity. This method works well when the background ROI is the perirenal or subrenal space. The suprarenal space contains the liver, and the activity in this region is not all extravascular, as is assumed in both the perirenal and subrenal regions. This results in an overestimation of the GFR because this region is not corrected for the intravascular activity. Russell (68) compared a method that used cardiac activity as the background correction to one that used a deconvoluted least-square technique. He found that the cardiac correction had a standard deviation of 18.9 mL/minute as compared with the plasma clearance method, whereas the least-square technique had a standard deviation of 14.5 mL/minute.

Differential ERPF can also be measured with a gamma-camera technique following either ^{131}I-OIH or ^{99m}Tc-MAG3 injection. Fine et al. (69) compared several gamma-camera techniques to two plasma clearance techniques using ^{131}I-OIH. The three gamma-camera methods differed only in the ROI chosen to correct for background. The regions were either between the lower poles, upper poles, or crescents lateral to the kidneys. A two-plasma sample method was used as the reference with samples drawn at 20 and 45 minutes. An additional plasma method was included that required one blood sample at 45 minutes. The ERPF measured with the reference method and the one plasma sample method was 384 mL/minute and 319 mL/minute, respectively. None of the gamma-camera techniques were as accurate as the plasma methods.

The reproducibility of manually drawn ROIs was also examined and was found to be very high (correlation coefficient regardless of the observer was greater than 0.98). Fine et al. suggested using either ultrasound or lateral scintigrams to correct for tissue depth because the ERPF was not altered by more than 1% as a result of depth correction in any patient in this study. The algorithm developed by Schlegel (57) was used.

Tondeur et al. (70) examined ERPF gamma-camera clearance with ^{99m}Tc-MAG3. Tc-MAG3 is significantly protein bound and therefore has a smaller extravascular component (71). It also has a higher renal clearance than ^{131}I-OIH. This was expected to result in a more accurate time activity curve by the gamma-camera and a higher target-to-background ratio. In this study, the ERPF was calculated by the double correction method discussed previously, and lateral scintigrams were used to correct for tissue depth. Cardiac activity was used to estimate plasma activity and a 20-minute plasma sample was drawn for the renal clearance calculation. Three different areas were used to correct for background: suprarenal, perirenal, and subrenal regions. The clearance calculated by suprarenal correction was repeatedly higher than clearances calculated with the other two regions. This was felt to be secondary to the unaccounted intravascular component in the suprarenal region. The cardiac plasma activity was also compared with plasma sample activity in 6- and 20-minute samples and was found to be lower with a mean difference of 19.2%. Even though the high protein binding of ^{99m}Tc-MAG3 was expected to diminish the error associated with extravascular activity in the precordium, the faster clearance of ^{99m}Tc-MAG3 produced rapidly decreasing plasma activity and may have made the precordial activity inaccurate except at very early measurements.

REFERENCES

1. Preuss H. Basics of renal anatomy and physiology. *Clin Lab Med* 1993; 13:2–10.
2. Guyton AC. Formation of urine by the kidney: glomerular filtration, tubular function, and plasma clearance. In: Preuss H, ed. *Textbook of medical physiology*. Philadelphia: WB Saunders, 1986:393–400.
3. Blaufox MD, Hollenberg NK, Raynaud C, eds. The radionuclide renal scan: past, present and future radionuclides in nephro-urology. *Contrib Nephrol (Basel)* 1990;79:87–98.
4. Saha GB. Uses of radiopharmaceuticals in nuclear medicine. In: Saha GB, ed. *Fundamentals of nuclear pharmacy,* 3rd ed. New York: Springer-Verlag, 1992:263–271.
5. Eshima D, Taylor A. Tc-MAG3: update on the new Tc renal tubular function agent. *Semin Nucl Med* 1992;22:61–73.
6. Arnold RW, Gopal SS, McAfee JG et al. Comparison of 99m-Tc complexes for renal imaging. *J Nucl Med* 1975;16:357–367.
7. Stabin M, Taylor T Jr, Eshima D et al. Radiation dosimetry for techne-

tium-99m-MAG3, technetium-99m-DTPA, and iodine-131-OIH

based on human biodistribution studies. *J Nucl Med* 1992;33:33–40.

8. Lee HB, Blaufox MD. Mechanism of renal concentration of technetium-99m glucoheptonate. *J Nucl Med* 1985;26:1308–1313.

9. Yee CA, Lee HBL, Blaufox MD. Tc-99m DMSA renal uptake: influence of biochemical and physiologic factors. *J Nucl Med* 1981;22:1054–1058.

10. Majd M, Rushton HG. Renal cortical scintigraphy in the diagnosis of acute pyelonephritis. *Sem Nucl Med* 1992;10:98–111.

11. Shapiro E, Slovis TL, Perlmutter AD et al. Optimal use of 99m-technetium-glucoheptonate scintigraphy in the detection of pyelonephritic scarring in children: a preliminary report. *J Urol* 1988;140:1175–1177.

12. Siegel A, Weiss D, Reilley J. Biliary excretion of glucoheptonate. *Sem Nucl Med* 1992;22:49–50.

13. Tyler JL, Powers TA. Gallbladder visualization with technetium-99m glucoheptonate: concise communications. *J Nucl Med* 1982;23:870–871.

14. Hladik WB, Ponto JA, Lentle BC et al. Iatrogenic alterations in the biodistribution of radiotracers as a result of drug therapy: reported instances. In: Hladik WB, Saha GB, Study KT, eds. *Essentials of nuclear medicine science.* Baltimore: Williams & Wilkins, 1987:197.

15. Blaufox MD. Procedures of choice in renal nuclear medicine. *J Nucl Med* 1991;32:1301–1309.

16. Older RA, Korobkin M, Workman J et al. Accuracy of radionuclide imaging in distinguishing renal masses from normal variants. *Radiology* 1980;136:443–448.

17. Leonard JC, Allen EW, Goin J et al. Renal cortical imaging and the detection of renal mass lesions. *J Nucl Med* 1979;20:1018–1022.

18. De Lange MJ, Piers DA, Kosterink JGW et al. Renal handling of technetium-99m DMSA: evidence for glomerular filtration and peritubular uptake. *J Nucl Med* 1989;30:1219–1223.

19. Peters AM, Jones DH, Evans K et al. Two routes for 99m-Tc-DMSA uptake into the renal cortical tubular cell. *Eur J Nucl Med* 1988;14:555–561.

20. Quinn RJ, Elder GJ. Poor technetium-99m-DMSA renal uptake with near normal technetium-99m-DTPA uptake caused by tubulointerstitial renal disease. *J Nucl Med* 1991;32:2273–2274.

21. Provoost AP, Van Aken M. Renal handling of technetium-99m DMSA in rats with proximal tubular dysfunction. *J Nucl Med* 1985;26:1063–1067.

22. Bingham JB, Maisey MN. An evaluation of the use of 99m-Tc dimercaptosuccinic acid (DMSA) as a static renal imaging agent. *Br J Radiol* 1978;51:559–607.

23. Elison BS, Taylor D, Van Der Wall H et al. Comparison of DMSA scintigraphy with intravenous urography for the detection of renal scarring and its correlation with vesicoureteric reflux. *Br J Urol* 1992;69:294–302.

24. Rossleigh MA, Wilson MJ, Rosenber AR et al. DMSA studies in infants under one year of age. *Contrib Nephrol (Basel)* 1990;79:166–169.

25. Gordon I. Indications for 99m-technetium dimercapto-succinic acid scan in children. *J Urol* 1987;137:464–467.

26. Shanon A, Feldman W, McDonald P et al. Evaluation of renal scars by technetium-labeled dimercaptosuccinic acid, intravenous urography, and ultrasonography: a comparative study. *J Pediatr* 1992;120:399–403.

27. Goldraich NP, Ramos OL, Goldraich IH. Urography versus DMSA in children with vesicoureteric reflux. *Pediatr Nephrol* 1989;3:1–5.

28. Groshar D, Embon OM, Frenkel A et al. Renal function and technetium-99m-dimercaptosuccinic acid uptake in single kidneys: the value of in vivo SPECT quantitation. *J Nucl Med* 1991;32:766–768.

29. Al-Naihas A, Jafri RA, Britton KE et al. Clinical experience with 99m-Tc-MAG3, mercaptoacetyltriglycine, and a comparison with 99m-Tc-DTPA. *Eur J Nucl Med* 1988;14:453–462.

30. Fritzberg AR, Kasina S, Eshima D et al. Synthesis and biological evaluation of technetium-99m-MAG3 as a hippuran replacement. *J Nucl Med* 1986;27:111–116.

31. Taylor A Jr, Eshima D, Fritzberg AR et al. Comparison of iodine-131-OIH and technetium-99m-MAG3 renal imaging in volunteers. *J Nucl Med* 1987;27:795–803.

32. Bubeck B, Brandau W, Eisenhut N et al. The tubular extraction rate

33. (TER) of MAG3: a new quantitative parameter of renal function. *Nucl Compact* 1987;18:260–267.

33. Bubeck B, Brandau W, Weber E et al. Pharmacokinetics of technetium-99m-MAG3 in humans. *J Nucl Med* 1990;31:1285–1293.

34. Jafri RA, Britton KE, Nimmon CC et al. Technetium-99m MAG3, a comparison with iodine-123 and iodine-131 orthoiodohippurate, in patients with renal disorders. *J Nucl Med* 1988;29:147–158.

35. Muller-Suur R, Muller-Suur C. Renal and extrarenal handling of a new imaging compound (99m-Tc-MAG-3) in the rat. *Eur J Nucl Med* 1986;12:438–442.

36. Russell CD, Thorstad BL, Stutzman ME et al. The kidney: imaging with Tc-99m mercaptoacetyltriglycine, a technetium-labeled analog of iodohippurate. *Radiology* 1989;172:427–430.

37. Taylor A Jr, Eshima D, Christian PE et al. Technetium MAG3 kit formulation: preliminary results in normal volunteers and patients with renal failure. *J Nucl Med* 1988;29:616–622.

38. Stadalnik RC, Vogel JM, Jansholt AL et al. Renal clearance and extraction parameter of ortho-iodohippurate (I-123) compared with OIH (I-131) and PAH. *J Nucl Med* 1980;21:168–170.

39. Eshima D, Taylor A Jr. Technetium-99m (99mTc) mercaptoacetyltriglycine: update on the new 99mTc renal tubular function agent. *Sem Nucl Med* 1992;22:61–73.

40. Zuckier LS, Axelrod MS, Wexler JP et al. The implications of decreased performance of new generation gamma-cameras on the interpretation of I-131 hippuran renal images. *Nucl Med Commun* 1987;8:49–61.

41. Russell CD, Thorstad BL, Yester MV et al. Quantitation of renal function with technetium-99m MAG3. *J Nucl Med* 1988;29:1931–1933.

42. Gordon I, Anderson PJ, Lythgoe MF et al. Can technetium-99m-mercaptoacetyltriglycine replace technetium-99m-dimercaptosuccinic acid in the exclusion of a focal renal defect? *J Nucl Med* 1992;33:2090–2093.

43. Dubovsky EV, Russell SD, Yester MV et al. Will 99mTc-MAG3 replace 131-I-OIH and 99mTc-DTPA in the follow-up of renal transplants? In: Blaufox MD, Hollenberg NK, Raynaud C, eds. Radionuclides in nephro-urology. *Contrib Nephrol (Basel)* 1990;79:118–122.

44. Peters AM. Quantification of renal haemodynamics with radionuclides. *Eur J Nucl Med* 1991;18:274–286.

45. Russell CD, Bischoff PG, Kontzen F et al. Measurement of glomerular filtration rate using 99m-Tc-DTPA and the gamma-camera: a comparison of methods. *Eur J Nucl Med* 1985;10:519–521.

46. Russell CD, Dubovsky EV. Measurement of renal function with radionuclides. *J Nucl Med* 1989;30:2053–2057.

47. Klopper JF, Hauser W, Atkins HL et al. Evaluation of 99mTc-DTPA for the measurement of glomerular filtration rate. *J Nucl Med* 1972;13:107–110.

48. Waller DG, Keast CM, Fleming JS et al. Measurement of glomerular filtration rate with technetium-99m DTPA: comparison of plasma techniques. *J Nucl Med* 1987;28:372–377.

49. Fawdry RM, Gruenewald SM. Three-hour volume of distribution method: an accurate simplified method of glomerular filtration rate measurement. *J Nucl Med* 1987;28:510–513.

50. Mulligan JS, Blue PW, Hasbargen JA. Methods for measuring GFR with technetium-99m-DTPA: an analysis of several common methods. *J Nucl Med* 1990;31:1211–1219.

51. Russell CD. Optimum sample times for single-injection, multisample renal clearance methods. *J Nucl Med* 1993;34:1761–1765.

52. Chachati A, Meyers A, Rigo P et al. Validation of a simple isotopic technique for the measurement of global and separated renal function. *Uremia Invest* 1986;9:177–179.

53. Gates GF. Glomerular filtration rate: estimation from fractional renal accumulation of 99mTc-DTPA. *AJR* 1981;138:565.

54. Russell DC, Bischoff PG, Rowell KL et al. Quality control of Tc-99m DTPA for measurement of glomerular filtration: concise communication. *J Nucl Med* 1983;24:722–727.

55. Lear JL, Feyerabend A, Gregory C. Two-compartment, two-sample technique for accurate estimation of effective renal plasma flow: theoretical development and comparison with other methods. *Radiology* 1989;172:431–436.

56. Russell CD, Dubovsky EV, Scott JW. Estimation of ERPF in adults from plasma clearance of I-131-hippuran using a single injection and

one or two blood samples. *Int J Radiat Appl Instrum Part B Nucl Med Biol* 1989;16:381–383.

57. Schlegel JU, Hamway SA. Individual renal plasma flow determination in 2 minutes. *J Urol* 1976;116:282–285.

58. Russell CD, Thorstad B, Yester MV et al. Comparison of technetium-99m MAG3 with iodine-131 hippuran by a simultaneous dual channel technique. *J Nucl Med* 1988;29:1189–1193.

59. Russell CD, Thorstad BL, Yester MV et al. Quantitation of renal function with technetium-99m MAG3. *J Nucl Med* 1988;29:1931–1933.

60. Russell CD, Taylor A, Eshima D. Estimation of technetium-99m-MAG3 plasma clearance in adults from one or two blood samples. *J Nucl Med* 1989;30:1955–1959.

61. Muller-Suur R, Magnusson G, Bois-Svensson I et al. Estimation of technetium-99m mercaptoacetyltriglycine plasma clearance by use of one single plasma sample. *Eur J Nucl Med* 1991;18:28–31.

62. Mettler FA, Guiberteau MJ, eds. *Essentials of nuclear medicine imaging,* 3rd ed. Philadelphia: WB Saunders, 1991.

63. Piepsz A, Dobbeleir A, Erbsmann R. Measurement of separate kidney clearance by means of 99m-Tc DTPA complex and a scintillation camera. *Eur J Nucl Med* 1977;2:173–177.

64. Rutland A. Comprehensive analysis of DTPA renal studies. *Nucl Med Commun* 1985;6:11–30.

65. Rehling M, Moller ML, Lund GO et al. Tc-99m DTPA gamma camera renography: normal values and rapid determination of single kidney glomerular filtration rate. *Eur J Nucl Med* 1985;11:1–6.

66. Bell SD, Peters AM. Extravascular chest wall technetium-99m diethylene triamine penta-acetic acid: implications for the measurement of renal function during renography. *Eur J Nucl Med* 1991;18:87–90.

67. Piepsz A, Dobbeleir A, Ham HR. Effect of background correction on separate technetium-99m-DTPA renal clearance. *J Nucl Med* 1990;31:430–435.

68. Russell CD. Estimation of glomerular filtration rate using 99m Tc-DTPA and the gamma-camera. *Eur J Nucl Med* 1987;12:548–552.

69. Fine EJ, Axelrod M, Gorkin J et al. Measurement of effective renal plasma flow: a comparison of methods. *J Nucl Med* 1987;28:1393–1400.

70. Tondeur M, Piepsz A, Dobbeleir A et al. Technetium-99m mercaptoacetyltriglycine gamma-camera clearance calculations: methodological problems. *Eur J Nucl Med* 1991;18:83–86.

71. Bubeck B, Brandau W, Weber E et al. Pharmacokinetics of technetium-99m-MAG3 in humans. *J Nucl Med* 1990;31:1285–1293.

Diagnostic Nuclear Medicine, Fourth Edition. Edited by M.P. Sandler, R.E. Coleman, J.A. Patton, F.J.Th. Wackers, A. Gottschalk. Lippincott Williams & Wilkins, Philadelphia 2003.

42

RENAL NUCLEAR MEDICINE

BRUCE J. BARRON
E. EDMUND KIM
LAMK M. LAMKI

Technical advances have increased the value of radionuclide study in evaluating the patient with suspected disease of the genitourinary tract. However, the progress in renal nuclear medicine during the last several years has been relatively slow. The introduction of ^{99m}Tc-mercaptoacetyltriglycine (MAG$_3$) and captopril renography provided significant progress with the phase of refining techniques. The actual performance of a renal radionuclide study varies greatly from institution to institution. There is a need for some guidance in setting up a more standardized approach. This chapter provides a broad overview for renal physiology, radiopharmaceuticals, and measurement of renal function. Practical applications of the principles are divided into sections reviewing radionuclide renography, renal vascular disorders, and trauma.

RENAL PHYSIOLOGY AND RADIOPHARMACEUTICALS

Renal Therapy

The human kidney performs three essential functions for the maintenance of life. The excretory function, by which the kidney excretes into the urine substances that are either unnecessary or foreign to the body, depends on the regulatory function by which the kidney maintains homeostasis of the internal environment. Electrolytes and acid-base balance, pH, and extracellular fluid volume are all regulated by the kidney. The endocrine function contributes to homeostasis by secreting or activating hormones or by turnover of various hormones. The renal excretory function involves three discrete processes: glomerular filtration, tubular secretion and reabsorption, and tubular fixation.

The structural and functional unit of the kidney is the nephron, which is composed of the glomerulus and the tubule. The capillaries that form the glomerular tuft are enclosed by an epithelial Bowman's capsule. The normal adult kidney receives approximately 20% to 25% of the cardiac output per minute. The arterial blood that enters the kidney normally traverses the glomerulus, where it is subjected to ultrafiltration, producing over 180 L/day of essentially protein-free filtrate. This filtrate is transferred to the lumen of the nephron where the tubules selectively process the filtrate, and approximately 99% of the filtered water is reabsorbed. The tubular reabsorption and secretion result in the daily excretion of 1 to 1.5 L of urine. The passive process of glomerular filtration does not require local expenditure of metabolic energy and may be quantitated by measurement of the renal clearance filtered at the glomerulus. Molecular charge and shape play an important role as determinants of the glomerular permeability of macromolecules (1). The pressure and rate with which blood is delivered to the kidneys determine the absolute glomerular filtration rate (GFR), although the GFR is constant over a wide range of changes in arterial pressure and renal blood flow (autoregulation). The average GFR values in men and women are 124 + 26 and 109 + 14 mL/minute/1.73 m^2, respectively. It is quite low in infants and also reduced as a result of the loss of functioning nephrons with advancing age.

The tubular secretory process involves the transport of substances from the peritubular fluid into the tubular lumen by active and/or passive mechanisms. The site of active secretion is the proximal tubule, and a continuous supply of energy is necessary to move the transported substances from the blood to the urine. The tubular reabsorption mechanism is responsible for transporting a number of solutes from the tubular lumen into the peritubular capillary fluid by very discrete active or passive processes. Many organic acids, bases, and compounds undergo passive tubular reabsorption to a slight extent. Certain substances undergo prolonged retention in the kidneys because of high binding affinity for sites in either proximal or distal tubules (2). Binding sites in the renal tubules include the thiol and disulfide moieties that have high affinity for heavy metal cations. The fixation processes allow the evaluation of renal morphology with radiopharmaceuticals that have these tubular binding properties.

Radiopharmaceuticals

To date no compound has been found that is completely extracted by the kidneys, and only para-aminohippuric acid (PAH)

B.J. Barron: Department of Radiology, University of Texas Medical School-Houston, Houston, TX.

E.E. Kim: Department of Nuclear Medicine and Radiology, University of Texas and Department of Nuclear Medicine, U.T.M.D. Anderson Cancer Center, Houston, TX.

L.M. Lamki: Department of Radiology, Division of Nuclear Medicine, University of Texas Medical School-Houston, Houston, TX.

comes close. Measurement of effective renal plasma flow (ERPF) using PAH is a time-consuming procedure that requires complex separation methods. Labeling orthoiodohippuric acid (OIH) with ^{123}I results in a better imaging than that with ^{131}I, but the cost and availability of ^{123}I makes a practical problem (Fig. 42.1). Over the last 25 years there has been considerable effort to develop the ideal agent to measure ERPF and perform renal imaging. Most research has been directed towards the development of ^{99m}Tc-labeled compound because of the favorable physical properties of ^{99m}Tc with low cost and easy availability. Technetium generally forms stable complexes with ligands that contain functional groups such as -COOH, -OH, -NH$_2$, and -SH. Attempts to develop a ^{99m}Tc-labeled analog of PAH by incorporation of an iminodiacetic acid (IDA) moiety yielded p-[(biscarboxymethylaminomethyl)carbamino] hippuric acid (PAHIDA), which showed a clearance of less than 50% of OIH (3). The most successful triamide mercaptide (N$_3$S) ligand to date is MAG$_3$, but MAG$_3$ is not an ideal replacement for OIH because of high (60% to 80%) plasma protein binding and only 60% to 65% clearance of OIH, making determination of ERPF complicated (4). However, ^{99m}Tc MAG$_3$ is currently the agent of choice for the evaluation of renal function.

An ideal renal imaging agent would be one that achieves a concentrated, homogeneous distribution of radioactivity throughout the renal parenchyma in a short interval of time prior to excretion of radioactivity into the renal pelvis. This would permit a high target-to-background ratio with detailed information about renal parenchymal integrity. The properties of polarity and molecular weight, strength of protein binding, and functional status of the principal organ decide the fate of excretion of most compounds. Compounds that are in the molecular weight range of 300 to 500 are efficiently extracted in both the urine and the bile, whereas those in the molecular range of 300 or lower are preferentially excreted in the urine. Highly polar substances and their metabolites are usually excreted

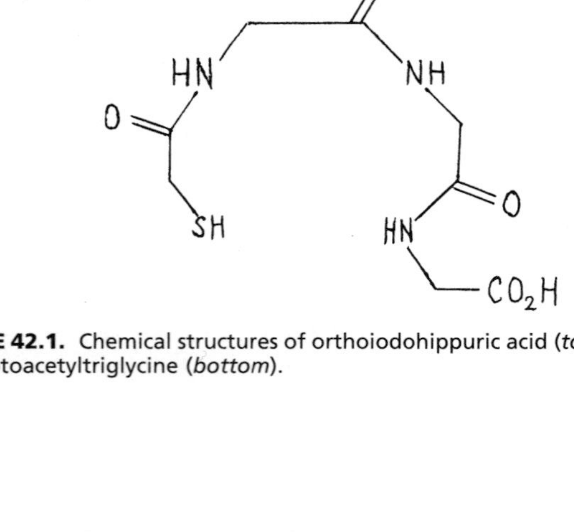

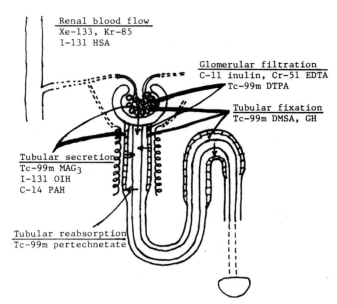

FIGURE 42.2. Nephron segments with different excretion of various radiopharmaceuticals.

chiefly by the kidneys. The loss of the functional integrity of one route of excretion generally results in compensatory excretion via the other route for most substances.

The radiopharmaceuticals for assessing renal function and anatomy can be grouped into those excreted by glomerular filtration, those excreted primarily by tubular excretion, and those retained in the renal tubules for long periods (Fig. 42.2). ^{99m}Tc-diethylenetriaminepentaacetic acid (DTPA) is almost completely filtered by the glomerulus and available for routine renography and for measuring GFR (Fig. 42.3). The extraction fraction of DTPA (the percentage extracted with each pass through the kidney) is approximately 20% in normal subjects. This extraction fraction is relatively low compared with MAG$_3$ (40% to 50%) (5). MAG$_3$ is highly protein bound and cleared in the kidney almost exclusively by the proximal renal tubules (5) (Fig. 42.1). Because of its more efficient extraction, MAG$_3$ is preferred over DTPA, particularly in patients with suspected urinary obstruction or impaired renal function (6). The MAG$_3$ clearance averages about 300 mL/minute/1.73 m^2 in adults under the age of 40, and it decreases at a rate of 3 to 4 mL/year after age 40 (7). MAG$_3$ is more highly protein bound than OIH and tends to remain in the intravascular compartment. The clearance of MAG$_3$ is only 50% to 60% that of OIH. However, the renogram curves of MAG$_3$ and OIH are almost identical due to the similar rates of excretion. In normal subjects, approximately 0.5% of the injected dose of MAG$_3$ accumulates in the gallbladder by 30 to 60 minutes, and 1% of the dose is present in the intestinal tract by 3 hours (8). The rapid voiding schedule reduces the radiation dose to the bladder and gonads by a factor of two to three and to the kidneys by 10%. The radiation doses to the kidneys, assuming no renal clearance, are 13 rads with ^{99m}Tc-DTPA and 15 rads with ^{99m}Tc MAG$_3$ (9). [99m]Tc L or D, D ethylenedicysteine (EC) is an excellent renal radiopharmaceutical with clearances slightly higher than MAG$_3$ (10), and its renal

FIGURE 42.1. Chemical structures of orthoiodohippuric acid (*top*) and mercaptoacetyltriglycine (*bottom*).

each kidney is performed. Significant urinary tract obstruction causing renal impairment requires surgery, the nature of which often depends on the individual performance of each kidney. Split-function studies have been useful in determining the degree of improvement in patients with renovascular hypertension (RVH) following bypass surgery or angioplasty. A DTPA scan can be combined with GFR measurement, and a MAG_3 scan can be combined with a MAG_3 clearance measurement. The most widely used techniques to measure the clearance of DTPA and MAG_3 are plasma-sample and camera-based clearances. Clearance measurements based on plasma samples are more accurate than camera-based ones, but plasma-sample clearance requires meticulous techniques, without contamination by saline, heparin, or plasma from an earlier time. Standards must be prepared accurately, dilutions made carefully, and ^{99m}Tc samples corrected for decay. Because DTPA is cleared more slowly than MAG_3, its clearance (GFR) is estimated from the dose injected and the activity in one or more plasma samples obtained 1 and 3 hours after injection (14). A single-sample technique (45-minutes postinjection) is used in transplant patients.

Camera-clearance methods also have problems related to estimation of renal depth and background substraction. The integral method requires a measurement of the counts in the kidney at an interval from 1- to 2-, 1- to 2.5-, or 2- to 3-minutes postinjection. The renal-to-background ratio is much higher for MAG_3 than DTPA, and potential error by oversubtraction or undersubstraction of background is significantly reduced. These methods provide at least as good a measurement of renal function as the creatinine clearance (15). Renal depth is usually estimated from a nomogram based on height and weight. Commercial camera-based techniques are currently available for measuring GFR (DTPA) and MAG_3 clearance. The average difference in renal depth between the two kidneys was 0.61 cm (15). Differences in the renal depth of the two kidneys can affect the relative uptake or function because of differences in attenuation, but this is rarely a clinically important problem (16). Relative uptake from 50/50 to 56/44 is considered as normal, 57/43 to 59/41 as borderline, and 60/40 or greater as abnormal.

RADIONUCLIDE RENOGRAPHY

General Technique

The various analytic methods for analyzing the radionuclide renogram reflect different approaches to complex renal physiologic events, which are represented by time-activity curves of renal radioactivity following bolus injection of a radiopharmaceutical with high renal clearance. Because the two kidneys normally receive approximately 20% of the cardiac output, a large fraction of the radiopharmaceutical reaches the kidney in the first passage through the circulation. About 20% of the amount reaching the kidney is trapped in the glomerular filtrate, or about 4% of the injected dose. If the compound is filtered and secreted, about 90% can be extracted during a single pass (this is approximately 18% of the injected dose). Various analyses of blood and tissue radioactivity curves indicate that they may be well fitted by the sum of three exponentials, suggesting three exchange compartments. After serial images are obtained, portions of kidney or

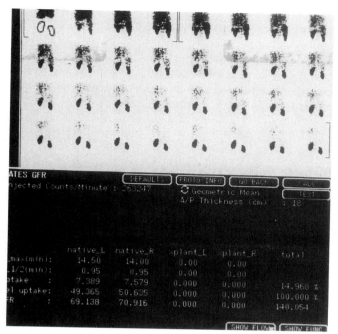

FIGURE 42.3. Glomerular filtration rate (GFR) measurement by modified Gates method: Total GFR is 140 mL/minute/1.73 m² (70.9 for right and 29.1 for left kidney).

clearance more closely approaches that of OIH (75.4% of OIH clearance). Glucoheptonate (GH) is cleared from the blood stream at a rate comparable to that of DTPA, but only 39% is excreted in the urine in 1 hour. It is 50% protein bound, with a hepatic uptake of 1.1% to 1.5%. Approximately 20% to 25% of the injected dose remains concentrated in the cortical parenchyma at 1 hour after injection. ^{99m}Tc-GH is satisfactory for renal imaging with about 5% to 10% of the dose fixed in each renal cortex for up to 24 hours (11). Dimercaptosuccinic acid (DMSA), which is approximately 50% protein bound, has a biodistribution similar to chlormerodrin, with 15% localizing in the liver and 7% to 14% excreted in the urine (12). Forty percent to 50% of the injected dose localizes in the renal cortex by 3 hours after injection, binding to the proximal tubules. Because blood clearance is slow, kidney to background activity ratio is similar to that of GH in spite of greater fractional renal uptake. In the presence of renal failure, the activity is shifted to the liver, gallbladder, and gut.

Measurement of Renal Function

An assessment of renal function is often critical in the treatment of renal disease. Renal function has been measured traditionally by creatinine clearance. However, creatinine clearance is not an accurate measure of the GFR because creatinine is also excreted by the tubules. Creatinine clearance overestimates GFR in patients with chronic renal disease, and patients with decreased muscle mass resulting from spinal cord injury have been found to have subnormal levels of serum creatinine and normal creatinine clearance with renal impairment (13). Creatinine clearance does not measure individual renal function unless catheterization of

the entire kidney may be outlined. Computer-generated curves permit the identification of unilateral pathology more clearly where subtle differences in the images are not readily appreciated (Fig. 42.4**A** and **B**). No significant difference has been demonstrated between ^{99m}Tc-MAG$_3$ and ^{131}I-OIH in the differential uptake, time to maximal activity, residual renal activity, or rate of emptying after furosemide injection at 20 minutes (17).

Analysis of renogram curves is usually done in three phases (Fig. 42.5). Within 15 to 20 seconds following the injection of the radiopharmaceutical, there is a rapidly rising slope, which at about 20 to 40 seconds reaches an inflection point. This rapid initial rise has been called the first phase of the renogram. Although the rate of perfusion primarily affected the initial phase, the slope is also affected by changes in renal tubular function. The second phase of the renogram is represented by a less rapid increase in activity, which reaches a peak normally at 3 to 5 minutes. During the second phase, the tubular secretory accumulation of radioactivity dominates. By about 3 to 5 minutes, the renal activity begins to leave the kidney via the collecting system and reaches the bladder. Thereafter, the tubular excretory curve is represented by a rapidly falling slope. The renogram curve is affected by the state of hydration of the patient, renal position, area of interest, and background chosen.

Dehydration can prolong the excretory phase of the renogram curve. Patients should be given 5 to 10 mL water/kg immediately on arrival, preferably 30 to 60 minutes before the examination. A specific gravity greater than 1.015 suggests dehydration. The time to the peak height on the renogram curve is a useful measurement, particularly for patients with suspected RVH. The peak should occur by 5 minutes after injection. As renal function deteriorates, there is often an abnormal prolongation of the excretory phase of the renogram. The degree of abnormality can be quantitated by a measurement of residual cortical activity (RCA) using the ratio of the counts at 20 or 30 minutes to the peak (maximum) counts (18). In a series of potential renal donors studied with MAG$_3$, the 20-minute-to-max ratio for background subtracted parenchymal regions-of-interest (ROIs) was 0.18 ± 0.06 (19).

Diuretic Renography

Obstruction to urinary outflow may lead to obstructive uropathy (dilation of calices, pelvis, or ureters), obstructive nephropathy (renal dysfunction resulting from obstructive uropathy), and hydronephrosis (dilated renal collecting system regardless of the etiology). The frequent clinical question is whether there is any renal damage from known obstructive uropathy (obstructive nephropathy). The most common error is equating hydroureteronephrosis with obstructive uropathy. There are nonobstructive causes of hydroureteronephrosis such as vesicoureteral reflux, postureteral reimplantation, high urine flow state, inflammation, drugs, lax pelvoureteral muscle, and relieved obstruction. Diuretic renography is the only study that can evaluate renal function and urodynamics in a single test. The Whitaker test remains the standard for the determination of obstruction. However, this procedure is generally considered too invasive for routine use. If the infusion requires pressures greater than 22 cm H$_2$0 to achieve a pelvoureteral flow rate of 10 mL/minute, the study is

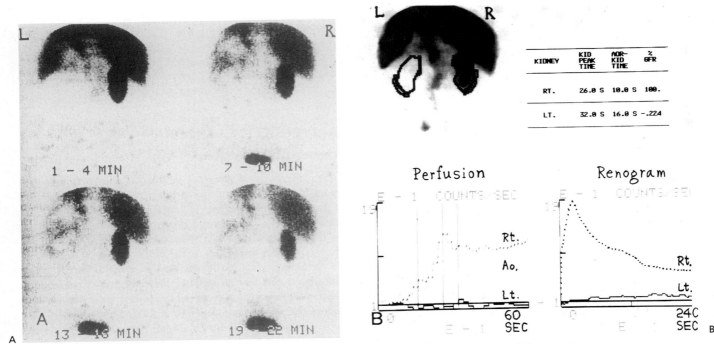

FIGURE 42.4. A: Serial static images of posterior abdomen using ^{99m}Tc-mercaptoacetyltriglycine show prompt uptake and excretion of the activity from the right kidney. No significant uptake of the activity is noted in the left kidney. **B:** Computer-generated perfusion and renogram curves show normal slopes from the right kidney.

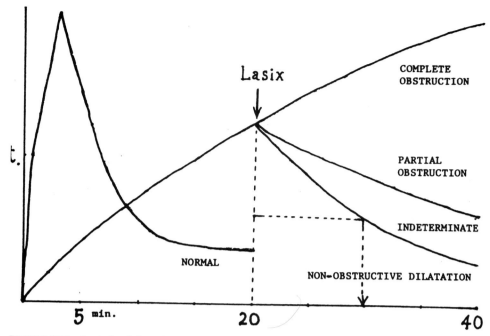

FIGURE 42.5. Analysis of diuretic renogram to differentiate urinary obstruction from nonobstructive dilatation.

considered diagnostic for obstruction, whereas pressures less than 15 cm H_2O exclude obstruction. Intermediate values are indeterminate.

The principle of diuretic renography can be understood by the following equation: $F = V/T$ where F is the rate of fluid flow through the renal pelvis, V is the pelvic volume, and T is the mean transit time of flow through the pelvis. A dilated, but nonobstructed, system is characterized by unchanged flow (F) despite a higher volume (V). This occurs when pelvic fluid takes a longer time (T) to transit across the pelvis. The increased T will appear as delayed washout of the renal pelvis, just as in obstruction. The flow rate (F) can be increased with a diuretic, causing the transit time across the pelvis (T) to decrease, resulting in rapid washout of the tracer. In complete urinary obstruction, F will not increase with a diuretic, so washout will not be observed (Fig. 42.5).

Angiotensin Converting Enzyme Inhibitor Renography

RVH is estimated to affect less than 1% to 3% of the unselected hypertension population. RVH is part of the spectrum of renovascular disease including renal artery stenosis (RAS) and ischemic nephropathy. RVH appears to depend on secretion of renin from the juxtaglomerular apparatus of the underperfused stenotic kidney. Angiotensin converting enzyme (ACE) inhibition interrupts the renin-angiotensin system by preventing the conversion of angiotensin I to angiotensin II, so that the vasoconstrictor and aldosterone-stimulating effects of angiotensin II are blocked. Within the stenotic kidney, inhibition of the enzyme reduces the angiotension II-dependent construction of the postglomerular arterial and thereby lowers the transcapillary

forces that maintain glomerular filtration. Because ACE inhibition decreases the glomerular filtration in the affected kidney, the renal uptake of DTPA is also decreased. A change in relative uptake or a decrease in absolute uptake of MAG3 or OIH by the affected kidney occurs. The cortical retention of MAG3 or OIH is secondary to the decrease in glomerular filtration induced by ACE inhibition. It can be quantitated by measuring the Tmax and the 20- or 30-minute-to-max ratio. With the decrease in GFR, there is decreased flow in the renal tubules and delayed washout of the radionuclide from the tubules. Chronic ACE inhibition may reduce the sensitivity (98% to 75%) in detecting RAS. Captopril (25 to 50 mg orally) peak activity does not occur until approximately 60 minutes after ingestion of radiopharmaceuticals. A second approach is to inject enalaprilat (Vasotec 40 mg/kg intravenously (IV) over 3 to 5 minutes), wait at least 15 minutes, and then inject the agent. Enalaprilat avoids the possibility of false-negative tests resulting from delayed gastric emptying in diabetic patients or from poor absorption.

Aspirin Renography

Prostaglandins have a role in regulation of renal blood flow and GFR. The synthesis of prostaglandin E_2 (PGE_2) is increased during reduction in renal blood flow, and increased PGE_2 stimulates renin release. It has been hypothesized that inhibition of prostaglandin synthesis would decrease renin and, therefore, might have an effect similar to captopril. In many respects, aspirin renography (AR) represents an intervention similar to ACE inhibitor renography, and it is used to diagnose RVH. The reported sensitivity of 25% to 28% (captopril renography) is not statistically different from 25% to 27% (AR) (20). Unilateral

RVH demonstrated ^{123}I-OIH retention and prolongation of Tmax on renogram curves 1 hour after oral aspirin (20 mg/kg).

Exercise Renography

Renal ischemia has been suspected of playing a role in human hypertension. Transplantations of kidneys from normotensive donors to patients with end-stage renal failure and a history of essential hypertension results in remission of the hypertension (21). In individuals without hypertension, renal ischemia results in increased sodium and water reabsorption without resultant reduction in urine flow and increased filtration fraction (ratio of GFR to renal blood flow). Consequently, renal solute excretion is delayed, or there is prolongation in the parenchymal transit time (PTT) of solute through the kidney. In 1983, Clorius and Scvhmidlin described the exercise renogram in which participants were injected twice with ^{131}I OIH, once prone at rest and on a second day after bicycle exercise sufficient to raise the heart rate at least 20 beats per minute over baseline values. In this study, 29 of 51 (57%) participants demonstrated exercise-induced prolonged parenchymal transit (EIPPT) with early essential hypertension. All prolongations in transit in the participant's recent studies were bilateral, suggesting a general dysregulation of GFR and ERPF. The data support a role for a bilateral renal perfusion abnormality in the maintenance phase of fixed RVH.

VASCULAR DISORDERS OF THE KIDNEYS

Congenital Anomalies

Renal scintigraphy is often used to locate or determine the presence of a functioning kidney in cases of nonvisualization by other imaging modalities, such as intravenous pyelogram (IVP) or ultrasound. Nuclear medicine is not the best method of evaluating renal arterial anatomic anomalies. However, congenital anomalies such as duplication of the renal artery, or less commonly an arteriovenous malformation or renal artery aneurysm, may be detected on renal scintigraphy. Disorders involving the arterial supply to or venous drainage from the kidneys can occur at any age. Although there are many variations of arterial supply and vascular drainage of the kidney, the most common variation from normal is a duplicated renal artery, and renal nuclear scanning is often of value because it can detect segmental renal perfusion abnormalities in these patients. Both the "flow" and the "functional" components of the renogram curve and images may show the segmental renal perfusion. Another abnormality, which is not uncommon, is renal artery aneurysm that can be either congenital or acquired. In these cases the nuclear "flow" study may demonstrate a focal area of increased activity at the site of the aneurysm (Fig. 42.6). Other congenital vascular anomalies such as aberrant renal arterial flow may be seen as part of the anomalies such as crossed, fused renal ectopia, in which both renal arteries arise from the same side of the aorta. Other congenital vascular anomalies, such as stenosis, may manifest themselves later in life when various nuclear provocative or stimulatory tests may be employed to detect the lesions.

Acquired vascular disorders include renal artery occlusion or stenosis, renal vein thrombosis (RVT), renal infarction, trauma,

(accidental or iatrogenic), dissection of an aortic aneurysm, and renal cortical necrosis.

Renal Artery Occlusion: Thrombosis and Embolism

Interruptions in vascular supply to the kidney may be acute or chronic and are most often because of trauma, dissection of an abdominal aortic aneurysm (e.g., from severe atherosclerotic disease), or in patients with malignancy. Other causes include RAS, instrumentation, umbilical artery catheterization, embolization from atherosclerotic plaques, or intraoperative coil or balloon placement. Thromboembolic disorder is another cause of vascular interruption that is of particular relevance in renal transplants. Spontaneous thrombosis has been associated with the use of oral contraceptives and blood dyscrasias (22).

The diagnosis of renal artery embolism is often delayed or missed and is a rare cause of renal infarction (23). More than 55% of patients evaluated had atrial fibrillation and 30% had cardiac valvular disease. Patients with renal artery embolus experience flank and abdominal pain, acute in onset and sharp and severe in quality. Early diagnosis is essential for appropriate therapy, such as lysis with streptokinase. As with other causes of renal artery occlusion, no flow is seen on renal scintigraphy (22). In patients with a renal allograft, acute renal artery thrombosis may be seen soon after the transplant surgery related to primary thrombosis or poor anastomosis, or even hyperacute rejection, resulting in loss of arterial flow. Acute rejection also involves a cellular response in the renal arteries, causing diminished or absent flow. In patients with severe stenosis, thrombosis of the vessel after angioplasty has been described (23). Thrombosis of a segmental branch may also cause decreased flow and eventual infarction (Fig. 42.7). Occlusion of the renal artery or its branches usually develops as a result of arterial embolism and rarely because of thrombosis (24–28). Those neonates who had an umbilical artery catheterization may develop aortic thrombosis, which may cause propagation of thrombus into the renal artery or impingement of thrombus against the ostium (28). Renal artery dissection can occur spontaneously, but more often it is the result of extension of abdominal aortic dissection or secondary to abdominal trauma or catheter. A renal function study after surgical repair of a dissected aneurysm is often useful to help in patient management (Fig. 42.8).

Renal Vein Thrombosis

RVT is a relatively uncommon disease, but may be seen with a host of clinical appearances. RVT is not uncommon in the neonatal population and in patients experiencing surgery or trauma. In children, RVT occurs 74% of the time in the first month of life (26). The cause of RVT at any age is usually related to a dehydrated state, immunologic renal disease, circulatory disorders, or birth trauma (27). Other causes include congestive heart failure, retroperitoneal fibrosis, abscess, tumor, lymphoma, and primary renal tumors. It can also be seen in various systemic diseases (29). In neonates, the disease is often bilateral. In renal transplants, RVT is noted in 1% to 4% of patients and usually occurs within the first few days or weeks of the transplant.

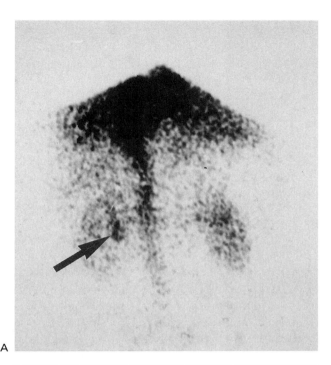

A

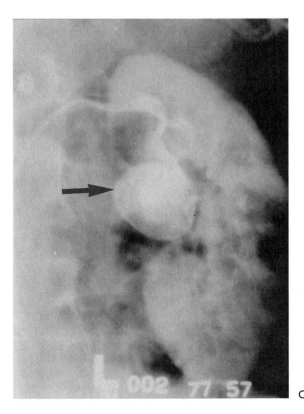

C

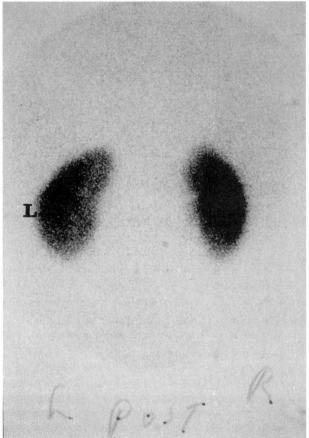

B

FIGURE 42.6. Renal perfusion study showing a focal area of increased flow in the region of the **(A)** renal artery aneurysm (*arrow*). This activity is seen early in the sequence and washes out by the end of the flow study. **B:** A static image showing diminished tracer uptake by the left kidney. **C:** A left renal arteriogram demonstrating the aneurysm (*arrow*).

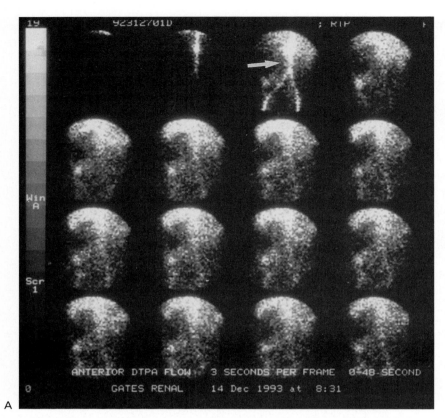

A

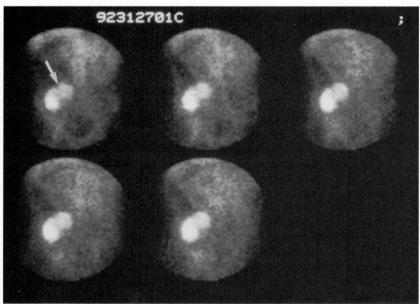

B

FIGURE 42.7. **A:** A renal perfusion study with ^{99m}Tc-diethylenetriaminepentaacetic acid showing decreased flow to the superior pole of a renal transplant (*arrow*) resulting from presumed thrombosis of a branch artery. **B:** A static ^{99m}Tc-mercaptoacetyltriglycine image showing decreased function in the superior pole of the transplant (*arrow*). Subsequent studies demonstrated persistent decrease in function of the superior pole.

Possible causes for renal allograft venous thrombosis include surgical technique, acute rejection, platelet dysfunction, cyclosporine, glomerulonephritis, lower extremity phlebothrombosis with extension, and renal vein compression by hematoma or urinoma (29). RVT is perhaps one of the hardest disorders to diagnose, in part because of its variable clinical presentation and radiographic findings (28). The progression of disease may be rapid or insidious. In the adult, acute onset of RVT is usually associated with flank pain and hematuria. In neonates, it is suspected in a child with a palpable mass and renal failure. The pathophysiologic response of the kidney depends on the acuteness and degree of occlusion. In acute RVT, the kidney becomes edematous. There is a transient increase in blood pressure associated with initial gross hematuria. If there is an acute partial thrombosis, the degree of collaterals will determine the level of function. A cortical "rim" of ^{99m}Tc-DTPA) may be seen in the

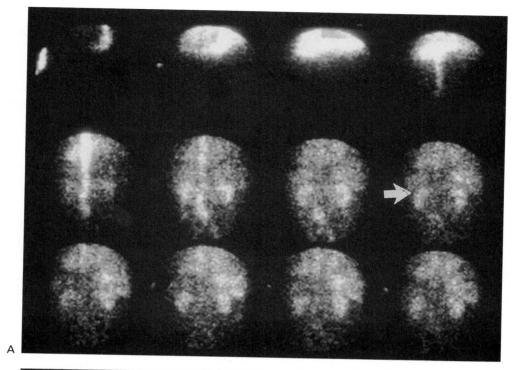

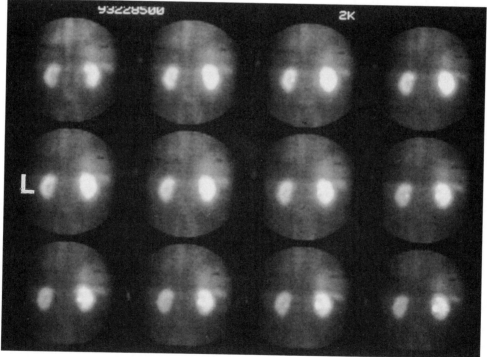

FIGURE 42.8. **A** and **B:** Postsurgical evaluation of a 65-year-old patient with a dissection of an abdominal aortic aneurysm. There is decreased flow (a) and function (b) (*arrow*) resulting from extension of the aneurysm to involve the left renal artery.

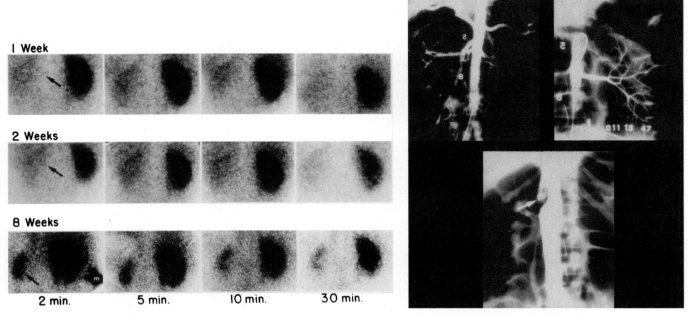

FIGURE 42.9. A: Sequential ⁹⁹ᵐTc-DTPA renal function studies in a 32-year-old woman demonstrate slight improvement of renal function and decreased size 8 weeks after presenting with a renal vein thrombosis. Note the better definition of the kidney with time (*arrows*). **B:** A renal arteriogram shows a flow void in the left renal vein.

nonfunctioning kidney and is indicative of perirenal capsular collateral drainage circulation (26). Nuclear medicine studies, although often helpful, are neither sensitive nor specific enough to be used as the only diagnostic tool. More commonly, renal scintigraphy is used to assess the level of renal function and possibly determine which kidney may be involved. Scintigraphy is also useful in tracking the progress of renal function recovery or deterioration after RVT has been diagnosed (Figs. 42.9 and 42.10). RVT usually results in diminished or absent flow to the involved kidney(s). When ⁹⁹ᵐTc-DTPA is used, one usually sees poor flow and delineation of the kidney. With ⁹⁹ᵐTc-MAG₃, one would expect to see poor excretion of tracer. The usual diagnostic workup also includes magnetic resonance imaging (MRI), color flow Doppler, and intravenous urography. Arteriography may detect a flow void in the renal vein. RVT may also involve a segmental renal vein.

Renal Artery Stenosis

Renal vascular diseases can be divided into those entities that cause hypertension and those that do not. Hypertension is one of the most common medical problems, with more than 60 million Americans classified as hypertensive (30–31) A curable form of hypertension is that caused by renovascular disease, which is a general term encompassing RVH and RAS (32). However, this entity occurs in only a small percent of the population, with an estimated prevalence of between 1% to 2%. The true incidence is probably in the range of 1%, with ranges up to 33% reported in selective groups (33–36). In childhood, RAS is bilateral in 35% to 71% of the patients (36). Hypertensive renovascular disease has been defined as stenotic lesions of the

main or segmental (branch) renal arteries that induce chronically elevated blood pressure and potentially improve after revascularization (31). However, not all stenotic lesions induce hypertension and nonrenal causes of hypertension may also be present. In addition, 45% of normotensive patients were demonstrated to have significant stenoses by arteriography. Holly et al. (37) performed an autopsy study that showed RAS in 49% of normotensive patients and 77% of hypertensive patients. Therefore, the presence of anatomic stenosis does not necessarily imply causation of hypertension (38). It is estimated that up to 1 million Americans have hypertension that could be improved or cured with revascularization (39–40). The place for renal scintigraphy with captopril (CRS) is to determine which patients have hemodynamically significant stenoses enough to cause hypertension. It has been shown that a stenosis of between 60% to 70% is needed to become hemodynamically significant. By identifying these patients, unnecessary arteriograms may be avoided. In addition, the response to captopril may also identify those patients who would benefit from ACE inhibition. The presence of a captopril-induced change predicts a good response to revascularization and may avoid unneeded angioplasty (41). There has been a deluge of RAS imaging protocols. Before delving into the specifics of the protocols a review of the etiologies of RAS and the effects of the renin-angiotensin on homeostasis of blood pressure will be addressed.

Etiologies of Renal Artery Stenosis

Hypertension secondary to a significant stenosis of the main or branch renal artery may be due to numerous disease entities including atherosclerosis and fibromuscular dysplasia and more

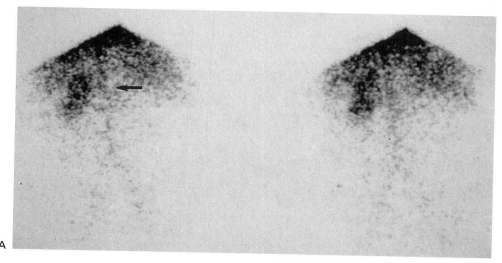

A

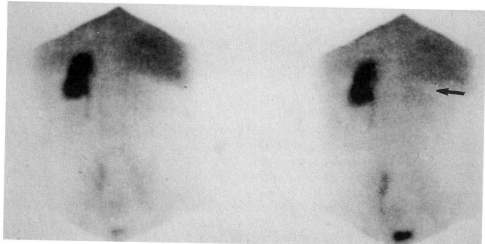

B

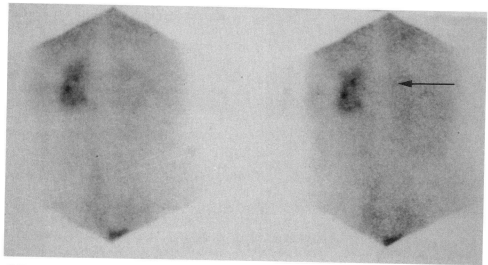

C

FIGURE 42.10. A: A 22-year-old with a history of mitral insufficiency, atrial fibrillation, and biventricular heart failure presented with flank pain. A renal perfusion study with ^{99m}Tc-diethylenetriaminepentaacetic acid (DTPA) shows decreased flow to the right kidney (*arrow*). **B:** Early ^{99m}Tc-DTPA function images show poor resolution of the right kidney (*arrow*). **C:** Delayed images demonstrate faint, ill-defined uptake in the region of the right kidney (*arrow*).

rare entities such as arteritis, dissection of an aortic or renal artery aneurysm, aortic coarctation, renal artery thrombosis, compression secondary to neurofibromatosis, abdominal trauma with intimal tears, iatrogenic (42), congenital RAS (39), or radiation injury (43). Diseases of renal main or branch arteries with secondary hypertension are listed later.

Atherosclerotic Disease

Approximately two thirds of all renovascular lesions in adults are due to atherosclerosis. More than one half of atherosclerotic stenoses involve the ostium. Bilateral disease is noted in 30% to 60% and there is a 2:1 male predominance (43). There is an increased prevalence in aged patients with generalized atherosclerosis (44). In addition, the finding of renal artery narrowing can also be seen in over a third of patients with atherosclerosis and no hypertension (38,44). Approximately 50% of cases involve the ostium, and osteal lesions have a poorer response to angioplasty (30%) when compared with nonosteal lesions (45). Lesions may be bilateral in 20% of lesions and may not be associated with significant atherosclerotic disease elsewhere (31).

Fibromuscular Disease

Fibromuscular dysplasia accounts for 25% of all cases of RVH and is the most common cause of this RVH in young patients, with a female predominance. Although the pathogenesis of the disorder is unknown, fibromuscular dysplasia may be classified as intimal fibroplasia, medial fibroplasia, arteriovenous malformations, medial fibroplasia with aneurysms, and perimedial fibroplasia. Most cases (60% to 85%) are of the medial fibroplasia with aneurysm type. This usually manifests as focal dilatations alternating with constrictions and is usually bilateral. It commonly involves the mid and distal portions of the renal artery, and in about 20% there may be progression leading to diminished renal function (45). The perimedial type is common in young women (43). In fibromuscular dysplasia, there is diminution of renal size in 62% of patients during subsequent follow-up and total occlusion developing in 25% (46).

Other

The other 7% to 8% of RAS may be due to the miscellaneous causes listed previously. It is beyond the scope of this chapter to review each in detail.

DETECTION OF DISEASE

Selection of Patients

By definition, the diagnosis of RVH can be made only after the patient responds to revascularization. A method of identifying patients with probable RVH is, therefore, of extreme importance. The diagnostic workup for RVH is not advisable for all patients with hypertension, because these tests cannot be used as screening tests. There are several reasons for this, but the primary concern is explained by Bayes' theorem. The incidence

of RVH is so low among hypertensives (pretest prevalence of only 1% to 2%), and, therefore, posttest probability of a positive test (predictive value of a positive result) still has a low probability of RVH. There are certain parameters that increase the likelihood of finding RVH. They are

1. Grade II or III retinopathy
2. Recent onset hypertension (<2 years)
3. Accelerated or malignant hypertension
4. Refractory hypertension
5. Age younger than 25 years or older than 50 years
6. Epigastric or flank bruit
7. Previous hypertensive urogram suggestive of RAS (47)
8. Unilateral small kidney discovered by any other study
9. Sudden development or worsening of hypertension
10. Sudden worsening of renal function in a hypertensive patient
11. Hypertension refractory to an appropriate three-drug regimen
12. Hypertension and extensive arterial occlusive disease (48)

Abdominal bruit is the most reliable indicator, 55% of patients with abdominal or flank bruits have renovascular disease (49).

Methods of Detection

Despite the numerous methods of detection, selection of patients who would benefit from revascularization remains difficult. Treatment intervention in patients with RAS does not guarantee improvement in blood pressure, and there is a failure rate as high as 45% (41). The challenge is to identify patients most likely to improve (i.e., those with unilateral stenosis and a normal contralateral kidney). Those with unilateral stenosis in a solitary kidney or bilateral disease will not respond as well. An intermediate stage occurs that represents a transition from a responsive to a refractory physiologic state (40,41). Traditional tests to detect renovascular disease, such as IVP, renal vein renin assays, and digital subtraction angiography may be useful but have been found lacking when looked at independently (32). Selective renal vein renin assays are invasive procedures and are not good predictors when used alone, and 65% of those with nonlateralizing renins will also have a clinical response to revascularization (41). In 15% to 20% of patients with elevated renal vein renin levels and significant RAS remain hypertensive following surgical revascularization (49–51). There is a significant morbidity from renal artery angioplasty or revascularization and, therefore, methods of more precise detection are needed. Numerous diagnostic algorithms have been suggested and tried with varied successes. When a hypertensive patient is evaluated for possible RVH, a functional diagnosis is needed before proceeding with therapy (52). Hypertensive urography, which was commonly used in the 1960s and 1970s was not sensitive enough to allow for its use as a radiographic screen for RVH.

Determination of flow velocity by color Doppler is highly operator dependent and requires meticulous positioning of the transducer over the renal arteries and is currently not the ideal screen. Sonography, which is primarily an anatomic study, does not diagnose RVH but may detect severe RAS. Duplex sonography has not been shown to be as sensitive or specific as arteriography (39). In addition, visualization of double renal arteries and branch vessels is problematic (36,53). In experienced hands, sensitivities of between 84% to 100% have been achieved (32). Gadolinium-enhanced magnetic resonance (MR) angiography is available on high-field-strength imaging systems. The protocols used are beyond the scope of this chapter but are available in the referenced articles. Most reported series have shown excellent correlation between conventional angiography and MR angiography (sensitivity greater than 95% and specificity greater than 90%) for detection of RAS of greater than 50% stenosis. Limitations of MR angiography include evaluation of branched vessels, presence of a metallic stent, detection of accessory arteries, and evaluation of small arteries (48,54,55). However, MR angiography is still an anatomic tool and faces the same difficulty in determining functionally significant disease.

Initial results of the use of MRI in the detection of significant RAS are not yet complete but are promising. In one study two-dimensional MRI had a sensitivity of 100% and a specificity of 94% in predicting RAS of 50% or greater (54–56). Furthermore, this method may not prove to be cost effective, especially in the era of health care reform. In Dunnick's series, using digital subtraction renal arteriography, they obtained 100% sensitivity and 93% specificity, and Svetkey (56) achieved 100% sensitivity and 71% specificity for RVH using intravenous digital subtraction. In general, the sensitivity and specificity is in the range of 90% (53). However, fibromuscular dysplasia may be missed by this method. Angiography detects vessels with significant stenoses and will detect most patients who improve after intervention. Some have proposed digital subtraction renal angiography as the primary method for workup (57). Although risk of intervention in patients diagnosed angiographically but without hemodynamically significant lesions may not be excessive, a method to further screen these patients is needed. Radionuclide renography without captopril is not a good screening test for RAS. Although one might identify patients with asymmetric renal size, it is not useful for predicting those patients that have hemodynamically significant disease.

There are several nuclear medicine studies that are useful for the detection of functionally significant RAS, namely, CRS, AR, and exercise renography. Each of these will be addressed.

Captopril-Enhanced Renal Scintigraphy

CRS has been shown to be a sensitive test in detecting those patients who will benefit from revascularization or angioplasty and those that might benefit from captopril therapy. In addition, segmental branch RAS may also be detected (Fig. 42.11**A–D**) (58). The various protocols in use have demonstrated good sensitivity. However, this method has been questioned in children and adolescents because those with false-positive CRS tended to be younger. In 1996, a consensus report on the use of CRS for detecting RVH was published (59). An enhanced version was reported as procedure guidelines for diagnosing RVH (60).

Angiotensin Converting Enzyme Inhibitor Scintigraphy

One of the most controversial current topics in nuclear medicine is the optimal method for performing angiotensin converting enzyme inhibitor (ACEI) scintigraphy. Numerous imaging protocols have been proposed with various combinations of radiopharmaceuticals and other variables discussed later. To understand how ACEI scintigraphy works, it is important to understand the pathophysiology of RAS and the mechanisms of action of the ACE inhibitors.

Pathophysiology of Renal Artery Stenosis

Goldblatt et al. coined the term "renovascular hypertension" (RVH) to explain a causative relationship between RAS and hypertension (61–63). A renewed interest in the renin-angiotensin system, which was discovered by Tigerstedt and Bergman in 1898, led to an understanding of the pathogenesis of RVH (64). Under normal circumstances the intraglomerular pressure and renal blood flow is maintained by various homeostatic mechanisms. There must be a balance between afferent arteriolar tone and efferent arteriolar tone. The former is influenced by calcium entry into the smooth muscle cells, and the latter is modulated by angiotensin II. A decrease in blood pressure detected by baroreceptors in the juxtaglomerular apparatus or a decrease in serum $NaCl^-$ or K^+ levels will trigger the renin-angiotensin cascade to bring about the conversion of angiotensin I to angiotensin II, via ACE, causing vasoconstriction and thus restoring blood pressure and renal blood flow and hence glomerular filtration (Fig. 42.12). A poststenotic decrease in pressure is seen after the narrowing exceeds 50% from normal (63). When the stenosis reaches 80%, the poststenotic pressure falls more precipitously (49). Renin also causes an increase in the secretion of aldosterone, which increases sodium and potassium reabsorption by the kidney, again helping to increase intraglomerular pressure (64). When there is normal function by the contralateral kidney there is increased sodium excretion by that kidney. Failure to preserve flow to the kidney will cause a decreased glomerular filtration. When a critical, functionally significant level of stenosis is reached, afferent arteriolar pressure is reduced and glomerular filtration may not be sustained. The renin-angiotensin system is then activated, and the effect of increased angiotensin II helps maintain intraglomerular hydrostatic pressure by virtue of increasing efferent arteriolar tone. However, this compensatory mechanism can help only to certain extent and only in some cases is it fully restored. The ability to restore GFR is dependent on the level of function of the kidney and is markedly decreased with increasing renal disease.

Thus, the best chance for improvement after intervention is early in the course of disease when the hypertension is due to elevated renin levels and there is not much deterioration in function of the involved or contralateral kidney (49). When the blood pressure and glomerular filtration is restored, the system is deactivated (52). However, in patients with significant RAS, the increased angiotensin II may improve glomerular filtration, but not necessarily renal blood flow. In 1983, Majd et al. (66) suggested the combination of captopril inhibition of renal function and separate renography (65). The addition of an ACEI

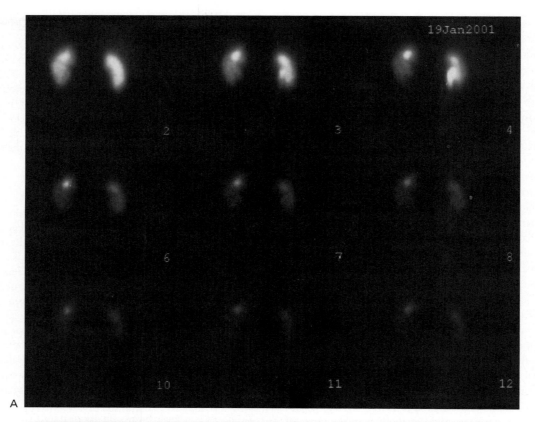

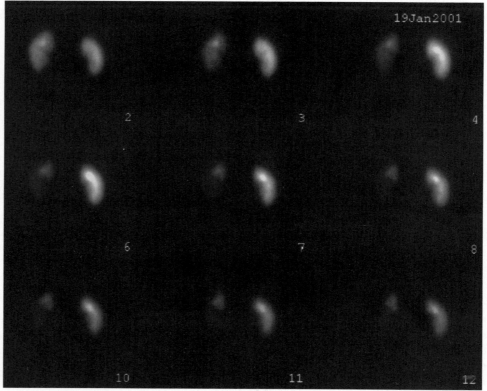

FIGURE 42.11.   Captopril augmented renal scan in a 2-year-old boy. **A:** Pre-captopril renal scan showing slight retention in left upper pole. **B:** Post-captopril scan showing delayed washout of the right kidney and upper pole of the left. Arteriography supported right renal artery stenosis and branched stenosis on the left. *(Figure continues.)*

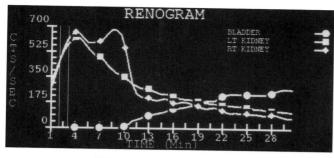
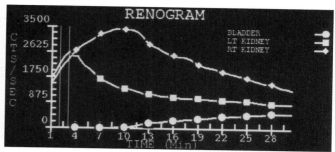

FIGURE 42.11. *Continued.* **C** and **D:** Pre-captopril and post-captopril renogram curves showing prolonged drainage time for the right kidney.

blocks the formation of angiotensin II and, thereby, disrupts the balance that previously existed. The decreased efferent arteriolar tone caused by the ACEI diminishes renal flow and glomerular function. By discriminating the subsequent renal flow and function after ACEI administration against that of the contralateral, presumed normal kidney before and after ACEI administration, a diagnosis of RVH can be made. However, the problem arises when both kidneys are involved or in the case of a transplanted kidney. These issues will be addressed later. Another problem exists when baseline renal function is poor. In these patients, the effect of ACEI on renal function may not be a valid indicator of RVS (66). When the baseline study demonstrates a 20 minute to peak value of greater than 30%, the validity of the study comes into question. As mentioned previously, there are numerous ways of conducting ACEI augmented renal scintigraphy.

Although there is no one protocol that is universally accepted or even accepted by a majority, the variables are presented and two sample protocols proposed (67,68).

The most commonly used ACEI clinically, are oral captopril and injectable enalaprilat. The adult oral dose of captopril is between 25 and 50 mg (69). In our institution we use a dose of 37.5 mg (1½ tablets), which are crushed and made into a slurry by adding water. This is given orally 1 hour before the renal scanning (70).

Eggli et al. reported no serious drops in blood pressure after intravenous infusion of enalaprilat. However, this drug may cause severe hypotension in normotensive patients with congestive heart failure (70). Hansen et al. (71) suggested that caution be used in patients with universal arteriosclerosis because of the risks of cerebral complications. In all patients undergoing this

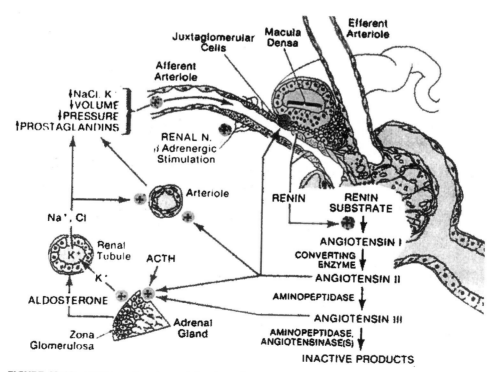

FIGURE 42.12. Diagram of renin-angiotensin pathway. (From Wyngaarden JB, Smith LH, Bennett JC, eds. *Cecil textbook of medicine*, vol 2, 19th ed. Philadelphia: WB Saunders, with permission.)

test, however, we recommend the maintenance of an intravenous line to enable a rapid infusion of normal saline should the blood pressure drop precipitously.

The following discussion looks at the variables in ACEI renal scintigraphy:

A. Patient Preparation
 1. Blood pressure medication
    There is some disagreement as to whether the patient must be off of ACEI before the day of the study. We currently recommend that the patient discontinue captopril 3 days before and enalaprilat 5 days before the study. However, it appears that the trend is to keep the patient on all antihypertensive medications until the day of the study. The patient should be off these medications for about 10 hours, the exception being beta blockers, which are not withheld (72–74). When a patient's systolic blood pressure is below 130 mmHg and the antihypertensive medication is withheld, the patient is asked to walk around the department or wait until the blood pressure rises again before receiving captopril.
 2. State of hydration
    The state of hydration is also a point of disagreement. We recommend adequate hydration with oral or intravenous hydration, with fluid volumes determined on an individual basis. Patients should be instructed to drink only water before the procedure. An alternative is providing the patient 7 mL water per kilogram body weight orally approximately 30 to 60 minutes before the study (60). Patients otherwise receive nothing by mouth (NPO) for at least 4 hours before the study. Some protocols do not recommend any extra hydration. However, Kubo et al. (74), in their enalaprilat protocol, recommend bladder catheterization to prevent the discomfort caused after furosemide injection. In our experience, using a captopril protocol and having the patient void just before the injection of furosemide has limited the amount of discomfort (45).
 3. Intravenous line
    Although establishing venous access is not proposed by all, we do start an intravenous line on all patients undergoing CRS as discussed previously. This is especially important in high-risk patients, those receiving furosemide, and those receiving intravenous enalaprilat. In low-risk patients, a heparin lock should be used.
 4. One- or 2-day protocol
    Either a 1- or 2-day protocol can be performed. However, when the patient is taken off of maintenance antihypertensive medications, it is preferable to do the test as a 1-day protocol. If the patient is not taken off the ACEI, the study should be timed, so that the peak action of the dose taken coincides with the time of injection of radiopharmaceutical.
B. Choice of Radiotracer
    Although Shamlou et al. propose the combined use of ^{99m}Tc-DTPA and ^{131}I-Hippuran, especially in transplant patients, we have been using ^{99m}Tc-MAG$_3$. The basis for the combined isotope study is to demonstrate the uncoupling of glomerular filtration and tubular function after ACEI adminis-

tration (75). We have been using a single day protocol with injection of doses of 1.5-mCi ^{99m}Tc-MAG$_3$ for the baseline study and 7.5 mCi for the portion after ACEI. ^{99m}Tc-DTPA, although used by many sites, has a lower sensitivity for RAS detection than a tubular agent, ^{99m}Tc-MAG$_3$. However, several centers do still use ^{99m}Tc-DTPA (76). The differences in results must be viewed with some caution, because one must take into account the variance of protocols. In fact, Itoh et al. (77), in his review, showed an overall sensitivity with ^{99m}Tc-DTPA of 90% and 87% for tubular agents. The tubular agents, ^{123}I or ^{131}I-Hippuran are also used by some, but neither is believed to be superior to ^{99m}Tc-MAG$_3$ when used alone. Because of higher extraction efficiencies, ^{99m}Tc-MAG$_3$ or ^{123}I-OIH are preferred over ^{99m}Tc-DTPA in patients with elevated creatinine levels (60). If ^{123}I or ^{131}I-hippuran is used, a dose of 2 mCi and 300 μCi, respectively, has been suggested (60,76).

C. Choice of ACEI Agent
    The two agents used most often are captopril and enalaprilat, both discussed previously. Our preference is for captopril in adults and enalaprilat in pediatric patients. The recommended doses of captopril for ACEI renal scintigraphy vary from 25 to 50 mg orally (75,77). We prescribe 37.5 mg crushed tablet because we have had two patients significantly drop their blood pressure from the 50-mg captopril dose. This is a problem, particularly when furosemide is given as well, and, therefore, blood pressure drop is more likely to occur. For patients with renal transplants our dose of captopril is reduced to 25 mg. The pediatric dose is 1 mg/kg body weight. The radiotracer is injected 1 hour after ingestion of the captopril because this time matches the onset of action. Enalaprilat has the advantage of an intravenous dose form and allows a much more rapid onset of action and no problem of absorption. However, its half-life is longer. The dose of enalaprilat varies among investigators but some recommend a dose of 0.04 to 0.05 mg/kg with a maximum dose of 2.5 mg, injected 15 minutes before the injection of radiotracer. In our experience, both of these drugs have been relatively safe. However, they should be used in caution in patients who are experiencing diarrhea or other symptoms that cause loss of body fluids. We have had one case of bilateral renal shutdown after a single dose of captopril.

D. Diuretic Usage
    There has been much discussion regarding the potential benefits of using a diuretic agent to empty the collecting systems and allowing the cortical clearance index to be more accurate. When using captopril one may give an injection of diuretic before or after the baseline and/or post-captopril injection. Our current procedure is to inject 40-mg furosemide IV at 2 minutes after ^{99m}Tc-MAG$_3$ injection. When using enalaprilat, one may inject the furosemide just before the radiopharmaceutical injection. This is thought to help clear tracer from the upper collecting system and to reduce interference with calculations of cortical index (45) or the 20-minute-to-peak count ratio. There is also evidence that furosemide may improve the sensitivity of renography for RAS (78). The dose should be titered from between 20 mg to 60 mg based on the serum creatinine level and on the patient's maintenance

furosemide dose, if any. One disadvantage of the use of furosemide is the potential for volume depletion. For this reason, an intravenous line for potential supplemental hydration is suggested.

Hypotension

Because of the potential for ACEI and furosemide to induce hypotension, regular blood pressure monitoring should occur and be recorded every 5 to 10 minutes. Significant drops in blood pressure give rise to a scan that is falsely positive for bilateral RAS. To reverse the hypotension, elevation of the patient's legs and supplemental fluids is usually all that is necessary.

Acquisition Parameters

The images should be acquired in the posterior projection on a digital scintillation gamma-camera. Several protocols recommend sitting or semisupine position (Table 42.1). However, more commonly, the patient is imaged in the supine position. Depending on the computer capacity, a 64×64 or 128×128 matrix word mode is recommended. We use a single dynamic acquisition divided into a flow phase of 60 one-second images followed by the second phase of 15-second images for 30 minutes. For the 1-day protocol we use a dose of 1.5 mCi ^{99m}Tc-MAG$_3$ for the baseline study and 7.5 mCi ^{99m}Tc-MAG$_3$ for the post-ACEI study. For patients who are currently on ACEI therapy one may do the ACEI challenge test first, and, if it is abnormal, the baseline can be performed after discontinuing captopril for 3 days or enalaprilat for 1 week.

Data Analysis–Criteria

Numerous factors are examined to decide which scans are suggestive of RAS (47,67,79,80). These include differential function, MAG$_3$ clearance, cortical clearance, time to peak, or mean parenchymal transit times (MPTTs). Although some rec-

Table 42.1. *Recommended Protocols*

ACEI	Captopril	Enalaprilat
Route	PO	IV
Dose	37.5 mg	0.04 mg/kg
Prep	Adequate hydration	NPO 4 hrs
	No Foley	Foley
IV 0.5 NS	75 ml/hr	75 ml/hr
Withholding of		
ACEI	2–5 days	9–10 hrs
Anti-HTN meds	9–10 hrs	9–10 hrs
Baseline:		
Furosemide dose	+2 min	−10 min
	none	40;60 mg
		Cr <3;>3
^{99m}TcMAG	1.5 mCi	2.0 mCi
Time	30 min	30 min
ACEI Challenge:		
Furosemide	+2 min	−10 min
Time for ACEI	30 min	90 min
Time of ^{99m}TcMAG$_3$	90 min	100 min
Dose of ^{99m}TcMAG$_3$	7.5 mCi	8.0 mCi

ACEI, angiotensin converting enzyme inhibitor; PO, by mouth; IV, intravenous; NS, normal saline; HTN, hypertension; MAG$_3$, mercaptoacetyltriglycine.

ommend visual inspection without quantitation, we believe that quantitation is needed to standardize interpretation. There has been some disagreement when it comes to drawing the ROI, and the collecting system should probably be excluded when looking at cortical clearance. Based on the consensus report, test results should be interpreted as indicating low, intermediate, or high probability of RAS. Normal findings on the renogram suggests a low probability for disease (<10%). Abnormal baseline findings (Grade I renogram) that improve after ACE inhibition also suggest a low probability for RVH. In addition, in a kidney with greater that 30% relative uptake and a Grade I renogram that does not change is also of low probability for RVH (<20%). Those included in the intermediate probability have abnormal baseline findings suggesting reduced renal function, with an unchanged renogram post-ACEI challenge (60).

As mentioned previously, bilateral worsening of the renogram curves may be due to hypotension during the study, salt depletion, poor hydration status, and distended bladder (81,82). A high probability for RVH exists when there is marked deterioration of the renogram curve. For ^{99m}Tc-DTPA, the deterioration in glomerular function is manifest by a decrease in relative contribution to function. For the tubular agents, increased cortical retention at 20 minutes versus the peak is noted. A normal cortical retention index is less than 0.3. When there is a rise of more than 0.15 post ACEI, the change is felt to be significant. A 0.1 to 0.15 change is borderline. The confidence level is improved when the retained tracer is not present in the pelvocalyceal system. It is also advisable to use parenchymal ROIs rather than whole kidney regions (83,84). Other parameters used are discussed in the following.

Criteria of Positivity

1. Baseline function: If the baseline "cortical retention ratio" (20-minute-to-peak counts) is more than 30%, some feel that renal function is severe enough to preclude a valid test result. In reality, however, a large number of patients have ratios greater than 30% and still respond well to ACEI.
2. Flow curves: The flow curves have not been very useful in evaluating the presence of RAS. They may be of some benefit when used to evaluate for segmental RAS. In this case, ROI curves for various parts of the kidney may be reviewed.
3. Shape of curve: Nally has constructed five curve patterns based on the upslope, peak activity, and downslope portions of an excretion curve. Assuming the curves represent renal cortical activity, the different curves corresponding to different functional states are numbered grades 0, 1, 2a, 2b, and 3, with 0 being normal (Fig. 42.13). When using a glomerular agent, two additional curve grades are used. The baseline and post-ACEI curves are compared, and when there is worsening of at least one grade, there is a high probability of hemodynamically significant RAS. An indeterminate probability is assigned if there is an abnormal baseline of 2b or lower which remains unchanged post-ACEI. If the grade improves, the probability is low. Using this method, there is a 93% sensitivity when looking at improvement postrevascularization (76,77). In Svetkey's (46) series a normal renogram or a normal renal vein renin was associated with a 97% likeli-

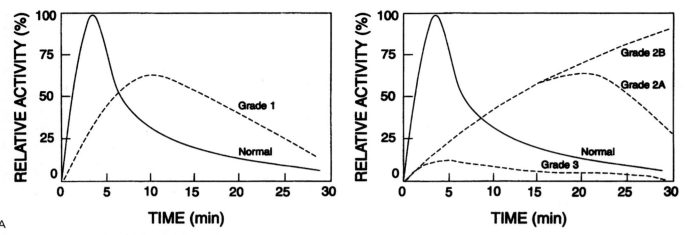

FIGURE 42.13. **A** and **B:** Normal and abnormal renogram curve patterns observed in either the pre-captopril or post-captopril renal studies. Described by Nally, a worsening in grade of the renogram curve is one positive criteria for functionally significant renal artery stenosis. (From Nally JV et al. Diagnostic criteria of renovascular hypertension with captopril renography: a consensus statement. *Am J Hypertens* 1991;4:750–751S, with permission.)

hood that the patient does not have RAS (Figs. 42.14 to 42.16).

4. Cortical retention ratio: The amount of activity remaining in the renal cortex as compared with peak activity is the RCA. This index applies when a tubular agent is used. If the RCA is less than 30% at baseline, a 10% rise with an absolute value of more than 30% is a positive finding. Those kidneys with an RCA greater than 30% at baseline have abnormal function and a further rise of more than 15% is also suggestive of RAS (83,84).

5. Time to peak (Tmax): A change in the time to peak is not as useful of an indicator as is a change in the RCA (76). An increase in Tmax of 2 minutes or 40% is considered significant. However, in our experience, RAS is usually not present when there is improvement in the time to peak.

6. Differential function (split renal function): Comparing radioactivity accumulated between 1 to 2 minutes or 1 to 3 minutes in each kidney gives the relative ratio that each kidney contributes to the function. Normal value is 50% + 5% for each kidney. A baseline differential function of less than 42% for one kidney raises the suspicion of RAS. Itoh considers a split renal function of less than 42% as positive for unilateral RAS. With 42% as the critical value, the sensitivity and specificity were both 63% for the diagnosis of RVH. However, if less than 45% was used, the sensitivity was increased to 88%, but the specificity was only 46%. A further worsening of more than 10% after ACEI and an associated delay in Tmax by more than 120 seconds is likely to represent RAS Concerning tubular agents, a change in relative uptake of more than 10% (i.e., from 50/50 to 60/40) indicates a high probability but is uncommon in patients with RVH (85).

7. GFR: Itoh used a captopril-induced reduction rate (CRR) to look at the effect of captopril on GFR. Using a criterion of a reduction of less than −20% for CRR, the sensitivity was 56% and specificity was 76%. This was improved when used in combination with a change in renogram curve type (77).

8. Rising baseline renogram: Patients with a high-grade RAS and sufficient collaterals may demonstrate a rising baseline renogram with ^{99m}Tc-MAG$_3$ and a slight worsening or no change after ACEI (52).

9. MPTT: Datseris uses the MPTT instead of the usual criteria. As renal function deteriorates, the changes produced by ACEI are less reliable. We looked at the MPTT to determine which patients may benefit from ACEI therapy. It is difficult to use the standard parameters in patients with severe renal disease. However, in these patients, the MPTT is still useful in detecting RAS. In patients in whom the MPTT was reduced after captopril and in whom ACEI therapy was continued, renal function showed improvement or no change. However, when MPTT decreased after captopril, no ACEI therapy was initiated. This set of patients was felt to have angiotensin II–dependent renovascular dysfunction. In a more recent study, however, Fine et al. (87,88) demonstrated the MPTT analysis of captopril ^{99m}Tc-DTPA renography is not more accurate and "offers no advantages compared with qualitative renography or with more commonly used measures." This was thought to be due in part to the high prevalence of underlying renal disease in their population.

In conclusion, ACEI renal scintigraphy appears to have promise in detecting functionally significant RAS. However, because of the varied protocols further refinements are necessary to arrive at an optimal protocol and evaluation criteria.

Aspirin Renography

AR has been shown to have similar sensitivities to ACEI scintigraphy. Aspirin reduces both renal blood flow and glomerular filtration and more effectively impairs the excretion of a tracer whose excretion depends on both filtration and tubular secretion. The rationale for AS is that there is increased dependence of the circulation of stenotic kidneys on prostaglandins. Prostaglandins have an acknowledged role in regulation of renal blood

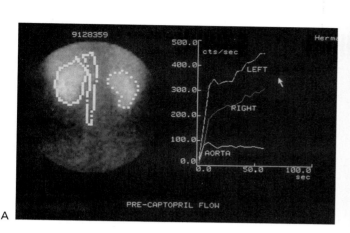

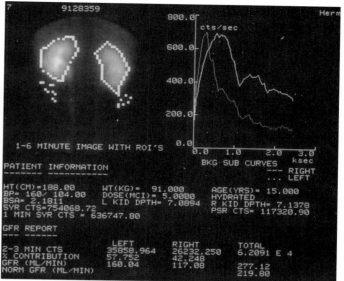

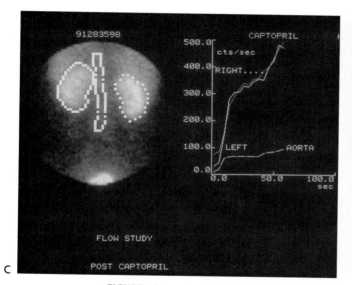

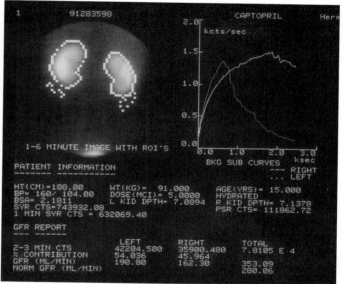

FIGURE 42.14. A: This patient is a 15-year-old with neurofibromatosis and hypertension. A baseline renal flow curves with ^{99m}Tc-mercaptoacetyltriglycine (MAG3) shows relatively decreased flow to the right kidney. **B:** Baseline renogram demonstrates relatively good excretion but slightly worse on the right. The numbers listed next to glomerular filtration rate actually reflect the ^{99m}Tc-MAG3 clearance. The differential function is 58% from the left and 42% from the right. The 42% differential and the asymmetry in flow suggested renal artery stenosis (RAS). **C:** Post-captopril renal flow curves demonstrating relatively symmetric flow. **D:** This post-captopril renogram shows a worsening of the right kidney curve, although the differential improves to 46%. This change in curve pattern is the major criterion met for a diagnosis of RAS. The angiogram demonstrated right RAS in addition to a right renal artery aneurysm. The involved kidney subsequently was autotransplanted.

flow and GFR (90). The synthesis of PGE$_2$ is increased during reduction of blood flow, such as stenosis, and an increase of this substance stimulated renin release (89). Elevated angiotensin II levels in the poststenotic kidney cause constriction mostly in the postglomerular arteriole. The preglomerular arteriole is kept open by increased amounts of vasodilating prostaglandins, which are inhibited by aspirin. On this basis, Japanese investigators thought that this inhibition of prostaglandin synthesis would produce preglomerular vasoconstriction, with the effect of de-

creasing glomerular capillary pressure and GFR, similar to the effects of captopril (90). The changes also occur in the contralateral kidney but to a much less extent (91–93). In the Dutch protocol, AR was performed at least 5 days after captopril renography. In addition to discontinuing ACEIs as in most protocols, nonsteroidal antiinflammatory drugs were also discontinued 14 days before the study. One hour before renal scintigraphy the patient receives 20-mg aspirin per kg orally. At that dose aspirin strongly decreases PGE$_2$ in renal venous plasma within 45 min-

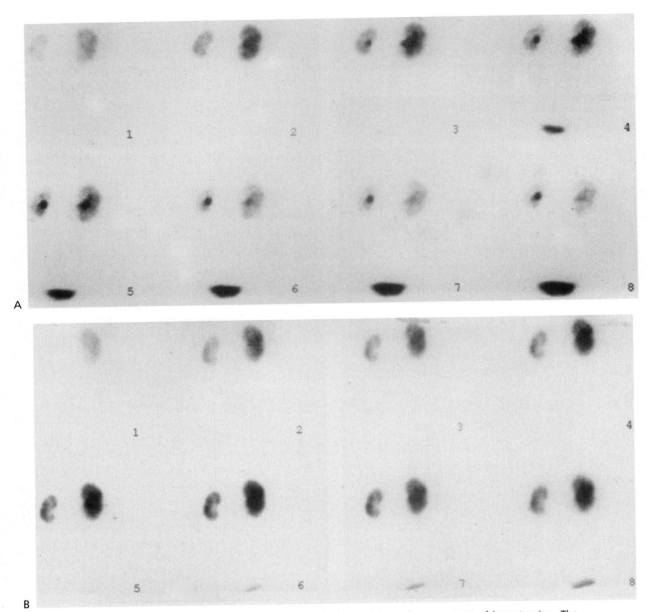

FIGURE 42.15. A: This patient is a 55-year-old with a history of recent onset of hypertension. The baseline ^{99m}Tc-mercaptoacetyltriglycine dynamic function images demonstrate a small left kidney with slightly delayed excretion bilaterally. A mildly dilated collecting system is noted on the left. **B:** The post-captopril study demonstrates worsening of cortical retention and a further delay in excretion. Furosemide was not given as part of this study. *(Figure continues.)*

utes after ingestion. Parameters for diagnosis of RAS used were similar for diagnosis of RAS using captopril scintigraphy. Although there were hopes that the sensitivity for the aspirin study would be better than captopril scintigraphy, the results demonstrated no improved sensitivity (91).

Exercise Renography

Exercise renography has been proposed as another method of evaluating patients with essential hypertension. Renal ischemia has been implicated in human hypertension, but RAS does not explain hypertension in most of these patients. Some investiga-

tors suggest corticomedullary diversion of renal blood flow as a cause (94). Exercise renography has been proposed as a method to differentiate patients with essential hypertension from normal patients. Several hypotheses suggest a subpopulation of nephrons in patients with essential hypertension that is not present in normal patients. These nephrons are the ones responsible for excess salt and water reabsorption seen in essential hypertension. Renal ischemia in nonhypertensive patients results in increased salt and water reabsorption and increases the filtration fraction. This results in prolongation of PPT (89). Early work by Clorius and Schmidlin described the "exercise renogram". Participants underwent two renal scans using ^{131}I-OIH. One dose was ad-

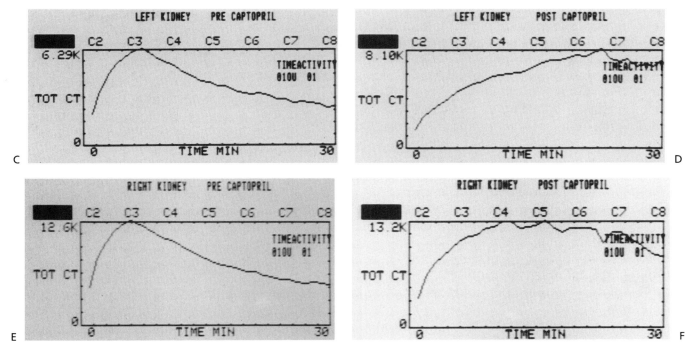

FIGURE 42.15. *Continued.* **C–F:** The renogram curves demonstrate mildly delayed excretion on the pre-captopril study. **(C),** left; **(E),** right kidney. The post captopril renograms **(D, F)** show marked worsening of renogram pattern consistent with bilateral functionally significant renal artery stenosis (RAS). Bilateral RAS was diagnosed on renal arteriogram, and the patient's hypertension did respond to revascularization. Although baseline function in this patient was minimally diminished, captopril-enhanced renal scintigraphy was able to diagnose bilateral disease. (Images provided by Dr. Ramesh Dhekne, St. Luke's Episcopal Hospital, Houston, Texas.)

ministered prone at rest. The second injection was after bicycle exercise. Fifty-seven percent of patients exhibited exercise-induced PPT. Normal volunteers did not demonstrate this phenomenon (95). This technique has been further evaluated in patients with RAS. Clorius examined 23 such patients with exercise renography. Nine of the 23 had normal baseline and exercise renography. Fourteen had bilateral PPT on exercise, which was not noted on baseline examinations. In addition, GFRs diminished in these patients. There is difficulty in excluding RAS in one kidney and essential hypertension in the other. As yet, this technique has not been accepted as a clinical tool. However, as work with this technique continues, new refinements may show this to be a useful diagnostic tool (96).

OBSTRUCTIVE UROPATHY

Hydronephrosis (distension of the pelvicalyceal system) or hyperureteronephrosis (distension of the pelvicalyceal system and ureter) is a common finding in the workup of patients with urinary tract symptomatology and is not limited to the pediatric population. There are multiple causes including congenital malformations, vesicoureteral reflux, urinary tract infection, noncompliant bladder, and urinary tract obstruction (congenital stenosis, tumor, lithiasis). Its diagnosis is relatively easy using standard IVP or ultrasound. However, the functional significance of urinary tract dilatation is more difficult to define because IVP only reflects relative estimates of renal function and

ultrasound does not reflect function at all. These modalities cannot reliably differentiate obstructive from nonobstructive causes. With partial obstruction, loss of function may be negligible. With complete obstruction, there may be no hydronephrosis (97). Early operative intervention in the functionally impaired obstructed kidney may lead to preservation or improvement of renal function. Another study, the pressure perfusion study (Whitaker test) measures collecting system pressures but is considerably more invasive.

Renal radionuclide scintigraphy has been employed in the context of urinary tract obstruction for diagnosis, assessment of parenchymal damage, determination of interval deterioration in function, determination of the appropriate time for surgical intervention, and postsurgical evaluation. With technical advances in computer technology, computer-assisted camera studies have refined the assessment of renal function from the realm of whole-kidney, dual-probe studies with hippuran to the present state of the art in which functionally distinct portions of the kidney (cortex, pelvis) can be isolated and independently analyzed (fractional renogram) (98). These refinements have significantly enhanced the utility of such studies in the noninvasive evaluation of urinary tract obstruction.

Pathogenesis of Obstruction

In adults, calculi and neoplasms are common causes of obstruction, which most often occurs at the ureterovesicular junction, the pelvic brim, or the ureteropelvic junction. Although more

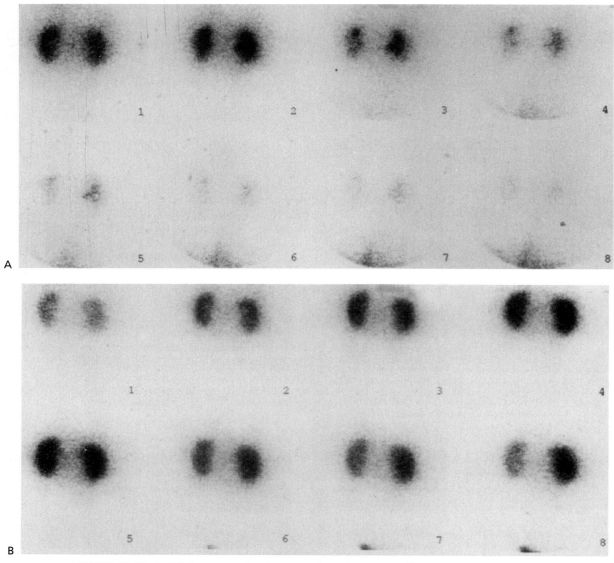

FIGURE 42.16. **A:** This is an example of a captopril renal scan using ¹³¹I-orthoiodohippuric acid. This patient also presented for evaluation of hypertension. The baseline study shows relatively good excretion bilaterally (A). **B:** After captopril administration, there is worsening of function bilaterally, right worse than left as seen by increased cortical retention. *(Figure continues.)*

than 80% of stones pass without need for intervention, secondary scarring and stricture formation may nevertheless cause clinically significant obstruction. Noncalculous obstruction most often results from prostate carcinoma or hypertrophy in men and from cervical carcinoma in women. Duplications of the urinary tract have a high association with obstruction. In cases of complete duplication, there is an increased incidence of ureterovesicular junction obstruction of the ureter to the upper portion of the duplex kidney. Typically the point of insertion into the bladder is medial and inferior to that of the ureter serving the lower portion of the kidney, which is usually unobstructed.

In contrast, obstruction in pediatric patients occurs most often at the ureteropelvic junction secondary to compression from crossing branches of the renal artery, fibrous bands, mu-

cosal folds, high insertion of the ureter, or an abnormal shape of the renal pelvis. Bladder abnormalities and infection can also be contributing factors. Embryonic failure to completely recanalize the ureter has also been cited to explain the high frequency of bilaterality and the wide spectrum of severity. Urinary stasis secondary to obstruction facilitates bacterial growth, which accelerates the destructive process and, in cases of complete obstruction, may constitute the predominant loss of renal function.

Radionuclide Scan Findings

Obstruction affects glomerular function earlier than tubular function, but the deterioration of tubular function appears to be more persistent. This was observed in parallel urographic

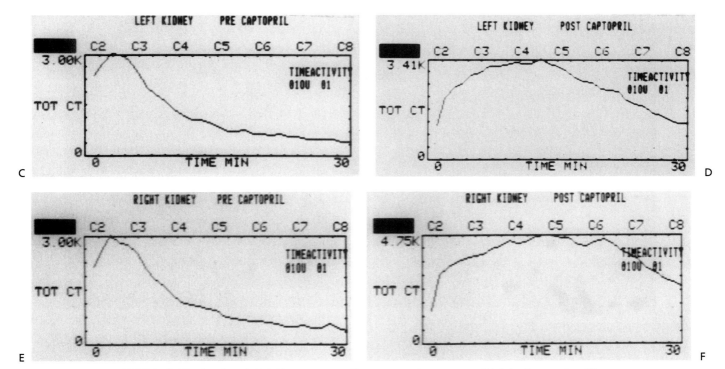

FIGURE 42.16. *Continued.* **C–F:** The pre-captopril renograms show a very mild delay in excretion (**C**), left; (**E**), right. After captopril, the left renogram shows a change to a Type I curve pattern (**D**). The pattern seen on the right is slightly worse than that seen of the left. This patient also had bilateral renal artery stenosis diagnosed on arteriography. No furosemide was given. (Images provided by Dr. Ramesh Dhekne, St. Luke's Episcopal Hospital, Houston, Texas.)

and radionuclide studies using ^{230}Hg, performed in dogs whose ureters were surgically ligated. Contrast excretion was absent after 4 days, whereas tracer uptake persisted for 7 days. After release of the ligature, however, contrast excretion (glomerular function) returned more promptly (99).

Obstruction can be evaluated by means of radionuclide imaging combined with time-activity curve (renogram) analysis using any of the ^{99m}Tc-labeled tracers or OIH. ^{99m}Tc-MAG$_3$ has become the most popular renal imaging agent. The specific findings of obstruction on radionuclide imaging vary as a function of duration and degree. In general, perfusion-phase images can be expected to show some degree of delay and diminished intensity on the affected side with a relatively hypoperfused central region in the presence of significant calyceal and pelvic dilatation. Early parenchymal phase (cortical) images will continue to show this pattern, and there will be a delay in the appearance of tracer in the collecting structures relatively proportional to the severity of the obstruction. Sufficiently delayed images should indicate the level of obstruction in a manner analogous to intravenous urography. Placing the patient in the upright position before delayed images may facilitate this demonstration, by allowing for gravitational drainage. Administration of 500 mL of water before evaluation will lessen the chance of pelvicalyceal retention secondary to dehydration.

In obstruction, the second phase of the renogram is prolonged, indicating impaired cortical transit, and the third, or excretory phase, either fails to fall at the normal rate or, in more severe obstruction, demonstrates a persistently ascending slope (Figs. 42.17 and 42.18).

Acute Versus Chronic Obstruction

In acute obstruction, the perfusion phase of the radionuclide study may show only mildly to moderately delayed and diminished blood flow. Parenchymal-phase images will demonstrate diminished early cortical uptake and a prolonged nephrogram phase. The intensity of cortical activity may eventually equal or exceed the normal. In acute obstruction of brief duration, there may be no appreciable dilatation of the collecting structures, even on sonographic examination. Filling of the collecting structures is delayed in proportion to the severity of obstruction, but these structures should ultimately appear intensely defined.

Prolonged obstruction will result in a progressive loss of renal function. The functional consequences of chronic obstruction are mirrored in sequential radionuclide studies. The perfusion phase will show further delay and even more pronounced diminution of blood flow. Atrophic changes begin in the distal nephron so that the glomerulus is the last portion of the nephron to show histologic damage secondary to obstruction. As chronic damage to the parenchyma progresses, the intensity of activity ultimately reaching the collecting structures diminishes. These findings are clearly mirrored on sequential renograms of severe obstruction, which should show progressive loss of amplitude proportional to the loss of functioning parenchyma (100).

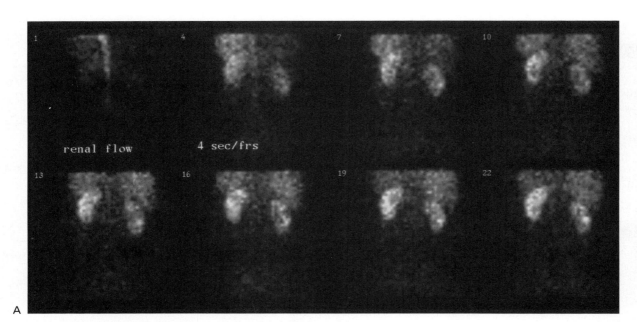

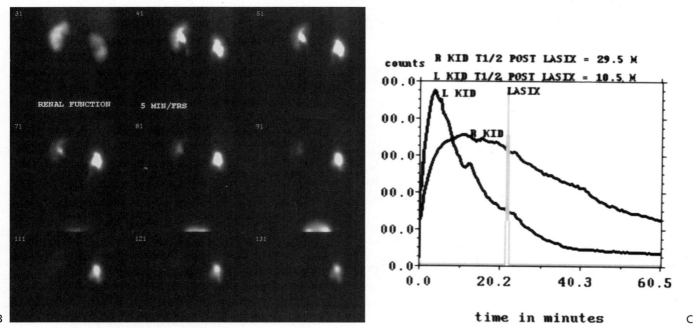

FIGURE 42.17. A–C: Diuretic renal scan demonstrates decreased flow initially to the left kidney and decreased activity in the right collecting system with moderate delay in drainage. The T½ for emptying is 29 minutes and is suggestive of infection.

Complete Versus Incomplete Obstruction

In cases of partial obstruction, renal parenchymal function may be largely preserved even after considerable time. The findings on the perfusion and parenchymal phases of renal imaging will closely approximate normal, although the excretory phase, particularly to the extent that it includes collecting structures, will be prolonged. ERPF may be normal or even increased.

As obstruction becomes more severe, there will be evidence of delayed and diminished blood flow on the perfusion phase of the study and progressively prolonged parenchymal and excretory phases as previously described. The specific characteristics

of the study are a function of both duration and severity. ERPF will diminish with increasingly severe obstruction, and diuretic agents will be progressively less able to accelerate emptying. In rare cases of acute, complete obstruction, the increased intraluminal pressure may cause extravasation and urinoma formation (101).

Nonobstructive Dilatation

Congenital megacalyces, extrarenal pelvis, pelvic duplication, and dilatation from chronic reflux or previous obstruction may

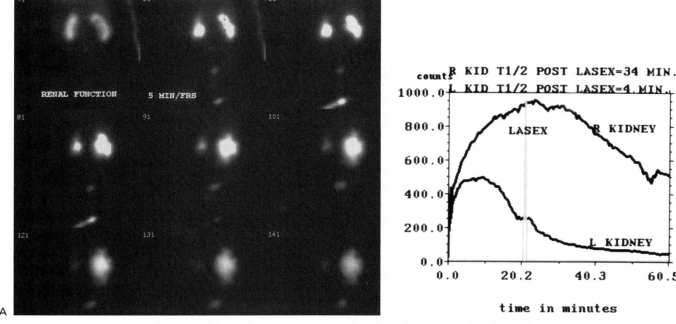

FIGURE 42.18. **A** and **B:** Scan of renogram in a 3-month-old boy with a history of Grade IV hydronephrosis. The renal scan demonstrates initial decrease in the right renal collecting system with markedly delayed washout (*arrow*).

all mimic obstruction on radionuclide images. The pooling of urine in these dilated structures may cause an apparent prolongation of transit time of OIH, a phenomenon that is most often observed in a relatively dehydrated patient, i.e., one whose urine excretion is approximately 0.5 mL/minute and whose urine specific gravity exceeds 1.018. Emptying is characteristically accelerated by diuretics in these patients.

Nonobstructive dilation is characterized by no delay in blood flow to the affected kidney on the perfusion phase of the study, although the amount of cortical perfusion may be reduced proportionally to the amount of parenchymal damage. Cortical transit time is normal, confirming the preservation of parenchymal function. Diuretic renography can successfully distinguish extrarenal pelvis and congenital, postinflammatory, or postobstructive ureterectasis from clinically significant obstruction, as well as evaluate newly reimplanted ureters for postoperative dilatation versus stricture. In the presence of cortical disease severe enough to impair response to the diuretic, however, reliance on conventional delayed imaging may suffice to distinguish obstructive from nonobstructive prolonged drainage (102,103).

INFLAMMATORY LESIONS

A number of unrelated insults to the kidneys result in impaired renal function with or without irreversible parenchymal damage through the mechanism of immunologic or inflammatory response. These insults include infectious processes (pyelonephritis), autoimmune processes (glomerulonephritis), and toxic chemical substances. The resulting renal impairment may be acute or chronic, diffuse or focal, unilateral or bilateral. The fact that alterations in renal function generally precede changes in renal morphology in these processes suggests that radionuclide renal evaluation should be particularly well suited to their early diagnosis. The fact that these processes are mediated through the inflammatory response suggests a complementary role for specialized radiopharmaceuticals (^{67}Ga-citrate, ^{111}In-labeled leukocytes) in both diagnosis and follow-up.

Pyelonephritis and Renal Scarring

Acute pyelonephritis is a major cause of morbidity in children with urinary tract infection, and it can result in irreversible renal scarring, hypertension, hyposthenuria, proteinuria, and chronic renal failure. Hypertension has been reported in 10% to 18% of patients with renal scarring, and renal scarring associated with vesicoureteral reflux accounts for 10% to 20% of patients with end-stage renal disease (104,105). Reflux nephropathy has been used interchangeably with chronic atrophic pyelonephritis and renal scarring. Renal scarring can be prevented or diminished by early diagnosis and treatment of acute pyelonephritis.

The diagnosis of acute pyelonephritis has been traditionally made on the basis of clinical signs and symptoms of fever and flank pain associated with pyuria and positive urine culture. Split ureteral catheterization or bladder washout studies may accurately localize infection to the urinary tract, but they are invasive and do not differentiate pyelitis from parenchymal involvement. Computed tomography (CT) is probably a sensitive and effective technique for documenting the parenchymal involvement. Imaging procedures using ^{67}Ga-citrate or ^{111}In-leukocytes may be reliable in the diagnosis of acute pyelonephritis and may also be helpful in the diagnosis of perinephric abscesses. However, they are not suited for routine use in the evaluation of children. Studies have shown that renal cortical scintigraphy using ^{99m}Tc-DMSA and to a lesser extent GH are significantly more sensitive than intravenous urography and renal sonography in the detection of renal parenchymal involvement (106). The sensitivity and specificity of the DMSA scan for the diagnosis of acute pyelonephritis in piglets were 91% and 99%, respectively, with an overall 97% agreement between the scintigraphic and histopathologic findings (107). Acute pyelonephritis is usually manifested as a single area or multiple areas of varying degrees of decreased cortical uptake of DMSA (Fig. 42.19) with or without bulging contour. Diminished uptake of DMSA in areas of acute inflammation probably reflects both focal tubular cell dysfunction and ischemia. The defect in uptake is not associated with loss of volume, and the lesion occurs mostly in the upper or lower poles. A less common pattern is one of diffusely decreased uptake in an enlarged kidney. Renal cortical scarring is usually the sequela of upper urinary tract infection. Vesicoureteral uptake is often a predisposing factor, although infection of the upper pole may occur in the absence of reflux. Accurate diagnosis of scarring is extremely important to reduce the risk of subsequently developing systemic hypertension and possibly renal impairment (108). A mature cortical scar is usually associated with contraction and loss of volume of the involved cortex. A mature cortical scar has marked reduction in activity as compared with active disease. The DMSA scan may be useful in the acute setting to detect relapse of acute pyelonephritis. Once detected and treatment initiated, however, a follow-up scan should not be performed for 3 to 6 months after initiation of therapy (109). DMSA scans showed acute pyelonephritis in 62 (55%) of 94 patients, and bilateral changes were noted in 12 patients Cortical scarring was present in 14 (15%) patients, and vesicoureteral reflux was demonstrated in 29 (31%) patients.

The Scientific Committee of Radionuclides in Nephrourology surveyed 30 international experts and developed a consensus report (110). This report reinforced the opinion that ^{99m}Tc-MAG$_3$ was the agent of choice for renal cortical scintigraphy. Although Tc-DTPA is not recommended, other tracers such as

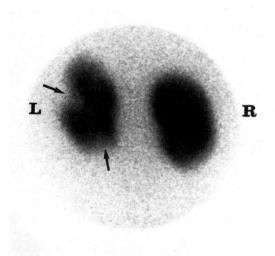

FIGURE 42.19. Dimercaptosuccinic acid scan in a 2-year-old girl with a history of two recent urinary tract infections. The scan shows areas of decreased activity suggesting active infection.

^{99m}Tc-GH and ^{99m}Tc-MAG$_3$ are less favored options. However, a recent study has shown the utility of injection of ^{99m}Tc-MAG$_3$ and furosemide in the detection of focal parenchymal abnormalities. A fast (25 minute) planar dynamic MAG$_3$-furosemide study was found to be as sensitive at depicting focal parenchymal abnormalities in acute pyelonephritis as the 3- to 4-hour routine DMSA scan (111). The recommended minimum dose of ^{99m}Tc-DMSA is 15 to 20 MBq (0.4 to 0.5 mCi) with a maximum adult dose of 110 MBq (3 mCi). Delayed scintigraphy, including differential function determination, is performed at about 3-hours postinjection. The utility of adding single photon emission computed tomography (SPECT) to the imaging protocol has been debated (112). In our experience, SPECT yields an increased number of false positives. This has been supported by a recent study in which DMSA SPECT alone was not shown to be preferable to the established planar methods. A DMSA study is considered abnormal if there is reduced relative function of a kidney and/or decreased or absent uptake of tracer in the renal cortex (111–113).

Glomerulonephritis

Glomerulonephritis is a term applied to a family of diseases that result from antigen-antibody reactions involving the kidneys. Acute glomerulonephritis is predominantly a disease of childhood, usually occurring one to several weeks following a group A β-hemolytic streptococcal infection. It may progress through a nephritic stage to chronic glomerulonephritis or may resolve completely. The kidneys are symmetrically enlarged by interstitial edema, with smooth, hemorrhagic surfaces. In the mild form, GFR, MAG$_3$ clearance, and ERPF may be slightly depressed, ^{99m}Tc-DTPA uptake may be mildly diminished, with prolonged transit time. In the severe and often rapidly progressive form, these changes will be proportionately magnified.

Chronic glomerulonephritis is characterized by renal decompensation and, usually, by hypertension. Most cases are not preceded by documented acute glomerulonephritis. The kidneys are symmetrically small and scarred, with destruction of both glomeruli and tubules, but grossly normal pelvis and calyces. Lymphocytes crowd the interstitium. The radionuclide renal study typically reveals small kidneys with poor perfusion and uptake and strikingly prolonged OIH transit times. ERPF is markedly depressed. ^{111}In-leukocytes are not useful, and ^{67}Ga-citrate imaging has produced variable results.

Interstitial Nephritis

Interstitial nephritis is a nonbacterial inflammatory process that, in its chronic form, is characterized by focal or diffuse fibrosis and that progresses to atrophy of renal tubules. It is a nonspecific reaction to a variety of insults, including analgesic abuse, lead and cadmium toxicity, nephrocalcinosis, urate nephropathy, radiation nephritis, sarcoidosis, Balkan nephritis, and, occasionally, obstructive uropathy. An acute form associated with systemic infections and drug sensitivity may resolve completely. Renal flow is generally well preserved. In addition to the anticipated loss of function on conventional renal imaging, interstitial nephritis has been shown to accumulate ^{67}Ga-citrate or ^{111}In-leukocytes (114).

Pyonephrosis

Pyonephrosis is the end stage of a long-standing obstruction complicated by infection, resulting in total destruction of renal function. The renal scan will show no significant uptake of renal agent.

Furthermore, there may be insufficient viable tissue to accumulate ^{67}Ga, creating the potential for a "false-negative" result.

Abscess

A renal abscess or carbuncle may appear on radionuclide cortical imaging as a focal defect similar to focal pyelonephritis. However, the perfusion phase may show increased activity in the region of an abscess, and either CT or ultrasound will demonstrate a space-occupying lesion. If the abscess is associated with obstruction, there may be diminished ERPF or MAG$_3$ clearance. Abscesses will generally demonstrate focal (possibly peripheral) uptake of gallium on delayed images. Abscess can also occur in renal transplant allografts, and, in these cases, ^{67}Ga-citrate can be extremely useful.

Acute Tubular Necrosis

Acute tubular necrosis (ATN) is an acute form of renal failure that may result from ischemia, circulatory insufficiency, trauma, or exposure to nephrotoxic agents. ATN is associated with generally preserved perfusion but decreased DTPA uptake and prolonged retention of OIH. The pattern seen with MAG$_3$ imaging is generally preservation of flow but prolonged retention and an upsloping renogram (Fig. 42.20). A characteristic disassociation between the handling of DTPA and OIH has been described. Radionuclide imaging is reported to surpass urography in the demonstration of functional impairment in ATN and other causes of acute renal failure.

RENAL TRAUMA

Renal trauma is most commonly the result of blunt or penetrating abdominal trauma, usually as a result of a motor vehicle accident, direct blow, or fall (115).

In approximately 4% of individuals who sustain blunt abdominal trauma, there is associated renovascular injury. The most commonly seen result of trauma is thrombosis. Although hematuria, flank pain, and tenderness are often present, these findings are not always reliable indicators of renal injury. Of patients with gross hematuria after trauma, 25% will have significant renal injuries. However, 24% of patients with renal pedicle injuries do not have gross hematuria. Injuries may result from a direct blow to the kidney, laceration by lower ribs, or tears from rapid acceleration or deceleration. Associated injuries to other organs may be seen in approximately 20% of patients with abdominal trauma (118) (Figs. 42.21 and 42.22).

Previously, diseased kidneys appear to have a higher likelihood of injury. With the advent of percutaneous transluminal angioplasty of the renal arteries, iatrogenic injury to the kidney is seen not infrequently.

Federle has stratified renal injuries into four categories. Category I, which represents about 75% to 85% of all injuries, includes contusions and small corticomedullary lacerations. Category II includes cases with parenchymal lacerations that communicate with the collecting system and are manifested by extravasation of urine. Category III comprises about 5% of renal injuries and includes shattered or fractured kidneys or injuries to the renal pedicle. The final group, Category IV, includes cases with ureteral pelvic junction avulsion and laceration of the renal pelvis. In cases of multiple findings, the category of the most severe finding is presumed (117).

Evaluation of the kidneys in cases of blunt abdominal trauma is important to detect vascular or parenchymal injury. Diagnostic imaging is needed to define the vascular integrity, the extent of renal damage, and associated injuries. For the most part, evaluation of the patient with suspected renal injury is performed in the trauma center setting and includes urography, angiography, or CT (118–120). Renal scintigraphy has some advantages including the speed at which it can be performed, the lack of need for patient preparation, and absence of interference by bowel gas. However, it has generally been replaced by newer technologies in the acute setting. Although many nuclear departments are equipped to do portable renal scans, renal scintigraphy is not commonly performed in the acute setting, because CT, for example, can detect associated injuries in other organs. However, for those patients with mild injury or those with renal fragments who do not undergo surgery, renal scintigraphy provides an excellent vehicle for determining the level of function and the presence of a leak or significant vascular compromise. As differential function and perfusion can be quantitated, renal scintigraphy has advantages in the follow-up assessment. Because Category III and IV patients and those with uncontrolled bleeding usually undergo surgery, Category I patients, and in some instances Category II patients, are ideal candidates for renal scintigraphic evaluation. Flow and function studies using preferably ^{99m}Tc-GHA provide a rapid method for demonstrating the presence and nature of the injury and assessing function. Scintigraphy is also useful in documenting the functioning status of the contralateral kidney, because clinical decisions may be guided by these findings. Another use of renal scintigraphy is in differentiating the causes of abnormalities seen on urography. For example, minor contusions and major vessel occlusions may have similar urographic appearance but markedly different scintigraphic findings. In a series of 24 trauma patients who had both studies, radionuclide imaging demonstrated a sensitivity of 94% with a specificity of 87%, compared with a sensitivity of only 64% (IBP showed 64% sensitivity for detection of renal injury) (122).

Because of the high incidence of associated splenic injuries, some authors recommend the addition of a liver/spleen flow after completion of the renal scan. Although several agents are useful for renal scintigraphy, ^{99m}Tc-GHA has been the most popular because of its ability to detect cortical lesions. ^{99m}Tc-DTPA is fixed less to the cortex and may miss small abnormali-

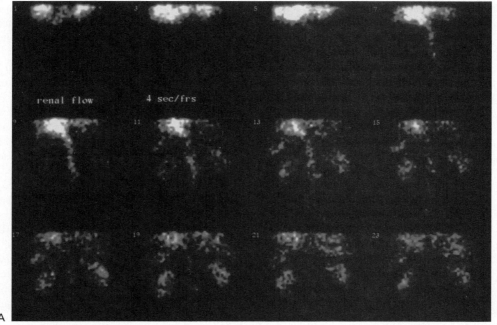

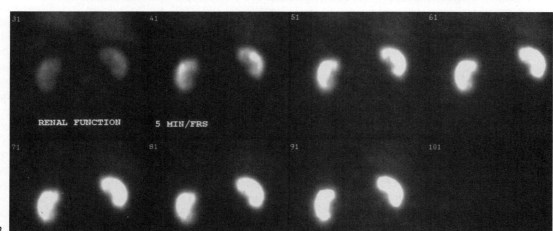

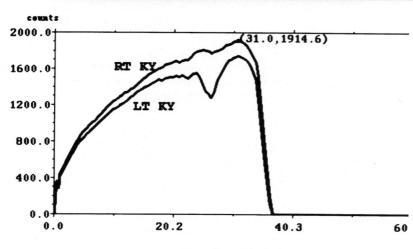

FIGURE 42.20. The flow study demonstrates persistent flow to the kidneys (A) and increasing activity with time on the dynamic images (B). The renogram (C) demonstrates increasing activity within the kidneys.

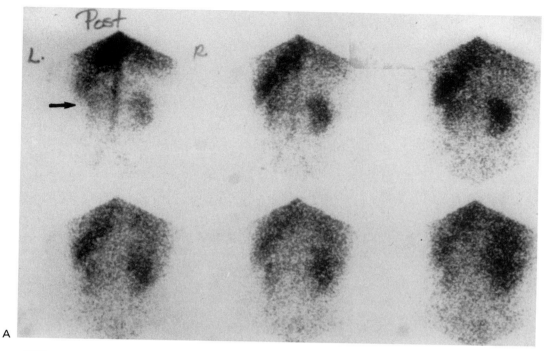

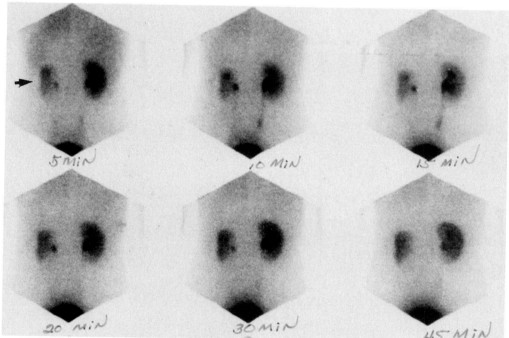

FIGURE 42.21. A: A ^{99m}Tc-diethylenetriaminepentaacetic acid renal flow study showing decreased flow to the shattered left kidney in a patient sustaining a fall. **B:** Dynamic functional images show decreased function of the left kidney. In addition, a small band of decreased activity representing a hematoma is noted (*arrow*). (*Figure continues.*)

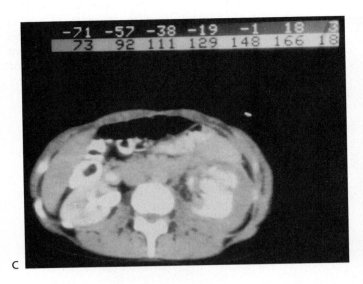

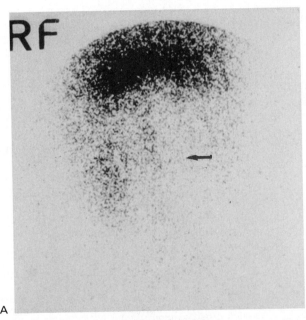

C

FIGURE 42.21. *Continued.* **C:** A computed tomography scan demonstrates the fractured kidney and hematoma (*arrow*).

FIGURE 42.22. **A:** Absence of ^{99m}Tc-diethylenetriaminepentaacetic acid renal perfusion to the right kidney in a child sustaining an intimal tear after a motor vehicle accident. **B:** Absence of function of the right kidney is seen. Note the rim of activity most likely secondary to collateral flow to the renal capsule (*arrows*).

A

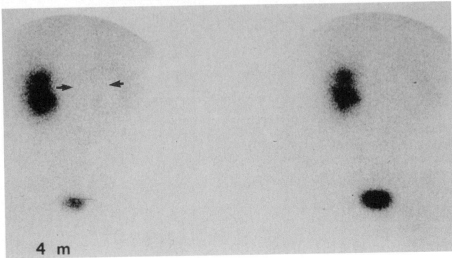

B

ties. Our experience with ^{99m}Tc-MAG$_3$ is mixed. Although cortical defects are readily detected, the relative increase in renal uptake has made detection of leaks more difficult. However, ^{99m}Tc-MAG$_3$ does have its place in imaging of the trauma patient, as discussed later.

A recommended procedure involves placing the camera beneath a patient in the supine position. Images with the patient in the lateral or prone position may also be tried but are generally less informative. An intravenous bolus of 15 mCi ^{99m}Tc-GHA is injected. Sequential flow and static images are obtained. Differential perfusion and function should be determined. The study should be continued until the kidneys, collecting systems, ureters, and bladder have been identified. Anterior images should be obtained to detect anteriorly displaced kidneys, leaks, or hematomas. If the patient is not going immediately to surgery, delayed images should also be obtained. For those patients who cannot be moved or turned, we have found imaging in the anterior projection with ^{99m}Tc-MAG$_3$ somewhat useful in documenting the presence of flow. In addition, in some cases, liver injury may also be detected because this agent often has a fair amount of liver uptake.

Vascular and Parenchymal Injury

Avulsion of the Renal Artery

Avulsion injury to the renal artery or one of its major intrarenal branches must be identified early to prevent loss of the kidney or segment served by the involved branch. In 24% of patients with renal pedicle avulsion, there was no associated gross hematuria (121). If the left kidney is involved, associated injuries to the splenic pedicle are common. In renal vascular pedicle injuries one sees no flow to the kidney. Although any ^{99m}Tc agent will detect absent flow, ^{99m}Tc-GHA is useful in detecting segmental renal artery injury. An extrarenal collection of tracer seen on the perfusion images likely represents bleeding.

Hematoma

Demonstrating the presence of a hematoma may be difficult because typically there is no tracer accumulation in the hematoma unless there is active bleeding during the study, which is very rare. However, unexplained photopenic regions or displacement of the kidney, ureter, or bladder on either the flow or functional images may indicate a hematoma. An intrarenal hematoma presents as a photopenic region within the parenchyma, often with displacement of the collecting system. An anterior or lateral image will help determine the presence of anterior displacement as a cause of poor visualization. A subcapsular hematoma or perirenal hematoma may cause tamponade with resultant nonvisualization; retroperitoneal hematomas can also be detected. Hematoma as a result of an angioplasty attempt may appear as an intrarenal hematoma with displacement or obstruction of the collecting system (Fig. 42.23). A bladder hematoma appears as a "cold" lesion within the bladder. Depending on its size or location within the bladder, it may cause obstruction of the ureter.

Contusion

Contusion can be defined as a bruise or subcapsular hematoma associated with an intact renal capsule. The process involved in contusion may yield significant edema, which may compromise renal function and perfusion. Depending on the severity of contusion varying degrees of decreased global or regional flow or function may be noted (Fig. 42.24). Severe contusion may demonstrate a small functioning kidney, whereas mild contusion may show an enlarged kidney. Cortical defects may be noted in segmental contusion and usually resolve after 3 days. Persistent focal defects are seen in infarction.

Ureteral and Bladder Injury

Avulsion of the ureteropelvic junction is the most common ureteral injury in blunt trauma, with most of these injuries occurring in children and adolescents (118,119). Ureteral injuries can be caused by shearing forces or penetrating injuries or may be iatrogenic as a complication of abdominal surgery. Extravasation of urine is better detected with ^{99m}Tc-GHA or ^{99m}Tc-DTPA. Subtle extravasation may be missed with ^{99m}Tc-MAG$_3$. In addition, excretion of this tracer via the gastrointestinal tract may make identification of a leak difficult. A well-defined extrarenal collection of tracer activity, which appears better visualized with time, is the most current finding. An initial decrease in activity in the involved kidney may be caused by attenuation by nonradioactive urine; as with other renal imaging, anterior and oblique views are often helpful.

Extravasation of urine can be seen anywhere along the urinary tract. There is usually good contrast between the activity in the leak and the peritoneal cavity. Bladder rupture is an uncommon result of trauma and is demonstrated by free activity in the pelvis. With penetrating injury, extravasated activity from the bladder may be seen in scrotum or colon. The good target-to-background ratio provides a potential advantage over urographic contrast studies (120). Tumor may also cause flow abnormalities to a kidney. Focal increased flow may be seen in renal carcinoma. Decreased flow may be seen if there is tumor compression of the renal artery or direct extension of tumor into the vessel (Fig. 42.25).

Radiation Nephritis

The kidney is a radiosensitive organ, and, thus, the dose of radiotherapy to abdominal tumors must be limited. In mouse studies, the LD$_{50}$ for kidneys had been difficult to determine. However, if accumulated deaths up to 16 months are counted, the LD$_{50}$ is about 1,300 rads (122). The major pathologic changes identified are hyperemia and increased capillary permeability with interstitial edema. In humans, up to 6 months from the time of completion of a standard course of radiotherapy, the renal function remains normal. A reduction in renal plasma flow may occasionally occur at doses of 450 rad. Glomerular filtration may be affected when levels exceed 2,000 to 2,400 rads (123). Clinical manifestations of acute radiation nephritis become apparent at 6 to 12 months posttherapy. The pathologic process is actually a nephrosclerosis (124). Symptoms include edema,

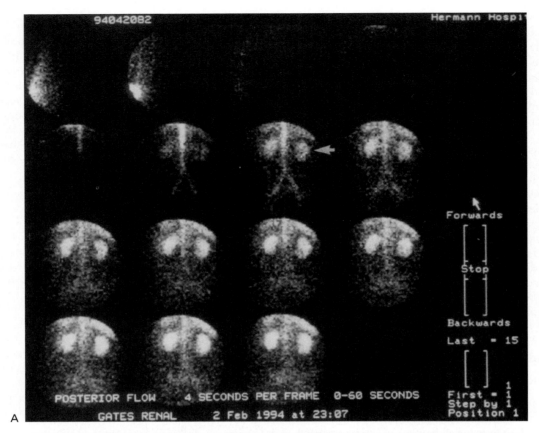

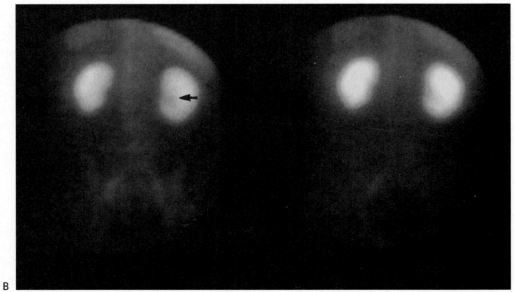

FIGURE 42.23. **A:** This patient was a 65-year-old man in whom incidental renal artery stenosis was discovered during cardiac catheterization. A renal perfusion study with ^{99m}Tc-mercaptoacetylglycine demonstrates decrease right kidney as a complication of percutaneous renal artery angioplasty. **B:** Static images demonstrating a defect resulting from an intrarenal hematoma caused during angioplasty (*arrow*). *(Figure continues.)*

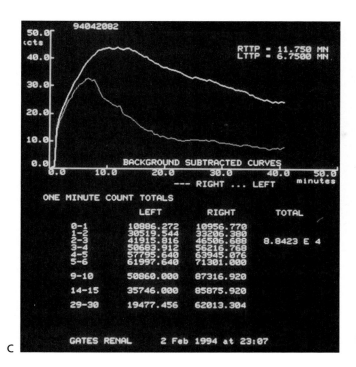

C

FIGURE 42.23. *Continued.* C: Renogram curves showing relatively delayed right renal excretion.

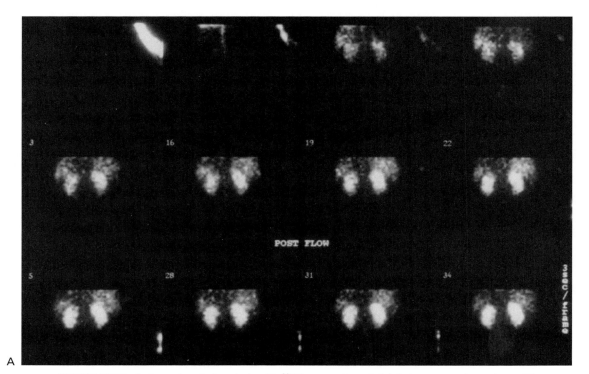

A

FIGURE 42.24. **A:** A renal perfusion study with ^{99m}Tc-mercaptoacetyltriglycine was performed on a 16-year-old boy presenting with hematuria after an auto accident. The renal flow images demonstrates relatively symmetrical flow. However, the flow curve shows a mild decrease in flow to the right kidney. *(Figure continues.)*

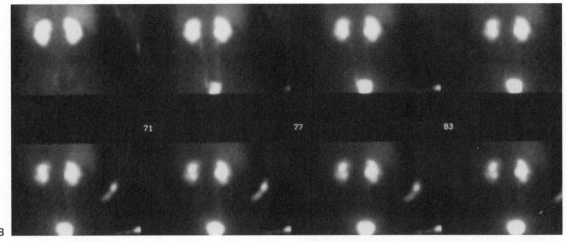

FIGURE 42.24. *Continued.* **B:** Sequential renal function images demonstrate mildly diminished function of the right kidney as evidenced by increasing cortical activity and relatively delayed excretion. A computed tomography scan showed a right psoas abscess and renal contusion.

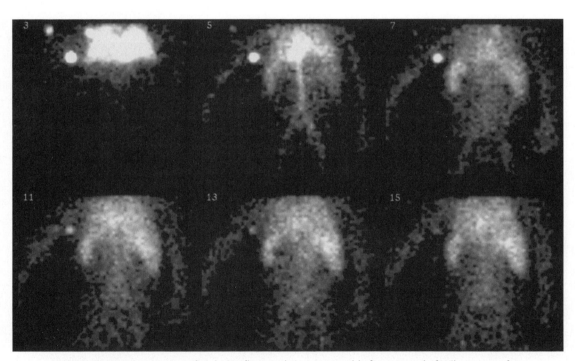

FIGURE 42.25. Mercaptoacetyltriglycine flow study in a 2-year-old after removal of Wilm's tumor from the left kidney. Study demonstrates poor flow to each kidney and near absent function. A tumor mass was removed from the left kidney, but the rest of the kidney was left intact. Reexploration revealed tumor invading the left renal artery but not the right.

hypertension, and proteinuria. The resultant hypertension is responsible for many of the early deaths. The tolerance dose for the adult kidney is in the range of 2,300 rads in 5 weeks to the parenchyma of both kidneys (123,124). Renal damage has been observed, however, after a dose of 1,500 rad over 18 days. Diminished uptake of renal radionuclide tracers has been observed. In addition, retention of bone tracers may also be seen in affected kidneys (125). Chronic nephritis involves anemia, hypertension, and diminution of renal function. Acute cystitis may also develop and may be seen 4 to 6 weeks after radiotherapy. In these cases, renal scanning may show hydroureter. Cystitis is expected after higher doses of radiation such as seen with implants. We have noted several patients with vesicocolic fistulae after bladder radiation.

ACKNOWLEDGMENT

We would like to extend our appreciation to our staff assistants, Catherine Yarborough and Bonnie Schroeder, for their diligence and assistance in the preparation of this chapter.

REFERENCES

1. Brenner BM, Hostetter TH, Humes HD. Molecular basis of proteinuria of glomerular origin. *N Engl J Med* 1978;298:826.
2. Raynaud C. Study of renal cell function by radiotracer fixation. In: Colombetti LG, ed. *Principles of radiopharmacology*, Vol. 3. Boca Raton, FL: CRC Press, 1978:89.
3. Chervu LR, Sandro BM, Blaufox MD. Technetium-99m labeled p-aminohippuric acid analog: A new renal agent. *J Nucl Med* 1984;25:1111–1115.
4. Moran JK. Technetium–99m-EC and other potential new agents in renal nuclear medicine. *Semin Nucl Med* 1999;29:91–101.
5. Bubeck B, Brandau W, Weber E, et al. Pharmacokinetics of Tc-99m MAG_3 in humans. *J Nucl Med* 1990;31:1285–1293.
6. O'Reilly P, Aurell M, Britton K, et al. Consensus on diuresis renography for investigating the dilated upper urinary tract. *J Nucl Med* 1996;37:1872–1876.
7. El-Galley R, Clarke HS, O'Brien DP, Taylor A. Normal parameters for Tc-99m MAG_3 renography. *J Nucl Med* 1998;39:87.
8. Russell CD, Taylor T, Dubovsky EV. Measurement of renal function with Tc-99m MAG_3 in children and adults. *J Nucl Med* 1996;37:588–593.
9. Stabin M, Taylor T Jr, Eshima D, Wooter W. Radiation dosimetry for Tc-99m MAG_3, Tc-99m DTPA, and I-131 OIH based on human biodistribution studies. *J Nucl Med* 1992;33:33–40.
10. Kabasakal L, Atay S, Vural AV, et al. Evaluation of Tc-99m L, L-ethylenedicysteine in renal disorders and determination of extraction ratio. *J Nucl Med* 1995;36:1398–1403.
11. Kahn PC, Dewanjec MK, Brown SS. Routine renal imaging after ^{99m}Tc-glucoheptonate brain scans. *J Nucl Med* 1976;17:786.
12. Valic-Razumenic N, Petrovic J. Biochemical studies of the renal radiopharmaceutical compound dimercaptosuccinate. II. Subcellular localization of the Tc-99m DMS complex in the rat kidney in vivo. *Eur J Nucl Med* 1982;7:304.
13. Bueschen AJ, Witten DM. Radionuclide evaluation of renal function. *Urol Clin North Am* 1979;6:307.
14. Blaufox MD, Aurell M, Bubeck B, et al. Report of the radionuclides in nephrology committee on renal clearance. *J Nucl Med* 1996;37:1883–1890.
15. Klingensmith WC, Briggs DE, Smith WI. Tc-99m MAG_3 renal studies: normal range and reproducibility of physiologic parameters as a function of age and sex. *J Nucl Med* 1994;35:1612–1617.
16. Taylor A, Lewis C, Giacometti A, et al. Improved formulas for the estimation of renal depth in adults. *J Nucl Med* 1993;34:1766–1769.
17. Hvid-Jacobsen K, Thomsen HS, Nielsen SL. Diuresis renography. A simultaneous comparison between ^{131}I-hippuran and $^{99}Tc^m$-MAG_3. *Acta Radiol* 1990;31:83–86.
18. Li Y, Russell CD, Palmer-Lawrence J, Dubovsky EV. Quantitation of renal parenchymal retention of Tc-99m MAG_3 in renal transplants. *J Nucl Med* 1994;35:846–850.
19. El-Galley R, Clarke HS, O'Brien DP, Taylor A. Normal parameters for Tc-99m MAG_3 renography. *J Nucl Med* 1998;39:87.
20. DeKlerk JMH, Beutler JJ, Van Isselt JW, et al. Aspirin versus captopril renography in the diagnosis of renal artery stenosis. *J Nucl Med* 1996;37:289 (abst).
21. Curtis JJ, Lupe RG, Dustan HP, et al. Remission of essential hypertension after renal transplantation. *N Engl J Med* 1983;309:1009–1015.
22. Pinea GF, Thorndyke WC, Steed BL. Spontaneous renal artery thrombosis: successful lysis with a streptokinase. *J Urol* 1987;138:1223–1225.
23. Gasparini M, Hofman R, Stoller M. Renal artery embolism: clinical features and therapeutic options. *J Urol* 1992;147:567–572.
24. Theiss MP, Dolken W et al. Spontaneous thrombosis of the renal vessels. *Urol Int* 1992;48:441–445.
25. Wiggelinkhuizen J, Oleszczuk-Raszke K, Nagel FO. Renal venous thrombosis in infancy. *S Afr Med J* 1989;75:413–416.
26. Petronis J. Renal Imaging findings in renal vein thrombosis: a note of caution. *Clin Nucl Med* 1989;14:654–656.
27. Keating MA and Althausen AF. The clinical spectrum of renal vein thrombosis. *J Urol* 1985;133:938–945.
28. Sfakianakis GN, Sfakianakis ED. Nuclear medicine in pediatric urology and nephrology. *J Nucl Med* 1988;29:1287–1300.
29. Delbeke D, Sacks GA, Sandler MP. Diagnosis of allograft renal vein thrombosis. *Clin Nucl Med* 1989;14:415–420.
30. Working Group on Renovascular Hypertension. Detection, evaluation and treatment of renovascular hypertension. *Arch Int Med* 1987;147:80–89.
31. Davidson RA, Wilcox CS. Newer tests for the diagnosis of renovascular disease. *JAMA* 1992;268:3353–3358.
32. Baldwin DS, Van den Brock H, Harnes JR et al. Renovascular hypertension in unselected patients. *Arch Intern Med* 1967;120:176–179.
33. Horvath JS, Waugh RC, Tiller DJ et al. The detection of renovascular hypertension: A study on 490 patients by renal angiography. *Q J Med* 1982;51:139–146.
34. Dean RH. Renovascular hypertension. *Curr Prob Surg* 1985;22:6–67.
35. Katial R, Zeissman HA. Segmental branch renal artery stenosis diagnosed with captopril renography. *J Nucl Med* 1992;33:266–268.
36. Guzetta PC, Davis CF, Ruley EJ. Experience with bilateral renal artery stenosis as a cause of hypertension in childhood. *J Ped Surg* 1991;26:532–534.
37. Holly KE, Hunt JC, Brown AL et al. Renal artery stenosis: a clinical pathologic study of normotensive and hypertensive patients. *Am J Med* 1964;37:14–22.
38. Dunnick NR, Sfakianakis GN. Screening for renovascular hypertension. *Radiol Clin North Am* 1991;29:497–510.
39. Roubidoux MA, Dunnick NR, Klotman PE et al. Renal vein renins: inability to predict response to revascularization in hypertensive patients. *Radiology* 1991;178:819–822.
40. Meier GH, Sumpio B, Setaro JF et al. Captopril renal scintigraphy: a new standard for predicting outcome after renal revascularization. *J Vasc Surg* 1993;17:280–287.
41. Larar GN, Treves ST. Accelerated renovascular hypertension following angioplasty: Assessment of therapy by 99m-Tc-DMSA imaging. *Clin Nucl Med* 1993;18:278–280.
42. Helmchen U, Ulrich O. Benign and malignant nephrosclerosis and renovascular disease. In: Tisher CC, Brenner BM, eds. *Renal pathology: with clinical and functional correlations*. Philadelphia: JB Lippincott, 1994:1223–1225.
43. Lewin A, Blaufox D, Castle H. Apparent prevalence of curable hypertension in the hypertension detection and follow-up program. *Arch Intern Med* 1985;245:424–427.
44. Tulchinsky M, Eggli DF, Waybill PN et al. Diagnosis of renovascular

hypertension: nuclear medicine techniques. *Appl Radiol* 1993;22: 13–20.

45. Goncharenko V, Gerlock AJ, Shaff MI et al. Progression of renal artery fibromuscular dysplasia in 42 patients as seen on angiography. *Radiology* 1981;139:45–51.
46. Svetkey LP, Wilkinson R, Dunnick NR et al. Captopril renography in the diagnosis of renovascular disease. *AJH* 1991;4:711S–715S.
47. Soulez G, Oliva VL, Turpin S et al. Imaging of renovascular hypertension: respective values of renal scintigraphy, renal Doppler US and MR angiography. *RadioGraphics* 2000;20:1355–1368.
48. Nortier J, Wautrecht JC, Delcour C et al. Role of the captopril test in renovascular hypertension: A case report. *Angiol* 1992;43:939–945.
49. Brown JJ, Davies DL, Morton JJ et al. Mechanisms of renal hypertension. *Lancet* 1976;1:1219–1221.
50. Foster JH, Dean RH, Pinkerton JA et al. Ten years' experience with the surgical management of renovascular hypertension. *Ann Surg* 1973;177:755–766.
51. Dean RH, Kreuger TC, Whiteneck JM et al. Operative management of renovascular hypertension: results after a follow-up of fifteen to twenty-three years. *J Vasc Surg* 1984;1:234–242.
52. Sfakianakis GN, Bourgoignie JJ, Georgiou M et al. Diagnosis of renovascular hypertension with ACE inhibition scintigraphy. *Radiol Clin North Am* 1993;31:831–848.
53. Hillman BJ. Imaging advances in the diagnosis of renovascular hypertension. *Am J Radiol* 1989;153:5–14.
54. Leung DA, Hoffman U, Pfammatter T et al. Magnetic resonance angiography versus duplex sonography for diagnosing renovascular disease. *Hypertension* 1999;33:726–731.
55. Kent KC, Edelman R, Kim D et al. Magnetic resonance imaging: a reliable test for the evaluation of proximal atherosclerotic renal artery stenosis. *J Vasc Surg* 1991;13:311–318.
56. Svetkey LP, Himmelstein SI, Dunnick NR et al. Prospective analysis of strategies for diagnosing renovascular hypertension. *Hypertension* 1989;14:247–257.
57. Kim D, Edelman RR, Kent KC et al. Abdominal aorta and renal artery stenosis: evaluation with MR angiography. *Radiology* 1990;174: 727–731.
58. Pape JF, Gudmundsen TE, Pedersen HK. Renal angiography may be used originally in the diagnosis of renovascular hypertension. *Scan J Urol Nephrol* 1988;22:41–44.
59. Taylor A, Nally J, Aurell M et al. Consensus report on ACE inhibitor renography for detecting renovascular hypertension. *J Nucl Med* 1996; 37:1876–1882.
60. Taylor A, Fletcher JW, Nally JV et al. Procedure guidelines for diagnosis of renovascular hypertension. *J Nucl Med* 1998;39:1297–1302.
61. Goldblatt H, Lunch J, Henzel RG et al. Studies on experimental hypertension: the production of persistent elevation of systolic blood pressure by means of renal ischemia. *J Exp Med* 1934;59:347–380.
62. Tigerstedt R, Bergman P. Nieure und Kreislauf. *Arch Physiol* 1898; 8:223–271.
63. Gauthier B, Trachtman H, Frank R et al. Inadequacy of captopril challenge test for diagnosing renovascular hypertension in children and adolescents. *Pediatr Nephrol* 1991;5:42–44.
64. Katial R, Ziessman HA. Segmental branch renal artery stenosis diagnosed with captopril renography. *J Nucl Med* 1992;33:266–268.
65. Majd M, Potter BM, Guzzetta PC et al. Effect of captopril on efficacy of renal scintigraphy in detection of renal artery stenosis. *J Nucl Med* 1983;24:23(abst).
66. Mann SL, Pickering TG, Sos TA et al. Captopril renal scintigraphy in the diagnosis of renal artery stenosis: accuracy and limitations. *Am J Med* 1991;90:30.
67. Datseris IE, Bomani JB, Brown EA et al. Captopril renal scintigraphy in patients with hypertension and chronic renal failure. *J Nucl Med* 1994;5:521–524.
68. Blaufox MD. The role and rationale of nuclear medicine procedures in the differential diagnosis of renovascular hypertension. *Nucl Med Biol* 1991;18:583–587.
69. Sfakianakis GN, Bourgoignie JJ. Renographic diagnosis of renovascular hypertension with angiotensin-converting enzyme inhibition and furosemide. *Am J Hypertens* 1991;4:70S–71S.
70. Eggli DF, Tulchinsky M. Scintigraphic evaluation of pediatric urinary tract infection. *Semin Nucl Med* 1993;23:199–218.
71. Hansen PB, Garsdal P, Fruergaard P. The captopril test for identification of renovascular hypertension: value and immediate adverse effects. *J Int Med* 1990;228:159–163.
72. Erbsloh-Moller B, Dumas A, Roth D et al. Furosemide-131-1-hippuranrenography after angiotensin-converting enzyme inhibition for diagnosis of renovascular hypertension. *Am J Med* 1991;90:23–29.
73. Kubo SH, Cody RJ, Laragh JH et al. Immediate converting-enzyme inhibition with intravenous enalapril in chronic congestive heart failure. *Am J Cardiol* 1985;55:122–126.
74. Setaro JF, Chen CC, Hoffer PB et al. Captopril renography in the diagnosis of renal artery stenosis and prediction of improvement with revascularization. *Am J Hypertens* 1991;4:S698–S705.
75. Shamlou KK, Drane WE, Hawkins IF et al. Captopril renography and the hypertensive renal transplantation patient: a predictive test of therapeutic outcome. *Radiology* 1994;190:153–159.
76. Sakianakis GN, Bourgoignie JJ, Jaffe D et al. Single dose captopril scintigraphy in the diagnosis of renovascular hypertension. *J Nucl Med* 1987;28:1383–1392.
77. Itoh K, Tsukamoto E, Nagao K et al. Captopril renal scintigraphy with 99m-Tc DTPA in patients with suspected renovascular hypertension: prospective and retrospective evaluation. *Clin Nucl Med* 1993;18:463–471.
78. Meier GH, Sumpio B, Black HR et al. Captopril renal scintigraphy—an advance in the detection and treatment of renovascular hypertension. *J Vasc Surg* 1990;11:770–777.
79. Kopecky RT, Thomas FD, McAfee JG. Furosemide augments the effects of captopril on nuclear studies in renovascular stenosis. *Hypertension* 1987;10:181–188.
80. Oei HY. Captopril renography. Early observations and diagnostic criteria. *Am J Hypertens* 1991;4:678S.
81. Nally JJ, Chen C, Fine E et al. Diagnostic criteria of renovascular hypertension with captopril renography. A consensus statement. *Am J Hypertens* 1991;4:749S–752S.
82. Roccatello D, Picciotto G, Rabbia C et al. Prospective study on captopril renography in hypertensive patients. *Am J Nephrol* 1992;12: 406–411.
83. Patrois F, Hignette C, Froissart M et al. Interpretation de la scintigraphy renale avec prise de captopril: a propos d'un faux positif bilateral. *Med Nucl* 1995;13:303–313.
84. Taylor A, Nally JV. Clinical applications of renal scintigraphy. *Am J Roentgenol* 1995;164:31–41.
85. Klingensmith WC III, Briggs DE, Smith WI. Technetium 99m-MAG$_3$ renal studies: normal range and reproducibility of physiologic parameters as a function of age and sex. *J Nucl Med* 1994;35: 1612–1617.
86. Chen CC, Hoffer PB, Vahjen G et al. Patients at high risk for renal artery stenosis: a simple method of renal scintigraphic analysis with 99m-DTPA and captopril. *Radiology* 1990;176:365–370.
87. Fine EJ, Li Y, Blaufox MD. Parenchymal mean transit time analysis of 99mTc-DTPA captopril renography. *J Nucl Med* 2000;41: 1627–1631.
88. Henrich WL. Role of prostaglandins in renin secretion. *Kidney Int* 1981;19:822–830.
89. Fine EJ. Interventions in renal scintirenography. *Semin Nucl Med* 1999;29:128–145.
90. Imanishi M, Kawamura M, Akabane S et al. Aspirin lowers blood pressure in patients with renovascular hypertension. *Hypertension* 1989;14:461–468.
91. van de Ven PJG, de Klerk JMH, Mertens JR et al. Aspirin renography and captopril renography in the diagnosis of renal artery stenosis. *J Nucl Med* 2000;41:1337–1342.
92. Olsen ME, Hall JE, Montani JP, Cornell JE. Interaction between renal prostaglandins and angiotensin I in controlling glomerular filtration in the dog. *Clin Sci* 1878;72:429–436.
93. Milot A, Lambert R, Lebel M et al. Prostaglandins and renal function in hypertensive patients with unilateral renal artery stenosis and patients with essential hypertension. *J Hypertens* 1996;14:765–771.
94. Gruenwald SM, Nimmon CC, Nawaz MK et al. A non-invasive

gamma camera technique for the measurement of intrarenal blood flow distribution in man. *Clin Sci* 1981;61:385–389.

95. Clorius JH, Schmidlin P. The exercise renogram: a new approach documents renal involvement in systemic hypertension. *J Nucl Med* 1987;10:280–286.

96. Clorius JH, Reingold F, Hupp T et al. Renovascular hypertension: a perfusion disturbance that escaped recognition. *J Nucl Med* 1993; 34:48–56.

97. Naidich JB, Rackson, ME, Mossey RT et al. Nondilated obstructive uropathy: percutaneous nephrostomy performed to reverse renal failure. *Radiology* 1986;160:653–657.

98. Dowling KH, Harmon EP, Ortenberg J et al. Ureteropelvic junction obstruction: the effect of pyeloplasty on renal function. *J Urol* 1988; 140:1227–1230.

99. Fujita K, Nakuchi K, Matsumoto K. Correlation between radioisotope renographic findings and results after relief of ureteral obstruction. *J Urol* 1972;107:23.

100. Bueschen AJ, Lloyd LK, Dubovsky E. Radionuclide kidney function evaluation in the management of urolithiasis. *J Urol* 1978;120:16.

101. Powers TA, Grove, RB, Bauriedel JK. Detection of uropathy using 99mtechnetium diethylenetriamine penta-acetic acid. *J Urol* 1980; 120:16.

102. Thrall JH, Koff SA, Keyes JW. Diuretic radionuclide renography and scintigraphy in the differential diagnosis of hydroureteronephrosis. *Semin Nucl Med* 1981;11:89.

103. Kroger RP, Ash JM, Silver M. Primary hydronephrosis: assessment of diuretic renography, pelvis perfusion pressure, operative findings, and renal and ureteral history. *Urol Clin North Am* 1980;7:231.

104. Jacobson SH, Eklof O, Eriksson CG et al. Development of hypertension and uremia after pyelonephritis in childhood: 27-year followup. *Br Med J* 1989;299:703.

105. Senekjian HO, Suki WN. Vesicoureteral reflux and reflux nephropathy. *Am J Nephrol* 1982;2:245.

106. Sty JR, Wells RG, Starshak RJ et al. Imaging in acute renal. Infection in children. *AJR* 1987;148:471–477.

107. Rossleigh MA. Renal cortical scintigraphy and diuresis renography in infants and children. *J Nucl Med* 2001;42:91–95.

108. Piepsz A, Blaufox MD, Gordon I et al. Consensus on renal cortical scintigraphy in children with urinary tract infection. *Semin Nucl Med* 1999;29:160–174.

109. Goldraich NP, Goldraich IH. Update on DMSA renal scanning in children with urinary tract infection. *Pediatr Nephrol* 1995;9: 221–226.

110. Sfakianakis GN, Cavagnaro F, Zilleruelo G et al. Diuretic MAG$_3$ scintigraphy (Fo) in acute pyelonephritis: regional parenchymal dysfunction and comparison with DMSA. *J Nucl Med* 2000;41: 1955–1963.

111. Majd M, Rushton HG, Chandra R et al. Technetium 99m-DMSA renal cortical scintigraphy to detect experimental acute pyelonephritis in piglets: a comparison of planar (pinhole) and SPECT imaging. *J Nucl Med* 1996;37:1731–1734.

112. Craig JC, Wheeler DM, Irwig L et al. How accurate is dimercaptosuccinic acid scintigraphy for the diagnosis of acute pyelonephritis? A meta-analysis of Experimental Studies. *J Nucl Med* 2000;41;986–993.

113. Wiyanto R, Testa HJ, Shields RA et al. Assessment of renal function and scarring: is a DMSA scan always necessary? *Contrib Nephrol* 1987; 56:250–255.

114. Wood BC, Sharma JN, Germann DR. Gallium citrate GA-67 imaging in noninfectious interstitial nephritis. *Arch Intern Med* 1978;138: 1665.

115. Rosenthal L, Ammann W. Renal trauma. *Sem Nuc Med* 1983;XIII: 238–244.

116. Kaufman JJ, Dinerstein, CR, Shah DM et al. Renal artery intimal flaps after blunt trauma: Indications for nonoperative therapy. *Urology* 1989;34:62–64.

117. Federle M. Evaluation of renal trauma. In: Pollack HM, ed. *Clinical urography.* Philadelphia: WB Saunders, 1989:1472–1494.

118. Flax S, McLorie G, Churchill BM et al. A comparative study of intravenous urograms and radionuclide renal scans in diagnosis of renal trauma. *Urology* 1989;34:62–64.

119. Pjura GA, Lowry P, Kim EE. Radiologic imaging of the upper urinary tract. In: Gottschalk A, ed. *Diagnostic nuclear medicine.* Baltimore: Williams & Wilkins, 1983:657–658.

120. Toporoff B, Scalea TM, Abramson D et al. Ureteral laceration caused by a fall from a height: Case report and review of the literature. *J Trauma* 1993;34:164–166.

121. Chopp RT, Hekmat-Ravan H, Mendez R. Technetium-99m-glucoheptonate renal scan in the diagnosis of acute renal injury. *Urology* 1980;15:201–206.

122. Hall EJ. Dose-response relationships for normal tissues. In: Hall EJ, ed. *Radiobiology for the radiobiologist,* 3rd ed. Philadelphia: JB Lippincott, 1988:64.

123. Mettler FA, Moseley RD. In: Mettler and Moseley, eds. *Medical effects of Ionizing radiation.* Orlando, FL: Grune & Stratton, 1985:155–156.

124. Fajardo LF. *Pathology of radiation injury.* New York: Masson, 1982.

125. Luxton RW, Kunkler PB. Radiation nephritis. *Acta Radiol* 1964;2: 169–178.

43

SCROTAL SCINTIGRAPHY

JOHN E. FREITAS

Since its introduction in 1973, scrotal scintigraphy (SS) has proven clinically useful in the evaluation of acute scrotal pain, a potential urologic emergency requiring accurate diagnosis and possible, prompt surgical management (1). The differential diagnosis of acute scrotal pain is broad, but a focused, simultaneous history and physical examination and subsequent urinalysis allow the definitive diagnosis to be made quickly in most patients. However, if the patient's presentation is nonspecific and his physical examination is limited by pain, tenderness, and swelling, the clinician finds SS useful in the differential diagnosis.

How common are testicular disorders? Surprisingly, there is a dearth of information. Testicular torsion incidence is approximately 1 in 4,000 males less than age 25 years with a peak incidence at puberty, but testicular torsion is seen in early childhood and in adults (2–4). By comparison, inflammatory scrotal disorders are at least three to five times more common than torsion. Although testicular trauma is said to be common, a 2-year national sample of 6,229 college football players noted only 4 testicular injuries out of 2,820 injuries, and another sports injury study of 7,468 school children (ages 8 to 18 years) noted no scrotal or testicular injuries (5,6). The yearly incidence of testicular cancer in the United States is only 3.4 per 100,000 men with the peak occurring between 25 to 30 years of age, but it can be difficult to distinguish from the more common benign scrotal mass, which may be intratesticular or extratesticular in location (7). To achieve the best interpretive accuracy, the imager must understand scrotal anatomy, physiology, and optimal scintigraphic technique.

ANATOMY

The scrotum is a two compartment cutaneous pouch composed of skin, a firmly adherent smooth muscle layer (dartos), and a connective tissue layer containing some striated muscle (cremaster). The scrotum is divided into its two compartments by a dartos septum with each compartment containing an ovoid testis

approximately 3 cm in diameter and 4 cm in length (Fig. 43.1). Each testis is enclosed by the tunica albuginea, a dense fibrous capsule, which radiates septa that divide the testis into roughly 250 lobules containing three to four seminiferous tubules each. These tubules coalesce to form the rete testis, a network of channels contained within the testicular mediastinum. The rete testis is connected by 10 to 15 efferent ducts to the epididymis, a semilunar structure firmly attached to the posterolateral testicular surface by the mesorchium and continuous inferiorly with the ductus deferens (spermatic duct). The anterior and lateral surfaces of the testis are enveloped by the tunica vaginalis comprised of two opposing tissue layers that form a serous cavity about the testis. Normally, the epididymis is firmly adherent to the scrotal wall between the reflections of the tunica vaginalis and is suspended with the testis in the scrotum by the spermatic cord containing the testicular blood supply and the spermatic duct (Fig. 43.2). However, if the tunica vaginalis completely envelopes the testis and epididymis ("bellclapper" anomaly), their more transverse orientation allows rotation freely around the axis of the spermatic cord and predisposes to spermatic cord torsion. Two of the four testicular appendages, the appendix testis and epididymis, are pedunculated and can torse mimicking testicular torsion.

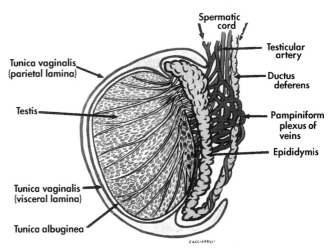

FIGURE 43.1. Anatomy of the normal testicle. (From Noujaim SE, Nagel CE. Acute scrotal injuries in athletes: evaluation by diagnostic imaging. *Phys Sports Med* 1989;17:125–133, with permission. Illustration by Alexander Cacciarelli, MD.)

J.E. Freitas: Radiology Department, University of Michigan Medical School, Ann Arbor, MI, and Radiology Department, St. Joseph Mercy Hospital, Ypsilanti, MI.

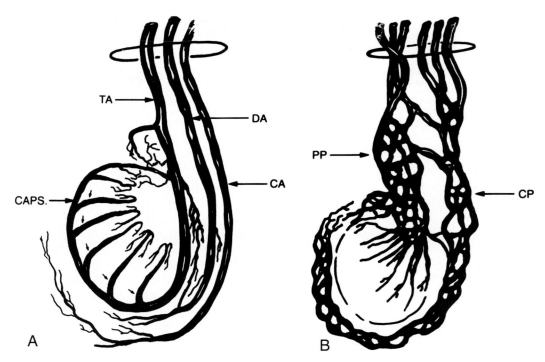

FIGURE 43.2. **A:** Arterial supply to the scrotum. **B:** Venous drainage of the scrotum. TA, testicular artery; DA, deferential artery; CA, cremasteric artery; CAPS, capsular artery; PP, pampiniform venous plexus; CP, cremasteric venous plexus. (From Nagle CE, Freitas JE: Scrotal imaging. In: Sandler MP, Patton JA, Gross MD, et al., eds. *Endocrine imaging.* Norwalk, CT: Appleton & Lange, 1992:377–403, with permission.)

The testicular artery arises from the abdominal aorta just distal to the renal arteries and joins the spermatic cord at the deep inguinal ring. Within the spermatic cord, the testicular artery parallels the ipsilateral cremasteric and deferential arteries before penetrating the tunica albuginea to form the capsular artery and its centripetal branches that course in the interlobular septa to the mediastinum. Although anastomoses exist, the testicular artery supplies primarily the testis, the deferential artery supplies the spermatic duct and epididymis, and the cremasteric artery supplies the tunica vaginalis. Scrotal venous outflow is through the pampiniform plexus and cremasteric plexus draining into the ipsilateral testicular vein. The right testicular vein empties directly into the inferior vena cava, and the left testicular vein drains into the left renal vein. Testicular innervation derives from the internal spermatic plexus consisting of sympathetic postganglionic fibers and visceral afferent fibers accompanying the testicular artery. Sensory nerve endings are present in the scrotum, tunica albuginea, epididymis, and spermatic cord contents.

SCROTAL SCINTIGRAPHY

SS is a rapid, noninvasive, highly accurate technique for evaluation of acute scrotal presentations if there is careful positioning of the scrotum and acquisition of motion-free high quality images and the images are correlated with palpatory findings (8). The patient lies supine, legs slightly abducted, with his scrotum elevated on a tape sling or towel between the legs. The penis is taped cephalad to remove its vascularity from the scrotal images. If there is marked asymmetric scrotal swelling, realignment of the median raphe of the scrotum by gentle traction using paper tape applied to the enlarged hemiscrotum and ipsilateral thigh is important (9). For pediatric patients, a gamma-camera with a converging collimator is preferred but a parallel-hole collimator should suffice if a magnification mode acquisition is performed. Most centers perform SS as a dynamic flow study followed by static images. With the camera positioned over the scrotum, 15 to 20 mCi of ^{99m}Tc pertechnetate is bolus injected intravenously in adults with proportional fractionation for pediatric patients. Sequential 2- to 5-second flow images are obtained for the first 60 seconds, followed by an immediate static image (300,000 to 500,000 counts/image). Before acquiring the static images, some centers use lead shields to narrow the field of interest surrounding the genitalia, to block bladder activity, or, when placed beneath the scrotum, to block underlying thigh activity. A thin, metal strip may be placed over the median raphe to delineate the right and left hemiscrotum (Fig. 43.3). Pinhole static images in prepubertal boys magnify the scrotal contents for better interpretation, but any motion markedly degrades image quality. Any delay in obtaining the static image should be avoided because of increasing bladder activity and body background. A typical study can be completed in 20 minutes.

CLINICAL APPLICATION

Acute scrotal disorders can be divided into those that involve the sac and those that involve scrotal contents (Table 43.1) (10).

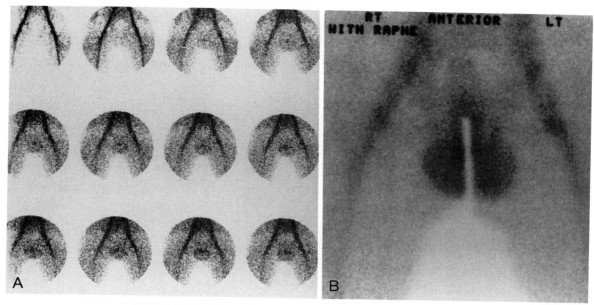

FIGURE 43.3. **A:** Normal testicular flow study. **B:** Normal static image.

Testicular torsion is the most common disorder evaluated by SS. Other acute disorders causing immediate anatomic changes, such as testicular fracture, hematoma, hydrocele, or other traumatic injuries, are best evaluated by real-time ultrasound (RTUS) or magnetic resonance imaging, whereas inflammatory processes, such as epididymitis or orchitis, may be diagnosed by SS, RTUS, or color doppler ultrasound. The SS patterns in the angiogram flow and static tissue phases are well established for most acute scrotal disorders.

Testicular Torsion

Most patients with acute torsion have a congenital anomaly of testicular suspension or attachment that allows the spermatic cord to twist on itself, occluding initially venous outflow and then arterial inflow (11). Testicular edema and congestion rapidly develop, followed by hemorrhage, and finally infarction if the torsion persists. The degree of pampiniform plexus twisting

Table 43.1. *Acute Scrotal Disorders*[a]

Scrotal Sac Lesions	Intrascrotal Lesions
Hematoma	Acute hydrocele
Idiopathic edema	Hemorrhagic testicular infarction
Scrotitis	Intravaginal spermatic cord torsion
Scrotal gangrene	Testicular appendage torsion
Scrotal peritonitis	Acute viral orchitis
Henoch-Schonlein purpura	Acute bacterial epididymitis
	Testicular tumor
	Testicular trauma
	Incarcerated scrotal hernia
	Testicular vasculitis
	Scrotal vein thrombosis
	Varicocele

[a]Modified from Witherington R. The acute scrotum: lesions that require immediate attention. *Postgrad Med* 1987;82(1):207–216, with permission.

and the duration of impaired blood flow are the major determinants of testicular viability. With three or more complete spermatic cord rotations, testicular infarction ensues within 2 hours, whereas a single 360-degree twist permits testicular viability for 12 to 24 hours. Surgical testicular salvage rates vary from 20% to 90% and are inversely related to symptom duration. Experimentally, there is 100% testicular viability if detorsion occurs within 3 hours, 10% to 20% viability at 24 hours or less, and rare viability beyond 24 hours (11,12). Although testicular viability is present, ischemic injury results in volume loss in the affected testicle and a decrease in spermatogenesis in greater than 50% of affected men (13,14).

The patient with testicular torsion most often presents with abrupt, severe hemiscrotal pain associated with nausea and vomiting but without fever or urinary tract symptoms. Mild discomfort lasting 1 to 3 days is more suggestive of testicular appendage torsion but should not exclude testicular torsion with spontaneous detorsion. Physical examination usually reveals an edematous hemiscrotum with an enlarged, tender testis that may be high in the scrotum, but these findings are not pathognomonic. At least half of the patients have had a previous similar episode that spontaneously resolved, and more than half of the patients demonstrate an elevated transverse-positioned testis in the contralateral hemiscrotum when examined in the erect position. If the diagnosis of testicular torsion is established, immediate surgical intervention is warranted without waiting for confirmatory imaging studies. When the diagnosis is uncertain and surgical intervention is questioned, imaging studies should be rapidly obtained.

The SS pattern of testicular torsion varies with symptom duration. In those symptomatic for a few hours, the flow study may or may not show decreased perfusion to the symptomatic testicle but testicular nonperfusion is confirmed on the static images by the presence of a photopenic defect (Fig. 43.4). If untreated, infarction (early missed torsion) occurs and induces

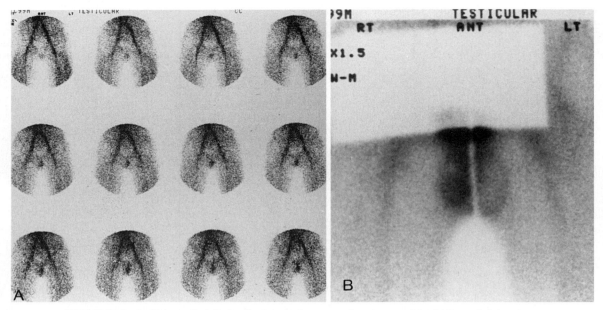

FIGURE 43.4. **A:** Abnormal testicular flow study demonstrating decreased perfusion to left hemiscrotum. **B:** Abnormal static image demonstrating decreased tracer localization in left testis indicative of acute testicular torsion. Lead sheet screens bladder activity.

a hyperemic, inflammatory scrotal response seen as a hot rim around the photopenic testis on the immediate static image. This scrotal "bull's eye" intensifies with time so that it is present on both the flow and static images (late missed torsion) (Fig. 43.5) (15). Once considered pathognomonic of delayed torsion, we now know that the bull's eye can also be seen with abscess, hematoma, suppurative orchitis, necrotic neoplasm, and other entities. SS sensitivity and specificity for acute testicular torsion exceeds 95% with false negatives occurring in patients with spontaneous detorsion, incomplete twists, or inguinal testis (9, 16–21). As the duration of symptoms exceeds 12 to 24 hours,

the specificity falls because missed torsion, abscess, and necrotic tumor give similar findings.

Testicular Trauma

Traumatic testicular injuries are seen as contusion, hemorrhage, laceration, or avulsion with a variable effect on tracer perfusion to the involved hemiscrotum. Contusion induces testicular edema with hemorrhage, but the capsule remains intact (Fig. 43.6). Laceration or rupture disrupts the tunica albuginea and blood fills the tunica vaginalis. An inflammatory reaction ensues

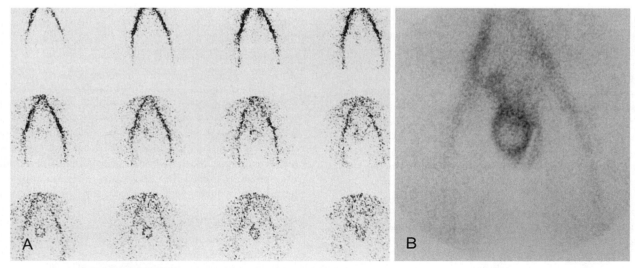

FIGURE 43.5. **A:** Abnormal testicular flow study demonstrating peripheral increased perfusion with photopenic center in right hemiscrotum. **B:** Static image shows "bull's eye" sign of 7 days missed torsion.

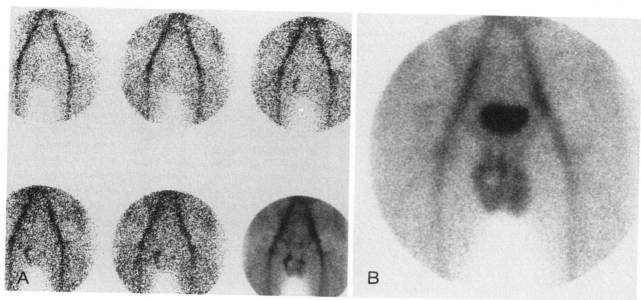

FIGURE 43.6. A: Abnormal testicular flow study with hyperperfusion to traumatized right hemiscrotum. **B:** Static image demonstrates photopenic testicular hematoma.

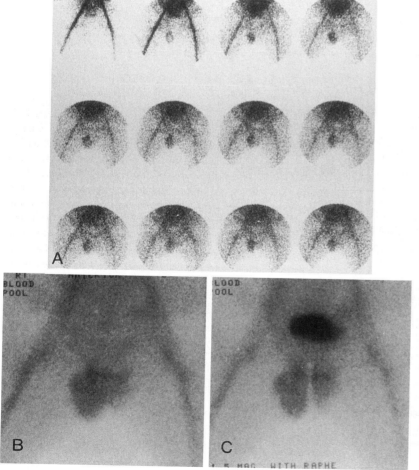

FIGURE 43.7. A: Abnormal testicular flow study demonstrating hyperperfusion to right hemiscrotum. **B:** Static image demonstrates diffuse increased tracer localization in right epididymo-orchitis. **C:** Static image with radhe marker added.

yielding a bull's eye sign usually indistinguishable from missed torsion. Early surgical intervention within 72 hours is associated with 90% salvageability, as compared with only 55% when surgical intervention is further delayed (22). Similarly, injury-induced torsion must be corrected within 4 hours to improve the likelihood of testicular survival.

Acute Epididymitis and Orchitis

Acute scrotal pain and swelling in the postpubertal patient younger than 20 years has a 3:2 ratio of epididymitis to torsion, whereas a similar presentation in a man older than 20 years is 9 times more likely to be epididymitis than torsion (23). Acute epididymitis is characterized by epididymal pain, inflammation, and swelling, whereas chronic epididymitis generally presents with pain only. Acute epididymitis is most often caused by infectious agents with the sexually transmitted pathogens, *Neisseria gonorrhoeae* and *Chlamydia trachomatis*, the most common etiologic agents in men 35 years or younger. Urinary tract pathogens in men with obstructive uropathy are more frequent in older patients. Epididymitis is uncommon in prepubertal males and usually occurs in response to generalized sepsis or urinary tract anomalies with associated infection. Epididymitis is commonly complicated by orchitis, but orchitis without accompanying epididymitis is uncommon and usually is viral, posttraumatic in nature, or due to bacteremia (24,25). Prompt treatment of epididymitis often prevents infectious extension into the testis.

SS is useful in the diagnosis of epididymitis and orchitis (21, 26). If the probability of epididymo-orchitis is high, then diagnostic confirmation is usually sufficient to initiate therapy. Imaging presumed inflammatory disease distinguishes surgically remediable disease such as testicular torsion, abscess, or tumor from medically treated inflammatory processes. Findings depend on the degree of inflammatory hyperemia and swelling present. Increased tracer perfusion on the flow study and comma-shaped peripheral localization on the static images are proportionate to inflammatory hyperemia (Fig. 43.7). If the inflammatory process progresses, an epididymal or testicular abscess may develop and can be visualized on SS as a photopenic area that is often eccentrically located in the hemiscrotum with an asymmetric hyperemic rim (15). SS can usually not determine whether the photopenic region is intratesticular or extratesticular.

Other Entities

Testicular appendage torsion usually demonstrates a normal pattern, but mild hyperemia with a small cold or hot spot has been reported (27). Testicular tumors can present acutely but give a variable nondiagnostic scan pattern. Reactive hydrocele can present acutely usually associated with epididymitis or testicular torsion (Fig. 43.8).

SUMMARY

SS has proved useful in the diagnosis of acute scrotal disorders for more than 25 years. It accurately depicts the perfusion status of the scrotal contents allowing prompt diagnosis and triage of patients with potentially emergent surgical presentations.

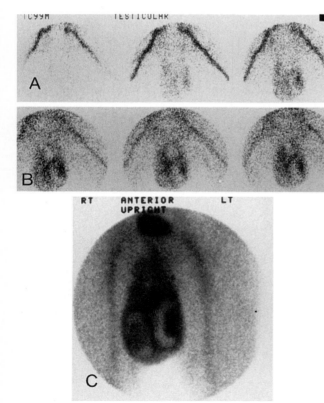

FIGURE 43.8. A: Abnormal early testicular flow study shows hyperperfusion to left lateral hemiscrotum indicative of epididymitis. **B:** Abnormal late testicular flow study shows photopenic left hydrocele. **C:** Static image demonstrating left epididymo-orchitis with sympathetic hydrocele and right hydrocele. A photopenic spermatocele is seen superiorly.

REFERENCES

1. Nadel NS, Jitter MH, Hahn LC et al. Pre-operative diagnosis of testicular torsion. *Urology* 1973;1:478–479.
2. Williamson RCN. Torsion of the testis and allied conditions. *Br J Surg* 1976;63:465–476.
3. Anderson JB, Williamson RCN. Testicular torsion in Bristol: a 25-year review. *Br J Surg* 1988;75:988–992.
4. Sharer WC. Acute scrotal pathology. *Surg Clin North Am* 1982;62:955–970.
5. Zemper ED. Injury rates in a national sample of college football teams: a two-year prospective study. *Phys Sports Med* 1989;17(11):100–113.
6. Backx FJG, Erich WBM, Kemper ABA et al. Sports injuries in schoolaged children: an epidemiological study. *Am J Sports Med* 1989: 17:234–240.
7. Haughey BP, Graham S, Brasure J et al. The epidemiology of testicular cancer in upstate New York. *Am J Epidemiol* 1989;130:25–36.
8. ACR Standard for the performance of scrotal scintigraphy. In: *Standards 2000–2001*. Reston, VA: American College of Radiology, 2000: 297–298.
9. Lutzker LG, Zuckier LS. Testicular scanning and other applications of radionuclide imaging of the genital tract. *Semin Nucl Med* 1990; 20:159–188.
10. Witherington R. The "acute" scrotum: lesions that require immediate attention. *Postgrad Med* 1987;82(1):207–216.

11. Sonda LP, Wang S. Evaluation of male external genital diseases in the emergency room setting. *Emerg Med Clin North Am* 1988;6:473–486.

12. Sonda LP, Lapides J. Experimental torsion of the spermatic cord. *Surg Forum* 1961;12:502–505.

13. Bartsch G, Frank S, Marberger H et al. Testicular torsion: late results with special regard to fertility and endocrine function. *J Urol* 1979; 124:375–378.

14. Thomas WEG, Crane GA, Cooper MJ et al. Testicular exocrine malfunction after torsion. *Lancet* 1984;2:1357–1359.

15. Konez O. The ring sign. *Radiology* 1998;207:439–441.

16. Chen DCP, Holder LE, Melloul M. Radionuclide scrotal imaging: further experience with 210 patients. 1. Anatomy, pathophysiology, and methods. *J Nucl Med* 1983;24:735–742.

17. Chen DCP, Holder LE, Melloul M. Radionuclide scrotal imaging: further experience with 210 patients. 2. Results and discussion. *J Nucl Med* 1983;24:841–853.

18. Mendel JB, Taylor GA, Treves S et al. Testicular torsion in children: scintigraphic assessment. *Pediatr Radiol* 1985;15:110–115.

19. Paltiel HJ, Connolly LP, Atala A et al. Acute scrotal symptoms in boys with an indeterminate clinical presentation: comparison of color doppler sonography and scintigraphy. *Radiology* 1998;207:223–231.

20. Melloul M, Paz A, Lask D et al. The value of radionuclide scrotal imaging in the diagnosis of acute testicular torsion. *Br J Urol* 1995: 76;628–631.

21. Flores LG II, Shiba T, Hoshi H et al. Scintigraphic evaluation of testicular torsion and acute epididymitis. *Ann Nucl Med* 1996:10;89–92.

22. Del Villar RG, Ireland GW, Cass AS. Early exploration following trauma to the testicle. *J Trauma* 1973;13:600–613.

23. Cass AS, Cass BP, Veeraraghavan K. Immediate exploration of the unilateral acute scrotum in young male subjects. *J Urol* 1980;124: 829–832.

24. Mittenmeyer BT, Berger RE, Borsai AA. Epididymitis: a review of 610 cases. *J Urol* 1966;95:390–398.

25. Freton RC, Berger RE. Prostatitis and epididymitis. *Urol Clin North Am* 1984;11:83–94.

26. Holder LE, Martire JR, Holmes ER III et al. Testicular radionuclide angiography and static imaging: anatomy, scintigraphic interpretation, and clinical indications. *Radiology* 1977;125:739–752.

27. Melloul M, Pal A, Lask D et al. The pattern of radionuclide scrotal scan in torsion of testicular appendages. *Eur J Nucl Med* 1996;23: 967–970.

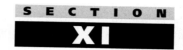

ONCOLOGY

44

GALLIUM-67 IMAGING FOR DETECTION OF MALIGNANT DISEASE

STANLEY J. GOLDSMITH
RACHEL BAR-SHALOM
LALE KOSTAKOGLU
RONALD D. NEUMANN
JOHN D. KEMP
RONALD E. WEINER

^{67}Ga citrate scintigraphy for the detection of tumors has been a component of nuclear medicine practice for more than 30 years. After the initial reports of ^{67}Ga imaging of Hodgkin's and non-Hodgkin's lymphoma by Randle and Hayes in 1969 (1), the technique was reported to help identify many other tumors, including carcinoma of the lung, mesothelioma, melanoma, head and neck tumors, testicular and other genitourinary tumors, hepatoma, a variety of gastrointestinal adenocarcinomas, soft-tissue sarcoma, and a variety of relatively rare tumors, including parathyroid and adrenal carcinoma (2,3).

Despite these reports, ^{67}Ga scintigraphy has not found widespread acceptance as a tumor imaging agent within the oncology community. This is due in part to the many problems associated with the use of ^{67}Ga as an imaging agent. These problems include the less than ideal physical properties for imaging, the lack of a clearly recognized mechanism by which ^{67}Ga localizes in tumor, a complex biodistribution pattern with nonspecific uptake in normal organs, intestinal excretion that clears slowly and complicates interpretation, and the development of computed tomography (CT) and eventually magnetic resonance imaging (MRI) that provided consistent diagnostic images with good anatomic detail. Throughout this period, nuclear medicine physicians and scientists continued to develop scintigraphic techniques to improve image quality. They sought to demonstrate the incremental diagnostic and management advantages of ^{67}Ga scintigraphy as a technique for characterizing tissue biochemistry associated with viable tumor rather than simply imaging anatomic changes such as lymph-node enlargement or identifying a mass. Nevertheless, the inherent limitations of ^{67}Ga as an imaging agent and the variable techniques and instrumentation used by different nuclear medicine practitioners have hampered widespread clinical use of ^{67}Ga scintigraphy as a tumor-imaging agent.

The goal of clinical acceptance has been achieved best in the care of patients with non-Hodgkin's lymphoma and Hodgkin's disease. Whereas the ability to identify tumor viability, rather than simply image a mass, has only limited advantages in the initial evaluation of patients (staging of disease), it is of particular value in characterizing persistent masses after therapy, in the early detection of disease recurrence, and, more recently, in prediction of long-term response. The ability to predict response to therapy is of particular value because therapy for lymphoma and Hodgkin's disease is prolonged. It may be advantageous to move on to an alternative therapeutic approach if it can be determined that the initial course is not likely to produce a prolonged remission.

Although ^{67}Ga scintigraphy is now performed at a higher level of technical excellence than ever before and is used in many centers in the treatment of patients with lymphoma and Hodgkin's disease, the recent development and availability of positron emission tomography (PET) fluorodeoxyglucose (FDG) imaging is likely to render ^{67}Ga scintigraphy obsolete as a tumor-imaging technique in the near future (4). Indeed, the initial recognition by the Health Care Finance Administration of the merit of ^{18}F-FDG coincidence imaging to assess Hodgkin's disease and non-Hodgkin's lymphoma came at the expense of ^{67}Ga scintigraphy; that is, ^{18}F-FDG imaging, even with dual-detector coincidence imaging systems, can be reimbursed as an alternative to ^{67}Ga scintigraphy (5).

Historical Note: Gallium-67 citrate became available in the early 1970s as a radioactive imaging agent for the detection

S.J. Goldsmith: Director, Nuclear Medicine, and Professor, Radiology and Medicine, New York Presbyterian Hospital—Weill Cornell Medical Center, New York, NY.

R. Bar-Shalom: Nuclear Medicine Physician, Department of Nuclear Medicine, Rambam Medical Center, Haifa, Israel.

L. Kostakoglu: Assistant Attending in Nuclear Medicine and Assistant Professor of Radiology, New York Presbyterian Hospital—Weill Cornell Medical College, New York, NY.

R.D. Neumann: Chief, Department of Nuclear Medicine, The National Institutes of Health, Bethesda, MD.

J.D. Kemp: Professor, Department of Pathology, Microbiology, and Immunology, University of Iowa College of Medicine, and Associate Director, Department of Immunopathology Laboratory, University of Iowa Hospitals, Iowa City, Iowa.

R.E. Weiner: Division of Nuclear Medicine, University of Connecticut Health Center, Farmington, CT.

and localization of tumors after the serendipitous observation reported by Randle and Hayes in 1969 that ^{67}Ga localized in Hodgkin's and non-Hodgkin's lymphoma as well as other tumors in patients who had volunteered to receive the tracer to evaluate its utility as a bone-imaging agent (1). At the time, bone imaging was performed in the evaluation of patients for malignant disease. ^{85}Sr was used in low doses because of its 64-day half-life. Ironic was that ^{18}F, as the fluoride ion, also had been evaluated for bone scintigraphy in the noncoincident mode but the 2-hour half-life was poorly suited to the radiopharmaceutical distribution system available at that time. Earlier investigations had shown that gallium tracers localized in bone. Because ^{67}Ga had a shorter half-life and lower-energy γ emissions than did ^{85}Sr, there was reason to believe that ^{67}Ga would be a better bone imaging agent than would ^{85}Sr.

MECHANISMS OF GALLIUM LOCALIZATION

Although there is an abundant body of research identifying various aspects of gallium ion biochemistry in both *in vitro* and *in vivo* biologic systems and disease states, the mechanism of tracer gallium tumor uptake remains unresolved to this day.

After intravenous injection of sterile ^{67}Ga citrate, ^{67}Ga is bound tightly to the serum iron-transport protein transferrin (6, 7). It also has a high affinity to a variety of other iron-binding molecules: the tissue proteins lactoferrin (8) and ferritin (9,10) and the bacterial iron-transport molecules called *siderophores* as well as desferrioxamine (11–12), a therapeutic agent used to remove excess tissue iron from patients with hemosiderosis and hemochromatosis. Despite these similarities between gallium and iron ionic species, animal (13) and human (14) studies have shown great disparity in biodistribution between ^{59}Fe and ^{67}Ga. ^{67}Ga apparently is not incorporated into the iron-containing heme portion of the hemoglobin molecule because it does not undergo reduction to the +2 valence state under physiologic conditions, whereas iron shuttles back and forth between the +2 and +3 state as it is absorbed, processed, and incorporated into the porphyrin ring to form heme.

In the first decade after ^{67}Ga became available as a tumor-imaging agent, Larson et al. (15–17) proposed that a tumor-associated transferrin receptor is the functional unit responsible for the affinity of gallium for certain neoplasms. This hypothesis was consistent with the observation that transferrin receptors are regulated to meet the need for iron in the enzyme ribonucleotide reductase that catalyzes the rate-limiting step in DNA synthesis—conversion of ribonucleotides to deoxyribonucleotides. In rapidly proliferating tumor cells with a high level of DNA synthesis, up-regulation of the surface transferrin receptors would promote increased ^{67}Ga uptake. Indeed, transferrin receptors have been identified in hepatic cells, in which transferrin is normally catabolized, and increased expression of transferrin receptors has been demonstrated in a variety of tumor cells (16,18, 19). There is good evidence that some tumors, particularly lymphoma and hepatoma, have transferrin receptors. In those instances, the ^{67}Ga transferrin complex probably directly participates in the delivery of gallium species to the intracellular environment through endocytosis. In the cell it binds intracellular proteins in lysosomes and in the cytosol.

There are substantial data, however, that not all ^{67}Ga uptake depends on binding to transferrin. Chitambar and Zibkovic (20) showed ^{67}Ga uptake increased as a function of time as did ^{67}Ga concentration in cells in culture without transferrin in the medium. This uptake constituted approximately 10% of transferrin-stimulated uptake evaluated over the same time frame. Chan et al. (21), using a nude-mouse tumor model, found that an antitransferrin receptor monoclonal antibody reduced the percentage injected dose per gram (%ID/g) of ^{67}Ga in tumors to 25% of control values but did not eliminate it.

^{67}Ga binding to transferrin ensures slower elimination from plasma than if ^{67}Ga were to circulate simply as an ionic species or a small-molecular-weight complex with citrate ion. Receptor uptake alone, however, does not appear to explain all of the observed biodistribution and pharmacologic properties of ^{67}Ga citrate. In the early 1980s, Vallabhajosula et al. (22) described a more generic phenomenon: the dissociation of ^{67}Ga from the ^{67}Ga-transferrin complex under conditions of reduced pH, such as those associated with accelerated anaerobic tumor metabolism (Fig. 44.1). Other investigators had previously reported decreased pH in the peritumoral extracellular environment in tumor-bearing animals and humans under certain conditions. Instead of the usual physiologic pH values of 6.8 to 7.0, values of 6.4 to 6.5 were recorded after glucose administration. This finding has been interpreted to be the result of increased intracellular lactic acid levels with diffusion of hydrogen ions into the peritumoral environment. Vallabhajosula et al. correlated a decrease in intratumoral pH in animal tumor models with proportional increases in tumor ^{67}Ga uptake. In rats bearing Walker-256 carcinosarcoma, ^{67}Ga content increased 29% after glucose infusion. In another experiment, rats bearing Murphy-Sturm lymphosarcoma had a 24% increase in ^{67}Ga content. Both results were statistically significant. The investigators hypothesized that tumor anaerobic metabolism resulted in dissociation of ^{67}Ga from transferrin to enable the free ^{67}Ga moiety to enter the cell by means of passive diffusion (no active process has been identified) whereby it binds to intracellular proteins (lactoferrin) or other compounds.

Both ^{67}Ga dissociation from carrier transferrin and ^{18}F-FDG cell uptake are directly proportional to anaerobic glucose metabolism (Fig. 44.1). Although a component of ^{67}Ga localization in some tumors is probably a function also of transferrin receptor binding, ^{67}Ga localization in many tumors is probably a reflection of accelerated anaerobic glucose metabolism. The differences observed between ^{67}Ga scintigraphy and ^{18}F-FDG PET may be caused by the more advantageous physical characteristics and instrumentation involved in ^{18}F-FDG PET rather than by basic differences in the mechanism of tracer localization.

Iosilevsky et al. (23) compared uptake of ^{3}H deoxyglucose with that of ^{67}Ga in an animal tumor model after local irradiation and chemotherapy. They found that both ^{67}Ga and ^{3}H deoxyglucose uptake declined in proportion to the amount of viable tumor, from control values of 10.0% ± 1.5%ID/g for ^{67}Ga and 9.1% ± 1.5%ID/g for ^{3}H deoxyglucose to 5.6% ± 1.5% and 6.0% ± 1.8% in partially viable tumors and to 2.0% ± 0.5% and 3.2% ± 0.7% in nonviable treated tumors. In 1991, Kubota et al. (24) found almost identical decreases in both ^{3}H deoxyglucose and ^{67}Ga in a rat tumor model after

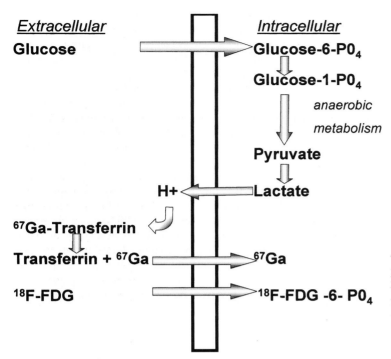

FIGURE 44.1. Schematic shows possible relation between anaerobic glucose metabolism and ^{67}Ga uptake. As anaerobic metabolism increases, hydrogen ion is generated. This reaction leads to dissociation of ^{67}Ga from the gallium-transferrin complex. The schematic provides a unifying hypothesis for tumor accumulation of ^{67}Ga and ^{18}F fluorodeoxyglucose uptake in tumor cells. This hypothesis suggests that the differences in overall accuracy between ^{67}Ga scintigraphy and ^{18}F-FDG PET may have more to do with the improved resolution of PET and the greater photon flux of ^{18}F than with inherent differences in the mechanism of tumor tracer accumulation. In certain instances, such as lymphoma, Hodgkin's disease, and hepatoma, ^{67}Ga accumulation is likely promoted additionally by tumor cell transferrin receptor binding of ^{67}Ga transferrin.

incremental doses of radiation. ^{67}Ga activity initially was slightly disparate from ^{3}H deoxyglucose values in that the ^{67}Ga showed a slight increase after irradiation. This observation has been attributed to infiltration of inflammatory cells but may be consistent with a pH-dependent mechanism, because pH decreases after irradiation are expected.

BIODISTRIBUTION AND PATTERNS OF GALLIUM LOCALIZATION

Although there is disagreement about the role of transferrin receptor in tumor localization, there is general agreement on the pivotal role of transferrin in delivering ^{67}Ga to normal tissue. After injection as ^{67}Ga citrate, the ^{67}Ga moiety binds to transferrin, the iron-binding plasma protein. Given the observation that free gallium species is more rapidly excreted by the kidneys and intestine and the relative insolubility of gallium ion at physiologic pH, the gallium-transferrin complex serves to maintain ^{67}Ga in the circulation. This allows time for transport of a greater fraction to tissue and tumor sites, where it is exposed to processes that either decrease transferrin binding (reduced pH) or to other metalloproteins that have greater binding affinity or capacity (ferritin and lactoferrin) or specific uptake mechanisms for either ^{67}Ga (iron) or ^{67}Ga transferrin. Under conditions such as recent transfusion, iron injection, or experimental administration of transferrin receptor antibodies or other class III metals, normal tissue (liver, spleen, bone marrow) uptake of ^{67}Ga is depressed and whole-body excretion is enhanced. ^{67}Ga activity in bone is unaffected or increases, however, in accordance with the observation of bone uptake of gallium when it is administered in pharmacologic (nontracer) amounts or under conditions that exceed transferrin-binding capacity (25–31).

^{67}Ga normally localizes principally in the liver (site of transferrin metabolism) and bone marrow (ferritin binding). Bone uptake, characteristic of metal ions, is not usually observed with diagnostic doses of ^{67}Ga citrate in which only trace amounts of gallium are present. Spleen uptake is variable despite the dense population of lymphocytes; factors relating to the degree of uptake have not been characterized (Figs. 44.2, 44.3). Uptake is found in tissues with increased lactoferrin content: the breasts of women, salivary and lacrimal glands, nasal mucosa, and external genitalia. Breast uptake is variable depending on the degree of estrogen or other stimulation. In particular, there is a marked increase in ^{67}Ga uptake in lactating breasts. Activity in salivary glands usually is faint or undetectable but increases with inflammation and can become very prominent after radiation therapy to the head and neck and, occasionally, after chemotherapy. Prominent salivary gland uptake can persist and may represent a challenge in terms of differential diagnosis (differentiation between recurrent tumor and simply postradiation response). Mediastinal uptake may be observed in normal children owing to gallium accumulation in normal thymic tissue. Prominent thymic uptake after chemotherapy, a phenomenon known as *thymic rebound,* should be recognized as a consequence of recent therapy rather than as disease recurrence (32). Faint hilar activity occasionally occurs in patients without known pulmonary disease. Whether this is caused by a mild, subclinical response to infectious agents is not known. It is often useful to contrast pulmonary activity to cardiac blood-pool activity. Absolute increased pulmonary activity that is not simply caused by the ^{67}Ga in the pulmonary blood pool is characterized by visualization of the "clear" cardiac blood pool and provides contrast to the pulmonary activity.

Variable degrees of gastric activity sometimes are discernible

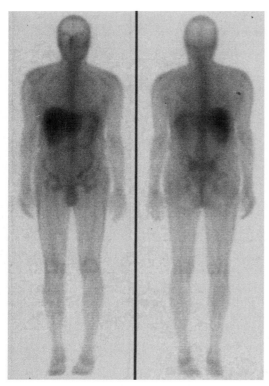

FIGURE 44.2. Normal biodistribution of ^{67}Ga injected as gallium citrate. Images were obtained 48 hours after injection with a contemporary dual-head whole-body scanner (Millenium VG3; General Electric Medical Systems, Milwaukee, WI). Activity is most prominent in the liver; lesser amounts are present in the spleen and active bone marrow with minimal soft-tissue background activity. (Courtesy of Division of Nuclear Medicine, Department of Radiology, New York Presbyterian Hospital–Weill Cornell Medical Center, New York, NY.)

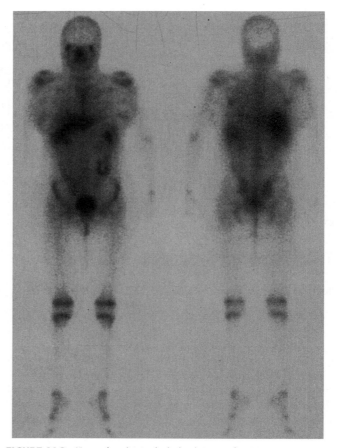

FIGURE 44.3. Normal variant whole-body scan of a young woman currently with no symptoms with a diagnosis of lymphoma in the past. The minimal increase in soft-tissue activity in the breasts and in the epiphyseal growth plates is in accordance with the findings for the patient's age group and sex. Bilateral lacrimal gland activity is another variant that is within normal limits. Focal accumulations throughout the abdomen suggest intestinal contents. The activity in the bladder occurs more than usual 48 hours after injection but also is an acceptable variant if clinical correlation excludes concern in this area. (Courtesy of Division of Nuclear Medicine, Department of Radiology, New York Presbyterian Hospital–Weill Cornell Medical Center, New York, NY.)

on 48- to 72-hour images. This is usually a consequence of variable degrees of hyperemia rather than of primary gastric tumor.

Renal activity can be moderately prominent on images obtained within the first 24 to 48 hours after injection, but it is usually faint or absent by 48 to 72 hours after injection. Prominent renal activity also can be seen in patients with iron overload or hepatic failure; it occasionally is associated with coincident treatment with Cyclophosphamide (Cytoxan) and vincristine. The following agents or conditions can alter the normal patterns of gallium uptake: stable gallium sometimes given in chemotherapy, gadolinium used as an MRI contrast agent, altered serum iron levels, and previous radiation therapy or chemotherapy.

Intestinal gallium activity represents a challenge in diagnosis and management. On the one hand, it is well known that ^{67}Ga is excreted into the intestine. Remarkable is that in some patients, even without supplemental bowel cleansing, no activity is visualized. In other patients, intense diffuse or focal activity is visualized. Even when this activity is confidently identified as intestinal contents, the potential to obscure underlying abdominal tumor or involved lymph nodes remains an obstacle to accurate detection of abdominal disease (Fig. 44.4).

In infants, prominent activity often is observed in the base of

the skull. Epiphyseal activity is prominent in children. Surgical wounds can show activity for several weeks after surgery, although faint wound activity can persist for a month or more. Localized activity in the bone may occur after bone marrow biopsy, fractures, or surgical manipulation.

Finally, ^{67}Ga localization is not specific for tumor activity but can be seen in a variety of inflammatory conditions, infectious and otherwise. Correlation with clinical history and a sophisticated awareness of potential coincident disease is necessary for accurate interpretation of ^{67}Ga scintigraphic and single photon emission computed tomography (SPECT) images.

Historical Note: Chen et al. (33) showed that the small intestine was the major (60%) source of ^{67}Ga excretion in the gastrointestinal tract, possibly by the mechanism involved in iron excretion (34); 20% is excreted in the bile. Increasing transferrin saturation (reducing the unsaturated iron binding capacity

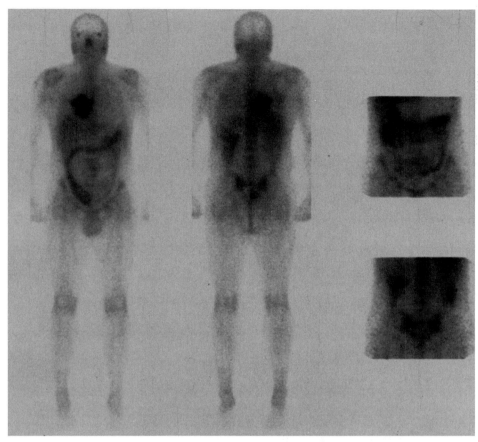

FIGURE 44.4. Large mass in the right hemithorax of a man represents Hodgkin's disease. On 48-hour whole-body images, there is accumulation of considerable activity in the large intestine from the cecum to the splenic flexure. Anterior and posterior views of the abdomen were obtained 72 hours after injection for evaluation of the intestinal activity pattern. Although there is still considerable activity, the alteration in the distribution confirms that the activity represents physiologic intestinal contents rather than inflammatory disease or tumor. (Courtesy of Division of Nuclear Medicine, Department of Radiology, New York Presbyterian Hospital–Weill Cornell Medical Center, New York, NY.)

[UIBC]) before ^{67}Ga administration substantially reduces excretion in the gastrointestinal tract. Renal excretion probably depends on dissociation of the metal ion from transferrin. Factors associated with decreased transferrin binding tend to increase the fraction excreted in urine. Engelstad et al. (35) presented ^{67}Ga scintigrams of four patients who had undergone repeated blood transfusions, which saturated their transferrin with iron. Kidney and bladder activity increased with decreased liver and colon activity. Whether the saturation affected abscess or tumor uptake was not resolved because in one patient, a very large area of osteomyelitis was easily detected but in another patient a normally ^{67}Ga-avid tumor was missed. Similar biodistributions were reported by others with increased saturation of transferrin (36,37) and with chemotherapy, which likely increases transferrin saturation (38). Desferrioxamine given to reduce iron overload in a patient with sickle cell anemia substantially increased ^{67}Ga excretion so that only the kidneys were visualized; skeletal, liver, and spleen uptake were minimal, and a lesion was missed (39). Another patient, to whom desferrioxamine was given for aluminum toxicity, showed similar biodistribution (40).

IMAGING TECHNIQUE

^{67}Ga is an accelerator product, produced from a zinc target, and is available as a radioactive tracer for diagnostic use as ^{67}Ga citrate. A 10 mCi (370 MBq) dose of ^{67}Ga citrate is recommended for use in adults. This dose, although higher than doses used initially, allows improved detection of disease in oncology patients who are at much greater risk from their underlying disease and therapy than from the incremental radiation absorbed dose.

10 mCi of ^{67}Ga citrate is injected intravenously, and the patient is scheduled for imaging approximately 48 hours later. After intravenous injection of ^{67}Ga citrate, the ^{67}Ga moiety binds to the serum protein transferrin. Accordingly, ^{67}Ga clears slowly from the blood pool. This phenomenon allows accumula-

tion in poorly perfused sites but reduces lesion-to-background contrast. Imaging usually is performed 48 to 72 hours after administration of ^{67}Ga to allow clearance of background activity from the blood pool. Bowel activity may be reduced with the use of cathartics, enemas, or both before imaging or after detection of abdominal activity that interferes with interpretation. Delayed scans can be performed to determine whether abdominal and pelvic activity has changed, indicating physiologic excretion into the intestine as opposed to persistent accumulation compatible with tumor or inflammation.

^{67}Ga decays by means of electron capture with the emission of a spectrum of γ photons with energy peaks at 93 keV, 184 keV, 296 keV, and 394 keV. Each peak is emitted in relatively low yield: 37%, 21%, 17% and 5%, respectively. As γ photons undergo Compton scatter, each of the three more abundant lower-energy windows contains signal that represents scatter from the higher energy peaks.

Imaging currently is performed with three distinct 15% to 20% energy windows centered on the three principal energy peaks. The highest energy peak, 394 keV, has only a 5% yield and is not included. A so-called medium energy collimator is used, but there is considerable difference in image quality from manufacturer to manufacturer. The difference exists in part because collimator specifications have variable degrees of septal penetration of the 394 and 296 keV photon peaks. Because the final electronic image used for interpretation is a summed image of images obtained from each of the energy windows, it is important that the image obtained from each energy window have precisely the same electronic dimensions so that alignment of the several images is precise. With the current wide use of digitized images, this is generally no longer a problem.

Current imaging techniques entail use of large-field gamma cameras, often with dual heads, which have the advantage of simultaneous acquisition of anterior and posterior images. In addition, when dual-head systems are used for SPECT imaging, greater acquisition time (40 seconds) can be spent at each angular stop with acquisition of more counts because only 60 stops per head are necessary (as opposed to the 120 stops required if a single-head camera is used). The greater count acquisition allows acquisition of SPECT images of finer matrix elements (128 × 128) and improved visual (and presumably) diagnostic quality compared with images obtained with earlier methods with a single-head camera and lower doses of ^{67}Ga citrate (Fig. 44.5).

Planar gamma-camera imaging can be performed in either the nonscanning or scanning (whole body) mode. In the nonscanning mode, images should be obtained for at least 10 minutes per view. The total number of counts varies with the size of the imaging field and the area imaged. Current large-field-of-view technique in examinations of adults patients receiving 10-mCi doses usually includes approximately 2,000-K counts in the thoracic view that usually include some liver activity. In the whole-body mode, the scan speed should be selected to ensure adequate information content. It is recommended that an information density greater than 450 counts per square centimeter be obtained. In addition, SPECT imaging of the thorax, abdomen, or both is recommended. SPECT imaging improves anatomic localization and detection of deep structures (e.g., paraaortic lymph nodes) (41–43). McLaughlin et al. (41) found

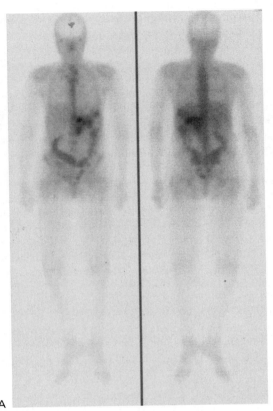

A

FIGURE 44.5. High-quality ^{67}Ga whole-body scintigraphic and SPECT images of in a patient with non-Hodgkin's lymphoma. **A:** Planar images show accumulation of ^{67}Ga in the left upper quadrant, a small-focus left paratracheal region, and a left inguinal region. *(Figure continues.)*

that in the evaluation of patients with lymphoma, SPECT scintigraphy improved lesion detection to 89% compared with that of planar imaging, which had a sensitivity of only 48% in the same series. Specificity decreased from 83% with planar imaging to 65% with SPECT imaging. Nevertheless, the overall accuracy increased with SPECT scintigraphy from 62% to 80% (42). Similar results have been reported by others (44). A variety of SPECT reconstruction methods have been used. Dillehay and Papatheofanis (45) indicated that a Henning filter with a 0.75 cutoff is used most commonly. At the New York Presbyterian Hospital, a Hann filter with a 0.7 to 0.9 cutoff is used because of the manufacturer's recommendation and physician preference. The use of a new technique, fusing CT images acquired in the same sitting as ^{67}Ga scintigraphy, allows precise registration of data to more accurately differentiate physiologic and tumoral accumulation of ^{67}Ga. This method improves specificity, which is essential in assessing response to treatment (Fig. 44.6).

CLINICAL APPLICATIONS

The role of ^{67}Ga scintigraphy in diagnosis and management of suspected or known tumors has evolved over the past 25 years. Even within the past 6 years, the Society of Nuclear Medicine

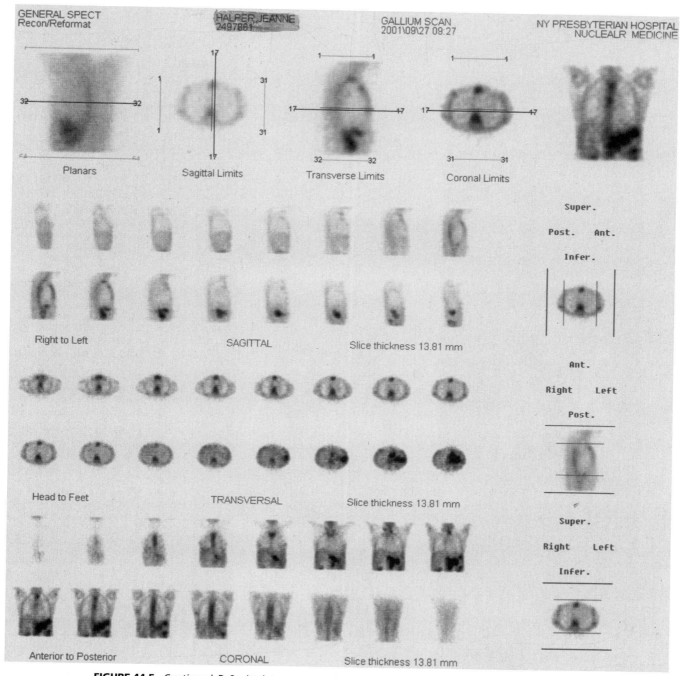

FIGURE 44.5. *Continued.* **B:** Sagittal, transverse and coronal SPECT images are of greater contrast and more clearly show (the coronal image in particular) right cervical, left paratracheal, and mediastinal lymphadenopathy and better definition of left upper quadrant paraaortic and splenic bed lymphadenopathy. (Courtesy of Division of Nuclear Medicine, Department of Radiology, New York Presbyterian Hospital–Weill Cornell Medical Center, New York, NY.)

has twice revised the *Procedure Guideline for Gallium Scintigraphy.* The current guideline (under review at the time of this writing) indicates that ^{67}Ga has proved useful in the management of lymphoma in (a) staging extent of disease, (b) determining response to therapy, (c) detecting relapse or progression of disease, and (d) predicting outcome. The proposed guideline goes on to indicate that other tumors have been shown to be gallium-avid, but no statement is made concerning the clinical utility of ^{67}Ga scintigraphy in the care of patients with these tumors. The tumors cited are lung cancer, melanoma, hepatocellular carcinoma, sarcoma, testicular tumors, multiple myeloma, head and neck tumors, and neuroblastoma. [67]Ga accumulation has been observed in mesothelioma involving the pleura or peritoneum. The significance of these observations is that ^{67}Ga local-

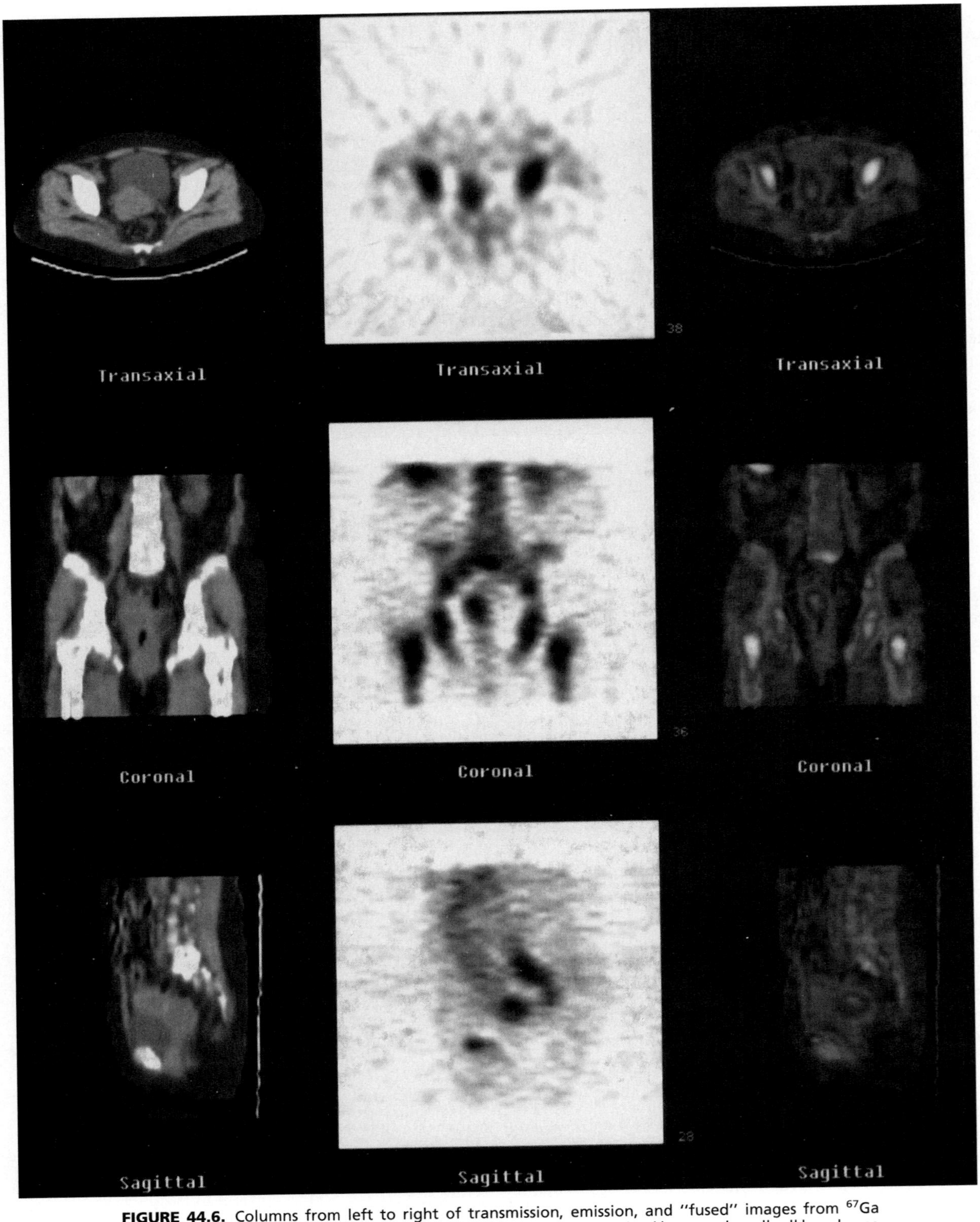

FIGURE 44.6. Columns from left to right of transmission, emission, and "fused" images from ^{67}Ga scintigraphy. Biopsy image of ^{67}Ga-positive focus represents diffuse mixed large and small cell lymphoma involving the body of the uterus in a woman who had recently had the unexpected finding of lymphoma after resection of the uterine cervix. Images show improved specificity of "fused" images as a result of assigning observed ^{67}Ga focus to the uterus as opposed to bladder or rectal activity. (Images courtesy of Dr. Ora Israel, Rambam Medical Center, Haifa, Israel, from Khalikhali I, Maublant JC, Goldsmith SJ. *Nuclear oncology.* Philadelphia: Lippincott Williams & Wilkins, 2000, with permission.)

izes in these tumors and can frequently be seen during scintigraphy but that ^{67}Ga scintigraphy has not been found as accurate as other diagnostic imaging techniques, including ^{18}F-FDG, and therefore is not used in management decisions affecting patients with these malignant lesions. Physicians interpreting ^{67}Ga scintigraphic images need to be aware of the potential for identification of these other tumors when interpreting ^{67}Ga images performed for any reason.

Lymphoma and Hodgkin's Disease

^{67}Ga scintigraphy has found its greatest clinical application and success in the imaging of lymphoma. During the early years of availability of ^{67}Ga scintigraphy, the sensitivity and specificity of the technique were assessed without regard to the tumor type, location, or histologic features or to the relevance of findings to patient care. It is now appreciated that the ability to detect lymphoma and Hodgkin's disease depends on all of these factors. The clinical utility is greatest for the assessment of response to therapy and the early detection of recurrence of disease because identification of tumor viability as opposed to simple visualization of a mass is essential for these applications. It has come to be appreciated that ^{67}Ga scintigraphy provides useful information in predicting response to therapy. This area is of great significance, because a variety of therapeutic interventions now are available. Because of potential hazards and toxicities, it is particularly useful to be able to assess therapeutic efficacy as early as possible in the course of disease.

Staging Extent of Disease

In the late 1970s, two cooperative studies appeared that showed patient and site sensitivity for ^{67}Ga scintigraphy as high as 88% for detection of disease per patient and 69% per site in patients with untreated Hodgkin's disease. Patient sensitivity of 76% and site sensitivity of 53% were reported for non-Hodgkin's lymphoma (46,47). These results were generally higher than had been previously reported when less optimal techniques were used. Subsequently, Front et al. (43) reported that the overall sensitivity for ^{67}Ga scintigraphy as a staging procedure increased from 78% with planar scintigraphy to 85% with SPECT (Fig. 44.5). It was soon appreciated that the sensitivity of ^{67}Ga scintigraphy was related to size and location of lesions and to the histologic type of disease as well as to technical factors. Sensitivity as high as 96% has been reported in the mediastinum, whereas for lesions in the abdomen and pelvis, a sensitivity of only 60% has been observed (48).

The histologic features of lesions are important. In Burkitt's lymphoma, it is rare for a lesion in any location not to be detected at ^{67}Ga scintigraphy. Sites of Hodgkin's disease and high-grade non-Hodgkin's lymphoma are highly gallium-avid and therefore usually identified with ^{67}Ga scintigraphy (48,49). Low-grade non-Hodgkin's lymphoma usually is less ^{67}Ga-avid, and the results, particularly for sensitivity for detection of disease, are therefore more dependent on technique. The sensitivity in any given series depends on the equipment and tracer amount used as well as the effort and determination of the investigator-clinician. A range of results are achieved depending on histologic

subtype. In one series of patients with low-grade lymphoma, a patient sensitivity of 89% was observed for histiocytic non-Hodgkin's lymphoma whereas only 59% sensitivity was recorded for well-differentiated lymphocytic non-Hodgkin's lymphoma (47). ^{67}Ga scintigraphy was helpful in identification of only 41% of nodal sites detected with CT or clinical examination in another series, but SPECT was performed in only selected cases (50). In evaluation of a series of 57 patients with low-grade non-Hodgkin's lymphoma, Ben Haim et al. (51) performed ^{67}Ga scintigraphy at initial diagnosis or during treatment. They reported an overall patient sensitivity of 79% and site sensitivity of 69%. In this series, ^{67}Ga scintigraphy sensitivity was much higher for the more common histologic subtypes of low-grade non-Hodgkin's lymphoma than for the rare types—91% for follicular mixed small and large cell and 84% for follicular small cleaved non-Hodgkin's lymphoma. Although these results compare favorably with results obtained in the care of series of patients with Hodgkin's disease and high-grade non-Hodgkin's lymphoma, the results with the series confirm the overall dependency of ^{67}Ga scintigraphy on technique and clinical and histologic subtype. It is only with meticulous technique and persistence that such good results are obtained in some subgroups of patients with low-grade non-Hodgkin's lymphoma.

Although ^{67}Ga scintigraphy performed before treatment may be of added value in identifying a site suitable for biopsy when there is a strong clinical suspicion of lymphoma but no adenopathy at physical examination and in finding additional, previously unknown sites, it has not been used nor encouraged as a staging method because of the convenience and established role of CT as well as the closer to uniform quality and overall reliability of CT. The principal value of ^{67}Ga scintigraphy before therapy is in characterizing baseline gallium avidity of the lymphoma so that ^{67}Ga scintigraphy can be used to evaluate response to treatment during or after therapy (48).

Evaluating Response to Treatment and Assessing the Nature of a Residual Mass

A significant role for ^{67}Ga scintigraphy has emerged in the evaluation of patients after therapy. Despite successful chemotherapy or radiation therapy, large lymphomatous masses frequently undergo tumor necrosis and fibrosis without complete resolution of the mass found at CT. Despite the resolution of symptoms, uncertainty persists about whether further therapy is indicated. In these instances, ^{67}Ga scintigraphy is an excellent means of assessing whether residual viable tumor is present on the basis of detection of ^{67}Ga uptake in masses with residual tumor activity. For greatest accuracy, many institutions perform baseline whole-body ^{67}Ga scintigraphy to detect ^{67}Ga avidity before therapy for comparison with the posttherapy images (Figs. 44.7, 44.8).

The value of ^{67}Ga scintigraphy in the assessment of response to management of lymphoma is based on the observation that gallium is a tumor-viability agent. The important distinction between a mass seen at CT or another anatomic imaging modality and viable tumor is expressed by the statement "residual mass may not be a residual disease" (52). Hence, characterizing a

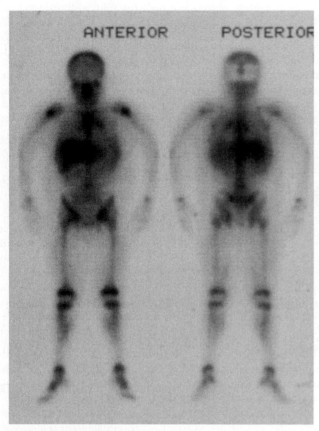

FIGURE 44.7. ^{67}Ga planar scintigraphy of an adolescent with a history of nasopharyngeal non-Hodgkin's lymphoma. Nearly symmetric mediastinal findings are most compatible with thymic rebound after therapy. There is no evidence of disease. (Courtesy of Division of Nuclear Medicine, Department of Radiology, New York Presbyterian Hospital–Weill Cornell Medical Center, New York, NY.)

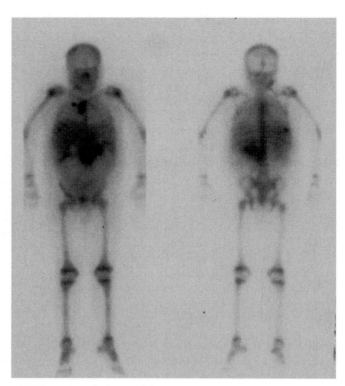

FIGURE 44.8. Relapse in adolescent depicted in Fig. 44.7. In addition to probable recurrence at the primary site, there are now well-defined right cervical, right paratracheal, and infraclavicular lymphadenopathy, a right upper quadrant focus, and a large left periaortic mass in the abdomen. (Courtesy of Division of Nuclear Medicine, Department of Radiology, New York Presbyterian Hospital–Weill Cornell Medical Center, New York, NY.)

residual mass after therapy with ^{67}Ga scintigraphy rather than CT to evaluate response to treatment has become the standard of practice (41,44,53–60).

The biodistribution of ^{67}Ga and hence the sensitivity of ^{67}Ga scintigraphy for detection of viable tumor after treatment depends on when the procedure is performed relative to chemotherapy. (48,61,62). The commonly accepted empiric rule is to allow 2 to 3 weeks from the previous treatment and a 24- to 48-hour interval between injection of gallium and the start of the next cycle (48,63–65).

Israel et al. (53) found that positive results of ^{67}Ga scintigraphy at the end of treatment of patients with gallium-avid lymphoma were an accurate predictor of complete remission in 95% of patients, whereas results of CT at the end of treatment were positive in only 57% of patients who would achieve complete remission. Results of ^{67}Ga scintigraphy remained positive in the four patients who did not achieve remission. The predictive value of abnormal scan results is similarly high.

In Hodgkin's disease, 89% of patients with positive results of ^{67}Ga scintigraphy at the end of treatment either died or had tumor progression; 88% of patients with negative results of post-treatment ^{67}Ga scintigraphy went on to achieve complete remis-

sion (54). In another series of 77 patients with Hodgkin's disease and non-Hodgkin's lymphoma, the value of gallium SPECT in excluding disease in residual masses after treatment was confirmed (43). The sensitivity and specificity of ^{67}Ga scintigraphy after treatment were 92% and 99%. Kostakoglu et al. (44) found that the sensitivity of ^{67}Ga scintigraphy was superior to that of CT in the detection of residual mediastinal disease. In 30 adult patients with Hodgkin's disease who underwent mediastinal biopsy, ^{67}Ga scintigraphy had a sensitivity of 96%, whereas CT had a sensitivity of only 68%. The specificity of ^{67}Ga was 96%, whereas that of CT was only 60%. Initial data on the use of fused ^{67}Ga scintigraphy and transmission images in evaluation of patients with lymphoma have confirmed the potential of this technique in improving specificity in characterizing focal accumulations of activity as physiologic and thus in excluding the presence of active disease (66).

Current opinion within the nuclear medicine community accepts the notion that results of ^{67}Ga scintigraphy are a better predictor of response to therapy than are results of alternative methods of assessment of response because of the failure of CT or other radiologic procedures to allow differentiation of residual disease (viable tumor) from nontumoral fibrotic masses. Evidence of persistent activity is an indication of residual disease. This finding is associated with a high frequency of clinical relapse. Failure to identify foci of ^{67}Ga activity after completion of therapy (a negative study), however, is less predictive of a long-term successful outcome; that is, the negative predictive value of ^{67}Ga scintigraphy after therapy is less than the positive predictive value. This clinical issue is discussed in detail later (see Prediction of Response to Therapy and of Long-term Outcome).

The predictive value of posttreatment ^{67}Ga scintigraphy is somewhat different in Hodgkin's disease and non-Hodgkin's lymphoma. In one report of 43 patients with Hodgkin's disease, the negative and positive predictive values of ^{67}Ga scintigraphy for response to treatment were 84% and 80% (59). In comparison, the negative and positive predictive values for CT were 88% and 29%. There is a significant difference in disease-free and overall survival rate among patients with Hodgkin's disease depending on whether they have positive or negative results of ^{67}Ga scintigraphy at the end of treatment. No such difference was found between patients with positive and negative CT results at the end of treatment (59,60). Despite this impressive result, patients with negative results of ^{67}Ga scintigraphy after treatment, however, do undergo relapse, especially if they have advanced Hodgkin's disease (60,61–64). The negative predictive value of posttherapy ^{67}Ga scintigraphy is higher among patients with limited disease (92%) than among those with advanced Hodgkin's disease (65%) (61). In a retrospective assessment of 48 patients with mediastinal Hodgkin's disease, a positive ^{67}Ga scintigraphic result at the end of treatment was highly predictive of poor prognosis. Nevertheless, 27% of patients with a negative result of ^{67}Ga scintigraphy had a relapse (63).

High predictive values have been reported for ^{67}Ga scintigraphy after therapy for non-Hodgkin's lymphoma (67,68). Front et al. (67) found that ^{67}Ga scintigraphy at the end of therapy for non-Hodgkin's lymphoma had a negative predictive value of 84% (the value for CT was 80%) and a positive predictive value of 73% (the value for CT was 35%). There was a significant difference in disease-free and overall survival rates between patients with positive and negative results of ^{67}Ga scintigraphy after treatment. No such difference was found between patients with negative and positive results of CT after treatment (67). In a series of 143 patients with aggressive non-Hodgkin's lymphoma, ^{67}Ga scintigraphy performed after high-dose chemotherapy and bone marrow transplantation was found highly predictive of outcome (68).

Detection of Recurrence

Sixty-five percent of patients with large cell non-Hodgkin's lymphoma and as many as 80% of patients with Hodgkin's disease initially achieve complete remission (69,70). However, disease may eventually recur and necessitate an aggressive second line regimen, such as high-dose chemotherapy and bone marrow transplantation (Figs. 44.7, 44.8). Because salvage therapy appears more effective when the tumor load is small, it is presumed to be worthwhile in the detection of recurrence at an early stage. Accordingly, periodic reexamination with ^{67}Ga scintigraphy of patients who have achieved complete remission to detect recurrent lymphoma early may improve long-term survival (63,71, 72). There are limited data, however, on the value of ^{67}Ga scin-

tigraphy in the detection of recurrence (61,69,73). Weeks et al. (69) assessed the sensitivity of various follow-up procedures for the detection of relapse of large cell non-Hodgkin's lymphoma. In 90% of 51 patients evaluated, relapse was identified only when clinically evident because of the presence of symptoms or palpatory findings. CT had a low sensitivity of 45% for recurrent disease in the chest and 55% for the detection of abdominal disease. ^{67}Ga scintigraphy was performed on 10 patients with relapse, but the results were positive for 9 of the 10. Front et al. (73) reported the sensitivity of ^{67}Ga scintigraphy in the detection of relapse to be 95% and the specificity to be 89%. In 27% of patients, relapse occurred at new sites of disease. This finding emphasized the importance of a whole-body screening procedure. In 12 events of recurrence, results of ^{67}Ga scintigraphy were abnormal an average of 6.8 months before the appearance of clinical symptoms or radiologic abnormalities.

Prediction of Response to Therapy and of Long-term Outcome

Accurate definition of remission at the end of treatment is important to avoid unnecessary toxic treatment or to indicate early the need for second-line chemotherapy. At the end of treatment, ^{67}Ga scintigraphy reflects not only the state of disease at that specific time point but also long-term prognosis. There is considerable evidence that ^{67}Ga scintigraphy is useful as a prognostic indicator of long-term response to therapy.

Although negative results of ^{67}Ga scintigraphy at the completion of therapy are a favorable finding, a large fraction of these patients do not have durable remissions, and relapse occurs after a disease-free period (Figs. 44.7, 44.8). It has been found that results of ^{67}Ga scintigraphy performed after only one cycle of therapy are more predictive of prolonged remission of both non-Hodgkin's lymphoma and Hodgkin's disease than are results of ^{67}Ga scintigraphy performed after completion of an entire therapeutic regimen, which often involves 6 to 9 months of chemotherapy. This seemingly counterintuitive observation is further confirmation of the sensitivity of ^{67}Ga uptake as a marker of tumor viability and aggressiveness. Patients with tumors who respond rapidly to chemotherapy are more likely to have prolonged and durable remissions than are patients in whom the response is observed only after prolonged therapy that interferes with tumor viability. The value of predicting long-term outcome is that the clinician can consider alternative management approaches earlier in the course of the disease and avoid the toxicity of prolonged therapies that ultimately are unsuccessful.

The development of new aggressive regimens for salvage therapy has increased the survival rate among patients with a poor prognosis but has also increased the risk of treatment-related toxicity. Stratification of patients according to long-term prognosis may enable optimization of treatment protocols. Patients at low risk with favorable response to initial treatment should be spared further aggressive toxic treatment. Unsuccessful therapy should be stopped and replaced by aggressive therapy as early as possible when tumor load is small and beneficial therapeutic effect is still possible.

Several sets of investigators have used ^{67}Ga scintigraphy for the early assessment of response to treatment (74–78). In a study with 30 patients with aggressive non-Hodgkin's lymphoma, Janicek et al. (75) showed that positive results of ^{67}Ga scintigraphy after two cycles of high-dose chemotherapy were predictive of treatment failure in 82% of patients. Negative results of ^{67}Ga scintigraphy during treatment were predictive of prolonged response in 94% of patients. CT was not of value in differentiating patients according to outcome. In a study with 118 patients with aggressive non-Hodgkin's lymphoma who underwent prospective assessment, a negative result of ^{67}Ga scintigraphy after the first cycle of chemotherapy was predictive of long-term continuous complete remission in 82% of patients (78). There was a statistically significant difference in disease-free survival rate between patients with a negative or positive result of ^{67}Ga scintigraphy after one cycle of chemotherapy. No such difference was found between negative or positive results of CT mid treatment (78). Positive results of ^{67}Ga scintigraphy after one cycle were predictive of treatment failure in 71% of patients. In 98 patients with Hodgkin's disease, a negative result of ^{67}Ga scintigraphy after the first cycle of treatment was predictive of prolonged complete remission in 92% of patients (77). Positive results of ^{67}Ga scintigraphy performed early in the course of therapy were less predictive of outcome; treatment failure was predicted in only 57% of these patients. A significant number of patients with positive ^{67}Ga scintigraphy achieved complete remission. Front et al. (77,78) suggested that a reduced course of chemotherapy could be used without affecting survival in the treatment of patients with Hodgkin's disease who had negative results of ^{67}Ga scintigraphy after one cycle. Patients with non-Hodgkin's lymphoma with positive results of ^{67}Ga scintigraphy early during treatment should be considered for more aggressive therapy. In children with early-stage lymphoma and negative results of ^{67}Ga scintigraphy after two cycles of chemotherapy, the dose of chemotherapy has been decreased with apparent satisfactory results (79,80).

The important potential role of ^{67}Ga scintigraphy in determining long-term outcome needs to be assessed with larger groups of patients and in various types and stages of disease to determine whether early modification of treatment on the basis of results of ^{67}Ga scintigraphy performed early during treatment will improve overall patient outcome.

Other Tumors

For the most part, ^{67}Ga scintigraphy has no current clinical role in the assessment of patients with other tumors. It does, however, have an interesting history in evaluation for lung carcinoma, malignant tumors of the head and neck, genitourinary tract tumors, mesothelioma, hepatoma, and malignant melanoma. When ^{67}Ga scintigraphy was introduced, it was the first imaging technique to show tumor activity and location. Despite the early recognition that ^{67}Ga localization was not tumor-specific and had limited sensitivity, ^{67}Ga scintigraphy provided an interesting and unique opportunity for tumor detection and determination of extent of involvement. Although the technical quality and sensitivity improved steadily, advances in other diagnostic imaging techniques, particularly CT, eclipsed ^{67}Ga scintigraphy for most indications except focused applications in non-Hodgkin's lymphoma and Hodgkin's disease.

Melanoma

Most malignant melanomas and metastatic lesions are sufficiently gallium-avid to be detected with ^{67}Ga scintigraphy when the tumor mass exceeds 1 cm in diameter. In a prospective study of 67 patients with metastatic melanoma who underwent ^{67}Ga scintigraphy with 10-mCi (370-MBq) doses of ^{67}Ga citrate with an early tomographic instrument (Pho/Con), Kirkwood et al. (81) reported an overall sensitivity and specificity of 82% and 99%. Nevertheless, ^{67}Ga scintigraphy is infrequently used in the care of patients with this malignant tumor. Kogan et al. (82) confirmed the accuracy of ^{67}Ga scintigraphy for detection of melanoma but did not find that additional clinical benefit was obtained by adding ^{67}Ga scintigraphy to the routine evaluation of patients with melanoma. The primary lesions of malignant melanoma usually are detected by means of physical examination. Although ^{67}Ga scintigraphy may be a method for long-term evaluation of patients after initial diagnosis and may be a means to assess response after therapy, there are no reports of its utility in this application.

Hepatoma

Most hepatocellular carcinomas (hepatomas) are gallium-avid. By contrast, in cirrhosis, zones of fibrosis or regenerating hepatic tissue representing the so-called pseudotumor of cirrhosis rarely display gallium uptake (83–93). Thus ^{67}Ga scintigraphy is useful in differentiating pseudotumor and hepatoma in patients with known cirrhosis who have signs of hepatic decompensation and are found to have masses at MRI, CT, or ultrasound examination. Cornelius and Atterbury (94) reviewed the pre-1984 literature on ^{67}Ga scintigraphy of hepatoma. In 164 patients described in nine articles, 63% of hepatomas concentrated more gallium than did the host liver tissue, 25% of the hepatomas had ^{67}Ga uptake approximately equal to the surrounding liver tissue, and only 12% of hepatomas showed radiogallium uptake less than that of the host liver. Thus approximately 88% of hepatomas are gallium-avid with reference to normal liver. However, exceptional care must be used in interpreting radiogallium scans of the liver. Many other hepatic lesions (abscess or gallium-avid metastatic disease) are positive at ^{67}Ga scintigraphy. The scintigraphic diagnosis of hepatoma can be made only in the correct clinical setting. Biopsy confirmation of this serious diagnosis usually is performed in any event. The findings at ^{67}Ga scintigraphy can serve to identify the site most likely to lead to the diagnosis.

Lung Carcinoma

^{67}Ga accumulates to a very high degree in primary tumors of the lung. The sensitivity of gallium scans in the detection of lung cancer is affected by the histologic features of the tumor and depends on tumor size. Tumors must be 1 cm or greater in diameter for reliable detection, even with current instruments and techniques (95). Gallium scintigraphy, however, is neither more sensitive nor more specific than simple chest radiography for detection of primary lesions of lung cancer. Gallium scans have been advocated, however, for evaluation of mediastinal metastatic disease, because detection of hilar and mediastinal lymph-node involvement is critical in determining prognosis and treatment of lung cancer patients. Small cell tumors usually are not managed surgically, but tumors of other cell types typically are managed by means of resection of the primary lesion. In the absence of hilar or mediastinal node involvement, the posttreatment survival rate approaches 50% at 5 years for patients with squamous cell cancer. However, if lymph nodes of the hilum and mediastinum are involved, the probability of disease-free survival decreases to less than 10% at 5 years, and thoracotomy usually is not indicated (96).

Mediastinoscopy is the procedure of choice for detection of mediastinal metastatic lesions, but it is a complex surgical procedure in and of itself, and lesions are not detected in a small percentage of cases (97). Alazraki et al (98) initially advocated gallium scanning as a screening method for detection of mediastinal involvement. In their early study, ^{67}Ga scanning was highly sensitive, although it suffered from relatively poor specificity. Thus these authors recommended preoperative mediastinoscopy only for patients with mediastinal uptake of gallium. Fosberg et al. (99) and Lesk et al. (100), in a retrospective study, confirmed these findings. Lunia et al. (101) in a prospective comparison, found that ^{67}Ga scanning was more accurate than chest radiography in the assessment of regional node involvement. DeMeester et al. (102), however, found radiogallium to be relatively insensitive as a detector of mediastinal lymph-node involvement. The false-negative rate was approximately 33% for paramediastinal primary lesions. In our experience (103), non-SPECT gallium scanning was neither sensitive nor specific for detection of mediastinal involvement in carcinoma of the lung.

A prospective study (104) with 75 patients with lung cancer who underwent ^{67}Ga scanning followed by thoracotomy with total mediastinal node dissection showed a very low sensitivity of 23%, specificity of 82%, and overall accuracy of only 63% for ^{67}Ga scintigraphy. The low sensitivity was attributed the inability of ^{67}Ga scanning to depict microscopic metastases in mediastinal lymph nodes. The specificity was diminished by gallium uptake in enlarged reactive nodes that contained no metastatic lesion. These results reinforce our earlier findings that gallium scintigraphy is not accurate enough to allow determination of which patients have metastatic lung carcinoma of hilar or mediastinal lymph nodes. A similar conclusion was published later by one of the groups who was initially very enthusiastic about ^{67}Ga scanning of the mediastinum (105). At present, conventional ^{67}Ga nuclear medicine techniques should not be relied on for preoperative staging of mediastinal lymph node metastasis in patients with lung cancer.

Gallium scanning has been evaluated for the detection of extrathoracic spread of lung carcinoma. The economy and logistic simplicity of evaluating local and distant metastatic lesions with a single imaging procedure are attractive, especially because symptoms may not lead to correct identification of the organ system affected by metastasis (106).

In one study of patients with small cell carcinoma, only 7% of extrathoracic metastatic lesions were found, although 84% of cases of mediastinal disease were identified (107). Another study, which included tumors of all cell types, showed that 75% of metastatic sites found with all other clinical methods (radionu-

clide scans of individual organs, CT, and clinical examination) were detected with whole-body gallium scanning. Whole-body gallium scans accurately depicted or excluded extrathoracic metastatic disease in 11 of 12 patients described in a separate report (102) on whom autopsy was performed within 3 months of the scan. However, the evidence currently available is insufficient for conclusive determination of the value of whole-body gallium scans in efficient and accurate detection of metastatic lung cancer.

Mesothelioma

[67]Ga scintigraphy has been reported to be useful in evaluation of the local extent of disease and distant metastasis for patients with pleural mesothelioma (108,109). The clinical experience with ^{67}Ga scintigraphy in this instance is very limited. However, the authors cited found gallium scans more sensitive than chest radiography in defining sites of malignant mesothelioma from benign pleural thickening.

Head and Neck Tumors

The utility of ^{67}Ga scanning in the staging and follow-up evaluation of head and neck tumors has been the subject of several reports with varying results. Kashima et al. (110) found positive results of ^{67}Ga scans in 86% of patients with primary tumors of the head and neck. All of the lesions detected were 2 cm or more in diameter. These results are not competitive, however, with current CT or MRI, which can usually depict primary lesions of the head and neck at a smaller size. Teates et al. (111) reported the data from a cooperative group study that analyzed ^{67}Ga scans on a site-by-site basis for patients with head and neck tumors. The overall sensitivity was only 56%. Of interest, previous surgery or irradiation of the primary or metastatic head and neck tumors did not seem to affect the tumor detection rate with ^{67}Ga scanning. Thus gallium scintigraphy may be of occasional use to such patients in the detection of recurrent tumor after therapy when the anatomic planes and landmarks are too obscure to allow accurate CT. Silverstein et al. (112) reported a poor prognosis for patients with tumors of the head and neck whose studies showed uptake in recurrent tumor as compared with patients who had "gallium-negative" residual masses. Finally, Higashi et al. (113) have used ^{67}Ga scans to differentiate malignant tumors of the maxillary sinus, which were strongly gallium-avid, and chronic sinusitis which was only faintly gallium-avid. This use treads a fine line, however, because active sinusitis could presumably be strongly gallium-positive.

Tumors of the Abdominal and Pelvic Organs

Primary and metastatic tumors involving the abdominal and pelvic organs can be detected with ^{67}Ga scintigraphy with varying accuracy. Several reports have indicated that ^{67}Ga scans were useful in detecting metastases, particularly to regional nodes, from some histologic types of malignant testicular tumors (114–117). Pinsky et al. (117) described a series of 36 patients with surgically proven testicular tumors with intraabdominal lymph node metastasis who underwent ^{67}Ga scanning. ^{67}Ga scintigraphy was 92% accurate in the detection of nodal metastases. Patterson et al. (115) found 13 of 15 ^{67}Ga scintigraphic examinations of patients with disseminated seminoma in relapse gave good images of the areas involved in metastatic disease. This group found a correlation between gallium uptake and histologic tumor type. All seminomas studied were detected with ^{67}Ga scintigraphy, but only approximately one fifth of the teratomas scanned accumulated sufficient gallium to be detected. ^{67}Ga uptake by metastatic lesions from testicular carcinoma thus seems to vary with the histologic type of the primary tumor. Approximate sensitivity determined in the previous reports was 75% for metastatic embryonal cell carcinoma, 57% to 90% for metastatic seminoma, approximately 25% for teratoma of the testis, and 93% to 100% for primary extragonadal seminoma.

Poor results have discouraged the use of ^{67}Ga scintigraphy for most gynecologic tumors (116–120). It is not completely clear why this should be the case because some tumors of the ovaries are counterparts to gallium-avid testicular tumors, and one would expect a similar degree of gallium uptake. The number of patients with ovarian carcinoma who have undergone ^{67}Ga scintigraphy, particularly with current techniques, is extremely small. Therefore reliable data on the utility of this test in these patients is difficult to assess. For example, one report found a slight improvement in the diagnostic utility of x-ray CT scans of patients with ovarian carcinoma when ^{67}Ga scintigraphy was performed as an additional test (120). It is doubtful, however, that gallium scintigraphy at present significantly affects the clinical use of CT, MRI, or ultrasonography in the evaluation of ovarian neoplasia.

Tumors of the gastrointestinal tract and pancreas, chiefly adenocarcinoma, are not usually evaluated with ^{67}Ga scintigraphy, again because of the poor accuracy reported in most published studies. Langhammer et al. (121) found that only 14 of 33 tumors of the gastrointestinal tract were showed positive results on ^{67}Ga scans. A 1974 review by Silberstein (122) showed only 10 instances of gallium-positive tumors of gastrointestinal tract. In a later review by Hauser and Alderson (123), there is a tabulation of only seven individual reports in the literature before 1978 with a combined sensitivity in the detection of nonlymphomatous gastric tumors of 47%; of colonic neoplasm, 25%; and of pancreatic tumors, only 15%. This reported low incidence of positive results of gallium scans in the detection of gastrointestinal tract and pancreatic tumors, with the exception of lymphoma, has not been challenged by recent reports. One problem is that although some types of gastrointestinal tract tumors can accumulate sufficient gallium, the normal intestinal excretion of this radionuclide combined with the relatively large amount of gallium normal in the liver and spleen make ^{67}Ga scintigraphy of abdominal tumors at best tedious and fraught with difficulty in interpretation. Gallium scans seem impractical in this application, in which other methods of imaging have established themselves.

Malignant Soft-tissue Tumors

Schwartz and Jones (124) reported very high sensitivity and good specificity for the use of gallium scans to detect soft-tissue sar-

coma, including occult metastatic lesions. The results of this prospective study were better than those in previous reports of this use of gallium (125,126).

CONCLUSION

^{67}Ga scintigraphy has evolved over the past 25 years. The results are an indicator of tumor viability based on metabolic activity rather than size. Thus the method is more specific than is anatomic imaging, such as CT and MRI or other radiologic procedures. ^{67}Ga scintigraphy has an established role in the care of patients with lymphoma and Hodgkin's disease because of its greater sensitivity and specificity in the detection of viable tumor than those of the radiologic procedures. In this disease group, imaging has replaced surgical intervention for staging and follow-up evaluation. Although ^{67}Ga scintigraphy also helps identify tumors such as lung carcinoma and melanoma, surgical assessment for staging and evaluation of possible recurrence has remained the standard of practice for these malignant diseases. ^{67}Ga scintigraphy has not become a reliable substitute for direct assessment of tumor viability of these and other neoplasms. Ironic is that ^{67}Ga scintigraphy, including SPECT imaging, has reached its highest state of technical quality. Oncologists have begun to recognize and use ^{67}Ga scintigraphy as a technique to assess response to therapy, for the more accurate detection of recurrent disease, and as a prognostic indicator of response to therapy among patients with lymphoma and Hodgkin's disease. ^{18}F-FDG PET has emerged as a likely replacement for ^{67}Ga scintigraphy in each of these indications. The physical characteristics of ^{18}F as a imaging agent are markedly superior to those of ^{67}Ga, and ^{18}F-FDG appears to be a sensitive tracer of the increased metabolism associated with tumors. For these reasons, it is not surprising that comparative studies confirm the previous good performance of ^{67}Ga scintigraphy and demonstrate the superiority of ^{18}F-FDG PET as a diagnostic imaging technique for each of the possible clinical indications in lymphoma management as well as for management of other types of tumors in which ^{67}Ga scintigraphy had shown early promise.

REFERENCES

1. Edwards CL, Hayes RL. Tumor scanning with gallium citrate. *J Nucl Med* 1969;10:103–105.
2. Hoffer PB. Status of gallium-67 in tumor detection. *J Nucl Med* 1980; 21:394–398.
3. Bekerman C, Hoffer PB, Bitran JD. The role of gallium-67 in the clinical evaluation of cancer. *Semin Nucl Med* 1984;14:296–323.
4. Kostakoglu L, Leonard J, Kuji I, et al. Comparison of fluorine-18 fluorodeoxyglucose positron emission tomography and ^{67}Ga scintigraphy in evaluation of lymphoma. *Cancer* 2002;94:879–888.
5. HCFA. Positron Emission Tomography Scans [50–36] in Coverage Issues Manual, Part 50 [available at http://cms.hhs.gov/manuals/cmtoc.asp.
6. Gunsekerra SW, King LJ, Lavender PJ. The behavior of tracer gallium-67 towards serum proteins. *Clin Chim Acta* 1972;39:401–406.
7. Vallabhajosula SR, Harwig JF, Siemsen JK, et al. Radiogallium localization in tumors: blood binding, transport and the role of transferrin. *J Nucl Med* 1980;21:650–656.
8. Hoffer PB, Huberty J, Khayam-Bashi H. The association of ^{67}Ga and lactoferrin. *J Nucl Med* 1977;18:713–717.

9. Clausen J, Edeling CJ, Fogh J. [67]Ga binding to human serum proteins and tumor components. *Cancer Res* 1974;34:1931–1937.

10. Hegge FN, Mahler DJ, Larson SM. The incorporation of ^{67}Ga into the ferritin fraction of rabbit hepatocytes in vivo. *J Nucl Med* 1977; 18:937–939.

11. Larson SM, Rasey JS, Grunbaum Z, et al. Pharmacologic enhancement of ^{67}Ga tumors to blood ratios for EMT-6 sarcoma. *Radiology* 1979;130:241–243.

12. Hoffer PB, Samuel A, Bushberg JT, et al. Effect of desferrioxamine on tissue and tumor retention of [67]Ga: concise communication. *J Nucl Med* 1979;26:248–251.

13. Sephton RG, Hodgson GS, De Abrew S, et al. [67]Ga and Fe-59 distributions in mice. *J Nucl Med* 1978;19:930–935.

14. Logan KJ, Ng PK, Turner CJ, et al. Comparative pharmacokinetics of ^{67}Ga and Fe-59 in humans. *Int J Nucl Med Biol* 1981;8:271–276.

15. Larson SM, Rasey JS, Allen DR, et al. Common pathway for tumor cell uptake of ^{67}Ga and iron-59 via a transferrin receptor. *J Natl Cancer Inst* 1980;64:41–53.

16. Larson SM, Rasey JS, Nelson NJ, et al. The kinetics of uptake and macromolecular binding of ^{67}Ga and Fe-59 by the EMT-6 sarcoma–like tumor of Balb/c mice. In: *Radiopharmaceuticals II: proceedings of the second international symposium on radiopharmaceuticals.* New York: Society of Nuclear Medicine, 1979:277–308.

17. Larson SM, Rasey JS, Allen DR, et al. A transferrin-mediated uptake of ^{67}Ga by EMT-6 sarcoma, II: studies in vivo (BALB/c mice)—concise communication. *J Nucl Med* 1979;20:843–846.

18. DeAbrew S. Assays for transferrin and transferrin receptors in tumor and other mouse tissues. *Int J Nucl Med Biol* 1981;8:217–221.

19. Ennis CA, Shindelman JE, Tonik SE, et al. Radioimmunochemical measurement of the transferrin receptor in human trophoblast and reticulocyte membranes with a specific anti-receptor antibody. *Proc Natl Acad Sci U S A* 1981;78:4222–4225.

20. Chitambar CR, Zivkovic Z. Uptake of ^{67}Ga by human leukemic cells: demonstration of transferrin receptor–dependent and transferrin-independent mechanisms. *Cancer Res* 1987;47:3929–3924.

21. Chan SM, Hoffer PB, Maric N, et al. Inhibition of gallium-67 uptake in melanoma by an anti-human transferrin receptor monoclonal antibody. *J Nucl Med* 1987;28:1303–1307.

22. Vallabhajosula SR, Harwig JF, Wolf W. Effect of pH on tumor cell uptake of radiogallium in vitro and in vivo. *Eur J Nucl Med* 1982; 7:462–468.

23. Iosilevsky G, Front D, Betman L, et al. Uptake of gallium-67 citrate and (2 H-3) deoxyglucose in the tumor model following chemotherapy and radiotherapy. *J Nucl Med* 1985;26:278–282.

24. Kubota K, Ishiwata K, Kubota R, et al. Tracer feasibility for monitoring tumor radiotherapy: a quadruple tracer study with fluorine-18–fluorodeoxyglucose or fluorine-18–fluorodeoxyuridine, L-[methyl-^{14}C] methionine, [6-^{3}H]thymidine, and gallium-67. *J Nucl Med* 1991;32:2118–2123.

25. Sohn ME, Jones BJ, Whiting JH, et al. Distribution of ^{67}Ga in normal and hypotransferrinemic tumor-bearing mice. *J Nucl Med* 1993;34: 2135–2143.

26. Bradley WP, Alderson PO, Eckelman WC, et al. Decreased tumor uptake of gallium-67 in animals after whole-body irradiation. *J Nucl Med* 1978;19:204–209.

27. Chilton HM, Witcofski RL, Watson NE, et al. Alteration of gallium-67 distribution in tumor-bearing mice following treatment with methotrexate: concise communication. *J Nucl Med* 1981;22: 1064–1068.

28. Scheffel U, Wagner Jr. HN, Klein JL. Gallium-67 uptake by hepatoma: studies in cell cultures, perfused livers, and intact rats. *J Nucl Med* 1985;26:1438–1444.

29. Sephton RG. *Factors affecting ^{67}Ga distribution: frontiers in nuclear medicine.* New York: Springer-Verlag, 1980:154–161.

30. Hayes RL, Rafter JJ, Byrd BL, et al. Studies of the in vivo entry of ^{67}Ga into normal and malignant tissue. *J Nucl Med* 1981;22:325–332.

31. Hayes RL, Rafter JJ, Carlton JE, et al. Studies on the in vivo uptake of ^{67}Ga by an experimental abscess: concise communication. *J Nucl Med* 1982;23:8–14.

32. Donahue DM, Leonard JC, Basmadjian GP, et al. Thymic ^{67}Ga in pediatric patients on chemotherapy. *J Nucl Med* 1981;22:1043–1048.

33. Chen DC, Scheffel U, Camargo EE, et al. The source of gallium-67 in gastrointestinal contents: concise communication. *J Nucl Med* 1980;21:1146–1150.

34. Crichton RR. *Inorganic chemistry of iron metabolism.* New York: Ellis Horwood, 1990:90–91.

35. Englestad B, Luk SS, Hattner RS. Altered ^{67}Ga citrate distribution in patients with multiple red blood cell transfusions. *Am J Radiol* 1982;139:755–759.

36. Loesberg AC, Martin WB. Altered biodistribution of ^{67}Ga citrate in an iron-overloaded patient with sickle cell disease. *Clin Nucl Med* 1994;19:157–159.

37. Hattner RS, White DL. Gallium-67/stable gadolinium antagonism: MRI contrast agent markedly alters the normal biodistribution of [67]Ga. *J Nucl Med* 1990;31:1844–1846.

38. Bekerman C, Pavel DG, Bitran J, et al. The effects of inadvertent administration of antineoplastic agents prior to ^{67}Ga injection: concise communication. *J Nucl Med* 1984;25:430–435.

39. Baker DL, Manno CS. Rapid excretion of ^{67}Ga isotope in an iron-overloaded patient receiving high-dose intravenous desferrioxamine. *Am J Hematol* 1988;29:230–232.

40. Brown SJ, Slizofiski WJ, Dadparvar S. Altered biodistribution of ^{67}Ga in a patient with aluminum toxicity treated with desferrioxamine. *J Nucl Med* 1990;31:115–117.

41. McLaughlin AF, Magee MA, Greenough R, et al. Current role of gallium scanning in the management of lymphoma. *Eur J Nucl Med* 1990;16:755–771.

42. Tumeh SS, Rosenthal DS, Kaplan WD, et al. Lymphoma: evaluation with ^{67}Ga SPECT. *Radiology* 1987;164:111–114.

43. Front D, Israel O, Epelbaum R, et al. [67]Ga SPECT before and after treatment of lymphoma. *Radiology* 1990;175:515–519.

44. Kostakoglu L, Yeh SD, Portlock C, et al. Validation of gallium-67–citrate SPECT in biopsy-confirmed residual Hodgkin's disease in the mediastinum. *J Nucl Med* 1992;33:345–350.

45. Dillehay GL, Papatheofanis F. Gallium Imaging of Tumors. In: Henkin RE, Boles MA, Dillebing GL, et al: *Nuclear medicine.* St. Louis: Mosby, 1996, pp. 1463–1492.

46. Johnson GS, Go MF, Benua RS, et al. Gallium-67 citrate imaging in Hodgkin's disease: final report of cooperative group. *J Nucl Med* 1977;18:692–698.

47. Andrews GA, Hubner KF, Greenlaw RH. [67]Ga citrate imaging in malignant lymphoma: final report of cooperative group. *J Nucl Med* 1978;19:1013–1019.

48. Bekerman C, Hoffer PB, Bitran JD. The role of gallium-67 in the clinical evaluation of cancer. *Semin Nucl Med* 1985;15:72–103.

49. Glass RB, Fernbach SK, Conway JJ, et al. Gallium scintigraphy in American Burkitt lymphoma: accurate assessment of tumor load and prognosis. *Am J Roentgenol* 1985;145:671–676.

50. Gallamini A, Biggi A, Fruttero A, et al. Revisiting the prognostic role of gallium scintigraphy in low-grade non-Hodgkin's lymphoma. *Eur J Nucl Med* 1997;24:1499–1506.

51. Ben-Haim S, Bar-Shalom R, Israel O, et al. Utility of gallium-67 scintigraphy in low-grade non-Hodgkin's lymphoma. *J Clin Oncol* 1996;14:1936–1942.

52. Canellos GP. Residual mass in lymphoma may not be residual disease [editorial]. *J Clin Oncol* 1988;6:931–933.

53. Israel O, Front D, Lam M, et al. Gallium-67 imaging in monitoring lymphoma response to treatment. *Cancer* 1988;61:2439–2443.

54. Wylie BR, Southee AE, Joshua DE, et al. Gallium scanning in the management of mediastinal Hodgkin's disease. *Eur J Haematol* 1989; 42:344–347.

55. Israel O, Front D, Epelbaum R, et al. Residual mass and negative gallium scintigraphy in treated lymphoma. *J Nucl Med* 1990;31: 365–368.

56. Drossman SR, Schiff RG, Kronfeld GD, et al. Lymphoma of the mediastinum and neck: evaluation with ^{67}Ga imaging and CT correlation. *Radiology* 1990;174:171–175.

57. Weiner M, Leventhal B, Cantor A, et al. Gallium-67 scan as an adjunct to computed tomography scans for the assessment of a residual

mediastinal mass in pediatric patients with Hodgkin's disease. *Cancer* 1991;68:2478–2480.

58. Karimjee S, Brada M, Husband J, et al. A comparison of gallium-67 single photon emission computed tomography and computed tomography in mediastinal Hodgkin's disease. *Eur J Cancer* 1992;28A: 1856–1857.

59. Front D, Israel O, Ben-Haim S. The dilemma of a residual mass in treated lymphoma: the role of gallium-67 scintigraphy. In: Freeman L, ed. *Nuclear medicine annual.* New York: Raven Press, 1991.

60. Ionescu I, Brice P, Simon D, et al. Restaging with gallium scan identifies chemosensitive patients and predicts survival of poor-prognosis mediastinal Hodgkin's disease patients. *Med Oncol* 2000;17: 127–134.

61. Salloum E, Brandt DS, Caride VJ, et al. Gallium scans in the management of patients with Hodgkin's disease: a study of 101 patients. *J Clin Oncol* 1997;15:518–527.

62. Bogart JA, Chung CT, Mariados NF, et al. The value of gallium imaging after therapy for Hodgkin's disease. *Cancer* 1998;82: 754–759.

63. Cooper DL, Caride VJ, Zloty M, et al. Gallium scans in patients with mediastinal Hodgkin's disease treated with chemotherapy. *J Clin Oncol* 1993;11:1092–1098.

64. Kaplan WD. Residual mass and negative gallium scintigraphy in treated lymphoma: when is the gallium scan really negative [editorial]? *J Nucl Med* 1990;31:369–371.

65. Front D, Israel O. The role of ^{67}Ga scintigraphy in evaluating the results of therapy of lymphoma patients. *Semin Nucl Med* 1995;25: 60–71.

66. Israel O, Yefremov N, Mor M, et al. A new technology of combined transmission (CT) and emission (^{67}Ga) tomography (TET) in the evaluation of patients with lymphoma. *J Nucl Med* 2000;41:70P(abst).

67. Front D, Ben-Haim S, Israel O, et al. Lymphoma: predictive value of ^{67}Ga scintigraphy after therapy. *Radiology* 1992;182:359–363.

68. Vose JM, Bierman PJ, Anderson JR, et al. Single-photon emission computed tomography gallium imaging versus computed tomography: predictive value in patients undergoing high-dose chemotherapy and autologous stem-cell transplantation for non-Hodgkin's lymphoma. *J Clin Oncol* 1996;14:2473–2479.

69. Weeks JC, Yeap BY, Canellos GP, et al. Value of follow-up procedures in patients with large-cell lymphoma who achieve a complete remission. *J Clin Oncol* 1991;9:1196–1203.

70. DeVita VT, Hellman S, Jaffe ES. Hodgkin's disease. In: DeVita VT, Hellman S, Rosenberg SA, eds. *Cancer: principles and practice of oncology,* 4th ed. Philadelphia: Lippincott–Raven, 1993.

71. Armitage JO, Weisenburger DD, Hutchins M, et al. Chemotherapy for diffuse large-cell lymphoma: rapidly responding patients have more durable remissions. *J Clin Oncol* 1986;4:160–164.

72. Vose JM, Armitage JO, Bierman PJ, et al. Salvage therapy for relapsed or refractory non-Hodgkin's lymphoma utilizing autologous bone marrow transplantation. *Am J Med* 1989;87:285–288.

73. Front D, Bar-Shalom R, Epelbaum R, et al. Early detection of lymphoma recurrence with gallium-67 scintigraphy. *J Nucl Med* 1993; 34:2101–2104.

74. Kaplan WD, Jochelson MS, Herman TS, et al. Gallium-67 imaging: a predictor of residual tumor viability and clinical outcome in patients with diffuse large-cell lymphoma. *J Clin Oncol* 1990;8:1966–1970.

75. Janicek M, Kaplan W, Neuberg D, et al. Early restaging gallium scans predict outcome in poor-prognosis patients with aggressive non-Hodgkin's lymphoma treated with high-dose CHOP chemotherapy. *J Clin Oncol* 1997;15:1631–1637.

76. Gasparini M, Bombardieri E, Castellani M, et al. Gallium-67 scintigraphy evaluation of therapy in non-Hodgkin's lymphoma. *J Nucl Med* 1998;39:1586–1590.

77. Front D, Bar-Shalom R, Mor M, et al. Hodgkin disease: prediction of outcome with Ga67 scintigraphy after one cycle of chemotherapy. *Radiology* 1999;210:487–491.

78. Front D, Bar-Shalom R, Mor M, et al. Aggressive non-Hodgkin lymphoma: early prediction of outcome with Ga67 scintigraphy. *Radiology* 2000;214:253–257.

79. Link MP, Shuster JJ, Donaldson SS, et al. Treatment of children and

young adults with early-stage non-Hodgkin's lymphoma. *N Engl J Med* 1997;337:1259–1266.

80. Magrath I. Limiting therapy for limited childhood non-Hodgkin's lymphoma. *N Engl J Med* 1997;337:1304–1305.

81. Kirkwood JM, Myers JE, Vlock DR, et al. Tomographic ^{67}Ga citrate scanning: useful new surveillance for metastatic melanoma. *Ann Intern Med* 1982;97:694–699.

82. Kogan R, Witt T, Bines S, et al. ^{67}Ga scanning for malignant melanoma. *Cancer* 1988;61:272–274.

83. Suzuki T, Honjo I, Hamamoto K, et al. Positive scintiphotography of cancer of the liver with ^{67}Ga citrate. *Am J Roentgenol* 1971;113: 92–103.

84. Lomas FR, Dibos PE, Wagner HN. Increased specificity of liver scanning with the use of ^{67}Ga citrate. *N Engl J Med* 1972;286:1323–1329.

85. James O, Wood J, Maze M, et al. ^{67}Ga citrate liver scanning: evaluation of its use in 80 patients and evidence of intrahepatic distribution by autoradiography. *Gut* 1974;15:342.

86. Blazek G. Mastnak C, Kahn P, et al. ^{67}Ga scintigraphy as an auxiliary method for differentiation of mass lesions of the liver. *Wien Klin Wochenschr* 1975;87:77–81.

87. Levin J, Kew MC. ^{67}Ga citrate scanning in primary cancer of the liver: diagnostic value in the presence of cirrhosis and relation to alpha-fetoprotein. *J Nucl Med* 1975;16:949–951.

88. Buraggi GL, Laurini R, Rodari A, et al. Double-tracer scintigraphy with ^{67}Ga citrate and ^{99m}Tc sulfur colloid in the diagnosis of hepatic tumors. *J Nucl Med* 1976;17:373–396.

89. Moreau R, Soussaline F, Chauvaud S, et al. Detection of hepatoma in liver cirrhosis. *Eur J Nucl Med* 1977;2:183.

90. Yeh S, Leeper R, Benau R. A study of filling defects in the liver and spleen with multiple radionuclides. *Clin Bull* 1977;7:3.

91. Waxman AD, Richmond R, Juttner H, et al. Correlation of contrast angiography and histologic pattern with gallium uptake in primary liver-cell carcinoma: noncorrelation of alpha-fetoprotein. *J Nucl Med* 1980;21:324–327.

92. Broderick TW, Gosink B, Menuck L, et al. Echographic and radionuclide detection of hepatoma. *Radiology* 1980;135:149–151.

93. Negasue N. Gallium scanning in the diagnosis of hepatocellular carcinoma: a clinicopathological study of 45 patients. *Clin Radiol* 1983; 34:139–142.

94. Cornelius EA, Atterbury CE. Problems in the imaging diagnosis of hepatoma. *Clin Nucl Med* 1984;9:30–38.

95. Abdel-Dayem HM, Scott A, Macapinlac H, et al. Tracer imaging in lung cancer. *Eur J Nucl Med* 1994;21:57–81.

96. Mountain CF. Biologic, physiologic and technical; determinants in surgical therapy for lung cancer. In: Strauss MJ, ed. *Lung cancer: clinical diagnosis and treatment.* New York: Grune & Stratton, 1977: 185–198.

97. Goldberg EM. Mediastinoscopy in assessment of lung cancer. In: Strauss MJ, ed. *Lung cancer: clinical diagnosis and treatment.* New York: Grune & Stratton, 1977:113–128.

98. Alazraki NP, Ramsdell JW, Taylor A, et al. Reliability of gallium scan, chest radiography compared to mediastinoscopy for evaluating mediastinal spread in lung cancer. *Am Rev Respir Dis* 1978;117: 415–420.

99. Fosburg RG, Hopkins GB, Kan MK. Evaluation of the mediastinum by ^{67}Ga scintigraphy in lung cancer. *J Thorac Cardiovasc Surg* 1979; 77:76–82.

100. Lesk DM, Wood TE, Carrol SE, et al. The application of ^{67}Ga scanning in determining the operability of bronchogenic carcinoma. *Radiology* 1978;128:707–709.

101. Lunia SL, Ruckdeschel JC, McKneally MF. Noninvasive evaluation of mediastinal metastases in bronchogenic carcinoma: a prospective comparison of chest radiography and ^{67}Ga scanning. *Cancer* 1981; 47:672–679.

102. DeMeester TR, Golumb HM, Kirchner P, et al. The role of ^{67}Ga scanning in the clinical staging and preoperative evaluation of patients with carcinoma of the lung. *Ann Thorac Surg* 1979;18:451–464.

103. Neumann RD, Hoffer PB, Merino MJ, et al. Clinical value of ^{67}Ga in imaging patients with lung carcinoma and melanoma. In: *Medical radionuclide imaging 1980.* Vol II. Vienna: IAEA, 1981.

104. McKenna RJ, Haynie TP, Libshitz HI, et al. Critical evaluation of the ^{67}Ga scan for surgical patients with lung cancer. *Chest* 1985;87: 428–431.
105. Friedman PJ, Feigin DS, Liston SE, et al. Sensitivity of chest radiography, computer tomography and gallium scanning to metastasis of lung carcinoma. *Cancer* 1984;54:1300–1306.
106. Hooper RG, Beechler CR, Johnson MC. Radioisotope scanning in the initial staging of bronchogenic carcinoma. *Am Rev Resp Dis* 1978; 118:279–286.
107. Brereton HD, Line BR, Londer HN, et al. Gallium scans for staging small cell lung cancer. *JAMA* 1978;240:666–667.
108. Sorek M, Teirstein AS, Goldsmith SJ, et al. ^{67}Ga citrate uptake in benign and malignant pleural disease. *Clin Res* 1979;27:491A.
109. Wolk RB. ^{67}Ga scanning in the evaluation of mesothelioma. *J Nucl Med* 1978;19:808–809.
110. Kashima H, Mckusick K, Malmed L, et al. ^{67}Ga scanning in patients with head and neck cancer. *Laryngoscope* 1974;84:1078–1089.
111. Teates CD, Preston DF, Boyd CM. ^{67}Ga citrate imaging in head and neck tumors: report of the cooperative group. *J Nucl Med* 1980;21: 622–627.
112. Silverstein EG, Kornblut A, Shumrich DA, et al. ^{67}Ga as a diagnostic agent for detection of head and neck tumors and lymphoma. *Radiology* 1974;110:605–608.
113. Higashi T, Auyama W, Mori Y, et al. ^{67}Ga scanning in the differentiation of maxillary sinus carcinoma from chronic maxillary sinusitis. *Radiology* 1977;123:117–122.
114. Jackson FI, Dietrich HC, Lentle BC. ^{67}Ga citrate scintiscanning in testicular neoplasia. *J Can Assoc Radiol* 1976;27:84–88.
115. Patterson AH, Peckham MJ, McCready VR. Value of gallium scanning in seminoma of the testis. *Br Med J* 1976;1:1118–1121.
116. Sauerbrunn B, Andrews G, Hubner K. ^{67}Ga citrate imaging in tumors of the genitourinary tract: report of cooperative study. *J Nucl Med* 1978;19:470–475.
117. Pinsky SM, Bailey TB, Blom J, et al. ^{67}Ga citrate in the staging of testicular malignancies. *J Nucl Med* 1973;14:439.
118. Symmonds RE, Tauke WN. ^{67}Ga scintigraphy of gynecologic tumors. *Am J Obstet Gynecol* 1972;114:356–369.
119. Pelosi MA, D'Amico RJ, Apuzzio J. Combined use of ultrasonography and gallium scanning in the diagnosis of pelvic pathology. *Surg Gynecol Obstet* 1980;150:331.
120. Okamura S. Diagnosis of ovarian tumors by CT and ^{67}Ga citrate scintigraphy. *Nippon Sanka Fujinka Gakkai Zasshi* 1983;35:805.
121. Langhammer H, Glaubitt G, Grebe SF, et al. ^{67}Ga for tumor scanning. *J Nucl Med* 1972;13:25–30.
122. Silberstein EB. Cancer diagnosis: the role of tumor imaging radiopharmaceuticals. *Am J Med* 1974;60:226–237.
123. Hauser MF, Alderson PO. ^{67}Ga imaging in abdominal disease. *Semin Nucl Med* 1978;8:251–270.
124. Schwartz HS, Jones CK. The efficacy of gallium scintigraphy in detecting malignant soft tissue neoplasias. *Ann Surg* 1992;215:78–82.
125. Kaufman JH, Cedermark BJ, Parthasarathy KL, et al. The value of ^{67}Ga scintigraphy in soft tissue sarcoma and chondrosarcoma. *Radiology* 1977;123:131–134.
126. Bitran JD, Bekerman C, Golomb HM, et al. Scintigraphic evaluation of sarcomata in children and adults by ^{67}Ga citrate. *Cancer* 1978;42: 1760–1765.

Diagnostic Nuclear Medicine, Fourth Edition. Edited by M.P. Sandler, R.E. Coleman, J.A. Patton, F.J.Th. Wackers, A. Gottschalk. Lippincott Williams & Wilkins, Philadelphia 2003.

45

THALLIUM-201 AND TECHNETIUM-99M METHOXYISOBUTYL ISONITRILE (MIBI) IN NUCLEAR ONCOLOGY

ALAN D. WAXMAN

[201]Tl scintigraphy is well established in its utility as a marker of myocardial perfusion and viability. The role of ^{201}Tl chloride as an effective radiopharmaceutical in nuclear oncology is less well known, although a large number of reports have described its role in this area (1–28). [99m]Tc methoxyisobutyl isonitrile (MIBI) has supplanted ^{201}Tl chloride in many nuclear cardiology applications because of certain desirable imaging and biologic characteristics. An increasing number of reports are being published and presented that suggest an important role for ^{99m}Tc MIBI in nuclear oncology (29–55).

MECHANISM OF UPTAKE

[201]Tl

[201]Tl administered as a chloride behaves similarly to potassium chloride in most biologic systems (56–59). Many studies have shown the importance of the adenosine triphosphatase (ATPase)–mediated sodium-potassium pump within cell membranes that transports the potassium ion into intact cells in high concentration relative to the extracellular space. Because of the physical and biologic similarities of thallium and potassium, thallium is concentrated in a similar manner (60). Tumors also concentrate potassium ions and thallium in a similar manner (61,62).

Sessler et al. (62) developed a model for studying cellular uptake of ^{201}Tl with Ehrlich ascites tumor cells. Using this model, these investigators found that uptake of ^{201}Tl by tumor cells was inhibited by ouabain, which is known to inhibit the ATPase-sodium-potassium pump. Of great interest was the finding that furosemide also inhibited thallium uptake by tumor cells. Furosemide is known to inhibit a cotransport system involving transport of potassium and sodium, as well as chloride, ions into the cell. This study showed an additive effect of furosemide and ouabain on the inhibition of thallium uptake. It was postulated that at least two transport systems are involved in the

uptake of thallium by tumor cells. The cotransport system for thallium demonstrated a significant increase from 6-day-old Ehrlich cells to 12-day-old Ehrlich cells. In contrast, the ATPase level decreased as the cells became older. It was believed that the cotransport system played a dominant role in ^{201}Tl uptake by tumor cells. Also of interest was the discovery that after inhibition of the ATPase system and the cotransport system, a minimal resting flow for ionic transport was still preserved. This flow was attributed to a calcium-dependent ion channel system (62).

Ando et al. (63) evaluated the biodistribution of ^{201}Tl in tumor-bearing animals and found that thallium was mainly accumulated by viable tumor, less well accumulated in connective tissue that contained inflammatory cells, and barely detectable in necrotic tumor tissue. Ando et al. also determined that regardless of the length of time after administration, ^{201}Tl mainly exists in the free form in the fluid of a tumor. A small fraction of thallium was localized in the nuclear, mitochondrial, and microsomal fractions of these tissues, and ^{201}Tl was bound to protein in these fractions.

Table 45.1 lists factors thought to influence uptake of ^{201}Tl by tumor cells. Blood flow to tumor tissue appears important for delivery purposes (2,8,59,61). Poor vascularization of a tumor suggests that thallium accumulation is less than in a highly vascularized tumor. This finding has been clearly demonstrated in tumors with a significant degree of necrosis; however, no conclusive studies have compared the vascularity of tumors with the degree of thallium uptake.

Waxman et al. (14,23,28) found that in lymphoma the degree of ^{201}Tl uptake was more closely related to cell type than to any other single factor. In this series, highly vascular, aggressive tumors were actually found to have less ^{201}Tl activity than did slower growing, relatively nonaggressive tumors. In a later study, similar findings were demonstrated for ^{99m}Tc MIBI (50).

[99m]Tc MIBI

The exact mechanism of ^{99m}Tc MIBI uptake by tumor cells is not yet defined. Table 45.2 lists some characteristics of MIBI that may be responsible for uptake within tumor cells. Many of the proposed mechanisms are derived from studies of myocardial tissue; therefore extrapolation to tumor cells is speculative.

A.D. Waxman: Department of Radiology. University of Southern California, and Nuclear Medicine, Cedars-Sinai Health System, Los Angeles, CA.

Table 45.1. *Factors Affecting Tumor Uptake of ^{201}Tl*

Blood flow
Adenosine triphosphatase sodium potassium pump
Chloride cotransport system
Calcium ion channel
Leakage of immature tumor blood vessels

Unlike the active transport involved in thallium accumulation within the myocardium, the fundamental mechanism of myocellular accumulation of ^{99m}Tc MIBI most likely involves passive diffusion across the sarcolemmal and mitochondrial membranes in response to transmembrane potentials (64–71). ^{99m}Tc MIBI is considered a lipophilic cation greatly influenced by the negative charges on the mitochondria and the increased mitochondrial density present in tumors (66).

As with thallium accumulation in the myocardium or in tumors, adequate blood flow must be present for uptake to occur. Thus in tumors as in the myocardium, limitation of blood supply can result in decreased ^{99m}Tc MIBI uptake. Extraction, however, appears to depend on the transmembrane potential difference developed by tumors and on mitochondrial density (64–71).

Mechanism of MIBI Uptake in Cancer

Chiu et al. (65,67) suggest the driving force of MIBI accumulation in tissue culture cells is a strong electrostatic attraction between the positive charge of the lipophilic ^{99m}Tc MIBI molecule and the negative charge of the mitochondria. Carvalho et al. (68) found that approximately 90% of ^{99m}Tc MIBI activity occurs within the mitochondria. Results of additional studies appear to confirm a relation between cellular uptake of MIBI and mitochondrial activity or density (69).

Other factors that regulate the washout of MIBI from tumor cells have been observed. The multidrug-resistant P-glycoprotein system has MIBI as a substrate and effectively transports it out of tumor cells (67). This may prove to be an important factor in the evaluation of patients undergoing chemotherapy in whom resistance to medication may be developing. Additional factors such as angiogenesis, mitotic activity, and cell type may affect MIBI activity (70,71).

The overall concentration of ^{99m}Tc MIBI in tumors appears to be a function of many variables, including factors that affect the rate of uptake and factors that determine washout or excretion from the cell. Thus the relations between the multidrug resistant system and mitochondrial factors as well as factors not

Table 45.2. *Factors Affecting Tumor Uptake of ^{Tc99m}Sestamibi*

Blood flow
Lipophilic molecule
Net positive molecular charge
Mitochondrial negative charge (transmembrane potential effect)
Mitochondrial density
Leakage of immature tumor blood vessels
Multidrug resistant P-glycoprotein system activity

yet defined ultimately will determine the tumor concentration at a given point in time.

TUMORS OF THE CENTRAL NERVOUS SYSTEM

Evaluation with ^{201}Tl

Ancri et al. (4) evaluated 103 patients with confirmed cerebral lesions. Using 1.5 to 2.0 mCi of ^{201}Tl, these investigators determined that the optimal time for imaging cerebral tumors was approximately 30 minutes after injection. In most cases, however, the initial 0- to 5-minute image also gave excellent results; this finding suggested rapid uptake of ^{201}Tl in brain tumors. In this series, all cases of proven cerebral tumors, including primary glioma of the brain, metastatic lesions of the brain, and some cases of cerebral infarctions or cerebral hematoma, gave positive results within 10 minutes of injection. Despite the evaluation of 45 patients with glioma, the paper did not attempt to characterize thallium uptake according to tumor grade.

Several groups attempted to define indices of thallium uptake in brain tumors to grade the tumor and relate thallium uptake to histologic grade (11,16,20). Mountz et al. (11) developed a tumor-to-cardiac ratio from planar imaging to estimate the presence of astrocytoma after therapy. A baseline value was obtained, and serial repetitive studies were done after chemotherapy to assess the remaining viable tumor tissue.

Black et al. (16) and Kim et al. (20) used single photon emission computed tomography (SPECT) of the brain to calculate a relative thallium index to compare the tumor with the contralateral normal area of the brain. With the SPECT technique, it was possible to separate high-grade from low-grade tumors successfully. Some centers have suggested using ^{201}Tl for evaluating the presence of viable tumor after radiation therapy or chemotherapy. The technique has been difficult to use for low-grade glioma because these tumors often are not ^{201}Tl-avid and may not be detected. Conversely, we have found false-positive results in patients with severe radiation necrosis in which thallium levels have been low or moderate with no tumor found at repeated biopsy. In general, however, moderate or greater ^{201}Tl accumulation in sites of previous radiation indicate the presence of recurrent glioma. An example of recurrent glioma found with ^{201}Tl SPECT is shown in Fig. 45.1A. The results of magnetic resonance (MR) spectroscopy suggested radiation necrosis. The MR images were equivocal, and biopsy showed recurrent tumor.

Waxman et al. (72) evaluated an intraoperative technique for assessing extent of tumor removal. The study showed that a ^{201}Tl-avid brain tumor can be imaged with a portable camera in the operating room; the results aid in successful prediction of the amount of tumor removed during the operation. With this technique, it was possible to direct the neurosurgeon to areas of tumor still in the operative field that were not visually detected.

Kaplan et al. (8) conducted a study with 29 patients who had grades 3 and 4 malignant glioma over an 18-month period. These patients had undergone extensive chemotherapy followed by autologous bone marrow transplantation. A disparity was found between brain-scan findings and the patients' perfor-

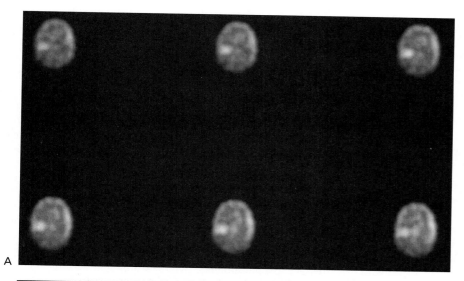

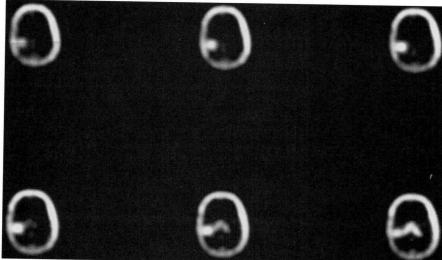

FIGURE 45.1. A: Axial SPECT images of a patient with recurrent glioma show intense focal increase in the right parietal region. This area on magnetic resonance (MR) images did not provide enough information for a diagnosis of recurrent tumor. The patient had undergone radiation therapy with a differential diagnosis of radiation necrosis or recurrent tumor. The findings at MR spectroscopy favored radiation necrosis. The clinical course and subsequent biopsy showed recurrent tumor. **B:** ^{99m}Tc MIBI axial SPECT image obtained as part of a dual-isotope simultaneous acquisition for the patient described in **A.** The exceptionally high tumor to brain ratio is evident. The choroid plexus normally is depicted and may be difficult to differentiate from tumor in patients undergoing ^{99m}Tc MIBI studies of the brain.

mance scores. Many patients were found to be in stable condition, and they experienced clinical improvement, despite the presence of an unchanging intracerebral mass defined at computed tomography (CT). Radionuclide brain scans, including ^{201}Tl studies, were performed to determine whether a better correlation could be obtained. Seven patients in this series died and had neuropathologic data available in relative proximity to the time of radionuclide scanning. Brain sections were reconstructed to match the radionuclide images. For the seven patients with autopsy data, ^{201}Tl imaging offered the most accurate information with regard to tumor viability. In addition to showing that ^{201}Tl imaging more accurately depicted viable tumor burden than did CT, ^{201}Tl imaging was compared with ^{67}Ga citrate and ^{99m}Tc pertechnetate imaging. The authors concluded that ^{201}Tl imaging more accurately reflected tumor viability than did either ^{99m}Tc pertechnetate or ^{67}Ga citrate imaging.

Kaplan et al. (8) suggested that ^{201}Tl accumulation by primary brain tumor was a function of blood flow and tissue viability. Although alteration in blood-brain barrier was probable, it was not considered the main explanation for abnormal ^{201}Tl uptake in tumor because several studies showed results of ^{99m}Tc glucoheptonate scanning were positive and that ^{201}Tl accumulation was negative.

Evaluation with ^{99m}Tc MIBI

MIBI has been found effective in the detection of brain tumors. O'Tuama et al. (52) reported on a comparison of ^{99m}Tc MIBI and ^{201}Tl in evaluation of a pediatric brain tumor with SPECT. Tumor-to-normal cortex ratios were 132:1 for ^{99m}Tc MIBI and 80:1 for ^{201}Tl. The authors considered MIBI to show great promise in the evaluation patients for cerebral tumors. Baillet et al. (36) also suggested a role of MIBI SPECT in the monitoring of adult patients with glioma.

The advantage of ^{99m}Tc MIBI over ^{201}Tl SPECT in the detection of brain tumors is the higher photon flux, which allows a greater amount of statistical certainty in image reconstruction. The disadvantage of ^{99m}Tc MIBI appears to be rather intense uptake in some patients in the ventricular regions, presumably within the choroid plexus of the ventricular system. Separation of tumor from choroid plexus accumulation can be difficult. Additional large-scale studies are needed to further evaluate the clinical utility of ^{99m}Tc MIBI in the evaluation of intracerebral tumors. Fig. 45.1B is the MIBI brain study performed simultaneously with the ^{201}Tl study shown in Fig. 45.1A.

BONE AND SOFT-TISSUE SARCOMA

The diagnosis, management, and follow-up evaluation of bone and soft-tissue sarcoma rely mainly on information obtained with imaging techniques with plain radiographs, CT, or MR imaging. ^{201}Tl and ^{99m}Tc MIBI have been used as metabolic markers of sarcoma. Imaging with these agents has been shown to give important information regarding tumor viability. Especially useful information is obtained in the care of patients with primary tumors of the bone (6,19,24,30,33,73–78).

^{201}Tl

Ramanna et al. (19) found findings at bone scintigraphy correlated poorly with chemotherapeutic effectiveness among patients undergoing chemotherapy before limb salvage. The investigators determined that for more than 80% of the patients in the study, the bone scan gave erroneous information in the assessment of chemotherapeutic effectiveness. The bone scan findings often were associated with an increase in radiopharmaceutical accumulation after chemotherapy that was shown to be associated with healing. Therefore, within 6 weeks of chemotherapy, the bone scan had no useful role, because increasing activity on the bone scan simply reflected healing and not necessarily aggressive tumor growth. The study also showed that an abnormality on ^{67}Ga citrate images was a relatively poor correlate; only 50% of patients successfully treated with chemotherapy had improvement on the ^{67}Ga scintigraphic study. Findings at ^{201}Tl imaging were found to have excellent correlation with therapeutic success. Nearly 100% of patients had significant improvement at ^{201}Tl scintigraphy when chemotherapy was found successful. Patients with more than 95% tumor necrosis had minimal or no ^{201}Tl uptake over pretreatment baseline ^{201}Tl value. The study showed that ^{201}Tl images were able to show tumor burden as well as tumor activity and were not affected by local healing of bone. The authors recommended ^{201}Tl scintigraphy as the test of choice in determining the effectiveness of chemotherapy before limb salvage.

Similar findings were obtained by Rosen et al. (76). Studies were performed before and during preoperative therapy for osteosarcoma and malignant fibrohistiocytoma. Twenty-seven patients were evaluated before and after chemotherapy with biopsy and ^{201}Tl studies. Excellent correlation of histologic evidence of necrosis was obtained with ^{201}Tl scintigraphy. When ^{201}Tl activity diminished to barely detectable or no detectable uptake, patients were found to have 95% necrosis or greater. Conversely, when ^{201}Tl scintigraphy showed no change or increasing activity after extensive chemotherapy, necrosis was far less than 95%.

The study also showed that relapse rates were higher among patients in whom only minimal improvement was found at ^{201}Tl scintigraphy than among patients in whom ^{201}Tl activity was not detected after chemotherapy.

Menendez et al. (75) had similar findings. This group evaluated sequential ^{201}Tl scintigraphy before and after a period of preoperative chemotherapy in the care of 16 patients with high-grade sarcoma of the bone or soft tissue. These investigators found that changes in ^{201}Tl accumulation correlated extremely well with histologic findings. When no improvement in abnormal accumulation on ^{201}Tl imaging was found, there was a poor histologic response to chemotherapy. When there was a decrease in ^{201}Tl accumulation after chemotherapy, there was a good or excellent histologic response to chemotherapy (with one exception). The degree of reduced ^{201}Tl accumulation correlated with increasing amounts of tumor necrosis.

Figures 45.2 and 45.3 are examples of ^{201}Tl, ^{67}Ga, and ^{99m}Tc methylene diphosphonate (MDP) scintigraphy before and after chemotherapy for osteosarcoma. The percentage necrosis was greater than 98% after therapy. Figure 45.4 is a ^{201}Tl, ^{67}Ga, ^{99m}Tc MDP comparison in the management of osteosarcoma with mild clinical improvement with the initial chemotherapy regimen. There is clinical correlation with improvement on ^{201}Tl but not on ^{67}Ga or MDP images.

^{99m}Tc MIBI

Findings similar to those obtained with ^{201}Tl have been reported for MIBI imaging. Caner et al. (30) found MIBI to accumulate

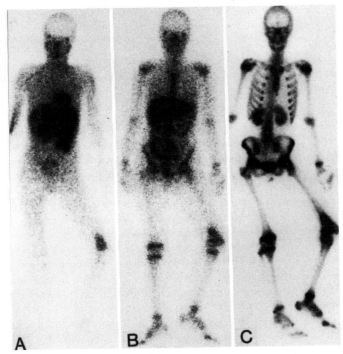

FIGURE 45.2. Comparison of **(A)** ^{201}Tl, **(B)** ^{67}Ga, and **(C)** ^{99m}Tc MDP images of a patient with osteosarcoma of the distal femur. Increased activity is evident in the region of the tumor in all three studies.

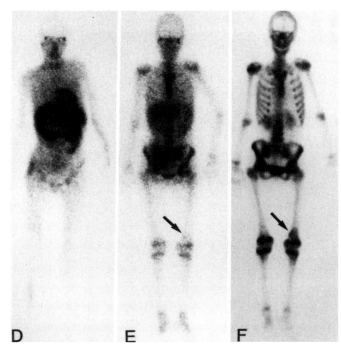

FIGURE 45.3. Same patient as in Fig. 45.2 after 8 weeks of chemotherapy The clinical status of the patient was normal, and the patient was able to straighten the left knee. At surgery, there was greater than 98% tumor necrosis. There is complete absence of ^{201}Tl activity **(D)**, which ^{67}Ga imaging showed as a small residual focus. The bone scan result remained strongly positive.

in an osteogenic sarcoma of the right proximal tibia. Abnormal accumulation also was found in a right inguinal lymph node that was proven by biopsy to be malignant. In a separate study, Caner et al. (33) demonstrated the potential of ^{99m}Tc MIBI for imaging of patients with primary bone tumors. In this study, 10 patients with malignant tumors underwent a pretherapy and posttherapy ^{99m}Tc MIBI evaluation. Radiation therapy or chemotherapy significantly inhibited ^{99m}Tc MIBI uptake. The study showed that posttherapy ^{99m}Tc MIBI uptake was a good reflection of the effectiveness of therapy as confirmed at histologic evaluation.

Ashok et al. (77,78) compared ^{201}Tl with ^{99m}Tc MIBI imaging in the evaluation of patients with soft-tissue as well as osteogenic sarcoma. For 19 patients with a history of osteosarcoma, ^{201}Tl and ^{99m}Tc MIBI scintigraphic studies were performed on the same day. With a semiquantitative rating system, a site comparison was performed on each patient. ^{201}Tl images had a rating of 2+ or greater in 12 of 15 sites proved to be tumor. ^{99m}Tc MIBI had a 2+ or greater tumor rating in all 15 sites. Response to chemotherapy also was compared in the study. In five patients, both tracers gave information concordant with findings in biopsy specimens evaluated for percentage necrosis. The authors concluded that the sensitivity of ^{99m}Tc MIBI detection of primary bone cancer is the same as that of ^{201}Tl detection. However, additional abnormal sites were better detected with ^{99m}Tc MIBI. Findings with both ^{201}Tl and ^{99m}Tc MIBI gave excellent correlation with biopsy information in evaluating tumor response to chemotherapy before limb-salvage procedures.

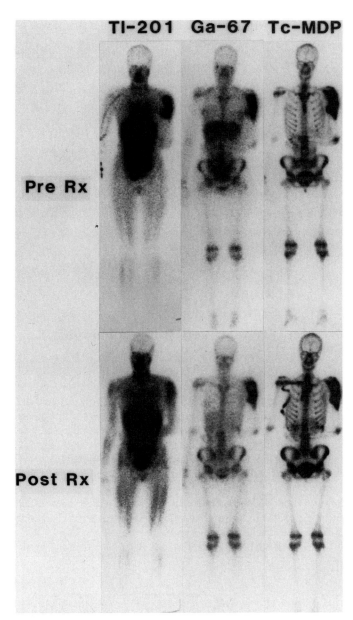

FIGURE 45.4. Patient with osteosarcoma of the left proximal humerus. Pretherapy studies with ^{201}Tl, ^{67}Ga, and ^{99m}Tc MDP show extensive activity in the left proximal humeral and soft-tissue regions. The posttherapy images show moderate improvement in the thallium study and no change in the gallium and bone scans. The patient had clinically evident mild to moderate improvement with reduction of pain, swelling, and tenderness. The thallium scan most closely reflects the clinical response to chemotherapy. Gallium and bone scan studies after therapy reflect healing and bony repair as well as residual tumor. Correlation with clinical response and biopsy with a gallium or bone scan may lead to underestimation of therapeutic benefit.

^{201}Tl and ^{99m}Tc MIBI Scan Patterns in Sarcoma

Ramanna et al. (73,74), evaluated ^{201}Tl scans in 105 patients with bone and soft tissue sarcomas. All of the patients demonstrated a moderate to marked increase in ^{201}Tl activity. The tumors which were considered high grade demonstrated a pattern of central lucency with a peripheral zone of intense ^{201}Tl uptake. This "donut" pattern was highly specific for high grade sarcomas. Greater than 95% of the high grade sarcomas presented with the donut sign. Low-grade sarcomas presented as solid areas of increase with no donut signs present.

Ashok et al. (77,78), demonstrated similar findings for ^{99m}Tc MIBI. These findings appear to parallel the natural course of sarcoma in which tumors grow extremely rapidly with the more central areas demonstrating necrosis as the tumor outgrows its blood supply. The peripheral areas of the tumor maintain adequate vascular perfusion and have pathological evidence of areas of active growth with little necrosis present. A positive result of a ^{99m}Tc MIBI or ^{201}Tl scan with a "doughnut" pattern indicates high-grade sarcoma until proved otherwise.

Figure 45.5 is a ^{99m}Tc MIBI study before and after chemotherapy in the care of a patient with high-grade malignant histiocytoma of the left superior gluteal region. The doughnut appearance of the tumor is evident.

Differentiation of Benign from Malignant Bone Lesions

Ramanna et al. (74) using ^{201}Tl categorized multiple lesions on bone. Sixteen patients with biopsy-proven benign bone lesions were included in the study. [201]Tl activity in the bony lesions was graded as marked, mild, or normal. Four patients with benign abnormalities had a marked increase in ^{201}Tl uptake. Among the diagnoses in this group were Paget's disease of bone, fibrous dysplasia, trauma, and ossifying fibroma. Five patients had mild but definite ^{201}Tl uptake. The diagnoses in this group included benign fibrous histiocytoma, benign fibrous myxoma, and three cases of Paget's disease. Seven patients with benign disease had entirely normal findings. The study showed that ^{201}Tl uptake in bone abnormalities is not specific for tumor and can be seen in a variety of benign abnormalities. A negative test result, how-

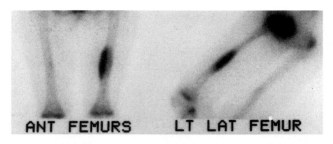
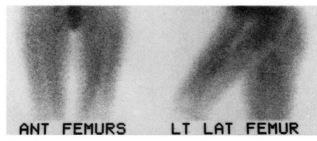

FIGURE 45.6. Computed tomographic (CT) scan shows a large calcific mass in the left mid femur. Patient was believed to have osteogenic sarcoma because of the CT findings and inconclusive biopsy results. The ^{99m}Tc MDP bone scan (*top row*) has markedly positive results, but the ^{201}Tl study (*bottom row*) had normal results. Repetition of the CT examination showed a stress fracture of the left mid femur that healed completely within 6 months.

ever, is significant in that the probability that primary bone tumor exists is minimal.

Figure 45.6 is a comparison of ^{99m}Tc MDP and ^{201}Tl images of a patient with the CT diagnosis of possible osteosarcoma of the left femur. The biopsy findings were inconclusive. A bone scan with MDP had strongly positive results, but results of ^{201}Tl imaging were negative. Repetition of CT of the area showed a stress fracture. The patient was a competitive gymnast who resumed high-bar competition within 1 year of the study.

Caner et al. (33) evaluated ^{99m}Tc MIBI uptake in benign and malignant lesions. Results with ^{99m}Tc MIBI were positive in 36 of 42 malignant tumors (86%), and 11 of 31 patients (35%) with benign disease had ^{99m}Tc MIBI uptake. The investigators concluded that malignant lesions tend to have higher overall ^{99m}Tc MIBI uptake than do benign lesions but that a significant overlap between benign and malignant bone abnormalities existed.

Summary

Bone and soft-tissue sarcoma is readily detected with both ^{99m}Tc MIBI and ^{201}Tl imaging. Significantly higher count rates are achieved with a 30-mCi dose of ^{99m}Tc MIBI than with the 3-mCi dose of [201]Tl. Because of the higher photon flux and more desirable imaging characteristics of ^{99m}Tc, a higher degree of resolution is achieved. Comparative studies show the sensitivity for detecting the primary sarcoma to be similar for ^{201}Tl and ^{99m}Tc MIBI at presentation; however, ^{99m}Tc MIBI appears somewhat superior in the detection of distant metastasis, including small lymph nodes within the drainage pattern of the tumor.

Both ^{201}Tl and ^{99m}Tc MIBI were found to concentrate in a

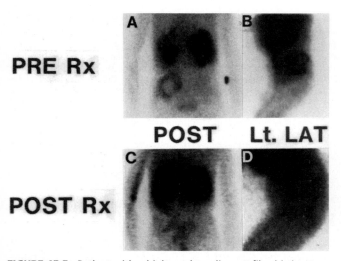

FIGURE 45.5. Patient with a high-grade malignant fibrohistiocytoma of the left gluteal region. **A, B:** Doughnut sign in the gluteal region on ^{99m}Tc MIBI image. **C, D:** Marked improvement after chemotherapy.

variety of benign lesions. However, because of the high sensitivity of ^{99m}Tc MIBI imaging, it may be possible to establish a diagnosis of benign disease detected with plain radiography or MR imaging when the results of the ^{99m}Tc MIBI study are negative. Both ^{201}Tl and ^{99m}Tc MIBI imaging give excellent correlative results in establishing the effectiveness of chemotherapy or radiation therapy. Significant improvement from baseline scans after tumor therapy generally indicate a good therapeutic effect. When tumor activity is minimal or undetectable on the follow-up study, necrosis of greater than 95% usually is present. Correlation with degree of improvement and survival suggests an important role for nuclear medicine techniques in the care of patients with bone and soft-tissue sarcoma.

EVALUATION OF CHEST TUMORS

^{201}Tl

Salvatore et al. (1) initially used ^{201}Tl to evaluate 43 patients with primary lung carcinoma, including 23 patients who had hilar masses and 20 patients who had peripheral abnormalities. Of the 23 patients with hilar abnormalities, 20 had accumulation of ^{201}Tl in the lesion. Of the 20 peripheral masses, 18 were detected. Kinetic evaluation of lung tumors also was undertaken by this group. Maximum accumulation of ^{201}Tl occurred between 30 and 60 minutes after injection. Tonami and Hisada (2) also found ^{201}Tl accumulation in 5 of 6 patients with carcinoma of the lung. They did not determine sensitivity or specificity of ^{201}Tl imaging in the evaluation of intrathoracic metastasis to the hilar or mediastinal nodes.

Tonami et al. (17) performed SPECT on patients with suspected lung cancer. All patients were examined with a high dose of ^{201}Tl (8 to 10 mCi). All studies were performed with a dual-headed SPECT camera 15 minutes after injection and again 3 hours after injection. Of 23 patients with proven malignant primary lesions, all had abnormal results at ^{201}Tl SPECT. The smallest detectable malignant lesion was a 1.5-cm × 1.0-cm adenocarcinoma of the lung. Among seven patients with benign pulmonary lesions, including tuberculosis, bronchopneumonia, hemorrhagic infarction, and a pulmonary scar, only two had abnormal results of a ^{201}Tl study. A small number of patients underwent evaluation of the hilar and mediastinal lymph nodes. Seven patients in this series were proved at surgery to have mediastinal involvement by tumor. Two of the seven did not have abnormal ^{201}Tl activity. Conversely, two studies had false-positive results. In this limited series, the sensitivity in the detection of malignant tumors of the mediastinum was reported to be 71% and the specificity 80%. The smallest mediastinal metastasis detected was 1.5 cm. in diameter. The two patients with false-negative findings of mediastinal metastasis had lesions measuring less than 1.0 cm in diameter.

The authors concluded from this small group of patients that lesions larger than 1.5 cm in diameter that did not accumulate ^{201}Tl most likely were benign. Abnormalities that were less intense on the 3-hour study than on the immediate image most likely were benign. Despite this enthusiastic report, it has not been shown that the use of ^{201}Tl for detecting or staging bronchogenic carcinoma has been helpful. The 8- to 10-mCi ^{201}Tl

dose used in this study could not be used at our center (maximum allowable, 4 mCi ^{201}Tl). This lower dose precludes accurate SPECT evaluation because of poor photon yield.

Several publications suggest a potential use for ^{201}Tl or ^{99m}Tc MIBI imaging in the evaluation of patients for hilar or mediastinal tumor (9,14,18,27,79,80). Many patients after having undergone chemotherapy or radiation therapy have low-grade inflammation of the lymph nodes in the hilum and mediastinum. ^{67}Ga imaging shows nonspecific uptake, which at times can be quite intense. Results with ^{201}Tl and ^{99m}Tc MIBI are most often negative in patients in whom no residual tumor is present or in whom the adenopathy is secondary to other diseases, such as sarcoidosis (9).

^{99m}Tc MIBI

^{99m}Tc MIBI has been evaluated for imaging of patients with pulmonary tumors. Hassan et al. (29) evaluated the uptake and kinetics of ^{99m}Tc MIBI in benign and malignant lesions of the lung. Using 10 to 15 mCi of ^{99m}Tc MIBI, they performed dynamic studies on 19 patients with lung abnormalities. Eleven patients had primary carcinoma of the lung and underwent the study before any form of therapy.

One patient with poorly differentiated squamous cell carcinoma underwent the study after chemotherapy, and one patient with a lung metastasis did so after radiation therapy. Of the six patients with benign disease, four were found to have nonmalignant lesions, including one patient each with hydatid cyst, lung abscess, bronchiectasis, and pneumonitis. Two patients had fibrosing alveolitis. Among the 11 patients with untreated carcinoma of the lung, 10 had abnormal results of MIBI studies. Of the patients with tumors of the lung who had received chemotherapy, two had negative and one had slightly positive results. Among those with benign lesions, both patients with fibrosing alveolitis had positive findings, and the others had negative results.

The kinetics of accumulation of MIBI in tumors showed slow but steady washout of MIBI from tumors that appeared to parallel the washout from the heart and contralateral normal lung. The authors also found reduced or absent uptake in tumors subjected to previous chemotherapy or radiation therapy.

Kao et al. (42) used ^{99m}Tc MIBI imaging and SPECT of the chest to differentiate lung carcinomas of various histologic types. Fifty-four patients with single, solid lung masses were evaluated in this series. The study gave disappointing results, showing a sensitivity of 65% (30/46) and a specificity of 25% (2/8). Fifteen malignant tumors greater than 30 mm in diameter had no abnormal ^{99m}Tc MIBI accumulation. Of interest, the authors stated that they administered 500 mg of perchlorate orally to all patients to prevent abnormal uptake from free pertechnetate. This procedure was unnecessary. Administration of perchlorate during a MIBI study is unusual, and it is not clear whether perchlorate has an adverse affect on the uptake of ^{99m}Tc MIBI in tumors.

Waxman et al. (79) evaluated the role of ^{99m}Tc MIBI SPECT in the evaluation of primary carcinoma of the lung. The main purpose of the study was to determine the effectiveness of MIBI SPECT with a multidetector high-resolution SPECT imaging system in characterizing both primary and metastatic lesions in patients with primary lung cancer. The investigators evaluated 18 patients with biopsy-proven primary lung cancer. Thirty millicuries of ^{99m}Tc MIBI was used in all cases, and SPECT was performed with a three-headed SPECT system. Comparison was with planar images. The study showed that 13 of 18 pulmonary nodules were detected with a planar imaging technique (72%) and that 18 of 18 (100%) were detected with SPECT. The smallest pulmonary nodule detected was 11 mm in greatest diameter. In 10 patients with hilar or mediastinal disease confirmed at biopsy, planar imaging showed 5 of 10 (50%) lesions whereas SPECT showed 10 of 10 (100%). The study showed SPECT to have an excellent sensitivity for the detection of primary as well as of metastatic lung cancer. Specificity determinations were less promising. Two patients had intense activity in radiographic nodules and had active granulomatous disease. One patient had an 18-mm subpleural nodule that at pathologic examination was found to be necrotizing granulomatous inflammation, which was caseating contained rare, acid-fast bacilli. It was believed that this patient had an active focus of tuberculosis. The other patient had a benign nodule that showed multiple granulomas of unknown causation.

Other ^{99m}Tc MIBI SPECT studies have consistently shown a high sensitivity for the detection of primary or metastatic lung cancer. However, specificity is of some concern for both the primary and the hilar and mediastinal regions. Figure 45.7 is a coronal SPECT ^{99m}Tc MIBI study of a patient with a mass in the upper part of the left lung. At thoracotomy, the patient was found to have adenocarcinoma with hilar and mediastinal metastasis.

In summary, ^{201}Tl and ^{99m}Tc MIBI imaging show promise in the evaluation of primary as well as metastatic intrathoracic tumors. High-quality SPECT images can be obtained with 30 mCi of ^{99m}Tc MIBI in conjunction with multidetector SPECT instruments. High sensitivity can be obtained with this technology, although more data are needed to evaluate specificity before these radiopharmaceuticals can be expected to play a significant role in the evaluation of patients with suspected intrathoracic tumors.

BREAST CANCER

Breast cancer in women is second only to lung cancer with respect to cancer deaths. Early detection of this cancer is believed to improve patient survival and to prevent metastasis, as long as early removal is accomplished. Mammography is a radiologic technique that relies on structural changes within the breast to detect abnormalities with a sensitivity of 70% to 90% (81–104). However, it has been shown that even palpable cancers may not be evident on mammographic studies (88,89). Mammography,

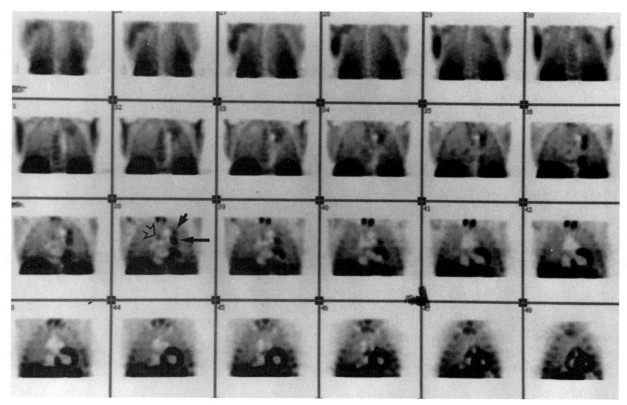

FIGURE 45.7. Patient with left upper lung small cell carcinoma with metastasis to the hilum and mediastinum identified at thoracotomy. The coronal SPECT images represent 6-mm sections from back (*upper left*) to front (*lower right*). *Open arrow,* 1.4-mm mediastinal node. *Long closed arrow,* hilar nodes. *Short closed arrow,* anterior tip of the mass in the upper part of the left lung. The study was performed with 30 mCi of ^{99m}Tc MIBI and a triple-head SPECT camera.

although accurate in the evaluation of low-density fatty breasts, has been less reliable for the detection of abnormalities in dense or dysplastic breasts. It has also been found that management of palpable breast masses may be adversely affected when the clinician delays biopsy, thus the need for rapid and accurate assessment of breast masses.

Mann et al. (88) found that false-negative results of a mammogram can cause considerable delay in the decision to perform biopsy on a patient subsequently shown to have carcinoma of the breast. Patients at high risk of the development of breast cancer, that is, patients with a strong family history of breast cancer, with previous histologic evidence of cellular atypia, with a history of breast cancer who have undergone lumpectomy, or who have undergone radiation therapy either for previous breast cancer or for other tumors, may be difficult to follow mammographically because of the dense fibroglandular tissue and physical changes often caused by irradiation of the breast. Currently, the only established method to solve the problem is random tissue sampling, which is usually attended by a high nonmalignant to malignant biopsy ratio.

Many studies have shown the lack of specificity of mammography; specificity is in the 15% to 25% range. This means that for every 100 patients who undergo biopsy because of a mammographic abnormality, approximately 20 patients are found to have cancer. Functional imaging techniques with ^{201}Tl or ^{99m}Tc MIBI, which generally rely on differential metabolic function of tumors for detection, have been suggested as possible methods for detection of breast cancer and metastasis.

^{201}Tl

In 1978, Hisada et al. (3) reported ^{201}Tl to be an effective tumor-seeking agent. Among 173 patients with malignant tumors, 2 patients with primary carcinoma of the breast were shown to have positive results of ^{201}Tl scintigraphy. Sehweil et al. (22) studied ^{201}Tl kinetics in malignant tumors. In this series, 18 patients with carcinoma of the breast had ^{201}Tl accumulation in the primary lesions. This study showed that the highest tumor to background ratio occurs within 15 minutes after injection.

Sluyser and Hoefnagel (27) found ^{201}Tl uptake in patients with primary tumors of the breast and in metastatic lesions in patients with advanced disease. Although these investigators examined a total of 15 patients, no statistics were given with regard to sensitivity or specificity.

Waxman et al. (26) performed ^{201}Tl studies on 81 women with palpable breast masses, all of whom subsequently underwent biopsy for determination of the disease process. The results of this study are shown in Table 45.3. This study included only patients with palpable masses. Of 43 proven primary tumors of the breast, 41 were detected with ^{201}Tl, for a sensitivity of 95%. Of great importance was the fact that 19 patients with fibrocystic disease were examined and that none had ^{201}Tl uptake. Two patients with fat necrosis also had negative results, whereas 3 of 13 adenomas were detected. All detectable adenomas were highly cellular. The overall specificity in this study was 91% (31/34). In addition to the patients with breast masses for whom specificity calculations were made, 30 patients in this series were referred for ^{201}Tl imaging for reasons other than evaluation of breast

Table 45.3. ^{201}Tl Sensitivity in Mass Abnormalities of the Breast

	True-positive result total with disease	Sensitivity (%)
Malignancy	45/47	96
Primary carcinoma	41/43	95
Other	3/3	100
Fibrocystic disease	0/19	0
Fat necrosis	0/2	0
Adenoma	3/13	23

cancer. There were no false-positive readings in this patient group, indicating the specificity for the general population would be extremely high. In addition to the primary tumors, 21 cases of axillary metastasis were found at surgery. Of these cases, 12 were detected with ^{201}Tl, for sensitivity of 57%. Of the 12 patients with positive results who underwent studies for axillary metastases, only 5 had palpable axillary lymph nodes. Thus it was shown that ^{201}Tl is of value in the detection of nonpalpable metastatic axillary disease. However, the 57% sensitivity was somewhat disappointing. One of the main disadvantages of the use of ^{201}Tl for breast scintigraphy was the inability to administer more than 3 mCi of ^{201}Tl because of excessive radiation burden. Thus count rates were limited and the detection of small lesions was impaired. The smallest lesion detected in this series was a 1.3 cm × 1.1 cm × 0.9 cm adenocarcinoma of the breast.

^{99m}Tc MIBI

^{99m}Tc MIBI has been found to be a potentially important radiopharmaceutical for the evaluation of primary breast cancer (39, 43–49,80,105–119). ^{99m}Tc has excellent characteristics for imaging with an Anger camera. A favorable radiation burden allows for doses of approximately 30 mCi of ^{99m}Tc MIBI compared with a 3-mCi dose of ^{201}Tl. The higher photon flux improves imaging the soft tissues of the breast.

Improvement in sensitivity over ^{201}Tl imaging has been reported for the evaluation of primary breast cancer when MIBI is used (30–34). Specificity concerns must be addressed, especially in the care of patients with hyperproliferative breast disorders. Figure 45.8 is a comparison of ^{201}Tl and ^{99m}Tc MIBI imaging in the care of a patient with multifocal cancer of the left breast. Better lesion detection with ^{201}Tl than with MIBI is probably due to the higher number of events detected.

Positioning Protocols for Sestamibi Breast Imaging

Initial breast imaging protocols with ^{201}Tl relied on techniques in which the patient was positioned supine with the arms raised to evaluate both the breast and axilla (26). The supine techniques consisted of an anterior view and several oblique projections, including anterior and posterior oblique views. It was believed that the breast was adequately evaluated because several projections covered the entire breast volume. A long imaging time was required because image were obtained at 10 minutes per view.

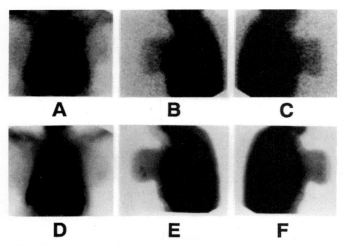

FIGURE 45.8. Comparison of ²⁰¹Tl **(A, B, C)** and ^{99m}Tc MIBI **(D, E, F)** breast imaging of a patient with multicentric adenocarcinoma of the left breast. Anterior views **(A, D)** were obtained with the patient in the supine position with the arms up. Lateral views **(B, C, E, F)** were obtained with the patient in the prone position. Better depiction of the tumor of the left breast is achieved with ^{99m}Tc MIBI than with ²⁰¹Tl.

Use of a multidetector camera may improve throughput, but the risk of not localizing a deep lesion against the chest wall theoretically was of concern when the supine-only technique was used. Khalkali et al. (46) developed a prone technique in which MIBI was used with a specially designed table to allow a patient to be placed in the prone position with the breast in a dependent position.

Most centers performing MIBI breast imaging rely on a prone technique. Some groups use a special table, imaging one breast at a time. Others use a modified MR imaging breast holder or other methods to allow imaging of both breasts simultaneously.

When imaging both breasts simultaneously, one must be sure that the breasts are separated by an appropriate thickness of lead to prevent "shine through" from the opposite breast. The throughput advantages of dual breast imaging may be offset if appropriate breast shielding is not used.

A combination of prone and supine imaging currently is the method of choice. Lateral prone imaging allows separation of the chest wall from lesions deep within the breast. One can separate the breast from the liver and heart when the appropriate prone technique is used. A potential disadvantage of the lateral view is the possibility of missing a small or low-intensity medial lesion because of attenuation.

Breast Imaging Protocol

Patients are given an intravenous injection of 20 to 30 mCi of ^{99m}Tc MIBI. The radiopharmaceutical may adhere to the regional veins after injection; this makes evaluation of the axilla and upper breast somewhat difficult. Performing the injection into the arm opposite the breast being evaluated reduces this risk. A 20-mL saline flush after injection is suggested to further clear the vessels.

Imaging can be instituted within 2 or 3 minutes after injection if the lateral projections are obtained first. Because of the high lung background, the anterior supine image is obtained after the lateral images.

A single detector camera is used, and the patient is placed on the imaging table in a prone position. If a special table with a breast cut-out along the lateral border of the table is used, the breast is inserted in the cut-out, and the detector is brought as close as possible to the lateral surface of the breast. The breast is imaged in its entirety. At facilities that do not have a specially constructed table, the patient can be moved to the edge of the imaging table and the breast placed in a dependent position so that it can be elongated by gravity. Care must be taken to ensure that the patient will not be placed at risk if this technique is chosen. After imaging of the breast in question the opposite breast is imaged with the same technique. When the single breast–single detector approach is used, one must be sure that the opposite breast is compressed by the patient's position during imaging of the uncompressed breast. High-quality images can be obtained in 10 minutes per view.

After the two 10-minute lateral breast images are obtained, an anterior supine arms-up view is obtained to evaluate both breasts simultaneously as well as the axillary regions bilaterally. If only a small-field-of-view camera is available, two independent, overlapping views of the axillary regions and breast may be obtained.

Multiview supine imaging of the breast with the arms above the head can be done effectively when patients cannot undergo prone imaging. When supine imaging is performed, acquisition of lateral views is not suggested because the breast often falls to the lateral aspect of the torso. Anterior and posterior oblique views are effective for evaluation of each breast. An advantage of supine imaging with oblique views is effective evaluation of the medial aspect of the breast with the anterior oblique projections. The disadvantages of use of oblique views is the inability to closely approximate the entire breast to the collimator surface.

When a triple-detector camera is used, throughput for a breast examination, including marker views, can be shortened to 20 minutes. An anterior and two posterior oblique views can be obtained simultaneously. If necessary, a posterior and two anterior oblique views can be obtained simultaneously. Figure 45.9 is a normal study (A, B, C) with marker views (D, E, F). The study was completed in less than 20 minutes.

Marker Views

Nipple markers are used in examinations of all patients. Markers can be placed on breast abnormalities in either the lateral or the anterior view by means of superimposition of an external source on the palpable breast abnormality or focus of increased isotope accumulation as noted on the persistence scope. Thus when the radioactive marker appears to coincide with an area of increased activity as noted on the persistence scope, one assumes the source is perpendicular to the lesion. With the appropriate amount of ^{99m}Tc within the source marker, it is possible to mark the lesion (with persistence scope assistance) and both nipples during the 5-minute marker view.

At the time of marking, an ink mark can be placed on the breast on the skin overlying the lesion at a right angle to the detector in both the lateral and anterior projections. These marks

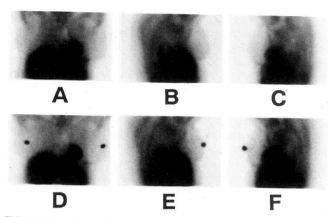

FIGURE 45.9. Normal MIBI study (**A, B, C**) of a patient with biopsy-proven fibrocystic changes in the breast. Nipple markers were imaged (**D, E, F**). The study was completed within 20 minutes with a triple-detector camera with the detector heads placed in the anterior and posterior oblique positions.

can serve as orthogonal vectors for triangulation purposes if the patient is to undergo biopsy. If the markers are to be used for biopsy, it is important to have the arms at the same position in which the biopsy is to be performed. In most studies, the arms are at a 90-degree angle to the trunk in the same plane as the trunk.

Delayed Imaging (Kinetics of MIBI Breast Imaging)

The kinetics of MIBI in breast cancer imaging may have clinical importance. Images obtained more than 1 hour after injection may show significant washout of MIBI from the tumor. We have observed a varying pattern of MIBI washout in imaging of patients at both early and delayed periods after injection. At times, benign abnormalities may appear to have greater activity 60 to 90 minutes after injection, whereas tumors may be less active 60 to 90 minutes after injection than on the early study. This pattern is inconsistent and needs further work to delineate the basis for the findings.

Ciarmiello et al. (111) attempted to correlate clearance rates of MIBI from a breast tumor before new adjuvant therapy. Patients who had the greatest rate of tumor clearance tended to have a histologic pattern consistent with lack of response to chemotherapy. Patients with slow clearance of MIBI from the breast tumor tended to have a favorable histologic pattern after chemotherapy. The overall conclusion was that rapid tumor clearance of MIBI was predictive of poor tumor response to chemotherapy.

SPECT of the Breast

SPECT in conjunction with planar imaging may give useful information regarding localization of the primary breast abnormality and information regarding the axilla. SPECT currently is done in the supine position with the arms up. Successful prone SPECT is limited by geometric constraints of the patient, imaging table, and gantry and by insufficient counts if short

imaging times are used. A multidetector system is helpful in ensuring adequate counts are obtained.

We have investigated SPECT for breast imaging and believe there is significant potential in breast imaging; however, the study is somewhat technically difficult to perform (48). A multidetector camera with imaging times of 30 to 45 minutes is required for optimal visualization of abnormalities. Although more abnormalities generally are detected, they may not be of a malignant nature. SPECT often brings out the nonhomogenous characteristics often seen in patients with fibroglandular changes; the result is a false-positive interpretation. Spatial localization and evaluation of the axilla have improved.

Caution must be used in the interpretation of SPECT images. When the technique is used appropriately, valuable information can be obtained. Figure 45.10 shows a focal malignant lesion of the right breast and axillary metastasis. The findings are more evident with SPECT.

Clinical Applications of MIBI Breast Scintigraphy

For a new test to be selected for use in a clinical setting, it must show incremental improvement of a significant degree over existing procedures. A definition of *significant* is related not only to a statistical comparison of efficacy but also to cost-effectiveness.

Screening of the general population for early diagnosis of breast cancer is currently being accomplished with screening mammography. This is a relatively low-cost, safe examination with a modestly high sensitivity for detection of early breast cancer. The overall sensitivity varies depending on population selection but is approximately 70% to 90% (81–104). Mammography appears to be more reliable for the older population

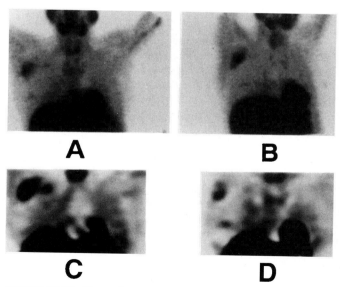

FIGURE 45.10. The patient presented with a right axillary mass and no abnormality at mammography or palpation of the right breast. Both MIBI planar (**A, B**) and SPECT (**C, D**) images show the axillary abnormality and a lesion in the right breast. SPECT of the breast improves sensitivity slightly. This advantage, however, is offset by a decline in specificity.

than for young women with dense breasts (94,95). Mammography is capable of depicting lesions of very small size, especially when calcifications appear to be present (99). Mammography has a relatively low positive predictive value and results in a high percentage of biopsy results negative for malignant growth. However, because of the low cost and high sensitivity, mammography is considered an excellent screening tool for the general population at this time. MIBI imaging does not appear to be competitive with mammography in either cost-effectiveness or sensitivity for screening purposes.

Diagnostic mammography and ultrasonography together have been the tools of the mammographer in evaluating patients for suspicious abnormalities at screening mammography, palpation, or other studies. Whether a patient should undergo biopsy often is determined by the outcome of mammography or ultrasound examination, expertise of the mammographer, the relation of the mammographer to the surgical community, and the practice standards of that community. With conventional imaging techniques for breast evaluation firmly established in the medical community, it is necessary to demonstrate that MIBI should be used because of improved efficacy and cost-effectiveness in the evaluation of suspicious abnormalities of the breast.

Evaluation of ^{99m}Tc MIBI Breast Imaging: Clinical Efficacy

Several studies have been published regarding the use of MIBI in the evaluation of breast cancer. Some of these results are summarized in Table 45.4. Table 45.4 shows a range of overall sensitivity for breast cancer detection from 84% to 94%. Overall specificity varies from 72% to 94%. Not all reports separate the statistics from the palpable and nonpalpable groups. It is evident that sensitivity for palpable abnormalities is considerably higher than that for nonpalpable abnormalities.

Factors That May Affect Efficacy

The variation in sensitivity and specificity in these reports may be due to several factors. These include patient referral bias, variable standards in defining abnormalities, acquisition techniques, display techniques, and variable reader experience. Table 45.4 indicates the variability in the type of abnormalities referred for evaluation. Although most groups had a high prevalence of palpable abnormalities, the DuPont study (119) showed a larger number of nonpalpable abnormalities. The cancer prevalence rate varied from 41% for Khalkhali et al. (106) to 84% for Kao et al. (108). Study populations with a large number of patients with proliferative breast disorders such as fibrocystic disease more likely have a relatively high false-positive rate.

Lack of standardization for defining whether the results of a study are positive or negative has a significant bearing on sensitivity and specificity. Small lesions that appear focal but faint on scans may be considered by one group as positive for small cancers, whereas other investigators may consider the findings normal variation. Quantitation has been suggested to aid in the differentiation of benign and malignant abnormalities (105). We have found that numerous benign abnormalities have target to background ratios greater than 1.4, whereas many malignant tumors, especially if small, have ratios of less than 1.4.

Acquisition techniques can vary. Instrumentation differences and positional differences can influence the results. Display techniques can affect results considerably. If the intensity is set at a high level more "abnormalities" are found within the breast. Reducing intensity or subtracting background can leave a small tumor undetectable.

Patient referral bias from the medical community also can influence results. If clinicians refer only "difficult" cases for study, then both sensitivity and specificity figures may not be reflective of the pool of patients who may benefit from the study. If clinicians do not perform a biopsy because results of a MIBI study are negative, those patients are unavailable for data analysis. Most studies with negative results would most likely reflect a nonmalignant outcome, causing a greater number of persons with normal levels than persons with abnormal levels to be removed from the data pool. This generally tends to lower specificity.

The DuPont Merck study consisted of 673 patients; 286 of these patients had palpable abnormalities and 387 had nonpalpable mammographically detected abnormalities. The studies were representative of a broad community experience—more than 30 institutions participated in the trial. The study by Kao et al. (108) included only palpable breast lesions, whereas the studies by Khalkhali et al. (106), Taillefer et al. (105), Waxman et al. (110), and DuPont Merck (119) included both palpable and nonpalpable breast masses.

Table 45.4. *Sensitivity and Specificity of MIBI in the Evaluation of Malignant Tumors of the Breast*

	Overall		Palpable		Nonpalpable		Abnormal		
	Sensitivity	Specificity	Sensitivity	Specificity	Sensitivity	Specificity	Palpable	Nonpalpable	Malignant
Reference	(%)	(%)	(%)	(%)	(%)	(%)	(%)	(%)	(overall %)
Taillefer et al (105)	92	94	NA	NA	NA	NA	44	21	72
Khalkhali et al (106)	94	88	NA	NA	NA	NA	85	21	41
Kao et al (108)	84	87	84	87	NA	NA	38	0	84
Waxman et al (110)	89	72	98	68	57	89	116	33	44
Khalkali et al (DuPont Merck) (119)	85	81	95	74	72	86	286	387	39
Palmedo et al (107)	88	83	100	80	25	90	40	14	44

NA, not available.

Lesion size seems to be a key factor in determining whether results of a study are positive or negative. Waxman et al. (120) found lesions larger than 12 mm in diameter had an extremely high sensitivity (>92%) whereas lesions between 7 and 11 mm in diameter were detected only 50% of the time (121). The smallest lesion detectable was 7 mm. Khalikhali et al. (106) have suggested that lesions less than 10 mm in diameter are difficult to evaluate. Studies in which patient referral is biased to larger lesions will have more favorable sensitivity than will studies in which the bias is toward smaller lesions. Technique was not standardized. The images obtained by Kao et al. (106) may have been displayed at a lesser intensity than those shown by Taillefer et al. (105,108). Increasing intensity depicts smaller lesions; conversely, specificity may be significantly affected.

Study populations with large numbers of patients with hyperproliferative breast disorders may have relatively high rates of false-positive results (47). The increase in MIBI activity that often occurs in patients with hyperproliferative breast disease most likely reflects higher than normal mitochondrial activity and increased mitochondrial density in areas found histologically to be abnormal. Although these areas are considered nonmalignant, it has been found that patients with hyperproliferative breast disease have a higher relative risk of development of breast cancer than do patients with nonproliferative benign breast disorders (121,122). Patients with typical hyperplasia associated with atypia were shown to have a relative risk of breast cancer higher than that among patients with proliferative changes with no atypia. The risk of breast cancer increases among patients found to have atypia and a first-degree relative with breast cancer (122).

Gupta et al. (123) found MIBI uptake in benign breast disease to be highly associated with the presence of proliferative changes. A negative result of a MIBI breast study significantly reduced the probability for the presence of proliferative breast disease. False-positive results of a MIBI breast examination actually may be a reflection of premalignant potential. Additional work in this area is needed to confirm these speculations.

Practical Considerations

If one considers the DuPont Merck trial results with 673 patients to be highly representative of the general medical community, then MIBI breast imaging would have an overall sensitivity of 80% and a specificity of 81%. For the data to be used effectively, the individual statistics for palpable and nonpalpable lesions must be separated because management strategy may differ, especially in determining whether biopsy should be performed. In most instances, palpable breast masses are subjected to biopsy if results at mammography or ultrasonography suggest the lesions to be suspicious.

The DuPont Merck study of MIBI imaging in the detection of nonpalpable lesions showed a blinded sensitivity of 55% and a specificity of 91% (119). The blinded figures from the Cedars-Sinai Medical Center were 51% and 89%. Unblinded figures for the DuPont Merck study were 72% sensitivity and 86% specificity (119). The medical community must decide whether these are acceptable results to justify use of MIBI in the care of patients with nonpalpable breast lesions. Conversely, in the DuPont Merck study, MIBI imaging had a sensitivity of 95% and a specificity of 74% in the detection of palpable lesions. These figures are close to those generated at Cedars-Sinai Medical Center, where a large population of patients with fibrocystic disease were seen. To decide whether a patient should forgo biopsy of a palpable breast mass, most surgeons require a test that has a negative predictive value approaching 100%.

Potential Role of ^{99m}Tc MIBI in Breast Imaging

The results generated by the aforementioned studies and by others indicate that ^{99m}Tc MIBI breast imaging is not a screening procedure. Sensitivity for lesions smaller than 10 mm in diameter is poor with almost no lesion detection at less than 6 mm. The test also is relatively expensive compared with screening mammography. The DuPont Merck statistics (119) suggest that among every 100 patients with palpable lesions that are later shown to be malignant, 5 lesions would be missed with the MIBI test. Currently, this is unacceptable in most medical communities. Therefore the use of MIBI imaging of palpable lesions may not be effective for purposes of reducing the number of unnecessary biopsies. Potential areas of clinical utility are suggested in Table 45.5.

Patients with mammograms that do not provide enough in-

Table 45.5. *Potential Role of MIBI in the Evaluation of Breast Cancer*

Patient at high risk with breast difficult to image with mammography[a]
  Genetic predisposition (*BRCA*-1,2)
  Familial predisposition (mother, sister with breast cancer)
  Previous malignant disease of the breast
  Hyperproliferative breast at previous biopsy
  Previous radiation to breast
    Breast cancer
    Lymphoma
    Other
Psychologically motivated patient with breast difficult to image with mammography[a]
  Ancillary test for establishing level of aggressiveness for pursuing biopsy
Mammographic scar from previous biopsy or lumpectomy
  Especially relevant when previous biopsy shows malignant growth or hyperproliferative breast tissue
Mass abnormalities of breast
  Poorly defined breast mass not detected at mammography or ultrasonography
  Breast mass in patients who delay biopsy because of patient reluctance or health care delivery system reluctance (triage for biopsy)
  Lumpectomy candidate who may have mammographically undetectable multifocal disease
Evaluation of therapeutic response
  Chemotherapy before excisional biopsy or lumpectomy in patients with breast cancer subtypes (viability assessment)
  Prediction of neoadjuvant effectiveness
Patients with axillary adenocarcinoma of unknown primary origin
  Presence of focal breast abnormality
Postlumpectomy residual
  Evaluate residual not removed
  Evaluate multifocal residual

[a]Includes patients with dense breasts, architectural distortions or scar.

formation for a diagnosis, especially those with dense breasts or architectural distortion who are at a high risk of harboring malignant lesions, may benefit from a test that is independent of breast density or distortion. The DuPont Merck multicenter trial convincingly showed that the results of MIBI breast imaging were independent of breast density (119). Mammography was performed on all patients entered into the study. Breast density was stratified into two groups consisting of subjects with fatty breasts and those with heterogenously dense breasts. The data showed that the sensitivity and specificity of MIBI breast scintigraphy for detection of malignant disease were identical for both groups. The conclusion was that comparable diagnostic accuracy of MIBI breast imaging in patients with dense and fatty breasts indicates that MIBI breast imaging may have advantages over mammography in the evaluation patients with dense breasts. Therefore this modality can make a significant contribution to clinical care of patients with suspected abnormalities of the breast. Figure 45.11 shows a patient with mammographically dense breasts and a palpable mass in the right breast. The mammogram did not provide enough information for a diagnosis. Before a scheduled lumpectomy, a MIBI study showed multiple abnormal foci. A mastectomy was performed, and multifocal invasive ductile cancer was found.

Identification of a high risk itself is insufficient reason to refer patients for MIBI breast studies unless these patients have mammograms that are difficult to interpret. The definition of *difficult* is subjective and variable within the breast imaging community. It must be demonstrated to the appropriate medical community, such as mammographers and surgeons, that the efficacy of MIBI breast scintigraphy is sufficient for detection of unsuspected breast cancer in this population with a frequency that warrants its use.

The presence of a "scar" within the breast from a previous biopsy often makes mammographic interpretation difficult as to whether malignant growth is present. Ultrasonography is generally of no benefit in this situation. A potential role for MIBI may be in the differentiation of benign from malignant findings on a mammogram that shows a scar pattern.

Patients may have a perceived breast mass that cannot be detected with mammography or ultrasonography. If the mass is larger than 10 mm in diameter, a MIBI study may be helpful because a positive test result would encourage a biopsy, whereas a negative result would most likely indicate a benign basis of the perceived palpable findings.

Patients who have suspicious breast abnormalities may be in situations in which biopsy may be delayed for reasons beyond the their control. Because delay in biopsy has been shown to have a high association with subsequent axillary metastasis, these patients may benefit from a MIBI study. Positive results would indicate the necessity for immediate biopsy.

A potentially large number of patients may benefit from a MIBI study before lumpectomy if mammography shows increased breast density. Lumpectomy followed by radiation therapy is an acceptable means of treatment; however, if considerable tumor burden is found outside the primary palpable mass, the treatment of choice would be mastectomy. In several instances, we have detected larger than expected tumor burden distant from the primary lesion with MIBI (Fig. 45.11).

To justify MIBI before lumpectomy, it would be important to determine whether radiation therapy is effective in the subgroup of patients who have unsuspected multifocal disease. Patients undergoing lumpectomy who have undetectable multifocal disease may be patients with early recurrence of breast cancer.

Patients with an axillary mass found to be adenocarcinoma most likely have primary breast cancer as the basis of the axillary mass. At times, these carcinomas are difficult to locate with mammography or ultrasonography. Imaging with MIBI may be of benefit to this population. Patients undergoing chemotherapy or radiation therapy for masses not surgically resectable may benefit from a MIBI examination. Results of MIBI imaging have been found to correlate well with tumor viability and can be used to evaluate the benefit of chemotherapy (65).

Localization

To date there has been great difficulty in successfully localizing radiopharmaceutical-avid areas within the breast. Use of orthogonal localization from an anterior and lateral projection is imprecise. With this technique, a large volume of breast tissue has to

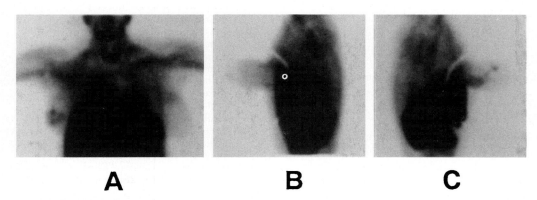

A   **B**   **C**

FIGURE 45.11. MIBI study of a patient with multifocal disease in the right breast. The breast appeared dense on a mammogram, and only one lesion was detected. The patient was scheduled for mastectomy before the MIBI study. After additional biopsy, the patient underwent mastectomy and was found to have extensive multifocal disease of the right breast.

be removed and examined by a pathologist for tumor content. More precise localization techniques are needed to evaluate focal findings on radiopharmaceutical breast studies.

Evaluation of the Axilla

Use of mammography, CT, ultrasonography, or MR imaging has proved difficult for the evaluation of breast cancer metastasis to the axilla. Physical examination in general is less than 50% effective in the detection of lymph nodes harboring breast cancer metastasis. Taillefer reported a sensitivity of 84% for the detection of axillary nodes with a specificity of 91% (105). The current sensitivity figures at Cedars-Sinai Medical Center for MIBI detection of axillary metastasis were somewhat lower at 55%; however, the specificity was 91%. SPECT may further improve the axillary node statistics.

Summary and Conclusions

Radiopharmaceuticals characterization of carcinoma of the breast has been reasonably well defined in the literature; results of biopsy of more than 1,000 lesions have been reported. MIBI and fluorodeoxyglucose (FDG) are most widely used. The U.S. Food and Drug Administration has approved MIBI for clinical use.

There are limitations of this test in respect to both sensitivity and specificity. Lesions smaller than 6 to 8 mm are extremely difficult to detect. Specificity is a problem in the evaluation of patients with hyperproliferative breast disorders; many benign abnormalities demonstrate activity. Although many of these patients may have a premalignant histologic pattern, current medical practice is not to aggressively treat these patients until a definite malignant tumor is found.

The clinical application of radiopharmaceutical imaging in evaluation of breast cancer appears limited; however, specific populations, especially those with high-risk factors and breasts difficult to image with mammography, may benefit from this technology. Improvement in localization of MIBI-avid areas is required before a wider use of this test is forthcoming. Techniques that allow fusion of radiopharmaceutical findings with findings at MR imaging or mammography may eventually prove useful in determining which patients should proceed to biopsy.

Improvement in instrumentation, possibly in the form of a dedicated breast detector or higher-resolution systems, may facilitate both detection and localization. The feasibility of use of nuclear medicine techniques to evaluate breast cancer has been clearly demonstrated. Further improvements in instrumentation and radiopharmaceuticals may eventually allow functional breast imaging to have a key role in the evaluation of breast cancer.

LYMPHOMA

^{201}Tl

Positron emission tomography (PET) with ^{18}F FDG in evaluation for lymphoma is rapidly replacing imaging with ^{67}Ga. Visualization of low-grade lymphoma is still difficult. Before the

development of PET, gallium citrate had been the main radiopharmaceutical used in evaluation of lymphoma. Several studies have addressed the issue of ^{67}Ga uptake in lymphoma according to tumor grade or lymphoma type. Recent reports on ^{201}Tl indicate uptake within lymphoma depends largely on tumor grade. Waxman et al. (14) found ^{201}Tl scintigraphy to be a promising tracer in the evaluation of low-grade lymphoma. The study compared the relation of ^{67}Ga to ^{201}Tl in lymphoma. Whereas ^{67}Ga citrate demonstrated poor uptake in low-grade lymphoma, ^{201}Tl had marked avidity. Kaplan et al. (18) used ^{67}Ga and ^{201}Tl imaging to evaluate patients with low-grade and patients with high-grade non-Hodgkin's lymphoma. The findings for the two groups were similar findings, and low-grade lymphoma was readily detected with ^{201}Tl but poorly detected with ^{67}Ga.

In a study performed at the Cedars-Sinai Medical Center, (14) 36 patients underwent both ^{67}Ga and ^{201}Tl scintigraphy. With a semiquantitative rating system, statistical comparisons were performed for ^{201}Tl versus ^{67}Ga in all lymphoma subgroups. Also of interest was a statistical comparison of ^{201}Tl with itself in all lymphoma subgroups. This statistical analysis also was performed for ^{67}Ga. The results of this study showed that patient sensitivity for ^{67}Ga citrate was 56% and site sensitivity was 32% among patients with low-grade lymphoma. Among the same patients, ^{201}Tl sensitivity was 100% on a patient basis and 100% on a site basis. The difference between ^{201}Tl and ^{67}Ga sensitivity among patients with low-grade lymphoma was statistically significant. Also noticed in the low-grade lymphoma group was that ^{201}Tl compared with itself in lymphoma subgroups was statistically more avid for low-grade lymphoma than for intermediate-, high-grade, and Hodgkin's lymphoma. Conversely, the sensitivity of ^{67}Ga for low-grade lymphoma was significantly less than for Hodgkin's lymphoma and intermediate-grade lymphoma. No significant differences were found between ^{201}Tl and ^{67}Ga in the intermediate-grade, high-grade, or Hodgkin's lymphoma subgroups.

The investigators concluded that ^{201}Tl studies had a significantly greater tumor to background ratio among patients with low-grade lymphoma than did ^{67}Ga citrate studies performed on the same patients. Conversely, ^{67}Ga citrate appeared to lack avidity for low-grade lymphoma when compared with ^{201}Tl and was statistically inferior in the detection of low-grade lymphoma than it was in the detection of intermediate-grade or high-grade lymphoma. It was concluded that ^{67}Ga citrate was not dependable in the evaluation of patients with low-grade lymphoma and perhaps accounted for much of the disagreement in the literature concerning the role of ^{67}Ga imaging for lymphoma, because previous studies made little effort to separate ^{67}Ga avidity in lymphoma according to tumor grade (28).

Figure 45.12 is a comparison of ^{201}Tl and ^{67}Ga images of a patient with low-grade lymphoma of the right inguinal and pelvic regions. The ^{201}Tl-avid nodes and less-avid ^{67}Ga nodes are evident. Both ^{201}Tl imaging and ^{67}Ga imaging are less accurate in the evaluation of low-grade lymphoma within the abdomen because ^{67}Ga avidity for low-grade lymphoma is extremely low, and gastrointestinal excretion of ^{201}Tl interferes with interpretation of findings in the abdomen or pelvis. Figure 45.13 compares

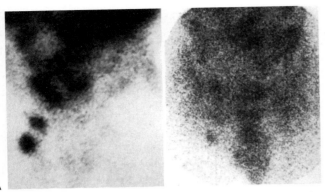

FIGURE 45.12. Comparison of ^{201}Tl **(A)** and ^{67}Ga **(B)** studies of a patient with a low-grade lymphoma of the inguinal and pelvic region. The uptake of ^{99m}Tc MIBI in the inguinal and inferior pelvic nodes is markedly greater than that of ^{67}Ga. ^{201}Tl and ^{99m}Tc MIBI show a marked increase in low-grade lymphoma, whereas the sensitivity of ^{67}Ga is extremely poor.

^{201}Tl with ^{67}Ga images of a patient with Hodgkin's lymphoma of the axilla and hilar-mediastinal region.

^{99m}Tc MIBI

Waxman et al. (50) reported on a series of patients with lymphoma and compared uptake of ^{99m}Tc MIBI with that of ^{67}Ga with respect to tumor detection. The study showed that low-grade lymphoma is readily detected with MIBI. In this study, five patients with low-grade lymphoma had excellent ^{99m}Tc MIBI uptake, whereas ^{67}Ga activity was either negative (two patients) or significantly less than that of ^{99m}Tc MIBI (three patients). These findings were similar to those with ^{201}Tl. The investigators concluded that MIBI has great potential for the detection of low-grade lymphoma in the neck, chest, and inguinal areas.

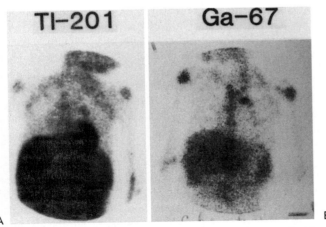

FIGURE 45.13. A patient with Hodgkin's lymphoma has a marked increase in activity on the ^{201}Tl study in the pulmonary, hilar, and mediastinal regions as well as the axillary areas bilaterally. ^{67}Ga image shows a solitary focus to the left of the sternum.

Summary

^{201}Tl and ^{99m}Tc MIBI have similar spectra of tumor avidity in lymphoma. Low-grade lymphoma is readily detected with either ^{201}Tl or ^{99m}Tc MIBI. Higher-grade lymphoma is better detected with ^{67}Ga citrate imaging or FDG PET. Neither ^{201}Tl nor ^{99m}Tc MIBI can be used effectively in the abdomen or pelvis because of the unpredictable gastrointestinal excretion. Monitoring of response to therapy for low-grade lymphoma in the neck, chest, or inguinal area is better accomplished with ^{201}Tl or ^{99m}Tc MIBI than with ^{67}Ga.

THYROID CARCINOMA

Differentiated Thyroid Cancer

The follow-up evaluation of patients with differentiated thyroid cancer who have undergone total thyroidectomy consists mainly of diagnostic body scans with 2 to 10 mCi of ^{131}I. The introduction of tumor markers such as thyroglobulin has been integrated with the diagnostic ^{131}I scans to best determine whether thyroid cancer has spread to regional or distant sites or whether tumor recurrence is present in the thyroid bed.

To prepare a patient properly for ^{131}I therapy, it is necessary to withdraw all exogenous thyroid hormone. Withdrawal of exogenous thyroid hormone promotes a significant rise in the level of thyroid-stimulating hormone, which results in greater uptake of iodine into residual iodine-avid tissue, which consists of either normal residual thyroid or differentiated thyroid cancer. Withdrawal of exogenous thyroid hormone for an extended period is an exceedingly stressful experience for the patient, often resulting in many days of extreme fatigability, impaired cognitive functioning, and other symptoms resulting from a hypothyroid state.

In 1986, Hoefnagel et al. (12) suggested a role of ^{201}Tl body scintigraphy in the follow-up evaluation of patients with thyroid carcinoma. This group performed ^{201}Tl total body scintigraphy on 326 patients. Histologic tumor types included papillary carcinoma in 191 patients, follicular carcinoma in 110 patients, medullary carcinoma in 18 patients, anaplastic carcinoma in 6 patients, and giant cell carcinoma in 1 patient. In 303 patients, the results were correlated with those of ^{131}I total body scintigraphy. Another 275 patients had ^{201}Tl scintigrams correlated with results of tumor marker assays. Thyroglobulin assays were performed for patients with papillary or follicular carcinoma, and levels of calcitonin and carcinoembryonic antigen were determined for patients with medullary carcinoma of the thyroid.

Twenty-four patients underwent both ^{201}Tl and ^{131}I studies, and the results were positive. All of these patients were confirmed to have metastatic carcinoma of the thyroid. Seven patients in this group had normal tumor markers. In 8 patients, ^{201}Tl scintigraphy revealed more metastatic lesions than did the ^{131}I study. In six patients, ^{131}I scintigraphy revealed more abnormalities than did ^{201}Tl scintigraphy. In 39 patients, results of ^{201}Tl scintigraphy were positive, whereas those of ^{131}I scintigraphy were negative. Thirty of these patients had differentiated thyroid cancer, 8 had medullary carcinoma, and 1 patient had a giant cell carcinoma. All 8 cases of medullary thyroid carcinoma were detected with ²⁰¹Tl. The authors concluded that ²⁰¹Tl scintigraphy was far more sensitive than ¹³¹I scintigraphy in the detection of metastasis from differentiated thyroid cancer. The sensitivity of ¹³¹I scintigraphy alone in the detection of recurrent or metastatic differentiated thyroid cancer was only 48%, and the specificity was 99%. The sensitivity and specificity with ²⁰¹Tl alone were 94% and 97%. ²⁰¹Tl and thyroglobulin levels in combination had a sensitivity of 98% and a specificity of 90%.

Because of their findings, Hoefnagel et al. instituted a new program for the postoperative care of patients with thyroid carcinoma. After surgery or ¹³¹I therapy, all patients with differentiated thyroid carcinoma undergo screening with both 5 mCi ¹³¹I and 3 mCi ²⁰¹Tl scintigraphy. When the results are negative, further follow-up evaluation depends on the results of both yearly ²⁰¹Tl and twice-yearly tumor marker assays. ¹³¹I scintigraphy is suggested only when either test or any other clinical or radiologic information suggests metastasis. The main objective is to determine whether the tumor is amenable to ¹³¹I treatment.

Ramanna et al. (25) and Lida et al. (124) confirmed the findings of Hoefnagel et al. (12) that showed increased sensitivity for detection of residual thyroid cancer or metastasis with ²⁰¹Tl and thyroglobulin serum levels when compared with a 5-mCi diagnostic ¹³¹I scan. Figure 45.14 shows the superiority of ²⁰¹Tl in the detection of neck and chest metastasis in a patient with differentiated thyroid cancer who has reduced ability to concentrate ¹³¹I.

The study by Ramanna et al. (25) showed the superiority of ¹³¹I in the detection of normal residual thyroid tissue when compared with ²⁰¹Tl. The overall study indicated that if ¹³¹I accumulation was moderate to intense and ²⁰¹Tl accumulation was absent to mild, the findings correlated well with the presence of normal residual thyroid tissue. However, when ²⁰¹Tl accumulation was moderate or marked and ¹³¹I accumulation was absent to mild, the findings most often represented thyroid cancer. Charles et al. (125) found that ²⁰¹Tl SPECT increased the ability to detect metastasis of thyroid cancer compared with conventional planar imaging. In 20 patients with known metastatic disease, planar ²⁰¹Tl images had positive findings in 60% of patients, whereas results of SPECT were positive in 85%. SPECT foci as small as 10 mm in the neck and 1.5 cm in the lungs were detected. Although some pitfalls in interpretation of the tomographic reconstructions were found, ²⁰¹Tl SPECT imaging was believed to be a marked improvement over planar imaging in the detection of metastasis of differentiated thyroid cancer.

Summary

²⁰¹Tl scintigraphy for detection of recurrent thyroid cancer is provocative in that recent studies indicate a high sensitivity for detection of recurrence of differentiated thyroid cancer without withdrawal of thyroid hormone when used in conjunction with thyroglobulin levels. ²⁰¹Tl may play a role in the follow-up care of patients with differentiated thyroid cancer. We have generally had mixed experience with ²⁰¹Tl for this purpose, except in the care of patients with pulmonary or abdominal metastasis. Where ²⁰¹Tl is not recommended currently, ¹³¹I with human recombinant thyroid-stimulating hormone for differentiated thyroid cancer is used for diagnostic testing. If undifferentiated thyroid cancer is suspected, PET FDG is used.

REFERENCES

1. Salvatore M, Carratti L, Porta E. Thallium-201 as a positive indicator for lung neoplasms: preliminary experiments. *Radiology* 1976;21: 487–488.
2. Tonami N, Hisada K. Clinical experience of tumor imaging with thallium-201 chloride. *Clin Nucl Med* 1977;2:75–81.
3. Hisada K, Tonami H, Miyamae T, et al. Clinical evaluation of tumor imaging with thallium-201 chloride. *Radiology* 1978;129:497–500.
4. Ancri D, Basset JY, Lonchampt MD, et al. Diagnosis of cerebral lesions by thallium-201. *Radiology* 1978;128:417–422.
5. Tonami N, Hisada K. Thallium-201 scintigraphy in postoperative detection of thyroid cancer: a comparative study with I-131. *Radiology* 1980;136:461–464.
6. Stoller DW, Waxman AD, Rosen G, et al. Comparison of thallium-201, gallium-67, technetium 99m MDP and magnetic resonance imaging of musculoskeletal sarcoma. *Clin Nucl Med* 1986;12[Suppl]: 15(abst).
7. Winzelberg GG, Melada GA, Hydrovitz JD. False-positive thallium-201 parathyroid scan of the mediastinum in Hodgkin's lymphoma. *Am J Roentgenol* 1986;147:819–821.
8. Kaplan WD, Takvorian T, Morris JH, et al. Thallium-201 brain tumor imaging: a comparative study with pathological correlation. *J Nucl Med* 1987;28:47–52.
9. Waxman AD, Goldsmith MS, Greif PM, et al. Differentiation of tumor versus sarcoidosis using thallium-201 in patients with hilar mediastinal adenopathy. *J Nucl Med* 1987;28:561(abst).
10. Ramanna L, Waxman AD, Binney G, et al. Increasing specificity of brain scintigraphy using thallium-201. *J Nucl Med* 1987;28:658(abst).
11. Mountz JM, Stafford-Schuck K, Mcleever P, et al. The tumor/cardiac ratio: a new method to estimate residual high grade astrocytoma using thallium-201. *J Nucl Med* 1987;28:706(abst).
12. Hoefnagel CA, Delprat CC, Marcus HR, et al. Role of thallium-201 total body scintigraphy in follow-up of thyroid carcinoma. *J Nucl Med* 1988;27:1854–1857.
13. Lee VW, Rosen MP, Baum A, et al. AIDS-related Kaposi sarcoma: findings on thallium-201 scintigraphy. *Am J Roentgenol* 1988;151: 1233–1235.
14. Waxman AD, Ramanna L, Said J. Thallium scintigraphy in lymphoma: relationship to gallium-67. *J Nucl Med* 1989;30:915(abst).
15. Waxman AD, Ramanna L, Brachman MB, et al. Thallium scintigraphy in primary carcinoma of the breast: evaluation of primary and axillary metastasis. *J Nucl Med* 1989;30:844(abst).

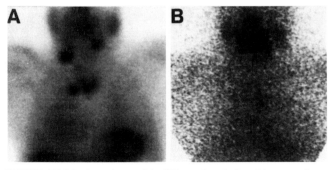

FIGURE 45.14. A patient with differentiated thyroid cancer has a marked increase in ²⁰¹Tl accumulation in the neck and chest **(A)**, whereas a 5-mCi ¹³¹I diagnostic scan was normal. Serum thyroglobulin levels in this patient were markedly increased.

16. Black KL, Hawkins R, Kit KT, et al. Use of thallium-201 SPECT to quantitate malignancy grade of gliomas. *J Neurosurg* 1989;71:342–346.

17. Tonami N, Shuke N, Yokoyama K, et al. Use of thallium-201 single photon emission computed tomography in the evaluation of suspected lung cancer. *J Nucl Med* 1989;30:997–1004.

18. Kaplan WD, Southee LM, Annese MS, et al. Evaluating low and high grade non-Hodgkin's lymphoma (NHL) with gallium-67 (Ga) and thallium-201 (Tl) imaging. *J Nucl Med* 1990;31:793(abst).

19. Ramanna L, Waxman AD, Binney G, et al. Thallium-201 scintigraphy in bone sarcoma: comparison with gallium-67 and technetium-MDP in evaluation of chemotherapy response. *J Nucl Med* 1990;31:567–572.

20. Kim KT, Black KL, Marciano D, et al. Thallium-201 SPECT imaging of brain tumors: methods and results. *J Nucl Med* 1990;31:965–969.

21. Waxman AD, Ramanna L, Memsic A, et al. Thallium scintigraphy in differentiating malignant from benign mass abnormalities of the breast. *J Nucl Med* 1990;31:747(abst).

22. Sehweil AM, McKillop JH, Milroy R, et al. Thallium scintigraphy in the staging of lung cancer, breast cancer and lymphoma. *Nucl Med Commun* 1990;11:263–269.

23. Waxman AD, Ramanna L, Eller D. Characterization of lymphoma grade using thallium (Tl) and gallium (Ga) scintigraphy. *J Nucl Med* 1991;32:917–918.

24. Waxman AD. Thallium-201 in nuclear oncology. In: Freeman LM, ed. *Nuclear medicine annual.* New York: Raven Press, 1991:193–209.

25. Ramanna L, Waxman AD, Braunstein G. Thallium-201 scintigraphy in differentiated thyroid cancer: comparison with radioiodine scintigraphy and serum thyroglobulin determination. *J Nucl Med* 1991;32:441–446.

26. Waxman AD, Ramanna L, Memsic LD, et al. Thallium scintigraphy in the evaluation of mass abnormalities of the breast. *J Nucl Med* 1993;34:18–23.

27. Sluyser M, Hoefnagel CA. Breast carcinomas detected by thallium-201 scintigraphy. *Cancer Lett* 1988;40:161–168.

28. Waxman AD, Eller D, Ashook G, et al. Comparison of gallium-67 citrate and thallium-201 scintigraphy in peripheral intrathoracic lymphoma. *J Nucl Med* 1996;37:46–50.

29. Hassan I, Sahweel C, Constantinides A, et al. Uptake and kinetics of ^{99m}Tc hexakis 2-methoxy isobutyl isonitrile in benign and malignant lesions in the lungs. *Clin Nucl Med* 1989;14:333–340.

30. Caner B, Kitapci M, Aras T, et al. Increased accumulation of hexakis (2-methoxyisobutylisonitrile) technetium(I) in osteosarcoma and its metastatic lymph nodes. *J Nucl Med* 1991;32:1977–1978.

31. Aktolun C, Demirel D, Kir M, et al. Unexpected uptake of technetium 99m hexakis-2-methoxy-isobutylisonitrile in grant lymph node hyperplasia of the mediastinum (Castleman's disease). *Eur J Nucl Med* 1991;18:856–859.

32. Briele B, Hotze A, Kropp J, et al. Vergleich von 201Tl und 99mTc-MIBI in der machsorge des differenzierten schilddrusenkarzinoms. [A comparison of 201Tl and 99mTc-MIBI in the follow-up of differentiated thyroid carcinomas.] *Nuklearmedizin* 1991;30:115–124.

33. Caner B, Kitapci M, Unlu M, et al. Technetium-99m-MIBI uptake in benign and malignant bone lesions: a comparative study with technetium-99m-MDP. *J Nucl Med* 1992;33:319–324.

34. Caner B, Kitapci M, Erbengi G, et al. Increased accumulation of ^{99m}Tc MIBI in undifferentiated mesenchymal tumor and its metastatic lung lesions. *Clin Nucl Med* 1992;17/2:144–145.

35. Albuquerque L, Baillet G, Delattre JY, et al. MIBI cerebral tomoscintigraphy for monitoring adult gliomas. *J Med Nucl Biophys* 1992;16:185.

36. Baillet G, Albuquerque L, Delattre JY, et al. MIBI uptake by supratentorial gliomas in adults. *J Med Nucl Biophys* 1992;16:185.

37. Campeau RJ, Kronemer KA, Sutherland CM. Concordant uptake of ^{99m}Tc sestamibi and Tl-201 in unsuspected breast tumor. *Clin Nucl Med* 1992;17:936–937.

38. Aktolun C, Bayhan H, Kir M. Clinical experience with ^{99m}Tc MIBI imaging in patients with malignant tumors: preliminary results and comparison with Tl-201. *Clin Nucl Med* 1992;17:171–176.

39. Waxman A, Ashook G, Kooba A, et al. The use of ^{99m}Tc-methoxy isobutyl isonitrile (MIBI) in evaluation of patients with primary carcinoma of the breast: comparison with Tl-201 (Tl). *Clin Nucl Med* 1992;17:761.

40. Kao CH, Wang SJ, Lin WY, et al. Detection of nasopharyngeal carcinoma using 99mTc methoxyisobutylisonitrile SPECT. *Nucl Med Commun* 1993;14:41–46.

41. Kitapci MT, Tastekin G, Turgut M, et al. Preoperative localization of parathyroid carcinoma using ^{99m}Tc MIBI. *Clin Nucl Med* 1993;18:217–219.

42. Kao CH, Wang SJ, Lin WY, et al. Differentiation of single solid lesions in the lungs by means of single photon emission tomography with technetium-99m methoxyisobutylisonitrile. *Eur J Nucl Med* 1993;20/3:249–254.

43. Khalkhali I, Mena 1, Jouanne E, et al. ^{99m}Tc-sestamibi prone breast imaging in patients (PTS) with suspicion of breast cancer (Ca). *J Nucl Med* 1993;34:140P.

44. Waxman A, Ashook G, Kooba A, et al. The use of ^{99m}Tc-methoxy isobutyl isonitrile (MIBI) in evaluation of patients with primary carcinoma of the breast: comparison with Tl-201 (Tl). *J Nucl Med* 1993;34:139P.

45. Khalkhali I, Mena I, Diggles L. Review of imaging techniques for the diagnosis of breast cancer: a new role of prone scintimammography using technetium-99m sestamibi. *Eur J Nucl Med* 1994;21:357–362.

46. Khalkhali I, Mena I, Jouanne E, et al. Prone scintimammography in patients with suspicion of carcinoma of the breast. *J Am Coll Surg* 1994;178:491–497.

47. Waxman A, Nagaraj N, Ashook S, et al. Sensitivity and specificity of ^{99m}Tc methoxyisobutyl isonitrile (MIBI) in the evaluation of primary carcinoma of the breast: comparison of palpable and nonpalpable lesions with mammography. *J Nucl Med* 1994;35[Suppl 5]:22P(abst).

48. Nagaraj N, Waxman A, Ashok S, et al. Comparison of SPECT and planar ^{99m}Tc sestamibi imaging in patients with carcinoma of the breast. *J Nucl Med* 1994;35[Suppl 5]:229P(abst).

49. Nagaraj N, Waxman A, Silverman J, et al. Comparison of ^{99m}Tc sestamibi (MIBI) and MRI in patients with dense breasts. *J Nucl Med* 1994;35[Suppl 5]:908(abst).

50. Waxman A, Nagaraj N, Khan S, et al. ^{99m}Tc sestamibi (MIBI) in the evaluation of lymphoma: comparison with gallium-67 citrate (Ga-67). *Clin Nucl Med* 1994;19:843.

51. Waxman A, Rosen G, Ramanna L, et al. Comparison of thallium-201 and ^{99m}Tc hexakis-2-methoxy-2-methylpropyl isonitrile (MIBI) in patients with neoplasia. *Clin Nucl Med* 1991;76:716.

52. O'Tuama LA, Packard AB, Treves ST. SPECT imaging of pediatric brain tumor with hexakis (methoxybutylisonitrile) technetium (I). *J Nucl Med* 1990;31:2040–2041.

53. O'Driscoll CM, Baker F, Casey MJ, et al. Localization of recurrent medullary thyroid carcinoma with technetium-99m-methoxyisobutylnitrile scintigraphy: a case report. *J Nucl Med* 1991;32:2281–2283.

54. Medolgao G, Virotta G, Pita A, et al. Abnormal uptake of technetium-99m hexakis-2-methoxyisobutylisonitrile in a primary cardiac lymphoma. *Eur J Nucl Med* 1992;19/3:222–225.

55. Waxman A. Nuclear oncology. *Curr Opin Radiol* 1991;3:871–876.

56. Gehring PJ, Hammand PB. The interrelationship between thallium and potassium in animals. *J Pharmacol Exp Ther* 1967;155:187–201.

57. Lebowitz E, Greene MW, Green R, et al. Thallium-201 for medical use, I. *J Nucl Med* 1975;16:151–155.

58. Bradley-Moore PR, Lebowitz E, Greene MW, et al. Thallium-201 for medical use, II: biological behavior. *J Nucl Med* 1975;16:156–160.

59. Atkins HL, Budinger TF, Lebowitz E, et al. Thallium-201 for medical use, III: human distribution and physical imaging properties. *J Nucl Med* 1977;18:133–140.

60. Britten JS, Blank M. Thallium activation of the (Na$^+$, K$^+$) activated ATPase of rabbit kidney. *Biochem Biophys Acta* 1968;15:160–166.

61. Muranake A. Accumulation of radioisotopes with tumor affinity, II: comparison of the tumor accumulation of Ga-67 citrate and thallium-201 chloride in vitro. *Acta Med Okayama* 1981;35:85–101.

62. Sessler MJ, Geek P, Maul FD, et al. New aspects of cellular Tl-201 uptake T + Na + -2Cl-cotransport is the central mechanism of ion uptake. *J Nucl Med* 1986;25:24–27.

63. Ando A, Ando I, Katayama M, et al. Biodistribution of Tl-201 in tumor bearing animals and inflammatory lesion induced animals. *Eur J Nucl Med* 1987;12:567–572.

64. Maublant JC, Gachon P, Moins N. Hexakis (2-methoxy isobutylisonitrile) technetium-99m and thallium-201 chloride: uptake and release in cultured myocardial cells. *J Nucl Med* 1988;29:48–54.

65. Chiu ML, Kronauge JF, Piwnica-Worms D. Effect of mitochondrial and plasma membrane potentials on accumulation of hexakis (2-methoxyisobutylisonitrile) technetium (I) in cultured mouse fibroblasts. *J Nucl Med* 1990;31:1646–1653.

66. Delmon-Moingeon LI, Piwnica-Worms D, Van den Abbeele AD, et al. Uptake of the cation hexakis (2-methoxyisobutylisoniitrile)-technetium-99m by human carcinoma cell lines in vitro. *Cancer Res* 1990;50:2198–2202.

67. Chiu ML, Herman LW, Kronauge JF, et al. Comparative effects of neutral dipolar compounds and lipophilic anions on technetium 99m-hexakis (2-methoxyisobutyl isonitrile) accumulation in cultured chick ventricular myocytes. *Invest Radiol* 1992;27:1052–1058.

68. Carvalho PA, Chtu ML, Kronauge JF, et al. Subcellular distribution and analysis of technetium-99m-MIBI in isolated perfused rat hearts. *J Nucl Med* 1992;33:1516–1621.

69. Crane P, Laliberte R, Heminway S, et al. Effect of mitochondrial viability and metabolism on technetium-99m-sestamibi myocardial retention. *Eur J Nucl Med* 1993;20:20–25.

70. Chernoff DM, Strichartz GR, Piwnica-Worms D. Membrane potential determination in large unilamellar vesicles with hexakis (2-methoxyisobutylisonitrile) technetium (I). *Biochim Biophys Acta* 1993;1147:262–266.

71. Maublant JC, Moins N, Gachon P, et al. Uptake of technetium-99m-teboroxime in cultured myocardial cells: comparison with thallium-201 and technetium-99m-sestamibi. *J Nucl Med* 1993;34:255–259.

72. Waxman AD, Grode M, Ashok G, et al. Intraoperative assessment of brain malignancies using Tl-201 (Tl). *J Nucl Med* 1993;34:37P(abst).

73. Ramanna L, Waxman AD, Weiss A, et al. Thallium-201 (Tl-201) scan patterns in bone and soft tissue sarcoma. *J Nucl Med* 1992;33:843.

74. Ramanna L, Waxman AD, Rosen, G. Evaluation of Tl-201 (Tl) uptake pattern in bone lesions: differentiation of benign from malignant processes. *J Nucl Med* 1992;33:869.

75. Menendez L, Fideler B, Mirra J. Thallium-201 scanning for the evaluation of osteosarcoma and soft-tissue sarcoma. *J Bone Joint Surg Am* 1993;4:527–531.

76. Rosen G, Loren G, Brien E, et al. Serial thallium-201 scintigraphy in osteosarcoma: correlation with tumor necrosis after preoperative chemotherapy. *Clin Orthop* 1993;293:302–306.

77. Ashok G, Waxman AD, Kooba A, et al. Comparison of Tl-201 (T1) and ^{99m}Tc methoxyisobutylisonitrile (MIBI) in the evaluation of patients with osteogenic sarcoma. *Clin Nucl Med* 1992;9:761(abst).

78. Ashok G, Waxman AD, Kooba A, et al. Comparison of Tl-201 (Tl) and ^{99m}Tc methoxyisobutylisonitrile in the evaluation of patients with non-osseous sarcomas. *Clin Nucl Med* 1992;9(abst).

79. Waxman AD, Khan S, Julien P, et al. Methoxyisobutalisonitrile in the evaluation of primary carcinoma of the lung: comparison of planar and SPECT techniques. *Clin Nucl Med* 1993;18:926(abst).

80. Burak Z, Argon M, Memix A. et al. Evaluation of palpable breast masses with ^{99m}Tc MIBI: a comparative study with mammography and ultrasonography. *Nucl Med Commun* 1994;15:604–612.

81. Rogers JV, Powell RW. Mammographic indications for biopsy of clinically normal breasts: correlation with pathologic findings in 72 cases. *Am J Roentgenol* 1972;115:794–800.

82. Homer MJ. Nonpalpable breast abnormalities: a realistic view of the accuracy of mammography in detecting malignancies. *Radiology* 1984;153:831–832.

83. Sickles EA. Mammographic features of 300 consecutive nonpalpable breast cancers. *Am J Roentgenol* 1986;146:661–663.

84. Pollei SR, Mettler FA, Bartow SA, et al. Occult breast cancer: prevalence and radiographic detectability. *Radiology* 1987;163:459–462.

85. Stomper PC, Davis SP, Weidner N, et al. Clinically occult, non-calcified breast cancer: serial radiologic-pathologic correlation in 27 cases. *Radiology* 1988;169:621–626.

86. Basset LW, Liu TH, Giuliano AE, et al. The prevalence of carcinoma in palpable versus impalpable, mammographically detected lesions. *Am J Roentgenol* 1991;157:21–24.

87. Kopans, D. B. The positive predictive value of mammography. *Am J Roentgenol* 1992;158:521–526.

88. Mann BD. Giuliano AE. Bassett LW, et al. Delayed diagnosis of breast cancer as a result of normal mammograms. *Arch Surg* 1983:118:23–25.

89. Holland R, Jan HC, Hendricks L, et al. Mammographically occult breast cancer: apathologic and radiologic study. *Cancer* 1983;52:1810–1819.

90. Feig SA, Shaber GA, Patchefskly A. Analysis of clinically occult and mammographically occult breast tumors. *Am J Roentgenol* 1977;128:403–408.

91. Kalisher L. Factors influencing false negative rates in xeromammography. *Radiology* 1979;133:297–301.

92. Burns PE, Grace MG, Lees AW, et al. False-negative mammography delay diagnosis of breast cancer. *N Engl J Med* 1978;299:201.

93. Burns PE, Grace MG, Lees AW, et al. False-negative mammograms causing delay in breast cancer diagnosis. *J Can Assoc Radiol* 1979;30:74–77.

94. Sickles EA. Mammographic features of early breast cancer. *Am J Roentgenol* 1984;143:461–464.

95. Moskowitz M. The predictive value of certain mammographic signa in screening for breast cancer. *Cancer* 1983;51:1007–1011.

96. Sadowsky N, Kopans DB. Breast cancer. *Radiol Clin North Am* 1983;21:51–65.

97. Niloff PH, Sheiner NM. False-negative mammograms in patients with breast cancer. *Can J Surg* 1981;24:50–52.

98. Spivey GH, Perry BW, Clark VA, et al. Predicting the risk of cancer at the time of breast biopsy: variation in the benign to malignant ratio. *Am Surg* 1982;48:326–332.

99. Mills RR, Davis R, Stacey AJ. The detection and significance of calcifications in the breast: radiologic and pathological study. *Br J Radiol* 1976;49:12–26.

100. Sickles EA. Breast Calcifications: mammographic evaluation. *Radiology* 1986;160:289–293.

101. Homer MJ. Nonpalpable mammographic abnormalities: timing the follow-up studies. *Am J Roentgenol* 1981;136:923–926.

102. Meyer JE, Sonnenfeld MR, Greenes RA, et al. Preoperative localization of clinically occult breast lesions; experience at a referral hospital. *Radiology* 1988;169:627–628.

103. Hermann G, Janus C, Schwartz IS, et al. Nonpalpable lesions: accuracy of pre-biopsy mammographic diagnosis. *Radiology* 1987;165:323–326.

104. Hall FM, Storella JM, Silverstone DZ, et al. Nonpalpable breast lesions: recommendations for biopsy based on suspicion of carcinoma at mammography. *Radiology* 1988;167:353–368.

105. Taillefer R, Robidoux A, Lambert R, et al. Technetium-99m sestamibi prone scintimammography to detect primary breast cancer and axillary lymph node involvement. *J Nucl Med* 1995;36:1758–1765.

106. Khalkhali I, Cutrone JA, Mena I, et al. Technetium-99m sestamibi scintimammography of breast lesions: clinical and pathological follow-up. *J Nucl Med* 1995;36:1784–1789.

107. Palmedo H, Schomburg A, Grunwald F, et al. Technetium-99m sestamibi scintimammography for suspicious breast lesions. *J Nucl Med* 1996;37:626–630.

108. Kao CH, Wang SJ, Liu TJ. The use of technetium-99m methoxyisobutylisonitrile breast scintigraphy to evaluate palpable breast masses. *Eur J Nucl Med* 1994;21:5.

109. Nguyen K, Waxman A, Gupta P, et al. Comparison of ^{99m}Tc methoxyisobutylisonitrile (MIBI) and MRI in breast malignancy: the significance of concordant and discordant findings. *J Nucl Med* 1996;37:75P(abst).

110. Waxman AD. The role of Tc99m methoxyisobutylisonitrile in imaging breast cancer. *Semin Nucl Med* 1997;27:40–54.

111. Ciarmello A, Del Vecchio S, Potena MI, et al. Tumor clearance of

technetium 99m–sestamibi as a predictor of response to neoadjuvant chemotherapy for locally advanced breast cancer. *J Clin Oncol* 1998; 16:1677–1683.

112. Khalkali I, Villanueva-Meyer J, Edell S, et al. Impact of breast density on the diagnostic accuracy of ^{99m}Tc sestamibi breast imaging in the detection of breast cancer. *J Nucl Med* 1996;288:74.

113. Omar WS, Eissa S, Moustafa H, et al. Role of thallium 201 chloride and ^{99m}Tc methoxy-isobutyl-isonitrile sestamibi in evaluation of breast masses: correlation with immunohistochemical characteristic parameters Ki-63 PCNA, BCI-2 and angiogenesis in malignant lesions. *Anticancer Res* 1997;17:1639.

114. Piwnica-Worms D, Luker G, Fracasso P, et al. Detection of MDR with ^{99m}Tc sestamibi. *J Nucl Med* 1997;38:369.

115. Mankoff D, Dunnwald L, Gralow J, et al. Monitoring the response of patients with locally advanced breast carcinoma to neoadjuvant chemotherapy using (technetium 99m) sestamibi scintimammography. *Cancer* 1999;85:2410.

116. Cutrone J, Yospur L, Khalkhali I, et al. Immunohistologic assessment of technetium 99m MIBI uptake in benign and malignant breast lesions. *J Nucl Med* 1998;39:449.

117. Cutrone J, Khalkhali I, Yospur L, et al. [99m]Tc sestamibi scintimammography for the evaluation of breast masses in patients with radiographically dense breasts. *Breast J* 1999;5:383.

118. Howarth D, Sillar R, Clark D, et al. Technetium-99m sestamibi scintimammography: the influence of histopathological characteristics, lesion size, and the presence of carcinoma in situ in the detection of breast carcinoma. *Eur J Nucl Med* 1999;26:1475.

119. Khalkali I, Villanueva-Meyer M, Edell S, et al. Diagnostic accuracy of ^{99m}Tc sestamibi breast imaging: multicenter trial results. *J Nucl Med* 2000;41:1973–1979.

120. Waxman A, Nagaraj N, Kovalevsky M, et al. Detection of primary breast malignancy with ^{99m}Tc methoxyisobutylisonitrile (MIBI) in patients with non-palpable primary malignancies: the importance of lesion size. *J Nucl Med* 1995;36:877–194(abst).

121. Black MM, Barclay THC, Culter SJ, et al. Association of atypical characteristics of benign breast lesions with subsequent risk of breast cancer. *Cancer* 1972;29:338–343.

122. Dupont WD, Page DL. Risk factors for breast cancer in women with proliferative breast disease. *N Engl J Med* 1985;312:146–151.

123. Gupta P, Waxman A, Nguyen K, et al. Correlation of Tc99m sestamibi uptake with histopathologic characteristics in patients with benign breast disease. *J Nucl Med* 1996;37:250.

124. Lida Y, Hidaka A, Hatabu H, et al. Follow-up study of postoperative patients with thyroid cancer by thallium-201 scintigraphy and serum thyroglobulin measurement. *J Nucl Med* 1991;32:2098–2100.

125. Charles ND, Vitti RA, Brooks K. Thallium-201 SPECT increases detectability of thyroid cancer metastases. *J Nucl Med* 1990;31: 147–153.

Diagnostic Nuclear Medicine, Fourth Edition. Edited by M.P. Sandler, R.E. Coleman, J.A. Patton, F.J.Th. Wackers, A. Gottschalk. Lippincott Williams & Wilkins, Philadelphia 2003.

46

CLINICAL APPLICATIONS OF MONOCLONAL ANTIBODY IMAGING

LIONEL S. ZUCKIER
ALDO N. SERAFINI

HISTORIC DEVELOPMENT OF RADIOIMMUNOSCINTIGRAPHY

The technique of co-opting the humoral immune system to selectively target radionuclides to sites of disease within the body was first used in 1948 in the prescient work of Pressman and Keighley (1), who targeted rat renal tissue with radiolabeled polyclonal antibodies derived from rabbit immune serum. Conceptually, the strategy of using therapeutic agents that selectively discern between pathogen and self was most clearly formulated by Paul Ehrlich in the early 1900s in his quest for "magic bullets" (2,3). Ehrlich's paradigm for selective therapy was administration of immune serum, which was toxic to the disease-causing agent but sparing of normal tissue.

Despite significant efforts over many decades, it has proved difficult to harness the immune system to produce optimal antibodies of high affinity and specificity to antigens of interest and particularly challenging to effectively direct these radiolabeled compounds to their intended targets in vivo. Goldenberg et al. (4) were the first to show that affinity-purified radiolabeled antibodies injected into patients with neoplasms could be detected with external imaging. These polyclonal antibodies, derived from immune serum, were not practical for widespread use. Through immunization, it is difficult to generate large amounts of high-affinity antibody to a given antigen and almost impossible to replicate similar responses when additional supplies are needed. This issue of availability and consistency of substrate, necessary requisites of a well-manufactured product, was solved only after Kohler and Milstein (5) described the hybridoma technique in 1975. This milestone in the production of antibodies finally allowed immunologic targeting to evolve into a commercially viable technique.

Successful realization of radioimmunotargeting has gradually

been achieved through these and numerous other developments in cell biology, molecular biology, and immunology that have revolutionized our understanding of the immune response, tumor biology, and antibody structure-function relations (6). Although a large number of monoclonal antibodies have been raised against a wide variety of antigens in the laboratory and investigated in the clinic, the number of agents approved by the U.S. Food and Drug Administration (FDA) for clinical use remains surprisingly small (Table 46.1). Only three of the five FDA-approved diagnostic radiolabeled antibodies are still being marketed in the United States. Combined usage most recently was estimated at only 6,000 kits per year (7).

Molecular biologic techniques are being used to improve the capacity of immunologic agents to serve as targeting vehicles for both diagnosis and therapy. Ongoing discoveries in the laboratory are actively being incorporated into second and third generations of radioimmunologic agents. It is therefore important for the nuclear medicine practitioner to appreciate the theoretic and biologic principles relevant to antibody targeting to understand the evolution of trends that will affect these new molecules.

ANTIBODIES: BASIC STRUCTURE AND FUNCTION

Specific immunity is the result of effector mechanisms mediated by antibodies and specific cellular elements of the lymphatic system (8). An immunologic response is therefore either humoral or cell-mediated. The former arm is mediated by antibodies, also called *immunoglobulins,* which are proteins produced by B cells or their progeny plasma cells, generally in response to foreign macromolecules called *antigens.* Antibodies have the potential to bind the specific antigen that stimulated their production; the result is neutralization or elimination. The specific region of the antigen molecule to which an antibody binds is called an *epitope*; antigen molecules generally possess numerous epitopes, both identical and disparate, to which subsets of antibodies can bind.

In the course of normal development, the immune system in humans produces a large variety of antibodies, all of which share a basic underlying structure. A greater degree of homology

L.S. Zuckier: Department of Radiology, New Jersey Medical School and University Hospital, Newark, NJ.
A.N. Serafini: Nuclear Medicine Division, University of Miami School of Medicine, Miami, FL.

Table 46.1. *Diagnostic Radiolabeled Antibodies in FDA-Sponsored Trials*

Generic name (trade name, company)	Antibody (mg)	Antigen	Description	Label (mCi)	FDA approved (date), investigational use
Satumomab pendetide (OncoScint CR/OV, Ctyogen)	B72.3 (1)	TAG-72	Whole murine IgG1	^{111}In (5)	Colorectal and ovarian carcinoma (12/29/92)
Capromab pendetide (ProstaScint, Cytogen)	7E11-C5.3 (0.5)	100-kd glycoprotein	Whole murine IgG1	^{111}In (5)	Prostate carcinoma (10/28/96)
Arcitumomab (CEA-Scan, Immunomedics)	IMMU-4 (1)	Carcinoembryonic antigen	Fab' murine IgG1	^{99m}Tc (20–25)	Colorectal (6/28/96), breast, small cell lung carcinoma
Imciromab pentetate (Myoscint, Centocor)	(0.5)	Heavy-chain cardiac myosin	Fab murine IgG2a	^{111}In (2)	Myocardial necrosis (7/3/96)
Nofetumomab merpentan (Verluma, NeoRx)	NR-LU-10 (5–10)	40-kd gycoprotein	Fab murine IgG2b	^{99m}Tc (15–30)	Small cell (8/20/96), non–small cell lung carcinoma
Sulesomab (LeukoScan, Immunomedics)	(0.25)	NCA-90	Fab' murine IgG1	^{99m}Tc (20–30)	Osteomyelitis, appendicitis, inflammatory bowel disease
(LymphoScan, Immunomedics)	LL2 (0.5)	CD22	Fab' murine IgG2a	^{99m}Tc (20–25)	Non-Hodgkin lymphoma
Votumumab (HumaSPECT, Intracel)	88BV59 (10)	Altered cytokeratins	Whole human IgG3	^{99m}Tc (30–35)	Colorectal, ovarian, breast carcinoma
LeuTech (Palatin Tech.)	—	CD15	Whole murine IgM	^{99m}Tc	White blood cells, infection
(AFP-Scan, Immunomedics)	(1)	Human α-fetoprotein	Fab' murine IgG1	^{99m}Tc (20–25)	Primary liver, germ cell carcinoma
(Myeloscan, Immunomedics)	—	NCA-90	Fab' murine IgG1	^{99m}Tc (20–25)	Bone marrow metastasis of solid tumors

Imaging for dosimetry only not included.
List derived from www.ndapipeline.com.

exists within specific subgroups of antibodies, which are called *classes* and *subclasses*. In both humans and mice, five distinct classes exist (IgG, IgM, IgE, IgA, and IgD). The most abundant class, IgG, is subdivided into four subclasses (numbered 1, 2, 3 and 4 in humans and 1, 2a, 2b and 3 in mice). Individual immunoglobulins within each class and subclass share a similarity of functional and structural properties.

The IgG molecule consists of two identical light (L) and two identical heavy (H) polypeptide chains covalently attached by disulfide bonds to form a Y-shaped structure with paired antigen-binding arms (Fig. 46.1). Heavy and light chains of immunoglobulins are divided into relatively compact globular regions approximately 110 amino acids long, called *domains*. Those located at the end of the antigen-binding arms are considerably more variable in composition than elsewhere in the molecule and are therefore called the *variable-heavy* (V_H) and *variable-light* (V_L) domains, in contrast to the remaining constant domains. In particular, three specific regions within each of V_H and V_L are especially varied, or hypervariable, and are interspersed between more-constant framework regions. The framework residues interact and fold in such as manner as to assemble the 6 hypervariable regions into a contiguous antigen-binding groove. Because the hypervariable regions determine the epitope to which the antibody will bind, they are also known as *complementarity-determining regions* (CDRs).

In the IgG heavy chain, in addition to V_H there are three constant-region domains, labeled C_H1, C_H2, and C_H3, and a hinge that provides segmental flexibility between C_H1 and C_H2. A carbohydrate moiety, which is used in some commercial products as a site on which to label the antibody (9), is attached to

the C_H2 region. Both IgD and IgA resemble IgG in that the heavy chain comprises one variable and three constant domains, whereas IgE and IgM include an additional fourth heavy domain (C_H4) that contributes to a higher molecular weight. All light chains are composed of a single constant-region domain C_L in addition to V_L.

IgA and IgM are secreted from B cells with an attached joining, or J, chain which leads to assembly of the IgA molecules into bimeric or trimeric forms and IgM into pentamers. With these multimeric antibodies, avidity of binding, referring to the sum total of interactions between the immunoglobulin and antigen, is markedly increased in the presence of adequate antigen density (10). By definition, the affinity of binding, which refers to the interaction between a single binding site and antigen, is unaffected by multivalency. The increased avidity of binding afforded by multivalency is crucial in the course of a normal immune response. IgM molecules initially formed in response to infection or antigenic challenge have not yet undergone affinity maturation and are of low affinity, yet they are able to bind effectively because of their multimeric nature.

The composition of the heavy-chain constant domains determines the class and subclass of the immunoglobulin. The heavy-chain constant domains of the antibody therefore are identical for all antibodies of a given class or subclass and are encoded by a specific heavy-chain immunoglobulin gene. The heavy-chain constant domains link the antibody to other molecules of the immune response and confer specific effector functions to each class and subclass, including binding to Fc receptors and phagocytic cells and activation of the complement cascade (11–13). Regulation of the catabolic rate of the immunoglobulin molecule

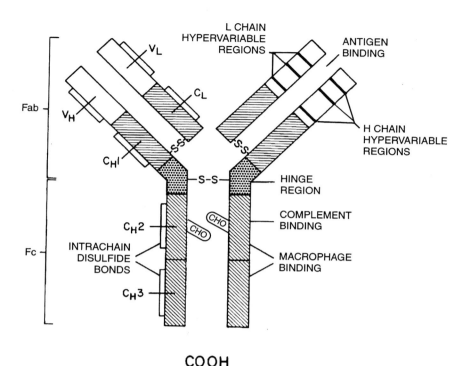

FIGURE 46.1. Structure of an IgG molecule. Interchain and intrachain disulfide bonds (—S—S—) and the C_H2 region carbohydrates (*CHO*) are indicated schematically on the molecule. (From Zuckier LS. Monoclonal Antibodies in Oncology. In: Aktolun C, Tauxe WN, eds. *Nuclear oncology.* New York: Springer Verlag, 1999:359–369, with permission.)

is determined by the constant region (14,15) and is mediated, at least in part, by the recently characterized FcRB, or Brambell, receptor (16).

When the IgG molecule is modified for imaging or therapy, it is important that the integrity of the variable regions be maintained. Modifications induced by radiolabeling or purification, which interfere with the binding site, reduce uptake at the targeted antigen. In contrast, the constant region of the molecule is not needed for antigen binding, and it may elicit undesirable host reactions. The constant portion of a murine antibody may trigger specific human immune responses when injected into patients. The result is production of human antimurine antibodies directed against the foreign proteins, commonly abbreviated HAMA. HAMA usually are detected within the first 12 weeks after exposure to murine antibodies, appear to be dose-related, and occur to varying degrees with different agents (17–20). They occur more frequently with whole antibodies and less frequently with fragments. Titers are not necessarily sustained, and serum HAMA levels generally decrease over several months. The potential consequence of developing HAMA is that they may interfere with subsequent use of the same, or even different, diagnostic or therapeutic murine-based immunologic agents. After binding to an injected immunoconjugate, the HAMA complex is rapidly removed from circulation, primarily by the reticuloendothelial system. The result is poor targeting and an ineffective diagnostic study or therapeutic effect. Techniques to make the antibody appear more human-like are being implemented to overcome this problem. HAMA also may cause interference with murine-

based immunoassays; however, this is a phenomenon that is being circumvented in newer immunoassay designs.

ANTIBODY PRODUCTION AND HYBRIDOMA TECHNOLOGY

Production of monoclonal antibodies involves immunization of a subject (usually a mouse) with a specific tumor-associated antigen or tumor cell. This results in a number of clones of B lymphocytes and plasma cells that secrete a mixture of antibodies of different classes, affinities, and binding specificities. Serum from the immunized animals may be affinity purified; however, this does not fully overcome poor specificity of the antibodies and the lack of antibody consistency from immunization to subsequent immunization.

Many of these shortcomings were solved with the introduction of hybridoma technology in 1975 (5). In this method, antibody-forming B cells from an immunized subject are fused to tissue culture–adapted malignant plasma cells to make hybrids that retain the properties of both the immunized antibody-forming cells and the immortal myeloma fusion partners (Fig. 46.2). Single-cell clones are then cultured into homogeneous antibody-producing cell lines that can be individually characterized and selected. Because they originate from single clones, antibodies produced from these cell lines are called *monoclonal*, unlike the *polyclonal* antibodies obtained from immunized serum that are derived from multiple B cells within an immunized host. Mono-

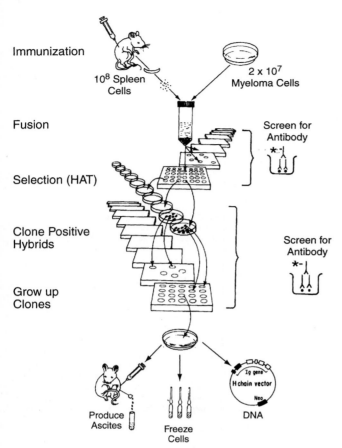

FIGURE 46.2. Production of mouse monoclonal antibodies. The labor-intensive steps of immunization, fusion, selection of fused cells with heterophil antibody titer medium, and screening are illustrated. Once a specific clone of cells has been characterized and selected, the clone is grown in culture and secretes antibody into the medium, which can be purified. Cells also can be used to produce ascites in mice that contain higher titers of antibody, can be frozen for future use, or can be used as a source of DNA for recombinant antibody engineering. (From Zuckier LS, Rodriguez LD, Scharff MD. Immunologic and pharmacologic concepts of monoclonal antibodies. *Semin Nucl Med* 1989;19:166–186, with permission.)

clonal antibodies have universally replaced pooled serum as the vehicle for targeting radionuclides to tumors. Unlimited amounts of homogeneous reagent can be produced from the cell line, making production of monoclonal antibodies economically feasible (21). Reagents can be selected on the basis of their attributes, including the class and subclass of the antibody (which determine half-life and bioavailability), the epitope to which the antibody binds, and the affinity of interaction between the antibody and the antigen. Finally, monoclonal antibodies, unlike polyclonal serum, are amenable to antibody engineering (22–26). This characteristic allows production of novel constructs, as described later.

MODIFICATION OF THE ANTIBODY MOLECULE

With greater understanding of the molecular biologic characteristics and structure-function relations of immunoglobulin, ef-

forts have been made to improve on its use as vehicle for radionuclide targeting. This has led to development of optimized second- and third-generation molecules designed for specific applications in radioimmunotargeting that have in common the following specific themes.

Size and Valence

The first generation of modified monoclonal antibodies consisted of well-defined subunits of the molecule obtained by means of enzymatic digestion (Fig. 46.3). Digestion by papain results in cleavage of the heavy chains above the inter–heavy chain disulfide bonds. The resultant univalent Fab fragment consists of the V_H, V_L, C_L, and C_H1 domains. The remaining duplicated C_H2 and C_H3 domains are called the Fc (crystallizable) fragment and do not bind antigen. The enzyme pepsin cleaves the heavy chains of the immunoglobulin molecule below their interchain disulfide bonds. The result is a bivalent $F(ab')_2$ fragment and small polypeptides derived from the Fc region. $F(ab')_2$ may be further chemically reduced into two Fab' fragments, each univalent and slightly larger than the Fab fragments. As shown in Table 46.1, both intact antibodies and fragments have been used in FDA-approved radioimmunoscintigraphic reagents.

The Fab, Fab' and $F(ab')_2$ fragments penetrate the interstitial spaces more readily than does the larger intact IgG molecule. Because much or all of the immunogenic Fc fragment has been deleted, the remaining antibody-binding portions of these molecules are also less likely to result in the formation of HAMA than are intact antibodies (27). The fragments also clear faster from the vascular system than does intact immunoglobulin. The result is a superior and more quickly attained tumor to background ratio (14). Because of the shortened bioavailability, the absolute amount of antibody associated with the tumor usually is decreased. Another potential disadvantage of the presence of Fab and Fab' fragments is a decrease in valence that results in decreased avidity and binding (28,29).

In addition to enzymatic digestion, recombinant DNA techniques, including the phage display library method (see later), can be used to produce Fab fragments (30,31) or even smaller immunologically active reagents (32). Single-chain Fv fragments (33) are composed of the heavy- and light-chain variable regions attached by linker peptides (Fig. 46.3). These small peptides have been shown to exhibit more rapid and homogeneous penetration of tumor than do larger immunoglobulin forms; the tumor to normal tissue ratios are equal or superior to those of larger fragments (34,35). Elevated kidney uptake, which occurs with Fab and $F(ab')_2$ fragments, is not found (35).

Even smaller molecules, such as variable-domain antibodies (dAbs), which consist of only single heavy-chain variable regions (36–38), or molecular recognition units (MRU), which consist of single hypervariable regions, have been described. One of the major advantages of small peptides such as MRUs is that they can be chemically synthesized *de novo* without the complexity and regulatory difficulties inherent in use of biologic cell lines for production. Disadvantages of MRUs are that binding is limited to a single hypervariable region, whereas in a native immunoglobulin molecule, the six hypervariable regions within each

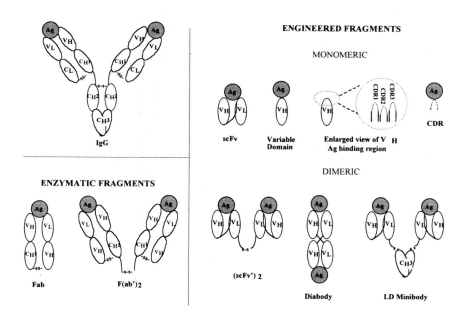

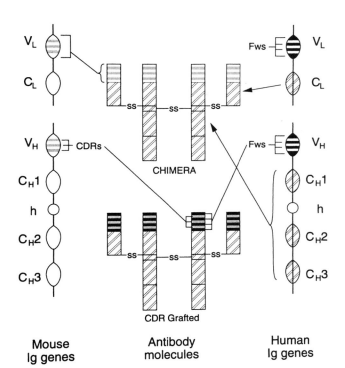

FIGURE 46.3. Structure of various antibody-based derivatives. Intact IgG molecules (*upper left panel*) can be enzymatically digested to yield Fab and F(ab')$_2$ fragments (*lower left panel*). With antibody-engineering techniques, a variety of monomeric and dimeric molecules have been produced (*right panel*). (From Adams GP. Improving the tumor specificity and retention of antibody-based molecules. *In Vivo* 1998; 12:11–22, with permission.)

Fab contribute jointly to binding with the epitope. It is therefore unlikely that a typical MRU will exhibit strong binding to the antigen. In certain cases, low affinity can be overcome by tandem repeats of the MRU-binding sequence, which increases avidity (39,40). Taking the hypervariable regions out of their normal context may render them conformationally altered. In this case, the peptides can be engineered to be conformationally constrained to resemble the native conformation of the immunoglobulin (39).

In contrast to the trend of miniaturizing binding agents, which often leads to a reduction in valence, there has been interest in generating larger multimeric antibodies to increase the avidity of binding (41). This is especially true in the case of small peptides, such as the univalent single-chain Fv, in which various dimeric constructs have been created to restore bivalence, including diabodies, (ScFv')$_2$, and minibodies (Fig. 46.3). With methods of antibody engineering, recombinant polymeric immunoglobulins have been constructed from IgG to produce supernormal valences (42,43).

Humanization

The obvious solution of decreasing HAMA by replacing murine immunoglobulins with human antibodies has been limited by ethical problems in obtaining immunized human lymphocytes and by intrinsic technical difficulties in the human hybridoma process (44,45). As an alternative, researchers have developed methods for combining murine-derived binding specificity with the constant-region structure of human immunoglobulins (Fig. 46.4). Initially, murine DNA coding for the variable region was spliced onto human DNA coding for the constant region and expressed in previously nonsecreting lymphocytes to produce *chimeric antibodies* (46,47). Although functionally similar to human antibodies (48), the murine-derived variable regions can elicit an immune response (49). To minimize this problem, humanized or CDR-grafted antibodies have been constructed

FIGURE 46.4. Chimeric and humanized antibodies. Mouse and human immunoglobulin (*Ig*) genes are represented on the *left* and *right* of the figure, respectively. Genes coding for the antibodies consist of exons, depicted as *oval*, with intervening introns, shown as *lines*. Corresponding antibody molecules (*center*) are made up of two light chains, each composed of a variable (V_L) and a constant (C_L) region attached by disulfide (−SS−) bonds to the two heavy chains, which are composed of a variable region (V_H), three constant regions (C_H1 through C_H3), and a hinge (*h*). Chimeric antibodies are composed of murine variable regions combined with human-derived constant regions. CDR grafted (humanized) antibodies are composed of human-derived constant and framework (*Fw*) regions, and only the complementarity defining regions (*CDRs*) are taken from the mouse. (From Pirofski LA, Casadevall A, Scharff MD. Current state of hybridoma technology. *ASM News* 1992; 58:613–617, with permission.)

whereby both the constant regions and framework portion of the variable regions are derived from human immunoglobulins; only the hypervariable regions are cloned from the immunized mouse (23,50,51). These antibodies often have diminished antigen binding because of altered interactions between the native framework regions and the grafted murine hypervariable regions (52,53). To compensate, modeling (53,54) and labor-intensive substitution of flanking amino acids (53,55) have been used to restore affinity.

Progress in human hybridoma technology has led to greater ease in directly generating human monoclonal antibodies by means of Epstein-Barr virus transformation (56–58) or human-mouse or human-human fusion (59,60). These methods were used to generate hu-mAb 88BV59, an antibody in trials for colorectal, ovarian, and breast carcinoma (6) (Table 46.1). Transgenic mice carrying human immunoglobulin genes have been developed as a means of generating human antibodies from an animal (61–63). These animals, endowed genetically with a functional human humoral immune system, can be immunized with a given antigen and their B cells used for subsequent hybridoma production.

An additional method of producing small antigen-binding proteins, mentioned earlier, entails use of immunoglobulin genes expressed in bacteria. Use of this method circumvents the need for immunization of live subjects. In this method, the *phage display library* (14,30,36,64), hundreds of thousands of variable region–derived amino-acid sequences are expressed or displayed on the surface of filamentous phages, which are then screened for binding to the antigen of interest. By use of multiple rounds of panning with the phage-display library, sequences that bind are retained and enriched, making it ultimately possible to isolate peptides with desired specificity.

Other Recombinant and Chemically Modified Proteins

In addition to modifications of size and immunogenicity, described earlier, numerous other changes to the antibody have been described, including those performed to add or alter functionality of the immunoglobulin molecule. For example, mutating critical amino-acid residues to improve binding can be performed on the basis of specific details of antibody and antigen structure (65). The function of an additional biologic agent, such as a cytokine (66), hormone (67), or ligand (68) can be chemically or genetically engineered into the antibody molecule. Alteration of an isoelectric point of the antibody has been used to modify pharmacokinetics and to improve tumor targeting (69). By somatic cell or chemical means, it is possible to construct antibodies with dual-binding specificity; one of the Fab fragments binds a given antigen and the second binds another (70–76). Bifunctional antibodies that bind two distinct antigens that coexist only in a given tumor tissue may be a means of increasing the specificity of tumor targeting.

Bifunctional monoclonal antibodies, or antibodies to which avidin or biotin has been attached (77–80), can be used in strategies of pretargeting, whereby the immunologic moiety is initially administered without the radiolabel (81,82). After a period sufficient to ensure adequate localization of this large molecule, ra-

dionuclide is administered attached to a small moiety that rapidly combines with the pretargeted molecule and is cleared from background. Pretargeting strategies have shown promise in improving localization of radionuclide to the tumor site (83).

There may be a role for biologic response modifiers as adjuvants to monoclonal antibody–based procedures (84), and these biologically active proteins can be directly attached to the antibody by chemical (85) or genetic (66) means. A modifier can be used to increase capillary permeability, resulting in greater tumor accretion of antibody (84), or to increase antigen expression on the tumor, leading to increased antibody binding (86, 87). Because the blood–brain barrier is generally impervious to systemically administered antibodies, ligands that are actively transported through the blood–brain barrier, such as transferrin, may be attached to the immunoglobulin molecule and act to ferry the antibody across (68).

There have been major advances in the understanding of structural factors that govern antibody catabolism (16). There is a threefold variation in serum half-life within the four subclasses of human IgG. The range is approximately 3 weeks for IgG1, IgG2, and IgG4 to 1 week for IgG3 (14,15). Half-lives of the non-IgG antibody classes are considerably shorter. Hybridomas can be switched in culture by means of somatic mutation to specific downstream antibody classes or can be altered with recombinant DNA techniques to produce antibodies of any selected class or subclass. By means of selection of novel heavy-chain domain sequences not normally present in nature, it may be possible to create immunoglobulins with prolonged (88) or shortened (89) serum half-lives.

RADIOLABELED ANTIBODIES

Various factors enter into the choice of an optimal radiolabel. These include suitability for imaging, physical half-life, biologic handling of the radioconjugate, radiation to the patient and family, and ease of labeling. Disposition and metabolic fate of the radioconjugate must be considered because the radiolabel can persist in altered radiochemical forms after breakdown and metabolism of the originally administered agent. Optimal choice of radionuclide also depends on the nature of the compound being labeled and its biologic behavior. For example, longer-lived radiolabels are better suited for use with whole antibodies, which have a prolonged intravascular clearance and are best imaged after several days. In contrast, antibody fragments and other small derivatives, which clear quickly from the blood, should be labeled with radionuclides with shorter physical half-lives, thereby reducing patient exposure. Although iodine isotopes historically were used in the development of radioimmunoimaging because of their availability and ease of use, at present, commercially available products are labeled with either ^{111}In or ^{99m}Tc (Table 46.1). These are believed to represent a more ideal combination of efficacy and radiation dosimetry, as discussed later.

^{111}In-labeled Antibodies

^{111}In decays through electron capture with the emission of 173-keV and 247-keV γ photons that are very suitable for imaging, typically performed with dual 20% symmetric energy windows centered on the photopeaks. The 2.8-day physical half-life of ^{111}In dovetails nicely with the biologic clearance of intact immunoglobulins. Imaging typically is performed for several days after injection.

The chemistry with which to attach indium to proteins has been developed with chelators such as diethylenetriaminepenta-acetic acid (DTPA) and tetraazacyclododecanetetraacetic acid (DOTA) (90). In two commercially available ^{111}In-labeled antibodies (Table 46.1), ^{111}In is attached by the linker-chelator glycyl-tyrosyl-(N,-DTPA)-lysine hydrochloride (GYK-DTPA-HCl) to the carbohydrate of the C_H2 region (9), thereby minimizing stearic interference with the distant binding sites. A limitation of ^{111}In-labeled antibodies is that they are metabolized with release of free ^{111}In, which accumulates in the reticuloendothelial cells within the liver and contributes to high liver background activity. To decrease this phenomenon, improved metal-binding chelators (91), such as isothiocyanatobenzyl-methyl DTPA (92), are being developed. As an alternative approach, peptide chelators designed to be metabolized by hepatic enzymes have been used to decrease nonspecific liver accretion (93). ^{111}In-labeled antibodies are currently best suited for the detection of extrahepatic lesions and are less well-suited for the detection of intrahepatic disease because liver lesions, such as metastasis, can appear photopenic or isointense to the liver.

^{99m}Tc-labeled Antibodies

The more-rapid localization and clearance of antibody fragments made it preferable to use shorter-lived radionuclides, and various techniques for ^{99m}Tc labeling have therefore been developed (90,94). ^{99m}Tc decays through isomeric transition with a 140-keV photopeak that is typically imaged with a single 20% symmetric window. ^{99m}Tc has no particulate radiation and a 6-hour physical half-life, leading to a low radiation burden to the patient (94). ^{99m}Tc in its pertechnetate form is readily eluted from a ^{99}Mo generator and is inexpensive. Early imaging usually is performed between 4 and 8 hours after injection. Later images should not be delayed beyond 24 hours because of the short physical half-life of the radiolabel. Use of technetium-labeled antibodies therefore requires a rigorous acquisition protocol and scrupulous attention to detail because patients cannot be recalled for additional views at a later time.

In "direct" methods of labeling, the ^{99m}Tc is believed to be attached to reduced sulfhydryl groups directly on the antibody molecule. In "indirect" methods of labeling, an exogenous chelating group is covalently linked to the antibody (95,96). One particular advantage of direct methods of radiolabeling with ^{99m}Tc is that high specific activities can be achieved in a very short time with readily formulated kit preparations. Two FDA-approved agents involve direct labeling with ^{99m}Tc (Table 46.1).

Other Diagnostic Labels

Positron-emitting tracers, such as ^{64}Cu, ^{68}Ga, and ^{124}I, have been used to label antibodies for imaging on positron emission tomography (PET) systems (97,98). A major advantage of PET is that is allows true quantitation of the radiopharmaceutical distribution; however, the slow biologic clearance of antibodies and requirement for delayed imaging limit the choice of suitable positron emitters.

CLINICAL RADIOIMMUNOSCINTIGRAPHY

At present, five radiolabeled monoclonal antibodies are FDA-approved for radioimmunoscintigraphy, and a small number of additional imaging agents are in FDA-monitored trials (Table 46.1). Two of the FDA-approved agents are no longer being marketed by their sponsors owing to economic considerations—nofetumomab merpentan (Verluma) indicated for the staging of small cell lung carcinoma (HBB93A) and imciromab pentetate (Myoscint), used for identifying the presence and location of myocardial necrosis (99,100). That the number of antibodies available for radioimmunoscintigraphy is small is the result of both intrinsic limitations in current antibody technology and vigorous competition by other imaging modalities, including ^{18}F fluorodeoxyglucose (FDG) PET and high-resolution computed tomography (CT) and magnetic resonance imaging (MRI). Discussion of clinical applications of radioimmunoimaging in this chapter concentrates on the three currently available FDA-approved products.

As with all nuclear medicine techniques, attention to detail is important in ensuing success. Before injection, a careful patient history should be obtained to exclude previous hypersensitivity. Patients with a history of injection of murine monoclonal antibodies, exposure to mice, or allergies to materials used in the preparation are at increased risk of adverse reactions. Blood tests to screen for the presence of HAMA are available and can be used as clinically indicated. Drugs, including epinephrine, diphenhydramine preparations, and hydrocortisone, should be available on an emergency cart in the event of a hypersensitivity reaction.

With the history and physical examination, miscellaneous causes of increased antibody accumulation should be identified to avoid false-positive results, including the presence of a colostomy and recent surgical incisions. Areas of hyperemia related to joint disease, aneurysms, inflammatory tissue, surgery, or radiation also can give false-positive localization and are likewise of importance.

Before imaging, patients should be asked to empty their bladder. Imaging should be performed in a standardized manner, especially if repeat acquisitions will be performed later. Standard imaging should include both planar and single photon emission computed tomography (SPECT) acquisitions. Care must be exercised to process the study in an appropriate manner designed to compensate for excessive activity in the liver (^{111}In-labeled antibodies) or kidneys (^{99m}Tc-labeled fragments), which should not unduly depress the gray scale. It is optimal to review the studies in digital format so that the intensity window can be appropriately varied and three-dimensional spatial relations can be investigated. Three-dimensional SPECT information also allows immunoscintigraphy to be compared and even fused with conventional radiographic imaging modalities such as CT and MRI (101,102). A commercially available gamma camera that incorporates a basic CT scanner can produce inherently fused images and has proved very promising in clinical practice (103, 104).

Each radiolabeled monoclonal antibody has its own unique biodistribution pattern. Many factors affect the normal biodistribution of an antibody. Familiarity with normal biodistribution as a function of time and the various factors that alter biodistribution is therefore of paramount importance. With ^{111}In-labeled intact antibodies, the liver, spleen, bone marrow, blood pool, genitalia, and breasts are visualized, as are to a lesser degree the kidneys and intestines (105,106). Blood-pool and renal activity is greatest on the images obtained during the first 1 to 2 days. When intact antibodies labeled with ^{111}In are used, imaging is best performed 72 to 96 hours after injection. Bone marrow uptake varies depending on the amount of reticuloendothelial activity (either suppressed or stimulated). Intestinal activity also varies among patients, and is usually greatest at the early imaging times, varies in position between imaging sessions, and becomes less intense on delayed imaging, especially after appropriate bowel cleansing. Intense liver activity may preclude visualization of hepatic lesions. Colostomy sites, degenerative joint disease, abdominal aneurysms, postoperative intestinal adhesions, and local inflammatory lesions can demonstrate nonspecific antibody localization. Antibody can appear to localize in tortuous blood vessels. Correlation with medical history and other imaging examinations can aid in the interpretation of images (106).

With ^{99m}Tc-labeled antibody fragments, clearance from the blood is much more rapid than with ^{111}In-labeled whole-antibody agents. Liver and blood-pool activity tends to be slightly less and renal activity slightly greater than with ^{111}In-labeled whole-antibody agents. The high counts found in the kidneys make the search for small tumor foci in the retroperitoneum difficult.

Prostate Carcinoma

Background

Prostate cancer is the most frequently diagnosed noncutaneous cancer in men. An estimated 198,000 new cases were detected in the United States in 2001 (107). It is the second leading cause of death of cancer with approximately 32,000 men dying from prostatic cancer per year. When they come to medical attention, 24% of patients with newly diagnosed cases have distant metastasis detected on a radionuclide bone scan.

Although surgical and radiation therapy frequently are used for curative intent, a large number of patients undergo primary therapy that fails, even though these patients were initially thought to have organ-confirmed early-stage disease. Conventional clinical and radiographic diagnostic methods, including CT, are unreliable for staging primary or recurrent disease (108). Metastasis to organs such as the skeletal system is most frequently identified; however, other sites of disease progression include spread to extrapelvic lymph nodes (29% of cases), lung (24% to 38%), and liver (20%). FDG PET, which is exquisitely sensitive in the staging of many cancers, is relatively less so in the detection of prostate carcinoma (109,110), preserving a clinical niche for antibody imaging.

Two major applications of radioimmunoscintigraphy have

emerged in the management of prostate carcinoma—presurgical staging and the evaluation of patients who have undergone prostatectomy and have a high likelihood of recurrence. In the former group, a major variable that determines prognosis and therapy is extension of the tumor beyond the capsule either locally (T3 or T4), into pelvic nodes (N1 to N3), or distally (N4 or M1). Immunoscintigraphy has the potential of providing a method to image both soft-tissue and bony metastasis and avoids the morbidity associated with surgical staging of pelvic lymph nodes. In the case of recurrent disease, evaluation of disease outside the pelvis helps determine whether systemic (hormonal) or local (radiation therapy or salvage surgery) therapy is most appropriate for treatment. Use of radioimmunoscintigraphy for planning conformal external beam radiation therapy (111) or prostatic brachytherapy (112) for recurrent pelvic disease is also an area of growth and interest. It allows intensified therapy to be directed to areas of cancer with relative sparing of normal tissues (Fig. 46.5).

Capromab Pendetide

Historically, antibodies against prostate-specific antigen (PSA) and prostatic acid phosphatase (PAP) were evaluated clinically. These methods however, were found to have poor sensitivity in the detection of bone and soft-tissue disease, and there was a high incidence of HAMA formation (113–115). At present, one FDA-approved antibody is approved for imaging of carcinoma of the prostate. ^{111}In-labeled capromab pendetide (ProstaScint; Cytogen, Princeton, NJ), also known as CYT-356 (116), is an ^{111}In labeled whole murine IgG1 antibody shown to have acceptable imaging characteristics and mild immunogenicity (117) (Table 46.1). The component antibody (7E11-C5.3) reacts with cytoplasmic membrane–rich fragments of the human prostatic carcinoma cell line LNCaP but not with soluble cytosol or secretory glycoproteins, such as PAP or PSA (116). The antibody is believed to target the intracellular domain of human prostate-specific membrane antigen (PSMA) (118), a 120-kd transmembrane glycoprotein expressed by prostate epithelial cells (119). Unlike the well-known PSA, which often wanes on dedifferentiation of the tumor, PSMA is maximally expressed in poorly differentiated and metastatic carcinoma, and hormone deprivation therapy does not appear to cause a decrease in antigen expression (120). In vitro immunohistologic studies show that 7E11-C5.3 was immunoreactive with more than 95% of adenocarcinomas of the prostate evaluated (106). PSMA is found in much lower concentrations in cells of the normal or hypertrophied prostate gland and to a small degree in the brain, salivary glands, and small intestine (111). Preliminary results suggest that the antibodies specific for extracellular epitopes of PSMA may be more useful that 7E11-C5.3, which targets an intracellular epitope (118).

For imaging, the linker-chelator GYK-DTPA-HCl is conjugated to the carbohydrate of the C_H2 region; the carbohydrate then chelates [111]In (9). Stearic interference with the distant binding sites is minimal. According to data obtained from clinical studies, clearance of the radiolabeled antibody from the blood follows a monoexponential elimination pattern with a terminal-phase half-life of 67 ± 11 hours. In addition to diagnostic use

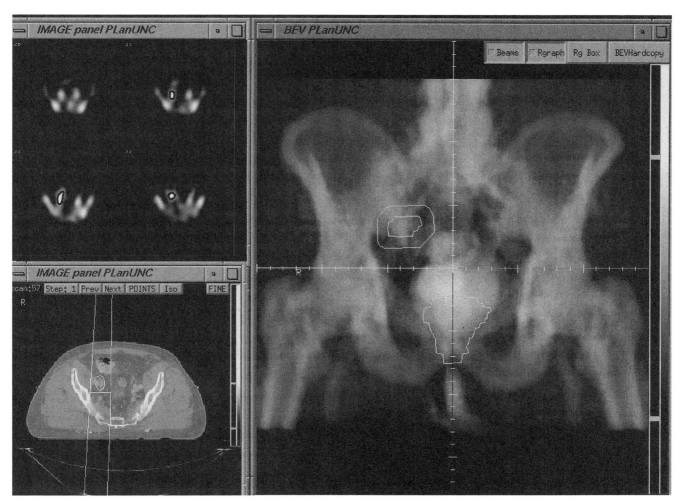

FIGURE 46.5. Use of antibody uptake to direct radiation therapy. *Upper left panel,* Transaxial ^{111}In images from dual-isotope ProstaScint study show an area of increased uptake, greater than that expected from blood-pool images alone, which has been thresholded (*black ROI*) (^{99m}Tc red blood cell data not shown). *Lower left panel,* Coregistered blood-pool images have been used to align the antibody images with the patient's therapy-planning computed tomographic (CT) scan. The area of antibody uptake on the ProstaScint study has been used to identify a lymph node suspect for harboring carcinoma of the prostate (*white ROI*). Two *white rays* entering the anterior abdomen show the location of a planned radiation port. *Right panel,* on the therapy planning CT scan, the prostatic fossa, identified in the lower pelvis, has been identified to receive a "boost" dose of radiation therapy greater than that delivered to the rest of the pelvis. The location of the suspect node has also been marked over the right pelvis (*inner white contour*), to which an additional boost will be administered within the indicated port (*outer white contour*). (Images courtesy of Dr. R.J. Hamilton, University of Chicago and University of Illinois, and Dr. M. J. Blend, University of Illinois.)

as ^{111}In-labeled 7E11-C5.3, this antibody has been labeled with ^{99m}Tc for diagnostic use (121) or with ^{90}Y, a high-energy β emitter, for tumor therapy (122).

ProstaScint is dispensed as a clinical kit containing 0.5 mg of capromab pendetide to which 6 to 7 mCi of ^{111}In chloride in sodium acetate buffer is added. After 30 minutes of reaction at room temperature, the mixture is diluted, filtered, and assayed in a dose calibrator. Instant thin-layer chromatography can be performed before administration, and the radiolabeled antibody is stable to be used within 8 hours of reconstitution.

According to the package insert (106), a final dose of 0.5 mg of antibody labeled with 5 mCi of ^{111}In is administered intravenously over 5 minutes and should not be mixed with any other medication during administration. SPECT and planar imaging are performed 72 to 120 hours after injection. SPECT within 30 minutes of administration is recommended, before any significant accretion in antigenic sites has occurred, and represents one of the methods of obtaining a blood-pool map, which aids in localization of blood vessels and tumor at subsequent imaging (106,111). Administration of a cathartic and an enema is recommended before delayed imaging, which according to the package insert is to be performed with a bladder catheter and irrigation. To further resolve potential ambiguities resulting from activity in the blood pool, stool, or urinary bladder, follow-up imaging with full patient preparation is recommended (106).

Because these recommendations are arduous for staff and uncomfortable for the patient, compliance is incomplete in common practice. Several modifications of the protocol designed to ease performance have been suggested. Most noteworthy is replacement of the initial 30-minute SPECT image acquisition with dual-energy acquisition during the delayed imaging session (123). In this technique, 5 mCi of autologous ^{99m}Tc red-blood cells are injected immediately after planar ^{111}In imaging at 72 to 120 hours. Dual-isotope ^{99m}Tc and ^{111}In SPECT acquisition is performed, which intrinsically coregisters the blood-pool and antibody images and allows blood vessels to be accurately identified and discounted on the ^{111}In antibody images (Figs. 46.6, 46.7). By assuring coregistration, this method was shown to accurately increase both the number of cases of disease identified and the total number of lesions visualized (111). In an innovative method, Blend and Sodee (111) used the blood-pool map as an internal marker to align the antibody scan with CT images for display of fused images (Fig. 46.5).

Clinical Validation

In a study of the efficacy of ProstaScint in the presurgical staging of prostate cancer, antibody was administered to 152 patients with clinically localized prostate cancer who were at high risk of lymph-node metastases and were scheduled for pelvic lymph-node dissection before prostatectomy (6,124). Sixty-four patients had histologically proven lymph-node metastasis at surgery, and of these, 40 had at least one lymph-node metastatic lesion detected with radioimmunoscintigraphy (sensitivity, 63%); only 4% were detected with CT. Twenty-five patients had lymph-node localization on a scan that was not confirmed at surgery, but among 21 of these patients who underwent follow-up evaluation, 14 had recurrent disease. Results of a relative risk analysis suggested that ProstaScint imaging provided strong and independent evidence, over and above serum PSA and Gleason sum, for prediction of extraprostatic disease in pelvic lymph nodes (125). Because of the inability of radioimmunoscintigraphy to depict microscopic metastatic lesions, a negative scan result did not eliminate the need for staging lymphadenectomy (111). Published results with several series of patients have confirmed the effectiveness of ProstaScint in initial staging (117, 126). Bone scans were more sensitive in the detection of osseous metastasis than was ProstaScint imaging (106).

The value of ProstaScint imaging after prostatectomy was assessed for a group of 181 patients with increasing PSA levels and negative results of bone scans. Results of radioimmunoscin-

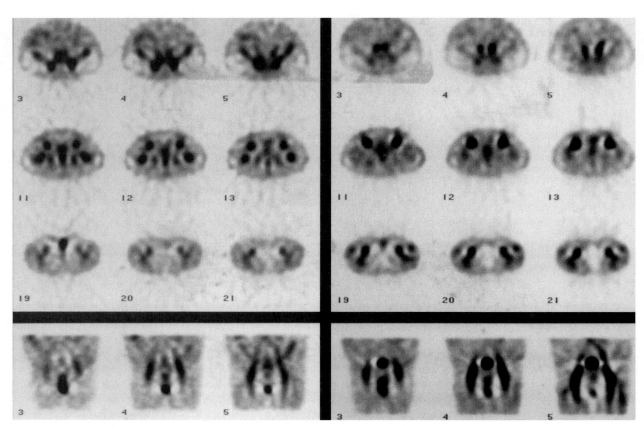

FIGURE 46.6. Selected images from a normal dual-isotope ProstaScint examination of a 65-year-old man acquired 72 hours after injection of ^{111}In antibody. Matching 72-hour ^{111}In antibody data (*left panels*) and ^{99m}Tc red blood cell data (*right panels*) are displayed in transaxial (*upper three-row panel*) and coronal (*lower panel*) projections. The perfectly coregistered blood-pool map is helpful in identification of normal vessels on the ^{111}In antibody study. (Images courtesy of Montefiore Medical Associates, Bronx, NY.)

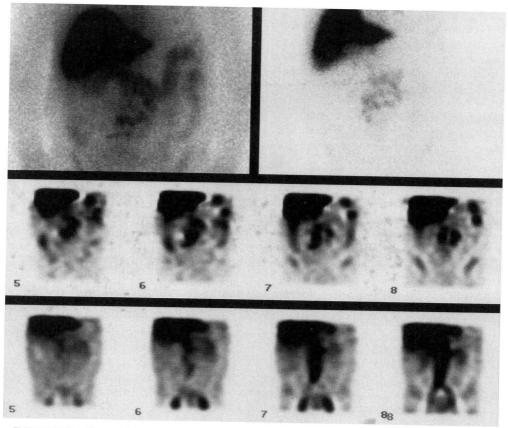

FIGURE 46.7. Abnormal dual-isotope ProstaScint examination. Patient is a 74-year-old man with 5-year history of carcinoma of the prostate. He was previously treated with radiation therapy and had prostate-specific antigen (PSA) levels near 0 ng/mL. After PSA level increased to 17 ng/mL, the study was performed to identify recurrence. Planar ProstaScint images obtained on day 3 (*upper left*) and day 7 (*upper right*) show multiple midabdominal paraaortic lymph nodes. Laxative administration resulted in clearing of bowel activity before day 7. Coronal ^{111}In ProstaScint (*second row*) and matching ^{99m}Tc red blood cell images (*third row*) clearly show retroperitoneal lymph nodes adjacent to the great vessels. (Images courtesy of Montefiore Medical Associates, Bronx, NY.)

tigraphy were positive in 108 cases, including 32 with localization in the prostatic fossa alone, 46 in extra-fossa sites, and 30 in both sites (125). Forty-two patients had evidence of disease in abdominal lymph nodes. It was not generally possible to perform biopsy on lymph-node metastasis in these patients, and CT evidence can lag behind radioimmunoscintigraphic abnormalities by several years. For these reasons, confirmation was obtained by means of evaluation of durable PSA response in 44 patients who underwent radiation therapy to the prostatic fossa. Only 3 of 12 patients with positive results of antibody scans outside the radiation field had durable PSA responses. Two of these patients had progressive disease on repeated scans despite the absence of PSA. Thirteen of 20 patients with positive results of antibody scans limited to the prostatic fossa had durable PSA responses after pelvic radiation therapy. Additional smaller studies confirmed the usefulness of ProstaScint imaging in restaging of disease after prostatectomy (117,127).

According to the ProstaScint package insert (106), scans that show metastatic disease should be confirmed histologically for patients who are otherwise candidates for surgery or radiation therapy. Scans that do not show metastatic disease should not

be used in lieu of histologic confirmation in light of the inability of the technique to depict microscopic disease (111). When possible, patient treatment should not be based on scan results without appropriate confirmatory studies. In the pivotal trials, there was a high rate of false-positive and false-negative image interpretation.

According to the package insert, HAMA (at levels greater than 8 ng/mL) were present in 8% of patients after single infusion and in 19% of patients after repeated infusion. The incidence of generally mild adverse reactions after repeated infusions was 5%, comparable with the 4% ratio observed after single infusion (106). Biodistribution was unaltered on 65 of the 70 (93%) repeated scans that could be evaluated; however, the efficacy of repeated studies was not evaluated.

Colorectal Carcinoma

Colon and rectal carcinoma together represent the third most common cause of new malignant disease among both men and women (estimated as 67,000 and 68,000 new cases per year, respectively) (107). Two murine antibodies are FDA-approved for imaging of adenocarcinoma (Table 46.1); Satumomab pendetide (OncoScint) is a whole ^{111}In-labeled murine antibody that has received approval for imaging of both colorectal and ovarian carcinoma. Arcitumomab (CEA-Scan) is a ^{99m}Tc-labeled murine Fab' fragment approved for imaging of colorectal carcinoma alone. Although a number of other antibodies have been in trials to target ovarian and colon carcinoma (113,128), they have not achieved FDA approval to date. OncoScint and CEA-Scan have been studied for targeting other types of adenocarcinoma, including tumors of the breast and lung, and these investigational applications have been reviewed elsewhere (6).

Satumomab Pendetide

Satumomab pendetide (OncoScint) is produced by the same manufacturer, using similar technology, as ^{111}In-labeled capromab pendetide (ProstaScint; Cytogen). Its component antibody, B72.3, targets the glycoprotein TAG-72 (129), which is present on approximately 83% of colorectal, 97% of common epithelial ovarian, and most breast, non–small cell lung, pancreatic, gastric, and esophageal cancers evaluated (130). There may be reactivity with salivary gland ducts, postovulatory endometrium, and some benign ovarian and fetal gastrointestinal tumors (131). Clearance of labeled OncoScint is either monoexponential or biexponential with a terminal half-life of 56 ± 14 hours (131). The indium chelator GYK-DTPA HCl is attached to carbohydrate on the constant region of the whole antibody by a site-specific method (9). Preparation is similar to that of capromab pendetide (ProstaScint). One milligram of antibody is labeled with 5 mCi of ^{111}In chloride and the antibody and is stable for use within 8 hours of radiolabeling. Planar imaging and SPECT are optimally performed between 48 and 72 hours after injection (131). A cathartic may be helpful in eliminating stool, and follow-up imaging is performed on subsequent days.

In the management of colon carcinoma, suggested indications for imaging with satumomab pendetide have included increasing serum tumor markers in the absence of a known source, known solitary disease in patients for whom curative resection is being considered, and equivocal lesions imaged with conventional methods (132). Pivotal phase III trials (133) clearly showed superior sensitivity of imaging with this agent over conventional imaging for detection of pelvic (74% versus 57%, $P = .035$) and extrahepatic intraabdominal disease (66% versus 34%, $P < 0.001$). In the liver, conventional imaging proved superior to OncoScint imaging in sensitivity (84% versus 41%, $P < .001$), likely because of the nonspecific accumulation of indium in hepatic parenchyma (134,135). Because the negative predictive value of the examination is low, the package inserts suggests that a negative scan result should not be relied on to alter clinical practice (131). Estimates of the overall effect of this examination on patient care for colon carcinoma has varied from moderate (beneficial or very beneficial in 26% of patients studied; negative or very negative in 3%) (136) to low (beneficial or very beneficial for 2 of 15 patients studied; negative or very negative for 3 of 15 patients) (137), although imaging in the latter study appears to have been suboptimal.

OncoScint induced HAMA against murine IgG after single administration in approximately 55% of patients undergoing

trials. Levels reverted to negative in one third of such patients within 6 months (131). OncoScint has been approved for repeated administration in HAMA-negative patients, which is important in the serial monitoring of patients with colorectal carcinoma and increasing levels of tumor markers in the serum. Because patients with HAMA have an altered distribution of antibody, screening for HAMA is vital before repetition of a study. Readministration can be performed if the HAMA level is less than 50 µg/mL and should not be done if levels and are greater than 400 µg/mL. Levels between 50 and 400 µg/mL have an intermediate incidence of altered distribution. After repeated administration to patients with negative results for HAMA, plasma clearance was similar to that obtained in single-dose trials. Overall sensitivity was similar to results in single-dose trials. Surgical confirmation was not obtained for most patients, however; therefore sensitivity and specificity could not be verified (131).

Arcitumomab

Arcitumomab (CEA-Scan; Immunomedics, Morris Plains, NJ) targets the colorectal cancer tumor marker carcinoembryonic antigen (CEA) and is a radiolabeled Fab' fragment derived from the murine monoclonal antibody formerly known as NP-4 or IMMU-4 (138,139) (Table 46.1). It is labeled with ^{99m}Tc, the result being less nonspecific liver accumulation and potentially better detection of hepatic metastasis. Each vial of CEA-Scan, which contains 1.25 mg of the antibody fragment, is reconstituted with 30 mCi of [99m]TcO$_4^-$ and should be used between 5 minutes and 4 hours after reconstitution. Radiochemical purity must be greater than 90% according to results of instant thin-layer chromatography, and the solution should not be particulate or discolored (140). Suggested imaging includes whole-body planar images at 2 to 5 hours after injection and 18 to 24 hours after injection. SPECT is performed 2 to 5 hours after injection (Fig. 46.8). The initial half-life of clearance was approximately 1 hour with a terminal half-life of 13 ± 4 hours (140). Results of analysis of multicenter arcitumomab trial data have suggested a sensitivity for imaging liver metastasis equivalent to that of conventional diagnostic modalities (63% versus 64%, respectively, not significant). The sensitivity of imaging of lesions elsewhere in the abdomen (55% versus 32%, $P = .007$) and pelvis (69% versus 48%, $P = .005$) was superior (141), although the specificity was lower (140). There was a trend suggesting that arcitumomab was more accurate than CT for predicting resectability of locally recurrent or metastatic colorectal cancer (57% versus 47%), including a subset of cases of hepatic metastasis (43% versus 33%) (142). In conjunction with CT, arcitumomab imaging was shown both to potentially double the number of patients who could avoid unnecessary abdominopelvic surgery and to increase 40% the detection of lesions in patients most likely to benefit from curative resection (142). A management paradigm was developed to evaluate the utility of CEA-Scan as an adjunct to CT in the analysis of possible curative resection of limited metastatic disease. In cases in which CT and CEA-Scan imaging were discordant, biopsy is required (140).

A comparison of FDG PET and CEA-Scan imaging in the care of 28 patients with suspected recurrence of colorectal cancer

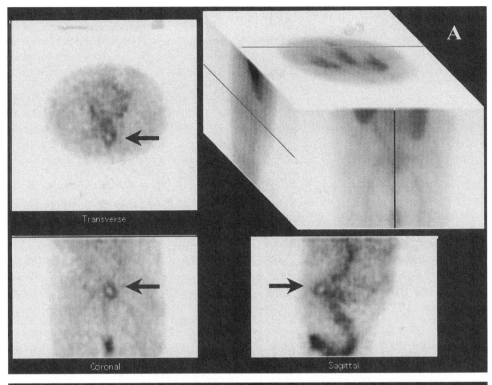

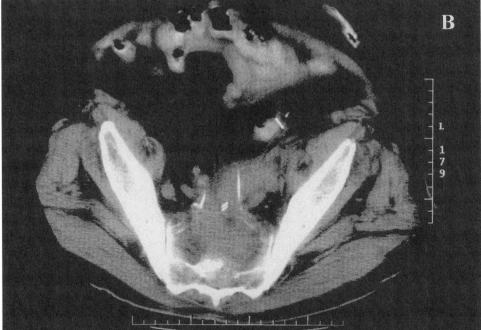

FIGURE 46.8. A 77-year-old man who had undergone resection of rectal carcinoma had local recurrence removed 2 years previously. Computed tomography (CT) of the pelvis performed because of increasing levels of carcinoembryonic antigen showed a presacral density interpreted as compatible with surgical scarring. **A:** Concurrent CEA-Scan imaging of this region showed a rounded focus of increased uptake with central photopenia highly suggestive of necrotic local recurrence. **B:** Although results of needle biopsy were negative, presumably because of sampling error, a repeated CT scan obtained 6 months thereafter showed unequivocal growth of the presacral mass, which was invading bony structures. (Images courtesy of Dr. Nicholas Hoff, St. Joseph's Hospital, Nashua, NH.)

indicated that both methods were suitable for diagnosis of local recurrence; however, FDG PET was clearly superior in the detection of distant metastasis, including metastasis to the liver (143). Anecdotal case reports suggest a possible role for CEA-Scan imaging in the evaluation of mucinous adenocarcinoma (144), which may have less avid FDG uptake than other histologic types (145).

Adverse effects have been rare. Among more than 500 patients whose cases have been studied, there has been only one report of an apparent grand-mal epileptic seizure that was thought to be "possibly related" to infusion of CEA-Scan. Other self-limited adverse effects were likewise unusual. After administration of the CEA-Scan Fab' fragment, fewer than 1% of patients had induction of HAMA (140). The package insert (140) indicates that in a small fraction of patients who received repeated injections, the pattern of CEA-Scan distribution after second administration differed slightly from that of the initial administration, even though HAMA titers were not elevated. In a study of the safety and efficacy of arcitumomab imaging after repeated administration (146), none of 35 patients available for evaluation had a HAMA response after a second administration of antibody. Three patients received a third injection and likewise remained HAMA-negative. In 1 patient who had a HAMA response after the initial administration of CEA-Scan, HAMA titers had reverted to negative by the time of second administration 1 year thereafter, and HAMA did not recur on readministration (146). Imaging efficacy after the second injection was similar to that obtained in the phase III trials.

Ovarian Carcinoma

Ovarian carcinoma is the sixth most common cause of new cases of carcinoma among women (23,000 cases per year) (107). Second-look surgery is routinely used to diagnose residual neoplasia after initial chemotherapy. Standard diagnostic tests such as MRI, CT, and ultrasonography lack sufficient specificity and sensitivity to obviate repeated exploration (113). Use of an imaging test to reduce unnecessary second-look surgery would avoid considerable expense and morbidity.

Satumomab Pendetide

OncoScint CR/OV, discussed previously as an agent for imaging colorectal carcinoma, also is approved for use in ovarian carcinoma because of a high frequency of TAG-72 expression (130) (Table 46.1). A multicenter trial of OncoScint CR/OV for ovar-

ian carcinoma was performed with 108 patients at 18 study sites (147–149). One hundred three patients underwent follow-up surgery or biopsy. Ninety-eight patients who could be evaluated underwent imaging with both radioimmunoscintigraphy and CT. Antibody imaging was more sensitive (69% versus 44%) but less specific (54% versus 79%). Antibody imaging led to detection of tumors in 19 patients with normal CT scans, whereas findings on CT scans were abnormal for only 2 patients with normal findings on antibody images (147). The ability of the agent to depict carcinomatosis was considered significant in light of the limitation of other diagnostic tests in this situation (71% versus 45% for CT) (Fig. 46.9). The sensitivity has been slightly lower in the upper abdomen owing to interference by physiologic uptake in the liver and spleen. In detection of disease in the lower abdomen the sensitivity of radioimmunoscintigraphy surpassed that of CT and MRI (150). The sensitivity is lower among patients with suspected recurrence than among those with primary disease. The low negative predictive value for this group has suggested to some experts that negative results of radioimmunoscintigraphy should not preclude second-look surgical exploration (147). The product insert therefore states that "a negative scan is not informative about disease and should not be used to guide clinical practice." Furthermore, low overall specificity of OncoScint CR/OV suggests that a positive test result is not useful in differentiating a malignant from a benign pelvic mass (131) and that expression of TAG-72 by benign ovarian tumors may at least partially account for this phenomenon.

OncoScint CR/OV imaging was believed beneficial or very beneficial to the care of 27% of patients with ovarian cancer and to have a negative or very negative effect in only 2% (147, 149). The utility of the agent included initial identification of occult tumor lesions and confirmation of findings initially identified with other diagnostic tests. Otherwise-occult lesions were found in 20 of 71 patients with surgically confirmed ovarian carcinoma (147). The incidence of HAMA is discussed earlier in the context of colorectal carcinoma.

Future Applications and Perspective

Monoclonal antibody imaging has achieved a measure of objective scientific validation, as measured by FDA approval of five radiopharmaceuticals. Nonetheless, the clinical use of the technique has been very limited—only three antibodies are commercially available in the United States at present. It is likely that more antibodies have not been developed because of the enor-

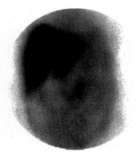
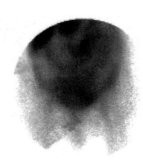

FIGURE 46.9. OncoScint CR/OV images of a 77-year-old woman with previously resected ovarian carcinoma. Planar images show several areas of increased uptake throughout the abdomen consistent with the presence of widespread intraabdominal tumor. Exploratory laparotomy revealed malignant ascites and diffuse metastatic disease. The tissue diagnosis was poorly differentiated papillary adenocarcinoma.

mous expenses involved in obtaining FDA approval and the limited financial returns ultimately envisioned (6). Antibody imaging must compete with new and effective modalities, such as FDG PET and high-resolution anatomic examinations; thus the potential market is severely limited.

As a functional imaging agent, radioimmunoscintigraphy retains an important role in several clinical niches, many of which relate to tailoring of therapy. One of the greatest impetuses to radioimmunoscintigraphy will be the successful development of radioimmunotherapy, whereby imaging may ultimately have a role in pretherapy staging and dosimetry. A role for these antibodies in assessing tumor response to therapy also may emerge. An additional area of potential growth of radioimmunoscintigraphy is in nononcologic applications, such as imaging of infection, as represented by the two antigranulocyte antibodies that are in FDA trials (151–155) (Table 46.1). With introduction of engineered imaging agents and improved strategies for antibody targeting, it is hoped that radioimmunoscintigraphy will reach its potential of contributing unique information to patient care.

REFERENCES

1. Pressman D, Keighley G. The zone of activity of antibodies as determined by the use of radioactive tracers; the zone of activity of nephrotoxic antikidney serum. *J Immunol* 1948;59:141–146.
2. Baumler E. *In search of the magic bullet: great adventures in modern drug research.* Dusseldorf, Germany: Econ-Verlag, 1965.
3. Fjermedal, G. *Magic bullets.* New York: Macmillan, 1984.
4. Goldenberg DM, DeLand F, Kim E, et al. Use of radiolabeled antibodies to carcinoembryonic antigen for the detection and localization of diverse cancers by external photoscanning. *N Engl J Med* 1978; 298:1384–1386.
5. Kohler G, Milstein C. Continuous cultures of fused cells secreting antibodies of predefined specificity. *Nature* 1975;256:295–297.
6. Zuckier LS, DeNardo GL. Trials and tribulations: oncological antibody imaging comes to the fore. *Semin Nucl Med* 1997;27:10–29.
7. Arlington Medical Resources, Inc. Written communication. Malvern, PA: July 3, 2001.
8. Abbas AK, Lichtman AH, Pober JS. *Cellular and molecular immunology,* 4th ed. Philadelphia: WB Saunders, 2000.
9. Rodwell JD, Alvarez VL, Lee C, et al. Site-specific covalent modification of monoclonal antibodies: in vitro and in vivo evaluations. *Proc Natl Acad Sci U S A* 1986;83:2632–2636.
10. Zuckier LS, Berkowitz EZ, Sattenberg RJ, et al. Influence of affinity and antigen density on antibody localization in a modifiable tumor targeting model. *Cancer Res* 2000;60:7008–7013.
11. Winkelhake JL. Immunoglobulin structure and effector functions. *Immunochemistry* 1978;15:695–714.
12. Burton DR. Immunoglobulin G: functional sites. *Mol Immunol* 1985; 22:161–206.
13. Ward ES, Ghetie V. The effector functions of immunoglobulins: implications for therapy. *Ther Immunol* 1995;2:77–94.
14. Zuckier LS, Rodriguez LD, Scharff MD. Immunologic and pharmacologic concepts of monoclonal antibodies. *Semin Nucl Med* 1989; 19:166–186.
15. Waldmann TA, Strober W. Metabolism of immunoglobulins. *Progr Allergy* 1969;13:1–110.
16. Junghans RP. Finally: the Brambell receptor (FcRB)—mediator of transmission of immunity and protection from catabolism for IgG. *Immunol Res* 1997;16:29–57.
17. Losman MJ, Dejager RL, Monestier M, et al. Human immune response to anticarcinoembryonic antigen murine monoclonal antibodies. *Cancer Res* 1990;50[Suppl]:1055–1058.
18. Massuger LF, Thomas CM, Segers MF, et al. Specific and non-specific immunoassays to detect HAMA after administration of indium-111-labeled OV-TL3 F(ab')₂ monoclonal antibody to patients with ovarian cancer. *J Nucl Med* 1992;33:1958–1963.
19. Ferroni P, Milenic DE, Roselli M. Potential artifacts for the increase of tumor associated antigens in serum samples from patients injected with monoclonal antibodies. *Intl J Rad Appl Instrum B* 1991;18: 383–387.
20. Tjandra JJ, Ramadi L, McKenzie IF. Development of human antimurine antibody (HAMA) responses in patients. *Immunol Cell Biol* 1990; 68:367–376.
21. Bogard WC Jr., Dean RT, Deo Y, et al. Practical consideration in the production, purification, and formulation of monoclonal antibodies for immunoscintigraphy and immunotherapy. *Semin Nucl Med* 1989;19:202–220.
22. Neuberger MS, Williams GT, Fox RO. Recombinant antibodies possessing novel effector functions. *Nature* 1984;312:604–608.
23. Winter G, Milstein C. Man-made antibodies. *Nature* 1991;349: 293–299.
24. Morrison SL. In vitro antibodies: strategies for production and application. *Annu Rev Immunol* 1992;10:239–265.
25. Wright A, Shin SU, Morrison SL. Genetically engineered antibodies: progress and prospects. *Crit Rev Immunol* 1992;12:125–168.
26. Hand PH, Kashmiri SVS, Schlom J. Potential for recombinant immunoglobulin constructs in the management of carcinoma. *Cancer* 1994; 73[Suppl]:1105–1113.
27. Goldenberg DM, Goldenberg H, Sharkey RM, et al. Clinical studies of radioimmunodetection with carcinoembryonic antigen monoclonal antibody fragment labeled with ¹²³I or ⁹⁹ᵐTc. *Cancer Res* 1990; 50[Suppl]:909s–921s.
28. Adams GP, McCartney JE, Tai MS, et al. Highly specific in vivo tumor targeting by monovalent and divalent forms of 741F8 Anti-c-*erb* B-2 single-chain Fv. *Cancer Res* 1993;53:4026–4034.
29. Adams GP, Schier R, McCall AM, et al. Tumor targeting properties of anti-C-ERB-2 single-chain Fv molecules over a wide range of affinities for the same epitope. *Tumor Target* 1996;2:154.
30. Huse WD, Sastry L, Iverson SA, et al. Generation of a large combinatorial library of the immunoglobulin repertoire in phage lambda. *Science* 1989;246:1275–1281.
31. Kang AS, Barbas CF, Janda KD, et al. Linkage of recognition and replication functions by assembling combinatorial antibody Fab libraries along phage surfaces. *Proc Natl Acad Sci U S A* 1991;88: 4363–4366.
32. Adams GP. Improving the tumor specificity and retention of antibody-based molecules. *In Vivo* 1998;12:11–22.
33. Huston JS, Levinson D, Mudgett-Hunter M, et al. Protein engineering of antibody binding sites: recovery of specific activity in an anti-digoxin single-chain Fv analogue produced in *Escherichia coli. Proc Natl Acad Sci U S A* 1988;85:5879–5883.
34. Milenic DE, Yokota T, Filpula DR, et al. Construction, binding properties, metabolism, and tumor targeting of a single-chain Fv derived from the pancarcinoma monoclonal antibody CC49. *Cancer Res* 1991;51:6363–6371.
35. Yokota T, Milenic DE, Whitlow M, et al. Rapid tumor penetration of a single-chain Fv and comparison with other immunoglobulin forms. *Cancer Res* 1992;52:3402–3408.
36. Ward ES, Gussow D, Griffiths AD, et al. Binding activities of a repertoire of single immunoglobulin variable domains secreted from *Escherichia coli. Nature* 1989;341:544–546.
37. Williams WV, Moss DA, Kieber-Emmons T, et al. Development of biologically active peptides based on antibody structure. *Proc Natl Acad Sci U S A* 1989;5537–5541.
38. Taub R, Gould RJ, Garsky VM, et al. A monoclonal antibody against the platelet fibrinogen receptor contains a sequence that mimics a receptor recognition domain in fibrinogen. *J Biol Chem* 1989;264: 259–265.
39. Williams WV, Kieber-Emmons T, VonFeldt J, et al. Design of bioactive peptides based on antibody hypervariable region structures: development of conformationally constrained and dimeric peptides with enhanced affinity. *J Biol Chem* 1991;266:5182–5190.
40. Knight LC, Radcliffe R, Maurer AH, et al. Thrombus imaging with technetium-99m synthetic peptides based upon the binding domain

of a monoclonal antibody to activated platelets. *J Nucl Med* 1994;
35:282–288.

41. Pollock RR, French DL, Gefter ML, et al. Identification of mutant monoclonal antibodies with increased antigen binding. *Proc Natl Acad Sci U S A* 1988;85:2298–2302.

42. Smith RIF, Morrison SL. Recombinant polymeric IgG: an approach to engineering more potent antibodies. *Biotechnology (N Y)* 1994;12: 683–688.

43. Poon PH, Morrison SL, Schumaker VN. Structure and function of several anti-dansyl chimeric antibodies formed by domain interchanges between human IgM and mouse IgG2b. *J Biol Chem* 1995; 270:8571–8577.

44. James K, Bell GT. Human monoclonal antibody production: current status and future prospects. *J Immunol Methods* 1987;100:5–40.

45. James K. Human monoclonal antibodies and engineered antibodies in the management of cancer. *Semin Cancer Biol* 1990;1:243–253.

46. Morrison SL, Johnson MJ, Herzenberg LA, et al. Chimeric human antibody molecules: mouse antigen-binding domains with human constant region domains. *Proc Natl Acad Sci U S A* 1984;81: 6851–6855.

47. Morrison SL. Generations of human monoclonal antibodies reactive with cellular antigens. *Science* 1985;229:1202–1207.

48. Bruggemann M, Williams GT, Bindon CI, et al. Comparison of the effector functions of human immunoglobulins using a matched set of chimeric antibodies. *J Exp Med* 1987;166:1351–1361.

49. Bruggemann M, Winter G, Waldmann H, et al. The immunogenicity of chimeric antibodies. *J Exp Med* 1989;170:2153–2157.

50. Jones PT, Dear PH, Foote J, et al. Replacing the complementarity-determining regions in a human antibody with those from a mouse. *Nature* 1986;321:522–525.

51. Riechmann L, Clark M, Waldmann H, et al. Reshaping human antibodies for therapy. *Nature* 1988;332:323–327.

52. Verhoeyen M, Milstein C, Winter G. Reshaping human antibodies: grafting an antilysozyme activity. *Science* 1988;239:1534–1536.

53. Queen C, Schneider WP, Selick HE, et al. A humanized antibody that binds to the interleukin 2 receptor. *Proc Natl Acad Sci U S A* 1989;86:10029–10033.

54. Roberts S, Cheetham JC, Rees AR. Generation of an antibody with enhanced affinity and specificity for its antigen by protein engineering. *Nature* 1987;328:731–734.

55. Co MS, Queen C. Humanized antibodies for therapy. *Nature* 1991; 351:501–502.

56. Steinitz M, Klein G, Koskimies S, et al. EB virus–induced B lymphocytic cell lines producing specific antibody. *Nature* 1977;269: 420–422.

57. Nakamura M, Burastero SE, Ueki Y, et al. Probing the normal and autoimmune B cell repertoire with Epstein-Barr virus: frequency of B cells producing monoreactive high affinity autoantibodies in patients with Hashimoto's disease and systemic lupus erythematosus. *J Immunol* 1988;141:4165–4172.

58. Kozbor D, Lagarde AE, Roder JC. Human hybridomas constructed with antigen-specific Epstein-Barr virus–transformed cell lines. *Proc Natl Acad Sci U S A* 1982;79:6651–6655.

59. Ostberg L, Pursch E. Human X (mouse X human) hybridomas stably producing human antibodies. *Hybridoma* 1983;2:361–367.

60. Cote RJ, Morrissey DM, Houghton AN, et al. Specificity analysis of human monoclonal antibodies reactive with cell surface and intracellular antigens. *Proc Natl Acad Sci U S A* 1986;83:2959–2963.

61. Mosier DE, Gulizia RJ, Baird SM, et al. Transfer of a functional human immune system to mice with severe combined immunodeficiency. *Nature* 1988;335:256–259.

62. McCune JM, Namikawa R, Kaneshima H, et al. The SCID-hu mouse: murine model for the analysis of human hematolymphoid differentiation and function. *Science* 1988;241:1632–1639.

63. Bruggemann M, Neuberger MS. Strategies for expressing human antibody repertoires in transgenic mice. *Immunol Today* 1996;17: 391–397.

64. Wells JA, Lowman HB. Rapid evolution of peptide and protein binding properties in vitro. *Curr Opin Biotechnol* 1992;3:355–362.

65. Riechmann L, Weill M, Cavanagh J. Improving the antigen affinity of an antibody Fv-fragment by protein design. *J Mol Biol* 1992;224: 913–918.

66. Fell HP, Gayle MA, Grosmaire L, et al. Genetic construction and characterization of a fusion protein consisting of a chimeric F(ab′) with specificity for carcinomas and human IL-2. *J Immun* 1991;146: 2446–2452.

67. Shin SU, Morrison SL. Expression and characterization of an antibody binding specificity joined to insulin-like growth factor 1: potential applications for cellular targeting. *Proc Natl Acad Sci U S A* 1990; 87:5322–5326.

68. Shin SU, Friden P, Moran M, et al. Transferrin-antibody fusion proteins are effective in brain targeting. *Proc Natl Acad Sci U S A* 1995; 92:2820–2824.

69. Sharifi J, Khawli LA, Hornick JL, et al. Improving monoclonal antibody pharmacokinetics via chemical modification. *Q J Nucl Med* 1998;42:242–249.

70. Suresh MR, Cuello AC, Milstein C. Bispecific monoclonal antibodies from hybrid hybridomas. *Methods Enzymol* 1986;121:210–228.

71. Clark M, Gilliland L, Waldmann H. Hybrid antibodies for therapy. *Progr Allergy* 1988;45:31–49.

72. Phelps JL, Beidler DE, Jue RA, et al. Expression and characterization of a chimeric bifunctional antibody with therapeutic applications. *J Immunol* 1990;145:1200–1204.

73. Moran TM, Usuba O, Shapiro E, et al. A novel technique for the production of hybrid antibodies. *J Immunol Methods* 1990;129: 199–205.

74. Stickney DR, Anderson LD, Slater JB, et al. Bifunctional antibody: a binary radiopharmaceutical delivery system for imaging colorectal carcinoma. *Cancer Res* 1991;51:6650–6655.

75. LeDoussal J-M, Chetanneau A, Gruaz-Guyon A, et al. Bispecific monoclonal antibody–mediated targeting of an indium-111-labeled DTPA dimer to primary colorectal tumors: pharmacokinetics, biodistribution, scintigraphy and immune response. *J Nucl Med* 1993;34: 1662–1671.

76. Peltier P, Curtet C, Chatal JF, et al. Radioimmunodetection of medullary thyroid cancer using a bispecific anti-CEA/anti-indium-DTPA antibody and an indium-111-labeled DTPA dimer. *J Nucl Med* 1993; 34:1267–1273.

77. Paganelli G, Magnani P, Siccardi AG, et al. Clinical application of the avidin-biotin system for tumor targeting. In: Goldenberg DM, ed. *Cancer therapy with radiolabeled antibodies*. Boca Raton, FL: CRC Press, 1995: 239–254.

78. Paganelli G, Malcovati M, Fazio F. Monoclonal antibody pretargetting techniques for tumour localization: the avidin-biotin system. *Nucl Med Commun* 1991;12:211–234.

79. Kalofonos HP, Rusckowski M, Siebecker DA, et al. Imaging of tumor in patients with indium-111-labeled biotin and streptavidin-conjugated antibodies: preliminary communication. *J Nucl Med* 1990;31: 1791–1796.

80. Hnatowich DJ, Virzi F, Rusckowski M. Investigations of avidin and biotin for imaging applications. *J Nucl Med* 1987;28:1294–1302.

81. Goodwin DA. Tumor pretargeting: almost the bottom line. *J Nucl Med* 1995;36:876–879.

82. Stoldt HS, Aftab F, Chinol M, et al. Pretargeting strategies for radioimmunoguided tumour localisation and therapy. *Eur J Cancer* 1997; 33:186–192.

83. Axworthy DB, Reno JM, Hylarides MD, et al. Cure of human carcinoma xenografts by a single dose of pretargeted yttrium-90 with negligible toxicity. *Proc Natl Acad Sci U S A* 2000;97:1802–1807.

84. Guadagni F, Roselli M, Nieroda C, et al. Biological response modifiers as adjuvants in monoclonal antibody-based treatment. *In Vivo* 1993; 7:591–599.

85. LeBerthon B, Khawli LA, Alauddin M, et al. Enhanced tumor uptake of macromolecules induced by a novel vasoactive interleukin 2 immunoconjugate. *Cancer Res* 1991;51:2694–2698.

86. Greiner JW, Guadagni F, Noguchi P, et al. Recombinant interferon enhances monoclonal antibody–targeting of carcinoma lesions in vivo. *Science* 1987;235:895–898.

87. Greiner JW, Ullmann CD, Nieroda C, et al. Improved radioimmunotherapeutic efficacy of an anticarcinoma monoclonal antibody (^{131}I-

CC49) when given in combination with gamma-interferon. *Cancer Res* 1993;53:600–608.

88. Zuckier LS, Chang CJ, Scharff MD, et al. Chimeric human-mouse IgG antibodies with shuffled constant region exons demonstrate that multiple domains contribute to in vivo half-life. *Cancer Res* 1998;58:3905–3908.

89. Pollock RR, French DL, Metlay JP, et al. Intravascular metabolism of normal and mutant mouse immunoglobulin molecules. *Eur J Immunol* 1990;20:2021–2027.

90. Hnatowich DJ. Recent developments in the radiolabeling of antibodies with iodine, indium, and technetium. *Semin Nucl Med* 1990;20:80–91.

91. Fritzberg AR, Wilbur DS. Radiolabeling of antibodies for targeted diagnostics. In: Torchilin VP, ed. *Handbook of targeted delivery of imaging agents.* Boca Raton, FL: CRC Press, 1995:83–101

92. Brechbiel MW, Gansow OA, Atcher RW, et al. Synthesis of 1-(p-isothiocyanatobenzyl) derivatives of DTPA and EDTA: antibody labeling and tumor-imaging studies. *Inorg Chem* 1986;25:2772–2781.

93. DeNardo SJ, Zhong GR, Salako Q, et al. Pharmacokinetics of chimeric L6 conjugated to indium-111– and yttrium-90–DOTA-peptide in tumor-bearing mice. *J Nucl Med* 1995;36:829–836.

94. Hnatowich DJ. Is technetium-99m the radioisotope of choice for radioimmunoscintigraphy? *J Nucl Biol Med* 1994;38[Suppl]:22–32.

95. Lin MS. Labeling proteins with ^{99m}Tc. In: Subramanian G, Rhodes BA, Cooper FJ, et al, eds. *Radiopharmaceuticals.* New York: Society of Nuclear Medicine Press, 1975:36–48

96. Fritzberg AR, Abrams PG, Beaumier PL, et al. Specific and stable labeling of antibodies with technetium-99m with a diamide dithiolate chelating agent. *Proc Natl Acad Sci U S A* 1988;85:4025–4029.

97. Kairemo KJA. Positron emission tomography of monoclonal antibodies. *Acta Oncol* 1993;32:825–830.

98. Philpott GW, Schwarz SW, Anderson CJ, et al. RadioimunoPET: detection of colorectal carcinoma with positron-emitting copper-64-labeled monoclonal antibody. *J Nucl Med* 1995;36:1818–1824.

99. Johnson LL, Seldin DW. The role of antimyosin antibodies in acute myocardial infarction. *J Nucl Med* 1987;28:1671–1678.

100. Johnson LL, Seldin DW, Becker LC, et al. Antimyosin imaging in acute transmural myocardial infarctions: results of a multicenter clinical trial. *J Am Coll Cardiol* 1989;13:27–35.

101. Kramer EL, Noz ME. CT-SPECT fusion for analysis of radiolabeled antibodies: applications in gastrointestinal and lung carcinoma. *Nucl Med Biol* 1991;18:27–42.

102. Weber DA, Ivanovic M. Correlative image registration. *Semin Nucl Med* 1994;24:311–323.

103. Bocher M, Balan A, Krausz Y, et al. Gamma camera–mounted anatomical x-ray tomography: technology, system characteristics and early images. *Eur J Nucl Med* 2000;27:619–627.

104. Israel O, Keidar Z, Iosilevsky G, et al. The fusion of anatomic and physiologic imaging in the management of patients with cancer. *Semin Nucl Med* 2001;31:191–205.

105. Maguire RT. OncoScint image atlas. In: Maguire RT, Van Nostrand D, eds. *Diagnosis of colorectal and ovarian carcinoma: application of immunoscintigraphic technology.* New York: Marcel Dekker, 1992:141–175

106. Cytogen Corporation. ProstaScint Kit package insert, 1997

107. Greenlee RT, Hill-Harmon MB, Murray T, et al. Cancer statistics, 2001. *CA Cancer J Clin* 2001;51:15–36.

108. Babaian RJ, Murray JL, Lamki LM, et al. Radioimmunological imaging of metastatic prostatic cancer with ^{111}indium-labeled monoclonal antibody PAY-276. *J Urol* 1987;137:439–443.

109. Haseman MK, Reed NL, Rosenthal SA. Monoclonal antibody imaging of occult prostate cancer in patients with elevated prostate-specific antigen: positron emission tomography and biopsy correlation. *Clin Nucl Med* 1996;21:704–713.

110. Shreve PD, Grossman HB, Gross MD, et al. Metastatic prostate cancer; initial findings of PET with 2-deoxy-2-[F-18]fluoro-D-glucose. *Radiology* 1996;199:751–756.

111. Blend MJ, Sodee DB. ProstaScint: an update. In: Freeman LM, eds. *Nuclear medicine annual 2001.* Philadelphia: Lippincott Williams & Wilkins, 2001:109–138.

112. Ellis RE, Sodee DB, Spirnak JP, et al. Feasibility and acute toxicities of radioimmunoguided prostate brachytherapy. *Int J Radiat Oncol Biol Phys* 2000;48:683–687.

113. Neal CE, Swenson LC, Fanning J, et al. Monoclonal antibodies in ovarian and prostate cancer. *Semin Nucl Med* 1993;23:114–126.

114. Babaian RJ, Lamki LM. Radioimmunoscintigraphy of prostate cancer. *Semin Nucl Med* 1989;19:309–321.

115. Abdel-Nabi H, Wright GL, Gulfo JV, et al. Monoclonal antibodies and radioimmunoconjugates in the diagnosis and treatment of prostate cancer. *Semin Urol* 1992;10:45–54.

116. Horoszewicz JS, Kawinski E, Murphy GP. Monoclonal antibodies to a new antigenic marker in epithelial prostatic cells and serum of prostatic cancer patients. *Anticancer Res* 1987;7:927–936.

117. Burgers JK, Hinkle GH, Haseman MK. Monoclonal antibody imaging of recurrent and metastatic prostate cancer. *Semin Urol* 1995;13:102–112.

118. Holmes EH. PSMA specific antibodies and their diagnostic and therapeutic use. *Exp Opin Invest Drugs* 2001;10:511–519.

119. Lamb HM, Faulds D. Capromab pendetide: a review of its use as an imaging agent in prostate cancer. *Drugs Aging* 1998;12:293–304.

120. Schellhammer PF, Wright GL Jr. Biomolecular and clinical characteristics of PSA and other candidate prostate tumor markers. *Urol Clin North Am* 1993;20:597–606.

121. Chengazi VU, Feneley MR, Ellison D, et al. Imaging prostate cancer with technetium-99m-7E11-C5.3 (CYT-351). *J Nucl Med* 1997;38:675–682.

122. Deb N, Goris M, Trisler K, et al. Treatment of hormone-refractory prostate cancer with ^{90}Y-CYT-356 monoclonal antibody. *Clin Cancer Res* 1996;2:1289–1297.

123. Quintana JC, Blend MJ. The dual-isotope ProstaScint imaging procedure clinical experience and staging results in 145 patients. *Clin Nucl Med* 2000;25:33–40.

124. Manyak MJ. Clinical applications of radioimmunoscintigraphy with prostate-specific antibodies for prostate cancer. *Cancer Control* 1998;5:493–499.

125. *Immunoscintigraphy of primary and recurrent prostate cancer.* East Princeton, NJ: Cytogen, 1996.

126. Babaian RJ, Sayer J, Podoloff DA, et al. Radioimmunoscintigraphy of pelvic lymph nodes with ^{111}indium-labeled monoclonal antibody CYT-356. *J Urol* 1994;152:1952–1955.

127. Kahn D, Williams RD, Seldin DW, et al. Radioimmunoscintigraphy with ^{111}indium labeled CYT-356 for the detection of occult prostate cancer recurrence. *J Urol* 1994;152:1490–1495.

128. Thor AD, Edgerton SM. Monoclonal antibodies reactive with human breast or ovarian carcinoma: in vivo applications. *Semin Nucl Med* 1989;19:295–308.

129. Johnson VG, Schlom J, Paterson AJ, et al. Analysis of a human tumor-associated glycoprotein (TAG-72) identified by a monoclonal antibody B72.3. *Cancer Res* 1986;46:850–857.

130. Thor A, Ohuchi N, Szpak CA, et al. Distribution of oncofetal antigen tumor-associated glycoprotein-72 defined by monoclonal antibody B72.3. *Cancer Res* 1986;46:3118–3124.

131. Cytogen Corporation. OncoScint CR/OV package insert, 1996.

132. Markowitz A, Saleemi K, Freeman LM. Role of In-111 labeled CYT-103 immunoscintigraphy in the evaluation of patients with recurrent colorectal carcinoma. *Clin Nucl Med* 1993;18:685–700.

133. Collier BD, Abdel-Nabi H, Doerr RJ, et al. Immunoscintigraphy performed with In-111-labeled CYT-103 in the management of colorectal cancer: comparison with CT. *Radiology* 1992;185:179–186.

134. Perkins AC, Pimm MV. Differences in tumour and normal tissue concentrations of iodine- and indium-labelled monoclonal antibody, 1: the effect on image contrast in clinical studies. *Eur J Nucl Med* 1985;11:295–299.

135. Shochat D, Sharkey RM, Vattay A, et al. In-111 chelated by DTPA-antibody is retained in the liver as a small molecular weight moiety. *J Nucl Med* 1986;27:943(abst).

136. Doerr RJ, Abdel-Nabi H, Krag D, et al. Radiolabeled antibody imaging in the management of colorectal cancer. *Ann Surg* 1991;214:118–124.

137. Dominguez JM, Wolff BG, Nelson H, et al. ^{111}In-CYT-103 scanning in recurrent colorectal cancer: does it affect standard management? *Dis Colon Rectum* 1996;39:514–519.

138. Gold P, Freedman SO. Specific carcinoembryonic antigens of the human digestive system. *J Exp Med* 1965;122:467–481.

139. Primus FJ, Newell KD, Blue A, et al. Immunological heterogeneity of carcinoembryonic antigen: antigenic determinants on carcinoembryonic antigen distinguished by monoclonal antibodies. *Cancer Res* 1983;43:686–692.

140. Immunomedics. CEA-Scan (Arcitumomab) package insert, 1999.

141. Moffat FL Jr, Pinsky CM, Hammershaimb L, et al. Clinical utility of external immunoscintigraphy with the IMMU-4 technetium-99m Fab′ antibody fragment in patients undergoing surgery for carcinoma of the colon and rectum: results of a pivotal, phase III trial. *J Clin Oncol* 1996;14:2295–2305.

142. Hughes K, Pinsky CM, Petrelli NJ, et al. Use of carcinoembryonic antigen radioimmunodetection and computer tomography for predicting the resectability of recurrent colorectal cancer. Unpublished, 1996.

143. Willkomm P, Bender H, Bangard M, et al. FDG PET and immunoscintigraphy with ^{99m}Tc-labeled antibody fragments for detection of the recurrence of colorectal carcinoma. *J Nucl Med* 2000;41:1657–1663.

144. Thropay JP, Colletti PM, Barragan A. Radiologic case of the month. *Appl Radiol* 2001;43–45.

145. Whiteford MH, Whiteford HM, Yee LF, et al. Usefulness of FDG-PET scan in the assessment of suspected metastatic or recurrent adenocarcinoma of the colon and rectum. *Dis Colon Rectum* 2000;759:767.

146. Wegener WA, Petrelli N, Serafini A, et al. Safety and efficacy of arcitumomab imaging in colorectal cancer after repeated administration. *J Nucl Med* 2000;41:1016–1020.

147. Surwit EA, Childers JM, Krag DN, et al. Clinical assessment of ^{111}In-CYT-103 immunoscintigraphy in ovarian cancer. *Gynecol Oncol* 1993;48:285–292.

148. Gallup DG. Multicenter clinical trial of ^{111}In-CYT-103 in patients with ovarian cancer. In: Maguire RT, Van Nostrand D, eds. *Diagnosis of colorectal and ovarian carcinoma.* New York: Marcel Dekker, 1992:111–124.

149. Surwit EA. Impact of ^{111}In-CYT-103 on the surgical management of patients with ovarian cancer. In: Maguire RT, Van Nostrand D, eds. *Diagnosis of colorectal and ovarian carcinoma.* New York: Marcel Dekker, 1992:125–140.

150. Low RN, Carter WD, Saleh F, et al. Ovarian cancer: comparison of findings with perfluorocarbon-enhanced MR imaging, In-111-CYT-103 immunoscintigraphy, and CT. *Radiology* 1995;195:391–400.

151. Becker W, Bair J, Behr T, et al. Detection of soft-tissue infections and osteomyelitis using a technetium-99m-labeled antigranulocyte monoclonal antibody fragment. *J Nucl Med* 1994;35:1436–1443.

152. Becker W, Goldenberg DM, Wolf F. The use of monoclonal antibodies and antibody fragments in the imaging of infectious lesions. *Semin Nucl Med* 1994;24:142–153.

153. Barron B, Hanna C, Passalaqua AM, et al. Rapid diagnostic imaging of acute, nonclassic appendicitis by leukoscintigraphy with sulesomab technetium 99m-labeled antigranulocyte antibody Fab′ fragment. LeukoScan Appendicitis Clinical Trial Group. *Surgery* 1999;125:288–296.

154. Kipper SL, Rypins EB, Evans DG, et al. Neutrophil-specific 99mTc-labeled anti-CD15 monoclonal antibody imaging for diagnosis of equivocal appendicitis. *J Nucl Med* 2000;41:449–455.

155. Thakur ML, Marcus CS, Kipper SL, et al. Imaging infection with LeuTech. *Nucl Med Commun* 2001;22:513–519.

47

RADIOLABELED MONOCLONAL ANTIBODY THERAPY

RICHARD L. WAHL

Radiolabeled antibody therapy, commonly known as *radioimmunotherapy* (RIT) for cancer is an emerging therapeutic approach to several types of cancer and potentially other conditions. The rationale for this form of therapy is the expectation that a radiolabeled antibody will specifically target and selectively irradiate antigen-positive tumors to a much greater extent than would nonspecific delivery of radioantibody to normal tissues. From fundamental radiation biology considerations, it is expected that the higher the radiation absorbed dose (radiation energy deposited to a given tissue) to a tumor, the greater is the likelihood that a tumor will respond to treatment. Similarly, if the radiation energy is delivered to normal tissues, the higher is the radiation absorbed dose to normal tissue, the greater is the probability of toxicity. As with external beam radiation, for treatment to be effective, efforts must be made to maximize tumor radiation dose while keeping normal tissue dose below toxic levels.

The concept of specific delivery of treatments to disease was first envisioned by Ehrlich (1), who mainly focused on therapy for infectious disease. The first RIT in the care of humans was performed more than 50 years ago by Beierwaltes, who used ^{131}I-labeled polyclonal antibodies raised against melanoma to treat several patients with metastatic melanoma, one of whom achieved a complete response. RIT also was used separately by Order (2). Early studies of RIT were performed with polyclonal antibodies. The invention of somatic cell fusion (hybridoma) techniques to make monoclonal antibodies greatly increased interest in the use of radiolabeled antibodies for treatment. Almost all antibodies used in current studies are monoclonal in nature.

Radioimmunoimaging, or radioimmunodiagnosis, is generally performed with radioactive isotopes that emit γ rays and is often an important component of the RIT process. The γ rays in radioimmunodiagnosis can be detected with a gamma camera and can allow estimation of the location and quantity of radioactivity in the body and in specific tissues in the body. The field of imaging with radiolabeled antibodies, or radioimmunoimaging (see Chapter 46), has been limited to date in applicability. It is used in the care of some patients with colorectal or prostate cancer. However, pure γ emitters are not generally good choices for treatment because they deposit only modest energy in tumors. Particle emitters or particle and γ photons, such as radioisotopes emitting β or α particles or auger electrons, are more commonly used.

The potential of RIT is considerable, but although it has for a long time been an attractive concept, only more recently has its promise begun to be realized in practice, especially in management of the more radiosensitive hematologic neoplasms (3,4). The promise of this therapy for other types of cancer has yet to be fully realized, in part because of inadequate targeted radiation delivery to most types of solid tumors. Varying aspects of RIT are reviewed in this chapter.

PRINCIPLES OF RADIOLABELED ANTIBODY THERAPY

Antigen

Tumor-specific or Tumor-associated

The use of radiolabeled antibodies in cancer therapy is based on the concept that antibodies are capable of high affinity and specific binding to unique antigenic targets. An antibody molecule is highly specific for its antigenic target; however, the choice of antigenic target must be carefully made for RIT to have the potential to succeed.

Tumor immunologists hoped there would be unique antigenic sites on all cancers that would help differentiate them in an absolute manner from all normal nontarget tissues. Such major structural differences between malignant and normal tissues appear to be the exception and not the rule. Only the antigen-variable region (idiotype) of the antibodies made by malignant human B-cell lymphoma and myeloma has been identified as a truly specific antigenic target. Such a specific target is appealing in concept, but from a drug-development standpoint, tumor-specific antigens are quite impractical. The impracticality stems from the fact that if radioantibody therapy could be developed for each specific tumor antigen (idiotype), there would be a different and patient-specific drug for each patient. Although this sounds intrinsically appealing, it would be very difficult in most countries to develop, commercialize, and market such a

R.L. Wahl: Division of Nuclear Medicine and Technology and Business Development, Johns Hopkins Medicine, Baltimore, MD.

970 *Oncology*

therapy owing to logistical, regulatory and economic considerations. Thus even if successful RIT could be developed for a specific idiotype of a B-cell neoplasm, it would be difficult to make into a legitimate therapeutic agent at a realistic cost.

If there were true tumor-specific antibodies that were present across a wide variety of tumors, that is, tumor- but not patient-specific, it would be far easier to develop and manufacture such a therapy. To date, such antigens have not been recognized. However, there are antigenic determinants which are preferentially, but not uniquely, displayed on tumors in excess of the level of their expression on normal tissues. Such antigens are known as *tumor-associated antigens.* These tumor-associated antigens have been the major targets for RIT to date. On first principles, it may seem unrealistic to consider tumor-associated antigens potentially useful targets for RIT; however, the greatest success in RIT has been achieved with such targets. Often the antigens are present on malignant and mature cells of a given type but are not expressed on normal tissues, such as stem cells. This is the case in the use of anti-CD20 antibodies in therapy for lymphoma (Fig. 47.1)—maturation of CD20 expression. If there is quantitative overexpression of the antigen in tumor as opposed to normal tissues, effective therapy may still be delivered.

Although it seems logical that most useful antigenic targets would be on cancer cell surfaces, and they are, there are other targets in the tissues immediately surrounding the tumor cells. For example, although carcinoembryonic antigen (CEA) is produced and on the surface of colon cancer cells, there are also high CEA levels in the tissues immediately surrounding the tumor, that is, the interstitial fluid, peritumoral compartments around the tumor. There also are other antigenic targets in the extracellular matrix surrounding the tumor and possibly in the blood vessels surrounding and supplying the tumor. Thus although tumor antigens classically are the target for RIT, other targets in the region of the tumor may be equally or more important as therapeutic opportunities.

This chapter discusses many of the antigenic targets used in RIT. A full description of each of these antigenic targets is be-

yond the scope of this chapter, although the targets of clinical relevance are emphasized.

Internalizing or Not

If a large molecule like a monoclonal antibody is to successfully interact with an antigen, the antigen must be physically accessible to the radioantibody. This generally means the antigen should be on the cell surface of the cancer cell and the extracellular portion of the antigen recognized by the targeting antibody. In general, intracellular targets or antigens are not as effective as extracellular targets because they are largely inaccessible to the large protein molecule. However, in some situations, intracellular antigens can serve as useful targets, if the intracellular antigen is somehow accessible to the antibody. This can occur in permeant cells that are dying or in dead cancer cells.

Some antigens, such as CD20, are firmly fixed on the cell surface and do not modulate when antibody binding occurs. Other antigens, such as CD22, detach from the cell when antibody binds, or are internalized with the antibody after binding. Antigens that detach are not good choices for targeting because the antibody and target will not remain localized to the tumor; however, antigens that internalize can be good choices for RIT if the proper radiolabel is chosen. For RIT to be most effective, the radiolabel must continue to be intracellular after internalization. Radiometals generally are better retained than is radioiodine, for example.

Circulating or Not

The ideal tumor antigen for RIT would be only on the tumor or the tissues immediately surrounding the tumor, and nowhere else. However, such ideal tumor antigens are rare. For example, the truly tumor-specific antigen from the idiotype of lymphoma cells is on the lymphoma cell surfaces, but is also secreted into the circulation. While in the circulation, the antigen is far from the tumor and can represent a barrier to the delivery of radioantibody to the tumor, because the radioantibody can interact with the circulating antigen and be diverted from targeting to the

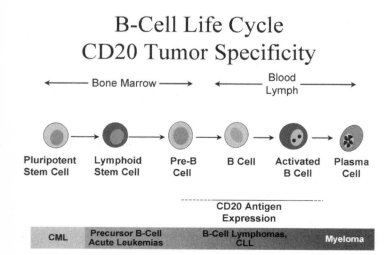

FIGURE 47.1. CD20 antigen expression. Despite being a tumor-associated antigen, CD20 represents a suitable target for radioimmunotherapy studies because it is not expressed on hematopoietic stem cells.

tumor. There are methods to deal with this problem, such as administering unlabeled antibody before the radiolabeled material, to complex and occupy the circulating antigenic sites.

Although circulating antigen can be troublesome, it is also clear that it is not an absolute barrier to the success of RIT. For example, imaging with anti-CEA antibodies is possible despite the presence of circulating CEA; similarly, therapy with anti-CD20 antibodies is feasible despite the presence of large populations of CD20-positive cells in the blood (3). The latter is feasible, in part, because unlabeled antibody predosing is often given to block the potential binding sites on the circulating CD20-positive B cells.

Antibody

Size and Species of Antibody Molecules

The choice of antibody for RIT is clearly that of a monoclonal antibody, that is, an antibody of uniform purity and consistency in production. Early attempts to image and treat with radiolabeled antibodies were with polyclonal reagents. However, such reagents, drawn from the blood of immunized animals such as sheep and goats, were simply not reproducible or easily scaled up to pharmacologic quality. Most studies with monoclonal antibodies in the late 1980s through the mid 1990s were performed with murine-origin monoclonal antibodies.

Because monoclonal antibodies are large-protein molecules, (150 kd for an intact monoclonal antibody), it is likely that they are treated as foreign materials in the patient receiving them. The development of human anti-mouse antibodies (HAMA) is quite common when immunocompetent patients receive murine monoclonal antibodies as therapy. More than one half of untreated patients with lymphoma develop HAMA when given murine antibody RIT (4). Such HAMA can limit subsequent administration of RIT and thus can be quite troublesome. Newer antibody reagents are more human-like, either having fully human constant regions (fully humanized) or being partly humanized (chimeric). The trend to a more human framework in the antibodies is based on a desire to minimize the likelihood of an anti-antibody response in the patient. With improved recombinant DNA techniques and better understanding of production methods, the human and humanized antibodies are becoming more generally available.

Murine antibodies typically have shorter half-lives in vivo than do humanized antibodies (mouse antibody typically clears from the bloodstream more rapidly than does human antibody, in a human), and this may be advantageous in some settings. Humanized antibodies often have more potent effector function (immunologic function) than do mouse antibodies. These properties of longer half-life, potentially greater effector function, and less incidence of anti-antibody response make humanized antibodies the clear choice for *unlabeled* antibody therapy. In RIT, both murine and humanized antibodies are used. The shorter half-life in the serum of murine antibody and the lesser immune effector function of murine antibodies are properties that may make the murine reagents superior because they are often better matched to the half-lives of the radioisotopes chosen and may cause less immune-related toxicity. If repeated adminis-

trations are given, murine antibodies are less likely to be good choices because of the risk of development of HAMA.

Almost all RIT is performed with intact monoclonal antibodies. Smaller pieces of the antibody molecule, either enzymatically produced or produced by means of molecular engineering often have preserved targeting and superior target to background ratios than intact antibodies. However, these agents additionally have high-level renal excretion, which can be troublesome and generally are retained in the tumor for a significantly shorter period than are intact antibodies (5). To date, antibody fragments have been used far less often than have intact monoclonal antibodies for tumor targeting. Although the superior tumor targeting properties of monoclonal antibodies as opposed to antibody fragments have been used in diagnosis with radiolabeled antibodies, the preferred carrier molecule to date for direct radioantibody targeting is the intact antibody molecule.

Direct Targeting or Pretargeting

When intact radiolabeled antibodies or antibody fragments are injected intravenously, there is an immediate distribution of the antibody throughout the circulatory system. This is necessary for the antibody to reach all potential sites of tumor. Intact monoclonal antibodies are quite large and only gradually develop high tumor to background uptake ratios. This is in part because blood clearance is slow and because permeation of the large antibody molecule into tumors is a gradual process. This slow rate of accumulation into tumors and a relatively slow disappearance of radioactivity from the bloodstream means that there is considerable irradiation of normal tissue during the uptake phase of the antibody into tumor and during the gradual process of radioantibody clearance from normal tissue. This relatively slow and relatively modest targeting of radioantibody to the tumor is a fundamental limitation of most RIT approaches to date. It makes it challenging in many instances to deliver sufficient radioactivity to the tumor to allow a sufficient radiation dose to control the tumor while sparing normal tissues (5).

A variety of approaches have been tried to enhance delivery of radioantibody to a tumor or to accelerate clearance from the blood. The use of immunoadsorbent columns, plasma exchange or pheresis, or second anti-antibodies to form immune complexes that would then be delivered to the liver are approaches that have been tested in preclinical and clinical systems (6–8). However, all these approaches suffer from the relatively slow uptake phase of the radioantibody into the tumor (at least after intravenous delivery) and from the overall underlying issue that the antibody is required to do two things well, that is, target the antigenic site and carry the radioactivity. Approaches in which these tasks are separated into two distinct steps, such as pretargeting approaches to radioactivity delivery (9), are attracting interest.

Pretargeting can be done in several ways, but the most common and widely applied approach has been the use of biotin-avidin conjugates for targeting. Biotin has a very high affinity for avidin or streptavidin and can be attached to an antitumor antibody. This antibody with biotin attached can be reacted with avidin or streptavidin so that avidin or streptavidin binding sites are exposed. Biotin is monovalent whereas avidin and streptavidin are tetravalent. Further, biotin binds to streptavidin with *very* high affinity. The biotin-avidin conjugated antibody can be injected intravenously and then allowed to localize to tumor while being allowed to slowly clear from the circulation. The clearance rate of the antibody-biotin-streptavidin complex then can be accelerated with a dose of anti-antibody or another agent, such as a biotinylated liver targeting molecule, to clear blood-pool radio activity. A radiolabeled small molecule, such as radiobiotin, then can be given. This agent either localizes to antibody targeted to the tumor or because of its low molecular weight clears rapidly through the kidneys. This type of approach is quite complex but can give higher levels of tumor targeting and lower background radioactivity levels than achieved by giving intact radioantibody intravenously. In preclinical model systems with the same antibody, the pretargeting approach has given better tumor dosimetry and therapeutic efficacy than has one performed with direct targeting in preclinical models (10). The disadvantage of this approach is its complexity and the relatively common incidence of development of host antibodies against the streptavidin molecule. Some experts give biotinylated antibody (step 1), avidin (step 2), and radiolabeled biotin (step 3), the so called three-step approach (11).

Another pretargeting approach that is under study is the affinity-enhancing system. This involves the use of bifunctional, anti-tumor–anti-hapten (anti-radioconjugate) antibodies, for example. This approach may be less complex than the biotin-streptavidin approach (e.g., a bifunctional antibody reactive with tumor and with a hapten can be given first, and the radiolabeled hapten can be given to deliver the radiation). This approach appears superior to use of antibody fragments for tumor therapy in animal models and has entered clinical trials (12). For the present, direct antibody localization to tumor and antibody therapy is most commonly performed. In the future, the pretargeting approaches may be more common, but the complexity of this approach and the immunogenicity of approaches with streptavidin are major impediments (see later).

Human Anti-mouse Antibodies

When immunocompetent patients receive mouse antibody, the host immune system views it as a foreign protein and responds with an antibody response of varying strength. Many patients with cancer have undergone extensive chemotherapy and are incapable of mounting a vigorous immune response. Thus a small number of HAMA reactions are present in patients who have undergone murine antibody therapy for lymphoma after undergoing extensive chemotherapy. HAMA ideally should be avoided, because host antibodies against infused antibodies can alter biodistribution of the infused radioantibody and immune complexes, and complement activation can lead to potentially serious toxicity in the presence of HAMA. HAMA are not an all-or-none phenomenon, and a very low-level HAMA response is of doubtful clinical importance.

Radioisotope

Type of Radioactive Decay

For most imaging, either γ emitters or isotopes that decay through positron emission are used. For therapy, radioisotopes

Table 47.1. *Properties of Several Therapeutic Radionuclides*

Colloid	T$_{1/2}$ (days)	Energy (MeV)		Range in water (mm)	
		Maximum	Mean	Maximum	Mean
^{33}P	14.29	1.710	0.695	8.0	3.2
^{90}Y	2.67	2.28	0.93	11.0	3.6
^{186}Re	3.7	1.08	0.349	3.7	1.2
^{131}I	8.04	0.59	0.190	0.8	0.27
^{177}Lu	6.7	0.497	0.133	0.7	0.23
^{211}At	0.3	α = 5.8, 7.5	6.8	0.065	—

that emit particles as a large portion of their decay, such as γ rays, although important for imaging, do not deposit sufficient energy into the tumor. Several of the major radioisotopes for RIT and their energy and half-lives are listed in Table 47.1. Other radioisotopes are possible but not all have been explored to date. The half-lives of these therapeutic radioisotopes often are much longer than are those used in diagnosis.

β Emitters, either mixed with γ emitters or pure, are the radioisotopes most commonly used for RIT. The particulate radiation of the β particle delivers energy sufficient to kill tumors in many instances. There are a variety of β emitters, some pure β emitters, such as ^{90}Y, and others mixed γ and β emitters, such as ^{131}I. The half-life, chemical properties, and energy of β particles differentiate the isotopes. Results of theoretical studies indicate that high-energy β emitters are better suited to larger tumors and that lower-energy β emitters are more suitable for smaller tumors (13). In addition, α emitters, which delivery higher linear energy transfer (and high lethality) particles to tumors are attractive possible choices but have been used only infrequently to date. α Emitters are well suited to killing small clusters of tumor cells if delivery of the radiopharmaceutical is reasonably uniform. Auger emitters, low-energy electrons, can be used in treatment. In general, however, β or mixed β emitters have been used to the greatest extent. The distribution of energy deposition on a microscopic level is important to the likelihood of success of RIT. Higher-energy β emitters have less heterogenous dose distribution but at the cost of depositing energy remote from tumor foci in some instances and difficulty in curing smaller tumors, because most emitted energy is deposited beyond the location of the primary lesion (14,15). It is clear that some tumors with major inhomogeneity are unlikely to be cured with low-energy β emitters, because the radiation dose is not uniformly distributed. Toxicity is predicted to increase, but response is not expected to improve if higher doses of radiopharmaceutical therapy are given in such tumors (16).

Low-energy βγ emitters such as ^{125}I have shown some promise in RIT studies. They have had a higher therapeutic index than has ^{131}I in preclinical studies (17). ^{111}In also may have potential as a therapeutic agent because of its Auger emissions of low energy. Isotopes with low-energy β emissions and, more notably, Auger emitters must enter the cell and localize near the nucleus to achieve optimal cell killing efficacy. To date, however, the most commonly used isotopes for RIT have been ^{131}I and ^{90}Y (Table 47.1).

α Emitters are very promising for RIT but have been used

only to a limited extent (18). These agents have tremendous killing ability but are limited in availability. ^{212}Bi, ^{211}At, ^{212}Pb, and ^{225}Ac are in early but promising phases of evolution (19).

Half-life

The half-life of the radioactive isotope chosen for therapy should be properly matched to the biokinetics of the targeting antibody. If it takes several days for the antibody to develop optimal targeting, it seems clear that an isotope with a half-life of a few hours would be poorly matched. Most of the radiation energy would have been deposited into nontarget locations before the antibody reached and was selectively retained at its target. However, for isotopes with an extremely long half-life, such as ^{125}I (half-life, 60 days), although much of the radiation energy is delivered after the radioantibody has targeted well to tumor, the dose rate can be quite low. This may allow tumor regrowth to occur at a rate faster than tumor cell kill. A reasonably high dose rate ideally is delivered, but not with all the energy being deposited owing to a short half-life before the selective targeting has occurred.

Properties of Localization

Radioisotopes used for treatment have included radiometals, halogens, and other isotopes. The typical radiometal is not directly bound to the antibody but is *chelated,* or attached by an intermediary molecule called a *chelator.* A common chelator in RIT is tetraazacyclododecanetetraacetic acid (DOTA). Ideally, the radiolabel remains tightly bound to the antibody and mimics its biodistribution in vivo. However, the chelator can retain radiometals with varying degrees of success. If the radiometals are released in vivo, they can become retargeted to a variety of normal tissue. For example, radiometals such as ^{90}Y, which is commonly used in therapy, accumulate substantially into normal bone. ^{131}I, which is covalently attached to antibody molecules, is accumulated in the thyroid, stomach, salivary glands, and excreted in the urine if it is liberated in vivo through the action of dehalogenases.

Intracellular trafficking and retention of radiolabels vary as well. For example, radiometals such as ^{90}Y often are retained in tumor cells if the antigen is internalized and targets to the lysosome. In contrast, most formulations of ^{131}I are not selectively retained in tumor cells but can be if they are attached to a positively charged moiety that has a better likelihood of retention in the lysosomes (20). Such considerations can make a great difference in radiation absorbed dose to tumor cells. At present, the optimal radioisotope for RIT is unknown; it may in fact vary by antibody target (21). For example, in some settings, ^{90}Y is clearly superior to ^{131}I, but this is not consistently the case (22). It is clear that radioiodine is generally a poor choice in the management of tumors that have antigenic modulation or internalization (if the labeling is through the typical tyrosine iodination process), because the iodine is rapidly cleaved from the antibody molecule and lost from the tumor. In contrast, iodine attached by an alternative method to enhance residualization of the tracer in tumor cells can be effective in such tumors. ^{131}I can be an effective choice for targeting stable antigens, such

as CD20, on the surface of tumors. Isotopes such as ^{131}I, ^{186}Re, and ^{177}Lu, which emit β emission that can be imaged, have the potential for precise dose quantitation in vivo, which is more difficult with pure β emitters.

Dosimetry of Radioimmunotherapy

Dosimetry in Radiopharmaceutical Therapy: Emerging Role

Once the choice of antibody and radioisotope is made, exactly how many radioactive molecules (millicuries) of a radiopharmaceutical should be given to properly treat a given patient is an important determination. It is increasingly apparent that a single administered millicurie-size dose for each patient may not be optimal. This is where the concept of dosimetry becomes critical. The concept of dosimetry is that a small amount of radioactive molecules attached to a targeting molecule can be administered to a patient and that the biodistribution and pharmacokinetics can be traced in vivo, often with a scanning device such as a gamma camera. This biodistribution is expected to be predictive of the biodistribution of a subsequently administered, much higher number of radioactive molecules a treatment dose. This tracer principle is key to much of nuclear medicine. Methods for dosimetry have evolved over the past several decades. A variety of centers routinely use dosimetric estimates to determine how many radioactive molecules (millicuries) of radioiodine should be used in the management of thyroid diseases such as Graves disease or thyroid cancer (23). Extending some of these concepts to radiopharmaceutical therapy is reasonable.

Many therapeutic drugs for cancer show variability in pharmacokinetics from patient to patient, and radiopharmaceuticals are not an exception to this. However, most cancer therapeutic drugs are not trace-imaged in vivo. Even when blood pharmacokinetics are determined for a cancer therapeutic agent, it is not generally possible to know its in vivo localization pattern. Radioactive drugs such as radioimmunoconjugates also show substantial variability in vivo biokinetics. With the proper radiolabel, they can be imaged in vivo and followed through the body by means of γ scanning. With such methods it is possible to measure reasonably accurately the accumulation of radioactivity and its time course and thus dosimetry in the entire body, in specific normal tissues, and in tumors (24). It is thus possible to plan the administered activity (the number of radioactive molecules given) for a specific patient. Such patient-specific dosing is possible with dosimetric methods (see Chapter 10).

In situations in which the therapeutic index of a drug is modest and there is interpatient variability in pharmacokinetics, the average dose of a drug may indeed prove to be an overdose in some patients and an underdose in others. This can lead to substantial variability in patient response, in both efficacy and toxicity. At least for radioactive drugs, dosimetry represents a method to correct for heterogeneity in the handling of drugs by individual patients to avoid overdosing and underdosing. In general, to determine radiation dose to a given tissue, sequential measurements of the radioactivity concentration in a given tissue must be made, a time–activity curve and area under this curve must be determined, the volume of the tissue and the predicted absorbed fraction of dose delivered determined, and the radiation absorbed energy calculated (24).

The simplest methods of dosimetry are those used in planning the treatment dose of ^{131}I tositumomab for RIT for non-Hodgkin's lymphoma (25). In this system, the predicted radiation dose to the whole body is determined after administration of a tracer dose of radioactivity, roughly 5 mCi of ^{131}I tositumomab. This is imaged with a gamma camera. The entire body is scanned immediately after tracer injection, 2 or 3 days after injection, and approximately 6 or 7 days after injection. These scans take only a few minutes with modern gamma cameras. With this reagent, clearance of ^{131}I from the body is monoexponential. When the rate of clearance of the radioactivity from the body, which is based on a plot of data from three time points, and the patient weight and intended therapeutic dose in centigrays to the entire body are known, therapeutic activity (number of radioactive molecules) of the same compound can be prescribed and administered a week or so after the tracer dose. The outline for patient-specific whole-body dosimetry for ^{131}I tositumomab therapy is shown in Fig. 47.2. This approach is not feasible when pure β emitters are used for treatment. This would include isotopes such as ^{90}Y or ^{32}P, which cannot be imaged well with gamma cameras.

Surrogates for ^{90}Y include [111]In (26). Although the biodistributions are similar, they are not identical, especially in bone and bone marrow. The discrepancy makes it difficult to perform reliable radiation dosimetry of bone and marrow with [111]In. Thus some of nonimaged therapeutic agents are dosed according to an average dose believed to be reasonably safe as opposed to an individualizing dose for specific patients.

Estimating radiation dose to organs, marrow, and tumor is more challenging and more prone to error than is whole-body dose estimation (see Chapter 10). Such estimates may be needed if bone marrow transplantation doses (high doses) of radioactivity are given or with newer investigative drugs. Current dosimetry techniques remain limited in their quality and ability to be used as predictors of toxicity. It is also clear that the extent of marrow reserve (which can be somewhat approximated with the white blood cell count and platelet count), extent of tumor involvement in the marrow, and history of recent chemotherapy are related to increased toxicity from a given radiation dose to the bone marrow (26,27).

Dosimetry and Toxicity

Toxicity due to RIT is expected to be positively correlated with the radiation absorbed dose to a tissue. However, it would be naive to expect that radiation dose alone would dictate toxicity. The intrinsic radiosensitivity of a tissue can vary from patient to patient. For example, it has been clearly shown that patients who have undergone extensive chemotherapy or bone marrow transplantation have greater toxicity from RIT than do patients who have not undergone treatment. Patients with more tumor involvement in the marrow also appear to have higher toxicity levels than do those without tumor involvement in the marrow. For this reason, it would not necessarily be expected that a strict linear correlation would occur with radiation absorbed dose. However, it is safe to say that in almost every RIT trial conducted, the number of radioactive molecules administered, the radiation absorbed dose in a given tissue, and toxicity are positively correlated. An example of the relation between toxicity and absorbed radiation dose to the total body predicted with dosimetric imaging studies is shown in Fig. 47.3. These results were achieved with ^{131}I tositumomab treatment.

Nonmyeloablative

At nonmyeloablative doses, toxicity to the bone marrow has generally been dose limiting for RIT. This is shown in Fig. 47.3 for ^{131}I tositumomab treatment. With this drug, the actual therapeutic radiation dose escalation study was conducted with patient-specific dosimetric methods. Generally, therapeutic indices are relatively modest for RIT. Thus the question should be asked how heterogeneous are the pharmacokinetics of a therapeutic radioconjugate. The variability in total-body residence time is shown in Fig. 47.4. The number of radioactive molecules (millicuries) needed to treat to a 75-cGy total body level is shown in Fig. 47.5 for ^{131}I tositumomab, in which there is a wide range of levels of radioactive molecules administered across patients. Calculation of number of radioactive molecules (millicuries) per square meter also can be a reasonable approach to therapy (28).

Treatment Regimen

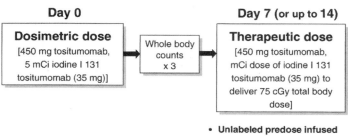

Day 0

Dosimetric dose
[450 mg tositumomab, 5 mCi iodine I 131 tositumomab (35 mg)]

Whole body counts × 3

Day 7 (or up to 14)

Therapeutic dose
[450 mg tositumomab, mCi dose of iodine I 131 tositumomab (35 mg) to deliver 75 cGy total body dose]

- Unlabeled predose infused over 1 hour
- Administered mCi activity determined by gamma counts

Thyroprotection (SSKI): Day -1 continuing through 14 days post-therapeutic dose

FIGURE 47.2. Dosimetric approach to ^{131}I tositumomab therapy. The concept is based on expectation and observations that tracer dose is an accurate predictor of the biodistribution and dosimetry of the therapeutic dose. Tracer dosimetry can be performed for therapeutics with a gamma or positron emitter of appropriate energy. Surrogate tracer dosimetry can be performed for β emitters. For example, a tracer study can be performed with ^{111}In before ^{90}Y therapy, if dosimetry is required. Organ dosimetry can be performed in a similar way, but more data points and more detailed imaging, often tomographic, may be required.

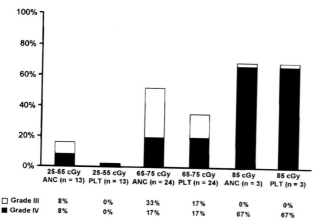

Hematologic Toxicity by Total Body Dose (TBD) Phase I/II Study*

	25-55 cGy ANC (n = 13)	25-55 cGy PLT (n = 13)	65-75 cGy ANC (n = 24)	65-75 cGy PLT (n = 24)	85 cGy ANC (n = 3)	85 cGy PLT (n = 3)
□ Grade III	8%	0%	33%	17%	0%	0%
■ Grade IV	8%	0%	17%	17%	67%	67%

*Patients without prior bone marrow transplant.
ANC = Absolute neutrophil count; PLT = Platelets.

FIGURE 47.3. Toxicity versus whole-body radiation absorbed dose (in centigrays) in a phase I-II dose escalation trial of ^{131}I tositumomab (30). Grade IV toxicity is common at the highest doses and indicates a dose-response relation for toxicity.

Myeloablative

The concept of myeloablative therapy means that an intentional decision has been made to give doses of radiation to the patient and the bone marrow that will prove sufficient to ablate clonogenic cells. The intention is to reinfuse stem cells or bone marrow cells some days after the therapeutic dose is administered so that the hematopoietic system is reconstituted successfully. In most instances, these research studies have been phase I dose escalations in which escalation is based on radiation dose to normal tissues, which are excepted to be the second organs to experience toxicity after bone marrow. For example, the liver, lungs, or kidneys may be expected to be organs of secondary radiation toxicity depending on the radioimmunoconjugate. In dose escalation trials conducted at the University of Washington by Press

et al (29), it was determined that the cardiopulmonary system was the organ of secondary toxicity after bone marrow. This was seen in a study in which dose escalation was based on results of dosimetry. A radiation dose of 27 cGy to the lungs exceeded the maximum tolerated dose (MTD) in their phase I study. [131]I tositumomab and doses of 25 cGy were better tolerated than the highest dose. Only through the use of organ dosimetry were the investigators able to ascertain the maximum tolerated radiation absorbed dose to the lung, heart, and kidney, for example (30). In other forms of radiopharmaceutical therapy, such as peptide-based RIT, the kidney can be dose limiting. Organ dosimetry is more challenging than is total-body dosimetry and is much less routinely performed in a prospective manner. It can be a powerful tool, however. Just as marrow reserve and extent

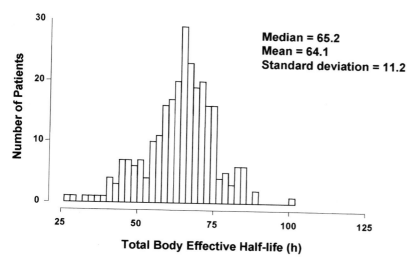

Variability in Total Body Half-life (TBHL)

Median = 65.2
Mean = 64.1
Standard deviation = 11.2

FIGURE 47.4. Variability in total-body half-life of ^{131}I tositumomab in patients referred for radioimmunotherapy. Rapid and slow outliers are shown from group mean data. Rapid clearance can result in an underdose of therapy versus that expected to be tolerable if average doses of radioactive molecules (millicuries) are infused. Similarly, an average dose would pose greater risk of toxicity in patients with long total-body half-lives.

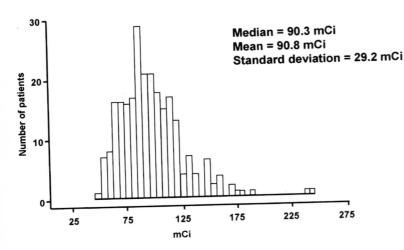

mCi to Deliver 75 cGy TBD (n = 262)

Median = 90.3 mCi
Mean = 90.8 mCi
Standard deviation = 29.2 mCi

FIGURE 47.5. Variability in number of radioactive molecules (millicuries) required to deliver 75-cGy total-body radiation dose of ^{131}I tositumomab to patients with lymphoma.

of tumor involvement can affect the likelihood of toxicity of anti-CD20 therapy or treatment with ^{131}I anti-CEA antibodies, treatment with other drugs may influence the radiosensitivity of nonmarrow target tissues. This is relevant especially if myeloablative therapy is combined with chemotherapy.

Dosimetry and Tumor Response

With dosimetry based on total-body dose or MTD to a given normal organ, the concept is to give as much radiation as possible to deliver as much as possible to the tumor. However, one might ask whether this is necessary. Because monoclonal antibodies have several mechanisms of action, is the radiation really needed? Although the answer would seem an intuitively obvious, "Yes," it also has been proved directly in clinical trials. Direct comparative trials of ^{90}Y anti-CD20 and unlabeled anti-CD20 have shown clear superiority of the labeled material to the unlabeled. Preliminary results with ^{131}I anti-CD20 have shown similar findings. Thus radioactivity is better than no radioactivity for antibody treatments.

Radiation absorbed doses to tumors are commonly sixfold to tenfold higher in myeloablative than in the nonmyeloablative trials. In the myeloablative trials, higher overall response rates and higher rates of complete remission are seen among patients for whom RIT has been unsuccessful than are seen in studies of nonmyeloablative dosing. Although it is difficult to make such comparisons across studies because of differing selection criteria, the data available suggest higher response rates the greater is the dose of radiation to tumor (29–33). It is clear that the histologic features and native radioresistance characteristics of the tumor make a major difference in the likelihood of response. For example, in patients with follicular non-Hodgkin's lymphoma, the response rates to ^{131}I tositumomab are much higher than in patients with diffuse or large cell tumor histologic features (30).

One might expect to see a dose-response relation across tu-

mors managed with RIT. In studies with patients with untreated non-Hodgkin's lymphoma who received ^{131}I RIT as initial treatment, my colleagues and I have observed considerable heterogeneity of dose and response. Most patients (>90%) respond to this treatment. However when we compared the percentage tumor shrinkage versus radiation absorbed dose to tumor; these parameters were only weakly correlated (32). Thus there is some evidence that absorbed dose to tumor and response are related, albeit weakly with ^{131}I anti CD-20 therapy.

Is Dosimetry Needed?

Total-body dosimetry is simple and appears to be a necessary and important component to optimize the treatment dose in specific patients with non-Hodgkin's lymphoma treated with ^{131}I tositumomab. However, it is not clear whether dosimetry is needed or feasible with each instance of RIT. Some experts have suggested that repeated small doses of radioactive molecules in RIT should be given over weeks to months. Some animal data support this concept and suggest higher efficacy for fractionated dosing. One could argue that dose fractions could be adjusted according to toxicity to a given test dose, to some extent as chemotherapy is administered. However, this often is not possible for RIT because some of the radioantibodies given are of murine origin or are mixed murine-human chimera. Such agents may be immunogenic and if given repeatedly may have varying rates of clearance of the radioantibody on later doses. Even fully humanized antibodies are potentially capable of generating an immune response. These sorts of responses are important, because they can change the pharmacokinetics of a radiolabeled compound. If this happens, prediction of toxicity and efficacy becomes difficult.

Summary of Dosimetry

Because of its simplicity, the "one dose fits all" concept of dose selection for RIT will be applied whenever it is feasible, safe, and effective. However, RIT with prospective patient-specific dosimetry is a required part of ^{131}I tositumomab therapy, which is emerging as a therapeutic agent for lymphoma. Not all therapeutic antibodies can be used to perform patient-specific dosimetry if they cannot be imaged. In such instances, a best-guess average dose may have to be given on the basis of weight or size of the patient and results of a standard phase I dose escalation trial. However, if there is considerable patient to patient pharmacokinetic variability, dosimetry will be essential for safe and successful therapy to be delivered to maximize tumor radiation dose and to minimize radiation absorbed dose to normal tissues. In cases in which bone marrow transplantation support is needed, it is also quite likely that dosimetry will be an essential element of therapeutic intervention and precede the treatment dose. In time, RIT may become as common and necessary as is treatment-planning dosimetry for external beam radiation. However, it must be realized that current methods are not optimal for assessing marrow dose and that even if doses could be assessed accurately, marrow radiosensitivity would still not be easily predicted.

CLINICAL STUDIES IN RADIOLABELED ANTIBODY THERAPY

Hematologic Malignant Disease

B-cell Lymphoma

Radiolabeled Antibodies

Several radiolabeled monoclonal antibodies have been evaluated since the technology to make monoclonal antibodies was reported about 25 years ago. Although promising, radioantibodies only slowly localize to tumor targets and deliver radiation to tumors. Thus the therapeutic margins for these methods have been relatively low between tumor and normal tissues. The more radiosensitive tumors have fared best in efforts to manage them with monoclonal antibodies. Progress has been made in the management of non-Hodgkin's lymphoma.

The limited radiation dose delivered to tumors by radioantibodies appears sufficient to have therapeutic efficacy in the management of lymphoma. In therapy for other solid tumors, however, the doses may be insufficient unless bone marrow or stem cell support is provided. At present, two radiolabeled antibodies are in advanced developmental stages. One of these was approved by the U.S. Food and Drug Administration (FDA) in February of 2002. Both these agents are reactive with CD20. CD20 is a marker of normal B cells that also is present on nearly all non-Hodgkin's lymphomas of B-cell histologic composition. The marker is B-cell lineage but not B-cell tumor-specific (Fig. 47.1). CD20 is not present on normal bone marrow stem cells; thus these cells are not necessarily ablated with RIT.

Unlabeled anti-CD20 (rituximab; Rituxan) has been approved for therapy for lymphoma (rituximab; MabThera). The unlabeled anti-CD20 used in therapy is a chimeric antibody with a genetically engineered human constant region and the mouse variable region. Such antibodies are less likely to generate HAMA responses than are pure mouse antibodies, although when this agent is given to patients with lymphoma, who are

typically immunosuppressed, HAMA are infrequent. Unlabeled anti-CD20 is an effective treatment, but only approximately 48% of patients respond to the treatment, and only a small percentage achieve a complete response to therapy (33). For this reason, a more potent version of the therapy is needed. Efforts are underway and appear promising to combine unlabeled antibody therapy with chemotherapy; however, radioactively labeling CD20 is an alternative approach, now approved by the FDA.

^{131}I Anti-CD20: Nonmyeloablative

^{131}I has been used in several clinical studies of radiolabeled anti-CD20. The radioantibody has been used in both nonmyeloablative and myeloablative doses. The nonmyeloablative studies were initially performed at the University of Michigan by Kaminski and Wahl but then disseminated to many sites as efforts to commercialize the technology were implemented (3). The higher-dose myeloablative approach was pioneered and investigated by Press et al at the University of Washington (29).

In brief, the studies with ^{131}I anti-CD20 (now known as *131I tositumomab*; Bexxar), were designed initially to establish an MTD of the radioantibody. However, rather than being dosed on a millicurie per kilogram, millicurie per square meter, or millicurie basis, dose escalation was based on total-body dose estimated from a tracer study performed 1 week before the therapy. This estimate was based on the expectation that the treatments would be variably cleared from the blood owing to cross reactivity of the anti-CD20 antibody with normal tissues (see earlier). However, patient to patient variability is common, and can be corrected for in this approach. A variety of clinical studies have now been completed.

In the phase I-II single-center studies at the University of Michigan, it was established that the MTD of the antibody in previously treated patients, who had not received a bone marrow transplant, was a total-body dose of 75 cGy (3,30). At this dose level, toxicity was quite acceptable and mainly hematopoietic and consisted of reversible reductions in platelet and white blood cell counts. Antitumor efficacy was clearly shown in the patients in the pilot study, especially those with low-grade lymphoma. Use of cold antibody dosing before dosing of the labeled antibody was assessed and shown useful for redirecting the targeting of the radiolabeled antibody.

In the phase I-II studies at the University of Michigan, a total of 59 patients were ultimately enrolled (30). Fifty-three patients received the therapeutic dose of radioantibody. In this group of patients, it was established that the MTD was lower, at approximately 45 cGy, in patients who had received stem cell transplants. Among the 59 patients enrolled, 71% responded to the treatment, 34% with complete response. Response rates were higher, 83% among patients with low-grade or transformed non-Hodgkin's lymphoma versus a 41% response rate among patients with de novo intermediate-grade non-Hodgkin's lymphoma ($P < .005$). These results indicated that the histologic composition of lesions was quite important to the likelihood of response. The responses among patients achieving complete remission were reasonably durable, a median of 20.3 months. HAMA were infrequent (17%), despite the use of mouse antibodies. Five of the patients eventually had elevated levels of thyroid-stimulating hormone. This finding suggested the presence of early hypothyroidism. Five patients eventually had myelodysplasia. A small number of patients had long-term complete remission, as long as nearly 6 years. Of some interest was the retreatment of 16 patients as part of this study. In this group, 9 patients responded and 5 had complete responses, a response rate grossly similar to that for the original treatment (30).

This same therapeutic approach was taken forward into a multicenter dosimetry validation phase II study performed at six medical centers. This study was designed to determine whether patient-specific dosimetry could be performed at major academic centers and to further refine the toxicity and efficacy profile of the agent. In this study, 47 patients were enrolled, and 45 were treated at a dose of 65 to 75 cGy to the entire body. The overall response rate was 57%, and the rate of complete remission was 32%. Toxicity was mainly hematopoietic and was generally reversible. The median duration of complete response was 19.9 months. The study showed that the method clearly could be disseminated to other sites and that the efficacy of the treatment was reasonably high. Only one patient in this group developed HAMA (34).

A phase III pivotal trial was performed in which 60 patients with low-grade (36 patients) or transformed low-grade (23 patients) non-Hodgkin's lymphoma and 1 patient with mantle cell non-Hodgkin's lymphoma refractory to chemotherapy were enrolled and treated with the 75-cGy dose. The patients had to have undergone at least two previous chemotherapy regimens and to have had either no response or a response of less than 6 months' duration with the last regimen. In this study, the efficacy of ^{131}I tositumomab therapy was compared with that of the preceding chemotherapy. The expectation in the management of non-Hodgkin's lymphoma is that subsequent therapies will be less efficacious than the initial treatment and that only 3% of the patients have a complete remission due to previous treatment. With RIT, 32 patients had a longer response than with their own previous treatment with chemotherapy. In contrast, only 9 patients had a longer response to previous chemotherapy than they did to RIT ($P < 0.001$). Thus RIT was more effective than the last qualifying chemotherapy (35).

An additional trial with ^{131}I tositumomab was conducted in which the efficacy of the unlabeled antibody component was compared with that of the labeled material in a crossover study. In brief, in a preliminary analysis of the study of 78 treated patients, 42 of whom received hot antibody and 36 the cold, complete remission occurred in 33% treated with hot and in 8% treated with cold antibody ($P < 0.05$). Overall response rates were higher in the radiolabeled than in the unlabeled groups, at 55% and 17%, respectively ($P < 0.01$) (36). Responses were common (42% rate of complete remission) among patients from the cold group who crossed over to hot salvage therapy. Thus the labeled material contributes significantly to the efficacy of RIT for lymphoma.

^{131}I tositumomab has been explored as primary therapy for newly diagnosed non-Hodgkin's lymphoma. In a preliminary report of a study with 76 patients conducted at the University of Michigan, well over 90% of patients responded to the treatment; approximately 75% of the responses were complete (4). Development of HAMA was far more common in this group of patients, however. Overall, these data indicate that nonmyeloabla-

tive doses of ^{131}I tositumomab have considerable therapeutic efficacy and are reasonably well tolerated. Reduced thyroid function and myelodysplasia, though infrequent, must be considered longer-term events associated with therapy in a small number of cases. Myelodysplasia, however, can occur after chemotherapy alone in the care of these patients.

Myeloablative ^{131}I Anti-CD20 Therapy

Nonmyeloablative therapy is attractive, but only a minority of heavily pretreated patients have achieved complete response. An alternative approach is to use stem cell or bone marrow transplantation support and deliver severalfold more radioactivity and dose to patients with a goal of ablating the marrow and giving sufficient dose to damage second organs. Press et al. (29) used this approach in a dose-escalation scheme. These investigators found that frequent tumor responses could be achieved. Among 24 patients who had "favorable" biodistributions on tracer scans, 19 received therapeutic infusions of 234 to 777 mCi (2 to 10 times higher than nonmyeloablative doses). In these patients, cardiopulmonary toxicity was dose limiting, but response rates were high, 16 of 19 patients achieving a complete response.

This group of investigators (37) followed up with a report on 25 patients treated with ^{131}I tositumomab. Twenty-one were treated, and 16 of these had complete remission. The progression-free survival rate was more than 60% for a 2-year period. Follow-up evaluation of 25 patients treated with ^{131}I tositumomab showed elevated levels of thyroid-stimulating hormone in 60% of subjects, and generally durable remissions as long as 7 years in duration (31). The same group then went on to combine chemotherapy and RIT with administration of ^{131}I anti-CD20. Fifty-two patients received myeloablative doses of ^{131}I tositumomab and then received etoposide and cyclophosphamide and underwent stem cell transplantation. This aggressive regimen was designed to use dosimetry to deliver not more than 27 cGy to lungs. The progression-free survival rate in this group was 83%, which was high for this group of patients. Several deaths were reported as a result of the treatment, which is a very aggressive form of therapy (38). Nonetheless, these data strongly suggest that the dose of ^{131}I tositumomab given is related to the likelihood of response and the probability of durable response. The logistics of myeloablative therapy are somewhat complex, but this approach is feasible in centers accustomed to transplantation support. With both nonmyeloablative and myeloablative approaches and patient-specific dosimetry, ^{131}I tositumomab therapy is feasible and reasonably efficacious.

^{90}Y Anti-CD20

CD20 is an attractive target for RIT. ^{131}I is a suitable label for treating this antigen, which is a substantially noninternalizing antigen, but other labels can be used. Considerable effort has been undertaken to make ^{90}Y anti-CD20 therapy feasible. This form of treatment takes advantage of the pure β emitter characteristics of ^{90}Y. ^{90}Y also has an energetic β particle and may be better suited to therapy for heterogeneous or large tumors than is the less energetic ^{131}I. However, ^{131}I may be better suited to the management of smaller tumor foci (39). Several studies have been performed with ^{90}Y anti-CD20 antibodies. This form of treatment is FDA approved.

A relative disadvantage of use of ^{90}Y is the lack of a γ emission. This is a disadvantage in the sense that it is not possible to precisely track the biodistribution of ^{90}Y directly in vivo. To track ^{90}Y with single photon emission computed tomography, a surrogate isotope must be used, often ^{111}In. This isotope traces reasonably well the biodistribution of ^{90}Y but does not exactly trace it because ^{90}Y is somewhat more bone-avid in some studies. In any case, ^{111}In is a reasonably good surrogate and has been used to estimate the dosimetry of ^{90}Y in vivo.

Using ^{90}Y anti-CD20 antibodies, Knox et al. (40) conducted a phase I-II study with 18 patients treated with doses of up to 50 mCi ^{90}Y anti-CD20. In this study, unlabeled anti-CD20 antibody improved radiolabeled antibody biodistribution. Myelosuppression was the main toxicity, and an overall response rate of 72% was achieved, with 6 cases of complete remission and 7 cases of partial remission. The doses in the study were not adjusted for body mass or size or for body surface area. Doses greater than 40 mCi were myeloablative. This study clearly showed feasibility and promise for the ^{90}Y approach.

Additional studies have been reported in which chimeric anti-CD20 was used before dosing and followed by ^{90}Y murine anti-CD20 RIT. The ^{90}Y agent, with ^{90}Y conjugated by the mitoxantrone–diethylenetriaminepentaacetic acid (MX-DTPA) chelator, is known as ibritumomab tiuxetan (Zevalin). In a phase I-II study (41) of the agent with 51 patients, the MTD was established to be 0.4 mCi/kg (0.3 mCi/kg in patients with platelet counts less than 150,000/μL). The overall response rate was 67% among the 51 patients for whom treatment was intended; 26% of the responses were complete remission. Fifty-six percent had complete remission in low-grade tumors. For intermediate-grade disease, the overall response rate was 43%. For mantle cell lymphoma (3 cases), no responses were seen. Toxicity was mainly hematopoietic and was correlated with the extent of marrow involvement with tumor (26,27,42,43).

A phase III study was initiated and accumulated 143 patients to compare unlabeled anti-CD20 and ^{90}Y anti-CD20. In this study, 80% of patients responded to ^{90}Y ibritumomab, although 44% responded to rituximab ($P < 0.05$). The latter finding supported the added value of the radiolabel for the treatment effect. Dosimetry was calculated for 72 patients. The investigators were unable to clearly define a relation between red marrow dose estimated with ^{111}In ibritomomab tiuxetan and toxicity, which was mainly hematopoietic (42). There was a better relation in this study between bone marrow reserve and fractional involvement with tumor than between bone marrow reserve and radiation dose. This finding shows that both the marrow and the radiation dose to the marrow are key elements in determining whether a given treatment will be myelotoxic. It may be that ^{111}In is simply inadequate as a surrogate for ^{90}Y, and this is why the predictive value of the assays is modest. It also clearly indicates that marrow status is important in predicting toxicity (an ^{111}In scan is required before dosing with ^{90}Y agent, however). Toxicity with these agents is not trivial, and grade III and IV hematopoietic toxicity has been commonly observed. Despite such concerns, an FDA advisory panel has given a favorable recommendation regarding limited approval of this agent for clinical use. On February 19, 2002, FDA approval was granted for Zevalin therapy.

Given the approval of Zevalin as a therapeutic agent, the following data are reported in the package labeling, as are some otherwise unpublished data (43). Specifically, Zevalin received two separate approvals, a full approval and an accelerated approval, on the basis of results of two major efficacy studies in the United States. Determination of the effectiveness of the Zevalin therapeutic regimen in a patient population with relapses or with refractory disease was based on overall response rate. The effects of the Zevalin therapeutic regimen on survival are not known. The first efficacy study, on which the full approval is based, was conducted with 54 patients with relapsed follicular lymphoma who no longer adequately responded to Rituxan. Seventy-four percent had an overall response to treatment with Zevalin, 15% of patients achieving complete remission with therapy, according to the International Workshop Response Criteria (IWRC). The second study, a phase III, randomized, controlled trial, the results of which support accelerated approval, was conducted with 143 patients with relapsed or refractory, low-grade or follicular non-Hodgkin's lymphoma or transformed B-cell non-Hodgkin's lymphoma. The 73 patients who received the Zevalin therapeutic regimen had an overall response rate of 80% compared with 56% among 70 patients who received Rituxan alone, according to the IWRC. Thirty percent of patients given Zevalin achieved a complete remission, and 4% achieved an unconfirmed complete remission with therapy, compared with 16% of patients given Rituxan who achieved complete remission and 4% who achieved unconfirmed complete remission, according to the IWRC. In safety data based on the records of 349 patients, the most serious adverse reactions of the Zevalin therapeutic regimen included severe infusion reactions (hypotension, angioedema, hypoxia, or bronchospasm) and severe and prolonged cytopenia, including thrombocytopenia (61% of patients with platelet counts less than 50,000/μL) and neutropenia (57% of patients with absolute neutrophil counts less than 1,000/μL) in patients with a platelet count of 150,000/μL or less before treatment. Severe infections (predominately bacterial in origin) and hemorrhage, including fatal cerebral hemorrhage, have occurred in a minority of patients in clinical studies. Myeloid malignant disease and dyscrasia (myelodysplastic syndrome) also occurred. The most common toxicities reported were neutropenia, thrombocytopenia, anemia, gastrointestinal symptoms (nausea, vomiting, abdominal pain, and diarrhea), increased cough, dyspnea, dizziness, arthralgia, anorexia, and ecchymosis. Hematologic toxicity often was severe and prolonged, whereas most nonhematologic toxicity was mild.

The following boxed warning label appears on the Zevalin product label:

> Boxed Warning Summary: Zevalin should only be used by health care professionals qualified by training and experience in the safe use of radionuclides. Fatal Infusion Reactions: Deaths have occurred within 24 hours of Rituximab infusions. These fatalities were associated with an infusion reaction symptom complex that included hypoxia, pulmonary infiltrates, acute respiratory distress syndrome, myocardial infarction, ventricular fibrillation, or cardiogenic shock. Prolonged and Severe Cytopenias: Yttrium-90 Zevalin administration results in severe and prolonged cytopenias in most patients.

Thus two CD20-based agents have been subjected to phase III studies and appear to demonstrate efficacy and known toxicity profiles. Direct comparative studies between the two agents have not yet been performed to compare safety and efficacy profiles. The ^{131}I agent offers the distinct advantage of individualized dosing, which may be safer. The ^{90}Y agent, however, offers greater simplicity of administration. In most states in the United States, both agents can be administered to outpatients at nonmyeloablative dose levels.

Pretargeted Anti-CD20 Therapy

The biotin-streptavidin pretargeting approach has been evaluated in preclinical models and in the clinic with anti-CD20. In the preclinical model systems, pretargeting is more effective than direct radioantibody targeting, having a greater therapeutic index and lesser toxicity (10). Pilot studies have been performed with 10 patients. In these studies, Rituximab was conjugated to streptavidin and given intravenously; 34 hours later, a preclearing agent, biotinylated galactosamine, was given. This agent targets the liver and removes intact radioantibody from the bloodstream. [111]In or ^{90}Y DOTA biotin was given. A dose of 30 to 50 mCi/m² of ^{90}Y DOTA biotin was given and showed overall excellent tumor targeting with tumor and whole-body uptake ratios of approximately 38:1. This ratio seems higher than those reported for ^{131}I anti-CD20, which have been approximately 10:1 to 15:1. Among the 7 patients who received 30 mCi/m² or more ^{90}Y DOTA biotin, 4 achieved responses. Three of the responses were complete, and one was partial (44). Development of human anti-streptavidin antibodies was the rule and may preclude retreatment. No grade IV toxicity was seen, including in the marrow. This approach is quite promising (44).

Anti CD-22

CD22 is another B-cell marker being used as a target for RIT studies. Although this reagent is earlier in the development process, this agent targets an internalizing pan–B-cell antigen. Unlabeled anti-CD22 appears to have antitumor activity. Both ^{131}I and ^{90}Y anti-CD20 have been shown to have antitumor activity when conjugated to the humanized anti CD22 monoclonal antibody. Juweid et al. (45) reported on 14 patients treated with ^{131}I LL2 (anti-CD22) at doses designed to deliver 50 to 100 cGy to the marrow. These doses resulted in myelosuppression and some antitumor response (2 of 13 patients treated with ^{131}I LL2). When ^{90}Y anti-CD22 was used, 2 of 7 patients responded. Given that CD22 internalizes and that ^{90}Y is better retained in the cells than is ^{131}I, ^{90}Y anti-CD22 is being carried forth in additional clinical trials of therapy for non-Hodgkin's lymphoma. Studies with myeloablative doses of anti-CD22 have shown even higher response rates and rates of complete remission (46).

Lym 1

The first radioantibody used to treat B-cell non-Hodgkin's lymphoma was the Lym 1 antibody, pioneered by DeNardo et al. (47). This agent, which binds to a variant HLA subclass on B-cell lymphoma, has been used in several trials of treatment. [131]I, ^{90}Y, and [67]Cu have been evaluated as radiolabels. It is clear that there are partial and complete responses to this form of therapy. In a study with 21 patients, those who received multiple fractionated doses of [131]I Lym 1 had the greatest probability of response,

and those receiving 100 mCi/m² (n = 3) all achieved complete response. This finding is consistent with the general concept that patients receiving the highest radiation dose are most likely to achieve complete response (48). Although [131]I Lym 1 was a pioneering reagent, the anti-CD20 reagents are now used far more often. Lym 1 is not likely to be commercialized in the near term.

Other Therapeutic Radioantibodies for Non-Hodgkin's Lymphoma

Several other antibodies have been used in the management of non-Hodgkin's lymphoma. For example, the OKB7 antibody, which is reactive with CD21, was evaluated in a phase I dose-escalation trial with 19 patients. Despite dose levels up to 200 mCi, only 1 partial response was observed (49). Results with anti-CD37 were only slightly better. In 11 patients treated with ^{131}I anti-CD37, the MTD proved to be approximately 40 cGy total-body dose. One complete response and one partial response were achieved. Thus activity of the agent was modest, and toxicity was consistently hematopoietic (50). Additional therapeutic efforts have been devoted to use of antiidiotype antibodies for management of non-Hodgkin's lymphoma. This approach is complex but was tested in 9 patients given 10 to 54 mCi of ^{90}Y antiidiotype antibody. These studies were complicated by idiotype circulating in the blood, which had to be cleared before RIT could be given. Nonetheless, 2 of 9 patients achieved a complete response and 1 of 9 a partial response (51). Logistical considerations of a unique antibody for each patient make such an approach unlikely to be commercially viable.

T-cell Lymphoma

The minority of non-Hodgkin's lymphomas are T-cell in histologic composition. There are T cell–associated differentiation antigens that have served as targets for RIT. This area has been less extensively studied than has B-cell non-Hodgkin's lymphoma, but some results have been promising. As early as 1987, Rosen et al. (52) used ^{131}I antibody T-101 (anti-CD5) to treat 5 patients with cutaneous T-cell lymphoma; they were given approximately 100 to 150 mCi of radioantibody. All of the patients responded, although responses were brief. These patients were immunocompetent and developed HAMA, which limited the effectiveness of additional therapy. This same antibody labeled with ^{90}Y was used to treat 10 patients with advanced chronic lymphocytic leukemia and cutaneous T-cell lymphoma. Imaging was done with ^{111}In-labeled antibody, and many lesions were detected. [90]Y had greater bone targeting than did ^{111}In, however. Partial responses occurred in 5 patients and lasted a median of 23 weeks. All patients developed HAMA. Myelosuppression was dose limiting (53). Thus RIT for T-cell non-Hodgkin's lymphoma lags RIT for B-cell disease at present.

Hodgkin's Lymphoma

Hodgkin's lymphoma is highly curable with chemotherapy or radiation therapy in many cases. However, recurrences are troublesome and can be incurable. There is a need for additional therapies for recurrent Hodgkin's lymphoma. Hodgkin's differs from other lymphomas in that the cell of origin often is not of a clear B- or T-cell lineage. Most therapeutic efforts to date have centered on the use of a radiolabeled polyclonal antibody reactive with ferritin. Herpst et al. (54) reported on the treatment of 87 patients with Hodgkin's disease. A response rate greater than 60% was reported with an average duration of approximately 6 months. This form of therapy is promising, but polyclonal antibodies are logistically extremely difficult to take forward as commercial therapeutic agents because of their considerable variability in affinity and composition from lot to lot.

Leukemia

Leukemia spans a broad range of cells of origin. Some are of B-cell histologic derivation, others T-cell, and others of a more primitive lineage. B-cell chronic lymphocytic leukemia has been managed in some studies with radiolabeled pan–B-cell antibodies. For example, DeNardo et al. (47) reported on the use of Lym 1 in therapy for B-cell chronic lymphocytic leukemia. Some patients treated with anti-CD20 have had circulating tumor cells present along with solid tumor foci (30,47). Clear evidence of antitumor efficacy has been shown, but the role of RIT in the care of these patients is undefined at present.

T-cell leukemia has been managed with ^{90}Y-labeled anti-Tac monoclonal antibody reactive with the interleukin-2 receptor. High-affinity interleukin-2 receptor is expressed on many of these tumors. Eighteen patients were treated with ^{90}Y anti-Tac, and 9 responded, two of whom had complete responses (55). This form of treatment is encouraging, but matching the particle path length to the disease volume is an important consideration. ^{90}Y may be a suboptimal choice for small or isolated tumors.

Acute leukemia has been managed with RIT. Two general approaches have been investigated—myeloablative and nonmyeloablative. The former approach is used with a plan to achieve bone marrow and tumor ablation, although the latter is used to achieve tumor kill while preserving marrow function. The most extensively evaluated approach has been use of the M-195 (anti-CD33) antibody. A dose-escalation trial with ^{131}I in the treatment of 24 patients showed clear targeting to tumor foci within the marrow in 22 patients, although in 23 patients, decreases in blood cell counts were achieved (56). Severe pancytopenia was achieved at doses of 135 mCi/m^2 or higher, and 3 of 8 patients had sufficient marrow cell kill to undergo transplantation, and 3 achieved marrow remission. Development of HAMA was common. This same agent has been humanized, and this reagent labeled with ^{131}I has been combined with chemotherapy before bone marrow transplantation. In such an algorithm, doses of up to 230 mCi/m^2 have been given, and complete remission has been commonly achieved (in 18 patients) with some durability of response. The radioantibody also has been given to patients who had achieved complete remission. In this group, some brief conversion of marrow polymerase chain reaction from positive to negative was achieved, and some durability of response has been observed (57). The α emitter Bi-213 has been used as a radiolabel and pilot studies of therapy (18). α Emitters may be of particular value in this type of application because of their short path length.

Some investigators have assessed use of *131*I anti-CD45 (BC8) therapy before transplantation. This treatment was evaluated in the care of 23 patients and combined with cyclophosphamide (Cytoxan) therapy and total-body irradiation. No excess toxicity was seen over that expected for the chemotherapy and total-body irradiation, and a substantial number of patients responded to the treatment, which delivered 4 to 30 Gy to the bone marrow (58). Another bone marrow conditioning approach has been studied, specifically the use of ^{188}Re-labeled anti-CD66 monoclonal antibody in the treatment of patients with acute myeloid leukemia and myelodysplastic syndrome. This treatment delivered, on average, 15.3 cGy to the marrow and 7.4 Gy to the kidneys. RIT was followed by chemotherapy, total-body irradiation to 12 Gy, and marrow transplantation. The regimen was associated with a 6% treatment-related death rate 100 days after treatment and a 22% treatment-related death rate 18 months after therapy. The relapse rate was 20% to 30%. Renal toxicity occurred in 17% of patients (59). Another approach to these treatments is the use of ^{188}Re anti–NCA-95, which has been preliminarily explored for dosimetric feasibility (60). The data suggest that marrow conditioning regimens that include radiolabeled monoclonal antibodies are quite promising but are in the early stages of clinical evaluation.

Solid Tumors
Colon Carcinoma

Carcinoma of the colon was the first tumor for which monoclonal antibody imaging was approved for clinical use. Therapy for this disease is more challenging than is imaging owing to the radioresistance of the lesions and the only modest tumor to background ratios achieved. Several monoclonal antibodies have been used for therapy, including those reactive with CEA, tumor-associated glycoprotein-72 (TAG-72), and other tumor-associated glycoproteins. Although some antitumor responses have occurred, the therapy has not yet been particularly effective. For example, when the ^{125}I-labeled 17-1A antibody was used, no objective responses occurred in 28 patients (61). When the ^{131}I CC49 antibody was used in 24 patients, there were no major responses (62). When the same antibody was used after interferon therapy to enhance antigen expression, no major responses were observed in 14 patients (63). When NP4 immunoglobulin G1 monoclonal antibody labeled with ^{131}I was used to treat 29 patients with colorectal cancer, no complete responses occurred (64). F(ab')$_2$ fragments of anti-CEA were given in higher doses for RIT, but responses were rare—one partial response at high dose (65). When ^{125}I A33 antibody was used to treat 21 patients, no partial or complete responses were observed (66). The best responses in management of this disease have been seen with pretargeting with the NR-LU-10 (anti–Ep-CAM) antibody but with considerable toxicity to the intestine owing to antigenic cross-reactivity (67). This pre-targeting approach delivers higher radiation doses to tumor than do conventional targeting approaches. Thus although colorectal cancer can be imaged reasonably well with monoclonal antibodies, it cannot be effectively controlled with this approach with the technologies evaluated to date.

Ovarian Carcinoma

Ovarian carcinoma is somewhat similar to colorectal cancer in its biologic characteristics. Because ovarian cancer often initially distributes intraperitoneally, regional (intraperitoneal) delivery approaches have been used to enhance delivery of radioantibody to intraperitoneal tumor foci. Intraperitoneal administration of ^{131}I-labeled monoclonal antibodies in the treatment of 29 patients showed no response in larger tumor foci. There were responses in lesions 2 cm or less in diameter or in patients with positive intraperitoneal tumor cells; 3 of 5 patients with positive intraperitoneal washings had a clearing of the positive cells after therapy (68). [90]Y antibodies appeared slightly more active (69). Intraperitoneal delivery of the MOv 18 antibody labeled with *131*I in low-tumor-volume intraperitoneal disease resulted in complete responses in 5 of 16 patients treated after positive results were obtained at second-look surgery. These patients had short responses in general, a mean of 10.5 months (70). In 17 patients treated with [186]Re NR-LU-10, tumor size decreased in several of the patients with primary tumors less than 1 cm in diameter (71). Studies with OC 125 antibody F(ab′)₂ did not have major responses (72). After intraperitoneal treatment with Lu-177 CC49 anti–TAG-72 antibody, 1 of 13 patients with large scale disease had a partial response, and patients with small tumors with positive cytologic results had only reasonably good disease-free survival rates (73). This same radioantibody combined with intraperitoneal paclitaxel (Taxol) has shown promise in RIT studies; 2 of 12 patients have had a partial response (74). Longer survival periods have been reported by Epenetos et al (68), who evaluated 52 patients after RIT. The treatment was associated with the longest survival period among patients who had achieved complete remission after standard chemotherapy. After such therapy, 78% of patients survived more than 10 years. These data suggest that RIT for ovarian carcinoma can be somewhat effective, especially if tumor volumes are low.

Breast Carcinoma

Only a limited amount of RIT has been performed for breast cancer. Challenges include identifying the proper antigenic target for therapy. Chimeric L6 antibody labeled with ^{131}I has been used in such treatments. Several patients were reported to have partial tumor responses (75). RIT for breast cancer with the [90]Y BrE-3 antibody has been reported. Six patients had no partial or complete response, and development of HAMA was common (76). Although data are limited, breast cancer is somewhat radiosensitive, and it is possible that higher-dose myeloablative regimens to manage breast cancer with RIT may be efficacious. To date, however, RIT for breast cancer is not routinely effective or performed, except in research trials.

Brain Tumors

Brain tumors are a locally aggressive and often lethal disease. Patients have been treated in experimental studies locoregionally with radiolabeled monoclonal antibodies. At present, this remains a research application, and several approaches have been tried. Riva et al. (77) reported on intralesional delivery to 111 patients with brain tumors managed with ^{131}I BC2 and BC4 anti-tenascin antibodies. Of this group, 74 patients participated in a phase II arm of the study. One of these patients had a complete response, 9 had partial responses, and the survival rate was 18 to 25 months, with better results for smaller tumors. Brown et al. (78) used 81C6 anti-tenascin monoclonal antibody in RIT for brain tumors after regional delivery. They were able to establish an intracavitary MTD of 120 mCi of antibody, which averaged a dose of approximately 43 Gy to the cyst wall of the brain tumor. Partial responses have occurred among some patients treated with this approach (79). In the phase I-II trial, investigators treated 42 patients with ^{131}I-labeled 81C6 monoclonal antibody in administered doses up to 180 mCi. Dose-limiting toxicity was observed at doses greater than 120 mCi and consisted of delayed neurotoxicity. None of the patients had major hematologic toxicity. The median survival time for patients with glioblastoma multiforme was 69 weeks and for all patients was 79 weeks. This result was considered encouraging.

Another approach to brain tumor therapy has been the biotin-streptavidin approach. With the three-step approach—biotinylated anti-tenascin antibody, streptavidin, and ^{90}Y biotin—in that order, the MTD was determined for 24 patients with recurrent or persistent high-grade glioma. An objective response rate of approximately 25% was reported, but only two partial responses and no complete responses occurred (80). This approach is early in the evaluative phase.

Other Tumors

Several other types of cancer have been studied with RIT with varying, though limited, results. Early evaluative studies of therapy for head and neck cancer have been conducted with the U36 monoclonal antibody labeled with [186]Re (81). Medullary cancer of the thyroid, which makes high levels of CEA, has been treated with anti-CEA antibodies, F(ab′)₂ fragments, or hybrid chimeric antibodies and radiohapten (82,83). Preliminarily encouraging results have been observed, but no complete responses. Although renal cancer and prostate cancer have been managed with RIT, responses rates have been low or absent, and currently there is not effective RIT for these cancers (84,85). Data on hepatoma have been somewhat encouraging, but therapy for these tumors is complicated by combination of the therapy with chemotherapy (86). Nonetheless, some hepatomas appear to respond well to anti-ferritin therapy and therapy with other antibodies in pilot studies (86). Some of the earliest RIT was performed with polyclonal antibodies by Order et al. (87) to manage hepatoma. Neuroblastoma also has been managed with radioantibodies in limited trials, and the therapy has shown promise (88).

PRACTICAL CONSIDERATIONS FOR ADMINISTRATION OF THERAPY

Revised Nuclear Regulatory Commission Rules Allowing Outpatient Therapy

Traditionally, patients treated with ^{131}I for thyroid cancer were hospitalized for a few days until radioactivity levels cleared from the body to less than 30 mCi. The rules governing release of patients after radioactive therapy were changed by the Nuclear Regulatory Commission (NRC) in the past several years in recognition of the low risk such patients present to society. It is possible in all NRC states and in some "agreement" states to treat cancer patients with ^{131}I in an outpatient setting if specific written instructions for patient education and patient-specific or drug-specific calculations are made. This change is logistically important because it decreases the resources required for delivery of this form of treatment. Several studies have shown this approach to be feasible and safe (89,90).

Implementation of Radioimmunotherapy in Practice

RIT should not be used in the care of patients with cancer unless the treatment is carefully integrated into the overall treatment plan for the patient. A medical oncologist usually is involved in the decisions about whether the therapy is appropriate, as is a nuclear medicine physician, often a radiation oncologist, in close association with pathology, radiology, and radiation safety and physics colleagues. Having a close working relationship and open communication is key to the success of such endeavors.

Radioantibodies can be expected to be the most expensive radiopharmaceuticals yet developed, on the basis of the costs of unlabeled antibody therapy for cancer. Drug costs will represent a large fraction of the overall cost of RIT. Costs associated with radiation safety, dosimetry, and pharmacy dispensing also are expected to be greater than currently faced, but the high costs are needed for effective care delivery. The approaches to treatment are fundamentally the same as those to other radiopharmaceutical therapies in nuclear medicine. With FDA approval of ^{90}Y anti-CD20 RIT, RIT is now established as an important part of the treatment of patients with cancer.

REFERENCES

1. Ehrlich P. In: Himmelweit F, ed. *Immunology and cancer research.* Vol 2. London: Pergamon Press, 1957.
2. Order SE. The history and progress of serologic immunotherapy and radiodiagnosis. *Radiology* 1976;118:219–223.
3. Kaminski MS, Zasadny KR, Francis IR, et al. Radioimmunotherapy of B-cell lymphoma with [131I]anti-B1 (anti-CD20) antibody. *N Engl J Med* 1993;329:459–465.
4. Wahl RL, Zasadny KR, Estes J, et al. Single center experience with iodine I 131 tositumomab radioimmunotherapy for previously untreated follicular lymphoma. *J Nucl Med* 2000;41:78p–79p.
5. Wahl RL, Parker CW and Philpott GW. Improved radioimaging and tumor localization with monoclonal F(ab')2. *J Nucl Med* 1983;24:316–325.
6. Wahl RL, Liebert M. Improved radiolabeled monoclonal antibody uptake by lavage of intraperitoneal carcinomatosis in mice. *J Nucl Med* 1989;30:60–65.
7. Wahl RL, Fisher S. Intraperitoneal delivery of monoclonal antibodies: enhanced regional delivery advantage using intravenous unlabeled anti-mouse antibody. *Nucl Med Biol* 1987;14:611–615.
8. Wahl RL, Piko CR, Beers BA, et al. Systemic perfusion: a method of enhancing relative tumor uptake of radiolabeled monoclonal antibodies. *Nucl Med Biol* 1988;15:611–616.
9. Goodwin DA. A new approach to the problem of targeting specific monoclonal antibodies to human tumors using anti-hapten chimeric antibodies. *Int J Rad Appl Instrum B* 1989;16:645–651.

10. Press OW, Corcoran M, Subbiah K, et al. A comparative evaluation of conventional and pretargeted radioimmunotherapy of CD20-expressing lymphoma xenografts. *Blood* 2001;98:2535–2543.
11. Cremonesi M, Ferrari M, Chinol M, et al. Three-step radioimmunotherapy with yttrium-90 biotin: dosimetry and pharmacokinetics in cancer patients. *Eur J Nucl Med* 1999;26:110–120.
12. Gruaz-Guyon A, Janevik-Ivanovska E, Raguin O, et al. Radiolabeled bivalent haptens for tumor immunodetection and radioimmunotherapy. *Q J Nucl Med* 2001;45:201–206.
13. O'Donoghue JA. Implications of nonuniform tumor doses for radioimmunotherapy. *J Nucl Med* 1999;40:1337–1341.
14. Flynn AA, Pedley RB, Green AJ, et al. Optimizing radioimmunotherapy by matching dose distribution with tumor structure using 3D reconstructions of serial images. *Cancer Biother Radiopharm* 2001;16:391–400.
15. Rayman RR and Wahl RL. Magnetically-enhanced protection of bone marrow from beta particles emitted by bone-seeking radionuclides: theory of application. *Med Phys* 1995;22:1285–1292.
16. O'Donoghue JA, Sgouros G, Divgi CR, et al. Single-dose versus fractionated radioimmunotherapy: model comparisons for uniform tumor dosimetry. *J Nucl Med* 2000;41:538–547.
17. Barendswaard EC, Humm JL, O'Donoghue JA, et al. Relative therapeutic efficacy of (125)I- and (131)I-labeled monoclonal antibody A33 in a human colon cancer xenograft. *J Nucl Med* 2001;42:1251–1256.
18. Yao Z, Garmestani K, Wong KJ, et al. Comparative cellular catabolism and retention of astatine-, bismuth-, and lead-radiolabeled internalizing monoclonal antibody. *J Nucl Med* 2001;42:1538–1544.
19. McDevitt MR, Ma D, Lai LT, et al. Tumor therapy with targeted atomic nanogenerators. *Science* 2001;294:1537–1540.
20. Sharkey RM, Behr TM, Mattes MJ, et al. Advantage of residualizing radiolabels for an internalizing antibody against the B-cell lymphoma antigen, CD22. *Cancer Immunol Immunother* 1997;44:179–188.
21. DeNardo GL, DeNardo SJ, O'Donnell RT, et al. Are radiometal-labeled antibodies better than iodine-131-labeled antibodies: comparative pharmacokinetics and dosimetry of copper-67-, iodine-131-, and yttrium-90-labeled Lym-1 antibody in patients with non-Hodgkin's lymphoma. *Clin Lymphoma* 2000;1:118–126.
22. Cardillo TM, Ying Z, Gold DV. Therapeutic advantage of (90)yttrium-versus (131)iodine-labeled PAM4 antibody in experimental pancreatic cancer. *Clin Cancer Res* 2001;7:3186–3192.
23. Harbert JC. Radioiodine therapy of differentiated thyroid cancer. In: Harbert JC, ed. *Nuclear medicine therapy* New York: Thieme Medical Publishers, 1986:37–89.
24. Robertson JS. Absorbed dose calculations. In: Harbert JC, ed. *Nuclear medicine therapy.* New York: Thieme Medical Publishers, 1986:285–296.
25. Wahl RL, Kroll S, Zasadny KR. Patient-specific whole-body dosimetry: principles and a simplified method for clinical implementation. *J Nucl Med* 1998;39[8 Suppl]:14S–20S.
26. Wiseman GA, White CA, Stabin M, et al. Phase I/II 90Y-Zevalin (yttrium-90 ibritumomab tiuxetan, IDEC-Y2B8) radioimmunotherapy dosimetry results in relapsed or refractory non-Hodgkin's lymphoma. *Eur J Nucl Med.* 2000;27:766–777.
27. Juweid ME, Zhang CH, Blumenthal RD, et al. Prediction of hematologic toxicity after radioimmunotherapy with (131)I-labeled anticarcinoembryonic antigen monoclonal antibodies: *J Nucl Med* 1999;40:1609–1616.
28. Liu T, Meredith RF, Saleh MN, et al. Correlation of toxicity with treatment parameters for 131I-CC49 radioimmunotherapy in three phase II clinical trials. *Cancer Biother Radiopharm* 1997;12:79–87.
29. Press OW, Eary JF, Appelbaum FR, et al. Radiolabeled-antibody therapy of B-cell lymphoma with autologous bone marrow support. *N Engl J Med* 1993;329:1219–1224.
30. Kaminski MS, Estes J, Zasadny KR, et al. Radioimmunotherapy with iodine (131)I tositumomab for relapsed or refractory B-cell non-Hodgkin lymphoma: updated results and long-term follow-up of the University of Michigan experience. *Blood* 2000;96:1259–1266.
31. Liu SY, Eary JF, Petersdorf SH, et al. Follow-up of relapsed B-cell lymphoma patients treated with iodine-131-labeled anti-CD20 anti-

body and autologous stem-cell rescue. *J Clin Oncol* 1998;16:3270–3278.

32. Koral KF, Dewaraja Y, Clarke LA, et al. Tumor-absorbed-dose estimates versus response in tositumomab therapy of previously untreated patients with follicular non-Hodgkin's lymphoma: preliminary report. *Cancer Biother Radiopharm* 2000;15:347–355.
33. IDEC Pharmaceuticals, Inc. Rituximab package insert.
34. Vose JM, Wahl RL, Saleh M, et al. Multicenter phase II study of iodine-131 tositumomab for hemotherapy-relapsed/refractory low-grade and transformed low-grade B-cell non-Hodgkin's lymphomas. *J Clin Oncol* 2000;18:1316–1323.
35. Kaminski MS, Zelenetz AD, Press OW, et al. Pivotal study of iodine I 131 tositumomab for chemotherapy-refractory low-grade or transformed low-grade B-cell non-Hodgkin's lymphomas. *J Clin Oncol* 2001;19:3918–3928.
36. Davis TA, Kaminski MS, Leonard JP, et al. Results of a randomized study of Bexxar™ (tositumomab and iodine I 131 tositumomab) vs. unlabeled tositumomab in patients with relapsed or refractory low-grade or transformed non-Hodgkin's lymphoma (NHL). Presented at the 43rd Annual Meeting of the American Society of Hematology, Orlando, FL, December 7–1, 2001.
37. Press OW, Eary JF, Appelbaum FR, et al. Phase II trial of 131I-B1 (anti-CD20) antibody therapy with autologous stem cell transplantation for relapsed B cell lymphomas. *Lancet* 1995;346:336–340.
38. Press OW, Eary JF, Gooley T, et al. A phase I/II trial of iodine-131-tositumomab (anti-CD20), etoposide, cyclophosphamide, and autologous stem cell transplantation for relapsed B-cell lymphomas. *Blood* 2000;96:2934–2942.
39. O'Donoghue JA, Bardies M, Wheldon TE. Relationships between tumor size and curability for uniformly targeted therapy with beta-emitting radionuclides. *J Nucl Med* 1995;36:1902–1909.
40. Knox SJ, Goris ML, Trisler K, et al. Yttrium-90-labeled anti-CD20 monoclonal antibody therapy of recurrent B-cell lymphoma. *Clin Cancer Res* 1996;2:457–470.
41. Witzig TE, White CA, Wiseman GA, et al. Phase I/II trial of IDEC-Y2B8 radioimmunotherapy for treatment of relapsed or refractory CD20(+) B-cell non-Hodgkin's lymphoma. *J Clin Oncol* 1999;17:3793–3803.
42. Witzig TE. Radioimmunotherapy for patients with relapsed B-cell non-Hodgkin lymphoma. *Cancer Chemother Pharmacol* 2001;48[Suppl 1]:S91–S95.
43. IDEC Pharmaceuticals. Zevalin package insert.
44. Weiden PL, Breitz HB. Pretargeted radioimmunotherapy (PRIT) for treatment of non-Hodgkin's lymphoma (NHL). *Crit Rev Oncol Hematol* 2001;40:37–51.
45. Juweid M, Sharkey RM, Markowitz A, et al. Treatment of non-Hodgkin's lymphoma with radiolabeled murine, chimeric, or humanized LL2, an anti-CD22 monoclonal antibody. *Cancer Res* 1995;55[23 Suppl]:5899s–5907s.
46. Behr TM, Wormann B, Gramatzki M, et al. Low- versus high-dose radioimmunotherapy with humanized anti-CD22 or chimeric anti-CD20 antibodies in a broad spectrum of B cell-associated malignancies. *Clin Cancer Res* 1999;5[10 Suppl]:3304s–3314s.
47. DeNardo GL, O'Donnell RT, Rose LM, et al. Milestones in the development of Lym-1 therapy. *Hybridoma* 1999;18:1–11.
48. DeNardo GL, DeNardo SJ, Goldstein DS, et al. Maximum-tolerated dose, toxicity, and efficacy of (131)I-Lym-1 antibody for fractionated radioimmunotherapy of non-Hodgkin's lymphoma. *J Clin Oncol* 1998;16:3246–3256.
49. Czuczman MS, Straus DJ, Divgi CR, et al. Phase I dose-escalation trial of iodine 131-labeled monoclonal antibody OKB7 in patients with non-Hodgkin's lymphoma. *J Clin Oncol* 1993;11:2021–2029.
50. Kaminski MS, Fig LM, Zasadny KR, et al. Imaging, dosimetry, and radioimmunotherapy with iodine 131-labeled anti-CD37 antibody in B-cell lymphoma. *J Clin Oncol* 1992;10:1696–1711.
51. White CA, Halpern SE, Parker BA, et al. Radioimmunotherapy of relapsed B-cell lymphoma with yttrium 90 anti-idiotype monoclonal antibodies. *Blood* 1996;87:3640–3649.
52. Rosen ST, Zimmer AM, Goldman-Leikin R, et al. Radioimmunodetection and radioimmunotherapy of cutaneous T cell lymphomas using an 131I-labeled monoclonal antibody: an Illinois Cancer Council Study. *J Clin Oncol* 1987;5:562–573.
53. Foss FM, Raubitscheck A, Mulshine JL, et al. Phase I study of the pharmacokinetics of a radioimmunoconjugate, 90Y-T101, in patients with CD5-expressing leukemia and lymphoma. *Clin Cancer Res* 1998;4:2691–2700.
54. Herpst JM, Klein JL, Leichner PK, et al. Survival of patients with resistant Hodgkin's disease after polyclonal yttrium 90-labeled antiferritin treatment. *J Clin Oncol* 1995;13:2394–2400.
55. Waldmann TA, White JD, Carrasquillo JA, et al. Radioimmunotherapy of interleukin-2R alpha–expressing adult T-cell leukemia with yttrium-90-labeled anti-Tac. *Blood* 1995;86:4063–4075.
56. Schwartz MA, Lovett DR, Redner A, et al. Dose-escalation trial of M195 labeled with iodine 131 for cytoreduction and marrow ablation in relapsed or refractory myeloid leukemias. *J Clin Oncol* 1993;11:294–303.
57. Sgouros G, Ballangrud AM, Jurcic JG, et al. Pharmacokinetics and dosimetry of an alpha-particle emitter labeled antibody: 213Bi-HuM195 (anti-CD33) in patients with leukemia. *J Nucl Med* 1999;40:1935–1946.
58. Matthews DC, Appelbaum FR, Eary JF, et al. Development of a marrow transplant regimen for acute leukemia using targeted hematopoietic irradiation delivered by 131I-labeled anti-CD45 antibody, combined with cyclophosphamide and total body irradiation. *Blood* 1995;85:1122–1131.
59. Bunjes D, Buchmann I, Duncker C, et al. Rhenium 188-labeled anti-CD66 (a, b, c, e) monoclonal antibody to intensify the conditioning regimen prior to stem cell transplantation for patients with high-risk acute myeloid leukemia or myelodysplastic syndrome: results of a phase I-II study. *Blood* 2001;98:565–572.
60. Reske SN, Bunjes D, Buchmann I, et al. Targeted bone marrow irradiation in the conditioning of high–risk leukemia prior to stem cell transplantation. *Eur J Nucl Med* 2001;28:807–815.
61. Meredith RF, Khazaeli MB, Plott WE, et al. Initial clinical evaluation of iodine-125-labeled chimeric 17-1A for metastatic colon cancer. *J Nucl Med* 1995;36:2229–2233.
62. Divgi CR, Scott AM, Dantis L, et al. Phase I radioimmunotherapy trial with iodine-131-CC49 in metastatic colon carcinoma. *J Nucl Med* 1995;36:586–592.
63. Meredith RF, Khazaeli MB, Plott WE, et al. Phase II study of dual 131I-labeled monoclonal antibody therapy with interferon in patients with metastatic colorectal cancer. *Clin Cancer Res* 1996;2:1811–1818.
64. Behr TM, Sharkey RM, Juweid ME, et al. Phase I/II clinical radioimmunotherapy with an iodine-131-labeled anti-carcinoembryonic antigen murine monoclonal antibody IgG. *J Nucl Med* 1997;38:858–870.
65. Ychou M, Pelegrin A, Faurous P, et al. Phase-I/II radio-immunotherapy study with iodine-131-labeled anti-CEA monoclonal antibody F6 F(ab')₂ in patients with non-resectable liver metastases from colorectal cancer. *Int J Cancer* 1998;75:615–619.
66. Welt S, Scott AM, Divgi CR, et al. Phase I/II study of iodine 125-labeled monoclonal antibody A33 in patients with advanced colon cancer. *J Clin Oncol* 1996;14:1787–1797.
67. Knox SJ, Goris ML, Tempero M, et al. Phase II trial of yttrium-90–DOTA–biotin pretargeted by NR-LU-10 antibody/streptavidin in patients with metastatic colon cancer. *Clin Cancer Res* 2000;6:406–414.
68. Epenetos AA, Hird V, Lambert H, et al. Long term survival of patients with advanced ovarian cancer treated with intraperitoneal radioimmunotherapy. *Int J Gynecol Cancer* 2000;10[Suppl 1]:44–46.
69. Stewart JS, Hird V, Snook D, et al. Intraperitoneal radioimmunotherapy for ovarian cancer: pharmacokinetics, toxicity, and efficacy of I-131 labeled monoclonal antibodies. *Int J Radiat Oncol Biol Phys* 1989;16:405–413.
70. Crippa F, Bolis G, Seregni E, et al. Single-dose intraperitoneal radioimmunotherapy with the murine monoclonal antibody I-131 MOv18: clinical results in patients with minimal residual disease of ovarian cancer. *Eur J Cancer* 1995;31A:686–690.
71. Jacobs AJ, Fer M, Su FM, et al. A phase I trial of a rhenium 186-labeled monoclonal antibody administered intraperitoneally in ovarian carcinoma: toxicity and clinical response. *Obstet Gynecol* 1993;82:586–593.

72. Mahe MA, Fumoleau P, Fabbro M, et al. A phase II study of intraperitoneal radioimmunotherapy with iodine-131-labeled monoclonal antibody OC-125 in patients with residual ovarian carcinoma. *Clin Cancer Res* 1999;5[10 Suppl]:3249s–3253s.

73. Alvarez RD, Partridge EE, Khazaeli MB, et al. Intraperitoneal radioimmunotherapy of ovarian cancer with 177Lu-CC49: a phase I/II study. *Gynecol Oncol* 1997;65:94–101.

74. Meredith RF, Alvarez RD, Partridge EE, et al. Intraperitoneal radioimmunochemotherapy of ovarian cancer: a phase I study. *Cancer Biother Radiopharm.* 2001;16:305–315.

75. DeNardo SJ, O'Grady LF, Richman CM, et al. Radioimmunotherapy for advanced breast cancer using I-131-ChL6 antibody. *Anticancer Res* 1997;17:1745–1751.

76. Schrier DM, Stemmer SM, Johnson T, et al. High-dose 90Y Mx-diethylenetriaminepentaacetic acid (DTPA)-BrE-3 and autologous hematopoietic stem cell support (AHSCS) for the treatment of advanced breast cancer: a phase I trial. *Cancer Res* 1995;55[Suppl 23]:5921s–5924s.

77. Riva P, Franceschi G, Riva N, et al. Role of nuclear medicine in the treatment of malignant gliomas: the locoregional radioimmunotherapy approach. *Eur J Nucl Med* 2000;27:601–609.

78. Brown MT, Coleman RE, Friedman AH, et al. Intrathecal 131I-labeled antitenascin monoclonal antibody 81C6 treatment of patients with leptomeningeal neoplasms or primary brain tumor resection cavities with subarachnoid communication: phase I trial results. *Clin Cancer Res* 1996;2:963–972.

79. Cokgor I, Akabani G, Kuan CT, et al. Phase I trial results of iodine-131-labeled antitenascin monoclonal antibody 81C6 treatment of patients with newly diagnosed malignant gliomas. *J Clin Oncol* 2000;18:3862–3872.

80. Paganelli G, Bartolomei M, Ferrari M, et al. Pre-targeted locoregional radioimmunotherapy with 90Y-biotin in glioma patients: phase I study and preliminary therapeutic results. *Cancer Biother Radiopharm* 2001;16:227–235.

81. Colnot DR, Quak JJ, Roos JC, et al. Radioimmunotherapy in patients with head and neck squamous cell carcinoma: initial experience. *Head Neck* 2001;23:559–565.

82. Kraeber-Bodere F, Faibre-Chauvet A, Sai-Maurel C, et al. Bispecific antibody and bivalent hapten radioimmunotherapy in CEA-producing medullary thyroid cancer xenograft. *J Nucl Med* 1999;40:198–204.

83. Juweid ME, Hajjar G, Swayne LC, et al. Phase I/II trial of (131)I-MN-14F(ab)2 anti-carcinoembryonic antigen monoclonal antibody in the treatment of patients with metastatic medullary thyroid carcinoma. *Cancer* 1999;85:1828–1842.

84. Divgi CR, Bander NH, Scott AM, et al. Phase I/II radioimmunotherapy trial with iodine-131-labeled monoclonal antibody G250 in metastatic renal cell carcinoma. *Clin Cancer Res* 1998;4:2729–2739.

85. Slovin SF, Scher HI, Divgi CR, et al. Interferon-gamma and monoclonal antibody 131I-labeled CC49: outcomes in patients with androgen-independent prostate cancer. *Clin Cancer Res* 1998;4:643–651.

86. Zeng ZC, Tang ZY, Liu KD, et al. Improved long-term survival for unresectable hepatocellular carcinoma (HCC) with a combination of surgery and intrahepatic arterial infusion of 131I-anti-HCC mAb: phase I/II clinical trials. *J Cancer Res Clin Oncol* 1998;124:275–280.

87. Stillwagon GB, Order SE, Haulk T, et al. Variable low dose rate irradiation (131I-anti-CEA) and integrated low dose chemotherapy in the treatment of nonresectable primary intrahepatic cholangiocarcinoma. *Int J Radiat Oncol Biol Phys* 1991;21:1601–1605.

88. Cheung NK, Kushner BH, LaQuaglia M, et al. N7: a novel multimodality therapy of high risk neuroblastoma (NB) in children diagnosed over 1 year of age. *Med Pediatr Oncol* 2001;36:227–230.

89. Gates VL, Carey JE, Siegel JA, et al. Nonmyeloablative iodine-131 anti-B1 radioimmunotherapy as outpatient therapy. *J Nucl Med* 1998;39:1230–1236.

90. Rutar FJ, Augustine SC, Colcher D, et al. Outpatient treatment with (131)I-anti-B1 antibody: radiation exposure to family members. *J Nucl Med* 2001;42:907–915.

48

APPLICATIONS OF PET IN ONCOLOGIC IMAGING

VAL J. LOWE
DOMINIQUE DELBEKE
R. EDWARD COLEMAN

An understanding of tumor physiology is necessary to appreciate the potential role of positron emission tomography (PET) in evaluating patients with suspected malignancy. The physiologic and biochemical properties that differentiate normal cells from malignant cells have been the subject of extensive studies for many years. Multiple processes in malignant cells are different from the processes in normal cells and provide unique opportunities and challenges for the development of PET imaging techniques to detect malignancy. The differences in metabolism of glucose, amino acids, and nucleic acids and in blood flow between malignant and normal tissues permit the differentiation of these tissues by using specifically designed physiologic imaging tracers labeled with appropriate positron emitting radionuclides.

Multiple studies have demonstrated the utility of PET in oncologic imaging. The advantages of improved spatial resolution and sensitivity over other nuclear medicine techniques; the availability of labeling simple metabolic substrates with ubiquitous biologic atoms like carbon, oxygen, and nitrogen; and the ability to obtain physiologic information that cannot be afforded by anatomic imaging make PET imaging attractive. The initial oncologic studies of PET were primarily performed in the brain, and data are now available from many other organ systems to demonstrate the importance of PET in characterizing malignancy. Whole-body imaging of ^{18}F-fluorodeoxyglucose (FDG) has become widely available and is now used routinely to diagnose, stage, and restage many malignancies. FDG PET is also being used in radiation therapy (XRT) planning and in monitoring the effect of therapy.

PET RADIOPHARMACEUTICALS

Cancer cells typically have increased metabolism and more rapid cell proliferation than normal cells. In the 1930s, malignant cells were shown to have increased glucose metabolism (1,2). Their increased metabolism appears to be related to increased levels of glucose transport protein messenger ribonucleic acid (RNA) and glucose transport proteins (3). Malignant cells also have larger amounts of hexokinase than is present in normal cells. The increased accumulation of glucose in malignant cells and the similarity of glucose and the ^{18}F-labeled analogue FDG (4) permit the identification of malignancy using PET imaging. After phosphorylation, FDG-6-PO$_4$ does not proceed further in the metabolic pathway and remains trapped within the tumor cells (Fig. 48.1). ^{11}C-glucose and other analogs of glucose have also been used to study glucose metabolism in tumors (5). The 20-minute half-life of ^{11}C and the rapid metabolism of the ^{11}C-glucose to carbon dioxide limit the use of this agent. Abnormalities in the transport of amino acids and in protein synthesis have been demonstrated in tumor cells (6). Several different labeled amino acids and amino acid derivatives have been used to study tumors including ^{11}C-methionine, ^{18}F-fluorophenylalanine, ^{18}F-fluorotyrosine, and others (7–9). Tumor cell proliferation that is greater than normal cell proliferation allows imaging with nucleic acid radiotracers specific to replication such as ^{11}C-thymidine (10). More recently, ^{18}F-fluorothymidine (FLT) has been used for imaging cellular proliferation *in vivo* (11). The ability to study polyamine metabolism in tumor cells has been demonstrated using ^{11}C-putrescine (12). ^{18}F-fluorocholine appears to be a promising agent for imaging membrane synthesis. Initial studies in prostate cancer are promising (13).

Because blood flow and blood volume are often increased in tumors compared with normal tissue, several radiopharmaceuticals have been used to study these parameters (14,15). Blood flow can be evaluated either qualitatively or quantitatively by the intravenous administration of ^{15}O-water. The blood volume within tumors can be measured using [15]O- or ^{11}C-carbon monoxide, which labels the hemoglobin in red blood cells. The [15]O- or ^{11}C-carbon monoxide can be administered by inhalation, and the labeling of the red blood cells occurs in the lungs. Oxygen utilization can be measured by the inhalation of ^{15}O-oxygen.

In addition to studying the physiologic and biochemical abnormalities of cancer, PET has also been used to study the distribution of chemotherapeutic agents in malignancy and to charac-

V.J. Lowe: Department of Radiology, Mayo Clinic, Rochester, MN.
D. Delbeke: Department of Radiology and Radiological Sciences, Vanderbilt University Medical Center, Nashville, TN.
R.E. Coleman: Department of Radiology, Division of Nuclear Medicine, Duke University Medical Center, Durham, NC.

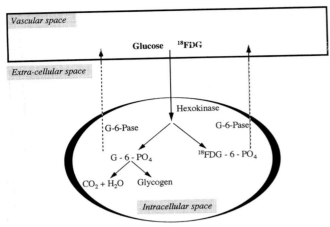

FIGURE 48.1. Cellular uptake of fluorodeoxyglucose (FDG). After the FDG is phosphorylated, it is not further metabolized like glucose.

terize the antigens on tumor cells. ^{18}F-5-fluorouracil (16), ^{13}N-cisplatin (17), and ^{11}C-carmustine (BCNU) (18) have been shown to localize in certain malignant cells and not in normal tissue. Data suggest that the amount of accumulation in malignancy is predictive of the response to therapy of the drug. A few studies have been performed that demonstrate the ability to label monoclonal antibodies with positron emitting radionuclides such as ^{18}F, ^{68}Ga, and [124]I. PET imaging permits accurate kinetic studies of the distribution of the monoclonal antibodies. The short half-lives of [18]F (110 minutes) and [68]Ga (68 minutes) limit the usefulness of these radionuclides for monoclonal antibody studies. However, the use of fragments of monoclonal antibodies and the use of genetically engineered portions of monoclonal antibodies that clear more rapidly from the blood pool increase the potential usefulness of these short half-life radionuclides. The 4.2-day half-life of [124]I makes possible the imaging of the distribution of the antibodies for several days.

PET IMAGING IN ONCOLOGY

The use of PET radiopharmaceuticals may require specific patient preparation depending on the physiologic mechanisms of uptake and distribution of the agent. For example, FDG imaging of tumors is performed in the fasting state to minimize competitive inhibition of FDG uptake by serum glucose. The effect of diabetes on the uptake of FDG is not fully elucidated, but elevated serum glucose levels result in decreased FDG accumulation in cancer cells.

The time course of accumulation of the PET tracer in the tissue of interest and the clearance from the blood pool are important in determining the appropriate time for the acquisition of emission information for each PET agent. Because uptake of FDG continues to increase even up to 2.5 hours after injection in some tumors, delayed imaging has been shown to increase lesion-to-background ratios and produce different results than early imaging. FDG emission scans should not be performed until at least 45 minutes after the intravenous administration of FDG for body tumor studies and 30 minutes after injection for

brain tumor studies (19,20). A dose range of 10 to 20 mCi of FDG is used for adult subjects. The dose may be based on administering 140 μCi/kg with a minimum of 10 mCi and a maximum of 20 mCi. Patient hydration should be used before and after FDG injection to minimize renal and bladder activity. Some facilities perform bladder catheterization in patients with suspected pelvic pathology. Other facilities have not found bladder catheterization necessary.

Whole-body scans are typically performed on oncology patients. For systems using bismuth germanate detectors, iterative reconstruction algorithms, and segmented attenuation, the two-dimensional (2D) emission scans are 3 to 6 minutes and the transmission scans are 2 to 5 minutes at each bed position. For three-dimensional (3D) acquisitions, the imaging time per bed position is decreased compared with the 2D acquisitions. The whole-body scan is performed from the base of the skull through the proximal femurs and requires five to seven bed positions. The transmission scan using rotating [68]Ge pin sources can be obtained before or after the emission scan or can be interlaced with the emission scan. The new combined PET and computed tomography (CT) scanners use the CT scan as the transmission scan and have shorter imaging times.

PET imaging provides qualitative, semiquantitative, and quantitative information about tumor physiology. Clinical FDG studies are generally analyzed using semiquantitative and qualitative data. Quantitative studies of glucose metabolic rates are too invasive and time consuming for routine oncologic studies. A standardized uptake value (SUV) is a semiquantitative index of glucose utilization that is obtained by normalizing the accumulation in the region-of-interest (ROI) to the injected dose and patient body weight. The abnormality of interest is identified on the PET scan. A ROI is placed on the abnormality. The mean activity (mCi per mL) is measured in the ROI. The decay corrected activities are then used to compute an SUV according to the following formula.

$$SUV = \frac{\text{mean ROI activity (mCi/ml)}}{\text{injected dose(mCi)/body wt(g)}}$$

Zasadny et al. (22) suggested that the SUV should be based on lean body weight and not the patient body weight. Other investigators have suggested a correction for serum glucose levels. Perhaps the use of the pixel with the greatest amount of activity would be more appropriate than the use of the mean activity of several pixels. In the evaluation of pulmonary lesions, a mean SUV value that is more than 2.5 is indicative of a malignant or an active infectious process (23). Because of the effects of resolution, measured uptake values in lesions less than 1.5 cm in diameter may need to be corrected for measurement losses by using recovery coefficients. In a chest phantom, the mean measured activity of an 8-mm diameter nodule is only approximately 60% of the actual activity.

Another method for evaluating FDG uptake in a lesion is the determination of an activity ratio. An activity ratio is generated by comparing FDG uptake in the lesion to an area in the contralateral normal tissue. Our experience with this method demonstrates that activity ratio analysis provides equivalent sensitivity and specificity when compared with SUV data in the evaluation of pulmonary abnormalities.

LUNG CANCER

Cancer is a close second to ischemic heart disease as a leading cause of mortality in the United States (24). Lung cancer claims 145,000 lives in the United States each year. Although cancer therapy has advanced, the death rate from cancer has not been reduced as much as anticipated (25). Lung cancer death rates have fluctuated in recent years, and, not surprisingly, the changes parallel the regional trends in cigarette smoking (26). Mortality rates from lung cancer for women older than 55 years have increased over fourfold in the last 20 years, probably reflecting changes in smoking habits that occurred decades ago (25). Today, lung cancer is responsible for 32% of all cancer deaths in men and 25% in women (27). In 1997, smoking rates among high school students in the United States were 32% higher compared with 1991 (28). Thus, advances in lung cancer detection and treatment must continue.

Lung Nodules

Lung cancer commonly presents as a focal lung abnormality or solitary pulmonary nodule. Imaging with chest radiography or CT cannot definitively differentiate benign from malignant focal lung abnormalities. With the advent of more sensitive, higher resolution CT, it is becoming more obvious that the solitary nodule may be a misnomer. More commonly, multiple nodules are being detected on high-resolution CT when only a single nodule was seen on chest x-ray film. These multiple nodules may be very tiny, and the appropriate clinical assessment, if any, of these tiny nodules is yet to be determined. The dilemma in evaluation now becomes increasingly more difficult as small size and multiplicity make biopsy decisions tricky. Large-nodule evaluation trials are being contemplated and will hopefully help to answer some of these clinical questions.

Several invasive modalities are available to assist in the diagnosis of the lung nodules that are large enough to be evaluated. However, negative results from either transbronchial or transthoracic biopsies cannot be accepted as reliable negatives (29). Most studies report a sensitivity of 75% to 86% sensitivity for malignancy in transthoracic needle aspiration (TTNA) of lung nodules (30,31). PET has been shown to compare favorably with these invasive techniques (32).

An accurate, noninvasive test for evaluating indeterminate pulmonary lesions would avoid considerable patient morbidity and potentially reduce cost from invasive procedures. In many cases, patients would probably opt for such a procedure, if the accuracy and risks of all available procedures were thoroughly explained to the patient.

Published data have demonstrated the ability of PET to accurately characterize lung abnormalities and have been particularly encouraging (33–41). After the identification of a pulmonary abnormality by an anatomic study such as a chest x-ray film, FDG PET imaging can be performed to evaluate the metabolic activity of the lesion in an attempt to distinguish a benign from

a malignant process. The data show that PET performs well in this group with an average sensitivity and specificity of 95% and 81% for the detection of malignancy in lung nodules (Figs. 48.2 and 48.3).

The sensitivity of PET is high enough that negative results on PET scan is reasonably considered to rule out malignancy in a population of low to moderate risk for malignancy. Depending on the population studied, some false-positive studies will be encountered. It would not, for example, be unexpected to find many false-positive PET studies in a community in which a high likelihood for pulmonary infection [e.g., tuberculosis (TB)] is encountered. The clinical setting the test is used in, as is true for all diagnostic tests, will determine its clinical value. A recent meta-analysis also concluded that this is true (40). In this meta-analysis the authors concluded that the sensitivity of PET is such that, in a low-risk population (20% risk), the posttest probability of malignancy after negative findings on PET scan is about 1%.

Lung Cancer Staging

Tumor

Lung cancer staging is based on the TNM system and requires accurate characterization of the primary tumor (T), regional lymph nodes (N), and distant metastasis (M). The appropriate categorization of stage presently relies on the information that can be obtained clinically. Traditionally, this information has been obtained by CT. PET is not used to assess T stage. Certainly, when a lesion is surrounded by lung and no other disease is detected, PET can rule out higher stage disease. However, when a tumor is directly adjacent to vital mediastinal structures, PET cannot clearly determine the extent of invasion. Invasion of the tumor directly into thoracic structures is often evaluated best in surgery, although CT can at times be helpful. There are occasional situations in which PET may be of help in T staging, but this will be the exception.

Lymph Nodes

Advancing nodal involvement correlates closely with worsening survival. The assessment of mediastinal nodes is relatively difficult. The nodal size criteria of 1 cm used in CT imaging is only reliable in about ⅔ of patients. Alternatively, invasive sampling with mediastinoscopy can be performed to assess lymph node status. However, the sensitivity of mediastinoscopy is imperfect—it is reported to be about 90% (42,43).

PET has produced an improvement in the accuracy of detecting lymph node disease or other metastasis. The average sensitivity and specificity for nodal disease is 88% and 91% for PET and 63% and 76% for CT in reports comparing the two modalities (44–55). This average sensitivity of PET for nodal disease is the same as that reported for mediastinoscopy. Examples are seen in Fig. 48.4.

Staging the mediastinum with PET also appears to be cost effective as a routine procedure. Gambhir et al. (41) evaluated the cost effectiveness of FDG PET staging of lung cancer. They showed that one can save $1154 per patient by including PET.

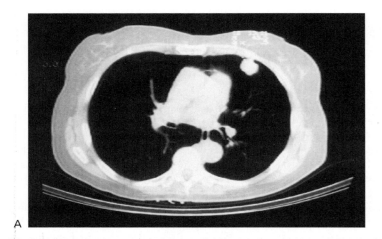

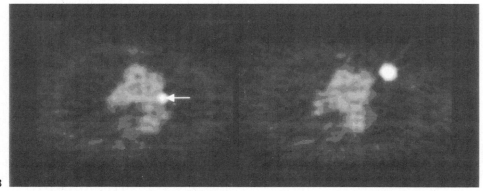

FIGURE 48.2. Computed tomography scan showing a left anterior lung nodule **(A)** that was hypermetabolic on fluorodeoxyglucose positron emission tomography (PET). **(B)** A small left hilar lymph node (*arrow*) was also hypermetabolic on PET. This patient had adenocarcinoma of the lung with a hilar metastasis.

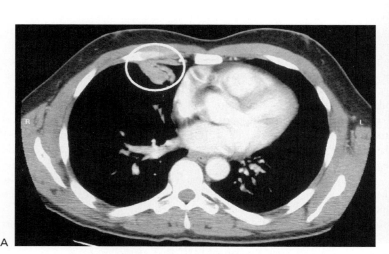

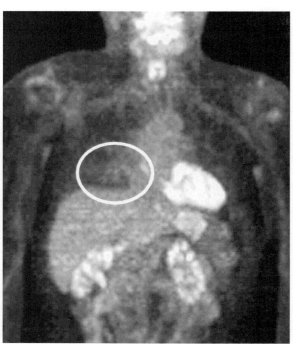

FIGURE 48.3. Computed tomography scan showing a right lung nodule (oval) **(A)** that was hypometabolic (oval) on fluorodeoxyglucose positron emission tomography **(B)**. This patient had a hamartoma.

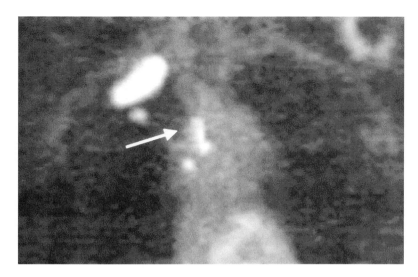

FIGURE 48.4. Positron emission tomography (PET) scan of a patient with a right lung mass on computed tomography that showed no adenopathy. PET shows hypermetabolism in the right lung mass and in mediastinal lymph nodes (*arrow*). Metastatic disease was confirmed in right paratracheal lymph nodes.

Distant Metastasis

PET has not been shown to be effective in screening patients for brain metastases, especially when they are asymptomatic (35). Many authors have reported that PET has the ability to detect distant disease that may otherwise be undetectable (50,57,58). These studies have shown that at a minimum, 11% of the patients who have PET are shown to have a distant metastasis that was not detected by CT or other imaging methods. Unsuspected disease identified on PET, thus, resulted in up-staging. The results imply that adding PET data will impact information regarding advisability of tumor resection. In the study by Lewis et al., the PET findings resulted in patient management changes in 41% of the cases.

PET imaging has been shown to distinguish benign adrenal enlargement from metastatic disease. Boland et al. (59) demonstrated that PET imaging showed a statistically significant differ-ence in lesion metabolism between benign, enlarged adrenal glands and those with malignancy. A study by Erasmus et al. (60) showed that in 27 patients (33 enlarged adrenal glands) with bronchogenic carcinoma, PET correctly identified all adrenal glands that had metastatic disease (Fig. 48.5).

Bone scans are commonly ordered in lung cancer patients to rule out bone metastasis. The sensitivity of bone scanning is high but the specificity can be problematic because chronic bone or joint disease or trauma can cause false-positive studies. PET has been compared with bone scintigraphy, and although the tests are very similar in high sensitivity for metastasis, PET has a much higher specificity for disease than bone scintigraphy (61). Imaging the lower limbs with PET would need to be performed to get the same skeletal information provided by the bone scan. It is reasonable to consider PET as a substitute for bone scans if completed in this way.

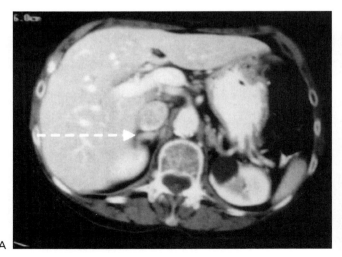
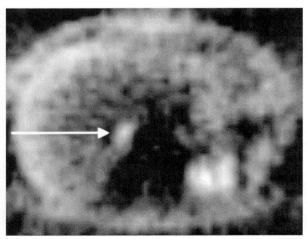

FIGURE 48.5. Computed tomography scan of the upper abdomen **(A)** demonstrating a normal right adrenal in a patient with a right lung cancer (*dashed arrow*). The fluorodeoxyglucose positron emission tomography scan **(B)** demonstrates hypermetabolism in the right adrenal lesion (*arrow*). Biopsy showed metastatic adenocarcinoma.

Evaluation of Therapy

XRT has been the treatment of choice for patients with unresectable non-small cell lung cancer. These patients have typically been treated with doses of 6,000 to 6,500 rads and have a median survival of 12 months. Patients with all types of lung cancer have a 5-year survival of 5% to 10% (62,63). The local control rates achieved in these patients have been difficult to assess but are generally poor (64). These results have prompted efforts to improve local control and possibly survival through dose escalation (65). The accurate assessment of the therapeutic effect of chemotherapy and XRT is of great importance if lung cancer survival is to be improved. The typical radiation dose for treating non-small cell carcinoma is 6,000 rads and not all non-small cell tumors respond to this amount of radiation. If the nonresponders could be identified, escalating the radiation dose could be considered.

FDG PET can identify changes in tumor glucose uptake after XRT (Fig. 48.6). Some investigators have concluded, however, that a decrease in FDG uptake did not necessarily indicate a good prognosis (66). FDG uptake decreases over time in some patients, but other patients do not have a similar response to XRT. Patient outcome data is needed to verify the potential impact that PET may have in predicting prognosis and therapeutic response to conventional therapy.

The determination of radiation treatment ports presently depends on the identification of tumor volume by anatomic imaging. Radiation ports encompass an area larger than the suspected tumor volume to compensate for error incurred by the insensitivity of anatomic imaging and variability of patient positioning. FDG PET can assist in XRT planning by focusing radiation ports to precise areas of tumor activity, preventing irradiation of uninvolved areas and omission of regions of active tumor from radiation ports.

Lung Cancer Recurrence Evaluation

Early diagnosis of recurrent lung cancer is another potential use of FDG PET. Radiologic changes such as scarring and necrosis

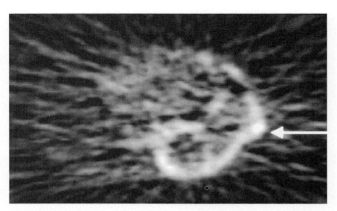

FIGURE 48.7. Fluorodeoxyglucose positron emission tomography image demonstrates hypermetabolism in the pleural region that was documented to be metastatic adenocarcinoma by biopsy.

that occur after therapy may obscure the identification of recurrent tumor unless significant volume changes occur over time. Unfortunately, a tissue biopsy that is negative for tumor is suspect because of the inherent difficulty in identifying and accurately sampling the areas of viable tumor in the midst of scar. A PET evaluation of tumor recurrence can potentially assist in this determination. Patients who have chest radiographic findings suspicious for tumor recurrence can be accurately characterized by FDG PET imaging as demonstrated in Fig. 48.7. The accuracy of differentiating treatment changes from recurrent disease with PET is high and is improved over CT in the same group of patients (34,67–71).

BRAIN TUMORS

FDG PET brain scans are performed using 3D acquisition and a calculated attenuation correction. The 3D acquisitions are for approximately 8 minutes. A uniform attenuation correction can

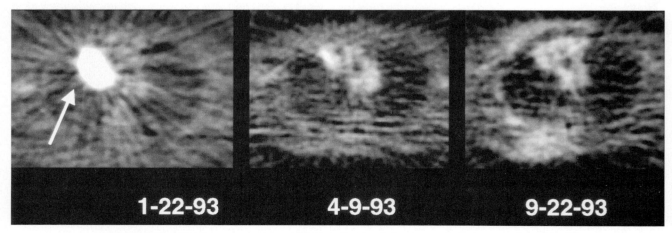

FIGURE 48.6. Serial fluorodeoxyglucose (FDG) positron emission tomography images of a non-small cell tumor in the right lung (*arrow*) that demonstrate steadily decreasing FDG accumulation in the tumor. Chest wall soft tissue uptake in the anterior and posterior right thorax that steadily increases over the same period is due to radiation therapy effects.

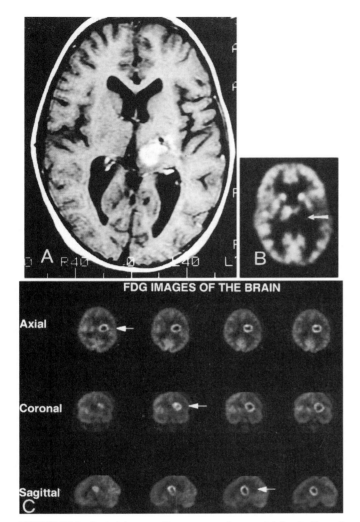

FDG IMAGES OF THE BRAIN

Axial

Coronal

Sagittal

FIGURE 48.8. A: Axial magnetic resonance image obtained after administration demonstrates gadolinium contrast enhancement in a left posterior thalamic region oligodendroglioma. **B:** Fluorodeoxyglucose (FDG) positron emission tomography (PET) image demonstrates hypometabolism in this region (*arrow*). **C:** Axial, coronal, and sagittal views of an FDG PET study demonstrating hypermetabolism (*arrow*) in a high-grade malignancy in the left subcortical region is also shown.

be used for the head because the tissues in the head have relatively uniform attenuation characteristics at 511 keV (72).

The feasibility of using PET to characterize tumors was first demonstrated for tumors of the brain. Many of the initial PET tomographs were able to image only the brain. Evaluation of tumors in the brain does not require whole-body imaging capability. Several applications of PET in brain tumors have been demonstrated (73). PET is used in determining the degree of malignancy of a tumor and in determining the prognosis of brain tumor patients. PET is useful in determining the appropriate biopsy site in patients with multiple lesions, large homogeneous lesions, and large heterogeneous lesions. PET is accurate in differentiating recurrent tumor from necrosis in patients who have undergone XRT and chemotherapy. We have found registration of FDG PET and magnetic resonance imaging (MRI) images extremely useful. Correlating small areas of abnormal

enhancement on the MRI with the PET scan is very difficult without registering the image.

Most studies of PET imaging in brain tumors have used FDG to characterize the metabolic activity of the cells. The brain tumors are qualitatively characterized as hypometabolic or hypermetabolic based on the amount of accumulation of FDG in the tumor compared with amount of FDG accumulation in normal white matter. Hypometabolic tumors have FDG accumulation equal to or less than normal white matter, whereas hypermetabolic tumors have accumulation greater than normal white matter. Hypometabolic tumors are generally proven to be astrocytomas and oligodendrogliomas, whereas hypermetabolic tumors are generally proven to be anaplastic astrocytomas or glioblastoma multiforme (Figs. 48.8 and 48.9). A good correlation has been demonstrated between increased FDG accumulation in the tumor and higher grade brain tumors (19). In a study of 100 patients, PET was able to separate high- and low-grade tumors by their glucose utilization (74). In a study of 72 patients by Patronas et al. (75), PET was more accurate than contrast CT in determining the grade of the tumor. PET appears to be able to differentiate the various grades of tumor by their metabolism (76).

The tumor grade can also be determined by L-(methyl-^{11}C) methionine accumulation (77,78). Fourteen patients with cerebral gliomas demonstrated accumulation of methionine. Differential absorption ratios (DARs), semiquantitative indices of radiopharmaceutical accumulation, were greater for higher grade tumors. No differences in DARs were seen between grade III and grade IV lesions. In another study of 22 patients with gliomas, methionine accumulation was found to correlate with tumor grade (79). By comparing the activity in the tumor to a normal contralateral ROI, the higher grade lesions had higher ratios. In 15 patients studied with both FDG and methionine, improved diagnostic accuracy in differentiating recurrent brain tumor from radiation injury could be obtained by using both tracers (80).

PET-MRI REGISTRATION

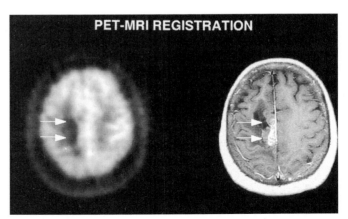

FIGURE 48.9. Axial magnetic resonance image (*right*) obtained after gadolinium administration demonstrates contrast enhancement (*arrows*) that precisely matches hypermetabolism (*arrows*) on fluorodeoxyglucose positron emission tomography (*left*). The two images are anatomically registered and the finding indicates high-grade tumor recurrence.

In addition to determining tumor grades using PET, patient outcome can be determined. Alavi et al. (81) showed that the mean survival of patients with hypermetabolic tumors was 7 months, whereas the mean survival with hypometabolic tumors was 33 months. The patients with a hypermetabolic tumor had a 1-year survival of 29%, and the patients with hypometabolic tumors had a 1-year survival of 78%. Schifter et al. (82) confirmed this finding and showed that patients with brain tumors that had low uptake of FDG (less than gray matter) had significantly longer survival. They demonstrated that serial scans provided more information than a single scan. The mean accumulation of FDG in the tumor changes little during the time of the study.

The histology of a brain tumor can change with time. For PET to be effective in evaluating these patients, it should be able to characterize the change in histology. Low-grade tumors are often followed without therapy, but aggressive therapy is given to these tumors when they degenerate to high-grade tumors. Francavilla et al. (83) reported the ability of PET to detect malignant degeneration in three patients who had premalignant and postmalignant degeneration PET studies. Enhance glucose accumulation was seen in the tumors after malignant degeneration had occurred.

PET is also useful in directing the neurosurgeon to the appropriate area to biopsy in patients with complicated anatomic lesions on CT studies or MRI. In these large and/or complex lesions, the differentiation of edema, tumor, and necrosis may be difficult. If the neurosurgeon biopsies the site of increased metabolism on the FDG study, a correct tissue diagnosis is more likely to occur (84).

The ability to detect persistent or recurrent tumor after surgery is difficult with CT and MRI. The postsurgical changes are similar to the changes seen with persistent tumor. Contrast enhancement of the perisurgical area is seen commonly and cannot be differentiated from tumor persistence (85). MRI also has nonspecific postsurgical changes that can make tumor identification unreliable (86). PET can reliably differentiate persistent or recurrent tumor after surgery. The results of a study comparing FDG PET imaging, CT scanning, and the surgeon's impression after having performed a subtotal resection or gross total resection demonstrated that the PET scan was most predictive of persistent tumor (87).

The effect of temporal lobectomy on FDG accumulation in the brain and of steroids on brain tumors has been studied. Surgery does not result in hypermetabolism at the surgical site (87). Furthermore, steroids do not have much of an effect on tumor accumulation of FDG (87). Because most patients with brain tumors are treated with steroids, the effect of steroids on FDG imaging must be known. Of five patients studied with FDG PET scans before and after receiving high doses of steroids, the PET imaging of FDG in the tumors was unchanged. Thus, steroid therapy does not affect tumor metabolism.

Patients with brain tumors often undergo surgery and receive chemotherapy and/or XRT. Subsequently, an increase in symptoms may be related to persistent tumor or necrosis from the chemotherapy or XRT. The changes from persistent tumor, scarring, and necrosis cannot be differentiated by CT or MRI (88, 89). Dooms et al. (89) showed that in 55 patients with gliomas proven by histology, MRI was unable to differentiate recurrent tumor from radiation necrosis. PET imaging can differentiate scar or necrosis from persistent or recurrent tumor. Investigators at the National Institutes of Health (NIH) have shown that PET could reliably differentiate cerebral necrosis (from radiation or chemotherapy) from brain tumors in 85 patients (90). Other studies have shown similar result in differentiating recurrent tumor from necrosis (91). Image registration techniques have allowed precise correlation of PET and MR or CT abnormalities (Fig. 48.9) for assessing tumor recurrence.

Thus, several studies have demonstrated the ability of PET to contribute to the clinical management of patients with brain tumors.

COLORECTAL CANCER

The American Cancer Society estimates that in the year 2001 there were 135,400 new cases of colorectal cancer in the United States; colorectal cancer is the third most common cause of cancer in men and women. In the year 2001 it is estimated that 56,700 patients died from this disease in the United States, representing 10% of all cancer deaths.

The diagnosis of colorectal carcinoma is based on colonoscopy and biopsy. The preoperative staging with imaging modalities is usually limited because most patients will benefit from colectomy to prevent intestinal obstruction. The extent of the disease can be evaluated during surgery. Therefore, although the sensitivity of FDG PET for the detection of a primary colon carcinoma is high (92,93), it has a limited role in the preoperative diagnosis or initial staging except in high-risk patients for which surgery can be avoided if metastases are identified.

One third of the 70% of patients treated with curative intent will have a recurrence in the first 2 years after resection. Twenty-five percent of these patients have recurrence limited to one site and are potentially curable by surgical resection. For example, about 14,000 patients per year present with isolated liver metastases at their first recurrence, and about 20% of these patients die with metastases exclusively to the liver. Therefore, accurate noninvasive detection of inoperable disease with imaging modalities plays a pivotal role in selecting patients who would benefit from surgery.

Conventional Modalities for Detecting and Staging Recurrent Colorectal Carcinoma

Detection of recurrence can be monitored with serum levels of carcinoembryonic antigen (CEA) in ⅔ of the patients with a sensitivity of 59% and specificity of 84%, but recurrent disease still must be localized (94). Barium studies have been used for detection of local recurrence with accuracy in the range of 80%. However, barium studies have been reported to be only 49% sensitive and 85% specific for overall recurrence (95).

CT is commonly used for localization but with a variable accuracy according to the site of recurrence. For example, metastases to the peritoneum, mesentery, and lymph nodes are commonly missed on CT, and the differentiation of postsurgical changes from tumor recurrence is often equivocal (96,97).

Among the patients with negative findings on CT, 50% will be found to have nonresectable lesions at the time of exploratory laparotomy. CT portography (superior mesenteric arterial portography) is more sensitive (80% to 90%) than CT (70% to 80%) for detection of hepatic metastases but has a considerable rate of false-positive findings, lowering the positive predictive value (98–101).

Radioimmunoscintigraphy is limited by difficulties with antigen modulation and variable depiction of tumor and nontumor cells, as well as by physiologic hepatic and bowel excretion. (102).

Detection and Staging Recurrent Colorectal Carcinoma with FDG PET Imaging

A number of studies have demonstrated the role of FDG PET imaging for detecting recurrent or metastatic colorectal carcinoma (103–124) (Fig. 48.10). Overall, the sensitivity of FDG

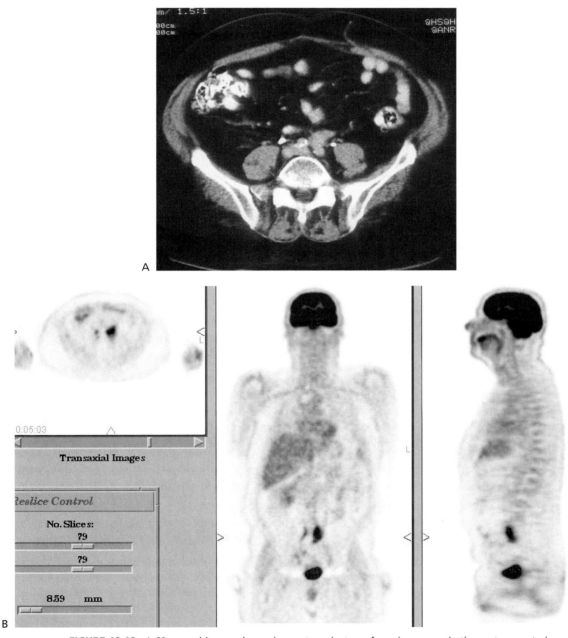

FIGURE 48.10. A 60-year-old man who underwent a colectomy for colon cancer in the past presented with elevated carcinoembryonic antigen levels and negative findings on computed tomography (CT). **A.** Orthogonal fluorodeoxyglucose (FDG) positron emission tomography (PET) images through the pelvis demonstrated a focal area of uptake in the region of the left ureter. **B.** Retrospective review of the CT revealed a corresponding soft tissue lesion. The patient underwent chemotherapy, and a follow-up FDG PET scan demonstrated residual but less intense uptake indicating a partial response to therapy.

PET imaging is in the 90% range and the specificity greater than 70%, both superior to CT. However, false-negative FDG PET findings have been reported with mucinous adenocarcinoma, the sensitivity is 40% to 60% according to the cellularity of these tumors (125,126).

For differentiation of scar from local recurrence, CT is equivocal in most cases, and the accuracy of FDG PET imaging is greater than 90% (104,105,109,110,114). In the largest study (76 patients) (110), the accuracy of FDG PET and CT were 95% and 65%, respectively. For detection of hepatic metastases, FDG PET is more accurate than CT and as good as CT portography because of the high rate of false-positive perfusion defects (110,111,113,114,116). In patients with unexplained elevation of serum CEA level and normal conventional workup including CT, FDG PET correctly demonstrates tumor in two thirds of patients with a sensitivity and specificity greater than 90% and 70%, respectively (115,116).

A comparison of the sensitivity and specificity of FDG PET and CT for specific anatomic locations found that FDG PET was more sensitive than CT in all locations except the lung, where the two modalities were equivalent (116). The largest difference between PET and CT was found in the abdomen, pelvis, and retroperitoneum, where over one third of PET-positive lesions were negative by CT. PET was also more specific than CT at all sites except the retroperitoneum, but the differences were smaller than the differences in sensitivity. Other studies (112,113) support these data concluding that outside the liver, FDG PET was especially helpful in detecting nodal involvement, differentiating local recurrence from postsurgical changes, and evaluating the malignancy of indeterminate lesions such as pulmonary nodules—indications for which CT has known limitations. In addition, because FDG PET imaging is a whole-body technique, it allowed identification of metastatic disease in the chest, abdomen, or pelvis, guiding subsequent CT examination of these regions to evaluate the exact anatomic location and potential resectability of any extrahepatic lesions.

A meta-analysis of 11 clinical reports and 577 patients determined that the sensitivity and specificity of FDG PET for detecting recurrent colorectal cancer were 97% and 76%, respectively (127). A comprehensive review of the PET literature (2,244 patient's studies) has reported weighted average for FDG PET sensitivity and specificity of 94% and 87%, respectively, compared with 79% and 73% for CT (128).

Impact of FDG PET Imaging on Patient Management

The greater sensitivity of PET compared with CT in diagnosis and staging of recurrent tumor results from two factors: early detection of abnormal tumor metabolism, before changes have become apparent by anatomic imaging, and the global nature of whole-body PET imaging, which permits diagnosis of tumor when it occurs in unusual and unexpected sites. A number of studies reported a change in management in patients referred for evaluation of recurrent colorectal carcinoma ranging from 14% to 44% with a weighted average of 36% (109,110, 112–116,118,122–124). In a survey-based study of 60 referring oncologists, surgeons, and generalists, FDG PET performed at

initial staging had a major impact on the management of colorectal cancer patients and contributed to a change in clinical stage in 42% (80% upstaged and 20% downstaged) and a change in the clinical management in more than 60%. As a result of the PET findings, physicians avoided major surgery in 41% of patients for whom surgery was the intended treatment (129). The meta-analysis of the literature determined that FDG PET changed the management in 29% (102/349) patients (127). The comprehensive review of the PET literature has reported a weighted-average change of management related to FDG PET findings in 32% of 915 patients (128).

Although survival is not an end point for a diagnostic test, Strasberg et al. (130) have estimated the survival of patients who underwent FDG PET imaging in their preoperative evaluation for resection of hepatic metastases. The Kaplan-Meier test estimate of the overall survival at 3 years was 77% and the lower confidence limit was 60%. These percentages are lower than those in previously published series that ranged from 30% to 64%. The 3-year disease-free survival rate was 40%.

Including FDG PET in the evaluation of patients with recurrent colorectal carcinoma has been shown to be cost effective in a study using clinical evaluation of effectiveness with modeling of costs (131) and studies using decision tree sensitivity analysis (116,132).

Monitoring Therapy of Colorectal Carcinoma with FDG PET Imaging

FDG PET can differentiate local recurrence from scarring after XRT (133). However, increased FDG uptake immediately following radiation may be due to inflammatory changes and is not always associated with residual tumor. The time course of postirradiation FDG activity has not been studied systematically; it is generally accepted that FDG activity present 6 months after completion of XRT most likely represents tumor recurrence.

There are preliminary reports suggesting that the response to chemotherapy in patients with hepatic metastases can be predicted with PET. Responders may be discriminated from nonresponders after 4 to 5 weeks of chemotherapy with 5-fluorouracil by measuring FDG uptake before and during therapy (134). A pilot study of 15 patients with primary rectal carcinoma demonstrated that FDG PET imaging adds incremental information for assessing the response to preoperative radiation and 5-fluorouracil-based chemotherapy (135).

Limitations of FDG PET Imaging for Evaluation of Colorectal Carcinoma

Tumor detectability depends on both the size of the lesion and the degree of uptake. False-negative lesions can be due to partial volume averaging, leading to underestimation of the uptake in small lesions (<1 cm) or in necrotic lesions with a thin viable rim. In the experience of Vitola et al. (111) for example, approximately half of the hepatic lesion that were less than 1 cm in size had FDG uptake that could be easily identified visually. The sensitivity of FDG PET for detection of mucinous tumors is lower than for nonmucinous tumors probably because of their relative hypocellularity (124,125).

In view of the known high uptake of FDG by activated macrophages, it is not surprising that inflamed tissue demonstrates FDG activity. Mild to moderate FDG activity seen along recent incisions, infected incisions, biopsy sites, drainage tubing, and catheters, as well as colostomy sites, can lead to errors in interpretation if the history is not known. Some inflammatory lesions, especially granulomatous ones, can accumulate FDG significantly including diverticulitis and inflammatory bowel disease.

FDG uptake normally present in the gastrointestinal tract can occasionally be difficult to differentiate from a malignant lesion, but the linear pattern of uptake, characteristic of bowel, is usually easily recognizable and is best seen on coronal views. The clinical history, physical examination, pattern of uptake, and correlation with anatomy as seen in the CT scan are more helpful in avoiding false-positive interpretations than semiquantitative evaluation by SUV.

Summary of the Indications for FDG PET Imaging in Patients with Colorectal Cancer

Evaluation of patients with known or suspected recurrent colorectal carcinoma is now an accepted indication for FDG PET imaging. FDG PET does not replace imaging modalities such as CT for preoperative anatomic evaluation but is indicated as the initial test for diagnosis and staging of recurrence and for preoperative staging (N and M) of known recurrence that is considered to be resectable. FDG PET imaging is valuable for differentiation of posttreatment changes from recurrent tumor, differentiation of benign from malignant lesions (indeterminate lymph nodes, hepatic and pulmonary lesions), and evaluation of patients with rising tumor markers in the absence of a known source. Addition of FDG PET to the evaluation of these patients reduces overall treatment costs by accurately identifying patients who will and will not benefit from surgical procedures.

Although initial staging at the time of diagnosis is often performed during colectomy, FDG PET imaging is recommended for a subgroup of patients at high risk (with elevated CEA levels) and normal CT and for whom surgery can be avoided if FDG PET shows metastases. Screening for recurrence in patients at high risk has also been advocated.

LYMPHOMA

The incidence of Hodgkin's disease (HD) and non-Hodgkin's lymphoma (NHL) is only 8% of all malignancies, but they are potentially curable malignancies. One of the most important factors influencing relapse-free and total survival of lymphoma patients (in addition to histologic appearance) is extent of disease, and accurate initial staging is essential for optimizing patient therapy and determining prognosis (136,137). Patients diagnosed with stage I or II HD and some subgroups of NHL may receive local external radiotherapy alone or in combination with chemotherapy; whereas those with stage III or IV disease are typically treated with chemotherapy (137). Prognostic implications are equally important; stage is consistently identified as a major prognostic factor in all lymphomas and HD.

Conventional Modalities for Detecting and Staging Lymphoma

Conventional modalities for staging lymphoma include physical examination; CT of the chest, abdomen and pelvis; bone scintigraphy; and bone marrow biopsy. Although CT is the best imaging technique to provide detailed information about the relationship between organs and vascular structures, CT criteria for pathologic adenopathy are based on size alone, which is a major limitation. In addition, CT has limited sensitivity for detection of spleen, liver, and bone marrow involvement.

^{67}Ga plays a role in the evaluation of residual posttherapy masses for the presence of viable tumor, but it is not superior to CT in initial staging of untreated lymphoma. ^{67}Ga has many limitations: suboptimal photon energy leading to noisy images; variable uptake of gallium by tumor, particularly low grade NHL; limited detection of abdominal disease secondary to marked physiologic hepatic and colonic activity; and multiple visits to the imaging facility on consecutive days. FDG PET has replaced the use of ^{67}Ga imaging for lymphoma in most institutions.

The sensitivity of bone scintigraphy for detection of bone marrow involvement is relatively poor (138–141); therefore, staging the bone marrow requires invasive biopsy and aspiration, but the sensitivity for detecting bone marrow disease is limited by sampling error (142–145). Although MRI appears to be the most sensitive imaging technique, whole-body MRI is not practical as a screening technique and should be reserved for areas that are clinically suspect (146,147).

Staging Lymphoma with FDG PET Imaging

Both HD and NHL exhibit marked FDG uptake, and FDG imaging is useful both for staging and monitoring therapy (148–161) (Fig. 48.11). Compared with ^{67}Ga, FDG is avidly trapped by virtually all lymphomas, although the degree of FDG uptake does seem to correlate with the histologic grade of malignancy and proliferation rate (150,153). There is, however, a large overlap between low- and high-grade lymphoma. The degree of FDG uptake in untreated patients seems to be a better prognostic factor than the degree of ^{67}Ga uptake (149,162) . Although physiologic gastrointestinal activity does occur with FDG, the better quality of the images usually allows differentiation of physiologic activity in the bowel from abdominal and pelvic lesions. With FDG PET imaging most of the skeleton is imaged during scanning, enabling noninvasive detection of focal bone marrow disease that may be missed through sampling error with standard iliac crest biopsy.

The high accuracy of FDG PET imaging for staging lymphoma, including low-grade (163,164), has been demonstrated in several studies evaluating the extent of lymphoma in nodal stations (155), extranodal sites (156), and bone marrow (157, 158). These studies demonstrated that both CT and FDG PET imaging detect additional nodal sites involved compared with each modality alone. However, FDG PET imaging is superior to CT for detection of extranodal lymphoma. FDG PET is also suitable for identifying bone marrow involvement (except in low-grade lymphoma) with a high positive predictive value and

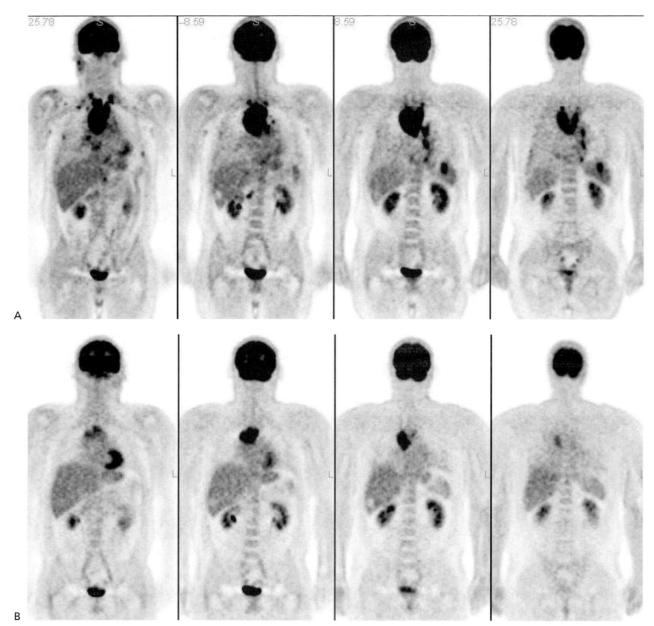

FIGURE 48.11. A 48-year-old man underwent resection of a right supraclavicular lymph node, and a diagnosis of B-cell non-Hodgkin's lymphoma was made. Computed tomography (CT) scan revealed a right parotid mass, a large mass in the mediastinum, a lesion in the spleen, and a lesion in the liver. The patient was referred for fluorodeoxyglucose (FDG) positron emission tomography (PET) imaging at initial staging **(A)** and after completion of therapy when the CT revealed a residual mass in the mediastinum **(B). A:** The FDG PET images obtained at the time of diagnosis revealed stage 4 widespread lymphomatous involvement of the right parotid, the large mediastinal mass extending to the base of the neck bilaterally, and the splenic lesion seen on CT. FDG PET images revealed additional foci of uptake in the mesentery, retroperitoneum, and in the ribs bilaterally. The hepatic lesions seen on CT appeared photopenic supporting the diagnosis of hepatic cysts. **B:** The FDG images obtained after completion of chemotherapy demonstrated marked improvement, but residual uptake in the mediastinal mass indicated partial response to therapy and residual tumor in the mediastinum.

is more sensitive and specific than bone scintigraphy (165). Compared with bone marrow biopsy, FDG PET imaging can detect bone marrow involvement when the posterior iliac crest biopsy is normal (157,158).

In these studies, FDG PET led to a change in staging and management in 7% to 22% of patients (155,158,160,161,164, 166). A survey-based study of referring physicians reported that FDG PET imaging contributed to a change of clinical stage and major management decisions in more than 40% of the patients (167). An overall review of the literature including 1,796 patients concluded that the sensitivity and specificity of FDG PET imaging for staging lymphoma was 90% and 93%, respectively, compared with 81% and 69% for CT. In that review, FDG PET imaging led to a change in management in 21% of the patients (168).

Monitoring Therapy and Detection of Persistent or Recurrent Lymphoma with FDG PET

In patients with NHL, standard chemotherapy causes a rapid decrease in tumor FDG uptake as early as 7 days after treatment and continues to decline during therapy (Fig. 48.11). The uptake at 42 days was superior to the uptake at 7 days posttherapy in predicting the long-term outcome (169). A study of 28 patients evaluated with FDG early during chemotherapy have demonstrated that the progression free survival at 1 and 2 years was 20% and 0%, respectively, for FDG-positive patients and 87% and 68% for FDG-negative patients (170).

Although the sensitivity of CT and FDG imaging may be comparable in staging untreated lymphoma, CT is unable to distinguish between active or recurrent disease and residual scar tissue after therapy. FDG PET is clearly superior to CT in that regard: Approximately 90% of patients with positive findings on PET relapse compared with less than 10% of patients with negative findings on PET (171–174), including patients with abdominal lymphomas (175). A larger study on 91 patients has demonstrated the excellent prognostic value of FDG PET imaging for prediction of relapse-free survival after completion of first-line therapy (176).

The overall review of the literature included 581 patients evaluated for recurrence; the sensitivity and specificity of FDG PET imaging was 87% and 93%, respectively, compared with 92% and 10% for CT. In that group of patients, FDG PET imaging led to a change in management in 10% of the patients (168).

Summary of the Indications of FDG PET Imaging for Patients with Lymphoma

FDG PET imaging is recommended for staging lymphoma in addition to CT and other conventional staging modalities, because it can detect additional nodal and extranodal lymphomatous lesions, as well as bone marrow involvement even when the bone marrow biopsy is for tumor. During chemotherapy, FDG PET imaging can identify the responders early in the course of treatment, allowing alterations in the chemotherapy regimen as indicated. Finally, FDG PET can differentiate scarring from persistent or recurrent tumor in residual masses after the end of treatment. FDG PET imaging after completion of therapy can accurately predict relapse-free survival. Because of the superior resolution of FDG images compared with ^{67}Ga scintigraphy, FDG imaging is replacing ^{67}Ga for evaluation of patients with lymphoma.

MELANOMA

The classification of melanomas is based on the depth of invasion in the dermis, as well as the thickness of the tumor (177,178).

The incidence of metastases and, therefore, the prognosis is related to the depth of invasion. The peak time for the development of metastases is during the first and second year after diagnosis. Melanoma can metastasize to virtually any organ; the most frequent metastatic sites are the skin and lymph nodes, lungs, liver, brain, and skeleton. The presence of systemic metastases is associated with a very poor prognosis and a mean survival of less than 6 months. Accurate staging of disease extent in malignant melanoma remains problematic.

Early-Stage Melanoma

For low-risk melanoma (thickness <1 mm), there is only 2% to 3% lymph node involvement, and there is no difference in survival whether observation or elective lymph node dissection is performed. For intermediate-risk melanoma (thickness 1 to 3 mm), there is a 20% to 50% risk of lymph nodes involvement, and staging of regional lymph nodes is critical for determining the prognosis and therapy. FDG PET has well-known limitations for detection of microscopic metastases, FDG PET sensitivity is ~90% for detection of metastatic deposits greater than 80 mm^3 but decreases rapidly for smaller volumes (179,180). A direct comparison of sentinel node biopsy and FDG PET in 50 patients with intermediate-risk melanoma confirmed the limitations of FDG PET (181). Therefore, identification and pathologic examination of the sentinel lymph node is the standard of care for patients with intermediate-risk melanoma.

High-Risk Melanoma

In patients with high-risk melanoma (thickness >3 mm), the incidence of metastases at the time of diagnosis is 50% to 70%, and FDG PET imaging is useful in detecting subclinical lymph node involvement noninvasively, as well as metastases to other organs (182) (Fig. 48.12). Subsequent studies have demonstrated the high accuracy of FDG PET to identify both nodal and visceral metastases from melanoma (183–192). False-positive findings have included other malignancies and inflammatory lesions; false negatives have included skin lesions without mass effects and lesions smaller than 5 mm in size. In a prospective study of 100 patients with high-risk melanoma (thickness >1.5 mm) comparing FDG PET imaging and conventional diagnostic methods, FDG PET was superior in staging melanoma at primary diagnosis and during follow-up both on a patient basis and a lesion basis (188). Although controversy still exists, combining sentinel lymph node localization and biopsy with whole-body FDG PET imaging may optimize initial staging of high-risk melanoma.

Cost-benefit and outcome analyses have not yet been reported. However, a 1996 to 1997 retrospective study of the inclusion of FDG PET in the staging of patients with suspected or metastatic melanoma demonstrated a saving of $1,800 per patient, a net savings-to-cost ratio of more than two (193).

A meta-analysis of 89 studies, of which 13 were selected for analysis, reported a sensitivity and specificity of FDG PET imaging for detection of lesions of 92% and 90%, respectively, leading to a change of management in 22% of patients (194). Another meta-analysis whose criteria included only six studies

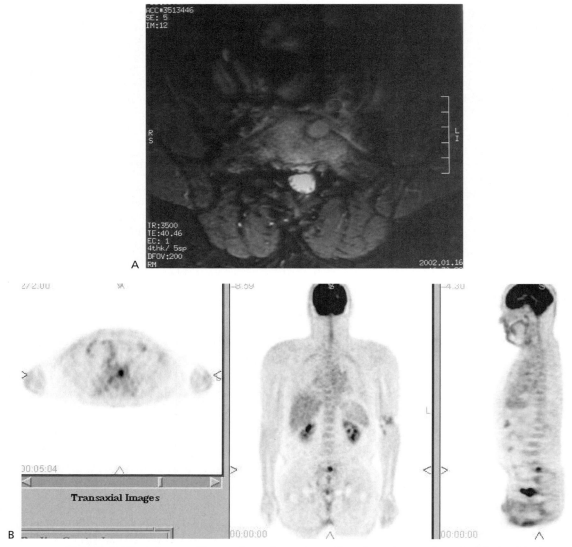

FIGURE 48.12. A 46-year-old man who underwent resection of a melanoma from the left shoulder 2 weeks earlier was referred for staging. **A:** Orthogonal fluorodeoxyglucose positron emission tomography images through the sacrum revealed a solitary focus of uptake in the sacrum. **B:** A magnetic resonance imaging confirmed the lesion and a biopsy confirmed a metastasis.

reported a pooled sensitivity and specificity of 79% and 86%, respectively. A subgroup analysis revealed that PET was more accurate for systemic staging than regional staging, and, when used for regional staging, FDG PET imaging performed better for patients with stage 3 disease than for patients with stage 1 and 2 disease (195). A extensive review of the literature including 888 patients reported a sensitivity and specificity of 83% and 91%, respectively, and a change of management in 26% of the patients (196).

Summary of the Indications of FDG PET Imaging for Patients with Melanoma

FDG PET imaging has proven beneficial in the assessment of patients with high-risk melanoma and in patients with suspected recurrent or metastatic disease. At present, it is not typically used in the initial evaluation of patients with low-to-intermediate-risk melanoma.

BREAST CANCER

Primary and metastatic breast cancer have been studied with PET imaging. Evaluations have demonstrated increased metabolic activity in both the primary tumors and metastatic lesions (Fig. 48.13). A recent meta-analysis of the PET literature in the diagnosis of breast cancer demonstrated sensitivity of 88% and a specificity of 79% using data from 606 patients (197). The role of PET in diagnosis of breast cancer is still being determined. New devices for breast imaging of FDG are being developed and may result in improved lesion detection accuracy The initial studies that evaluated the accuracy of PET in staging the axilla

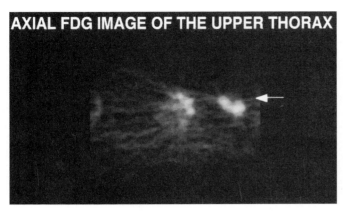

FIGURE 48.13. Fluorodeoxyglucose positron emission tomography image of the upper thorax in a woman with breast cancer demonstrates hypermetabolism in left axillary lymph nodes (*arrow*) and in the anterior mediastinum indicating metastatic disease.

were very promising (198,199). More recent studies have been mixed with sensitivities ranging from 70% to 100% and specificities ranging from 60% to 90%. Most centers do not consider PET to be a replacement for sentinel lymph node studies.

[18]F-labeled estrogen compounds can be used to image breast cancer cells with estrogen receptors (200). In 93% of metastatic lesions that were identified in 16 patients, 16 α-[^{18}F]fluoro-17 β-estradiol (FES) imaging showed increased uptake. The uptake diminished with antiestrogen therapy, demonstrating the specificity of the technique for imaging estrogen receptors.

Initial evaluation of breast cancer therapy response has been performed with both FDG and ^{11}C-methionine (201,202). After chemohormonotherapy, breast tumors larger than 3 cm in diameter have shown sequential decreases in FDG accumulation in partial and complete response patients, whereas nonresponding patients showed no decrease. Decreased ^{11}C-methionine has been shown to correspond with clinical stability or regression of disease. A recent study using FDG PET in 22 patients demonstrated that PET correctly identified responses to systemic therapy following the first course with a sensitivity of 100% and specificity of 85% (203). A metabolic response was defined as a decrease in the tumor SUV to a level below 55% of baseline.

Studies using whole-body imaging have demonstrated the ability of FDG PET to accurately stage breast malignancy. FDG PET is complementary to other imaging techniques in detecting occult distant metastatic disease (204,205). In patients who have both FDG PET scans and radionuclide bone scans, PET detects a greater fraction of osteolytic lesions, and bone scans detect more osteoblastic lesions.

BONE AND SOFT TISSUE TUMORS

Bone and soft tissue tumors are like brain tumors in that they exist in multiple grades of aggressivity. PET has been able to accurately identify the grades of different soft tissue tumors. In musculoskeletal tumors, the glucose utilization rate as identified by quantitative FDG PET correlates to the grade of the tumor

(206). Semiquantitative assessment of FDG accumulation by uptake ratio calculation has been demonstrated as a means of distinguishing benign and malignant soft tissue masses (207) and correlates with the grade of musculoskeletal tumors (208). ^{13}N-labeled glutamate evaluation of osteogenic sarcoma (209) and [13]N L-glutamate imaging of Ewing sarcoma (210) have demonstrated increased uptake in the tumors. ^{11}C-α-aminoisobutyric acid imaging of malignant fibrous histiocytoma (211) has also been reported.

Identification of the effect of therapy on these tumors has been the subject of investigation with PET. Animal models have demonstrated that PET regional oxygen utilization decreases after irradiation to 30% of that initially in the tumor and that regional blood flow increases in the tumor initially and then decreases 1 week after irradiation (212). Combined hyperthermia and irradiation protocols have been evaluated using FDG PET; after therapy, a very hypometabolic central area of necrosis (Fig. 48.14) that is surrounded by a hypermetabolic pseudocapsule (213) is demonstrated. These findings indicate that PET

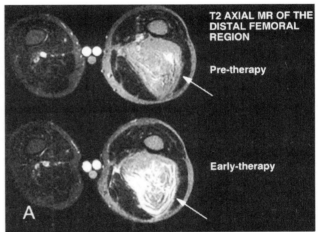

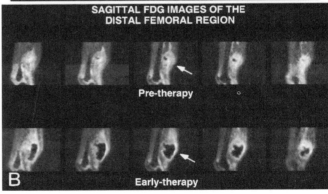

FIGURE 48.14. A: T2-weighted magnetic resonance images of a distal femoral region liposarcoma (*arrow*) before (*upper images*) and 1 week after beginning (*lower images*) therapy demonstrating an increase in T2 signal intensity in the early therapy study. **B:** Fluorodeoxyglucose positron emission tomography images demonstrate hypermetabolism in the distal femoral region (*arrow*) corresponding to the mass on magnetic resonance imaging on the pretherapy study (*upper images*) and an ametabolic central area of necrosis on the early-therapy study (*lower images*) with a hypermetabolic rim that represents a nontumorous pseudocapsule.

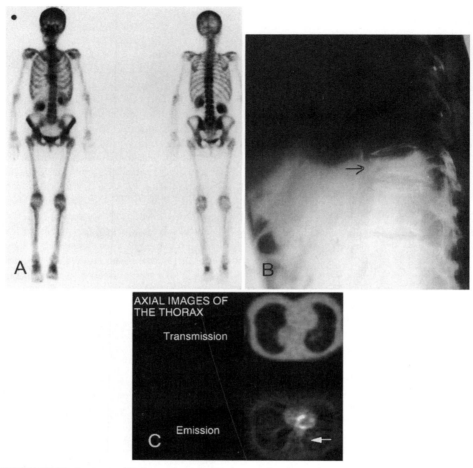

FIGURE 48.15. Bone scan **(A)** demonstrates a T9 abnormality that is shown to be a compression fracture on plain film (*arrow*) **(B)**. The fluorodeoxyglucose positron emission tomography image **(C)** is hypometabolic in this region (*arrow*). Pathology identified the abnormality as a benign compression fracture.

may be useful in assessing the effect of therapy. The utility of PET in identifying recurrent disease has yet to be evaluated.

Metastatic disease to the bones occurs commonly with prostate, breast, and lung cancer. Cancer patients will commonly present with back pain and be found to have vertebral body abnormalities on plain films, CT, MRI, or bone scan. The abnormality can often have a component of vertebral body compression, and it is impossible to differentiate malignant from benign causes on the imaging studies. FDG PET can differentiate benign vertebral pathology from malignant disease (214) (Fig. 48.15). Increased FDG uptake may occur in acute compression fractures and in osteomyelitis. Tissue biopsy of vertebral body lesions is difficult and subject to sampling error. FDG PET can direct needle biopsy to locations of tumor and allow an accurate diagnosis to be obtained (Figs. 48.15 and 48.16).

HEAD AND NECK CANCER

Head and neck cancer represents about 5% of all malignancies diagnosed annually. Greater than 90% of these tumors have squamous cell pathology. Risk factors for head and neck squamous cell cancer (HNSCC) are classically reported as prolonged tobacco and ethanol abuse. The prognosis for most subsites and stages of HNSCC has remained unchanged over the last 40 years. Organ-sparing approaches (chemotherapy and radiation) have gained an increased acceptance as a therapeutic modality but are still considered an alternative to surgery with postoperative radiotherapy. An exception to this statement would be tumors of the larynx in which an organ-sparing approach is first attempted at most cancer centers (215,216).

PET Imaging Techniques for the Head and Neck

Head and neck PET images should include at least regions from the inferior orbits to the lower abdomen. The emission data should be corrected using measured attenuation correction when performing head and neck imaging. The acute curvature around the mouth, nose, mandible, and neck results in severe edge artifacts when PET studies are performed without attenuation correction. Neck lymph nodes can lie near the skin surface and edge artifacts created without attenuation correction can hamper

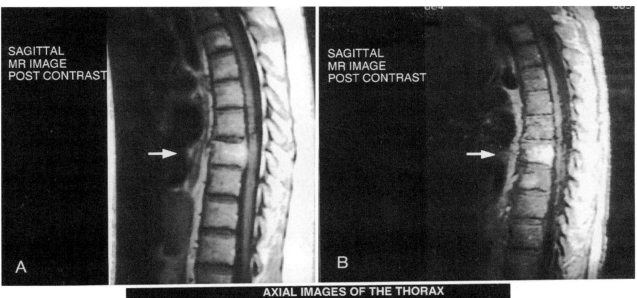

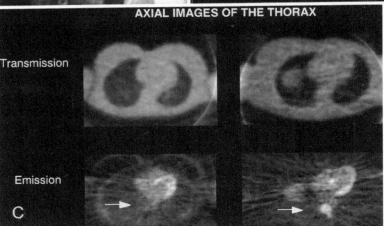

FIGURE 48.16. Sagittal magnetic resonance (MR) images obtained after gadolinium administration show enhancement of vertebral bodies with some degree of compression abnormality (*arrow*). MR image **(A)** corresponds to the positron emission tomography (PET) images on the right **(C)** that demonstrate hypermetabolism (*arrow*) and were found to be pathologic from metastatic breast cancer. MR image **(B)** corresponds to the PET images on the left **(C)** that demonstrate hypometabolism (*arrow*) and were found to be benign.

their identification. The anatomic relationships of airways and bony structures to soft tissue can also be more reliably assessed when an attenuation map is available for comparison.

Imaging the head and neck region presents unique challenges for PET. The region has substantial normal variation in uptake that can present dilemmas in the identification of pathologic conditions (Fig. 48.17). Uptake in adenoidal, palatine, and lingual tonsil tissue is a normal variant that must be recognized. Uptake in floor of mouth and laryngeal and neck musculature are also commonly seen findings. Taking steps to reduce or eliminate muscle uptake is crucial. Making sure that patient is not chewing gum, reading, or talking during the uptake phase is important. Some have advocated the use of diazepam (Valium) to suppress muscle uptake. This appears to work well but deserves an extra note of caution in head and neck cancer patients because of existing airway compromise. Technical attention to

the position of the patient's head during the uptake phase is of prime importance. Experimenting with chair designs and pillow placement to ensure slight head flexion and complete head relaxation is essential to obtaining a scan without muscle uptake interference. Also, with 3D surface projections and careful examination of all three orthogonal views, most muscle uptake can be differentiated from disease by its anatomic pattern of distribution. This cannot, however, replace proper patient preparation.

Staging Head and Neck Cancer

Accurate staging is the single most important factor in patient assessment, treatment planning, and survival prognostication (217,218). The most commonly used imaging modality for HNSCC is CT with intravenous iodinated contrast. Lymph nodes greater than 1 cm in diameter (1.5 cm for jugulodigastric

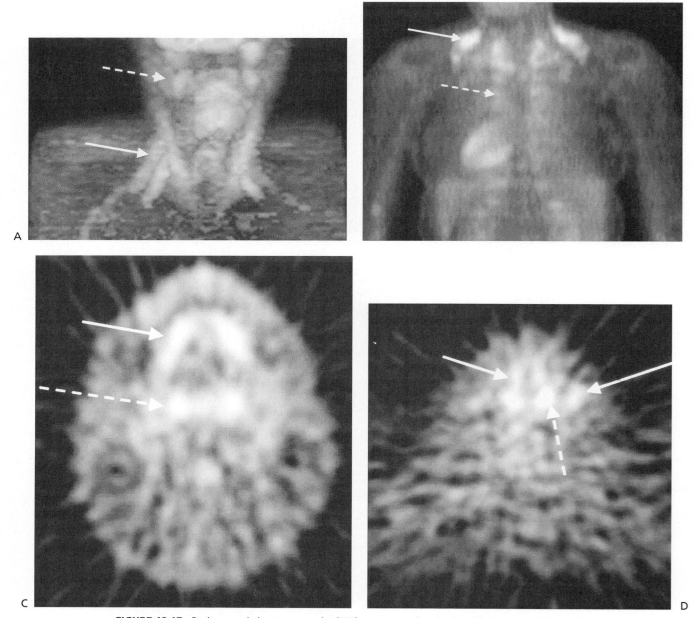

FIGURE 48.17. Positron emission tomography (PET) scan coronal projection **(A)** showing high metabolism in neck muscles, probably scalene and sternocleidomastoid muscles (*arrow*). Pterygoid muscle uptake is also seen (*dashed arrow*). PET scan coronal projection **(B)** showing high metabolism at neck muscle insertions (*arrow*) and at costovertebral articulations (*dashed arrow*). PET scan axial view **(C)** showing high metabolism in floor of mouth muscles, probably mylohyoid (*arrow*), and at palatine tonsils (*dashed arrow*). PET scan axial view **(D)** showing high metabolism probably in vocalis muscles (*short arrow*), cricoarytenoid posterior muscle (*dashed arrow*), and the inferior margin of a tumor-bearing lymph node (*long arrow*).

nodes) or with central necrosis are considered abnormal and suspicious for metastasis.

Standard assessment for distant metastases in HNSCC, which is uncommon for patients presenting with a new tumor, can include chest x-ray film and liver function tests. CT of the chest or abdomen is most commonly used to evaluate abnormalities found on the preceding two studies.

Staging of the primary tumor (T stage) using PET has been described in several published articles (219,220). When the primary was seen by conventional techniques, PET did not show an advantage over conventional techniques. Primary tumor staging with PET will likely contribute little over conventional staging in most patients. Standard tumor staging using CT and physical examination with endoscopy will provide more tumor staging anatomic information than PET. In about 5% of cases, however, the primary may not be identified by standard techniques. PET

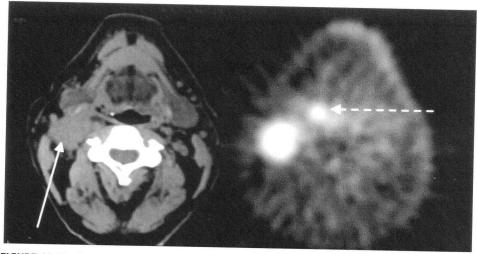

FIGURE 48.18. Computed tomography (CT) and positron emission tomography (PET) images of a patient with a right neck mass showing squamous cell cancer on biopsy (*arrow*) and an unknown primary even after review of the CT, physical examination, and panendoscopic biopsies that were negative for tumor. Thereafter, PET showed a right base of tongue primary (*dashed arrow*).

may identify the unknown primary in about 20% to 50% of cases as reported by several authors (221–226) (Fig. 48.18). There is some evidence that PET should only be performed after clinical assessment because routine panendoscopy and physical examination will identify some small lesions that may not be seen by PET (227).

Previous authors have described the high accuracy of FDG PET in local nodal staging of head and neck cancer (219,220, 228–233) (Fig. 48.19). All studies have shown PET to be equivalent or superior to anatomic methods of nodal staging. In a study by Adams et al. (228) about 1,400 lymph nodes were sampled in 60 patients, and PET had a 10% advantage in sensitivity for local nodal disease over CT, MRI, or ultrasound (US). The specificity was also 10% higher for PET. The authors showed highly statistically significant differences in the performance of these modalities. Metastatic disease to distant regions may also be better evaluated by PET, although distant metastasis are somewhat less common with head and neck cancer than with other malignancies.

Evaluation of Therapy of Head and Neck Cancer

PET's potential role in evaluating tumor response to nonoperative therapies is promising. Many times, artifact produced by chemotherapy or XRT (fibrosis, erythema, edema) may confound the practitioner's ability to evaluate tumor response to therapy either by physical examination or anatomic imaging. Standard anatomic imaging using CT or MRI has limited ability to evaluate the effect of radiation or chemotherapy on malignancy. This is most commonly true because of contrast enhancement and/or soft tissue distortion that is apparent in posttherapy regions seen on conventional imaging. Changes in tumor size may also lag behind metabolic effects of therapy. Because PET is a functional study, persistence of tumor in the setting of no

anatomic abnormality, or absence of tumor in the setting of persistent anatomic abnormality, can be assessed.

Significantly increased FDG uptake can be seen in soft tissue regions that have been recently irradiated. Commonly, uptake will be seen in tissues that are more intensely exposed. Some normal deep structures may not show radiation-related changes

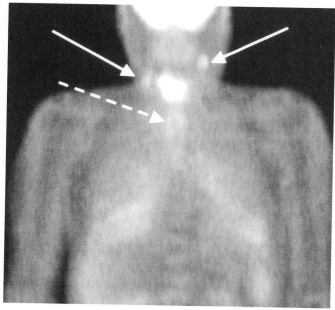

FIGURE 48.19. Positron emission tomography (PET) image demonstrating improved staging with PET of a patient with laryngeal cancer who had a computed tomography (CT) scan showing a laryngeal mass and left neck and subcarinal adenopathy. The PET showed bilateral neck disease (*arrows*), the laryngeal primary, and no subcarinal disease. A tracheostomy site is also faintly seen secondary to inflammation (*dashed arrow*). Bilateral neck dissections confirmed bilateral neck disease and a follow-up CT showed resolution of the subcarinal adenopathy.

in metabolism (234). The duration following XRT during which increased uptake occurs is of interest for study interpretation. Increased FDG accumulation in regions of XRT can be statistically significant at least 12 to 16 months after treatment in some body regions (235). Radiation-related uptake is generally less than what is found in recurrent tumor. Nevertheless, FDG uptake from radiation effects can occasionally be in a range that is worrisome for malignancy and must be recognized.

Metabolic changes in tumor occurring during chemotherapy may be somewhat more specific to tumor response. Some tumors demonstrate a significant reduction in metabolism that is associated with good pathologic response. Hypermetabolism secondary to inflammation does not appear to be a significant problem in contrast to radiation-treated tissue. Tumor metabolism can be at baseline soft tissue levels as early as 1 week after therapy in responding patients (236). PET has 90% sensitivity and specificity in detecting residual disease after chemotherapy in this

setting. Lowe et al. (236) and Greven et al. (237) used pathologic standards to assess the use of PET in the posttherapy evaluation of residual disease. Lowe et al. described PET to be as sensitive as needle biopsy (90%) in detecting residual disease after therapy and to have an 83% specificity (Fig. 48.20).

Assessment of Recurrent Head and Neck Cancer

All HNSCC patients are at high risk for recurrence and second primary disease. Most recurrences occur in the first 24 months following therapy for HNSCC. Later occurring lesions (lesions at different locations and with distinct histology) are probably second primaries. Local recurrences can present many challenges but, when detected early, can often be reexcised. Reexcision will further compromise any preexisting dysfunction (speech, voice, swallowing, or airway) and will negatively impact on a patient's

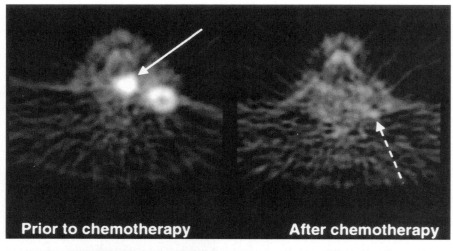

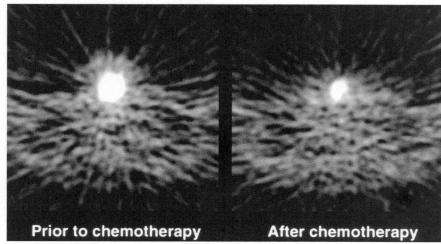

FIGURE 48.20. A: Positron emission tomography (PET) images demonstrating hypermetabolism in a base of tongue cancer (*arrow*) and a left jugulodigastric lymph node before therapy and resolution of all abnormalities after neoadjuvant chemotherapy except for minimal activity in the lymph node posttherapy (*dashed arrow*). Postchemotherapy neck dissection documented residual disease in the lymph node. PET images demonstrating hypermetabolism in a larynx cancer **(B)** before therapy and reduction but persistent activity after neoadjuvant chemotherapy. Needle biopsy failed to document residual disease but salvage laryngectomy confirmed residual disease.

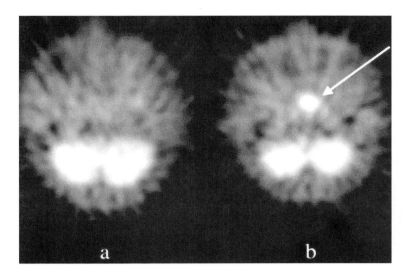

FIGURE 48.21. Positron emission tomography (PET) images of a patient with a history of nasopharynx cancer showing no disease 2 months after completion of chemotherapy and radiation therapy **(A)** but showing high nasopharynx recurrence (*arrow*) at the 9 month posttherapy scan **(B)**. Computed tomography showed stable posttherapy abnormalities at these times not indicative of recurrence. Biopsy was difficult given the location and was negative 2 months after the second PET. Disease was not confirmed pathologically until 1 year after the initially positive findings on PET and had continued to enlarge on PET during this time.

quality of life. Distant recurrences are more common in patients with locally recurrent disease than are distant metastasis at initial staging. The lungs are the most common site of distant recurrence. Before embarking on therapy of locally recurrent disease, distant disease recurrence should be excluded, because it would obviate the need for any attempt at curative resection of locally recurrent disease.

PET is clearly superior to other modalities in identifying recurrence of head and neck cancer after therapy. The use of PET for deciding if head and neck cancer has recurred has been described by several authors (220,232,237–243). The data show improved detection of recurrence by PET with the exception that Lapela et al. showed slightly higher sensitivity of CT (difference of 4%) for recurrence in their series (PET had a 36% higher specificity in this group). When PET is used in surveillance of patients who have completed treatment for head and neck cancer, PET can identify nearly twice as many cases of recurrent tumor as regular physical examination or routine CT imaging (242). Most of these recurrences are understandably small, and they may require repeated biopsies to confirm. If an initial biopsy is not positive for tumor when PET shows an abnormality, repeat biopsy or close follow-up should be undertaken. Surgical exploration should also be considered if the PET results are impressive because they are rarely incorrect (Figs. 48.21 and 48.22).

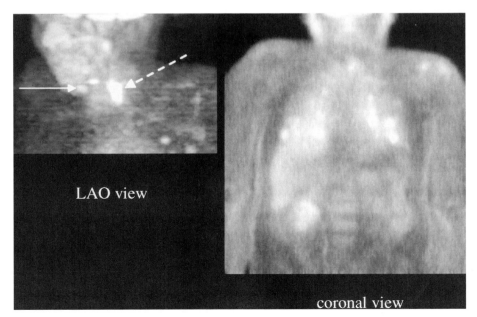

LAO view

coronal view

FIGURE 48.22. Positron emission tomography (PET) images of a patient who had a prior laryngectomy and radiation treatment for larynx cancer who presents with difficulty swallowing and a "suspicious" needle aspirate of a submental lymph node. Computed tomography imaging showed only postoperative changes in the head and neck. The PET showed nodal disease (*arrow*), local larynx recurrence (*dashed arrow*), and lung metastasis.

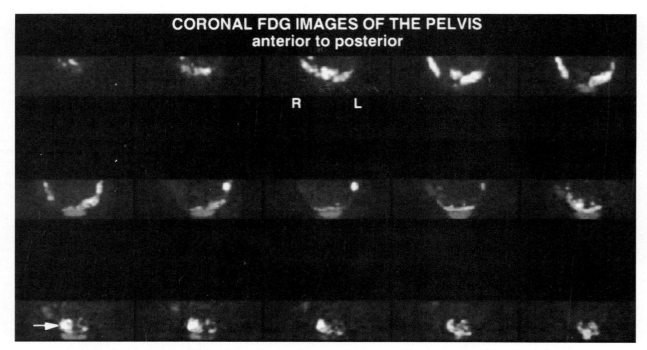

CORONAL FDG IMAGES OF THE PELVIS
anterior to posterior

R L

FIGURE 48.23. Coronal fluorodeoxyglucose positron emission tomography images of the pelvis demonstrating hypermetabolism in a right ovarian malignancy (*arrow*) with diffuse peritoneal and pelvic involvement.

OTHER CANCER

FDG PET is used to assess pelvic malignancy (Fig. 48.23). PET has been demonstrated to be superior to conventional imaging modalities in patients with cervical cancer. PET may be a useful adjunct to conventional imaging in the staging and restaging of ovarian cancer, but its low sensitivity for detection of occult disease limits its usefulness.

FDG PET is used for the detection of metastatic disease in patients who have had well-differentiated thyroid cancer and elevated levels of thyroglobulin but negative findings on ^{131}I sodium iodide scans. FDG PET has also been shown to detect metastatic lesions in patients who have had medullary carcinoma of the thyroid and elevated serum levels of calcitonin.

SUMMARY

PET imaging in oncology relies on specific differences between tumor and normal cell physiology. By capitalizing on these differences, numerous radiotracers can be used to image cancer in the body. Many cancers can be imaged successfully by PET, and the use of whole-body scanners enables complete evaluation of tumors that often have systemic involvement. PET scanning in the future may more fully use these capabilities, as well as perform diagnostic functions that are poorly performed by other imaging modalities today.

REFERENCES

1. Warburg O. *The metabolism of tumors.* London: Constable, 1930.
2. Weber G. Enzymology of cancer cells. Part I. *N Engl J Med* 1977; 296:468–492.
3. Flier JS, Mueckler MM, Usher P et al. Elevated levels of glucose transport and transporter messenger RNA are induced by ras or src oncogenes. *Science* 1987;235:1492–1495.
4. Gallagher BM, Fowler JS, Gutterson NI et al. Metabolic trapping as a principle of radiopharmaceutical design: some factors responsible for the biodistribution of [18F] 2-deoxy-2-fluoro-D-glucose. *J Nucl Med* 1978;19:1154–1161.
5. Blomqvist G, Stone-Elander S, Halldin C et al. Positron emission tomographic measurements of cerebral glucose utilization using [1-C-11]D-glucose. *J Comput Assist Tomogr* 1991;15:796–801.
6. Isselbacher KJ. Sugar and amino acid transport by cells in culture: differences between normal and malignant cells. *N Engl J Med* 1972; 286:929–933.
7. Bolster JM, Vaalburg W, Paans AM et al. Carbon-11 labelled tyrosine to study tumor metabolism by positron emission tomography (PET). *Eur J Nucl Med* 1986;12:321–324.
8. Lilja A, Bergstrom K, Hartvig P et al. Dynamic study of supratentorial gliomas with L-methyl-11C-methionine and positron emission tomography. *Am J Neuroradiol* 1985;6:505–514.
9. Mineura K, Kowada M, Shishido F. Brain tumor imaging with synthesized 18F-fluorophenylalanine and positron emission tomography. *Surg Neurol* 1989;31:468–469.
10. Conti PS, Grossman SA, Wilson AA et al. Brain tumor imaging with C-11-labeled thymidine and PET. *Radiology* 1990;177P:234.
11. Guerson JR, Shields AR. Radiosynthesis of 3'-deoxy-3'- [18F] fluorothymidine: [18F] FLT for imaging of cellular proliferation in vivo. *Nucl Med Biol* 2000;27:143–156.
12. Hiesiger EM, Fowler JS, Logan J et al. Is [1-11C]putrescine useful as a brain tumor marker? *J Nucl Med* 1992;33:192–200.
13. DeGrado TR, Reiman RE, Liao RP et al. Pharmacokinetics and radiation dosimetry of [18F]Fluorocholine (FCH). *J Nucl Med* 2002;43: 92–99.
14. Tyler JL, Diksic M, Villemure JG et al. Metabolic and hemodynamic evaluation of gliomas using positron emission tomography. *J Nucl Med* 1987;28:1123–1133.
15. Ogawa T, Uemura K, Shishido F et al. Changes of cerebral blood flow, and oxygen and glucose metabolism following radiochemotherapy of gliomas: a PET study. *J Comput Assist Tomogr* 1988;12:290–297.

16. Strauss LG, Conti PS. The applications of PET in clinical oncology. *J Nucl Med* 1991;32:623–648.
17. Ginos JZ, Cooper AJ, Dhawan V et al. [13N]cisplatin PET to assess pharmacokinetics of intra-arterial versus intravenous chemotherapy for malignant brain tumors. *J Nucl Med* 1987;28:1844–1852.
18. Tyler JL, Yamamoto YL, Diksic M et al. Pharmacokinetics of superselective intra-arterial and intravenous [11C]BCNU evaluated by PET. *J Nucl Med* 1986;27:775–780.
19. Di Chiro G, DeLaPaz RL, Brooks RA et al. Glucose utilization of cerebral gliomas measured by [18F] fluorodeoxyglucose and positron emission tomography. *Neurology* 1982;32:1323–1329.
20. Lowe VJ, Delong DM, Hoffman JM et al. Dynamic FDG-PET imaging of focal pulmonary abnormalities to identify optimum time for imaging. *J Nucl Med* 1994;35:225P.
21. Turkington TG, Coleman RE, Schubert SF et al. An evaluation of post-injection transmission measurement in PET. *IEEE Trans Nucl Sci* 1994;41:1538–1544.
22. Zasadny KR, Wahl RL. Standardized uptake values of normal tissues at PET with 2-[fluorine-18]fluoro-2-deoxy-D-glucose: variations with body weight and a method for correction. *Radiology* 1993;189:847–850.
23. Patz EJ, Lowe VJ, Hoffman JM et al. Focal pulmonary abnormalities: evaluation with F-18 fluorodeoxyglucose PET scanning. *Radiology* 1993;188:487–490.
24. Beckett WS. Epidemiology and etiology of lung cancer. *Clin Chest Med* 1993;14:1–15.
25. Bailar JC III, Gornik HL. Cancer undefeated. *N Engl J Med* 1997;336:1569–1574.
26. Devesa SS, Grauman DJ, Blot WJ et al. Cancer surveillance series: changing geographic patterns of lung cancer mortality in the United States, 1950 through 1994. *J Natl Cancer Inst* 1999;91:1040–1050.
27. Prager D, Cameron R, Ford J et al. Bronchogenic carcinoma. In: Murray JF, Nadel JA, eds. *Textbook of respiratory medicine.* Philadelphia: WB Saunders, 2000:1415–1448.
28. Smith RA, Glynn TJ. Epidemiology of lung cancer. *Radiol Clin North Am* 2000;38:453–470.
29. Winning AJ, McIvor J, Seed WA et al. Interpretation of negative results in fine needle aspiration of discrete pulmonary lesions. *Thorax* 1986;41:875–879.
30. Odell MJ, Reid KR. Does percutaneous fine-needle aspiration biopsy aid in the diagnosis and surgical management of lung masses? *Can J Surg* 1999;42:297–301.
31. Tsukada H, Satou T, Iwashima A et al. Diagnostic accuracy of CT-guided automated needle biopsy of lung nodules. *Am J Roentgenol* 2000;175:239–243.
32. Dewan NA, Reeb SD, Gupta NC et al. PET-FDG imaging and transthoracic needle lung aspiration biopsy in evaluation of pulmonary lesions. A comparative risk-benefit analysis. *Chest* 1995;108:441–446.
33. Kubota K, Matsuzawa T, Fujiwara T et al. Differential diagnosis of lung tumor with positron emission tomography: a prospective study. *J Nucl Med* 1990;31:1927–1932.
34. Duhaylongsod FG, Lowe VJ, Patz EJ et al. Detection of primary and recurrent lung cancer by means of F-18 fluorodeoxyglucose positron emission tomography (FDG PET). *J Thorac Cardiovasc Surg* 1995;110:130–139.
35. Bury T, Dowlati A, Paulus P et al. Evaluation of the solitary pulmonary nodule by positron emission tomography imaging. *Eur Respir J* 1996;9:410–414.
36. Knight SB, Delbeke D, Stewart JR et al. Evaluation of pulmonary lesions with FDG-PET. Comparison of findings in patients with and without a history of prior malignancy. *Chest* 1996;109:982–988.
37. Gupta NC, Maloof J, Gunel E. Probability of malignancy in solitary pulmonary nodules using fluorine-18-FDG and PET. *J Nucl Med* 1996;37:943–948.
38. Lowe VJ, Duhaylongsod FG, Patz EF et al. Pulmonary abnormalities and PET data analysis: a retrospective study. *Radiology* 1997;202:435–439.
39. Lowe VJ, Fletcher JW, Gobar L et al. Prospective investigation of positron emission tomography in lung nodules. *J Clin Oncol* 1998;16:1075–1084.
40. Gould MK, Maclean CC, Kuschner WG et al. Accuracy of positron emission tomography in the diagnosis of pulmonary nodules and mass lesions: a meta-analysis. *JAMA* 2001;285:914–924.
41. Gambhir SS, Shepherd JE, Shah BD et al. Analytical decision model for the cost-effective management of solitary pulmonary nodules. *J Clin Oncol* 1998;16:2113–2125.
42. Van Schil PE, Van HRH, Schoofs EL. The value of mediastinoscopy in preoperative staging of bronchogenic carcinoma. *J Thorac Cardiovasc Surg* 1989;97:240–244.
43. Patterson GA, Ginsberg RJ, Poon PY et al. A prospective evaluation of magnetic resonance imaging, computed tomography, and mediastinoscopy in the preoperative assessment of mediastinal node status in bronchogenic carcinoma. *J Thorac Cardiovasc Surg* 1987;94:679–684.
44. Wahl RL, Quint LE, Greenough RL et al. Staging of mediastinal non-small cell lung cancer with FDG PET, CT, and fusion images: preliminary prospective evaluation. *Radiology* 1994;191:371–377.
45. Patz EJ, Lowe VJ, Goodman PC et al. Thoracic nodal staging with PET imaging with 18FDG in patients with bronchogenic carcinoma. *Chest* 1995;108:1617–1621.
46. Scott WJ, Schwabe JL, Gupta NC et al. Positron emission tomography of lung tumors and mediastinal lymph nodes using [18F]fluorodeoxyglucose. The members of the PET-Lung Tumor Study Group. *Ann Thorac Surg* 1994;58:698–703.
47. Sasaki M, Ichiya Y, Kuwabara Y et al. The usefulness of FDG positron emission tomography for the detection of mediastinal lymph node metastases in patients with non-small cell lung cancer: a comparative study with X-ray computed tomography. *Eur J Nucl Med* 1996;23:741–747.
48. Steinert HC, Hauser M, Allemann F et al. Non-small cell lung cancer: nodal staging with FDG PET versus CT with correlative lymph node mapping and sampling. *Radiology* 1997;202:441–446.
49. Sazon DA, Santiago SM, Soo HG et al. Fluorodeoxyglucose-positron emission tomography in the detection and staging of lung cancer. *Am J Respir Crit Care Med* 1996;153:417–421.
50. Valk PE, Pounds TR, Hopkins DM et al. Staging non-small cell lung cancer by whole-body positron emission tomographic imaging. *Ann Thorac Surg* 1995;60:1573–1581.
51. Vansteenkiste JF, Mortelmans LA. FDG-PET in the locoregional lymph node staging of non-small cell lung cancer: a comprehensive review of the Leuven lung cancer group experience. *Clin Pos Imag* 1999;2:223–231.
52. Pieterman RM, van Putten JW, Meuzelaar JJ et al. Preoperative staging of non-small-cell lung cancer with positron-emission tomography. *N Engl J Med* 2000;343:254–261.
53. Vansteenkiste JF, Stroobants SG, De LP et al. Mediastinal lymph node staging with FDG-PET scan in patients with potentially operable non-small cell lung cancer: a prospective analysis of 50 cases. Leuven Lung Cancer Group. *Chest* 1997;112:1480–1486.
54. Yasukawa T, Yoshikawa K, Aoyagi H et al. Usefulness of PET with 11C-methionine for the detection of hilar and mediastinal lymph node metastasis in lung cancer. *J Nucl Med* 2000;41:283–290.
55. Hara T, Inagaki K, Kosaka N et al. Sensitive detection of mediastinal lymph node metastasis of lung cancer with 11C-choline PET. *J Nucl Med* 2000;41:1507–1513.
56. Palm I, Hellwig D, Leutz M et al. Brain metastases of lung cancer: diagnostic accuracy of positron emission tomography with fluorodeoxyglucose (FDG-PET). *Medizinische Klinik* 1999;94:224–227.
57. Bury T, Dowlati A, Paulus P et al. Whole-body 18FDG positron emission tomography in the staging of non-small cell lung cancer. *Eur Respir J* 1997;10:2529–2534.
58. Lewis P, Griffin S, Marsden P et al. Whole-body 18F-fluorodeoxyglucose positron emission tomography in preoperative evaluation of lung cancer. *Lancet* 1994;344:1265–1266.
59. Boland GW, Goldberg MA, Lee MJ et al. Indeterminate adrenal mass in patients with cancer: evaluation at PET with 2-[F-18]-fluoro-2-deoxy-D-glucose. *Radiology* 1995;194:131–134.
60. Erasmus JJ, Patz EJ, McAdams HP et al. Evaluation of adrenal masses in patients with bronchogenic carcinoma using 18F-fluorodeoxyglucose positron emission tomography. *AJR* 1997;168:1357–1360.
61. Bury T, Barreto A, Daenen F et al. Fluorine-18 deoxyglucose positron

emission tomography for the detection of bone metastases in patients with non-small cell lung cancer. *Eur J Nucl Med* 1998;25:1244–1247.

62. Becker GL, Whitlock WL, Schaefer PS et al. The impact of thoracic computed tomography in clinically staged TI, NO, MO chest lesions. *Arch Int Med* 1990;150:557–559.

63. Recine D, Rowland K, Reddy S et al. Combined modality therapy for locally advanced non-small cell lung carcinoma. *Cancer* 1990;66:2270–2278.

64. Ginsberg RJ, Kris MG, Armstrong JG. Cancer of the lung. In: DeVita VT, Hellman S, Rosenberg SA, eds. *Cancer. Principles and practice of oncology,* 4th ed. Philadelphia: JB Lippincott, 1993:673–722.

65. Cox JD, Azarnia N, Byhardt RW et al. A randomized phase I/II trial of hyperfractionated radiation therapy with total doses of 60.0 Gy to 79.2 Gy: possible survival benefit with >69.9 Gy in favorable patients with Stage III non-small cell lung cancer: report of Radiation Therapy Oncology Group 83-11. *J Clin Oncol* 1990;8:1543–1555.

66. Ichiya Y, Kuwabara Y, Sasaki M et al. A clinical evaluation of FDG-PET to assess the response in radiation therapy for bronchogenic carcinoma. *Ann Nucl Med* 1996;10:193–200.

67. Lowe VJ, Patz EF, Harris L et al. FDG-PET evaluation of pleural abnormalities. *J Nucl Med* 1994;35:229P.

68. Patz EJ, Lowe VJ, Hoffman JM et al. Persistent or recurrent bronchogenic carcinoma: detection with PET and 2-[F-18]-2-deoxy-D-glucose. *Radiology* 1994;191:379–382.

69. Inoue T, Kim EE, Komaki R et al. Detecting recurrent or residual lung cancer with FDG-PET. *J Nucl Med* 1995;36:788–793.

70. Bury T, Corhay JL, Duysinx B et al. Value of FDG-PET in detecting residual or recurrent nonsmall cell lung cancer. *Eur Respir J* 1999;14:1376–1380.

71. Lowe VJ, Hebert ME, Anscher MS et al. Chest wall FDG accumulation in serial FDG-PET images in patients being treated for bronchogenic carcinoma with radiation. *Clin Positron Imag* 1998;1:185–191.

72. Wong TZ, Coleman RE. Brain tumors. In: Bender H, Palmedo H, Brersaik HJ et al., eds. *Atlas of clinical PET in oncology.* Berlin: Springer, 2000:153–170.

73. Coleman RE, Hoffman JM, Hanson MW et al. Clinical application of PET for the evaluation of brain tumors. *J Nucl Med* 1991;32:616–622.

74. Di Chiro G. Positron emission tomography using F[18F]-fluorodeoxyglucose in brain tumors: a powerful diagnostic and prognostic tool. *Invest Radiol* 1986;2:360–371.

75. Patronas NJ, Brooks RA, DeLaPaz RL et al. Glycolytic rate (PET) and contrast enhancement (CT) in human cerebral gliomas. *AJNR* 1983;4:533–553.

76. Kim CK, Alavi JB, Alavi A et al. New grading system of cerebral gliomas using positron emission tomography with F-18 fluorodeoxyglucose. *J Neurooncol* 1991;10:85–91.

77. Kameyama M, Shirane R, Itoh J et al. The accumulation of 11C-methionine in cerebral glioma patients studied with PET. *Acta Neurochir* 1990;104:8–12.

78. Ribon D, Eriksson A, Hartman M et al. Positron emission tomography [11}C-methionine and survival in patients with low-grade gliomas. *Cancer* 2001;92:1541–1549.

79. Derlon JM, Bourdet C, Bustany P et al. [11C]L-methionine uptake in gliomas. *Neurosurgery* 1989;25:720–728.

80. Ogawa T, Kanno I, Shishido F et al. Clinical value of PET with 18F-fluorodeoxyglucose and L-methyl-llC-methionine for diagnosis of recurrent brain tumor and radiation injury. *Acta Radiol* 1991;32:197–202.

81. Alavi JB, Alavi A. Chawluk J et al. Positron emission tomography in patients with glioma. A predictor of prognosis. *Cancer* 1988;62:1074–1078.

82. Schifter T, Hoffman JM, Hanson MW et al. Serial FDG-PET studies in the prediction of survival in patients with primary brain tumors. *J Comput Assis Tomogr* 1993;17:509–561.

83. Francavilla TL, Miletich RS, Di CG et al. Positron emission tomography in the detection of malignant degeneration of low-grade gliomas. *Neurosurgery* 1989;24:1–5.

84. Hanson MW, Glantz MJ, Hoffman JM et al. FDG-PET in the selec-

85. Laohaprasit N, Silbergeld DL, Ojemann GA et al. Postoperative CT contrast enhancement following lobectomy for epilepsy. *J Neurosurg* 1990;73:392–395.

86. Burke JW, Podrasky AE, Bradley WG. Meninges: benign postoperative enhancement on MR images. *Radiology* 1990;174:99–102.

87. Glantz MJ, Hoffman JM, Coleman RE et al. Identification of early recurrence of primary central nervous system tumors by [18F]fluorodeoxyglucose positron emission tomography. *Ann Neurol* 1991;29:347–355.

88. Chao ST, Sub JH, Raja S et al. The sensitivity and specificity of FDG PET in distinguishing recurrent brain tumor from radionecrosis in patients treated with stereotactic radiosurgery. *Int J Cancer* 2001;96:191–197.

89. Dooms GC, Hecht S, Brant-Zawadski M et al. Brain radiation lesions: MR imaging. *Radiology* 1986;158:149–155.

90. Di Chiro G, Oldfield E, Wright DC et al. Cerebral necrosis after radiotherapy and/or intra-arterial chemotherapy for brain tumors: PET and neuropathologic studies. *AJR* 1988;150:189–197.

91. Kim EE, Chung SK, Haynie TP et al. Differentiation of residual or recurrent tumors from post-treatment changes with F-18 FDG PET. *Radiographics* 1992;12:269–279.

92. Abdel-Nabi H, Doerr RJ, Lamonica DM et al. Staging of primary colorectal carcinomas with fluorine-18 fluorodeoxyglucose whole-body PET: correlation with histopathologic and CT findings. *Radiology* 1998;206:755–760.

93. Mukai M, Sadahiro S, Yasuda S et al. Preoperative evaluation by whole-body 18F-fluorodeoxyglucose positron emission tomography in patients with primary colorectal cancer. *Oncol Rep* 2000;7:85–87.

94. Moertel CG, Fleming TR, McDonald JS et al. An evaluation of the carcinoembryonic antigen (CEA) test for monitoring patients with resected colon cancer. *JAMA* 1993;270:943–947.

95. Cheu YM et al. Recurrent colorectal carcinoma: evaluation with barium enema examination and CT. *Radiology* 1987;163:307–310.

96. Sugarbaker PH, Grianola FJ, Dwyer S et al. A simplified plan for follow-up of patients with colon and rectal cancer supported by prospective studies of laboratory and radiologic test results. *Surgery* 1987;102:79–87.

97. Steele G Jr, Bleday R, Mayer R et al. A prospective evaluation of hepatic resection for colorectal carcinoma metastases to the liver: Gastrointestinal Tumor Study Group protocol 6584. *J Clin Oncol* 1991;9:1105–1112.

98. Soyer P, Levesque M, Elias D et al. Detection of liver metastases from colorectal cancer: comparison of intraoperative US and CT during arterial portography. *Radiology* 1992;183:541–544.

99. Nelson RC, Chezmar JL, Sugarbaker PH et al. Hepatic tumors: comparison of CT during arterial portography, delayed CT and MR imaging for preoperative evaluation. *Radiology* 1989;172:27–34.

100. Small WC, Mehard WB, Langmo LS et al. Preoperative determination of the resectability of hepatic tumors: efficacy of CT during arterial portography. *AJR* 1993;161:319–322.

101. Peterson MS, Baron RL, Dodd GD III et al. Hepatic parenchymal perfusion detected with CTPA: imaging-pathologic correlation. *Radiology* 1992;183:149–155.

102. Suckler LS, DeNardo GL. Trials and tribulations: oncological antibody imaging comes to the fore. *Semin Nucl Med* 1997;27:10–29.

103. Yonekura Y, Benua RS, Brill AB et al. Increased accumulation of 2-deoxy-2[18F]fluoro-D-glucose in liver metastases from colon carcinoma. *J Nucl Med* 1982;23:1133–1137.

104. Strauss LG, Clorius JH, Schlag P et al. Recurrence of colorectal tumors: PET evaluation. *Radiology* 1989;170:329–332.

105. Ito K, Kato T, Tadokoro M et al. Recurrent rectal cancer and scar: differentiation with PET and MR imaging. *Radiology* 1992;182:549–552.

106. Kim EE, Chung SK, Haynie TP et al. Differentiation of residual or recurrent tumors from post-treatment changes with F-18 FDG-PET. *Radiographics* 1992;12:269–279.

107. Gupta NC, Falk PM, Frank AL et al. Pre-operative staging of colo-

rectal carcinoma using positron emission tomography. *Nebr Med J* 1993;78:30–35.

108. Falk PM, Gupta NC, Thorson AG et al. Positron emission tomography for preoperative staging of colorectal carcinoma. *Dis Colon Rectum* 1994;37:153–156.

109. Beets G, Penninckx F, Schiepers C et al. Clinical value of whole-body positron emission tomography with [18F]fluorodeoxyglucose in recurrent colorectal cancer. *Br J Surg* 1994;81:1666–1670.

110. Schiepers C, Penninckx F, De Vadder N et al. Contribution of PET in the diagnosis of recurrent colorectal cancer: comparison with conventional imaging. *Eur J Surg Oncol* 1995;21:517–522.

111. Vitola JV, Delbeke D, Sandler MP et al. Positron emission tomography to stage metastatic colorectal carcinoma to the liver. *Am J Surg* 1996;171:21–26.

112. Lai DT, Fulham M, Stephen MS et al. The role of whole-body positron emission tomography with [18F]fluorodeoxyglucose in identifying operable colorectal cancer. *Arch Surg* 1996;131:703–707.

113. Delbeke D, Vitola J, Sandler MP et al. Staging recurrent metastatic colorectal carcinoma with PET. *J Nucl Med* 1997;38:1196–1201.

114. Ogunbiyi OA, Flanagan FL, Dehdashti F et al. Detection of recurrent and metastatic colorectal cancer: comparison of positron emission tomography and computed tomography. *Ann Surg Oncol* 1997;4: 613–620.

115. Flanagan FL, Dehdashti F, Ogunbiyi OA et al. Utility of FDG PET for investigating unexplained plasma CEA elevation in patients with colorectal cancer. *Ann Surg* 1998;227:319–323.

116. Valk PE, Abella-Columna E, Haseman MK et al. Whole-body PET imaging with F-18-fluorodeoxyglucose in management of recurrent colorectal cancer. *Arch Surg* 1999;134:503–511.

117. Ruhlmann J, Schomburg A, Bender H et al. Fluorodeoxyglucose whole-body positron emission tomography in colorectal cancer patients studied in routine daily practice. *Dis Colon Rectum* 1997;40: 1195–1204.

118. Flamen P, Stroobants S, Van Cutsem E et al. Additional value of whole-body positron emission tomography with fluorine-18-2-fluoro-2-deoxy-D-glucose in recurrent colorectal cancer. *J Clin Oncol* 1999; 1:894–901.

119. Akhurst T, Larson SM. Positron emission tomography imaging of colorectal cancer. *Semin Oncol* 1999;26:577–583.

120. Vogel SB, Drane WE, Ros PR et al. Prediction of surgical resectability in patients with hepatic colorectal metastases. *Ann Surg* 1994;219: 508–516.

121. Imbriaco M, Akhurst T, Hilton S et al. Whole-body FDG-PET in patients with recurrent colorectal carcinoma. A comparative study with CT. *Clin Positron Imag* 2000;3:107–114.

122. Imdahl A, Reinhardt MJ, Nitzsche EU et al. Impact of 18F-FDG-positron emission tomography for decision making in colorectal cancer recurrences. *Arch Surg* 2000;385:129–134.

123. Staib L, Schirrmeister H, Reske SN et al. Is (18)F-fluorodeoxyglucose positron emission tomography in recurrent colorectal cancer a contribution to surgical decision making? *Am J Surg* 2000;180:1–5.

124. Kalff VV, Hicks R, Ware R. F-18 FDG PET for suspected or confirmed recurrence of colon cancer. A prospective study of impact and outcome. *Clin Pos Imag* 2000;3:183.

125. Whiteford MH, Whiteford HM, Yee LF et al. Usefulness of FDG-PET scan in the assessment of suspected metastatic or recurrent adenocarcinoma of the colon and rectum. *Dis Colon Rectum* 2000;43: 759–767; discussion 767–770.

126. Berger KL, Nicholson SA, Dehadashti F et al. FDG PET evaluation of mucinous neoplasms: correlation of FDG uptake with histopathologic features. *Am J Roentgenol* 2000;174:1005–1008.

127. Huebner RH, Park KC, Shepherd JE et al. A meta-analysis of the literature for whole-body FDG PET detection of colorectal cancer. *J Nucl Med* 2000;41:1177–1189.

128. Gambhir SS, Czernin J, Schimmer J et al. A tabulated review of the literature. *J Nucl Med* 2001;42(Suppl):9S–12S.

129. Meta J, Seltzer M, Schiepers C et al. Impact of ^{18}F-FDG PET on managing patients with colorectal cancer: the referring physician's perspective. *J Nucl Med* 2001;42:586–590.

130. Strasberg SM, Dehdashti F, Siegel BA et al. Survival of patients evaluated by FDG PET before hepatic resection for metastatic colorectal carcinoma: a prospective database study. *Ann Surg* 2001;233: 320–321.

131. Gambhir SS, Valk P, Shepherd J et al. Cost effective analysis modeling of the role of FDG-PET in the management of patients with recurrent colorectal cancer. *J Nucl Med* 1997;38:90P.

132. Park KC, Schwimmer J, Sheperd JE et al. Decision analysis for the cost-effective management of recurrent colorectal cancer. *Ann Surg* 2001;233:310–319.

133. Haberkorn U, Strauss LG, Dimitrakopoulou A et al. PET studies of fluorodeoxyglucose metabolism in patients with recurrent colorectal tumors receiving radiotherapy. *J Nucl Med* 1991;31:1485–1490.

134. Findlay M, Young H, Cunningham D et al. Noninvasive monitoring of tumor metabolism using fluorodeoxyglucose and positron emission tomography in colorectal cancer liver metastases: correlation with tumor response to fluorouracil. *J Clin Oncol* 1996;14:700–708.

135. Guillem J, Calle J, Akhurst T et al. Prospective assessment of primary rectal cancer response to preoperative radiation and chemotherapy using 18-Fluorodeoxyglucose positron emission tomography. *Dis Colon Rectum* 2000;43:18–24.

136. Jotti G, Bonandonna G. Prognostic factors in Hodgkin's disease: implications for modern treatment. *Anticancer Res* 1998;8:749–760.

137. Armitage JO. Drug therapy: treatment of non Hodgkin's lymphoma. *N Engl J Med* 1993;328:1023–1030.

138. Landgren O, Axdorph U, Jacobson H et al. Routine bone scintigraphy is of limited value in the clinical assessment of untreated patients with Hodgkin's disease. *Leuk Lymph* 1998;29(Suppl 1): (abstr).

139. Orzel J, Sawaf NW, Richardson ML. Lymphoma of the skeleton: scintigraphic evaluation. *Am J Rehabil* 1988;150:1095–1099.

140. Schechter JP, Jones SE, Woolfenden JM et al. Bone scanning in lymphoma. *Cancer* 1976;38:1142–1146.

141. Ferrant A, Rodhain J, Michaux JL et al. Detection of skeletal involvement in Hodgkin's disease: a comparison of radiography, bone scanning, and bone marrow biopsy in 38 patients. *Cancer* 1975;35: 1346–1353.

142. Brunning RD, Bloomfield CD, McKenna RW et al. Bilateral trephine bone marrow biopsies in lymphoma and other neoplastic disease. *Ann Intern Med* 1975;82:375.

143. Ebie N, Loew JM, Gregory SA. Bilateral trephine bone marrow biopsies for staging non-Hodgkin's lymphoma: a second look. *Hematol Pathol* 1989;3:29.

144. Haddy TB, Parker RI, Magrath IT. Bone marrow involvement in young patients with non-Hodgkin's lymphoma: the importance of multiple bone marrow samples for accurate staging. *Med Pediatr Oncol* 1989;17:418.

145. Juneja SK, Wolf MM, Cooper IA. Value of bilateral bone marrow biopsy specimens in non-Hodgkin's lymphoma. *J Clin Pathol* 1990; 43:630.

146. Shields AF, Porter BA, Olson DO et al. The detection of bone marrow involvement by lymphoma using magnetic resonance imaging. *J Clin Oncol* 1987;5:225–230.

147. Altenhoefer C, Blum U, Bathmann J et al. Comparative diagnostic accuracy of magnetic resonance imaging and immunoscintigraphy for detection of bone marrow involvement in patients with malignant lymphoma. *J Clin Oncol* 1997;15:1754–1760.

148. Paul R. Comparison of fluorine-18-2-fluorodeoxyglucose and gallium-67 citrate imaging for detection of lymphoma. *J Nucl Med* 1987; 28:288–292.

149. Okada J, Yoshikawa K, Imazeki K et al. The use of FDG-PET in the detection and management of malignant lymphoma: correlation of uptake with prognosis. *J Nucl Med* 1991;32:686–691.

150. Okada J, Yoshikawa K, Imazeki K et al. Positron emission tomography using fluorine-18fluorodeoxyglucose in malignant lymphoma: a comparison with proliferative activity. *J Nucl Med* 1992;33:325–329.

151. Leskinen-Kallio S, Rudsalainen U, Nagren K et al. Uptake of carbon-11 methionine and fluorodeoxyglucose in non-Hodgkin's lymphoma: a PET study. *J Nucl Med* 1991;32:1211–1218.

152. Lapela M, Leskinen S, Minn HR et al. Increased glucose metabolism in untreated non Hodgkin's lymphoma: a study with positron emis-

sion tomography and fluorine-18 fluorodeoxyglucose. *Blood* 1995;86: 3522–3527.

153. Rodriguez M, Rehn S, Ahlström H et al. Predicting malignancy grade with PET in non-Hodgkin's lymphoma. *J Nucl Med* 1995;36: 1790–1796.

154. Hoh CK, Gaspy J, Rosen P et al. Whole body FDG-PET imaging for staging of Hodgkin's disease and lymphoma. *J Nucl Med* 1997; 38:343–348.

155. Moog F, Bangerter M, Diedrichs CG et al. Lymphoma: role of whole-body 2-deoxy-2-[F 18]fluoro D-glucose (FDG) PET in nodal staging. *Radiology* 1997;203:795–800.

156. Moog F, Bangerter M, Diedrichs CG et al. Extranodal malignant lymphoma: detection with FDG-PET versus CT. *Radiology* 1998; 206:475–481.

157. Carr R, Barrington SF, Madan B et al. Detection of lymphoma in bone marrow by whole-body positron emission tomography. *Blood* 1998;91:3340–3346.

158. Moog F, Bangerter M, Kotzerke J et al. 18-F fluorodeoxyglucose-positron emission tomography as a new approach to detect lymphomatous bone marrow. *J Clin Oncol* 1998;16:603–609.

159. Stumpe KD, Urbinelli M, Steinert HC et al. Whole-body positron emission tomography using fluorodeoxyglucose for staging of lymphoma: effectiveness and comparison with computed tomography. *Eur J Nucl Med* 1998;25:721–728.

160. Delbeke D, Martin WH, Morgan DS et al. 18F-fluorodeoxyglucose imaging with positron emission tomography for initial staging of Hodgkin's disease and lymphoma. *Mol Imag Biol* 2002;1:105–113.

161. Buchmann I, Reinhardt M, Elsner K et al. 2-(Fluorine-18)Fluoro-2-deoxy-D-glucose positron emission tomography in the detection and staging of malignant lymphoma. *Cancer* 2001;91:889–899.

162. Okada J, Oonishi H, Yoshikawa K et al. FDG-PET for predicting prognosis of malignant lymphoma. *Ann Nucl Med* 1994;8:187–191.

163. Najjar F, Hustinx R, Jerusalem G et al. Positron emission tomography (PET) for staging low-grade non-Hodgkin's lymphomas (NHL). *Cancer Biother Radiopharm* 2001;16:297–304.

164. Jerusalem G, Beguin Y, Najjar F et al. Positron emission tomography (PET) with 18F-fluorodeoxyglucose (18F-FDG) for the staging of low-grade non-Hodgkin's lymphoma. *Ann Oncol* 2001;12:825–830.

165. Moog F, Kotzerke J, Reske SN. FDG PET can replace bone scintigraphy in primary staging of malignant lymphoma. *J Nucl Med* 1999; 40:1407–1413.

166. Bangerter M, Moog F, Buchmann I et al. Whole-body 2-[18F]-fluoro-2-deoxy-D-glucose positron emission tomography (FDG PET) for accurate staging of Hodgkin's disease. *Ann Oncol* 1998;9:1117–1122.

167. Schoder H, Meta J, Yap C et al. Effect of whole-body 18F-FDG PET imaging on clinical staging and management of patients with malignant lymphoma. *J Nucl Med* 2001;42:1139–1143.

168. Gambhir SS, Czernin J, Schimmer J et al. A tabulated review of the literature. *J Nucl Med* 2001;42(Suppl):16S–20S.

169. Romer W, Hanauske AR, Ziegler S et al. Positron emission tomography in non-Hodgkin's lymphoma: assessment of chemotherapy with fluorodeoxyglucose. *Blood* 1998;91:4464–4471.

170. Jerusalem G, Beguin Y, Fassotte MF et al. Persistent tumor 18F-FDG uptake after a few cycles of polychemotherapy is predictive of treatment failure in non-Hodgkin's lymphoma. *Haematologica* 2000; 85:613–618.

171. de Wit M, Bumann D, Beyer W et al. Whole-body positron emission tomography (PET) for diagnosis of residual mass in patients with lymphoma. *Ann Oncol* 1997;8(Suppl 1):57–60.

172. Mikhaeel NG, Timothy AR, Hain SF et al. 18-FDG-PET for the assessment of residual masses on CT following treatment of lymphomas. *Ann Oncol* 2000;11(Suppl 1):147–150.

173. Jerusalem G, Beguin Y, Fassotte MF et al. Whole-body positron emission tomography using 18F-fluorodeoxyglucose for posttreatment evaluation in Hodgkin's disease and non-Hodgkin's lymphoma has higher diagnostic and prognostic value than classical computed tomography scan imaging. *Blood* 1999;94:429–433.

174. Michaeel NG et al. *Leuk Lymphoma* 2000;39:543–553.

175. Zinzani PL, Magagnoli M, Chierichetti F et al. The role of positron emission tomography (PET) in the management of lymphoma patients. *Ann Oncol* 1999;1181–1184.

176. Spaepen K, Stroobants S, Dupont P et al. Prognostic value of positron emission tomography (PET) with fluorine-18 fluorodeoxyglucose ([18F]FDG) after first-line chemotherapy in non-Hodgkin's lymphoma: is [18F]FDG-PET a valid alternative to conventional diagnostic methods? *J Clin Oncol* 2001;19:414–419.

177. Breslow A. Thickness, cross sectional areas and depth of invasion in the prognosis of cutaneous melanoma. *Ann Surg* 1970;172:902–908.

178. Clark WH, From L, Bernardino EA et al. The histogenesis and biologic behavior of primary human malignant melanoma of the skin. *Cancer Res* 1969;29:705–706.

179. Wagner JD, Schauwecker DS, Davidson D et al. FDG-PET sensitivity for melanoma lymph node metastases is dependent on tumor volume. *J Surg Oncol* 2001;77:237–242.

180. Crippa F, Leutner M, Belli F et al. Which kind of lymph node metastases can FDG PET detect? A clinical study in melanoma. *J Nucl Med* 2000;41:1491–1494.

181. Acland KM, Healy C, Calonje E et al. Comparison of positron emission tomography scanning and sentinel node biopsy in the detection of micrometastases of primary cutaneous malignant melanoma. *J Clin Oncol* 2001;19:2674–2678.

182. Gritters LS, Francis IR, Zasadny KR et al. Initial assessment of positron emission tomography using 2-fluoro-18-fluoro-2-deoxy-D-glucose in the imaging of malignant melanoma. *J Nucl Med* 1993;34: 1420–1427.

183. Steinert HC, Huch-Boni RA, Buck A et al. Malignant melanoma: staging with whole-body positron emission tomography and 2-[F-18]-fluoro-2-deoxy-D-glucose. *Radiology* 1995;195:705–709.

184. Boni R, Boni RA, Steinert H et al. Staging of metastatic melanoma by whole-body positron emission tomography using 2-fluorine-18-fluoro-2-deoxy-D-glucose. *Br J Dermatol* 1995;132:556–562.

185. Blessing C, Feine U, Geiger L et al. Positron emission tomography and ultrasonography. A comparative retrospective study assessing the diagnostic validity in lymph node metastases of malignant melanoma. *Arch Dermatol* 1995;131:1394–1398.

186. Damian DL, Fulham MJ, Thompson E et al. Positron emission tomography in the detection and management of metastatic melanoma. *Melanoma Res* 1996;6:325–329.

187. Wagner JD, Schauwecker D, Hutchins G et al. Initial assessment of positron emission tomography for detection of nonpalpable regional lymphatic metastases in melanoma. *J Surg Oncol* 1997;64:181–189.

188. Rinne D, Baum RP, Hor G et al. Primary staging and follow-up of high risk melanoma patients with whole-body 18F-fluorodeoxyglucose positron emission tomography: results of a prospective study of 100 patients. *Cancer* 1998;82:1664–1671.

189. Macfarlane DJ, Sondak V, Johnson T et al. Prospective evaluation of 2-[18F]-2-deoxy-D-glucose positron emission tomography in staging of regional lymph nodes in patients with cutaneous malignant melanoma. *J Clin Oncol* 1998;16:1770–1776.

190. Holder WD Jr, White RL Jr, Zuger JH et al. Effectiveness of positron emission tomography for the detection of melanoma metastases. *Ann Surg* 1998;227:764–769.

191. Steinert HC, Voellmy DR, Trachsel C et al. Planar coincidence scintigraphy and PET in staging malignant melanoma. *J Nucl Med* 1998; 39:1892–1897.

192. Wagner JD, Schauwecker D, Davidson D et al. Prospective study of fluorodeoxyglucose-positron emission tomography imaging of lymph node basins in melanoma patients undergoing sentinel node biopsy. *J Clin Oncol* 1999;17:1508–1515.

193. Valk PE, Segall GM, Johnson DL et al. Cost-effectiveness of whole-body FDG PET imaging in metastatic melanoma. *J Nucl Med* 1997; 38(Suppl):89P(abst).

194. Schwimmer J, Essner R, Patel A et al. A review of the literature for whole-body FDG PET in the management of patients with melanoma. *Q J Nucl Med* 2000;44:153–167.

195. Mijnhout GS, Hoekstra OS, van Tulder MW et al. Systematic review of the diagnostic accuracy of (18)F-fluorodeoxyglucose positron emission tomography in melanoma patients. *Cancer* 2001;91:1530–1542.

196. Gambhir SS, Czernin J, Schimmer J et al. A tabulated review of the literature. *J Nucl Med* 2001;42(Suppl):13S–15S.
197. Samson D, Flamm CR, Aronson N. *FDG positron emission tomography for evaluation of breast cancer.* Blue Cross and Blue Shield Association 2001:1–93.
198. Adler LP, Crowe JP, Al Kaisi NK et al. Evaluation of breast masses and axillary lymph nodes with [F-18] 2-deoxy-2-fluoro-D-glucose PET. *Radiology* 1993;187:743–750.
199. Nieweg OE, Kim EE, Wong WI et al. Positron emission tomography with fluorine-18-deoxyglucose in the detection and staging of breast cancer. *Cancer* 1993;71:3920–3925.
200. McGuire AH, Dehdashti F, Siegel BA et al. Positron tomographic assessment of 16 α-[18F] fluoro-17 p-estradiol uptake in metastatic breast carcinoma. *J Nucl Med* 1991;32:1526–1531.
201. Huovinen R, Leskinen KS, Nagren K et al. Carbon-11-methionine and PET in evaluation of treatment response of breast cancer. *Br J Cancer* 1993;67:787–791.
202. Wahl RL, Zasadny K, Helvie M et al. Metabolic monitoring of breast cancer chemohormonotherapy using positron emission tomography: initial evaluation. *J Clin Oncol* 1993;11:2101–2111.
203. Schelling M, Avid N, Nahrig J et al. Positron emission tomography using [18F] fluorodeoxyglucose for monitoring primary chemotherapy in breast cancer. *J Clin Oncol* 2000;18:1686–1695.
204. Schirrmeister H, Kuhn T, Guhlmann A et al. Fluorine-18 2-deoxy-2-fluoro-D-glucose PET in the preoperative staging of breast cancer: comparison with the standard staging procedures. *Eur J Nucl Med* 2001;28:351–358.
205. Avril N, Dose J, Janiicke F et al. Assessment of axillary lymph node involvement in breast patients with positron emission tomography using radiolabeled 2-(fluorine-18)-fluoro-2-deoxy-D-glucose. *J Natl Cancer Inst* 1996;88:1204–1209.
206. Kern KA, Brunetti A, Norton JA et al. Metabolic imaging of human extremity musculoskeletal tumors by PET. *J Nucl Med* 1988;29:181–186.
207. Griffeth LK, Dehdashti F, McGuire AH et al. PET evaluation of soft-tissue masses with fluorine-18 fluoro-2-deoxy-D-glucose. *Radiology* 1992;182:185–194.
208. Adler LP, Blair HF, Makley JT et al. Noninvasive grading of musculoskeletal tumors using PET. *J Nucl Med* 1991;32:1508–1512.
209. Gelbard AS, Benua RS, Laughlin JS et al. Quantitative scanning of osteogenic sarcoma with nitrogen-13-labeled L-glutamate. *J Nucl Med* 1979;20:782–784.
210. Reiman RE, Rosen G, Gelbard AS et al. Imaging of primary Ewing sarcoma with N-13-L glutamate. *Radiology* 1982;142:495–500.
211. Schmall B, Conti PS, Bigler RE et al. Imaging of patients with malignant fibrous histiocytoma using C-11α-aminoisobutyric acid (AIB). *Clin Nucl Med* 1987;1:22–26.
212. Kairento AL, Brownell GL, Elmaleh DR et al. Comparative measurement of regional blood flow, oxygen and glucose utilisation in soft tissue tumour of rabbit with positron imaging. *Br J Radiol* 1985;58:637–643.
213. Jones DN, Brizel DM, Charles HC et al. Monitoring of response to neoadjuvant therapy of soft tissue and musculoskeletal sarcomas using 18F FDG-PET. *J Nucl Med* 1994;35:38P.
214. Lowe VJ, Kallmes DF, Grey L et al. FDG-PET evaluation of vertebral compression fractures in cancer patients. *J Nucl Med* 1993;34:7P.
215. Kraus DH, Pfister DG, Harrison LB et al. Larynx preservation with combined chemotherapy and radiation therapy in advanced hypopharynx cancer. *Otolaryngol Head Neck Surg* 1994;111:31–37.
216. Spaulding MB, Fischer SG, Wolf GT. Tumor response, toxicity, and survival after neoadjuvant organ-preserving chemotherapy for advanced laryngeal carcinoma. The Department of Veterans Affairs Cooperative Laryngeal Cancer Study Group. *J Clin Oncol* 1994;12:1592–1599.
217. Bocca E, Calearo C, Marullo T et al. Occult metastases in cancer of the larynx and their relationship to clinical and histological aspects of the primary tumor: a four year multicentric research. *Laryngoscope* 1984;94:1086–1090.
218. Shuller DE, McGuirt WF, McCabe BF et al. The prognostic significance of metastatic cervical lymph nodes. *Laryngoscope* 1980;90:557–570.
219. Laubenbacher C, Saumweber D, Wagner MC et al. Comparison of fluorine-18-fluorodeoxyglucose PET, MRI and endoscopy for staging head and neck squamous-cell carcinomas. *J Nucl Med* 1995;36:1747–1757.
220. Wong WL, Chevretton EB, McGurk M et al. A prospective study of PET-FDG imaging for the assessment of head and neck squamous cell carcinoma. *Clin Otolaryngol Appl Sci* 1997;22:209–214.
221. Kole AC, Nieweg OE, Pruim J et al. Detection of unknown occult primary tumors using positron emission tomography. *Cancer* 1998;82:1160–1166.
222. Braams JW, Pruim J, Kole AC et al. Detection of unknown primary head and neck tumors by positron emission tomography. *Int J Oral Maxillofac Surg* 1997;26:112–125.
223. AAssar OS, Fischbein NJ, Caputo GR et al. Metastatic head and neck cancer: role and usefulness of FDG PET in locating occult primary tumors. *Radiology* 1999;210:177–181.
224. Lassen U, Daugaard G, Eigtved A et al. 18F-FDG whole body positron emission tomography (PET) in patients with unknown primary tumours (UPT). *Eur J Cancer* 1999;35:1076–1082.
225. Safa AA, Tran LM, Rege S et al. The role of positron emission tomography in occult primary head and neck cancers. *Cancer J Sci Am* 1999;5:214–218.
226. Jungehulsing M, Scheidhauer K, Damm M et al. 2[F]-fluoro-2-deoxy-D-glucose positron emission tomography is a sensitive tool for the detection of occult primary cancer (carcinoma of unknown primary syndrome) with head and neck lymph node manifestation. *Otolaryngol Head Neck Surg* 2000;123:294–301.
227. Greven KM, Keyes JJ, Williams DR et al. Occult primary tumors of the head and neck: lack of benefit from positron emission tomography imaging with 2-[F-18]fluoro-2-deoxy-D-glucose. *Cancer* 1999;86:114–118.
228. Adams S, Baum RP, Stuckensen T et al. Prospective comparison of 18F-FDG PET with conventional imaging modalities (CT, MRI, US) in lymph node staging of head and neck cancer. *Eur J Nucl Med* 1998;25:1255–1260.
229. Benchaou M, Lehmann W, Slosman DO et al. The role of FDG-PET in the preoperative assessment of N-staging in head and neck cancer. *Acta Oto Laryngol* 1996;116:332–335.
230. McGuirt WF, Williams DW 3rd, Keyes JJ et al. A comparative diagnostic study of head and neck nodal metastases using positron emission tomography. *Laryngoscope* 1995;105:373–375.
231. Myers LL, Wax MK, Nabi H et al. Positron emission tomography in the evaluation of the N0 neck. *Laryngoscope* 1998;108:232–236.
232. Rege S, Maass A, Chaiken L et al. Use of positron emission tomography with fluorodeoxyglucose in patients with extracranial head and neck cancers. *Cancer* 1994;73:3047–3058.
233. Kau RJ, Alexiou C, Laubenbacher C et al. Lymph node detection of head and neck squamous cell carcinomas by positron emission tomography with fluorodeoxyglucose F 18 in a routine clinical setting. *Arch Otolaryngol Head Neck Surg* 1999;125:1322–1328.
234. Rege SD, Chaiken L, Hoh CK et al. Change induced by radiation therapy in FDG uptake in normal and malignant structures of the head and neck: quantitation with PET. *Radiology* 1993;189:807–812.
235. Lowe VJ, Heber ME, Anscher MS et al. Chest wall FDG accumulation in serial FDG-PET images in patients being treated for bronchogenic carcinoma with radiation. *Clin Positron Imag* 1998;1:185–191.
236. Lowe V, Dunphy F, Varvares M et al. Evaluation of chemotherapy response in patients with advanced head and neck cancer using FDG-PET. *Head Neck* 1997;19:666–674.
237. Greven KM, Williams DW 3rd., Keyes JJ et al. Can positron emission tomography distinguish tumor recurrence from irradiation sequelae in patients treated for larynx cancer? *Cancer J Sci Am* 1997;3:353–357.
238. Anzai Y, Carroll WR, Quint DJ et al. Recurrence of head and neck cancer after surgery or irradiation: prospective comparison of 2-deoxy-

2-[F-18]fluoro-D-glucose PET and MR imaging diagnoses. *Radiology* 1996;200:135–141.

239. Lapela M, Grenman R, Kurki T et al. Head and neck cancer: detection of recurrence with PET and 2-[F-18]fluoro-2-deoxy-D-glucose. *Radiology* 1995;197:205–211.

240. Farber LA, Benard F, Machtay M et al. Detection of recurrent head and neck squamous cell carcinomas after radiation therapy with 2-18F-fluoro-2-deoxy-D-glucose positron emission tomography. *Laryngoscope* 1999;109:970–975.

241. Kao CH, ChangLai SP, Chieng PU et al. Detection of recurrent or persistent nasopharyngeal carcinomas after radiotherapy with 18-fluoro-2-deoxyglucose positron emission tomography and comparison with computed tomography. *J Clin Oncol* 1998;16:3550–3555.

242. Lowe VJ, Boyd JH, Dunphy FR et al. Surveillance for recurrent head and neck cancer using positron emission tomography. *J Clin Oncol* 2000;18:651–658.

243. Fischbein NJ, AAssar OS, Caputo GR et al. Clinical utility of positron emission tomography with 18F-fluorodeoxyglucose in detecting residual/recurrent squamous cell carcinoma of the head and neck. *Am J Neuroradiol* 1998;19:1189–1196.

49

SENTINEL NODE STAGING OF EARLY BREAST CANCER WITH LYMPHOSCINTIGRAPHY AND AN INTRAOPERATIVE GAMMA-DETECTING PROBE

JOHN AARSVOLD

NAOMI ALAZRAKI

SANDRA F. GRANT

SENTINEL LYMPH NODE STAGING OF CANCER

Background

As popularization of the sentinel node concept has taken hold, interest and enthusiasm for lymphoscintigraphy, the imaging of flow through lymphatic vessels to lymph nodes, has heightened. In 1977 Cabanas (1), a urologist, reported use of the sentinel node concept in a surgical approach to staging cancer of the penis. He performed intraoperative palpation along the expected course of lymphatic drainage from the penile tumor to the first palpated lymph node. He called the first node on the course the *sentinel lymph node* (SLN).

Dye staining of lymphatic drainage from the tumor site to the SLN was introduced by Morton et al. (2), oncologic surgeons, for surgical staging of melanoma. In the operating room, injections of isosulfan blue dye were given and nodes that were stained blue were identified as SLNs, excised, and sent for histopathologic examination. Validation of the reliability of SLN histopathologic results as an indicator of the presence or absence of tumor spread was reported, but problems in the use of blue dye, initially in melanoma cases, prompted Alex and Krag (3) to investigate the use of radiotracers for lymphatic mapping and SLN identification. Detection of the radioactive tracer within a SLN was achieved with a gamma-detecting probe, a small hand-held device with a sterile covering so that the surgeon could work with the probe in the operative field. Lymphoscintigraphy has been performed in the nuclear medicine departments for the past four to five decades, but imaging lymphatic drainage pathways did not in the past generate the interest the SLN concept has engendered.

Past applications of lymphoscintigraphy included localization of internal mammary lymph node chains for radiation therapy port assignments in breast cancer patients and investigation of the cause of lymphedema. Localization of the internal mammary nodal chain before radiation was accomplished by means of subcostal injection of radiolabeled colloid particles posterior to the rectus sheath. The injection was made 3 cm inferior to the xiphoid process and 1 to 2 cm medial to the midclavicular line of the breast under study. The colloid particles were absorbed into lymphatic channels and transported to internal mammary lymph nodes (4,5). Images of the internal mammary nodes were acquired with a scintillation camera, the locations of the nodes determined on the images, and the identified locations used to guide radiation therapists in the setting of ports to treat the internal mammary nodes. Kaplan (5) reported that information on 167 patients consecutively examined in this manner showed 75% of 5,768 nodes imaged were between the first and third ribs.

Another application of lymphoscintigraphy was to define the nature of the problem in patients with peripheral lymphatic dysfunction or idiopathic edema (6), including differentiating lymphatic and venous obstruction. In recent years, in addition to melanoma and breast cancer (the two cancers for which SLN staging has been used most), other cancers have been staged with SLN histopathologic examinations. These include cancer of the penis, vulva, uterine cervix, and head and neck. They also include other genitourinary cancers—some staged via definition of iliopelvic lymph drainage after perianal administration of tracer (7), colon cancer, and pancreatic cancer. Colorectal and pancreatic cancers have been investigated intraoperatively for identification of the SLN. Blue dye or radiocolloid is injected at the cancer site, and a sterile-sheathed, handheld gamma-detecting probe is used to find an SLN that contains deposits of the radiotracer (8–10).

J. Aarsvold: Nuclear Medicine Service, Veterans Affairs Medical Center, and Division of Nuclear Medicine, Department of Radiology, School of Medicine, Emory University, Atlanta, GA.

N. Alazraki: Nuclear Medicine Service, Veterans Affairs Medical Center, and Division of Nuclear Medicine, Department of Radiology, School of Medicine, Emory University, Atlanta, GA.

S. F. Grant: Nuclear Medicine Service, Veterans Affairs Medical Center, Atlanta, GA.

Lymphoscintigraphic Staging of Melanoma

Published reports (11–14) have shown that imaging with radio-labeled colloid particles commonly depicted unexpected lymphatic drainage pathways from cutaneous melanoma. Uren et al. (12) reported that in more than 10% of cases, lymphatic drainage from cutaneous melanoma went to three or more node groups in different anatomic regions. A tumor cell could travel down any of those lymph channels and arrive at any of one, two, three, or occasionally even more SLNs. Often, each lymph channel draining from the tumor leads to an independent SLN (Fig. 49.1). Not infrequently, an SLN with micrometastasis is not in a lymph node bed that would have been predicted, according to previous conventional estimates by surgeons, to receive lymphatic drainage from a primary cutaneous melanoma. Glass et al. (14) reported on 132 patients with intermediate-thickness (0.75 to 4.0 mm) cutaneous malignant melanoma. The patients underwent preoperative and intraoperative lymphatic mapping. SLNs were excised and examined for micrometastasis by means of light microscopy with conventional stains and immunocytochemical analysis for S-100 protein and HMB-45 antibodies. Only patients with micrometastasis underwent complete lymph-node dissection. The results showed that SLNs were identified in all patients. Micrometastasis was found in 23% of patients at selective lymphadenectomy, and an SLN was the only node

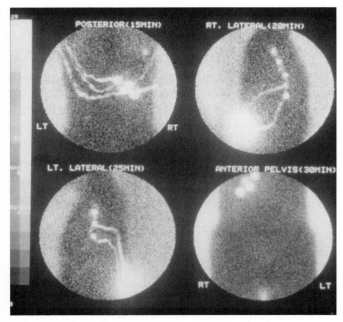

FIGURE 49.1. Images of a patient with truncal cutaneous melanoma. The body contour is outlined by the transmission scan of ^{57}Co photons in a flat flood source. The patient is positioned between the flood source and the camera. The four foci of activity to the right of midline in the posterior view (*upper left*) are the injection sites administered around the melanoma. At least three discrete lymphatic channels are depicted crossing the midline and coursing to the left axilla. At least two channels course to the right axilla. On the lateral views (*upper right, lower left*), sentinel lymph nodes (two on the right and two on the left) are present at the termination of the lymph channels. The two upper channels on the left (*upper left*) join as they approach the axilla; therefore only two channels terminate on two sentinel nodes. Secondary and tertiary nodes are superior to the sentinel nodes.

with tumor in 83% of those, according to results of subsequent complete nodal dissection. Current state-of-the-art practice is to perform SLN staging for intermediate-thickness cutaneous melanoma. One report, however, described an SLN positive for micrometastasis in a patient with a very thin tumor (<0.75 mm) one that was Clark level III (15). Perhaps the unpredictability with which melanoma metastasizes and as to which nodal groups it migrates are the only observations.

Data on outcome among patients who underwent SLN excisional biopsy years ago are now appearing in published reports. One recent multicenter study (15) confirmed that SLN positivity for tumor and Breslow and Clark levels were joint predictors of survival. Disease recurrence was found in 8.8% of patients with tumor-negative SLN. No patient with Clark level II primary tumors was found to have tumor-positive SLN or recurrence. SLN histopathologic findings were the most significant prognostic factor and were superior to measurement of the thickness of the primary melanoma. Other investigators (16) have shown that tumor thickness more than 1.5 mm ($P = 0.01$), ulceration of the primary tumor ($P < 0.01$), and presence of lymphovascular invasion ($P = 0.05$) were predictive of the presence of SLN micrometastasis.

Cutaneous melanoma can appear anywhere—on the trunk, head and neck, or extremities. One might believe that lymphoscintigraphy may not be warranted to localize drainage direction for extremity melanoma because lower-extremity tumors are expected to drain to inguinal nodes and upper-extremity tumors to axillary nodes. However, in approximately 6% of cases, an SLN is located in the epitrochlear or popliteal region (17). Such SLN sometimes are called *intercalated* or *in-transit* nodes (Fig. 49.2).

The success rate of imaging SLN in cutaneous melanoma has been high (93% to 100%) (18). The reproducibility of lymphoscintigraphy for lymphatic mapping of cutaneous melanoma is reported to be 85% to 88% (18–20). Often the difference between two studies of the same patient relates to visualization of additional secondary lymph nodes, although some SLNs may be missed. The method used in melanoma SLN studies is considerably more standardized than that for breast cancer SLN studies. There are, however, methodologic differences between institutions and centers around the world regarding methods for melanoma SLN studies. Causes of variations in results are likely multiple, including radiopharmaceutical particle size, injection dose and volume, melanoma location (head versus trunk versus extremities), camera acquisition and display parameters, timing of imaging, and variable disruption of lymphatic flow if very wide or deep excisional biopsy of the primary tumor had been performed.

Method

Four intradermal injections (raising a wheal) of 100 μCi in 0.1 mL of ^{99m}Tc sulfur colloid (filtered or unfiltered) are generally used with high success in truncal and extremity lesions. Careful attention must be paid to selecting the four sites for injection surrounding the tumor, or the excision site if the tumor has been previously removed for biopsy. In head and neck lesions, care must be taken not to obscure SLNs that may be very near the primary tumor. Because drainage from head and neck tumors

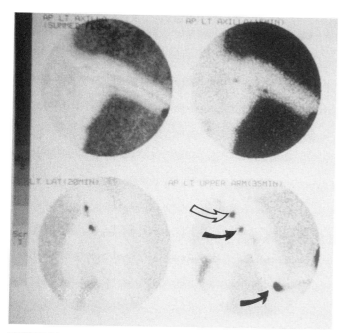

FIGURE 49.2. Cutaneous melanoma of the distal left forearm (*distal to the image field of view*). An epitrochlear sentinel node is present (*lower right, lower arrow*), as is a channel leading to it. The channel continues, as does a separate channel, to the axilla (*top and lower right*). Therefore the two axillary nodes (*two upper arrows*) may be sentinel nodes and should both be excised for histopathologic examination.

is generally in the caudal direction, it is advisable to avoid injection inferior to the tumor. After each intradermal injection, finger massage is applied. Imaging is performed immediately. The transmission source is placed so that the patient is between the source and the camera, to provide a reference outline of the body surface for better localization of the imaged activity in the injection sites, lymphatic channels, and SLNs or secondary lymph nodes. Imaging should be performed in more than one projection for optimum localization and is continued until satisfactory visualization of the SLNs is achieved (usually within 30 to 40 minutes). The patient may be scheduled to go to the operating room when imaging is completed or the next day (~18 hours after the injections). In protocols involving next day surgeries, when possible, images should be acquired immediately before surgery to assure the distribution of radioactivity in the SLNs is the same as that in the first day images.

CHANGES IN SURGICAL BREAST CANCER MANAGEMENT

The surgical management of breast cancer has become progressively less invasive. Breast-conserving lumpectomy has replaced simple mastectomy, which only 20 years ago, replaced radical mastectomy in the treatment of many patients. When it was introduced, simple mastectomy was considered revolutionary and was used only for patients with small tumors. Today we are witnessing a transition in the approach to the staging of this

disease as we watch staging procedures transition from axillary dissection and multiple node assessment to SLN excision and SLN only assessment. This transition is considered investigational by some, but it has become standard care in most centers.

The SLN concept applied to patients with breast lesions smaller than 5 cm, that at least one SLN will, show positive for metastasis if there has been lymphatic tumor spread. When the SLN is tumor-free, we can be sure with very high accuracy (98%) that tumor has not spread through the lymphatic vessels. The SLN imaging procedure may last 5 minutes to 1 hour or more; it shows the transport of radiolabeled colloid particles from a tumor to a lymph node (the SLN). In the course of breast cancer, the process by which tumor cells reach a lymph node can last years. There are many differences between the transport of a radiocolloid and that of a tumor cell from the tumor to the SLN, even in this oversimplified example. Perhaps one very important difference is the size of the much smaller radiolabeled colloid particle, approximately 1 μm, versus that of a tumor cell, approximately 16 μm. If we were to try to use a radiolabeled particle of comparable size to a tumor cell, that is, a macroaggregate, such as particles used for lung perfusion imaging, we probably would not see transport to the SLN during the time that can be allotted for a clinical study (several hours).

LYMPHATIC MAPPING IN BREAST CANCER

Two primary methods of lymphatic mapping to identify SLNs are used: the blue dye approach and the radiotracer approach. In the blue dye method, the patient is placed on the operating room table, anesthetized, and injected with isosulfan & blue dye. The injection is in the involved breast near the tumor. The breast is massaged for approximately 7 minutes (3–10 minutes depending on the distance between the tumor and the axilla). An incision is made just below the axillary hairline, and the surgeon visually searches for a blue-stained lymphatic channel leading to a blue-stained lymph node. With radiotracer methods, an appropriate radiopharmaceutical (usually a ^{99m}Tc-labeled colloid particle) is administered by means of peritumoral, subdermal, or periareolar injection (see later Injection Site). Injection is followed by imaging and intraoperative probe-guided localization of lymph nodes containing small amounts of radioactivity (identified as SLNs on images).

The sensitivity of SLN identification by various methods or combinations of methods applied by many investigations has been compiled by Nieweg et al. (21) and further analyzed by Alazraki et al. (18). Reported success in finding an SLN with the blue dye method ranges from 41% to 98% (22–28). A weighted average based on eight published reports of 734 patients in whom blue dye alone was used indicates that in 76.3% of cases, an SLN was found (Table 49.1).

In 5 studies with 649 patients (29–33) on which preoperative lymphoscintigraphy, intraoperative gamma probe, and blue dye were all used, the sensitivity of finding SLNs ranged from 87% to 98% with a weighted average of 94%. Using all available tools (blue dye, lymphoscintigraphic imaging before surgical incision, and gamma-detecting probe) achieves the highest and the tightest range of sensitivities for finding a SLN. Likewise, although the sensitivity of imaging and use of a probe (87.8%) (34–38)

Table 49.1. *Success Rate for Identifying Sentinel Node by Technique*

Technique	No. of patients/ No. of studies	% Weighted average sentinel nodes identified
Blue dye	667/8 (22–28)	76.3
Probe	635/6	91.5
Blue dye and probe	104/2	91.3
Imaging and probe	508/5 (34–38)	87.8
Imaging, probe, and blue dye	649/5 (29–33)	93.8

Numbers in parentheses are references.
From Alazraki N, Styblo T, Grant S, et al. Sentinel node staging of early breast cancer using lymphoscintigraphy and the intraoperative gamma-detecting probe *Semin Nucl Med* 2000;30:56–64 and Nieweg OE, Jansen L, Olmos RAV, et al. Lymphatic mapping and sentinel lymph node biopsy in breast cancer. *Eur J Nucl Med* 1999;26[Suppl]:S11–S16, with permission.

was higher than that of use of blue dye alone, there was a significant difference in favor of using all three techniques ($P < 0.0025$) (18). Scrutiny of the studies on which these sensitivity results are based reveals concerns that may have caused some compromises in the results, including the well-described learning-curve phenomenon (39).

Wide variation in results reported from different centers for the same methods may reflect learning-curve phenomena in some instances. Strategies have been suggested for surgeons to minimize failed procedures or the rate of false-negative results during the surgeon's learning phase (39). Early in the surgeon's experience, it is recommended that axillary dissection be performed in addition to excision of SLNs. During the training phase, SLN biopsy is reserved to be performed without axillary dissection only in the care of patients with low likelihood of having metastasis. Likewise, for radiologists or nuclear medicine physicians, an initial case experience (10 to 25 cases) to overcome learning-curve problems is advised. This initial experience should include marking the SLN on the patient's skin with a handheld gamma probe and following the patient to the operating room to work with the surgeon in localizing the SLN. This is particularly important when surgeons have had limited or no experience working with a probe. The imaging physician can educate the surgeon to understand that interference from non-SLN activity (i.e., the injection site) can affect the procedure, as can the method of handling the probe.

According to current information and informal discussions at meetings, imaging specialists are not succeeding as well as they should in finding SLNs on images, probably because of inexperience, lack of attention to detail, and lack of instruction. Many details can enhance success in imaging SLNs (see later, Imaging). In the operating room, the counts detected with the probe are recorded and should be included in the nuclear medicine report to document significance of counts in excised nodes. The number of counts detected in a lymph node is an area of extreme variability. It depends on the probe equipment (e.g., manufacturer, detecting elements), the angle of the probe relative to the node being counted (even if the probe is touching the node), and the injection dose. Some investigators define SLN on the basis of probe-detected counts. These counts, however, are inherently variable, and methods for counting are not standardized. In addition, there are physiologic and anatomic variabilities such that the SLNs (Figs. 49.3, 49.4) are not necessarily

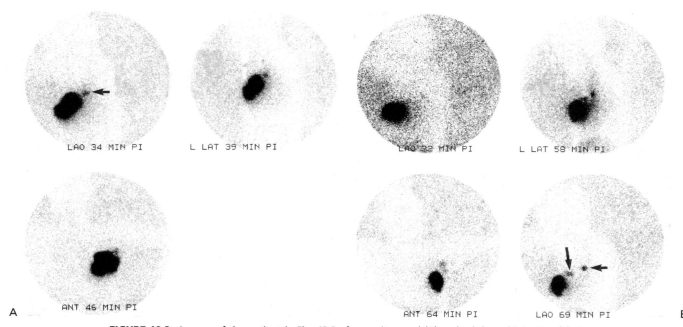

FIGURE 49.3. Images of the patient in Fig. 49.2 after peritumoral (**A**) and subdermal injection (**B**). **A:** The large black focus is the injection site. The sentinel node is evident in the left axilla (*arrow*). **B:** The same sentinel node as in **A** (*vertical arrow*) after subdermal injection. A secondary node also is present (*lower right, horizontal arrow*). The secondary node is hotter than the sentinel node. Data show that the sentinel node is not the hottest node in approximately 30% of cases.

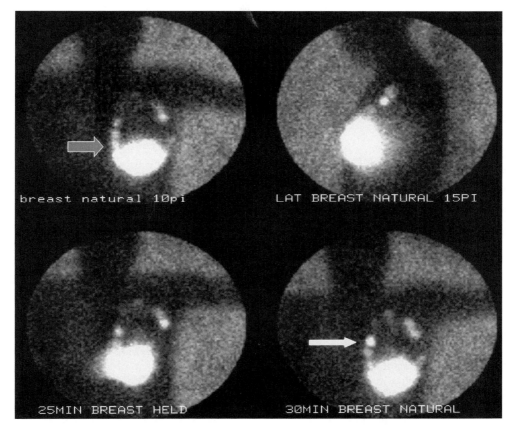

FIGURE 49.4. Chain of three internal mammary nodes. At 10 minutes, (*upper left*), the most inferior of the three nodes is hottest (*arrow*). At 30 minutes, the most superior of the three nodes is hottest (*lower right, arrow*). The most inferior node is the sentinel node (first to visualize). Axillary sentinel node is evident. This case demonstrates that intensity of activity in nodes can change over time.

the hottest nodes, nor are they necessarily the nodes closest to the tumor (40). We have found the hottest node is a SLN in 70% of patients (41). The counts detected in a SLN are ideally more than 10 times (ex vivo counts) the background count (non-SLN, ex vivo) (30). Lack of standardization of methods for counting with probes, including what is counted and how it is counted, may contribute to variations in reported results.

Sentinel Node: Standard of Care?

SLN biopsy is close to being accepted as the standard of care for early breast cancer. It already is the standard of care in the surgical management of melanoma. The following compelling facts favor SLN staging of the axilla in preference to axillary dissection: (a) axillary node dissection is recognized as a high-morbidity procedure that leaves women with sometimes painful arm edema, limited range of motion of the arm, and paresthesia, all of which can become chronic for some patients; (b) approximately 60% of women with early breast cancer have no tumor found at routine staging axillary dissection and do not need the procedure; (c) SLN biopsy shows micrometastasis more frequently than does axillary dissection because of the more careful, thorough histopathologic examination that can be performed (including immunohistochemical stains and multisectioning of

the nodes) on the one, two, or three SLNs removed during SLN lymphadenectomy and biopsy. Such thorough analysis generally cannot be performed on the 20 to 30 lymph nodes submitted to the pathologist from axillary dissection.

The primary reason for the delay in universal acceptance of axillary SLN staging of early breast cancer is that there is no consensus on (18,42) standardization of an optimum method for identification of SLNs. Identifications with radiotracers are being performed differently at centers throughout the world. The major variables are injection site, injection volume, injection activity, radiopharmaceutical, and use or non-use of imaging.

Injection Site

Four tracer injection sites have been used in patients with breast cancer: peritumoral, subdermal, intratumoral, and subareolar or periareolar. Investigators (35) in Milan, Italy, used subdermal injections of radiocolloid preparations (50 to 200 μm). In the first 163 patients, the SLN was found and excised according to results of imaging and probe detection in 98% of patients. The volume, 0.2 mL, containing 300 μCi was injected at one subdermal site near the tumor. As previously discussed by Keshtgar and Ell (42), subdermal injection is distinctly different from both intradermal and subcutaneous injection. Intradermal injections are important in melanoma, because cutaneous melanoma truly originates at intradermal sites. The subdermal level contains an abundance of lymph vessels, which are not present at the subcutaneous level. The interstitial tissues deep in the breast, compared with the subdermal level, are more sparsely populated by lymph vessels.

Peritumoral and Subdermal Injection

In studies performed in the United States (18,25,30), peritumoral injection of filtered sulfur colloid was used with high success in finding the SLNs with imaging, probe, and blue dye in 94% to 98% of patients. The techniques involved use of 4 to 8 mL sulfur colloid containing 400 μCi to 1 mCi injected in four to six 1-mL aliquots in separate sites at the periphery of the tumor or previous excisional biopsy site directed with palpation or ultrasound (36,41–43). Investigators at Emory University and the Veterans Affairs Medical Center, Atlanta (41,44,45), compared subdermal, peritumoral, and periareolar injections of filtered ^{99m}Tc sulfur colloid, two of which were administered to the same patient on separate days (Fig. 49.3). Results of 202 studies on 98 patients showed that imaging depicted axillary SLNs in 100% of patients; the SLNs were found at surgery with the probe and excised from 100% of patients. Subdermal injection followed by imaging resulted in identification of an axillary SLN in 96% of patients. Peritumoral injection followed by imaging resulted in identification of an axillary SLN in 94%. Periareolar injection (smaller numbers of patients studied) resulted in identification of a SLN in all patients (41). The main difference in results obtained from the use of varied injection sites was the degree of visualization of internal mammary SLNs. In addition to the axillary SLN, internal mammary node drainage was seen in 26% of patients who received peritumoral injections but was seen with subdermal injection in only 1% (1 of 95) of patients. Internal mammary SLN biopsy was performed on only a few patients; most had no metastasis in either axillary or internal mammary SLNs, but 2 had micrometastasis in axillary and internal mammary SLNs. We conclude that a combination of peritumoral and subdermal injections is the optimal method (41). Total activity administered should not exceed 500 to 600 μCi (100 μCi per peritumoral injection, two injections are adequate) plus 200 μCi per subdermal injection. Each injection should be followed by gentle massage for 30 to 60 seconds.

Intratumoral Injection

Most centers performing SLN detection do not inject radiotracer directly into the tumor. Although intratumoral injections have been reported to successfully lead to identification of SLNs in patients with early breast cancer (46), this method is not favored by most investigators, mainly for the following reasons: (a) intratumoral tissue has relatively high interstitial and intracellular pressures, and leakage of injectate out of the tumor into the peritumoral spaces occurs rapidly, (b) safety of intratumoral injection in regard to spreading tumor cells along the needle track is a concern, (c) there are no lymphatic vessels in tumor masses. However, Gennari et al. (47) described intratumoral injection of ^{99m}Tc albumin colloid for intraoperative localization of nonpalpable tumors with a probe and simultaneous SLN localization. This is a novel procedure that is less invasive than is wire localization. Results show the success of this technique for margin-free excision of small tumors is comparable with that of wire localization.

Radiopharmaceutical

Imaging lymphatic flow with a variety of radiopharmaceuticals has been a nuclear medicine procedure for the last 30 years. In the United States, gold-colloid particles initially were used. These were very small particles, which perhaps recorded different flow patterns on images than those seen with larger particles used today. In 1966, Vendrell-Torne et al. (48) used ^{198}Au colloid to define normal lymphatic drainage in the breast by quadrants. ^{99m}Tc sulfur colloid, filtered or unfiltered, is widely used in the United States. Other colloids of varying particle sizes (antimony sulfide colloid and albumin colloids), and ^{99m}Tc human serum albumin or technetium-labeled dextran (37,40) are used in Europe, Australia, South America, and elsewhere. The particle size (1,000 to 2,000 nm) of these radiopharmaceuticals is the major variable responsible for different behaviors in lymphatic mapping.

Particles smaller than 4 nm in diameter may penetrate capillary membranes and would be partially unavailable to migrate through lymphatic channels. Capillary blood uptake may add undesirable blood background counts to an image and to intraoperative probe detection of SLN. Radiolabeled dextran, however, has been successfully used in breast cancer lymphoscintigraphy (49,50). Nonetheless, logic dictates that the ideal particle size must be sufficiently small to facilitate rapid uptake into the lymphatic vessels and flow with lymph within the lymphatic vessels and be sufficiently large to not leak from lymphatic vessels and not pass through blood capillary membranes. Particles less than 100 nm (0.1 μm) in diameter satisfy the requirement of rapid transfer into lymphatic vessels, yet are retained for several hours in SLNs. Larger colloid particles (0.5 to 1.0 μm) have a much slower rate of clearance from the interstitial space and therefore likely slower accumulation into an SLN. In the United States, we have been using ^{99m}Tc sulfur colloid but have modified its preparation by means of microfiltration, with 0.1-μm and 0.22-μm filters (51–53).

Eshima et al. (52) have described mechanisms to decrease particle size of ^{99m}Tc sulfur colloid. They suggest, in addition to microfiltration, decreasing the heating time and using ^{99m}Tc pertechnetate derived from a generator with a longer time since last elution. Simply passing the ^{99m}Tc sulfur colloid through a 0.22-μm or 0.1-μm filter, or both, appears to give good results as well. Commercial radiopharmacies in the United States are using this modification to prepare ^{99m}Tc sulfur colloid for lymphoscintigraphy (Table 49.2)

A clinical analysis of the effect of microfiltration versus no filtration of ^{99m}Tc sulfur colloid on lymphoscintigraphic images of patients with melanoma was performed by Goldfarb et al. (54). They found significantly more frequent visualization of lymphatic channels leading to SLNs on images when 0.22-μm filters versus very coarse 5-μm filters (essentially no filter) were used in preparing ^{99m}Tc sulfur colloid. Thus the finer filtration provided clinically superior studies in visualization of lymphatic drainage pathways, more precise identification of SLNs, and

Table 49.2. *Classification of Lymphoscintigraphic Radiopharmaceuticals by Size*

Size	Radiocolloid
<4 nm	[99m]Tc dextran
<4 nm	[99m]Tc human serum albumin
1–15 nm	[198]Au colloid
15–50 nm	[99m]Tc antimony sulfide colloid
~80 nm	[99m]Tc nanocoll (albumin colloid)[a]
>50 nm	[99m]Tc sulfur colloid, depending on filtration and preparation
200–1000 nm	[99m]Tc albumin microcolloid (Albu-res)[a]
200–1000 nm	[99m]Tc sulfur colloid, conventional unfiltered preparation

[a]Available outside the United States from Amersham Health.
From Alazraki N, Styblo T, Grant S, et al. Sentinel node staging of early breast cancer using lymphoscintigraphy and the intraoperative gamma-detecting probe. *Semin Nucl Med* 2000;30:56–64, with permission.

better discrimination between secondary nodes and SLN in patients with melanoma.

In a National Cancer Institute–sponsored multicenter trial of SLN biopsy versus axillary node dissection in the evaluation of breast cancer, unfiltered ^{99m}Tc sulfur colloid and gamma probe–guided detection were used in the operating room with no imaging. SLN localization was reported in 93% of patients (55). A volume of 4.0 mL containing 1.0 mCi of unfiltered ^{99m}Tc sulfur colloid was injected in divided aliquots at four sites into interstitial tissue around the tumor. The imaging experience with unfiltered ^{99m}Tc sulfur colloid particles indicates poorer penetration into lymphatic vessels; the result is that smaller percentages of injected activity reach the SLNs. Perhaps to counter the disadvantage that a lower percentage of injected activity penetrates the lymphatic vessels when larger particles are used, higher activity levels have generally been administered for unfiltered colloid (1 mCi) than for filtered colloid (0.4 to 0.6 mCi).

Imaging

A question frequently asked by surgeons is: "What is the role of imaging?" The question is reasonable, because probe detection without imaging has succeeded in localization of the SLN at surgery in 91.5% of cases (18,21). Many surgeons prefer not to bother with imaging. Some surgeons argue that the negatives of the time needed preoperatively to perform imaging and the cost are not outweighed by benefits. Other surgeons counter that a lymphoscintigraphic image is a map that increases the level of confidence in calling a "hot" node a SLN, rather than a secondary or tertiary lymph node. Second, and more important, an image helps the surgeon with incision planning. The incision can be founded on knowledge of the location and number of SLNs or secondary nodes. A smaller incision can be made if the precise location of a SLN is known. Two images (two projections—anterior and lateral or oblique) clearly define the spatial relations of one node to another in the axilla (Fig. 49.3B), internal mammary chain, and supraclavicular and infraclavicular regions. Third, and perhaps most important, surgical time is shortened. Lymphatic mapping with a probe without image guidance takes about 20 minutes performed by the most experienced sur-

geons. Incision to SLN excision takes as little as 5 minutes when image guidance and skin markings of SLN locations are used in combination with a probe. Many surgeons also report high levels of confidence in having removed the true SLNs on the basis of image guidance. Fourth, clinical experience is that lower radioactivity levels (0.3 to 0.6 mCi) of smaller-particle radiocolloids can be used successfully with imaging. The disadvantage of using smaller particles is that more secondary lymph nodes are detected, because more tracer appears to flow through and beyond the SLNs. If lymphatic channels leading to nodes are visualized, there is greater certainty that the node seen at the end of the channel is the SLN. Similarly, the pattern of changes in the counts in nodes on sequential images in relation to other anatomically lined-up nodes gives information about the SLN of a given node versus secondary node status (Fig. 49.4). In the absence of images, a cautious surgeon should excise all hot nodes, because no information is available to the surgeon about SLN versus secondary node status. On images, if more than three nodes are hot, the images can provide guidance for selecting nodes with highest likelihood of being a SLN.

Attention to Details for Imaging Success

Successful node detection with imaging is directly related to experience and attention to detail. Massage after injections (at least 30 seconds after each injection) and moving the breast (Fig. 49.5) to optimally clear the axillary and internal mammary regions of overlying soft tissue are keys to successful imaging (56). Only approximately 1% of the injected dose (500 μCi) is in an SLN (~5 μCi). Such low-level activity is easily obscured by breast soft-tissue attenuation. It is important to minimize

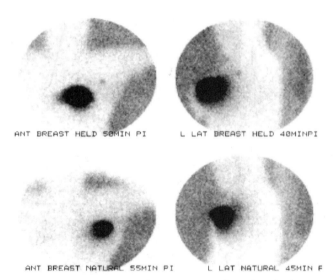

FIGURE 49.5. Images show the importance of moving the breast to minimize tissue attenuation that masks visualization of the sentinel lymph nodes. The anterior image at 50 minutes (*upper left*) and the lateral image at 40 minutes (*upper right*) were obtained with the breast moved and held inferiorly and medially during the 5 minutes of image acquisition. The anterior image at 55 minutes (*lower left*) and the lateral image at 45 minutes (*lower right*) were obtained with the breast in its natural position. The axillary sentinel node is not visible because of overlying tissue attenuation.

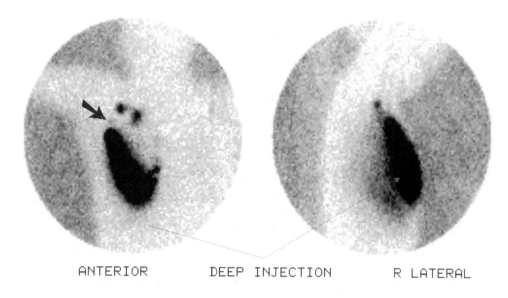

ANTERIOR   DEEP INJECTION   R LATERAL

ONE HOUR POST INJECTION

FIGURE 49.6. The patient had undergone excisional biopsy 2 weeks before sentinel node study. The technetium colloid was to have been injected peritumorally (around the site from which the cancer had been removed). The dose was unintentionally injected into the cavity that formed when the mass was excised. The cavity is evident on ultrasound scans but was not palpable. Ultrasound should be used to guide "peritumoral" injection when the mass has been excised. Three node-like foci are evident. The closest node to the site of the excised mass is the least hot (*arrow*) but is the sentinel node (the first node visualized after tracer injection). It is easy to see that a cavity injection (*large black activity, small arrowhead on lateral view*) can mask visualization of a sentinel lymph node. The lateral view does not show the true sentinel node.

overlying soft tissue in the axillary region by moving the breast caudad and medially. To image clearly the internal mammary region, the breast is moved laterally and a separate image is acquired. At least two projections, anterior and lateral or oblique, preferably with transmission to outline the body contour, should be obtained. Sometimes, a SLN is seen in one view and not the others, usually because of superimposition of regions of activity or because of attenuation (Fig. 49.6, Fig. 49.7). Success in imaging SLNs in patients with breast cancer is not difficult to attain but requires attention to detail, experience, and skillful, compassionate interaction with the patient.

Gamma-counting Probes

Gamma-counting probes were first developed and used in the late 1940s (57–60). The first were used to detect γ emissions from ^{32}P. Since then, numerous gamma probes have been developed—some simple, some complex (61,62). The counting probes used for detection and localization of SLN in patients with breast cancer are relatively simple. Most have scintillation detectors or ionization detectors. Most with scintillation technology have a scintillation crystal such as thallium-doped sodium iodide—NaI(Tl)—or thallium-doped cesium iodide—CsI(Tl)—optically coupled to a photomultiplier tube. Most probes with ionization technology have semiconductor detectors such as cadmium telluride (CdTe) or cadmium zinc telluride (CdZnTe).

A probe system is a 10- to 20-mm diameter, 200-mm long cylinder; a set of interchangeable tungsten apertures of varying

lengths and diameters; a control unit comprising pulse-height analysis electronics and a howler for audible count-rate tone presentation; and an electrical or optical cable that connects the probe and the control unit.

The tasks of detection and localization of radioactive lymph nodes necessitate that photopeak events emitted from the lymph nodes be differentiated from photopeak events emitted from injection sites. Detection and localization also necessitate that photopeak events from the lymph nodes be differentiated from photons that have scattered after being emitted from the nodes or injection sites. The source of origin of scattered photons cannot be easily determined. Thus detection of scattered photons is not generally useful in node detection and localization. Detector energy resolution, probe energy window settings, detector intrinsic and geometric sensitivity, probe shielding, probe aperture shape, and operator-controlled probe directionality are factors that affect success in detection and localization tasks. Probes with excellent sensitivity and energy resolution would be ideal for SLN localization, but such probes do not exist. Sensitivity and energy resolution are, at least to some degree, competing factors. As a result, the designs of commercially available probes are based on tradeoffs of numerous performance and practical-use factors, including sensitivity, energy resolution, probe weight, and frequency and pitch of audio signal.

Scintillation detectors tend to have higher sensitivity and better reliability than do ionization detectors. Ionization detectors tend to have better energy resolution and therefore better scatter rejection than do scintillation detectors. Performance differences exist suggest that "better" probes can be identified with objective

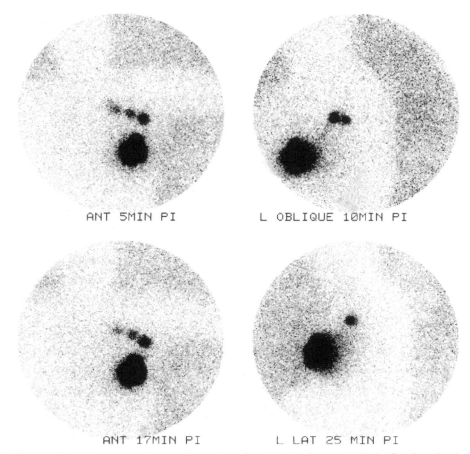

ANT 5MIN PI   L OBLIQUE 10MIN PI

ANT 17MIN PI   L LAT 25 MIN PI

FIGURE 49.7. Oblique view obtained 10 minutes after injection (*upper right*) clarifies that the single activity focus on the lateral view (*lower right*) at 25 minutes is two nodes superimposed. The third node (most medial, infraclavicular) is a tertiary node. A vague channel present on the oblique view only (*upper right*) identifies the true sentinel node as the most anterior node.

performance measures; this is not generally true. In practice, the differences between the technologies and thus the differences between probes do not translate to clear superiority of one technology or probe over another. This is particularly true when probe performance is assessed for detection of low-energy—as opposed to medium- or high-energy—emissions, such as those from the ^{99m}Tc-labeled colloids used for SLN localization in patients with breast cancer. As a result, a surgeon's choice of probe is seldom made strictly according to objective technical considerations about detector performance. It is instead almost always based on a combination of objective considerations and a variety of subjective considerations, such as probe ergonomics, howler tone, and the nature and speed of the response of a probe to the surgeon's manner of use of the probe.

Characterization of counting probes and their performances has not been standardized. Several authors have proposed tests to characterize and compare probes (63), but as of 2001, the nuclear medicine community had not adopted standards. In 2000, the National Electrical Manufacturers Association (NEMA) established a committee to develop a standards document for probes. It will probably be available in 2003. NEMA standards will make possible some objective comparison of probes, but such standards are not sufficient for predicting the

success of SLN localization by a specific surgeon. Successful probe use is highly dependent on a surgeon's ability to alter effectively and efficiently the orientation and position of a detector in response to detected counts communicated to the surgeon through the audible tones of the system howler. Assessment of a surgeon's success with a specific probe is subjective, not objective, and not easily codified.

Before each use, a quality control check of count rate constancy should be performed. This is generally done with a long-lived check source such as ^{57}Co. When the quality control check is complete, the user should confirm that the energy window is set correctly for ^{99m}Tc. Intraoperative use of probes necessitates that they be sterile. This is most often accomplished by use of a removable sterile sheath. Other methods can be used for some probes. Vendor restrictions and recommendations regarding a probe, such as calibration procedures, storage requirements, preventive maintenance, and cleaning, should be followed so that risk of damage to the probe is minimized.

Intraoperative Gamma Cameras

Breast cancer SLN protocols vary greatly. The protocols of some nuclear medicine–surgical teams include preoperative imaging with a conventional gamma camera and intraoperative node localization with a counting probe. The protocols of other teams include only intraoperative node localization with a counting probe. Preoperative imaging complicates preoperative procedures; but if it is done well it reduces the time of intraoperative probe use and increases surgeon confidence regarding SLN localization and removal.

Teams who use protocols with preoperative imaging and an intraoperative probe are not likely to markedly improve their success rate of SLN resection by addition of intraoperative imaging to their protocol. However, teams who do not use preoperative imaging, that is, teams who use protocols with only an intraoperative probe, might improve their SLN localization and resection rates if they modify their protocols to include intraoperative use of a small-field-of-view gamma camera. Investigations to develop such intraoperative imagers and to assess the value of such imagers are being pursued (62,64).

Histopathology

Pathologists who have studied SLN staging of early breast cancer have reported that for the detection of micrometastasis immunohistochemical stains are more sensitive that conventional hematoxylin and eosin stains and multisectioning of SLNs is more sensitive than conventional minimal sectioning of multiple removed node (65). There is documentation that micrometastasis is as important in prognosis as is macrometastasis. One study showed that women with micrometastasis had as many recurrences of metastatic cancer as did women with macrometastasis. Both groups had much higher rates of recurrence than did women with no metastasis (65). The presence of occult metastasis in two or more lymph nodes as an independent prognostic indicator has been associated with increases in 5-year mortality and disease recurrence rates (66).

The reported incidence of SLNs harboring micrometastasis identified with immunohistochemical stains but not with conventional hematoxylin and eosin stains is approximately 14% of all cases of metastasis (44). Other preliminary studies report similar results (55,56). Although data are not yet available to support any conclusions about recurrence and survival rates, observations suggest that higher rates of detection of micrometastasis with appropriate therapeutic management may lead to a decreased rate of recurrence and an increased survival rate among patients with breast cancer.

Radiation Safety

Nuclear medicine physicians, technologists, and scientists work with radiation daily and are knowledgeable about radiation safety, risks of radiation exposures, and the regulatory requirements designed to protect the general public and occupationally exposed personnel. Patients routinely undergo diagnostic nuclear medicine tests before surgical procedures, sometimes within 24 hours of going to the operating room. Patients also mix with the general public immediately after completion of diagnostic nuclear medicine studies without unwarranted concern for safety. Lymphatic mapping with radiotracers and portable intraoperative probe detectors has focused new attention on routine practices by persons who do not work with radiation. Therefore education of these persons about low-level radiation is needed.

Low-level radiation is a fact of our environment. Living on Earth, we all are exposed to radiation from cosmic and natural background sources. At sea level, this has been determined to be approximately 300 mrem per year. At higher altitudes (Denver, CO, for example) annual exposures are higher (~500 mrem). Compare this environmental exposure with that measured in the operating room during SLN excision with radiotracer-probe guidance: approximately 10 mrem to the hands of the surgeon per surgical procedure (67). The hands of a surgeon performing SLN excision on 30 patients per year would be exposed to 300 mrem per year, the same as the body exposure of a person living for 1 year at sea level. The pathologist usually spends less time than the surgeon handling the tissues. Because ^{99m}Tc decays to one half its activity every 6 hours, the pathologist is exposed to considerably less radioactivity than is the surgeon. There is no need to delay pathologic examination of tissues in SLN cases.

The foregoing considerations are based on the following:

1. Administered radioactivity is less than 600 to 1,000 μCi, of which approximately 1% (6 to 10 μCi) may migrate to an SLN.

2. The radiation dose to the hands of the surgeon has been estimated to be 0.5 to 5.0 mrem per melanoma SLN procedure (~400 to 1,000 μCi by intradermal administration). Doses to pathology personnel are less than or equivalent to the dose to the surgeons, because pathology personnel handle the radioactive tissues (SLNs and primary tumor specimens) for less time than do the surgeons.

Radioactive waste from the operating room (e.g., sponges) or pathology laboratory should be collected for disposal with other radioactive nuclear medicine waste. Institutional procedures should apply, that is, radioactive waste should be stored and decayed (67,68). Given the limited exposure that pathology personnel have, specimens can be processed for histopathologic diagnosis, without delay which is critical to patient care.

REFERENCES

1. Cabanas RM. An approach for the treatment of penile carcinoma. *Cancer* 1977;39:456–466.
2. Morton DL, Wen D, Wong JH, et al. Technical details of intra-operative lymphatic mapping for early stage melanoma. *Arch Surg* 1992; 127:392–399.
3. Alex JC, Krag DN. Gamma probe guided localization of lymph nodes. *Surg Oncol* 1993;2:137–143.
4. Ege GN: Internal mammary lymphoscintigraphy. *Radiology* 1976;118: 101–107.
5. Kaplan WD. Lymphoscintigraphy: importance to cancer detection and radiation treatment planning. *Front Radiat Ther Oncol* 1994;28:25–36.
6. Witte C, Witte M, Unger E, et al. Advances in imaging of lymph flow disorders. *Radiographics* 2000;20:1697–1719.
7. Alazraki NA: Lymphoscintigraphy and the intraoperative gamma probe. *J Nucl Med* 1995;36:1780–1783.
8. Waters G, Geisinger K, Garske D, et al. Sentinel lymph node mapping for carcinoma of the colon: a pilot study. *Am Surg* 2000;66:943–946.
9. Joosten JJ, Strobbe LJ, Wauters CA, et al. Intraoperative lymphatic mapping and the sentinel node concept in colorectal carcinoma. *Br J Surg* 1999;86:482–486.

10. Gervasoni JE Jr, Taneja C, Chung MA, et al. Biologic and clinical significance of lymphadenectomy. *Surg Clin North Am* 2000;80:1631–73.

11. Berman C, Norman J, Cruse CW, et al. Lymphoscintigraphy in malignant melanoma. *Ann Plast Surg* 1992;28:29–32.

12. Uren RF, Hofman-Giles RB, Shaw HM, et al. Lymphoscintigraphy in high risk melanoma of the trunk: predicting draining node groups, defining lymphatic channels and locating the sentinel node. *J Nucl Med* 1993;34:1435–1440.

13. O'Brien CJ, Uren RF, Thompson JF, et al. Predictions of potential metastatic sites in cutaneous head and neck melanoma using lymphoscintigraphy. *Am J Surg* 1995;170:461–466.

14. Glass LF, Fenske NA, Messina JL, et al. The role of selective lymphadenectomy in the management of patients with malignant melanoma. *Dermatol Surg* 1995;21:979–983.

15. Harlow SP, Krag DN, Ashikaga T, et al. Gamma probe guided biopsy of the sentinel node in malignant melanoma: a multicentre study. *Melanoma Res* 2001;11:45–55.

16. Nguyen CL, McClay EF, Cole DJ, et al. Melanoma thickness and histology predict sentinel lymph node status. *Am J Surg* 2001;181:8–11.

17. Roozendal GK, de Vries JDH, van Poll D, et al. Sentinel nodes outside lymph node basins in patients with melanoma. *Br J Surg* 2001;88:305–308.

18. Alazraki N, Styblo T, Grant S, et al. Sentinel node staging of early breast cancer using lymphoscintigraphy and the intraoperative gamma-detecting probe. *Semin Nucl Med* 2000;30:56–64.

19. Mudun A, Murray DR, Herda SC, et al. Early stage melanoma: lymphoscintigraphy, reproducibility of sentinel node detection, and effectiveness of the intraoperative gamma probe. *Radiology* 1996;199:171–175.

20. Kateijn BAE, Olmos V, Panday B, et al. Reproducibility of lymphoscintigraphy to identify the first draining lymph node in clinically localized melanoma of the skin: The Netherlands Cancer Institute. *J Nucl Med* 1995;36:223P.

21. Nieweg OE, Jansen L, Olmos RAV, et al. Lymphatic mapping and sentinel lymph node biopsy in breast cancer. *Eur J Nucl Med* 1999;26[Suppl]:S11–S16.

22. Kapteijn BAE, Nieweg OE, Petersen JL, et al. Identification and biopsy of the sentinel node in breast cancer. *Eur J Surg Oncol* 1998;24:427–430.

23. Koller M, Barsuk D, Zippel D, et al. Sentinel lymph node involvement: a predictor for axillary node status with breast cancer: has the time come? *Eur J Surg Oncol* 1998;24:166–168.

24. Guenther JM, Krishnamoorthy M, Tan LR. Sentinel lymphadenectomy for breast cancer in a community managed care setting. *Cancer J Sci Am* 1997;3:336–340.

25. Giuliano AE, Kirgan DM, Guenther JM, et al. Lymphatic mapping and sentinel lymphadenectomy for breast cancer. *Ann Surg* 1994;220:391–401.

26. Horgan K, Mancie-Jones B, Madan M, et al. Axillary sentinel node identification in breast cancer with dye injection alone. *Br J Surg* 1998;85[Suppl]:51–52(abst).

27. Flett MM, Going JJ, Stanton PD, et al. Sentinel node localization in patients with breast cancer. *Br J Surg* 1998;85:991–993.

28. Fölscher DJ, Langman G, Panieri E, et al. Sentinel axillary lymph node: helpful in axillary management in patients with breast cancer? *Br J Surg* 1997;84:1586(abst).

29. de Vries J de, Doting MHE, Nieweg OE, et al. *Combined detection technique of radioactive tracer and blue dye for sentinel lymph node biopsy in breast cancer.* Presented at the 51st Annual Meeting Society of Surgical Oncology and World Federation for Surgical Oncology Society Congress, San Diego, CA, March 26–29, 1998.

30. Cox CE, Pendas S, Cox JM, et al. Guidelines for sentinel node biopsy and lymphatic mapping of patients with breast cancer. *Ann Surg* 1998;226:645–653.

31. Van der Ent FW, Kengen RA, Van der Poll HAG, et al. Sentinel node biopsy in 70 unselected patients with breast cancer. *Ann Surg* 1998;226:645–653.

32. O'Hea BJ, Hill ADK, El-Shirbiny AM, et al. Sentinel lymph node biopsy in breast cancer: Initial experience at Memorial Sloan-Kettering Cancer Center. *J Am Coll Surg* 1998;186:423–427.

33. Schneebaum S, Stadler Y, Cohen M, et al. *Sentinel lymph node localization in breast cancer: a feasibility study.* Presented at the 49th Annual Meeting of the Society of Surgical Oncology, Atlanta, GA, March 21–24, 1996.

34. Roumen RHM, Valkenburg JGM, Geuskens LM. Lymphoscintigraphy and feasibility of sentinel node biopsy in 83 patients with primary breast cancer. *Eur J Surg Oncol* 1997;23:495–502.

35. Veronesi U, Paganelli G, Galimberti V, et al. Sentinel node biopsy to avoid axillary dissection in breast cancer with clinically negative lymphnodes. *Lancet* 1997;349:1864–1867.

36. Borgstein PJ, Pijpers R, Comans EF, et al. Sentinel lymph node biopsy in breast cancer: guidelines and pitfalls of lymphoscintigraphy and gamma probe detection. *J Am Coll Surg* 1998;186:275–283.

37. Gill PG, Hall VE, Kirkwood I, et al. Lymphoscintigraphy for locating the sentinel lymph node in patients with breast cancer. *Breast* 1997;6:225(abst).

38. Reuhl T, Kaisers H, Markwardt J, et al. Axillaausraumung bei klinisch nodal-negativem Mammakarzinom. Kann die Indikation durch "sentinel node" Nachweis individualisiert werden? *Dtsch Med Wochenschr* 1998;123:583–587.

39. Cody HS III, Hill ADK, Tran KN, et al. Credentialing for breast lymphatic mapping: how many cases are enough? *Ann Surg* 1999;229:723.

40. Taylor A, Murray D, Herda S, et al. Dynamic lymphoscintigraphy to identify the sentinel and satellite nodes. *Clin Nucl Med* 1996;21:755–758.

41. Alazraki NP, Styblo T, Grant S, et al. Optimum injection methods (peritumoral [PT] subdermal [SD] and periareolar [PA]) to image sentinel lymph nodes (SLNs) is breast cancer. *J Nucl Med* 2001;24:116P.

42. Keshtgar MRS, Ell PJ. Sentinel lymph node detection and imaging. *Eur J Nucl Med* 1999;26:57–67.

43. Giuliano AE, Jones RC, Brennan M et al. Sentinel lymphadenectomy in breast cancer. *J Clin Oncol* 1997;15:2345–2350.

44. Alazraki NA, Styblo T, Grant S, et al. Breast cancer sentinel lymph node lymphoscintigraphy: comparison of subdermal and peritumoral injections. *J Nucl Med* 1999;40:59P.

45. Alazraki NP, Styblo T, Grant SF, et al. Breast cancer (BRCA) sentinel lymph node (SLN) lymphoscintigraphy: comparison of subdermal and peritumoral injections. *J Nucl Med* 1999;40:59P.

46. Olmos RAV, Hoefnagel CA, Nieweg OE, et al. *Eur J Nucl Med* 1999;26[Suppl]:S2–S10.

47. Gennari R, Galimberti V, De Cicco C, et al. Use of technetium-99m-labeled colloid albumin for peroperative and intraoperative localization of nonpalpable breast lesions. *J Am Coll Surg* 2000;190:692–699.

48. Vendrell-Torne E, Setain-Quinquer J, Domenech-Torne FM. Study of normal lymphatic drainage using radioactive isotopes. *J Nucl Med* 1972;13:801–805.

49. Offodile R, Hoh C, Barsky SH, et al. Minimally invasive breast carcinoma staging using lymphatic mapping with radiolabeled dextran. *Cancer* 1998;82:1704–1708.

50. Henze E, Schelbert HR, Collins JD, et al. Lymphoscintigraphy with Tc-99m labeled dextran. *J Nucl Med* 1982;23:923–929.

51. Alazraki NP, Eshima D, Eshima LA, et al. Lymphoscintigraphy, the sentinel node concept, and the intraoperative gamma probe in melanoma, breast cancer and other potential cancers. *Semin Nucl Med* 1997;27:55–67.

52. Eshima D, Eshima L, Botti N, et al. Technetium 99m sulfur colloid for lymphoscintigraphy: effects of preparation parameters. *J Nucl Med* 1996;37:1575–1578.

53. Hung JC, Wiseman GA, Wahner HW, et al. Filtered technetium-99m-sulfur colloid evaluated lymphoscintigraphy. *J Nucl Med* 1995;36:1895–1901.

54. Goldfarb LN, Alazraki NP, Eshima D, et al. Lymphoscintigraphic identification of sentinel lymph nodes: clinical evaluation of 0.22 μm filtration of Tc-99m sulfur colloid. *Radiology* 1998;208:505–509.

55. Krag D, Weaver D, Ashikaga T, et al. The sentinel node in breast cancer: a multicenter validation study. *N Engl J Med* 1998;339:941–946.

56. Grant SF, Styblo T, Larsen T, et al. Technical factors which affect

success in imaging sentinel lymph nodes (SLNs) for breast cancer. *J Nucl Med Technol* 1999;27:162.

57. Low-Beer B. Surface measurements of radioactive phosphorus in breast tumors as a possible diagnostic method. *Science* 1946;104:399.

58. Moore GE. Use of radioactive diiodofluorescein in the diagnosis and localization of brain tumors. *Science* 1948;107:569–571.

59. Robinson CV, Selverstone B. Localization of brain tumors at operation with radioactive phosphorus. *J Neurosurg* 1958;15:76–83.

60. Selverstone B, Solomon AK. Radioactive isotopes in the study of intracranial tumors. *Trans Am Neurol Assoc* 1948;73:115–119.

61. Woolfenden JN, Barber HB. Design and use of radiation detector probes for intraoperative tumor detection using tumor-seeking radiotracers. In: Freeman LM, ed. *Nuclear medicine annual.* New York: Raven Press, 1990:151–173.

62. Hoffman EJ, Tornai MP, Janecek M, et al. Intraoperative probes and imaging probes. *Eur J Nucl Med* 1999;26:913–935.

63. Britten AJ. A method to evaluate intra-operative gamma probes for sentinel lymph node localisation. *Eur J Nucl Med* 1999;26:76–83.

64. Aarsvold JN, Mintzer RA, Greene C, et al. Sterile field imaging of sentinel nodes initial experience. *J Nucl Med* 2002;43:156P, 2002.

65. Gerber B, Krause A, Reimer T. Immunohistochemically detected lymph node micrometastases in breast cancer and their correlation with prognostic factors. *Breast J* 1997;3:106–111.

66. Hainsworth PJ, Tjandra JJ, Stillwall RG, et al. Detection and significance of occult metastases in node-negative breast cancer. *Br J Surg* 1993;80:459–463.

67. Miner TJ, Shriver CD, Flicek PR, et al. Guidelines for the safe use of radioactive materials during localization and resection of the sentinel lymph node. *Ann Surg Oncol* 1999;6:75–82.

68. Gulec SA, Moffat FL, Serafini AN, et al. Sentinel node localization in patients with breast cancer. *J Nucl Med* 1997;38:33P.

Diagnostic Nuclear Medicine, Fourth Edition. Edited by M.P. Sandler, R.E. Coleman, J.A. Patton, F.J.Th. Wackers, A. Gottschalk. Lippincott Williams & Wilkins, Philadelphia 2003.

50

TREATMENT OF PAIN FROM BONE METASTASES EMPLOYING UNSEALED SOURCES

EDWARD B. SILBERSTEIN

The scope of the problem of optimal treatment of pain from metastatic bone disease is enormous. Each year in the United States there are approximately 125,000 cases of cancer metastatic to bone. Approximately two thirds of these require an analgesic, often a narcotic, and quality of life can be severely affected by the lethargy and constipation that occur as side effects of the opiates employed. Other clinical effects of bone metastases include pathologic fracture, immobility, hypercalcemia, loss of independence, and tremendous emotional sequelae, including depression, fear, and isolation (1,2).

Metastases may reach bone by direct extension or, more commonly, through the hematogenous route, usually beginning in marrow. Of all patients with metastatic disease, 70% will have disease in the vertebrae and ribs, 40% in the pelvis, 25% in the femur, and 15% in the skull, often concurrently. Pathologic fracture occurs in approximately 10% of patients with bone metastases. Of these, 50% involve the femur and 15% the humerus. Breast cancer causes over half of all pathologic fractures, and renal, lung, and thyroid carcinomas each account for 5% to 10% of the total (3).

Of several nonnarcotic modalities available to treat the pain of osseous metastases, radiation therapy, both as teletherapy (external beam) and internal electron and β-emitting radiopharmaceuticals, has been proven efficacious over many years of clinical experience and research trials. The goal of externally or internally administered radiation therapy in these patients is not only pain relief or reduction but also improvement of functional status. To this we may add the possibility that electron or β-emitting radiopharmaceuticals may be able to prevent or delay the onset of new painful metastatic disease.

Bisphosphonates are newer additions to the clinician's armamentarium of pain-relieving agents, and this pharmacologic approach has become an important alternative to radiotherapy.

E.B. Silberstein: Departments of Radiology and Medicine, University of Cincinnati Medical Center, Cincinnati, OH.

EXTERNAL BEAM RADIOTHERAPY

Teletherapy may be given to focal sites of painful disease or as hemibody radiation to wider fields when there are multiple painful sites (4,5). There are many local radiotherapy fractionation schedules. Among the most common of these are the administration of 40 to 50 Gy in fractions of 180 to 200 cGy 5 days per week for 4 to 5 weeks, 20 to 40 Gy in doses of 250 to 400 cGy 5 days per week for 1 to 3 weeks, or single doses of 8 to 10 Gy (6). There are only a few studies comparing fractionation schedules for solitary or multiple metastatic disease. One of the best of these studies stratified patients by the primary site of metastasis, the presence of internal osseous fixation, and the medical center where the therapy was employed. For solitary osseous metastases, there was no difference in pain reduction between 20 Gy given over 1 week and 40.5 Gy over 3 weeks. With multiple sites of metastatic disease, the same large study showed no difference of pain reduction from 15 Gy in 1 week or 30 Gy given over 2 weeks (7). There appears to be little difference between delivering 8 Gy in a single fraction to a site of painful osseous metastasis and 30 Gy in 10 daily fractions over 2 weeks, as measured by the time to onset of relief, incidence of relief, duration of response, or survival (8). A more recent meta-analysis suggested that 20 Gy in 5 fractions, 30 Gy in 10 fractions, or 35 Gy in 14 fractions are acceptable. Daily doses in excess of 4 Gy were not commonly suggested (9).

Partial body radiation, involving 6 to 8 Gy to the upper hemibody, 8 Gy to the lower hemibody, or 6 to 8 Gy from neck to pubis, has been used successfully to ameliorate bone pain. From upper body hemiradiation not exceeding 8 Gy, significant toxicity has included severe nausea and vomiting in 16% of cases and clinically significant myelosuppression in about one third of patients. Radiation pneumonitis can be avoided with doses of 8 Gy or below. Lower hemibody radiation causes a low incidence of severe diarrhea, as well as nausea and vomiting, with about 10% of cases having severe myelosuppression. These techniques yield a complete response in 19% (elimination of pain), 47% partial response, and 34% of patients with some or no response. In this group, a better performance scale score predicted a greater chance for pain reduction with hemibody radiation (10).

RADIOPHARMACEUTICALS EMPLOYED FOR PAIN RELIEF

Bone-seeking radiopharmaceuticals play a significant role in the treatment of the pain of osteoblastic metastatic disease. These radiopharmaceuticals, called "unsealed sources" by the Nuclear Regulatory Commission of the United States, are β- or electron-emitters with a chemical affinity for sites of new bone formation by one of several mechanisms. These include direct substitution for stable analogs in hydroxyapatite (^{89}Sr for calcium and ^{32}P-orthophosphate for stable phosphate), chemisorption on the hydroxyapatite surface by the phosphate moiety of phosphonate chelates (^{186}Re, ^{188}Re, and possibly ^{153}Sm), or formation of insoluble salts with bone (trivalent ^{153}Sm and ^{117m}Sn). The uptake of these radiopharmaceuticals is greater where new reactive bone is being formed, because of increased blood flow to the site and increased surface area of calcium phosphate salts as they are secreted and become hydroxyapatite molecules (11).

Table 50.1 lists seven radiopharmaceuticals, ordered by half-lives, that were examined for the ability to reduce or relieve pain of osteoblastic metastatic disease. The range of physical properties of these radiopharmaceuticals is remarkable, with half-lives ranging from less than a day (^{188}Re) to 50.5 days (^{89}Sr), and mean particle energies as low as 0.13 MeV (the electrons of ^{117m}Sn) and as high as 0.79 MeV (the β of ^{188}Re). The mean range in soft tissue is proportional to energy so that the ^{117m}Sn electron range is only 0.2 mm, whereas that of the β of ^{188}Re exceeds 3 mm.

All the radiopharmaceuticals listed emit γ-rays, except for ^{32}P. ^{89}Sr has a γ-ray in very low abundance, which cannot be used for imaging, whereas the other radiopharmaceuticals do emit γ-rays that have been employed to document the localization of the injected radiopharmaceutical at precisely the sites of osteoblastic metastasis identified by a ^{99m}Tc-labeled diphosphonate.

One might predict differences in response to these radiopharmaceuticals because of the dramatically different dose rates implicit in their very short and very long half lives. Also, with a longer mean path of the electron or β particle in the marrow, one radiopharmaceutical might have a greater tumoricidal effect but also perhaps greater myelosuppression.

There are other variables determining the dose received by tumor from a given amount of administered activity. The intensity of uptake by reactive bone can vary dramatically. Although the usual ratio of abnormal to normal bone is 3:1 to 5:1, ratios as high as 13:1 to 15:1 have been noted (12). An extensive amount of reactive bone, as in a "superscan," could dilute the effect of an injected radiopharmaceutical, with fewer atoms per volume of tumor because of the widespread uptake within the marrow. Another variable determining the dose to individual lesions is the inhomogeneity in distribution of tumor, marrow, and trabecular bone within a given site of osteoblastic uptake seen scintigraphically. The greater the osteoblastic trabecular volume, the greater the deposition of these therapeutic agents with a resultant increase in tumor dose (13). The radiopharmaceuticals appearing in Table 50.1 all have significant renal excretion, so that altered renal function will lead to increased body and lesion retention.

MECHANISMS OF PAIN RELIEF

There is no question of the efficacy of external beam therapy or of intravenous β-emitting or electron-emitting radiopharmaceuticals (or oral ^{32}P-orthophosphate) in pain reduction. Bone pain may diminish after only a few days of teletherapy treatment or within a week of radiopharmaceutical administration, even when the total dose to the painful site is less than 10 Gy. In such a short period, it is clear that the tumor cells within the marrow have not disappeared and, in fact, there may be some edema surrounding these cells as they are radiated.

The neurons are radioresistant. Therefore, although pressure and mechanical stretch may be invoked as possible mechanisms of pain from osseous metastases, there must be other reasons for the efficacy of radiation. Besides the tumor cell, other target cells have been postulated (Table 50.2). One or more of these cell types may be responsible for producing chemical mediators that could modulate the pain response of the neuron (2). A list of possible pain mediators appears in Table 50.3. Intramedullary hypoxia has also been hypothesized as a source of pain. Thus, radiation to radiation-sensitive cells such as lymphocytes could lead to a decrease in cytokine-induced pain modulation.

Table 50.1. *Physical Properties of Radiopharmaceuticals used for Painful Osseous Metastases*

Radiopharmaceutical	$t_{1/2}$ (d.)	Maximum E_B(MeV)	Mean E_B(MeV)	Mean Range (mm)	Gamma MeV (% abundance)
^{188}Re(Sn)HEDP	0.7	2.12	0.73	2.7	0.155 (10%)
			0.79	3.1	
^{153}Sm-EDTMP	1.9	0.81	0.22	0.8	0.103 (28%), 0.041 (49%)
^{186}Re(Sn)HEDP	3.8	1.07	0.35	1.1	0.137 (9%)
^{131}I-BDP	8.1	0.81	0.19	0.8	0.374 (82%)
^{117m}Sn-DTPA			0.16	0.29	
	13.6	—	0.13	0.21	0.161 (86%)
^{32}P-phosphate	14.3	1.71	0.70	3.0	—
^{89}Sr-chloride	50.5	1.43	0.58	2.4	0.910 (0.01%)

Table 50.2. *Target Cells for Bone Pain Reduction*

Tumor cell	Lymphocyte
Osteoblast	Vascular epithelium
Osteoclast	Nocioreceptors
Macrophage	Nerve fibers
Mast cell	

Finally, as osseous metastases spread, there is destruction of trabecular and cortical bone. At what point does this destruction become an occult painful fracture?

RADIOPHARMACEUTICALS CURRENTLY EMPLOYED FOR THE TREATMENT OF BONE PAIN

^{32}P-Orthophosphate

^{32}P as the orthophosphate has been employed for approximately 5 decades, with at least 30 articles in the medical literature describing its efficacy in relieving pain from osseous metastases (14). ^{32}P-orthophosphate has a 14.3-day half-life, a maximum β-energy of 1.71 MeV, and a mean range in tissue of 3 mm. It has been given to thousands of patients with more than 850 reported in the medical literature. Eighty-five percent of an administered dose is incorporated into hydroxyapatite, but some 15% of this moiety is taken up by nonosseous tissues where it is, in fact, the major intracellular anion. Phosphate appears in molecules involved with energy storage, cell structure, intracellular messengers, and, most importantly, in the backbone of deoxyribonucleic acid (DNA) and ribonucleic acid (RNA) where, as a β-emitter, it may damage these nucleic acids. Bone marrow will, therefore, receive radiation from the ^{32}P that it takes up, as well as from the β particle of ^{32}P incorporated into surrounding bone.

^{32}P-orthophosphate has been administered as a single dose, with activities from 5 to 12 mCi, as well as in multiple doses over a period up to a month, with total activities as high as 24 mCi (14). There are no comparative studies to indicate the optimal activity for ^{32}P-orthophosphate administration, whether the activity should be given in single or multiple doses, and whether the oral route is as efficacious as intravenously administered ^{32}P-orthophosphate.

Based on a single abstract in the literature, ^{32}P-orthophosphate was often given in the past with androgens to stimulate bone uptake. Parathyroid hormone has been similarly employed, but there are no studies to indicate that these hormonal manipu-

Table 50.3. *Possible Chemical Mediators of Bone Pain from Metastatic Disease*

ATP	Substance P
Histamine	Serotonin
Lipidic acids	Bradykinin or its metabolites
Leukotrienes	Prostaglandins, especially PGE
Calcitonin	Interleukins 1 and 2

lations provide any therapeutic advantage over administration of intravenous ^{32}P-orthophosphate with no hormonal injection.

A review of at least 30 papers in print indicates that there is no relationship between the total administered activity and the percent of patients responding in the two tumors most commonly treated, prostate and breast carcinoma metastatic to bone. The overall response rate in the literature is approximately 80% (77% prostate, 84% breast). These data come from adding together series in which criteria for patients responding were not always clear and in which hormones were sometimes used (14). Nevertheless, the response rate is in the same range seen with external beam local or widefield radiation therapy. The mean reported duration of response to ^{32}P-orthophosphate is 5.1 ± 2.6 months, with the longest responses noted in multiple series as 16.8 ± 9.4 months. There may be some radiographic or scintigraphic improvement with ^{32}P-orthophosphate, as with the other radiopharmaceuticals employed. This does not correlate with pain reduction.

The side effects described with ^{32}P-orthophosphate were often actually from an androgen given for a week preceding ^{32}P-orthophosphate administration. Thus, an increase in bone pain (the "flare phenomenon") has been seen in as many as one half of the patients receiving androgen followed by ^{32}P-orthophosphate, whereas this number is generally lower with the other radiopharmaceuticals. Cord compression has resulted from androgen stimulated tumor growth. Nausea and vomiting are also caused by androgen administration and are not seen when ^{32}P-orthophosphate is administered without this hormone. Androgen administration is, in fact, contraindicated in prostate cancer.

Pancytopenia occurs with ^{32}P-orthophosphate and all of the electron or β-emitters, although in the published literature there is only one death that has been attributed to ^{32}P myelosuppression. An intracerebral hemorrhage in another patient in the literature is probably also related to ^{32}P-orthophosphate-induced marrow suppression, however.

^{32}P-orthophosphate has been employed for the treatment of myeloproliferative diseases (e.g., polycythemia vera, essential thrombocythemia) for many years, and there is, consequently, a bias that the degree of myelosuppression from this radiopharmaceutical is greater than that from the other agents in Table 50.1. The leukocyte and platelet counts return to normal by 8 weeks (15) after ^{32}P myelosuppression. A recent study planned by the International Atomic Energy Agency comparing ^{32}P given orally with intravenous ^{89}Sr indicated that in fact the two agents had equal efficacy of about 90% in pain reduction. With ^{32}P, 2 of 16 patients had grade 2 leukocyte toxicity and 6 of 16 had grade 2 platelet toxicity; none required therapy. The ^{89}Sr patients had only grade 1 toxicity (16).

^{32}P contained in polyphosphate (phosphate ester chains up to 50 or more), pyrophosphate, and bisphosphonate have all been employed. Polyphosphate and pyrophosphate labeled with ^{32}P are rapidly broken down in blood and tissues by phosphatases into the orthophosphate moiety. One series reported that ^{32}P-hydroxyethylidene diphosphate (HEDP) therapy caused significant myelosuppression from a low administered activity in five cases (17), so this approach was abandoned.

^{89}Sr-Strontium Chloride

^{89}Sr, injected as the chloride, substitutes for calcium in the hydroxyapatite molecule. It was first suggested for the palliation of bone pain from metastatic disease in 1942 (18), preceding the earliest reports of ^{32}P-orthophosphate for this purpose. After intravenous injection, strontium uptake in reactive bone surrounding tumor has been associated with abnormal to normal bone ratios of between 3:1 and 15:1 (12). It is excreted by both renal (80%) and fecal (20%) routes with a biologic half-life of 4 to 5 days. However, approximately 30% to 35% of the radiopharmaceutical remains in normal bone for 10 to 14 days with 20% retention at 3 months. The biologic half-life of ^{89}Sr in the woven, reactive bone around osteoblastic metastases is long, with retention of 89% to 90% of the injected dose described in involved sites at 3 months following injection.

The physical half-life of ^{89}Sr is 50.5 days with a maximal β energy of 1.43 MeV and a mean range in tissue of 2.4 mm. The γ-ray emitted at 0.910 MeV has only 0.01% abundance.

Intravenous injection of ^{89}Sr should be performed over a period of 60 to 120 seconds because the patient will experience a warm flushing feeling if a rapid bolus injection is attempted. The optimal activity to be administered is not clear. Over a threshold of 20 to 25 μCi/kg administered activity, it is likely that there is no increasing response with increasing administered activity, although with larger doses of strontium, more myelosuppression will result (19). Even in a patient with no previous chemotherapy, one cannot predict the degree of myelosuppression with a high degree of certainty, because with advanced marrow replacement by tumor and with fewer stem cells available to participate in recovery from the radiation-induced myelosuppression, one may see platelet and leukocyte nadirs that are only 25% to 30% of the initial counts. The more usual response is milder myelosuppression, with a decrease in these counts to approximately 60% to 70% of pretreatment levels with a nadir at 5 to 8 weeks and recovery by 10 to 16 weeks (16,19–21).

The response time to ^{89}Sr may occur as early as 3 days but is most commonly noted in the second week, with patients reporting a decrease in pain as late as 25 days following injection. In analyzing data on ^{89}Sr efficacy, one should, therefore, exclude patients who were treated but did not survive for 1 month. The published data on strontium response show a range of 65% to 90%, with complete relief of pain in 5% to 20% of patients injected (16,19–21). The mean duration of pain reduction is 3 to 6 months, and retreatment for responders is possible at approximately 3-month intervals, with about half of these also responding to a second treatment. It is not clear if patients who do not respond to the first injection will respond to a second injection, but a few such cases have been reported.

In the trans-Canadian study patients were randomized to receive teletherapy to painful sites or teletherapy plus an adjuvant dosage of 10.8 mCi of ^{89}Sr. This administered activity is two or three times greater than that currently used in the United States. In patients who received this activity of ^{89}Sr, however, there was a significant delay to recurrence of the painful site compared with patients who received teletherapy alone (22). The Canadian data, and those from the United Kingdom using 5.4 mCi, indicated that new sites of pain occurred less often in the patients who received ^{89}Sr (22,23). This effect may be related to the long physical and biologic half-life of the radiopharmaceutical. The Canadian study provided no evidence that ^{89}Sr prolonged life. A New Zealand report showed that those patients who had a prostate-specific antigen (PSA) fall after ^{89}Sr lived more than twice as long as those with no PSA response (24). However a drop in PSA did not correlate, in another study, with the clinical response (25), suggesting that death of tumor cells is not the only mechanism for pain reduction.

We are unable to predict which patients with osteoblastic metastases will have pain reduction with ^{89}Sr. The performance level, occurrence and degree of cytopenia, the presence of narcotic tolerance, and activity of ^{89}Sr have not been shown to be predictive of response.

^{186}Re-Etidronate

^{186}Re-HEDP (generic name—etidronate) has a 3.8-day half-life and a maximum β energy of 1.07 MeV with a mean range in soft tissue of 1.1 mm. Its β emission, with a photopeak of 0.137 MeV, can provide adequate bone imaging, although this has not proven to be helpful in the use of the radiopharmaceutical. ^{186}Re-etidronate, like the other bone-seeking radiopharmaceuticals, can only be used efficaciously in a patient whose ^{99m}Tc-diphosphonate bone scintigraph shows abnormal uptake. It is, therefore, unnecessary to give a tracer dose of ^{186}Re-etidronate preceding the therapeutic activity. The phosphonate moiety carrying rhenium is characterized by carbon-to-phosphorus bonds that cannot be hydrolyzed by phosphatases. The phosphate moiety of the rhenium diphosphonate chemisorbs to calcium atoms in bone hydroxyapatite. In fact, rhenium and technetium chemistry are similar, because both are members of Group VIIA of the Periodic Table.

Approximately 70% of administered ^{186}Re-etidronate activity is excreted in the urine by 72 hours in patients with a relatively small mass of osteoblastic metastases, although extensive body retention can occur, analogous to a ^{99m}Tc-diphosphonate superscan, with widespread metastatic disease. This radiopharmaceutical is retained longer in the reactive bone around metastases than in normal bone, similar to the behavior of ^{89}Sr. With doses of approximately 30 to 70 mCi, a response (PR plus CR) has been seen in about 55% to 75% of cases (26,27). The more carefully applied the pain reduction criteria are, with inclusion of effects of analgesics and changes in activities of daily living, the lower the response rate appears to be (27).

A flare response occurs from ^{186}Re-etidronate in approximately 10% of cases, similar to that noted with ^{89}Sr. Second (or more) treatments have been performed in responders with approximately 50% noting a further decrease in pain. Pain relief may occur within 1 to 3 weeks. Dose-escalation studies have not shown an increase in response, although more myelosuppression results. A radiation dose threshold of 2.10 Gy for ^{186}Re-etidronate has been calculated (28). No difference in response rates have been found in a small study of ^{89}Sr, ^{186}Re-etidronate, and ^{188}Re-etidronate (29).

^{153}Sm-Lexidronam

^{153}Sm has a 1.9-day half-life with a maximum β energy of 0.81 MeV and a mean range in tissue of 0.8 mm. It has two γ photo peaks, at 0.103 and 0.041 MeV. ^{153}Sm, like rhenium, has been chelated with bone-seeking polyphosphonates. The optimal combination of high bone uptake, rapid blood clearance, and renal excretion was found to be samarium chelated with ethylenediaminetetramethylenephosphonate (EDTMP), now called lexidronam (30). ^{153}Sm-lexidronam, clears more rapidly from the blood than the bone-imaging agent ^{99m}Tc-methylene diphosphonate (MDP), while providing identical scintigraphic and bone marrow ratios. In patients with very small tumor burdens in bone, 50% to 65% of the injected ^{153}Sm-lexidronam will be taken up by bone, with higher levels of retention in the presence of osteoblastic metastases. ^{153}Sm appears to form an insoluble oxide on the hydroxyapatite surface, and renal excretion is complete within about 8 hours. ^{153}Sm-lexidronam, given in activities of 0.5 to 1.5 mCi/kg, leads to pain reduction in 65% to 70% of evaluable patients, with a greater degree of myelosuppression from higher administered activities. As with the other radiopharmaceuticals, pain reduction or relief usually begins in 14 days and has lasted as long as 11 months. Response to a second treatment parallels that of ^{186}Re-etidronate, with about 50% of patients noting pain reduction from a second injection (30). No dose-response relationship has been seen to date with ^{153}Sm-lexidronam, again similar to the other bone-seeking radiopharmaceuticals previously discussed. Mild myelotoxicity occurs with a reduction in leukocyte and platelet counts of about 10% to 40%, and full recovery occurs in 6 to 8 weeks. No difference in response rates have been noted in a retrospective comparison of ^{89}Sr and ^{153}Sm-lexidronam (31).

^{117m}Sn-Pentetate

Pentetate (DTPA) is a widely employed chelating agent in nuclear medicine, which is excreted through glomerular filtration. It has been chelated to ^{117m}Sn and injected into patients, in whom the ^{117m}Sn moiety forms an insoluble salt with hydroxyapatite, localizing at areas of increased osteoblastic activity by a mechanism similar to that of ^{153}Sm. ^{117m}Sn, with the mean electron energies of 0.13 and 0.16 MeV, and a resultant mean range in tissue of about 0.2 mm, could theoretically have relatively less myelotoxicity, because of the reduced range of its electron emission relative to that of the β particles of the other radiopharmaceuticals reviewed. Clinical studies of ^{117m}Sn-pentetate suggest that this hypothesis may be true, although much more data are required. The response rate is 60% to 83% with only one case of grade 3 leukocyte toxicity (no grade 3 platelet toxicity) noted in 40 treatments (32).

^{188}Re-etidronate

Also of considerable interest is ^{188}Re-etidronate, with a half-life of only 0.7 days, because it can be administered at much larger activities than a radiopharmaceutical like ^{89}Sr with a 50.5-day half-life. Its efficacy is similar to that of ^{186}Re-etidronate and ^{153}Sm-lexidronam (29). If a dose rate effect can be observed with ^{188}Re-diphosphate, there could be a therapeutic advantage to employing this radiopharmaceutical.

CHOICE OF TELETHERAPY VERSUS INTERNAL β-EMITTERS

There are no clinical data yet available directly comparing teletherapy and intravenous radiopharmaceutical treatment, although both provide efficacious radiotherapy. There are certain circumstances under which teletherapy is clearly the treatment of choice. If the bone scan is negative at the tumor site, the radiopharmaceutical will not have adequate uptake to deliver a therapeutic dose. When there is impending pathologic fracture, with more than 50% of the cortex destroyed, teletherapy will usually be efficacious in prophylaxis (or treatment) of this condition, whereas the radiopharmaceutical will not deliver a sufficient dose rapidly enough to be as effective. In the presence of cord compression, teletherapy is the treatment of choice, because the extraosseous tumor will receive little radiation from radiopharmaceuticals localizing in bone. Teletherapy to a single site of pain will affect only the regional bone marrow in a patient who may have had previous chemotherapy, whereas the radiopharmaceuticals we have reviewed will cause mild to moderate myelosuppression that will not be observed with teletherapy. Pain relief is probably more prompt with teletherapy as well, although a blinded comparative study has not been performed to examine this point.

When there are multiple painful metastases in a patient whose ^{99m}Tc-MDP bone scan indicates that the osteoblastic lesions correspond to the painful sites, one of the internal emitters should be employed. There must be no cord compression and no large soft tissue mass extending to bone causing the patient's discomfort. Single vertebral lesions may lead to spinal cord compression and should receive teletherapy first, but when the cord has received 40 to 45 Gy, a β- or electron-emitting radiopharmaceutical is appropriate for such painful sites. When it is impossible for the patient and the family to return daily for a fractionated course of radiotherapy 5 days a week for 3 weeks, the intravenous radiopharmaceuticals provide a significant advantage, because only one injection is required.

ADMINISTRATION OF UNSEALED β-EMITTERS

Careful planning must precede the administration of these unsealed sources. The painful site must correspond to an area positive on a bone scan usually performed within the previous month or so. Radiographs of the site may be necessary to exclude a lytic lesion that is large enough to cause pathologic fracture.

The patient's platelet and leukocyte counts must be adequate, probably more than 100,000/μL for the former and 4,500/μL for the latter. Disseminated intravascular coagulation has been associated with severe or lethal thrombocytopenia and should be excluded. If the patient has received chemotherapy in the last 4 to 6 weeks, one must be certain that full recovery of the marrow has occurred. This is particularly important when long-acting agents such as nitrosoureas have been given. The patient must understand that the degree of myelosuppression is not entirely predictable and that there is a remote chance of a life-threatening drop in the patient's platelet and leukocyte counts. Azotemia requires some reduction in administered activity. An informed consent form should be employed before therapy.

Patients receiving these radiopharmaceuticals have often had multiple injections of chemotherapy or other drugs that may reduce the number of available veins. An intravenous line should be placed before the administration of the radiopharmaceutical, to ensure that there will be no infiltration of the injectate that could deposit significant energy in a small volume and also to reduce the radiation dose to the fingers of the physicians, which might become excessive if multiple attempts are made to insert the needle into a vein. A finger dosimeter is recommended for the injecting physician, and a plastic syringe shield should be employed. β-particles or electrons from these radiopharmaceuticals produce bremsstrahlung that is proportional to the atomic number of the material interacting with the particle. Therefore, a lead syringe shield is inappropriate.

These radiopharmaceuticals should be injected over at least 1 minute. ^{89}Sr, like its analog calcium, can cause vasodilatation and arrhythmia if injected rapidly. The phosphonate chelates can also chelate calcium and cause hypocalcemic symptoms if injected too rapidly.

MEDICAL ECONOMICS

There are data from several sources documenting that ^{89}Sr as an adjuvant to external radiotherapy can reduce patient management costs (33,34).

EMBALMING OR AUTOPSY IN A TREATED PATIENT

If a patient dies while there is a significant β- or electron-emitting radiopharmaceutical in that individual, embalming without opening the body yields minimal exposure. With the body open, these particles may radiate the hands and to a much less extent the body. Double gloving is recommended if an autopsy is necessary. With exposure to 10 mCi of ^{32}P on the surface of an area, the individual doing the autopsy will receive only 0.3 rem/mCi per hour to the hands. Goggles should be worn to protect from splashing and to reduce β exposure in the air. Further details appear in NCRP Report #37 (35).

FUTURE INVESTIGATION

There are three radiopharmaceuticals for pain therapy now commercially available in the United States, ^{32}P-orthophosphate, ^{89}Sr, and ^{153}Sm-lexidronam. ^{186}Re-etidronate is widely used in Europe. ^{117m}Sn-pentetate and ^{188}Re-etidronate have interesting physical properties, which may make them valuable in the treatment of pain from osteoblastic metastases.

The problem of determining the most effective radiopharmaceutical for pain relief with the least marrow toxicity is a difficult one. The response of all the radiopharmaceuticals studied to date lies in the range of 55% to 80%, and to find statistically significant differences of 5% or 10% between two agents will require hundreds or thousands of patients in each of two study groups if one is to avoid a Type II statistical error. The cost of such studies is enormous.

Other questions remain. Which is the best of these radiopharmaceuticals not only in efficacy but also for cost and safety? Do any of these agents really prolong life? Do these agents all reduce the incidence of new painful sites at the commonly used administered activities? Are combinations of short- and long-lived radiopharmaceuticals useful? Is split-dose therapy useful? Should painless osteoblastic metastases be treated? If the first treatment is not effective, should a second treatment be attempted? What about combinations of radiopharmaceuticals and chemotherapy? A recent report suggests improved survival with the addition of ^{89}Sr to four other drugs (36). Because unlabeled bisphosphonates are showing efficacy for reducing the incidence of pathologic fracture and preventing or reducing bone pain, good comparative studies are required to determine if the electron- or β-emitters can compete in efficacy, cost, and safety.

These questions make it clear that much work remains to be done in optimizing the use of radiopharmaceuticals for the relief of pain resulting from osteoblastic metastases.

REFERENCES

1. Foley KM. The treatment of cancer pain. *N Eng J Med* 1985;313: 84–95.
2. Nielsen OS, Munro AJ, Tannock IF. Bone metastases: pathophysiology and management policy. *J Clin Oncol* 1991;9:509–524.
3. Abrams HL, Spiro R, Goldstein N. Metastases in carcinoma. Analysis of 1000 autopsied cases. *Cancer* 1950;23:74–85.
4. Greenwald HP, Bonica JJ, Bergner M. The prevalence of pain in four cancers. *Cancer* 1987;60:2563–2569.
5. Poulson HS, Neilsen OS, Klee M et al. Palliative irradiation of bone metastases. *Cancer Treat Rev* 1989;16:41–48.
6. Hoskin PJ. Palliation of bone metastases. *Eur J Cancer* 1991;27: 950–951.
7. Tong D, Gillick L, Hendrickson FR. The palliation of symptomatic osseous metastases. Final results of the study by the Radiation Therapy Oncology Group. *Cancer* 1982;50:893–899.
8. Price P, Hoskin PJ, Easton D et al. Prospective randomized trial of single and multifraction radiotherapy schedules in the treatment of painful bony metastases. *Radiother Oncol* 1986;6:247–255.
9. Rose CM, Kagen AR. The final report of the expert panel for the radiation oncology bone metastases working group of the ACR. *Int J Radiat Oncol Biol Phys* 1998;40:117–120.
10. Salazar OM, Rubin P, Hendrickson FR et al. Single dose half-body irradiation for palliation of multiple bone metastases from solid tumors. Final Radiation Therapy Oncology Group Report. *Cancer* 1986;58: 29–36.
11. Volkert WA, Keutsch EA. Bone-seeking radiopharmaceuticals in cancer therapy. *Advances Metals Med* 1991;1:115–153.
12. Blake GM, Zivanovic MA, McEwan AJB et al. Sr-89 therapy: strontium kinetics in disseminated carcinoma of the prostate. *Eur J Nucl Med* 1986;12:447–454.
13. Samaratunga RC, Thomas SR, Hinnefeld JD et al. A Monte Carlo simulation model for radiation dose to metastatic skeletal tumor from rhenium-186 (Sn)-HEDP. *J Nucl Med* 1995;36:336–350.
14. Silberstein EB. The treatment of painful osseous metastases with phosphorus-32-labeled phosphates. *Sem Oncol* 1993;20(Suppl 2):10–21.
15. Sheh Syed GM, Maken RN, Muzzaffar N et al. Effective and economical option for pain palliation in prostate cancer with skeletal metastases: ^{32}P therapy revisited. *Nucl Med Commun* 1999;20:697–702.
16. Nair N. Relative efficacy of ^{32}P and ^{89}Sr in palliation in skeletal metastases. *J Nucl Med* 1999;40:256–261.

17. Potsaid MS, Irwin RJ, Castronovo FP et al. (32 P) diphosphonate dose determination in patients with bone metastases from prostate carcinoma. *J Nucl Med* 1978;19:98–104.
18. Pecher C. Biological investigations with radioactive calcium and strontium: preliminary report on the use of radioactive strontium in treatment of metastatic bone cancer. *U Cal Public Pharmacol* 1942;11:117–149.
19. Silberstein EB, Williams C. Strontium-89 therapy for the pain of osseous metastases. *J Nucl Med* 1985;26:345–348.
20. Robinson RG, Preston DF, Spicer JA et al. Radionuclide therapy of intractable bone pain: emphasis on strontium-89. *Sem Nucl Med* 1992;22:28–32.
21. McEwan AJB, Porter AT, Vennes DM et al. An evaluation of the safety and efficacy of treatment with strontium-89 in patients who have previously received wide field radiotherapy. *Antibody Immunoconjugates Radiopharm* 1990;3:91–98.
22. Porter AT, McEwan AJB, Powe JE et al. Results of a randomized phase III trial to evaluate the efficacy of strontium-89 adjuvant to local field external beam irradiation in the management of endocrine resistant metastatic prostate cancer. *Int J Rad Oncol Biol Phys* 1993;25:805–813.
23. Quilty PM, Kirk D, Bolger JJ et al. A comparison of the palliative effects of strontium-89 and external beam radiotherapy in metastatic prostate cancer. *Radiother Oncol* 1994;31:33–40.
24. Zyskowski A, Lamb D, Morum P et al. Strontium-89 treatment for prostate cancer bone metastases: Does a prostate-specific antigen response predict for improved survival? *Australas Radiol* 2001;45:39–42.
25. Turner SL, Gruenewald S, Spry N et al. Less pain does equal better quality of life following strontium-89 therapy for metastatic prostate cancer. *Br J Cancer* 2001;84:297–302.
26. Maxon HR, Thomas SR, Hertzberg VS et al. Rhenium-186 hydroxyethylidene diphosphonate for the treatment of painful osseous metastases. *Sem Nucl Med* 1992;22:33–40.
27. Quirijnen JMSP, Han SH, Zonnenberg BA et al. Efficacy of rhenium-186 etidronate in prostate cancer patients with metastatic bone pain. *J Nucl Med* 1996;37:1511–1515.
28. Israel O, Keidar Z, Rubinov R et al. Quantitative bone single-photon emission computed tomography for prediction of pain relief in metastatic bone disease treated with rhenium-186 etidronate. *J Clin Oncol* 2000;18:2747–2754.
29. Liepe K, Franke WG, Kropp J et al. Comparison of rhenium-188, rhenium-186-HEDP, and strontium-89 in palliation of painful bone metastases. *Nuklearmedizine* 2000;39:146–151.
30. Holmes RA. [153Sm] EDTMP: a potential therapy for bone cancer pain. *Sem Nucl Med* 1992;22:41–45.
31. Dickie GJ, Macfarlane D. Strontium and samarium therapy for bone metastases from prostate carcinoma. *Australes Radiol* 1999;43:476–479.
32. Srivastava SC, Atkins HL, Krishnamurthy GT et al. Treatment of metastatic bone pain with tin-117m stannic diethyltriaminepentaacetic acid: A phase I/II clinical study. *Clin Cancer Res* 1998;4:61–68.
33. McEwan AJB, Amyotte GA, McGowan DG et al. A retrospective analysis of the cost effectiveness of treatment with Metastron in patients with prostate cancer metastatic to bone. *Eur Urol* 1994;26(Suppl):26–31.
34. Malmberg I, Persson U, Ask A et al. Painful bone metastases in hormone-refractory prostate cancer: economic costs of strontium-89 and/or external radiotherapy. *Urology* 1997;50:747–753.
35. NCRP Report No. 37. *Precautions in the management of patients who have received therapeutic amounts of radionuclides.* Washington, DC: National Council on Radiation Protection and Measurements, 1978.
36. Tu SM, Millikan RE, Megistu B et al. Bone-targeted therapy for androgen-independent carcinoma of the prostate: a randomized Phase II trial. *Lancet* 2001;357:336–341.

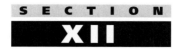

TRANSPLANTATION

51

EVALUATION OF RENAL AND PANCREATIC TRANSPLANTS

EVA V. DUBOVSKY
CHARLES D. RUSSELL

EVALUATION OF RENAL TRANSPLANTS

Since the first successful kidney grafting was performed 40 years ago between monozygotic twins (1), renal transplantation has become a procedure of choice for treatment of patients with end-stage renal disease. Because the survival of patients with renal transplants is significantly prolonged when compared with the patients treated by dialysis (2), the number of renal transplantation surgeries is increasing with steadily improving results. Based on the United Network for Organ Sharing (UNOS) 1999 report, the 1- and 3-year graft survival rates for living related donor (LRD) kidneys were 93% and 86%, respectively, with a half-life of 17 years. One-year graft survival rates were 96% for recipients of HLA-identical sibling-donor transplants (half-life 39 years) and 94% for recipients of one-haplotype matched donor grafts (half-life 16 years). The 1- and 3-year survival rates were 92% and 86% for living unrelated donor (LURD) and 87% and 76% for cadaveric grafts, respectively (3).

Advances have occurred in surgical techniques, in better understanding of the principles of immunologic tolerance (4), and in methodology for identifying tissue antigens and antibodies (5). New drugs have been developed to treat immunologic complications (6). Besides the standard antirejection triple therapy (prednisone, azathioprine, and cyclosporin), drugs blocking IL-2 production (tacrolimus and sirolimus) and affecting B- and T-cell proliferation and antibody production (mycophenolate mofetil) are widely used. Because rejection-free grafts have higher survival (3), antirejection therapy early after transplantation is a topic of active research. Monoclonal antibody against T cells (OKT3) and new anti-IL-2 antibodies dacliximab and chimeric basiliximab were approved by the Food and Drug Administration (FDA) as safe and effective (7).

Long-term results are affected by a large number of additional factors, such as the quality of the transplanted kidney (9) and the socioeconomic status, age, race, and general health of the recipient. Infections such as cytomegalovirus (CMV) and the more recently described polyoma viruses causing interstitial nephritis (6), hypertension (8), and poorly understood chronic allograft nephropathy [chronic rejection (CR)] limit graft survival. Furthermore, drugs given to control infection (nephrotoxic antibiotics), rejection, and hypertension (10) may profoundly affect renal function.

Complications of Renal Transplantation

Certain complications occur at fairly characteristic times following transplantation (11) (Table 51.1). Ischemic damage leading to acute tubular necrosis (ATN) is present in a large number of cadaveric transplants at the time of transplantation and results in delayed graft function. Some of the contributing factors include cold ischemia time (time between harvesting and implantation), donor age, and the use of kidneys from cerebrovascular accident donors. The damage usually is self-limited and resolves without specific therapy. Only very severe ischemia leading to cortical necrosis results in the irreversible loss of the function and the graft. ATN in LRD grafts is rare. It may occur after complicated surgery (multiple arteries) or hypotensive episode or as a reaction to radiologic contrast media.

Immunologic complications are best prevented by HLA-antigen matching of the donor with the recipient. Excellent results in HLA identical siblings and in zero (HLA A, B and DR) mismatched cadaver donors lead to mandatory sharing of six-antigen matched organs. With the exception of these two groups, acute rejection (AR) is still a very common complication after transplantation. It usually occurs at least 5 days after grafting and is more frequent in the first year but may develop at any time, especially when triggered by inadequate antirejection treatment, infection, or therapy noncompliance. Histologically, AR is characterized by interstitial mononuclear infiltration (grade I) with foci of severe tubulitis or mild-to-moderate intimal arteritis (grade II) and severe intimal arteritis with fibrinoid change, necrosis of medial smooth muscle cell leading to focal infarction, and interstitial hemorrhage (grade III) (12). Infiltration of the graft by lymphocytes results in swelling, pain, and fever. It develops rapidly and is usually successfully treated.

Hyperacute rejection (HR), presumed to be due to preformed antibodies, is extremely rare because all potential recipients are

E.V. Dubovsky: Department of Radiology, University of Alabama at Birmingham Medical Center and VA Medical Center, Birmingham, AL.

C.D. Russell: Department of Nuclear Medicine, Department of Radiology, Division of Nuclear Medicine, University of Alabama at Birmingham, University Hospital, and VA Medical Center, Birmingham, AL.

Table 51.1. *Complications after Transplantation Pertinent to Nuclear Medicine*

Complication	Most frequent time of occurrence	Comments
Surgical		
Wound infection	Within first few weeks	Surgical and medical treatment
Abscess	Few days/weeks	Drainage
Hematoma	Within hours to days	Drainage
Lymphocele	Second to fourth month	Drainage, sclerosing agents
Urine leak	Within hours to days	Surgical repair
Obstruction		
Intrinsic	Days, months, years	Clots, scars, calculi
Extrinsic pressure	Days, months, years	Surgical repair Lymphocele, hematoma Drainage
Renal artery stenosis	Anytime	Medical therapy, PTA, or surgery
Medical		
Ischemic damage (ATN)	Present at time of kidney transplantation	Cadaveric Tx— common
Immunologic		
Hyperacute	Within minutes to hours	Preformed antibodies, irreversible—rare
Acute	Rapid development after several days, most common during first 3 months	Predominantly cell mediated, reversible with therapy
Chronic	Usually after a few months or years, slowly developing	Humoral, irreversible
Other		
Cyclosporin	While on medication (high plasma levels)	Improvement after withdrawal
Recurrent disease	Anytime	Biopsy

carefully screened for their presence. HR is characterized by polymorphonuclear leukocyte accumulation in glomerular and peritubular capillaries starting during transplantation with subsequent endothelial damage and capillary thrombosis (12).

CR is a slow, irreversible process leading to gradual loss of graft function. Histologically, the typical finding is arterial fibrous thickening with resulting changes ranging from mild-to-moderate interstitial fibrosis and tubular atrophy (grades I and II) to severe fibrosis with tubular loss (grade III) (12). The mechanism is not well understood, and it was proposed that the interstitial fibrosis might result from two different pathogenetic mechanisms—the severity and frequency of AR and the use of cyclosporin. Because the presently available antirejection drugs are not effective in stopping the progression of CR, the trials concentrating on controlling early AR with new immunosuppressive agents are of paramount importance (6).

Surgical complications range from wound infections and perinephric fluid collections to obstruction and vascular complica-

tions. Some perinephric fluid collections are common, such as hematomas and lymphoceles, and some are uncommon, such as urinomas or abscesses (Table 51.1). Urine leaks are considered a surgical emergency (revision of ureterocystostomy). The other fluid collections are usually treated by drainage under ultrasound (US) guidance (13), especially if they exert pressure on the collecting system and cause obstruction. Intrinsic obstruction, resulting from clots, stones, or ureteral stenosis, requires urologic intervention such as ureterocystoscopy, stent placement, or surgery. Vascular complications comprise arterial and venous fistulas and pseudoaneurysms (14).

Impaired graft function is seldom caused by a single well-defined entity. More typically, several complications coincide. AR develops before the ATN has resolved. Obstruction caused by fluid collection or renal artery stenosis (RAS) may be present at the time of AR or CR. In addition, recurrent disease, such as immune complex glomerulonephritis, focal sclerosis, diabetic nephropathy, and hemolytic-uremic syndrome, or nephrotoxicity caused by high plasma levels of cyclosporine-A (CyA) complicate the clinical presentation, which is often nonspecific.

The selection of the best diagnostic procedure and appropriate therapy will determine the fate of the graft. Conventional sonography has proven to be an excellent tool for detection of perigraft fluid collections and obstruction, Color and duplex Doppler imaging has not fulfilled expectations as a reliable method to detect rejection but is helpful in the diagnosis of pseudoaneurysms and arteriovenous (AV) fistulae (15). Because conventional radiographic contrast media have been shown to impair renal function (16), intravenous urography for stone detection is performed with nonionic material. Arteriograms to detect vascular complications are usually performed with an intraarterial digital subtraction technique and dilute contrast material (14). Imaging with computed tomography (CT) and magnetic resonance imaging (MRI), although yielding excellent results especially in the differential diagnosis of surgical complications, presently play a limited role primarily because of their expense.

Nuclear Medicine Testing

Nuclear medicine tests are used by most transplantation centers because of their noninvasive nature and ability to quantitate renal function. The differential diagnosis of various complications requires correlation of scintigraphic findings with the patient's clinical course, physical findings, laboratory values, current therapy, prior scintigraphic findings, and results of other imaging tests.

A few important facts should be kept in mind. Many transplant recipients have more than one kidney. Besides the graft, they may have their native kidneys (three kidneys) and another, usually failing, older transplant (four kidneys). Two small pediatric kidneys may be transplanted en bloc (17). Occasionally, two kidneys from adult marginal donors were used (18). Bladder activity and plasma clearance will reflect total function of all kidneys not just the graft. Isolated graft function can be measured only by direct measurement of graft uptake.

Because many of the complications are diagnosed from the changes of tracer kinetics over time, it is important to obtain a baseline study soon after transplantation and use the same technical procedure for subsequent studies (19).

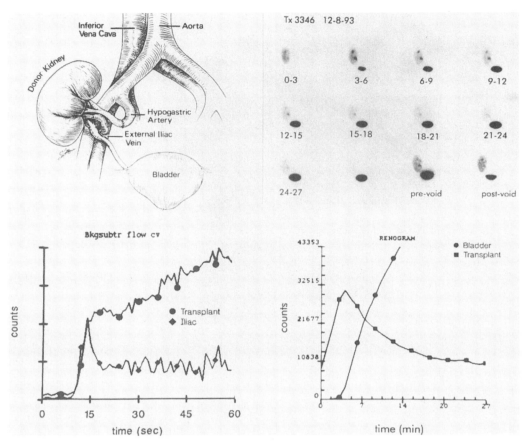

FIGURE 51.1. Normally functioning cadaveric graft 17 days after transplantation. *Upper right:* Study obtained with 3.5 mCi of ^{99m}Tc-mercaptoacetyltriglycine in nine 3-minute frames with 1-minute prevoid and postvoid images of the bladder (note the change in the intensity settings). *Lower left:* 60-second perfusion study comparing normal graft time-activity curve with iliac artery curve. *Lower right:* Renogram and bladder curve derived from their respective region-of-interest. Quantitation: Effective renal plasma flow—408 mL/minute; excreted activity at 30 minutes—58%; EI 0.85; Tmax—4 minutes; and 20/3 minutes—0.50.

Protocols vary, but in general two aspects of graft performance are studied, perfusion and excretory function (Fig. 51.1). In the past, the perfusion phase was studied with ^{99m}Tc-diethylenetriaminepentaacetic acid (DTPA) followed by the function phase study using ^{131}I-orthoiodohippurate (^{131}I-OIH). At present, the tubular agent ^{99m}Tc-mercaptoacetyltriglycine (MAG3) can be used for both phases (17–32). The ^{99m}Tc label permits a good quality perfusion phase and the high extraction rate of the tracer yields excellent images even in poorly functioning grafts. Its rapid excretion helps to evaluate the collecting system and rule out obstruction or urine leak.

Vascular problems (AV fistulae, pseudoaneurysm, arterial obstruction) are assessed during the first minute of the study. The anatomy of the graft (infarction, tumor, infection) (Fig. 51.2) is reliably evaluated during the first 5 minutes, whereas abnormalities of the ureter (obstruction, displacement) and the bladder (extrinsic pressure by fluid collections) (Figs. 51.3 and 51.4) are seen best later in the study. There are, however, important differences between ^{99m}Tc-MAG3 and the traditionally used radiotracers. Perfusion curves obtained with ^{99m}Tc-DTPA and ^{99m}Tc-MAG3 are different. This is caused by the difference in

the extraction rates. ^{99m}Tc-DTPA, a glomerular filtration rate (GFR) agent, has a low extraction rate, a high recirculation fraction, and, therefore, higher background relative to kidney activity than ^{99m}Tc-MAG3. ^{99m}Tc-labeled impurities and a small fraction of the ^{99m}Tc-MAG3 are excreted through the biliary system into the gallbladder and gastrointestinal tract. Such activity in the gastrointestinal tract may be confused with urine leaks on delayed images (11).

Evaluations of Graft Perfusion

Because normal perfusion of the graft is essential for normal function, several methods have been developed to assess blood flow through the transplant during the first pass of the bolus of ^{99m}Tc-labeled radiotracer. Visual inspection establishes arterial patency and excludes occlusion of the renal artery or one of its branches. A rare AV fistula or pseudoaneurysm may also be detected. Perfusion of other abdominal organs, such as the native kidneys, liver, spleen, and uterus, can also be assessed (Fig. 51.5). If a pancreatic graft is present, it too can be evaluated. Several semiquantitative (20,33–36) and quantitative (37–41) methods

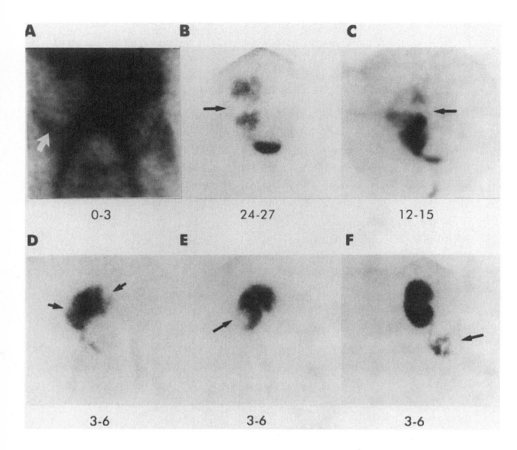

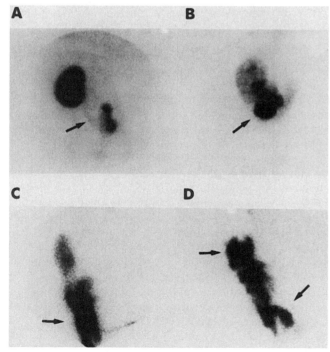

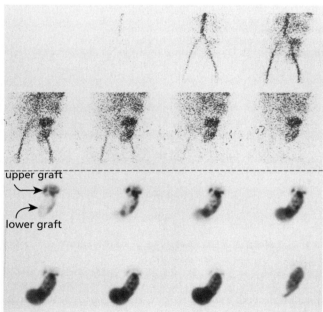

FIGURE 51.2. Selected frames from six different studies performed with 3 mCi of ^{99m}Tc-mercaptoacetyltriglycine; the acquisition time (in minutes) is indicated under the images. **A:** Infarcted graft—cold area with a hot rim. **B:** Large infarct in a chronically rejecting graft—wedge-shaped defect involving cortex. **C:** Graft with renal vein thrombosis in the upper pole. **D:** Graft with metastatic carcinoma—nonspecific presentation. **E:** Graft with an abscess, later drained and healed with a scar. **F:** Large clot in the bladder.

FIGURE 51.3. ^{99m}Tc-mercaptoacetyltriglycine blood flow and renogram obtained 66 days after transplantation of two pediatric en bloc kidneys. The upper graft shows good perfusion and rapid transit time and excretion. The lower graft shows poorer perfusion, prolonged transit time, and cortical and urinary stasis. Urinary obstruction can cause parenchymal graft retention. An echogram obtained on the same day showed hydronephrosis. (From Morin F, Côté I. Tc-99m MAG3 evaluation of recipients with en bloc renal grafts from pediatric cadavers. *Clin Nucl Med* 2000;25:579–584, with permission.)

FIGURE 51.4. Selected frames from four different studies demonstrating **A:** Displacement of the bladder by lymphocele. **B:** Urinoma. **C:** Urine leak in the scrotum. **D:** Urine leak around the graft and bladder.

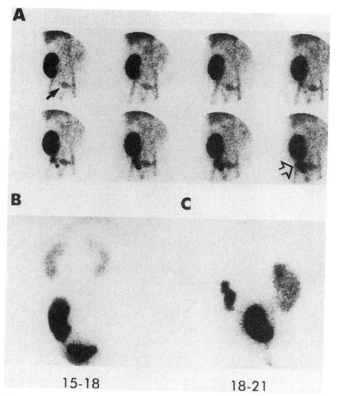

FIGURE 51.5. Examples of organs other than the graft of interest visualized during imaging. **A:** Third frame of the perfusion study [20-second frames demonstrates the uterus (*black arrow*); ureteral activity is not visualized until frame seven and bladder activity until frame 10 (*open arrow*]. **B:** Native kidneys. **C:** First graft (*left*) with chronic rejection, new graft (*right*) with good function. Note that the bladder is slightly displaced by a hematoma.

have been advocated to measure the blood flow. It has been reported that grafts with poor function caused by ATN have relatively better perfusion than those with AR (33,41). There have been occasional reports describing poor perfusion in patients with relatively good function (42,43), as in "Page kidney," caused by compression of the graft by lymphocele or hematoma (43).

A large-field-of-view (LFOV) camera with low-energy all-purpose (LEAP) collimator is placed over the anterior abdomen in such a way that the abdominal aorta, the graft, and both iliac arteries are included in the field-of-view. After a bolus injection of ^{99m}Tc-DTPA (5 to 15 mCi) or ^{99m}Tc-MAG3 (3 to 10 mCi), the images are acquired in 0.5- to 1.0-second frames (64 × 64 matrix) for 1 minute. The images are usually displayed by adding together two to five frames (Fig. 51.6) or as a functional image (44). Perfusion time-activity curves are generated from the region-of-interest (ROI) drawn around the graft.

The curves can be analyzed in several ways (39,41,45) and are often compared with curves derived from a ROI over the iliac artery or aorta. Hilson et al.'s (33) perfusion index and Kirchner et al.'s (34) kidney-to-aorta (K/A) ratio can be calculated with any ^{99m}Tc-labeled agent, because only that part of the curve before the peak is used (20) (Fig. 51.6). Quantitation of graft perfusion by calculating the vascular transit time (VTT)

(39,41) yields good separation between ATN (VTT = 5.4 seconds ± 3.1) and AR (20.6 seconds ± 6.4). Another concept (40) used in pediatric transplantation (37) is to measure graft blood flow as a percentage of the cardiac output. The value in normally functioning grafts is 20.6 ± 3.7% and in rejecting grafts, less than 5.2%.

Evaluation of Graft Function

^{99m}Tc-DTPA, OIH labeled with ^{123}I or ^{131}I, and ^{99m}Tc-MAG3 have been used for the assessment of allograft function. Acquisition in 20- to 60-second frames for 20 to 30 minutes, follows the perfusion phase obtained with ^{99m}Tc-labeled radiotracers, whereas imaging with ^{131}I-OIH requires a high-energy collimator. The time-activity curves are generated from graft and bladder ROI (with background subtraction) and the uptake, parenchymal transit, and excretion of tracer are analyzed. GFR can be quantitatively measured with ^{99m}Tc-DTPA (39), and effective renal plasma flow (ERPF) can be measured with OIH (46). ^{99m}Tc-MAG3 clearance is lower than OIH clearance, but ERPF can be calculated by proportion, using an empirical constant relationship between ^{131}I-OIH and ^{99m}Tc-MAG3 clearances (21,23,47,48). Parenchymal transit times derived from deconvolution analysis (49) are sometimes used, as are functional images (44).

The uptake and excretion of the radiotracer by normally functioning renal transplants are similar to those of normally functioning native kidneys. Scintigrams obtained with ^{99m}Tc-MAG3 show higher uptake with lower background than ^{99m}Tc-DTPA. They are of better quality because of the superior physical properties of ^{99m}Tc but otherwise resemble ^{131}I-OIH images (50).

Uptake, parenchymal transit, and excretion of ^{99m}Tc-MAG3 by a normal renal allograft are rapid. The peak activity in normally hydrated subjects is reached before 5 minutes (Tmax = 4.3 min. ± 1.1), and the fall to half the peak activity is around 5 to 6 minutes after that ($T_{1/2}$ = 6.6 min. ± 2.8). Thirty minutes after injection, most of the tracer is in the bladder with little background activity present (Fig. 51.1). Native kidneys and gallbladder are often seen in patients with poor graft function. Renal clearance of the tracer is proportional to, and can be evaluated by, the slope of the renogram or by the uptake of ^{99m}Tc-MAG3 at 2 minutes (19). Several indices have been developed to assess tubular transit. A simple index is the ratio of counts at 20 minutes to that at 3 minutes (20/3 minutes) (51), which is used in our laboratory. Interpretation of these parameters varies according to whether retention occurs in the parenchyma or in the collecting system, a distinction easily made by inspection of the images. More complicated measures are the mean parenchymal transit time (49,52,53), or the excretory index, which requires urine collection (43). Absolute quantitation of graft function is, in our opinion, very important. In acute disease, changes in GFR and ERPF precede changes in plasma creatinine levels. In chronic disease, plasma creatinine is an insensitive measure of disease progression until damage is severe.

ATN is present in most cadaveric grafts and it resolves spontaneously. The speed of recovery depends on the degree of ischemic insult. Perfusion of the kidney is relatively better than its function. Uptake of the tracer is impaired and tracer clearance is diminished. The most conspicuous finding with tubular agents

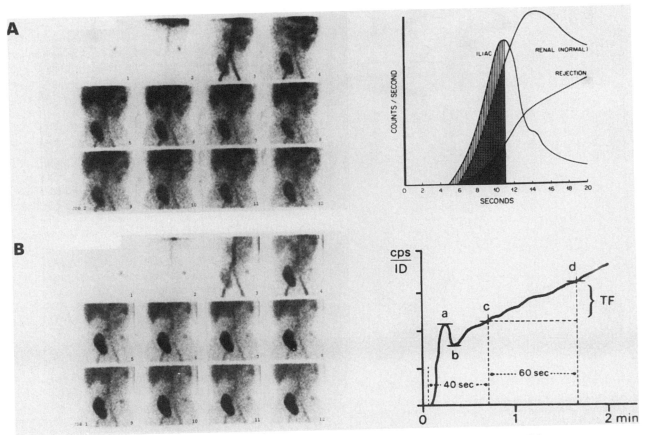

FIGURE 51.6. Perfusion study performed with ⁹⁹ᵐTc-diethylenetriaminepentaacetic acid (DTPA) (*upper left*) and ⁹⁹ᵐTc-mercaptoacetyltriglycine (*lower left*) demonstrating difference in extraction rate and background. This affects the shape of the perfusion curve. *Upper right:* Time-activity curves generated from graft and iliac region-of-interest (ROI) (schematically after Hilson) demonstrate well-defined peak of ⁹⁹ᵐTc-DTPA in normally functioning graft. *Lower right:* Normal time-activity curve from graft ROI (schematically after Bubeck). Such a curve can be analyzed for calculation of transplant perfusion (TP) and transplant function (7).

is delayed transit with delayed Tmax and $T_{1/2}$ and high 20/3 minute ratio. In anuric ATN, the curve rises continuously and Tmax is reached at the end of the study. On serial studies, improving uptake (increasing GFR, ERPF) and excretion (decreasing $T_{1/2}$, 20/3 minutes ratio) occur with resolution (Fig. 51.7). Changes in the opposite direction suggest superimposed AR (11). Continued low function without improvement is a poor prognostic sign and is suggestive of irreversible damage.

AR may develop before resolution of ATN. The graft is often enlarged with impaired perfusion, impaired tracer uptake, prolonged parenchymal transit, and decreased excretion (11) (Fig. 51.8). The images are similar to those with ATN. At our center, the distinction between ATN and AR is made by the time course on serial quantitative studies that routinely include an early post-transplant baseline (11,19).

In contrast to AR and ATN, the graft with stable CR has thinned cortex with mild hydronephrosis and demonstrates low uptake and normal parenchymal transit with absent or minimal cortical retention (normal Tmax with low GFR and ERPF) (49, 54) (Fig. 51.9).

The diagnosis of CyA toxicity is usually made by exclusion (55,56). Reversible vasoconstriction of the afferent arteriole causes a decrease in kidney perfusion (57) and is sometimes accompanied by newly developed nodular hyaline deposits. In patients with well-functioning grafts who received low doses of CyA, toxic plasma levels are relatively uncommon. This is not true in poorly functioning grafts in which toxic plasma levels can be easily reached. For this reason, CyA therapy is usually delayed in cadaver transplant recipients until the ATN has resolved. The scintigraphic pattern of mild CyA toxicity can resemble CR (57) or mild AR (55). It resolves rapidly with dose adjustment. Severe degrees of CyA toxicity cause tubular dysfunction resembling ATN (55,56) and are seen on the biopsy as vacuolization, eosinophilic inclusions, and microcalcifications (12). This pattern is often seen in children and in patients who have other complications. There is still no agreement on whether long-term CyA administration contributes to the chronic nephropathy characterized by striped and patchy fibrosis of the graft (6,12).

Renovascular hypertension caused by RAS often cannot be differentiated from CR unless challenged by angiotensin-converting enzyme (ACE) inhibitors (58–60). Hemodynamically

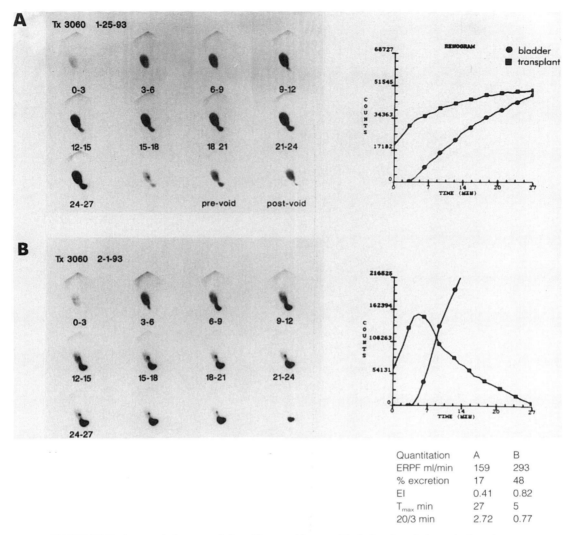

Quantitation	A	B
ERPF ml/min	159	293
% excretion	17	48
EI	0.41	0.82
T_{max} min	27	5
20/3 min	2.72	0.77

FIGURE 51.7. Acute tubular necrosis in a 33-year-old man with first cadaveric transplant on January 23, 1993, studied 2 days **(A)** and again 8 days **(B)** after grafting with 3 mCi ^{99m}Tc-mercaptoacetyltriglycine (MAG3). **A:** The first study (1/25/93) demonstrates low uptake with prolonged transit of the tracer indicated by prominent cortical retention at the end of the study and low excretion into the bladder. **B:** Follow-up study (2/1/93) demonstrates normal MAG3 kinetics.

significant RAS (or iliac artery stenosis proximal to the graft) is characterized by parenchymal retention of ^{99m}Tc-MAG3 after ACE inhibition (Fig. 51.10), hence the pattern of CR changes to a pattern of AR. Similar response was described after angiotensin-receptor blockade (61). In patients with segmental RAS, cortical retention is seen in the region of the graft supplied by the stenotic branch (62). For diagnosis, two studies are required, one with and one without ACE inhibition. Hemodynamically significant graft RAS can also be diagnosed with captopril-enhanced ^{99m}Tc-DTPA or ^{99m}Tc-2,3-dimercaptosuccinic acid (DMSA) (60,63) scintigraphy. ACE inhibition causes a fall in GFR by decreasing the filtration pressure in the glomeruli. This results in marked decrease in the uptake of filtered tracer, and the graft is poorly visualized (in contrast to the persistent parenchymal activity seen with tubular agents). After successful therapy, the graft function returns to normal.

^{99m}Tc-MAG3 images in combination with US usually yield definitive diagnoses of surgical complications, such as urine leaks, intrinsic obstruction, and mass lesions causing external pressure on the ureter and bladder (64,65). Some scintigraphic findings can be easily misinterpreted, if the patient's history and clinical status are unknown. Activity in a native contracted or large polycystic kidney, reflux into the native ureter or pancreatic graft, and gallbladder or gastrointestinal activity on delayed images (Fig. 51.11) may be confused with urine (11).

Obstruction in renal transplants is an important hazard leading to parenchymal damage and graft survival. It is important to differentiate obstruction from simple pelvocalyceal dilatation. Diuretic renography with furosemide (Lasix) yields this information (66). Additional images in an erect position after voiding are often helpful especially in pediatric transplants. Visual inspection of the images and time-activity curve is accurate in

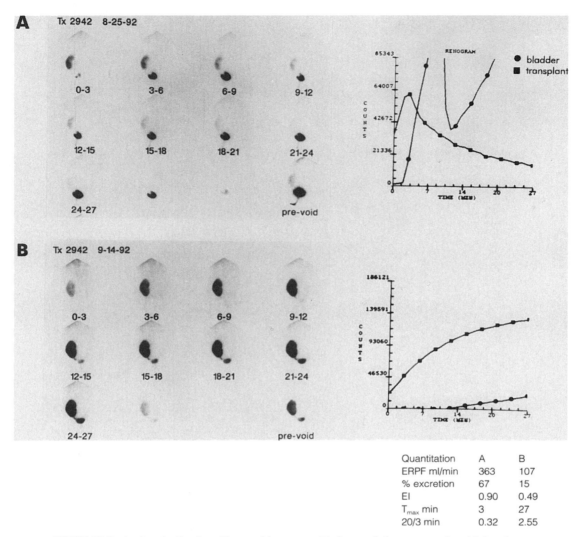

Quantitation	A	B
ERPF ml/min	363	107
% excretion	67	15
EI	0.90	0.49
T_{max} min	3	27
20/3 min	0.32	2.55

FIGURE 51.8. Acute rejection in a 45-year-old woman with first graft from an unrelated living donor on August 24, 1992. Scintigrams shown here were obtained on day one **(A)** and at the time of acute rejection **(B)**. **A:** First study (8/25/92) demonstrates rapid uptake and excretion of tracer into the bladder. Note the activity in the indwelling catheter on the prevoid frame and a small defect in the bladder caused by the tip of the catheter. **B:** Second study (9/14/92) shows enlarged graft with low uptake and markedly prolonged transit of the tracer resulting in high cortical activity.

majority of patients. The use of various washout indices is laboratory specific and varies with protocol and software. Alternative method to diagnose urinary tract obstruction using the quantitative parameter of output efficiency (67) has been validated in patients with renal transplants (68).

Cortical defects, although well seen on early images, are nonspecific and often require other imaging procedures or biopsy (69).

Tests to Diagnose Rejection

A number of other methods have been proposed for the diagnosis and confirmation of rejection. [125]I- or ^{131}I-labeled fibrinogen (70) and ^{67}Ga-citrate have only historical importance (71). ^{111}In-labeled leukocytes (72) and lymphocytes (73) localize in rejection grafts but are also in hematomas and infections. Good results have been obtained with ^{111}In-labeled platelets (74), but routine use is expensive.

AR can be demonstrated by imaging with ^{99m}Tc-sulfur colloid (SC). The mechanism of uptake, based on autoradiographic findings, is the trapping of SC particles in fibrin thrombi present in rejecting graft (75). Allografts with ATN have no such thrombi. A quantitative method comprising perfusion, blood pool activity image, and ^{99m}Tc-SC uptake at 20 minutes, was reported to have high sensitivity and specificity. False-positive findings were reported in patients with infections and, on occasion, in ATN, whereas false-negative results were found in patients with CR. Similar results were reported with ^{99m}Tc-tin colloid (76). In the pediatric population, a combination of ^{99m}Tc-DTPA and ^{99m}Tc-SC has been recommended for differential diagnosis of AR and CyA toxicity (77). Poor uptake and clearance with ^{99m}Tc-DTPA studies and high ^{99m}Tc-SC uptake

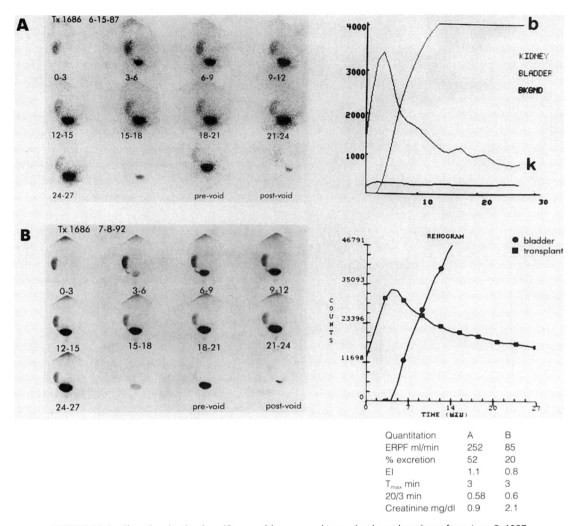

Quantitation	A	B
ERPF ml/min	252	85
% excretion	52	20
EI	1.1	0.8
T_{max} min	3	3
20/3 min	0.58	0.6
Creatinine mg/dl	0.9	2.1

FIGURE 51.9. Chronic rejection in a 43-year-old woman who received a cadaveric graft on June 8, 1987. **A:** Study performed on 6/15/87 (300 mCi of ^{131}I-orthoiodohippurate) demonstrates normal uptake and excretion of the tracer. **B:** Study dated 7/8/92 (3 mCi of ^{99m}Tc-mercaptoacetyltriglycine) shows low uptake but normal transit and excretion of the tracer. Images and time-activity curve appear normal.

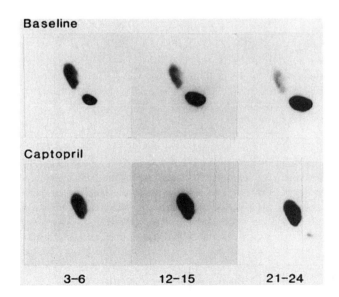

FIGURE 51.10. Renovascular hypertension diagnosed by angiotensin-converting enzyme inhibition scintigraphy. A 48-year-old woman with cadaveric transplant since June 28, 1986, was admitted with blood pressure 225/125 mm Hg. On July 17, 1990, baseline study [1 mCi ^{99m}Tc-mercaptoacetyltriglycine (MAG3)] and renogram (10 mCi ^{99m}Tc-MAG3) performed 1 hour after 25 mg of captopril, demonstrated prominent prolongation of parenchymal transit time of the tracer. Arteriogram demonstrated high-grade stenosis of the iliac artery above the renal artery anastomosis. Blood pressure normalized after successful angioplasty. (From Dubovsky EV, Diethelm AG, Keller F et al. Renal transplant hypertension caused by iliac artery stenosis. *J Nucl Med* 1992;33:1178–1180, with permission.)

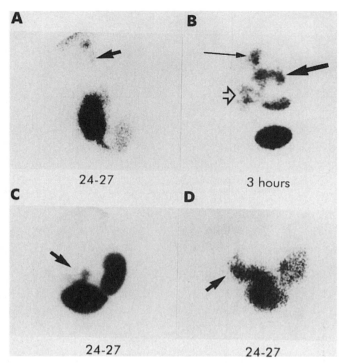

FIGURE 51.11. Examples of artifacts imitating urine leaks. **A:** Reflux into native ureter. **B:** A 3-hour delayed image demonstrates activity in the gallbladder (*small arrow*), in the gastrointestinal tract (*large arrow*), and residual activity in the collecting system of a normally functioning graft (*open arrow*). 99mTc-mercaptoacetyltriglycine (MAG3) impurities are excreted through the biliary tract, a normal finding. **C:** Reflux of 99mTc-MAG3, from the bladder in the anastomosis of the pancreatic transplant duct. **D:** More prominent reflux of 131I-orthoiodohippurate in the whole length of the pancreatic graft duct.

was found in most patients with AR, but the specificity of these findings has been low.

EVALUATION OF PANCREATIC TRANSPLANTATION

As of 1999, more than 13,000 pancreas transplants were reported to the International Pancreas Transplant Registry (IPTR). Of these, more than 9,000 were performed in the United States. The database classifies the pancreas transplants according to recipient category, donor source, and duct management technique. All recipients were insulin-dependent diabetics. The most common procedure is simultaneous kidney/pancreas (SPK), followed by pancreas after kidney (PAK) and pancreas alone (PTA) grafting. Technical failure rates have been on the decline and 1-year graft survival (defined as insulin independence) in the United States was 82% for SPK, 72% for PAK, and 62% for PTA (6). As expected, well-matched grafts had a lower rate of rejection. An increasing proportion of SPK transplants are being performed with primary enteric drainage, but in PTA and PAK, bladder drainage still predominates.

Complications seen after transplantation that require another laparotomy include thrombosis of the graft, infection, intraabdominal bleeding, and duodenal leak (6). With refinement of

surgical techniques and increased clinical experience, early diagnosis of AR remains a major challenge because there is no reliable method for its detection. In SPK, the therapy is guided by the symptoms of AR of the renal graft, because rejection seldom occurs in the pancreas alone. However, it has been reported that a pancreas allograft may reject alone. The diagnosis of AR is made based on increase of plasma creatinine, 50% reduction of urine amylase levels, biopsy, and urine cytology. Hyperglycemia is a late sign of rejection and usually indicates irreversible graft injury. The therapy with cyclosporin, tacrolimus, and mycophenolate mofetil resulted in decrease in the early immunologic graft loss to 2% for SPK, 9% for PAK, and 16% for PTA transplantation.

All imaging modalities have been evaluated for the diagnosis of pancreas graft rejection. These included US (78,79), CT (80), MRI (78), digital subtraction angiography (DSA) (81), and scintigraphy (81–95).

CT has been helpful in detection of postoperative complications (78,80) but not in assessment of parenchymal pathology. US has been effective in detection of perigraft and intragraft fluid collections and as a guide for biopsy. Duplex Doppler measurement of arterial resistive index has been recommended for the confirmation of rejection (91), whereas reversal of diastolic flow was found in patients with venous thrombosis (79). MRI has been found very sensitive in detection of rejection by demonstrating changes in organ size, tissue water content, vascular patency, intrapancreatic and extrapancreatic pathologic changes, and fluid collections (78).

Many radiopharmaceuticals have been used for imaging pancreatic grafts. These include 75Se-selenomethionine (84) and miscellaneous 99mTc-labeled agents (DTPA, glucoheptonate, or MAG3) to assess perfusion of the allograft (85–87,93) and 99mTc-SC (92), 99mTc-hexamethylpropylene amine oxime (HMPAO) (90,94), 99mTc-sestamibi (95), 201Tl-chloride (91), and 111In-labeled platelets (89).

It has been concluded by most investigators that a normal perfusion study of the pancreas graft performed with a bolus of 99mTc-labeled tracer is consistently found in the presence of good allograft function. Abnormal perfusion, however, does not differentiate AR from other parenchymal pathologic conditions such as pancreatitis.

The technique is similar to that of renal graft perfusion study, and both grafts are usually studied simultaneously. The ROI for the pancreas graft should exclude the underlying iliac artery. The time-activity curve generated from this ROI is often compared with the time-activity curve of the ipsilateral iliac artery (85) or abdominal aorta (86). The acquisition is performed in 1- to 2-second frames, and static images are obtained immediately afterwards. The graft time-activity curve in a normally functioning graft is sharply peaked similar to that derived from the iliac artery or aorta (Fig. 51.12). The image of the graft has well-defined edges and homogeneous distribution of activity. Sequential studies permit comparison of the height of the curve (relative to the aorta), the distribution of activity, and the size of the allograft. Decrease in the curve slope (relative to the aorta or iliac artery) is indicative of graft dysfunction. Enlarged grafts with poor edge definition and parenchymal defects are found in rejection and infected transplants. During the perfusion study, other complications such as hemorrhage are detected.

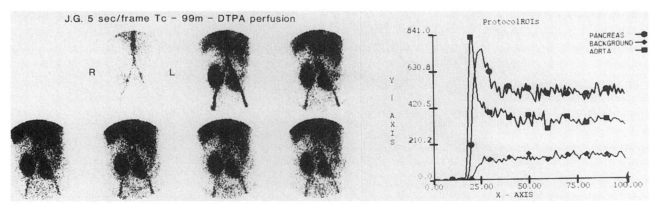

FIGURE 51.12. Perfusion study of the renal and pancreatic graft using 15 mCi of ^{99m}Tc-diethylenetri-aminepentaacetic acid. Time-activity curves generated from normalized region-of-interest over the abdominal aorta and pancreatic graft excluding the iliac artery demonstrate normal findings.

Pancreatic blood flow curves have the same appearance, regardless of which of the ^{99m}Tc-tracers (5 to 10 mCi) were used (pertechnetate, DTPA, glucoheptonate, MAG3, HMPAO, Sestamibi). Static scintigrams will, however, differ. ^{99m}Tc-MAG3, because of high protein binding in the circulation, will not define

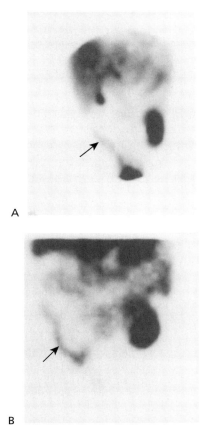

FIGURE 51.13. Scintigrams of pancreatic transplants (arrow) obtained with 20 mCi of ^{99m}Tc-sestamibi after the completion of the renal transplant scintigram with ^{99m}Tc-mercaptoacetyltriglycine. **A:** Pancreatic graft with the direct drainage into the bladder. **B:** Pancreatic graft with primary enteric drainage. Note the distance between the graft and the bladder activity.

the pancreatic graft as well as DTPA or glucoheptonate with their rapid distribution in the extravascular space. HMPAO (10 mCi, 3-minutes postinjection), a lipophilic compound, is taken up by the organs in proportion to the regional blood flow so that decrease in uptake on delayed static images parallels decrease in perfusion on flow images (90,94). ^{201}Tl, an indicator of cellular integrity, has demonstrated segmental necrosis of the pancreas (91). AR of the pancreatic graft is pathologically similar to that of the renal transplant with interstitial cellular infiltrates and thrombotic vasculitis, and these findings can be demonstrated with the same radiotracers that demonstrate AR in renal grafts: ^{99m}Tc-SC (92) and ^{111}In-platelets (89). Both agents seem to have high sensitivity, but false-positive studies can be expected in disorders such as thrombosis or hematomas.

The most commonly used radiotracer to image a pancreatic graft is ^{99m}Tc-sestamibi (95). The perfusion sequence (2-second frames for 1 minute) and static images (5 minutes for 30 minutes) are usually obtained early after SKP transplantation to demonstrate the integrity of the grafted organ (Fig. 51.13). Normal perfusion and high uptake exclude complications and correlate well with normal glucose and amylase levels. Poor uptake or nonvisualization of the transplanted pancreas can represent rejection, pancreatitis, or vascular problems such as thrombosis and cannot be differentiated by scintigraphy. US or CT is the next step in managing such patients.

REREFENCES

1. Merrill JP, Murray JE, Harrison JR et al. Successful homotransplantation of the human kidney between identical twins. *JAMA* 1956;160:277–282.
2. Port FK, Wolfe RA, Mauger EA et al. Comparison of survival probabilities for dialysis patients vs. cadaveric renal transplant recipients. *JAMA* 1993;270:1339–1343.
3. Cecka JM. The UNOS scientific renal transplant registry 1999. In: Cecka JM, Terasaki PI, eds. *Clinical transplants 1999*. Los Angeles: UCLA Immunogenetics Center, 2000:10–20.
4. Starzl TE, Demetris AJ. Transplantation milestones. Viewed with one- and two-way paradigms of tolerance. *JAMA* 1995;273:876–879.
5. Kasiske BL, Ramos EL, Gaston RS et al. The evaluation of renal transplant candidates. Clinical practice guidelines. *J Am Soc Nephrol* 1995;6:1–34.

6. Hirose R, Vincenti F. Review of transplantation—1999. In: Cecka JM, Terasaki PI, eds. *Clinical transplants 1999.* Los Angeles: UCLA Immunogenetics Center, 2000:295–315.

7. Harlan DM, Kirk AD. The future of organ and tissue transplantation. Can T-cell costimulatory pathway modifiers revolutionize the prevention of graft rejection? *JAMA* 1999;282:1076–1082.

8. Mange KC, Cizman B, Joffe M et al. Arterial hypertension and renal allograft survival. *JAMA* 2000;283:633–638.

9. Russell CD, Yang H, Gaston RS et al. Prediction of renal transplant survival from early postoperative radioisotope studies. *J Nucl Med* 2000; 41:1332–1336.

10. Abu-Romeh SH, El-Khatib D, Rashid A et al. Comparative effects of enalapril and nifedipine on renal hemodynamics in hypertensive renal transplant recipients. *Clin Nephrol* 1992;37:183–188.

11. Dubovsky EV, Russell CD, Erbas B. Radionuclide evaluation of renal transplants. *Semin Nucl Med* 1995;25:49–59.

12. Solez K, Axelsen RA, Benediktsson H et al. International standardization of criteria for the histologic diagnosis of renal allograft rejection: the Banff working classification of kidney transplant pathology. *Kidney Int* 1993;44:411–422.

13. Steem SB, Novick AC, Steinmuller DR et al. Percutaneous techniques for the management of urological renal transplant complications. *J Urol* 1986;135:456–459.

14. Dodd GD III, Tublin ME, Shah A et al. Imaging of vascular complications associated with renal transplants. *AJR* 1991;157:449–459.

15. Tublin ME, Dodd GD. Sonography of renal transplantation. *Radiol Clin North Am* 1995;33:447–459.

16. Rabito CA, Fang LS, Waltman AC. Renal function in patients at risk of contrast material induced acute renal failure: noninvasive, real-time monitoring. *Radiology* 1993;186:851–854.

17. Morin F, Côté I. Tc-99m MAG3 evaluation of recipients with en bloc renal grafts from pediatric cadavers. *Clin Nucl Med* 2000;25:579–584.

18. Dunn EK, Distant DA, Strashun AM. Tc-99m MAG3 evaluation of recipients with dual adult cadaveric renal allografts. Simultaneous transplantation of both kidneys from marginal donors. *Clin Nucl Med* 1999; 24:547–552.

19. Dubovsky EV, Russell CD, Bischof-Delaloye A et al. Report of the Radionuclides in Nephrourology committee for evaluation of transplanted kidney (review of techniques). *Semin Nucl Med* 1999;29: 175–188.

20. Al-Nahhas AA, Jafri RA, Britton KE et al. Clinical experience with 99mTc-MAG3, mercaptoacetyltriglycine, and a comparison with 99mTc-DTPA. *Eur J Nucl Med* 1988;14:453–462.

21. Russell CD, Thorstadt B, Yester MV et al. Quantitation of renal function with Tc-99m MAG$_3$. *J Nucl Med* 1988;29:1931–1933.

22. Fraile M, Castell J, Buxeda M et al. Transplant renography: 99mTc-DTPA versus 99mTc-MAG3. A preliminary note. *Eur J Nucl Med* 1989;15:776–779.

23. Bubeck B, Brandau W, Weber E et al. Pharmacokinetics of technetium-99m-MAG$_3$ in humans. *J Nucl Med* 1990;31:1285–1293.

24. Taylor A, Ziffer JA, Eshima D. Comparison of Tc-99m MAG$_3$ and Tc-99m DTPA in renal transplant patients with impaired renal function. *Clin Nucl Med* 1990;15:371–378.

25. Wellman HN, Milgrom M. Assessment of renal transplant patients with Tc-99m MAG3: case reports and review. *Dialysis Transplantation* 1992;21:720–736.

26. O'Malley JP, Ziessman HA, Chantarapitak N. Tc-99m MAG$_3$ as an alternative to Tc-99m DTPA and I-131 Hippuran for renal transplant evaluation. *Clin Nucl Med* 1993;18:22–29.

27. Kramer W, Baum RP, Scheuermann E et al. Verlaufskontrolle nach Nierentransplantation. Sequentielle Funktionsscintigraphie mit Technetium-99m-DTPA oder Technetium-99m-MAG3. *Urologie (A)* 1993;34:115–120.

28. Neubauer NJ, Johnson LJ, Lemmers MJ et al. Renal transplant nuclear tomography using Tc-99m MAG3. *Clin Nucl Med* 1996;21:851–854.

29. Lin E, Alavi A. Significance of early tubular extraction in the first minute of Tc-99m MAG3 renal transplant scintigraphy. *Clin Nucl Med* 1998;23:217–222.

30. El-Maghraby TAF, de Fijter JW, van Eck-Smit BLF et al. Renographic indices for evaluation of changes in graft function. *Eur J Nucl Med* 1998;25:1575–1586.

31. Tulchinski M, Dietrich TJ, Eggli DF et al. Technetium-99m-MAG3 scintigraphy in acute renal failure after transplantation: a marker of viability and prognosis. *J Nucl Med* 1997;38:475–478.

32. Müller-Suur R, Bois-Svensson, Mesko L. 99mTc-MAG$_3$ and 123I-hippurate in patients with renal disorders. *J Nucl Med* 1990;31: 1811–1817.

33. Hilson AJW, Maisey MN, Brown CB et al. Dynamic renal transplant imaging with Tc-99m DTPA(Sn) supplemented by a transplant perfusion index in the management of renal transplants. *J Nucl Med* 1978; 19:994–1000.

34. Kirchner PT, Goldman MH, Leapman SG et al. Clinical application of the kidney and aortic blood flow index (K/A ratio). *Contrib Nephrol* 1978;11:120–126.

35. Anaise D, Oster ZH, Atkins HL et al. Cortex perfusion index. A sensitive detector of acute rejection crisis in transplanted kidneys. *J Nucl Med* 1986;27:1697–1701.

36. Sfakianakis GN, Vuong H, Tapia M et al. A comprehensive technique for the evaluation of renal transplants with MAG$_3$. *J Nucl Med* 1997; 38:296P.

37. Ash J, DeSouza M, Peters M et al. Quantitative assessment of blood flow in pediatric recipients of renal transplants. *J Nucl Med* 1990;31: 580–585.

38. Lear JL, Raff U, Jain R et al. Quantitative measurement of renal perfusion following transplant surgery. *J Nucl Med* 1988;29:1656–1661.

39. Rutland MD. A comprehensive analysis of renal DTPA studies. II. Renal transplant evaluation. *Nucl Med Commun* 1985;6:21–30.

40. Peters AM, Gunasekera RD, Henderson BL et al. Noninvasive measurement of blood flow and extraction fraction. *Nucl Med Commun* 1987;8:823–837.

41. Chaiwatanarat T, Laorpatanaskul S, Poshyachinda M et al. Deconvolution analysis of renal blood flow; evaluation of post renal transplant complications. *J Nucl Med* 1994;35:1792–1796.

42. Herrman T, Granjon D, Decousus M et al. Mismatch between radionuclide and contrast angiography in the assessment of the perfusion of a transplanted kidney. *Clin Nucl Med* 1991;16:853–854.

43. Yussim A, Shmuely D, Levy J et al. Page kidney phenomenon in kidney allograft following peritransplant lymphocele. *Urology* 1988;31: 512–514.

44. Nicoletti R. Evaluation of renal transplant perfusion by functional imaging. *Eur J Nucl Med* 1990;16:733–739.

45. Baillet G, Ballarin J, Urdaneta N et al. Evaluation of allograft perfusion by radionuclide first-pass study in renal failure following renal transplantation. *Eur J Nucl Med* 1986;11:463–469.

46. Dubovsky EV, Logic JR, Diethelm AG et al. Comprehensive evaluation of renal function in transplanted kidney. *J Nucl Med* 1975;16: 1115–1120.

47. Taylor A, Eshima D, Fritzberg AR et al. Comparison of iodine-131 OIH and technetium-99m MAG$_3$renal imaging in volunteers. *J Nucl Med* 1986;27:795–803.

48. Russell CD, Taylor A, Eshima D. Estimation of technetium-99m-MAG$_3$ plasma clearance in adults from one or two plasma samples. *J Nucl Med* 1989;30:1955–159.

49. Piepsz A, Ham HR, Erbsmann F et al. A cooperative study on the clinical value of dynamic renal scanning with deconvolution analysis. *Br J Radiol* 1982;55:419–433.

50. Russell CD, Thorstadt BL, Stutzmann M et al. The kidney: imaging with Tc-99m-mercaptoacetyltriglycine, a technetium labelled analog of iodohippurate. *Radiology* 1989;172:427–430.

51. Li Y, Russell CD, Palmer-Lawrence J et al. Quantitation of renal parenchymal retention of Tc-99m MAG$_3$ in renal transplants. *J Nucl Med* 1994;35:846–850.

52. Russell CD, Yester MV, Dubovsky ED. Measurement of renal parenchymal transit time of 99mTc-MAG$_3$ using factor analysis. *Nuklearmedizin* 1990;29:170–176.

53. Bajén MT, Puchal R, González AJ et al. MAG3 renogram deconvolution in renal transplantation: utility of the measurement of initial tracer uptake. *J Nucl Med* 1997;38:1295–99.

54. Dubovsky EV, Diethelm AG, Tauxe WN. Differential diagnosis of cell-mediated and humoral rejection by orthoiodo-hippurate kinetics. *Arch Int Med* 1977;137:738–742.

55. Bellomo R, Berlangieri S, Wong C et al. Renal allograft scintigraphy with Tc-99m-DTPA—its role during cyclosporin therapy. *Transplantation* 1992;53:143–145.

56. Kim EE, Pjura G, Lowry P et al. Cyclosporin-A nephrotoxicity and acute cellular rejection in renal transplant recipients: correlation between radionuclide and histologic findings. *Radiology* 1986;159:443–446.

57. Curtis JJ, Luke RG, Dubovsky E et al. Cyclosporin in therapeutic doses increases renal allograft vascular resistance. *Lancet* 1986;2:477–479.

58. Dubovsky EV, Russell CD. Diagnosis of renovascular hypertension after renal transplantation. *Am J Hypertension* 1991;4:724–730S.

59. Dubovsky EV, Diethelm AG, Keller F et al. Renal transplant hypertension caused by iliac artery stenosis. *J Nucl Med* 1992;33:1178–1180.

60. Taylor A, Nally J, Aurell M et al. Consensus report on ACE inhibitor renography for detecting renovascular hypertension. *J Nucl Med* 1996;37:1876–1882.

61. Fuster D, Marco MP, Setoain FJ et al. A case of renal artery stenosis after transplantation: can Losartan be more accurate than captopril renography? *Clin Nucl Med* 1998;23:731–734.

62. Mousa D, Hamilton D, Hassan A et al. The diagnosis of segmental transplant artery stenosis by captopril renography. Clin Nucl Med 1999;24:504–506.

63. Kremer-Hovinga TK, de Jong PE, Piers DA et al. Diagnostic use of angiotensin converting enzyme inhibitors in radioisotope evaluation of unilateral renal artery stenosis. *J Nucl Med* 1989;30:605–614.

64. Beyga ZT, Kahan BD. Surgical complications of kidney transplantation. *J Nephrol* 1998;11:137–145.

65. Bybel B, Greenberg ID. Intraperitoneal leak following renal transplant. *Clin Nucl Med* 1998;23:411–413.

66. O'Reilly PH, Aurell M, Britton KE et al. Consensus on diuretic renography for investigating the dilated upper urinary tract. *J Nucl Med* 1996;36:1872–1876.

67. Britton KE, Nawaz MK, Whitfield HN et al. Obstructive nephropathy: comparison between parenchymal transit time index and frusemide diuresis. *Br J Urol* 1987;59:121–132.

68. Spicer ST, Ka-kit Chi, Nankivell BJ et al. Mercaptoacetyltriglycine diuretic renography and output efficiency measurement in renal transplant patients. *Eur J Nucl Med* 1999;26:152–154.

69. Lawrence SK, Van Buren DH, MacDonell RC Jr et al. Carcinoma in a transplanted kidney detected with MAG₃ scintigraphy. *J Nucl Med* 1993;34:2185–2187.

70. Yeboah ED, Chislom GD, Short MD. The detection and prediction of acute rejection episodes in human renal transplants using radioactive fibrinogen. *Br J Urol* 1073;45:273–280.

71. George EA, Codd JE, Newton WT et al. Comparative evaluation of renal transplant rejection with radioiodinated fibrinogen, ⁹⁹ᵐTc-sulfur colloid and ⁶⁷Ga-citrate. *J Nucl Med* 1984;25:156–159.

72. Forstram LA, Loken MK, Cook A et al. In-111-labeled leukocytes in the diagnosis of rejection and cytomegalovirus infection in renal transplant patients. *Clin Nucl Med* 1981;6:146–148.

73. Martin-Comin J. Kidney graft rejection studies with labeled platelets and lymphocytes. *Nucl Med Biol* 1986;13:173–181.

74. Tisdale PL, Collier BD, Kauffman HM et al. Early diagnosis of acute postoperative renal transplant rejection by Indium-111-labeled platelet scintigraphy. *J Nucl Med* 1986;27:1266–1272.

75. George EA, Meyerovitz M, Codd JE et al. Renal allograft accumulation of Tc-99m sulfur colloid: temporal quantitation and scintigraphic assessment. *Radiology* 1983;148:547–551.

76. Sundram FX, Edmondson RPS, Ang ES et al. ⁹⁹Tcᵐ-tin colloid scans in the evaluation of renal transplant rejection. *Nucl Med Commun* 1986;7:897–906.

77. Massengill SF, Pena DR, Drane WE et al. Technetium-99m sulfur colloid accumulation as a predictor of acute renal transplant rejection. *Transplantation* 1992;54:969–973.

78. Yuh WTC, Wiese JA, Abu-Yousef MM et al. Pancreatic transplant imaging. *Radiology* 1988;167:679–683.

79. Foshager MC, Hedlund LJ, Troppmann C et al. Venous thrombosis of pancreatic transplants: diagnosis by duplex sonography. *AJR* 1997;169:1269–1273.

80. Meador TL, Krebs TL, Wong You Cheong JJ et al. Imaging features of posttransplantation lymphoproliferative disorder in pancreas transplant recipients. *AJR* 2000;174:121–124.

81. Rasmussen K, Burcharth F, Thomsen HS et al. Monitoring of pancreas-graft perfusion by radionuclide and digital subtraction angiography. *Diabetes* 1989;38:21–23.

82. Patel B, Markivee CR, Mahanta B et al. Pancreatic transplantation: scintigraphy, US, and CT. *Radiology* 1988;167:685–687.

83. Batiuk TD, Carpenter HA, Morton MJ et al. Correlation of pancreas allograft biopsy with radionuclide and ultrasound imaging of pancreas allografts. *Transplant Proc* 1991;23:1606–1607.

84. Toledo-Pereyra LH, Kristen KT, Mittal VK. Scintigraphy of pancreatic transplants. *AJR* 1982;138:621–622.

85. Thompsen HS, Rasmussen K, Burcharth F et al. Monitoring of pancreatic graft perfusion by first passage radionuclide angiography. *Acta Radiologica* 1988;29:138–140.

86. Nghiem DD, Conrad GR, Rezai K et al. Diagnosis of pancreatic rejection with Tc-99m DTPA scintigraphy. *Transplant Proc* 1989;21:2791–2792.

87. Kuni CC, du Cret RP, Boudreau RJ. Pancreas transplants: evaluation using perfusion scintigraphy. *AJR* 1989;153:57–61.

88. Boiskin I, Sandler MP, Fleischer AC et al. Acute venous thrombosis after pancreas transplantation: diagnosis with duplex Doppler sonography and scintigraphy. *AJR* 1990;154:529–531.

89. Catafau AM, Lomena FJ, Ricart MJ et al. Indium-111-labeled platelets in monitoring human pancreatic transplants. *J Nucl Med* 1989;30:1470–1475.

90. Teule GJJ, Leunissen KML, Hakders SGEA et al. Serial radionuclide determinations of graft perfusion in pancreas transplantation. *Transplant Proc* 1989;21:2795–2796.

91. Hirsch H, Fernandez-Ulloa M, Munda R et al. Diagnosis of segmental necrosis in a pancreatic transplant by thallium-201 perfusion scintigraphy. *J Nucl Med* 1991;32:1605–1607.

92. George EA, Salami Z, Carney K et al. Radionuclide surveillance of the allografted pancreas. *AJR* 1988;150:811–816.

93. Shulkin BL, Dafoe DC, Wahl RL. Simultaneous pancreatic-renal transplant scintigraphy. *AJR* 1986;147:1193–1196.

94. Van der Hem LG, van der Linden CJ, Ticheler CHJM et al. Early detection of post-transplant pancreatic graft dysfunction with technetium-99m HMPAO scintigraphy. *J Nucl Med* 1994;35:1488–1490.

95. Elgazzar AH, Munda R, Fernandez-Ulloa M et al. Scintigraphic evaluation of pancreatic transplants using technetium-99m-sestamibi. *J Nucl Med* 1995;36:771–777.

Diagnostic Nuclear Medicine, Fourth Edition. Edited by M.P. Sandler, R.E. Coleman, J.A. Patton, F.J.Th. Wackers, A. Gottschalk. Lippincott Williams & Wilkins, Philadelphia 2003.

52

HEART AND LUNG TRANSPLANTATION

JEROEN J. BAX
DOMINIQUE DELBEKE
JOÃO VITOLA
DON POLDERMANS
ERIC BOERSMA
ERNST E. VAN DER WALL
MARTIN P. SANDLER

With the improvement of immunosuppressive therapy, heart, lung, and combined heart-lung transplantation have become accepted therapy for selected patients with end-stage cardiac or pulmonary disease. According to the registry of the International Society for Heart and Lung Transplantation, more than 25,659 transplant procedures have been performed worldwide in 229 transplant centers. In recent years, this represents more than 3,200 organ transplants per year, 83% of which are cardiac, 7% heart-lung, 7% single-lung, and 3% double-lung transplantation (1).

The indications for heart transplantation in adults are cardiomyopathy in 50%, coronary artery disease in 43%, valvular disease in 4%, and congenital heart disease in 2% of the cases.

Heart-lung transplantation is commonly performed for patients with end-stage heart disease resulting in pulmonary hypertension. Single-lung transplantation is a therapeutic option for patients with end-stage pulmonary fibrosis and emphysema. Single-lung transplantation is also available to patients with pulmonary hypertension because of recoverability of right ventricular function (2). Double-lung transplantation is performed for patients with bilateral pulmonary disease associated with chronic pulmonary sepsis, such as cystic fibrosis, bronchiectases, and emphysema. Patients with bilateral lung transplantation for emphysema are at greater risk for developing complications and have a worse survival rate than patients with single-lung transplantation (3). The survival rate is better for cardiac transplant recipients (79% at 1 year and 68% at 5 years) than for lung transplant recipients (60% at 1 year and 40% at 5 years following transplantation) (1).

CARDIAC TRANSPLANTATION

In the United States, over 2,000 cardiac transplant procedures are performed annually. However, because of the shortage of donors, only 10% of cardiac transplant candidates will actually undergo transplantation. Therefore, it is critical to understand the role of noninvasive imaging technology to evaluate which patients are most likely to benefit from transplantation. Although the long-term survival rate of cardiac transplant recipients is good, the care of these patients is extremely difficult. Infection and rejection are the major causes of death in the early postoperative period (during the first 3 months following transplantation) and allograft coronary disease is the major cause of death in long-term survivors. Knowledge of the pathology of transplantation is necessary to understand the role of the different diagnostic modalities available to assess the complications of transplantation.

Because of the number of patients affected, heart failure is becoming a major problem in clinical cardiology. The number has increased rapidly over the past decades. A recent National Institutes of Health (NIH) report has indicated that 4.7 million patients in the United States have chronic heart failure; 400,000 new cases are diagnosed each year with 1 million hospitalizations (4). As a consequence, the costs (diagnostic and therapeutic) are high, probably more than $11 billion per year (5,6). Different cardiomyopathies can result in heart failure, such as (idiopathic) dilated, hypertrophic, and ischemic. When data from recent ran-

J.J. Bax: Department of Cardiology, Leiden University Medical Center, Leiden, The Netherlands.

D. Delbeke: Department of Radiology and Radiological Sciences, Vanderbilt University Medical Center, Nashville, TN.

J. Vitola: Federal University of Parana Medical School, Curitiba, Parana, Brazil.

D. Poldermans: Department of Cardiology, Leiden University Medical Center and Department of Cardiology/Epidemiology, Thorax Center, Rotterdam, The Netherlands.

E. Boersma: Department of Cardiology, Leiden University Medical Center and Department of Cardiology/Epidemiology, Thorax Center, Rotterdam, The Netherlands.

E.E. van der Wall: Department of Cardiology, Leiden University Medical Center and Department of Cardiology/Epidemiology, Thorax Center, Rotterdam, The Netherlands.

M.P. Sandler: Department of Radiology and Radiological Sciences, Vanderbilt University Medical Center, Nashville, TN.

domized, multicenter heart failure trials were pooled (13 studies, more than 20,000 patients), it appeared that coronary artery disease was the underlying etiology of heart failure in almost 70% of the patients (4,5).

Medical therapy for heart failure has improved significantly in the last few years. Important clinical trials such as SAVE and SOLVD (6,7) have shown significant improvement in survival when angiotensin-converting enzyme (ACE) inhibitors are used. The ELITE II trial demonstrated a similar benefit with angiotensin-II receptor blockade (8). Furthermore, different trials with β-adrenergic blocking agents have shown a survival benefit in patients with ischemic cardiomyopathy (9). Despite all the advances in medical therapy, morbidity and mortality for patients with severe heart failure still remains high (10). The treatment of choice would be heart transplantation; however, the limited number of donor hearts is largely exceeded by the demand (11).

Myocardial revascularization, when feasible, may provide an alternative to medical therapy or transplant in patients with severe ischemic cardiomyopathy (12). Survival of patients with ischemic cardiomyopathy and depressed ejection fraction following coronary artery bypass grafting (CABG) has been reported to be 83% at 3 years (13), compared with 67.8% at 5 years for cardiac transplant recipients (1). Compared with medical therapy, a substantial survival benefit in patients with depressed left ventricular (LV) function following CABG has been shown (14). Revascularization procedures in heart failure patients are associated with a high mortality and morbidity risk. Thus, identification of patients (with viable but jeopardized myocardium at risk for adverse cardiac events or sudden death) who may demonstrate significant benefit from revascularization procedures appears critical.

Role of Imaging Modalities in the Pretransplant Evaluation

Myocardial Viability

Rahimtoola et al. (15) demonstrated that patients with ischemic cardiomyopathy may improve LV function following revascularization. Since this early experience, others have shown similar findings (16,17). These observations have led to the hypothesis that some dysfunctional myocardium in patients with chronic coronary artery disease may not be irreversibly damaged but may be still viable and may recover in function following adequate revascularization. This phenomenon was referred to as *hibernation* (18). Rahimtoola et al. (15) suggested that blood flow was reduced in the dysfunctioning myocardium, and some studies have indeed demonstrated a reduction in blood flow (19). However, other studies have demonstrated (near) normal resting flow in chronic dysfunctional myocardium that improved function after revascularization (20–22). Several studies indicated that flow reserve (and not resting flow) was impaired in chronic dysfunctional myocardium, and accordingly, the term *(repetitive) stunning* was proposed to describe these findings (23).

Is Assessment of Viability Clinically Relevant?

The presence of viable tissue has been related to a superior outcome after revascularization (24) (Table 52.1). If the extent of

Table 52.1. *Benefits of Viability in Relation to Outcome After Revascularization*

	Evidence
Improvement of regional LV function	+++
Improvement of global LV function	++
Improvement of heart failure symptoms	+
Improvement in exercise capacity	+
Reverse remodeling	+
Reduction of arrhythmias	−
Improvement of long-term prognosis	+

LV, left ventricular.

viable tissue is large, improvement of left ventricular ejection fraction (LVEF) can be anticipated (24). There are also relations between the presence of viable tissue and improvement of heart failure symptoms and/or exercise capacity after revascularization (24). Finally, various retrospective analyses have shown that patients with viable myocardium had an excellent long-term prognosis, whereas patients with viable tissue who did not undergo revascularization had a high event-rate over time (24).

Currently, the exact incidence of viable myocardium in patients with chronic ischemic LV dysfunction is not entirely clear. A few studies however have focused on this issue (25–28) (Table 52.2). Auerbach et al. (26) have evaluated 283 patients with ischemic cardiomyopathy (LVEF 26 ± 8%) with ^{18}F-fluorodeoxyglucose (^{18}F-FDG) and positron emission tomography (PET); 156 (55%) patients exhibited viable tissue. Three other studies identified viability in 37% to 57% of the patients studied (25,27,28). Beanlands et al. (29) evaluated 67 patients with ^{18}F-FDG PET while therapy was already established. Thus, 11 patients were scheduled for heart transplantation, 38 for revascularization, and 18 for medical treatment. Based on the presence or absence of myocardial viability, therapy was changed in 31 (46%) patients (Fig. 52.1).

The same group demonstrated that once viability has been detected, revascularization should follow as soon as possible (30). The authors evaluated 35 patients with ^{18}F-FDG PET; 18 patients underwent early revascularization (less than 12 ± 9 days) and 17 underwent late revascularization (145 ± 97 days). In the early revascularization group, the preoperative mortality was lower, more patients improved in LVEF postoperatively, and the event-free survival was higher (Fig. 52.2).

Schwartz et al. (31) reported similar findings. All these findings support the necessity and clinical relevance of viability as-

Table 52.2. *Prevalence of Viability in Patients with Ischemic Cardiomyopathy*

Author	No. patients	LVEF	Viability technique	Viability present
Fox[27]	27	NA	MPI	10 (37%)
Auerbach[26]	283	26 ± 8%	FDG PET	156 (55%)
Schinkel[25]	83	25 ± 7%	DSE	47 (57%)
Al-Mohammed[28]	27	19 ± 6%	FDG PET	14 (52%)

DSE, dobutamine stress echocardiography; FDG, fluorodeoxyglucose; LVEF, left ventricular ejection fraction; MPI, myocardial perfusion imaging; NA, not available; PET, positron emission tomography.

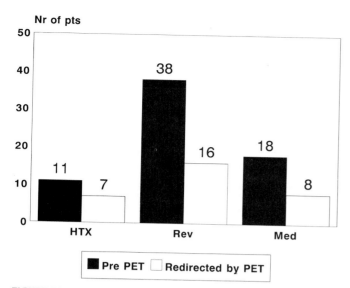

FIGURE 52.1. Bar graph illustrating the effect of fluorodeoxyglucose positron emission computed tomography (^{18}F-FDG PET) on patient management. The black bars indicate the number of patients and their planned treatment before ^{18}F-FDG PET was performed; the white bars demonstrate the number of patients in whom therapy was changed according to the ^{18}F-FDG PET results. HTX, heart transplantation; Med, medical treatment; Rev, revascularization. (From Beanlands RSB, De-Kemp R, Smith S et al. F-18-fluorodeoxyglucose PET imaging alters clinical decision making in patients with impaired ventricular function. *Am J Cardiol* 1997;79:1092–1095, with permission.)

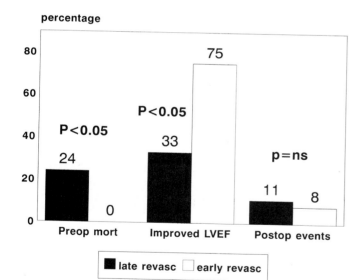

FIGURE 52.2. Bar graph showing the effect of delayed revascularization (*black bars*) versus timely revascularization (*white bars*) in patients with viable tissue on fluorodeoxyglucose positron emission tomography. Patients with delayed revascularization had a higher preoperative mortality rate, a higher postoperative event-rate, and a lower percentage of patients exhibiting improvement of left ventricular ejection fraction after revascularization. Mort, mortality; preop, preoperative; postop, postoperative. (From Beanlands RSB, Hendry PJ, Masters RG et al. Delay in revascularization is associated with increased mortality rate in patients with severe left ventricular dysfunction and viable myocardium on fluorine 18-fluorordeoxyglucose positron emission tomography. *Circulation* 1998;98:II-51–II-56, with permission.)

sessment in patients with ischemic cardiomyopathy. Currently, a variety of techniques has become available for the noninvasive assessment of myocardial viability.

Scintigraphic Imaging Modalities Available for Assessment of Myocardial Viability and Evaluation of Candidates for Revascularization Rather than Cardiac Transplantation

Dysfunctional but viable myocardium exhibits certain characteristics that form the basis for the imaging modalities that are currently available to assess myocardial viability (Table 52.3). These characteristics include cell membrane integrity, intact mitochondria, preserved glucose metabolism, intact resting perfusion, and contractile reserve (32).

Myocardial perfusion can be evaluated using radiopharmaceuticals such as ^{15}O-water, ^{13}N-ammonia, and ^{82}Rb. Glucose metabolism can be evaluated with ^{18}F-FDG, fatty acid metabolism with ^{11}C-palmitate, and oxidative metabolism with ^{11}C-acetate. Because of its long half-life of 120 minutes, ^{18}F-FDG is the most practical radiopharmaceutical for clinical studies, and ^{18}F-FDG PET has become the "gold standard" to evaluate myocardial viability. However, a variety of alternative procedures are available for assessing myocardial viability (33). Criteria have been developed to differentiate ischemic versus nonischemic cardiomyopathy. In patients with ischemic cardiomyopathy, criteria are available to identify viable jeopardized myocardium and to identify patients that would benefit from revascularization rather than cardiac transplantation (34,35).

^{18}F-FDG Imaging

^{18}F-FDG imaging can be used to assess glucose metabolism (24). ^{18}F-FDG closely resembles glucose, with the exception that one OH group has been replaced by a ^{18}F atom. Initial uptake of ^{18}F-FDG in the myocyte is similar to that of glucose; however, following phosphorylation, ^{18}F-FDG-PO^4 cannot be metabolized further and remains trapped in the myocardium, providing a strong signal for imaging. For optimal prediction of functional recovery, integration of perfusion and ^{18}F-FDG uptake is needed. Four patterns can be observed in dysfunctional myocardium (Table 52.4), representing the different myocardial states [stunning, hibernation, and (non-) transmural scar]. Regions with normal perfusion and ^{18}F-FDG uptake represent stunning, regions with reduced perfusion with (relatively) increased ^{18}F-FDG uptake (mismatch pattern) represent hibernation, and re-

Table 52.3. *Features versus Viability Techniques*

Feature	Technique
Glucose metabolism	^{18}F-FDG PET/SPECT
Intact cell membrane	^{201}Tl
Intact mitochondria	^{99m}Tc tracers
Intact perfusion	^{201}Tl/^{99m}Tc tracers
Contractile reserve	Dobutamine echo (MRI)

^{18}F-FDG, ^{18}F-fluorodeoxyglucose; MRI, magnetic resonance imaging; PET, positron emission tomography; SPECT, single photon emission computed tomography.

Table 52.4. *Myocardial Perfusion and ^{18}F-FDG Uptake Patterns in Dysfunctional Myocardium*

	Perfusion	FDG uptake
Repetitive stunning	Normal	Normal/increased
Hibernation	Reduced	Normal/increased
Transmural scar	Severely reduced	Severely reduced
Nontransmural scar	Mildly reduced	Mildly reduced

FDG, ^{18}F-fluorodeoxyglucose.

gions with concordantly reduced perfusion and ^{18}F-FDG uptake represent scar tissue (match pattern).

Because myocyte uptake of ^{18}F-FDG is similar to uptake of glucose, the metabolic conditions during the test are extremely important (36). Among the different metabolic substrates and hormones, free fatty acids and insulin may be the most important. High plasma levels of free fatty acids inhibit myocardial glucose and ^{18}F-FDG uptake; high plasma levels of insulin inhibit peripheral lipolysis (and thereby availability of free fatty acids) and stimulate glucose and ^{18}F-FDG uptake in the myocyte directly. Thus, low plasma levels of free fatty acids and high levels of insulin allow maximal glucose and ^{18}F-FDG uptake. Oral glucose loading is the simplest protocol to create these circumstances; however, in patients with (subclinical) diabetes the increase in insulin levels following glucose loading may be attenuated. Because diabetes is often present in patients with chronic coronary artery disease, alternative protocols have been proposed in these patients, including coadministration of insulin

Table 52.5. *Direct Comparative Studies between ^{18}F-FDG PET and ^{18}F-FDG SPECT/Gamma-Camera Coincidence Imaging*

Author	Agreement (%)	Pts (n)	LVEF (%)	Pts with MVD (%)	Pts with Previous MI
PET vs SPECT					
Burt[41]	93	20	NA	NA	NA
Martin[42]	100	9	NA	NA	NA
Bax[43]	76	20	39 ± 16	83	100
Chen[44]	90	36	NA	NA	NA
Srinivasan[45]	94	28	33 ± 15	93	64
PET vs gamma-camera coincidence imaging					
Hasegawa[46]	48	20	NA	80	100
De Sutter[47]	70	19	44 ± 13	63	100
Nowak[48]	74	21	41 ± 13	80	57

^{18}F-FDG, ^{18}F-fluorodeoxyglucose; LVEF, left ventricular ejection fraction; MI, myocardial infarction; MVD, multivessel disease; NA, not available; pts, patients; PET, positron emission tomography; SPECT, single photon emission computed tomography.

or hyperinsulinemic euglycemic clamping (36). Administration of a nicotinic acid derivative (Acipimox, Byk, The Netherlands) may offer another alternative; Acipimox does not influence insulin levels but lowers plasma levels of free fatty acids (37). To increase insulin levels, Acipimox is administered in combination with a small meal (38). Data obtained in small numbers of patients have demonstrated good image quality, but further studies are needed (37,38).

Because ^{18}F-FDG is a positron emitter, ^{18}F-FDG imaging is

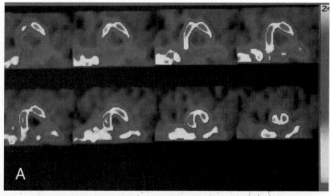
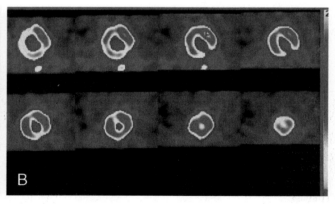
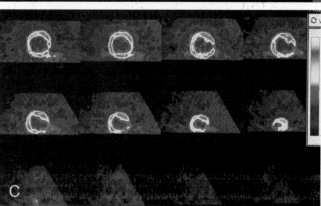

FIGURE 52.3. 51-year-old woman with unstable angina and congestive heart failure. ^{99m}Tc-sestamibi **(A)** and ^{18}fluorodeoxyglucose (^{18}F-FDG) single photon emission computed tomography (SPECT) **(B)** short-axis images of the heart show a large area of decreased perfusion and maintained metabolism in the inferolateral wall indicating jeopardized but viable myocardium. Only a small area demonstrates absent metabolism. ^{18}F-FDG positron emission tomography short-axis images **(C)** of the heart are virtually identical to the ^{18}F-FDG-SPECT images. The advantages of a single acquisition include patient convenience, shorter length of image acquisition, and perfect registration of the images.

performed with PET; PET, however, has limited availability for routine clinical use. Much effort has been invested in the development of 511 keV collimators to permit ^{18}F-FDG imaging with single photon emission computed tomography (SPECT), because of the increasing demand for viability studies (24,39,40). Five direct comparisons between ^{18}F-FDG PET and ^{18}F-FDG SPECT demonstrated excellent agreement for assessment of viability (24,41–45) (Table 52.5) (Fig. 52.3). More recently, gamma cameras with the option of coincidence imaging have been developed; this approach enhances resolution of the system but necessitates the use of attenuation correction (24). Three direct comparisons between ^{18}F-FDG PET and gamma camera coincidence imaging have shown suboptimal agreement (46–48) (Table 52.5); this agreement was even less when attenuation correction was not applied for coincidence imaging. Moreover, the segments with disagreement were located predominantly in the septum and inferior wall, suggesting the influence

of attenuation. Further studies, in particular with functional follow-up after revascularization, are needed. For ^{18}F-FDG SPECT imaging, studies in patients undergoing revascularization have demonstrated high accuracy in predicting outcome after revascularization (17).

Initial studies have also shown that ischemic cardiomyopathy can be differentiated from nonischemic cardiomyopathy with PET, using ^{13}N-ammonia to evaluate myocardial perfusion and ^{18}F-FDG to evaluate myocardial metabolism. An index has been developed that incorporates the number and severity of the defects from circumferential profile analysis; this index was significantly lower in patients with nonischemic versus ischemic cardiomyopathy. The sensitivity and specificity to differentiate the two patient groups was 100% and 80%, respectively (49–51).

Close correlation between a matched decrease in ^{13}N-ammonia and ^{18}F-FDG uptake and infarcted myocardium were demonstrated in two studies in which human explanted hearts were

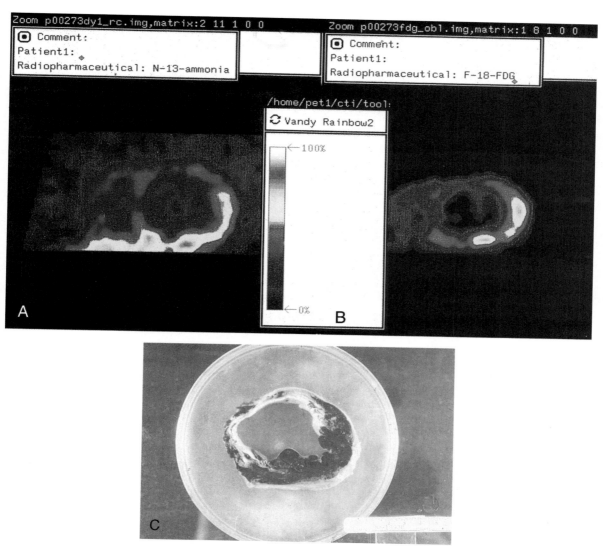

FIGURE 52.4. Positron emission tomography images from a 57-year-old man with a history of previous myocardial infarction and ischemic cardiomyopathy, These short-axis images from the midheart show a ^{13}N-ammonia **(A)** and ^{18}F-fluorodeoxyglucose defect **(B)** in the anterior wall of the left ventricle corresponding to a transmural old infarct seen on the pathologic specimen **(C)**.

examined pathologically at the time of transplantation (52,53) (Figs. 52.4 and 52.5).

²⁰¹Tl Imaging

²⁰¹Tl imaging can be used to assess perfusion and cell membrane integrity (16). Initial uptake of ²⁰¹Tl following tracer injection is dependent on regional perfusion, whereas prolonged tracer uptake is dependent on cell membrane integrity and, thus, myocardial viability. Two main protocols are currently being used for assessment of viability with ²⁰¹Tl: stress-redistribution-reinjection and rest-redistribution. When the clinical question concerns viability only, rest-redistribution provides adequate information. With rest-redistribution imaging, the initial data set is obtained directly following tracer injection, representing myocardial perfusion. Three to 4 hours later, the redistribution images are acquired, representing myocardial viability. Four patterns in regions with contractile dysfunction can be observed: (a) no defect in the dysfunctional region (indicating stunning), (b) initial defect with redistribution (representing hibernating myocardium), (c) initial defect without redistribution with tracer activity on the late images equal to or greater than 50% (subendocardial necrosis), and (d) initial defect without redistribution with activity on the late images less than 50%, (transmural scar). The available studies with ²⁰¹Tl rest-redistribution imaging in patients undergoing revascularization have shown an excellent sensitivity to predict improvement of function after revasculari-

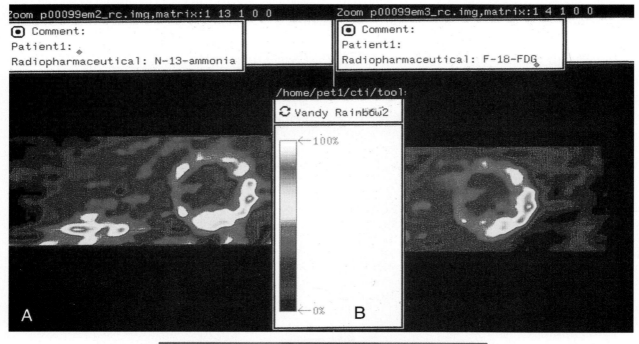

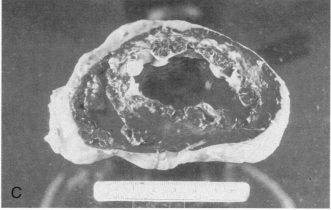

FIGURE 52.5. Positron emission tomography images from a 58-year-old man with a history of ischemic cardiomyopathy. These short-axis images from the midheart show globally decreased perfusion on the ¹³N-ammonia scan **(A)** and match decreased metabolism on the ¹⁸F-fluorodeoxyglucose scan **(B)** corresponding to patchy interstitial fibrosis on the pathologic specimen **(C)**. The patchy fibrosis is more prominent in the anterior wall of the left ventricle and extends circumferentially in most apical slices. The wall thickness is better preserved than in the patient in Fig. 52.4.

zation; however the specificity was somewhat less. The lower specificity is related to the viability criteria that are used (54). Previous studies have shown that segments with no initial defect (stunned myocardium) or an initial defect with redistribution (hibernation) have a high likelihood of recovery of function. Segments with a fixed defect and activity less than 50% (transmural scar) will virtually never recover in function. The problem is related to segments with a fixed defect with tracer activity equal to or greater than 50% (subendocardial scar); these do not often improve in function following revascularization and may (at least in part) explain the lower specificity. However, revascularization of these segments may prevent remodeling and be important for long-term prognosis.

The other ^{201}Tl protocol that is used frequently is stress-redistribution-reinjection (55). This protocol provides information on viability and stress-inducible ischemia. A higher specificity can be obtained using this protocol; Kitsiou et al. (56) have shown that segments with tracer activity equal to or greater than 50% on the reinjection images are likely to improve in function when superimposed ischemia is present (Fig. 52.6). Thus, the combination of viability and stress-inducible ischemia may allow more accurate prediction of recovery of function after revascularization.

^{99m}Tc-Labeled Agents

^{99m}Tc-labeled agents can be used to evaluate perfusion and intact mitochondria (57). Most experience has been obtained with ^{99m}Tc-sestamibi, whereas recent studies have also used ^{99m}Tc-tetrofosmin (58). The uptake and retention of these tracers is dependent on perfusion, cell membrane integrity, and mitochondrial function (membrane potential) (57). Over the past 15 years, the role of ^{99m}Tc-sestamibi for the assessment of viability has been debated (57). Several studies demonstrated that ^{99m}Tc-sestamibi underestimated the presence of viable myocardium, particularly in the inferior wall (58–61). However, Matsunari et al. (58) demonstrated the benefit of attenuation correction, in a comparative study between ^{18}F-FDG PET and ^{99m}Tc-tetrofosmin.

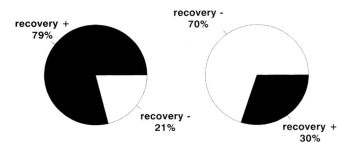

FIGURE 52.6. Improvement of function after revascularization in dysfunctional segments with ^{201}Tl activity ≥50% on the reinjection images. Improvement of function occurs often in the presence of superimposed ischemia but is rare in the absence of ischemia. (Data based on Kitsiou AN, Srinivasan G, Quyyumi AA et al. Stress-induced reversible and mild-to-moderate irreversible thallium defects: are they equally accurate for predicting recovery of regional left ventricular function after revascularization? *Circulation* 1998;98:501–508.)

In addition, Schneider et al. (62) have suggested a different threshold of activity in the inferior wall for the detection of viability: Using a cutoff value of 50% tracer uptake in the anterior region and a cutoff value of 35% tracer uptake in the inferior wall, the authors could reliably predict improvement of function after revascularization.

To further improve the detection of viability with sestamibi, additional modifications of the imaging protocol have been proposed. Originally, a resting image was performed.

Smanio et al. (63) have used gated sestamibi SPECT and combined the information of tracer uptake with the functional (wall motion) information.

Several groups have performed studies with ^{99m}Tc-sestamibi imaging following administration of nitrates (either orally or intravenously) (64,65). It is thought that nitrates enhance blood flow (and tracer uptake) to myocardial regions that are subtended by severely stenosed arteries. In most of these studies, two sets of images are obtained—a resting image and a nitrate-enhanced image—and these results are compared. Bisi et al. (64) have demonstrated excellent results with nitrate-enhanced sestamibi SPECT imaging for the detection of viable myocardium.

Assessment of myocardium viability using various single photon and positron-labeled imaging agents is also discussed in Chapter 16.

Pathologic Appearance of Ischemic Heart Disease and Limitations of Scintigraphic Techniques

The pathologic difference between acute and remote infarction with chronic ischemic disease should be emphasized. In acute myocardial infarction, the thickness of the myocardium is preserved, whereas in remote infarction, the infarcted tissue becomes a band of fibrosis with marked thinning of the myocardial wall (Fig. 52.4). In addition, in chronic ischemia the thickness of the myocardium can be relatively preserved with a pattern of patchy interstitial fibrosis (Fig. 52.5). When there is patchy fibrosis, it is difficult to delineate an abnormal area both pathologically and on scintigraphic images (52). The resolution of scintigraphic techniques does not allow differentiation of endocardial and epicardial regions of the myocardium, and the uptake of radiopharmaceuticals reflect average transmural distribution. In consequence, it should be kept in mind that a flow/metabolism match contains a mixture of scarred and normal myocardium and that a flow/metabolism mismatch contains some ischemic but salvageable myocardium in addition to the mixture of scarred and normal tissue. Therefore, a region of flow/metabolism match does not mean transmural infarction, and a region of flow/metabolism mismatch does not imply full recovery of the contractile function but rather that the contractile function is likely to improve following revascularization.

Dobutamine Stress Echocardiography

Dobutamine stress echocardiography can be used to assess contractile reserve. Experimental studies have shown that infusions of low-dose dobutamine (5 to 10 mcg/kg/minute) can increase contractility in dysfunctional but viable myocardium; this phe-

Table 52.6. *Different Responses to Dobutamine in Chronic Dysfunctional Myocardium*

	WM response at low-dose	WM response at high-dose	Representing
Biphasic reponse	Improved	Worsening	Viability and ischemia
Direct worsening	Worsening	Worsening	Ischemia
Sustained improvement	Improved	Improved	Subendocardial scar
No change	No change	No change	Transmural scar

WM, wall motion.

nomenon has been referred to as *contractile reserve*. Segments without viable myocardium do not exhibit this contractile reserve. Many studies in patients have demonstrated the value of dobutamine stress echocardiography to assess viable myocardium (66). More recently, the protocol has been modified into a low-high dose protocol. With this protocol, dobutamine is infused stepwise, starting at 5 mcg/kg/minute (with 5 to 10 mcg increments) until 40 mcg/kg/minute with, if necessary, the addition of 1 to 2 mg atropine. This protocol allows assessment of viability at low dose with assessment of ischemia at high dose. The safety of this protocol in patients with severely depressed LV function was demonstrated recently by Poldermans et al. (67) in 200 patients with depressed LVEF (<35%).

Four patterns in regions with contractile dysfunction can be observed (Table 52.6): (a) biphasic response (initial improvement followed by worsening of wall motion), (b) worsening (direct deterioration of wall motion without initial improvement), (c) sustained improvement (improvement of wall motion without subsequent deterioration), and (d) no change (no change in wall motion during the entire study). All patterns except the fourth pattern (which represents scar tissue) are related to the presence of viable myocardium.

Magnetic Resonance Imaging

Magnetic resonance imaging (MRI) has been also been used to detect viability (68) (Table 52.7). The first studies on myocardial viability used resting MRI and focused on the end-diastolic wall thickness (EDWT), systolic wall thickening (SWT) and signal intensity without contrast-enhancement (SI). Early observations revealed severely reduced EDWT, reduced or absent SWT, and decreased SI in patients with previous infarction. Baer et al. (69) compared MRI with ^{18}F-FDG PET and showed that segments without SWT and EDWT less than 5.5 mm were mainly nonvi-

able on ^{18}F-FDG PET. Moreover, segments with EDWT less than 5.5 mm virtually never showed recovery of function after revascularization (70). However, segments with EDWT equal to or greater than 5.5 mm did not always improve in function after revascularization, indicating the need for additional testing in segments with EDWT equal to or greater than 5.5 mm to accurately predict outcome after revascularization. Subsequently, Baer et al. demonstrated that the presence of contractile reserve during low-dose dobutamine MRI in segments with EDWT equal to or greater than 5.5 mm allowed accurate prediction of outcome after revascularization. The addition of tagging to dobutamine MRI may even further enhance the diagnostic accuracy of the technique because it enables distinction of responses to dobutamine by different myocardial layers (71).

The most recent studies concerning MRI have used contrast agents; Kim et al. (72) have demonstrated the use of contrast-enhanced MRI for the detection of viability and subsequent prediction of improvement of function in 50 patients with chronic ischemic LV dysfunction. Using this approach, hyperenhanced regions represent scar tissue, and, with the high resolution of MRI, it is possible to detect different stages of transmural infarct. The results showed nicely that the higher the transmurality, as evidenced by hyperenhancement, the lower the likelihood of recovery of function after revascularization. In contrast, segments without hyperenhancement had a high likelihood of recovery.

Prediction of Recovery of Function After Revascularization

Different end points have been used against which viability tests have been validated. The most frequently used end point is prediction of *improvement of regional function* following revascularization. Recently, an updated meta-analysis was published on the

Table 52.7. *Parameters Derived from Magnetic Resonance Imaging for the Assessment of Viability*

Technique	Parameters	Clinical Relevance
Resting MRI represents scar	End-diastolic wall thickness	EDWT <5.5 mm represents scar
	Systolic wall thickening	Absence of SWT represents scar
	Signal intensity (without contrast)	Decreased SI represents scar
Dobutamine MRI	Contractile reserve	CR represents viable tissue
Contrast-enhanced MRI	Hyper-enhancement	Hyper-enhanced is scar tissue

CR, contractile reserve; EDWT, end-diastolic wall thickness; SI, signal intensity; SWT, systolic wall thickening.

Table 52.8. *Pooled Data from Studies Focusing on Prediction of Recovery of Function Postrevascularization*

Technique	NPV (%)	PPV (%)	No. studies	No. pts	Sensitivity (%)	Specificity (%)
^{18}F-FDG PET	86	71	20	598	93	58
^{201}Tl	81	64	33	858	87	55
^{99m}Tc tracers	71	71	20	488	81	66
Dobutamine echo/MRI	85	77	32	1090	81	80

^{18}F-FDG, ^{18}F-fluorodeoxyglucose; MRI, magnetic resonance imaging; NPV, negative predictive value; PET, positron emission tomography; PPV, positive predictive value.

prediction of functional recovery after revascularization using one of the aforementioned techniques (66). Inclusion criteria for this meta-analysis included: (a) prospective study, patients with chronic coronary artery disease undergoing revascularization and (b) results should allow assessment of sensitivity and specificity to predict improvement of regional function. Accordingly, a MEDLINE search was conducted over the period 1980–2001. A total of 850 references were identified; a summary of the studies meeting the inclusion criteria is shown in Table 52.8. In total, 105 studies, with 3,034 patients were included. The incidence of recovery of regional function varied substantially between all studies (ranging from 16% to 91%), suggesting inclusion of different study populations. Still, when all studies were pooled, a sensitivity of 84% and a specificity of 69% were obtained (Fig. 52.7).

An important discrepancy was noted between the sensitivity and specificity of dobutamine stress echocardiography and nuclear imaging. When the meta-analysis was restricted to 11 studies with 325 patients who underwent both low-dose dobutamine echocardiography and some form of rest nuclear imaging (thus, both protocols only focusing on viability without ischemia), nuclear imaging appeared significantly more sensitive in the predic-

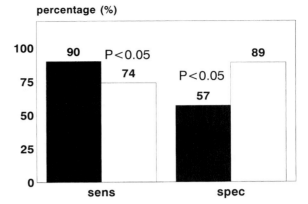

FIGURE 52.8. Prediction of improvement of regional functional following revascularization; comparison of nuclear imaging with dobutamine stress echocardiography; data obtained from 11 studies with 325 patients. (Data based on Bax JJ, Poldermans D, Elhendy A et al. Sensitivity, specificity, and predictive accuracies of various noninvasive techniques for detecting hibernating myocardium. *Curr Probl Cardiol* 2001;26:142–186.)

tion of functional recovery, whereas dobutamine echocardiography was more specific (Fig. 52.8). Recently, the use of sequential testing with ^{201}Tl imaging and low-dose dobutamine echocardiography has been suggested (73). Using this sequential approach (in which approximately 40% of the patients need a second test), the diagnostic accuracy could be improved as compared with using ^{201}Tl imaging or dobutamine echocardiography alone.

From a clinical point-of-view, improvement of global LV function may be more relevant than improvement of regional LV function. The number of studies focusing on improvement of global function after revascularization is significantly less than those focusing on improvement of regional LV function. A total of 29 studies, with 758 patients focused on prediction of improvement of global LV function; these studies were uniform in showing a significant improvement of LVEF in patients with viable myocardium, whereas patients without viable myocardium did not show improvement of LVEF. The results are summarized in Table 52.9. Importantly, the criteria to classify a

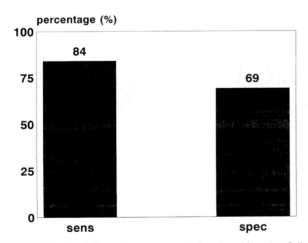

FIGURE 52.7. Prediction of improvement of regional function following revascularization using viability testing; data obtained from 105 studies with 3,034 patients. (Data based on Bax JJ, Poldermans D, Elhendy A et al. Sensitivity, specificity, and predictive accuracies of various noninvasive techniques for detecting hibernating myocardium. *Curr Probl Cardiol* 2001;26:142–186.)

Table 52.9. *Pooled Data from Studies Focusing on Prediction of Improvement of Global LV Function Postrevascularization*

Technique	Nonviable patients			Viable patients	
	LVEF pre	LVEF post	No. studies/ pts	LVEF pre	LVEF post
^{18}F-FDG PET	39	40	12/333	37	47
^{201}Tl	29	31	5/96	30	38
^{99m}Tc tracers	40	39	4/75	47	53
DSE	35	36	8/254	35	43

LVEF pre and post represent LVEF before and after revascularization, respectively.
DSE, dobutamine stress echocardiography; ^{18}F-FDG, ^{18}F-fluorodeoxyglucose; LVEF, left ventricular ejection fraction; PET, positron emission tomography; pts, patients.

patient as viable differed substantially among the different studies. Recently, receiver operating characteristic (ROC) curve analysis was applied and demonstrated that 25% dysfunctional but viable LV may be the optimal threshold to predict improvement of LVEF after revascularization (17).

Prediction of Improvement of Symptoms and Exercise Capacity After Revascularization

Another end point used in viability studies is prediction of improvement in heart failure symptoms and exercise capacity. Heart failure symptoms are difficult to assess; in the clinical setting, the New York Heart Association (NYHA) classification is frequently used. Currently, six studies have evaluated NYHA class before and after revascularization in patients evaluated for myocardial viability (74,75) (Table 52.10). These studies indicated that NYHA class improved significantly in patients with viable myocardium. One study has evaluated the relation between the extent of dysfunctional but viable tissue and the magnitude of improvement in heart failure symptoms (17,76). A more objective measure of functional capacity is exercise capacity. Three studies have analyzed improvement of exercise capacity in relation to viability (76–78). Marwick et al. (77) evaluated 23 patients with ^{18}F-FDG PET before revascularization and demonstrated that patients with extensive viability improved significantly in exercise capacity after revascularization (from 5.6 ± 2.7 metabolic equivalents (METS) to 7.5 ± 1.7 METS). Similar results were reported by DiCarli et al. (76) and Gunning et al. (78).

Viability Versus Long-Term Prognosis

Recently, viability studies have used long-term prognosis as an end point; this may be the most ideal end point in the clinical setting. Several studies are available that have related viability to long-term prognosis; it should be emphasized, however, that all of these studies were retrospective analyses. Haas et al. (79) evaluated 76 patients with chronic coronary artery disease and depressed LV function. Thirty-five patients underwent surgical

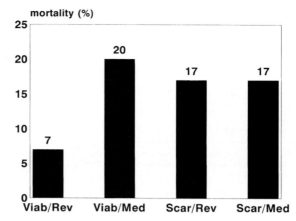

FIGURE 52.9. Mortality rate according to the presence/absence of viable tissue and the treatment (medical, Med; versus revascularization, Rev). Based on pooled data from 17 prognostic studies.

revascularization on clinical presentation and angiographic results. The remaining 41 patients underwent surgical revascularization only when substantial viable myocardium (assessed by ^{18}F-FDG PET) was present; if this was not the case, patients ($n = 7$) were treated medically or were referred for heart transplantation. The patients with viable myocardium who underwent revascularization had a lower perioperative event-rate and a lower short-term (30 days) and long-term (12 months) mortality rate. Other studies have evaluated long-term prognosis only; in these studies, the patients were grouped according to the presence or absence of viable tissue and treatment (medical versus revascularization). Currently, 17 prognostic studies are available (7 employing ^{18}F-FDG PET, 4 ^{201}Tl imaging, and 6 dobutamine echocardiography) (80–96). The results are displayed in Fig. 52.9, indicating a high mortality rate in all groups except in the group of patients with viable myocardium who underwent revascularization. As stated before, the main shortcoming of these studies is their retrospective, nonrandomized character. Clearly, a randomized, prospective study is needed to draw definitive conclusions concerning the prognostic value of viability assessment in treatment of patients with chronic coronary artery disease and depressed LV function.

Conclusions

The number of patients with heart failure secondary to chronic coronary artery disease is rising rapidly. Potential therapies include: medical treatment, heart transplantation, or revascularization. Revascularization may be considered one of the best options, when feasible and when viable myocardium is present. Different nuclear imaging techniques are available for the detection of viability, using ^{201}Tl-chloride, ^{99m}Tc-labeled tracers and ^{18}F-FDG. Dobutamine stress echocardiography and MRI may also provide alternative options for the assessment of viability. Viability has been related to improvement of regional and global function after revascularization, to improvement in heart failure symptoms and exercise capacity, and to a superior long-term prognosis. Thus, viability testing is an important part of the

Table 52.10. *Prediction of Heart Failure Symptoms Postrevascularization in Relation to Presence/Absence Viability*

Author	Technique	No. pts	NYHA pre	NYHA post
Haas[79]	FDG PET	34	3.0	1.6
Schwarz[31]	FDG PET	32	1.4 ± 1.2	0.1 ± 0.3
Beanlands[30]	FDG PET	18	3.0 ± 0.8	1.6 ± 0.7
Dreyfuss[74]	FDG PET	46	3.1 ± 0.3	2.0 ± 0
Bax[17]	FDG SPECT	47	3.4 ± 0.5	1.7 ± 0.8
Marwick[75]	DSE/FDG PET	63	2.6 ± 0.7	1.9 ± 0.7
Bax[93]	DSE	62	3.2 ± 0.7	1.6 ± 0.5
Gunning[78]	[201]Tl RR	19	2.7 ± 0.6	1.3 ± 0.7

NYHA pre and post represent NYHA before and after revascularization, respectively.
DSE, dobutamine stress echocardiography; ^{18}F-FDG, ^{18}F-fluorodeoxyglucose; NYHA, New York Heart Association classification; PET, positron emission tomography; SPECT, single photon emission computed tomography; ^{201}Tl RR, ^{201}Tl rest-redistribution.

diagnostic workup of patients with chronic ischemic LV dysfunction and may help to guide optimal treatment.

Role of Imaging Modalities After Cardiac Transplantation

Although there are significant perioperative problems, development of infections, and an increased incidence of tumors in cardiac transplant recipients, the major problems are acute rejection and the development of accelerated allograft vasculopathy.

Perioperative Changes

Rarely, hyperacute rejection may occur because of the presence of preformed recipient antibodies to donor antigens, mainly ABO mismatch. In hyperacute rejection, the myocardium shows marked global hemorrhage and is not functional without major support despite aggressive immunotherapy. The only treatment is retransplantation.

If there was a prolonged period of ischemia, ischemic changes and reperfusion injury may be present in the myocardium for about 2 weeks. Pathologically, in the early stage, myocyte damage is usually more prominent than the cellular infiltrate. Later, the ischemic area is replaced by granulation tissue. These changes can complicate interpretation of endomyocardial biopsies.

Infections

A recent study reported that 10% of cardiac transplant recipients develop lung nodules after cardiac transplantation and that 75% of these nodules are infectious. The most frequent pathogens are *Aspergillus,* in 32% of cases and *Nocardia,* in 25% of cases (97,98).

Malignant Tumors

Transplant recipients have a higher incidence of malignant tumors, probably related to their immunosuppression. The frequency varies between 1% and 12% in different studies. Non-Hodgkin's lymphomas and skin malignancies are most common and seem to be related to the presence of Epstein-Barr virus and cytomegalovirus (98,99).

Bone Morbidity

Osteoporosis, osteopenia, osteonecrosis, and associated pathologic fractures are known complications following organ transplantation (98,100–104). Disease processes before transplantation may also affect bone mineral metabolism and predispose recipients to bone disease. The pathogenesis of osteoporosis is not always clear but may be related to several factors such as malnutrition, inactivity, smoking, and prolonged diuretic use. Immunosuppressive therapy with glucocorticoids and cyclosporine may play a major role after transplantation (102–104).

Bone mineral density measurements can be used to monitor the development of osteoporosis (Fig. 52.10). Several radiographic methods are available to measure bone mineral density including quantitative computed tomography (QCT), single photon absorptiometry (SPA), dual photon absorptiometry (DPA), and dual-energy x-ray absorptiometry (DEXA). DEXA is the most recently developed technique and has several advantages over the other methods. An advantage of using an x-ray source rather than an isotope source is the production of a more intense beam and, therefore, a shorter scanning time, lower radiation dose, and increased patient throughput. DEXA was found to have a precision in the 0.5% to 2% range and an accuracy of 3% to 5%, better than that of SPA, DPA, and QCT (105). (See Chapter 33.)

Acute Cardiac Rejection

Pathology

Acute rejection occurs most often from 1 to 6 months after transplantation and involves cell-mediated immunity. Diagnosis of acute cardiac rejection is a significant limiting factor for survival of cardiac recipients. When patients are treated with cyclosporine, a biopsy specimen is necessary for accurate diagnosis.

Endomyocardial Biopsy

The technique of endomyocardial biopsy was developed at Stanford University and a four-step grading system was developed according to the severity of the histologic changes (lymphocyte infiltration and myocyte damage) that are present on the endomyocardial biopsy specimen. More recently, the International Society for Heart and Lung Transplantation has developed a seven-grade classification.

Mild rejection is usually not treated, but a follow-up biopsy should be performed within a week. It is important to treat the patient at the stage of moderate rejection because the conducting system is often involved and fatal arrhythmias can occur. Because of the high frequency of episodes of acute rejection during the first 3 months after transplantation, surveillance biopsies are performed at short intervals during that time and less often after 6 months posttransplantation.

Although endomyocardial biopsy is the gold standard to establish the presence of cell-mediated rejection, it is an expensive and invasive technique that is not free of complications. These occur in up to 1% of the patients and include right ventricular perforation and tamponade, arrhythmias, air embolus, pneumothorax, bleeding, and infection. Sampling error is common if the number of specimens is inadequate. With one biopsy, sampling error is approximately 80% and decreases to less than 5% with five biopsies (106). Another limitation of this technique is the tendency to sample previous biopsy sites, which results in interpretation difficulties. In addition, an endomyocardial biopsy cannot be used as a diagnostic standard for vascular rejection that is antibody-mediated and is more difficult to treat.

Cytoimmunologic monitoring of changes of helper/suppressor ratio is a noninvasive technique helpful in detecting acute cardiac rejection, but this technique has limitations in differentiating acute rejection from certain infections and changes in immunosuppressive therapy that can also alter lymphocyte subpopulations (107,108).

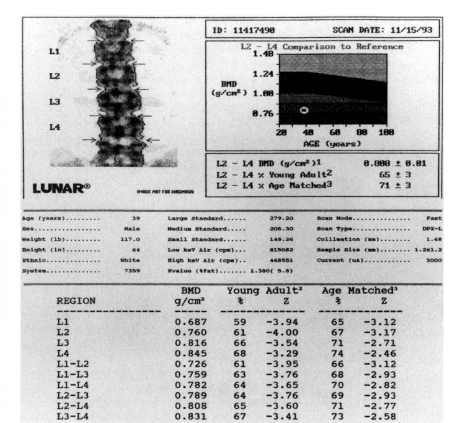

REGION	BMD g/cm²	Young Adult² %	Young Adult² Z	Age Matched³ %	Age Matched³ Z
L1	0.687	59	-3.94	65	-3.12
L2	0.760	61	-4.00	67	-3.17
L3	0.816	66	-3.54	71	-2.71
L4	0.845	68	-3.29	74	-2.46
L1-L2	0.726	61	-3.95	66	-3.12
L1-L3	0.759	63	-3.76	68	-2.93
L1-L4	0.782	64	-3.65	70	-2.82
L2-L3	0.789	64	-3.76	69	-2.93
L2-L4	0.808	65	-3.60	71	-2.77
L3-L4	0.831	67	-3.41	73	-2.58

FIGURE 52.10. Dual energy x-ray absorptiometry of the lumbar spine shows decreased bone mineral density in this 39-year-old patient, 3 years following a single-lung transplant.

Noninvasive Modalities to Detect Acute Rejection

Evaluation of Left Ventricular Function. Acute rejection with myocyte necrosis is associated with abnormalities of LV function. Changes in ventricular volumes measured by radionuclide ventriculography correlate with histologic findings of myocyte necrosis on endomyocardial biopsy. The highest correlation was found for a decrease in the stroke volume, followed by the end-diastolic volume and the end-systolic volume, respectively (109). Diastolic dysfunction has also been demonstrated in allografts with moderate rejection on biopsy with a decrease in end-diastolic volume and a reduction of the peak filling rate. The changes are similar to those seen in restrictive cardiomyopathy and may be related to changes in diastolic elastic properties of the myocardium resulting from edema and cellular infiltration. Although no correlation between histologic rejection and ejection fraction was found, a reduction of the ejection fraction below 50% is more common both with moderate and severe rejection than with mild rejection. Echocardiography with Doppler analysis can also show changes in LV systolic and diastolic dynamics associated with rejection (110–112).

Conventional Myocardial Imaging Agents. The possibility of detecting acute rejection was reported with several conventional radiopharmaceuticals in animal models. In these studies, rejecting cardiac transplants have shown increased ^{67}Ga uptake, presumably resulting from intramyocardial leukocyte infiltration, increased ^{99m}Tc-pyrophosphate uptake resulting from myocyte necrosis, and decreased ^{201}Tl uptake resulting from decreased perfusion. Despite these encouraging data in experimental studies, clinical studies in humans are less satisfactory, with a good specificity but poor sensitivity (113–115).

Labeled Antimyosin Antibodies. ^{111}In-labeled antimyosin monoclonal antibody is a marker that can identify myocyte necrosis directly, instead of cardiac dysfunction resulting from the injury. A multicenter trial documented the diagnostic utility of this agent to detect, localize, and quantify myocardial necrosis in acute myocardial infarction (116). This antibody can also be used to detect acute cardiac rejection. The heart/lung ratio at 48 hours after administration is the index that correlates the best with histologic criteria of rejection (117), but the response time is a concern with this modality that requires up to 48-hour imaging for a disease requiring a quick therapeutic response. Ballester et al. (118) found a correlation between the degree of myocytes necrosis indicated by heart/lung ratio of antimyosin antibody uptake and the Stanford biopsy grade classification. However, no correlation was found for the intermediate scores of the current International Society of Heart and Lung Transplantation (ISHLT) seven-grade classification suggesting that perhaps the current ISHLT classification does reflect the progressive severity of myocardial damage. There is also recent evidence that programmed cell death or apoptosis may contribute to myocardial damage determining the morbidity and outcomes in cardiac allograft rejection. This theory is supported by a study demonstrating antimyosin uptake in patients with no evidence of rejection on biopsy but with evidence of apoptosis (119). (See also the section on novel noninvasive approaches for acute rejection diagnosis.)

Labeled Lymphocytes. Although animal studies have shown the possibility of detecting acute rejection using ^{111}In-labeled lymphocytes, data in human cardiac recipients show only a 56% sensitivity and 36% specificity when correlated with biopsy specimens (120). Activated lymphocytes express somatostatin receptors, and results of a pilot study suggest that somatostatin receptor scintigraphy may predict impending cardiac rejection at least 1 week before endomyocardial biopsy (121).

Positron Emission Tomography. PET is an imaging technique that allows for correction of photon attenuation and, therefore, quantification of myocardial blood flow and metabolic status of the myocardium noninvasively by tracing the kinetics of radiolabeled physiologic substrates. Krivokapich et al. (122) quantified absolute myocardial perfusion with PET using ^{13}N-ammonia in normal volunteers, in patients with suspected y coronary artery disease, and in patients with cardiac transplantation. In cardiac transplants, blood flow at rest was significantly higher than in normal volunteers, and the response to exercise (122) or dipyridamole stress (123,124) of the coronary vasculature is preserved. The preservation of coronary blood flow reserve in cardiac transplant recipients without angiographic evidence of coronary artery disease was also demonstrated by Doppler flow velocity measurements at rest and following maximal vasodilation with papaverine (125).

During acute rejection, reversible abnormalities of the coronary vascular reserve occur and were demonstrated by intracoronary Doppler flow velocity measurements (126). Hoff et al. (127) used PET in a rat transplant model to show that ^{13}N-ammonia and ^{18}F-FDG could detect decreased perfusion and increased metabolism, respectively, in rejecting cardiac allografts. However, homogenously increased ^{18}F-FDG uptake has also been demonstrated in normally functioning nonrejecting heart transplants (128).

MRI and Magnetic Resonance Spectroscopy (MRS). The recent developments of cardiovascular MRI have widened the clinical applications of this imaging technique. The description of the complex sequences allowing evaluation of ventricular function and volumes, evaluation of coronary blood flow reserve, and evaluation of the coronaries arteries is beyond the scope of this chapter (129–131). A pilot study in rats suggests that MRI with ultra-small supermagnetic iron oxide particles can identify macrophage accumulation associated with acute cardiac allograft rejection (132).

Preliminary MRS results in experimental animal studies are promising. The role of phosphorus in muscle metabolism is well known. Adenosine triphosphate (ATP) is the energy currency of the body, phosphocreatine (PCr) is one of the chief reservoirs for ATP, and inorganic phosphate (Pi) is the product of ATP catabolism. Loss of ATP would decrease PCr, and although de-

creased PCr/ATP ratio has been reported in cardiac rejection compared with normal controls, the PCr/ATP ratios are not useful in assessing the level of rejection (133,134).

Vascular Rejection and Allograft Vasculopathy

Pathology

Long-term cardiac transplant survivors can still have episodes of acute rejection resulting from changes of immunosuppressive therapy or an infectious episode. However, the main problem is the development of accelerated graft vascular disease, which is seen in both cardiac and combined heart-lung transplantation, in addition to the development of normal nontransplant atherosclerosis with typical eccentric and focal lesions. Allograft vasculopathy is a diffuse process characterized by concentric intimal proliferation involving the entire length of the vessel (Fig. 52.11) that can progress to occlude the lumen of the vessel. It affects both epicardial arteries and small intramyocardial vessels and may occur as rapidly as 3 to 9 months following transplantation. Allograft vasculopathy develops in about 15% of cardiac transplants each year and affects about 40% of the patients 3 years after transplantation by angiographic criteria (135). Allograft vasculopathy does not correlate with age, sex, hypertension, or hypercholesterolemia, which are the usual risks of native coronary artery disease. There seems to be poor correlation between transplant risk factors such as episodes of acute rejection, HLA donor-recipient mismatch, immunosuppressive therapy, and allograft vasculopathy. Although its pathogenesis is not well understood, it is likely to be due to immune-mediated endothelial cell injury and related to episodes of acute humoral vascular rejection (136,137).

Invasive Procedures to Detect Allograft Vasculopathy

Because cardiac allografts are denervated, most patients do not experience chest pain, and allograft vasculopathy results in silent myocardial infarctions, congestive heart failure, ventricular arrhythmias, and sudden death. Because of the nature of the dis-

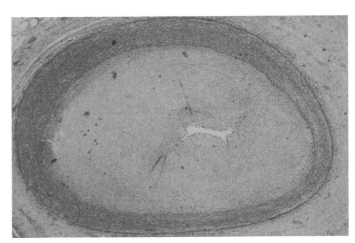

FIGURE 52.11. Histologic section of a coronary artery several years after transplantation shows concentric intimal proliferation, characteristic of allograft vasculopathy.

ease, detection of allograft vasculopathy remains problematic. Coronary angiography, the recognized gold standard for diagnosis of primary coronary artery disease, is usually performed annually to monitor the development of allograft coronary artery disease. A grading system has been developed to classify coronary artery disease (Table 52.11). However, the clinical utility of routine angiographic surveillance in the detection of cardiac allograft vasculopathy in transplant recipients appears low (138).

In naturally occurring coronary artery disease, most of the lesions are type A, but in transplant recipients, type B and C lesions predominate. Coronary angiography has been shown to be insensitive for detecting these smooth and diffuse lesions typical of allograft vasculopathy. Because coronary revascularization is of limited applicability, the only treatment is retransplantation. More reliable modalities to detect the development of allograft vasculopathy are clearly desirable.

Computerized quantitative coronary angiography allows measurement of arterial diameter and maximum percent diameter stenosis of epicardial vessels. A comparison of sequential measurements of coronary luminal size in cardiac transplant recipients and normal coronary segments in nontransplant patients with coronary artery disease shows a 20-fold more rapid rate of luminal reduction in the first year following transplantation, compared with the year follow-up in nontransplant patients (139).

Doppler flow velocity measurements can be obtained at rest and following maximal vasodilation with papaverine to measure the coronary blood flow reserve. It was suggested that microvascular involvement may alter the coronary blood flow reserve and that such measurements may help to detect allograft vasculopathy. Transplant recipients studied 6 to 67 months after transplantation, with no evidence of coronary artery disease or with mild-to-moderate diffuse atherosclerosis defined by 30% narrowing of epicardial vessel diameter on quantitative coronary angiography, have normal coronary blood flow reserve compared with normal volunteers as measured by Doppler flow velocity (125). However, there is progressive deterioration of coronary flow reserve over time after cardiac transplantation, as patients develop allograft vasculopathy (140,141).

Intracoronary ultrasound may be the best modality to detect allograft vasculopathy that is characterized by diffuse intimal thickening (Fig. 52.12). A group of researchers at Stanford University showed that most cardiac transplant recipients have ultrasound evidence of intimal thickening not apparent on arteriography, one or more years after transplantation (140). Thus, the

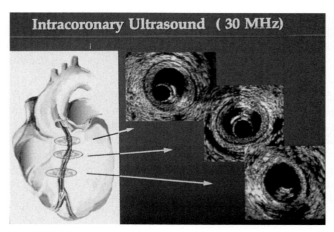

FIGURE 52.12. Intracoronary ultrasound image from the left anterior descending coronary artery of a patient 5 years after cardiac transplantation shows concentric intimal thickening, typical of allograft vasculopathy. (Courtesy of Dr Tim A. Fischell.)

use of intracoronary ultrasound provides a sensitive and relatively reliable method to quantify even minor changes in intimal hyperplasia in cardiac allograft recipients and allows monitoring of the incidence and progression of the disease (142). However, this is still an invasive and expensive procedure.

Noninvasive Procedures to Detect Allograft Vasculopathy

Multiple noninvasive tests have been used to investigate allograft vasculopathy including echocardiography, rest/exercise radionuclide blood pool scans, dipyridamole ^{201}Tl scans, and electrocardiographic monitoring for silent ischemia and arrhythmia. All these modalities have more than 75% specificity and negative predictive value; however, because of poor sensitivity and positive predictive value, they are not acceptable as screening tests for allograft vasculopathy (143). However stress/rest myocardial perfusion imaging is adequate as a screening method for detection of significant coronary artery stenosis suitable for coronary revascularization (144,145).

Several centers have investigated perfusion of cardiac allografts with PET using ^{13}N-ammonia. As discussed previously, measurements of coronary blood flow reserve in cardiac transplant recipients with no angiographic evidence of coronary artery disease confirm the data obtained with Doppler blood flow velocity measurements and show no significant difference compared with normal volunteers (122–125). When patients are followed longitudinally over years with multiple sequential quantitative perfusion measurements, the resting blood flow rate decreases over time in cardiac transplant recipients (146,147). In the study by Zhao et al. (146), a decrease in the resting myocardial blood flow was found in 62% of patients who survived more than a year after transplantation, yet coronary angiography demonstrated the presence of allograft vasculopathy in only 32% of the study population. The decrease in myocardial blood flow was more severe in patients who had angiographic evidence of vasculopathy. Quantitative perfusion measurements with PET may reflect more closely the true incidence of allograft vasculopathy than coronary angiography findings when compared with postmortem findings, although there is no established

Table 52.11. *Coronary Angiographic Abnormalities in Coronary Artery Disease*

(a) Normal
(b) Type A lesions
    Discrete or short tubular stenoses present in the proximal, mid or distal major epicardial coronary segments
(c) Type B lesions
    Diffuse concentric mid or distal luminal narrowings and minor luminal irregularities that do not qualify as type A lesions
(d) Type C lesions
    Narrow distal branches with loss of small branches

gold standard for the detection of allograft vasculopathy *in vivo*. The decrease in perfusion observed in patients over a period of time is consistent with the known progressive nature of allograft vasculopathy. The study of Allen-Auerbach et al. (147) demonstrated that dipyridamole-induced hyperemic flow measured by PET and the flow reserve normalized to the resting rate pressure product were lower in allograft 1 to 2 years after transplantation than in a healthy control. In addition, the flow reserve correlated with changes in total vessel area and lumen diameter measured by intracoronary ultrasound. These findings suggest that PET holds promise as a useful noninvasive modality for detecting the development and monitoring of allograft vasculopathy. Although, in the absence of a reference standard for detection of allograft vasculopathy *in vivo*, it is difficult to determine the diagnostic sensitivity, specificity and predictive accuracy of any single technique.

Innervation of the Transplanted Heart

After transplantation, the postganglionic fibers remain viable in the allograft. However, it may take several years before significant reinnervation by sympathetic nerves occurs (148). Because of the absence of vagal tone, the resting heart rate of the denervated heart is elevated (110 ± 10 beats per minute). The heart rate response to exercise is slower than in age-matched controls, and peak level during maximum exercise is not reached. Because of the loss of inhibitory parasympathetic innervation, transplanted denervated heart displays an exaggerated inotropic and chronotropic response to circulating catecholamine and to dobutamine (149).

Sympathetic innervation of the myocardium can be evaluated by PET imaging with ^{11}C-labeled epinephrine analogs. There is decreased retention of ^{11}C-hydroxyephedrine in recent cardiac transplant recipients compared with normal controls and reinnervation 2 years following transplantation. Schwaiger et al. (150,151) have studied extensively sympathetic innervation of the myocardium and have recently demonstrated that the restoration of sympathetic innervation in heart transplant recipients is associated with improved responses of heart rate and contractile function to exercise.

HEART-LUNG AND LUNG TRANSPLANTATION

Role of Imaging Modalities in Recipient Selection

Chest x-ray films and CT are helpful to evaluate the presence of underlying pulmonary disease resulting in a higher complication rate. For example, bleeding during heparinization can complicate implantation in patients with extensive hilar calcification or pleural scarring. Parenchymal masses may indicate the presence of opportunistic infections or lung tumors.

Ventilation and perfusion lung scans are useful to evaluate if pulmonary hypertension has developed secondary to pulmonary emboli. Quantitative differential lung function can be calculated from lung ventilation and perfusion scans and plays an important role in the decision of which lung to transplant. Generally, the lung demonstrating the worse function is replaced.

Role of Imaging Modalities After Lung Transplantation

Reimplantation Response

The reimplantation response refers to transient problems in pulmonary gas exchange, compliance, and vascular resistance, leading to noncardiogenic pulmonary edema seen on a standard chest x-ray film. The changes on the x-ray film can range from a perihilar haze to unilateral or bilateral consolidation involving the perihilar regions and lung bases. It usually occurs during the first 3 postoperative days but can last up to 3 weeks following lung transplantation (152). The pathogenesis of the reimplantation response is not well understood, but it is thought to represent reperfusion injury of postischemic lungs.

Bronchial Dehiscence

Bronchial dehiscence refers to disruption of the bronchial anastomosis, probably resulting from airway ischemia. This complication has caused or contributed to the death of most of the lung recipients in the early experience with lung transplantation. It usually occurs 1 to 3 weeks following transplantation (153). The bronchial anastomosis is usually located in a watershed area of perfusion between the tracheal blood supply and retrograde lung blood supply. Episodes of acute rejection may aggravate the ischemia, and several groups have noted a coincidence between parenchymal rejection and bronchial dehiscence. This complication occurs more often in double-lung transplants with tracheal anastomosis rather than those with bilateral bronchial anastomoses. In combined heart-lung transplantation, the coronary and bronchial anastomotic network is preserved, and bronchial dehiscence is less frequent. CT and bronchoscopy are the noninvasive imaging modalities performed for evaluation of bronchial dehiscence and should be performed emergently if the chest x-ray film shows a diverticulum of extraluminal air.

Bronchial stricture is a long-term complication of bronchial dehiscence. They can be treated by dilatation alone or stenting. The length of the stricture and condition of the distal airway are critical to the patient's management, and can be evaluated by bronchoscopy and CT (154,155).

Infections

In the immediate postoperative period, infections often affect the transplanted lung, probably related to aspiration in the donor or to prolonged intubation and the presence of drains. Impaired mucociliary transport in the denervated lung may also play a role. The organisms are often gram-negative bacteria and can be identified by multiple cultures (156).

After 4 to 6 weeks, these immunosuppressed patients tend to develop viral infections. The most common viral pathogen is cytomegalovirus, which can present as a diffuse or localized disease. If the patients had unrecognized dormant granulomas with the immunosuppressive therapy, they can develop disseminated disease, such as tuberculosis or coccidioidomycosis. Because of decreased lymphatic drainage, these infections can result in cavitary lesions, even when treated with adequate therapy. These infections can develop in the transplant, as well as the native lung, and careful comparison of the transplanted and native lung, respectively, must be done on sequential chest x-ray films. Transbronchial biopsy and bronchoalveolar lavage can help considerably for the diagnosis of these infections (156).

Acute Rejection

When combined heart-lung transplantation is performed, acute rejection of the myocardium is relatively rare (157). Pulmonary rejection occurs first, probably because the maximum donor-recipient interface is at the level of the lungs.

Acute rejection is a major concern in the first 3 months following transplantation and can be treated effectively with immunosuppression. The diagnosis is usually based on a drop in the arterial partial pressure in oxygen, with no evidence of infection, airway obstruction, or fluid overload. Blood gas abnormalities, however, can be absent in up to one third of the cases of acute rejection (158). Acute rejection produces a loss of compliance of the lung with a fall of forced expiratory volume (FEV_1) and vital capacity (VC). Pulmonary function monitoring is useful to detect acute rejection and to decide when to proceed with transbronchial biopsy (159).

Radiographic Appearance

On chest x-ray films, acute rejection can present as a diffuse process or a localized infiltrate, the presence of which are an indication for bronchoscopy and biopsy (160). Common radiographic findings are increasing septal lines and increasing pleural effusion without a concomitant increase in cardiac size, vascular pedicle width, and vascular redistribution. This pattern has been reported as 68% sensitive and 90% specific for acute pulmonary rejection (161), but it has not been confirmed by subsequent studies (162). As the chest x-ray film can be normal in 50% of cases of rejection, this is not a reliable modality to detect rejection. CT cannot differentiate infection from rejection but can help guide the biopsy (163).

Ventilation and Perfusion Scintigraphy

Although the detection of perioperative vascular complications and postoperative pulmonary emboli are the only established indications for ventilation and perfusion lung scintigraphy, quantitative differential lung perfusion scanning was used originally to better understand posttransplant physiology. For example, in patients with heart-lung transplantation and no evidence of obliterative bronchiolitis, lung scintigraphy demonstrates a similar pattern of ventilation and perfusion to that of normal individuals (164). In patients with single-lung transplantation, ventilation and perfusion scintigraphy has been used to monitor physiologic changes of the transplanted lung.

Patients with pulmonary fibrosis were originally identified as ideal candidates for single-lung transplantation because both ventilation and perfusion tend to be shifted to the transplanted lung (165). In general, the function and perfusion of the transplanted lung improves markedly over the initial 3 weeks after transplantation and continues to improve in the following 3 months. Because the transplanted lung receives most of the perfusion, administration of a reduced dose of ^{99m}Tc-macroaggregated albumin (MAA) particles is recommended.

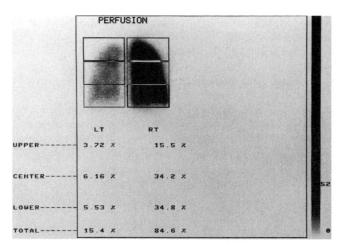

FIGURE 52.13. Quantitative perfusion lung scintigraphy of a patient immediately after right lung transplantation for pulmonary hypertension shows that most of the perfusion is shifted to the transplanted lung.

Theoretically, in patients with emphysema, the perfusion should be shifted to the transplanted lung and the ventilation to the native lung. Because of this conceptual ventilation/perfusion mismatch, patients with emphysema were thought to be unsuitable for single-lung transplantation. However, several reports have shown that single-lung transplantation can be successful in this group of patients and that even when this imbalance is present, it seems to have no significant functional impact (166–168).

In patients with primary pulmonary hypertension, most of the perfusion is shifted to the transplanted lung virtually immediately after transplant (Fig. 52.13), the ventilation is shifted to the transplanted lung also but to a lesser extent (165).

Relatively decreased perfusion to the transplanted lung has been associated with episodes of acute rejection. These changes can be monitored with sequential quantitative differential lung perfusion imaging (166).

Transbronchial Lung Biopsy

Because the radiographic appearance of rejection and opportunistic infections, such as *Pneumocystis* or cytomegalovirus, can be similar, more invasive techniques are needed for the differential diagnosis. Although transbronchial biopsy often presents sampling problems, sensitivity and specificity of 72% to 84% and 100%, respectively, were reported to detect acute rejection (158, 169). A working formulation for classification and grading of pulmonary rejection on transbronchial or open lung biopsy specimen was developed by the ISHLT.

Novel Noninvasive Approaches for the Diagnosis of Acute Rejection

Apoptosis is a set of cellular processes by which cells are eliminated from the body without harming adjacent healthy tissues. It is a form of programmed cell death. Apoptosis is characterized by activation of endonucleases that cleave DNA into oligonucleosomal fragments that can be identified by *in situ* terminal deoxyribonucleotide transferase-mediated dUTP nick-end labeling (TUNEL). Using the TUNEL technique, it has been shown that apoptosis contributes to cell death during acute pulmonary graft rejection and cytomegalovirus infection (170). Early during apoptosis, cells expose phosphatidylserine (PS) at their surface instead of in the membrane leaflets that face the cytosol. Annexin V is a protein that binds selectively to PS and, therefore, can identify apoptotic cells (171). ^{99m}Tc-Annexin is a new radiopharmaceutical that can image apoptosis and preliminary data suggest that it may be a promising agent for detection of rejection (172,173).

As for acute cardiac rejection, a pilot study in a rat model has demonstrated a novel approach for the detection of acute lung allograft rejection using MRI after administration of ultrasmall supermagnetic iron oxide particles (174).

Complications in Long-Term Survivors of Lung Transplantation

Bronchiolitis obliterans has emerged as the main long-term complication of heart-lung transplantation and can occur as early as 3 months following surgery. Although the etiology is still controversial, it seems that multiple episodes of acute rejection may contribute to its development. Bronchiolitis obliterans is a form of chronic rejection and is characterized by epithelial metaplasia, leading to denudation of the ciliated respiratory epithelium. When the disease progresses, there is ulceration of the epithelium and sloughing of the bronchial wall into the lumen, which partially occludes the bronchial lumen together with granulation tissue and fibrosis (175). These changes are irreversible and poorly responsive to therapy. Bronchiolitis obliterans is a major problem in lung transplantation with a high incidence (approximately 50% of lung transplants), rapid progression, and poor survival. It affects all type of lung transplantation, regardless of sex, age, or underlying diagnosis. Acute rejection and infections after bronchiolitis obliterans affects the progression and survival (176). The pediatric incidence of acute rejection and bronchiolitis obliterans is higher than that of adults (177).

On chest x-ray film and CT, there is progressive restriction in lung size, increase in interstitial markings, decrease in vascular markings, and postobstructive consolidation. In early obliterative bronchiolitis, chest x-ray film and CT are often normal (178). Pulmonary function tests are the most sensitive modality to detect this disease and show a constrictive pattern. A study suggests that quantitative perfusion lung scintigraphy 1 to 3 months after single-lung transplantation for emphysema and pulmonary fibrosis was predictive for the development of chronic rejection, whereas FEV_1 values were not (179).

In heart-lung transplant, rejection-mediated vasculopathy characterized by accelerated intimal hyperplasia occurs in all vessels of lung grafts but is usually less severe in the lungs than in the heart, although acute rejection is worse in lungs than heart (180).

SUMMARY

The role of nuclear medicine procedures is well established in the evaluation of cardiac and lung transplant recipients before transplantation. For example, metabolic cardiac imaging with PET or SPECT is the reference procedure to evaluate the presence of viable myocardium in patients with LV dysfunction and chronic ischemia, identifying patients that would benefit from revascularization procedures rather than cardiac transplantation. It also allows differentiation of ischemic versus nonischemic cardiomyopathy. ^{201}Tl myocardial scintigraphy with SPECT is more widely available and is performed for the same indications. Ventilation and perfusion lung scintigraphy can help to exclude pulmonary emboli as the etiology of pulmonary hypertension, and quantitative differential lung perfusion measurements can identify the lung with worse function that is to be replaced first.

After transplantation, however, nuclear medicine procedures are mainly used to understand physiologic changes in the transplanted organs. Endomyocardial and transbronchial biopsy remain the techniques of choice to diagnose acute rejection, and, although coronary artery angiography is the reference technique to diagnose coronary artery disease, it largely underestimates the presence of allograft vasculopathy that is characterized by small vessel disease. Intravascular ultrasound is the technique of choice to characterize small vessel disease.

REFERENCES

1. Bennett LE, Keck BM, Dailey OP et al. Worldwide thoracic organ transplantation: a report from the UNOS/ISHLT international registry for thoracic organ. *Clin Transpl* 2000;31–44.
2. Pasque MK, Kaiser LR, Dresler CM et al. Single lung transplantation for pulmonary hypertension. *J Thorac Cardiovascul Surg* 1992;103:475–482.
3. Low DE, Trulock EP, Kaiser LR et al. Morbidity, mortality, and early results of single versus bilateral lung transplantation for emphysema. *J Thorac Cardiovascul Surg* 1992;103:1119–1125.
4. Challapalli S, Bonow RO, Gheorghiade M. Medical management of heart failure secondary to coronary artery disease. *Coron Art Disease* 1998;9:659–674.
5. Gheorghiade M, Bonow RO. Chronic heart failure in the United States. A manifestation of coronary artery disease. *Circulation* 1998;97:282–289.
6. Pfeffer MA, Braunwald E, Moye LA et al. Effect of captopril on mortality and morbidity in patients with left ventricular dysfunction after myocardial infarction: results of the Survival and Ventricular Enlargement Trial. *N Engl J Med* 1992;327:669–677.
7. The SOLVD investigators. Effect of enalapril on survival in patients with reduced left ventricular ejection fractions and congestive heart failure. *N Engl J Med* 1991;325:293–302.
8. Pitt B, Poole-Wilso PA, Segal R et al. Effect of losartan compared with captopril on mortality in patients with symptomatic heart failure: randomized trial—The Losartan Heart Failure Study ELITE II. *Lancet* 2000;355:1582–1587.
9. Braunwald E. Expanding indications for beta-blockers in heart failure. *N Engl J Med* 2001;344:1711–1712.
10. Khand A, Gemmel I, Clark A et al. Is the prognosis of heart failure improving? *J Am Coll Cardiol* 2000;36:2284–2286.
11. Evans RW, Manninen DL, Garrison LP et al. Donor availability as the primary determinant of the future of heart transplantation. *JAMA* 1986;255:1892–1898.
12. Baker DW, Jones R, Hodges J et al. Management of heart failure. III. The role of revascularization in treatment of patients with moderate or severe left ventricular systolic dysfunction. *JAMA* 1994;272:1528–1534.
13. Kron IL, Flanagan TL, Blackbourne LH et al. Coronary revascularization rather than cardiac transplantation for chronic ischemic cardiomyopathy. *Ann Surg* 1989;210:348–354.
14. Pigott JD, Kouchoukos NT, Oberman A et al. Late results of surgical

and medical therapy for patients with coronary artery disease and depressed left ventricular function. *J Am Coll Cardiol* 1985;5: 1036–1045.

15. Rahimtoola SH. The hibernating myocardium. *Am Heart J* 1989; 117:211–221.

16. Bonow RO, Dilsizian V. Thallium-201 for assessing myocardial viability. *Semin Nucl Med* 1991;21:230–241.

17. Bax JJ, Visser FC, Poldermans D et al. Relationship between preoperative viability and postoperative improvement in LVEF and heart failure symptoms. *J Nucl Med* 2001;42:79–86.

18. Wijns W, Vatner SF, Camici PG. Hibernating myocardium. *N Engl J Med* 1998;339:173–181.

19. Tawakol A, Skopici HA, Abrahmam SA et al. Evidence of reduced resting blood flow in viable myocardial regions with resting asynergy. *J Am Coll Cardiol* 2000;36:2146–2153.

20. Mäki M, Luotolahti M, Nuutila P et al. Glucose uptake in the chronically dysfunctional but viable myocardium. *Circulation* 1996;93: 1658–1666.

21. Marinho NVS, Keogh BE, Costa DC et al. Pathophysiology of chronic left ventricular dysfunction. New insights from the measurement of absolute myocardial blood flow and glucose utilization. *Circulation* 1996;93:737–744.

22. Vanoverschelde JLJ, Wijns W, Depre C et al. Mechanisms of chronic regional postischemic dysfunction in humans. New insights from the study of noninfarcted collateral-dependent myocardium. *Circulation* 1993;87:1513–1523.

23. Braunwald E, Kloner RA. The stunned myocardium: prolonged postischemic ventricular dysfunction. *Circulation* 1982;66:1146–1148.

24. Bax JJ, Patton JA, Poldermans D et al. 18-Fluorodeoxyglucose imaging with PET and SPECT: cardiac applications. *Semin Nucl Med* 2000;30:281–298.

25. Schinkel AFL, Bax JJ, Boersma E et al. How many patients with ischemic cardiomyopathy exhibit viable myocardium? *Am J Cardiol* 2001;88:561–564.

26. Auerbach MA, Schöder H, Gambhir SS et al. Prevalence of myocardial viability as detected by positron emission tomography in patients with ischemic cardiomyopathy. *Circulation* 1999;99:2921–2926.

27. Fox KF, Cowie MR, Wood DA et al. Coronary artery disease as the cause of incident heart failure in the population. *Eur Heart J* 2001; 22:221–236.

28. Al-Mohammad A, Mahy IR, Norton MY et al. Prevalence of hibernating myocardium in patients with severely impaired ischaemic left ventricles. *Heart* 1998;80:559–564.

29. Beanlands RSB, DeKemp R, Smith S et al. F-18-fluorodeoxyglucose PET imaging alters clinical decision making in patients with impaired ventricular function. *Am J Cardiol* 1997;79:1092–1095.

30. Beanlands RSB, Hendry PJ, Masters RG et al. Delay in revascularization is associated with increased mortality rate in patients with severe left ventricular dysfunction and viable myocardium on fluorine 18-fluorodeoxyglucose positron emission tomography. *Circulation* 1998; 98:II-51–II-56.

31. Schwartz ER, Schoendube FA, Kostin S et al. Prolonged myocardial hibernation exacerbates cardiomyocyte degeneration and impairs recovery of function after revascularization. *J Am Coll Cardiol* 1998; 31:1018–1026.

32. Bax JJ, Van Eck-Smit BLF, Van der Wall EE. Assessment of tissue viability: clinical demand and problems. *Eur Heart J* 1998;19: 847–858.

33. Dilsizian V, Borrow RO. Current diagnostic techniques for assessing myocardial viability in patients with hibernating and stunned myocardium. *Circulation* 1993;87:1–20.

34. Louie HW, Laks H, Milgalter E et al. Ischemic cardiomyopathy. Criteria for coronary revascularization and cardiac transplantation. *Circulation* 1991;84:III290–III295.

35. Gropler RJ. Methodology governing the assessment of myocardial glucose metabolism by positron emission tomography and fluorine 18-labeled fluorodeoxyglucose. *J Nucl Cardiol* 1994;1:S1–S14.

36. Dilsizian V, Bacharach SL, Khin MM et al. Fluorine-18-deoxyglucose SPECT and coincidence imaging for myocardial viability: clinical and technologic issues. *J Nucl Cardiol* 2001;8:75–88.

37. Knuuti MJ, Yki-Järvinen H, Voipio-Pulkki LM et al. Enhancement of myocardial [fluorine-18] fluorodeoxyglucose uptake by a nicotinic acid derivative. *J Nucl Med* 1994;35:989–998.

38. Bax JJ, Veening MA, Visser FC et al. Optimal metabolic conditions during fluorine-18 fluorodeoxyglucose imaging; a comparative study using different protocols. *Eur J Nucl Med* 1997;23:35–41.

39. Sandler MP, Patton JA. Fluorine 18-labeled fluorodeoxyglucose myocardial single-photon emission computed tomography: an alternative for determining myocardial viability. *J Nucl Cardiol* 1996;3:342–349.

40. Delbeke D, Videlefsky SW, Patton JA et al. Rest myocardial perfusion/metabolism imaging using simultaneous dual-isotope acquisition SPECT with Technetium-99m-MIBI and fluorine-18-FDG. *J Nucl Med* 1995;36:2110–2119.

41. Burt RW, Perkins OW, Oppenheim BE et al. Direct comparison of fluorine-18-FDG SPECT, fluorine-18-FDG PET and rest thallium-201 SPECT for the detection of myocardial viability. *J Nucl Med* 1995;36:176–179.

42. Martin WH, Delbeke D, Patton JA et al. FDG-SPECT: correlation with FDG-PET. *J Nucl Med* 1995;36:988–995.

43. Bax JJ, Visser FC, Blanksma PK et al. Comparison of myocardial uptake of F18-fluorodeoxyglucose imaged with positron emission tomography and single photon emission computed tomography. *J Nucl Med* 1996;37:1631–1636.

44. Chen EQ, MacIntyre J, Go RT et al. Myocardial viability studies using fluorine-18-FDG SPECT: a comparison with fluorine-18-FDG PET. *J Nucl Med* 1997;38:582–586.

45. Srinivasan G, Kitsiou AN, Bacharach SL et al. [¹⁸F]fluorodeoxyglucose single photon emission computed tomography. Can it replace PET and thallium SPECT for the assessment of myocardial viability? *Circulation* 1998;97:843.

46. Hasegawa S, Uehara T, Yamaguchi H et al. Validity of F-18 fluorodeoxyglucose imaging with a dual-head coincidence gamma camera for detection of myocardial viability. *J Nucl Med* 1999;40: 1884–1892.

47. De Sutter J, de Winter F, Van de Wiele C et al. Cardiac fluorine-18 fluorodeoxyglucose imaging using a dual-head gamma camera with coincidence detection: a clinical pilot study. *Eur J Nucl Med* 2000; 27:676–685.

48. Nowak B, Zimny M, Schwarz ER et al. Diagnosis of myocardial viability by dual-head coincidence gamma camera fluorine-18 fluorodeoxyglucose positron emission tomography with and without nonuniform attenuation correction. *Eur J Nucl Med* 2000;27:1501–1508.

49. Mody FV, Brunken RC, Stevenson LW et al. Differentiating cardiomyopathy of coronary artery disease from nonischemic dilated cardiomyopathy utilizing positron emission tomography. *J Am Coll Cardiol* 1991;17:373–383.

50. Gellman JD, Smith JL, Beecher D et al. Altered regional myocardial metabolism in congestive cardiomyopathy detected by positron emission tomography. *Am J Med* 1983;74:773–785.

51. Eisenberg JD, Sobel BE, Gellman EM. Differentiation of ischemic from non-ischemic cardiomyopathy with positron emission tomography. *Am J Cardiol* 1987;59:1410–1414.

52. Delbeke D, Lorenz CH, Silveira ST et al. ¹³N-ammonia PET estimation of left ventricular mass and infarct size validated with pathological examination of explanted human hearts. *J Nucl Med* 1992;33: 826–838.

53. Berry JJ, Hoffman JM, Steenbergen C et al. Human pathologic correlation with PET in ischemic and nonischemic cardiomyopathy. *J Nucl Med* 1993;34:39–47.

54. Bax JJ, Visser FC, Van Lingen A et al. Comparison between 360° and 180° data sampling in thallium-201 rest-redistribution single-photon emission tomography to predict functional recovery after revascularization. *Eur J Nucl Med* 1997;24:516–522.

55. Dilsizian V, Rocco TP, Freedman NMT et al. Enhanced detection of ischemic but viable myocardium by the reinjection of thallium after stress-redistribution imaging. *N Engl J Med* 1990;323:141–146.

56. Kitsiou AN, Srinivasan G, Quyyumi AA et al. Stress-induced reversible and mild-to-moderate irreversible thallium defects: are they equally accurate for predicting recovery of regional left ventricular function after revascularization? *Circulation* 1998;98:501–508.

57. Bonow RO, Dilsizian V. Thallium-201 and technetium-99m-sestamibi for assessing viable myocardium. *J Nucl Med* 1992;33:815–818.

58. Matsunari I, Böning G, Ziegler SI et al. Attenuation-corrected ⁹⁹ᵐTc-tetrofosmin single-photon emission computed tomography in the de-

tection of viable myocardium: comparison with positron emission tomography using ^{18}F-fluorodeoxyglucose. *J Am Coll Cardiol* 1998; 32:927–935.

59. Soufer R, Dey HM, Ng CK et al. Comparison of sestamibi single-photon emission computed tomography with positron emission tomography for estimating left ventricular myocardial viability. *Am J Cardiol* 1995;75:1214–1219.

60. Sawada S, Allman KC, Muzik O et al. Positron emission tomography detects evidence of viability in rest technetium-99m sestamibi defects. *J Am Coll Cardiol* 1994;23:92–98.

61. Altehoefer C, Vom Dahl J, Biedermann M et al. Significance of defect severity in technetium-99m-MIBI SPECT at rest to assess myocardial viability: comparison with fluorine-18-FDG PET. *J Nucl Med* 1994; 35:569–574.

62. Schneider CA, Voth E, Gawlich S et al. Significance of rest technetium-99m sestamibi imaging for the prediction of improvement of left ventricular dysfunction after Q wave myocardial infarction: importance of infarct location adjusted thresholds. *J Am Coll Cardiol* 1998;32:648–654.

63. Smanio PEP, Watson DD, Segalla DL et al. Value of gating of technetium-99m sestamibi single-photon emission computed tomographic imaging. *J Am Coll Cardiol* 1997;30:1687–1692.

64. Bisi G, Sciagra R, Santoro GM et al. Rest technetium-99m sestamibi tomography in combination with short-term administration of nitrates: feasibility and reliability for prediction of postrevascularization outcome of asynergic territories. *J Am Coll Cardiol* 1994;24:1282–1289.

65. Sciagra R, Pellegri M, Pupi A et al. Prognostic implications of Tc-99m sestamibi viability imaging and subsequent therapeutic strategy in patients with chronic coronary artery disease and left ventricular dysfunction. *J Am Coll Cardiol* 2000;36:739–745.

66. Bax JJ, Poldermans D, Elhendy A et al. Sensitivity, specificity, and predictive accuracies of various noninvasive techniques for detecting hibernating myocardium. *Curr Probl Cardiol* 2001;26:142–186.

67. Poldermans D, Rambaldi R, Bax JJ et al. Safety and utility of atropin addition during dobutamine stress echocardiography for the assessment of viable myocardium in patients with severe left ventricular dysfunction. *Eur Heart J* 1998;19:1712–1718.

68. Van der Wall EE, Bax JJ. Current clinical relevance of cardiovascular magnetic resonance and its relationship to nuclear cardiology. *J Nucl Cardiol* 1999;6:462–469.

69. Baer FM, Voth E, Schneider CA et al. Comparison of low-dose dobutamine-gradient-echo magnetic resonance imaging and positron emission tomography with [18F]fluorodeoxyglucose in patients with chronic coronary artery disease. A functional and morphological approach to the detection of residual myocardial viability. *Circulation* 1995;91:1006–1015.

70. Baer FM, Theissen P, Schneider CA et al. Dobutamine magnetic resonance imaging predicts contractile recovery of chronically dysfunctional myocardium after successful revascularization. *J Am Coll Cardiol* 1998;31:1040–1048.

71. Geskin G, Kramer CM, Rogers WJ et al. Quantitative assessment of myocardial viability after infarction by dobutamine magnetic resonance tagging. *Circulation* 1998;98:217–223.

72. Kim RJ, Wu E, Rafael A et al. The use of contrast-enhanced magnetic resonance imaging to identify reversible myocardial dysfunction. *N Engl J Med* 2000;343:1445–1453.

73. Bax JJ, Maddahi J, Poldermans D et al. Enhanced diagnostic accuracy to predict improvement of LVEF post-revascularization by sequential thallium-201 imaging and dobutamine echocardiography. *J Nucl Med* 1999;40:1P(abst).

74. Dreyfus GD, Duboc D, Blasco A et al. Myocardial viability assessment in ischemic cardiomyopathy: benefits of coronary revascularization. *Ann Thorac Surg* 1994;57:1402–1408.

75. Marwick TH, Zuchowski C, Lauer MS et al. Functional status and quality of life in patients with heart failure undergoing coronary bypass surgery after assessment of myocardial viability. *J Am Coll Cardiol* 1999;33:750–758.

76. DiCarli MF, Asgarzadie F, Schelbert HR et al. Quantitative relation between myocardial viability and improvement in heart failure symp-

toms after revascularization in patients with ischemic cardiomyopathy. *Circulation* 1995;92:3436–3444.

77. Marwick TH, Nemec JJ, Lafont A et al. Prediction by postexercise fluoro-18 deoxyglucose positron emission tomography of improvement in exercise capacity after revascularization. *Am J Cardiol* 1992; 69:854–859.

78. Gunning MG, Chua TP, Harrington D et al. Hibernating myocardium: clinical and functional response to revascularisation. *Eur J Cardio-Thorac Surg* 1997;11:1105–1112.

79. Haas F, Haehnel CJ, Picker W et al. Preoperative positron emission tomographic viability assessment and perioperative and postoperative risk in patients with advanced ischemic heart disease. *J Am Coll Cardiol* 1997;30:1693–1700.

80. Di Carli M, Davidson M, Little R et al. Value of metabolic imaging with positron emission tomography for evaluating prognosis in patients with coronary artery disease and left ventricular dysfunction. *Am J Cardiol* 1994;73:527–533.

81. Eitzman D, Al-Aouar ZR, Kanter HL et al. Clinical outcome of patients with advanced coronary artery disease after viability studies with positron emission tomography. *J Am Coll Cardiol* 1992;20:559–565.

82. Vom Dahl J, Altehoefer C, Sheehan FH et al. Effect of myocardial viability assessed by technetium-99m-sestamibi SPECT and fluorine-18-FDG PET on clinical outcome in coronary artery disease. *J Nucl Med* 1997;38:742–748.

83. Yoshida K, Gould KL. Quantitative relation of myocardial infarct size and myocardial viability by positron emission tomography to left ventricular ejection fraction and 3-year mortality with and without revascularization. *J Am Coll Cardiol* 1993;22:984–987.

84. Lee KS, Marwick TH, Cook SA et al. Prognosis of patients with left ventricular dysfunction, with and without viable myocardium after myocardial infarction. Relative efficacy of medical therapy and revascularization. *Circulation* 1994;90:2687–2694.

85. Pagano D, Lewis ME, Townend JN et al. Coronary revascularization for postischemic heart failure: how myocardial viability affects survival. *Heart* 1999;82:684–688.

86. Tamaki N, Kawamoto M, Takahashi N et al. Prognostic value of an increase in fluorine-18 deoxyglucose uptake in patients with myocardial infarction: comparison with stress thallium imaging. *J Am Coll Cardiol* 1993;22:1621–1627.

87. Gioia G, Powers J, Heo J et al. Prognostic value of rest-redistribution tomographic thallium-201 imaging in ischemic cardiomyopathy. *Am J Cardiol* 1995;75:759–762.

88. Pagley PR, Beller GA, Watson DD et al. Improved outcome after coronary bypass surgery in patients with ischemic cardiomyopathy and residual myocardial viability. *Circulation* 1997;96:793–800.

89. Zafrir N, Leppo JA, Reinhardt CP et al. Thallium reinjection versus standard stress/delay redistribution imaging for prediction of cardiac events. *J Am Coll Cardiol* 1998;31:1280–1285.

90. Cuocolo A, Petretta M, Nicolai E et al. Successful coronary revascularization improves prognosis in patients with previous myocardial infarction and evidence of viable myocardium at thallium-201 imaging. *Eur J Nucl Med* 1998;25:60–68.

91. Chaudhry FA, Tauke JT, Alessandrini RS et al. Prognostic implications of myocardial contractile reserve in patients with coronary artery disease and left ventricular dysfunction. *J Am Coll Cardiol* 1999;34: 730–738.

92. Senior R, Kaul S, Lahiri A. Myocardial viability on echocardiography predicts long-term survival after revascularization in patients with ischemic congestive heart failure. *J Am Coll Cardiol* 1999;33: 1848–1854.

93. Bax JJ, Poldermans D, Elhendy A et al. Improvement of left ventricular ejection fraction, heart failure symptoms and prognosis after revascularization in patients with chronic coronary artery disease and viable myocardium detected by dobutamine stress echocardiography. *J Am Coll Cardiol* 1999;34:163–169.

94. Afridi I, Grayburn PA, Panza J et al. Myocardial viability during dobutamine echocardiography predicts survival in patients with coronary artery disease and severe left ventricular systolic dysfunction. *J Am Coll Cardiol* 1998;32:921–926.

95. Meluzin J, Cerny J, Frelich M et al. Prognostic value of the amount of dysfunctional but viable myocardium in revascularized patients

with coronary artery disease and left ventricular dysfunction. *J Am Coll Cardiol* 1998;32:912–920.

96. Williams MJ, Odabashian J, Laurer MS et al. Prognostic value of dobutamine echocardiography in patients with left ventricular dysfunction. *J Am Coll Cardiol* 1996;27:132–139.

97. Hamarati LB, Schulman LL, Austin JHM. Lung nodules and masses after cardiac transplantation. *Radiology* 1993;188:491–497.

98. Knollmann FD, Hummel M, Hetzer R et al. CT of heart transplant recipients: spectrum of disease. *Radiographics* 2000;20:1637–1648.

99. Mattila PS, Aalto SM, Heikkila L et al. Malignancies after heart transplantation: presence of Epstein-B virus and cytomegalovirus. *Clin Transplant* 2001;15:337–342.

100. Leidig-Bruckner G, Hosch S, Dodidou P et al. Frequency and predictors of osteoporotic fractures after cardiac or liver transplantation: a follow-up study. *Lancet* 2001;357:342–347.

101. Shane E, Rivas MDC, Silverberg SJ et al. Osteoporosis after cardiac transplant. *Am J Med* 1993;94:257–263.

102. Cremer J, Wagenbreth I, Demertzis S et al. Progression of steroid associated osteoporosis following heart transplant. *J Heart Transplant* 1993;12:588.

103. Shane E, Rivas M, McMahon DJ et al. Bone loss and turnover after cardiac transplantation. *J Clin Endocrinol Metab* 1997;82:1497–1506.

104. Thiebaud D, Krieg MA, Gillard-Berguer D et al. Cyclosporine induces high bone turnover and may contribute to bone loss after heart transplantation. *Eur J Clin Invest* 1996;26:549–555.

105. Blake GM, Fogelman I. Bone densitometry and the diagnosis of osteoporosis. *Semin Nucl Med* 2001;31:69–81.

106. Spiegelhalter D, Stovin P. An analyses of repeated biopsies following cardiac transplantation. *Stat Med* 1983;2:33.

107. Wijngaard PL, Doornewaard H, van der Meulen A et al. Cytoimmunologic monitoring as an adjunct in monitoring rejection after heart-transplantation: results of a 6-year follow-up in heart transplant recipients. *J Heart Lung Transplant* 1994;13:869–875.

108. Hammer C, Klanke D, Lersch C et al. Cytoimmunologic monitoring (CIM) for the differentiation between cardiac rejection and viral, bacterial, or fungal infection: its specificity and sensitivity. *Transplant Proc* 1989;21:3631–3633.

109. Iturralde M, Novitzky D, Cooper DK et al. The role of nuclear cardiology procedures in the evaluation of cardiac function following heart transplantation. *Semin Nucl Med* 1988;18:221–240.

110. Hershberger RE, Ni H, Toy W et al. Distribution and declines in cardiac allograft radionuclide left ventricular ejection fractions in relation to late mortality. *J Heart Lung Transplant* 2001;20:417–424.

111. Amende I, Simon R, Seegers A et al. Diastolic dysfunction during acute cardiac allograft rejection. *Circulation* 1990;81(Suppl 3):66–70.

112. Moidl R, Chevtchik O, Simon P et al. Noninvasive monitoring of peak filling rate with acoustic quantification echocardiography accurately detects acute cardiac allograft rejection. *J Heart Lung Transplant* 1999;18:194–201.

113. Yamamoto S, Bergsland J, Michalek SM et al. Uptake of myocardial imaging agents by rejecting and nonrejecting cardiac transplants. A comparative clinical study of thallium-201, technetium-99m, and gallium-67. *J Nucl Med* 1989;30:1464–1469.

114. Addonizio LJ. Detection of cardiac allograft rejection using radionuclide techniques. *Prog Cardiovascul Dis* 1990;33:73–83.

115. Bocchi EA, Mocelin AO, de Moraes AV et al. Comparison between two strategies for rejection detection after heart transplantation: routine endomyocardial biopsy versus gallium-67 cardiac imaging. *Transplant Proc* 1997;29:586–588.

116. Johnson LL, Seldin DW, Becker LC et al. Antimyosin imaging in acute transmural infarctions: results of a multicenter clinical trial. *J Am Coll Cardiol* 1989;13:27–35.

117. Ballester M, Obrador D, Carrio I et al. Indium-111 monoclonal antimyosin antibody studies after the first year of heart transplantation. *Circulation* 1990;82:2100–2108.

118. Ballester M, Bordes R, Tazelaar HD et al. Evaluation of biopsy classification for rejection: relation to detection of myocardial damage by monoclonal antibody imaging. *J Am Coll Cardiol* 1998;31:1357–1361.

119. Puig M, Ballester M, Matias-Guiu X et al. Burden of myocardial damage in cardiac allograft rejection: scintigraphic evidence of myocardial injury and histologic evidence of myocyte necrosis and apoptosis. *J Nucl Cardiol* 2000;7:132–139.

120. Rubin PJ, Hartman JJ, Hasapes JP et al. Detection of cardiac transplant rejection with 111In-labeled lymphocytes and gamma scintigraphy. *Circulation* 1996;94:(9 Suppl):II298–303.

121. Aparici CM, Narula J, Puig M et al. Somatostatin receptor scintigraphy predicts impending cardiac allograft rejection before endomyocardial biopsy. *Eur J Nucl Med* 2000;27:1754–1759.

122. Krivokapich J, Stevenson L, Kobashigawa J et al. Quantification of absolute myocardial perfusion at rest and during exercise with positron emission tomography after human cardiac transplantation. *J Am Coll Cardiol* 1991;18:512–517.

123. Rechavia E, Araujo L, De Silva R et al. Dipyridamole vasodilator response after human orthotopic heart transplantation: quantification by oxygen-15-labeled water and positron emission tomography. *J Am Coll Cardiol* 1992;19:100–106.

124. Senneff MJ, Hartman J, Sobel BE et al. Persistence of coronary vasodilator responsivity after cardiac transplantation. *Am J Cardiol* 1993;71:333–338.

125. McGinn AL, Wilson RF, Olivari MT et al. Coronary vasodilator reserve after orthotopic cardiac transplantation. *Circulation* 1988;78:1200–1209.

126. Nitenberg A, Tavolaro O, Benvenuti C et al. Recovery of a normal coronary vascular reserve after rejection therapy in acute human cardiac allograft rejection. *Circulation* 1990;81:1312–1318.

127. Hoff SJ, Stewart JR, Frist WH et al. Non-invasive detection of heart transplant rejection with positron emission scintigraphy. *Ann Thorac Surg* 1992;53:572–577.

128. Rechavia E, de Silva R, Kushwaha SS et al. Enhanced myocardial 18F-2-fluoro-2-deoxyglucose uptake after orthotopic heart transplantation assessed by positron emission tomography. *J Am Coll Cardiol* 1997;30:533–538.

129. Beckmann N, Hof RP, Rudin M. The role of magnetic resonance imaging and spectroscopy in transplantation: from animal models to man. *NMR Biomed* 2000;13:329–348.

130. Schwitter J, DeMarco T, Kneifel S et al. Magnetic resonance-based assessment of global coronary flow and flow reserve and its relation to left ventricular functional parameters: a comparison with positron emission tomography. *Circulation* 2000;101:2696–2702.

131. Bellenger NG, Marcus NJ, Davies C et al. Left ventricular function and mass after orthotopic heart transplantation: a comparison of cardiovascular magnetic resonance with echocardiography. *J Heart Lung Transplant* 2000;19:444–452.

132. Kanno S, Wu YJ, Lee PC et al. Macrophage accumulation associated with rat cardiac allograft rejection detected by magnetic resonance imaging with ultrasmall superparamagnetic iron oxide particles. *Circulation* 2001;104:934–938.

133. Buchtal SD, Noureuil TO, den Hollander JA et al. 31P-magnetic resonance spectroscopy studies of cardiac transplant patients at rest. *J Cardiovasc Magn Reson* 2000;2:51–56.

134. Pohost GM, Meduri A, Razmi RM et al. Cardiac MR spectroscopy in the new millennium. *Rays* 2001;26:93–107.

135. Johnson DE, Gao SZ, Schroeder JS et al. The spectrum of coronary artery pathological findings in human cardiac allografts. *J Heart Lung Transplant* 1989;8:349–359.

136. Behrendt D, Ganz P, Fang JC. Cardiac allograft vasculopathy. *Curr Opin Cardiol* 2000;15:422–429.

137. Weis M, Pehlivanli S, von Scheidt W. Heart allograft endothelial cell dysfunction. Cause, course and consequences. *Z Kardiol* 2000;89(Suppl 9):X/58–62.

138. Clague JR, Cox ID, Murday AJ et al. Low clinical utility of routine angiographic surveillance in the detection and management of cardiac allograft vasculopathy in transplant recipients. *Clin Cardiol* 2001;24:459–462.

139. Gao SZ, Alderman EL, Schroeder JS et al. Progressive coronary luminal narrowing after cardiac transplantation. *Circulation* 1990;82(Suppl 4):IV269–IV275.

140. Valantine H, Pinto FJ, St Goar FG et al. Intracoronary ultrasound imaging in heart transplant recipients: the Stanford experience. *J Heart Lung Transplant* 1992;11:S60–S64.

141. Mazur W, Bitar JN, Young JB et al. Progressive deterioration of coronary flow reserve after heart transplantation. *Am Heart J* 1998;136:504–509.

142. Julius BK, Attenhoffer JCH, Sutsch G et al. Incidence, progression and functional significance of cardiac allograft vasculopathy after heart transplantation. *Transplantation* 2000;69:847–853.

143. Rodney RA, Johnson LL. Myocardial perfusion scintigraphy to assess heart transplant vasculopathy. *J Heart Lung Transplant* 1992;11:S74–S78.

144. Elhendy A, Sozzi FB, van Domburg RT et al. Accuracy of dobutamine tetrofosmin myocardial perfusion imaging for the noninvasive diagnosis of transplant coronary artery stenosis. *J Heart Lung Transplant* 2000;19:360–366.

145. Carlsen J, Toft JC, Mortensen SA et al. Myocardial perfusion scintigraphy as a screening method for significant coronary artery stenosis in cardiac transplant recipients. *J Heart Lung Transplant* 2000;19:873–878.

146. Zhao XM, Delbeke D, Sandler MP et al. N-13-ammonia positron emission tomography (PET) to detect allograft coronary artery disease after heart transplantation: comparison with coronary angiography. *J Nucl Med* 1995;36:982–987.

147. Allen-Auerbach M, Schoder H, Johnson J et al. Relationship between coronary function by positron emission tomography and temporal changes in morphology by intravascular ultrasound (IVUS) in transplant recipients. *J Heart Lung Transplant* 1999;18:211–219.

148. Rowan RA, Billingham ME. Myocardial innervation in long-term cardiac transplant survivors: a quantitative ultrastructural survey. *J Heart Transplant* 1988;7:448–452.

149. Gerber BL, Bernard X, Melin JA et al. Exaggerated chronotropic and energetic response to dobutamine after orthopic cardiac transplantation. *J Heart Lung Transplant* 2001;20:824–832.

150. Schwaiger M, Hutchins GD, Kalff V et al. Evidence for regional catecholamine uptake and storage sites in the transplanted human heart by positron emission tomography. *J Clin Invest* 1991;87:1681–1690.

151. Bengel FM, Ueberfuhr P, Schiepel N et al. Effect of sympathetic reinnervation on cardiac performance after heart transplantation. *N Engl J Med* 2001;345:731–738.

152. Khan SU, Salloum J, O'Donovan PB et al. Acute pulmonary edema after lung transplantation: the pulmonary reimplantation response. *Chest* 1999;116:187–194.

153. Alvarez A, Algar J, Santos F et al. Airway complications after lung transplantation: a review of 151 anastomoses. *Eur J Cardiothorac Surg* 2001;19:381–387.

154. McAdams HP, Palmer SM, Erasmuss JJ et al. Bronchial anastomotic complications in lung transplant recipients: virtual bronchoscopy for non-invasive assessment. *Radiology* 1998;209:689–695.

155. Schlueter JJ, Semenkovich JW, Glazer HS et al. Bronchial dehiscence after lung transplantation: correlation of CT findings with clinical outcome. *Radiology* 1996;199:849–854.

156. Alexander BD, Tapson VF. Infectious complications of lung transplantation. *Transpl Infect Dis* 2001;3:128–137.

157. Glanville AR, Imoto E, Billingham ME et al. The role of right ventricular endomyocardial biopsy in the long-term management of heart-lung transplant recipients. *J Heart Transplant* 1987;6:357–360.

158. Sleiman C, Groussard O, Mal H et al. Clinical use of transbronchial biopsy in single-lung transplantation. *Transplantation* 1991;51:927–929.

159. Ottulana BA, Higenbottam JP, Scott JP et al. Pulmonary function monitoring allows diagnosis of rejection in heart-lung transplant recipients. *Transplant Proc* 1989;21:2583–2584.

160. Herman SJ, Weisbrod GL, Weisbrod GA et al., The Toronto Lung Transplant Group. Chest radiographic findings after bilateral lung transplantation. *AJR* 1989;153:1181–1185.

161. Bergin CJ, Castellino RA, Blank N et al. Acute lung rejection after heart-lung transplantation: correlation of findings on chest radiographs with lung biopsy results. *AJR* 1990;155:23–27.

162. Kundu S, Herman SJ, Larhs A et al. Correlation of chest radiographic findings with biopsy-proven acute lung rejection. *J Thorac Imaging* 1999;14:178–184.

163. Gotway MB, Dawn SK, Sellami D et al. Acute rejection following lung transplantation: limitations in accuracy of thin-section CT for diagnosis. *Radiology* 2001;221:207–212.

164. Lisbona R, Hakim TS, Dean GW et al. Regional pulmonary perfusion following human heart-lung transplantation. *J Nucl Med* 1989;30:1297–1301.

165. Kramer MR, Marshall SE, McDougall IR et al. The distribution of ventilation and perfusion after single-lung transplantation in patients with pulmonary fibrosis and pulmonary hypertension. *Transplant Proc* 1991;23:1215–1216.

166. Stevens PM, Johnson PC, Bell RL et al. Regional ventilation and perfusion after lung transplantation in patients with emphysema. *N Engl J Med* 1970;282:245–249.

167. Veith FJ, Koerner SK, Siegelman SS et al. Single lung transplantation in experimental and human emphysema. *Ann Surg* 1973;178:463–475.

168. Mal H, Andreassian B, Pamela F et al. Unilateral lung transplantation in end-stage pulmonary emphysema. *Am Rev Respir Dis* 1989;140:797–802.

169. Trulock EP, Ettinger NA, Brunt EM et al. The role of transbronchial lung biopsy in the treatment of lung transplant recipients: an analysis of 200 consecutive procedures. *Chest* 1992;102:1049–1054.

170. Hansen PR, Holm AM, Svendsen UG et al. Apoptosis in acute pulmonary allograft rejection and cytomegalovirus infection. *APMIS* 1999;107:529–533.

171. Kemerink GJ, Liem IH, Hofsra L et al. Patient dosimetry of intravenously administered ^{99m}Tc-annexin V. *J Nucl Med* 2001;42:382–387.

172. Blankenberg FG, Robbins RC, Stoot JH et al. Radionuclide imaging of acute lung transplant rejection with annexin V. *Chest* 2000;117:834–840.

173. Blankenberg FG, Strauss HW. Non-invasive diagnosis of acute heart- or lung-transplant rejection using radiolabeled annexin V. *Pediatr Radiol* 1999;29:299–305.

174. Kanno S, Lee PC, Dodd SJ et al. A novel approach with magnetic resonance imaging used for the detection of lung allograft rejection. *J Thorac Cardiovasc Surg* 2000;120:923–934.

175. Yousem SA, Burke CM, Billingham ME. Pathologic pulmonary alterations in long-term human heart-lung transplantation. *Hum Pathol* 1985;16:911.

176. Heng D, Sharples LD, McNeil K et al. Bronchiolitis obliterans syndrome: incidence, natural history, prognosis, and risk factors. *J Heart Lung Transplant* 1998;17:1255–1263.

177. Scott JP, Whitehead B, de Leval M et al. Pediatric incidence of acute rejection and obliterative bronchiolitis: a comparison with adults. *Transpl Int* 1994;7(Suppl 1):S404–S406.

178. Morrish WF, Herman SJ, Weisbrod GL et al. Bronchiolitis obliterans after lung transplantation: findings at chest radiography and high-resolution CT. The Toronto Lung Transplant Group. *Radiology* 1991;179:487–490.

179. Hardoff R, Steinmetz AP, Krausz Y et al. The prognostic value of perfusion lung scintigraphy in patients who underwent single-lung transplantation for emphysema and pulmonary fibrosis. *J Nucl Med* 2000;41:1771–1776.

180. Radio S, Wood S, Wilson J et al. Allograft vascular disease: comparison of heart and other grafted organs. *Transplant Proc* 1996;28:496–499.

Diagnostic Nuclear Medicine, Fourth Edition. Edited by M.P. Sandler, R.E. Coleman, J.A. Patton, F.J.Th. Wackers, A. Gottschalk. Lippincott Williams & Wilkins, Philadelphia 2003.

53

LIVER TRANSPLANTATION

ROBERT J. BOUDREAU
CHRISTOPHER C. KUNI

The first human liver transplantation was performed in 1963 by Starzl (1). Initial attempts at liver transplantation were unsuccessful, and the procedure did not gain widespread acceptance until the 1980s. Since that time more than 18,000 liver transplantations have been performed in approximately 160 centers worldwide (2). Improved surgical techniques and effective immunosuppression led to improved patient and graft survival (3, 4). The rate of rejection has been reduced to 10% to 15% (5).

Although acute rejection is a serious problem, the liver is unique among solid organ allografts in its long-term behavior. If liver recipients survive with well-functioning grafts until the end of the second postoperative year, they tend to stabilize for the long term (6). Chronic rejection, a lingering problem for kidney, heart, and pancreas grafts, is less commonly seen. However, the biggest problem facing liver organ transplantation is neither rejection nor technical problems. The pool of recipients expands while the availability of organs declines because of improved road safety standards. Organ availability has now become the limiting factor for liver transplantation (4). The use of marginal donors and reduced size or split grafts has temporarily alleviated some of the organ shortage, but it is unlikely that organ supply will be able to keep pace with the long-term demand (7). Because there is no end-stage life-support mechanism for liver failure analogous to renal dialysis, organ availability problems will likely restrict liver transplantation for the foreseeable future (8). Approximately 20 transplants per year are necessary to maintain institutional competence. This requirement, coupled with economic pressures, will likely restrict the procedure to specialized centers in the future (9).

Currently, most appropriate liver transplant candidates are patients with end-stage liver disease that is not secondary to a malignancy and that is unlikely to improve. These criteria make cirrhosis the main indication for the procedure, followed by other pediatric liver diseases and malignancy (8). In the pediatric age group, the major indication for liver transplantation is extrahepatic biliary atresia, which constitutes 50% of the referrals in children. Less common pediatric indications include acute hepatitis, cirrhosis, and tyrosinemia (9). In adults, the most common diseases leading to liver transplantation are primary biliary cirrhosis, chronic hepatitis, sclerosing cholangitis, acute hepatic failure, and metabolic disorders (10,11). In recent years, the number of patients receiving transplants for fulminant hepatitis and retransplantation has increased, with a smaller increase for alcoholic cirrhosis. Hepatocellular and metastatic malignancies have shown a small decline in the number of patients.

Even though liver transplantation is an uncommon procedure, patients undergoing the procedure are frequently imaged. Physicians interpreting these studies must understand the procedure and its complications so that they can make a meaningful contribution to the subspecialized team managing these patients. In this chapter, the surgical procedure and its complications are discussed. The role of radionuclide imaging is to identify the complications of the procedure so that they can be effectively treated. Table 53.1 lists the commonly observed complications of liver transplantation.

SURGICAL TECHNIQUE

The liver transplantation procedure has been previously described in some detail elsewhere (10–12), and only the commonest techniques are described here. In Figure 53.1 an orthotopic liver transplantation using a choledochojejunostomy is shown. Figure 53.2 shows the alternate biliary reconstruction,

Table 53.1. *Complications Among 56 Liver Graft Recipients*

Item	No. of occurrences[a]	No. of deaths[b]
Rejection	30	5
Infection	27	12
Vascular compromise	7	3
Bile duct stenosis	6	2
Tumor (recurrent)	2	2
Biliary leak	2	1
Hemorrhage	1	0

[a]Most patients had more than one complication.
[b]Indicates principal cause of death.
From Loken MK, Ascher NL, Boudreau RJ, Najarian JS. Scintigraphic evaluation of liver transplant function. *J Nucl Med* 1986;27:451–459, with permission.

R.J. Boudreau: Radiology, Division of Nuclear Medicine, University of Minnesota, MN.
C.C. Kuni: Department of Radiology, University of Colorado Health System, University Hospital, Denver, CO.

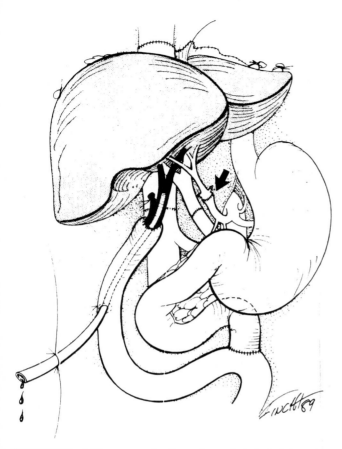

FIGURE 53.1. A biliary reconstruction using a choledochojejunostomy is shown. This type of anastomosis is used when the recipient's common bile duct is diseased or absent. The donor bile duct is anastomosed over a drainage tube that is externalized through the Roux-en-Y limb of jejunum. (From Letourneau JG, Hunter DW, Payne WD et al. Pictorial essay. Imaging of and intervention for biliary complications after hepatic transplantation. *AJR* 1990;154:729–733, with permission.)

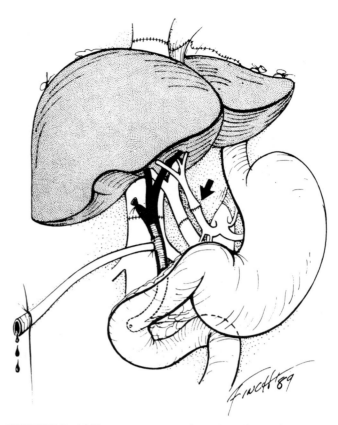

FIGURE 53.2. A biliary tract reconstruction using a duct to duct anastomosis is shown. This type of anastomosis is also called a choledochocholedochostomy. It is used when the recipient common bile duct is not diseased. (From Letourneau JG, Hunter DW, Payne WD et al. Pictorial essay. Imaging of and intervention for biliary complications after hepatic transplantation. *AJR* 1990;154:729–733, with permission.)

a choledochocholedochostomy. The choledochojejunostomy is more commonly performed in children, and it is used when the recipient common bile duct is diseased or absent. The duct-to-duct anastomosis shown in Fig. 53.2 can be used only when the recipient has a bile duct that is not diseased (11). In the early 1980s, other types of anastomoses were performed, including those using the gallbladder as a conduit. The arterial and venous anastomoses can be surgically challenging because of limited exposure. Recognizing and treating vascular complications is an important part of the management of these patients postoperatively.

A recent development is the use of split or partial organ grafts that are primarily used in children (8,9,13). Split grafts refer to the use of one liver for two recipients. Reduced-size grafts are used when the liver is too large for the recipient. Obviously, if a partial or reduced-size allograft is used, it will have an unusual appearance scintigraphically. The exact surgical procedure should be discussed with the team before making an evaluation of an unusual appearing graft. Results of split organ grafting do not appear as favorable as results with whole organs at this time

(4,6,8). Recent reductions in surgical risk have allayed ethical objections to harvesting a portion or the entire left hepatic lobe from living donors (14). Another variation that may be encountered is a heterotopic liver transplant, also termed an auxiliary partial liver transplantation (15,16).

Currently, patient survival following whole organ transplantation is good, with an adult rate now approaching or surpassing 80% at 1 year (2,9). In the pediatric age group, normal growth and development patterns can occur following transplantation, including catch-up growth (9). However, more data and long-term follow-up are needed in this area. The 1-year pediatric survival figures range between 60% and 80% at active centers.

NUCLEAR MEDICINE TECHNIQUES

The contribution of nuclear medicine to these patients' management is extremely important and perhaps not widely appreciated. With the exception of the anatomic surgical variations described earlier, the performance and interpretation of radionuclide hepatobiliary imaging studies in liver allograft recipients do not differ significantly from patients with other vascular, hepatocellular, or biliary tract diseases. Several radiopharmaceuticals have been used historically for the evaluation of liver transplants (1).

---

^{99m}Tc-diisopropyliminodiacetic acid (DISIDA) or ^{99m}Tc-mebrofenin are the radiopharmaceuticals of choice. Both of these tracers show a high affinity for the hepatocyte uptake mechanism and provide useful information about the hepatobiliary system even when liver function is marginal.

Anterior images are obtained at 5, 10, 15, 30, 45, and 60 minutes after injection of 6 mCi of ^{99m}Tc-DISIDA. Oblique views are optional because the gallbladder is not present in a transplanted liver. When severe cholestasis exists, delayed images are obtained as late as 24-hours postinjection. One million counts should be obtained for the first image, and subsequent images are acquired for the same duration as the first image. This protocol allows adequate assessment of the changes in liver parenchymal intensity with time. Several authors have advocated the use of quantitative techniques (1,17–20). These methods may be useful, but whether they offer significant advantage over nonquantitative or semiquantitative approaches remains to be seen. The complexity of the transplanted liver, in which hepatocellular diseases ranging from rejection to hepatitis can be intermingled with both intrahepatic and extrahepatic cholestasis, confounds the ability to differentiate pathologic conditions based on quantitative analysis alone. The primary pathologic processes being imaged affect either initial uptake (hepatocellular blood flow and function) or transit time (tracer excretion through the biliary system), both of which can be visually assessed. Adequate clinical results can be obtained by visual analysis of the images, and sophisticated quantitative analysis is not essential for patient management (1,10,21–24).

NORMALLY FUNCTIONING TRANSPLANT

The integrity of the hepatocytes can be estimated by examination of the 5-minute image. If hepatocyte function is normal, the 5-minute image will not reveal any cardiac blood pool activity. This guideline assumes that the image is properly exposed and that the image contrast is appropriately adjusted for hepatic scintigraphy (11). The hepatic parenchyma reaches its maximum intensity 12 ± 2 minutes following radiopharmaceutical administration in a fasting subject, and one third or less of the activity remains 1-hour postinjection. The large intrahepatic bile ducts, common bile duct, or intestine are usually visualized within 12 ± 6 minutes following radiopharmaceutical administration in the fasting subject. Excretion is somewhat faster postprandial. Thus, by examining the images carefully, one can extract useful semiquantitative measures of hepatocyte function and biliary excretion (23,24). A normal study is illustrated in Fig. 53.3.

SURGICAL COMPLICATIONS

Vascular

Because of the complexity of the vascular supply of the liver, it is at risk for several complications including hepatic artery thrombosis or stenosis, portal vein thrombosis or stenosis, and rarely inferior vena cava occlusion (1,25). Vascular compromise was the third most common cause of complications in the pa-

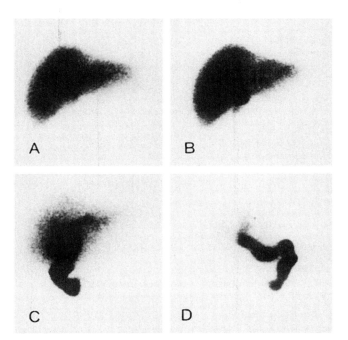

FIGURE 53.3. Normally functioning transplant at **(A)** 5 minutes (*anterior*), **(B)** 10 minutes (*anterior*), **(C)** 30 minutes (*anterior*), and **(D)** 30 minutes (*right lateral*). The cardiac blood pool is invisible at 5 and 10 minutes, indicating normal extraction. Radioactive bile is first seen outside the liver by 10 minutes. Parenchymal intensity decreases appropriately with time.

tients studied at the University of Minnesota (Table 53.1). Dominguez et al. (26) reported a 20% frequency of vascular complications in their experience. Hepatic artery thrombosis is the most common and serious vascular complication that occurs in the early postoperative course (25). In the allograft, the bile duct is totally dependent on the donor hepatic artery for its blood supply. Unless retransplantation occurs, the resulting mortality from hepatic artery thrombosis because of common duct necrosis and sepsis is high. Portal venous and inferior vena cava complications are less frequent, although they can occur. Scintigraphy of these complications will depend on the distribution of the vascular compromise and consists of decreased tracer uptake in regions of decreased perfusion. The diagnosis is often made through a combination of ultrasonic, angiographic, and scintigraphic examinations. Doppler ultrasound is an excellent method to screen for the presence of hepatic artery thrombosis or other vascular complications, although all imaging modalities are capable of identifying the secondary parenchymal manifestations of necrosis (25,27,28).

The sensitivity of duplex sonography for the diagnosis of hepatic artery thrombosis has been challenged. McDiarmid et al. (29) reported that only 7 of 13 grafts with hepatic artery thrombosis would have been diagnosed if only the duplex sonogram results were considered. They hypothesize that duplex ultrasound signals were detected from a network of collaterals and misinterpreted as hepatic arterial flow. This problem occurs more often in the pediatric than in the adult population because these collaterals do not form in the older age groups (30). Thus, there still is a role for the scintigraphic examination in suspected high-risk patients. In addition, the scintigraphic examination will provide information concerning the integrity of the common bile duct.

Scintigraphic findings for vascular compromise may be focal or regional and may result in nonspecific hepatocyte dysfunction. The situation is confounded by the dual blood supply of the liver. Nevertheless, the demonstration of reasonably good hepatocyte uptake is a very good indicator of intact vascular grafts and patients routinely have one postoperative ^{99m}Tc-DISIDA study for this purpose. In Figure 53.4, a hepatobiliary study following transplantation shows multiple focal defects. The patient eventually died and autopsy revealed both hepatic artery and portal vein thrombosis along with regional hepatic necrosis.

Biliary Leakage and Obstruction

Hepatobiliary scintigraphy is an exquisitely sensitive method to detect leakage of radioactive material outside the liver and bile ducts (31). Although the detection of the leak is straightforward, its localization is much more difficult and often requires special views. Scintigraphy reveals egress of tracer to either a loculated nonphysiologic location or freely into the peritoneal space (32). Often, delayed imaging is necessary to differentiate excretion into the gut from leakage into the peritoneal cavity. Causes of leakage include breakdown of the common bile duct anastomosis and removal of T-tubes. A case of scintigraphic detection of

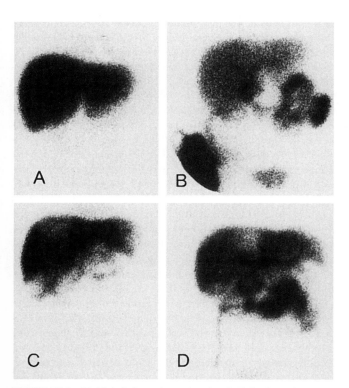

FIGURE 53.4. Multiple infarcts (*anterior views*). Eight days after transplantation, acquisitions at **(A)** 5 minutes and **(B)** 60 minutes show normal extraction and mild intrahepatic cholestasis. **(C)** 5-minute and **(D)** 60-minute images done 6 days later show several regions of decreased uptake.

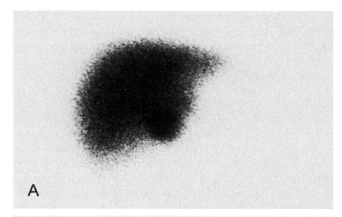

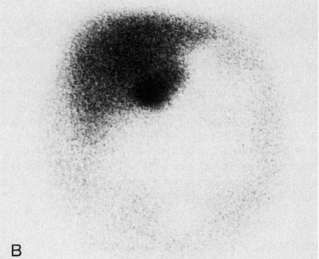

FIGURE 53.5. Bile leak at **(A)** 5 minutes and **(B)** 60 minutes (*anterior views*). Radioactivity is entering ascites in the peritoneum from an anastomotic leak near the liver hilum.

bile leakage is shown in Fig. 53.5. Invasive techniques such as cholangiography are usually necessary to define the exact anatomic location and etiology of the problem.

Biliary obstruction occurs secondary to stricture, T-tube kinking, or occlusion of a biliary stent. If a T-tube is in place, a T-tube cholangiogram is usually the method of choice to evaluate the biliary tract. However, scintigraphy is the only physiologic method that evaluates bile flow without the artifacts associated with injection of contrast under pressure. Scintigraphy can be performed either with or without the T-tube clamped to determine the preferential physiologic drainage route. The T-tube should not be clamped without discussing the case with the referring surgeon, because the integrity of the common bile duct could be compromised. A case of biliary tract obstruction is shown in Fig. 53.6. Hepatobiliary imaging also plays an important role following the interventional management of bile strictures by dilatation or stenting. The sensitivity and specificity of scintigraphy in diagnosing posttransplant biliary strictures are 62% and 64% when retrograde cholangiography is used as the gold standard (33). These somewhat disappointing figures are

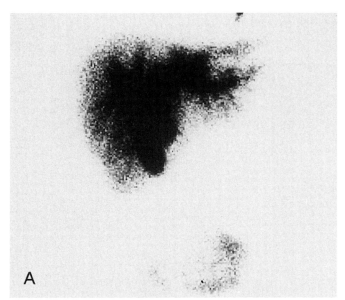

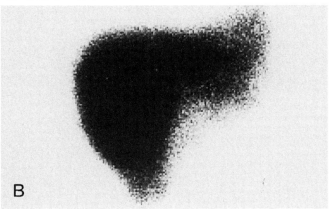

documented episode (Table 53.1). Acute rejection is also a common serious complication (28). Differentiation of rejection from other causes of allograft dysfunction based on scintigraphic criteria alone may be difficult (23,24). The scintigraphic evaluation of hepatocyte uptake and biliary excretion correlates well with the histopathologic findings of hepatocyte damage and cholestasis, respectively. Different histologic findings in rejection (portal inflammation, bile duct damage, and endotheliitis) versus intrahepatic cholestasis (bile collections in Kupffer cells, hepatocytes, bile ductules, and bile ducts) raised hopes that scintigraphy might distinguish between these conditions. Unfortunately, excretion on scintigraphy is abnormal in both rejection and intrahepatic cholestasis without rejection, whereas hepatocyte uptake tends to be relatively normal in both conditions (Fig. 53.7). Scintigraphy is useful, however, in differentiating rejection or intrahepatic cholestasis from other causes of liver failure, such as vascular insufficiency and extrahepatic partial biliary obstruction.

The literature does not support any other imaging modality as being specific for the diagnosis of rejection. Doppler ultrasonography was initially promoted as being able to diagnose rejection based on the loss of diastolic flow. Longley et al. (38) found that there was no significant difference in the proportion of acute allograft rejection present in a group lacking diastolic flow, compared with those with normal diastolic flow. They concluded that loss of hepatic artery diastolic flow has no clinical application for the diagnosis of acute hepatic allograft rejection. Others have confirmed these poor results (39,40). Similarly, the CT finding of a low attenuation periportal collar has been found to be an unreliable indicator of acute allograft rejection (41).

The lack of a sufficiently accurate imaging test to diagnose rejection has left the liver biopsy as the procedure of choice for the management of these patients. The difficulties that diagnostic imaging encounters in diagnosing acute rejection are probably related to the fact that both hepatocyte damage and intrahepatic cholestasis are histopathologic features of acute and chronic rejection. The cholestatic component is often the most prominent finding that leads to the scintigraphic pattern, albeit nonspecific, of decreased uptake with prolonged parenchymal transit. In contrast, purely hepatocellular diseases such as hepatitis usually spare the excretory function and have a relatively normal transit time, despite the reduced uptake. The situation is always complex in the liver allograft in which superimposed drug effects, along with the previously mentioned common bile duct complications, can all coexist. An example of a hepatobiliary study showing rejection is shown in Fig. 53.8.

HEPATIC INFECTION AND ABSCESS

Infection is a common problem in any transplant patient and is related to effective immunosuppression. Computed tomography (CT) or ultrasound examinations are the initial procedures of choice for a patient with a suspected infection because they can readily detect abscess formation and are helpful in definitive management by aspiration and culture (25,42,43). The role of nuclear medicine in the investigation of these patients is secondary. Infection must be considered in the differential diagnosis

FIGURE 53.6. Biliary obstruction. Anterior views at **(A)** 5 minutes and **(B)** 60 minutes show normal extraction, dilated intrahepatic bile ducts, and delayed appearance of radioactivity outside the liver.

misleading in that scintigraphy estimates bile flow rather than anatomic detail. Scintigraphy augmented by challenge with amyl nitrate or nifedipine can be used to more accurately distinguish anatomic stricture from Oddi's sphincter dysfunction caused by denervation (34,35). In fact, it is one of the more common indications for hepatobiliary imaging at our institution.

Although sonography is helpful in the evaluation of biliary tract complications, it is limited in the early detection of these abnormalities after liver transplantation. In one report, sonography was only abnormal in 22 of 41 cases with biliary tract abnormalities (36). Morton et al. (37) also found that ultrasound was more helpful in evaluating vascular flow than biliary tract complications.

REJECTION

Rejection is a common complication observed after transplantation, with approximately 50% of the patients experiencing one

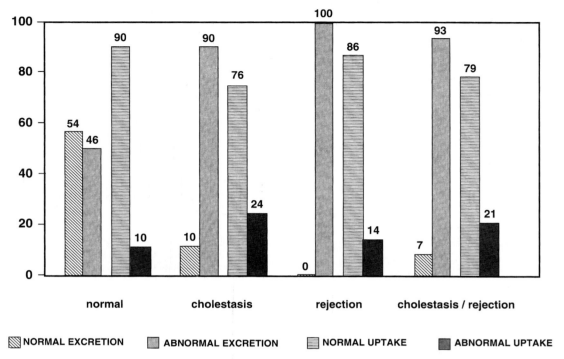

BIOPSY RESULTS

FIGURE 53.7. Biopsy results in a series of liver transplant patients. The bars indicate percentages of scintigraphic findings of normal or abnormal uptake and excretion for each biopsy result. Scintigraphy is a sensitive, but nonspecific, indicator of transplant pathology. Rejection and other causes of cholestasis show relatively normal uptake and abnormal excretion. Biopsy failed to reveal the cause of abnormal excretion in a significant fraction of cases.

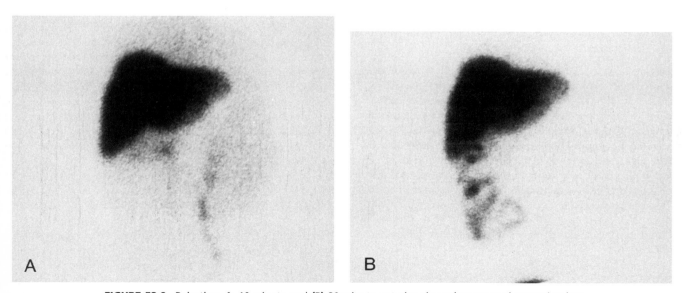

FIGURE 53.8. Rejection. **A:** 10-minute and **(B)** 30-minute anterior views show normal extraction but delayed appearance of extrahepatic radioactive bile along with abnormal retention of parenchymal radioactivity. These findings are identical to those of intrahepatic cholestasis of other causes. (From Kuni CC, Engeler CM, Nakhleh RE et al. Correlation of technetium-99m-DISIDA hepatobiliary studies with biopsies in liver transplant patients. *J Nucl Med* 1991;32:1545–1547, with permission.)

of a parenchymal defect in the liver, which may also be related to an abscess (44), hematoma, or vascular compromise. If a photon-deficient defect fills with tracer, it is more likely to be a biloma than an abscess. The findings of diffuse liver infection are related to abnormal hepatocyte function that usually manifests itself as reduced initial uptake with a relatively normal parenchymal transit time. The use of ^{111}In-labeled white blood cells for these patients has not been evaluated, but the results would likely be similar to other patient groups.

SUMMARY

Liver transplantation is used for the treatment of life-threatening, irreversible liver failure. The most common diseases leading to transplantation are cirrhosis in adults and extrahepatic biliary atresia in children. Knowledge of the surgical technique and its complications are important in the interpretation of scintigrams. Most liver transplantations use whole cadaveric organs with a choledochocholedochostomy or choledochojejunostomy. Imaging with ^{99m}Tc-DISIDA or ^{99m}Tc-mebrofenin is used to evaluate hepatocyte function and perfusion and biliary excretion, but accurate differentiation of rejection from intrahepatic cholestasis without rejection is not yet possible. Scintigraphy is very sensitive in the detection of bile leaks and obstruction, but the precise localization of a leak may be difficult to determine.

REFERENCES

1. Hawkins RA, Hall T, Gambhir SS et al. Radionuclide evaluation of liver transplants. *Semin Nucl Med* 1988;18:199–212.
2. Höckerstedt K. Liver transplantation: present results and problems. *Ann Med* 1992;24:325–328.
3. Ascher NL. Immunosuppression and rejection in liver transplantation. *Transplant Proc* 1993;25:1744–1745.
4. Shorrock C, Neuberger J. The changing face of liver transplantation. *Gut* 1993;34:295–298.
5. Stieber AC, Gordon RD, Galloway JR. Orthotopic liver transplantation. In: Zakim D, Boyer TD, eds. *Hepatology. A text book of liver disease.* Philadelphia: WB Saunders, 1996:1759–1780.
6. Sheil AG. Quandaries and controversies in liver transplantation. *Transplant Proc* 1992;24:2375–2378.
7. Bronsther O, Fung JJ, Izakis A et al. Prioritization and organ distribution for liver transplantation. *JAMA* 1994;271:140–143.
8. Bismuth H, Azoulay D, Dennison A. Recent developments in liver transplantation. *Transplant Proc* 1993;25:2191–2194.
9. Superina RA. Liver transplantation in children: an update. *Surg Ann* 1992;24:195–226.
10. Loken MK, Ascher NL, Boudreau RJ et al. Scintigraphic evaluation of liver transplant function. *J Nucl Med* 1986;27:451–459.
11. Letourneau JG, Day DL, Ascher NL, eds. *Radiology of organ transplantation.* St. Louis: Mosby Year Book, 1991:159–225.
12. Letourneau JG, Hunter DW, Payne WD et al. Pictorial essay. Imaging of and intervention for biliary complications after hepatic transplantation. *AJR* 1990;154:729–733.
13. Zonderland HM, Lameris JS, Terpstra OT et al. Auxiliary partial liver transplantation: imaging evaluation in 10 patients. *AJR* 1989;153:981–985.
14. Kawasaki S, Makuuchi M, Matsunami H et al. Living related liver transplantation in adults. *Ann Surg* 1998;227:269–274.
15. Blankensteijn JD, Schalm SW, Terpstra OT. New aspects of heterotopic liver transplantation. *Transpl Int* 1992;5:43–50.
16. Sudan DL, Shaw BW Jr, Fox IJ et al. Long-term followup of auxiliary

17. Woodle ES, Ward RE, Stadalnik RC et al. Tc-NGA imaging in liver transplantation: preliminary clinical experience. *Surgery* 1989;1050:401–407.
18. Brown PH, Juni JE, Lieberman DA et al. Hepatocyte versus biliary disease: a distinction by deconvolutional analysis of technetium-99m IDA time-activity curves. *J Nucl Med* 1988;29:623–630.
19. Brunot B, Petras S, Germain P et al. Biopsy and quantitative hepatobiliary scintigraphy in the evaluation of liver transplantation. *J Nucl Med* 1994;35:1321–1327.
20. Erkman M, Fjalling M, Friman S et al. Liver uptake function measured by IODIDA clearance rate in liver transplant patients and healthy volunteers. *Nucl Med Commun* 1996;17:235–242.
21. Rossleigh MA, McCaughan GW, Gallagher ND et al. The role of nuclear medicine in liver transplantation. *Med J Aust* 1988;148:561–563.
22. Brown RK, Memsic LD, Busuttil RW et al. Accurate demonstration of hepatic infarction in liver transplant recipients. *J Nucl Med* 1986;27:1428–1431.
23. Kuni CC, Engeler CM, Nakhleh RE et al. Correlation of technetium-99m-DISIDA hepatobiliary studies with biopsies in liver transplant patients. *J Nucl Med* 1991;32:1545–1547.
24. Engeler CM, Kuni CC, Nakhleh RE et al. Liver transplant rejection and cholestasis: comparison of technetium 99m-diisopropyl iminodiacetic acid hepatobiliary imaging with liver biopsy. *Eur J Nucl Med* 1992;19:865–870.
25. Davis PL, Van Thiel DH, Zajko AB et al. Imaging in hepatic transplantation. *Semin Liver Dis* 1989;9:90–101.
26. Dominguez R, Young LW, Ledesma-Medina J et al. Pediatric liver transplantation. Part II. Diagnostic imaging in postoperative management. *Radiology* 1985;157:339–344.
27. Pariente D, Rion JY, Schmit P et al. Variability of clinical presentation of hepatic artery thrombosis in pediatric liver transplantation: role of imaging modalities. *Pediatr Radiol* 1990;20:253–257.
28. Oliver JH, Federle MP, Campbell WL et al. Imaging the hepatic transplant. *Radiol Clin North Am* 1991;29:1285–1298.
29. McDiarmid SV, Hall TR, Grant EG et al. Failure of duplex sonography to diagnose hepatic artery thrombosis in a high-risk group of pediatric liver transplant recipients. *Transplant Proc* 1990;22:1529–1530.
30. Hall TR, McDiarmid SV, Grant EG et al. False-negative duplex Doppler studies in children with hepatic artery thrombosis after liver transplantation. *AJR* 1990;154:573–575.
31. Sandoval B, Goettler C, Robinson A et al. Cholescintigraphy in the diagnosis of bile leak after laparoscopic cholecystectomy. *Am Surg* 1997;63:611–616.
32. Scott-Smith W, Raftery AT, Wright EP et al. Tc-99m labeled HIDA imaging in suspected biliary leaks after liver transplantation. *Clin Nucl Med* 1983;8:478–479.
33. Kurzawinski T, Selves L, Farouk M et al. Prospective study of hepatobiliary scintigraphy and endoscopic cholangiography for the detection of early biliary complications after orthotopic liver transplantation. *Br J Surg* 1997;84:620–623.
34. Madacsy L, Velosy B, Lonovics J et al. Differentiation between organic stenosis and functional dyskineasia of the sphincter of Oddi with amyl nitrite-augmented quantitative hepatobiliary scintigraphy. *Eur J Nucl Med* 1994;21:203–208.
35. Bhatnagar A. Nifedipine interventional cholescintigraphy. A new method for assessing sphincter of Oddi? *Indian J Nucl Med* 1997;12:93–96.
36. Zemel G, Zajko AB, Skolnick ML et al. The role of sonography and transhepatic cholangiography in the diagnosis of biliary complications after liver transplantation. *AJR* 1988;151:943–946.
37. Morton MJ, James EM, Wiesner RH et al. Applications of duplex ultrasonography in the liver transplant patient. *Mayo Clin Proc* 1990;65:360–372.
38. Longley DG, Skolnick ML, Sheahan DG. Acute allograft rejection in liver transplant recipients: lack of correlation with loss of hepatic artery diastolic flow. *Radiology* 1988;169:417–420.
39. Marder DM, DeMarino GB, Sumkin JH et al. Liver transplant rejec-

tion: value of the resistive index in Doppler US of hepatic arteries. *Radiology* 1989;173:127–129.

40. Kubota K, Billing H, Eriezon BG et al. Duplex Doppler ultrasonography for monitoring liver transplants. *Acta Radiol* 1990;31:279–283.

41. Stevens SD, Heiken JP, Brunt E et al. Low-attenuation periportal collar in transplanted liver is not reliable CT evidence of acute allograft rejection. *AJR* 1991;157:1195–1198.

42. Dupuy D, Costello P, Lewis D et al. Abdominal CT findings after liver transplantation in 66 patients. *AJR* 1991;156:1167–1170.

43. Letourneau JG. Radiology of hepatic transplantation. *Crit Rev Diagn Imaging* 1990;30:281–315.

44. Brown RK, Memsic LD, Pusey EJ et al. Hepatic abscess in liver transplantation. Accurate diagnosis and treatment. *Clin Nucl Med* 1986; 11:233–236.

Diagnostic Nuclear Medicine, Fourth Edition. Edited by M.P. Sandler, R.E. Coleman, J.A. Patton, F.J.Th. Wackers, A. Gottschalk. Lippincott Williams & Wilkins, Philadelphia 2003.

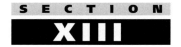

PEDIATRICS

54

NUCLEAR MEDICINE IN PEDIATRIC NEPHROLOGY AND UROLOGY

MASSOUD MAJD

Nuclear medicine plays a primary role in the diagnosis and management of a variety of congenital and acquired disorders of the genitourinary systems in infants and children. Nuclear medicine procedures are generally noninvasive and require little or no preparation. Radiopharmaceuticals have no systemic pharmacologic effects and do not cause any allergic reaction. Absorbed radiation doses from the radionuclide studies are low. Most important, radionuclide studies offer quantitative functional information currently not available with other imaging modalities. Furthermore, they lend themselves to a variety of physiologic and pharmacologic interventions that can enhance their diagnostic accuracy. Many disorders of the genitourinary system in children are part of a dynamic process that requires serial assessment. Noninvasive radionuclide studies are an optimal means of evaluating and following the course of such disorders. The following is a review of the principles of nuclear medicine as they apply to the evaluation and management of urogenital disorders in children.

EVALUATION OF RENAL FUNCTION AND STRUCTURE

Radiopharmaceuticals

Radionuclide renal studies are used to assess renal perfusion and certain aspects of renal function and structure. The information provided depends on the radiopharmaceutical used. The radiopharmaceuticals discussed here are currently available for evaluation of the kidneys.

^{99m}Tc-diethylenetriaminepentaacetic acid (DTPA) is almost exclusively cleared by glomerular filtration with no significant tubular secretion or cortical retention. It is mainly used for calculation of glomerular filtration rate (GFR) in children undergoing chemotherapy with nephrotoxic drugs. It can also be used for dynamic renal imaging in the evaluation of hydronephrosis or hypertension (Fig. 54.1).

^{99m}Tc-mercaptoacetyltriglycine (MAG3) is rapidly cleared by

tubular secretion and is not retained in the parenchyma of normal kidneys. The quality of ^{99m}Tc-MAG3 images is superior to the quality of ^{99m}Tc-DTPA images. This is primarily because MAG3 is highly protein bound, and most of the injected dose remains in the intravascular compartment and is available for renal clearance. This smaller volume of distribution results in faster clearance and a higher target to background ratio (Fig. 54.2). Therefore, ^{99m}Tc-MAG3 is superior to ^{99m}Tc-DTPA for use in the pediatric age group particularly for certain applications such as diuresis renography. There is often some hepatobiliary excretion of MAG3 resulting in visualization of the tracer in the gallbladder and/or in the intestinal tract on the delayed images.

^{99}Tc-glucoheptonate (GHA) is cleared by a combination of glomerular filtration and tubular fixation. Most of the tracer is rapidly excreted in the urine, allowing moderately good visualization of the pelvicaliceal system, ureters, and bladder. Approximately 20% of the administered dose of GHA remains in the renal cortex, firmly bound to the tubular cells. Therefore, delayed imaging at 2 to 3 hours provides visualization of renal cortex. Hepatobiliary excretion of GHA, with visualization of the tracer in the gallbladder and/or intestine, occurs often, particularly in infants (Fig. 54.3).

^{99m}Tc-dimercaptosuccinic acid (DMSA) is the best cortical imaging agent currently available. Approximately 60% of the administered dose is tightly bound to the proximal tubular cells, and the remaining dose is gradually excreted in the urine in a low concentration. Unlike GHA, there is no hepatobiliary excretion of DMSA (Fig. 54.4). Therefore, DMSA allows excellent visualization of the renal parenchyma without interference from retention of tracer in the pelvicaliceal systems, gallbladder, or intestines and is recommended for detection of cortical lesions such as acute pyelonephritis, cortical scars, or infarcts.

Procedures

Dynamic Renal Imaging

The conventional radionuclide renal study usually consists of a radionuclide angiogram followed by sequential functional images of the kidneys, ureters, and bladder. After the rapid intravenous administration of an appropriate radioactive dose of tracer (DTPA, GHA, or MAG3) (Table 54.1), digital images are acquired on a computer at the rate of one image per second for

M. Majd: Radiology and Pediatrics, George Washington University School of Medicine and Radiology, Children's National Medical Center, Washington, DC.

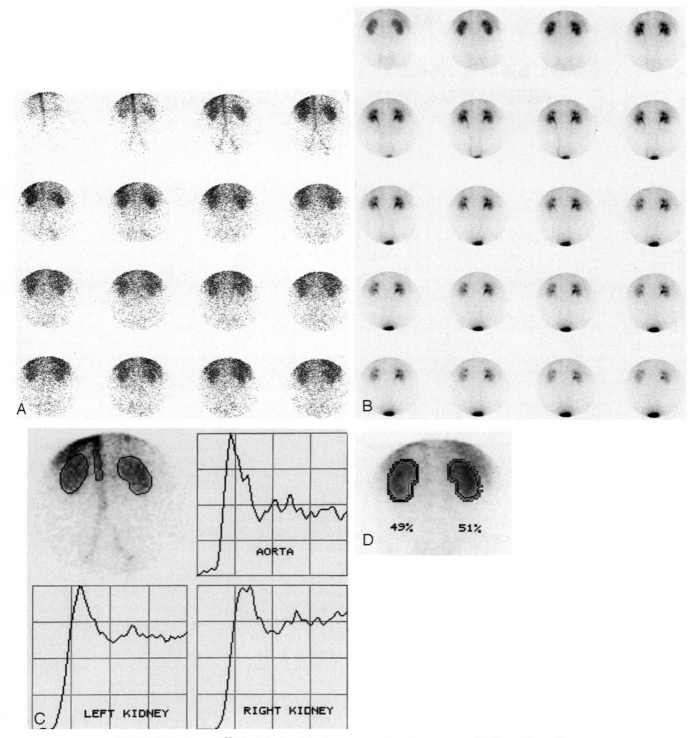

FIGURE 54.1. Normal ^{99m}Tc-diethylenetriaminepentaacetic acid renal scan. Radionuclide angiogram **(A)** and functional images **(B)** demonstrate normal perfusion, function, and drainage bilaterally. **C:** Time-activity curves of the first transit of the tracer through the abdominal aorta and the kidneys show similar slopes. **D:** Differential renal function based on the relative accumulation of the tracer in each kidney between 1 and 3 minutes after injection is similar. Note the region-of-interest (ROI) chosen for background subtraction is 1-pixel wide and 1-pixel away from the renal ROI.

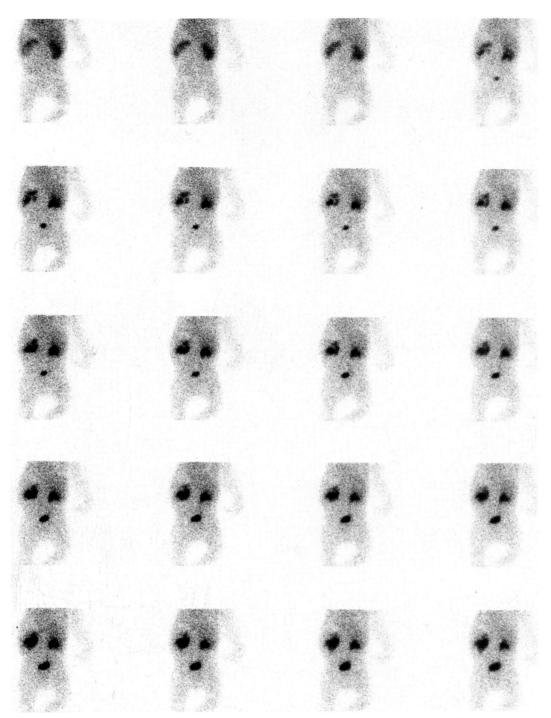

FIGURE 54.2. 99mTc-mercaptoacetyltriglycine renal scan in a 5-day-old infant with left hydronephrosis diagnosed on perinatal sonogram. There is prompt extraction of the tracer bilaterally. The right kidney is normal. There is left hydronephrosis with preserved function.

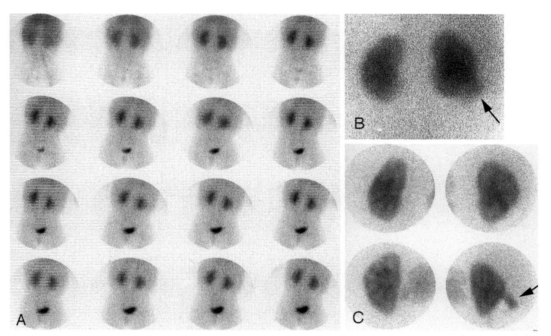

FIGURE 54.3. Normal ^{99m}Tc-glucoheptonate renal scan. **A:** Early images show prompt function and normal drainage bilaterally. Delayed posterior image **(B)** and magnified posterior and posterior oblique images **(C)** show normal cortical uptake. There is hepatobiliary excretion of the tracer with accumulation in the intestinal tract and the gallbladder (*arrows*).

60 seconds (angiographic images), followed by a series of 15-second images for 20 to 30 minutes (functional images). The angiographic images are used for evaluation of renal perfusion. Regions-of-interest (ROIs) are placed over the abdominal aorta and the kidneys. Time-activity curves are generated from these ROIs. The slopes of the time-activity curves of the kidneys are then compared with one another and with the aortic curve. The early functional images, after the angiographic phase and before accumulation of the tracer in the collecting systems, are used to calculate relative renal function (Fig. 54.1).

Renal Cortical Imaging

Renal cortical scintigraphy is accomplished by delayed imaging 2 to 3 hours after intravenous administration of either ^{99m}Tc-GHA or ^{99m}Tc-DMSA. ^{99m}Tc-GHA imaging has the advantage of providing visualization of the renal collecting systems. However, retention of GHA in the collecting systems may interfere with the evaluation of the renal cortex particularly with single photon emission computed tomography (SPECT). There is often some hepatobiliary excretion of GHA with visualization of the tracer in the gallbladder and/or intestine (Fig. 54.3). ^{99m}Tc-DMSA imaging provides excellent visualization of the renal parenchyma without interference from retention of tracer in the pelvicaliceal systems, gallbladder, or intestine (Fig. 54.4). Radiation to the cortex of the kidneys per millicurie administered dose is three times higher with DMSA as compared with GHA because of the cortical accumulation of a larger fraction of the administered dose of DMSA. Therefore, the administered dose of DMSA can be reduced to one third that of GHA (50 μCi/

kg vs. 150 μCi/kg). With this adjustment in the administered dose, the total DMSA tracer retained in the kidneys and resultant renal radiation doses are equal to those of GHA. However, because a lesser amount of DMSA accumulates in the bladder, the gonadal radiation dose is significantly less. Therefore, we prefer to use DMSA for cortical imaging, particularly in infants and young children.

A posterior image of the kidneys using a parallel-hole collimator is obtained for calculation of differential renal function (Fig. 54.4A). Magnified high resolution images of each kidney, in posterior and posterior oblique projections, are then obtained using a pinhole collimator with 3-mm aperture (Fig. 54.4B). SPECT images of the kidneys are obtained in selected cases. In patients with severe spinal deformity or with ectopic kidney, simultaneous anterior and posterior images of the kidneys are obtained for the generation of a geometric mean image and more accurate calculation of the relative function of the kidneys.

Relative Renal Function

The differential or relative function of each kidney can be calculated by determining the accumulation of the tracer in each kidney between 1 and 3 minutes after injection of DTPA, MAG3 or GHA. During this period all the radioactivity within the kidney is confined to the vessels and functioning renal parenchyma, because the tracer has not yet reached the collecting system. ROIs are selected for each kidney and its background. Background activity is then subtracted from corresponding renal activity. The net counts within each kidney are expressed as a percentage of the total renal counts (Fig. 54.1**D**). The same

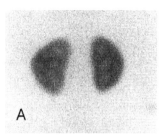

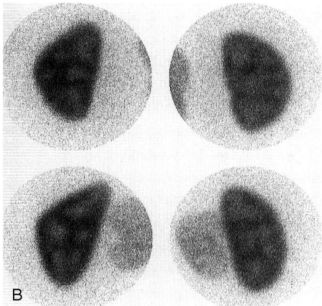

FIGURE 54.4. Normal ^{99m}Tc-dimercaptosuccinic acid renal scan. Posterior image obtained with a parallel-hole collimator **(A)** and magnified images of the kidneys in posterior (*upper*) and posterior-oblique (*lower*) projections using pinhole collimator **(B)** show normal cortical uptake of the tracer bilaterally. Central areas of lower concentration of the tracer correspond to the collecting systems and medulla.

principle can be used in calculating the relative contribution of the upper and lower moieties of a duplex kidney to its total function. There are several pitfalls in the differential function analysis based on the early images. The technique is operator dependent, and selection of the frames and the ROIs affects the results. This is particularly critical for the background ROIs. We use a 1-pixel wide background ROI drawn automatically or manually around and 1-pixel away from the renal ROI (Fig. 54.1**D**). This method is probably the most reproducible tech-

Table 54.1. *Radiopharmaceutical Doses for Renal Imaging in Children*

Radiopharmaceutical	Dose (mCi/kg)	Minimum dose (mCi)
^{99m}Tc-DTPA	0.100	1
^{99m}Tc-MAG3	0.050	0.500
^{99m}Tc-GHA	0.150	1
^{99m}Tc-DMSA	0.050	0.500

DMSA, 2,3-dimercaptosuccinic acid; DTPA, diethylenetriaminepentaacetic acid; GHA, glucoheptonate; MAG3, mercaptoacetyltriglycine.

nique and facilitates detection of change in renal differential function on serial examinations. The results may also be invalid in the presence of extreme hydronephrosis. When the cortex is thin and poorly functioning, selecting an area of interest is difficult. Attenuation of the counts from the anterior parenchyma, which is widely displaced by the dilated urine-filled pelvicaliceal system, will result in inaccurate calculation of the total activity contained in the entire renal parenchyma.

The relative renal function can be reliably calculated on delayed DMSA images. The background activity is negligible by that time, and, thus, one source of potential error is eliminated. Both anterior and posterior images can be obtained from which a geometric mean value can be calculated. The geometric mean may be more reliable than the count ratios from posterior images alone, particularly when the kidneys are at different depths. Cortical uptake of GHA in each kidney on the delayed images can also be used for calculation of renal differential function provided that there is no retention of the tracer in the pelvicaliceal system, gallbladder, or intestine overlying the kidneys.

Total and Separate GFR

Because ^{99m}Tc-DTPA is excreted almost exclusively by glomerular filtration, its rate of clearance from blood is an accurate measure of GFR. ^{51}Cr-ethylenediaminetetraacetic acid (EDTA) may provide more accurate values for GFR than ^{99m}Tc-DTPA, but it is not commercially available in the Unites States. A variety of methods may be used to calculate GFR (see chapter 41). A reliable method, which employs three blood samples drawn between 2 and 3 hours after injection, is based on a modified compartmental analysis of the plasma clearance of DTPA. After intravenous injection of DTPA, the tracer clears from the plasma in two phases. In the first phase, there is rapid decrease in the plasma concentration because of a combination of glomerular filtration and redistribution of the tracer between the intravascular and extravascular spaces. Once the exchange of tracer between these compartments reaches equilibrium, the gradual decrease in plasma concentration of tracer is related directly to GFR. Although GFR is calculated from plasma samples only, concomitant renal imaging provides information about morphologic features and relative function of the kidneys, as well as drainage of the tracer. Absolute GFR of each kidney can then be calculated by multiplying the total calculated GFR in milliliters per minute by the percentages obtained from the renal differential function. Other methods of calculating GFR based on external counting without blood samples or with a single blood sample have become popular in adult nuclear medicine, but their reliability for use in children remains uncertain.

Pharmacologic Interventions in Renal Scintigraphy

Diuresis renography and captopril renography are two modified techniques of renal scintigraphy that use pharmacologic intervention and are discussed in the clinical applications section.

Clinical Applications

Although the radionuclide renal study does not provide the anatomic resolution of the intravenous urogram (IVU), it has several advantages, including quantitative assessment of renal function, independence of image quality from overlying bowel contents and bony structures, and ability to visualize renal tissue with a very low level of function. These advantages are particularly important in neonates. GFR at birth is about 20% of the corrected adult value and reaches only 45% by 2 weeks of age (1). Adult levels are reached at 6 to 12 months of age. GFR in very low birth weight premature infants is even lower (10% of normal) with a slower rise to normal level (2). The low GFR, together with overlying bowel gas, generally results in poor visualization of kidneys on the IVU. Radionuclide imaging, which is limited only by severe renal dysfunction, is superior to IVU for localization and functional analysis of the kidneys in all ages, particularly the newborn (Fig. 54.2). Almost all of the congenital and acquired renal disorders in children can be adequately evaluated by renal scintigraphy alone or in combination with renal sonography. On rare occasions, IVU may be necessary for better anatomic evaluation of the collecting systems and ureters.

Acute Pyelonephritis and Renal Scarring

Urinary tract infection (UTI) is a common problem in children. Infection may be limited to the bladder (cystitis) or upper collecting systems (ureteritis, pyelitis) or it may involve the renal parenchyma (pyelonephritis). Infections confined to the bladder and the upper collecting systems usually have a benign clinical course and are treated easily without any sequelae. Acute pyelonephritis on the other hand can result in irreversible damage (scarring) leading to hypertension and/or chronic renal failure (3,4). Experimental and clinical studies have shown that renal scarring can be prevented or minimized by early effective antimicrobial therapy (5–7). Therefore, early and accurate diagnosis of acute pyelonephritis has clinical relevance. Prospective clinical studies have shown that commonly used clinical and laboratory findings are unreliable in differentiating acute pyelonephritis from lower UTI in infants and children, and the use of diagnostic imaging is often necessary. Contrary to common assumptions, most cases of acute pyelonephritis occur in the absence of demonstrable vesicoureteral reflux. Furthermore, once acute pyelonephritis occurs, the subsequent development of renal scarring is independent of the presence or absence of reflux (8,9). Therefore, it seems unwise to limit evaluation of cortical integrity in urinary tract infection only to those patients with proven vesicoureteral reflux.

Several imaging techniques have been evaluated as a means of differentiating acute pyelonephritis from lower urinary tract infection. IVU has a very low sensitivity for the diagnosis of pyelonephritis. Radionuclide imaging procedures using ^{67}Ga-citrate or ^{111}In-labeled leukocytes may be very reliable in the diagnosis of acute pyelonephritis. These imaging procedures, however, result in a high radiation absorbed dose, require 24 to 48 hours to perform, and do not provide any information about the function and morphology of the kidneys.

Clinical studies have shown renal cortical scintigraphy using ^{99m}Tc-DMSA or ^{99m}Tc-GHA to be significantly more sensitive than IVU and renal sonography (10,11) in the detection of acute pyelonephritis. ^{99m}Tc-DMSA renal cortical scintigraphy using either planar or SPECT imaging has been shown to have both

sensitivity and specificity of better than 90% in the diagnosis of experimentally induced acute pyelonephritis in piglets, using strict histopathologic criteria as the standard of reference (12, 13).

Uptake of DMSA in normal kidneys reflects the morphology of renal cortex. High-resolution magnified images show the details of the cortex and cortical columns with good differentiation from the collecting systems and medulla (Fig. 54.4). Flattening of the anterolateral aspect of the upper pole of the left kidney by the spleen may be seen. On the posterior image, this flattening may mimic pathologic decreased uptake, but on the posterior-oblique image, the cortical thickness and tracer uptake are normal (Fig. 54.5). Irregularities in the contour of the kidneys resulting from fetal lobulation may be present. The indentations that result from fetal lobulation are clearly between the medullary pyramids and can be differentiated from cortical scars that are over the pyramids. A transverse band of cortex separating the upper and lower moieties of a duplex collecting systems may be seen (Fig. 54.6).

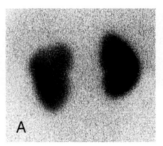

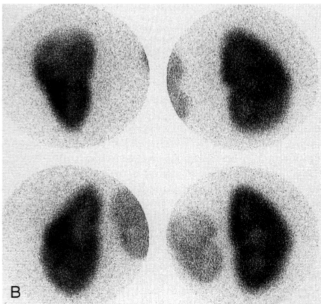

FIGURE 54.5. Splenic impression on the left kidney. ^{99m}Tc-dimercaptosuccinic acid renal scan in a 5-year-old child with history of febrile urinary tract infection shows apparent enlargement of the upper pole of the left kidney with decreased uptake on the posterior planar image **(A)** and on the magnified posterior image (*left upper* image on **B**) mimicking acute pyelonephritis. The posterior-oblique image of the left kidney (*left lower* image on **B**), however, shows flattening of the left upper pole with normal cortical uptake of the tracer.

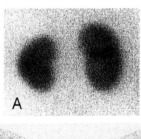

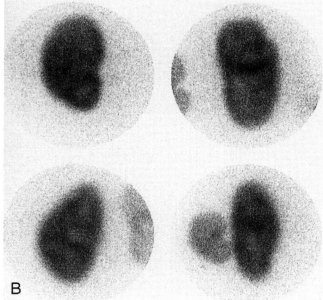

FIGURE 54.6. Duplication of the collecting system and fetal lobulation of the right kidney. **A:** Posterior planar image shows the right kidney to be bigger than the left with a transverse band of normal cortex at the junction of the upper 2/5 and lower 3/5. **B:** The magnified images also shows the transverse band of cortex separating the upper and lower moieties of a duplex right kidney. There is also an indentation on the lateral aspect of the upper pole of the right kidney from fetal lobulation.

Acute pyelonephritis usually appears as a single area or multiple areas of varying degrees of decreased cortical uptake of the tracer without deformity of renal outline or loss of volume. In some cases, the decreased uptake is even accompanied by increase in volume of the affected area (Figs. 54.7 and 54.8). Although most lesions occur in the upper and lower poles, the midzone of the kidney is often involved. A less common scintigraphic pattern of acute pyelonephritis is one of diffusely decreased tracer uptake in an enlarged kidney (Fig. 54.9). Acute pyelonephritis may resolve completely and the scintigram return to normal within a few months (Fig. 54.10), or it may evolve into permanent damage and scar formation (Fig. 54.11).

The pathophysiology that accounts for the decreased uptake of DMSA in acute pyelonephritis is probably multifactorial. Cortical uptake of DMSA is primarily determined by intrarenal blood flow and proximal tubular cell membrane transport function. Any pathologic process that alters either or both of these parameters may result in focal or diffuse areas of decreased uptake. Experimental studies, using ^{51}Cr microspheres in the piglet model, suggest that focal ischemia is an early event that precedes tubular damage (14). Therefore, the DMSA image may become

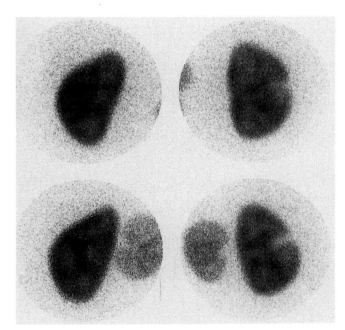

FIGURE 54.7. Focal acute pyelonephritis involving the midzone of the right kidney.

positive in a very early stage of parenchymal inflammatory response to invasion by bacteria. It is reasonable to assume that adequate treatment of acute pyelonephritis in this very early stage would result in complete resolution without progression to scar formation.

A mature cortical scar is usually associated with contraction and loss of volume of the involved cortex. This may manifest as cortical thinning, flattening of the renal contour, or a wedge-

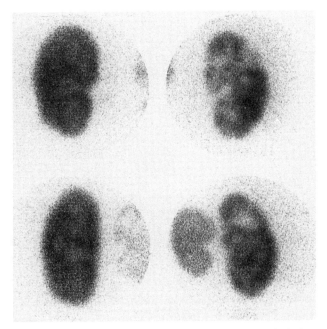

FIGURE 54.8. Multifocal acute pyelonephritis of the right kidney.

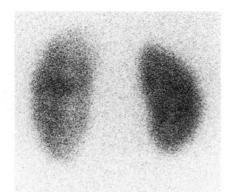

FIGURE 54.9. Diffuse acute pyelonephritis of the left kidney.

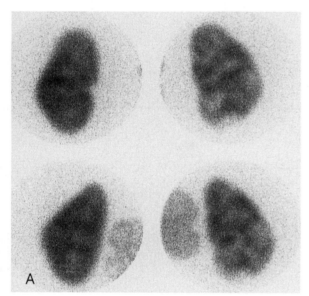

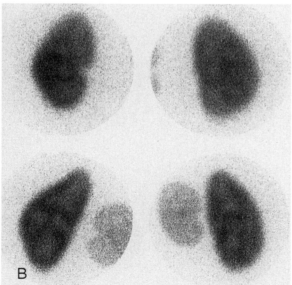

FIGURE 54.10. Resolution of acute pyelonephritis. **A:** The initial ^{99m}Tc-dimercaptosuccinic acid images obtained at the time of acute febrile urinary tract infection demonstrates multiple areas of decreased tracer uptake. **B:** Follow-up scan 11 months later shows complete resolution.

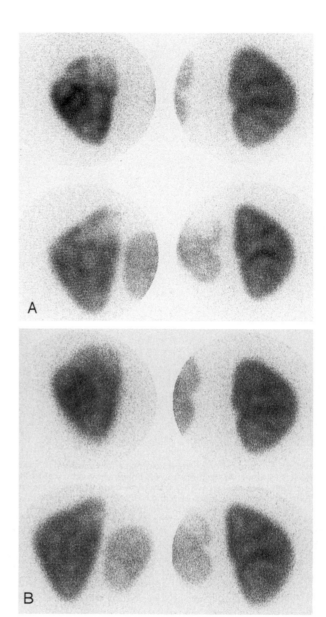

FIGURE 54.11. Progression of acute pyelonephritis to cortical scar. **A:** Initial ^{99m}Tc-dimercaptosuccinic acid scan obtained at the time of acute febrile urinary tract infection shows acute pyelonephritis involving the upper pole of the left kidney. **B:** Follow-up scan 1 year later shows contraction and loss of volume of the left upper pole.

shaped defect (Fig. 54.12). The defect of a mature scar may gradually become more prominent because of the growth of surrounding normal renal cortex. The scintigraphic pattern of a maturing scar varies and depends on the severity, age, and location of the lesion, as well as the rate of growth of surrounding normal tissues.

Renal sonography is commonly used in the evaluation and management of infants and children who have UTI. It is truly a noninvasive imaging technique that is highly reliable for the detection of hydronephrosis and some of the congenital anomalies that may be associated with UTI. It is also useful in the detection of renal abscesses, pyonephrosis, and abnormalities of

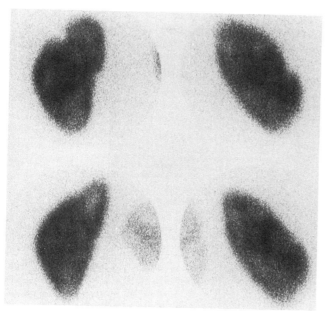

FIGURE 54.12. Cortical scars. ^{99m}Tc-dimercaptosuccinic acid images obtained 1 year after scintigraphically documented bilateral acute pyelonephritis demonstrate a wedge-shaped cortical defect in the lateral aspect of the upper pole of the left kidney, best seen on the posterior image (*upper left* image). There is also cortical thinning in the medial aspect of the right upper pole and indentation on the lateral aspect of the right midzone (*upper right* image).

the perinephric space. Changes secondary to acute pyelonephritis may also be recognized on renal sonogram as either hyperechoic or hypoechoic foci, loss of corticomedullary differentiation, focal or diffuse renal enlargement, and mild to moderate dilatation of renal pelvis. However, renal sonography has proved to have a low sensitivity for the detection of acute inflammatory changes of renal cortex. (11). Power Doppler has improved the sensitivity of sonography for the detection of pyelonephritis by demonstrating focal ischemia. However, in an experimental study, it proved to be significantly less sensitive and specific than ^{99m}Tc-DMSA SPECT (13).

Computed tomography (CT), particularly spiral CT, is an effective technique for documenting the nature of parenchymal involvement and for the evaluation of the perinephric space. The lesions of acute pyelonephritis typically appear as wedge-shaped, ill-defined, or striated areas of decreased attenuation. Spiral CT is highly sensitive and specific for the detection of acute pyelonephritis. However, it requires rapid intravenous injection of a large volume of contrast agent and is associated with high radiation dose (13). Therefore, its routine use in the evaluation of children with UTI is not practical and should be reserved for complicated cases.

Magnetic resonance imaging (MRI) with the fast inversion recovery sequence and intravenous administration of gadolinium has been shown to be highly sensitive and specific for the detection of acute pyelonephritis (13). The fast inversion recovery markedly reduces the signal intensity of normal renal parenchyma and allows pyelonephritic lesions to be seen as focal zones of medium or high signal intensity against the background low

signal intensity of low normal renal tissue (Fig. 54.13). MRI has the advantages of not using ionizing radiation and allowing evaluation of the perinephric space. However, its routine use is not practical because of limited availability, need for sedation and high cost.

At present, renal cortical scintigraphy is the most reliable and practical imaging technique for routine use in the initial evaluation and follow-up of children with febrile urinary tract infection. Renal sonography plays a complementary role to scintigraphy.

Hydronephrosis

The patient with hydronephrosis or hydroureteronephrosis may present with UTI or an abdominal mass. With the increasing use of antenatal sonography, however, renal anomalies, including hydronephrosis, are being diagnosed much earlier and with greater frequency. Assessment of renal function and differentiation between obstructive and nonobstructive hydronephrosis are essential in the management of these patients. The conventional renal scan demonstrates the presence, extent, and severity of hydronephrosis and allows quantitative assessment of residual renal function. Associated anomalies, such as duplication, are also detected. Conventional renal scintigraphy, however, does not differentiate obstructive from nonobstructive hydronephrosis. For this purpose, diuresis renography is of special value.

The causes of hydronephrosis and hydroureter include vesicoureteral reflux, ureteropelvic junction (UPJ) obstruction, ureterovesical junction obstruction, posterior urethral valve, ectopic ureter with or without duplication, ectopic ureterocele, primary nonobstructive megaureter, and prune belly syndrome.

Multicystic dysplastic kidney and hydronephrosis resulting from congenital UPJ obstruction are the two most common flank masses in the neonatal period. Depending on the number of functioning nephrons remaining, a multicystic dysplastic kidney may show minimal or no function (Fig. 54.14). On the other hand, a kidney with congenital UPJ obstruction without dysplasia of the renal parenchyma usually retains significant function, unless prolonged obstruction has existed or infection has supervened. The salvageable hydronephrotic kidney demonstrates a cap of functioning cortex of varying thickness at the periphery on the early static images, whereas the delayed images show significant accumulation of the tracer in the dilated pelvicaliceal system.

Duplication of the collecting system may be partial or complete. In a completely duplicated system, the ureter draining the upper moiety usually inserts in the bladder more caudally and more medially than the lower moiety ureter and may be associated with ectopic ureterocele and obstruction (Fig. 54.15). There is often reflux into the lower moiety ureter. A less common form of complicated duplex system is UPJ obstruction of the lower moiety. Occasionally, a dysgenetic, nonfunctioning whole kidney, or one moiety of a duplex kidney, is visualized on renal scan by reflux of the tracer from the bladder into the corresponding ureter and pelvicaliceal system.

Diuresis Renography

Diuresis renography is a safe and valuable method for the evaluation and management of hydronephrosis in infants and children.

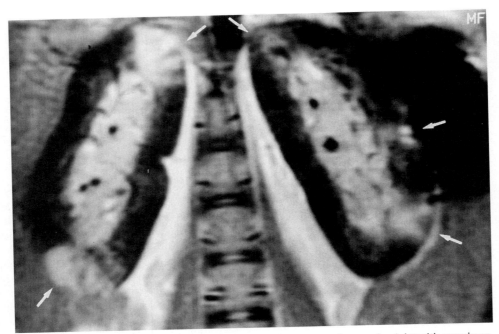

FIGURE 54.13. Coronal gadolinium-enhanced fast inversion recovery image of a piglet with experimentally induced acute pyelonephritis demonstrates foci (*arrows*) of high signal intensity in the upper and lower poles of the right kidney and the lower pole of the left kidney.

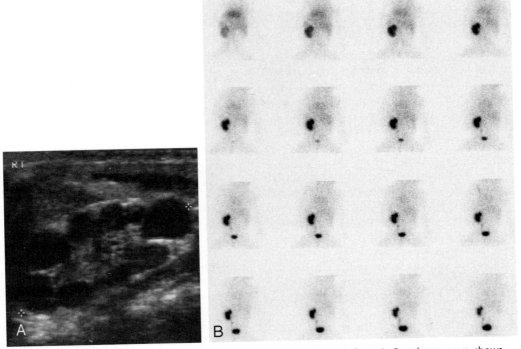

FIGURE 54.14. Multicystic dysplastic right kidney in a 3-week-old infant. **A:** Renal sonogram shows that the kidney is replaced by many cysts of varying size without a central pelvic structure. **B:** ^{99m}Tc-mercaptoacetyltriglycine renal scan shows photon deficiency in the right renal region with no demonstrable function. The left kidney is normal.

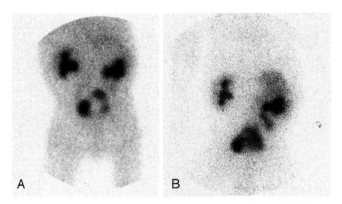

FIGURE 54.15. Ectopic ureterocele. Selected **(A)** early and **(B)** delayed posterior images of a ^{99m}Tc-diethylenetriaminepentaacetic acid renal scan demonstrate duplication of the right renal collecting system. The upper pole is hydronephrotic and shows delayed and decreased function. The collecting system of the lower pole of the right kidney is tilted. There is a filling defect in the bladder. This constellation is characteristic of ectopic ureterocele. The left kidney is normal.

This provocative test is based on the hypothesis that the prolonged retention of the tracer in the nonobstructed dilated upper urinary tract is caused by a reservoir effect and that increased urine flow following diuretic administration should result in prompt washout of the tracer; whereas, in obstructive hydronephrosis, there should not be any significant washout. The techniques and analytic methods used by different investigators vary widely. Diuresis renography is dependent on several physiologic, mechanical, and technical factors. Understanding the principles of the test, its limitations, and the sources of error are essential in the interpretation of the results and in effective use of the test. The following technique has evolved at our institution and has been used effectively for the past 23 years.

Technique of Diuresis Renography

The patient is positioned supine on the scanning table, which is placed above the gamma-camera. A venous line is established, and an indwelling bladder catheter is inserted. The patient is hydrated by intravenous administration of 5% dextrose in 0.03% saline during the test. The total intravenous fluid volume is about 15 mL/kg, one third of which is usually given before the intravenous administration of the tracer. A conventional renal study using either ^{99m}Tc-DTPA (100 μCi/kg; minimum 1 mCi) or preferably ^{99m}Tc-MAG3 (50 μCi/kg; minimum 500 μCi) is obtained. Accumulation of the tracer is continuously monitored and when the dilated system is entirely filled with tracer, furosemide is administered intravenously in a dose of 1 mg/kg up to 40 mg. Higher doses are used in obese patients and in those who have been on diuretics. Digital images are stored on a computer at the rate of 4 frames/minute from the time of administration of the tracer until 30 minutes after administration of furosemide. Urine output is measured at 10-minute intervals during the period before injection of furosemide and afterward. If drainage is markedly delayed during the first 30 minutes after diuretic injection, the patient is placed in the prone position and additional images are obtained for 15 minutes. Alternatively, static renal images may be obtained before

and after the patient is kept in upright position for 15 minutes. The computer data are then processed for generation of the renogram curve and calculation of the clearance of the tracer from the dilated upper urinary tract (Figs. 54.16 and 54.17).

Analysis and Interpretation of Diuretic Renogram

There are basically two methods to analyze a diuresis renogram curve: (a) pattern recognition and (b) quantitative analysis. The pattern recognition method is based on the subjective analysis of the shape of the curve. There is a spectrum of responses ranging from a very rapid drainage to no drainage (Fig. 54.18). Characteristic patterns, which are easily recognizable, are seen at the ends of the spectrum for nonobstructed hydronephrosis and for high-grade obstruction. Most often, however, the curves demonstrate an intermediate response, which may suggest mild to moderate obstruction. Determination of the significance of obstruction, if any, based on the subjective interpretation of the shape of the intermediate curves is often impossible. Quantitative analysis methods based on the washout half-time or some other measures of the washout rate help to reduce subjectivity in the interpretation of the curve and to decrease the number of indeterminate results. This analysis is particularly helpful when comparing serial examinations.

In addition to the washout half-time, the shape of the curve should also be considered in the analysis of the diuretic renogram. The curve may show an initial rapid decline with a short, calculated, washout half-time, but instead of continuing to drop exponentially to a low level of residual activity, it may plateau at a high level of activity or it may even rise. These biphasic curves are almost always caused by flow dependent obstruction (Fig. 54.18).

Limitations and Pitfalls

Understanding the principles of the test, its limitations, and the sources of error is essential in the interpretation of the results and effective use of diuresis renography. The physiologic, mechanical, and technical factors that affect the rate of the washout of the tracer and the shape of the renogram curve include the following.

Variable Grades of Obstruction. Practically all cases of obstruction are partial with varying degrees of severity and, in some cases, are intermittent. It is often difficult to predict what degree of obstruction will lead to deterioration of renal function. Furthermore, the obstructive process, particularly in a young infant, may be progressive. Therefore, definition of significant obstruction remains imprecise.

Variable Impairment of Renal Function. The rate of accumulation of radionuclide in the dilated collecting system, as well as the response to diuretic, are dependent on renal function. Therefore, in the presence of poor renal function the test is unreliable. Unfortunately, the level of renal function below which the diuresis renogram becomes unreliable is not clearly defined. Our experience suggests that when the collecting system does not completely fill within 1 hour after injection of the tracer or if the affected kidney has less than 20% of the total

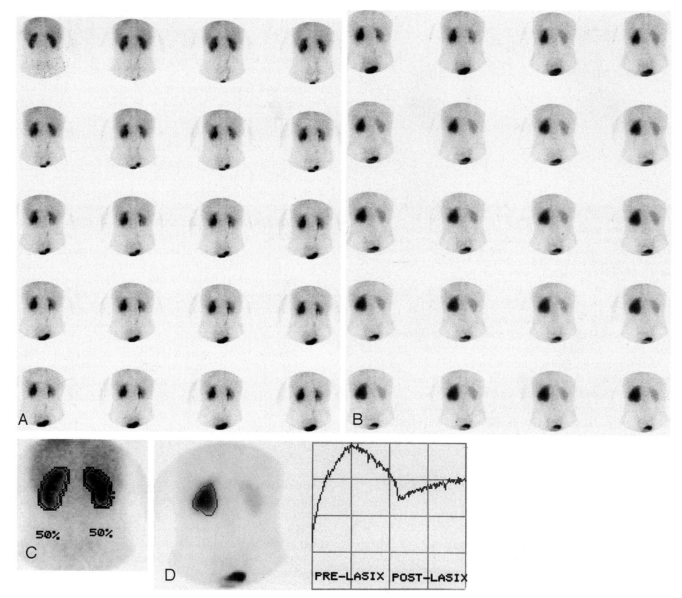

FIGURE 54.16. Diuresis renogram in a 7-year-old girl with left ureteropelvic junction obstruction. **A:** Sequential 1-minute images obtained after administration of ^{99m}Tc-diethylenetriaminepentaacetic acid show hydronephrosis of the left kidney with poor drainage of the tracer. **B:** Sequential 90-second images after administration of furosemide show gradual distention of the left renal pelvis and marked retention of the tracer. **C:** The renal differential function is divided equally. **D:** The time-activity curve of the maximally distended left renal pelvis demonstrates peak activity at about 15 minutes after injection of the tracer and slow washout for the next 15 minutes. After administration of furosemide, there is an initial washout for a few minutes after which the curve rises continuously. This pattern is characteristic of flow-dependent high-grade obstruction.

renal function, a prolonged washout may not be associated with obstruction.

Capacity and Compliance of the Dilated System.
In the presence of massive hydroureteronephrosis, even a very good response to furosemide may have little effect on the washout of tracer from the huge pool of retained tracer and may cause false-positive results. Distensibility or compliance of the dilated collecting system also plays a role.

State of Hydration.
Adequate hydration is essential for diuresis. In addition to oral intake of fluid before the test, we routinely hydrate the patient with intravenous infusion of 5% dextrose in 0.03% saline. This hydration improves excretion of the tracer, enhances the response to furosemide, and prevents dehydration.

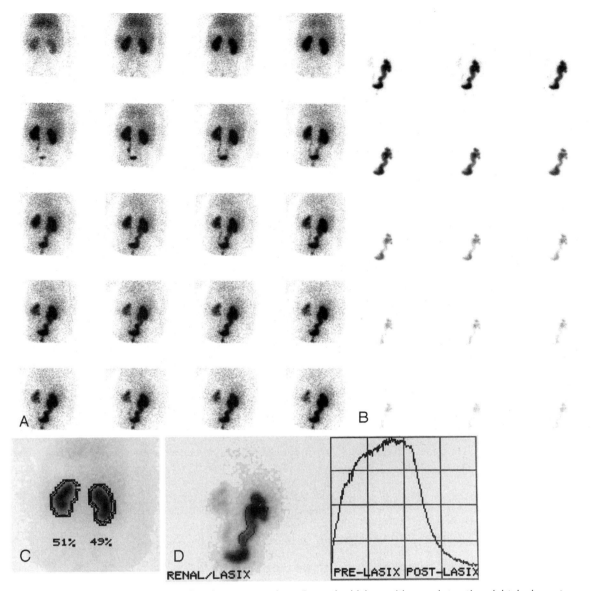

FIGURE 54.17. Diuresis renogram in a 5-month-old boy with nonobstructive right hydroureteronephrosis. **A:** Sequential 60-second images after administration of 99mTc-mercaptoacetyltriglycine show markedly dilated right pelvicaliceal system and ureter. **B:** Sequential 90-second images obtained after injection of furosemide show rapid clearance of the tracer. **C:** The renal differential function is symmetric. **D:** The time-activity curve of the entire dilated system, including ureter, shows continuous rise before and rapid fall after administration of furosemide.

Dose of Diuretic. The response to furosemide is dose dependent. A dose of 1 mg/kg appears to be both effective and safe.

Time of Diuretic Injection. Maximum diuresis in a well-hydrated child usually occurs within a few minutes after injection of furosemide. Therefore, the optimal time for administration of furosemide is when most of the tracer has cleared from the blood and the entire dilated system is completely filled with the tracer. In well-hydrated patients with normal renal function, this occurs at about 20 to 30 minutes after administration of the tracer. Administration of furosemide before or shortly after (2 to 3 minutes) administration of the tracer may not adversely

affect the washout curves of the mildly dilated systems, but more severely dilated systems will probably remain incompletely filled during the acquisition of the computer data and the washout will appear falsely prolonged.

Fullness of the Bladder. Increased intravesical pressure associated with a full bladder may significantly affect the drainage from the upper urinary tract. The routine use of an indwelling catheter for continuous drainage of urine from the bladder has these advantages: (a) it eliminates the effect of a full bladder on the washout, (b) it allows measurement of the urine output at

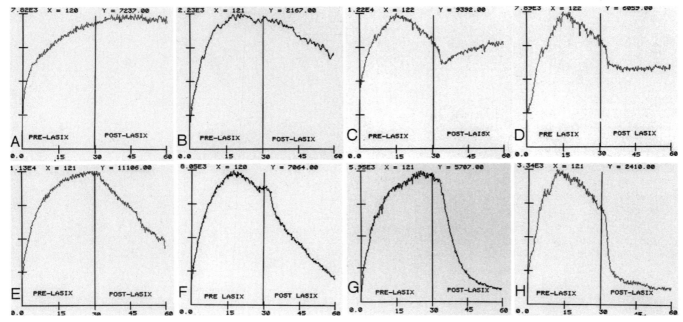

FIGURE 54.18. Spectrum of diuresis renogram curves. Examples of actual time-activity curves of hydro-nephrotic kidneys with diuretic injection at the midpoint of a 60-minute acquisition. Patterns **A** and **B** indicate high-grade obstruction. Patterns **C** and **D** are characteristic of flow-dependent obstruction. Patterns **E** and **F** are equivocal. Patterns **G** and **H** are seen in nonobstructed hydronephrosis.

any chosen intervals before and after injection of furosemide, (c) it eliminates the discomfort of a full bladder that can cause the patient to move during acquisition of computer data, (d) it decreases radiation dose to the gonads by continuous drainage of the radioactive urine, and (e) it eliminates the effect of vesicoureteral reflux should reflux exist.

Patient Position. Washout of the retained tracer is occasionally affected by the position of the patient. The easiest and most practical position for immobilization and observation of the patient and for performance of diuresis renography in the pediatric age group is supine with the camera positioned underneath the patient. If drainage is markedly delayed during the first 30 minutes after diuretic injection, additional images should be obtained with the patient in the prone or upright position. Markedly improved drainage in the prone or upright position makes high-grade obstruction less likely and is usually associated with preservation of renal function.

Radiopharmaceutical. The ideal radiopharmaceutical for diuresis renography should have rapid blood clearance, a short physical half-life, and radiation characteristics suitable for imaging and should be readily available at a reasonable cost. At present, either DTPA or MAG3 can be used. The advantage of MAG3 is its faster and better clearance from the renal cortex, particularly in the first 2 weeks of life.

Region-of-Interest. Appropriate ROI should be chosen for generation of the curves. The changes in the amount of tracer in a portion of a dilated system may not be representative of the drainage from the entire system. After injection of diuretic, the renal pelvis may distend gradually. Therefore, the image with maximum distension of the pelvis should be chosen for generation of the time-activity curve. In the presence of both pelvic and ureteral dilatation, the ureter can function as a reservoir for the tracer drained from the renal pelvis. Therefore, the ROI should include the entire dilated system.

Hypertension

Hypertension in children is often of renal origin. Therefore, radionuclide renal studies play an important role in the evaluation and management of hypertension in infants and children. Some of the renal causes of hypertension such as infarction, postpyelonephritic cortical scarring, and posttraumatic injuries are easily diagnosed by conventional radionuclide renal imaging. These methods, however, are less reliable in the diagnosis of renal artery stenosis, which is the cause of approximately 5% of all cases of childhood hypertension. The prevalence is considerably higher when the hypertension occurs in association with neurofibromatosis or aortic anomalies. Stenosis of the renal artery is usually an isolated lesion secondary to fibromuscular dysplasia. In the presence of unilateral renal artery stenosis, conventional radionuclide imaging and renography may show evidence of decreased renal perfusion and function on the affected side. The kidney with a stenotic artery, however, may remain adequately perfused, and, owing to the autoregulation mechanism, the radionuclide renal studies may remain normal or near normal. Therefore, the conventional radionuclide studies are not reliable screening tests for detection of renovascular hypertension, particularly in the presence of bilateral or segmental renal artery stenosis. The efficacy of renal scintigraphy for the diagnosis of renovascular hypertension, however, is markedly improved by the use of angiotensin-converting enzyme (ACE) inhibitors.

Captopril-Enhanced Renal Scintigraphy and Renography

In the presence of renal artery stenosis, the intrarenal perfusion pressure is decreased and there is a tendency for GFR to fall. However, within a wide range of perfusion pressure, GFR is maintained at a normal level by an autoregulation mechanism mediated by the renin-angiotensin system. A major factor in maintaining GFR is the transcapillary pressure gradient across the glomerulus, related to the difference in resistance at the level of the afferent and efferent arterioles, which is regulated by angiotensin II-induced selective constriction of the efferent arterioles. ACE inhibitors, such as captopril or enalaprilat, block the formation of angiotensin II, which results in dilatation of the efferent arterioles and decreased transcapillary pressure gradient. This decrease in the gradient leads to a significant, but reversible, decrease in GFR of the kidney with a stenotic artery, which can be easily detected by renal scintigraphy and renography.

The choice of radiopharmaceutical, ACE inhibitor, and technique of examination varies among investigators. In the original studies in pediatric patients, ^{99m}Tc-DTPA was used (15). Subsequent experience has shown that either glomerular filtration or tubular secretion agents can be used (16–18). Either captopril or enalaprilat can be used as the choice of ACE inhibitor. To ensure absorption of captopril, the patient should not eat solids for approximately 4 hours before the examination. The advantage of enalaprilat is that it is administered intravenously and,

unlike oral captopril, its effect is not dependent on variable rate of absorption through the gastrointestinal tract.

Blood pressure may significantly fall even after a single dose of captopril. The probability of severe hypotension is even greater with intravenous enalaprilat. Therefore, the patient should be well hydrated and an intravenous access maintained throughout the study. Diuretics may exaggerate the hypotensive effect of ACE inhibitors. Their use in conjunction with captopril renography is not advised in infants and children.

A baseline study is obtained followed by a repeat study either 1 hour after oral administration of captopril (1 mg/kg; maximum 50 mg) or 10 minutes after intravenous administration of enalaprilat (0.03 mg/kg). An alternative technique is to obtain the initial study with the use of ACE inhibitor and to repeat the study later without the use of an ACE inhibitor only if the first study is abnormal.

The scintigraphic manifestations of decreased renal function induced by ACE inhibitor in the presence of hemodynamically significant renal artery stenosis depends on which radiopharmaceutical is used. The primary effect of ACE inhibitor is decreased GFR. Therefore, on a ^{99m}Tc-DTPA study, it will manifest as varying degrees of decreased extraction and delayed appearance of the tracer in the collecting systems (Fig. 54.19), whereas with the use of tubular agents prolonged parenchymal retention of the tracer is seen (Fig. 54.20). Because it is easier to detect cortical retention of tracer than it is to appreciate its focal decreased extraction, ^{99m}Tc-MAG3 is probably more effective than ^{99m}Tc-DTPA for the detection of segmental renal artery stenosis.

In the presence of bilateral renal artery stenosis, narrowing is usually asymmetric, as is the effect of captopril on the function of each kidney. A symmetric decrease in renal function is usually associated with either dehydration or severe hypotensive crisis and should not be misinterpreted as bilateral renal artery stenosis.

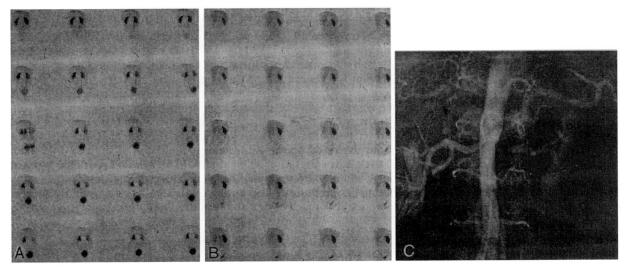

FIGURE 54.19. Captopril-enhanced ^{99m}Tc-diethylenetriaminepentaacetic acid renal study in a 7-year-old boy with hypertension. **A:** Baseline study demonstrates slightly delayed function on the left associated with relative hyperconcentration of the tracer in the collecting systems consistent with renal artery stenosis. The right kidney is normal. **B:** Post-captopril study shows marked deterioration of renal function bilaterally, more severe on the left side. **C:** Renal arteriogram shows bilateral renal artery stenosis more severe on the left.

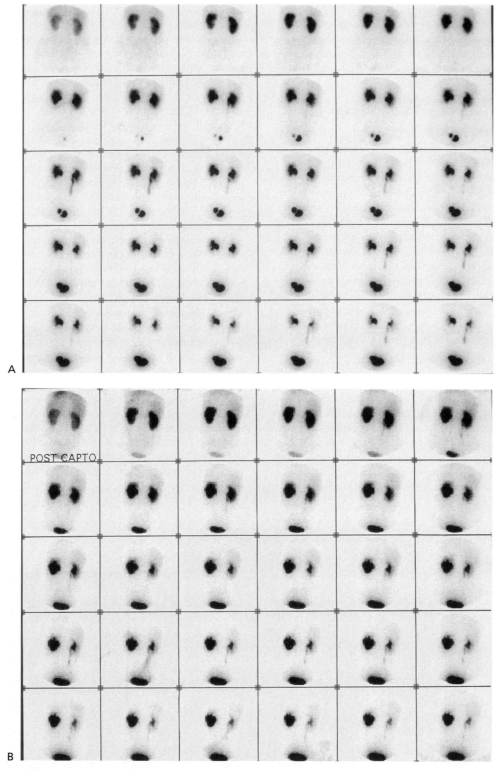

FIGURE 54.20. Captopril-enhanced mercaptoacetyltriglycine renal study in a 12-year-old girl with hypertension. **A:** Baseline study is essentially normal. **B:** Post-captopril study shows marked cortical retention of the tracer in the lower ½ of the left kidney consistent with segmental renal artery stenosis. Renal arteriogram showed two left renal arteries. *(Figure continues.)*

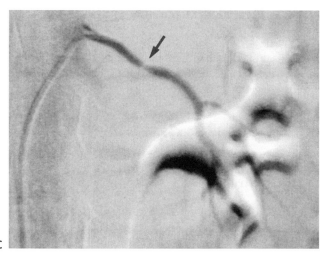

FIGURE 54.20. *Continued.* **C:** Selective arteriogram of the artery supplying the lower part of the kidney demonstrates stenosis.

Renal Artery Thromboembolism

Occlusion of the renal artery by thrombus or embolism in the newborn is an uncommon but well-recognized disorder, is almost always unilateral, and is observed most often as a complication of umbilical artery catheterization. The disorder is also found in infants of diabetic mothers and in infants with sepsis; hypotension; and hemoconcentration from diarrhea, blood loss, or other causes. Severe systemic hypertension is the main clinical manifestation of the disorder. Proteinuria and microscopic hematuria are common. Renal sonogram shows cortical hyperechogenicity in a kidney that is either normal or decreased in size. Depending on the site and severity of arterial occlusion, conventional radionuclide renal imaging may show decreased perfusion and function of the kidney or it may remain normal. In patients who have a normal baseline study, captopril renography may show deterioration of renal function.

Renal Vein Thrombosis

Renal vein thrombosis occurs most often in neonates and is usually unilateral. Thrombotic changes start in arcuate and interlobar veins and propagate to the main renal vein. Occasionally, the thrombus starts in the main renal vein or inferior vena cava. Decreased renal blood flow and venous stasis associated with dehydration and hemoconcentration from diarrhea, blood loss, or other causes are the main predisposing factors. Infants of diabetic mothers are also prone to develop renal vein thrombosis. The affected kidney becomes hemorrhagic, necrotic, and usually enlarged. Renal vein thrombosis and adrenal hemorrhage may coexist, probably as a result of propagation of thrombus from renal to adrenal vein, and are more common on the left side.

A rapidly enlarging kidney, hematuria, and falling hematocrit are the main clinical manifestations of renal vein thrombosis. The natural course of renal vein thrombosis depends on the extent of the thrombosis and potential for collateral circulation. Partial or complete return of function with a normal or slightly decreased renal size may be observed, but more often the kidney atrophies within a few weeks to a few months.

The diagnosis is often suspected on clinical grounds and is confirmed by renal sonography and/or scintigraphy. In the early stages, the sonogram shows enlargement of the kidney associated with increased echogenicity resulting from edema and hemorrhage. After 1 to 2 weeks, the kidney becomes hypoechoic with poor corticomedullary differentiation. A thrombus in the main renal vein or inferior vena cava may be seen. Coexisting adrenal hemorrhage is also detected. Color Doppler sonography shows absence of blood flow in the intrarenal branches of the renal vein.

Radionuclide renal imaging in the early stages shows both decreased perfusion and function in an enlarged kidney. In the later stages, a small, poorly functioning kidney may be identified. Scintigraphic findings of renal vascular occlusion are nonspecific and should be interpreted in the clinical context.

Renal Ectopia and Fusion Anomalies

Any functioning renal tissue, irrespective of its location, can be visualized by radionuclide renal imaging. Ectopic kidneys, which are often superimposed on bones and may remain obscure on an IVU, can be easily demonstrated and differentiated from renal agenesis (Fig. 54.21). This is particularly important in the evaluation of girls with paradoxical enuresis secondary to ectopic insertion of the ureter of a small poorly functioning ectopic kidney (19). The horseshoe kidney and other variants of fused kidneys are also often better evaluated on a renal scintigram than on an IVU (Figs. 54.22 and 54.23). In patients with meningomyelocele and severe spinal deformity, the kidneys may be malpositioned and mimic horseshoe kidney. This "pseudo-horseshoe" kidney can be differentiated from true horseshoe kidney by magnified cortical images in oblique projection.

Renal Trauma

Renal injuries are often caused by blunt abdominal trauma or, less commonly, by penetration. Iatrogenic injuries may also

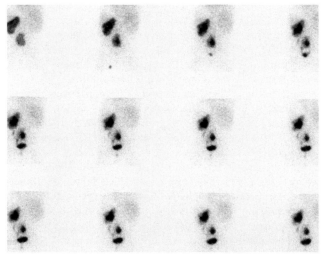

FIGURE 54.21. Ectopic kidney. Sequential posterior images after injection of ^{99m}Tc-mercaptoacetyltriglycine demonstrate a small pelvic right kidney with normal function and drainage. The hydronephrotic left kidney is in normal location.

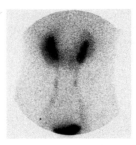

FIGURE 54.22. Horseshoe kidney. Anterior image of a ^{99m}Tc-diethyl-enetriaminepentaacetic acid scan demonstrates fusion of the lower poles of the kidneys.

occur as a result of surgical intervention, renal biopsy, retrograde pyelography, or interventional radiographic procedures. Diagnostic imaging procedures used in the evaluation of renal trauma include excretory urography, sonography, CT, radionuclide studies, and arteriography. The role of these imaging modalities in the diagnostic algorithm depends on the patient's condition and associated injuries, as well as the availability of equipment and expertise.

Excretory urography, the most readily available procedure, is sensitive in the detection of renal pedicle injuries but underestimates minor renal injuries. It has a low sensitivity for the detection of urinary leakage and does not provide information about injury to the other organs.

Renal sonography is useful in the detection of subcapsular and perirenal hematomas, lacerations, blood clots in the renal pelvis, and urinary tract obstruction. The use of Doppler allows evaluation of the renal blood flow. Renal sonography, however, does not provide any information about the renal function, which may be a critical factor in the acute management of the patient. Nonvisualization of a kidney on an excretory urogram or radionuclide renal study may be due to renal agenesis, and, unless a renal silhouette is observed on the plain abdominal radiograph, ultrasound may be required to differentiate renal pedicle injury from renal agenesis.

CT of the abdomen with intravenous contrast enhancement provides superior anatomic detail, which allows accurate evaluation of the extent of renal trauma, as well as simultaneous evaluation of other organs, the peritoneal cavity, and the retroperitoneum. It may be regarded as the single most informative imaging procedure in the evaluation of abdominal trauma.

Angiography is the best method of demonstrating vascular injury directly and also offers an opportunity to control active hemorrhage by selective arterial embolization. It is, however, invasive and is not suitable for screening and serial evaluation.

Radionuclide renal imaging provides information about overall and regional perfusion and function of the kidneys. It is extremely sensitive in detecting renal pedicle injuries, segmental infarctions, contusions, lacerations, and urine extravasation. Preexisting congenital anomalies, such as fusion, ectopia, and hydronephrosis, which make the kidneys more susceptible to trauma, are easily detected. Radionuclide renal studies in conjunction with ultrasound are particularly useful in follow-up assessment of healing of traumatic injuries to the urinary tract and detection of secondary complications.

RADIONUCLIDE CYSTOGRAPHY

The conventional method for diagnosing vesicoureteral reflux is the radiographic voiding cystourethrography (VCUG), which provides excellent delineation of bladder and urethral anatomy and allows grading of the reflux using international grading criteria (20). An alternative method for the detection of reflux is radionuclide cystography, of which there are two types: direct (retrograde) and indirect (intravenous).

Direct (Retrograde) Radionuclide Cystography

Technique

Direct radionuclide cystography has replaced radiographic VCUG in many situations. The techniques used in different institutions vary. Basically it involves urethral catheterization; retrograde filling of the bladder with normal saline mixed with tracer; and imaging the bladder and upper abdomen during filling, during voiding, and after voiding. The following technique is used in our institution.

No preparation or sedation is used. The patient is positioned supine on the table with the gamma-camera underneath. A plastic-lined absorbent pad is placed under the patient to prevent contamination of the table. Following aseptic preparation, the urethra is catheterized with an 8-Fr Foley catheter or infant feeding tube. The bladder is emptied, and a urine sample is collected in a sterile bottle for culture. The catheter is connected to a bottle of normal saline by a regular intravenous infusion tubing set. The bottle of saline is placed 100 cm above the table top. After the flow of normal saline is established, 1 mCi of ^{99m}Tc-pertechnetate (0.5 mCi in neonates) is injected into the stream of saline through the injection site of the infusion tube. An alternative technique is to mix the tracer with the saline in the bottle and infuse a constant concentration of the tracer into the bladder. The patient is positioned with the bladder on the lower edge of the field of view of the gamma-camera. While the

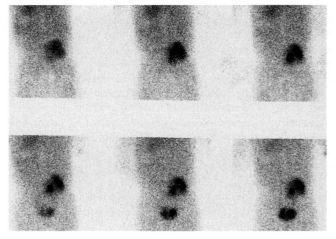

FIGURE 54.23. Crossed fused ectopia. The left kidney has crossed the midline and is fused to the right kidney that is low in position.

bladder is filling, it is continuously monitored on the persistence scope of the gamma-camera. When reflux is seen, the volume of instilled saline (the bladder volume at the time of reflux) is recorded. If bilateral reflux is observed, flow of normal saline is immediately discontinued. If no reflux is seen or only unilateral reflux occurs, the bladder is filled to capacity. Functional bladder capacity has a nonlinear relationship with age (21). However, the expected minimum capacity of the bladder in children can be estimated from the following formula: bladder capacity = (Age [yr] + 2) × 30 mL. The capacity of a hypertonic bladder may be as low as 10 to 20 mL, whereas, in those who void infrequently, the capacity may be greater than 500 mL. The resting pressure of a full bladder is about 30 cm of water. Therefore, in a quiet child, if the flow of saline solution ceases when the bottle is lowered to 30 cm above the level of the bladder, it must be assumed that the bladder is full. When the bladder is filled to its capacity, voiding is usually initiated. The infants are allowed to void on the table, around the catheter. The older patient is seated on a bedpan in front of the gamma-camera, which has been placed in a vertical position. The catheter is removed and the patient is encouraged to void. Dynamic 10-second images are acquired during filling, during voiding, and after voiding (Figs. 54.24 to 54.26).

Advantages

The most important advantage of direct radionuclide cystography is its extremely low radiation dose. With 1 mCi of ^{99m}Tc-pertechnetate in 200 mL of saline, the dose to the bladder wall during direct radionuclide cystography is about 1 mrad per minute of contact. The average length of bladder exposure is only about 15 minutes, which results in a radiation dose of about 15 mrad to the bladder wall. The dose to the ovary is less than 5 mrad. The testicular dose is probably less than 2 mrad. On the other hand, gonadal dose with standard x-ray VCUG ranges from 75 mrad to several rads, depending on the fluoroscopy time and the number of films taken. Therefore, on average, the gonadal dose is about 1/50 that of standard x-ray VCUG. In

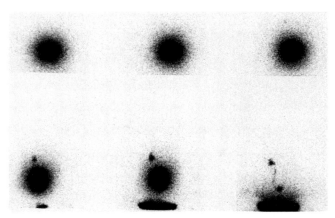

FIGURE 54.25. Direct radionuclide cystogram. Serial images show reflux occurring only during voiding.

some centers, ^{99m}Tc-DTPA or ^{99m}Tc-sulfur colloid is used to prevent absorption of the tracer through the bladder mucosa. However, the total body radiation that may result from possible absorption of a minimal amount of ^{99m}Tc-pertechnetate through the bladder mucosa is negligible.

Reflux is often intermittent and may vanish within a matter of seconds. Such reflux may be missed on standard x-ray VCUG but is detected with radionuclide cystography, which allows continuous monitoring of the urinary tract during filling, during voiding, and after voiding with no increase in the amount of radiation. In addition, reflux is more easily detected by this method because overlying bowel contents and bones do not interfere with its detection as they may do during standard x-ray VCUG. The exception is minimal reflux to the distal ureter, which may be obscured by the radionuclide-filled bladder. Direct radionuclide cystography is more sensitive than x-ray cystography in detecting vesicoureteral reflux. Furthermore, it provides the opportunity to calculate residual urine volume, bladder volume at the time of reflux, volume, and rate of clearance of reflux. Bladder volume at the time of reflux appears to have a prognostic significance. If the bladder volume at the time of demonstration of reflux increases on annual serial examinations, it may indicate a better prognosis for spontaneous cessation of reflux.

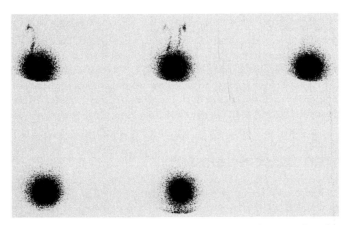

FIGURE 54.24. Direct radionuclide cystogram. Serial images show bilateral mild vesicoureteral reflux during filling phase that clears rapidly. There is no evidence of reflux during voiding.

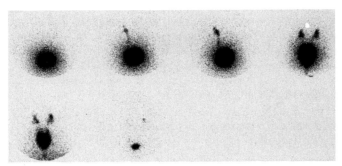

FIGURE 54.26. Direct radionuclide cystogram. Serial images show left reflux during bladder filling and right reflux during voiding.

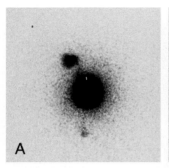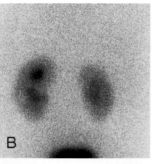

FIGURE 54.27. Reflux into the lower moiety of a duplicated system. **A:** Direct radionuclide cystogram shows left vesicoureteral reflux. **B:** The "drooping lily" appearance of the collecting system is suggestive of duplication with reflux into the lower moiety. Duplication of the left renal collecting system is confirmed on the ^{99m}Tc-glucoheptonate renal scan.

Disadvantages

The major disadvantage of direct radionuclide cystography is its unsuitability for evaluation of the male urethra. Therefore, its use for the initial study in boys is not advised unless the urethra is adequately evaluated on a voiding film obtained as part of an excretory urogram. Urethral anomalies, however, are practically nonexistent in girls. Therefore, radionuclide cystography can be safely used for the initial evaluation of girls with UTI.

Because the anatomic resolution of direct radionuclide cystography is not as good as that of x-ray VCUG, reflux cannot be graded accurately. The extremes of the spectrum (grades I, II, and V) can be differentiated, but grades III and IV cannot be accurately separated. It is, however, possible to grade reflux as mild (corresponding to grades I and II on VCUG), moderate (grade III on VCUG), and severe (grades IV and V on VCUG).

Major abnormalities such as large filling defects in the bladder (ureterocele), distortion and displacement of the bladder, and most duplications associated with reflux, can be appreciated on radionuclide cystography (Fig. 54.27), but minor abnormalities of the bladder wall such as diverticula will be missed. These minor abnormalities, however, are usually of no clinical significance.

Clinical Applications

Because of its sensitivity and minimal radiation dose, direct radionuclide cystography is the method of choice for (a) follow-up examinations in patients with known reflux who are on medical management or who have had antireflux surgery, (b) a screening test to detect reflux in asymptomatic siblings of children with known reflux, (c) serial evaluation of children with neuropathic bladder who are at-risk to develop reflux, and (d) initial screening to detect reflux in girls with UTI.

Indirect (Intravenous) Radionuclide Cystography

Technique

Indirect radionuclide cystography is a means of identifying reflux without urethral catheterization. It is based on the ideal condi-

tion of rapid and complete renal clearance of an intravenously injected radiopharmaceutical. The patient is normally hydrated (oral fluids). Following intravenous administration of 100 μCi/kg of ^{99m}Tc-DTPA, or preferably 50 μCi/kg of ^{99m}Tc-MAG3, a conventional renal scintigram is obtained. The patient is instructed not to void and is monitored intermittently. When the upper urinary tract is drained and most of the tracer is contained in the bladder, the child is placed in front of the gamma-camera in a sitting or standing position, and images are obtained before, during, and after voiding. A sudden increase in radioactivity over a kidney or ureter indicates vesicoureteral reflux (Fig. 54.28).

Advantages

The theoretical advantages of indirect radionuclide cystography are that unpleasant catheterization is avoided, voiding may be more normal because the urethra is not irritated, the study is performed without overdistending the bladder, and renal function and morphology, as well as reflux, may be evaluated simultaneously.

Disadvantages

The disadvantages of the indirect method include its dependence on renal function and adequate drainage, as well as on cooperation by the patient who must be able to void on request. The study is not practical in children who have a neuropathic bladder and in those who are not toilet trained. The radiation dose is higher than that of the direct cystogram and may become considerable if the child withholds urine for a protracted period.

Although some reports indicate good correlation between the indirect radionuclide cystography and x-ray VCUG (22), our study comparing the two radionuclide methods in 120 children with known reflux showed that the indirect technique using ^{99m}Tc-DTPA had a low sensitivity with an overall false-negative rate of 41% (23). The use of ^{99m}Tc-MAG3, which is cleared faster than ^{99m}Tc-DTPA, has not improved the accuracy of the indirect radionuclide cystograph (24).

Clinical Applications

Because of its low sensitivity for detection of reflux, indirect radionuclide cystography should not be used as an initial screening test. In children with known reflux, if renal scanning with DTPA or MAG3 is part of the follow-up evaluation, an indirect cystogram may be obtained. A positive study is reliable, but a negative study should be confirmed by direct cystography.

SCROTAL SCINTIGRAPHY

Radionuclide scrotal imaging has been refined and has proved very useful in differentiating surgical from nonsurgical disorders of the scrotal contents. This study, if performed properly in patients presenting with an acutely enlarged and painful hemiscrotum, may drastically decrease the number of unnecessary surgical explorations.

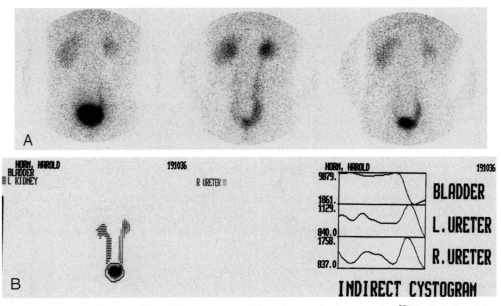

FIGURE 54.28. Indirect radionuclide cystogram. Delayed posterior images of a ^{99m}Tc-diethylenetri-aminepentaacetic acid renal scan before voiding, during voiding, and after voiding **(A)** and corresponding time-activity curves of the ureters and the bladder **(B)** show marked increase in the amount of tracer in both ureters and pelves during voiding and return of refluxed urine into the bladder after voiding.

Technique

The patient's thyroid is blocked by oral administration of potassium perchlorate in a dose of 5 mg/kg immediately before the test. The child is positioned supine on the imaging table. The penis is taped up over the pubis and the scrotum is supported by towels. The scrotum is positioned under the center of a gamma-camera equipped with converging collimator or electronic magnification capability. After rapid intravenous injection of ^{99m}Tc-pertechnetate in a dose of 200 μCi/kg, multiple 3-second dynamic images (perfusion images) are obtained. Immediately after the perfusion phase, early static images (blood pool or tissue phase) are obtained. This is usually followed by the use of a pinhole collimator to obtain high-resolution magnified static images. Lead shielding under the scrotum is not recommended for the perfusion phase of the examination, but for the static images, particularly in younger children, a lead shield under the scrotum facilitates detection of areas of decreased blood flow. Physical examination of the scrotum and accurate localization of the testicles by the nuclear medicine physician is crucial in correct interpretation of the scintigraphic findings.

Scintigraphic Patterns

Basic knowledge of the vascular anatomy of the scrotal contents is essential for understanding the scintigraphic findings. The scrotal contents have a dual blood supply. The first pathway is composed of the vessels entering the spermatic cord: the testicular artery, which supplies the testicle, epididymis, and tunica vaginalis; the deferential artery; and the cremasteric artery. These three vessels enter the spermatic cord at different levels and usually anastomose at the testicular mediastinum. The cremasteric artery forms a network over the tunica vaginalis and also participates in anastomoses with vessels supplying the scrotal wall. The second pathway is composed of the vessels that do not enter the spermatic cord. These include the internal pudendal artery and the superficial and deep external pudendal arteries. These arteries supply the scrotum and penis.

Normal Scrotal Scintigram

In a normal scrotal scintigram, the iliac arteries are well visualized, but, because of their size and the relatively small amount of blood flow, the vessels supplying the scrotal contents are ill defined and the scrotum and its contents blur into a homogeneous area of tracer accumulation slightly more intense than the soft tissues of the thigh. Dartos activity cannot be separated from testicular or epididymal activity.

Testicular Torsion

The scintigraphic pattern in testicular torsion depends on the duration of torsion. In the early phase of acute torsion (probably within the first 6 hours), the perfusion images may show decreased blood flow to the hemiscrotum or may appear normal. Blood flow to the hemiscrotum is never increased at this stage. The static images (tissue phase) show decreased accumulation of the tracer in the testicle without the reactive surrounding halo of increased activity seen in the later phases (Fig. 54.29). After a few hours, there is reactive hyperemia in the region supplied by the pudendal arteries. The perfusion images shows increased blood flow to the dartos, and the early static images show a halo of mildly increased activity around a photopenic center. The halo of increased activity may gradually disappear on the subsequent images. If the patient does not seek immediate medical

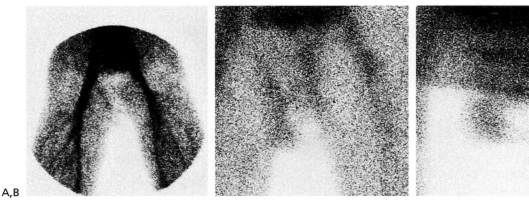

A,B

C

FIGURE 54.29. Early-phase testicular torsion. This 8-year-old boy presented with a 6-hour history of pain and swelling of the left hemiscrotum. **A:** Composite of the dynamic blood flow images shows decreased blood flow to the left hemiscrotum. The static images without **(B)** and with **(C)** a lead shield under the scrotum demonstrate markedly decreased accumulation of the tracer in the left hemiscrotum.

attention or is erroneously diagnosed (late phase), irreversible testicular infarction occurs. The pain and swelling will resolve in a few days to weeks with subsequent atrophy of the testicle. It is important to diagnose late phase testicular torsion to remove the necrotic testicle and to perform orchiopexy on the contralateral side. In the late phase of torsion, the perfusion images show marked increased blood flow to the dartos, and static images reveal a complete rim or halo of increased activity around a photopenic center. The halo persists throughout the examination, which usually takes about 10 to 15 minutes (Fig. 54.30).

Spontaneous Detorsion

A torsed testicle may undergo spontaneous detorsion in the early phases of torsion before severe reactive changes have occurred. The testicular scan may appear normal or may show slightly and diffusely increased scrotal activity if obtained shortly after detorsion, a pattern similar to that of nonsurgical causes of swollen hemiscrotum. The diagnosis is best made on the basis of clinical history if examination has not been carried out before the detorsion. Demonstration of an intact blood supply to the testicle obviates only the need for emergency surgery. If the history is typical of intermittent torsion, but physical examination shows the testis to be normally positioned and the scrotal scan shows intact perfusion and slightly increased activity, elective orchiopexy may be indicated.

Acute Epididymitis

In acute epididymitis, the perfusion images show markedly increased blood flow to the area corresponding to the epididymis. The tissue phase images also show increased accumulation of the tracer in the epididymis or diffusely in the hemiscrotum, if epididymo-orchitis is present (Fig. 54.31). Epididymitis in infants and young children may be secondary to an underlying anatomic abnormality such as an ectopic ureter and warrants complete investigation of the genitourinary system.

Torsion of the Testicular Appendages

Torsion of the appendix testis or appendix epididymis may be visualized as a focal area of increased blood flow and blood pool

activity probably secondary to reactive hyperemia around the torsed appendix. The ischemic appendix itself is too small to be resolved on the images.

A more common scintigraphic pattern is that of mild, generalized, increased blood flow and blood pool activity indistinguishable from epididymitis. This differentiation is of no surgical significance, because both epididymitis and torsion of the appen-

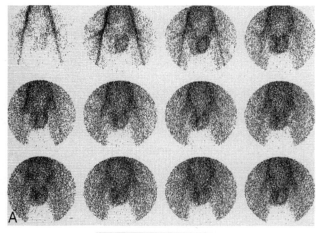

A

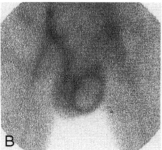

B

FIGURE 54.30. Late-phase testicular torsion. This 15-year-old boy presented with a 24-hour history of pain and swelling of the left hemiscrotum. The dynamic blood flow images **(A)** and the unshielded static image **(B)** of the scrotum show decreased blood flow to the left testicle, with a surrounding halo of reactive hyperemia.

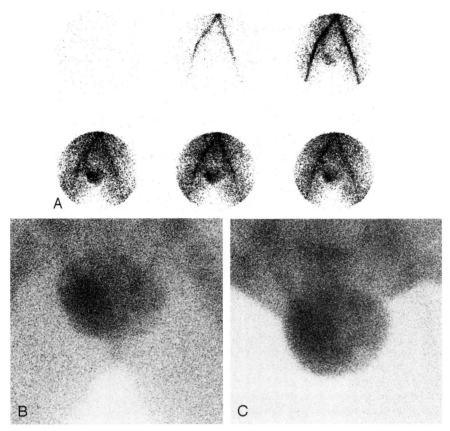

FIGURE 54.31. Epididymitis. This 15-year-old boy presented with a 24-hour history of pain and swelling of the right hemiscrotum. **A:** Radionuclide angiogram shows marked increased blood flow to the right hemiscrotum. Static tissue phase images without **(B)** and with **(C)** a lead shield also show diffuse increased accumulation of the tracer on the right.

dix testis are generally considered to be nonsurgical problems. Radionuclide studies in the early phase of torsion of the appendix testis, before a significant inflammatory response, may be normal.

Scrotal Trauma

The scintigraphic pattern following scrotal trauma depends on the extent of injury, as well as the time elapsed between the trauma and the examination. Mild traumatic changes may appear as slightly to moderately diffuse increased tracer accumulation. Testicular or intrascrotal hematoma may appear as a cold lesion with or without a surrounding halo of increased activity similar to testicular torsion. Testicular rupture is also a surgical problem. Ultrasound may be a useful adjunct in localizing a hematoma in relation to the testicle.

Hydrocele

The diagnosis of a simple hydrocele is made by physical examination and transillumination. In secondary hydrocele, which is seen in association with torsion, epididymitis, trauma, or following herniorrhaphy, scintigraphic findings reflect the underlying condition. Hydrocele often appears as a horseshoe or a crescentic photon deficiency surrounding the testicle (Fig.54.32).

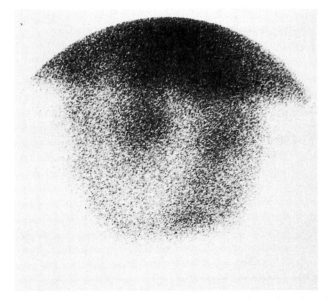

FIGURE 54.32. Hydrocele in a neonate. There is a horseshoe-shaped area of decreased accumulation of the tracer in the right hemiscrotum surrounding the normally perfused right testicle.

Testicular or Intrascrotal Abscess

Scrotal scintigraphy in these lesions demonstrates a cold center surrounded by a rim of increased activity similar to that of late phase torsion. The diagnosis is usually made in the context of the clinical history.

Basic Scintigraphic Patterns

There are four basic scintigraphic patterns in the acute hemiscrotum:

1. Diffuse increased blood flow and blood pool activity without any photopenic component (excluding typical secondary hydrocele) (Fig. 54.31). This pattern is seen in patients with epididymitis, torsion of the appendix testis, minor posttraumatic abnormalities, and spontaneous detorsion. Except for spontaneous detorsion, these are nonsurgical conditions. The problem of differentiating spontaneous detorsion is usually solved on the basis of clinical history and findings on physical examination.
2. Focal increased blood flow and blood pool activity. This pattern is characteristic of torsion of the testicular appendage.
3. Diffuse decreased blood flow and blood pool activity (Fig. 54.29). This pattern is seen in the early phase of testicular torsion, the early phase of large testicular or intrascrotal hematoma, and in large tense hydrocele.
4. Photopenic center with a surrounding rim of increased activity (Fig. 54.30). This doughnut-shaped pattern is seen in late phase testicular torsion, late phase hematoma, and abscess.

Clinical Applications

When the clinical presentation and physical findings are typical of the early phase of acute testicular torsion, surgery should be performed immediately without delaying for a testicular scan. When the clinical presentation suggests inflammatory disease or conditions other than acute torsion or when the patient cannot be properly examined because of extreme swelling and tenderness, testicular scanning is indicated and can reliably differentiate the surgical from the nonsurgical conditions.

REFERENCES

1. McCrory WW. *Develpemental nephrology.* Cambridge, MA: Harvard University Press, 1972:96.
2. Vanpee M, Blennow M, Linne T et al. Renal function in very low birth weight infants: normal maturity reached during early childhood. *J Pediatr* 1992;121:784–788.
3. Jacobson HSH, Eklöf O, Eriksson CG et al. Development of hypertension and uremia after pyelonephritis in childhood: 27-year follow up. *Br Med J* 1989;299:703–706.
4. Alexander SR, Arbus GS, Butt KMH et al. The 1989 report of the North American Pediatric Renal Transplant Cooperative Study. *Pediatr Nephrol* 1990;4:542–553.
5. Miller T, Phillips S. Pyelonephritis: the relationship between infection, renal scarring, and antimicrobial therapy. *Kidney Int* 1981;19:654–662.
6. Ransley PG, Risdon RA. Reflux nephropathy: effect of antimicrobial therapy on the evolution of the early pyelonephritic scar. *Kidney Int* 1981;20:733–742.
7. Slotki IN, Asscher AW. Prevention of scarring in experimental pyelonephritis in the rat by early antibiotic therapy. *Nephron* 1982;30:262–268.
8. Majd M, Rushton HG, Jantausch B et al. Relationship among vesicoureteral reflux, P-fimbriated Escherichia coli and acute pyelonephritis in children with febrile urinary tract infection. *J Pediatr* 1991;119:578–585.
9. Rushton HG, Majd M, Jantausch B et al. Renal scarring following reflux and nonreflux pyelonephritis in children: evaluation with 99mTc-DMSA scintigraphy. *J Urol* 1992;147:1327–1332.
10. Sty JR, Wells RG, Starshak RJ et al. Imaging in acute renal infection in children. *AJR* 1987;148:471–477.
11. Björgvinsson E, Majd M, Eggli K. Diagnosis of acute pyelonephritis in children: comparison of sonography and 99mTc-DMSA scintigraphy. *AJR* 1991;157:539–543.
12. Majd M, Rushton HG, Chandra R et al: 99mTc-DMSA renal cortical scintigraphy for the detection of experimental acute pyelonephritis in piglets: comparison of planar (pinhole) and SPECT imaging. *J Nucl Med* 1996;37:1731–1734.
13. Majd M, Nussbaum Blask AR, Markle BM et al. Acute pyelonephritis: comparison of diagnosis with 99mTc-DMSA SPECT, spiral CT, MRI, and power Doppler sonography in an experimental pig model. *Radiology* 2001;218:101–108.
14. Majd M, Rushton HG. Renal cortical scintigraphy in the diagnosis of acute pyelonephritis. *Semin Nucl Med* 1992;22:98–111.
15. Majd, Potter BM, Guzzeta PC et al. Effect of captopril on efficacy of renal scintigraphy in detection of renal artery stenosis. *J Nucl Med* 1983;24:23(abst).
16. Sfakianakis GN, Bourgoignie JJ, Jaffe D et al. Single-dose captopril scintigraphy in the diagnosis of renovascular hypertension. *J Nucl Med* 1987;28:1383–1392.
17. Hovinga TKK, de Jong PE, Piers DA et al. Diagnostic use of angiotensin converting enzyme inhibitors in radioisotope evaluation of unilateral renal artery stenosis. *J Nucl Med* 1989;30:605–614.
18. Dondi M, Franchi R, Levorato M et al. Evaluation of hypertensive patients by means of captopril enhanced renal scintigraphy with technetium-99m DTPA. *J Nucl Med* 1989;30:615–621.
19. Pattaras JG, Rushton HG, Majd M. The role of 99mTechnetium dimercapto-succinic acid renal scans in the evaluation of occult ectopic ureter in girls with paradoxical incontinence. *J Urol* 1999;162:821–825.
20. International Reflux Study Committee. Medical versus surgical treatment of primary vesicoureteral reflux. *Pediatrics* 1981;67:392–400.
21. Treves ST, Zurakowski D, Bauer SB et al. Functional bladder capacity measured during radionuclide cystography in children. *Radiology* 1996;198:269–272.
22. Gordon I, Peters AM, Morony S. Indirect radionuclide cystography: a sensitive technique for the detection of vesico-ureteral reflux. *Pediatr Nephrol* 1990;4:604–606.
23. Majd M, Kass EJ, Belman AB. Radionuclide cystography in children: comparison of direct (retrograde) and indirect (intravenous) techniques. *Ann Radiol* 1985;28:322–328.
24. DE Sadeleer C, De Boe V, Keuppens F et al. How good is technetium-99m mercaptoacetyltriglycine indirect cystography? *Eur J Nucl Med* 1994;21:223–227.

55

SPECIFIC PROBLEMS AND MUSCULOSKELETAL IMAGING IN CHILDREN

DAVID L. GILDAY

HANDLING CHILDREN (OR HOW TO GET A QUALITY STUDY)

Performing effective nuclear medicine procedures in children requires certain modifications of the techniques that are used when studying adult patients. These modifications can be categorized under the following headings: child-parent-staff interaction, injection techniques, radiopharmaceutical dose, and sedation.

Child-Parent-Staff Interaction

The reaction and response of a child to a nuclear medicine procedure is largely dependent on the attitude of the staff toward that child, the technique used in performing the study, and the general environment of the department. All staff members dealing with the child should have a calm, relaxed demeanor and a kind, confident, and sympathetic approach. It is important to gain parental understanding and cooperation.

A child old enough to understand (as young as 3 years) should have all aspects of the study explained in appropriate words. Positive aspects of the study should be emphasized and negative aspects minimized. However, it is crucial never to mislead the child about what is to happen. A child's trust in the staff may be difficult to obtain, and once obtained it is easily jeopardized.

Allowing a parent to maintain close physical contact and to talk with the child while the study is being performed distracts the child's attention from the procedure and often gains greater cooperation. Encouraging the child to watch a child-oriented video or to listen to a personal cassette player is distracting and relieves the boredom of lying still for a total body scan or single photon emission computed tomography (SPECT). Providing toys and soothers goes a long way toward achieving a successful study. We give each younger child a colorful sticker or "bubble pen," after the injection, as a reward for being cooperative.

D.L. Gilday: Medical Imaging, University of Toronto, Department of Diagnostic Imaging, The Hospital for Sick Children, Toronto, Ontario, Canada.

To minimize movement, a parent is encouraged to participate in monitoring the child. It has been our experience that with well-trained staff and parental involvement, it is rare not to obtain a successful study. Children who are a disciplinary problem are often more uncooperative when parents are present, and in this case the presence of a parent should be reconsidered and the parent encouraged to voluntarily retire.

Careful restraint is often necessary in the younger child but should be used in moderation because excessive use can result in the child struggling against it. Babies should be restrained by wrapping them in a sheet. This provides adequate restraint without causing discomfort. Uncooperative children or infants may be immobilized with restrainers strapped around the stretcher top with Velcro straps.

Injection Techniques

Injection of radiopharmaceuticals in small children presents several minor problems, all of which are easily surmounted by a few modifications. Because very small children will be completely covered by the head of a large-field-of-view camera, we place the child supine on the pallet with the camera underneath. This decreases the child's anxiety and makes the injection much easier.

Finding a suitable site for intravenous injections is rarely a problem, if several points are remembered. Although the antecubital fossa often has the largest vein, the elbow is less easily immobilized than the hand or foot, and the latter is often a preferable injection site. Scalp veins are also easily accessible but are used only as a last resort because a small area of hair must be shaved away to find them. Jugular vein injections are mandatory for left-to-right shunt evaluations and are also useful in procedures in which multiple blood samples are required (e.g., glomerular filtration rate determination) and when the child's other veins have been used for repeated venipunctures in the past. Central lines may be used for venous access, using the appropriate sterile precautions.

Our injection apparatus is a 6- or 12-mL syringe of saline connected with extension tubing to a three-way stopcock that is also connected to the syringe containing the radiopharmaceutical and a 23- or 25-gauge butterfly needle. This allows the dose syringe to be completely isolated from the saline while the needle is inserted into the vein. Once the needle is properly positioned (confirmed by injecting some saline into the vein), the injection is carried out. The bolus of radiopharmaceutical is pushed through the butterfly needle by injecting the saline.

Radiopharmaceutical Dose

The amount of radioactivity can be readily calculated by referring to a graph. The percentage of the standard adult dose is determined according to the child's body surface area. This dose calculation permits distribution of tracer per unit area of organ rather than per kilogram of body weight. It is important to establish a minimum dose for each radiopharmaceutical. To get an adequate study, especially a dynamic one, there has to be enough photons detected per unit time to adequately assess the child's problem. It is better to have a slightly higher delivered radiation dose than to have an uninterpretable study. The risk of the higher radiation dose is negligible, especially if we have helped the child.

Sedation

If moderate restraint is not likely to be successful, then sedation is necessary to obtain a technically satisfactory study. Sedation is recommended in overly anxious children who refuse to cooperate, as well as in the very young (6 months to 5 years of age), in hyperactive children who are unable to remain still, and, especially, in patients who lack the mental capacity to follow simple instructions.

In the correct setting, sedation with intravenous pentobarbital sodium (Nembutal) is the most effective. Using a dose of 5 to 6 mg/kg^{-1} (to a maximum of 100 mg), we administer half the volume rapidly, wait 60 seconds, and then administer a quarter of the dose. This usually puts the child to sleep in about 2 to 3 minutes. If not, then the remaining quarter dose is given. The child remains asleep for about 45 to 60 minutes. The advantages of this technique are that the child falls asleep very quickly, the effect is more reliable than with intramuscularly injected pentobarbital sodium, and the child recovers faster.

Pentobarbital sodium is contraindicated in neonates younger than 2 months. They lack adequate levels of the liver enzymes to metabolize pentobarbital sodium before it acts *in vivo*. In place of pentobarbital sodium we use chloral hydrate, 30 to 45 minutes before scanning. The effect is less pronounced than with pentobarbital sodium, but it is usually adequate and the child arouses readily.

When children are sedated, their cardiac and respiratory status must be closely monitored by appropriately trained individuals. We currently use an automated pulse oximeter attached to a first toe. The digital readout is easy to read and an alarm is available if the readings go outside of preset limits.

MUSCULOSKELETAL SCINTIGRAPHY

Other than malignancy, the two major indications for scanning the osseous system are investigation of pain or fever/infection.

This is usually done after plain film examination or computed tomography (CT) has failed to detect a lesion. Our standard technique is a two-part study consisting of blood pool; delayed planar images and, when indicated, static SPECT images. The highest resolution system available is necessary to obtain adequate images in small children and infants, and magnification with a pinhole or converging collimator is often necessary (1).

Osteomyelitis

Often, the diagnosis of osteomyelitis in children is difficult. The child may present with bone pain, joint tenderness, soft tissue swelling, erythema, fever, and bacteremia. The clinical differentiation of osteomyelitis from pure cellulitis may be difficult. Unfortunately, the radiologic examination can yield a wide range of findings: normal, soft tissue swelling, and, in a few, the frank bone changes of osteomyelitis. Using combined blood pool and bone imaging, we found it possible to differentiate osteomyelitis from cellulitis very early in the course of the child's illness. Bone scintigraphy has its greatest value in assessing areas difficult to evaluate by standard radiologic means, such as the pelvis and spine. These areas do not have the easily seen fat planes of the long bones and, therefore, the early diagnosis of osteomyelitis is best made by bone scintigraphy.

The typical bone scan appearance of osteomyelitis is a well-defined focus of increased radioactivity within bone, associated with an identical area of hyperemia in the blood pool images. This is usually located in the metaphysis of long bones in the acute case and is highly distinctive (Fig. 55.1) (2). Occasionally, the focal increase is superimposed on a more diffuse bone increase secondary to hyperemia. This appears to be specific for osteomyelitis and is readily differentiated from the patterns of cellulitis and septic arthritis. There is an unusual presentation of osteomyelitis when thromboses occur at the site, which results in a photopenic defect without hyperemia. In these instances, gallium scintigraphy is useful.

The blood pool images are rarely of value in the spine because of radiotracer in the blood in the underlying abdominal and thoracic organs. Planar images or SPECT of the spine readily

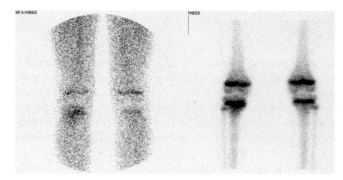

FIGURE 55.1. Metaphyseal osteomyelitis. There is focal increased activity in the proximal right tibial metaphysis with hyperemia on the blood pool image. Delayed anterior views of the right knee show increased activity in the right tibial metaphysis that obscures the distal aspect of the physis.

demonstrate the abnormal vertebral bodies involved, usually confirming the radiologic diagnosis of discitis and/or osteomyelitis. Bone scintigraphy can be positive as early as 24 hours after the onset of symptoms and is always positive by 3 days, well before any bony changes are evident in the x-ray films. Occasionally, however, soft tissue swelling or indistinct fat lines permit the presumptive radiologic diagnosis of osteomyelitis several days after the onset of symptoms. Children who have middle ear infections are prone to develop mastoiditis. Planar scanning is notoriously poor at detecting mastoiditis, whereas SPECT is very good.

It is important to differentiate cellulitis and septic arthritis from the presence of associated osteomyelitis, because either of the former may mask the latter. Cellulitis appears as diffuse increase in radioactivity involving the soft tissues and bone that is readily apparent in both the blood pool and delayed bone images. Septic arthritis has a similar appearance because of the hyperemia involving the joint. The subchondral bone on either side of the affected joint has increased tracer metabolism.

In some unusual cases, the scan will be normal despite definite clinical signs. In such cases, ^{67}Ga citrate imaging has proven useful in differentiating osteomyelitis from soft tissue inflammation. This is especially true in early osteomyelitis when the only abnormality may be hyperemia. The gallium scan is usually positive and confirms the suspected osteomyelitis.

If a child has clinical symptoms suggesting osteomyelitis and a normal x-ray film, then the examination that can most readily give the correct answer is bone scintigraphy. This is especially true early in the illness or if the axial skeleton is involved. However, in some unusual cases (less than 5%), the scan may be normal despite definite clinical signs, in which case gallium citrate imaging has proven useful in detecting occult osteomyelitis. We do not use gallium as the primary test because of its higher radiation dose and 24-hour delay in getting good images.

Chronic multifocal recurrent osteomyelitis is an indolent form of osteomyelitis that occurs in older children and lasts for several years (3). It is characterized by the following: A detectable organism is lacking, antibiotics are ineffective, pain is prominent, and the disease is self-limiting with few if any sequelae.

The infant, who is less than 6 weeks of age at the time of onset of osteomyelitis, often has a very aggressive, destructive type of osteomyelitis. There are usually multiple sites (40%) of osteomyelitis, involving the epiphysis, as well as the metaphysis. In the infant, the x-ray film usually becomes abnormal by the time the disease is suspected clinically. The gross destruction of the bone is evident radiologically, and, unfortunately, it is more difficult to diagnose than osteomyelitis in older children. This very destructive lesion, which does not allow a bony reaction in this phase, is seen as a photopenic area (4).

Septic Arthritis of the Hip

Septic arthritis of the hip can often cause symptoms of severe hip pain associated with clinical and hematologic changes of infection. The important feature of this entity is that it can cause compression of the blood supply to the femoral capital epiphysis. Ultrasound examination can determine whether fluid is present in the hip joint. The proper course of action is to aspirate the hip joint promptly, which relieves the pressure and makes the diagnosis. If one were to image before drainage, there would be decreased blood flow and decreased tracer accumulation within the femoral head. With magnification the abnormality is seen as a reduction of activity in the femoral capital epiphysis and the adjacent growth zone (Fig. 55.2). Normally, bone scanning is done postoperatively to determine whether a concomitant osteomyelitis is present. This is of concern because part of the femoral neck (noncartilage-covered bone) is within the hip joint. Subsequently, the scan will show hyperemia of the hip, which is the normal response to inflammation and infection.

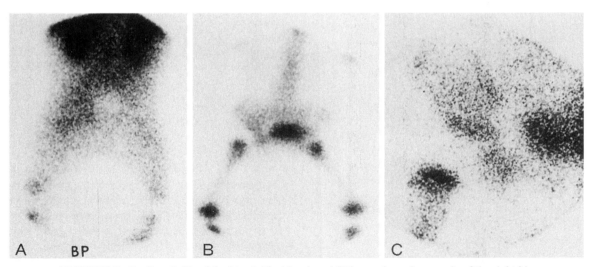

FIGURE 55.2. Septic arthritis of the hip. **A:** The blood pool (BP) scan shows hyperemia of the right hip, but the delayed **(B)** and pinhole magnification **(C)** images show reduction of activity in the femoral capital epiphysis. This is an example of septic arthritis with compromised blood supply to the femoral head.

Ischemic Bone Disease

Legg-Perthes Disease

Avascular necrosis of the femoral head (e.g., Legg-Perthes disease) is usually detected radiographically or by magnetic resonance imaging (MRI). In the few equivocal cases, bone scintigraphy can be used to detect avascular necrosis in the presence of an inconclusive MRI study. Bone scintigraphy, especially when using pinhole magnification, remains an excellent technique for detecting avascularity of the femoral capital epiphysis (5,6).

Osteonecrosis

Osteonecrosis usually causes an intense reactive (healing) response. This is usually hyperemic. Children treated with steroids or anti-autoimmune drugs develop a form of osteoporosis that probably results in cortical microfractures. The bone scan (Fig. 55.3) always shows increased activity, which is often intense, and usually hyperemia. The commonest sites are the femoral head and condyles and proximal tibia, and less common sites are the talus, calcaneus, and distal tibia.

Sickle Cell Disease

The child who has sickle cell disease often presents to the emergency room with pain and sometimes fever. The dilemma is to determine whether the child has a sickle cell crisis with possible marrow infarction or has osteomyelitis, which is relatively rare. The imaging scheme we use is to assess the marrow with ^{99m}Tc-sulfur colloid, then to inject ^{99m}Tc-methylene diphosphonate (MDP), and, after the bone scan is finished, to inject ^{67}Ga citrate

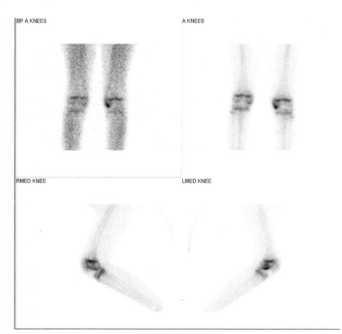

FIGURE 55.3. Osteonecrosis of the left medial femoral condyle. The blood pool image shows hyperemia, and the bone scan shows increased metabolism of the bone tracer in the right medial femoral condyle subchondrally. Medial view confirms location of the osteonecrosis.

if needed. The marrow scan is often abnormal at the site of the pain indicating marrow dysfunction, which could be due to a sickle crisis or secondary to osteomyelitis (7). If the bone scan is normal, then the diagnosis is ischemia (Fig. 55.4), and the gallium scan is not needed. If the bone scan is abnormal and the gallium is normal, then the diagnosis is most likely postischemic healing. If the bone and gallium scans are abnormal in the pattern seen in osteomyelitis, then that is the diagnosis.

Trauma

Most bone trauma circumstances are readily evaluated by plain x-ray films. Occasionally, the fracture may not be evident and then a bone scan can yield the diagnosis, because it will become abnormal in 24 hours (often earlier).

Stress Injury

Stress injury usually consists of a focal area of bone injury that results from repetitive stress to a portion of bone. Because muscular contraction causes stress at tendon insertions, this is the site of many stress-related bony injuries. Forceful repetitive trauma, especially among athletes, results in varying degrees of injury—from reactive periosteal new bone formation to a true stress fracture with transcortical injury. In the case of simple periosteal injury, often known as "shin splints," the trauma probably causes disruption of the subperiosteal vessels and bleeding. A true stress fracture occurs as the result of repeated severe trauma and involves at least 50% of the cortex. It is often seen in the tibia or a metatarsal. A favorite location is at the site where supporting footgear stops, such as the boot top of a skate. These injuries are most common in runners, ballet dancers, skaters, and gymnasts (also prone to spinal and wrist stress injuries).

Bone scanning is very sensitive in detecting stress fractures and for distinguishing between osseous and muscular injury. The bone scan is abnormal at the time of presentation (Fig. 55.5), whereas the x-ray film, if it becomes abnormal, does so some weeks later. The clinical importance of this differentiation is that periosteal stress reaction heals much more rapidly than true stress fractures, and patients with periosteal stress reaction can be allowed to return to athletic activity more quickly. Clinically, most patients with uncomplicated periosteal stress reaction will have resolution of pain within 2 weeks of cessation of the offending activity and will remain pain free following gradual resumption of activity.

Toddler's Fracture

Greenstick or toddler's fractures are usually seen as a relatively faint increase in activity in a linear or spiral appearance along the tibia (Fig. 55.6). They are important to differentiate from the periosteal reaction commonly associated with nonaccidental trauma (8).

Nonaccidental Trauma

The estimated incidence of reported child abuse increased by 50% from 1985 to 1992. The incidence of skeletal injury in

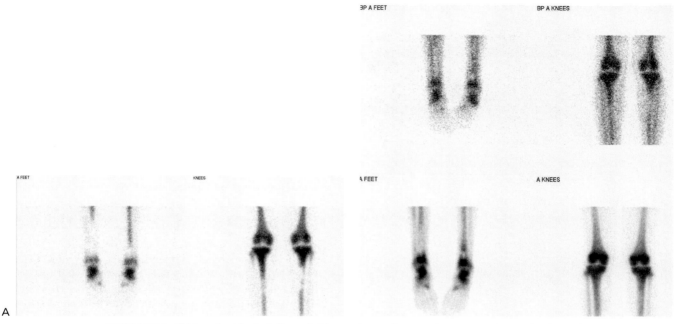

FIGURE 55.4. Sickle cell crisis. **A:** Sulfur colloid scan shows absence of marrow activity in both distal tibia and right proximal tibia. **B:** Bone scan shows decreased metabolic activity in same locations. There is one-to-one correlation of the two studies indicating a crisis rather than osteomyelitis.

these children is approximately 20% and is more common among those younger than 1 year. Children older than 3 years tend to have predominantly soft tissue injury. Cerebral injury is common at any age. The fractures are usually multiple, involving the long bones, skull, vertebrae, ribs, and facial bones and usually show different stages of healing.

Radiographic skeletal survey and MDP bone scintigraphy are complementary procedures for diagnosing and documenting this type of injury. In experienced hands, the bone scan is more sensitive, with a false-negative rate of 0.8% compared with 12.3% with x-ray films. The bone scan may be positive as early as 7 hours after injury, although the child is usually not brought to hospital immediately so there is time for bone repair to start. Knowledge of the normal bone scan appearance for the age of the child is mandatory to assess developmental variation. Particular attention should be paid to skeletal asymmetry, focal abnormality, and extraosseous and renal accumulation of tracer.

Metaphyseal-epiphyseal injury is common. Careful positioning and correct windowing are important to avoid obscuring a minimal abnormality. Accurate interpretation will depend on assessment of the intensity and shape of abnormality. The bone scan is especially useful detecting injury in the ribs, costoverte-

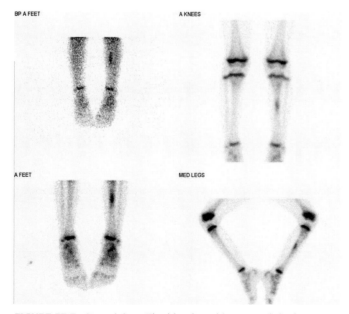

FIGURE 55.5. Stress injury. The blood pool image and the bone scan show the presence of a linear increase in activity involving the posterior cortex of the mid diaphysis of the left tibia.

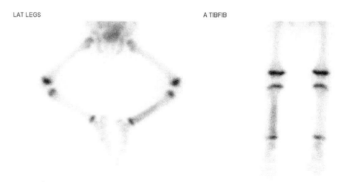

FIGURE 55.6. Toddler's fracture. The bone scan demonstrates a diffuse mild increase in metabolic activity along the distal two thirds of the right tibia.

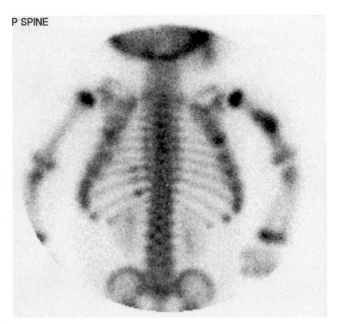

P SPINE

FIGURE 55.7. Nonaccidental trauma. Bone scans show a fracture involving the right humerus and fractures of the left seventh, eighth, and ninth ribs.

bral junctions, hands, feet, spine, and diaphyses of long bones (9,10) (Fig. 55.7).

Classic Patterns

Skull injuries are best evaluated by radiography because they are poorly detected by the bone scan. We believe that if the bone scan is normal 3 days or more after injury, then there is no evidence for acute bony injury. Disadvantages of the bone scan include inability to determine the type, extent, and age of each injury; poor bone accumulation of the ^{99m}Tc-MDP compound in cases of severe malnutrition; inability to differentiate systemic and metabolic disorders associated with trauma from trauma alone; and nondetection of the completely healed fracture or hairline fracture of the skull. Consequently, radiologic workup of suspected child abuse usually includes immediate x-ray films of the clinically obvious fractures; bone scan; skull x-ray films to document the extent of skeletal injury; and other tests, such as ultrasound, MRI, and CT, to document visceral and soft tissue injury based on clinical suspicion.

Spondylolysis

Spondylolysis is a common congenital abnormality. The break in the pars interarticularis is often secondary to trauma. Therefore, if the bones are close together, they will attempt to reunite. The lack of integrity of the neural arch results in extra stresses being placed on the facet joints, which react by becoming hypermetabolic. In many cases, the pars interarticularis defect may not be easily identified on the spinal x-ray films. SPECT bone imaging has the advantage of being able not only to detect the reparative attempts of the defect but also to show the increased bone stress at the articular facets. In addition, SPECT can locate the abnormality spatially, so that facet stress can be distinguished from the healing pars interarticularis (11–13). Intriguingly, there are four patterns of reaction. The first pattern is the healing one in which the increased activity is more centrally located in the neural arch. The second pattern is when the increased activity is at one facet joint on the same side as the interrupted pars

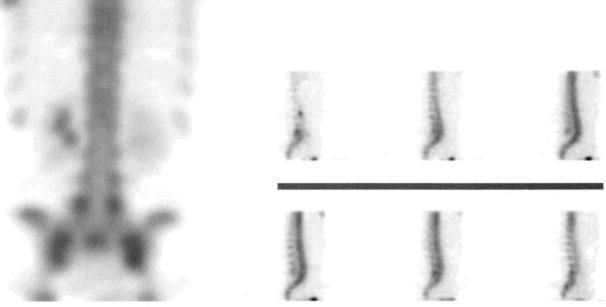

A   B

FIGURE 55.8. Spondylolysis. **A:** Coronal and **(B)** sagittal images demonstrate bilateral reaction to the spondylolysis at the articular facets. This is a typical case in which the localization needs multiple projections.

interarticularis; sometimes it is on the contralateral side, which is presumably secondary to the stress reaction. The third pattern is bilateral reaction (Fig. 55.8). The last pattern is when there is only stress injury; stress injury alone without disruption of the neural arch, usually involving the par interarticularis, will result in a picture that can look similar to the first pattern described above. At this point, CT is needed to confirm that the neural arch is intact and possibly to see the bony reaction to the stress.

MUSCULOSKELETAL TUMORS

Neuroblastoma

Neuroblastoma is the commonest solid nonneurologic tumor in childhood, and it often metastasizes to bone. The radionuclide scans are more sensitive than radiographic skeletal survey. From 30% to 70% of the lesions seen on radionuclide scans are normal on x-ray film. A radionuclide skeletal survey should, therefore, be the primary investigation. The bony involvement is usually seen as multiple foci of increased activity in the metaphysis; is usually asymmetric; and usually involves skull, vertebrae, ribs, pelvis, and long bones (14). Often, symmetric metaphyseal involvement is seen, especially around the knees (Fig. 55.9). The physis is normally slightly elliptic in infants younger than 18 months and is plate-like in older children. The metaphyseal border is always well demarcated. When the uptake in the physis is wedge shaped or globular, or if there is blurring of the metaphyseal border, metastasis should be suspected even if the involvement is symmetric (Fig. 55.9). Occasionally, if the tumor is very destructive, the metaphysis may be photon deficient.

At the time of diagnosis, the primary tumor will accumulate the ^{99m}Tc-MDP 50% to 60% of the time for abdominal tumors and 80% of the time for tumors in the thorax. The mechanism of uptake is as yet unknown and may be related to dystrophic calcification in the tumor. When the primary tumor is intraabdominal, renal abnormalities such as nonfunction, obstruction, or inferior and/or lateral displacement are commonly seen. Blood pool and sequential renal scans should be performed during the first 15 minutes after injection of the ^{99m}Tc-MDP in any child suspected of having neuroblastoma or abdominal tumor.

^{131}I-metaiodobenzylguanidine (^{131}I-MIBG) was first de-scribed in 1983. It was rapidly and enthusiastically adopted for both the investigation and therapy of neuroblastoma in children (15). It was subsequently replaced by ^{123}I-MIBG because of the better imaging characteristics of ^{123}I. Before this, the ^{99m}Tc-MDP bone scan was the only way to determine whether a child had skeletal involvement by neuroblastoma. The problem with ^{99m}Tc-MDP bone scanning is that the studies require great care to avoid false-negative interpretations even though the skeletal lesions have a significant lesion-to-background activity level. It was because of this and the generally poor ability to detect soft tissue or marrow neuroblastoma lesions that ^{131}I and then ^{123}I-MIBG were so quickly adopted. However, Gordon et al. (16) bring a strong concern forward about the use of MIBG scanning as the sole test for the detection of skeletal neuroblastoma lesions. They found that ^{123}I-MIBG revealed more extensive skeletal disease than ^{99m}Tc-MDP, but all had abnormal bone scans. On the other hand, five patients had normal ^{123}I-MIBG with abnormal ^{99m}Tc-MDP studies of the skeleton.

In view of the inability of ^{123}I or ^{131}I-MIBG scanning to detect all neuroblastoma bony lesions, all children with a diagnosis of neuroblastoma must have both the ^{123}I/^{131}I-MIBG and ^{99m}Tc-MDP scan to stage and monitor their neuroblastoma involvement.

During the last 10 years a number of centers have started to treat neuroblastoma with ^{131}I-MIBG, more recently in conjunction with enhancers such as vitamin C or retinoic acid.

Osteogenic Sarcoma

Osteogenic sarcomas usually occur in the metaphyses of long bones, a common site being the distal femur or proximal tibia. They have a peak incidence between 10 and 17 years of age. Occasionally, they may involve several sites at time of presentation. The plain film always is abnormal but the appearance can mimic other diseases such as chronic osteomyelitis.

The untreated osteogenic sarcoma has a typical MDP scan appearance. The bone scan demonstrates an inhomogeneous, intensely increased distribution of tracer in the metaphysis usually with photopenic components. The blood pool image shows increased blood volume within the tumor, which may or may not mimic the appearance of the bone scan (Fig. 55.10). The radionuclide angiogram has a markedly increased blood flow compared with that expected from the blood pool image. This is due to the presence of arteriovenous malformations with direct arteriovenous shunting, which also causes early venous return.

Recently, there have been attempts to determine the potential response to chemotherapy by measuring the washout of ^{99m}Tc-sestamibi from the tumor. P-Glycoprotein is present in cell membranes. Tumor cells with a high P-glycoprotein content will washout chemotherapeutic agents. ^{99m}Tc-sestamibi washout is also facilitated by P-glycoprotein, and hence the measurement of ^{99m}Tc-sestamibi washout during the 3 hours after injection can provide an index of P-glycoprotein levels and the likelihood of multiple drug resistance. In a study of 11 children, Nadel et al. (17) showed that there was good correlation between the histologic response to chemotherapy and the retention of the thallium in the untreated tumor.

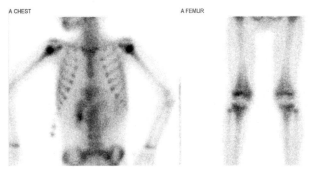

FIGURE 55.9. Neuroblastoma. The primary tumor accumulates methylene diphosphonate. Metastases have occurred in both distal femoral and proximal tibial metaphyses. The normal physeal metaphyseal interface is lost.

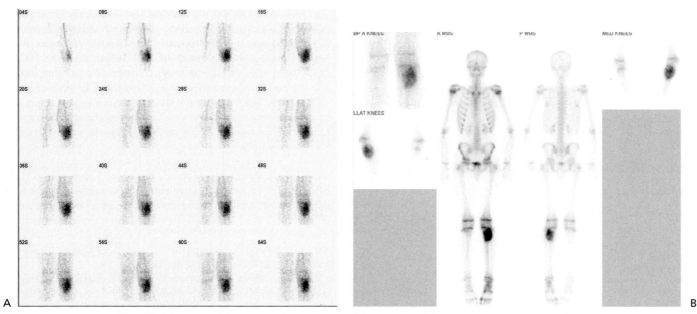

FIGURE 55.10. Osteogenic sarcoma. **A:** The radionuclide angiogram shows more flow to the neoplasm than would be expected from the blood pool image and the methylene diphosphonate bone scan. **B:** There is increased activity in the left proximal tibia, which is homogeneous.

Ewing's Sarcoma

Ewing's sarcoma has several differences from osteogenic sarcoma. First, the site is usually not metaphyseal but rather diaphyseal or in flat bones. An isolated rib Ewing's sarcoma is an especially common presentation (Fig. 55.11). There is no arteriovenous shunting and usually little hyperemia. The distribution of the radiotracer is usually inhomogeneous.

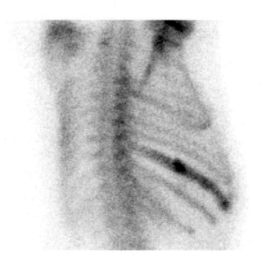

FIGURE 55.11. Ewing's sarcoma. There is increased activity involving the whole of the right ninth rib, which is a classic presentation.

Lymphoma

Gallium scanning plays a major role in the evaluation of children with lymphoma. MDP scanning has no place in the evaluation of childhood lymphoma unless it is being used to evaluate an orthopedic problem (18). Hodgkin's lymphoma, non-Hodgkin's lymphoma, and Burkitt's lymphoma are gallium avid in children. Both the presenting site and metastases are readily identified. The 72-hour scan, performed after bowel cleansing with laxatives, readily shows abdominal node involvement (Fig. 55.12). SPECT can be added to better depict lesions in the abdomen when colonic activity remains.

The mediastinum is often a difficult area to evaluate because of the presence of the thymus. The thymus may enlarge in viral illnesses and by rebound after radiation therapy. SPECT imaging of the chest can help in differentiating the thymus from recurrent lymphoma. The timing of the gallium scan is important. If it is performed too close to either radiation therapy or chemotherapy, the resultant pneumonitis will cause diffuse gallium accumulation in the lungs mimicking the appearance of an opportunistic infection.

Langerhans Cell Histiocytosis

Langerhans cell histiocytosis (formerly called histiocytosis X) is the term used to describe three diseases that all have histiocytic hyperproliferation: eosinophilic granuloma, Hand-Schuller-Christian disease, and Letterer-Siwe disease. These diseases present in many variations from a solitary mass or painful lesion in bone to a disseminated disease that is very aggressive and is usually fatal. Approximately 50% of the children present with only bone lesions. The preferred method of investigation is the

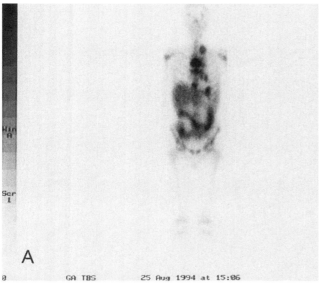

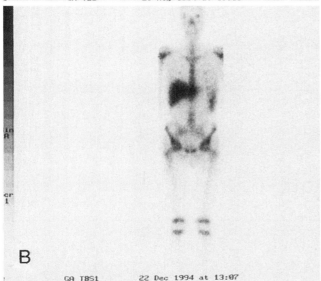

FIGURE 55.12. Lymphoma. **A:** Initial study shows multiple lymphomatous lesions in the mediastinum and upper abdomen, in addition to the presenting left neck mass. **B:** Four months later all the lesions have resolved in response to therapy.

radiographic skeletal survey. However, the radiographic study can miss up to 20% to 30% of bone lesions that can be seen on the MDP total body scan (19). Because the MDP scan also misses a number of lesions seen on the x-ray films, the two should be used together.

The bone scan typically demonstrates focal areas of increased activity at the lytic sites. These lesions are characterized by a photopenic center. However, there can be false-negative scans with the rapidly destructive lesions. Therefore, we perform both bone scans and x-ray films in all children suspected of having histiocytosis X. It is important to correlate all modalities, especially CT, if the face is involved.

REFERENCES

1. Mandell GA. Nuclear medicine in pediatric orthopedics. *Semin Nucl Med* 1998;28:95–115.
2. Gilday D, Paul D, Patterson J. Diagnosis of osteomyelitis in children by combined blood pool and bone imaging. *Radiology* 1975;117:331.
3. Howman-Giles R, Uren R. Multifocal osteomyelitis in childhood, review by radionuclide bone scan. *Clin Nucl Med* 1992;17:274–278.
4. Bressler E, Conway J, Weiss S. Neonatal osteomyelitis examined by bone scintigraphy. *Radiology* 1984;152:685–688.
5. D'Angilelis J et al. 99m Tc-pertechnetate bone imaging in Legg-Perthes disease. *Radiology* 1975;115:407.
6. Conway J, Weiss S, Maldonadov U. Scintigraphic patterns in Legg-Calvé-Perthes disease. *Radiology* 1983;149:102.
7. Kim H et al. Differentiation of bone and bone marrow infarcts from osteomyelitis in sickle cell disorders. *Clin Nucl Med* 1989;15:249–254.
8. Englaro EE, Gelfand MJ, Paltiel HJ. Bone scintigraphy in preschool children with lower extremity pain of unknown origin. *J Nucl Med* 1992;33:351–354.
9. Conway JJ et al. The role of bone scintigraphy in detecting child abuse. *Semin Nucl Med* 1993;23:321–333.
10. Smith F et al. Unsuspected costovertebral fractures demonstrated by bone scanning in the child abuse syndrome. *Pediatr Radiol* 1980;10(B):103–106.
11. Sty JR, Wells RG, Conway JJ. Spine pain in children. *Semin Nucl Med* 1993;23:296–320.
12. van Den Oever M, Merrick M, Scott J. Bone scintigraphy in symptomatic spondylolysis. *J Bone Surg Br* 1987;69:453–456.
13. Bellah R et al. Low-back pain in adolescent athletes: detection of stress injury to the pars interarticularis with SPECT. *Radiology* 1991;180:509–512.
14. Howman-Giles R, Gilday D, Ash J. Radionuclide skeletal survey in neuroblastoma. *Radiology* 1979;131:497–502.
15. Hoefnagal C et al. Radionuclide diagnosis and therapy of neural crest tumors using iodine 131 metaiodobenzylguanidine. *J Nucl Med* 1987;28:308–314.
16. Gordon I et al. Tc-99m bone scans are more sensitive than I-123 MIBG scans for bone imaging in neuroblastoma. *J Nucl Med* 1990;31:129–143.
17. Nadel HR. Thallium-201 for oncological imaging in children. *Semin Nucl Med* 1993;23:243–254.
18. Mouratidis B, Gilday DL, Ash JM. Comparison of bone and 67Ga scintigraphy in the initial diagnosis of bone involvement in children with malignant lymphoma. *Nucl Med Commun* 1994;15:144–147.
19. Schaub T, Ash JM, Gilday DL. Radionuclide imaging in histiocytosis X. *Pediatr Radiol* 1987;17:397–404.

56

SCINTIGRAPHY OF CHILDHOOD MALIGNANCIES

JOHN H. MILLER

Although cancer cure rates have greatly increased over the past 25 years, the incidence of cancer in children younger than 15 years has also increased (1). Various imaging modalities that are used for diagnosis, staging, and evaluation of progression and therapy play a vital role in the care and management of childhood cancer patients. The unique characteristics of nuclear imaging studies often play a pivotal role in the evaluation of pediatric oncologic disorders.

Nuclear medicine procedures are safe and well tolerated by children. Administered doses of radioactivity are determined at a level that will yield adequate diagnostic results but minimize the patient's radiation exposure. Pediatric dose is usually determined based on body surface area or weight using simple formulas or nomograms (2).

STATISTICS OF CHILDHOOD MALIGNANCIES

Between 1973 and 1988, cancer among children younger than 15 years increased in incidence equally among whites and blacks of both sexes, from 12 to nearly 14 cases per 100,000 per year (1). In the pediatric Caucasian population, an increased incidence of acute lymphoblastic leukemia (ALL) and tumors of the central nervous system (CNS) has been noted (1). However, there is no significant increase in the incidence of common childhood malignancies such as lymphoma and Hodgkin disease (HD) (1). Cancer mortality in children younger than 15 years has dropped 38%, despite a 4% increase in incidence of malignancy between 1973 to 1988 (3). The current overall cure rate for childhood malignancies in the United States is between 70% and 90% (3). At least some part of these improvements can be credited to improvements in diagnostic imaging of childhood cancer patients, which allows earlier and more accurate diagnosis, staging, and evaluation.

IMAGING CONSIDERATIONS IN INFANTS AND CHILDREN

The pediatric population is unique and distinct from adults in its psychosocial behavior and encompasses a spectrum from neo-

nates to near-adult adolescents. The spectrum of pediatric disorders is different from those affecting adults, and the level of comprehension that a child may have of his or her disability varies widely. All of these factors affect the way children react and their ability and willingness to cooperate with the imaging procedures. The physician and technologist must be skilled enough to be aware of and tend to the psychologic needs of the child. In addition, they must be able to communicate with the child and the parents effectively to ward off anxieties as much as possible and to make the child's stay as comfortable as possible, while obtaining the best possible images (2,4). Nuclear medicine personnel should create a favorable atmosphere for parents, who usually have unspoken anxieties of their own. The parents should be kept with their children as much as possible, because it comforts parent and child and facilitates the imaging procedure.

Restraint and positioning of the patient are extremely important for optimal image acquisition. Children differ anatomically from adults in that they are disproportionately smaller, so great care must be taken to position the patient so that the various structures are optimally displayed. Some patients, especially children younger than 5 years and physically and/or mentally challenged children, may require sedation (2,4). Because of longer imaging procedures there is a need for procedural sedation, often under the supervision of the nuclear physician. Usually the anesthesia service will have a teaching module that will provide the basic procedures and guidelines for patient supervision during procedural sedation. One will also feel more secure in the management of sedation in sick children if a course in pediatric advanced life support (PALS) is attended and repeated on a recurring basis.

In most instances, radionuclide imaging of children should begin with an evaluation of perfusion, or scintiangiography, of the region-of-interest. The immediate postflow tissue phase images assess the relative vascularity of the organs concerned. Delayed static images are obtained when optimal target-to-background radioactivity is attained. Because of the relatively small size of the various organs in children, carefully positioned high-resolution, high-count density images should be obtained. Computer acquisition of images enables manipulation of data for better visualization of subtle abnormalities in tracer uptake. Better gamma-cameras, double- and triple-headed single photon emission computed tomography (SPECT) and now coincidence

J.H. Miller: Department of Nuclear Radiology, Children's Hospital, Los Angeles, CA.

2-[^{18}fluorine]-fluoro-2-deoxy-D-glucose (FDG) imaging have given the pediatric nuclear physician much improved contrast and spatial resolution, as well as the opportunity to perform true metabolic imaging. FDG imaging offers same-day imaging similar to skeletal scintigraphy and allows for whole-body evaluation, especially with coincidence FDG studies. A study comparing conventional skeletal scintigraphy, whole-body magnetic resonance imaging (MRI), and FDG positron emission tomography (PET) found that of the three modalities FDG whole-body PET had the highest sensitivity for the detection of bone marrow metastases. (5,6). There is a caveat of caution when evaluating bone marrow involvement by malignancy in patients who have received granulocyte-colony stimulating factor (G-CSF) because G-CSF has been shown to stimulate metabolism to such extent that marrow involvement is simulated (7,8). In general the use of whole-body FDG PET in a variety of childhood neoplasms has been shown to be very efficacious (9). Similar results have been seen in whole-body FDG coincidence imaging as well (10). The radiation delivered dose is miniscule as compared with many imaging modalities or scintigraphic studies. The short half-life of ^{18}F provides the ability to perform the study and to minimize radiation exposure to other family members and nursing personnel. The prolonged biologic and physical halftimes of ^{67}Ga and ^{131}I have always presented problems for parents, other siblings, and nursing personnel who are either pregnant or hoping to become pregnant. The lack of ne-

cessity for body fluid precautions following FDG imaging has been a boon in this latter regard.

CENTRAL NERVOUS SYSTEM

Brain

Primary intraaxial malignant tumors of the brain are the second most common pediatric malignancy (1). Approximately 55% to 60% of brain tumors in children are infratentorial, and most are in the posterior fossa. They include cerebellar astrocytoma, primitive neuroectodermal tumor (PNET), brainstem glioma, and ependymoma (11–13). Most supratentorial tumors are cerebral astrocytomas and ependymal tumors, which are far less frequent than astrocytomas (11,12). Sellar tumors account for 15% to 20% of primary intracranial tumors and include craniopharyngioma, hypothalamic glioma, chiasmatic optic glioma, and suprasellar germinoma (14). Other primary intracranial tumors, such as neuroblastoma (NBL), may also occur. Meningiomas and primary lymphomas are rare. However, metastatic disease to the dura is often encountered in the neural crest tumors.

Various radiopharmaceuticals are used for brain tumor imaging. FDG PET has been shown to be more accurate than either computed tomography (CT) or MRI for evaluation of high-grade tumors (15–18). High-grade cerebral gliomas show intense FDG uptake, whereas areas of radiation necrosis free of

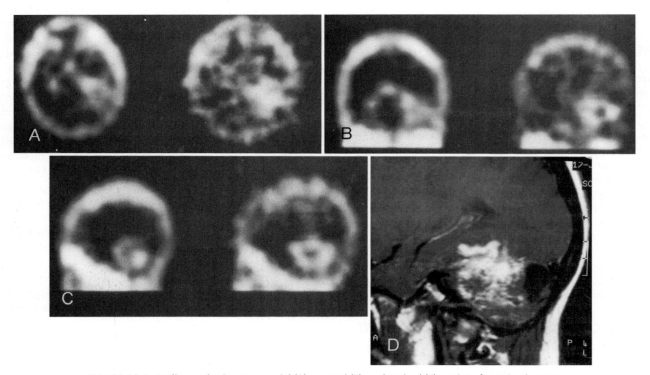

FIGURE 56.1. Malignant brain tumor. Axial (**A**), coronal (**B**), and sagittal (**C**) sections from simultaneous ^{99m}Tc-sestamibi (MIBI) (*left side*) and ^{201}Tl (*right side*) brain single photon emission computed tomography reveal extensive tumor arising in the cerebellum. This tumor has been previously treated with resection and radiation. This study was performed to assess for the presence of viable tumor. Better definition of tumor margins is seen in the MIBI study, but uptake is noted in the choroid plexus of the opposite lateral ventricle and in the peripineal vascular structures. **D**: Sagittal magnetic resonance imaging section reveals this inhomogeneously enhancing mass lesion.

neoplasm showed little tracer uptake (15–19). This differentiation aids in the medical management of children afflicted with these neoplasms. Many pediatric supratentorial tumors are low grade. FDG and ^{201}Tl accumulate in PNETs, but often ependymomas have poor uptake of the tracer agents. [201]Tl or ^{67}Ga-citrate may be used for evaluation of metastatic disease to the brain. Nadel (20) reported that ^{201}Tl imaging offers a distinct advantage over gallium tumor imaging with a short total imaging time. Sensitivity and specificity of ^{201}Tl for pediatric brain tumors have been reported to be 77% and 93%, respectively (21). Comparison of ^{201}Tl and ^{99m}Tc-labeled sestamibi brain imaging yielded similar results for tumor avidity of both tracers (Fig.

56.1). However, clearer identification of tumor boundaries by sestamibi may be an advantage for treatment planning when using modalities such as radiotherapy (22). Pituitary tumors, especially those associated with multiple endocrine neoplasia (MEN) syndromes, may be detected by somatostatin receptor imaging (23,24) (Fig. 56.2).

Retinoblastoma

Retinoblastoma, a highly malignant but readily treatable cancer of the retina, occurs with an incidence of 1 per 20,000 live births (25). It occurs bilaterally in about 60% to 80% of cases and is the

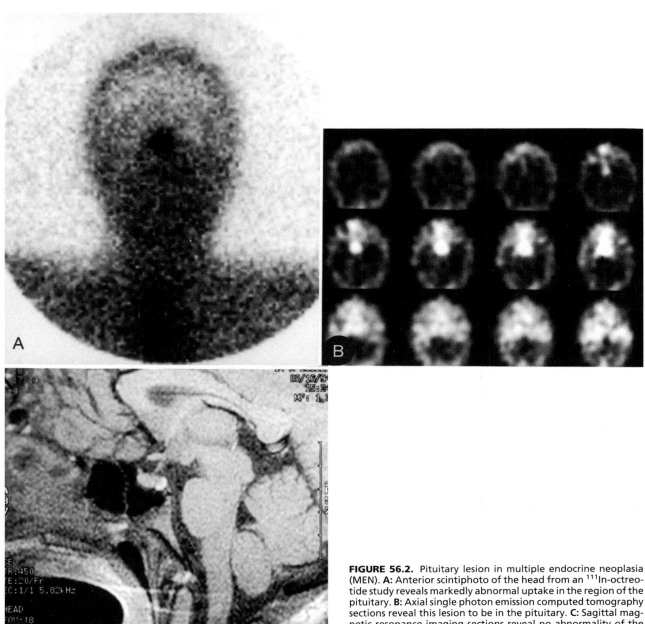

FIGURE 56.2. Pituitary lesion in multiple endocrine neoplasia (MEN). **A:** Anterior scintiphoto of the head from an ^{111}In-octreotide study reveals markedly abnormal uptake in the region of the pituitary. **B:** Axial single photon emission computed tomography sections reveal this lesion to be in the pituitary. **C:** Sagittal magnetic resonance imaging sections reveal no abnormality of the pituitary. This constellation of findings suggests the presence of a microadenoma in this patient with MEN syndrome.

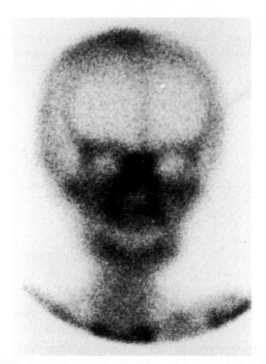

FIGURE 56.3. Retinoblastoma. Anterior RNSS scintiphoto of the head reveals increased activity in the right periorbital structures. This is a common finding following enucleation and is related to bony growth secondary to the absence of the globe. This does not represent orbital recurrence of tumor. Increased uptake noted over the calvarium on the right side is abnormal and was found to represent tumor involvement of the meninges.

eighth most common childhood malignancy (1). In the United States, the average age at diagnosis is 18 months (26). There are no gender or race differences, and both eyes are at equal risk.

The imaging method of choice for intraocular retinoblastoma is MRI. This tumor may metastasize by access to the cerebrospinal fluid (CSF), directly to the CNS via the optic nerve or direct orbital extension, or by lymphatic or hematogenous routes. This is best defined with MRI with contrast enhancement. Distant metastases may occur to the skeletal system, liver, bone marrow, lymph nodes, or facial structures. Whole-body radionuclide skeletal scintigraphy (RNSS) will effectively detect osseous metastatic disease but cannot be relied on to assess local orbital disease (Fig. 56.3) (27). This caveat is also true for patients who develop a second neoplasm in the orbital region after radiation therapy (28).

Spinal Cord

Primary intraaxial spinal cord tumors are rare and account for less than 1% of malignancies in childhood. Astrocytomas and ependymomas are the most frequent primary tumors in the spinal cord. Skeletal metastases to the spine from NBL, osteosarcoma, rhabdomyosarcoma, Ewing sarcoma, and other childhood malignancies occur much more often than primary spinal tumors. Non-Hodgkin lymphoma or leukemia may present, either at diagnosis or as a site of relapse, as a symptomatic extradural mass. This may be a tumor mass and/or hemorrhage secondary to altered blood coagulation. Patients with neoplastic involvement of the spinal cord may present with varying, and sometimes vague, symptoms, including urinary dysfunction, gait disturbance, sensory deficits, spastic or flaccid paralysis, pain in various parts of the body, and torticollis (29,30). Imaging of spinal cord

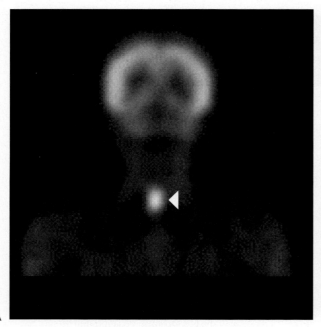

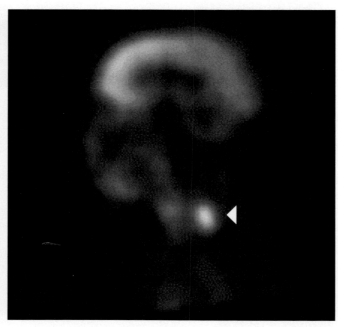

A   B

FIGURE 56.4. Metastatic primitive neuroectodermal tumor to spine on 2-[¹⁸fluorine]-fluoro-2-deoxy-D-glucose coincidence imaging. Coronal (**A**) and sagittal (**B**) section reveals intense uptake at the site of a metastatic focus. Magnetic resonance imaging only revealed nonspecific swelling of the cord and was felt to represent a radiation effect.

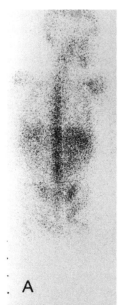

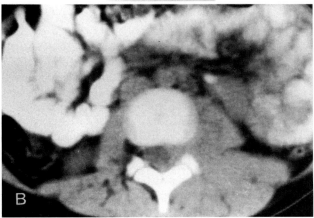

FIGURE 56.5. Lymphoma of the spine. **A:** Posterior whole-body scinti-photo reveals abnormally increased uptake of ⁶⁷Ga in the spine in a patient with Hodgkin disease. **B:** Computed tomography section reveals extensive involvement of the spinal canal and paraspinous structures.

tumors, primary or metastatic, involves MRI with contrast (31). FDG may offer another method of investigation of primary or secondary spinal cord tumors (Fig. 56.4), although this has received little attention. Skeletal scintigraphy is extremely accurate in assessing osteoblastic foci involving vertebral bodies, posterior elements, and transverse processes (32). Photopenic foci resulting from osteolytic activity may be identified in cases of Langerhans cell histiocytosis (LCH) and NBL. Possible lymphomatous involvement of the spine warrants ⁶⁷Ga-citrate imaging, and abnormal tracer accumulation in the paraspinous region (Fig. 56.5) mandates other radiographic studies, such as CT or preferably contrast enhanced magnetic resonance (MR) to evaluate for neoplastic involvement of the spinal cord.

HEAD AND NECK

The head and neck region is frequently involved by neoplasm in childhood with the incidence of primary tumors in this region

placed at 19.6% in a large retrospective study (33). Lymphomas, usually HD, are the most common head and neck tumors (34, 35). Lymphadenopathy secondary to HD or other types of lymphomas may first present as masses in the head and neck region (35–37). Other tumors, which involve the head and neck region, include rhabdomyosarcoma, fibrosarcoma, neurofibrosarcoma, thyroid malignancies, primary NBL, and squamous cell carcinoma. The type of tumor most frequently encountered varies with age (38). Head and neck tumors present with nonspecific symptoms and may sometimes remain innocuous, necessitating a detailed and careful clinical and imaging workup.

Paranasal sinus tumors, which are usually rhabdomyosarcoma, grow silently and are often difficult to detect clinically until they reach an advanced stage when patients may complain of nasal congestion, ear infection, rhinorrhea, and epistaxis. Rhabdomyosarcoma is the most common nonocular tumor of the orbit. Vision disturbances may occur if the orbital wall is involved, because of pressure on the contents of the orbit. Tumors of the middle ear cavity are usually rhabdomyosarcoma arising in the stapedius muscle. Tumors of the oropharynx are more easily diagnosed. Rhabdomyosarcoma of the head, neck, or nasopharynx are often embryonal and tend to spread to the cervical lymph nodes and to the meninges (39–42). Other tumors, which involve these regions, are HD, other lymphomas, fibrosarcoma, neurofibrosarcoma, and lymphoepithelioma. Nasopharyngeal carcinoma is rare in the pediatric population (43, 44). Metastases may also occur from Ewing sarcoma, renal clear cell carcinoma, eosinophilic granuloma, osteosarcoma, and other malignant tumors (45).

In general, high-resolution computed tomography (HRCT) and MR imaging are the primary modalities used for most lesions. Skeletal scintigraphy should be used to assess for osseous involvement, whereas gallium imaging of the head and neck may yield vital information on soft tissue neoplasia that has spread to adjacent bony structures or regional lymph nodes (46,47). However, radionuclide examinations generally yield poor results in cases of tumors involving the base of the skull. FDG imaging of lesions near the skull base has been limited by the proximity to the brain. Primary tumors or metastases from NBL may be detected by bone scans and metaiodobenzylguanidine (MIBG) scans (discussed later). ⁹⁹ᵐTc bone scans allow assessment of the extent of osseous involvement, as well as distant metastases, which may not be revealed by clinical examination or other diagnostic modalities. Gallium scintigraphy is useful for detecting nodal lesions. FDG imaging has been helpful for the evaluation of tumors in the lower cervical region and may allow the identification of masses that may not be identified on cross-sectional imaging. Distant metastases may also be identified by this methodology as well (Fig. 56.6).

Thyroid

Scintigraphy of the thyroid allows classification of tumors as cold, warm, or hot nodules based on the degree of tracer accumulation. A cold nodule in a child is more likely malignant than a similar lesion in an adult. Rarely, well-differentiated thyroid carcinomas may reveal accentuated tracer uptake (48,49). Benign tumors include adenoma and the rare teratoma. Papillary

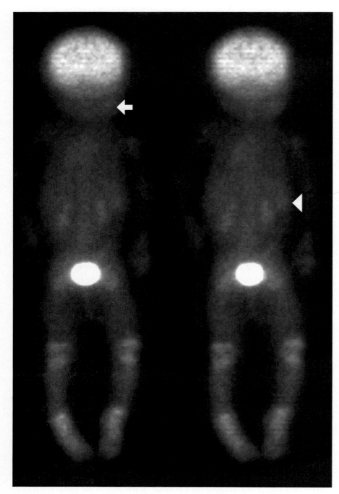

FIGURE 56.6. Scalp melanoma in an infant. Whole-body ¹⁸F-FDG coincidence imaging of a child with a scalp melanoma. The primary tumor overlying the brain is difficult to resolve. However, a metastatic lymph node in the left neck (*arrow*) and a splenic metastasis (*arrowhead*) were identified. Both were unsuspected before the ¹⁸F study.

thyroid carcinomas are the most common thyroid malignancies, whereas follicular carcinomas account for less than 5% of pediatric thyroid tumors (48,50–52).

¹²³I and ¹³¹I-MIBG have been reported to be taken up by sporadic cases of medullary thyroid carcinoma (MTC) and carcinomas associated with Sipple syndrome (53,54). Somatostatin receptor imaging has also been reported to be successful in the evaluation of MTC (23,24).

Thyroid malignancy in children appears to be more aggressive than that in adults and is treated by thyroidectomy with preservation of the parathyroid gland. Residual tumor following surgery may be ablated with ¹³¹I therapy (55,56). Follow-up ¹³¹I scans are useful for evaluation of local recurrence or metastatic disease to the lungs (Fig. 56.7) or bones.

CHEST, MEDIASTINUM, AND HEART

Lymphoma is the most common neoplasm involving the thoracic region in children. Ganglioneuromas and ganglioneu-

roblastomas may occur in the paraspinous region and cervical sympathetic ganglia. Other tumors that may involve the musculoskeletal structures of the thorax are rhabdomyosarcoma and other soft tissue or osseous malignancies. Primary abdominal tumors and metastases from other sites may also invade the thoracic region.

HRCT with contrast enhancement is the method of choice for evaluation of tumors involving the pulmonary parenchyma, pulmonary vasculature, and mediastinum.

Radionuclide ventilation-perfusion (V/Q) lung scanning provides little information regarding primary or secondary neoplasm, although it may reveal microscopic tumor emboli, lymphangitic carcinomatosis, or pulmonary emboli that occur as a complication of malignancy or treatment (57–59). The V/Q scan may also be performed to assess pulmonary reserve in patients who have had prior resection of metastatic nodules. Radionuclide venography using a peripheral arm vein may be used to evaluate for superior vena cava (SVC) obstruction (60).

⁶⁷Ga-citrate scintigraphy, although sensitive for the detection of tumor involvement of the mediastinum, does not distinguish between neoplasia and infection and hence should be used in conjunction with HRCT of the chest (61,62). Thymic uptake of gallium may be increased after chemotherapy, or occur as a "rebound" phenomenon (63,64) (Fig. 56.8). ²⁰¹Tl may be used to assess this difficult problem. In the usual circumstance, nontumor conditions will not have ²⁰¹Tl uptake (20). ⁹⁹ᵐTc-sestamibi imaging has also been used for this purpose as well. Because of superior imaging characteristic of the ⁹⁹ᵐTc-based compound, the images may have greater anatomic resolution and lend themselves to SPECT imaging. Unfortunately, FDG imaging has not allowed a differentiation between recurrent tumor and rebound hypertrophy (Fig. 56.9).

Multiple-gated acquisition (MUGA) determinations of the left ventricular ejection fraction of the heart allow for assessment of cardiac function when cardiotoxic drugs are used, as well as for assessment of tumor involvement of the myocardial wall (20). ²⁰¹Tl may be useful in evaluating primary cardiac tumors (65), which are extremely rare; most cases are cardiac myxomas and rhabdomyomas (66,67). ²⁰¹Tl scintigraphy may also reveal myocardial photopenic defects (68,69).

Primary lung tumors are extremely uncommon in childhood (70). Both primary and metastatic pulmonary blastoma, an embryonal tumor, are gallium avid (71,72). Various tumors may have metastatic nodules in the lungs, which may be evaluated with ²⁰¹Tl, ⁹⁹ᵐTc-sestamibi, ⁶⁷Ga scintigraphy, or more recently FDG imaging (73–76).

ABDOMEN, LIVER, AND SPLEEN

Liver

Primary hepatic malignancies are an uncommon pediatric malignancy (77,78). Malignant hepatic tumors are more frequent than benign tumors (79). Hepatoblastoma (HBL) presents in the neonatal period or infancy, and hepatic cell carcinoma (HCC) occurs in late childhood or adolescence. These neoplasms may be associated with defined syndromes (80,81). Vascular origin tumors and a number of other primary nonhepatocyte primary tumors may also occur (80). Malignant liver tumors often metas-

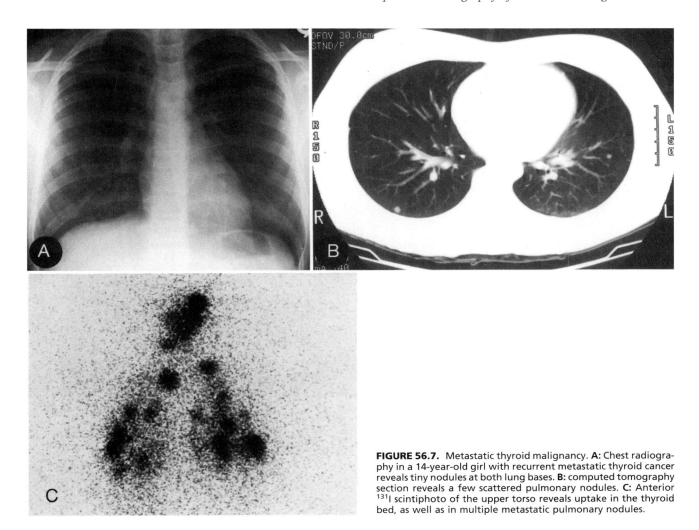

FIGURE 56.7. Metastatic thyroid malignancy. **A:** Chest radiography in a 14-year-old girl with recurrent metastatic thyroid cancer reveals tiny nodules at both lung bases. **B:** computed tomography section reveals a few scattered pulmonary nodules. **C:** Anterior ^{131}I scintiphoto of the upper torso reveals uptake in the thyroid bed, as well as in multiple metastatic pulmonary nodules.

tasize to the lungs, regional lymph nodes, and the brain. Hepatic metastases, both by direct extension or hematogenous spread, are far more common than primary hepatic malignancies and may occur in Wilms tumor, NBL, lymphoma, leukemia, and rhabdomyosarcoma.

The primary imaging modality for hepatic tumors is HRCT or MR with magnetic resonance angiography (MRA). Radionuclide imaging plays only an ancillary role but often allows the correct characterization of lesions because of definition of the physiologic nature of the lesion (81,82). ^{99m}Tc-sulfur colloid studies in HBL and HCC usually show an avascular defect, which appears as a photopenic region on static images (81,83, 84). ^{99m}Tc-dimethyl iminodiacetic acid (IDA) scans also reveal similar photopenic defects. However, ^{99m}Tc-IDA uptake helps to differentiate HCC from regenerative or other benign functioning nodules (81,82). ^{99m}Tc-labeled red blood cell (RBC) studies enable very reliable differentiation between vascular origin lesions of the liver and other tumors, such as HBL and mesenchymal hamartoma (85,86) (Fig. 56.7). Gallium is avidly taken up by HCC in 90% of cases (87,88). However, gallium is nonspecific and intrahepatic metastases from HCC often show poor gallium uptake. Occasionally, ^{99m}Tc-methylene diphosphonate (MDP) uptake is seen in necrotic tumors. Primary he-

patic rhabdomyosarcoma and monotypic small cell sarcomas rarely occur. They have the scintigraphic appearance of photopenic defects with the exception of gallium uptake in rhabdomyosarcoma. The two vascular origin tumors of infancy, capillary hemangioma and cavernous hemangioendothelioma can be accurately identified using ^{99m}Tc-RBCs, as can mesenchymal hamartoma (86). Capillary hemangioma, analogous to the cutaneous strawberry hemangioma, usually presents as a solitary palpable liver mass (Fig. 56.10). This lesion has dramatically increased flow on ^{99m}Tc-RBC perfusion imaging and immediate pooling of ^{99m}Tc-labeled RBCs within the lesion. The infant with cavernous hemangioendothelioma, a lesion which produces giant vascular lakes within the liver, usually presents with hepatomegaly and some degree of high-output cardiac state because of the shunting of blood through the multiple liver lesions (Fig. 56.10). This lesion causes an apparent diffuse increase in flow throughout the liver, but on delayed static images multiple intrahepatic sites containing ^{99m}Tc-RBC activity will be seen that represent dilated vascular lakes of this tumor.

Biliary System and Gallbladder

The most common primary biliary malignancy in children is rhabdomyosarcoma, which causes obstructive jaundice (89).

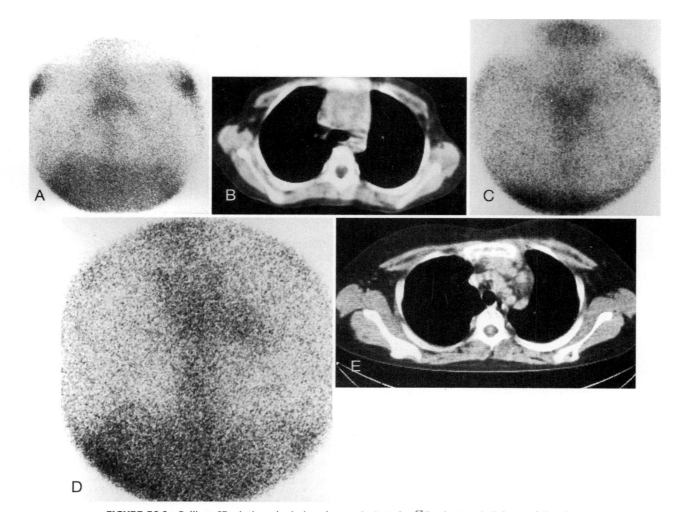

FIGURE 56.8. Gallium-67 scintigraphy in lymphoma. **A:** Anterior ^{67}Ga-citrate scintiphoto of the chest reveals marked thymic prominence. **B:** Computed tomography (CT) section reveals fullness in the anterior mediastinum. This was a manifestation of the "rebound" phenomenon, and on a subsequent examination the thymus had decreased to normal size. Note in this patient that the thymus has a relatively normal, bilobed configuration. **C:** Anterior gallium scintiphoto of the chest in another patient reveals prominent thymic uptake with a slight left predominance. A marked prominence of the left side of the thymus was noted on the next sequential gallium scintiphoto (**D**). **E:** CT section reveals fullness in the anterior mediastinum without evidence of a discrete mass. This was subsequently proven to be recurrent disease. In this example, the thymus does not have a normal contour or configuration.

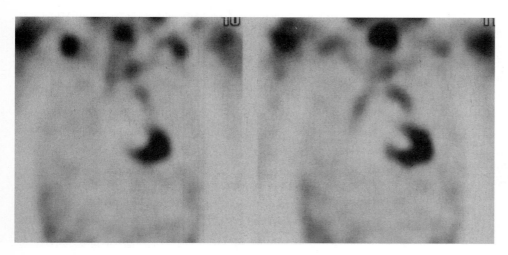

FIGURE 56.9. Thymic rebound. Coronal section from a ^{18}F-FDG coincidence study reveals marked enlargement on the thymus in a patient who had been treated for cervical region lymphoma. Biopsy was needed to prove that this was benign thymic hypertrophy following chemotherapy.

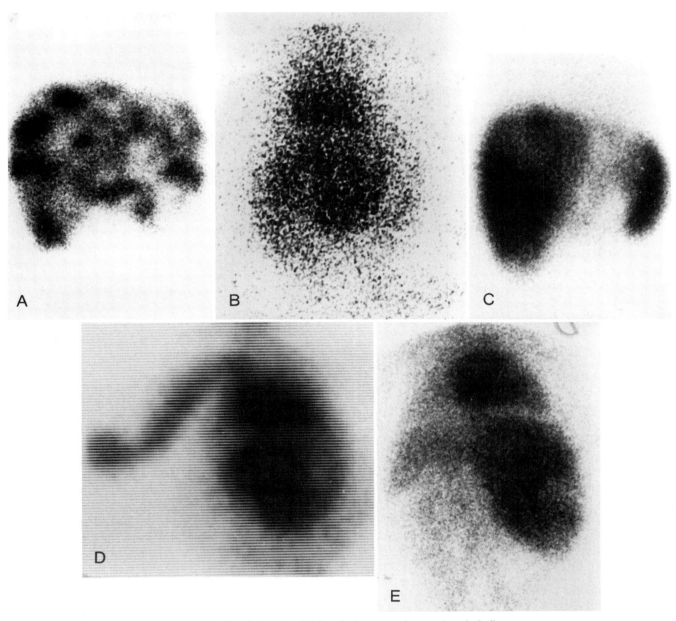

FIGURE 56.10. Vascular liver lesions in childhood. Cavernous hemangioendothelioma appears as a "Swiss cheese" liver on conventional ^{99m}Tc-sulfur colloid scintigraphy (**A**), but on ^{99m}Tc-red blood cell (RBC) scintigraphy (**B**) these lesions are seen to fill in. Capillary hemangioma is seen, as on this anterior ^{99m}Tc-sulfur colloid scintiphoto (**C**) of the liver, as a space-occupying lesion replacing the left lobe and a portion of the right lobe of the liver. A computer-summed perfusion scintiphoto (**D**) reveals this process to have markedly increased blood flow, and on ^{99m}Tc-RBC scintigraphy (**E**) a large vascular lesion is seen arising from the left lobe of the liver. Activity within this lesion must be equal to the activity within the heart blood pool to allow the diagnosis of vascular origin tumor. *(Figure continues.)*

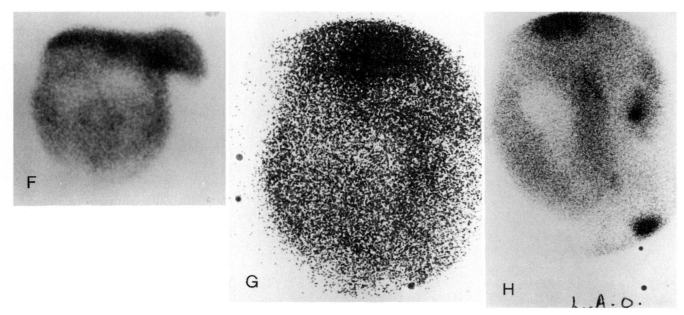

FIGURE 56.10. *Continued.* Mesenchymal hamartoma of the liver is seen on this anterior ^{99m}Tc-sulfur colloid scintiphoto (**F**) as a large lesion replacing most of the right lobe of the liver. ^{99m}Tc-RBC perfusion scintigraphy (**G**) reveals increased blood flow in the margins of the lesion with a central colder photopenic area. On the delayed static ^{99m}Tc-RBC scintiphoto (**H**) the lesion has mixed components, some of which are greater in activity than that of the uninvolved liver but less than the heart blood pool. The only liver lesion of childhood that has this scintigraphic appearance is a mesenchymal hamartoma.

Other types of primary biliary tumors are rare in childhood. ^{99m}Tc-sulfur colloid studies demonstrate a hypovascular intrahepatic or extrahepatic mass (90). ^{99m}Tc-IDA is helpful if biliary system involvement is suspected (91,92). Gallium uptake may be seen in the primary tumor (90).

Spleen

Secondary involvement of the spleen by lymphoma may appear as photopenic defects on ^{99m}Tc-sulfur colloid scans. However, splenic photopenic defects in leukemic patients are more likely clues to infectious processes (Fig. 56.11) or hematoma rather than leukemic infiltrate (90). On the other hand, photopenic defects seen in patients with non-Hodgkin lymphoma are most often due to the presence of the disease (90). Increased uptake of FDG may suggest the presence of diffuse lymphomatous involvement of the spleen when seen on FDG imaging (Fig. 56.12). Comparison between FDG, ^{67}Ga, and CT found that increased uptake of FDG, when compared with the liver uptake, was indicative of HD involving the spleen and was decidedly more accurate than CT (93,94).

Splenic involvement by extrasplenic abdominal malignancies such as Wilms tumor and NBL can be evaluated by ^{99m}Tc-sulfur colloid studies. Reduced or delayed perfusion in a significantly enlarged spleen (as compared with the liver) may be noted (90). ^{99m}Tc-sulfur colloid and gallium scintigraphy are somewhat nonspecific in cases of splenic abscess. Often a defect will be visualized on sulfur colloid scintigraphy, which is either warm or cold on gallium scintigraphy (95).

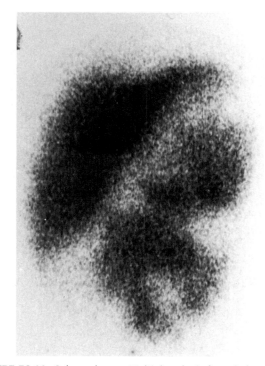

FIGURE 56.11. Spleen abscess. Multiple splenic fungal abscesses in a patient with leukemia are revealed on this left lateral ^{99m}Tc-sulfur colloid scintiphoto of the spleen. Multiple cold defects are seen within an enlarged spleen.

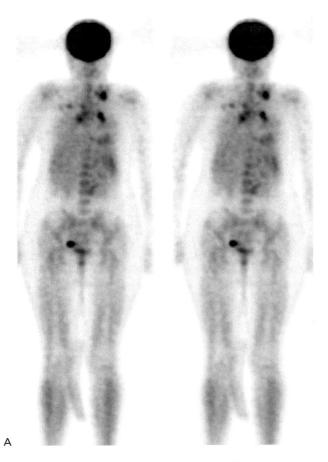

A

FIGURE 56.12. 2-[18fluorine]-fluoro-2-deoxy-D-glucose imaging of lymphoma with splenic involvement. Whole-body (**A**) 18F-FDG coincidence imaging of a patient with lymphoma reveals multiple sites of abnormal uptake of tracer. These include supraclavicular, mediastinal, and prevertebral nodes. There is significantly increased uptake of tracer in the spleen. This is seen to better advantage on axial sections (**B**). The spleen (*closed arrowhead*) and multiple prevertebral nodes (*open arrowhead*) are "hot."

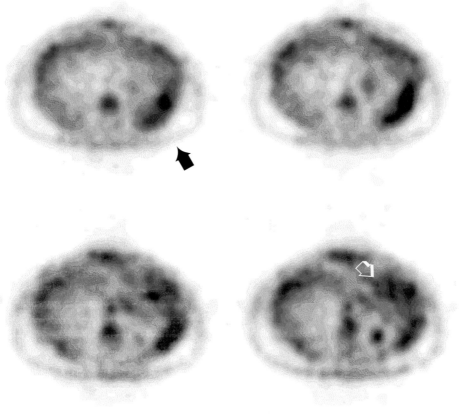

B

GASTROINTESTINAL TRACT, PANCREAS, AND RETROPERITONEUM

Primary gastrointestinal (GI) tumors account for less than 1% of pediatric malignancy (96). Malignant gastric neoplasms of childhood include adenocarcinomas, lymphomas, or soft tissue sarcomas and may accumulate gallium. However, benign processes involving the stomach may have increased gallium uptake (76,97,98). Gastric teratoma may have uptake of skeletal tracer within the tumor. Colonic and pancreatic adenocarcinomas occur, but in most other GI sites sarcomas are more common (99). Primary pancreatic tumors are very rare but may occur in association with MEN syndrome or von Hippel-Lindau disease. Extramural tumor involvement and nodal metastases may be detected using gallium scintigraphy (100,101).

The most common malignancy involving the small bowel in childhood is lymphoma, which may involve the distal ileum, cecum, appendix, and the ascending colon. ^{67}Ga-citrate scintigraphy is valuable for the initial evaluation and staging of small bowel lymphomas (Fig. 56.13), because it may reveal the extent of abdominal involvement by tumor and also distant metastases (102). Carcinoid tumors, which rarely occur in children, may be visualized using ^{111}In-octreotide scintigraphy (23,24).

Mucinous colloid adenocarcinoma accounts for most cases of colon carcinoma in children (96). Familial polyposis or antecedent ulcerative colitis are predisposing factors (103,104). Radionuclide evaluations play a less important role when compared with other modalities in the evaluation of colonic tumors. Adenocarcinoma and lymphoma involving the colon are gallium avid (105,106), but gallium uptake may be present in both benign and malignant tumors (107). Hepatic and skeletal metastases may be identified with either gallium or ^{99m}Tc-MDP scintigraphy.

GENITOURINARY TRACT

Most solid tumors found in the pediatric age group are those arising in the abdomen from the kidneys and the adrenal glands. A palpable abdominal mass is a frequent mode of presentation of genitourinary tumors in childhood.

Scintigraphic evaluation of the genitourinary tract plays an ancillary role to other radiographic modalities; the exception is evaluation for skeletal metastases in NBL. Gallium scintigraphy has limited use in abdominal scintigraphy, although it may be employed in the initial evaluation, staging, and follow-up of patients with germ-cell tumors and NBL (87,108–111). ^{123}I-MIBG or ^{131}I-MIBG is used primarily in patients with the neural crest tumors of childhood and aids in the detection of metastatic NBL and pheochromocytomas, especially in children with the MEN syndromes. Because MIBG is a catecholamine analog, it concentrates in the catecholamine neurotransmitter vesicles and allows the intraadrenal and extraadrenal localization of tumors with high accuracy (112,113). There may be a role for somatostatin receptor imaging as well (23,24). Limited experience also indicates a role for FDG in the evaluation of these patients (10,114,115).

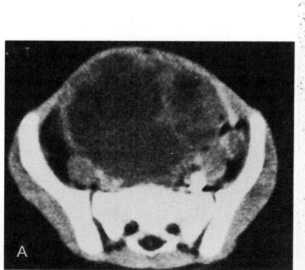 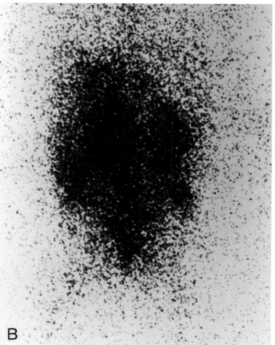

FIGURE 56.13. Abdominal non-Hodgkin lymphoma. Non-Hodgkin lymphoma arising from the distal small bowel is seen as low-density masses in the pelvis on computed tomography (**A**), whereas gallium scintigraphy (**B**) of the torso reveals extensive involvement of the entire abdomen.

Kidney

Wilms tumor is the fifth most common pediatric tumor, the most common pediatric genitourinary neoplasm, and the most common intraabdominal solid tumor in childhood (1,3). Most of these tumors develop by age 6 years (116). Bilateral tumors occur in 5% to 10% of children and may be synchronous or metachronous in occurrence. Patients may present with an asymptomatic abdominal mass, hypertension, hematuria, dysuria, or renal failure. Radionuclide assessment of the kidneys using cortical imaging agents, such as ^{99m}Tc-glucoheptonate (GH) or dimercaptosuccinic acid (DMSA), will usually demonstrate an intrarenal mass lesion. The renal scan may reveal renal parenchymal distortion but allows an assessment of renal function (Fig. 56.14). This also enables assessment of the unaffected kidney, because sometimes small lesions involving this kidney may be missed by other modalities. Therefore, the planned surgical approach may be influenced by this modality. Cortical scintigraphy may be useful in the evaluation of residual renal parenchyma following a partial renal resection for Wilms tumor. Skeletal involvement by clear cell or anaplastic Wilms tumor is best assessed with radionuclide skeletal scintigraphy.

Renal cell carcinoma is very rare in children younger than 10 years but is more common among older children and adolescents (117–121). Radionuclide imaging plays an ancillary role in the evaluation and follow-up of these patients.

Retention of gallium within the kidneys on 48- and 72-hour scintiphotos is characteristic of infectious processes such as *Candida* and *Torulopsis* (122). In renal failure secondary to malig-

nancy, radionuclide studies may be used to identify an obstructive uropathy or quantify the degree of renal failure. Unilateral or bilateral toxic renal disease secondary to radiation therapy may be adequately evaluated with ^{99m}Tc-mercaptoacetyltriglycine (MAG3) scans.

Congenital mesoblastic nephroma, usually discovered in the first year of life, may show skeletal tracer uptake in portions of the benign tumor. In nephroblastomatosis, ^{99m}Tc-GH scintigraphy may reveal nephromegaly with uniformly reduced uptake of tracer and delayed excretion. Radionuclide studies are not routinely used in the evaluation of angiomyolipoma, renal cysts, and multilocular cystic nephromas.

Collecting System

Transitional cell carcinoma, rhabdomyosarcoma, and leiomyosarcomas of the collecting system rarely occur (120). Primary tumors of the lower genitourinary tract are most often rhabdomyosarcoma of the urogenital sinus. Approximately 15% of all rhabdomyosarcomas in children arise in the vagina, prostate, or bladder. Primary bladder tumors, however, are very rare in the pediatric age group (123). Radionuclide studies play a secondary role in evaluating these tumors.

Gonadal

Gonadal tumors and teratomas, although infrequent, are an important group of childhood malignancies. Testicular tumors are

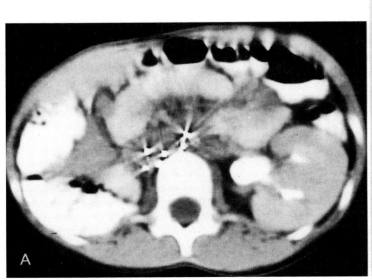
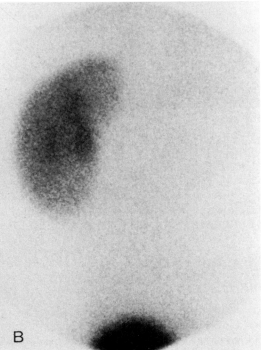

FIGURE 56.14. Renal hypertrophy. **A:** Contrast-enhanced computed tomography following resection of the right kidney for Wilms tumor reveals distortion of the left renal pelvis by an apparent mass. **B:** ^{99m}Tc-glucoheptonate scintigraphy reveals uniform uptake of tracer throughout this mass lesion indicating that it represents a hypertrophied column of Bertin.

the seventh most common neoplasms in childhood (124). Sixty percent of all pediatric patients with testicular tumors are younger than 2 $\frac{1}{2}$ years at the time of diagnosis. The remaining cases are almost exclusively diagnosed during late adolescence. Eighty percent of all testicular tumors in children are malignant (125). Seminoma is the most common tumor associated with cryptorchidism (126). However, this is rare, and endodermal sinus tumor is the most common childhood testicular tumor (127,128). Two thirds of testicular tumors in children are of germ-cell origin, and 40% are endodermal sinus tumor. Embryonal carcinomas, teratomas, and tumors of the mixed cell type are rare but do occur (119,122,126,129). The testicle may be a site for involvement with leukemic and lymphomatous infiltrates. Relapse may occur within the testicles of these children.

Paratesticular tumors include intrascrotal tumors involving the epididymis, the spermatic cord, or its covering. Rhabdomyosarcoma is the most common paratesticular tumor in childhood. These tumors may present as a unilateral mass, but an occasional associated finding is a hydrocele.

More than 50% of testicular tumors, with the exception of seminomas, demonstrate increased ^{67}Ga activity in the primary lesion (87,108,130). Gallium scans are also useful in detecting testicular involvement by lymphoma in the prepubescent male. In the postpubescent male, slightly increased gallium accumulation in the scrotal contents precludes a reliable assessment of lymphomatous involvement. There has been a report of abnormal gallium accumulation in a testicle, which was enlarged as a result of leukemic infiltrate (131). Gallium is also effective in detecting abdominal metastases secondary to embryonal carcinoma and malignant teratomas (87,108,131).

Ovarian tumors account for 1% of all childhood tumors, and approximately 20% to 30% of these are malignant. They tend to be more common at the onset of puberty (87,126). Presenting characteristics include abdominal pain, ascites, precocious puberty, vaginal bleeding, or masculinization (87,132,133). In children, most tumors are of germ-cell origin and include teratomas, dysgerminomas, embryonal carcinomas, endodermal sinus tumors, and choriocarcinomas. Epithelial tumors of the ovary, stromal tumors, and gonadoblastomas rarely occur in childhood. The ovaries may be the sites of metastases in acute leukemia and disseminated non-Hodgkin lymphoma (134–136). Many of the primary ovarian neoplasms are gallium-avid (87,108), but, because of their proximity to the colon, abnormal uptake may be difficult to visualize. FDG imaging can be helpful, often allowing assessment of areas that are indeterminate on sectional imaging (Fig. 56.15). Osseous metastases may be detected by conventional bone scintigraphy.

Adrenal Gland

NBL originates from the primitive sympathetic neuroblasts, which later in life contribute to the development of sympathetic ganglia. Overall, it is the fourth most common childhood cancer (1,124,137). Fifteen percent of all cancer deaths in childhood are due to NBL (137). There are three pediatric neural crest tumors: NBL, ganglioneuroblastoma, and ganglioneuroma can be differentiated by their degree of cellular maturation. Patient age and stage of disease at diagnosis are important prognostic features. Younger children (younger than 14 to 24 months) statistically have a better chance for survival than older children (138). The most common site of origin is in the abdomen (54% to 68%); two thirds of these tumors are of adrenal origin, and 15% of cases arise in the thorax. Much less frequently, tumors are encountered in the pelvis, neck, and head (139–141). Tumors arising in the abdomen have the poorest prognosis, with adrenal primaries faring the worst (142,143).

Staging is done at the time of presentation with a radionuclide skeletal survey, and high-resolution contrast-enhanced CT of the site of origin of the tumor (Fig. 56.16). Extraosseous skeletal tracer uptake by neural crest tumors is high (144–146). Demonstration of tracer uptake in paraspinous tissues raises the possibility of intraspinal neoplastic involvement and warrants a follow-up CT scan. An assessment of the relative function of both kidneys may be performed using ^{99m}Tc-MAG3 when nephrectomy is considered a therapeutic option, in case of tumoricidal radiation therapy, or in patients with increased blood pressure or renal failure without an apparent cause. Gallium scintigraphy in patients with NBL may give an indication of prognosis (147).

Ganglioneuroblastoma involving the thorax usually occurs in older children, and ganglioneuromas typically occur in adulthood (148). Demonstrable calcification is more frequent in these tumors than in thoracic NBL (148). These tumors may present as apical thoracic masses in infants and children and may be associated with Horner syndrome, heterochromia of the iris, and watery diarrhea resulting from hypersecretion of vasoactive intestinal polypeptide (VIP) (138). Radionuclide skeletal tracer uptake may be less apparent compared with that of abdominal tumors; however, this modality is of prime importance in excluding the presence of sites of osseous metastatic disease.

Primary intracerebral NBL, which belongs to the group of PNETs, may occur in three distinct forms: (a) resembling a peripheral NBL, (b) a desmoplastic type tumor with marked proliferation of connective tissue stroma, or (c) a mixed tumor in which both of the previous elements are present (149).

Metastatic involvement of the skeletal system and liver is very common in NBL (150). Approximately 70% of skeletal lesions are osteoblastic, as evidenced by increased skeletal tracer uptake in the lesion (146) (Fig. 56.17). Lesions with a mixed scintigraphic appearance (osteoblastic and osteolytic) may be visualized in the remainder of the patients with skeletal involvement. Demonstration of abnormal tracer activity in the vertebrae necessitates further evaluation with other imaging modalities. Metastatic involvement of the calvarium, evidenced by increased activity in the skull and abnormal orbital region activity, is an early sign of disease spread. Bone marrow scintigraphy with ^{99m}Tc-sulfur colloid may reveal replacement of marrow in the regions of tumor deposit, which will be visualized as a photopenic region. In children younger than 1 year, NBL is the most common cause of hepatic metastases (150), which may be partly due to fetal circulation.

The sequential evaluation of patients with NBL can be problematic. Routine RNSS is performed, as are CT and MR of the primary lesion site. However, residual tumor mass may be seen on sectional imaging and persistent abnormalities on the RNSS.

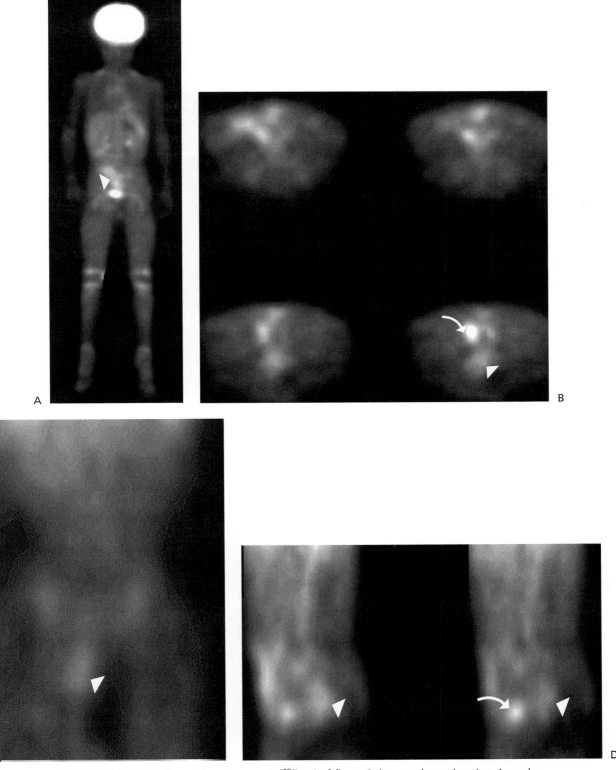

FIGURE 56.15. Endodermal sinus tumor on 2-[18fluorine]-fluoro-2-deoxy-D-glucose imaging. An endodermal sinus tumor had been resected from the right ovary 6 months before this posttherapy examination. Recurrent tumor (*arrowhead*) is seen on whole-body (**A**), axial (**B**), coronal (**C**), and sagittal (**D**)
sections. The patient had increasing alpha-fetoprotein levels, and the computed tomography examination was compatible with postoperative reaction. The whole-body study could be confused with physiologic bowel activity, but on the reconstructions tumor uptake is seen posterior to the bladder (*curved
arrow*) extending into the pelvis arising from the pelvic floor.

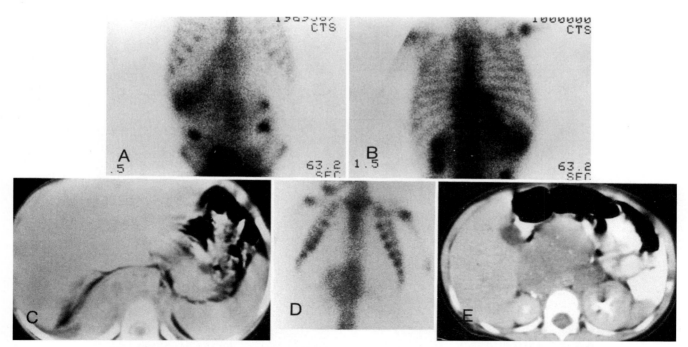

FIGURE 56.16. Abdominal neuroblastoma. Extensive abdominal neuroblastoma is revealed on anterior (**A**) and posterior (**B**) ⁹⁹ᵐTc-methylene diphosphonate scintiphotos. The kidneys are inferiorly displaced, and there is abnormal extraosseous uptake in the right paraspinous structures extending from the abdomen into the chest. This finding is confirmed on contrast-enhanced computed tomography (CT) (**C**) of the lower chest. A large paraspinous mass is seen insinuated behind the posterior crura of the hemidiaphragm. **D:** A localized abdominal neuroblastoma is revealed on this anterior scintiphoto of the upper torso by abnormal extraosseous uptake in the midline. **E:** Contrast-enhanced CT section reveals a large mass in the abdomen.

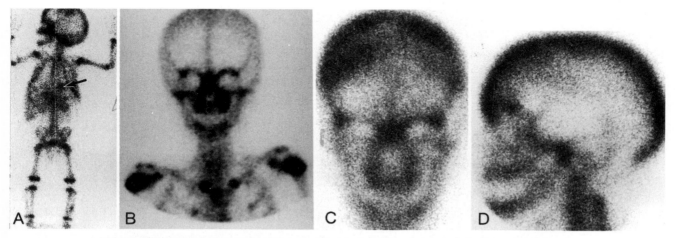

FIGURE 56.17. Skeletal involvement by neuroblastoma. **A:** Extensive metastatic disease involving the skeleton is revealed on this anterior whole-body scintiphoto. Extensive uptake in liver metastases and a left adrenal primary (*arrow*) is seen as well. **B:** Calvarial and orbital disease is seen in another patient on an anterior scintiphoto of the head and neck. Extensive calvarial disease is seen on anterior (**C**) and left lateral (**D**) ⁹⁹ᵐTc-methylene diphosphonate scintiphotos of the head.

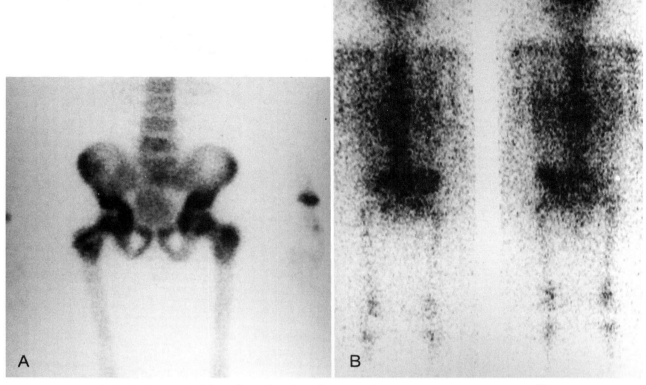

FIGURE 56.18. Metaiodobenzylguanidine (MIBG) scintigraphy in neuroblastoma. **A:** Anterior ⁹⁹ᵐTc-methylene diphosphonate scintiphoto of the pelvis reveals slightly increased activity in the right ilium. **B:** Posterior (*left*) and anterior (*right*) whole-body ¹³¹I-MIBG scintigraphy reveals extensive disease in the right ilium, as well as definite evidence of bone marrow metastases involving both femoral shafts and both proximal tibiae.

To determine if these abnormalities represent persistent or recurrent tumor has always posed problems. Therefore, MIBG (Fig. 56.18) and FDG (Figs. 56.19 and 56.20) imaging have been used (151,152).

MIBG is taken up in tumor, which may not be identified by RNSS or CT (153). This is particularly true of ¹²³I-MIBG imaging (Fig. 56.21), alone or accompanied by SPECT imaging (154,155). We have observed many instances of negative or equivocal RNSS findings with an area of uptake of MIBG clearly identified. The converse has also been observed in a case of an adrenal NBL tumor mass with significant MIBG uptake, which was found to be a mature ganglioneuroma on biopsy. The MIBG imaging procedure is very expensive in imaging time and material cost. We, therefore, do not use MIBG on a routine basis but reserve it for problem cases or before bone marrow transplantation (BMT), using the RNSS and sectional imaging to follow these children (156). However, other authors use MIBG scintigraphy in a routine manner with excellent results.

Adrenal carcinoma has a definite female preponderance and is more common than adrenal adenoma (157–159). Cushing syndrome in children is most often due to adrenal carcinoma (158). Nonfunctioning adrenocortical carcinomas account for only 10% of adrenal cortical tumors (159–162). Adrenal scintigraphy with 6-iodomethyl-19-norcholesterol (NP-59), often used in adults, is not warranted in childhood for the evaluation of

an adrenal tumor. Gallium may be taken up by metastatic or recurrent disease (163).

Pheochromocytoma arises from neural crest cells wherever chromaffin cells are present (thoracic and abdominal sympathetic chain, organ of Zuckerkandl, bladder wall, and ureters) (157). Fewer than 5% of pheochromocytomas occur in the pediatric age group (164). Two percent of these tumors are malignant in children (157,164–166). Metastases may occur to local lymph nodes, liver, lung, or bone (157,166,167). Most cases of malignancy occur in extraadrenal sites (163). Intermittent or sustained hypertension is present in approximately 90% of children with pheochromocytoma (167,168). There is an increased incidence of pheochromocytoma in MEN IIA (II) and IIB (III) syndromes, neurofibromatosis, and von Hippel-Lindau syndrome. There is also a sporadic and familial incidence of these tumors (169–171).

The currently used compound, MIBG labeled with ¹²³I or ¹³¹I, is a norepinephrine precursor, which is taken up by adrenergic tissues and directly incorporated into catecholamine neurotransmitter vesicles (112,172,173). MIBG scans are useful in the care of patients with strong clinical or familial suspicion of pheochromocytoma but with equivocal findings on CT and ultrasound (112,173). Somatostatin imaging may also be valuable in the evaluation of pheochromocytoma.

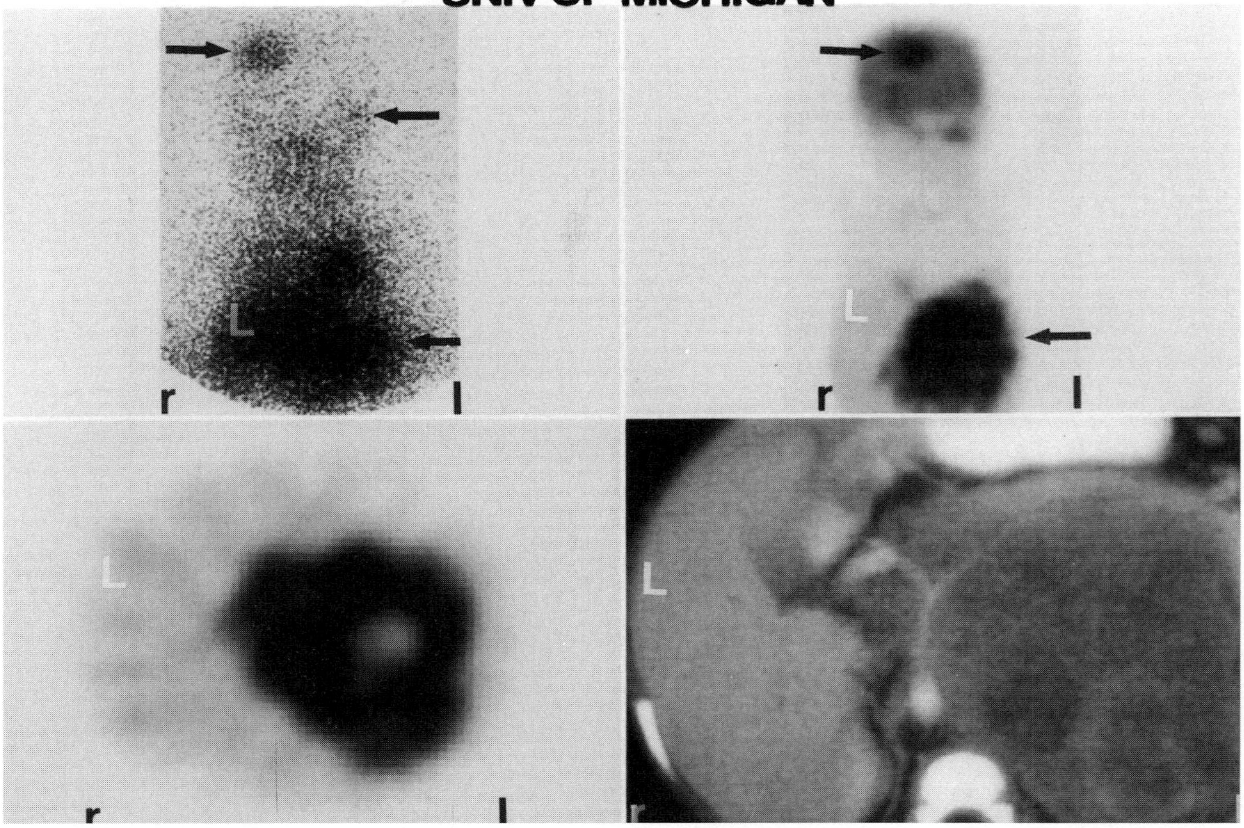

FIGURE 56.19. 2-[^{18}fluorine]-fluoro-2-deoxy-D-glucose (FDG) scintigraphy of neuroblastoma. **A:** Anterior ^{131}I-metaiodobenzylguanidine scintiphoto reveals abnormal uptake in the right skull and left orbit and extensive abnormality involving the abdomen. **B:** FDG positron emission tomography (PET) projection view reveals abnormality in the skull, orbits, and in an abdominal lesion. **C:** Axial FDG PET image reveals dramatic uptake within the left-sided neuroblastoma, with central areas of reduced FDG activity. **D:** Computed tomography (CT) of this patient revealed a large left-sided mass with mixed attenuation in the central portion of the tumor. Liver (*L*). The findings of the CT and PET indicate a central necrosis within this large abdominal neuroblastoma. (Courtesy of Barry Shulkin, MD, University of Michigan Medical Center, Ann Arbor, MI.)

MUSCULOSKELETAL AND SOFT TISSUE

In tumors of the musculoskeletal system, a conventional radiographic examination is a prerequisite to imaging evaluation. Appropriate radionuclide evaluation can consist of skeletal, bone marrow, thallium, sestamibi or FDG scintigraphy.

Skeletal scintigraphy has high sensitivity and low specificity (174,175). It may be used (a) to define the extent of osseous tumor involvement, (b) to identify osseous involvement by an extraosseous malignancy, and (c) to assess therapeutic response. In general, however, bone scans overestimate the extent of osseous involvement by tumor. Gallium scintigraphy has been used extensively in the evaluation of soft tissue malignancies (87,109, 174). It shows the extent of primary tumor involvement and clinically occult involvement of regional lymph nodes. Bone marrow scintigraphy with ^{99m}Tc-sulfur colloid provides useful information regarding intramedullary extension of primary bone tumors, as well as metastatic spread to the marrow from various neoplasms. Although highly sensitive, a diffusely abnormal bone

marrow scan may not be a reliable indicator of metastatic disease (176). Radiation-induced vascular compromise of a limb may be evaluated by the use of ^{99m}Tc-labeled RBCs.

Rhabdomyosarcoma

Soft tissue tumors are the sixth most common neoplasm of childhood, and rhabdomyosarcoma is the most frequent pediatric soft tissue tumor (4% to 5% of all tumors in children younger than 15 years) and is highly malignant (177–180). The tumor may have as its primary site the head and neck (including the orbit), genitourinary tract, extremities, trunk, retroperitoneum, or hepatobiliary region (181). Embryonal rhabdomyosarcoma is the most common form of this tumor (177,180,182), followed by the alveolar histologic type.

The head and neck are the most common sites of rhabdomyosarcoma in the pediatric age group. The orbit, nasopharynx, paranasal sinuses, oral cavity, middle ear cavity or mastoid cells, temporal bone, soft tissues of the face and neck, and the larynx

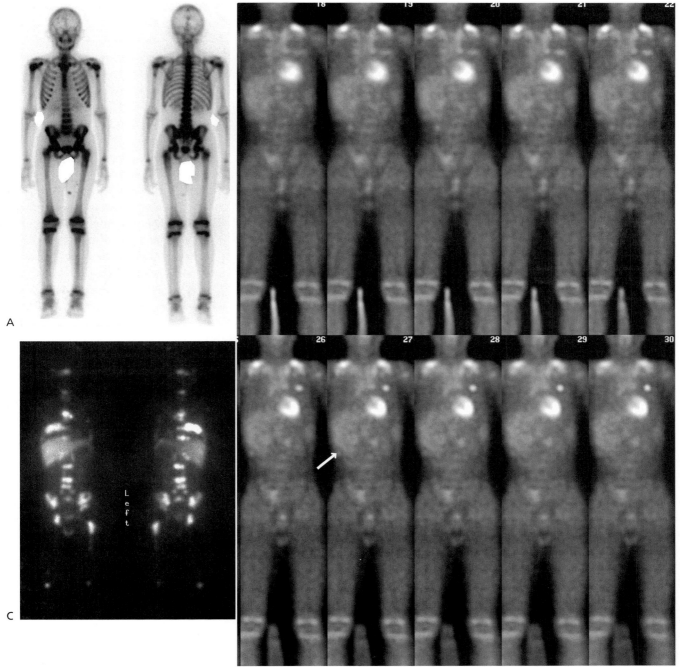

FIGURE 56.20. Coincidence 2-[^{18}fluorine]-fluoro-2-deoxy-D-glucose (FDG) imaging in recurrent neuroblastoma. **A:** Whole-body bone scintigraphy with ^{99m}Tc-methylene diphosphonate reveals multiple sites of abnormal uptake in the appendicular skeleton and pelvis. It is not possible to assess tumor activity on this study. **B:** Whole-body FDG coincidence study reveal multiple sites of abnormal uptake in mediastinum, abdomen, and pelvis. A small metastatic nodule on the inferior aspect of the liver (*arrow*) was biopsied with a laparoscope and proven to be recurrent neuroblastoma. **C:** Posttherapy ^{131}I-metaiodobenzylguanidine (MIBG) study reveals many of the sites that were revealed on the FDG study, but the lesions in the long bones were not seen. Prior imaging with a diagnostic dose (380 μCi) of ^{131}I-MIBG had not revealed the extra abdominal sites of uptake.

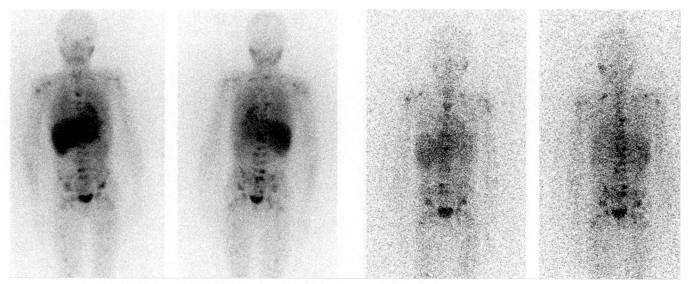

FIGURE 56.21. ¹²³I-metaiodobenzylguanidine (MIBG) study. Whole-body scintigraphy at 4 hours and 24 hours reveals multiple sites of abnormal uptake of ¹²³I-MIBG, primarily involving the axial skeleton. ¹²³I-MIBG is a much more favorable imaging compound than ¹³¹I-MIBG. This is due to higher allowable doses and more favorable imaging characteristics. There is less injury to the thyroid from free iodine. Excellent imaging can be obtained at 4 hours, which should be continued through 24 hours. (Courtesy of Dr. Fred Mishkin, Harbor UCLA Medical Center, Los Angeles, CA.)

(in decreasing order of frequency) may be involved (Fig. 56.22). Recurrence at the primary site, distant metastases, and direct perineural extension into the CNS occur with equal frequency (182,183). The trigone of the bladder, the prostate, the seminal vesicles, spermatic cord, vagina, uterus, and parametric structures may be involved by the tumor (179). It is often difficult to determine the site of origin of the neoplasm because extensive disease may be present at the time of presentation. Specific symptoms include dysuria, hematuria, lower abdominal mass, obstructive uropathy, vaginal discharge, or vaginal mass. Testicular or spermatic cord rhabdomyosarcoma may present as a testicular mass. Thoracic rhabdomyosarcoma may arise from the chest wall, hemidiaphragm, heart, mediastinum, or pulmonary parenchyma, whereas abdominal tumor may arise in the abdominal wall or retroperitoneal structures. Rhabdomyosarcoma involving the extremities and CNS have also been well documented (184). Because this tumor is a sarcoma, it tends to metastasize to local nodes first and then systemically to the lungs and other viscera.

HRCT and MRI allow exquisite definition of tumor extension and margins. Skeletal scintigraphy reveals evidence of osseous involvement and may also reveal signs of meningeal infiltration. Gallium scans are helpful in detecting metastatic spread to regional lymph nodes, as well as systemic dissemination. Because of normal accumulation of tracer in the nasopharyngeal and facial structures, evaluation of the structures of the head and neck may prove difficult with gallium scintigraphy, as is evaluation of the extent of disease in the pelvis secondary to bowel activity (178). FDG imaging may offer a method superior to ⁶⁷Ga because physiologic uptake is less and a whole-body survey may be performed.

Fibromatous tumors, such as desmoid tumors, aggressive ju-

venile fibromatosis, congenital generalized fibromatosis, fibrosarcoma, and malignant fibrous histiocytoma, are commonly seen in childhood (180). Some of these tumors are locally aggressive and have a tendency toward local recurrence following surgery. Both benign and malignant tumors take up skeletal tracer and the RNSS provides useful information regarding presence of tumor and determination of tumor resectability (185). Gallium scintigraphy may be the best modality in the detection of recurrent and metastatic disease in cases of malignant fibrous histiocytoma (109,186,187). FDG imaging may now offer a method of evaluation of these tumors.

Osteosarcoma

Osteosarcoma is the most common primary malignant bone tumor in the pediatric and adolescent age groups (124) and is the seventh most frequent childhood malignancy (1). Approximately 50% of the cases occur during the second decade, and osteosarcoma is slightly more common in males (188). The proximal humerus, ilium, proximal femur, facial bones, skull, spine, ribs, and other sites may be involved (188,189). Multicentric osteosarcoma, which may be synchronous or metachronous, occurs occasionally (190–192). Osteosarcoma is highly malignant and has rapid hematogenous spread. The lungs are the most common sites of both metastatic and recurrent disease. Radionuclide skeletal scintigraphy and HRCT of the lungs should be the initial imaging modalities for the evaluation of a child presenting with radiographic findings of osteosarcoma (Fig. 56.23). FDG imaging will provide an assessment of local disease and allow evaluation of skip lesions and may also provide information on the metabolic activity of pulmonary nodules (Fig.

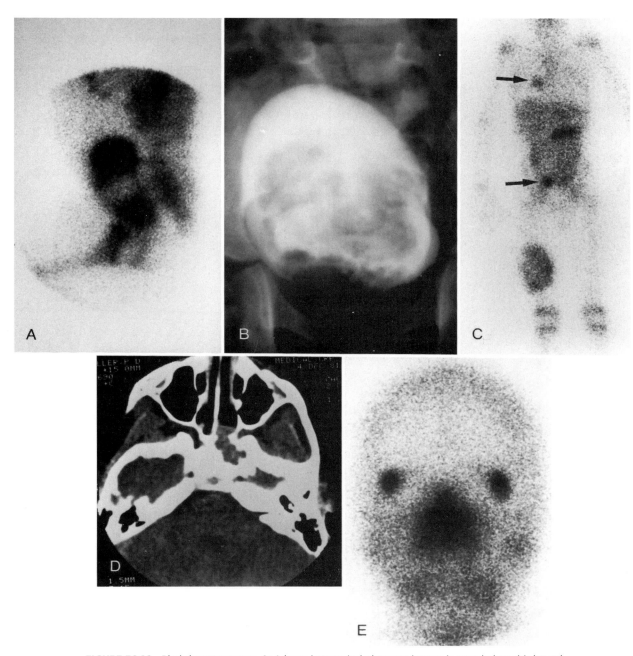

FIGURE 56.22. Rhabdomyosarcoma. **A:** A large intravesical photopenic mass is revealed on this lateral ^{99m}Tc-methylene diphosphonate scintiphoto of the pelvis in a 14-month-old boy being evaluated for possible discitis. **B:** Subsequent contrast cystogram reveals an extensive intraluminal tumor, compatible with rhabdomyosarcoma. **C:** Rhabdomyosarcoma arising in the right thigh is seen on this anterior whole-body ^{67}Ga-citrate scintiphoto. Metastatic nodes (*arrows*) in the right inguinal area and in the right chest are also revealed. **D:** Abnormal soft tissue density is seen involving the high nasopharynx on computed tomography, in a patient presenting with epistaxis. **E:** Gallium scintigraphy reveals extensive uptake in the nasal region in this patient with nasopharyngeal rhabdomyosarcoma.

56.24). This is particularly important during the treatment phases of this disease and for the evaluation of limb salvage patients.

The perfusion phase images of RNSS assess the extent of any hyperemic response and may help define the extent of an associated soft tissue mass, as does a tissue phase scintiphoto.

Following an appropriate delay, skeletal whole-body scintigraphy is performed. This modality has 100% sensitivity for the primary tumor and sites of skeletal metastases. Skeletal scintigrams may be used to assess extent of disease in the involved bone and are used as a rough guide for the level of surgical amputation, but the exact level is usually established by MRI.

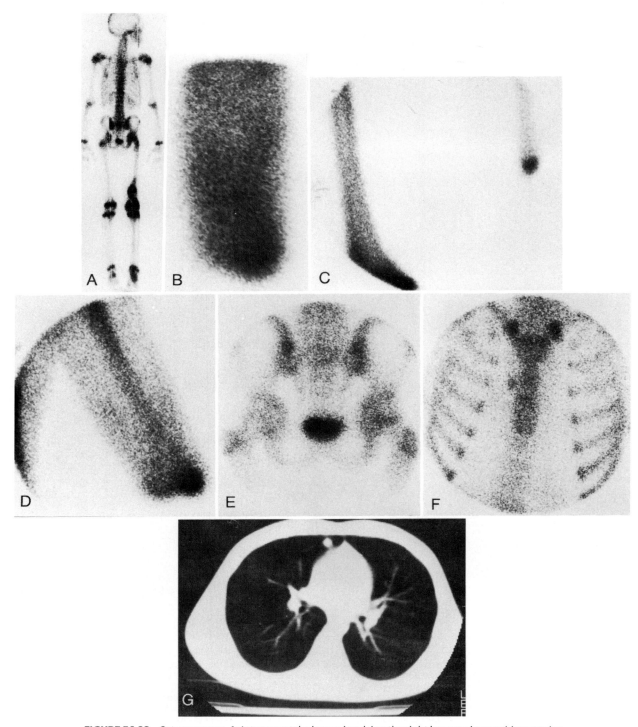

FIGURE 56.23. Osteosarcoma. **A:** Intense uptake is seen involving the right knee region on this posterior whole-body scintiphoto. Note the dramatically increased uptake in the remainder of the extremity, which represents "extended uptake" secondary to disuse. Extensive uptake is seen on tissue phase 99mTc-methylene diphosphonate (MDP) scintigraphy (**B**) with a focal area of increased uptake seen on delayed scintigraphy (**C**) in a patient with reactive changes secondary to a poorly fitting prosthesis. **D:** Focal increased activity is seen on a 99mTc-MDP scintiphoto in a distal humerus secondary to an infection. **E:** A photopenic process is noted on a posterior 99mTc-MDP scintiphoto of the pelvis in the left femoral neck in a patient with left hip pain. Note the physis is absent. This was a "cold" osteosarcoma. **F:** An area of abnormal 99mTc-MDP uptake is noted on an anterior 99mTc-MDP scintiphoto of the chest in the right parasternal area in a patient evaluated for osteosarcoma. This represented a tiny metastatic nodule seen on computed tomography section (**G**) of the chest.

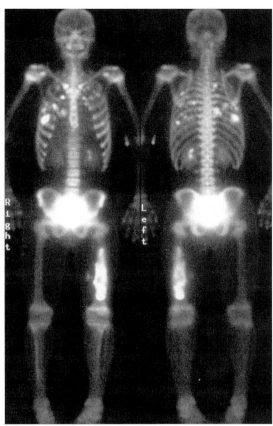

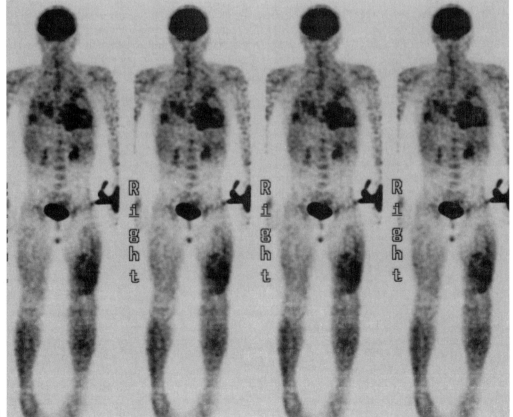

FIGURE 56.24. Pulmonary metastasis on 2-[18fluorine]-fluoro-2-deoxy-D-glucose (FDG). **A:** Whole-body 99mTc-methylene diphosphonate study reveals extensive uptake of tracer in a primary osteosarcoma involving the distal left femoral shaft. Uptake of skeletal tracer is also seen in the lung compatible with calcified pulmonary metastases. Uptake of skeletal tracer does not connote metabolic activity but rather calcific deposit. **B:** Whole-body FDG coincidence imaging reveals uptake in the extraosseous soft tissue component of the tumor and in multiple sites throughout the lungs. The uptake of FDG in the marrow of the spine is a common finding in young adults.

Extended areas of increased skeletal tracer uptake proximal to the site of tumor involvement may be secondary to bone marrow hyperemia and medullary reaction or periosteal new bone formation secondary to the presence of neoplasm (193–195). Extended uptake may also be seen in an extremity distal to a primary malignancy. This uptake may be due to disuse, gait sparing, or the hyperemic effect of a proximal tumor. It is important to recognize these changes, because many children are now treated by limb salvage following resection of the primary tumor. If the most proximal extent of abnormal osteoblastic activity is taken, the bone margins will be free of tumor and that information is of paramount importance in limb salvage procedures. MRI allows an accurate evaluation of proximal extent of tumor with greater accuracy than RNSS (196). However, FDG imaging should be performed to assess tumor extent that may not be revealed on MR or HRCT imaging. This methodology may have efficacy for the evaluation of pulmonary metastases before resection of pulmonary nodules.

Intense extended uptake of bone tracer agent associated with the presence of a malignant tumor may mask the presence of skip metastases within the medullary canal (193). FDG will provide an excellent definition of the extent of medullary involvement and will also allow detection of skip lesions proximal to a primary extremity osteosarcoma (Fig. 56.25).

Metastatic disease to the skeletal system from osteosarcoma is best detected by radionuclide skeletal scintigraphy, with conventional radiography and MRI used to evaluate areas of abnormality detected on scintigraphy (197–199). Because of the biomechanics of an abnormal gait following an amputation or limb salvage for osteosarcoma, abnormal skeletal tracer disposition may be seen in the sacroiliac joints, the acetabular region, and in any remaining portion of an involved limb. Abnormally increased uptake of skeletal tracer will be seen in the wrists and shoulders of children who are crutch gaited and should not be mistaken for metastatic disease. Chronic osteomyelitis or a poorly fitting prosthesis may result in abnormal osteoblastic activity simulating persistent or recurrent neoplasm. ^{61}Ga-citrate or ^{111}In-labeled white blood cell (WBC) scintigraphy may aid in the detection of inflammatory foci (200,201). Thallium scintigraphy has proven to be a very good method of assessing both the therapeutic response of osteosarcoma and local recurrence of disease (202). ^{99m}Tc-sestamibi imaging may prove to be as efficacious as ^{201}Tl scintigraphy (203) (Fig. 56.26). Localization of recurrent foci of tumor may be done using a hand-held intraoperative probe. This allows the surgeon to resect only the area of suspicion and to avoid a wide dissection in search of the recurrent neoplasm. Following local radiation, all scintigraphic modalities may be unreliable in the detection of abnormal foci.

Ewing and Other Osseous Origin Sarcomas

Ewing sarcoma, a primitive primary sarcoma of bone, has a wide range of clinical and radiographic presentations. It causes significant morbidity and mortality in the pediatric population. It is the second most common malignant bone tumor of children and young adults (204). Nearly 50% of cases occur between the ages of 10 and 20 years, and 70% occur in patients younger than 20 years (124,205). The femur and pelvic bones are the most common sites of tumor origin. However, any bone in the skeletal system may be affected, including ribs, skull, or scapula.

The presenting symptoms may include persistent bone pain, soft tissue mass, fever, malaise, anorexia, and/or other specific symptoms, depending on the systems involved. Metastatic disease is present at the time of diagnosis in approximately 20% of patients. If Ewing sarcoma is left untreated, or is inadequately treated, at least 90% of patients will develop metastases within 1 year of diagnosis. Multiple sites of skeletal involvement without pulmonary metastases is a common finding at the time of initial evaluation of a patient with Ewing sarcoma. The lungs and bone are the usual initial sites of metastases, and the tumor may later spread to any organ, including lymph nodes, bone marrow, liver, spleen, and brain.

Radionuclide skeletal scintigraphy is usually the diagnostic modality used after conventional radiography (Fig. 56.27). Skeletal scintigrams cannot effectively differentiate between malignant and benign lesions of bone, which result in increased tracer uptake (206). Scintigraphically, Ewing sarcoma is a very vascular soft tissue mass with evidence of increased bone turnover. The extent of bone tracer deposition in Ewing sarcoma is less than that of osteosarcomatous lesions. The presence of lytic and blastic lesions and intramedullary extension of tumor, often in a serpiginous manner, favor the diagnosis of Ewing sarcoma. Metastatic disease may be evaluated with radionuclide skeletal scintigraphy and bone marrow scintigraphy (207). ^{99m}Tc-sulfur colloid scintigraphy may detect areas of bone marrow involvement undetected by skeletal scintigraphy or conventional radiography and provides a total body survey (208). However, this modality is less reliable after chemotherapy or radiation therapy (206). FDG evaluation may offer a new method of evaluation of these lesions, because they are often very active metabolically.

A rare extranodal presentation of non-Hodgkin lymphoma is primary disease in bone. Less than 10% of all cases of primary skeletal lymphoma occur in childhood (209), although it is the third most common pediatric neoplasm (1,210). Clinically it presents as a painful diaphyseal mass in the long bones, and the femur is most commonly affected, although flat bones may also be affected. It usually arises within and spreads through the medullary canal. Infiltration and destruction of the cortical bone with periosteal involvement and extension into soft tissues may be seen. Regional lymph nodes are commonly involved, and hematogenous spread may occur to the lung, liver, spleen, other viscera, and meninges. Conventional skeletal scintigraphy reveals increased activity on blood-pool and delayed-phase images in patients with this disease. Gallium scintigraphy provides valuable information regarding the extent of disease and is more effective for imaging of non-Hodgkin lymphoma than for other primary bone tumor (200).

Synovial cell sarcomas are rare in childhood; less than 10% of cases occur in the pediatric population (211,212). They arise as painless masses in the extremities, most often in the lower limbs, and are the most common soft tissue tumors of the hands and feet (180). Metastases may occur in the lungs, regional lymph nodes, bone and other organs.

Chondrosarcoma accounts for less than 5% of primary bone tumors in childhood and often arises in the trunk and the proximal ends of the humerus and femur (211). It is a slow-growing

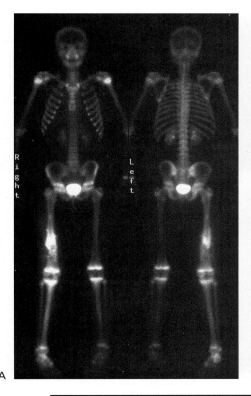

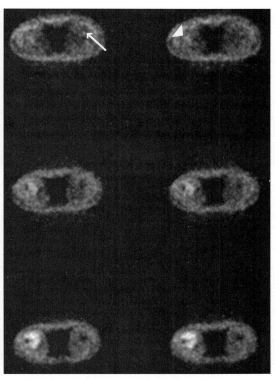

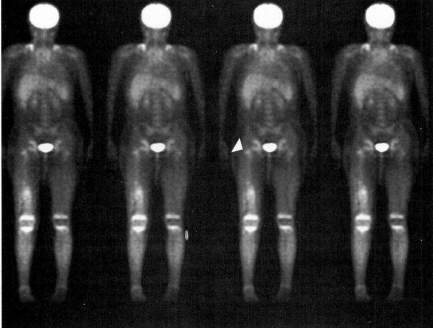

FIGURE 56.25. Locally aggressive osteosarcoma with intramedullary extension on 2-[¹⁸fluorine]-fluoro-2-deoxy-D-glucose (FDG) imaging. **A:** Whole-body ⁹⁹ᵐTc-methylene diphosphonate scintigraphy reveals and extensive osteoblastic tumor involving the distal right femur. There is increased uptake in the femoral shaft proximal to the tumor. This could be an example of "extended uptake," as is seen in the right lower leg, and not tumor extension. Magnetic resonance imaging revealed abnormal signal in the proximal femur to the subtrochanteric region but did not indicate tumor extension into the intertrochanteric region. This is a very important site if a limb salvage procedure is contemplated. **B:** Whole-body FDG coincidence imaging reveals a metabolically active tumor arising in the distal half of the right femur. Normal thymic uptake of FDG is seen in this patient. There is abnormal uptake of tracer in the intertrochanteric region (*white arrowhead*). **C:** Axial sections at the tumor level reveal an extensive extraosseous component with extension into the soft tissues. The highest sections reveal normal marrow (*white arrow*) on the left with tumor activity in the medullary canal on the right (*white arrowhead*). (*Figure continues.*)

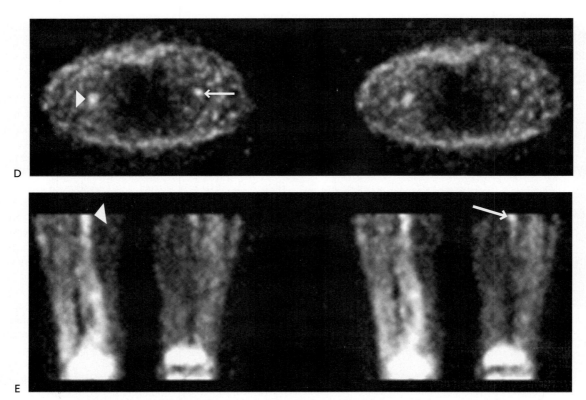

FIGURE 56.25. *Continued.* **D:** Axial section at the intertrochanteric level of the FDG study reveals normal marrow uptake on the left (*white arrow*) and tumor uptake on the right (*arrowhead*). **E:** Coronal section also reveals cephalad extension of tumor (*white arrowhead*), whereas normal marrow is seen on the left (*white arrow*).

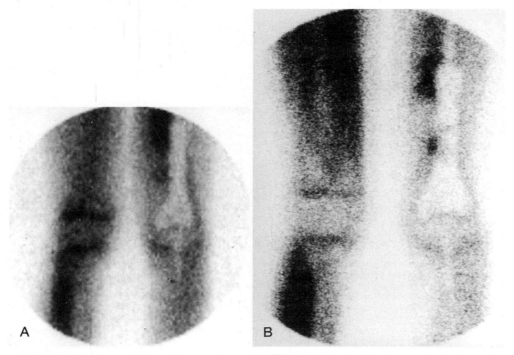

FIGURE 56.26. Recurrent osteosarcoma. **A:** Anterior ^{201}Tl scintiphoto of the knees reveals abnormal uptake along the medial aspect of prosthesis in a child with recurrent osteosarcoma. **B:** ^{99m}Tc-sestamibi scintiphoto reveals these lesions more clearly.

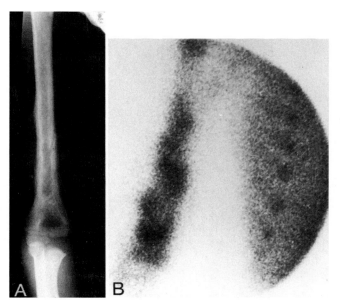

FIGURE 56.27. Ewing sarcoma. **A:** Conventional radiograph reveals an extensive lytic and blastic process involving the distal humerus. **B:** Anterior ^{99m}Tc-methylene diphosphonate scintiphoto of the right humerus reveals an extensive mixed osteolytic and osteoblastic process involving the humeral shaft in a serpiginous manner.

tumor and presents as a painless mass. The possibility of metastasis is high only in the histologically high-grade tumor.

Fibrosarcoma, chordoma, malignant fibrous histiocytoma, and desmoplastic fibroma of bone are very rare skeletal tumors and have all the characteristics of other primary skeletal neoplasm except that they do not form calcifications. Skeletal tracer agent may be taken up by the neoplastic mass and adjacent bone (193). Abnormal deposition of gallium may be seen on gallium scintigraphy in these neoplasms (87,186,206,213).

MULTIPLE SYSTEM MALIGNANCIES

Leukemia

Leukemia is the most common of the pediatric malignancies (1, 214). Its classification is based on morphologic evaluation of bone marrow aspirates. ALL is the most common form of childhood leukemia, accounting for 80% to 85% of cases (215). Chronic leukemia in the pediatric population is uncommon and chronic myelogenous leukemia (CML) is the only significant type found in childhood (216).

Osseous disease is infrequent in leukemia. Skeletal scintigraphy accurately depicts the extent of bone involvement, which may be diffuse or localized and symmetric or asymmetric (Fig. 56.28A–C). However, symmetric, uniform, or asymmetric bone involvement makes interpretation of these scans difficult. The most common sites of leukemic skeletal involvement are those with the greatest blood supply, such as the metaphyses of long bones, which can mimic an acute osteomyelitis. Complications secondary to acute leukemia may be evaluated by all modalities (174). Routine gallium scintigraphy is not recommended because of low yield (200,216) (Fig. 56.28**D**).

Hepatosplenomegaly occurs in 70% to 80% of patients at the time of initial diagnosis and is one of the initial prognostic factors (214). Diffuse leukemic infiltration of these organs usually occurs; however, enlargement may occur that is not due to tumor involvement (217). The liver and spleen may remain enlarged during remission because of hepatic fatty metamorphosis secondary to hyperalimentation, anemic heart failure, Budd-Chiari syndrome (thrombosis of hepatic veins), hepatotoxicity secondary to chemotherapy, viral infections, splenic vein thrombosis, or an immunologic reaction against leukemia (218–220). In benign hepatosplenomegaly, there is normal ^{99m}Tc-sulfur colloid uptake by these viscera. ^{99m}Tc-sulfur colloid scintigraphy may reveal reduced tracer uptake in both organs in the presence of leukemic infiltrate (150). The findings of focal intrahepatic and intrasplenic defects are nonspecific but rarely represent focal leukemic infiltrate; they more often represent complications of the disease, such as fungal abscess (217). There may be a reduction in ^{99m}Tc-sulfur colloid extraction by the liver on patients after chemotherapy or on hyperalimentation (221).

Leukemic renal involvement may manifest as nephromegaly and reduced renal function (122), which results in delayed excretion of chemotherapeutic agents and increased systemic toxicity (222). Nephromegaly in these patients may also be due to other causes (223), such as uric acid nephropathy in poorly hydrated patients with excess leukocyte breakdown (224), or may be part of the benign panorganomegaly seen in children with acute leukemia (217). Nephrotoxicity may also be secondary to chemotherapy and radiation therapy (215,216). ^{99m}Tc-MAG3 imaging assists in evaluation of renal function in these patients. Parenchymal transit time is prolonged in cases of leukemic infiltrates, whereas clearance of ^{99m}Tc-MAG3 is reduced in nephrotoxicity.

Testicles are recognized as a sanctuary for leukemia, and 10% to 15% of cases of relapse occur in this region in children on maintenance therapy and in more than 15% of children who had discontinued maintenance therapy for 2 to 3 years (225–227). This is often followed by bone marrow or CNS relapse despite aggressive therapy (226,227). Testicular enlargement suggests leukemic involvement, which may appear photopenic on testicular scintigraphy.

Mediastinal and hilar lymphadenopathy occur in approximately 10% of leukemic children (228,229). Mediastinal lymphadenopathy correlates with T-cell leukemia and denotes an unfavorable prognosis (214). Thymic involvement, pleural effusions, respiratory compromise, and SVC obstruction may also occur (228–230). A radionuclide superior vena cavagram may be used to assess flow through the SVC.

Intercurrent infection, which results in 80% of all mortality in leukemic children, requires a multimodal approach for detection (231,232). Gallium scintigraphy is an excellent screening modality with which to localize and direct further diagnostic procedures even in the absence of WBCs because of the multiple mechanisms of uptake of this tracer agent.

Abnormal accumulation of tracer in the mastoid region (because of otitis media), chest (resulting from pneumonic infiltrates), and heart (because of endocarditis) may be clinically undetected. In candidal esophagitis and fungal renal infections, increased gallium uptake is noted (233). Hepatic candidiasis may give variable scintigraphic appearances on gallium scintigraphy

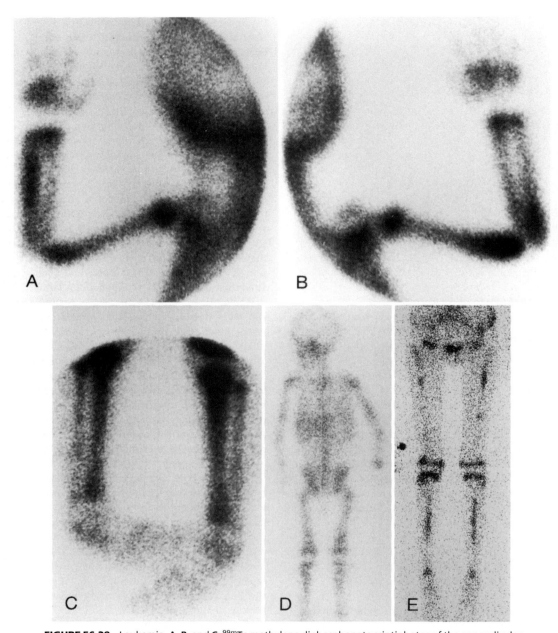

FIGURE 56.28. Leukemia. **A, B,** and **C:** ^{99m}Tc-methylene diphosphonate scintiphotos of the appendicular skeleton of a 2-year-old child with symptoms suggesting an infection of the right elbow. Increased activity is noted in the region of the right elbow on the posterior scintiphoto (**B**). However, focal areas of increased activity are also noted on the left ulna scintiphoto (**A**) and involving the left tibia and fibula (**C**). This scintigraphic appearance is very typical of leukemia with multiple sites of osseous involvement. **D:** Gallium scintigraphy in another patient with leukemia reveals diffuse uptake in the skeletal system. **E:** ^{99m}Tc-sulfur colloid bone marrow scintigraphy following bone marrow transplantation reveals multiple sites of implantation of the bone marrow.

(95,234,235). Candidiasis may produce gallbladder wall thickening and failure to fill during ^{99m}Tc-IDA scintigraphy. Abnormal gallium accumulation in infected central venous catheters has been observed on whole-body scintigraphy for unexplained fever (236).

BMT has had increasing success in the therapeutic management of leukemia (237,238). Morbidity and mortality from BMT occurs as a result of infection, interstitial pneumonitis,

and graft-versus-host disease (GVHD) (237). Complications associated with BMT are due to the complete suppression of the patient's hematopoietic system. Infections resulting from rare organisms such as *Mycobacteria kansasii, Aspergillus* sp., *Torulopsis glabrata,* cytomegalovirus, and herpes zoster virus and gastrointestinal GVHD, hepatosplenomegaly, Budd-Chiari syndrome, nephromegaly, and migratory arthritis may develop after BMT (237,239–245). Migratory arthritis may cause increased skeletal tracer uptake in the juxtaarticular bones, and sites of bone marrow implantation may be detected with ^{99m}Tc-sulfur colloid imaging (Fig. 56.28**E**).

Lymphoma

HD and non-Hodgkin lymphoma constitute the third most common pediatric malignancy (1). Non-Hodgkin lymphoma is very similar to ALL and differs markedly from the adult forms of non-Hodgkin lymphoma. This malignancy represents approximately 6% of all childhood cancers and more than 60% of pediatric lymphoma (246). Childhood non-Hodgkin lymphoma is often widely disseminated at the time of presentation and is a rapidly progressing tumor. Approximately one third of patients will have grossly localized, predominantly extranodal disease, which is in contrast to adult lymphomas and HD. The abdomen accounts for approximately 50% of sites of presentation, and the mediastinum is the second most common site. It is at this latter site where the most dangerous involvement is found. Mediastinal non-Hodgkin lymphoma may have a doubling time of hours and can produce the SVC syndrome or potentially fatal airway compromise. Presentation of non-Hodgkin lymphoma in the mediastinum is virtually indistinguishable from ALL, particularly the T-cell variety.

HD presents most often in adolescents and is similar to adult HD (246). The presenting site is usually nodal and often associated with cervical lymphadenopathy. Supraclavicular, mediastinal, axillary, intraabdominal, and inguinal primary sites may be identified. The usual sequence of disease is progression by lymphatic pathways to contiguous lymph node groups and the spleen. It is this frequency of nodal groups that further contrasts with non-Hodgkin lymphoma. Approximately one third of HD patients with mediastinal involvement will have associated hilar lymphadenopathy, which increases the risk of direct spread to the lungs.

Although non-Hodgkin lymphoma and HD are distinct and unrelated entities, they share similar imaging features (246). Nuclear imaging of these tumors consists primarily of gallium scintigraphy used both at the time of initial diagnosis and as a method of follow-up (Fig. 56.29). High-quality images are required for accurate evaluation. A maximum dose of 10 mCi is recommended; delayed images are obtained at 168 hours. Earlier imaging may be performed to assist with staging. The tracer should be administered before any chemotherapy or radiation. Bowel cleansing using oral cathartics and enemas is particularly important, because this will improve imaging and decrease body burden. FDG imaging has provided a new method of evaluation of lymphoma with excellent results (247,248). Lesions may be detected that are impalpable clinically or that can be detected by any other methodology (Fig. 56.30) (10).

For sequential evaluation, gallium remains an excellent imaging modality, which can be augmented by ^{201}Tl or ^{99m}Tc-sestamibi or FDG imaging (247–249). This is particularly true in the patient with thymic rebound following the discontinuance of chemotherapy. In this setting, ^{201}Tl or ^{99m}Tc-sestamibi scintigraphy has been particularly valuable, revealing minimal or no uptake in the mediastinum in patients with thymic rebound, whereas marked uptake is usually seen in those patients with

recurrent malignancy (250,251). The identification of new or occult sites of disease in patients in relapse has been particularly valuable, allowing early intervention. The addition of SPECT has further increased the value of gallium scintigraphy at the time of diagnosis and in sequential evaluation (200). Focal areas of involvement, which may vary in size from a lymph node to a retroperitoneal mass virtually filling the abdomen, may be seen. In the untreated stage, uptake in the dominant mass approaches 100% in childhood (246). Lymphoma in bone, a very rare occurrence at the time of presentation but more often seen at the time of relapse, may be evaluated by conventional skeletal scintigraphy. However, gallium offers a detection rate for bone involvement similar to that of skeletal scintigraphy and has the added advantage of multiorgan assessment, as well as assessment of soft tissues. Unless a specific area of skeletal involvement is questioned, routine skeletal scintigraphy in patients with lymphoma is not generally recommended. Although difficult to document by site positivity (to obtain an absolute sensitivity or true-positive ratio to be ascribed), we, like others, believe that childhood lymphoma has a greater propensity for uptake of gallium than does adult lymphoma (200). Site-specific imaging, however, is similar to that seen in adult tumors.

Histiocytosis

LCH, or histiocytosis X, is a group of rare syndromes of uncertain etiology (252). These syndromes range in severity from an evanescent maculopapular rash to a neoplastic-like fatal systemic illness. There exists a histologic link between solitary eosinophilic granuloma, multifocal systemic eosinophilic granuloma with diabetes insipidus (Hand-Schuller-Christian syndrome) or only skeletal involvement, and some cases of Letter-Siwe syndrome (253). Clinical abnormalities in patients with the most severe form of histiocytosis X include seborrheic hemorrhagic rash, hepatosplenomegaly, lymphadenopathy, anemia, and thrombocytopenia. Death usually occurs from sepsis. These tumors arise from histiocytes, which in turn originate from pluripotent bone marrow stem cells (254). The abnormal histiocytes may spread to the skeletal system. Solitary eosinophilic granulomas of bone tend to be age related, because older children and adults do not usually develop systemic disease. For children younger than 2 years, however, there is a higher likelihood of systemic spread (255). Hepatosplenomegaly may result from involvement of these organs by histiocytosis and is a grave prognostic sign in children younger than 2 years (255).

Histiocytosis X often affects the CNS, causing a significant percentage of these patients to suffer from diabetes insipidus and other cerebellar tract involvement (255,256). The bone marrow is also commonly affected, and many patients with the systemic disease suffer from anemia and thrombocytopenia. Lymphadenopathy, abdominal visceromegaly, and nephromegaly may also occur (257). Hepatic sinusoidal infiltration by histiocytes and lymphocytes in the lymphohistiocytic disorders may result in nodular lymphocytic infiltrates and endothelial cell hypertrophy of the hepatic central veins, which may, in turn, result in cholestatic jaundice (252,258). Hepatocellular dysfunction, reduction in hepatic coagulation factors, and hypoproteinemia follow. Portal hypertension and cirrhotic changes secondary to histiocytic

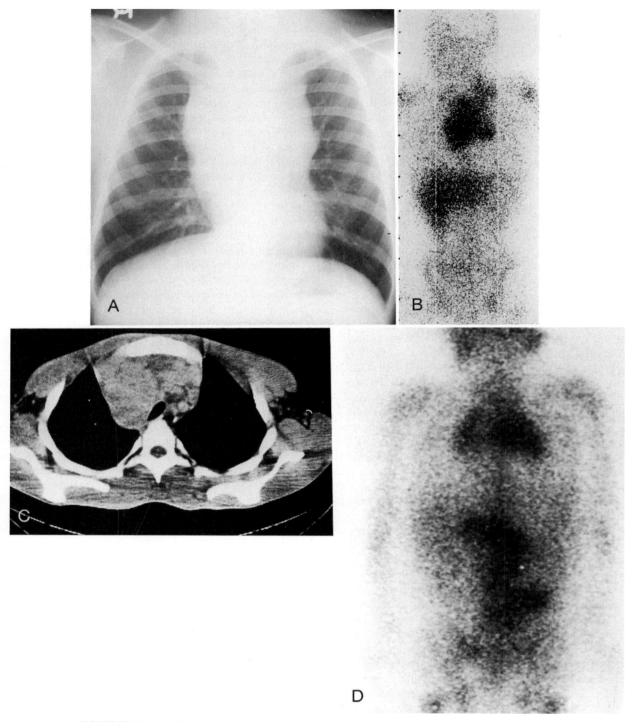

FIGURE 56.29. Lymphoma. Hodgkin disease involving the mediastinum is seen on this chest radiograph (**A**), ⁶⁷Ga scintiphoto (**B**), and computed tomography (CT) section (**C**). There is supraclavicular extension of tumor revealed on the gallium study. **D:** Hodgkin disease involving the mediastinum and abdomen in a 14-month-old boy is evidenced by abnormal uptake in the mediastinum and at multiple sites in the abdomen on whole-body ⁶⁷Ga scintigraphy. *(Figure continues.)*

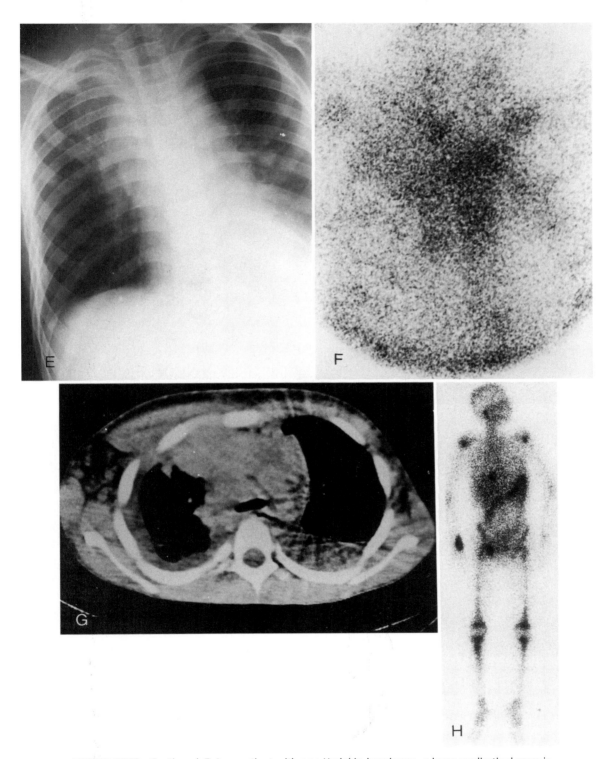

FIGURE 56.29. *Continued.* **E:** In a patient with non-Hodgkin lymphoma, a large mediastinal mass is seen on conventional radiography associated with bilateral pleural effusions. **F:** Gallium scintigraphy reveals an extensive process in the upper chest with involvement of the anterior mediastinum, supraclavicular region, and chest wall as well. **G:** CT section reveals extensive mediastinal processes with malignant involvement through the chest wall. **H:** Recurrent non-Hodgkin lymphoma in another patient is revealed on this whole-body scintiphoto by abnormal uptake in the right groin and at the right lung base. Neither of these sites of recurrence was suspected by clinical evaluation.

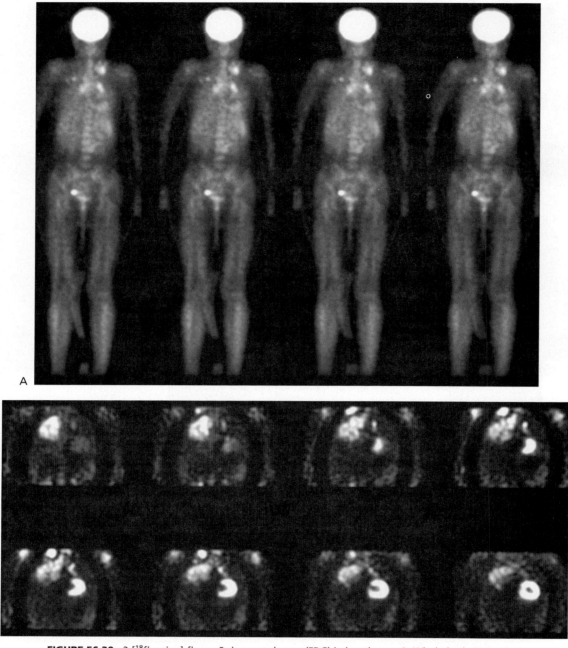

FIGURE 56.30. 2-[18fluorine]-fluoro-2-deoxy-D-glucose (FDG) in lymphoma. **A:** Whole-body FDG coincidence scintigraphy reveals extensive mediastinal and hilar lymphadenopathy in a patient with Hodgkin lymphoma. There is left supraclavicular and right pectoral lymphadenopathy as well. Extensive nodal disease is also seen in the upper abdomen. **B:** Coronal section of the chest reveals how well individual nodes can be seen in what may appear on gallium scintigraphy as an aggregate mass. Note the left hilar lymph node immediately above the left ventricle. Demonstration of involvement of hilar lymph nodes can have significant therapeutic import.

infiltration have also been reported (259). Pulmonary fibrosis resulting from infiltration of histiocytes has a grim prognosis (260).

Nuclear imaging studies are helpful indirect methods for assessment of the extent of disease. Most osseous histiocytic lesions are osteoblastic and hence show up as foci of abnormally increased tracer uptake (Fig. 56.31). About 10% to 15% of these lesions are purely osteolytic and, thus, photopenic. Vertebra plana may be perceived scintigraphically as loss of height of an involved vertebral body, usually without increased osteoblastic activity. Hence, lateral scintiphotos of the spine should be obtained if vertebral involvement by histiocytosis is suspected. Involvement of the base of the skull, the maxilla, and the mandible are best evaluated by other modalities. However, RNSS may reveal subclinical involvement of the mastoid region; thus, a true posterior skull scintiphoto in children suspected of having

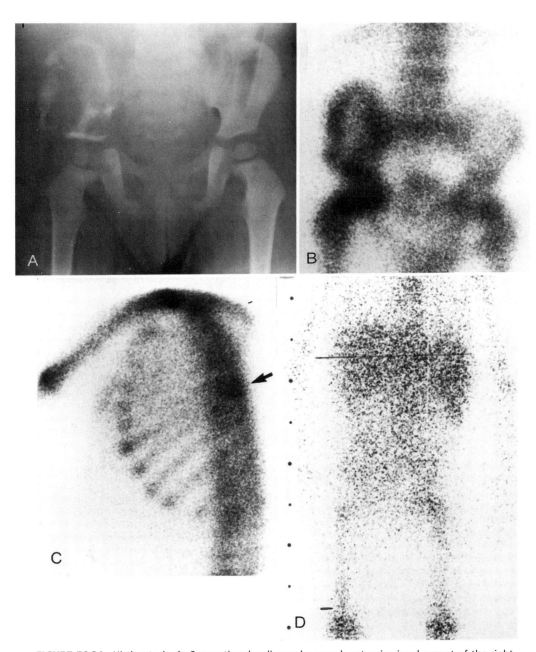

FIGURE 56.31. Histiocytosis. **A:** Conventional radiography reveals extensive involvement of the right ilium by an osteolytic process. **B:** Abnormal osteoblastic activity is appreciated in the right ilium and the right proximal femur on an anterior skeletal scintiphoto. **C:** A lateral scintiphoto of the spine in this patient reveals increased uptake in the midthoracic spine (*arrow*). This was due to vertebra plana. Note the loss of height of the posterior rib interspaces indicating collapse of the vertebral body. **D:** [67]Ga scintigraphy in this patient revealed decreased uptake in the right pelvis and proximal femur. *(Figure continues.)*

osseous histiocytosis should always be obtained (261). This method of evaluation is superior to conventional x-ray evaluation, having a much higher sensitivity and specificity (262). Hepatosplenomegaly occurs secondary to histiocytic infiltration in some patients. Reduced radionuclide tracer uptake associated with hepatosplenomegaly is indicative of histiocytic involvement (263). Follow-up evaluation of patients with histiocytosis is achieved best by an alternating series of conventional skeletal radiographic and scintigraphic evaluation (262).

COMPLICATIONS OF CANCER THERAPY

The nuclear physician must be aware of the protean effects of chemotherapy and/or radiation therapy on growing organ systems. In the brain, the need for differentiation between radiation necrosis and recurrent malignancy is not unique to the pediatric patient. Both FDG and conventional nuclear imaging with ^{201}Tl and ^{99m}Tc-sestamibi imaging are helpful in this regard. A more important sequela that is seen with increased frequency is the

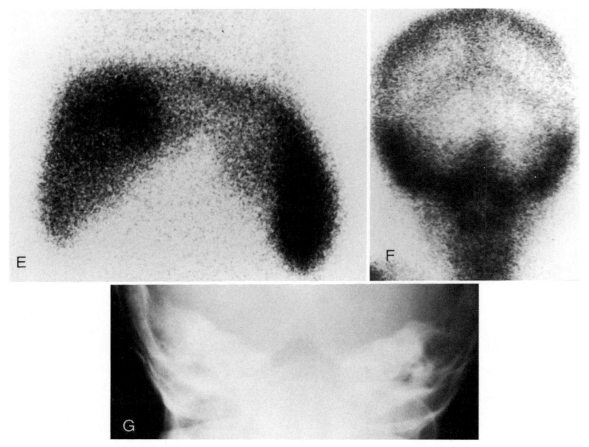

FIGURE 56.31. *Continued.* **E:** Hepatosplenomegaly is seen on an anterior ^{99m}Tc-sulfur colloid scinti-photo of the liver and spleen. The liver uptake is relatively inhomogeneous and the spleen is enlarged. These findings indicate the presence of histiocytic involvement of the liver and spleen. **F:** Involvement of the left mastoid region is seen on a posterior scintiphoto of the head. **G:** This correlated with conventional radiography.

remote effects of radiation therapy of intraaxial neoplasms in early childhood. Both stroke and impaired cognitive function have been well-recognized sequelae (264–268). However, affective disorders may also be seen. Imaging with brain perfusion compounds often reveals dramatic areas of reduction in uptake at some distance from the site of the primary tumor (269). This is felt to be due to an obliterative vasculitis produced by scattered primary beam therapy.

An increase in thyroid nodules could be anticipated in children who have received radiation therapy to the head and neck. We have not, however, encountered any thyroid malignancies in children who have received radiation therapy to this area, even at a young age.

The growing heart is particularly vulnerable to the effects of either radiation or chemotherapy. This is particularly true of the cardiotoxic drugs, which apparently produce myocardial fibrosis. This is manifest by a reduction in ejection fraction, which does not fully recover with the cessation of therapy. A normal child's ejection fraction is usually around 65%. Chemotherapy and/or radiation therapy to the chest should be discontinued if the ejection fraction falls below 50%. To allow the ejection fraction to decrease to 40% will almost certainly produce irreversible damage to the myocardium and may compromise a person's later life. The radiation effects on the lungs are similar to those seen in adults.

GI tract abnormalities associated with therapy are usually related to immunocompromise. These include esophagitis and typhlitis. Liver complications include the "recall reaction" and intrahepatic cholestasis. The recall reaction can be documented by conventional ^{99m}Tc-sulfur colloid scintigraphy (Fig. 56.32), and intrahepatic cholestasis may be addressed using the ^{99m}Tc-IDA compounds. IDA scans may provide false results for acute cholecystitis in patients on total parenteral nutrition, because there may be delayed filling of the gallbladder. An ultrasound may be useful in confirming the diagnosis. Following biliary tract surgery, functional assessment of the biliary tract along with exclusion of biliary leaks can be accomplished with ^{99m}Tc-IDA scintigraphy. Renal injury may be seen particularly with chemotherapy with the platin-based compounds, which have a distinct nephrotoxicity. Glomerular filtration rate is used to follow patients undergoing these therapies and is apparently a good measure of renal injury. Retention of skeletal tracer may be identified in the kidneys diffusely in the presence of nephrotoxicity and in focal areas included in radiation therapy fields. Diminu-

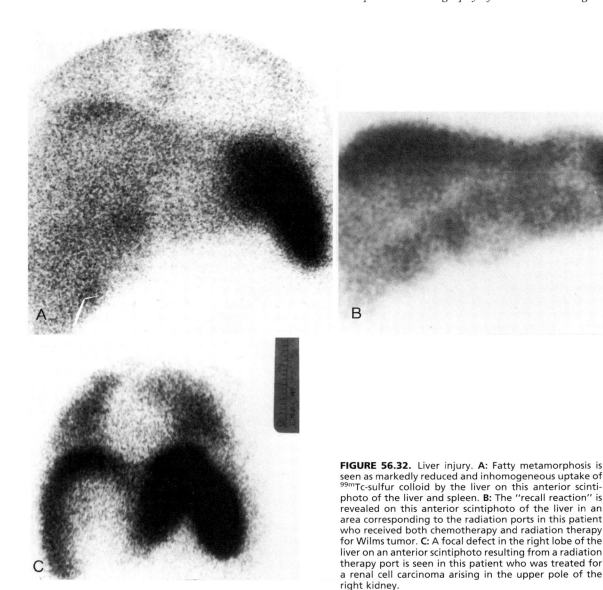

FIGURE 56.32. Liver injury. **A:** Fatty metamorphosis is seen as markedly reduced and inhomogeneous uptake of ^{99m}Tc-sulfur colloid by the liver on this anterior scintiphoto of the liver and spleen. **B:** The "recall reaction" is revealed on this anterior scintiphoto of the liver in an area corresponding to the radiation ports in this patient who received both chemotherapy and radiation therapy for Wilms tumor. **C:** A focal defect in the right lobe of the liver on an anterior scintiphoto resulting from a radiation therapy port is seen in this patient who was treated for a renal cell carcinoma arising in the upper pole of the right kidney.

tion in parenchymal handling of ^{99m}Tc-MAG3 may be seen. This is manifest by prolongation of the parenchymal transit time and a generalized flattening and broadening of the renogram curve.

The musculoskeletal system is susceptible to radiation injury. Second malignancies occur with increasing frequency. Most of these second primary tumors are osteosarcoma, which arise within the radiation treatment field. Benign tumors may also develop. These are usually osteochondromas, which apparently do not have a propensity for malignant degeneration (270). In addition, there is always the possibility of reduction in somatic growth when the spine or an extremity receives radiation therapy (Fig. 56.33).

The imaging of infectious complications of chemotherapy is the most important imaging that will likely be encountered in the evaluation of children who are actively treated for childhood malignancy. The malignancy often produces a relative compro-

mise because of replacement of bone marrow or tumor effect on the immune system. ALL and myelocytic leukemia may produce a granulocytopenia because of replacement of marrow or may incite abnormal granulocyte bacteriocidal activity resulting from tumor effects (271). Lymphoma and lymphocytic leukemia have a direct effect on the immune system, which produces a decrease in circulating antibody, whereas HD causes a reduction in cell-mediated immunity. The cytotoxic chemotherapeutic agents, such as cyclophosphamide, chlorambucil, and mercaptopurine, kill tumor cells, as well as the normal host cells in the bone marrow. Neutrophil phagocytosis and migration may be inhibited by treatment with corticosteroids. Both steroids and cytotoxic agents may impair immunoglobulin synthesis, azathioprine and methotrexate may suppress antibody formation during the induction of the primary immune response, and cyclophosphamide will reduce antibody formation (271). The single most important immune deficiency in children with cancer is neutro-

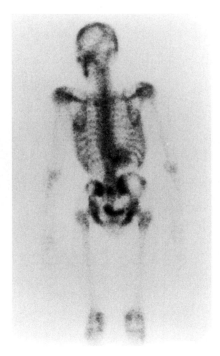

FIGURE 56.33. Radiation injury to bone. A posterior whole-body scintiphoto reveals dramatic shortening of the lumbar spine and hypoplasia of the left hemipelvis in an adult who had received radiation therapy as a child for a Wilms tumor.

penia. If the absolute granulocyte count falls below 500 WBCs/μL, there is a decided risk of either bacterial or fungal infection, which increases during the period of granulocytopenia (271).

Any organ system can be infected by either a bacterial or a fungal process. Ultrasound, CT, or MRI is often used to evaluate specific organs suspected of harboring an occult infection. Nuclear imaging is often used in the childhood cancer patient with unexplained fever. The radioisotope used most often in this regard is ^{67}Ga-citrate; however, FDG imaging may offer a new method of detection of these abnormalities (Fig. 56.34) (272). In a few patients in whom infection of a specific intraabdominal site was suspected, matched donor ^{111}In-labeled WBCs may be used.

In a child with unexplained fever and granulocytopenia, 24- and 48-hour imaging may be performed. Oral cathartic agents may be used to facilitate bowel cleansing, but enemas should not be given, because there is an obvious risk of inducing a perirectal abscess. On the gallium scintigraphic study, particular emphasis should be placed on observing sites of infection in children, which may produce fevers and may not be readily discernible to clinical or other imaging method evaluation. In the head and neck, increased uptake in the mastoid region may be identified, as well as necrotizing gingivitis or retropharyngeal abscess (Fig. 56.35). In the lungs, opportunistic infections such as cytomegalovirus or *Pneumocystis* pneumonia may be seen. Uptake in the distal esophagus may be seen in *Candida* or *Pseudomonas* esophagitis. Certainly, a bacterial pneumonia may be detected by a focal area of increased uptake. In the abdomen, liver abscess, splenic abscess, or pyelonephritis may be detected. One of the more common findings is a focal area of abnormality in the abdomen caused by a necrotizing transmural granulocytopenic

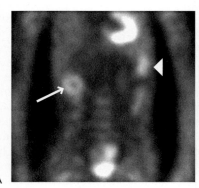

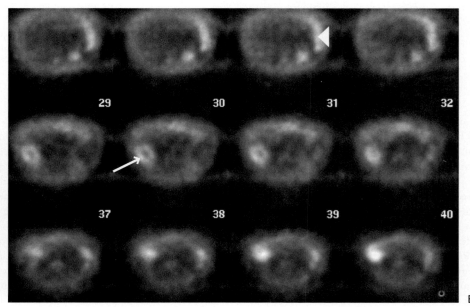

A   B

FIGURE 56.34. Superinfection with *Aspergillus* was serendipitously discovered on 2-[^{18}fluorine]-fluoro-2-deoxy-D-glucose coincidence whole-body scintigraphy in a patient being followed for neuroblastoma. At the time of the initial scan the patient was completely asymptomatic. The fungal involvement of the right suprarenal region (*arrow*) and of the spleen (*arrowhead*) were well seen on the reconstructed coronal sections (**A**). The lesions were delineated on axial reconstructions (**B**) as well. *(Figure continues.)*

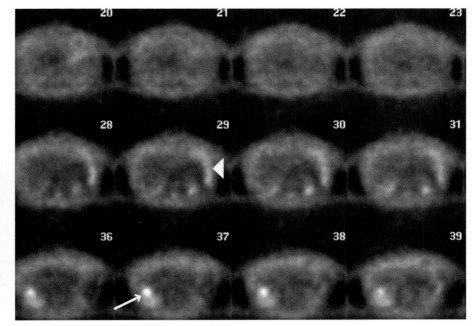

FIGURE 56.34. *Continued.* The suprarenal region was biopsied, because the lesion was expected to be recurrent neuroblastoma. However, it was found to be fungal hyphae compatible with *Aspergillus* infection. Six weeks following appropriate antifungal therapy the patient had only small residual foci seen on whole-body and coronal sections (**C**) and axial reconstructions (**D**). The patient underwent splenectomy because the splenic lesions had less demonstrable response than did the suprarenal mass.

enterocolitis, also known as typhlitis. This is believed to arise primarily in the region of the cecum, although it has occurred at most sites of reflection or angulation of the colon and is particularly frequent at the flexures. Typhlitis may be seen scintigraphically as an early and persistent focal area of gallium retention. This is even more problematic in that these areas are diffi-

cult to image by any modality other than barium enema. Soft tissue and musculoskeletal infections are well imaged by gallium. Even when osteomyelitis is suspected in an immunocompromised patient, gallium scintigraphy offers a better method of imaging than does conventional skeletal scintigraphy because of its ability to demonstrate soft tissue components (273). Gallium

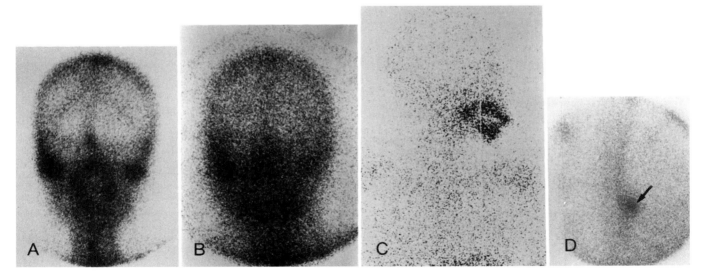

FIGURE 56.35. Infectious complications of cancer chemotherapy in various patients. Mastoiditis is revealed as abnormal increased uptake in the left mastoid as seen on these posterior ^{99m}Tc-methylene diphosphonate (**A**) and ^{67}Ga scintiphotos (**B**). **C:** Necrotizing gingivitis is revealed on a lateral ^{67}Ga scintiphoto of the head and neck. **D:** Fungal ulcer of the distal esophagus is seen as a focal area of abnormal gallium uptake (*arrow*) on a scintiphoto of the torso. *(Figure continues.)*

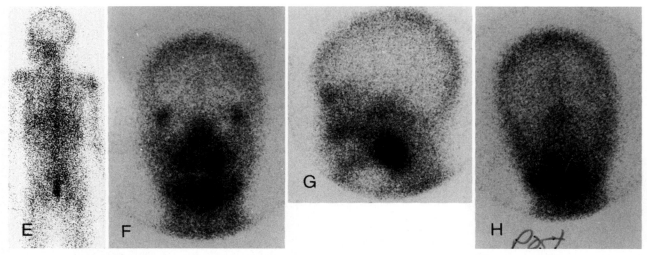

FIGURE 56.35. *Continued.* E: A perirectal abscess is seen as a focal area of abnormal activity in the midpelvis on a posterior whole-body gallium scintiphoto. A retropharyngeal abscess is seen as abnormally increased uptake in the peripharyngeal area on these anterior (F), left lateral (G), and posterior (H) ^{67}Ga scintiphotos of the head.

may be more reliable than CT imaging, which relies on an inflammatory response for the detection of possible abscesses in children who are markedly granulocytopenic. Infection around long-term indwelling catheters or infected thrombophlebitis may be identified as well (236).

SUMMARY

The nuclear physician can play a pivotal role in the initial evaluation and subsequent care of children with cancer. Imaging of the patients must be done in a careful manner with attention to good anatomic positioning and to the needs of children with cancer and their families. By performing examinations in this manner, the nuclear physician will have the satisfaction of being a valued member of the therapeutic team.

REFERENCES

1. Bleyer WA. The impact of childhood cancer on the United States and the world. *CA Cancer J Clin* 1990;40:355–371.
2. Conway JJ. Practical considerations in radionuclide imaging of pediatric patients. In: Freeman LM, ed. *Freeman and Johnson's clinical radionuclide imaging*, 3rd ed, vol I. Orlando, FL: Grune & Stratton, 1984:329–359.
3. Foley GV, Whittam EH. Care of the child dying of cancer: part I. *CA* 1990;40:327–354.
4. Neel HL, Becerra DM. The nuclear imaging technologist and the pediatric patient. In: Miller JH, Gelfand MJ, eds. *Pediatric nuclear imaging*. Philadelphia: WB Saunders, 1994:1–10.
5. Daldrup-Link HE, Franzius C, Link TM et al. Whole-body MR imaging for detection of bone metastases in children and young adults: comparison with skeletal scintigraphy and FDG PET. *AJR* 2001;177:229–236.
6. Alnafisi N, Whang J, Yun M et al. 18F FDG PET for the detection of bone marrow infiltration with lymphoma. *J Nucl Med* 2001;42:32P.
7. Li PY, Zhang LY. Evaluation of bone marrow infiltration in lymphoma patients with FDG PET. *J Nucl Med* 2001;42:32P.
8. Kim YK, Chung JK, Yeo JS et al. Differential features between the hypermetabolic bone marrow mediated by G-CSF and diffuse bone marrow metastases on FDG PET. *J Nucl Med* 2001;42:271P.
9. Porn U, Rossmueller B, Fischer S et al. Diagnosis of pediatric tumors with FDG PET. *J Nucl Med* 2001;42:39P.
10. Miller JH. Whole body FDG coincidence imaging in infants and children with malignant tumors. *Radiology* 1999;213(P):325.
11. Hooper R. Intracranial tumors in childhood. *Childs Brain* 1975;1:136–140.
12. Heiskanen O. Intracranial tumors of children. *Childs Brain* 1977;3:69–78.
13. Weinblatt ME, Ortega JA, Miller JH et al. The reliability of noninvasive diagnostic procedures in children with brain tumors. *Am J Pediatr Oncol* 1982;4:367–373.
14. Miller JH, Peña A, Segall HD. Radiological investigation of sellar region masses in childhood. *Radiology* 1980;134:81–87.
15. Patronas NJ, DiChiro G, Brooks, RA et al. Progress. [18F] fluorodeoxyglucose and positron emission tomography in evaluation of radiation necrosis of the brain. *Radiology* 1982;144:885–889.
16. Francavilla TL, Miletich RS, DiChiro G et al. Positron emission tomography in the detection of malignant degeneration of low-grade gliomas. *Neurosurgery* 1989;24:1–5.
17. DiChiro G, Oldfield E, Wright DC et al. Cerebral necrosis after radiation therapy and/or infra-arterial chemotherapy for brain tumors: PET and neuropathologic studies. *AJR* 1988;150:189–197.
18. Alan JB, Alan A, Chawluk J et al. Positron emission tomography in patients with glioma: a predictor of prognosis. *Cancer* 1988;62:1074–1078.
19. DiChiro G, Brooks RA, Patronas NA et al. Issues in the in vivo measurement of human central nervous system tumors. *Ann Neurol* 1984;15:5138–5146.
20. Nadel HR. Thallium-201 for oncologic imaging in children. *Semin Nucl Med* 1993;23:243–254.
21. O'Tuama LA, Janicek MJ, Barnes PD et al. 201-Tl/99m-Tc-HMPAO SPECT imaging of treated childhood brain tumors. *Pediatr Neurol* 1991;7:249–257.
22. O'Tuama LA, Treves ST, Larar JN et al. Thallium-201 versus technetium-99m MIBI SPECT in evaluation of childhood brain tumors: a within-subject comparison. *J Nucl Med* 1993;34:1045–1051.
23. Krenning EP, Kwekkeboom EJ, Renbi JC et al. [111In-DTPA-D-Phe1]-octreotide on somatostatin receptor scintigraphy. Orlando, FL:

The Society of Nuclear Medicine Correlative Imaging Council, June 1994.

24. Krenning EP, Kwekkeboom DJ, Bakker WHY et al. Somatostatin receptor scintigraphy with [111In-DTPA-D-Phe1]- and [123I-Tyr3]-octreotide: the Rotterdam experience with more than 1000 patients. *Eur J Nucl Med* 1993;20:716–731.

25. Hong F, Lee WH. Sequence similarity between part of human retinoblastomic susceptibility gene product and a neurofilament protein subunit. *Biosci Rep* 1991;11:159–163.

26. Ellsworth RM. The practical management of retinoblastoma. *Trans Am Ophthalmol Soc* 1969;67:462–534.

27. White L, Miller JH. Falsely positive periorbital bone scans in retinoblastoma patients. *Cancer* 1991;4:254–256.

28. Paganic JJ, Bassett LW, Winter J et al. Osteogenic sarcoma after retinoblastoma radiotherapy. *AJR* 1979;133:699–702.

29. Desousa AL, Kalsbeck JE, Mealey J et al. Intraspinal tumors in children. A review of 81 cases. *J Neurosurg* 1979;51:437–445.

30. Zwatveerce FL, Kaplan AM, Hart MC et al. Meningeal sarcoma in the spinal cord in a newborn. *Arch Neurol* 1978;35:844–846.

31. Nakagawa H, Huang YP, Malls LI et al. Computed tomography of intraspinal and paraspinal neoplasms. *J Comput Assist Tomogr* 1977;1:377–390.

32. Miller JH, Fishman LS. Spinal cord tumors. In: Miller JH, ed. *Imaging in pediatric oncology.* Philadelphia: Williams & Wilkins, 1985:101–105.

33. Suttow WW. Cancer of the head & neck in children. *JAMA* 1963;190:414–416.

34. Jaffe BF, Jaffe N. Head and neck tumors in children. *Pediatrics* 1973;51:731–740.

35. Jaffe BF. Pediatric head and neck tumors: a study of 178 cases. *Laryngoscope* 1973;83:1644–1651.

36. Butler J. Hodgkin's disease in children. In: *Neoplasms of childhood: 12th annual clinical conference on cancer.* Chicago: Yearbook, 1969:267–279.

37. Ziegler JL. Burkitt's lymphoma. *N Engl J Med* 1981;305:735–745.

38. Jaffe BF. Malignant neoplasm. In: Strome M, ed. *Differential diagnosis in pediatric otolaryngology.* Boston: Little, Brown and Company, 1975:201–209.

39. Donaldson SS, Castro JR, Wilbur JR et al. Rhabdomyosarcoma of head and neck in children. *Cancer* 1973;31:26–35.

40. Maurer HM, Moon T, Donaldson M et al. The intergroup rhabdomyosarcoma study: a preliminary report. *Cancer* 1977;40:2015–2026.

41. Gerson JM, Jaffe N, Donaldson MH et al. Meningeal seeding from rhabdomyosarcoma of the head and neck with back of the skull invasion: recognition of the clinical evaluation and suggestions for management. *Med Pediatr Oncol* 1978;5:137–144.

42. Raney BR. Spinal cord "drop" metastases from head and neck rhabdomyosarcomas: proceedings of the tumor board of the Children's Hospital of Philadelphia. *Med Pediatr Oncol* 1978;4:3—9.

43. Jenkin RD, Anderson JR, Jacob B et al. Nasopharyngeal carcinoma: a retrospective review of patients less than thirty years of age. *Cancer* 1981;47:146–152.

44. Lombardi F, Gasparint M, Gianni C et al. Nasopharyngeal carcinoma in childhood. *Med Pediatr Oncol* 1982;10:243–250.

45. Schenk Z, Osuch WE, Janczewski G. The head and neck metastases from clear cell carcinoma of the kidney. *Otolaryngol Polska* 1994;48:203–208.

46. Gates GF, Goris ML. Maxillary-facial abnormalities assessed by bone imaging. *Radiology* 1976;121:677–682.

47. Bergstedt HF, Loud MG. Facial bone scintigraphy: diagnostic potential in neoplastic and inflammatory lesions. *Acta Radiol (Diag) (Stockh)* 1978;36:993–1006.

48. Hung LO, August GP, Randolph JG et al. Solitary thyroid nodules in children and adolescents. *J Pediatr Surg* 1982;17:225–229.

49. Naga GR, Pitts WC, Basso L et al. Scintigraphic hot nodules and thyroid carcinoma. *Clin Nucl Med* 1987;12:123–127.

50. Reiter EO, Root AW, Retting K et al. Childhood thyromegaly: recent developments. *J Pediatr* 1981;99:507–518.

51. Jereb B, Lorohagen T. Carcinoma of the thyroid in children and young adults. *Acta Radiol Suppl (Stockh)* 1972;11:411–421.

52. DeKeyser LFM, Van Herle AJ. Differentiated thyroid cancer in children. *Head Neck Surg* 1985;8:100–114.

53. Pedisot R, Rohmee V, Lejenne JJ et al. Thyroid uptake of MIBG in Sipple's syndrome. *Eur J Nucl Med* 1988;14:37–38.

54. Ansari AN, Siegel ME, DeQuattro V et al. Imaging of medullary thyroid carcinoma and hyperfunctioning adrenal medulla using iodine-131 metaiodobenzylguanidine. *J Nucl Med* 1986;27:1858–1860.

55. Ramanna L, Waxman AD, Brachman MB et al. Treatment rationale in thyroid carcinoma: effect of scan dose. *Clin Nucl Med* 1985;10:687–689.

56. Freitas JE, Gross MD, Ripley S et al. Radionuclide diagnosis and therapy of thyroid cancer: current status report. *Semin Nucl Med* 1985;15:106–131.

57. Sty JR, Starshak RJ, Miller JH. Pulmonary scintigraphy. In: *Pediatric nuclear medicine.* Norwalk, CT: Appleton-Century-Crofts, 1983:159–166.

58. Fanta CH, Compton CC. Microscopic tumor emboli to the lungs: cause of dyspnea and pulmonary hypertension. *Thorax* 1980;43:794–795.

59. Sostman HD, Brown M, Toole A et al. Perfusion scan in pulmonary vascular/lymphangitic carcinomatosis: the segmental contours pattern. *AJR* 1981;137:1072–1074.

60. Wells RG, Sty JR, Miller JH. Vascular scintigraphy. In: Miller JH, Gelfand MJ, eds. *Pediatric nuclear imaging.* Philadelphia: W.B. Saunders, 1994:287–308.

61. Siemsen JK, Grebe SF, Sargent EN et al. Gallium-67 scintigraphy of pulmonary disease as a complement to radiography. *Radiology* 1976;118:371–375.

62. Gupta SM, Sziklas JJ, Spencer RP et al. Significance of diffuse pulmonary uptake via radiogallium scans: concise communication. *J Nucl Med* 1980;21:328–332.

63. Cohen M, Hill CA, Cangir A et al. Thymic rebound after treatment of childhood tumors. *AJR* 1980;135:151–156.

64. Donahue DM, Leonard JC, Basmadjian GP et al. Thymic gallium-67 localization in pediatric patients on chemotherapy: concise communication. *J Nucl Med* 1981;22:1043–1048.

65. Treves ST, Hill TC, Van Praagh R et al. Computed tomography of the heart utilizing thallium-201 in children. *Radiology* 1979;133:707–710.

66. Schmaltz AA, Aptz J. Primary heart tumors in infancy and childhood: report of four cases and review of literature. *Cardiology* 1981;67:12–22.

67. Silverman NA. Primary cardiac tumors. *Ann Surg* 1980;191:127–138.

68. Caralis DG, Kennedy HL, Bailey I et al. Primary right cardiac tumor: detection by echocardiographic and radioisotopic studies. *Chest* 1980;77:100–102.

69. Starshak RJ, Sty JR. Radionuclide angiocardiography: use in the detection of myocardial rhabdomyosarcoma. *Clin Nucl Med* 1978;3:106–107.

70. Lowman GT, Trueworthy RC, Vats TS. Tumors of the respiratory tract. In: Sutow WW, Vietti TJ, Fernback DJ, eds. *Clinical pediatric oncology,* 2nd ed. St. Louis: CV Mosby, 1977:698–711.

71. Weinblatt ME, Siegel SE, Isaacs H. Pulmonary blastoma associated with cystic lung disease. *Cancer* 1982;49:669–671.

72. Sumnee TE, Phelps CR, Crowe JE et al. Pulmonary blastoma in a child. *AJR* 1979;133:147–148.

73. Hisada K, Tonami N, Miyamae T et al. Clinical evaluation of tumor imaging with 201Tl chloride. *Radiology* 1978;129:497–500.

74. Cox JN. Respiratory system. In: Berry CL, ed. *Pediatric pathology.* Berlin: Springer-Verlag, 1981:299–394.

75. Caner B, Kitapa M, Aras T et al. Increased accumulation of hexakis (2-methoxyosisobutylisonitrile) technetium (1) in osteosarcoma and its metastatic lymph nodes. *J Nucl Med* 1991;32:1977–1978.

76. Sty JR, Starshak RJ, Miller JH. Gallium-67 imaging. In: *Pediatric nuclear medicine.* Norwalk, CT: Appleton-Century-Crofts, 1983:121–135.

77. Wallace S. Primary liver tumors. In: Parker BR, Castellino RA, eds. *Pediatric oncologic radiology.* St. Louis: CV Mosby, 1977:301–335.

78. Kompo DM, Rogers PCJ. Tumors of the gastrointestinal tract. In: Sutow WW, Vietti TJ, Fernback DJ, eds. *Clinical pediatric oncology,* 2nd ed. St. Louis: CV Mosby, 1977:712–719.

79. Fraumeni JF, Miller RW, Hill JA. Primary carcinoma of the liver in childhood: an epidemiologic study. *J Natl Cancer Inst* 1968;40: 1087–1099.

80. Landing BH. Tumors of the liver in childhood. In: Okuda B, Peters RL, eds. *Hepatocellular carcinoma.* New York: Wiley, 1976:205–226.

81. Miller JH, Greenspan BS. Integrated imaging of hepatic tumors in childhood. Part I. Malignant lesions (primary and metastatic). *Radiology* 1985;154:83–90.

82. Miller JH, Greenspan BS. Integrated imaging of hepatic tumors in childhood. Part II. Benign lesions (congenital, reparative, and inflammatory). *Radiology* 1985;154:91–100.

83. Miller JH, Gates GF, Stanley P. The radiologic investigation of hepatic tumors in childhood. *Radiology* 1977;124:451–458.

84. Gates GF, Miller JH, Stanley P. Scintiangiography of hepatic masses in childhood. *JAMA* 1978;239:2667–2670.

85. Rabinowitz SA, McKusick KA, Strauss HW. Tc-99m red blood cell scintigraphy in evaluating focal liver lesions. *AJR* 1984;143:6368.

86. Miller JH. Technetium-99m labeled red blood cells in the evaluation of hemangiomas of the liver in infants and children. *J Nucl Med* 1987; 29:1412–1418.

87. Teates CD, Bray ST, Williamson BRJ. Tumor detection with 67Ga-citrate: a literature survey (1970-1978). *Clin Nucl Med* 1978;3: 456–460.

88. Hoffer P. Status of gallium-67 in tumor detection. *J Nucl Med* 1980; 21:394–398.

89. Lee FA. Rhabdomyosarcoma. In: Parker BR, Castellino RA, eds. *Pediatric oncologic radiology.* St. Louis: CV Mosby, 1977:407–436.

90. Miller JH, Weinberg K. Liver and spleen. In: Miller JH, ed. *Imaging in pediatric oncology.* Baltimore: Williams & Wilkins, 1985:164–215.

91. Weissmann WH, Sugerman LA, Frank MS et al. Serendipity in Tc-99m dimethyl iminodiacetic acid cholescintigraphy. *Radiology* 1980; 135:449–454.

92. Bown ML, Frietas JE, Wahner HW. Useful hepatic parenchymal imaging in hepatobiliary scintigraphy. *AJR* 1981;136:893–895.

93. Rini JN, Manalili EY, Mehrota B et al. The utility of 18FDG, 67Ga and CT for detecting splenic involvement in Hodgkin's disease. *J Nucl Med* 2001;42:271P.

94. Rini JN, Manalili EY, Hoffman MA et al. Splenic uptake of 18FDG and 67 Ga in Hodgkin's lymphoma: a comparison of baseline and post-chemotherapy studies in patients with and without splenic disease. *J Nucl Med* 2001;42:271P.

95. Miller JH, Greenfield LD, Wald BR. Candidiasis of the liver and spleen in childhood. *Radiology* 1982;142:375–380.

96. Miller JH, Lammers PJ. Gastrointestinal tract, pancreas, and retroperitoneum. In: Miller JH, ed. *Imaging in pediatric oncology.* Baltimore: Williams & Wilkins, 1985:216–240.

97. White L, Miller JH, Reid BS. Preoperative ultrasound and gallium-67 assessment of abdominal non-Hodgkin lymphoma in childhood. *Am J Dis Child* 1984;138:740–745.

98. Miller JH, Hindman BW, Lam AHK. Ultrasound in the evaluation of small bowel lymphoma in children. *Radiology* 1980;135:409–414.

99. Ariel IM, Pack GT. Uncommon tumors of childhood. In: Ariel IM, Pack GT, eds. *Cancer and allied diseases of infancy and childhood.* Boston: Little, Brown and Company, 1960:517–537.

100. Kondo M, Hashimoto S, Kubo A et al. 67Ga scanning in the evaluation of esophageal carcinoma. *Radiology* 1979;131:723–726.

101. Pearlman AW. Gallium imaging in cancer of the esophagus. *Clin Nucl Med* 1981;6:380–383.

102. King DJ, Dawson AA, McDonald AF. Gallium scanning in lymphoma. *Clin Radiol* 1980;31:729–732.

103. Devroede GJ, Taylor WF, Sauer WG et al. Cancer risk and life expectancy of children with ulcerative colitis. *N Engl J Med* 1971;285: 17–21.

104. Kottmeier PK, Clatworthy HW. Intestinal polyps and associated carcinoma in childhood. *Am J Surg* 1965;110:709–716.

105. O'Connell DJ, Thompson AJ. Lymphoma of the colon: spectrum of radiologic changes. *Gastrointest Radiol* 1978;2:377–385.

106. Douds HN, Berens SV, Long RF et al. 67Ga-citrate scanning in gastrointestinal malignancies. *Clin Nucl Med* 1978;3:179–183.

107. Pechman R, Tatelman M, Athonmattei S et al. Diagnostic significance of persistent colonic gallium activity: scintigraphic patterns. *Radiology* 1978;128:691–695.

108. Sauerbrunn VJL, Andrews GA, Hubner KF. 67Ga citrate imaging in tumors of the genitourinary tract: report of cooperative study. *J Nucl Med* 1978;10:470–475.

109. Bekerman C, Port RB, Pang E et al. Scintigraphic evaluation of childhood malignancies by 67Ga-citrate. *Radiology* 1978;127:719–731.

110. Edeling CJ. Tumor visualization using 67gallium scintigraphy in children. *Radiology* 1978;127:727–731.

111. Yang SL, Alderson PO, Kaizer HA et al. Serial 67Ga citrate imaging in children with neoplastic disease: concise communication. *J Nucl Med* 1979;20:210–214.

112. Valk TW, Frager MS, Gross MD et al. Spectrum of pheochromocytoma in multiple endocrine neoplasia: a scintigraphic portrayal using 131I metaiodobenzylguanidine. *Ann Intern Med* 1981;94:762–767.

113. Sisson JC, Frager MS, Valk TS et al. Scintigraphic localization of pheochromocytoma. *N Engl J Med* 1981;305:12–17.

114. Shulkin BL, Chang E, Strouse PJ et al. PET FDG studies of Wilms tumors. *J Pediatr Hematol/Oncol* 1997;19:334–338.

115. Shulkin BL, Hutchinson RJ, Castle VP et al. Neuroblastoma: positron emission tomography with 2-[fluorine-18]-fluoro-2-deoxy-D-glucose. *Radiology* 1996;199:743–750.

116. Beckwith JB. *Renal tumors of children: pathologic considerations relevant to diagnostic imaging.* The EBD Neuhauser Lecture. 26th annual meeting of the Society for Pediatric Radiology, Atlanta, GA, April 16, 1983.

117. Delmer LP, Leestung JE, Price EB. Renal cell carcinoma in children: a clinicopathologic study of 15 cases and review of the literature. *Pediatrics* 1970;76:358–368.

118. Castellanos RD, Aron BS, Evans AT. Renal adenocarcinoma in children: incidence, therapy and prognosis. *J Urol* 1974;111:534–538.

119. Nygaard KK, Simon BH. Hypernephroma in children: review and case report. *Arch Surg* 1974;108:97–100.

120. Donaldson M, Duckett JW. Malignant genitourinary tumors. In: Sutow WW, Vietti TJ, Ferbach DJ, eds. *Clinical pediatric oncology,* 2nd ed. St. Louis: CV Mosby, 1977:636–653.

121. MacArthur CA, Isaacs H Jr, Miller JH et al. Pediatric renal cell carcinoma: a complete response to recombinant interleukin-2 in a child with metastatic disease at diagnosis. *Med Pediatr Oncol* 1994;23: 365–371.

122. Sty JR, Starshak R, Miller JH. Genitourinary imaging. In: *Pediatric nuclear medicine.* Norwalk, CT: Appleton-Century-Crofts, 1983: 167–199.

123. Duckett JW, Cromie WB, Vongiovanni AM. Genitourinary tumors in children. *Semin Oncol* 1974;1:71–75.

124. Young JL Jr, Heise HW, Silverberg E et al. *Cancer incidence, survival and mortality under 15 years of age.* Professional education publication no. 3022-PE. American Cancer Society, 1978.

125. Colodny AH, Hopkins TB. Testicular tumors in infants and children. *Urol Clin North Am* 1977;4:347–358.

126. Altman AJ, Schwartz AD. *Malignant disease of infancy, childhood and adolescence.* Philadelphia: WB Saunders, 1978:427–474.

127. Exelby PR. Testicular cancer in children. *Cancer* 1980;20: 1803–1809.

128. Exelby PR. Testis cancer in children. *Semin Oncol* 1979;6:116–120.

129. Javadpour N. Germ cell tumor of the testes. *CA Cancer J Clin* 1980; 20:242–255.

130. Holder LE, Melloul M, Chen D. Current status of radionuclide scrotal imaging. *Semin Nucl Med* 1981;11:232–249.

131. Jackson FI, Dietrich HC, Lentle BC. Gallium-67 citrate scintigraphy in testicular neoplasia. *J Can Assoc Radiol* 1976;27:84–88.

132. Barber HRK. Ovarian cancers in childhood. *Int J Radiat Oncol Biol Phys* 1982;8:1427–1430.

133. Smith JP. Malignant gynecologic tumors. In: Sutow WW, Vietti TJ,

Fernback DJ, eds. *Clinical pediatric oncology,* 2nd ed. St. Louis: CV Mosby, 1977:654–663.

134. Cecalupo AJ, Frankel LS, Sullivan MP. Pelvic and ovarian extramedullary leukemic relapse in young girls: a report of four cases and review of the literature. *Cancer* 1982;50:587–593.

135. Zarrouk SO, Kim TH, Hargreaves HK et al. Leukemic involvement of the ovaries in childhood acute lymphocytic leukemia. *J Pediatr* 1982;100:422–424.

136. Reid H, Marsden HB. Gonadal infiltration in children with leukemia and lymphoma. *J Clin Pathol* 1980;33:722–729.

137. Evans AE. Natural history of neuroblastoma. In: Evans AE, ed. *Advances in neuroblastoma research.* New York: Raven Press, 1980:3–12.

138. Miller JH, Sato JK. Adrenal origin tumors. In: Miller JH, ed. *Imaging in pediatric oncology.* Baltimore: Williams & Wilkins, 1985:305–340.

139. Jaffe N. Neuroblastoma: review of the literature and an examination of factors contributing to its enigmatic character. *Cancer Treat Rev* 1976;3:61–82.

140. Sutow WW. Neuroblastoma. In: Sutow WW, ed. *Malignant solid tumors in children: a review.* New York: Raven Press, 1981:75–103.

141. Pochedly C. Neuroblastoma in the neck, chest, abdomen and pelvis. In: Pochedly C, ed. *Neuroblastoma.* Acton, MA: Publishing Sciences Group, 1976:59–92.

142. Kinnier-Wilson L, Draper G. Neuroblastoma, its natural history and prognosis: a study of 487 cases. *Br Med J* 1974;3:301–307.

143. Fortner J, Nicastri A, Murphy ML. Neuroblastoma: natural history and results of treating 133 cases. *Ann Surg* 1968;167:132–142.

144. Sty JR, Babbitt DP, Casper JT et al. 99mTC diphosphonate imaging in neural crest tumors. *Clin Nucl Med* 1979;4:12–17.

145. Smith FW, Gilday DL, Ash JM et al. Primary neuroblastoma uptake of 99-technetium methyl diphosphonate. *Radiology* 1980;137:501–504.

146. Heisel MA, Miller JH, Reid BS et al. Radionuclide bone scan in neuroblastoma. *Pediatrics* 1983;71:206–209.

147. Bidani N, Moohr JW, Kirchner P et al. Gallium scanning as prognostic indicator in neuroblastoma. *J Nucl Med* 1978; 19:692(abst).

148. Reed JC, Kagan-Hallet K, Feigen DS. Neural tumors of the thorax: subject review from the AFIP. *Radiology* 1978;126:9–17.

149. Chambers EF, Turski PA, Sobel D et al. Radiologic characteristics of primary cerebral neuroblastomas. *Radiology* 1981;139:101–104.

150. Sty JR, Starshak R, Miller JH. Gastrointestinal nuclear medicine. In: *Pediatric nuclear medicine.* Norwalk, CT: Appleton-Century-Crofts, 1983:53–82.

151. Shulkin BL, Mitchell DS, Ungar DR et al. Neoplasms in a pediatric population: 2-[F-18]-fluoro-2-deoxy-d-glucose PET studies. *Radiology* 1995;194:495–500.

152. Beierwaltes WH. Update on basic research and clinical experience with metaiodobenzylguanidine. *Med Pediatr Oncol* 1987;15:158–163.

153. Gelfand MJ, Hoefnagel CA. Imaging with tumor-specific radiopharmaceuticals. In: Miller JH, Gelfand MJ, eds. *Pediatric nuclear imaging.* Philadelphia: WB Saunders, 1994:309–322.

154. Shapiro B, Gross MD. Radiochemistry, biochemistry, and kinetics of 131I-metaiodobenzylguanidine (MIBG) and 123I-MIBG: clinical implications of the use of 123I-MIBG. *Med Pediatr Oncol* 1987;15:170–176.

155. Gelfand MJ, Elgazzar AH, Kriss VM et al. Iodine-123-MIBG SPECT versus planar imaging in children with neural crest tumors. *J Nucl Med* 1994;35:1753–1757.

156. Miller JH, Allwright SJ, Villablanca JG et al. Comparison of conventional skeletal, bone marrow, and I-131 MIBG scintigraphy in the evaluation of skeletal metastases in patients with neural crest tumors. *Radiology* 1991;181(P):201(abst).

157. Friedland GW, Crowe JE. Neuroblastoma and other adrenal neoplasms. In: Parker BR, Castellino RA, eds. *Pediatric oncologic radiology.* St. Louis: CV Mosby, 1977:267–300.

158. Clayton GW, Holcom BE. Tumors of the endocrine gland. In: Sutow WW, Vietti TJ, Fernback DJ, eds. *Clinical pediatric oncology,* 2nd ed. St. Louis: CV Mosby, 1977:682–697.

159. Danemen A, Chan HSL, Martin DJ. Adrenal carcinoma and adenoma in children: a review of 17 patients (1943–1981). *AJR* 1982;139:1031.

160. Gyepes MT, Lindstrom R, Merten D et al. Hormonally active adrenal adenomas and carcinomas in children. *Ann Radiol* 1977;20:123–131.

161. White L, Hughes DO. Non-hormonal adrenocortical tumor in childhood: case report. *Am J Pediatr Hematol/Oncol* 1981;3:310–312.

162. Suefczek DM, Bowen A, Young LW. Non-hormonal adrenocortical carcinoma-radiological case of the month. *Am J Dis Child* 1982;136;163–165.

163. Parthasarathy KL, Bakshi SP, Parikh S. Localization of metastatic adrenal carcinoma utilizing 67Ga citrate. *Clin Nucl Med* 1987;3:24–26.

164. Robinson MJ, Kent M, Stocks J. Pheochromocytoma in child-hood. *Arch Dis Child* 1993;48:137–142.

165. Stackpole RH, Melicow MM, Uson AC. Pheochromocytoma in children: report of nine cases and review of the first one hundred published cases with follow-up studies. *J Pediatr* 1963;63:314–330.

166. Phillipps AF, McMurtry RJ, Taubman J. Malignant pheochromocytoma in childhood. *Am J Dis Child* 1976;130:1252–1255.

167. Lorenzo RL. Malignant recurrent extra-adrenal pheochromocytoma in a child: case report. *Pediatr Radiol* 1976;5:175–177.

168. Hodgkinson DJ, Telander RL, Sheps SG et al. Extra-adrenal intrathoracic functioning paraganglioma (pheochromocytoma) in childhood. *Mayo Clin Proc* 1980;55:271–276.

169. Spring DB, Palubinskas AJ. Familial pheochromocytoma: a rare case of hydronephrosis and hydroureter in two generations. *Br J Radiol* 1977;50:596–599.

170. Kaufman JJ, Franklin S. Familial pheochromocytoma: a report of two cases in a kindred. *J Urol* 1979;121:801–804.

171. St. John Sutton MG, Sheps SG, Lie TJ. Prevalence of clinically unsuspected pheochromocytoma: review of a 50-year autopsy series. *Mayo Clin Proc* 1981;56:354–360.

172. Nakajo M, Shapiro B, Copp JE et al. The normal and abnormal distribution of the adrenomedullary agent m-[I-131] iodobenzylguanidine (I-131 MIBG) in man: evaluation by scintigraphy. *J Nucl Med* 1983;24:672–682.

173. Sisson JC, Frager MS, Valk TW et al. Scintigraphic localization of pheochromocytoma. *N Engl J Med* 1981;305:12–17.

174. Sty JR, Starshak RJ, Miller JH. Bone scintigraphy. In: *Pediatric nuclear medicine.* Norwalk, CT: Appleton-Century-Crofts, 1983:1–25.

175. Gilday DL, Ash JM, Reilly BJ. Radionuclide skeletal survey for pediatric neoplasms. *Radiology* 1977;123:399–406.

176. Shreiner DP, Hsuy Y. Comparison of reticuloendothelial scans with bone scans in malignant disease. *Clin Nucl Med* 1981;6:101–104.

177. Sutow WW. Childhood rhabdomyosarcoma. In: Sutow WW, ed. *Malignant solid tumors in children: a review.* New York: Raven Press, 1981:129–147.

178. Weinblatt ME, Miller JH. Radionuclide scanning in children with rhabdomyosarcoma. *Med Pediatr Oncol* 1981;9:293–301.

179. Lee FA. Rhabdomyosarcoma. In: Parker BR, Castellino RA, eds. *Pediatric oncologic radiology.* St. Louis: CV Mosby, 1977:407–436.

180. Ragab AH, Phelan ET, Razek AA. Malignant tumors of the soft tissues. In: Sutow WW, Vietti TJ, Fernback DJ, eds. *Clinical pediatric oncology,* 2nd ed. St. Louis: CV Mosby, 1977:569–604.

181. Maurer HM. *The intergroup rhabdomyosarcoma study: update November 1978.* NCI Monograph 56. Sarcomas of soft tissue and bone in childhood. April 1981:61–68.

182. Gaiger AM, Soule EN, Newton WA. *Pathology of rhabdomyosarcoma: experience of the intergroup rhabdomyosarcoma study, 1972–1978.* NCI Monograph 56. Sarcomas of soft tissue and bone in childhood. April 1981:19–27.

183. Raney RB, Donaldson M, Sutow WW et al. *Special consideration related to primary site in rhabdomyosarcoma: experience of the intergroup rhabdomyosarcoma study, 1972–1978.* NCI Monograph 56. Sarcomas of soft tissue and bone in childhood. April 1981:69–74.

184. Miller JH, Ortega JA. Rhabdomyosarcomas and soft tissue tumors. In: Miller JH, ed. *Imaging in pediatric oncology.* Baltimore: Williams & Wilkins, 1985:355–377.

185. Enneking WF, Chew FS, Springfield DS et al. The role of radionu-

clide bone scanning in determining the resectability of soft tissue sarcomas. *J Bone Joint Surg Am* 1981;63A:249–257.

186. Kaufman JH, Cedarmark BJ, Parthasarathy KL et al. The value of 67Ga scintigraphy in soft tissue sarcoma and chondrosarcoma. *Radiology* 1977;123:131–134.

187. Zazzaro PF, Bosworth JE, Schneider V et al. Gallium scanning in malignant fibrous histiocytoma. *AJR* 1980;135:775–779.

188. Dahlin DC, Coventry MB. Osteogenic sarcoma: a study of 600 cases. *J Bone Joint Surg* 1967;49A:101–110.

189. McKenna RJ, Schwinn CP, Soong KY et al. Sarcomata of the osteogenic series (osteosarcoma, fibrosarcoma, chondrosarcoma, parosteal osteogenic sarcoma and sarcomata arising in abnormal bone). *J Bone Joint Surg* 1966;48A:1–26.

190. Cremin BJ, Heselson NG, Webber BL. The multiple sclerotic osteogenic sarcoma of early childhood. *Br J Radiol* 1976;49:416–419.

191. Reider-Grosswasser I, Grunebaum M. Metaphyseal multifocal osteosarcoma. *Br J Radiol* 1978;51:671–681.

192. Mahoney JP, Spanier SS, Morris JL. Multifocal osteosarcoma. *Cancer* 1979;44:1897–1907.

193. Chew FS, Hudson TM. Radionuclide bone scanning of osteosarcoma: falsely extended uptake patterns. *AJR* 1982;139:49–55.

194. Thrall JH, Ghaed N, Geslien GE et al. Pitfalls in Tc-99m polyphosphate skeletal imaging. *AJR* 1974;121:739–747.

195. Thrall JH, Geslien GE, Corcoran RJ et al. Abnormal radionuclide deposition patterns adjacent to focal skeletal lesions. *Radiology* 1975; 115:659–663.

196. Padua EM, Miller JH. Use of imaging and scanning in diagnosis of cancer. In: Pochedly CA, ed. *Neoplastic diseases of childhood.* Lausanne, Switzerland: Harwood Academic Press 1991;240–275.

197. Damgaard-Pedersen K, Edeling CJ, Hertz H. CT whole-body scanning and scintigraphy in children with malignant tumors. *Pediatr Radiol* 1979;8:103–107.

198. Goldstein H, McNeil BJ, Zufall E et al. Changing indications for bone scintigraphy in patients with osteosarcoma. *Radiology* 1980;135: 177–180.

199. Siddiqui AR, Wellman HN, Weetman RM et al. Bone scanning in management of metastatic osteogenic sarcoma. *Clin Nucl Med* 1979; 4:6–11.

200. Howman-Giles R. Gallium-67 imaging in pediatrics. In: Miller JH, Gelfand MJ, eds. *Pediatric nuclear imaging.* Philadelphia: WB Saunders, 1994:323–370.

201. Gainey, MA. Radiolabeled leukocyte imaging. In: Miller JH, Gelfand MJ, eds. *Pediatric nuclear imaging.* Philadelphia: WB Saunders, 1994: 371–382.

202. Ramanna L, Waxman A, Binney G et al. Thallium-201 scintigraphy in bone sarcoma: comparison with gallium-67 and technetium-MDP in the evaluation of chemotherapeutic response. *J Nucl Med* 1990; 31:567–572.

203. Caner B, Kitapçl M, Unlü M et al. Technetium-99m-MIBI uptake in benign and malignant bone lesions: a comparative study with technetium-99m-MDP. *J Nucl Med* 1992;33:319–324.

204. Huvos AG. *Bone tumors, diagnosis, treatment and prognosis.* Philadelphia: WB Saunders, 1979.

205. Pritchard DJ, Dahlin DC, Dauphine RT et al. Ewing's sarcoma: a clinicopathological and statistical analysis of patients surviving five years or longer. *J Bone Joint Surg* 1975;57:10–16.

206. Miller JH, Ettinger LJ. Methods of evaluation of musculoskeletal tumors. In: Miller JH, ed. *Imaging in pediatric oncology.* Baltimore: Williams & Wilkins, 1985:342–354.

207. Jones GR, Miller JH, White L et al. Improved detection of metastatic Ewing's sarcoma utilizing bone marrow scintigraphy. *Med Pediatr Oncol* 1987;28:966–972.

208. Harcke HT, Mandell GA. Musculoskeletal scintigraphy. In: Miller JH, Gelfand MJ, eds. *Pediatric nuclear imaging.* Philadelphia: WB Saunders, 1994:253–286.

209. Dahlin DC. *Bone tumors: general aspects and data on 6,221 cases,* 3rd ed. Springfield, IL: Charles C Thomas, 1978.

210. Steinbach LH, Parker BR. Primary bone tumors. In: Parker BR, Castellino RA, eds. *Pediatric oncologic radiology.* St. Louis: CV Mosby, 1977:378–406.

211. Suit HD, Sutow WW, Martin RG. Primary malignant tumors of the bone. In: Sutow WW, Vietti TJ, Fernback DJ, eds. *Clinical pediatric oncology,* 2nd ed. St. Louis: CV Mosby, 1977:605–635.

212. Lee SM, Hajdu SI, Exelby PR. Synovial sarcoma in children. *J Surg Gynecol Obstet* 1974;138:701–794.

213. Simon MA, Kirchner PT. Scintigraphic evaluation of primary bone tumors: comparison of technetium-99m-phosphonate and gallium citrate imaging. *J Bone Joint Surg* 1980;62-A:758–764.

214. Miller DR. Acute lymphoblastic leukemia. *Pediatr Clin North Am* 1980;27:269–291.

215. Saller SE, Weinstein HJ. Childhood leukemia. In: Nathan DG, Oski FA, eds. *Hematology of infancy and childhood.* Philadelphia: WB Saunders, 1981:980–1087.

216. Cooke JV. Chronic myelogenous leukemia in children. *J Pediatr* 1953; 42:537–550.

217. Miller JH, Heisel MA. Leukemia. In: Miller JH, ed. *Imaging in pediatric oncology.* Baltimore: Williams & Wilkins, 1985:406–426.

218. Manoharan A, Goldman JH, Lampert IA et al., Significance of splenomegaly in childhood acute lymphoblastic leukaemia in remission. *Lancet* 1980;1:821.

219. Hardisty RM, Chessells J. Splenomegaly in childhood leukaemia [Letter]. *Lancet* 1980;1:821.

220. Tricot G, Boogaerts MA, van Camp B et al. Splenomegaly in childhood leukaemia [Letter]. *Lancet* 1980;1:821–822.

221. Kaplan WD, Drum DE, Lokich JJ. Effects of cancer chemotherapeutic agents on the liver-spleen scan. *J Nucl Med* 1980;21:84–87.

222. Frei E, Bentzel CJ, Rieselbach R et al. Renal complications of neoplastic disease. *J Chronic Res* 1963;16:757–776.

223. Zuehzer WW, Flatz G. Acute childhood leukemia, a ten-year study. *Am J Dis Child* 1960;100:886–907.

224. Pinkel D. Treatment of acute leukemia. *Pediatr Clin North Am* 1976; 23:117–130.

225. Baum E, Sather H, Nachman J et al. Relapse rates following cessation of chemotherapy during complete remission of acute lymphocytic leukemia. *Med Pediatr Oncol* 1979;7:25–34.

226. Land VJ, Berry DH, Herson J et al. Long-term survival in childhood acute leukemia: "late" relapses. *Med Pediatr Oncol* 1979;7:19–24.

227. Hustu HO, Aur RJA. Extramedullary leukemia. *Clin Haemotol* 1978; 7:19–24.

228. Gwinn JL. Leukemia. In: Parker BR, Castellino RA, eds. *Pediatric oncologic radiology.* St. Louis: CV Mosby, 1977:133–159.

229. Mishner DC, Weinstein HJ, Kirkpatrick JA. The radiologic diagnosis of leukemia and lymphoma in children. *Semin Roentgenol* 1980;15: 316–334.

230. Blank N, Castellino RA. The intrathoracic manifestations of the malignant lymphomas and leukemias. *Semin Roentgenol* 1980;15: 227–245.

231. Hughes WT. Fatal infections in childhood leukemia. *Am J Dis Child* 1971;122:283–287.

232. Simone JV, Holand E, Jonshon W. Fatalities during remission of childhood leukemia. *Blood* 1972;39:759–770.

233. Miller JH, Thomas DW. Uptake of gallium-67 in a fungal esophageal ulcer. *Clin Nucl Med* 1981;6:332–333.

234. Ho B, Cooperberg PL, Li DKB et al. Ultrasonography and computed tomography of hepatic candidiasis in immunosuppressed patients. *J Ultrasound Med* 1982;1:157–159.

235. Callen PW, Filly RA, Marcus FS. Ultrasonography and computed tomography in the evaluation of hepatic microabscesses in the immunosuppressed patient. *Radiology* 1980;136:433–434.

236. Miller JH. Detection of deep venous thrombophlebitis by gallium-67 scintigraphy. *Radiology* 1981;140:183–186.

237. Johnson FL. Marrow transplantation in the treatment of acute childhood leukemia. *Am J Pediatr Hematol/Oncol* 1981;3:389–395.

238. Gale RP. Autologous bone marrow transplantation in patients with cancer. *JAMA* 1980;243:540–542.

239. Katchel SJ, Rodriquez V. Acute infections in cancer patients. *Semin Oncol* 1978;5:167–169.

240. Cryer PE, Kissane JM. Pulmonary and hepatic disease after chemotherapy and bone marrow transplantation for acute leukemia. Clinico-

pathologic conference, Washington University School of Medicine. *Am J Med* 1979;66:484–494.

241. Scrota FT, Starr SE, Bryan CK et al. Acyclovir treatment of herpes zoster infections: use in children undergoing bone marrow transplantation. *JAMA* 1982;247:2132–2135.
242. Pagani JJ, Kangarloo H, Gyepes MT et al. Radiographic manifestations of bone marrow transplantation in children. *AJR* 1979;132:883–890.
243. Rosenberg HK, Scrota FT, Koch P et al. Radiographic features of gastrointestinal graft-vs.-host disease. *AJR* 1981;136:371–374.
244. Fisk JD, Shulman HM, Grenning RR et al. Gastrointestinal radiographic features of human graft-vs.-host disease. *AJR* 1981;136:329–336.
245. Pagani JJ, Kangarloo H. Chest radiography in pediatric allogeneic bone marrow transplantation. *Cancer* 1980;546:1741–1745.
246. Miller JH, White L. Lymphoma. In: Miller JH, ed. *Imaging in pediatric oncology.* Baltimore: Williams & Wilkins, 1985:427–460.
247. Newman JS, Francis IR, Kaminski MS et al. Imaging of lymphoma with PET with 2-[F-18]-Fluoro-2-deoxy-D-glucose: correlation with CT. *Radiology* 1994;190:111–116.
248. Moody R, Shulkin BL, Yanik G et al. PET FDG imaging in pediatric lymphomas. *J Nucl Med* 2001;42: 39P.
249. Front D, Israel O, Ben-Haim S. The dilemma of a residual mass in treated lymphoma: the role of gallium-67 scintigraphy. In: Freeman LM, ed. *Nuclear medicine annual.* New York: Raven Press, 1991:212–220.
250. Kostakoglu L, Yeh SDJ, Portlock C et al. Validation of gallium-67-citrate single-photon emission computed tomography in biopsy-confirmed residual Hodgkin's disease in the mediastinum. *J Nucl Med* 1992;33:345–350.
251. Waxman AD. Thallium-201 in nuclear oncology. In: Freddman LM, ed. *Nuclear medicine annual.* New York: Raven Press, 1991:193–209.
252. Lichenstein L. *Histiocytosis X. Arch Pathol* 1953;56:84–102.
253. Basset F, Nezelof C. Presence en microscopic electronique de structures filamenteuses originales dans les lesions pulmonaires et osseuses de l'histiocytose X. *Bull Soc Med Hop Paris* 1966;117:413–426.
254. Kline JH, Lehrer RI, Territo MC et al. Monocytes and macrophages: functions and disease. *Ann Intern Med* 1987;88:78–88.
255. Greenberger JS, Crocker AC, Gordon V et al. Results of treatment of 127 patients with systemic histiocytosis (Letterer-Siwe syndrome, Schuller-Christian syndrome and multifocal eosinophilic granuloma). *Medicine (Balt)* 1981;60:311–338.
256. Rube J, Tava SDL, Pickren JW. Histiocytosis X with involvement of brain. *Cancer* 1967;20:486–492.
257. Starling KA. Histiocytosis. In: Sutow WW, Vietti TJ, Fernback DJ, eds. *Clinical pediatric oncology*, 2nd ed. St. Louis: CV Mosby, 1977:467–486.

258. Leblanc A, Hadchouel M, Jehan P et al. Obstructive jaundice in children with histiocytosis X. *Gastroenterology* 1981:80:134–139.
259. Nesbit ME, Krivit W. Histiocytosis. In: Bloom HJG, Memerle J, Neidhard TMK, et al., eds. *Cancer in children.* New York: Springer-Verlag, 1975:193–199.
260. Lahey ME. Prognosis in reticuloendotheliosis in children. *J Pediatr* 1962;60:664–671.
261. Siddiqui AR, Tashjian JH, Lazarus K et al. Nuclear medicine studies in evaluation of skeletal lesions in children with histiocytosis. *Radiology* 1981;140:787–789.
262. Dogan S, Bhattathiry MM, Grier D et al. Histiocytosis x: radiography versus scintigraphy. *Am J Pediatr Hematol/Oncol* 1996;18:51–58.
263. Miller JH, Shore NA. Histiocytosis. In: Miller JH, ed. *Imaging in pediatric oncology.* Baltimore: Williams & Wilkins, 1985:461–470.
264. Fogarty K, Volonino V, Caul J et al. Acute leukemia. Learning disabilities following CNS irradiation. *Clin Pediatr (Phila)* 1988;27:524–528.
265. Perani D, Di Piero V, Gucignani G et al. Remote effects of subcortical cerebrovascular lesions: a SPELT cerebral perfusion study. *J Cerebral Blood Flow Metabol* 1988;8:560–567.
266. Paakko E, Vainionpaa L, Lanning M et al. White matter changes in children treated for acute lymphoblastic leukemia. *Cancer* 1992;70:2728–2733.
267. Brouwers P, Poplack D. Memory and learning sequelae in long-term survivors of acute lymphoblastic leukemia: association with attention deficits. *Am J Pediatr Hematol/Oncol* 1990;12:174–181.
268. Kramer JH, Crittenden MR, Halberg FE et al. A prospective study of cognitive functioning following low-dose cranial radiation for bone marrow transplantation. *Pediatrics* 1992;90:447–450.
269. Curran JC, Miller JH, Allwright SJ et al. Evaluation of adverse effects of radiation therapy in children treated for primary brain tumors: comparison of imaging methods. *Radiology* 1990;177(P):143–144.
270. Moskowitz PS, Parker BR. Complications of cancer therapy. In: Miller JH, ed. *Imaging in pediatric oncology.* Baltimore: Williams & Wilkins, 1985:472–499.
271. Miller JH, Mason WH. Imaging of infectious complications. In: Miller JH, ed. *Imaging in pediatric oncology.* Baltimore: Williams & Wilkins, 1985:500–522.
272. Dreyer M, Borgwrdt L, Reichnitzer C et al. The role of whole body FDG PET in pediatric patients with fever of unknown origin. *J Nucl Med* 2001;42:38P.
273. Miller JH, Ettinger LJ. Gallium-67 scintigraphic detection of chronic osteomyelitis in children with leukemia. *Am J Dis Child* 1986;140:230–232.

Diagnostic Nuclear Medicine, Fourth Edition. Edited by M.P. Sandler, R.E. Coleman, J.A. Patton, F.J.Th. Wackers, A. Gottschalk. Lippincott Williams & Wilkins, Philadelphia 2003.

57

CARDIOPULMONARY STUDIES IN PEDIATRIC NUCLEAR MEDICINE

MARCELO F. DICARLI,
VICTOR H. GERBAUDO,
T.P. SINGH,
S. TED TREVES

Congenital heart disease (CHD) affects 8 per 1,000 live births. Approximately one third of these children require catheter or surgical intervention usually within the first year of life (1) (Fig. 57.1). Significant advances in echocardiography, diagnostic and interventional catheterization, cardiac intensive care, and cardiac surgery have occurred during the past decades. Corrective operations can now be performed in even the smallest neonates (2). Nuclear medicine offers several methods, including myocardial perfusion scintigraphy, first-pass radionuclide angiocardiography, gated blood-pool angiocardiography, pulmonary scintigraphy, and radionuclide venography that are applicable to the diagnosis and assessment of cardiopulmonary disorders in children. In this chapter, we focus on the clinical applications of nuclear medicine and its imaging tools that are relevant in contemporary pediatric cardiology practice and that offers insights that may not be available using other imaging modalities.

ASSESSMENT OF MYOCARDIAL PERFUSION

Clinical Applications

Coronary abnormalities are rare in children (3). However, children and adolescents with congenital or acquired abnormalities of the coronary arteries may be at risk of myocardial ischemia, arrhythmia, and even sudden death during strenuous activity (4). Myocardial perfusion scintigraphy provides important information in children suspected of having coronary abnormalities. It assists the clinician with decisions regarding patient participation in sports and need for coronary angiography to further

delineate the coronary anatomy. Myocardial perfusion scintigraphy has a role in a child with a known coronary abnormality to assess its hemodynamic significance. Examples of such patients include children with Kawasaki disease, children who have undergone coronary translocation surgery during neonatal arterial switch operation (ASO) for d-transposition of the great arteries (d-TGA) survivors of surgical repair of anomalous left coronary artery arising from the pulmonary artery, children following chest trauma, children with chest pain, and children with post-transplant coronary vasculopathy. Some of these patient groups are discussed in this chapter. Myocardial perfusion scintigraphy with exercise or pharmacologic challenge may also provide useful physiologic information in children with congenital coronary artery fistula, those with hypertrophic cardiomyopathy, and in children with myocardial bridging of the left anterior descending coronary artery.

Mucocutaneous Lymph Node Syndrome (Kawasaki Disease)

Acquired coronary artery disease in pediatric patients is very rare and in this population is often seen in the mucocutaneous lymph node syndrome (Kawasaki disease). Kawasaki disease is an acute vasculitis that occurs predominantly in infancy and early childhood. In the United States, Kawasaki disease is the leading cause of acquired heart disease in children. The cause of Kawasaki disease is unknown, although an infectious agent seems likely, because there is a seasonal incidence with a peak in the winter and spring and cases are usually clustered geographically. The highest incidence of Kawasaki disease is in the toddler age group (85% of cases are in children younger than age 5 years), and it is very rare in adults. The fatality rate of Kawasaki disease is approximately 0.3% with virtually all deaths occur from the cardiac sequelae of this disease.

The incidence of coronary artery involvement decreased fourfold in patients with Kawasaki disease during the mid-1980s when intravenous immunoglobulin treatment was introduced. Coronary artery aneurysms develop in approximately 5% of chil-

M.F. DiCarli: Radiology, Harvard Medical School, Division of Nuclear Medicine, Brigham and Women's Hospital, Boston, MA.

V.H. Gerbaudo: Radiology, Harvard Medical School, Division of Nuclear Medicine, Brigham and Women's Hospital, Boston, MA.

T.P. Singh: Pediatrics, Wayne State University School of Medicine, Pediatric Heart Transplant Program, Children's Hospital of Michigan, Detroit, MI.

S. Ted Treves: Radiology, Harvard Medical School, Division of Nuclear Medicine, Children's Hospital and Brigham and Women's Hospital, Boston, MA.

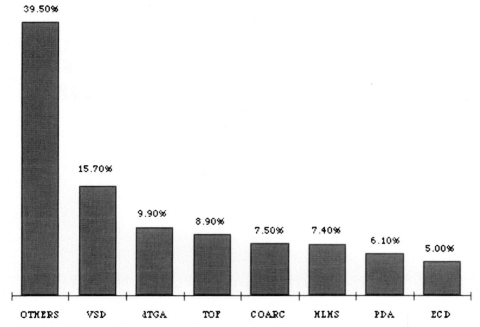

FIGURE 57.1. Relative incidence of critical congenital heart disease as determined by the New England Regional Infant Cardiac Program. Nuclear medicine methods are applicable in the preoperative or postoperative evaluation of nearly all these lesions. *VSD*, ventricular septal defect; *dTGA*, d-transposition of the great arteries; *TOF*, tetralogy of Fallot; *COARC*, coarctation; *HLHS*, hypoplastic left heart syndrome; *PDA*, patent ductus arteriosus; *ECD*, endocardial cushion defect. (From Fyler DC. Report of the New England Regional Infant Cardiac Program. *Pediatrics* 1980;65[Suppl]:377, with permission.)

dren with the disease and may lead to infarction, sudden death, or chronic coronary artery insufficiency (5).

The cardiac lesions in Kawasaki occur in four stages. Stage 1 (0 to 9 days) is characterized by acute perivasculitis and vasculitis of the microvessels and small arteries. In stage 2 (12 to 25 days) there is panvasculitis of the coronary arteries and aneurysms with thrombosis. Aneurysms can be small or can be centimeters in diameter (giant aneurysms). Myocarditis, pericarditis, and endocarditis may be present in this phase as well. In stage 3 (28 to 31 days) there is granulation of the coronary arteries and disappearance of inflammation in the microvessels. Stage 4 (40 days to 4 years) is characterized by myocardial scarring with severe stenosis in the major coronary arteries.

Echocardiography is useful during the acute and subacute phases of the disease for the assessment of ventricular function and to delineate coronary artery ectasia or aneurysms. Myocardial perfusion scintigraphy has been widely used during follow-up of patients with known coronary artery involvement to assess perfusion during stress (6–9) (Fig. 57.2). In the past, children with a previous history of Kawasaki disease, but no detectable coronary abnormalities during the acute or subacute phase, were thought not to be at risk for myocardial ischemia. More recent studies have reported reversible perfusion abnormalities in asymptomatic children with a previous history of Kawasaki disease and normal coronary arteries (10). The clinical significance of these reversible perfusion defects in myocardial territories supplied by normal epicardial coronary arteries is unknown. Pathophysiologically, they may indicate the presence of luminal narrowing and/or thickening of the wall in the coronary microvasculature as a result of a previous inflammatory process.

It has been suggested that the alteration in myocardial perfusion seen in asymptomatic children who have presumably recovered from Kawasaki disease and who have no gross coronary sequelae seems to be a more diffuse process than previously thought (11). Muzik et al. (11) reported that maximal vasodilator reserve, as measured by positron emission tomography (PET) during adenosine-induced hyperemia, was diffusely impaired in children with a history of Kawasaki disease despite the absence of abnormalities in the epicardial coronary arteries. These findings agree with pathologic observations at the acute stage of Kawasaki disease, which demonstrate a diffuse coronary vasculitis. Evidence provided by Suzuki et al. (12) demonstrates a modest increase in intimal thickness, as assessed by intravascular ultrasonography, with impaired endothelium-dependent vasodilatation in angiographically normal coronary arteries of children with previous Kawasaki disease. The abnormality of endothelial dysfunction in these patients appears to be generalized as demonstrated by abnormal endothelium-dependent vasodilation of brachial arteries in patients with previous Kawasaki disease (13). Together, these data demonstrate the potential late effects of Kawasaki disease on the coronary circulation, even in children without anatomic abnormalities in their coronary arteries (Fig. 57.3). These abnormalities are modest and do not appear to diminish exercise performance in these patients. It, therefore, seems acceptable to allow these children to perform unrestricted exercise activities (10). However, the findings can have implications later in life, because they may affect the severity of flow abnormalities in the event of coronary artery disease during adulthood. Thus, myocardial perfusion imaging seems well suited to diagnose and monitor these coronary flow abnormalities. For children who

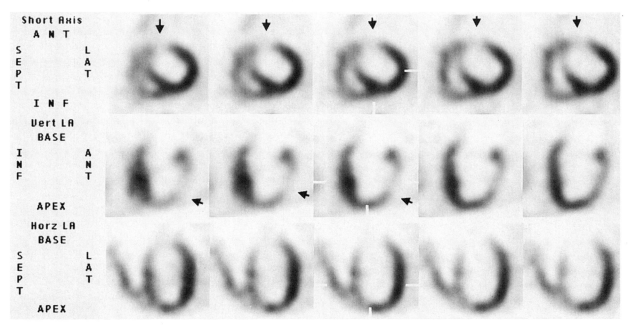

FIGURE 57.2. Kawasaki disease and myocardial infarction. Exercise myocardial perfusion single photon emission computed tomography with ^{99m}Tc-sestamibi shows a perfusion defect in the anterior wall of the left ventricle (*arrows*). The right ventricular wall is visualized. The ventricular chambers are enlarged with thin ventricular walls.

have coronary artery ectasia or aneurysm following Kawasaki disease, the findings of stress myocardial perfusion scintigraphy may be useful in making recommendations regarding participation in sports.

Transposition of the Great Arteries after Arterial Switch Operation

In children with TGA, the aorta (and the coronary arteries) arises from the right ventricle. The ASO translocates coronary arteries from the anterior semilunar root to the reconstructed neo-aorta (14). The long-term success of this operative approach depends principally on the continued patency and adequate functioning of the coronary arteries (15–18). Vogel et al. (19) have reported areas of myocardial hypoperfusion following the ASO. At Children's Hospital-Boston, Weindling et al. (20) found regional perfusion abnormalities, as assessed by exercise ^{99m}Tc-sestamibi (MIBI) single photon emission computed tomography (SPECT) in 22 of 23 patients following ASO. Most of these perfusion abnormalities were considered fixed and a

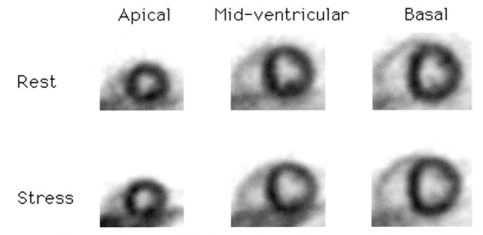

FIGURE 57.3. Stress and rest myocardial perfusion positron emission tomography (PET) images in short-axis views obtained in corresponding apical, midventricular, and basal levels in a patient with a previous history of Kawasaki disease. The images show relatively homogenous distribution of ^{13}N activity at rest and during adenosine-stress in all left ventricular regions. The global quantitative myocardial blood flow by PET was 56 ml/100 g/minute at rest and 251 ml/100 g/minute during hyperemia, with a coronary vasodilator reserve of 2.61.

STRESS

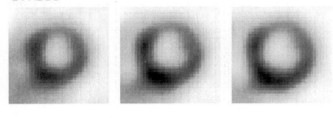

REST

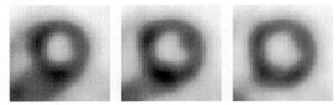

FIGURE 57.4. Stress and rest myocardial perfusion positron emission tomography images in short-axis views in a patient with d-transposition of the great arteries after arterial switch operation. The images show a moderately severe and partially reversible defect in the anterior and anterolateral walls. (Courtesy of Dr. Frank Bengel, Munich, Germany.)

small proportion were interpreted as reversible (3.7%). However, these perfusion abnormalities did not correlate with echocardiographic indices of wall-motion abnormalities and most likely were related to small areas of hypoperfusion perhaps resulting from aortic cross-clamping at surgery (20). Bengel et al. (21) reported a lower incidence of regional perfusion defects, using adenosine ^{13}N-ammonia PET. They found reversible perfusion defects in 5 of 22 (23%) patients after ASO, and fixed defects

in 2 additional patients. Maximal myocardial blood flow (MBF) and coronary flow reserve in response to adenosine were significantly lower in the patients after ASO compared with young healthy controls (21). Thus, it appears that reimplantation of the coronary arteries during ASO leads to a modest degree of diffuse coronary vascular dysfunction that may be regionally more severe in some patients (Fig. 57.4). In our experience, the lack of ischemic symptoms or electrocardiogram (ECG) changes during exercise suggest that myocardial perfusion is adequate during physiologic stress in children up to 8 years after ASO (20). Further follow-up and investigation should help determine whether the reported abnormalities in regional and/or global MBF have long-term implications in these patients.

Myocardial perfusion and/or metabolic imaging can also be useful to determine coronary artery patency and the extent and magnitude of myocardial viability in the event that a patient develops significant cardiac dysfunction after ASO (Fig. 57.5). Rickers et al. (22) reported their experience with fluorodeoxyglucose (FDG) PET to determine myocardial viability in a small group of infants and children presenting with regional and/or global left ventricular (LV) dysfunction after ASO. They reported that this approach was useful in guiding subsequent management in these patients (i.e., those with evidence of viable myocardium underwent revascularization, whereas those showing nonviable myocardium were treated medically).

Anomalous Origin of the Left Coronary Artery from the Pulmonary Artery

Origin of the left coronary artery from the pulmonary artery results in severe myocardial dysfunction and ischemia in early infancy (23,24). A number of surgical techniques have been used

Rest N-13 ammonia

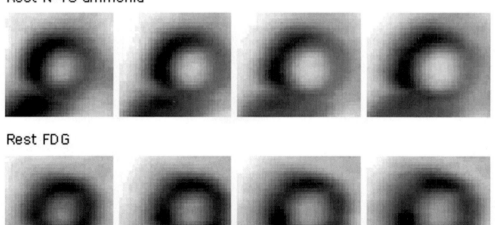

Rest FDG

FIGURE 57.5. Rest myocardial perfusion and glucose metabolism positron emission tomography images in short-axis views in an infant with d-transposition of the great arteries 10 days after arterial switch operation. The images show a large and severe perfusion defect in the anterolateral, inferolateral, and inferior walls, with preserved fluorodeoxyglucose uptake (perfusion-metabolic mismatch) consistent with viable but hibernating myocardium. Follow-up coronary angiography demonstrated a severe stenosis of the left coronary artery.

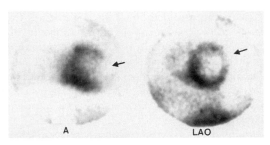

FIGURE 57.6. Anomalous coronary artery from the pulmonary artery. ²⁰¹Tl pinhole magnification scintigraphy reveals a focal perfusion defect in the anteroapical and lateral walls of the left ventricle (*arrows*). *A*, anterior; *LAO*, left anterior oblique. (From Treves ST, Hurwitz RA, Kuruc A et al. Heart. In: Treves ST, ed. *Pediatric nuclear medicine.* New York: Springer-Verlag, 1985:245–287, with permission.)

in the treatment of this disorder (25,26). The diagnosis can usually be readily made from the history, physical examination, ECG, and echocardiogram with color Doppler. Myocardial perfusion SPECT is helpful in assessing the severity of hypoperfusion and also to evaluate recovery of function and perfusion following repair (27) (Fig. 57.6).

Following surgical repair to establish blood flow to the left coronary arteries from the aorta, LV function recovers and usually normalizes within 2 to 3 years. However, perfusion abnormalities in long-term survivors are common and are typically located in the anterior and anterolateral ventricular walls (Fig. 57.7). These regions, which are supplied by the surgically repaired left coronary artery, may have low coronary flow reserve when compared with the myocardium supplied by the right coronary artery (28). Although these perfusion abnormalities may be worse in patients who have developed an occlusion of the left coronary connection to the aorta and, therefore, are dependent on collateral supply from the right coronary artery, they are also seen in patients with patent left coronary arteries.

Patients with severely reduced regional coronary flow reserve may be at risk of exercise-induced ischemic events. Identification of these patients by myocardial perfusion SPECT can help the clinician to guide recommendations regarding physical activity, antiischemic measures, and revascularization.

Cardiac Transplantation

Pediatric orthotopic heart transplantation is the treatment of choice for children with cardiac disease that is refractory to medical therapy or for whom other surgical approaches would be of no benefit. CHD accounts for approximately 78% of pediatric transplants in infants younger than 12 months. In children between the ages of 1 and 5 years, cardiomyopathy and CHD are the main indications, and after 6 years of age dilated cardiomyopathy accounts for 60% of cardiac transplantations (29). The 1-year survival rate for orthotopic heart transplant recipients is approximately 85%, with a 5-year survival rate greater than 70%. Transplant recipients surviving 5 years have an 80% actuarial 10-year survival rate and a 67% 15-year survival rate (30). However, the short- and long-term threats for survival continue to be allograft rejection and transplant vasculopathy, processes that can be evaluated with nuclear medicine techniques.

Acute allograft rejection is the most common cause of death during the first 12 months after heart transplantation in children (31). Most episodes occur within the first 3 months, and the incidence decreases 6 months after surgery. Many rejections are asymptomatic, or only characterized by nonspecific symptoms such as fever and lethargy. Physical signs include tachycardia, tachypnea, gallop rhythm, supraventricular and ventricular tachyarrhythmias, jugular venous distension, and hypotension. The onset of infection could present with the same nonspecific symptoms. Endomyocardial biopsy is considered the "gold standard" for allograft rejection surveillance, especially during the first year after heart transplantation. Typically, biopsies are ob-

Stress Myocardial Perfusion

Basal Myocardial Perfusion

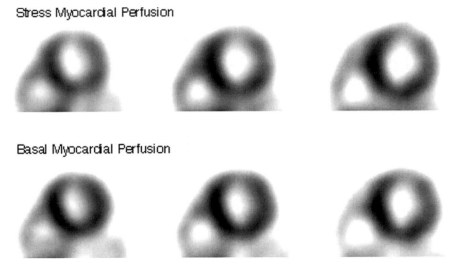

FIGURE 57.7. Stress and rest myocardial perfusion positron emission tomography images in short-axis views in a 17-year-old patient with a history of a corrected anomalous left coronary artery arising from the pulmonary artery. The images show a modest and reversible perfusion defect in the anterior and anterolateral walls. Follow-up coronary angiography demonstrated normal coronary arteries.

tained at short intervals during the first 3 months after surgery and gradually decrease to a 6-month schedule. However, controversy exists regarding the usefulness of surveillance endomyocardial biopsies late after heart transplantation. Early acute rejection in children affects diastolic function, and, as the process becomes more severe, systolic dysfunction follows. Echocardiography, magnetic resonance imaging (MRI), and radionuclide angiography have all been used with varying degrees of success for detecting acute rejection. These methods may be useful as well for monitoring the response to therapy (32–38).

The lymphocytic infiltrate present during rejection consists of activated lymphocytes that express upregulated somatostatin receptors, which can be imaged with radiolabeled somatostatin receptor analogues. Preliminary results with ^{111}In-pentetreotide demonstrated that cardiac uptake at 4-hours postinjection appears to correlate well with histopathologic evidence of rejection (39). Newer ligands using technetium chemistry such as ^{99m}Tc-depreotide (40) have been developed, but more study is needed to determine if they will be useful in this setting. Programmed cell death, or apoptosis, contributes to cardiac allograft rejection and can be detected using ^{99m}Tc-annexin V scintigraphy. This approach has been used successfully to detect allograft rejection and to monitor response to therapy in animal models (41,42). Clinical trials are currently under way to study the potential clinical role of ^{99m}Tc-annexin V in human cardiac allograft rejection and therapy. PET assessments of MBF have also been used to evaluate allograft rejection (43,44). During acute transplant rejection, resting MBF increases and hyperemic flow decreases leading to an impaired coronary vasodilator reserve. These changes in coronary dynamics improve following antirejection therapy and can be accurately measured with PET (43).

Transplant coronary artery disease (Tx-CAD) is the leading cause of death 1-year after transplantation. It may affect patients of any age, including neonates. Although its etiology remains elusive, it is clearly different from that of traditional atherosclerosis (45). It appears that the process is the result of immunologic injury to the coronary endothelial cells, and it may be related to chronic rejection. In a study of 210 children who survived more than 1 year posttransplantation, Mulla et al. (46) showed that the frequency and severity of late rejection were independent predictors of Tx-CAD. Tx-CAD affects the intramyocardial and epicardial coronary circulation, and it manifests as a progressive, concentric myointimal proliferation throughout the entire vascular structure (47). In children, the incidence is lower than in adults, in whom Tx-CAD is present in approximately 50% of transplant recipients 5 years after surgery (48). The clinical manifestations of Tx-CAD include silent myocardial infarction, congestive heart failure, and/or sudden death (49). Its detection is affected by the absence of angina pectoris resulting from the lack of innervation of the transplanted heart. Because of its diffuse nature, coronary angiography alone underestimates the presence and severity of Tx-CAD. This procedure is often used in combination with intravascular ultrasound (IVUS) (50). Although elegant, these procedures are invasive, expensive, and risky. In addition, they are limited for the evaluation of allograft vasculopathy in the distal and intramyocardial coronary vessels (51). Noninvasive methods are always preferred; however, vari-

able sensitivity and specificity limit their usefulness (52). Attempts to overcome these limitations have been made with pharmacologic stress imaging such as dobutamine echocardiography and radionuclide myocardial perfusion techniques.

Dobutamine stress echocardiography has good specificity but low sensitivity for the detection of Tx-CAD. Higher sensitivity values have been achieved when combining echocardiographic results with those obtained with thallium scintigraphy. Bacal et al. (53) demonstrated an increase in sensitivity from 64% to 71% with the combination of these two methods for the detection of Tx-CAD in asymptomatic transplant recipients with normal ventricular function.

Although earlier studies using planar imaging for the detection of Tx-CAD showed suboptimal results (54), reports using myocardial SPECT appear more promising (55). Early after transplantation ^{201}Tl SPECT shows inhomogeneous radiotracer uptake, including areas with fixed defects, redistribution, or reverse redistribution, that do not correlate with the affected coronary territories detected by IVUS (55). One year after transplantation, there is significant progression of scintigraphic abnormalities without a significant increase in vascular alterations. These findings may be secondary to the diffuse pattern of allograft vasculopathy and suggest progressive small vessel disease not represented by the degree of involvement of the epicardial coronary circulation (56). No significant difference has been found between ^{201}Tl and ^{99m}Tc-MIBI SPECT for the detection of Tx-CAD (57). By multivariate analysis, a normal stress ^{201}Tl study has been reported as the only significant predictor of survival at 5 years. Quantitative determinations of MBF and coronary vasodilator reserve with PET are potentially very useful and more suitable for the evaluation of diffuse Tx-CAD (43).

Methods

Radiopharmaceuticals

Myocardial perfusion SPECT in children is obtained using a variety of blood flow tracers including ^{99m}Tc-MIBI, (Cardiolite, Dupont Pharmaceuticals) ^{99m}Tc-tetrofosmin, (Myoview, Nycomed Amersham), or [201]Tl. Because of higher photon flux, more ideal imaging characteristics of the tracer, and lower radiation exposure, at present, the radiopharmaceuticals of choice for myocardial perfusion scintigraphy in children are the ^{99m}Tc-labeled compounds. The administered dose of ^{99m}Tc-MIBI or tetrofosmin are adjusted based on whether a single study or both rest and exercise studies are performed on the same day (Table 57.1). In our laboratory for a single study (rest or exercise), a dose of 0.25 mCi (9.25 MBq) per kilogram with a minimum total dose of 4 mCi (148 MBq) and a maximum dose of 10 mCi (370 MBq) is used. If rest and exercise studies are performed on two separate days, the same dose of ^{99m}Tc-MIBI or tetrofosmin can be used. In PET studies, MBF is most commonly evaluated using [134]N-ammonia or [82]Rb.

Stress Protocols

As in adults, myocardial perfusion SPECT can be performed in combination with graded exercise or pharmacologic stress,

Table 57.1. *Pediatric Nuclear Cardiopulmonary Studies and Usual Radiopharmaceutical Doses*[a]

Procedure	Radiopharmaceutical	Dose/kg		Minimal total dose		Dose/70 kg	
		mCi	MBq	mCi	MBq	mCi	MBq
Radionuclide angiocardiography	99mTc-pertechnetate	0.2	7.4	2.0	74	10–20	370–740
Myocardial perfusion scintigraphy	99mTc-MIBI	0.4	14.8	2.0	74	10–30	370–110
Myocardial perfusion scintigraphy	201Tl as thallous chloride	0.003	1.11	0.15	5.55	2.0	74
Gated blood-pool angiocardiography	99mTc-labeled red blood cells	0.2	7.4	2.0	7.4	10–20	370–740
Pulmonary perfusion scintigraphy	99mTc-MAA	0.05	1.85	0.2	7.4	3	111
Right-to-left shunts	99mTc-MAA[b]	0.02	0.74	0.1	3.7	1	37
Pulmonary perfusion scintigraphy	133Xe on saline	0.3	11.1	5	185	30	1110
Ventilation	133Xe gas	Total dose: 8–30 mCi—inhalation/ [296–1110 MBq]					

MAA, macroaggregated albumin; MIBI, sestamibi.
[a]Usual doses at Children's Hospital, Boston.
[b]>10,000 particles.

depending on the clinical situation, the age of the patient, and the imaging method that is used (SPECT or PET). Pharmacologic stress in children can be performed using vasodilators such as dipyridamole (0.56 mg/kg over 4 minutes) or adenosine (0.14 mg/kg/min over 4 or 6 minutes) or beta agonists such as dobutamine.

Imaging

SPECT is the standard method in the assessment of regional myocardial perfusion. The available imaging protocols, as well as the acquisition and processing parameters, are described in detail elsewhere in this book. Appropriate magnification should be used depending on the patient's heart size (Fig. 57.8).

DETECTION AND QUANTITATION OF CARDIOVASCULAR SHUNTS

Clinical Applications

First-pass radionuclide angiography is used in the detection and quantitation of cardiovascular shunts and in the evaluation of

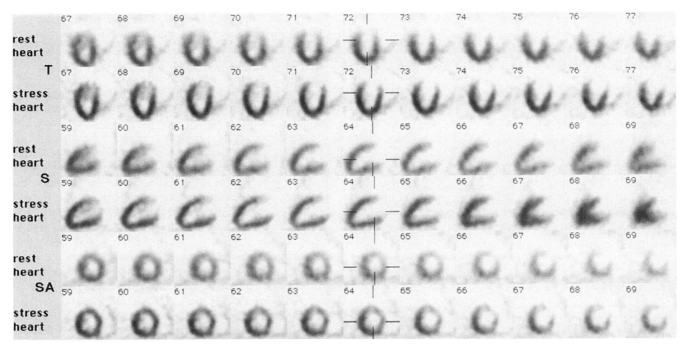

FIGURE 57.8. Normal myocardial perfusion. Rest and exercise 99mTc-sestamibi myocardial perfusion single photon emission computed tomography from a 5-year-old with Kawasaki disease. There are no perfusion defects. *T*, transverse horizontal long-axis; *S*, sagittal vertical long-axis; *SA*, short axis.

Table 57.2. *Comparison of ECG-Gated Blood Pool Scan and First-Pass Radionuclide Angiography*

	Gated blood pool scan	First-pass radionuclide angiography
ECG computer interface	Yes	No
Injection technique importance	No	Yes
Counting statistics and spatial resolution	Good	Fair
Shunt quantitation	No	Yes
Temporal separation of structures	No	Yes
Background	High (60–80%)	Low (≤20%)
Recording time	20–30 min	<30 sec
Multiple studies within a short time	Yes	Yes
Quantitation of valvular insufficiency	Yes	Maybe
Transit times	No	Yes

ventricular function. This method is accurate and ideally suited for children because it can be performed in just a few seconds and, therefore, does not require prolonged immobilization or sedation (Table 57.2).

Left-To-Right Shunts

Radionuclide angiocardiography is an accurate imaging tool for detecting and assessing the magnitude of left-to-right or right-to-left intracardiac shunts in certain congenital lesions (Table 57.3).

Right-To-Left Shunts

Examples of congenital lesions with right-to-left shunts are listed in Table 57.4.

Methods

Radiopharmaceuticals

^{99m}Tc-pertechnetate is the most commonly used radiopharmaceutical for first-pass radionuclide angiocardiography. ^{99m}Tc-labeled radiopharmaceuticals with a rapid blood disappearance rate, such as ^{99m}Tc-mercaptoacetyltriglycine (MAG3) or ^{99m}Tc-diethylenetriaminepentaacetic acid (DTPA), can also be used for serial radionuclide angiocardiography. When using ^{99m}Tc-

Table 57.3. *Left-to-Right Shunt Lesions*

Arterial septal defect
Ventricular septal defect
Truncus arteriosus
Patent ductus arteriosus
Complete atrioventricular canal
Aortopulmonary collaterals

Table 57.4. *Right-to-Left Shunt Lesions*

Tetralogy of Fallot
Tricuspid atresia
Pulmonary atresia/intact ventricular septum
Tetralogy of Fallot with pulmonary atresia

pertechnetate, the patient should be premedicated with sodium [intravenous (IV)] or potassium (oral) perchlorate to reduce thyroid uptake of the tracer. (See Table 57.1 for usual administered doses.)

Generator-produced ultrashort-lived radionuclides have advantages over ^{99m}Tc for radionuclide angiocardiography, including higher photon flux from higher administered doses and lower patient radiation exposure. In addition, their short half-lives allows serial studies to be acquired within a short period to assess the cardiovascular changes that result from exercise, drugs, or catheter interventions. The group of ultrashort-lived radionuclides includes ^{195m}Au, ^{191m}Ir, and ^{178}Ta (58–65). At present, generator-produced ultrashort-lived radionuclides are not widely available.

A simple, accurate, and effective method for the detection and quantitation of *left-to-right shunts* using first-pass radionuclide angiography was developed in our laboratory in 1973 and it is now used widely (66). For left-to-right shunt assessment, the patient is imaged in the supine position. The gamma-camera is equipped with a high-sensitivity parallel-hole collimator, which is positioned in front of the patient's chest. The field-of-view should include the entire cardiopulmonary volume. A framing rate of two to four frames per second provides adequate temporal resolution for left-to-right shunt assessment. If, in addition to shunt assessment, evaluation of ventricular ejection fraction is desired, the radionuclide angiogram should be recorded at 25 frames per second. Recording begins with the rapid intravenous injection of the tracer in an antecubital vein. Following the acquisition, the study is evaluated on a cine loop for a general assessment of the study. Left-to-right shunts can be diagnosed visually as persistence of tracer in the lung fields because of premature return of tracer into the pulmonary arterial circulation and by relatively poor visualization of the left ventricle and aorta at the normally expected times. These characteristic angiographic findings are easier to recognize in shunts of pulmonary-to-systemic flow ratios (Qp:Qs) greater than 2.0. Detection and quantitation of left-to-right shunts is aided by analysis of the pulmonary time-activity curve (Fig. 57.9). The normal time-activity curve reveals an initial peak resulting from the first pass of the radiotracer through the pulmonary circulation. As the tracer leaves the lungs, the peak is followed by a rapid exponential descent almost reaching the baseline. A second peak that is wider and of lesser amplitude follows as the tracer returns to the lung following systemic circulation. In left-to-right shunts, the exponential descent following the initial peak on the pulmonary time-activity curve is interrupted by tracer returning prematurely to the lungs through the shunt, which occurs irrespective of the shunt level (atrial, ventricular, or extracardiac). Quantitative analysis of the pulmonary time-activity curve using the γ-variate analysis provides a direct measurement of the pulmonary-to-

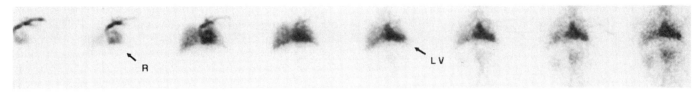

1 Frame per Second

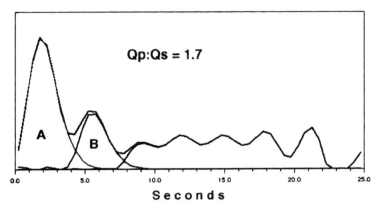

FIGURE 57.9. Left-to-right shunt. First-pass radionuclide angiography in a patient with a left-to-right shunt. The images displayed at one frame per second reveal persistence of radiotracer in the lungs because of premature recirculation through the shunt. The right (*R*) and left (*LV*) ventricular blood pools are well seen. Analysis of the pulmonary time-activity curve using γ-variate analysis reveals a pulmonary-to-systemic flow ratio (Qp:Qs) of 1.7. Area A, pulmonary flow; area B, shunt flow. Qp:Qs = A/A-B. Curve analyzed following deconvolution. (From Maltz DL, Treves S. Quantitative radionuclide angiocardiography: determination of Qp:Qs in children. *Circulation* 1973;47:1049–1056, with permission.)

systemic flow ratio (66–69). The γ-variate is used to define two areas under the pulmonary time-activity curve. The first area (A) is due to the initial passage of tracer through the lungs and the second area (B) is due to the premature recirculation of the tracer through the left to-right shunt. A ratio of A:A-B provides the Qp:Qs (Fig. 57.9). The normal value of Qp:Qs is 1.0. The γ-variate technique is accurate in the Qp:Qs range of 1.2 to 3.0. It is sometimes difficult to differentiate the absence of a left-to-right shunt from a very small one (Qp:Qs < 1.2). Shunts larger than Qp:Qs greater than 3.0 cannot be accurately calculated with this technique. However, the presence of a Qp:Qs greater than 3.0 signifies a shunt large enough to necessitate correction. Quantitation of left-to-right shunting with radionuclide angiography requires meticulous attention to detail with particular care to the injection technique, region-of-interest (ROI) selection, and curve fitting. The time-activity curve over the superior vena cava should demonstrate a single peak of duration of less than 3 seconds [full width at half maximum (FWHM)]. Fragmented or prolonged boluses are not acceptable because they may yield erroneous results. Deconvolution analysis, however, corrects for most bolus inadequacies and should be employed routinely (70, 71). Several investigators have published modifications of our method for the estimation of Qp:Qs from pulmonary time-activity curves (72–77).

A technique for evaluation of *right-to-left t shunts* uses ^{99m}Tc-macroaggregated albumin (MAA). After intravenous administration of radioactive particles in right-to-left shunting, the ratio of particles that enter the pulmonary and systemic circulations

equals the ratio of pulmonary-to-systemic blood flow. Tracer activity in the whole body is compared with that in the lungs (78,79). No adverse reactions have been reported from the intravenous administration of particles in patients with right-to-left shunting. Nevertheless, one is reminded that these particles produce systemic microembolization, including in the brain and the kidneys. In patients with right-to-left shunts, we empirically employ a small number of particles (<10,000) to reduce systemic embolization.

In right-to-left shunting, the first-pass radionuclide angiogram reveals rapid appearance of the tracer in the left atrium and/or the left ventricle and the aorta, which appears to occur at the same time or before the tracer reaches the lungs. The time-activity curve from a small ROI over the left ventricle reveals a first peak of activity, resulting from blood shunted from the right to the left side of the heart, which is followed by a second peak of activity resulting form the radioactive blood that has circulated through the lungs. Using an exponential extrapolation of the downslope following these peaks, shunt flow can be estimated as the ratio of the area under the first peak to the whole area under both peaks (80–82).

ASSESSMENT OF VENTRICULAR FUNCTION AND VALVULAR REGURGITATION

Clinical Applications

Two-dimensional echocardiography and cardiac catheterization are currently the most widely used techniques for the quantitative assessment of ventricular function (23,83–86). However, the ability of echocardiography to quantitate LV ejection fraction and load-independent measures of contractility is limited to patients with (a) two ventricles of normal size, (b) ventricles in the normal anatomic location, and (c) normal interventricular pressure relationships (84,87–89). In clinical practice, qualitative assessment of systemic ventricular function [of right ventricular (RV) or LV morphology] is usually sufficient for management decisions and clinical follow-up. Radionuclide ventriculography may be helpful in patients with more complex heart disease when quantitative measures of cardiac function are desired, and the clinician does not wish to pursue cardiac catheterization (90–95) (Fig. 57.10). There are a number of anatomic abnormalities (Table 57.5) in which the morphologic right ventricle is the systemic pumping chamber and, thus, it is connected to the aorta. These include d-TGA following atrial level (Mustard or Senning) repair in which the right ventricle is anterior and rightward, as well as the l-TGA ("congenitally corrected") in which the morphologic right ventricle is posterior and leftward. Standard echocardiographic estimates of ejection fraction are unreliable in these patients because of the shape and contraction pattern of the right ventricle (83,89,96). Radionuclide ventriculography is helpful in quantitating ventricular function in these patients (69,90,92,94,95). Fontan's palliation for

a variety of *single ventricle lesions* has been used with increasing frequency over the past two decades (97–99). Following this surgical repair, the venous return is directed (by direct anastomosis or conduit) into the pulmonary arteries, bypassing the heart. The single (right, left, or common) ventricular mass ejects oxygenated blood to the body. As with morphologic right ventricles, standard echocardiographic measurements are unreliable in this patient group for *quantitative* assessment of ventricular function. Radionuclide ventriculography may be valuable in the evaluation of these patients both preoperatively and postoperatively (99–101).

Radionuclide assessment of valvular heart disease has been used for quantitative evaluation of aortic and/or mitral regurgitation (102). In current clinical practice, however, this method has been largely replaced by two-dimensional and Doppler echocardiography, which allow a reliable assessment of the degree of valvular regurgitation and resultant cardiac chamber dilation.

Methods

Determination of Ventricular Ejection Fraction

Early studies in our laboratory have demonstrated a good correlation in the determination of ventricular function from first-pass

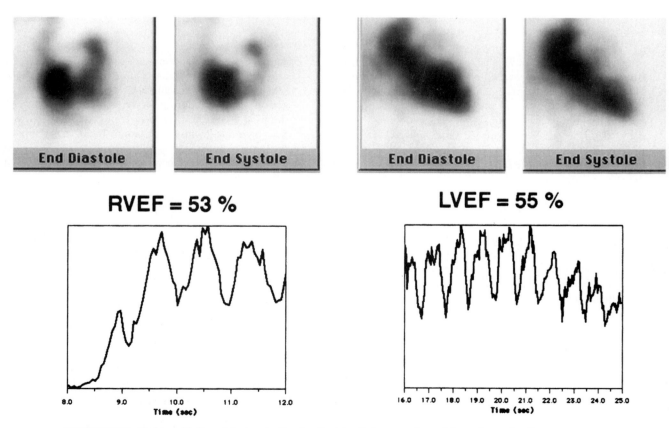

FIGURE 57.10. Right and left ventricular ejection fractions by first-pass radionuclide angiography. On the top are selected images depicting the right and left ventricular diastole and systole obtained in the right anterior oblique projection. Time-activity curves during the right and left ventricular phases of the angiogram are shown on the bottom. Right ventricular ejection fraction (*RVEF*) equals 53%; left ventricular ejection fraction (*LVEF*) equals 55%.

Table 57.5. *Uses of Radionuclide Angiography for Quantitative Assessment of Ventricular Function*

Ventricular morphology	Physiology	Location	Clinical examples
Right	Pulmonary ventricle	Anterior/rightward	Tetralogy of Fallot Truncus arteriosis Valvar pulmonary stenosis Cystic fibrosis
Right	Systemic ventricle	Anterior/rightward Posterior/leftward	D-TGA L-TGA
Left	Systemic ventricle	Posterior/leftward	Kawasaki disease After chemotherapy After transplantation After corrective cardiac surgery
Left	Pulmonary ventricle	Anterior/rightward	L-TGA
Variable	Pulmonary ventricle	Variable	After Fontan surgery

TGA, transposition of the great arteries.

radionuclide angiocardiography and biplane angiocardiography (103). In addition, normal values of RV and LV ejection fractions in children are available (Table 57.6) (104).

Gated Blood-Pool Angiography

Reports on the technique and application of gated blood-pool angiography have been extensively published. Gated blood-pool angiography requires synchronizing scintigraphic recording with an indicator of cardiac contraction such as the electrocardiogram, pulse wave tracing, or heart sounds (105,106). This technique permits repetitive sampling of a specific phase of the cardiac cycle from each of many cycles until an image of appropriate count density is recorded (Table 57.2). Either *in vivo* or *in vitro* methods may be used for ^{99m}Tc red blood cell (RBC) labeling (107). Generally, no patient preparation is needed for this study, but young children may require sedation for the 20 to 30 minutes that are necessary to acquire the data. The study is viewed in a cinematic mode to assess global cardiac function and chamber sizes and to detect abnormal wall motion. Analysis of the radionuclide ventriculogram can be performed manually or by several available automated methods. Global and regional ventricular ejection fraction, ejection rate, filling rate, and valvular regurgitation can be calculated (Fig. 57.10). Details regarding imaging agents, labeling techniques, acquisition parameters, and data analysis can be found elsewhere in this book.

Table 57.6. *Right and Left Ventricular Ejection Fractions in Children*

Age (years)	Patients	RVEF	Patients	LVEF
<1	5	0.54 ± 0.09	5	0.68 ± 0.13
1–5	12	0.53 ± 0.07	11	0.62 ± 0.09
6–10	16	0.52 ± 0.05	15	0.69 ± 0.08
11–15	19	0.54 ± 0.03	18	0.65 ± 0.09
16–20	22	0.53 ± 0.06	23	0.70 ± 0.08
Totals/M	**74**	**0.53 ± 0.06**	**72**	**0.68 ± 0.09**

RVEF, right ventricular ejection fraction; LVEF, left ventricular ejection fraction.

PULMONARY SCINTIGRAPHY FOR THE EVALUATION OF CONGENITAL AND ACQUIRED ANOMALIES OF THE HEART AND GREAT VESSELS

Clinical Applications

Pulmonary studies using radionuclides often complement the assessment of children with congenital cardiac disorders. At present, the most frequent indication for pulmonary scintigraphy with ^{99m}Tc-MAA at Children's Hospital-Boston is for the assessment of regional pulmonary blood flow (rPBF) in patients with congenital or acquired (surgically induced) abnormalities of pulmonary blood flow. The technique is rapid, safe, and easy to perform and provides useful information about the regional distribution of total pulmonary blood flow. Pulmonary scintigraphy is the only quantitative method of assessing the results of interventional procedures designed to relieve obstruction to pulmonary blood flow. Although echocardiography has assumed an increasingly prominent role in assessment of congenital anomalies of the heart, the distal pulmonary arteries remain inaccessible to investigation because of the overlying lungs. Pulmonary perfusion scintigraphy is, therefore, useful in the overall assessment of patients before and after catheter or surgical arterioplasty, intravascular stent placement, and coil occlusion of unwanted vascular communications (Fig. 57.11).

Peripheral Pulmonary Stenosis

Stenosis of the major branches of the pulmonary arterial tree can occur congenitally (especially in patients with tetralogy of Fallot and pulmonary atresia) or can be acquired following surgically created shunts (e.g., Blalock-Tausig or Waterston shunts). Asymmetric distribution of pulmonary blood flow can result in abnormal angiogenesis and alveologenesis and can lead to pulmonary hypertension in the contralateral lung without stenoses. Balloon angioplasty, with or without intravascular stent placement, has become the procedure of choice for the relief of these obstructions. Pulmonary perfusion scintigraphy is often used before and after these procedures to assess results.

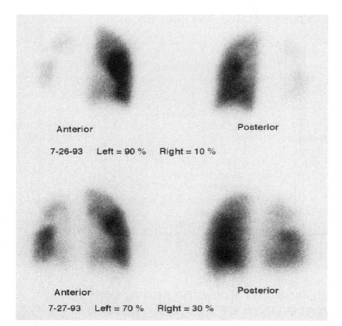

Anterior   Posterior

7-26-93   Left = 90 %   Right = 10 %

Anterior   Posterior

7-27-93   Left = 70 %   Right = 30 %

FIGURE 57.11. Regional pulmonary blood flow before and after balloon angioplasty. Ten-year-old boy born with tetralogy of Fallot had a complete surgical repair at age 2 years and had residual right pulmonary stenosis with asymmetric pulmonary flow. A precatheterization ^{99m}Tc-MAA pulmonary scintigram reveals only 10% of the total pulmonary blood flow to the right lung. Cardiac catheterization revealed proximal right pulmonary artery and severe right upper pulmonary artery stenosis. These stenoses were dilated and a postcatheterization study reveals an improvement of right pulmonary flow to 30% of the total.

Pulmonary Vein Stenosis

Obstruction to pulmonary venous outflow from the lungs can also lead to asymmetric pulmonary blood flow and pulmonary hypertension. Unilateral pulmonary vein stenosis may be associated with complex CHD; left pulmonary vein stenosis has been rarely reported in patients with TGA. Pulmonary vein stenosis may be difficult to detect echocardiographically and angiographically but may be identified by pulmonary scintigraphy by demonstrating regions of low perfusion in the lung in the absence of pulmonary artery stenoses.

Pulmonary Arteriovenous Malformations

Pulmonary arteriovenous malformations are congenital or acquired anomalies with direct connections between the pulmonary arteries and veins. Acquired arteriovenous malformations are typically associated with hepatic disease or systemic venous to pulmonary shunts (Glenn or Fontan procedures). The abnormalities are usually cavernomatous and cause physiologic right-to-left shunting and arterial desaturation. These lesions can be solitary, multiple, diffuse (telangiectatic), or mixed. More than 60% are solitary, and most occur in the lower lobes. In approximately one half of patients with pulmonary arteriovenous malformations, there is associated familial telangiectasis and hemangiomas of the skin and mucous membranes. Clinical symptoms are secondary to abnormal oxygenation related to the right-to-

left shunt (cyanosis, dyspnea, hemoptysis, epistaxis, and exercise intolerance) and secondary embolic pneumonia. Physical examination of patients with pulmonary arteriovenous malformations reveals conjunctival hemorrhages, digital clubbing, or murmur. Polycythemia or cerebrovascular accidents may occur. Radiographs of the chest show single or multiple lesions with linear, vascular shadows. Pulmonary angiography is diagnostic. Detection with radionuclide angiography depends on the size and location of the lesion. The appearance on radionuclide angiography is that of a distinct and localized "blush" of tracer activity within a lung field immediately after appearance of tracer in the right side of the heart.

Surgery and Changes in Regional Pulmonary Blood Flow

In patients with a single ventricle, the staged surgical repair connects the systemic venous return to the pulmonary arteries and provides more effective pulmonary blood flow. In the classic Glenn shunt, the superior vena cava is directly connected to the right pulmonary artery, with ligation of the connection between the cardiac end of the superior vena cava and the right atrium and division of the connection between the right pulmonary artery and the main pulmonary artery. This shunt results in all the systemic venous return from the head, neck, and arms entering the right lung. However, the "bidirectional" Glenn shunt does not result in pulmonary vascular discontinuity; injection into the upper extremity veins in these patients will accurately reflect the distribution of pulmonary blood flow. In patients who have had a classic Glenn shunt, injection of ^{99m}Tc-MAA into a vein of the upper body will concentrate nearly entirely in the right lung, thereby making calculations of asymmetric pulmonary veins blood flow difficult or impossible. If the injection is made in the lower extremity, most of the tracer will enter the left lung, and a larger right-to-left shunt will be detected. It is, therefore, extremely important that the precise surgical anatomy of these patients be determined for proper interpretations of results.

Methods

Of the available techniques for the assessment of regional pulmonary function, perfusion scintigraphy using ^{99m}Tc-MAA is the technique most frequently used. Table 57.7 lists the available

Table 57.7. *Method for Radionuclide Assessment of the Pulmonary System in Children*

Assessment	Radiopharmaceuticals
Regional pulmonary flow	^{99m}Tc-MAA, ^{133}Xe in saline
Regional ventilation	^{133}Xe gas, ^{81m}Kr gas, Technegas
Fluid transport	Aerosolized ^{99m}Tc-DTPA
Mucociliary clearance	Aerosolized ^{99m}Tc-sulfur colloid
Aspiration	Oral ^{99m}Tc-sulfur colloid
Parenchymal diseases	^{67}GA, ^{201}Tl, ^{99m}Tc-MIBI, ^{123}I, or ^{131}I

DTPA, diethylene triamine pentaacetic acid; MAA, macroaggregated albumin; MIBI, sestmibi.

Table 57.8. *Indications for Pulmonary Scintigraphy in Children*

Cystic fibrosis	Arteriovenous malformation
Pneumonia, inflammation, infection	HIV-related pathology
Cyanosis	Pectus excavatum
Lobar emphysema	Pulmonary sequestration
Assessment of pulmonary artery angioplasty or surgery	Sarcoidosis
Congenital diaphragmatic hernia and repair	Evaluation of pulmonary transplants
Bronchopulmonary dysplasia	Effects of irradiation
Foreign body	
Aspiration	
Asthma	
Pulmonary hypoplasia, stenosis, aplasia, agenesis	
Pulmonary sequestration	
Pulmonary embolism	
Pulmonary valve stenosis	

HIV, human immunodeficiency virus.

radionuclide methods for the assessment of the pulmonary system in children. Indications for pulmonary scintigraphy in pediatric patients are listed in Table 57.8. Abnormalities of pulmonary artery blood flow and distribution are extremely common in complex CHD. A number of complex lesions require the combined surgical and catheter intervention approaches (108–113).

Radiopharmaceuticals

After intravenous injection, ^{99m}Tc-MAA particles temporarily embolize arterioles in the lungs in a distribution proportional to regional arterial pulmonary blood flow. The number of arterioles occluded with one typical intravenous injection of ^{99m}Tc-MAA is relatively small and without physiologic significance. Once lodged in the pulmonary arterioles, the ^{99m}Tc-MAA particles are degraded into smaller particles and polypeptides, which are taken up by the liver and eliminated in the bile. The biologic half-life of ^{99m}Tc-MAA in the lungs is 6 to 8 hours. The minimum toxic dose for albumin is 20 mg/kg, which exceeds the usual adult imaging dose of less than 10 μg of albumin by a factor of 1,000 (78,100). In newborns and young children whose pulmonary vasculature is immature, a small number of particles should be used. In the human infant, the number of alveoli increases rapidly during the first year of life and gradually reaches adult levels at approximately 8 years of age (78,101,114). Although the precise age at which alveolar multiplication ceases is

not known with certainty, one study shows a rapid increase from approximately one tenth to one third of adult values during the first year of life and to one half the adult number by 3 years of age. The number of injected particles should not exceed 50,000 in the newborn or 165,000 at 1 year of age. We recommend that a small number of particles (<10,000) be used in neonates and patients with severe pulmonary disease. For quantitation of right-to-left shunting, a small number of particles (i.e., <10,000) are sufficient. Table 57.9 lists the suggested number of injected particles and usual administered doses for patients at various ages. SPECT can be performed in about the same time as planar imaging and offers obvious advantages.

VENOGRAPHY AND ASSESSMENT OF CENTRAL VENOUS LINES

Clinical Applications

Radionuclide venography employs very small volumes of material and can be performed using simple intravenous needles. Radionuclide venography is a very sensitive, rapid, safe, and effective technique. Radionuclide venography can be used to evaluate venous drainage in patients that have had multiple central venous lines to determine venous patency and to help decide a site for the placement of a new line. Also, this technique is indicated to evaluate venous drainage in patients with suspected superior vena cava syndrome. A left-hand injection can detect a left superior vena cava, which is common in certain complex CHD and may not be visible on the transthoracic echocardiogram.

Methods

Radiopharmaceuticals and Imaging

^{99m}Tc-pertechnetate is commonly used, although other radiopharmaceuticals including ^{99m}Tc-DTPA and ^{99m}Tc-MAG3, which have a more rapid blood disappearance rate, can be used as well. When evaluating venous drainage from a single extremity, the imaging method is very simple. Once venous access has been gained as described earlier, the gamma-camera equipped with a high-resolution collimator is positioned anteriorly over the patient covering an area including the injection site, the extremity, and the heart. The tracer is injected as a bolus as described earlier. The venogram is recorded beginning at the time of injection at a rate of two frames per second for 60 seconds on a 64 × 64 or 128 × 128 matrix. Recommended administered dose for a single study is 0.03 mCi (11.1 MBq)/

Table 57.9. *Usual Administered Doses of ^{99m}Tc-MAA*

	Newborn	1 yr	5 yrs	10 yrs	15 yrs	Adult
Body weight (kg)	3.5	12.1	20.3	33.5	55.0	70.0
Administered dose (mCi)	0.2	0.5	1.0	1.5	2.5	3.0
Range of particles administered (×100)	10–50	50–150	200–300	200–300	200–700	200–700

MAA, macroaggregated albumin.

Table 57.10. *Recommended Administered Doses for Three Sequential Doses for Radionuclide Venography*

First injection	0.03 mCi [11.1 MBq]/kg, minimum 1 mCi [37 MBq], maximum 2 mCi [74 MBq]
Second injection	0.06 mCi [22.2 MBq]/kg, minimum 2 mCi [74 MBq], maximum 4 mCi [148 MBq]
Third injection	0.12 mCi [44.4 MBq]/kg, minimum 4 mCi [148 MBq], maximum 8 mCi [296 MBq]

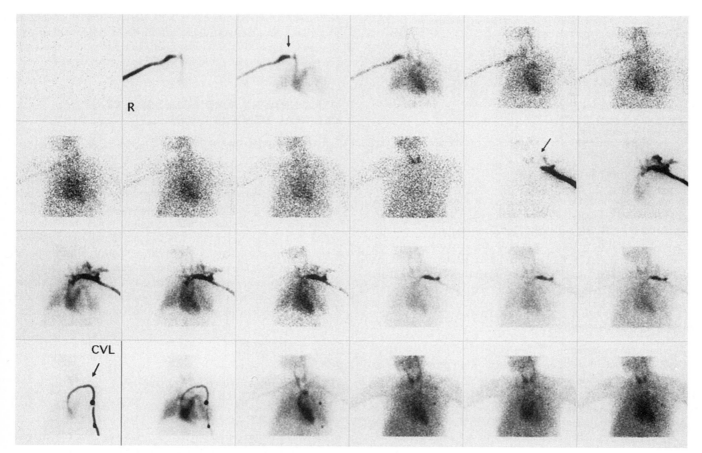

FIGURE 57.12. Radionuclide venography and assessment of central venous line. Study done in a young patient who had several previous central venous lines with a question of patency of his current left central line (*CVL*). Three sequential injections of ^{99m}Tc-pertechnetate. The first injection done in a right antecubital vein (*R*) reveals tracer flowing into the superior vena cava and the right side of the heart. There is some delay in flow into the thoracic inlet but no obstruction. The second injection in a left antecubital vein reveals a significant obstruction to venous flow. Tracer reaches the right heart by a combination of innominate vein and by collateral venous circulation. The third injection into the central venous line reveals rapid flow into the right side of the heart.

kg, with a minimum of 1 mCi (37 MBq) and a maximum of 2 mCi (74 MBq). Patients with central venous lines are best evaluated using three injections: one in the right arm, one in the left arm, and one in the central line (Table 57.10). Clotting and other complications may occur in the proximal veins and not in the central venous line. Three sequential recording phases, each at a rate of two frames per second for 60 seconds, are preset. First, the arms are injected in sequence (right, then left, or vice versa), and the central line is injected last. Once the venogram is completed, it is evaluated by viewing it on cinematic mode on the computer monitor (Fig. 57.12).

ACKNOWLEDGMENT

We are indebted to Nancy Ralph and Elisa Ortiz for their invaluable help in the preparation of this manuscript.

REFERENCES

1. Report of the New England Regional Infant Cardiac Program. *Pediatrics* 1980;65:375–461.
2. Castaneda AR, Mayer JE Jr, Jonas RA et al. The neonate with critical

congenital heart disease: repair—a surgical challenge. *J Thorac Cardiovasc Surg* 1989;98:869–875.

3. Davis JA, Cecchin F, Jones TK et al. Major coronary artery anomalies in a pediatric population: incidence and clinical importance. *J Am Coll Cardiol* 2001;37:593–597.

4. Taylor AJ, Rogan KM, Virmani R. Sudden cardiac death associated with isolated congenital coronary artery anomalies. *J Am Coll Cardiol* 1992;20:640–647.

5. Dajani AS, Taubert KA, Takahashi M et al. Guidelines for long-term management of patients with Kawasaki disease. Report from the Committee on Rheumatic Fever, Endocarditis, and Kawasaki Disease, Council on Cardiovascular Disease in the Young, American Heart Association. *Circulation* 1994;89:916–922.

6. Kondo C, Hiroe M, Nakanishi T et al. Detection of coronary artery stenosis in children with Kawasaki disease. Usefulness of pharmacologic stress 201Tl myocardial tomography. *Circulation* 1989;80:615–624.

7. Kondo C, Nakanishi T, Sonobe T et al. Scintigraphic monitoring of coronary artery occlusion due to Kawasaki disease. *Am J Cardiol* 1993;71:681–685.

8. Nakanishi T, Takao A, Kondoh C et al. ECG findings after myocardial infarction in children after Kawasaki disease. *Am Heart J* 1988;116:1028–1033.

9. Tatara K, Kusakawa S, Itoh K et al. Collateral circulation in Kawasaki disease with coronary occlusion or severe stenosis. *Am Heart J* 1991;121:797–802.

10. Paridon SM, Galioto FM, Vincent JA et al. Exercise capacity and incidence of myocardial perfusion defects after Kawasaki disease in children and adolescents. *J Am Coll Cardiol* 1995;25:1420–1424.

11. Muzik O, Paridon SM, Singh TP et al. Quantification of myocardial blood flow and flow reserve in children with a history of Kawasaki disease and normal coronary arteries using positron emission tomography. *J Am Coll Cardiol* 1996;28:757–762.

12. Suzuki A, Miyagawa-Tomita S, Komatsu K et al. Active remodeling of the coronary arterial lesions in the late phase of Kawasaki disease: immunohistochemical study. *Circulation* 2000;101:2935–2941.

13. Dhillon R, Clarkson P, Donald AE et al. Endothelial dysfunction late after Kawasaki disease. *Circulation* 1996;94:2103–2106.

14. Castaneda AR, Mayer JE Jr, Jonas RA et al. Transposition of the great arteries: the arterial switch operation. *Cardiol Clin* 1989;7:369–376.

15. Arensman FW, Sievers HH, Lange P et al. Assessment of coronary and aortic anastomoses after anatomic correction of transposition of the great arteries. *J Thorac Cardiovasc Surg* 1985;90:597–604.

16. Day RW, Laks H, Drinkwater DC. The influence of coronary anatomy on the arterial switch operation in neonates. *J Thorac Cardiovasc Surg* 1992;104:706–712.

17. Goor DA, Shem-Tov A, Neufeld HN. Impeded coronary flow in anatomic correction of transposition of the great arteries: prevention, detection, and management. *J Thorac Cardiovasc Surg* 1982;83:747–754.

18. Tsuda E, Imakita M, Yagihara T et al. Late death after arterial switch operation for transposition of the great arteries. *Am Heart J* 1992;124:1551–1557.

19. Vogel M, Smallhorn JF, Gilday D et al. Assessment of myocardial perfusion in patients after the arterial switch operation. *J Nucl Med* 1991;32:237–241.

20. Weindling SN, Wernovsky G, Colan SD et al. Myocardial perfusion, function and exercise tolerance after the arterial switch operation. *J Am Coll Cardiol* 1994;23:424–433.

21. Bengel FM, Hauser M, Duvernoy CS et al. Myocardial blood flow and coronary flow reserve late after anatomical correction of transposition of the great arteries. *J Am Coll Cardiol* 1998;32:1955–1961.

22. Rickers C, Sasse K, Buchert R et al. Myocardial viability assessed by positron emission tomography in infants and children after the arterial switch operation and suspected infarction. *J Am Coll Cardiol* 2000;36:1676–1683.

23. Rein AJ, Colan SD, Parness IA et al. Regional and global left ventricular function in infants with anomalous origin of the left coronary artery from the pulmonary trunk: preoperative and postoperative assessment. *Circulation* 1987;75:115–123.

24. Sauer U, Stern H, Meisner H et al. Risk factors for perioperative mortality in children with anomalous origin of the left coronary artery from the pulmonary artery. *J Thorac Cardiovasc Surg* 1992;104:696–705.

25. Bunton R, Jonas RA, Lang P et al. Anomalous origin of left coronary artery from pulmonary artery. Ligation versus establishment of a two coronary artery system. *J Thorac Cardiovasc Surg* 1987;93:103–108.

26. Vouhe PR, Tamisier D, Sidi D et al. Anomalous left coronary artery from the pulmonary artery: results of isolated aortic reimplantation. *Ann Thorac Surg* 1992;54:621–626; discussion 627.

27. Hurwitz RA, Caldwell RL, Girod DA et al. Clinical and hemodynamic course of infants and children with anomalous left coronary artery. *Am Heart J* 1989;118:1176–1181.

28. Singh TP, Di Carli MF, Sullivan NM et al. Myocardial flow reserve in long-term survivors of repair of anomalous left coronary artery from pulmonary artery. *J Am Coll Cardiol* 1998;31:437–443.

29. Boucek MM, Faro A, Novick RJ et al. The Registry of the International Society for Heart and Lung Transplantation: Fourth Official Pediatric Report—2000. *J Heart Lung Transplant* 2001;20:39–52.

30. Hosenpud JD, Novick RJ, Bennett LE et al. The Registry of the International Society for Heart and Lung Transplantation: thirteenth official report—1996. *J Heart Lung Transplant* 1996;15:655–674.

31. Shaddy RE, Naftel DC, Kirklin JK et al. Outcome of cardiac transplantation in children. Survival in a contemporary multi-institutional experience. Pediatric Heart Transplant Study. *Circulation* 1996;94:II69–73.

32. Boucek MM, Mathis CM, Boucek RJ Jr et al. Prospective evaluation of echocardiography for primary rejection surveillance after infant heart transplantation: comparison with endomyocardial biopsy. *J Heart Lung Transplant* 1994;13:66–73.

33. Boucek MM, Mathis CM, Kanakriyeh MS et al. Serial echocardiographic evaluation of cardiac graft rejection after infant heart transplantation. *J Heart Lung Transplant* 1993;12:824–831.

34. Santos-Ocampo SD, Sekarski TJ, Saffitz JE et al. Echocardiographic characteristics of biopsy-proven cellular rejection in infant heart transplant recipients. *J Heart Lung Transplant* 1996;15:25–34.

35. Mannaerts HF, Balk AH, Simoons ML et al. Changes in left ventricular function and wall thickness in heart transplant recipients and their relation to acute rejection: an assessment by digitised M mode echocardiography. *Br Heart J* 1992;68:356–364.

36. Donofrio MT, Clark BJ, Ramaciotti C et al. Regional wall motion and strain of transplanted hearts in pediatric patients using magnetic resonance tagging. *Am J Physiol* 1999;277:R1481–1487.

37. Follansbee WP, Kiernan JM, Curtiss EI et al. Changes in left ventricular systolic function that accompany rejection of the transplanted heart: a serial radionuclide assessment of fifty-three consecutive cases. *Am Heart J* 1991;121:548–556.

38. Valette H, Bourguignon MH, Desruennes M et al. Ventricular function during the acute rejection of heterotopic transplanted heart: gated blood-pool studies. *Eur J Nucl Med* 1991;18:879–884.

39. Aparici CM, Narula J, Puig M et al. Somatostatin receptor scintigraphy predicts impending cardiac allograft rejection before endomyocardial biopsy. *Eur J Nucl Med* 2000;27:1754–1759.

40. Virgolini I, Traub T, Novotny C et al. New trends in peptide receptor radioligands. *J Nucl Med Allied Sci* 2001;45:153–159.

41. Vriens PW, Blankenberg FG, Stoot JH et al. The use of technetium Tc 99m annexin V for in vivo imaging of apoptosis during cardiac allograft rejection. *J Thorac Cardiovasc Surg* 1998;116:844–853.

42. Blankenberg FG, Strauss HW. Non-invasive diagnosis of acute heart- or lung-transplant rejection using radiolabeled annexin V. *Pediatr Radiol* 1999;29:299–305.

43. Chan SY, Kobashigawa J, Stevenson LW et al. Myocardial blood flow at rest and during pharmacological vasodilation in cardiac transplants during and after successful treatment of rejection. *Circulation* 1994;90:204–212.

44. Rechavia E, Araujo LI, De Silva R et al. Dipyridamole vasodilator response after human orthotopic heart transplantation: quantification by oxygen-15-labeled water and positron emission tomography. *J Am Coll Cardiol* 1992;19:100–106.

45. Billingham ME. Histopathology of graft coronary disease. *J Heart Lung Transplant* 1992;11:S38–44.
46. Mulla NF, Johnston JK, Vander Dussen L et al. Late rejection is a predictor of transplant coronary artery disease in children. *J Am Coll Cardiol* 2001;37:243–250.
47. McGiffin DC, Savunen T, Kirklin JK et al. Cardiac transplant coronary artery disease. A multivariable analysis of pretransplantation risk factors for disease development and morbid events. *J Thorac Cardiovasc Surg* 1995;109:1081–1088; discussion 1088–1089.
48. Ventura HO, Mehra MR, Smart FW et al. Cardiac allograft vasculopathy: current concepts. *Am Heart J* 1995;129:791–799.
49. Kuhn MA, Jutzy KR, Deming DD et al. The medium-term findings in coronary arteries by intravascular ultrasound in infants and children after heart transplantation. *J Am Coll Cardiol* 2000;36:250–254.
50. Jamieson SW. Investigation of heart transplant coronary atherosclerosis. *Circulation* 1992;85:1211–1213.
51. Fang JC, Rocco T, Jarcho J et al. Noninvasive assessment of transplant-associated arteriosclerosis. *Am Heart J* 1998;135:980–987.
52. Derumeaux G, Redonnet M, Mouton-Schleifer D et al. Dobutamine stress echocardiography in orthotopic heart transplant recipients. VA-COMED Research Group. *J Am Coll Cardiol* 1995;25:1665–1672.
53. Bacal F, Stolf NA, Veiga VC et al. Noninvasive diagnosis of allograft vascular disease after heart transplantation. *Arq Bras Cardiol* 2001;76:29–42.
54. Carlsen J, Toft JC, Mortensen SA et al. Myocardial perfusion scintigraphy as a screening method for significant coronary artery stenosis in cardiac transplant recipients. *J Heart Lung Transplant* 2000;19:873–878.
55. Puskas C, Kosch M, Kerber S et al. Progressive heterogeneity of myocardial perfusion in heart transplant recipients detected by thallium-201 myocardial SPECT. *J Nucl Med* 1997;38:760–765.
56. Rodney RA, Johnson LL, Blood DK et al. Myocardial perfusion scintigraphy in heart transplant recipients with and without allograft atherosclerosis: a comparison of thallium-201 and technetium 99m sestamibi. *J Heart Lung Transplant* 1994;13:173–180.
57. Verhoeven PP, Lee FA, Ramahi TM et al. Prognostic value of noninvasive testing one year after orthotopic cardiac transplantation. *J Am Coll Cardiol* 1996;28:183–189.
58. Franken PR, Dobbeleir AA, Ham HR et al. Clinical usefulness of ultrashort-lived iridium-191m from a carbon-based generator system for the evaluation of the left ventricular function. *J Nucl Med* 1989;30:1025–1031.
59. Heller GV, Treves ST, Parker JA et al. Comparison of ultrashort-lived iridium-191m with technetium-99m for first pass radionuclide angiocardiographic evaluation of right and left ventricular function in adults. *J Am Coll Cardiol* 1986;7:1295–1302.
60. Hellman C, Zafrir N, Shimoni A et al. Evaluation of ventricular function with first-pass iridium-191m radionuclide angiocardiography. *J Nucl Med* 1989;30:450–457.
61. Kipper SL, Ashburn WL, Norris SL et al. Gold-195m first-pass radionuclide ventriculography, thallium-201 single-photon emission CT, and 12-lead ECG stress testing as a combined procedure. *Radiology* 1985;156:817–821.
62. Lacy JL, Layne WW, Guidry GW et al. Development and clinical performance of an automated, portable tungsten-178/tantalum-178 generator. *J Nucl Med* 1991;32:2158–2161.
63. Lahiri A, Zanelli GD, O'Hara MJ et al. Simultaneous measurement of left ventricular function and myocardial perfusion during a single exercise test: dual isotope imaging with gold-195m and thallium-201. *Eur Heart J* 1986;7:493–500.
64. Treves S, Cheng C, Samuel A et al. Iridium-191 angiocardiography for the detection and quantitation of left-to-right shunting. *J Nucl Med* 1980;21:1151–1157.
65. Treves S, Fyler D, Fujii A et al. Low radiation iridium 191m radionuclide angiography: detection and quantitation of left-to-right shunts in infants. *J Pediatr* 1982;101:210–213.
66. Maltz DL, Treves S. Quantitative radionuclide angiocardiography: determination of Qp:Qs in children. *Circulation* 1973;47:1049–1056.
67. Askenazi J, Ahnberg DS, Korngold E et al. Quantitative radionuclide angiocardiography: detection and quantitation of left to right shunts. *Am J Cardiol* 1976;37:382–387.
68. Kuruc A, Treves S, Smith W et al. An automated algorithm for radionuclide angiocardiographic quantitation of circulatory shunting. *Comput Biomed Res* 1984;17:481–493.
69. Treves ST, Newberger J, Hurwitz R. Radionuclide angiocardiography in children. *J Am Coll Cardiol* 1985;5:120S–127S.
70. Ham HR, Dobbeleir A, Virat P et al. Radionuclide quantitation of left-to right cardiac shunts using deconvolution analysis: concise communication. *J Nucl Med* 1981;22:688–692.
71. Kuruc A, Treves S, Parker JA et al. Radionuclide angiocardiography: an improved deconvolution technique for improvement after suboptimal bolus injection. *Radiology* 1983;148:233–238.
72. Bourguignon MH, Links JM, Douglass KH et al. Quantification of left to right cardiac shunts by multiple deconvolution analysis. *Am J Cardiol* 1981;48:1086–1090.
73. Kveder M, Bajzer Z, Nosil J. A mathematical model for the quantitative study of left to right cardiac shunt. *Phys Med Biol* 1985;30:207–215.
74. Kveder M, Bajzer Z, Zadro M. Theoretical aspects of multiple deconvolution analysis for quantification of left to right cardiac shunts. *Phys Med Biol* 1987;32:1237–1243.
75. Madsen MT, Argenyi E, Preslar J et al. An improved method for the quantification of left-to-right shunts. *J Nucl Med* 1991;32:1808–1812.
76. Nakamura M, Suzuki Y, Nagasawa T et al. Detection and quantitation of left-to-right shunts from radionuclide angiocardiography using the homomorphic deconvolution technique. *IEEE Trans Biomed Eng* 1982;29:192–201.
77. Parker JA, Treves S. Radionuclide detection, localization, and quantitation of intracardiac shunts and shunts between the great arteries. *Prog Cardiovasc Dis* 1977;20:121–150.
78. Gates GF, Orme HW, Dore EK. Measurement of cardiac shunting with technetium-labeled albumin aggregates. *J Nucl Med* 1971;12:746–749.
79. Lin CY. Lung scan in cardiopulmonary disease. I. Tetralogy of Fallot. *J Thorac Cardiovasc Surg* 1971;61:370–379.
80. Riihimaki E, Heiskanen A, Tahti E. Theory of quantitative determination of intracardiac shunts by external detection. *Ann Clin Res* 1974;6:45–49.
81. Treves S. Detection and quantitation of cardiovascular shunts with commonly available radionuclides. *Semin Nucl Med* 1980;10:16–26.
82. Weber PM, Dos Remedios LV, Jasko IA. Quantitative radioisotopic angiocardiography. *J Nucl Med* 1972;13:815–822.
83. Borow KM, Keane JF, Castaneda AR et al. Systemic ventricular function in patients with tetralogy of Fallot, ventricular septal defect and transposition of the great arteries repaired during infancy. *Circulation* 1981;64:878–885.
84. Colan SD, Borow KM, Neumann A. Left ventricular end-systolic wall stress-velocity of fiber shortening relation: a load-independent index of myocardial contractility. *J Am Coll Cardiol* 1984;4:715–724.
85. Graham TP Jr, Jarmakani JM, Canent RV Jr et al. Left heart volume estimation in infancy and childhood. Reevaluation of methodology and normal values. *Circulation* 1971;43:895–904.
86. Sluysmans T, Sanders SP, van der Velde M et al. Natural history and patterns of recovery of contractile function in single left ventricle after Fontan operation. *Circulation* 1992;86:1753–1761.
87. Agata Y, Hiraishi S, Misawa H et al. Two-dimensional echocardiographic determinants of interventricular septal configurations in right or left ventricular overload. *Am Heart J* 1985;110:819–825.
88. Louie EK, Rich S, Brundage BH. Doppler echocardiographic assessment of impaired left ventricular filling in patients with right ventricular pressure overload due to primary pulmonary hypertension. *J Am Coll Cardiol* 1986;8:1298–1306.
89. Sholler GF, Colan SD, Sanders SP. Effect of isolated right ventricular outflow obstruction on left ventricular function in infants. *Am J Cardiol* 1988;62:778–784.
90. Baker EJ, Shubao C, Clarke SE et al. Radionuclide measurement of right ventricular function in atrial septal defect, ventricular septal

defect and complete transposition of the great arteries. *Am J Cardiol* 1986;57:1142–1146.

91. del Torso S, Milanesi O, Bui F et al. Radionuclide evaluation of lung perfusion after the Fontan procedure. *Int J Cardiol* 1988;20:107–116.
92. Hurwitz RA, Caldwell RL, Girod DA et al. Ventricular function in transposition of the great arteries: evaluation by radionuclide angiocardiography. *Am Heart J* 1985;110:600–605.
93. Hurwitz RA, Siddiqui A, Caldwell RL et al. Assessment of ventricular function in infants and children. Response to dobutamine infusion. *Clin Nucl Med* 1990;15:556–559.
94. Parrish MD, Graham TP Jr, Bender HW et al. Radionuclide angiographic evaluation of right and left ventricular function during exercise after repair of transposition of the great arteries. Comparison with normal subjects and patients with congenitally corrected transposition. *Circulation* 1983;67:178–183.
95. Rees S, Somerville J, Warnes C et al. Comparison of magnetic resonance imaging with echocardiography and radionuclide angiography in assessing cardiac function and anatomy following Mustard's operation for transposition of the great arteries. *Am J Cardiol* 1988;61:1316–1322.
96. Trowitzsch E, Colan SD, Sanders SP. Two-dimensional echocardiographic estimation of right ventricular area change and ejection fraction in infants with systemic right ventricle (transposition of the great arteries or hypoplastic left heart syndrome). *Am J Cardiol* 1985;55:1153–1157.
97. de Leval MR, Kilner P, Gewillig M et al. Total cavopulmonary connection: a logical alternative to atriopulmonary connection for complex Fontan operations. Experimental studies and early clinical experience. *J Thorac Cardiovasc Surg* 1988;96:682–695.
98. Fontan F, Kirklin JW, Fernandez G et al. Outcome after a "perfect" Fontan operation. *Circulation* 1990;81:1520–1536.
99. Parikh SR, Hurwitz RA, Caldwell RL et al. Ventricular function in the single ventricle before and after Fontan surgery. *Am J Cardiol* 1991;67:1390–1395.
100. Akagi T, Benson LN, Gilday DL et al. Influence of ventricular morphology on diastolic filling performance in double-inlet ventricle after the Fontan procedure. *J Am Coll Cardiol* 1993;22:1948–1952.
101. Akagi T, Benson LN, Green M et al. Ventricular performance before and after Fontan repair for univentricular atrioventricular connection:

angiographic and radionuclide assessment. *J Am Coll Cardiol* 1992;20:920–926.
102. Hurwitz RA, Treves S, Freed M et al. Quantitation of aortic and mitral regurgitation in the pediatric population: evaluation by radionuclide angiocardiography. *Am J Cardiol* 1983;51:252–255.
103. Kurtz D, Ahnberg DS, Freed M et al. Quantitative radionuclide angiocardiography. Determination of left ventricular ejection fraction in children. *Br Heart J* 1976;38:966–973.
104. Hurwitz RA, Treves S, Kuruc A. Right ventricular and left ventricular ejection fraction in pediatric patients with normal hearts: first-pass radionuclide angiocardiography. *Am Heart J* 1984;107:726–732.
105. Berman DS, Salel AF, DeNardo GL et al. Clinical assessment of left ventricular regional contraction patterns and ejection fraction by high-resolution gated scintigraphy. *J Nucl Med* 1975;16:865–874.
106. Strauss HW, Zaret BL, Hurley PJ et al. A scintiphotographic method for measuring left ventricular ejection fraction in man without cardiac catheterization. *Am J Cardiol* 1971;28:575–580.
107. Hegge FN, Hamilton GW, Larson SM et al. Cardiac chamber imaging: a comparison of red blood cells labeled with Tc-99m in vitro and in vivo. *J Nucl Med* 1978;19:129–134.
108. Driscoll DJ, Hesslein PS, Mullins CE. Congenital stenosis of individual pulmonary veins: clinical spectrum and unsuccessful treatment by transvenous balloon dilation. *Am J Cardiol* 1982;49:1767–1772.
109. Gentles TL, Lock JE, Perry SB. High pressure balloon angioplasty for branch pulmonary artery stenosis: early experience. *J Am Coll Cardiol* 1993;22:867–872.
110. O'Laughlin MP, Perry SB, Lock JE et al. Use of endovascular stents in congenital heart disease. *Circulation* 1991;83:1923–1939.
111. O'Laughlin MP, Slack MC, Grifka RG et al. Implantation and intermediate-term follow-up of stents in congenital heart disease. *Circulation* 1993;88:605–614.
112. Rothman A, Perry SB, Keane JF et al. Balloon dilation of branch pulmonary artery stenosis. *Semin Thorac Cardiovasc Surg* 1990;2:46–54.
113. Rothman A, Perry SB, Keane JF et al. Early results and follow-up of balloon angioplasty for branch pulmonary artery stenoses. *J Am Coll Cardiol* 1990;15:1109–1117.
114. Heyman S. Toxicity and safety factors associated with lung perfusion studies with radiolabeled particles. *J Nucl Med* 1979;20:1098–1099.

58

PEDIATRIC BRAIN IMAGING

MICHAEL J. GELFAND
DOMINIQUE DELBEKE
SANDRA K. LAWRENCE

TECHNICAL ASPECTS OF PEDIATRIC BRAIN IMAGING

The techniques used in brain imaging must be tailored to the needs of pediatric patients. Radiopharmaceutical doses are adjusted for the child's weight or body surface area. High-quality images, especially those obtained in tomographic formats, are obtained when the infant or child remains motionless throughout the time during which the patient is being imaged.

Radiopharmaceutical Dose

There are two widely used approaches in the determination of appropriate radiopharmaceutical dose in children. In both cases, the standard adult radiopharmaceutical dosage is reduced in proportion to the child's size. In the first case, the child's body surface area is determined from a standard nomogram, and the child's dose is calculated according to the equation

$$Child's\ dosage\ (mCi) = \frac{adult\ dosage\ (mCi) \cdot child's\ body\ surface\ area\ (sq\ m)}{1.73\ sq\ m}$$

Alternatively, the child's weight is used to determine the dose by the equation

$$Child's\ dosage\ (mCi) + \frac{adult\ dosage\ (mCi)\ -\ child's\ weight\ (kg)}{70\ kg}$$

When the body surface area-adjusted method is used, children will receive somewhat larger administered activities and the absorbed radiation dose will be somewhat higher than when the weight-adjusted method is used.

Radiopharmaceuticals used for brain imaging are listed in

M.J. Gelfand: Children's Hospital Medical Center of Cincinnati, Chief, Section of Nuclear Medicine, Cincinnati, OH.

D. Delbeke: Radiology and Radiological Sciences, Vanderbilt University Medical Center, Nashville, TN.

S.K. Lawrence: Department of Radiology and Radiological Sciences, Vanderbilt University Medical Center, Nashville, TN.

Table 58.1. Radiopharmaceutical selection is addressed as each clinical indication is discussed in the text. The administered activities of the ^{99m}Tc-labeled radiopharmaceuticals are large enough to permit the acquisition of first-transit flow images, but flow images are usually acquired only for blood–brain barrier leak studies and brain death studies.

Timing of Radiopharmaceutical Injection and Image Acquisition

Because regional brain metabolism and blood flow are affected by the sensory environment surrounding the patient and by the patient's motor activity at and shortly after the time of injection, one must plan the circumstances under which a child, especially an uncooperative child, is to be imaged. First, a secure intravenous line is established in the child. Then, the infant or child is allowed to regain his or her composure and rest quietly in a semidark room with low level "white noise" in the background. Without disturbing the child, the radiopharmaceutical is injected into the intravenous line, and the child continues to rest quietly until the radiopharmaceutical has localized in the brain. Finally, infants and small or uncooperative children are sedated, usually with an intravenously administered drug. Once the sedated child is asleep, monitoring equipment is attached and the child is positioned for imaging.

Positioning

Flexion of the neck may occlude the airway in an infant; therefore, care should be taken in positioning to ensure that an adequate airway is maintained at all times. If the result of less than optimal positioning is a set of tomographic sections that are oblique to or rotated from their optimal orientation, software designed for reorientation of axes of the heart can be used to eliminate any "pitch, roll, and yaw" and recreate a perfectly positioned study. Fiduciary markers may aid in reorientation of tomographic sections and permit registration fusion of the emission tomographic sections with images obtained from other modalities such as magnetic resonance imaging (MRI).

Sedation and Monitoring

Sedation must be done with caution and skill, or any of several adverse outcomes are possible. If the child is inadequately se-

Table 58.1. *Administered Activities and Imaging Times for Brain Imaging Radiopharmaceuticals in Children*

Radiopharmaceutical	Administered activity (mCi/kg)	Planar static or tomographic imaging time after injection
Blood-brain-barrier integrity		
^{99m}Tc-pertechnetate	0.285	2.0 hr
^{99m}Tc-gluceptate	0.285	1.5 hr
Regional cerebral blood flow (rCBF$_{glc}$)		
^{99m}Tc-HMPAO	0.285	1.0 hr[a]
^{123}I-iofetamine (IMP)	0.070	0.33 hr
^{123}I-HIPDM	0.070	0.33 hr
^{99m}Tc-ECD	0.285	0.25 hr
Regional metabolic rate of glucose (rCMR$_{glc}$) ^{18}FDG	0.070–0.140	0.75 hr
Tumor uptake		
^{201}Tl	0.060	0.25–0.33 hr
^{99m}Tc-sestamibi[b]	0.0285	0.25–0.33 hr
Regional cerebral blood volume (rCBV)		
^{11}C-carbon monoxide	0.285	0.1 hr
^{99m}Tc-red blood cells	0.285	0.1 hr

ECD, ethyl cysteinate dimer; FDG, fluorodeoxyglucose.
[a]Images may be obtained as early as 5 minutes postinjection, especially in brain death studies.
[b]Choroid plexus uptake limits the utility of this agent for tumor detection in many cases.

dated, the study is unlikely to be of clinical utility, and the infant or child will receive exposure to ionizing radiation, albeit small in amount, without benefit. More ominous than inadequate sedation are other risks. The child should have nothing by mouth for a period that is adequate to insure that the stomach is empty and aspiration unlikely. Oversedation can lead to hypoventilation or even respiratory and cardiac arrest, the latter carrying a substantial risk of permanent neurologic injury, even if resuscitation is successful. Appropriate administration of sedative drugs and adequate monitoring by well-trained personnel significantly reduces the frequency and severity of sedation problems.

Sedation in children should be performed as part of an organized sedation program for imaging in children. Physicians should familiarize themselves with the doses of an oral hypnotic, such as chloral hydrate, and one or two drugs that can be used for intravenous sedation. The physician should be available immediately in case of emergency. A person who has demonstrated skill in monitoring and resuscitation should remain in the room with the patient at all times, and monitoring equipment, such as a pulse-oximeter, should be used in every case. All equipment, supplies, and drugs required for resuscitation should be available in the same room with the sedated patient.

Image Acquisition Protocols

For blood–brain barrier leak studies and brain death studies, flow images are obtained in rapid sequence as soon as activity appears in the neck vessels. If analog images are obtained, the flow images should also be acquired on a digital computer for backup purposes. Although posterior flow images are preferred, an anterior flow study is obtained if the patient cannot be moved onto an imaging table or if a frontal lobe lesion is suspected. Three to four orthogonal static blood-pool images are obtained immediately after injection. Delayed static images in four or-

thogonal projections are obtained at 90 to 120 minutes postinjection for blood–brain barrier leak studies. Single photon emission computed tomography (SPECT) imaging is preferred over orthogonal planar projections for delayed static images whenever feasible.

Regional cerebral blood flow (rCBF) and regional glucose metabolic rate (rCMR$_{glc}$) imaging studies are injected while the patient is awake and resting in a quiet environment, and sedation may be given through the same intravenous line when radiopharmaceutical localization in the brain is nearly complete. The minimum time from injection until sedation and imaging varies from 5 minutes for ^{99m}Tc-hexamethylpropyleneamine oxime (^{99m}Tc-HMPAO) to 45 minutes for ^{18}F-fluorodeoxyglucose (FDG) (Table 58.1). When ^{99m}Tc-HMPAO is used, sedation and imaging are best delayed until 1-hour postinjection, to allow a decrease in background activity in the scalp, skull, and meninges. ^{123}I-iodoamphetamine (^{123}I-IMP) partially redistributes with time into areas of ischemia, so the initial set of images at 20-minutes postinjection may be followed by "redistribution" images at 4-hours postinjection, particularly when there is a need to differentiate ischemia from infarction. Imaging of rCBF and rCMR$_{glc}$ should be performed with tomographic imaging equipment; only a few of the abnormalities detected by SPECT and positron emission tomography (PET) techniques can be appreciated on two-dimensional planar views. When compared with SPECT and PET, planar images are severely degraded by low-image contrast and superimposition of structures containing gray matter.

PET imaging of brain tumors with ^{18}FDG is performed in the manner described earlier, with imaging at 45 minutes after injection. SPECT imaging with ^{201}Tl or ^{99m}Tc-methoxyisobutylisonitrile (sestamibi) may begin 15 to 20 minutes after injection. Delayed ^{201}Tl SPECT, to evaluate washout of radiopharmaceutical from possible tumor sites, may yield additional diagnostic information.

^{201}Tl SPECT and ^{18}FDG PET images differ greatly in appearance. ^{201}Tl does not cross the intact blood–brain barrier; therefore, tumor uptake is seen on a background of low uptake. In contrast, ^{18}FDG is accumulated in metabolically active brain cells, with approximately threefold greater concentration in normal gray matter than in normal white matter. ^{18}FDG uptake in viable tumor may be identified when the tumor concentrates ^{18}FDG to a greater extent than white matter, but tumor uptake does not always exceed gray matter uptake. It is important to read each nuclear imaging study of the brain with an anatomic study [e.g., computed tomography (CT) or MRI] available for comparison. In brain tumor patients, it is critical that the interpretation of the ^{18}FDG study include a slice-by-slice comparison between the ^{18}FDG PET study and a recent MRI (or CT when a MRI study is not available).

^{99m}Tc-sestamibi is not used as often for brain tumor imaging as ^{18}FDG PET or ^{201}Tl SPECT. With ^{99m}Tc-sestamibi, there is choroid plexus uptake that is not blocked by potassium perchlorate. This choroid plexus uptake is more prominent than the very minimal, occasionally detectable, choroid plexus uptake of ^{201}Tl.

Cerebrospinal fluid (CSF) imaging studies should use a radiopharmaceutical, such as ^{111}In-diethylenetriaminepentaacetic acid (DTPA), that is sterile and pyrogen-free in a single-dose vial to minimize the risk of infection. ^{99m}Tc-DTPA, filtered through a 0.22-micron sterile filter, may be acceptable. The technique for injecting the radiopharmaceutical into CSF shunts that originate in the cerebral ventricles will vary according to the type of reservoir and valve used and according to whether there is a need to visualize the cerebral ventricles. Imaging is performed over 30 to 90 minutes and includes a sequence of images of the head and, in the typical case of a ventriculoperitoneal shunt, of the abdomen as well. The effect of placing the infant or child in a sitting position and pumping the shunt valve are also evaluated sequentially whenever appropriate. Lumboperitoneal shunts are imaged by obtaining sequential images of the lumbar region in the posterior projection for 30 minutes after lumbar intrathecal injection. Cisternography is performed in the same manner as in adults, but images are acquired earlier after injection because of more rapid cerebral blood flow (CBF) in infants and young children. In this age group, the first image should be performed at 2-hours postinjection, followed by images at 6-hours, 24-hours, and, if needed, 48-hours postinjection. SPECT imaging is optional.

BRAIN DEVELOPMENT IN THE NEONATAL PERIOD AND INFANCY

During the neonatal period and infancy, growth is more rapid than at any period during life, but the brain does not grow as fast as the rest of the body. The brain of a normal full-term neonate weighs an average of 335 g (10.4% of body mass), increasing to 691 g (9.2% of body mass) at 6 months and 1,141 g (7.9% of body mass) at 3 years. At age 9 years, the average brain mass is 1,275 g (4.5% of total body mass).

The neonatal brain has relatively high water content. Myelination is advanced in only a few locations. These include the

dorsal pons, cerebellar peduncles, lateral thalamus, posterior limb of the internal capsule, and paracentral gyri. Wherever gray matter is richly connected to other locations in the brain, already defined rCBF is the greatest. The distribution patterns of rCBF and rCMR$_{glc}$ are usually closely linked to each other, so that images of rCBF and rCMR$_{glc}$ obtained at the same spatial resolution are difficult to differentiate from each other.

At birth, rCBF and rCMR$_{glc}$ are greatest in the portions of the brain that are the most developed at that time, the cerebellum, the thalamus, midbrain, brainstem, and sensorimotor gray matter in the region of the central sulcus at the interface between the frontal and parietal lobes (1). Uptake of agents that demonstrate rCBF and rCMR$_{glc}$ is also relatively high in the visual cortex of the occipital lobes, but this is not true of premature infants in whom visual cortex uptake of these agents is relatively low. rCMR$_{glc}$ has been measured to be 13 to 25 μmol glucose/minute/100 g brain tissue in neonates.

As the brain develops in a normal infant, the patterns of rCBF and rCMR$_{glc}$ gradually approach the adult pattern (2). During the first few months of life, rCBF and rCMR$_{glc}$ increase in the basal ganglia and in the frontal lobes and parietal cortex adjacent to the sensorimotor cortex, and relative radiopharmaceutical uptake in these regions increases. At 6 months of age, there is still relatively reduced rCBF and rCMR$_{glc}$ in the anterior poles of the frontal lobes, but, by 1 year of age, the pattern of rCBF and rCMR$_{glc}$ closely resembles that seen in adults. Measured rCMR$_{glc}$ in the cerebral cortex continues to increase during early childhood, reaching 19 to 33 μmol glucose/minute/100 g at 2 years and rising further to 45 to 65 μmol glucose/minute/100 g at 3 to 4 years of age. rCMR$_{glc}$ begins to gradually decline at age 9 years, falling to adult values during late adolescence (2).

The development of PET has allowed study of a number of biochemical and biologic processes in the brain. For example, ^{11}C-L-methionine has been used to study amino acid transport at several stages of brain maturation (3).

Cerebral Palsy

Children with severe development delay continue to demonstrate patterns of rCBF and rCMR$_{glc}$ distribution that are similar to those seen in early infancy (1,4). However, less severe forms of cerebral palsy demonstrate a variety of rCBF and rCMR$_{glc}$. Decreased rCMR$_{glc}$ is present in the thalamus and lenticular nuclei in the choreoathetoid form of cerebral palsy, but no focal cortical abnormalities are seen. In spastic diplegia, there are areas of decreased rCMR$_{glc}$ that do not correspond to structural abnormalities on anatomic imaging examinations. In infantile hemiplegia, there is unilateral hypometabolism on the side contralateral to the clinical deficit, and no crossed cerebellar diaschisis is present.

Asphyxia and Hypoxic-Ischemic Brain Injury

The normal pattern of development must be taken into account in the interpretation of studies performed in infants with neurologic problems. An abnormal rCBF or rCMR$_{glc}$ imaging study in a neonate who has had birth asphyxia is highly predictive of later developmental problems. Infants damaged by neonatal asphyxia may demonstrate unilateral decreases in uptake in the sensorimotor cortex. However, the most damaged infants have demonstrated significantly enhanced uptake of rCBF radiopharmaceuticals in the frontal lobes anterior to the motor cortex, where cortical uptake in normal infants is relatively low. Some infants have demonstrated decreased rCBF in the watersheds between the anterior and middle cerebral arteries (5).

Measurement of rCBF with PET and $[^{15}O]H_2O$ in premature infants with intraventricular hemorrhage demonstrated reduced blood flow distant to the anatomic hemorrhage. The extent of the hypoperfused zone corresponded to the symptomatology of the patients (6). Although adult CBF values below 10 ml/100 g/minute occur only in infarcted brain (7), a mean CBF as low as 5 ml/100 g/minute in newborn infants can be associated with normal subsequent neurologic development and preservation of cerebral tissue (8).

In comparing different imaging modalities for prognostic predictive value in cases of perinatal asphyxia and hypoxic-ischemic brain injury, a study correlated the absence of localized echoes on ultrasound to a symmetric pattern or loss of architecture on PET and to hypodense areas of CT (9). However, another study did not confirm the predictive value of ultrasound. When abnormally developed infants have globally decreased CMR_{glc}, increasing CMR_{glc} on subsequent PET studies is a good predictive factor for normal development, whereas increasing or persistent hypometabolism is predictive of a poor prognosis (10).

CEREBROVASCULAR ANOMALIES, PERFUSION ABNORMALITIES, AND CEREBRAL INFARCTION

Stroke

Stroke is surprisingly common in children, with new cases occurring about as frequently as brain tumors. Cerebrovascular accidents (CVAs) in children are 55% ischemic and 45% hemorrhagic. Thirty percent of the ischemic CVAs are of indeterminate etiology, whereas hemorrhagic CVAs are more likely to result from a definable cause. Children with sickle cell disease and right-to-left intracardiac shunts are at increased risk for stroke. A number of other instigating factors have been described: craniospinal irradiation and intrathecal chemotherapy for malignancy (especially leukemia), occlusive vasculitis in systemic lupus erythematosus, trauma, and, occasionally, as a sequela of extracorporeal membrane oxygenation when a carotid artery is used as perfusion site (11). Anatomic patterns of brain injury typical of stroke are also seen in some asphyxiated neonates. Still, pediatric stroke often occurs without a known predisposing factor.

In children, the moyamoya phenomenon may occur as a reaction to focal cerebrovascular disease. In this condition, neovascularity develops distal to the narrowed major cerebral artery and is usually supplied by striatal vessels. The term moyamoya derives from the angiographic appearance of the multiple collateral vessels, described as a "puff of smoke" in Japanese.

rCBF SPECT imaging has almost completely replaced blood–brain barrier imaging for depiction of ischemic infarcted brain. The area of the stroke has decreased uptake when an iodoamine, ^{99m}Tc-HMPAO, ^{99m}Tc-ECD, or ^{18}FDG is used

(Fig. 58.1), although a few cases of increased uptake have been seen about 1 week after the stroke when ^{99m}Tc-HMPAO is used. In difficult cases of infantile brain infarction or porencephaly versus subtle closed-lip schizencephaly or cases of encephalitis with questionable ischemia on radiographic studies, ^{18}FDG imaging may help in the differential diagnosis (Figs. 58.2 and 58.3). When there is ischemic but still viable brain surrounding the stroke, the volume of decreased uptake may be larger than the volume of brain injury later delineated on CT (12,13). Ischemia surrounding the stroke is better depicted by the ^{123}I-iodoamines than by ^{99m}Tc-HMPAO.

Delineation of ischemic tissue at risk has been attempted with use of multiple PET tracers, that is, ^{18}FDG or $[^{15}O]O_2$ and $[^{11}C]CO_2$. A volume of tissue surrounding the stroke can be identified in which there is viable but ischemic brain. This penumbra of ischemic brain can be shown to have increased oxygen extraction and metabolic activity (14). Another approach to the imaging of ischemic brain in stroke patients uses the iodoamine tracers. Four-hour postinjection ^{123}I-iodoamine imaging sometimes demonstrates filling around the margins of the stroke, this phenomenon being attributed to movement of activity into ischemic but still viable brain. In some patients, decreased rCBF can be demonstrated in areas of relative ischemia where there is no evidence of brain infarction (Fig. 58.4). In patients with suspected ischemia, or in a stable patient after stroke, rCBF imaging may be performed before and after acetazolamide infusion to determine if there are any portions of the brain that lack perfusion reserve. Acetazolamide causes dilatation of those vessels that are able to dilate. Perfusion increases in well-perfused areas of the brain, increasing the differential uptake (and image contrast) between well-perfused and poorly perfused brain (15, 16).

Crossed cerebellar diaschisis is an interesting physiologic phenomenon seen on the rCBF and $rCMR_{glc}$ studies of patients with severe strokes. Loss of afferent input from the region of the stroke to the cerebellum contralateral to the stroke results in decreased cerebellar activity on that side. Reduced cerebellar activation results in decreased rCBF or $rCMR_{glc}$ in the contralateral cerebellum (12). Other structures distal to an infarct may also show hypometabolism resulting from deafferentiation such as in the thalamus following a cortical infarction (14).

In sickle cell disease, a vasculitis of the cerebral arteries is present in those patients who develop clinical evidence of cerebral ischemia or stroke. The decrease in perfusion in the portion of the brain supplied by these vessels may be demonstrated by rCBF or $rCMR_{glc}$ imaging (17). Treatment protocols that employ hypertransfusion can reverse the angiographic findings of vasculitis. An occlusive vasculitis also occurs in some patients with juvenile system lupus erythematosus. In these patients, rCBF SPECT can demonstrate the resulting perfusion abnormalities (18).

In addition to the effects of arterial stenosis and occlusion, other vascular abnormalities and their effects upon the brain can be recognized. An intravascular tracer such as ^{99m}Tc-red blood cells, in conjunction with SPECT imaging, may demonstrate abnormal uptake in the enlarged vessels of an arteriovenous malformation. Brain adjacent to the malformation is often poorly perfused as blood flows preferentially through the abnormally

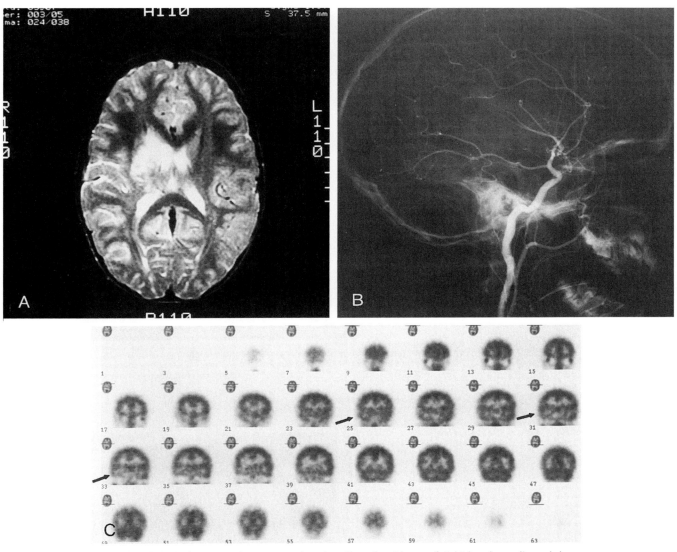

FIGURE 58.1. A: On magnetic resonance imaging, there is evidence of right basal ganglia and deep white matter infarction. **B:** The right middle cerebral artery is narrowed on cerebral angiography. **C:** Regional cerebral blood flow single photon emission computed tomography after injection of ^{99m}Tc-hexamethylpropyleneamine oxime shows only a slight decrease in right temporal lobe perfusion. (From Miller JH, Gelfand MJ. Central nervous system. In: Miller JH, Gelfand MJ, eds. *Pediatric nuclear imaging*. Philadelphia: WB Saunders, 1994:11–44, with permission.)

enlarged vessels of the malformation. This "steal" phenomenon may be demonstrated by rCBF or rCMR$_{glc}$ imaging (19). Brain perfusion and metabolism are decreased on rCBF and rCMR$_{glc}$ imaging, respectively, on the affected side in Sturge-Weber syndrome (31). Regional cerebral blood volume (rCBV) imaging may also demonstrate the great vein of Galen malformation in infants. Occlusion of the superior sagittal sinus may be seen as a discontinuity in that vessel on rCBV imaging. Cortical venous thrombosis may be associated with small areas of infarction. These areas may be depicted by blood–brain barrier imaging.

In asphyxiated infants, blood–brain barrier imaging may demonstrate three patterns of abnormal uptake. Infants may demonstrate abnormal uptake on delayed images in a pattern typical of stroke in a major cerebral artery distribution or abnor-

mal uptake may be seen in the watersheds between major cerebral artery distributions, where decreased blood flow has been confirmed by PET (5). The most severely affected infants will have increased uptake in a "skullcap-like" pattern and will demonstrate histologic evidence of laminar cortical necrosis.

In infants who have undergone extracorporeal membrane oxygenation with sacrifice of a carotid artery, decreased rCBF is often observed on SPECT studies (11,21).

Brain Death

Anoxic injury, some inflammatory and infectious processes, and trauma may cause the brain to swell. When marked swelling occurs within the closed calvarium, intracerebral pressure may

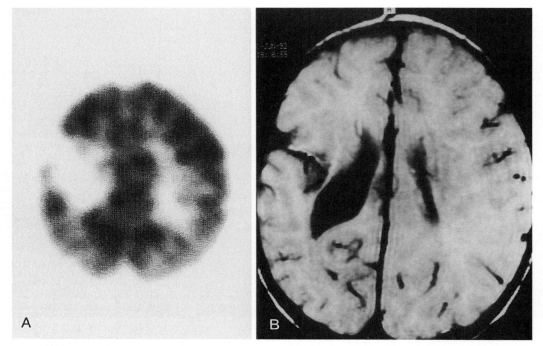

FIGURE 58.2. Cerebral infarct. A 6-month-old with right hemispheric infantile hemiplegia. **A:** The magnetic resonance image shows a defect in the right cerebral hemisphere. **B:** The [18]fluorodeoxyglucose positron emission tomography image shows a cortical-based area of marked decreased uptake, indicating a cerebral infarct.

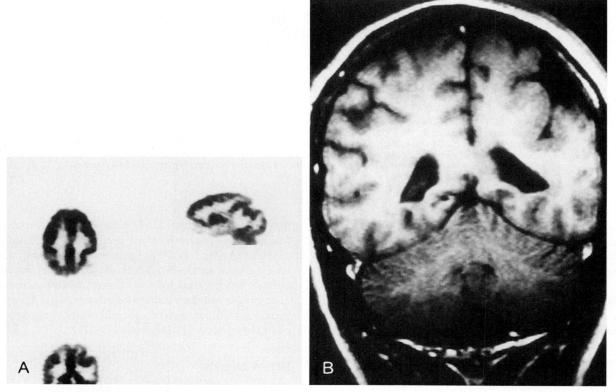

FIGURE 58.3. Schizencephaly. The [18]fluorodeoxyglucose (FDG) positron emission tomography image **(A)** shows [18]FDG uptake in the cortical lining of the defect seen on magnetic resonance imaging in the left hemisphere **(B)** confirming the diagnosis of schizencephaly.

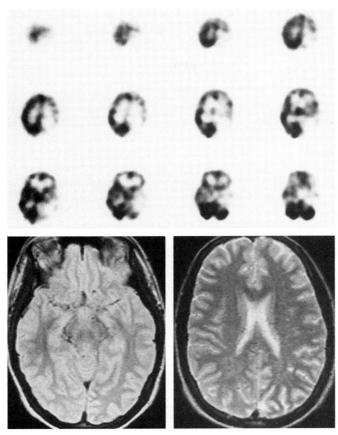

FIGURE 58.4. **A:** In this child with moyamoya disease, there is extensive hypoperfusion of the left hemisphere. **B** and **C:** The magnetic resonance imaging demonstrates abnormal cortical vessels around the brainstem and basal ganglia but only minimal cortical abnormality. (From Miller JH, Gelfand MJ. Central nervous system. In: Miller JH, Gelfand MJ, eds. *Pediatric nuclear imaging.* Philadelphia: WB Saunders, 1994:11–44, with permission.)

become high enough to cause a cessation of cerebral flow, followed by brain death. Scintigraphy with a portable gamma-camera is a simple bedside method for the determination of brain death. In some institutions it is routinely used for this purpose; in others it is reserved for cases in which the clinical picture is unclear.

Original descriptions of brain death used ^{99m}Tc-pertechnetate or various ^{99m}Tc-chelates and a sequence of first-pass flow images. When there is cessation of flow to the cerebrum, activity is seen in the carotid arteries, but not in the anterior or middle cerebral arteries. Activity may be seen in the skull-scalp-meningeal region. This extracerebral activity may be diminished by used of a tourniquet around the head above the ears. On immediate postinjection blood-pool images, activity is seen again in the skull-scalp-meningeal region. Activity in the superior sagittal sinus or transverse sinuses in the absence of cerebral blood flow is due to backflow rather than cerebral perfusion (22,23).

Availability of rCBF tracers such as ^{99m}Tc-HMPAO allow a look at cerebral flow, not only during the first-pass flow images but also during the series of immediate postinjection static images. When cerebral flow is absent, ^{99m}Tc-HMPAO and ^{99m}Tc-

pertechnetate first-pass flow images are identical. However, when ^{99m}Tc-HMPAO is used, the immediate postinjection static images clearly demonstrate whether cerebral perfusion is absent (Figs. 58.5 and 58.6). When cerebral perfusion is present, there is activity in the brain on static images, and planar images obtained at the bedside will indicate whether or not the cerebral hemispheres, basal ganglia, and cerebellum are perfused. In this situation, bedside planar imaging of an unstable patient is adequate for determination of brain death, and the high resolution rCBF mapping of SPECT imaging may be omitted. When cerebral perfusion is present, gross abnormalities and asymmetries of perfusion are sometimes seen on planar imaging. If there is increasing brain edema, cerebral perfusion may disappear from one day to the next on sequential scans (24–26).

Infants pose two special problems in the determination of brain death. Infants who have had anoxic brain damage may have preservation of brain perfusion despite overwhelming clinical evidence of brain death (27). In addition, the immature pattern of brain perfusion that is normal in infants younger than 6

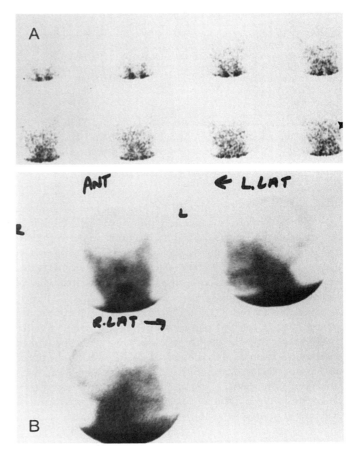

FIGURE 58.5. **A:** Brain death. The bedside ^{99m}Tc-hexamethylpropyleneamine oxime planar imaging study demonstrates absent flow to the cerebral hemispheres on the anterior first-pass flow study. The child was comatose due to a severe encephalopathy. **B:** There is absent perfusion of the cerebral hemispheres, basal ganglia, and cerebellum on the static images obtained a few minutes after injection. A tiny amount of backflow is noted in the area of the torcular herophili. (From Miller JH, Gelfand MJ. Central nervous system. In: Miller JH, Gelfand MJ, eds. *Pediatric nuclear imaging.* Philadelphia: WB Saunders, 1994:11–44, with permission.)

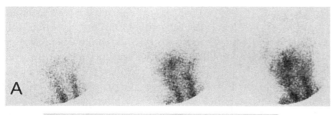

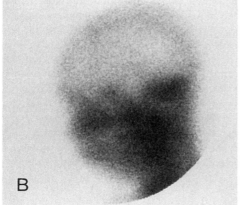

FIGURE 58.6. A: The anterior first-pass ^{99m}Tc-hexamethylpropyleneamine oxime flow study demonstrates no evidence of flow to the cerebral hemispheres. This adolescent was comatose after being struck by an automobile. **B:** Static images obtained a few minutes after injection demonstrate preservation of flow only to the cerebellum.

months of age may be seen on both planar and SPECT rCBF imaging and should not be confused with brain ischemia.

TRAUMA

Abnormalities of rCBF and rCMR$_{glc}$ are often present in severe head trauma. Regions of decreased perfusion or metabolism may be seen in areas of contusion and in the cortex underlying subdural or epidural hematoma (28,29). A few studies suggest that there is a correlation between the extent and persistence of perfusion abnormalities after head trauma and the eventual clinical outcome.

Severe head trauma may lead to extensive brain edema and compromise of cerebral perfusion. In these patients, a rCBF imaging study may be used to assess cerebral perfusion and to determine if brain death has occurred, as described in the previous section. Infants with severe head trauma, unlike those who have been asphyxiated, uncommonly have preservation of cerebral perfusion in the face of persistent and unequivocal clinical evidence of brain death (26).

NEOPLASM

In adults, there are several well-established applications for PET imaging with ^{18}FDG and SPECT imaging with ^{201}Tl (30–39) and ^{99m}Tc-sestamibi (40). These include

1. Determination of the histologic grade of astrocytomas before initial surgery or surgery for recurrence

2. Differentiation of recurrent or persistent tumor from radiation necrosis
3. Differentiation of viable tumor from edema surrounding the tumor
4. Differentiation of focal infection from focal lymphoma in acquired immune deficiency patients

These last three applications are likely to be as valid in children as in adults with astrocytomas. However, children present with a much wider variety of tumor histology than do adults, and the published experience with emission computed tomography in most tumor histologies is still limited. As a result, grading is reasonable at this time only in lesions with histology that resembles adult astrocytomas.

Astrocytomas

The 1993 World Health Organization grading system for central nervous system tumors include four grades of glioma (41):

1. Pilocystic and subependymal giant cell astrocytoma
2. Low-grade astrocytoma
3. Anaplastic astrocytoma
4. Glioblastoma multiform

In children, most low-grade gliomas occur in the optic pathway, cerebellar hemispheres, and brainstem. Tumors with high-grade histology are most common in the cerebral hemispheres.

Astrocytomas of the cerebral hemispheres comprise approximately 20% of brain tumors in children (42). Prognosis is determined by histologic grade and completeness of resection. In cerebral hemisphere astrocytomas, it appears that tumor imaging radiopharmaceuticals may be used in the same way in children as in adults. Although the number of pediatric patients studied with these tumors is relatively small, there is as yet no evidence to presume that results in adults and pediatric patients differ (43,44).

High-grade (histologic grade III and IV) astrocytomas will usually concentrate ^{18}FDG and ^{201}Tl, and low-grade tumors usually will not (31–37,45). A study evaluated primary cerebral tumors with biopsy proved histology to determine the optimal ^{18}FDG uptake cut-off level that would differentiate low-grade from high-grade tumors. A tumor/white matter ^{18}FDG uptake less than 1.5:1 ratio is indicative of low-grade glioma. In addition, the same cutoff level could be used when cerebral tumor of other histologic types is considered (46). When there is ^{18}FDG or ^{201}Tl uptake in a tumor of low-grade histology, the tumor usually behaves more aggressively than those low-grade tumors that do not concentrate these radiopharmaceuticals. ^{18}FDG PET or ^{201}Tl SPECT can aid the physician in predicting the histologic grade and biologic behavior before biopsy of new or recurrent tumor (32,47) (Fig. 58.7). Similarly, for high-grade astrocytomas, ^{18}FDG PET will aid in the differentiation of recurrent tumor from radiation necrosis (Fig. 58.8). ^{18}FDG rarely localizes in areas of tumor necrosis (31), and ^{201}Tl has a relatively low rate of localization in necrotic brain proven to be free of tumor (45,48).

In adults, labeled amino acids, particularly ^{11}C-methionine, have been shown to concentrate not only in high-grade astrocy-

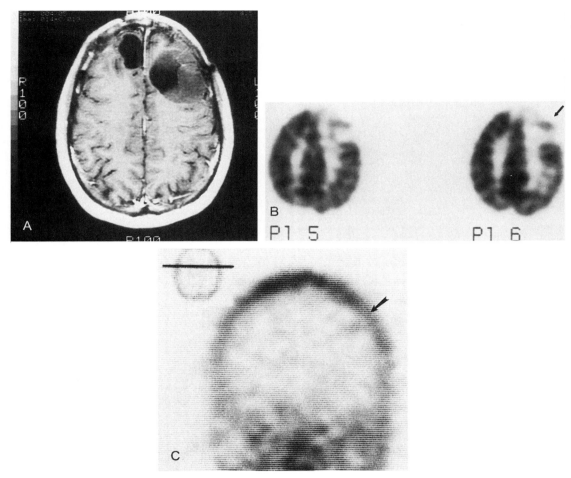

FIGURE 58. 7. A: Two years after resection of bilateral low-grade frontal lobe astrocytoma, a magnetic resonance image demonstrates possible tumor recurrence. **B:** An [18]fluorodeoxyglucose positron emission tomography image demonstrates a small focus (*arrow*) of increased radiopharmaceutical uptake at the same location. **C:** A ^{201}Tl single photon emission computed tomography image demonstrates slightly increased uptake at the same location. (From Miller JH, Gelfand MJ. Central nervous system; in Miller JH, Gelfand MJ, eds., *Pediatric nuclear imaging*. Philadelphia: WB Saunders, 1994:11–44, with permission. PET study courtesy of Martin Jacobs, MD, Kettering Medical Center, Dayton, OH.)

tomas but also in many grade II astrocytomas and in a number of other brain tumors (49–54). These agents also allow differentiation of recurrent brain tumor from radiation injury (55,56). These agents are potentially useful in tumors that do not concentrate [18]FDG or [201]Tl.

Pilocystic Astrocytoma

The histology and biologic behavior of pilocystic astrocytomas is distinct from that of other astrocytomas found in children. They comprise about 10% of pediatric brain tumors and are usually found in or near the posterior fossa, with a predilection for the cerebellar hemispheres. They may also occur in the optic pathway, hypothalamus, and less commonly in the ventricles or cerebral hemispheres. They are less aggressive than most astrocytomas and have the biologic behavior of a low-grade brain tumor.

Although these tumors behave as low-grade tumors, they usually demonstrate intense uptake of [18]FDG and ^{201}Tl, in marked contrast to other astrocytomas of low-histologic grade (42,57, 58).

Brainstem Glioma

Brainstem gliomas comprise 10% to 20% of pediatric central nervous system neoplasms. They are very difficult to treat adequately. Because of location, complete resection is very difficult to accomplish, and their biologic behavior may be aggressive.

Brainstem gliomas usually concentrate [18]FDG and [201]Tl. However, interpretation of [18]FDG PET requires some knowledge of normal distribution of gray matter in the brainstem. [201]Tl uptake in the tumor must be separated from normal uptake of thallium in the area of clivus.

Optic Glioma

Optic gliomas may occur in the optic nerves or optic chiasm. They are relatively uncommon, but occur in 5% to 15% of

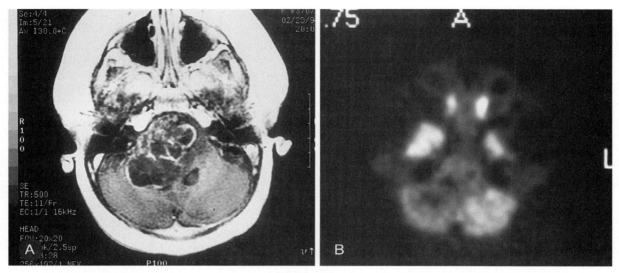

FIGURE 58.8. **A:** The brainstem glioma depicted in this contrast-enhanced T1-weighted magnetic resonance imaging has increased in size and in the amount of cystic change and enhancement. **B:** On an [18]fluorodeoxyglucose positron emission tomography image, the abnormally increased uptake along the margins of some of the cysts in consistent with high-grade tumor. (Courtesy of R.E. Coleman, MD, Duke University Medical Center, Durham, NC.)

patients with neurofibromatosis type 1 (NF-1). Relatively few optic gliomas have been studied with emission computed tomography, and ^{201}Tl uptake has been observed (Fig. 58.9). In neurofibromatosis, [18]FDG PET occasionally detects additional lesions before they are seen on a anatomic study (59) (Fig. 58.10).

Ependymoma

Ependymomas arise from the cells that form the ependymal lining of the ventricles. Most are located in or near the posterior

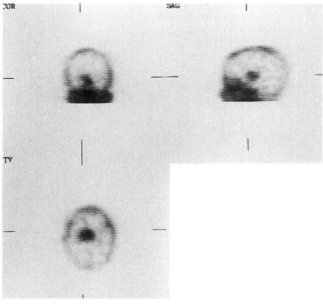

FIGURE 58.9. There is marked increased uptake of ^{201}Tl in a recurrent hypothalamic-optic glioma. (From Miller JH, Gelfand MJ. Central nervous system. In: Miller JH, Gelfand MJ, eds. *Pediatric nuclear imaging.* Philadelphia: WB Saunders, 1994:11–44, with permission.)

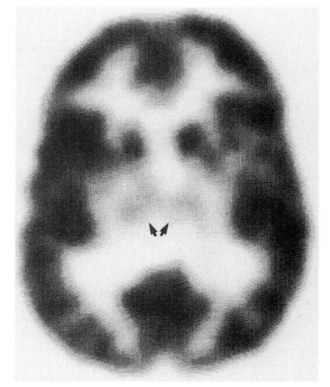

FIGURE 58.10. Neurofibromatosis. In this child with neurofibromatosis, the [18]fluorodeoxyglucose positron emission tomography image shows decreased uptake in both thalami (*arrows*). A magnetic resonance imaging (MRI) performed at the same time was normal, but thalamic lesions could be visualized on an MRI performed 1 year later.

fossa, with about 60% in an infratentorial location and 40% lying above the tentorium. They comprise approximately 2% to 8% of pediatric brain tumors.

These tumors are usually demonstrated on [18]FDG PET and ^{201}Tl SPECT, but the intensity of radiopharmaceutical uptake in the tumor varies from patient to patient (43,57).

Primitive Neuroectodermal Tumors

The term primitive neuroectodermal tumors (PNETs) is used by many pathologists to include medulloblastoma, ependymoblastoma, medulloepithelioma, primary cerebral neuroblastoma, and pineoblastoma. PNETs constitute 15% to 25% of all pediatric brain tumors. Medulloblastoma is an infratentorial PNET that occurs primarily in children. This form of PNET is the most common neoplasm in children younger than 10 years, and ranks with cerebellar astrocytoma as the most common posterior fossa neoplasm. These tumors are usually in the

midline, arising in the inferior cerebellar vermis and growing into the fourth ventricle. After resection they have a high rate of recurrence and metastasis. Medulloblastomas often metastasize early and extensively throughout the central nervous system. Metastases tend to occur along the surfaces of the central nervous system with many occurring as "drop metastases" within the spinal canal.

[18]FDG PET studies and ^{201}Tl SPECT studies demonstrate consistent localization of radiopharmaceutical in new or recurrent PNET (57,60,61) (Fig. 58.11). PET and SPECT tumor imaging are useful in intracranial lesions when the effects of treatment, especially radiation necrosis, are not clearly differentiated from recurrent or persistent tumor by CT or MRI.

Craniopharyngioma

Craniopharyngioma arises from rests of squamous epithelium lining the remnant of Rathke's pouch. More than 95% lie in

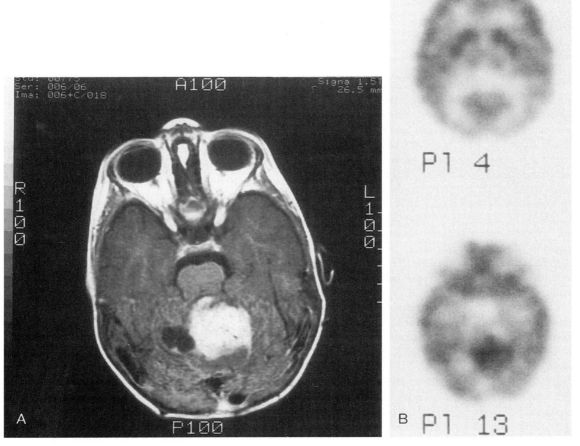

FIGURE 58.11. Primitive neuroectodermal tumor of the posterior fossa. **A:** On magnetic resonance imaging, there is a recurrent tumor nodule in the posterior fossa, in the midline extending to the left of midline. **B:** [18]fluorodeoxyglucose positron emission tomography demonstrates increased localization of the radiopharmaceutical in the tumor nodule but not in the cyst. (From Miller JH, Gelfand MJ. Central nervous system. In: Miller JH, Gelfand MJ, eds. *Pediatric nuclear imaging.* Philadelphia: WB Saunders, 1994:11–44, with permission. PET study courtesy of Martin Jacobs, MD, Kettering Medical Center, Dayton, OH.)

the suprasellar cistern, and the tumor is usually cystic in gross morphology. This tumor is more common in children than adults, with peak incidences at 8 to 12 years and again in mid-adult life. Craniopharyngiomas comprise about 7% of intracranial neoplasms.

Several radiopharmaceuticals have been shown to concentrate in pituitary tumors and hold promise for the imaging of craniopharyngioma. These include [18]FDG and ^{111}In-tyr-octreotide (62–64).

INFECTION

Meningitis, Subdural Empyema, and Effusion

In different age groups, bacterial meningitis is caused by different organisms. In neonates, meningitis is most often caused by Group B β-streptococcus, and *Escherichia coli* meningitis is also common. In late infancy and in toddlers, *Haemophilus influenza* infection becomes the most common cause of bacterial meningitis. In older children, meningococcal infection becomes a prominent cause of meningitis, as in adults. In infants and preschool children, bacterial meningitis is associated with a high rate of complications and neurologic residua. In *H. influenza* meningitis, neurologic residua, when they occur, are most often due to vasculitis and infarction. Persistent fevers with meningitis are associated with subdural effusions. Occasionally, ventriculitis complicates meningitis.

Radionuclide imaging with first-pass flow studies was once used to detect complications of meningitis. Abnormalities that can be seen include a "superficial" cortical decrease in flow in the area of a subdural effusion or a large flow defect in the area of a larger brain infarction. Flow may also be reduced in one hemisphere because of edema, vasculitis, or vasospasm. On immediate postinjection blood-pool images, benign subdural effusion is relatively "cold," whereas an inflammatory process such as subdural empyema usually has increased uptake. Delayed images with blood–brain barrier agents demonstrate ventricular uptake on the occasion when ventriculitis complicates meningitis. In most cases, patches of increased uptake are present because of uptake in areas of meningeal inflammation, but these focal areas of uptake rarely correspond to treatable complications of meningitis. As a result, first-pass flow studies and blood–brain barrier imaging are not often performed for the diagnosis of meningitis complications. CT, and especially MRI, identify subdural effusion and empyema and cerebral infarction more accurately than scintigraphy. The role of rCBF SPECT and [18]FDG PET has not been defined in this clinical setting.

Bacterial meningitis is usually associated with bacterial sepsis. When skeletal symptoms or persistent fevers are noted, whole-body imaging (bone, ^{67}Ga, or white blood cell imaging) in search of distant sites of infection is occasionally productive.

Viral Encephalitis

The blood–brain barrier scan is often abnormal in viral infections of the brain. The first-pass flow images may demonstrate increased flow to the involved hemisphere with slow transit activity peripherally in the hemisphere. Immediate postinjection blood-pool images may demonstrate a ring of increased uptake along the periphery of a hemisphere or, when infection is severe, multiple focal areas of abnormal uptake. Delayed static imaging may demonstrate focal, multifocal, or extensive areas of diffuse uptake.

The greatest imaging experience is in herpes encephalitis. In older children and adults, infection with herpes simplex virus type 1 (HSV-1) often involves the temporal lobes, and focal uptake is often seen in an involved temporal lobe (60,65). In this clinical setting, abnormalities are more often seen on blood–brain barrier imaging than on contrast-enhanced CT (Fig. 58.12) (60). In infants, infection with herpes simplex virus type 2 (HSV-2) typically involves the entire brain.

An alternative approach is to perform rCBF or rCMR$_{glc}$ imaging. Herpes encephalitis is effectively treated with antiviral drugs when treatment is started early in the disease; in contrast, devastating neurologic damage typically ensues when treatment is delayed. ^{99m}Tc-HMPAO and [18]FDG PET imaging demonstrate focally increased uptake in a high percentage of temporal lobes affected with herpes encephalitis and appear to be a more promising approach than blood–brain barrier imaging (66–68).

Human Immunodeficiency Virus Infection

Human immunodeficiency virus (HIV) infection of the brain has been shown to cause multiple foci of decreased rCMR$_{glc}$ and rCBF on emission computed tomography.

[18]FDG PET imaging has been employed in differentiating two relatively common opportunistic complications in the brain related to HIV immunodeficiency. In most cases, focal toxoplasma infection has not concentrated [18]FDG (Fig. 58.13), whereas lymphoma has concentrated the radiopharmaceutical (Fig. 58.14). In the same way, ^{201}Tl imaging may also be used in this setting (69,70).

Brain Abscess

Although blood–brain barrier imaging and ^{67}Ga imaging were effectively used in past years for the diagnosis of brain abscess, scintigraphy has been replaced by CT and MRI. In difficult diagnostic cases, labeled white blood cells appear to be sensitive and specific in the diagnosis of brain abscess (71,72), although high-dose steroid therapy may reduce the sensitivity of the examination (73).

EPILEPSY

In infants and small children, the progressive nature of epilepsy creates a risk of disruption of normal development and can lead to permanent cortical maldevelopment or focal sclerosis. In addition, the psychologic aspects increase the teenage suicide rate for adolescents with epilepsy.

Several technologic advancements have led to improved evaluation of surgical candidates. These include continued improvements in MRI and functional nuclear imaging techniques (PET

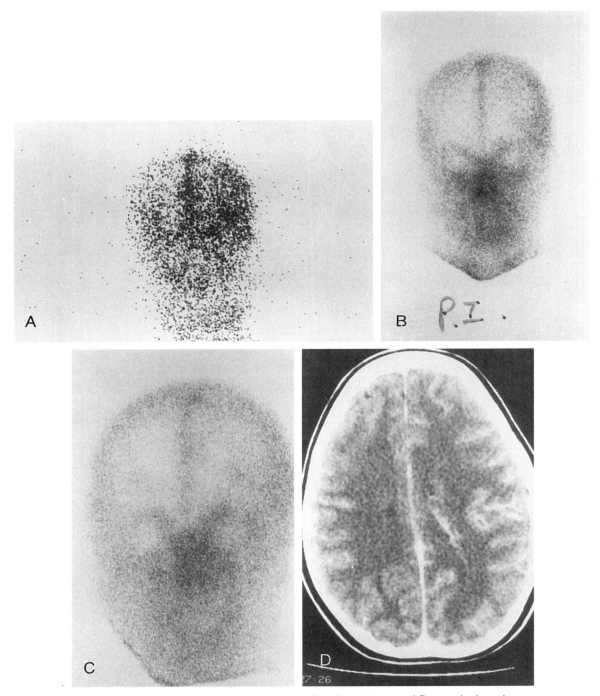

FIGURE 58.12. **A:** In a patient with herpes encephalitis, there is increased flow to the lateral aspects of the left hemisphere on the first-pass flow study. **B:** There is increased uptake on the immediate postinjection static image. **C:** The increase in uptake is more prominent in the left hemisphere, and especially in the left temporal lobe, on the delayed static blood–brain barrier images. **D:** On the contrast-enhanced computed tomography scan, there is increased gyral enhancement in the same location. (From Miller JH, Gelfand MJ. Central nervous system. In: Miller JH, Gelfand MJ, eds. *Pediatric nuclear imaging.* Philadelphia: WB Saunders, 1994:11–44.)

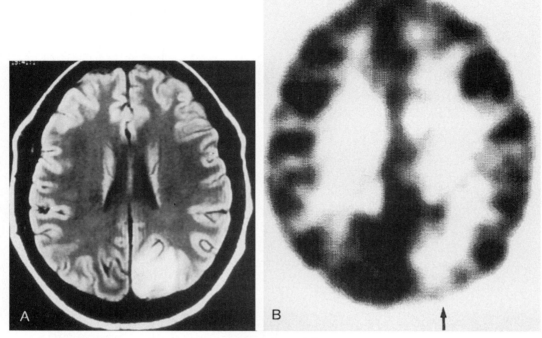

FIGURE 58.13. Human immunodeficiency virus immunodeficiency and toxoplasmosis. **A:** The magnetic resonance image shows a lesion in the posterior parietal region on the left. **B:** The [18]fluorodeoxyglucose image shows decreased metabolism indicating an infectious process.

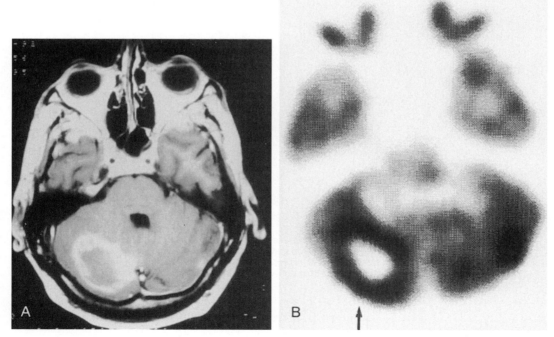

FIGURE 58.14. Human immunodeficiency virus and lymphoma. **A:** The magnetic resonance image shows a ring-enhancing lesion in the right cerebellum. **B:** The [18]fluorodeoxyglucose image shows a rim of increased metabolism with a hypometabolic center indicating a high-grade tumor with central necrosis (*arrow*).

and SPECT), better defined analysis of scalp/sphenoidal [electroencephalogram (EEG)] recorded ictal onsets, long-term monitoring of epileptic seizures, foramen ovale and epidural electrodes providing intermediate invasiveness of chronic monitoring, and use of subdural grid electrodes.

Newer surgical techniques with smaller standard resections are more widely used, such as amygdalohippocampectomy, modified anterior temporal lobectomy sparing most of the lateral cortex, hemispherectomies, computerized lesionectomy, subpial cortical transection, and corpus callosum partial or total transection. The criteria to select surgical candidates continue to evolve with more patients considered for surgical treatment. Infants and children with catastrophic secondary generalized seizures, extratemporal neocortical epileptogenic foci, hemimegaloencephaly with frequent drop attacks, Sturge-Webster syndrome, and infantile spasms are now considered for early surgical intervention in some institutions.

In 1939, Penfield et al. (74) observed hyperemia at the site of seizure foci at the time of craniotomy. Thirty years later, these observations were extended by Engel using noninvasive ^{18}FDG PET imaging (75–77). In partial continuous epilepsy, rCMR$_{glc}$ was demonstrated to be increased during seizure activity in the area of the seizure focus during clinical seizure activity and, in some cases, during subclinical seizure activity (Fig. 58.15). However, only a minority of patients with difficult to control epilepsy had increased rCMR$_{glc}$ at the seizure focus during the interictal period, when it was most feasible to study them. Rather, during the interictal period, seizure foci were most often characterized

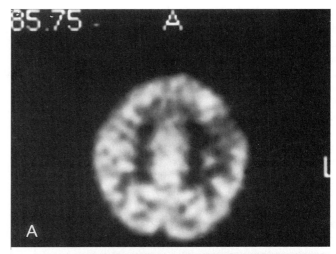

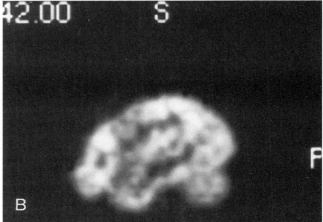

FIGURE 58.16. ^{18}Fluorodeoxyglucose positron emission tomography (FDG PET) axial (**A**) and sagittal images (**B**) in a child with partial recurrent seizures. There is an area of hypometabolism high in the left frontal lobe. Magnetic resonance imaging (MRI) was normal in this area. The temporal lobes were normal by ^{18}FDG PET and MRI. (Courtesy of R.E. Coleman, MD, Duke University Medical Center, Durham, NC.)

by decreased rCMR$_{glc}$ (Fig. 58.16), and, in the immediate postictal period, the volume of brain with decreased rCMR$_{glc}$ was often much greater in extent than in the interictal period. Subsequently, similar observations were made with rCBF SPECT. During the next decade, these observations were extended to several clinical types of epilepsy, and, in some cases, correlated with pathologic findings and the effects of therapy (77–82).

More recently, tracers of neurotransmitter function have been developed and have been used in clinical studies. ^{11}C-flumazil and ^{123}I-iomazenil are benzodiazepine receptor antagonists that have been used to localize seizure foci which have decreased concentration of benzodiazepine receptors (83,84).

PET is usually performed in the waking, resting state of normal or epileptic subjects. The latter are usually in their interictal state. Ictal scanning is difficult to obtain, given the relatively short half-life and expense of PET radiopharmaceuticals. However, ictal rCBF SPECT imaging is feasible, with ictal injection of radiopharmaceutical followed by imaging after the seizure.

Anatomic cross-sectional imaging methods will demonstrate

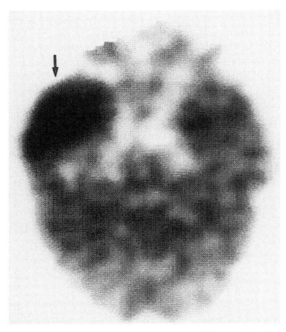

FIGURE 58.15. Ictal seizure focus. A 10-year-old boy with a history of complex partial seizures and multiple seizure spikes on electroencephalogram monitoring during the ^{18}fluorodeoxyglucose (FDG) uptake period. ^{18}FDG positron emission tomography image shows a marked increase in uptake in the right temporal lobe, consistent with an ictal seizure focus (*arrow*).

the site of the seizure focus in a minority of cases. CT will demonstrate small cortical neoplasms in a few cases, and MRI will demonstrate small cortical neoplasms or small regions of sclerosis in a larger number of cases. At surgery the cortical neoplasms are most often low-grade astrocytomas, hamartomas, or gangliogliomas and neuromas (85). Still, in more than one half of patients with difficult to control epilepsy, the anatomic site of the seizure focus is not identified. Because of the critical role of antiseizure surgery in patients with medically refractive seizures, accurate identification of the epileptogenic focus is often critical. Identification of one or more anatomic abnormalities does not prove that the anatomic abnormality is the site of origin of the patient's seizures.

Partial Continuous Epilepsy

Partial continuous epilepsy has been the form of epilepsy most extensively investigated with radionuclide imaging (75,76,78, 79,86,87). In this form of epilepsy, the temporal lobe is most often involved and the most common pathologic lesion is mesial temporal sclerosis. A minority of the seizure foci are located outside of the temporal lobe, usually in the frontal lobe (Fig. 58.16). Surgical resection of the seizure focus can eliminate or significantly reduce the frequency of seizures in patients in whom multiple attempts at drug therapy have been unsuccessful (88).

rCBF and rCMR$_{glc}$ imaging has been successful in identifying the seizure focus in 50% to 75% of patients who undergo interictal imaging. Metabolic studies using PET appear to identify the seizure focus in a higher percentage of patients than SPECT studies (75,89,90). In about 10% of those who have abnormal scans, the seizure focus will have increased rCBF or rCMR$_{glc}$. In the remainder of those who have abnormal scans, decreased rCBF or rCMR$_{glc}$ will be found. Imaging findings are closely correlated with invasive electrocorticographic findings (83). At some centers, rCBF or rCMR$_{glc}$ imaging in combination with other noninvasive techniques has made chronic intracranial electroencephalographic monitoring unnecessary in 50% or more of older children and adults with medically intractable temporal lobe epilepsy (91). A single focus of interictal temporal hypometabolism (15% to 20%) on ^{18}FDG PET is an excellent predictor of seizure control after surgery, whereas identification of multiple foci predicts a poorer postsurgical outcome.

Ictal Imaging

SPECT imaging with tracers of rCBF are better suited for ictal imaging than PET because of the short half-life of PET tracers and the relatively long uptake phase for ^{18}FDG compared with the transient duration of a seizure. Ictal injection of a rCBF radiopharmaceutical enhances the sensitivity of radionuclide imaging in the identification of seizure foci (86,91–93). Seizure medications are decreased or withdrawn, and the patient is observed in the hospital. The radiopharmaceutical is kept at the patient's bedside and injected into an intravenous line as soon as seizure activity is noted. The patient is then imaged after the conclusion of the seizure. The seizure focus is then identified as a focus of increased rCBF. This approach increases the sensitivity of radionuclide imaging by 25% to 50% over interictal imaging.

If interictal radiopharmaceutical injection and imaging are first performed and followed by imaging after ictal injection (in those cases in which a clear diagnosis is not available), the seizure focus will be identified in 75% to 85% of cases. Ictal SPECT is particularly valuable in evaluation of extratemporal epilepsy in which interictal PET appears less sensitive (94,95).

In addition to patients with partial continuous epilepsy, there are other patients in whom identification of an area of increased radiopharmaceutical localization can be invaluable. In patients in whom one or more regions of abnormal gray matter are identified as possible seizure foci by CT or MRI, for example, when evidence of cortical dysplasia or heterotopia has been noted, identification of a site of increased activity after radiopharmaceutical injection during a clinical interictal or ictal period can be extremely useful in the planning of antiseizure surgery (96,97). Ictal injection of radiopharmaceutical has been used to identify the seizure focus for subsequent surgical resection (98). PET after ictal injection of ^{18}FDG has also been used by Chugani et al. as part of an effort toward classification of seizure activation patterns according to ictal patterns of rCMR$_{glc}$, with comparison between rCMR$_{glc}$ imaging patterns and surgical outcome (99, 100).

rCBF and rCMR$_{glc}$ Imaging of Infants and Small Children with Seizures

Infantile Spasms

rCBF and rCMR$_{glc}$ imaging have also been used to study infants and small children with seizure disorders typical of those age groups. Infantile spasms are divided into two categories: (a) symptomatic with definable cause and (b) cryptogenic. Infantile spasms are usually refractory to medication, and the prognosis for intact neurologic function is extremely poor (101). Two patterns of abnormality have been found. In some infants, symmetric hypometabolism will be found in the lenticular nuclei and midbrain. Others will have asymmetric or multifocal decreases in rCMR$_{glc}$. Although initial data suggested that patients with symmetric hypometabolism had a better clinical prognosis, recent data suggest that infants with hypsarrhythmia and focal uptake abnormalities may demonstrate remarkable improvement after antiseizure surgery. In these children with cryptogenic-type infantile spasms and focal hypometabolism, unsuspected foci of cortical dysplasia have been found in the surgical specimen (102–105). A few infants were reported in whom ^{18}FDG PET was used to plan the surgical treatment of medically refractory seizures that had been present since the neonatal period (106).

Lennox-Gastaut Syndrome

The Lennox-Gastaut syndrome is defined by a triad of symptoms: 1 to 2.5 Hz spike-wave pattern on EEG, intellectual impairment, and multiple seizure types including minor-motor, tonic-clonic, atypical absence, and/or partial seizures.

In preschool children with Lennox-Gastaut syndrome, three patterns of metabolic abnormality have been described (107). The variety of imaging findings is not surprising given the varied

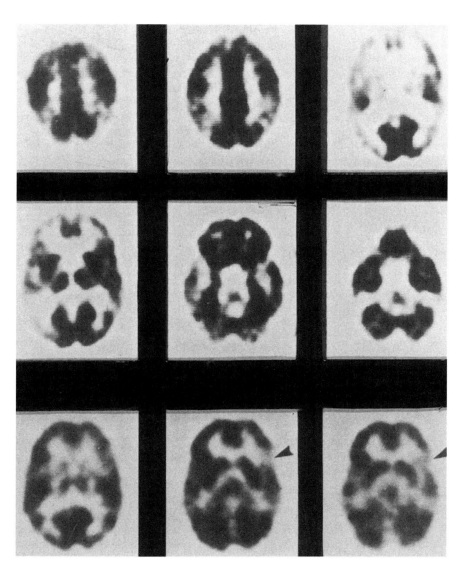

FIGURE 58.17. *Top* and *middle row:* In a child with Lennox-Gastaut seizures, the ¹⁸fluorodeoxyglucose positron emission tomography scan shows bilateral lateral diffuse hypometabolism in the frontal, temporal, and parietal cerebral cortex, when compared with the thalamus, basal ganglia, and cerebellum. *Bottom row:* In another child, there is only a single area of focal hypometabolism in the left frontal lobe (*arrows*). (From Chugani HT, Mazziotta JC, Engel J Jr et al. The Lennox-Gastaut syndrome: metabolic subtypes determined by 2-deoxy-2[¹⁸F] fluoro-D-glucose positron emission tomography. *Ann Neurol* 1987;21:4–13.)

seizure patterns in this syndrome; many clinicians feel that the Lennox-Gastaut syndrome is actually a heterogeneous group of seizure disorders. Some children have demonstrated unilateral focal decreased in rCMR$_{glc}$ (Fig. 58.17). Other children have had unilateral or bilateral diffuse reductions in rCMR$_{glc}$ (107). In another study, uptake patterns varied from patient to patient (108). In some institutions, the ^{18}FDG pattern of uptake can guide the type of surgical intervention performed (107). If there is a lateralized epileptiform discharge on EEG and unilateral diffuse hypometabolism on ^{18}FDG imaging, some have advocated cerebral hemispherectomy or corpus callosotomy, depending on the presence of hemiparesis. Patients with bilateral diffuse hypometabolism are only considered for corpus callosotomy if their seizure type is tonic or atonic drop attacks (91).

Other Pediatric Seizure Disorders

Landau-Kleffner Syndrome

In children with acquired epileptic aphasia (Landau-Kleffner syndrome), abnormalities in rCBF and rCMR$_{glc}$ have been

found most often in the temporal lobes and have been present unilaterally or more often both sides (109–111).

Epilepsy Associated with Tuberous Sclerosis

Tuberous sclerosis is an autosomal dominant disorder characterized by cutaneous abnormalities and tumors of the brain, eyes, heart, and kidneys. In the brain, abnormalities may include subependymal tubers (hamartomas), cortical tubers, heterotopic gray matter, and hypomyelination in white matter. MRI imaging often demonstrates multiple abnormalities of several types. Seizures are common and are often difficult to control.

^{18}FDG PET imaging demonstrates decreased uptake at sites where cortical tubers are seen on MRI (112). Multiple cortical tubers are typically present in patients with difficult to control seizures, and consequently the multiple areas of decreased ^{18}FDG uptake that are present fail to differentiate nonepileptogenic tubers from epileptogenic tubers. α-[^{11}C]methyl-L-tryptophan ([^{11}C]AMT), a radiopharmaceutical that accumulates in serotonergic terminals, has been used to identify epileptogenic tubers. The serotonin accumulates at the margin of the epileptogenic tubers. Resection of tubers and adjacent cortical margin, when increased [11C]AMT uptake and EEG abnormalities are present, has resulted in significantly improved seizure control in a small number of patients (112,113).

Partial or Complete Agenesis of the Corpus Callosum

In children with partial or complete agenesis of the corpus callosum and seizures, focal metabolic abnormalities can be present, regardless of whether electroencephalographic abnormalities are focal or widespread (114). Cortical abnormalities on MRI are present in only a minority of the patients studied.

Petit Mal Epilepsy

Petit mal epilepsy is associated with a normal interictal pattern of rCMR$_{glc}$, and the ictal change is a global increase in rCMR$_{glc}$ (115).

Sturge-Weber Syndrome

Sturge-Weber syndrome is characterized by a fifth cranial nerve distribution of a facial capillary nevus ("port-wine stain") and ipsilateral leptomeningeal angiomatosis. Other features that may be associated with Sturge-Weber syndrome are intracerebral calcifications, contralateral hemiparesis, hemiatrophy, glaucoma, and/or epilepsy. Mental retardation is felt to represent a sequela of long-term intractable epilepsy. Functional imaging demonstrates early functional cerebral changes before CT or MRI radiographic findings. 18FDG imaging reveals widespread unilateral cerebral hypometabolism ipsilateral to the facial nevus, except in infants younger than 1 year in whom interictal 18FDG PET imaging often shows a paradoxical hypermetabolism (20). In infants with early onset of intractable seizures and hemiparesis, hemispherectomy optimally performed in the first year of life can prevent progressive deterioration (91). Focal cortical resection may be beneficial for patients with more limited angioma and no hemiparesis (20).

DEVELOPMENTAL ANOMALIES

There is a definite role for functional imaging in developmental anomalies. The findings described in this section with 18FDG PET could also be evaluated with high-resolution SPECT.

Hemimegaloencephaly

Hemimegaloencephaly is a rare developmental brain malformation characterized clinically by varying degrees of developmental delay, hemiparesis, hemianopia, and neonatal epilepsy that often progresses to intractable epilepsy or status epilepticus. A subset of patients presents with body hemihypertrophy or an isolated unilateral somatic abnormality (116). Pathologically, there is congenital hypertrophy and hyperplasia of a cerebral

hemisphere, ipsilateral ventriculomegaly, lack of cortical neuronal layering, presence of giant neurons and neuronal heterotopias, and increased numbers of dendritic branches. Although seizure frequency usually decreases after surgical hemispherectomy, there often remains a poor developmental outcome. In children with hemimegaloencephaly and seizures, early evidence suggests that outcome after surgery may, in part, depend on the normality of the unaffected hemisphere on rCMR$_{glc}$ imaging (116).

Heterotopia

Heterotopia of gray matter is a rare embryologic developmental malformation in which ectopic cortex is found in the cerebral white matter secondary to migrational arrest of the neuroblasts as they move from mantle to the outer marginal layer of the neural tube. Agenesis of the corpus callosum, microgyria, congenital aqueduct stenosis, and cerebellar dysgenesis may be associated with gray matter heterotopia. Although in the past the diagnosis of cortical heterotopia was established with pneumoencephalography or CT, MRI is the current radiographic imaging choice. In difficult cases, functional imaging firmly establishes the diagnosis by demonstrating rCBF or rCMR$_{glc}$ uptake corresponding to the localization of the ectopic cortex (Fig. 58.18) (97, 117). Because many patients with cortical malformations have intractable seizures, if surgical resection is considered, functional imaging should be performed to evaluate for other functional areas of potential epileptogenic foci that could contraindicate surgery.

Successful drug therapy is reflected by improvement of the rCBF or rCMR$_{glc}$ imaging pattern (118).

Schizencephaly

Schizencephaly is another rare embryologic developmental malformation without gender predominance characterized by gross and microscopic structural defects of neural migration whereby a primitive four-layer cortical lamination lines a well-defined pial-ependymal cleft that extends from the pia arachnoid to the periventricular germinal area or ventricle primarily in the Rolandic and parasylvian areas. They are termed type 1 or "closed-lip" ("fused-lip") when the cleft edges are close together and type 2 or "open-lip" when the cleft edges are widely separated (Fig. 58.3). Although there was once debate in the literature as to the existence of unilateral schizencephalic clefts, it is now universally recognized that unilateral clefts are more common than bilateral clefts. Schizencephaly is associated with clinical manifestations, including mental retardation of varying severity, cerebral seizures, hemiparesis, hemiplegia, microgyria, agenesis of the pyramidal tracts, cerebellar hypoplasia, septo-optic dysplasia (Morsier syndrome), and other developmental abnormalities. However, clinical symptomatology depends upon the size, location, presence of other associated neuronal malformations, and whether there is a unilateral or bilateral cleft defect.

Although some patients with schizencephaly are asymptomatic, schizencephaly has been considered an area of primary epileptogenic focus. 18FDG PET imaging is helpful in the presurgical evaluation of these patients (119–122).

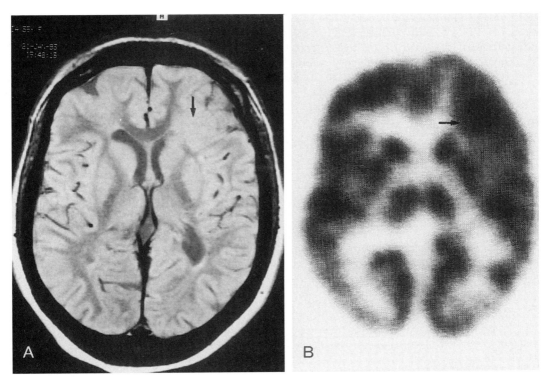

FIGURE 58.18. Heterotopia. **A:** The magnetic resonance image shows ectopic cortex in the white matter of the left frontal lobe (*arrow*). **B:** The ^{18}fluorodeoxyglucose (FDG) positron emission tomography image shows ^{18}FDG uptake (*arrow*) at the same level as normal cortex in the lesion seen on magnetic resonance imaging confirming the presence of ectopic cortex.

Porencephaly

Porencephalic cysts are encephaloclastic cavities developed in fetal life or early infancy that are believed to be secondary to ischemic insult to normal brain tissue. When a porencephalic cyst communicates with the subarachnoid space it can be confused with a schizencephalic cleft on MRI imaging. ^{18}FDG PET is helpful in identifying a gray-matter lining of the cleft and is critical in differentiating schizencephaly from porencephaly (Figs. 58.2 and 58.3). An accurate diagnosis of schizencephaly is important because of the poor prognosis and for genetic counseling, because the incidence of brain anomalies in subsequent siblings is increased and there are rare case reports of familial incidence.

BEHAVIORAL DISORDERS

A few reports of ^{18}FDG PET imaging have described investigations of children and adolescents with behavioral disorders. In infantile autism, most of the small number of children studied to date have had normal CT, MRI, and PET studies. However, neuronal migrational abnormalities (focal pachygyria) were demonstrated in some affected children associated with focal hypometabolism. In some cases, the MRI abnormalities were identified only after focal hypometabolism had been noted on PET (123).

In adolescents with attention deficit disorder (ADD) and

adults with ADD of childhood onset, rCMR$_{glc}$ is reduced in several areas of the brain. In adults, reductions in rCMR$_{glc}$ were noted in the premotor cortex and in the superior prefrontal cortex, which are areas considered to be in control of attention and motor activity (124). In teenagers, decreased metabolism in the left anterior frontal lobe was most closely correlated with the severity of symptoms (125). rCMR$_{glc}$ abnormalities on PET were not altered by acute stimulant therapy or clinically effective chronic stimulant therapy (126,127).

More interesting results have been obtained recently with SPECT, using radiopharmaceuticals that depict dopamine transporters, which were initially synthesized for the study of Parkinsonism. When adult patients with ADD were compared with control subjects, there was a 70% increase in striatal accumulation of an ^{123}I-labeled tropane derivative in the ADD patients (128). A ^{99m}Tc-labeled tropane derivative demonstrated a smaller increase in striatal uptake over controls, and this increase was blocked by methylphenidate (129).

GENETIC DISEASE AND INHERITED DISORDERS OF METABOLISM

Functional imaging studies with PET and SPECT are a useful research tool to investigate pathophysiologic mechanisms of these diseases and to detect and localize early changes in brain function before structural studies such as CT or MRI become abnormal. Preliminary PET studies were performed in some diseases affecting the brain: Huntington's disease (130–132), benign hereditary chorea (133), X-linked adrenoleukodystrophy (134), mitochondrial diseases (157), adenylsuccinase deficiency, and phenylalanine dehydrogenase deficiency or phenylketonuria (135).

IMAGING OF CEREBROSPINAL FLUID (CSF) SPACES

Imaging of CSF spaces has been discussed in Chapter 62.

ACKNOWLEDGMENT

The authors acknowledge the assistance of Bernadette Koch, MD, for her review of the original manuscript.

REFERENCES

1. Chugani HT, Phelps ME. Maturational changes in cerebral function in infants determined by ^{18}FDG positron emission tomography. *Science* 1986;231:840–843.
2. Chugani HT, Phelps ME, Mazziotta JC. Positron emission tomography study of human brain functional development. *Ann Neurol* 1987; 22:487–497.
3. O'Tuama LA, Phillips PC, Smith QR et al. L-Methionine uptake by human cerebral cortex: maturation from infancy to old age. *J Nucl Med* 1991;32:16–22.
4. Kerrigan JF, Chugani HT, Phelps ME. Regional cerebral glucose metabolism in clinical subtypes of cerebral palsy. *Pediatr Neurol* 1991; 7:415–425.
5. Volpe JJ, Herscovitch P, Perlman JM et al. Positron emission tomography in the asphyxiated term newborn: parasagittal impairment of cerebral blood flow. *Ann Neurol* 1985;17:287–296.
6. Volpe JJ, Herscovitch P, Perlman JM et al. Positron emission tomography in the newborn: extensive impairment of regional blood flow with intraventricular hemorrhage and hemorrhagic intracerebral involvement. *Pediatrics* 1983;72:589–601.
7. Powers WJ, Grubb RL, Darriet D et al. Cerebral blood flow and cerebral metabolic rate of oxygen requirements for cerebral function and viability in humans. *J Cereb Blood Flow Metab* 1985;5:600–608.
8. Altman DI, Powers WJ, Perlman JM et al. Cerebral blood flow requirement for brain viability in newborn infants is lower than in adults. *Ann Neurol* 1988;24:218–226.
9. Thorp PS, Levin SD, Garnett ES et al. Patterns of cerebral glucose metabolism using 18FDG and positron emission tomography in the neurologic investigation of the full term newborn infant. *Neuropediatrics* 1988;19:146–153.
10. Suhonen-Polvi H, Kero P, Korvenranta H et al. Repeated fluorodeoxyglucose positron emission tomography of the brain in infants with suspected hypoxic-ischaemic brain injury. *Eur J Nucl Med* 1993;20: 759–765.
11. Kumar P, Bederd MP, Shankaran S et al. Post extracorporeal membrane oxygenation single photon emission tomography (SPECT) as a predictor of neurodevelopmental outcome. *Pediatrics* 1994;93: 951–955.
12. Brott TG, Gelfand MJ, Williams CC et al. Frequency and patterns of abnormality detected by iodine-123 amine emission CT after cerebral infarction. *Radiology* 1986;158:729–734.
13. Feole JB, Ali A, Fordham EW et al. Serial SPECT imaging in moyamoya using I-123 IMP. A method of noninvasive follow-up and evaluation. *Clin Nucl Med* 1993;18:43–45.
14. Kuhl DE, Phelps ME, Kowell AP et al. Effects of stroke on local

15. Carter JC, Burt RW. Acetazolamide intervention for technetium-99m HMPAO SPECT brain imaging. *J Nucl Med Technol* 1992;20: 131–134.
16. Hoshi H, Ohnishi T, Jinnouchi S et al. Cerebral blood flow in patients with moyamoya disease evaluated by IMP SPECT. *J Nucl Med* 1994; 35:44–50.
17. Rodgers GP, Clark CM, Larson SM et al. Brain glucose metabolism in neurologically normal patients with sickle cell disease. Regional alterations. *Arch Neurol* 1988;45:78–82.
18. Szer IS, Miller JH, Rawlings DR et al. Cerebral perfusion abnormalities in children with central nervous system manifestations of lupus detected by single photon emission computed tomography. *J Rheumatol* 1993;20:2143–2148.
19. Homan RW, Devous MD Sr, Stokeley EM et al. Quantitation of intracerebral steal in patients with arteriovenous malformation. *Arch Neurol* 1986;43:779–785.
20. Chugani HT, Mazziota JC, Phelps ME. Sturge-Weber syndrome: a study of cerebral glucose utilization with positron emission tomography. *J Pediatr* 1989;114:244–253.
21. Park CH, Spitzer AR, Desai HJ et al. Brain SPECT in neonates following extracorporeal oxygenation: evaluation of technique and preliminary results. *J Nucl Med* 1992,33:1943–1948.
22. Mishkin F. Determination of cerebral death by radionuclide angiography. *Radiology* 1975;115:135–137.
23. Brill DR, Schwartz JA, Baxter JA. Variant flow patterns in radionuclide cerebral imaging performed for brain death. *Clin Nucl Med* 1985;10:346–352.
24. Spieth ME, Ansari AN, Kawada TK et al. Direct comparison of Tc-99m-DTPA and Tc-99m-HMPAO for the evaluating of brain death. *Clin Nucl Med* 1994;19:867–972.
25. Reid RH, Gulenchyn KY, Baillinger JR. Clinical use of technetium-99m HM-PAO for determination of brain death. *J Nucl Med* 1989; 30:1621–1626.
26. Laurin NR, Driedger AA, Hurwitz GA et al. Cerebral perfusion imaging with technetium-99m-HMPAO in brain death and severe central nervous system injury. *J Nucl Med* 1989;30:1627–1635
27. Reid RH, Gelfand MJ, Singh N. Tc-99m-HMPAO determination of brain death in children: uncoupling of flow and function. *J Nucl Med* 1993;34:52P(abst).
28. Abdel-Dayem HN, Sadek S, Kouris K et al. Changes in cerebral perfusion after acute head injury: comparison of CT with Tc-99m-SPECT. *Radiology* 1987;165:221–226.
29. Roper SN, Mena I, King WA et al. An analysis of cerebral blood flow in acute closed head injury using technetium-99m-HMPAO SPECT and computed tomography. *J Nucl Med* 1991;32:1684–1687.
30. Patronas NJ, DiChiro G, Brooks RA et al. Progress. [^{18}F]fluorodeoxyglucose and positron emission tomography in evaluation of radiation necrosis of the brain. *Radiology* 1982;144:885–889.
31. Francavilla TL, Miletich RS, DiChiro G et al. Positron emission tomography in the detection of malignant degeneration of low-grade gliomas. *Neurosurgery* 1989;24:1–5.
32. DiChiro G, Oldfield E, Wright DC et al. Cerebral necrosis after radiotherapy and/or intraarterial chemotherapy for brain tumors: PET and neuropathologic studies. *AJR* 1988;150:189–197.
33. Alavi JB, Alavi A, Chawluk J et al. Positron emission tomography in patients with glioma. A predictor of prognosis. *Cancer* 1988;62: 1074–1078.
34. DiChiro G, Brooks RA, Patronas NA et al. Issues in the in vivo measurement of glucose metabolism of human central nervous systems tumors. *Ann Neurol* 1984;15:5138–5146.
35. Kaplan WD, Takvorian T, Morris JH et al. Thallium-201 brain tumor imaging: a comparative study with pathological correlation. *J Nucl Med* 1987;28:47–52.
36. Kim KT, Black KL, Marciano D et al. Thallium-201 SPECT imaging of brain tumors: methods and results. *J Nucl Med* 1990;31:965–969.
37. Black KL, Hawkins RA, Kim KT et al. Use of thallium-201 SPECT to quantitate malignancy grade of gliomas. *J Neurosurg* 1989;71: 342–346.

38. Schwartz RB, Carvalho PA, Alexander E 3d et al. Radiation necrosis vs high-grade recurrent glioma: differentiation by using dual-isotope SPECT with 2°171 and 11-fc-HMPAO. *AJNR* 1991;12:1187–1192.
39. Burkard R, Kaiser KP, Wieler H et al. Contribution of thallium-201 SPECT to the grading of tumorous alterations of the brain. *Neurosurg Rev* 1992;15:265–275.
40. O'Tuama LA, Treves ST, Larar JN et al. Thallium-201 versus technetium-99m-MIBI SPECT in evaluation of childhood brain tumors: a within-subject comparison. *J Nucl Med* 1993;34:1045–1051.
41. Klethues P, Burger PC, Scheithauer BW. *The new WHO classification of brain tumors.* Berlin: Springer-Verlag, 1993.
42. Pollack IF. Brain tumors in children. *New Engl J Med* 1994;331:1500–1507.
43. Hoffman JM, Hanson MV, Friedman HS et al. FDG-PET in pediatric fossa brain tumors. *J Comput Assist Tomogr* 1992;16:62–68.
44. Holzer T, Hernoltz K, Jeske J et al. FDG-PET as a prognostic indicator in radiochemotherapy of glioblastoma. *J Comput Assist Tomogr* 1991;17:681–687.
45. Mountz JM, Stafford-Schuck K, McKeever PE et al. Thallium-201 tumor/cardiac ratio estimation of residual astrocytoma. *J Neurosurg* 1988;68:705–709.
46. Delbeke D, Meyerowitz C, Lapidus RL et al. Evaluation of brain tumors with ^{18}FDG-PET: optimal cut-off level for tumor/white matter FDG. *Radiology* 1995;195:47–51.
47. Schifter T, Hoffman JM, Hanson MW et al. Serial FDG-PET studies in the prediction of survival in patients with primary brain tumors. *J Comput Assist Tomogr* 1993;17:509–561.
48. Maria BL, Drane WE, Quisling RG et al. Value of thallium-201 SPECT imaging in childhood brain tumors. *Pediatr Neurosurg* 1994;20:11–18.
49. Ericsson K, Lilja A, Bergstrom M et al. (C-11-methyl)-L-methionine and C-11-diglucose in the diagnosis of intracranial tumors. *J Cereb Blood Flow Metab* 1985;5:551.
50. Biersack HJ, Coenen HH, Stöcklin G et al. Imaging of brain tumors with L-3-[″3I)iodo-methyltyrosine and SPECT. *J Nucl Med* 1989;30:110–112.
51. Mosskin M, von Holst H, Bergstrom M et al. Positron emission tomography with ^{11}C-methionine and computed tomography of intracranial tumours compared with histopathologic examination of multiple biopsies. *Acta Radiol* 1987;28:673–681.
52. Shishido F, Uemura K, Inugami A et al. Value of ^{11}C-methionine and PET in diagnosis of low grade gliomas. *Jpn J Nucl Med* 1990;27:293–302.
53. Wienhard K, Herholz L, Coenen HH et al. Increased amino acid transit transport into brain tumors measured by PET of L-(2-^{18}F)fluorotyrosine. *J Nucl Med* 1991;32:1338–1346.
54. Ogawa T, Shishido F, Kanno I et al. Cerebral glioma: evaluation with methionine PET. *Radiology* 1993;186:45–53.
55. Ogawa T, Kanno I, Shishido A et al. Clinical value of PET with ^{18}F-fluorodeoxyglucose and L-methyl-^{11}C-methionine for diagnosis of recurrent brain tumor and radiation injury. *Acta Radiol* 1991;32:197–202.
56. Ogawa T, Kanno I, Hatazawa J et al. Methionine PET for followup of radiation therapy of primary lymphoma of the brain. *Radiographics* 1994;14:101–110.
57. O'Tuama LA, Janicek MJ, Barnes PD et al. ^{201}Tl/^{99m}Tc HMPAO SPECT imaging of treated childhood brain tumors. *Pediatr Neurol* 1991;7:249–570.
58. Fulham MJ, Melisi JW, Nishimiya J et al. Neuroimaging of juvenile pilocytic astrocytomas: an enigma. *Radiology* 1993;189:221–225.
59. Chiron C, Ray N, Cusmai R et al. Morphological functional study in tuberous sclerosis: brain MRI/SPECT correlation. *Epilepsia* 1990;31:613–620.
60. Miller JH, Gelfand MJ. Central nervous system. In: Miller JH, Gelfand MJ, eds. *Pediatric nuclear imaging.* Philadelphia: WB Saunders, 1994:11–44.
61. Holthoff VA, Herholz K, Berthold F et al. In vivo metabolism of childhood posterior fossa tumors and primitive neuroectodermal tumors before and after treatment. *Cancer* 1993;72:1394–1403.
62. Lamberts SW, Hofland LJ, de Herder WW et al. Octreotide and

63. Bergstrom M, Muhr C, Lundberg PO et al. PET as a tool in the clinical evaluation of pituitary adenomas. *J Nucl Med* 1991;32:610–615.
64. De Souza B, Brunetti A, Fulham MJ et al. Pituitary microadenomas: a PET study. *Radiology* 1990;177:39–44.
65. Launes J, Nikkinen P, Lindroth L et al. Diagnosis of acute herpes encephalitis by brain perfusion single photon emission computed tomography. *Lancet* 1988;1:1188–1191.
66. Meyer MA, Hubner KF, Hunter K et al. Sequential positron emission tomographic evaluations of brain metabolism in acute herpes encephalitis. *J Neuroimaging* 1994;4:104–105.
67. Meyer MA. Focal high uptake of HM-PAO in brain perfusion studies: a clue in the diagnosis of encephalitis. *J Nucl Med* 1990;31:1094–1098.
68. Nara T, Nozaki H, Nishimoto H. Brain perfusion in acute encephalitis: relationship to prognosis studied using SPECT. *Pediatr Neurol* 1990;6:422–424.
69. O'Malley JP, Ziessman HA, Kumar PN et al. Diagnosis of intracranial lymphoma in patients with AIDS: value of ^{201}Tl single-photon emission tomography. *AJR* 1994;163:417–421.
70. Hoffman JM, Waskin HA, Schifter T et al. ^{18}FDG-PET in differentiating lymphoma from nonmalignant central nervous system lesions in patients with AIDS. *J Nucl Med* 1993;34:567–575.
71. Grimstead IA, Hirschberg H, Rootwelt K. ^{99m}Tc-hexamethylpropyleneamine oxime leukocyte scintigraphy and C-reactive protein levels in the differential diagnosis of brain abscesses. *J Neurosurg* 1992;77:732–736.
72. Palestro CJ, Swyer AJ, Kim CK et al. Role in In-111 labeled leukocyte scintigraphy in the diagnosis of intracerebral lesions. *Clin Nucl Med* 1991;16:305–308.
73. Schmidt KG, Rasmussen JW, Frederiksen PB et al. Indium-111-granulocyte scintigraphy in brain abscess diagnosis: limitations and pitfalls. *J Nucl Med* 1990;31:1121–1127.
74. Penfield W, von Santh K, Cipriani A. Cerebral blood flow during induced epileptiform, seizures in animals and man. *J Neurophysiol* 1939;2:257–267.
75. Engel J Jr, Kuhl DE, Phelps ME et al. Interictal cerebral glucose metabolism in partial epilepsy and its relation to EEG changes. *Ann Neurol* 1982;12:510–517.
76. Engel J Jr, Troupin AS, Crandall PH et al. Recent developments in the diagnosis and therapy of epilepsy. *Ann Intern Med* 1982;97:584–598.
77. Engel J Jr, Brown WJ, Kuhl DE et al. Pathologic findings underlying focal temporal lobe hypometabolism in partial epilepsy. *Ann Neurol* 1982;12:518–528.
78. Gelfand MJ, Stowens DW. I-123-iofetamine tomography in school age children with difficult to control epilepsy. *Clin Nucl Med* 1989;14:675–680.
79. Engel J Jr, Henry TR, Risinger MW et al. Presurgical evaluation for partial epilepsy: relative contributions of chronic depth electrode recordings versus FDG-PET and scalp-sphenoidal ictal EEG. *Neurology* 1990;40:1670–1677.
80. Mazziotta JC, Engel J Jr. The use and impact of positron computed tomography scanning in epilepsy. *Epilepsia* 1984;25:S86–S104.
81. Podreka I, Suess E, Goldenberg G et al. Initial experience with technetium-99m HM-PAO brain SPECT. *J Nucl Med* 1987;28:1657–1666.
82. Olson DM, Chugani HT, Shewmon DA et al. Electrocorticographic confirmation of focal positron emission tomographic abnormalities with intractable epilepsy. *Epilepsia* 1990;31:731–739.
83. Muzik O, Da Silva EA, Juhasz C et al. Intracranial EEG versus flumazenil and glucose PET in children with extratemporal epilepsy. *Neurology* 2000;54:171–179.
84. Van Huffelen AC, van Isselt JW, van Veeler CWM et al. Identification of the epileptic focus with [^{123}I]iomazenil SPECT. *Acta Neurochir* 1990;50(Suppl):95–99.
85. Adelson PD, Peacock WJ, Chugani HT et al. Temporal and extended

temporal resections for the treatment of intractable seizures in early childhood. *Pediatr Neurosurg* 1992;18:169–178.

86. Lee BI, Markand ON, Siddiqui AR et al. Single photon emission computed tomography (SPECT) brain imaging using N,N,N′-trimethyl-N′-trimethyl-N′-(2 hydroxy-3-methyl-5-[121]-iodobenzyl)1,3-propanediamine 2 HCl (HIPDM): intractable complex partial seizures. *Neurology (Minneap)* 1986;36:1471–1477.

87. Andersen AR, Rogvi-Hansen B, Dam M. Utility of SPECT of rCBF for focal diagnosis of the epileptogenic zones. *Acta Neurol Scand* 1994;152(Suppl):129–134.

88. Radtke RA, Hanson MW, Hoffman JM et al. Temporal lobe hypometabolism on PET: predictor of seizure control after temporal lobectomy. *Neurology* 1993;43:1088–1092.

89. Theodore WH, Dorwart R, Holmes M et al. Neuroimaging in refractory partial seizures: comparison of PET, CT, and MRI. *Neurology* 1986;36:750–759.

90. Latack J, Abou-Khalil BW, Siegel GJ et al. Patients with partial seizures: evaluation of MRI, CT, and PET imaging. *Radiology* 1986;159:159–163.

91. Chugani HT. The use of positron emission tomography in the clinical assessment of epilepsy. *Sem Nucl Med* 1992;22:247–253.

92. Rowe CC, Berkovic SF, Benjamin ST et al. Localization of epileptic foci with postictal single photon emission computed tomography. *Ann Neurol* 1989;26:660–668.

93. Rowe CC, Berkovic SF, McKay WJ et al. Patterns of postictal cerebral blood flow in temporal lobe epilepsy: qualitative and quantitative analysis. *Neurology* 1991;41:1096–1103.

94. Stefan H, Bauer J, Feistel H et al. Regional cerebral blood flow during focal seizures of temporal and frontocentral onset. *Ann Neurol* 1990;27:162–166.

95. Marks DA, Katz A, Hoffer P et al. Localization of extratemporal epileptic foci during ictal single photon emission computed tomography. *Ann Neurol* 1992;31:250–255.

96. Kuzniecky R, Mountz JM, Wheatley G et al. Ictal single photon emission computed tomography demonstrates localized epileptogenesis in cortical dysplasia. *Ann Neurol* 1993;34:627–631.

97. Henkes H, Hosten N, Cordes M et al. Increased rCBF in gray matter heterotopias detected by SPECT using ^{99m}Tc hexamethyl-propyleneamine oxime. *Neuroradiology* 1991;33:310–312.

98. Theodore WH, Sato S, Kufta C et al. Temporal lobectomy for uncontrolled seizures: the role of positron emission tomography. *Ann Neurol* 1992;32:789–794.

99. Chugani HT, Rintahaka PJ, Shewmon DA. Ictal patterns of cerebral glucose utilization in children with epilepsy. *Epilepsia* 1994;35:813–822

100. Chugani HT, Shewmon DA, Khanna DA et al. Interictal and postictal focal hypermetabolism on positron emission tomography. *Pediatr Neurol* 1993;9:10–15.

101. Shields WD, Shewmon DA, Chugani HT et al. Treatment of infantile spasms: medical or surgical? *Epilepsia* 1992;33(Suppl 4):526–531.

102. Chugani HT, Shields WD, Sherman DA et al. Infantile spasms: I. PET identifies focal cortical dysgenesis in cryptogenic cases for surgical treatment. *Ann Neurol* 1990;27:406–413.

103. Chugani HT, da Silva, Chugani DC. Infantile spasms: III. prognostic implications of bitemporal hypometabolism on positron emission tomography. *Ann Neurol* 1996;39:643–649.

104. Chugani HT, Shewmon DA, Shields WD et al. Surgery for intractable infantile spasms: neuroimaging perspectives. *Epilepsia* 1993;34:764–771.

105. Chugani HT, Conti VR. Etiologic classification of infantile spasms in 140 cases: role of positron emission tomography. *J Child Neurol* 1996;11:44–48.

106. Chugani HT, Shewmon DA, Peacock WJ et al. Surgical treatment of intractable neonatal-onset seizures: the role of positron emission tomography. *Neurology* 1988;38:1178–1188.

107. Chugani HT, Mazziotta JC, Engel J Jr et al. The Lennox-Gastaut syndrome: metabolic subtypes determined by 2-deoxy-2-[18F] fluoro-D-glucose positron emission tomography. *Ann Neurol* 1987;21:4–13.

108. Theodore WH, Rose D, Patronas N et al. Cerebral glucose metabolism in Lennox-Gastaut syndrome. *Ann Neurol* 1987;21:14–21.

109. Maquet P, Hirsch E, Dive D et al. Cerebral glucose utilization during sleep in Landau-Kleffner syndrome: a PET study. *Epilepsia* 1990;31:778–783.

110. Da Silva EA, Chugani DC, Chugani HT. Landau-Kleffner syndrome: metabolic abnormalities in temporal lobes are a common feature. *J Child Neurol* 1977;12:489–495.

111. O'Tuama LA, Urion DK, Janicek MJ et al. Regional cerebral perfusion in Landau-Kleffner syndrome and related childhood aphasias. *J Nucl Med* 1992;33:1758–1765.

112. Chugani DC, Chugani HT, Muzik O et al. Imaging epileptogenic tubers in children with tuberous sclerosis complex using beta-[11C]methyl-L-tryptophan positron emission tomography. *Ann Neurol* 1998;44:858–866.

113. Asano E, Chugani DC, Muzik O et al. Multimodality imaging for improved detection of epileptogenic foci in tuberous sclerosis complex. *Neurology* 2000;4:1976–1984.

114. Khanna S, Chugani HT, Messa C et al. Corpus callosum agenesis and epilepsy: PET findings. *Pediatr Neurol* 1994;10:221–227.

115. Engel JE Jr, Lubens P, Kuhl DE et al. Local cerebral metabolic rate for glucose during petit mal absences. *Ann Neurol* 1985;17:121–128.

116. Rintahaka PJ, Chugani HT, Messa C et al. Hemimegaloencephaly: evaluation with positron emission tomography. *Pediatr Neurol* 1993;9:21–28.

117. Bairamian D, Chiro GD, Theodore WH et al. MR imaging and positron emission tomography of cortical heterotopia. *J Comput Assist Tomogr* 1985;9:1137–1139.

118. Michihiro N, Ariizumi M, Shiihara H et al. Timecourse changes of regional cerebral blood flow by SPECT with N-isopropyl-p-[123]iodoamphetamine in childhood partial seizures. *Brain Dev* 1992;24:335–341.

119. Barkovich AJ, Norman D. MR of schizencephaly. *AJNR* 1988;9:297–302.

120. Barkovich AJ, Kjos B. Schizencephal: correlation of clinical findings with MR characteristics. *AJNR* 1992;13:85–94.

121. Leblanc R, Tampieri D, Robitaille Y et al. Surgical treatment of intractable epilepsy associated with schizencephaly. *Epilepsia* 1991;29:421–429.

122. Landy HJ, Ramsay E, Ajmone-Marsan C et al. Temporal lobectomy for seizures associated with unilateral schizencephaly. *Surg Neurol* 1992;37:477–481.

123. Schifter T, Hoffman JM, Haten HP Jr et al. Neuroimaging in infantile autism. *J Child Neurol* 1994;9:155–161.

124. Zametkin AJ, Nordahl TE, Gross M et al. Cerebral glucose metabolism in adults with hyperactivity of childhood onset. *N Engl J Med* 1990;323:1413–1415.

125. Zametkin AJ, Liebenbauer LL, Fitzgerald GA et al. Brain metabolism in teenagers with attention-deficit hyperactivity disorder. *Arch Gen Psychiatry* 1993;50:333–340.

126. Matochik JA, Liebenbauer LL, King AC et al. Cerebral glucose metabolism in adults with attention deficit hyperactivity disorder after chronic stimulant treatment. *Am J Psychiatry* 1994;151:658–664.

127. Matochik JA, Nordahl TE, Gross M et al. Effects of acute stimulant medication on cerebral metabolism in adults with hyperactivity. *Neuropsychopharmacology* 1993;8:377–386.

128. Dougherty DD, Bonab AA, Spencer TJ et al. Dopamine transporter density in patients with attention deficit hyperactivity disorder. *Lancet* 1999;354:2132–2133.

129. Dresel S, Krause J, Krause KH et al. Attention deficit hyperactivity disorder: binding of [99mTc]TRODAT-1 to the dopamine transporter before and after methylphenidate treatment. *Eur J Nucl Med* 2000;27:1518–1524.

130. Phelps ME, Mazziotta JC, Wapenski J et al. Cerebral glucose utilization and blood flow in Huntington's disease. *J Nucl Med* 1985;26:P47(abst).

131. Mazziotta JC, Phelps ME, Pahl JJ. Reduced cerebral glucose metabolism in asymptomatic subjects at risk for Huntington's disease. *N Engl J Med* 1987;316:357–362.

132. Sedvall G. Dopamine D1 receptor number–a sensitive PET marker for early brain deterioration in Huntington's disease. *Eur Arch Psychiatry Clin Neurosci* 1994;243:249–255.

133. Suchowersky O, Hayden MR, Martin WR et al. Cerebral metabolism of glucose in benign hereditary chorea. *Move Disord* 1986;1:33–44.

134. Berkovic SF, Carpenter S, Evans A et al. Myoclonus epilepsy and ragged-red fibers (MERRF). 1. A clinical, pathological, magnetic resonance spectrographic and positron emission study [Review]. *Brain* 1989;112:1231–1260.

135. De Volder AG, Jaeken J, Van den Berghe G et al. Regional brain glucose utilization in adenylosuccinase-deficient patients measured by positron emission tomography. *Pediatr Res* 1988;24:238–242.

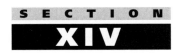

S E C T I O N

XIV

INFLAMMATION

59

GALLIUM-67 IMAGING IN INFECTION

RONALD D. NEUMANN
JOHN G. MCAFEE

MECHANISMS OF LOCALIZATION

[67]Ga acts biologically as an iron analog (1). When ^{67}Ga citrate is injected intravenously, the gallium is rapidly bound to transferrin (2,3). It was once thought that the major pathway of gallium localization in infection involved direct binding of radiogallium to circulating leukocytes (4,5), but this mechanism is now believed to play a relatively minor role (6). Nonetheless, leukocytes do play a significant role in gallium localization. Gallium, either bound to transferrin or in the ionic state in equilibrium with protein-bound gallium, probably diffuses through the loose endothelial junctions of capillaries at sites of inflammation and enters the extracellular fluid space (7). In inflammatory lesions, this space is rich in at least two types of iron-binding compounds. One is lactoferrin, which is elaborated primarily by leukocytes. The other is a class of low-molecular-weight compounds called *siderophores,* which are elaborated by bacteria (8).

Lactoferrin is contained within the specific granules of the leukocyte (9). When stimulated, the leukocyte either secretes the contents of the secondary granule into the extracellular space or disintegrates; the result is release of its contents (10). Lactoferrin has high affinity for ferric ion. Its physiologic role appears to be to bind any free ferric ion to inhibit bacterial growth (11). When lactoferrin is released at the site of inflammation, some becomes bound to the surface of lymphocytes and to tissue macrophages (12). Lactoferrin has a higher binding affinity for gallium than does transferrin at neutral and acid pH values. Thus gallium bound to transferrin will, in the presence of lactoferrin, preferentially bind to the latter (13). Lactoferrin-bound gallium may subsequently be transferred to other intracellular proteins, such as ferritin (11). Nonetheless, ^{67}Ga in inflammatory lesions is frequently found in the extracellular space in association with mucopolysaccharides (14). Pinocytosis and interaction of ^{67}Ga transferrin with specific cell-surface transferrin receptors may play a role in internalizing some of this extracellular gallium (15).

Secretory organs, such as the lacrimal glands, salivary glands, and breast, elaborate lactoferrin (16). Inflammatory processes in these organs may enhance lactoferrin production and result in increased gallium uptake, even in the absence of leukocytes. The female breast also produces large amounts of lactoferrin during milk production. Thus pregnancy and lactation usually are associated with markedly enhanced breast uptake of gallium (17).

Bacteria and other pathogenic microorganisms are capable of direct gallium uptake. This uptake is mediated through the action of siderophores, low-molecular-weight compounds that bind ferric ion and facilitate its intracellular incorporation. When iron binds to the siderophore, iron is transported into the cell, where it is subsequently released. Gallium also avidly binds to siderophores but is apparently not released once incorporated into the cell (18).

In summary, intravenous gallium leaks into areas of inflammation and becomes "bound" within these regions either by iron-binding proteins elaborated by inflammatory cells, siderophores produced by bacteria, or other metal-binding mucopolysaccharide proteins. The complex mechanism of gallium uptake in inflammatory lesions conveniently explains why gallium can be used in leukopenic patients (19) as well as in the detection of sterile abscesses (4).

Initially, after diffusion into inflammatory lesions, gallium is still in equilibrium with the blood pool. Within approximately 12 to 24 hours, the gallium becomes firmly bound within the lesion, and changes in gallium levels in the blood do not influence activity in the lesion (20). Investigators have attempted to use this tissue-binding effect to enhance clearance of gallium from the blood while not affecting activity in the lesion (20, 21). Unfortunately, gallium taken up by normal tissues also apparently becomes bound within 12 to 24 hours. Although techniques such as the use of desferrioxamine to stimulate urinary excretion of gallium do reduce the blood level, they do not significantly enhance detection of either inflammatory lesions or tumors.

TECHNIQUE

Authors generally recommend a dose of 5 mCi (185 MBq) of ^{67}Ga citrate for imaging of inflammatory lesions in adults. This dose provides high-count-density images at a reasonable radiation dose to the patient (22). Pediatric doses are proportionally smaller on the basis of the 5-mCi (185 MBq) dose to a 70-kg adult. When a specific anatomic region is to be examined,

R.D. Neumann: Chief, Nuclear Medicine Department Clinical Center, NIH, Bethesda, MD.
J.G. McAfee: Physician Emeritus, NMD Clinical Center, NIH, Bethesda, MD.

tomographic images are preferred (23). These are best obtained with single photon emission computed tomographic (SPECT) instruments and multiple energy windows (24). Triple windows centered on the 93-, 185-, and 296-keV peaks are generally used with medium- to high-energy collimators. Regional, whole-body, or SPECT images can be obtained depending on the clinical indication.

Although early imaging has been advocated (24), most clinics do not generally perform imaging sooner than 18 to 24 hours after administration of the radiogallium. Earlier images contain high background activity that can mask lesions to produce false-negative results. The major single problem with radiogallium imaging of the abdomen is differentiating normal bowel activity from inflammatory lesions. Bowel preparation does not always eliminate intraluminal gallium activity (25). If confusion exists in interpretation of the 24-hour image because of either high background activity or bowel activity, delayed images can be obtained up to 1 week or more after injection of the radiogallium. Activity in the intestinal lumen usually at least moves on delayed images, and background activity typically diminishes to a visual optimum within 72 to 96 hours.

If hepatic lesions are suspected, a ^{99m}Tc sulfur colloid liver scanning should be performed before the injection of radiogallium (22). Because the liver is gallium-avid, hepatic abscesses can have gallium uptake equal to but not exceeding that of normal liver. These lesions can produce a "normal"-appearing liver if only the gallium scan is viewed. The ^{99m}Tc colloid scan disclose lesions such as "cold" areas. Any cold lesion on a ^{99m}Tc colloid scan that fills in on a gallium scan should be considered positive with regard to gallium uptake (Fig. 59.1).

Abdomen

Although ^{67}Ga was first evaluated as a tumor-scanning agent (26), its value for detection of inflammatory lesions was soon recognized (27), especially for detecting otherwise occult abdominal infections (28). Early investigators achieved approximately 90% sensitivity and specificity with this method of detecting intraabdominal abscesses (28–30). In prospective series, the sensitivity was usually approximately 80% (31,32).

To interpret gallium scans of the abdomen most effectively, it is necessary that one have an appreciation of abdominal anatomy, especially the attachments of the intraabdominal organs and mesentery to the posterior abdominal wall. These attachments serve as natural barriers to the spread of intraabdominal infection. Meyers (33) carefully reviewed abdominal anatomy. He described the intraabdominal cavity as divided by the mesocolic ligament (which attaches the transverse colon to the posterior peritoneum) into supramesocolic and inframesocolic spaces. The inframesocolic space is further divided by the root of the mesentery and the posterior attachments of the ascending and descending colon into four regions. The regions between the colon and mesenteric root are referred to as the *right and left inframesocolic spaces,* and the regions between the colon and lateral abdominal wall are described as the paracolic gutters. All of the inframesocolic spaces communicate inferiorly with the paracolic pelvic space and the pouch of Douglas in women (Fig. 59.2). The superior extent of the left paracolic gutter is limited

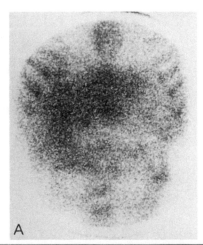

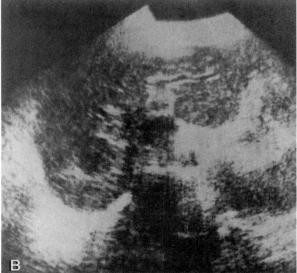

FIGURE 59.1. Hepatic abscess. **A:** Scintiphotograph of anterior abdomen shows relatively homogenous ^{67}Ga distribution in the liver except for the photopenic area near the confluence of the hepatic veins and inferior vena cava. The patient has diverticulitis of the colon with hepatic abscesses. One of the abscesses appears cold on this ^{67}Ga scan, whereas a second, located in the lower part of the right hepatic lobe **(B)**, fills in with activity similar to that of normal liver. No ^{99m}Tc sulfur colloid study was performed.

by the phrenicocolic ligament. No such anatomic barrier separates the right paracolic space from the supramesocolic region, and it often acts as a conduit for infection to spread from inframesocolic to supramesocolic areas. At its superior extent, the right paracolic gutter communicates freely with the posterior infrahepatic space, commonly called *Morrison's pouch.* The supramesocolic region is divided by midline structures, including the falciform ligament, into right and left regions.

The right supracolic space is occupied primarily by the liver, which is fixed posteriorly to the posterior peritoneum by a reflection of the hepatic capsule. There is no attachment between the liver and the superior aspect of the diaphragm. The peritoneal space of the right supramesocolic region is divided by the liver into a broad suprahepatic, subdiaphragmatic space and an anterior and posterior subhepatic space, the latter being Morison's

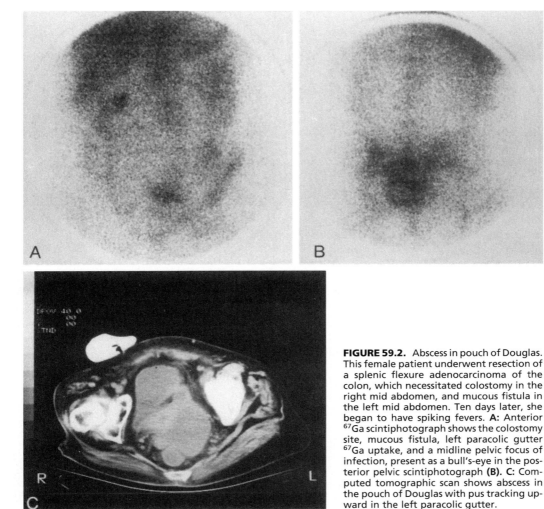

FIGURE 59.2. Abscess in pouch of Douglas. This female patient underwent resection of a splenic flexure adenocarcinoma of the colon, which necessitated colostomy in the right mid abdomen, and mucous fistula in the left mid abdomen. Ten days later, she began to have spiking fevers. **A:** Anterior ⁶⁷Ga scintiphotograph shows the colostomy site, mucous fistula, left paracolic gutter ⁶⁷Ga uptake, and a midline pelvic focus of infection, present as a bull's-eye in the posterior pelvic scintiphotograph **(B). C:** Computed tomographic scan shows abscess in the pouch of Douglas with pus tracking upward in the left paracolic gutter.

pouch and abutting the retroperitoneum over the superior pole of the right kidney. Morison's pouch, which is a dependent area when supine, communicates with the right paracolic gutter, suprahepatic space, and anterior subhepatic space. It is a major site of remote abscess formation.

The anterior infrahepatic space is adjacent to the gallbladder and has a potential communication with the lesser sac through the foramen of Winslow. This narrow communication site often is sealed off by tissue edema before infection can spread through it.

The left supramesocolic space includes anterior and posterior components, the latter usually referred to as the *lesser sac.* The two regions are separated in the subdiaphragmatic region by the coronary ligament, from which the left hepatic lobe (medial segment) is suspended and attached to the dome of the left hemidiaphragm. The anterior space is poorly defined, but the lesser sac is well demarcated by surrounding structures, which include the stomach, transverse mesocolon, posterior peritoneum, spleen and its ligamentous attachments, and posterior aspect of the left hemidiaphragm (Fig. 59.3).

There are three basic types of intraabdominal inflammatory

processes: abscesses, cellulitis (phlegmon), and peritonitis. An abscess is an anatomically well-demarcated lesion with a discrete wall and cavity containing microorganisms and, often, necrotic tissue debris. Abscesses are detectable with ultrasonography, computed tomography (CT), and magnetic resonance imaging as well as with gallium imaging, because they not only are "functional" lesions but also are anatomically defined. Abscesses can occur within intraabdominal organs or in the peritoneal spaces. They usually are confined to specific regions, as defined by the posterior peritoneal attachments.

Cellulitis (phlegmon) is an inflammatory lesion limited to a specific anatomic site but without a well-defined or circumscribed border. A phlegmon has no discrete central cavity but represents focal tissue inflammation. Such lesions may not be detectable with ultrasonography or CT because of the absence of discrete anatomic features.

Peritonitis is diffuse inflammation that involves the entire or large portions of the peritoneal cavity. It often cannot be detected with ultrasonography and CT and is not confined by the anatomic barriers of the posterior peritoneal attachments.

Because the gallium scan is a detector of microbial presence

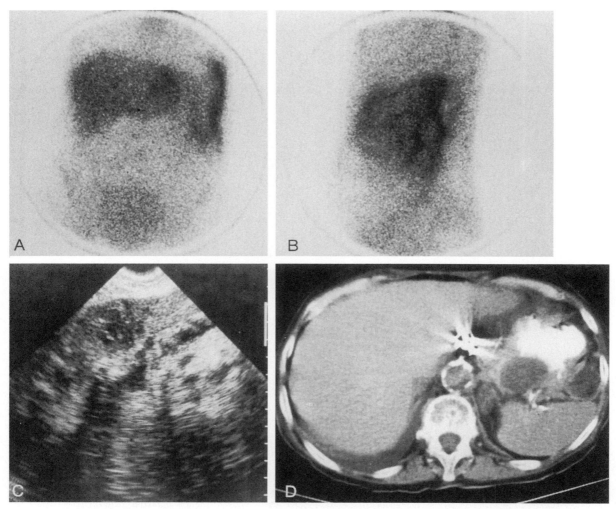

FIGURE 59.3. Infection of the anterior supramesocolic space. A 78-year-old woman presented with vague pain in the left upper quadrant of the abdomen. Anterior **(A)** and left lateral **(B)** ⁶⁷Ga scintiphotographs show intense ⁶⁷Ga concentration in the left upper quadrant of the abdomen, including the left lobe of the liver. At laparotomy a gastric ulcer was found that had perforated to produce infection of the lesser sac, peripancreatic retroperitoneum, and left paracolic gutter. Ultrasound **(C)** and computed tomographic images **(D)** show the ulcer also produced intrahepatic abscesses.

and the body's inflammatory response, it can be used to detect abscess, cellulitis, and peritonitis. These lesions can, however, be differentiated according to their appearance and correlative imaging information (34). Lesions that are confined to specific organs, regions, or peritoneal spaces usually are abscesses (Fig. 59.4). However, if the margins of such lesions are not defined by anatomic images, cellulitis should be suspected. Diffuse distribution of activity throughout the abdominal cavity, especially extending along the lateral border of the right lobe of the liver and into the right subdiaphragmatic region, should be considered peritonitis (34) (Fig. 59.5). Peritonitis in moribund patients occasionally produces a border-like pattern outlining the peripheral margins of the peritoneal cavity and leaving a central lucent area consisting primarily of dilated loops of intestine.

The limitations of gallium imaging include the 24-hour or more delay between injection and imaging, poor spatial defini-

tion of anatomically discrete lesions, and possible misinterpretation as a result of gallium uptake in adjacent organs, especially the liver, or failure to clear intraluminal gallium from the intestine. A ⁹⁹ᵐTc sulfur colloid liver-spleen scan is recommended if intrahepatic abscess is suspected, because the abscess can have gallium uptake equal to, but not exceeding, that of the liver and therefore be undetectable on a gallium scan alone. Although bowel preparation can minimize the amount of intraluminal gallium, it is not always effective or possible. ¹¹¹In-labeled leukocytes have the advantages of not localizing in normal intestine or in the normal urinary tract (see Chapter 60).

Abdominal gallium scans usually do not differentiate pancreatitis from focal pancreatic abscess formation. In both disorders, part or all of the pancreas localizes gallium (35). Abdominal gallium scanning can be helpful in the detection of acute cholecystitis and ascending cholangitis (Fig. 59.6). Gallium imaging

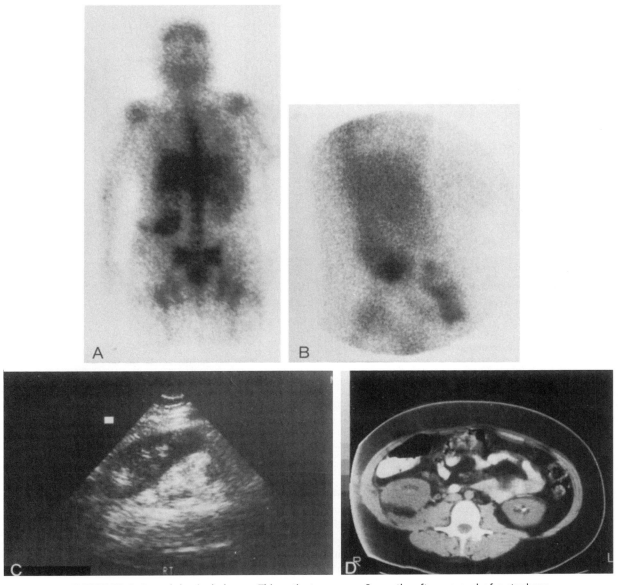

FIGURE 59.4. Intraabdominal abscess. This patient was seen 3 months after removal of a staghorn calculus of the right kidney. Fever prompted this ^{67}Ga study (posterior PhoCon image **[A]** and right lateral gamma-camera image **[B]**), which depicted a perinephric abscess adjacent to the inferior pole of the right kidney. **A:** A band of ^{67}Ga activity extends toward the right flank; this was a sinus track. Ultrasound **(C)** and computed tomographic **(D)** studies also depict this abscess.

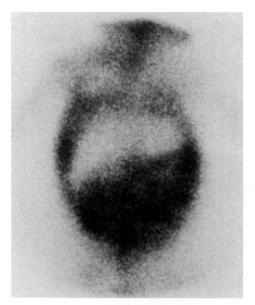

FIGURE 59.5. Peritonitis. Anterior ^{67}Ga gamma-camera image of a very ill child shows a dramatic example of diffuse peritonitis. Radiogallium is concentrated along the lateral and diaphragmatic borders of the liver, which appears "cold" in this image, along both paracolic gutters, and diffusely throughout the abdomen and pelvis.

also can be useful in the detection of abscess formation in Crohn's disease (36) (Fig. 59.7). Whereas a positive scan result is nonspecific, a negative result almost excludes the presence of an abscess.

Bone

Gallium scanning can be a useful adjunctive procedure in the diagnosis of both acute and "chronic" osteomyelitis (more accurately, osteomyelitis in traumatized bone) as well as joint and disk infections (37–41). Suspected acute osteomyelitis is best evaluated with radiography of the suspected site of infection followed by bone scanning. Radiography is insensitive in the detection of early lesions, but abnormal results establish the diagnosis. The bone scan is considerably more sensitive. It is also useful in the detection of unsuspected secondary sites of involvement, which occur in as many as 20% of patients with hematogenous spread of osteomyelitis. However, bone scan results are negative in 10% to 30% of infants and young children with acute osteomyelitis (42,43). In these cases, the ^{67}Ga scan is particularly useful in establishing the presence of infection (Fig. 59.8). The ^{67}Ga scan is very sensitive in the detection of acute osteomyelitis (40). The limitations for this application are the 24-hour delay required between administration of the radionuclide and imaging, occasional false-positive results due to inability to differentiate activity in bone and activity in adjacent joints or soft tissues, and a somewhat higher radiation dose delivered to the patient. We recommend, for the diagnosis of acute osteomyelitis, that radiographs and a bone scan be obtained first. In most cases, the results establish the diagnosis with minimum delay and expense. If the results of these studies are normal, but osteomyelitis is clearly present because of the clinical presentation, surgical

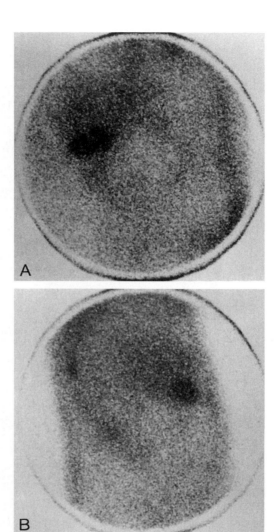

FIGURE 59.6. Cholecystitis. Anterior **(A)** and right lateral **(B)** gamma camera scintiphotographs show uptake of radiogallium 24 hours after administration in a patient with acute cholecystitis. This was an unsuspected finding because the patient had chronic alcoholism and presented with new onset of fever, ascites, and septicemia.

drainage and cultures should be considered (42). If the diagnosis is less clear and it is believed from a clinical standpoint that a 24-hour delay in starting treatment can be tolerated, a ^{67}Ga scan or radiolabeled leukocyte scan can be performed (44). Almost everything stated regarding acute osteomyelitis can be applied to the diagnosis of acute joint and disk infection (38,40). Unfortunately, results of a ^{67}Ga scan can be falsely positive in acute inflammatory joint disease of noninfectious origin (e.g., rheumatoid arthritis) (45).

^{67}Ga scintigraphy is useful in the diagnosis of chronic osteomyelitis, but the sensitivity and specificity are lower than in the diagnosis of acute osteomyelitis. Although radiographs and bone scans should be obtained for patients with suspected chronic osteomyelitis, results of these studies are invariably positive even when active infection is not present. However, the studies are necessary for interpretation of the ^{67}Ga scan. Rosenthall et al. (39) described two criteria for a positive result of a ^{67}Ga scan

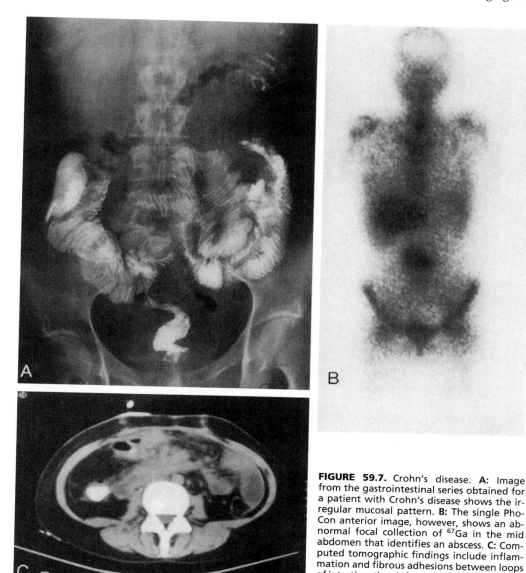

FIGURE 59.7. Crohn's disease. **A:** Image from the gastrointestinal series obtained for a patient with Crohn's disease shows the irregular mucosal pattern. **B:** The single PhoCon anterior image, however, shows an abnormal focal collection of ^{67}Ga in the mid abdomen that identifies an abscess. **C:** Computed tomographic findings include inflammation and fibrous adhesions between loops of intestine, the abdominal wall, and the posterior peritoneal surface.

in the presence of violated bone: The ^{67}Ga uptake must be either equal or greater in intensity than the uptake of radionuclide on a bone scan, and the pattern of ^{67}Ga uptake must be disparate from the pattern of uptake on a bone scan. Some physicians relax these criteria to include in the positive category ^{67}Ga uptake that is slightly less intense than that seen on a bone scan but still "significantly" hot. These criteria conform more or less to the patterns associated with active disease described by Tumeh et al. (46). Noninfected traumatized bone occasionally produces "false-positive" gallium scans.

The bone and ^{67}Ga scan combination is useful in evaluating suspected chronic osteomyelitis in patients with diabetes (39, 47), patients with fractures or recent surgical procedures involving bone, and patients with suspected reinfection. Some authors have advocated ^{67}Ga imaging for evaluation of infections associated with prostheses (41,48,49). ^{67}Ga imaging sometimes can be useful in gauging the adequacy of antibiotic therapy in eradi-

cating osteomyelitis (50). This is especially true when no radiographically detectable changes have occurred (51) (Fig. 59.9).

Pulmonary

Gallium is used in the evaluation of numerous pulmonary diseases with associated inflammation (52–56). In the evaluation of pulmonary uptake of ^{67}Ga, certain cautions should be observed. Faint ^{67}Ga uptake 24 hours after injection may be seen in healthy persons (57). The 48-hour postinjection image therefore should be used for quantitative assessment. Also, SPECT sometimes produces a "smear" of bone activity on some views that simulates increased pulmonary uptake. Bilateral breast uptake of gallium usually is normal; symmetric breast activity may occur in as many as 10% to 15% of premenopausal women. Increased breast uptake has been seen in patients taking a number of drugs or hormones (58).

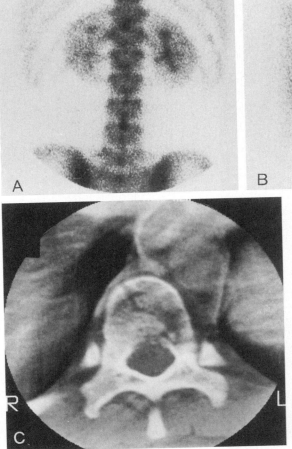

FIGURE 59.8. Osteomyelitis. These studies were performed on a 34-year-old man with persistent fever, anemia, and elevated leukocyte count who reported back pain. **A:** Posterior spinal image from a ^{99m}Tc methylene diphosphonate bone scan did not provide enough information for a diagnosis. The T11 and L3 spinous processes were found to have only minimally increased activity. Findings on thoracic and lumbar radiographs were normal. **B:** ^{67}Ga image shows increased activity in the body of T10. **C:** Computed tomographic scan shows abnormality in T10. Results of surgical biopsy confirmed the diagnosis of acute and chronic osteomyelitis in the body of T10, but no organism was identified in cultures.

In most circumstances, chest radiography is superior to ^{67}Ga imaging in detection of subtle anatomic changes that help in differentiation and staging of disease. However, there are some pulmonary diseases in which early or even chronic inflammatory conditions are not radiographically evident or in which chronic radiographic changes obscure assessment of the activity of the disease.

^{67}Ga imaging is particularly useful in the early diagnosis of opportunistic infections such as *Pneumocystis carinii* (53,59) and cytomegalovirus (60) infections in immunosuppressed hosts (Fig. 59.10). Such patients with clinical symptoms of upper respiratory infection may have significant pulmonary involvement in the absence of radiographic changes. Although a positive result of a ^{67}Ga scan in these circumstances is nonspecific (61) (e.g., it does not help differentiate one infection from another), it can be used as an early indicator or screen for such infections.

^{67}Ga uptake in the lung can occur in pulmonary toxicity caused by a number of chemotherapeutic agents as well as other drugs, including bleomycin, busulfan, nitrofurantoin, nitrosourea, cyclophosphamide, methotrexate, and amiodarone (61–64). This gallium uptake can occur in the absence of radiographic abnormalities.

^{67}Ga imaging has been investigated for the staging of idiopathic pulmonary fibrosis. The extent of ^{67}Ga uptake correlates well with the neutrophil content of bronchial lavage fluid (65) and presumably with the stage of activity of disease. Thus ^{67}Ga scanning has been advocated as a substitute for periodic lavage in the assessment of disease activity and effects of treatment. Unfortunately, the relative ^{67}Ga pulmonary uptake is not useful in the prediction of clinical outcome (65).

^{67}Ga imaging has been advocated for the assessment of the activity of disease in sarcoidosis (66). Most but not all investigators find good correlation between gallium lung uptake and lymphocyte content in lavage fluid (66,67). Thus gallium uptake presumably correlates with the level of active alveolitis. However, Abe et al. (68) found in a study with 26 patients who underwent transbronchial lung biopsy that quantitative assessment of pulmonary uptake of ^{67}Ga correlated primarily with granuloma formation rather than with alveolitis. Their data suggested that gallium uptake reflects more advanced, chronic changes. Nonetheless, Baughman et al. (69) and Lawrence et al. (70) reported that results of ^{67}Ga scanning are useful for predicting response to glucocorticoid therapy.

^{67}Ga imaging is useful in the early detection of inflammatory

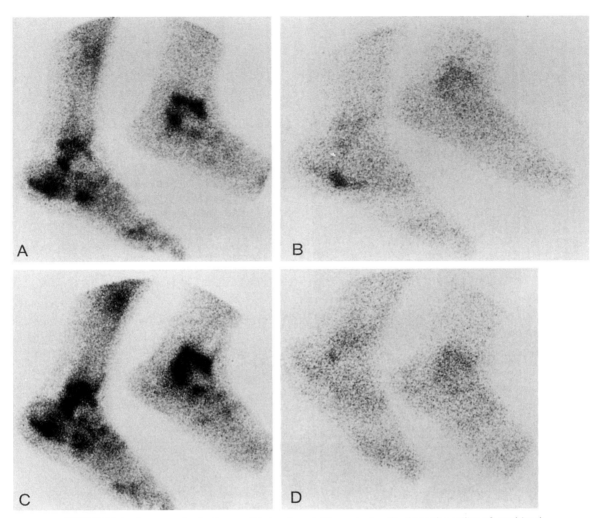

FIGURE 59.9. Assessment of osteomyelitis treatment. These studies illustrate the utility of combined 99mTc methylene diphosphonate (MDP) and 67Ga scintigraphy for monitoring osteomyelitis in patients with traumatized bone. In this case, the patient had attempted suicide by jumping from a building. **A:** MDP study performed at initial presentation. **B:** 67Ga image obtained 1 week later shows focal uptake in the right calcaneus representing a focus of osteomyelitis. The radiographs at this time showed the effects of multiple trauma to both ankles and feet. In the fifth week of antibiotic therapy, the scintigraphic studies were repeated. **C:** The first MDP image is technically slightly darker but continues to be abnormal in the multiple trauma sites and in the focus of osteomyelitis. **D:** 67Ga image obtained 2 days later indicates resolution of the calcaneal osteomyelitis.

changes of asbestosis (71). Gallium imaging has been described as useful in differentiating infiltrates due to pulmonary infarction from those due to pneumonia (72). ^{67}Ga uptake is rare in pure pulmonary infarction but common in pneumonia (73).

Renal Disease

Renal uptake of ^{67}Ga is a normal finding during the first 24 to 48 hours after administration of radionuclide because 10% to 25% of the activity is excreted in the urine (17). On images obtained with current ^{67}Ga scintigraphic methods 48 hours or more after injection, faint renal activity usually is present (74). However, unilateral or focal uptake in the kidneys almost always is associated with renal disease.

Increased ^{67}Ga localization in the kidneys is a nonspecific

finding that has been described in vicarious excretion, infection, acute tubular necrosis, nephritis, rejection, amyloidosis, and tumor infiltration (75–77). The nonspecificity of this finding, combined with the existence of alternative reliable methods of establishing specific diagnosis, limits this use of ^{67}Ga imaging.

In one form of renal infection, however, ^{67}Ga imaging has been useful (78). Acute focal bacterial nephritis, also known as acute lobar nephronia, is an inflammatory condition of bacterial origin that can be difficult to diagnose. The disease occurs most commonly among persons with diabetes and is believed to result from reflux of urine that contains bacteria into the renal papillae. The clinical manifestations vary from those of pyelonephritis to those of apparent renal abscess or tumor. Intravenous pyelography often shows a discrete mass, and ultrasonography may show only subtle changes such as loss of the corticomedullary border.

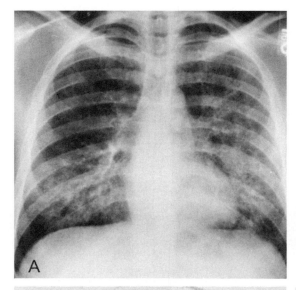

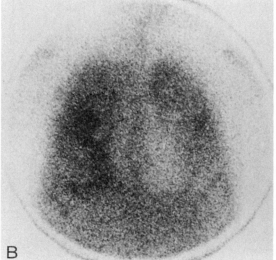

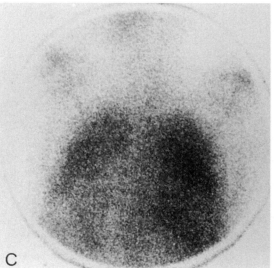

FIGURE 59.10. Opportunistic pulmonary infection. **A:** Chest radiograph of a patient with acquired immunodeficiency syndrome shows a reticular infiltrate that raised concern that an opportunistic pulmonary infection had developed. Anterior **(B)** and posterior **(C)** 48-hour ⁶⁷Ga scintiphotographs clearly show extensive involvement of both lungs by the infection.

At angiography, the renal arteries rarely are distorted, although the renal veins may be displaced. On ⁶⁷Ga scans, one of two patterns usually is observed (78). Either there is unilateral diffuse renal uptake (Fig. 59.11) or multifocal unilateral or bilateral uptake that is more extensive than the involvement suggested with other imaging modalities. The combination of ultrasound and ⁶⁷Ga scan findings usually establishes the diagnosis.

Acquired Immunodeficiency Syndrome

The diagnosis of human immunodeficiency virus infection is confirmed primarily by means of immunoassay, Western blot tests, and depression of the T-cell helper-suppressor lymphocyte ratio (CD4/CD8 ratio normally 0.8 to 2.9). Radionuclide imaging can be helpful in the diagnosis of many of the myriad complications of AIDS. Excellent reviews on this subject have been published by Vanarthos et al. (79) and Miller (80), but we high-

light some of the particular applications of gallium scintigraphy in this disease.

A common infectious complication of AIDS is *P. carinii* pneumonia (PCP), which typically causes diffuse bilateral increased uptake of ⁶⁷Ga (Fig. 59.10). Diffuse pulmonary infiltrates may or not be visible radiographically. When this infection is managed by means of inhalation of antimicrobial agents, follow-up gallium images may show increased uptake only in the upper lung fields, because the gas and aerosol exchange there is not as great as in the lower lung fields. ¹³³Xe ventilation and ⁹⁹ᵐTc macroaggregated albumin images sometimes show pneumatoceles associated with PCP.

Diffuse pulmonary uptake of ⁶⁷Ga in children with AIDS is frequently caused by lymphocytic interstitial pneumonitis (81). This condition usually has an insidious onset with salivary gland swelling, digital clubbing, extensive lymphadenopathy, frequent splenomegaly, and sometimes coarse nodular pulmonary inter-

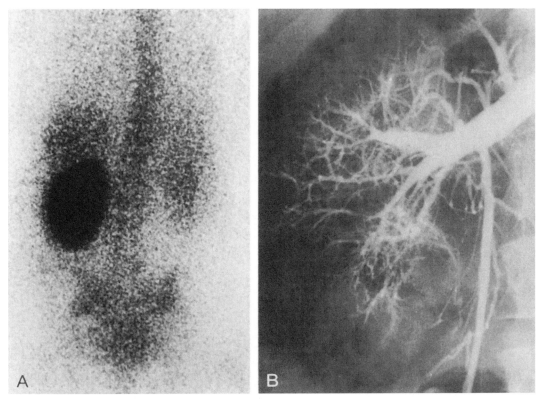

FIGURE 59.11. Acute focal bacterial nephritis. **A:** Posterior PhoCon image shows intense diffuse ^{67}Ga accumulation in the entire right kidney as described for acute lobar nephronia. **B:** Venous contrast image of the same kidney shows displaced veins; this finding suggests a more discrete inflammatory process.

stitial infiltrates on radiographs. Biopsy shows nodular peribronchial lymphocytic infiltration. There may be mediastinal widening and prominent hila in addition to the diffuse pulmonary parenchymal uptake of gallium. However, the pulmonary uptake tends to be not as marked as in PCP (79).

In cytomegalovirus infection, typically there is slight perihilar activity. Eye uptake can be the result of retinitis, and adrenal involvement not infrequently produces increased uptake. In PCP and other diffuse infections, hepatic uptake often is depressed and accompanied by increased pulmonary activity. As a result, lung-to-liver uptake ratios tend to be abnormally high.

Localized or regional increased lung uptake of gallium can be caused by bacterial pneumonia but sometimes occurs in PCP (82). Nodal or perihilar uptake is commonly caused by *Mycobacterium avium-intracellulare* infection but also can occur with *Mycobacterium tuberculosis* infection. These inflammatory nodes usually can be differentiated from the contiguous more bulky mass of lymphoma complicating AIDS. In infections associated with AIDS, findings on ^{201}Tl images typically are normal, and those on ^{67}Ga images are abnormal. However, in Kaposi sarcoma, results of gallium imaging typically are negative and those of thallium imaging typically are positive (83). AIDS-related myocarditis or pericarditis can produce increased cardiac gallium uptake.

Almost one half of all patients AIDS who have increased salivary uptake of gallium have diffuse infiltrative lymphocytosis

syndrome (DILS) (84). In the remaining patients, the increased uptake can be caused by undifferentiated salivary gland disease or AIDS itself. The increased uptake then is generally not as intense as in DILS. The CD8 cell counts are markedly elevated and the CD4 counts moderately reduced in DILS. In contrast, AIDS patients have normal CD8 counts and markedly reduced CD4 counts.

In AIDS nephropathy, bilateral diffusely increased uptake of gallium may be present in some patients (79) but not in others (85). Twelve percent to 55% of patients with AIDS (average, approximately 30%) have acute renal failure with a rapid progression of disease (86).

SUMMARY

A sound understanding of the mechanisms by which the various radiopharmaceutical preparations for the evaluation of inflammation localize such lesions is the best guide to proper application.

ACKNOWLEDGMENT

The authors wish to acknowledge their gratitude to Paul B. Hoffer, MD, for his role in exciting their interest in the role of gallium as a radiopharmaceutical. Dr. Hoffer was our mentor, collaborator, and coauthor on many occasions, and we miss him.

REFERENCES

1. Hoffer PB. Gallium: mechanisms. *J Nucl Med* 1980;21:282.
2. Hara T. On the binding of gallium to transferrin. *Int J Nucl Med Biol* 1974;1:152.
3. Hartman RE, Hayes RL. Gallium binding by blood serum. *Fed Proc* 1967;26:780(abst).
4. Burleson RL, Holman BL, Tow DE. Scintigraphic demonstration of abscesses with radioactive gallium labeled leukocytes. *Surg Gynecol Obstet* 1975;141:379.
5. Gelrud LG, Arseneau JC, Milder MS, et al. The kinetics of 67-gallium incorporation into inflammatory lesions: experimental and clinical studies. *J Lab Clin Med* 1974;83:489.
6. Tsan MF, Chen WY, Schefel U, et al. Studies on gallium accumulation in inflammatory lesions, I: gallium uptake by human polymorphonuclear leukocytes. *J Nucl Med* 1978;19:36.
7. Tzen KY, Oster ZH, Wagner HN Jr, et al. Role of iron binding proteins and enhanced capillary permeability on the accumulation of gallium-67. *J Nucl Med* 1980;21:31.
8. Nielands JB. Siderophores: biochemical ecology and mechanism of iron transport of enterobacteria. In: Raymond KN, ed. *Bioinorganic chemistry II: advanced chemistry series.* Vol. 162. Washington, DC: American Chemical Society, 1977:3.
9. Esaguy N, Aguas AP, Silva MT. High resolution localization of lactoferrin in human neutrophils. *J Leukoc Biol* 1989;46:51–62.
10. Wang-Iverson P, Prywansky KG, Spitznagel JK, et al. Bactericidal capacity of phorbol myristate acetate-treated human polymorphonuclear leukocytes. *Infect Immun* 1978;22:945.
11. Van Snick JL, Markowitz B, Masson PL. The ingestion and digestion of human lactoferrin by mouse peritoneal macrophages and the transfer of its iron into ferritin. *J Exp Med* 1977;146:817.
12. Bennett RM, Davis J. Lactoferrin binding to human peripheral blood cells: an interaction with a B-enriched population of lymphocytes and a subpopulation of adherent misonuclear cells. *J Immunol* 1981;127:1211.
13. Hoffer PB, Huberty JP, Khayan-Bashi H. The association of Ga-67 and lactoferrin. *J Nucl Med* 1977;18:713.
14. Ando A, Nitta K, Ando I, et al. Mechanisms of Ga-67 accumulation in inflammatory tissue. *Eur J Nucl Med* 1990;17:21.
15. Hoffer PB, Huberty J, Samuel A. Use of an affinity chromatographic method to determine relative binding of Ga-67 to lactoferrin and transferrin in tear fluid. *J Nucl Med* 1978;19:732.
16. Hayes RL. The interaction of gallium with biological systems. *Int J Nucl Med Biol* 1983;10:257.
17. Larson SM, Hoffer PB. Normal patterns of localization. In: Hoffer PB, Bekerman C, Henkin RE, eds. *Gallium-67 imaging.* New York: John Wiley & Sons, 1978:23.
18. Emery T, Hoffer PB. Gallium, a physiologic competitor of iron. *J Nucl Med* 1980;21:935.
19. Dhawan VM, Sziklas JJ, Spencer RP. Localization of Ga-67 in inflammations in the absence of circulating polymorphonuclear leukocytes. *J Nucl Med* 1978;19:292.
20. Hoffer PB, Samuel A, Bushberg JT, et al. Effect of desferoxamine on tissue and tumor retention of gallium-67: concise communication. *J Nucl Med* 1979;20:248.
21. Hoffer PB, Samuel A, Bushberg JT, et al. Desferoxamine mesylate (Desferal): a contrast-enhancing agent for gallium-67 imaging. *Radiology* 1979;131:775.
22. Hoffer PB. Gallium and infection. *J Nucl Med* 1980;21:484.
23. Hauser MF, Gottschalk A. Comparison of the Anger tomographic scanner and the 15-inch scintillation camera for Ga-67 imaging. *J Nucl Med* 1978;19:1074.
24. Hopkins GB, Mende CW. Gallium-67 and subphrenic abscesses-is delayed scintigraphy necessary? *J Nucl Med* 1975;16:609.
25. Silberstein EB, Fernandez-Ulloa M, Hall J. Are oral cathartics of value in optimizing the gallium scan? *J Nucl Med* 1981;22:424.
26. Edwards CL, Hayes RL. Tumor scanning with gallium citrate. *J Nucl Med* 1969;10:103.
27. Lavender JP, Lowe J, Barker JR, et al. Gallium-67 citrate scanning in neoplastic and inflammatory lesions. *Br J Radiol* 1971;44:361.
28. Littenberg RL, Taketa RM, Alazraki NP, et al. Gallium-67 for localization of septic lesions. *Ann Intern Med* 1973;79:403.
29. Kumar B, Coleman E, Alderson P. Gallium citrate (Ga-67) imaging in patients with suspected inflammatory processes. *Arch Surg* 1975;110:1237.
30. Harvey WC, Podoloff DA, Kopp DT. Gallium-67 in 68 consecutive infection lesions. *Radiology* 1975;16:2.
31. Kumar B, Alderson PO, Geisse G. The role of Ga-67 citrate imaging and diagnostic ultrasound in patients with suspected abdominal abscesses. *J Nucl Med* 1977;18:534.
32. McNeil BJ, Sanders R, Alderson PO, et al. A prospective study of computed tomography, ultrasound and gallium imaging in patients with fever. *Radiology* 1981;139:647.
33. Meyers MA. *Dynamic radiology of the abdomen.* New York: Springer-Verlag, 1976.
34. Myerson PJ, Myerson D, Spencer RP. Anatomic patterns of Ga-67 distribution in localized and diffuse peritoneal inflammation: case report. *J Nucl Med* 1977;18:877.
35. Hauser MF, Alderson PO. Gallium-67 imaging in abdominal disease. *Semin Nucl Med* 1978;8:251.
36. Goldenberg DJ, Russell CD, Mihas AA, et al. Value of gallium-67 citrate scanning in Crohn's disease: concise communication. *J Nucl Med* 1979;20:215.
37. Lewin JS, Rosenfield NS, Hoffer PB, et al. Acute osteomyelitis in children: combined Tc-99m and Ga-67 imaging. *Radiology* 1986;158:795–804.
38. Bruschwein DA, Brown ML, McLeod RA. Gallium scintigraphy in the evaluation of disk-space infections: concise communication. *J Nucl Med* 1980;21:925.
39. Rosenthall L, Kloiber R, Damtew B, et al. Sequential use of radiophosphate and radiogallium imaging in the differential diagnosis of bone, joint and soft tissue infection: quantitative analysis. *Diagn Imaging* 1982;51:249.
40. Handmaker H, Giammona ST. Improved early diagnosis of acute inflammatory skeletal-articular diseases in children: a two radiopharmaceutical approach. *Pediatrics* 1984;73:661.
41. Love C, Tomas MB, Marwin SE, et al. Role of nuclear medicine in diagnosis of the infected joint prosthesis. *Radiographics* 2001;5:1229.
42. Sullivan DC, Rosenfield NS, Ogden J, et al. Problems in the scintigraphic detection of osteomyelitis in children. *Radiology* 1980;135:731.
43. Harcke HT. Bone imaging in infants and children: a review. *J Nucl Med* 1978;19:324.
44. Turpin S, Lambert R. Role of scintigraphy in musculoskeletal and spinal infection. *Radiol Clin North Am* 2001;39:169.
45. Coleman RE, Samuelson CO, Baim S, et al. Imaging with Tc-99m MDP and Ga-67 citrate in patients with rheumatoid arthritis and suspected septic arthritis: concise communication. *J Nucl Med* 1982;23:479.
46. Tumeh SS, Aliabad P, Weissman BN, et al. Chronic osteomyelitis: bone and gallium patterns associated with active disease. *Radiology* 1986;158:685-688.
47. Forman A, Hoffer P. Limitations of three phase bone scintigraphy in suspected osteomyelitis. *J Nucl Med* 1983;23:P83.
48. Rosenthall L, Lisbona R, Hernandez M, et al. 99mTc-PP and 67-Ga imaging following insertion of orthopedic devices. *Radiology* 1979;133:717.
49. Rushton N, Coakley AJ, Tudor J, et al. The value of technetium and gallium scanning in assessing pain after total hip replacement. *J Bone Joint Surg Br* 1982;6413:313.
50. Kolyvas E, Rosenthall L, Ahronheim GA, et al. Serial Ga-67 citrate imaging during treatment of acute osteomyelitis in childhood. *Clin Nucl Med* 1978;3:461.
51. Graham GD, Lundy MM, Frederick RJ, et al. Predicting the cure of osteomyelitis under treatment: concise communication. *J Nucl Med* 1983;24:110.

52. Peters AM. Nuclear medicine imaging in fever of unknown origin. *Q J Nucl Med* 1999;42:61.
53. Palestro CJ, Torres MA. Radionuclide imaging of nonosseous infection. *Q J Nucl Med* 1999;43:46.
54. Thadepalli H, Rambhatla K, Mishkin FS, et al. Correlation of microbiological findings and 67-gallium scans in patients with pulmonary infections. *Chest* 1977;72:442.
55. Siemsen JK, Grebe SF, Waxman AD. The use of gallium-67 in pulmonary disorders. *Semin Nucl Med* 1978;8:235.
56. Bekerman C, Hoffer PH, Bittran JD, et al. Gallium-67 citrate imaging studies of the lung. *Semin Nucl Med* 1980;10:286.
57. Simon TR, Li J, Hoffer PB. The non-specificity of diffuse pulmonary uptake of 67-Ga on 24-hour images. *Radiology* 1980;135:455.
58. Hadik WB, Ponte JA, Lentle BC, et al. Iatrogenic alterations in the biodistribution of radiotracers as a result of drug therapy. In: *Essentials of nuclear medicine.* Baltimore: Williams & Wilkins, 1987:189.
59. Turbinger EH, Yeh SD, Rosen PP, et al. Abnormal gallium scintigraphy in *Pneumocystis carinii* pneumonia with a normal chest radiograph. *Radiology* 1978;127:437.
60. Hamed I, Wenzel J, Leonard J, et al. Pulmonary cytomegalovirus infections: detection by gallium-67 imaging in the transplanted patient. *Arch Intern Med* 1979;139:286.
61. McMahon H, Bekerman C. Diagnostic significance of gallium lung uptake in patients with normal chest radiographs. *Radiology* 1978;127:189.
62. Richman SD, Levenson SM, Bunn PA, et al. Gallium-67 accumulation in pulmonary lesions associated with bleomycin toxicity. *Cancer* 1976;36:1966.
63. Sostman HD, Gamsu G, Putnam CE. Diagnosis of chemotherapy lung. *Am J Roentgenol* 1981;136:33.
64. Crook MJ, Kaplan PD, Adatepe MH. Gallium-67 scanning in nitrofurantoin-induced pulmonary reaction. *J Nucl Med* 1982;23:690.
65. Gelb AL, Dreisen RB, Epstein JD, et al. Immune complexes, gallium lung scans and bronchoalveolar lavage in idiopathic interstitial pneumonitis fibrosis. *Chest* 1983;84:148.
66. Line BR, Hunninghake GW, Koegh BA, et al. Gallium-67 scanning to stage the alveolitis in sarcoidosis: correlation with clinical studies, pulmonary function studies, and bronchoalveolar lavage. *Am Rev Resp Dis* 1981;123:440.
67. Johnson DG, Johnson SM, Harris CC, et al. Ga-67 uptake in the lung in sarcoidosis. *Radiology* 1984;150:551.
68. Abe S, Munakata M, Nishimura M, et al. Gallium-67 scintigraphy bronchoalveolar lavage and pathologic changes in patients with pulmonary sarcoidosis. *Chest* 1984;85:650.
69. Baughman RP, Fernandez M, Bosken CH. Comparison of gallium-67 scanning bronchoalveolar lavage and serum angiotensin-converting enzyme levels in pulmonary sarcoidosis. *Am Rev Resp Dis* 1984;129:676.
70. Lawrence C, Teague MS, Gottlieb MS, et al. Serial changes in markers of disease activity with corticosteroid treatment in sarcoidosis. *Am J Med* 1983;74:747.
71. Begin R, Cantin A, Drapeau G, et al. Pulmonary uptake of gallium-67 in asbestos-exposed humans and sheep. *Am Rev Resp Dis* 1983;127:623.
72. Nidin AH, Mishkin FS, Khurana ML, et al. 67-Ga lung scan: an aid in the differential diagnosis of pulmonary embolism and pneumonitis. *JAMA* 1977;237:1206.
73. Brown JM, Moreno AJ, Weisman I, et al. Positive gallium-67 scintigraphy associated with pulmonary embolism. *Chest* 1983;84:233.
74. Garcia JE, Van Nostrand D, Howard WH, et al. The spectrum of gallium-67 renal activity in patients with no evidence of renal disease. *J Nucl Med* 1984;25:575.
75. Kumar B, Coleman RE. Significance of delayed 67-Ga localization in the kidneys. *J Nucl Med* 1976;17:872.
76. Fanwaz RA, Johnson PM. Renal localization of radiogallium: a retrospective study. *J Nucl Med* 1977;18:595.
77. Alazraki N, Sterkel B, Taylor A Jr. Renal gallium accumulation in the absence of renal pathology in patients with severe hepatocellular disease. *Cin Nucl Med* 1983;8:200.
78. Rosenfield AT, Glickman MG, Taylor KJ, et al. Acute focal bacterial nephritis (acute lobar nephronia). *Radiology* 1979;132:533.
79. Vanarthos WJ, Ganz WI, Vanarthos JC, et al. Diagnostic uses of nuclear medicine in AIDS. *Radiographics* 1992;12:731.
80. Miller RF. Nuclear medicine and AIDS. *Eur J Nucl Med* 1990;16:103.
81. Zuckier LS, Ongseng F, Goldfarb CR. Lymphocytic interstitial pneumonitis: a cause of pulmonary gallium-67 uptake in a child with acquired immunodeficiency syndrome. *J Nucl Med* 1988;29:707.
82. Kramer EL, Sanger JJ, Garay SM, et al. Gallium-67 scans of the chest in patients with acquired immunodeficiency syndrome. *J Nucl Med* 1987;28:1107.
83. Lee VW, Fuller JD, O'Brien MJ, et al. Pulmonary Kaposi sarcoma in patients with AIDS: scintigraphic diagnosis with sequential thallium and gallium scanning. *Radiology* 1991;180:409.
84. Rosenberg ZS, Joffe SA, Itescu S. Spectrum of salivary gland disease in HIV-infected patients: characterization with Ga-67 citrate imaging. *Radiology* 1992;184:761.
85. Bourgoignie JJ. Renal complications of human immunodeficiency virus type 1. *Kidney Int* 1990;37:1571.
86. Korbet SM, Schwrtz MM. Human immunodeficiency virus infection and nephrotic syndrome. *Am J Kidney Dis* 1992;20:97.

60

DETECTION OF INFLAMMATORY DISEASE WITH RADIOLABELED CELLS

R. EDWARD COLEMAN
FREDERICK L. DATZ

Investigators have used various techniques to label blood cells with radionuclides to study cell survival. In early studies ^{51}Cr chromate (1), ^{3}H thymidine (2), and ^{32}P diisofluorophosphate (3) were used to label human leukocytes for measuring cell survival by means of in vitro counting. External imaging could not be performed with these agents. Early attempts at labeling granulocytic leukocytes with γ-emitting radionuclides such as ^{67}Ga and ^{99m}Tc (4–6), which would allow external imaging, met with little success.

In 1976, McAfee and Thakur (7,8) found that the ^{111}In chelate of oxine was suitable for in vitro labeling of phagocytic leukocytes. ^{111}In emits γ photons that are within the range suitable for gamma camera imaging and thus allow visualization of cell distribution within the body. Since the original development of ^{111}In oxine, the clinical use of ^{111}In-labeled white blood cells for detection of inflammatory disease has greatly increased. The distribution of activity on images of ^{111}In-labeled leukocytes reflects the distribution of the labeled leukocytes within the body. Because an abscess consists primarily of leukocytes, leukocytes labeled with ^{111}In localize in the abscess and are detectable with imaging. ^{111}In is a cyclotron-produced radionuclide with a physical half-life of 67 hours. It emits two γ photons of 173 keV (89% abundance) and 247 keV (94% abundance) that are well suited for external detection with scintillation cameras.

For almost two decades, ^{111}In has been the primary radionuclide used to label leukocytes for imaging areas of suspected infection. More recently, techniques for radiolabeling leukocytes with ^{99m}Tc have become available and are being used in many centers.

LEUKOCYTES

Polymorphonuclear leukocytes (granulocytes), lymphocytes, and monocytes are the three types of leukocytes normally present in the blood. Although each of these elements has a somewhat different function, leukocytes are cells that circulate in the blood and are responsible for resisting infection and repairing damaged tissue.

Granulocytes

Neutrophilic granulocytes (neutrophils) are primarily responsible for defending the body against various noxious agents. Neutrophils are able to perform this function because of certain properties they exhibit in response to an acute inflammatory stimulus. These characteristics include chemotaxis, which is the unidirectional migration toward an attractant, phagocytosis, and killing of ingested microorganisms.

Granulocytes remain in the peripheral blood for 5 to 9 hours. Approximately one half of these cells are freely circulating, and one half are marginated near vessel walls (9). Once they leave the circulation, granulocytes remain in the tissues until they are either lost in body secretions or broken down.

Lymphocytes and Monocytes

Mononuclear leukocytes are important in defense against infection and tumors. Lymphocytes are principally involved with immune reactions and appear in the chronic phase of inflammatory responses, although the exact function and fate of lymphocytes that enter the bloodstream are not well understood. There are three subpopulations of lymphocytes: (a) thymus-dependent or T lymphocytes, (b) bursa-dependent or B lymphocytes, and (c) other lymphocytes that have characteristics of both. In general, T lymphocytes recirculate and have a life span of 100 to 200 days. B lymphocytes, on the other hand, do not usually recirculate and have a short turnover in the lymph nodes and spleen.

Monocytes, or mononuclear macrophages, are present normally in the blood, bone marrow, lymph nodes, and spleen. The half-life of these cells in the circulation is approximately 8 hours. Monocytes function in three general areas: phagocytosis, delayed hypersensitivity, and aid in antibody formation. Monocytes accumulate in an inflammatory response and transform into tissue macrophages.

R.E. Coleman: Department of Radiology, Division of Nuclear Medicine, Duke University Medical Center, Durham, NC.
F.L. Datz: Retired, Salt Lake City, UT.

RADIOPHARMACEUTICALS

Several initial attempts to develop a ^{99m}Tc radiopharmaceutical to label leukocytes to a degree adequate for imaging were not very successful (5,10–12). [67]Ga, another γ emitter, has been incorporated into leukocytes but has been found impractical for imaging because of poor labeling efficiency (13).

After surveying several radioactive soluble agents (7) and particles (8), McAfee and Thakur found ^{111}In oxine the most attractive agent for labeling leukocytes. ^{111}In-labeled leukocytes subsequently were shown to localize in experimental abscesses in dogs to a greater degree than did ^{67}Ga citrate (14). After these animal experiments, results of studies with patients (15,16) confirmed that ^{111}In-labeled leukocytes were effective for clinical imaging of abscesses.

Although other ^{111}In radiopharmaceuticals are being used for labeling blood cells, ^{111}In oxine is the agent most widely used. Oxine (8-hydroxyquinoline) is a lipophilic ligand that chelates certain metal ions, including [111]In. The ^{111}In-oxine complex is lipid soluble and readily diffuses through the cell membranes of all blood cells. Once inside the cell, ^{111}In separates from the oxine and is bound, whereas the oxine is eluted from the cell and can be removed from the material to be injected. [111]In oxine is available commercially as a U.S. Food and Drug Administration (FDA)-approved radiopharmaceutical for leukocyte imaging. A brief description of other ^{111}In radiopharmaceuticals that have been used for labeling leukocytes is included, and the labeling technique is described.

Other [111]In Radiopharmaceuticals

A possible limitation to the use of ^{111}In oxine is the necessity of having to wash the cells free of plasma before labeling because in the presence of plasma, ^{111}In binds avidly to transferrin. Leukocytes are extremely sensitive to manipulation, and additional steps such as washing can injure cells. Several studies (17–19) have shown that tropolone, another agent that binds ^{111}In, may be superior to oxine because tropolone can be used to label cells in plasma with high efficiency. It is not clear which of these two agents is the better because reports in the literature are conflicting. In one study (17), investigators found oxine labeling reduced polymorphonuclear cell chemotaxis and phagocytosis to 70% of control values, whereas tropolone decreased these same cell functions to 85% of control values. The labeling efficiency of both agents was similar. Gunter et al. (20), found that tropolone, at concentrations required for efficient labeling, markedly impaired neutrophil chemotaxis, whereas oxine caused no impairment of chemotaxis. In this study, the labeling efficiency of leukocytes with ^{111}In tropolone under optimal conditions was consistently less than with ^{111}In oxine. In another study (19) that showed the advantages of the use of ^{111}In tropolone, investigators found that the accuracy of abscess localization in 101 patients was excellent, but they did not compare ^{111}In tropolone with ^{111}In oxine. It appears that oxine should not be displaced as the agent of choice for the labeling of leukocytes.

Other proposed alternatives to ^{111}In oxine for labeling leukocytes are ^{111}In oxine sulfate (21) and ^{111}In acetylacetone (17, 22). Neither of these agents requires ethanol as a solvent because they are soluble in aqueous buffer solutions. The absence of alcohol as a solvent reduces the possibility of alcohol-induced damage to cells. [111]In acetylacetone offers other advantages: it is more easily prepared and it eliminates the potential toxic effects of oxine. This latter advantage, however, may not be important because it appears that there is no significant toxicity encountered with the microgram quantities used for cell labeling (14). However, there are conflicting reports in the literature regarding the amount of oxine required before toxicity to leukocytes is encountered (23–25).

In summary, neither ^{111}In oxine sulfate nor ^{111}In acetylacetone has been shown to offer any significant improvement in abscess detection over ^{111}In oxine (21,22). For now, ^{111}In oxine is the ^{111}In radiopharmaceutical of choice for autologous leukocyte labeling. In the quantities used for leukocyte labeling, ^{111}In oxine is nontoxic, labels cells with high efficiency, remains in association with cells in vivo, and requires that only 20 to 50 mL of blood be drawn from the patient. This agent is well suited for kinetics studies of inflammatory cells and external imaging of abnormal collections of such cells.

IN VIVO PREPARATION OF AUTOLOGOUS [111]IN-LABELED LEUKOCYTES

Because platelets and red blood cells are labeled with ^{111}In oxine, the leukocytes must be separated from red blood cells and platelets before labeling. Gravity sedimentation does not adequately separate leukocytes from platelets so differential centrifugation must be used. During the entire process of leukocyte separation, extreme care must be taken not to damage the cells. If damaged or excessively manipulated, leukocytes can lose their ability to migrate to areas of inflammation. Thus, in general, the fewer the manipulations, the better are the imaging results.

Blood Collection and Leukocyte Preparation

The leukocyte count should be greater than 5,000 cells/μL to obtain an adequate number of cells for labeling. Approximately 30 to 50 mL of venous blood is drawn from the patient into a syringe containing 1 mL (1,000 units) of heparin and taken to the laboratory. In the laboratory, the anticoagulated blood is allowed to stand vertically in the syringe with the needle end up for approximately 1 hour.

Sedimentation agents are not generally necessary because patients with abscesses or other inflammatory processes have elevated sedimentation rates (15). The upper layer, which is the leukocyte-rich plasma (LRP), contains 50% to 70% of the leukocytes in the whole blood. To avoid red blood cell contamination, the LRP is expressed through a butterfly catheter attached to the syringe into a centrifuge tube (16). The LRP is centrifuged at 300g to 350g for 5 minutes. The leukocytes form a white blood cell button or pellet at the bottom of the tube. The plasma is now free of leukocytes and is called *leukocyte-poor plasma* (LPP). This LPP is saved for later washing and resuspending. The leukocyte pellet is resuspended in 5 mL of normal saline solution and is ready for labeling with ^{111}In oxine.

The resulting leukocyte fraction contains granulocytes, lymphocytes, monocytes, and a few red blood cells (9). Because patients with suspended abscesses usually have a polymorphonuclear leukocytosis, this mixture of white blood cells usually is adequate for imaging, because few mononuclear cells are present for reinjection. Relatively pure granulocyte suspensions have been obtained with a density gradient technique with fewer than 1% mononuclear leukocytes and 5% red blood cells (26). Lymphocytes and monocytes also can be separated and labeled if desired (27).

Cell Labeling

Approximately 1.0 to 1.5 mCi (37.0 to 55.5 MBq) of ^{111}In oxine is added dropwise to the leukocyte-saline mixture and allowed to incubate for 30 minutes at room temperature (25°C). This suspension is then centrifuged at 300g to 350g for 5 minutes, and the saline supernatant is removed. To remove additional non–cell-bound ^{111}In oxine, some investigators recentrifuge at 300g to 350g for 5 minutes (16), although others (26) have not found this necessary.

Washing the pellet with 5 to 8 mL of LPP (saved from the first separation) is useful to remove free ^{111}In oxine before the second centrifugation. The resulting cell pellet is resuspended in LPP (5 to 8 mL), drawn into a syringe, and assayed for radioactivity. It is then ready for injection.

Labeling efficiency depends on the methods used and the leukocyte count. High leukocyte counts result in increasing labeling efficiency (14). Coleman et al. (15) reported an 87% labeling efficiency with a method similar to the one described earlier and found decreased labeling efficiency in the presence of plasma because ^{111}In combines with transferrin. Most investigators report labeling efficiencies of 75% to 95% (14,28,29). Separation of unlabeled activity is simple and efficient.

Function Analysis

Zakhireh et al. (23) reported that leukocytes labeled with ^{111}In oxine (in ethanol) have no abnormality of ultrastructure, function (random migration, chemotaxis, bactericidal capacity), or viability. It appears, then, that leukocytes are not damaged by the cell labeling technique. As discussed earlier, not all reports agree that the labeling technique is harmless to leukocytes.

Other tests of function can be used to test the in vivo behavior of cells (26). Recovery, an indirect indicator of cell function and viability, refers to the percentage of the administered dose circulating in the leukocytes soon after injection. Disappearance half-times can be obtained if serial blood samples are drawn. Disappearance half-time is approximately 7 hours (28,30) when a mixed population of leukocytes is used.

Leukocyte Dosimetry

Another major consideration when labeling cells with a radionuclide such as ^{111}In is the possible effect of radiation on the cell. [111]In, in addition to its emission of γ-rays, emits low-energy electrons (conversion electrons and Auger electrons of 0.6 to 25.4 keV), which have a very short range in tissue and can cause

excessive radiation to the labeled leukocytes (31). The radiation dose to neutrophils separated from 30 mL of blood and labeled with 1 mCi (37 MBq) of ^{111}In oxine is approximately 15,000 rad (32). It appears, however, that neutrophils are not damaged by the radiation exposure associated with standard labeling procedures (23).

Lymphocytes, on the other hand, are much more radiosensitive. It has been suggested that mutagenic and oncogenic effects may result from cell-labeling procedures (33). Whether these transformed lymphocytes proliferate into a malignant process is not known. Studies have shown that ^{111}In oxinate induces severe dose-dependent chromosomal alterations in labeled lymphocytes from human peripheral blood (33). These damaged chromosomes may still be able to proliferate. The hazard that transformed lymphocytes produce malignant growth has relevance in abscess imaging, because ^{111}In-labeled mixed leukocyte preparations may contain a large number of lymphocytes. Lymphocytes are relatively long-lived cells and the effects of radiation from ^{111}In are not well known. This issue is an important one, and more studies are needed to determine the limitations and possible deleterious effects of radionuclide-labeled cells.

Quality Control

Because of concern for the viability of the leukocytes if they are not immediately reinjected into the body, and because of the possibility that pathogens are already present in the blood, standard radiopharmaceutical quality control measures such as testing for sterility and pyrogenicity usually cannot be performed (16). The use of sterile centrifuge tubes, membrane filtration, and pyrogen-free glassware for leukocyte separation and labeling results in a final radiopharmaceutical preparation that is sterile.

Tests to evaluate function of the leukocytes before administration of the labeled leukocytes are not routinely performed. Several studies have shown that neutrophils do remain functional, as judged in vitro (23) and do retain their ability to accumulate in abscesses (14,15). Before injection, a small sample of labeled cells should be examined with a microscope. The final radiopharmaceutical preparation should be examined mainly for polymorphonuclear leukocytes with normal morphologic features and the absence of clumping of the cells.

Quality control of the study includes careful evaluation of each patient before the ^{111}In-labeled leukocyte study is begun. Care should be taken to assure that interfering radionuclides such as ^{67}Ga, ^{131}I, and ^{99m}Tc have not been recently administered (34).

Imaging Technique

Total-body images of leukocyte distribution are routinely obtained at our institution at approximately 18 to 24 hours after intravenous administration of the radiopharmaceutical. A large-field-of-view scintillation camera is used with both the 173- and 247-keV peaks of [111]In. The injected preparation has approximately 0.50 mCi (18.5 MBq) of ^{111}In, which is reported to deliver 3 to 9 rad to the spleen and 0.5 to 2.5 rad to the liver (28,29). Some abscesses are detected as early as 30 minutes after administration, and most are detected within 4 hours (15). Im-

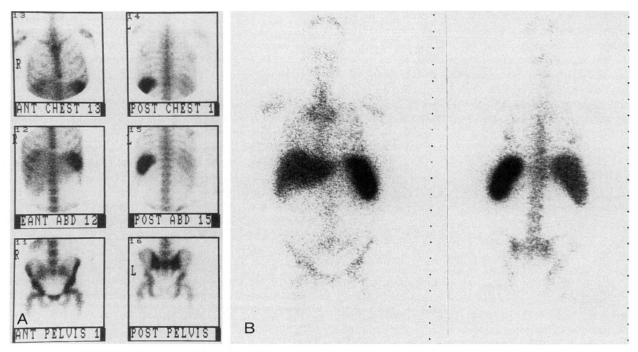

FIGURE 60.1. Normal ¹¹¹In-labeled leukocyte scan. Normal gamma-camera **(A)** and whole-body **(B)** images obtained 18 hours after administration of ¹¹¹In-labeled leukocytes. Activity is evident in the liver, spleen, and bone marrow.

ages obtained 18 to 24 hours after injection are needed to detect small collections of labeled leukocytes. Delayed images, obtained more than 24 hours after injection, do not usually add information (19). Routine views should include anterior and posterior views of the entire body with additional views of special areas of interest if needed.

Image Interpretation

Immediately after administration of the leukocytes, activity is seen in the lungs, liver, spleen, and blood pool. After several hours, less blood-pool and lung activity is present. A normal 18- to 24-hour image shows activity only in the liver, spleen, and bone marrow (Fig. 60.1). The presence of activity in another location is indicative of an abnormality. Abscesses are typically intense accumulations that are focal (Figs. 60.2, 60.3). Moderate activity, or uptake of the radiopharmaceutical of a degree equal to the liver, most likely represents a significant inflammatory response but not necessarily a localized, potentially drainable abscess. Tracer activity equal to or less than marrow uptake is unlikely to represent an abscess (29). Unlike ⁶⁷Ga citrate scans, normal ¹¹¹In-labeled leukocyte scans do not show activity within the urinary tract, small intestine, or colon. ¹¹¹In-labeled leukocytes typically do not localize in granulating, uninfected wounds.

¹¹¹IN-LABELED LEUKOCYTE SCANS FOR SUSPECTED ABSCESS

An abscess is a local collection of pus in a cavity that has formed through necrosis and destruction of tissues. The purulent con-

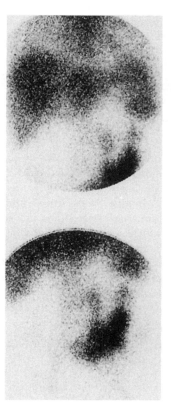

FIGURE 60.2. Intraabdominal abscess. A 61-year-old man had with left lower-quadrant pain and fever. ¹¹¹In-labeled leukocyte images show abnormal accumulations in the left lower quadrant extending into the gutter on the anterior abdomen (*top*) and pelvis (*bottom*).

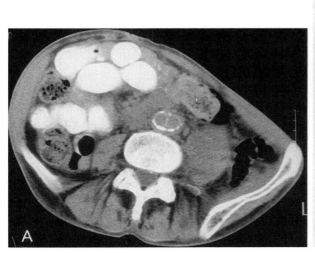
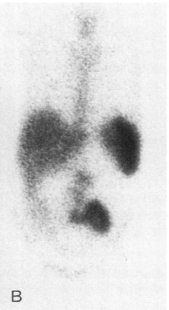
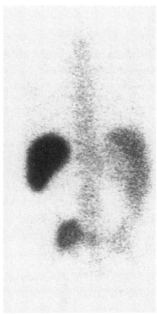

FIGURE 60.3. Aortic bifemoral graft abscess. A 72-year-old man presented with pain and fever 6 weeks after infection of an aortic bifemoral graft. **A:** Computed tomographic scan shows a soft-tissue mass adjacent to the left of the graft. **B:** Anterior (*left*) and posterior (*right*) whole-body ^{111}In-labeled leukocyte scans show abnormal accumulation in the left lower quadrant that corresponds to the abnormality in **A.** The mass was aspirated and found to be a perigraft abscess.

tents of an abscess are separated from the surrounding normal tissue by a tissue barrier or wall. An abscess is different from a phlegmon, which is an area of inflammation in tissue that is not walled-off and usually heals spontaneously. An abscess, on the other hand, must be drained surgically, and this should be done as early as possible because the mortality of undrained abscesses can be as high as 35% (35).

The origins of abscesses are diverse, but many abscesses occur postoperatively or after penetrating injury. Other causes include bacterial contamination from endogenous gastrointestinal flora, hematogenous dissemination from distant infected sites, and obstruction of ducts that drain an organ. Although local signs and symptoms usually are present, some abscesses, particularly those that are intraabdominal, may manifest as fever and sepsis and not have localized findings.

Abscesses can be solitary or multiple and can take several days to several years to form (36), depending on the inciting cause. The pathologic mechanism is the effects of bacterial or fungal infection. The body's natural defense mechanisms tend to try to contain infection; these defense mechanisms consist foremost of neutrophils aided by opsonins, which engulf and kill bacteria. Neutrophils that enter the abscess cavity cannot return to the bloodstream and die in 3 to 5 days (37). Lysosomal enzymes are released when the neutrophil dies and tend to liquefy the center of the abscess. As the contents of the abscess become higher in osmolarity, further growth of the abscess occurs as a result of fluid influx due to osmotic pressure.

Imaging Abscesses

Identification of an occult abscess remains a difficult clinical problem, and the search for more accurate, noninvasive means

of diagnosing such problems is continuing. Before the development of cell-labeled radiopharmaceuticals, ^{67}Ga citrate was the most common radiopharmaceutical for localization of inflammatory lesions. In recent years, computed tomography (CT) and ultrasonography have been used in the diagnosis of abscesses. The imaging specialist is, however, not limited to mere diagnosis of abscesses but now is able to aid in the management of abscesses. Percutaneous needle drainage of abscesses in almost any location has been successfully performed with the aid of fluoroscopic, CT, or ultrasound guidance.

[111]In-labeled Leukocyte Imaging

Imaging with ^{111}In-labeled white blood cells has been shown to be an accurate method of detecting abscesses. The sensitivity and specificity in identifying abdominal and pelvic abscesses have been reported to be approximately 90% and 95% (15,28, 38). In a study involving 542 patients over a 5-year period, investigators found the accuracy, sensitivity, specificity, and predictive values of negative and positive tests to be in the range of 91% to 93% (39).

Comparison with [67]Ga Citrate

[67]Ga citrate has been used for many years for localizing inflammatory lesions (40). [67]Ga scintigraphy, although sensitive, is not specific (41). Interpretation of ^{67}Ga scans is difficult, particularly for postoperative patients, because of normal excretion into the colon and accumulation in normally healing wounds. Clinical comparison of ^{111}In-labeled leukocytes and ^{67}Ga citrate imaging modalities is difficult because the γ photon energy emissions

and physical half-lives of ^{67}Ga and ^{111}In are similar. Earlier work with dogs (14,42) showed higher accumulation of ^{111}In-labeled leukocytes than of ^{67}Ga citrate in experimentally induced abscesses. More recently, clinical comparisons (14,43–45) showed that results of both ^{67}Ga and ^{111}In imaging procedures are generally abnormal for patients with abscesses. Results of ^{111}In leukocyte studies, however, appear to be easier to interpret because of the lack of uptake in the colon and normally healing, uninfected granulating wounds (15). ^{111}In-labeled leukocyte studies appear to be more specific than ^{67}Ga citrate studies (43,45). In a recent prospective study with 32 patients who underwent both ^{111}In-labeled leukocyte and ^{67}Ga scintigraphy, imaging with ^{111}In-labeled leukocytes was found more accurate for infections of short duration, whereas ^{67}Ga imaging was more accurate for prolonged or chronic infection (44). For a more thorough discussion of the use of ^{67}Ga imaging in the detection of inflammatory lesions, see Chapter 59.

Comparison with Ultrasonography and Computed Tomography

Imaging with ^{111}In-labeled leukocytes compares favorably with ultrasonography and CT in the detection of abscesses. In a study comparing the results of ultrasonography and ^{111}In-labeled leukocyte scintigraphy in the evaluation of 163 patients for suspected intraabdominal abscesses, both modalities were found approximately 95% specific, whereas leukocyte studies were slightly more sensitive than was sonography (46). The results of another study (47) comparing the accuracy of all three of these modalities in the evaluation of suspected abdominal abscesses led to the conclusion that CT was slightly more accurate (95%) than was ultrasonography (90%) or ^{111}In-labeled white blood cell procedures (92%). Thus the diagnostic accuracy of these three methods is similar in the evaluation of suspected intraabdominal abscess.

Pitfalls in ^{111}In Leukocyte Imaging

^{111}In-labeled leukocyte scans are highly specific, and few studies with false-positive results have been reported. Several causes of accumulation of leukocytes in areas that are not abscesses have been reported (29,48) and are listed in Table 60.1. Abnormal activity on the image should be intense (similar to or greater than liver activity) and focal to suggest an abscess. If clumping of white blood cells is a consideration, or if inflammatory disease is suspected in the chest (where clumping can cause confusion), images of the chest obtained immediately after injection help determine the time of the localization. ^{111}In-labeled leukocytes, unlike ^{67}Ga citrate labeled leukocytes, do not typically localize in neoplastic processes, although the presence of malignant growth has been reported to cause a positive focus on leukocyte scans (49).

Current Status of ^{111}In Leukocyte Scans for Abscesses

Because of the difficulty in evaluating patients with unexplained fever and suspected occult abscess, there is a need for noninvasive

Table 60.1. *Potential Causes of Positive Interpretations of ^{111}In-Labeled Leukocyte Scans*

Cause	Location
Accessory spleens	Left upper quadrant of abdomen
Clumping of leukocytes	Chest
Intestinal accumulation due to multiple enemas, vasculitis, or inflammatory bowel disease	Abdomen
Intestinal activity resulting from swallowed activity due to ear, nose, or throat or esophageal inflammation or bleeding	Abdomen
Activity in drains in abscesses	Any site
Infarcted organ (within 2–3 d of onset)	Heart, brain, intestine
Pulmonary embolism	Chest
Cystic fibrosis	Chest
Malignant tumor (rare)	Bone

imaging techniques to help localize or rule out an abscess. ^{111}In-labeled leukocyte scans are helpful because they are accurate and relatively easy to obtain for patients who are difficult to manipulate and who are unable to cooperate. A major advantage of ^{111}In-labeled leukocyte imaging is the whole-body survey of patients who do not have localizing signs or symptoms (47). Because CT and ultrasonography are more rapidly performed and can be used to guide percutaneous needle drainage, these modalities are particularly useful in the evaluation of patients who have localizing signs.

Finally, separation and labeling of leukocytes is time-consuming. The availability of the procedure became more widespread when ^{111}In oxine became an FDA-approved radiopharmaceutical. However, because of the necessity of handling blood for the preparation and the problems with HIV-positive blood, the procedure should be performed with particular attention to the safety of the patient and the persons handling the blood.

^{111}IN-LABELED LEUKOCYTES IN THE DETECTION OF OTHER INFLAMMATORY DISORDERS

A spectrum of inflammatory diseases can be evaluated with ^{111}In-labeled leukocyte scans. Although the most common clinical indication is localization of an occult abscess, usually intraabdominal or pelvic, white blood cell scanning has been used for many other indications. Unsuspected abscesses outside the abdomen are occasionally discovered, and the results of the study often direct the clinician toward proper therapy (Fig. 60.4).

Leukocyte scans are useful in differentiating abscess from other causes of space-occupying defects found at CT or ultrasonography. A specific use of leukocyte imaging has been in differentiating pancreatic abscesses from pseudocysts once a mass is discovered with another imaging modality (50). The leukocyte imaging procedure is a functional study and shows the presence or absence of white blood cells within the mass, whereas a purely

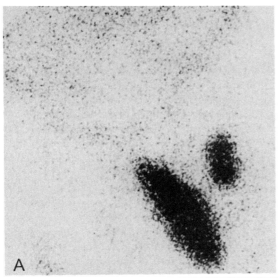

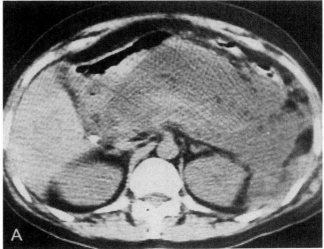

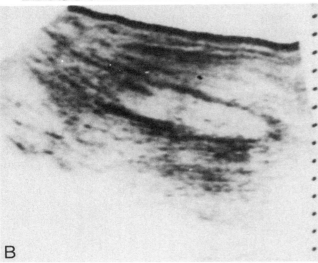

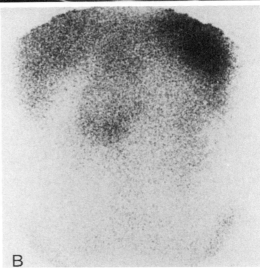

FIGURE 60.4. Extraabdominal abscess. **A:** Anterior image of left upper thigh 18 hours after administration of ^{111}In-labeled leukocytes to a 24-year-old man with *Staphylococcus aureus* bacterial endocarditis who continued to have a fever for 2 weeks after appropriate antibiotic therapy. The image shows two focal areas of abnormal accumulation that were not detected clinically. **B:** Ultrasound scan of the larger thigh abscess, which was subsequently drained.

FIGURE 60.5. Pancreatic mass lesion. A 45-year-old woman had fever and epigastric pain. Computed tomographic scan **(A)** shows a large pancreatic mass that was found to be an inflammatory mass on the ^{111}In-labeled leukocyte study **(B)**.

anatomic study such as CT or ultrasonography may not help differentiate infection from tumor or another sterile lesion (Fig. 60.5). In a study with 8 patients with a pancreatic mass lesion, leukocyte studies helped differentiate abscess from pseudocyst correctly in 7. There was one false-positive scan of diffuse pancreatitis (50).

Leukocyte scans have been used successfully for differentiation of hepatic abscess from tumor (51) and of perinephric abscess from pyelonephritis (52). Abscesses in the upper abdomen, particularly subphrenic abscesses, are less likely to be definitely positive because of normal liver and spleen activity. Computer subtraction techniques with ^{99m}Tc sulfur colloid have been shown useful in this area (53).

Bone and Joint Infections

[111]In-labeled leukocyte imaging is generally less accurate in the detection of skeletal infections than in detection of soft-tissue abnormalities. Two large studies (approximately 125 patients combined) of ^{111}In-labeled leukocyte imaging in the evaluation of suspected bone or joint infection resulted in a sensitivity of only 50%, whereas the specificity was approximately 90% (15, 54). The reasons for the low sensitivity in skeletal lesions are not known, but previous antibiotic therapy or the chronicity of the disease may be contributing factors (Fig. 60.6). In this regard, a study with rabbits showed that ^{111}In-labeled leukocyte scans were accurate in the diagnosis of acute osteomyelitis. Results of leukocyte scans were generally positive earlier than were those of ^{99m}Tc methylene diphosphonate bone scans in cases of acute infection (55). Results of a clinical study with a small

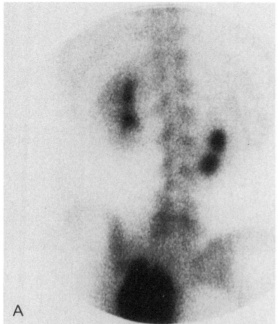

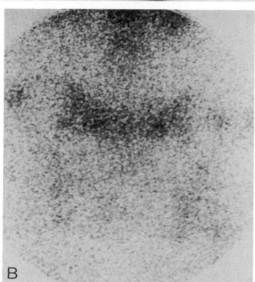

FIGURE 60.6. Suspected bone and joint infection. A 34-year-old woman had a history of disk surgery at L4-5 18 months earlier. She had intermittent pain and fever since then and was taking several antibiotics. **A:** Bone scan shows focal abnormal activity at the L4-5 level. **B:** ¹¹¹In-labeled leukocyte image of the lower lumbar spine and pelvis shows decreased activity in the L4-5 area. The patient subsequently underwent surgery and had chronic inflammatory changes, and the disk space was culture-positive.

group of patients suggested that ¹¹¹In-labeled leukocyte scans are accurate in the diagnosis of acute osteomyelitis but not that of chronic osteomyelitis (56). It is not clear whether ¹¹¹In-labeled leukocyte imaging is superior to ⁶⁷Ga imaging in the evaluation of suspected acute osteomyelitis, although ⁶⁷Ga imaging is probably more sensitive in the evaluation of chronic bone and joint infection (15).

The use of ¹¹¹In-labeled leukocyte imaging in the diagnosis of infection of total hip and knee prostheses is limited. In a study of 153 scans of 193 patients who underwent repeated surgery because of loose or painful joints or for resection arthroplasty, ¹¹¹In-labeled leukocyte scans had a 77% sensitivity and 86% specificity (57). The authors concluded that "negative indium scan results may be useful in suggesting the absence of infection." In another study of combined ⁹⁹ᵐTc sulfur colloid and ¹¹¹In-labeled leukocyte imaging in the evaluation of suspected infection of total hip or knee prostheses, the investigators concluded that the accuracy was too low for recommendation of routine use of these scans (58). Sequential radionuclide bone scans and ¹¹¹In-labeled leukocyte scans are not accurate enough to be useful in the management of suspected prosthetic joint infection (59).

Because ¹¹¹In-labeled leukocytes localize in the bone marrow to the degree that normal bony structures are visualized, this imaging study occasionally shows photopenic areas within the vertebral column or other skeletal structures (Fig. 60.7). Labeled white blood cells can, therefore, be used as a bone marrow imaging agent and often show unsuspected or incidental bone abnormalities when imaging is performed to search for an abscess or for other, unrelated reasons. Areas of decreased activity in the bone marrow have been seen after radiation therapy, in osteomyelitis, in compression fractures (Fig. 60.8), and in metastatic disease.

Inflammatory Bowel Disease

Reports indicate that ¹¹¹In-labeled leukocyte imaging accurately depicts areas of active ulcerative colitis or Crohn's disease (60).

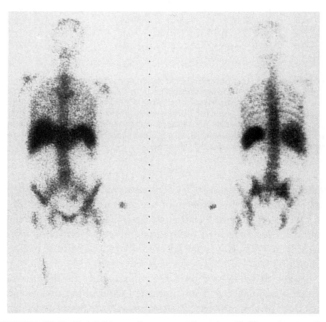

FIGURE 60.7. Total hip replacement. Anterior (*left*) and posterior (*right*) whole-body ¹¹¹In-labeled leukocyte images show no activity in the right proximal femur resulting from a femoral prosthesis. The radioactivity to the left of the pelvic area is a radioactive marker. The focus of abnormal accumulation in the left pelvis resulted from diverticulitis depicted on a computed tomographic scan.

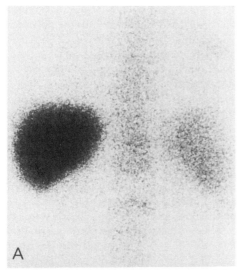

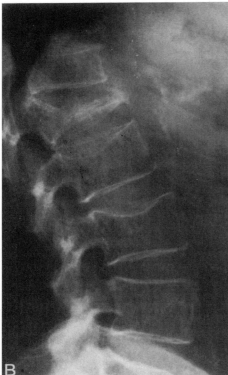

FIGURE 60.8. Compression fracture. A 64-year-old man with persistent fever after abdominal surgery. **A:** Posterior ^{111}In-labeled leukocyte image of the lower chest and upper abdomen shows decreased activity in a vertebral body. **B:** Lateral radiograph of the spine shows a collapsed vertebral body that corresponds to the abnormality on the leukocyte scan.

Results of leukocyte studies correlate well with those of double-contrast barium enema examination and colonoscopy (60). Findings on ^{111}In-labeled leukocyte scans usually cannot establish the diagnosis but may provide an accurate, noninvasive method with which to follow patients with known inflammatory bowel disease, particularly at times when patients are too ill to undergo barium enema or colonoscopy. However, studies to determine the role of ^{111}In-labeled leukocyte imaging in evaluating the extent or severity of the disease have been conducted with only a small number of patients (60).

[111]In-labeled leukocytes also accumulate in small-intestinal infarction (61), vasculitis involving the intestine (62), and gastrointestinal bleeding (63). Any of these abnormalities can be interpreted as active ulcerative colitis or Crohn's disease or as an abdominal abscess. In patients with intestinal bleeding, several imaging times reveal a distribution of activity that has changed because of movement of blood within the alimentary canal (63).

Other Potential Applications

Preliminary experience with labeled leukocytes in the evaluation of renal transplant rejection has shown that labeled leukocytes accumulate at the site of the renal transplant in all patients with acute rejection and in some patients with chronic rejection (64). We have seen accumulation of ^{111}In-labeled leukocytes in renal transplants that were normal at biopsy. ^{111}In-labeled leukocytes may be useful in the detection of rejection of cardiac allografts (65), but further studies are needed to determine the role of the radiolabeled cells in the evaluation of transplanted organs.

The inflammatory response to acute myocardial infarction has been studied in dogs with ^{111}In-labeled leukocytes (66). In these animals, images obtained 48 hours after coronary occlusion showed accumulation of activity in the region of infarction. In patients with acute myocardial infarction, ^{111}In-labeled leukocytes tend to accumulate in the infarct if administered within 24 hours of infarction (67).

[111]In-labeled leukocytes are useful in diagnosis of prosthetic graft infection (68–70). This imaging procedure is sensitive and specific because white blood cells do not tend to accumulate in uninfected grafts (70).

OTHER RADIOLABELED CELLS IN INFLAMMATORY CONDITIONS

Donor Leukocytes

Autologous leukocytes have been used in most ^{111}In-labeled leukocyte studies. In patients with severe leukopenia or who have abnormal leukocytes, labeling of autologous leukocytes is not practical. In such patients, ^{111}In-labeled donor leukocytes have been shown to be successful as a tracer of areas of inflammation, including abscesses (56,71,72). In patients undergoing granulocyte transfusion, it is easy to label the donor leukocytes with ^{111}In oxine (71).

Other Cells

[111]In oxine labels all cellular elements of the blood. Relatively pure platelet, granulocyte, lymphocyte, or monocyte preparations are possible with refinement of separation techniques. ^{111}In-labeled autologous lymphocytes have been shown suitable for the study of lymphocyte kinetics in a few healthy volunteers and in patients with Hodgkin's disease (27). However, the role that lymphocyte imaging will play in abnormalities such as lym-

phoma or transplant rejection is not known because these studies remain experimental. Radiolabeled lymphocytes and monocytes may prove useful in the evaluation of interstitial lung disease, such as sarcoidosis, rheumatic disorders, and vasculitis. The use of labeled eosinophils and their relation to allergic or parasitic disease is being explored.

99MTC-LABELED LEUKOCYTES

Early attempts to label leukocytes with ^{99m}Tc were unsuccessful, which is unfortunate because this isotope has a number of advantages over ^{111}In. The γ-photon energy of ^{99m}Tc is 140 keV, which is ideal for the current generation of gamma cameras. Because larger amounts of ^{99m}Tc than ^{111}In radioactivity can be administered, image quality is superior. Finally, because it is generator-produced, ^{99m}Tc is significantly less expensive than ^{111}In and always is available.

Initial Attempts to Label Leukocytes with ^{99m}Tc

Most early attempts to label leukocytes with ^{99m}Tc were based on phagocytosis of ^{99m}Tc-labeled particles such as ^{99m}Tc sulfur colloid (73,74). This approach was appealing because cell separation of whole blood was unnecessary—only the phagocytic cells would engulf the radioactive particles and bind with the label. However, two problems were found with this approach. First, phagocytosis induced metabolic changes in the leukocytes and resulted in decreased in vivo function compared with that of ^{111}In-labeled cells. Second, it was found that a separation step was still necessary. The combination of untagged activity from unengulfed ^{99m}Tc particles, as well as from radiolabel adhering to the surface of the cells, caused significant background activity to appear in the image. In addition, preparation times were long and labeling yields low.

^{99m}Tc Albumin-labeled Leukocytes

A phagocytic labeling technique developed by Marcus et al. (75) overcomes many of the problems mentioned earlier. Their technique involves use of ^{99m}Tc albumin colloid as the radiolabel. After the blood is centrifuged to obtain a white blood cell button, the cells are incubated with ^{99m}Tc albumin colloid for 15 minutes at 37°C. Approximately 50% of the activity is bound to leukocytes. Studies indicate that neutrophils lose activity over the next 2 to 3 hours, whereas monocytes continue to phagocytize particles for up to 4 hours. However, considering that monocytes account for one third of the cells in an average inflammatory exudate, this difference in activity is not as significant as it might seem. Some studies of drained pus have shown that the primary labeled cells are monocytes rather than neutrophils. Over time, the reduced ^{99m}Tc in the label is oxidized in vivo to free pertechnetate. Such oxidation can be explained partially by the presence of phagocytic cells capable of oxidizing the label. This process prevents delayed imaging at 24 hours (75).

Uptake of the agent in inflammatory sites has been recorded as early as 10 minutes after injection. This uptake may not represent migration of labeled leukocytes into the inflammatory site. Noncellularly bound ^{99m}Tc albumin in the preparation can reach sites through increased blood flow and leave the circulation as nanocolloids do. Initial uptake by the unbound activity appears to be augmented by cellular infiltration at a later time (75).

The primary application of ^{99m}Tc albumin–labeled cells has been in the noninvasive diagnosis of appendicitis (76,77). In a study with 100 patients with suspected appendicitis, imaging with ^{99m}Tc albumin colloid–labeled cells had a sensitivity of 89% and a specificity of 92% (78). Results were positive as early as 10 minutes after injection, most becoming positive within 1 hour. Among 17 patients with results interpreted as indeterminate for appendicitis, approximately one half were later proved to have the disease. The agent was not as accurate in women because of confusion with gynecologic disease. The scan also was not as useful in the evaluation of chronic infection as it was in that of acute infection, apparently because of slower uptake in such lesions and oxidative loss of the label with time.

99MTC HMPAO–LABELED LEUKOCYTES

Hexamethylpropyleneamine oxime (HMPAO) was originally developed for imaging cerebral blood flow (79). HMPAO is a small, neutral, and lipophilic complex that binds ^{99m}Tc. The lipophilicity of HMPAO allows it to cross the membrane of brain cells, where it remains fixed. This same mechanism has been applied to leukocyte labeling.

Labeling

After crossing the leukocyte cell membrane, the primary ^{99m}Tc HMPAO complex changes into a hydrophilic secondary complex that is trapped within the cell. The radioactivity is bound to intracellular organelles, primarily the mitochondria and nucleus (80). Mixed-cell labeling with ^{99m}Tc HMPAO produces a purer granulocyte preparation than does labeling with ^{111}In oxine, although this finding recently has been questioned. Unlike ^{111}In oxine, which indiscriminately labels all cell types, HMPAO has a predilection for labeling granulocytes (73,81–85). In addition, the ^{99m}Tc HMPAO label is more stable in granulocytes than in mononuclear cells. The label elutes from mononuclear cells five times more rapidly than from granulocytes.

^{99m}Tc HMPAO labeling can be performed with small amounts of plasma present (86,87). Studies indicate that leukocytes deprived of plasma for as little as 10 minutes have morphologic changes (73). Such cells have a greater tendency to aggregate and to stain with supravital stains. Studies of labeled platelets have shown that those labeled in saline solution have reduced in vitro function than do platelets labeled in plasma (88). Experimental studies of abscesses have indicated greater accumulation of cells labeled in plasma than of cells labeled out of plasma (88). ^{111}In oxine, however, cannot be used to label leukocytes in the presence of plasma; 90% of ^{111}In oxine added to whole blood binds to transferrin with only 4% of the dose binding to leukocytes (73). ^{111}In tropolone can be used in the presence of plasma and yields a higher labeling efficiency than does ^{99m}Tc HMPAO. The ^{99m}Tc label is not stable with time. Studies show that both circulating cells and leukocytes localized in sites of infection elute the label over time.

Viability, Kinetics, and Biodistribution

There is no evidence that the ^{99m}Tc HMPAO label damages the leukocytes. In vitro studies of ^{99m}Tc HMPAO–labeled cells have shown normal random migration, chemotaxis, phagocytosis, and intracellular killing capacity. No morphologic alterations have been found with electron microscopy (85). As many authors have pointed out, however, the best measure of cell viability is in vivo function (73). Studies have shown that neither in vivo percentage recovery rates nor liver transit times differ from those of other radiolabels (81). Organs with high concentrations of reticuloendothelial cells, such as the liver and spleen, have not shown increased uptake, as occurs with damaged radiolabeled cells. Finally, no increased lung uptake has been found; increased lung retention is seen with heat-damaged leukocytes. The blood disappearance half-time of ^{99m}Tc HMPAO–labeled leukocytes is 4 hours, compared with 6 hours for ^{111}In-labeled granulocytes (81). This discrepancy is caused by elution of ^{99m}Tc from circulating leukocytes. When corrected for elution, the blood half-time increases to 6 hours.

With intravenous administration, some ^{99m}Tc HMPAO leukocytes marginate in the lung. The activity decreases significantly by 4 hours after injection, as it does with leukocytes tagged with other radiolabels. Like ^{111}In-labeled cells, most ^{99m}Tc-labeled cells are in the spleen, liver, and bone marrow. In contrast to the situation with ^{111}In, however, genitourinary and gastrointestinal activity normally occurs. The kidneys and bladder appear as early as 1 hour after administration (74). Activity is primarily present in the urine, although there also is some parenchymal uptake. By 1 hour, the gallbladder appears in approximately 4% of patients. Over time it is visualized in approximately 10% of patients. Gastrointestinal activity is almost never seen before 2 hours after injection (81), but by 24 hours, bowel activity is seen in almost all patients (Fig. 60.9).

The cause of the gastrointestinal and genitourinary activity is not known with certainty. It is not caused by free ^{99m}Tc pertechnetate, however, because thyroid visualization does not occur. Gastrointestinal and urinary tract activity probably results from the formation of secondary complexes of ^{99m}Tc HMPAO. Urinary tract visualization is related to excretion of such secondary complexes through the kidneys. Gallbladder excretion causes the bowel activity. Gastrointestinal activity has been described in patients undergoing brain imaging with ^{99m}Tc HMPAO (81).

Comparison with Other Leukocyte Labels

In a study in which ^{99m}Tc HMPAO–labeled leukocytes and ^{111}In tropolone–labeled leukocytes were injected simultaneously into animals that had experimental abscesses, the mean concentration of ^{99m}Tc in the abscesses was only one-third that of ^{111}In 18 hours after injection (89). The abscess to blood and abscess to normal tissue ratios for ^{99m}Tc HMPAO also were significantly lower. In a second animal study, uptake of ^{99m}Tc HMPAO–labeled leukocytes was only 66% of the uptake of ^{111}In-labeled leukocytes (86,90).

Patient studies, on the other hand, consistently have shown that the results with ^{99m}Tc HMPAO–labeled leukocytes are equal or superior to those with either ^{111}In-labeled cells or ^{67}Ga citrate (74,87,91–97). The reported sensitivity of imaging with ^{99m}Tc HMPAO–labeled leukocytes has been between 92% and 100%. These studies are especially impressive because, in most

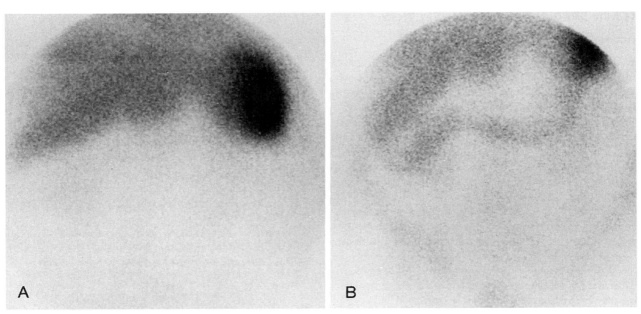

FIGURE 60.9. Normal ^{99m}Tc HMPAO leukocyte scan. **A:** Anterior abdominal image obtained 1 hour after injection shows the absence of bowel activity. **B:** Twenty-four-hour image shows normal colonic activity.

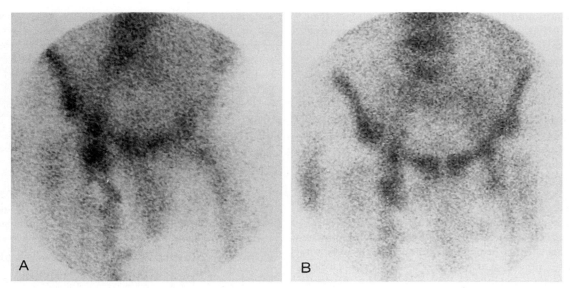

FIGURE 60.10. Graft infection. **A:** Image of the lower pelvis and legs obtained 1 hour after injection shows increased uptake in the region of the right limb of the graft. **B:** Image obtained 5 hours after injection shows persistence of the increased uptake.

cases, the two leukocyte labels were directly compared in the same patient by means of injection of double-labeled cells. This comparison is possible because of the different photopeaks of the two radionuclides. In addition, ^{99m}Tc-labeled leukocytes show maximal sensitivity as early as 30 minutes to 1 hour after injection (Fig. 60.10). Imaging with ^{111}In oxine–labeled leukocytes has a sensitivity of only 33% 1 to 4 hours after injection, although imaging ^{111}In tropolone–labeled cells may have a higher early sensitivity (98,99).

UTILITY IN SPECIFIC SITES OF INFECTION

Abdomen and Soft Tissue

Because of the normal excretion of activity into the gastrointestinal and urinary tracts, evaluating the abdomen can be more difficult with ^{99m}Tc HMPAO–labeled leukocytes than with ^{111}In-labeled cells (81). Studies indicate that performing abdominal imaging 4 hours after administration of the radiolabel causes a significant number of false-positive results. Such false-positive results can be prevented by obtaining images 1 hour after administration in addition to images 4 hours after administration, because gastrointestinal activity normally is not seen before 1 to 2 hours after administration.

The combination of early and delayed imaging can be useful in evaluation of the liver. Normal liver uptake of ^{99m}Tc HMPAO leukocytes decreases 1 to 4 hours after injection, whereas activity in sites of infection within the liver increases. The reason for the normal decrease in liver activity with time is not known, although it may be similar to the initial uptake and release of activated cells by the lungs (81). As with ^{111}In-labeled leukocytes images, ^{99m}Tc sulfur colloid liver-spleen scans can be performed and compared with labeled leukocyte scans to improve detection of upper-quadrant abscesses.

Genitourinary tract infections may be difficult to diagnose because of normal excretion of the label. Hepatobiliary inflammatory lesions such as acute cholecystitis also are difficult to diagnose because of the possibility of normal hepatobiliary excretion, although a negative study result is helpful in excluding disease.

Surprising is that ^{99m}Tc HMPAO–labeled leukocytes have been useful in the diagnosis and evaluation of inflammatory bowel disease (82). The better resolution obtained with ^{99m}Tc than with ^{111}In allows involved segments, especially of small intestine, to be identified more easily. The earlier imaging capability (one author reported ^{99m}Tc HMPAO leukocyte localization of inflammatory bowel disease within 2 minutes) and shorter imaging times, which reduce movement artifacts, also improve visualization of the small intestine. Early imaging is essential when leukocyte imaging is used in evaluation for suspected inflammatory bowel disease. The finding of segments with positive results at 1 hour with increasing uptake over the next 3 hours has a 97% positive predictive value; the value is 73% for segments with negative results at 1 hour but positive results at 4 hours.

Infected prosthetic vascular grafts can be detected with ^{99m}Tc HMPAO–labeled leukocytes (Fig 60.10). In a study with 129 consecutive patients with suspected prosthetic vascular graft infection, labeled leukocyte imaging had an accuracy of more than 95% (92).

Enteric fistula is difficult to diagnose with ^{99m}Tc HMPAO leukocytes. Because of the short half-life of ^{99m}Tc, quantification of leukocyte uptake is not possible.

Bone

The normal uptake of ^{99m}Tc HMPAO–labeled leukocytes in the bone marrow of the axial skeleton makes the diagnosis of osteomyelitis in this region difficult. Several techniques can be used to improve diagnostic accuracy (81). First, early images can be compared with images obtained 24 hours after injection. Bone uptake seen primarily on images obtained 1 hour after injection is caused by marrow activity in the sinusoids rather than by infection. With infection, activity should increase in the site with time.

A second technique is to combine a ^{99m}Tc sulfur colloid bone marrow scan with the leukocyte scan. This procedure is done easily with ^{111}In-labeled leukocytes because of the different energies of the two radioisotopes. Combining the two scans when ^{99m}Tc HMPAO leukocytes are used is much more difficult. A third alternative is to double-label the leukocytes with ^{99m}Tc and ^{111}In. Bone marrow is shown on the 1-hour ^{99m}Tc photopeak and can be compared with activity at 24 hours on the ^{111}In photopeak.

In the peripheral skeleton, bone marrow uptake is not a problem except in patients with expanded bone marrow (Fig. 60.11), and differentiating soft tissue from bone infection is the usual problem. Imaging with ^{99m}Tc HMPAO–labeled leukocytes has been shown accurate in the evaluation of osteomyelitis of the foot in patients with preexisting bony abnormalities and in patients with diabetes. In 27 patients who had preexisting bony abnormalities and suspected osteomyelitis, ^{99m}Tc HMPAO–labeled leukocyte imaging had an accuracy of 89%; the accuracy was 63% for bone scans and 55% for plain radiography (93). In a study of 56 foot ulcers in 42 patients, ^{99m}Tc HMPAO–labeled leukocyte imaging had an accuracy of 93%; the accuracy was 70% for radiography and 63% for three-phase bone scans (94).

Like ^{111}In-labeled leukocytes, ^{99m}Tc HMPAO–labeled leukocytes have decreased sensitivity for osteomyelitis in the spine (74,81). It is not known why this is the case. In addition, ^{99m}Tc HMPAO leukocytes are not as useful if the patient has chronic bone infection.

Acute versus Chronic Infection

The high sensitivity for infection of early postinjection ^{99m}Tc HMPAO–labeled leukocyte imaging makes this technique ideal for the detection of acute soft-tissue infection. HMPAO-labeled leukocytes are not as useful for the evaluation of chronic infection because the exchange of leukocytes slows in such sites (81). Elution of the radionuclide from both circulating leukocytes and those localized in the infection reduces the photon flux on 24-hour images.

^{99m}Tc versus ^{111}In-labeled Leukocytes

Peters (100) has offered advice on the best radiolabel to use in different clinical situations. If a rapid diagnosis is needed in a case of acute infection, use of ^{99m}Tc HMPAO leukocytes, with their superior early sensitivity, is indicated. In the evaluation of chronic infections, such as with fever of unknown origin, ^{111}In-labeled leukocytes are a better choice because 24-hour imaging is required. Suspected infection of the urinary tract should be imaged with ^{111}In-labeled cells. Although gastrointestinal inflammation can be imaged with either label, if quantification is needed, ^{111}In is the better choice. If exact localization of the inflammatory site is important, ^{99m}Tc-labeled cells should be used. In bone infections, the degree of acuteness is a guide to which technique to use. The higher photon flux of ^{99m}Tc-labeled leukocytes is an advantage in evaluation of peripheral bone infection, such as those in the hand or foot. If both bone and leukocyte scans are needed, however, ^{111}In may be a better choice because simultaneous imaging is possible.

SUMMARY

The ability to image labeled cellular components of blood has provided a rekindling of the interest in nuclear hematology. ^{111}In

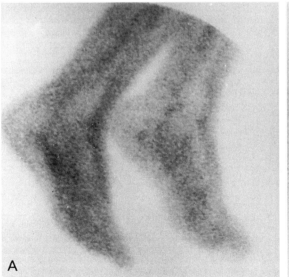 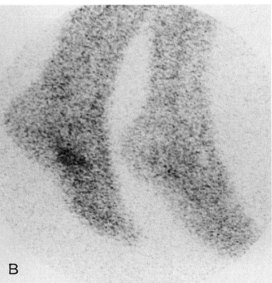

FIGURE 60.11. Osteomyelitis. **A:** Right lateral image obtained 1 hour after injection shows uptake in the midfoot. **B:** Image obtained 24 hours after injection shows increasing uptake.

oxine and ^{99m}Tc HMPAO are radiopharmaceuticals used to label cells involved in inflammatory processes. The radiolabeled autologous leukocytes have been particularly useful in the diagnosis of suspected abscesses.

^{111}In-labeled leukocyte scans are able to depict most abscesses within 4 hours of injection, although 18 to 24 hours may be necessary to depict smaller lesions. Normal images show only liver, spleen, and bone marrow. No colonic or renal activity is present on normal 18-hour images, and healing wounds normally do not accumulate ^{111}In-labeled leukocytes.

^{111}In-labeled leukocyte scans have been shown to be approximately 90% sensitive and specific in the diagnosis of intraabdominal abscesses and are supplementary to CT and ultrasound imaging. Perhaps the major advantage of radiolabeled leukocytes is in the evaluation of patients who have no localizing signs, because total-body imaging is easily performed.

^{111}In-labeled leukocyte scans are preferable to ^{67}Ga citrate scans in the evaluation of acute infection, but ^{67}Ga scans may be superior in the evaluation of chronic infection and of inflammatory conditions of the bones and joints. A major advantage of ^{111}In leukocyte imaging is the absence of normal radioactivity in the gastrointestinal tract and kidneys.

^{99m}Tc HMPAO–labeled leukocyte imaging shows activity in the gastrointestinal tract and genitourinary system as early as 1 hour after administration. Delayed imaging after 1 hour may have false-positive results. If a rapid diagnosis of an acute infectious process is needed, a ^{99m}Tc HMPAO–labeled leukocyte study may be preferred to a ^{111}In-labeled leukocyte study. However, in most other clinical situations, ^{111}In-labeled leukocyte imaging is the procedure of choice.

REFERENCES

1. Call MS, Sutherland DA, Eisentraut AM, et al. The tagging of leukemic leukocytes with radioactive chromium and measurement of the in vivo cell survival. *J Lab Clin Med* 1955;45:717.
2. Deubelbeiss KA, Dancey JT, Harker LA, et al. Neutrophil kinetics in the dog. *J Clin Invest* 1975;55:833.
3. Athens JW, Mauer AM, Ashenbrucker H, et al. Leukokinetic studies, I: a method for labeling leukocytes with diisopropyl fluorophosphate (DF32P). *Blood* 1959;14:303.
4. Burleson RL, Johnson MC, Head H. Scintigraphic demonstration of experimental abscesses with intravenous ^{67}Ga citrate and ^{67}Ga-labeled blood leukocytes. *Ann Surg* 1973;178:446.
5. English D, Andersen BE. Labeling of phagocytes from human blood with ^{99m}Tc-sulfur solloid. *J Nucl Med* 1975;16:5.
6. Anderson BR, English D, Akalin HE, et al. Inflammatory lesions localized with technetium Tc-^{99m}-labeled leukocytes. *Arch Intern Med* 1975;135:1067.
7. McAfee JG, Thakur ML. Survey of radioactive agents for in vitro labeling of phagocytic leukocytes, I: soluble agents. *J Nucl Med* 1976;17:480.
8. McAfee JG, Thakur ML. Survey of radioactive agents for in vitro labeling of phagocytic leukocytes, II: particles. *J Nucl Med* 1976;17:488.
9. Coleman RE. Radiolabeled leukocytes. In: Freeman LM, Weissman HS, eds. *Nuclear medicine annual 1982.* New York: Raven Press, 1982:119–141.
10. Linhart N, Bok B, Meignan M, et al. Technetium-^{99m} labeled human leukocytes: in vitro and animal studies. In: Thakur ML, Gottschalk A, eds. *Indium-111 labeled neutrophils, platelets, and lymphocytes.* New York: Trivirum, 1981:69.
11. Uchida T, Vincent PC. In vitro studies of leukocyte labeling with ^{99m}Tc. *J Nucl Med* 1976;17:730–736.
12. Uchida T, Nemoto T, Yui T, et al. Use of technetium-99m as a radioactive label to study migratory patterns of leukocytes. *J Nucl Med* 1979;20:1197.
13. Burleson RL, Holman BL, Tow DE. Scintigraphic demonstration of abscesses with radioactive gallium labeled leukocytes. *Surg Gynecol Obstet* 1975;141:379.
14. Thakur ML, Coleman RE, Welch MJ. Indium-111-labeled leukocytes for the localization of abscesses: preparation, analysis, tissue distribution, and comparison with gallium-67 citrate in dogs. *J Lab Clin Med* 1977;89:217.
15. Coleman RE, Welch DM, Baker WJ, et al. Clinical experience using indium-111 labeled leukocytes. In: Thakur ML, Gottschalk A, eds. *Indium-111 labeled neutrophils, platelets, and lymphocytes.* New York: Trivirum, 1981:103-118.
16. Beightol RW, Baker WJ. Labeling autologous leukocytes with indium-111 oxine. *J Hosp Pharm* 1980;37:847.
17. Burke JET, Roath S, Ackery D, et al. The comparison of 8-hydroxyquinoline, tropolone, and acetylacetone as mediators in the labeling of polymorphonuclear leukocytes with indium-111: a functional study. *Eur J Nucl Med* 1982;7:73.
18. Danpure HJ, Osman S, Brady F. The labeling of blood cells in plasma with In-111 tropolonate. *Br J Radiol* 1982;55:247.
19. Peters AM, Saverymuttu SH, Reavy HJ, et al. Imaging of inflammation with indium-111 tropolonate labeled leukocytes. *J Nucl Med* 1983;24:39.
20. Gunter KP, Lukens JN, Clanton JA, et al. Neutrophil labeling with indium-111: tropolone vs. oxine. *Radiology* 1983;149:563.
21. McAfee JG, Gagne GM, Subramanian G, et al. Distribution of leukocytes labeled with In-111 oxine in dogs with acute inflammatory lesions. *J Nucl Med* 1980;21:1059.
22. Sinn H, Sylvester DJ. Simplified cell labeling with indium-111 acetylacetone. *Br J Radiol* 1979;52:758.
23. Zakhireh B, Thakur ML, Malech HL, et al. Indium-111 labeled human polymorphonuclear leukocytes: viability, random migration, chemotaxis, bactericidal capacity and ultrastructure. *J Nucl Med* 1979; 20:741.
24. Segal AE, Deteix P, Garcia R, et al. Indium-111 labeling of leukocytes: a detrimental effect on neutrophil and lymphocyte function and an improved method of cell labeling. *J Nucl Med* 1978;19:1238.
25. Danpure HJ, Osman S. Cell labelling and cell damage with indium-111 acetylacetone: an alternative to indium-111 oxine. *Br J Radiol* 1981;54:597.
26. Weiblen BW, Forstrom L, McCollough J. Studies of the kinetics of ^{111}In-labeled granulocytes. *J Lab Clin Med* 1979;94:246.
27. Lavender JP, Goldman JM, Arnot RN, et al. Kinetics of indium-111 labeled lymphocytes in normal subjects and patients with Hodgkin's disease. *Br Med J* 1977;2:797.
28. Goodwin DA, Doherty PW, McDougall IR. Clinical use of indium-111 labeled cells: an analysis of 312 cases. In: Thakur ML, Gottschalk A, eds. *Indium-111 labeled neutrophils, platelets, and lymphocytes.* New York: Trivirum, 1981:131–145.
29. Kipper MS, Williams RJ. Indium-111 white blood cell imaging. *Clin Nucl Med* 1983;8:449.
30. Thakur ML, Lavender JP, Arnot RN, et al. Indium-111 labeled autologous leukocytes in man. *J Nucl Med* 1977;18:1012–1019.
31. Watson EE. Cell labeling: radiation dose and effects. *J Nucl Med* 1983;24:637.
32. Bassano DA, McAfee JG. Cellular radiation doses of labeled neutrophils and platelets. *J Nucl Med* 1979;20:255.
33. ten Berge RJM, Natarajan AT, Hardeman MR, et al. Labeling with indium-111 has detrimental effects on human lymphocytes: concise communication. *J Nucl Med* 1983;24:615.
34. Gobaty AH, Kim EE, Lazarre C. Technologic, clinical, and basic science considerations for In-111-oxine-labeled leukocyte studies. *J Nucl Med Technol* 1983;11:190.
35. Altemeir WA, Culbertson WR, Fuller WD. Intra-abdominal abscesses. *Am J Surg* 1973;125:76.

36. Hiatt JR, Williams RA, Wilson SE. Intra-abdominal abscess: etiology and pathogenesis. *Semin Ultrasound* 1983;4:71.
37. Murphy P. *The neutrophil.* New York: Plenum, 1976.
38. Forstrom LA, Weiblen BJ, Gomez L, et al. Indium-111-oxine labeled leukocytes in the diagnosis of occult inflammatory disease. In: Thakur ML, Gottschalk A, eds. *Indium-111 labeled neutrophils, platelets and lymphocytes.* New York: Trivirlum, 1981:123.
39. Goodwin DA. Clinical use of In-111 leukocyte imaging. *Clin Nucl Med* 1983;8:36.
40. Kumar B, Coleman RE, Alderson PO. Gallium citrate Ga-67 imaging in the evaluation of patients with suspected inflammatory processes. *Arch Surg* 1975;110:1237.
41. Biello DR, Levitt RG, Melson GL. The roles of gallium-67 scintigraphy, ultrasonography, and computer tomography in the detection of abdominal abscesses. *Semin Nucl Med* 1979;9:58.
42. Thakur ML, Coleman RE, Mayhall CG, et al. Preparation and evaluation of ^{111}In-labeled leukocytes as an abscess imaging agent in dogs. *Radiology* 1976;119:731.
43. Lantieri RL, Fawcett HD, McKillop JH, et al. Ga-67 or In-111 white blood cell scans for abscess detection: a case for In111. *Clin Nucl Med* 1980;5:185.
44. Sfakianakis GN, Al-Skeikh W, Heal A, et al. Comparison of scintigraphy with In-111 leukocytes and Ga-67 in the diagnosis of occult sepsis. *J Nucl Med* 1982;23:618.
45. McDougall IR, Goodwin DA. Gallium scan v. indium-111 labeled oxyquinoline WBC scan. *Arch Intern Med* 1982;142:1407.
46. Caroll B, Silverman PM, Goodwin DA, et al. Ultrasonography and indium-111 white blood cell scanning for the detection of intra-abdominal abscesses. *Radiology* 1981;140:155.
47. Knochel JQ, Koehler PR, Lee TG, et al. Diagnosis of abdominal abscesses with computed tomography, ultrasound, and ^{111}In-leukocyte scans. *Radiology* 1980;137:425.
48. Coleman RE, Welch D. Possible pitfalls with clinical imaging of indium-111 leukocyte scintigraphy in a skeletal metastasis. *Am J Roentgenol* 1982;139:601.
49. Chiu W, Amodio JB, Scharf SC, et al. Indium-111-oxine labeled leukocyte uptake in Ki-1-positive anaplastic large cell lymphoma. *Pediatr Radiol* 1999;29:31.
50. Bicknell TA, Kohatsu S, Goodwin DA. Use of indium-111 labeled autologous leukocytes in differentiating pancreatic abscess from pseudocyst. *Am J Surg* 1981;142:312.
51. Fawcett HD, Lantieri RL, Frankel A, et al. Differentiating hepatic abscess from tumor: combined ^{111}In white blood cell and ^{99m}Tc liver scans. *Am J Roentgenol* 1980;135:53.
52. Fawcett HD, Goodwin DA, Lantieri RL. In-111 leukocyte scanning in inflammatory renal disease. *Clin Nucl Med* 1981;6:237.
53. Rovekamp MH, van Royen EA, Folmer SCCR, et al. Diagnosis of upper-abdominal infections by In-111 labeled leukocytes with Tc-99m colloid subtraction technique. *J Nucl Med* 1983;24:212.
54. Wellman HN, Giorgi P, Sinn H, et al. Scintimaging of skeletal infectious processes with a new leukocyte labeling technique utilizing In-111 acetylacetone. *J Nucl Med* 1981;22:P27.
55. Raptopoulis V, Doherty PW, Goss TP, et al. Acute osteomyelitis: advantage of white cell scans in early detection. *Am J Roentgenol* 1982; 139:1077.
56. McDougall IR, Baumert JE, Lantieri RL. Evaluation of ^{111}In leukocyte whole-body scanning. *Am J Roentgenol* 1979;133:849.
57. Scher DM, Pak K, Lonner JH, et al. The predictive value of indium-111 leukocyte scans in the diagnosis of infected total hip, knee or resection arthroplasties. *J Arthroplasty* 2000;15:295.
58. Joseph TN, Miytaba M, Chen AL, et al. Efficacy of combined technetium-99m sulfur colloid/indium-111 leukocyte scans to detect infected total hip and knee arthroplasties. *J Arthroplasty* 2001;16:753.
59. Teller RE, Christie MJ, Martin W, et al. Sequential indium-labeled leukocyte and bone scans to diagnose prosthetic joint infection. *Clin Orthop* 2000;373:24.
60. Singleton JW, Klingensmith WC. Indium-111 leukocyte imaging study in inflammatory bowel disease. *Gastroenterology* 1983;84:426.
61. Gray HW, Cuthbert I, Richards JR. Clinical imaging with indium-111 leukocyte uptake in bowel infarction. *J Nucl Med* 1981;22:701.
62. Coleman RE, Black RE, Welch DM, et al. Indium-111 labeled leukocytes in the evaluation of suspected abdominal abscesses. *Am J Surg* 1980;139:99.
63. Fisher MF, Rudd TG. In-111 labeled leukocyte imaging: false-positive study due to acute gastrointestinal bleeding. *J Nucl Med* 1983;24: 803.
64. Erick MP, Henke CE, Forstrom LA, et al. Use of ^{111}In-labeled leukocytes in evaluation of renal transplant rejection: a preliminary report. *Clin Nucl Med* 1979;4:24.
65. Wang TST, Oluwole S, Fawwax RA, et al. Cellular basis for accumulation of In-111 labeled leukocytes and platelets in rejecting cardiac allografts: concise communication. *J Nucl Med* 1982;23:993.
66. Weiss ES, Ahmed SA, Thakur ML, et al. Imaging of the inflammatory response in ischemic canine myocardium with ^{111}In-labeled leukocytes. *Am J Cardiol* 1977;40:195.
67. Zaret BL, Davies RE, Thakur ML, et al. Imaging the inflammatory response to acute myocardial infarction. In: Thakur ML, Gottschalk A, eds. *Indium-111 labeled neutrophils, platelets and lymphocytes.* New York: Trivirum, 1981:151.
68. Stevick CP, Fawcett D. Aortoilic-graft infection. *Arch Surg* 1981;116: 939.
69. McKeown PP, Miller C, Jamieson SW, et al. Diagnosis of arterial prosthetic graft infection by indium-111 oxine white blood cell scans. *Circulation* 1982;66[Suppl I]:130.
70. Wilson DG, Seabold JE, Lieberman LM. Detection of aortoarterial graft infections by leukocyte scintigraphy. *Clin Nucl Med* 1983;8: 412.
71. Anstall HB, Coleman RE. Donor-leukocyte imaging in granulocytopenic patients with sustpected abscesses: concise communication. *J Nucl Med* 1982;23:319.
72. Dutcher JP, Schiffer CA, Johnston GS. Rapid migration of ^{111}In-labeled granulocytes to sites of infection. *N Engl J Med* 1981;304: 586.
73. Datz FL, Taylor AT. Cell labeling: techniques and clinical utility. In: Freeman LM, ed. *Freeman and Johnson's clinical radionuclide imaging,* 3rd ed. Orlando, FL: Grune & Stratton 1986:1785–1913.
74. Datz FL. Current status of radionuclide infection imaging. In: Freeman LM, ed. *Nuclear medicine annual.* New York: Raven Press, 1993: 47-76.
75. Marcus CS, Kuperus JH, Butler JA, et al. Phagocytic labeling of leukocytes with technetium-99m albumin colloid for nuclear imaging. *Nucl Med Biol* 1988;15:673.
76. Butler JA, Marcus CS, Henneman PL, et al. Evaluation of technetium-99m leukocyte scan in diagnosis of acute appendicitis. *J Surg Res* 1987;42:575.
77. Henneman PL, Marcus CS, Butler JA, et al. Appendicitis-evaluation of technetium-99m leukocyte scan. *Ann Emerg Med* 1988;17:111.
78. Henneman PL, Marcus CS, Inkelis SH, et al. Evaluation of children with possible appendicitis using technetium-99m leukocyte scan. *Pediatrics* 1988;85:838.
79. Kung HF, Ohmomo Y, Kung MP. Current and future radiopharmaceuticals for brain imaging with single photon emission computed tomography. *Semin Nucl Med* 1990;2:290.
80. Costa DC, Lui D, Ell PJ. White cells radiolabeled with indium-111 and technetium-99m: a study of relative sensitivity and in vivo viability. *Nucl Med Commun* 1988;9:725.
81. Peters AM. Utility of technetium-99m HMPAO leukocytes for imaging infection. *Semin Nucl Med* 1994;24:110.
82. Bennink R, Peeter M, D'Haens G, et al. Tc-99m HMPAO white blood cell scintigraphy in the assessment of the extent and severity of an acute exacerbation of ulcerative colitis. *Clin Nucl Med* 2001; 26:99.
83. Danpure HJ, Osman S, Carroll MJ. Development of a clinical protocol for radiolabeling of mixed leukocytes with technetium-99m hexamethylpropyleneamine oxime. *Nucl Med Commun* 1988;9:465.
84. Kelbaek H, Linde J, Nielsen SL. Evaluation of new leukocyte labeling procedure with technetium-99m HMPAO. *Eur J Nucl Med* 1988; 14:621.

85. Mortelmans L, Malbrain S, Stuyck J, et al. In vitro and in vivo evaluation of granulocyte labeling with [technetium-99m]d, 1-HMPAO. *J Nucl Med* 1989;30:2022.

86. Mock BH, Schauwecker DS, English D, et al. In vivo kinetics of canine leukocytes labeled with technetium-99m HMPAO and indium-111 tropolonate. *J Nucl Med* 1988;29:1246.

87. Ecclestone M, Proulx A, Ballinger JR, et al. In vitro comparison of HMPAO and gentisic acid for labeling leukocytes with technetium-99m. *Eur J Med* 1990;16:299.

88. Datz FL. Indium-111-labeled leukocytes for detection of infection: current status. *Semin Nucl Med* 1994;24:92.

89. McAfee JG, Subramanian G, Gagne G, et al. Technetium-99m HMPAO for leukocyte labeling: experimental comparison with indium-111 oxine in dogs. *Eur J Nucl Med* 1987;13:353.

90. McAfee JG. What is best method for imaging focal infections? *J Nucl Med* 1990;31:413.

91. Peters AM, Roddie ME, Danpure HJ, et al. Technetium-99m HMPAO-labeled leukocytes: comparison with indium-111-tropolonate-labeled granulocytes. *Nucl Med Commun* 1988;9:449.

92. Liberatore M, Iurilli AP, Ponzo F. Clinical usefulness of technetium-99m-HMPAO labeled leukocyte scan in prosthetic vascular graft infection. *J Nucl Med* 1998;39:875.

93. Blume PA, Arrighi JA, Dey HM, et al. Diagnosis of pedal osteomyelitis with Tc-99m HMPAO labeled leukocytes. *J Foot Ankle Surg* 1997;36:120.

94. Devillers A, Moisan A, Hennion F, et al. Contribution of technetium-99m hexamethylpropylene amine oxime labelled leukocyte scintigraphy to the diagnosis of diabetic foot injection. *Eur J Nucl Med* 1998;25:132.

95. Vorne M, Soini I, Lantto T, et al. Technetium-99m HMPAO-labeled leukocytes in detecting inflammatory lesions: comparison with gallium-67 citrate. *J Nucl Med* 1989;30:1332.

96. Mountford PJ, Kettle AG, O'Doherty MJ, et al. Comparison of technetium-99m HMPAO leukocytes with indium-111-oxine leukocytes for localizing intra-abdominal sepsis. *J Nucl Med* 1990;31:311.

97. Lindahl J, Ristkari SKK, Vorne M, et al. Technetium-99m HMPAO-labeled leukocytes in diagnosing acute colonic diverticulitis. *Acta Chir Scand* 1989;155:479.

98. Hallingsworth JW, Siegal ER, Creasy WQ. Granulocyte survival in synovial exudate of patients with rheumatoid arthritis and other inflammatory joint diseases. *Yale J Biol Med* 1967;39:289.

99. Datz FL, Bedont RA, Baker WJ, et al. No difference in sensitivity for occult infection between oxine- and tropolone-labeled indium-111 leukocytes when imaged early. *J Nucl Med* 1984;25:43.

100. Peters AM. Imaging inflammation: current role of labeled autologous leukocytes. *J Nucl Med* 1992;33:65.

Diagnostic Nuclear Medicine, Fourth Edition. Edited by M.P. Sandler, R.E. Coleman, J.A. Patton,
F.J.Th. Wackers, A. Gottschalk. Lippincott Williams & Wilkins, Philadelphia 2003.

61

DETECTION OF FOCAL INFLAMMATION USING RADIOLABELED, NONSPECIFIC HUMAN POLYCLONAL IMMUNOGLOBULIN-G

ALAN J. FISCHMAN
ROBERT H. RUBIN

Detection of the anatomic site and extent of inflammatory processes is a central issue in the effective clinical management of patients with infections and idiopathic conditions such as rheumatoid arthritis and inflammatory bowel disease. Defining the site of an inflammatory lesion is critical for precise diagnosis and therapy. Furthermore, quantifying the extent of the process offers important prognostic information, and serial examinations can be an effective method for assessing effectiveness of therapy (1).

Techniques such as conventional radiography, computed tomography, magnetic resonance imaging, and ultrasonography are highly effective for the detection of intraabdominal, intrathoracic, and intracranial infections in patients with normal anatomy (2–5). However, these methods are less reliable in the evaluation of patients with suspected focal infection of surgical sites or of elements of the cardiovascular or musculoskeletal systems, particularly when normal anatomic landmarks are distorted by trauma, surgery, or previous disease. Also, the sensitivity of these techniques is limited in acutely evolving processes and in immunocompromised patients (6,7). For these patients, and those with systemic evidence of inflammation without localizing signs or symptoms, total body inflammation imaging with radiopharmaceuticals such as ^{67}Ga citrate and ^{111}In- or ^{99m}Tc-labeled leukocytes has proved useful (8–17).

Although currently available radiopharmaceuticals have been useful in specific situations, each agent has disadvantages that limits its utility—nonspecific accumulation of ^{67}Ga citrate in the bowel, and the requirement for handling infected blood and complicated ex vivo processing with radiolabeled leukocytes (17). The ideal infection and inflammation imaging should have the following characteristics: (a) identification of focal inflammation should be reliable, and at least a semiquantitative assessment of disease activity should be possible; (b) preparation of the reagent should be straightforward and not require handling and reinjection of potentially contaminated blood; (c) there should be no side effects associated with the agent, and its radiation dosimetry characteristics should permit serial studies for assessing response to therapy ("proof of cure" studies); (d) nonspecific accumulation in background organs should be minimal; and (e) the results of the study should be available in a timely fashion that is meaningful for clinical decision making (18).

In this chapter, laboratory and clinical results with two new radiopharmaceuticals for inflammation imaging, ^{111}In-IgG and ^{99m}Tc-IgG, are presented, with particular emphasis on how well they fulfill the specifications of an ideal inflammation imaging agent.

PRECLINICAL STUDIES WITH RADIOLABELED IGG

The first indication for the use of radiolabeled IgG as an infection and inflammation imaging agent came from studies of specific radioimmunoimaging. In these investigations, a rodent model of focal Pseudomonas aeruginosa type 1 infection was used to compare the imaging properties of a radiolabeled, high-affinity monoclonal antibody specific for this organism with a monoclonal antibody directed against an arsenate haptene (19). The results of these investigations were striking. Although specific immune imaging could be clearly demonstrated, this was significant only at 48 or more hours after injection of the specific antibody. At earlier times, the site of the infection was equally well visualized with both the specific and nonspecific antibodies (Fig. 61.1). This finding suggested that nonspecific radiolabeled IgG might be a useful reagent for inflammation imaging (19),

A.J. Fischman: Radiology, Harvard Medical School, and Radiology Nuclear Medicine, Massachusetts General Hospital, Boston, MA.
R.H. Rubin: Radiology, Nuclear Medicine, Massachusetts General Hospital, Boston, MA.

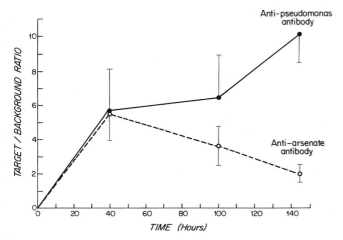

FIGURE 61.1. Time dependence of the target-to-background (T/B) ratios (infected/normal) for groups of rats with focal *Pseudomonas aeruginosa* type 1 thigh infections imaged with specific and nonspecific monoclonal antibodies. At 40 hours after injection, the T/Bs were not significantly different. At 100 and 144 hours, the T/B was significantly higher for the specific antibody (p <0.02 and p <0.0001, respectively).

and intensive laboratory studies to assess the mechanisms of nonspecific accumulation were initiated.

This experience also suggested that extreme caution should be used in evaluating the mechanism of localization of radiolabeled monoclonal antibodies. For example, ^{99m}Tc-labeled BW 250/183, a monoclonal antibody that binds to the NCA-95 epitope on human granulocytes, has been used to detect sites of inflammation (20–23). Perkins et al. (24) suggested that this reagent might be very useful for the evaluation of patients with idiopathic inflammatory bowel disease; however, less than 20% of the radioactivity in blood was associated with granulocytes, suggesting that a significant component of localization might be nonspecific. This result was very similar to our experience with specific anti-*Pseudomonas* antibodies. These observations indicate that rigid criteria must be fulfilled (e.g., Fab fragments should target, as well as intact antibody) before accepting that the inflammation imaging properties of an antibody are a result of specific antigen binding.

An important step in the application of ^{111}In-IgG for human imaging was the demonstration that radiolabeled nonspecific human polyclonal IgG provides images comparable to those from conventional imaging agents in a rodent model of focal infection. In these studies, ^{67}Ga citrate and ^{111}In-IgG were coinjected, and serial images of both radionuclides were acquired. The results of these investigations demonstrated that ^{111}In-IgG was both more sensitive and specific than ^{67}Ga citrate. The utility of ^{111}In-IgG for imaging various inflammatory processes was demonstrated by studies of focal inflammation caused by a wide array of initiating agents, including bacteria such as *P. aeruginosa, Staphylococcus aureus, Escherichia coli, Klebsiella pneumoniae,* and *Bacteroides fragilis;* fungi such as *Candida albicans* and *Pneumocystis carinii;* and sterile inflammation produced by turpentine (25,26,27). In addition, Breedveld et al. (28) demonstrated that nonspecific IgG may be useful in the evaluation of inflammatory arthritis. The nonspecificity of this approach was further vali-

dated when it was shown that radiolabeled Fc but not Fab fragments of IgG also localized at the site of inflammation to an extent sufficient for imaging (29). Also, it was demonstrated that pretreatment of animals with corticosteroids, indomethacin, or cyclophosphamide did not affect the ability of the ^{111}In-IgG to localize at sites of infection (30).

Although the possibility that the accumulation of radiolabeled IgG at sites of infection was related to binding to Fc receptors on inflammatory cells was attractive (19,20), several lines of evidence showed this hypothesis to be incorrect. Coadministration of ^{111}In-IgG with large amounts of unlabeled IgG had no effect on imaging, arguing against ligand-receptor interaction (31). Carefully performed autoradiographic studies showed that most radiolabeled IgG accumulated in the expanded extracellular space of inflammatory lesions but was not associated with inflammatory cells (32). Although ^{111}In-IgG has significant binding to Fc receptors *in vitro* and deglycosylation abolished this binding, the inflammation imaging properties of radiolabeled deglycosylated IgG were identical to the unmodified reagent (31). Finally, a series of studies by Oyen et al. (17,33,34), have shown that (a) radiolabeled IgA also accumulates at sites of inflammation although there are very low concentrations of specific receptors for this protein at sites of infection and (b) severe granulocytopenia does not prevent the localization of ^{111}In-IgG at sites of inflammation.

What then is the mechanism of localization of labeled IgG at the site of inflammation? Detailed studies of kinetics of IgG localization have demonstrated that the rate of entry of IgG into the expanded extracellular space of infected tissue is markedly elevated because of increased capillary permeability that results in the delivery of a variety of proteins, including albumin, IgG, and gallium bound to transferrin, into the inflammatory site. However, the rate of egress of IgG is significantly reduced, possibly resulting from abnormal lymphatic drainage (35). In addition, once present in the inflammatory exudate, *in vitro* studies suggested that physicochemical changes occur in IgG that enhance trapping (36).

CLINICAL APPLICATION OF [111]IN- AND [99M]TC-LABELED IGG

Although preclinical studies clearly demonstrated that a variety of radionuclides such as ^{111}In, ^{123}I, and ^{99m}Tc could be used to radiolabel IgG for inflammation imaging (19,25,26), the reasons for initially choosing ^{111}In for clinical use were threefold: (a) a reproducible method for labeling IgG with ^{111}In that provided a reagent that was suitable for use in humans was available. This method, in which IgG is conjugated with diethylenetriaminepentaacetic acid (DTPA) produces a stable reagent to which ^{111}In can be easily conjugated as needed; (b) the physical half-life of ^{111}In is well matched to the biologic half-life of IgG and is long enough for serial studies to be obtained over several days to determine the optimal times for imaging different disease processes (1,17); and (c) the ^{111}In-labeled agent has very low levels of accumulation in the bowel. Thus far, more than 2,000 humans with suspected or proven focal inflammation have been studied with this reagent, in the United States and Europe, and the following general points can be made.

1. There have been no significant side effects associated with the administration of radiolabeled human polyclonal IgG, even with repeated doses (as many as seven times over a 3-year period in a single patient) (1,17). Because the usual clinical dose of ^{111}In-IgG is 0.025 mg/kg of protein labeled with approximately 60 MBq of ^{111}In, the freedom from side effects is not surprising given the excellent safety record associated with multiple doses of 100 to 500 mg/kg of unlabeled IgG to patients requiring therapeutic IgG. However, because adverse reactions to therapy with IgG have been observed in patients with IgA deficiency, this condition may be a relative counterindication to the use of ^{111}In-IgG. Each dose of ^{111}In-IgG results in a radiation burden of 0.7 cGy to the whole body and 1.09 cGy to the kidneys, posing about one half of the radiation exposure of a barium series with fluoroscopy (1,17).

2. The normal distribution of ^{111}In-IgG is primarily intravascular; however, significant concentrations of the reagent accumulate in the liver, spleen, kidneys, bone marrow, and nasal mucosa but not in the gut. Images are interpreted as abnormal if focal zones of abnormal accumulation of tracer are visualized initially and become more intense over time. The physical half-life of ^{111}In lends itself to extremely delayed imaging. A clear-cut assessment of positivity or negativity can usually be made within 24 hours of injection (delayed imaging is used primarily in suspected vascular infection). Diagnostic quality images can often be acquired within 12 hours after injection of ^{111}In-IgG and even as early as 6 hours in some cases. Unfortunately, this time frame does not permit the evaluation of acutely evolving processes such as most cases of appendicitis (1,17,18,26).

3. Focal accumulation of ^{111}In-IgG occurs in patients with inflammation resulting from infection, inflammatory bowel disease, and rheumatoid arthritis. In addition, focal areas of ^{111}In-IgG accumulation have also been detected in patients with malignancies, such as gynecologic cancer, melanoma, lymphoma, and prostate cancer (1,17). Autoradiographic studies in animals with experimental tumors have shown that the reagent accumulates not in the tumor but in areas of inflammation that develop in response to the presence of the tumor. As in infections, ^{111}In-IgG accumulates in the extracellular portion of the inflammatory reaction and is not cell associated (unpublished results, author's laboratory).

Although ^{111}In-IgG has proven to be an extremely useful imaging agent, a ^{99m}Tc-labeled agent might have several important advantages. The more favorable radiation dosimetry of ^{99m}Tc would result in higher count density images that might allow earlier imaging particularly with single photon emission computed tomography (SPECT). In addition, the lower cost and wider availability of ^{99m}Tc would foster the application of IgG imaging. As previously indicated, until recently, the technology for labeling IgG with ^{111}In was more advanced than that for labeling with ^{99m}Tc. Currently, there are several methods for ^{99m}Tc labeling of IgG, including direct binding of technetium to donor atoms on the protein, conventional bifunctional chelating agents, and conjugation of a prelabeled ^{99m}Tc-4,5-bis (thioacetanido) pentanoate active ester to amino groups of lysine residues (N_2S_2 method). Unfortunately, none of these methods has been totally satisfactory for a number of reasons including (a) dissociation of the technetium-antibody complex with time, (b) accumulation of the radiolabel in bowel and the reticuloendothelial system, (c) unreliable yields of specifically bound technetium, (d) excessive complexity, and (e) marked discrepancy in biodistribution compared with indium and iodine-labeled IgG (37, 38).

To address these issues, we developed a method for labeling human polyclonal IgG with ^{99m}Tc via a hydrazino nicotinamide (HYNIC) derivative (39). Biodistribution studies in animals and humans that compared the indium and the technetium-labeled compounds showed them to be essentially identical (40–42). As expected, radiation absorbed dose was much lower with the technetium agent (43). In animal models of focal thigh infection, the imaging properties (target-to-background and percent residual activity) of the two compounds were nearly identical, with the increased photon flux of the technetium-labeled reagent being superior for detecting early accumulation (39,40). The availability of ^{99m}Tc labeled HYNIC-IgG has allowed the direct comparison of the infection imaging properties of radiolabeled IgG with ^{111}In leukocytes. In these studies, both radiopharmaceuticals were coinjected in groups of rabbits with focal *E. coli* infection and serial images were acquired (40). At all imaging times, excellent images of the infection sites were obtained with both agents. However, the target-to-background ratio was consistently higher and background accumulation lower with ^{111}In leukocytes. Although these results indicate that ^{111}In leukocyte is a generally superior imaging agent, the higher photon flux, ease of preparation, and lack of blood handling makes radiolabeled IgG (particularly when labeled with ^{99m}Tc) an attractive alternative. Recently, ^{99m}Tc-HYNIC-IgG was compared with ^{67}Ga citrate for detection of intraabdominal infections in rats with abscesses produced by the cecal ligation and puncture technique (44). With both agents the lesions were visualized by 4 hours, indicating that ^{99m}Tc-IgG performed at least as well as the standard agent, ^{67}Ga citrate, with obvious advantages of lower radiation exposure and more favorable physical properties.

Recently, the imaging properties of ^{99m}Tc-HYNIC-IgG and ^{111}In-IgG were directly compared in a prospective study of 37 patients with suspected infectious or inflammatory disease (45). After administration of ^{99m}Tc-HYNIC-IgG, imaging was performed at 4 and 24 hours. After acquisition of the final images, the patients were injected with ^{111}In-IgG and additional images were acquired at 4, 24, and 48 hours. Imaging results were confirmed by microbiologic, histologic, radiologic, and clinical methods. In all patients, the two radiopharmaceuticals showed 100% concordance.

In the following sections, specific applications of ^{111}In- and ^{99m}Tc-IgG for imaging a variety of types of infection are described.

Intraabdominal Infections

In our initial experience with ^{111}In-IgG, 21 true-positive and 30 true-negative results were obtained in patients with suspected

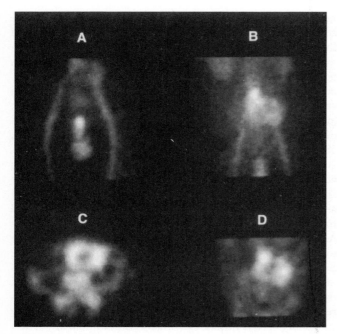

FIGURE 61.2. ^{99m}Tc-IgG images of the abdomen of a patient with acute sigmoid diverticulitis. **A:** Planar image 5 hours postinjection. **B:** Planar image 18 hours postinjection. **C and D:** Transverse and coronal single photon emission computed tomography images at 5 hours postinjection.

intraabdominal infection. False-negative results were obtained in three subjects: (a) a patient with focal intrahepatic infection following partial hepatectomy; (b) a patient with diverticulitis studied after 2 weeks of treatment with antibiotics who was found to have a tiny (<1 cm^2) residual focus of inflammation at surgery; and (c) a patient with low-grade infection of a peripancreatic fluid collection, which on culture was found to contain small amounts of lactobacilli (gram stain was negative) (1). Since that time, we have studied more than 400 additional patients with sensitivity and specificity of greater than 90%. Figure 61.2 illustrates the results of ^{99m}Tc-IgG imaging at 5 and 8

hours after injection in a patient with a diverticular abscess. Although the lesion was detectable in the 5-hour planar image, lesion definition was much better at 18 hours. However, superb images were obtained at 6 hours using SPECT. These results suggest that the time required to acquire diagnostic quality images can be significantly reduced by SPECT imaging of ^{99m}Tc-IgG.

The greatest difficulty in interpreting IgG images occurs in patients with suspected infection in and around the liver because of high physiologic concentrations of tracer and in patients with recent surgery. In the latter group, IgG imaging has been found to be at least as sensitive as computed tomography (CT), with serial scans being particularly useful (Fig. 61.3). ^{111}In-IgG imaging provided accurate information in five patients with focal inflammation that was missed by CT and ultrasonography because previous surgery and disease made these studies extremely difficult to interpret (1,17,28).

Although the largest experience with ^{111}In-IgG imaging has been in patients with diverticulitis and diverticular abscesses, positive results have also been obtained in periappendiceal abscesses, deep surgical wound infections, and diffuse colitis in patients with enterocolitis from *E. coli* and *Campylobacter jejuni* infection (as well as in several patients with idiopathic ulcerative colitis) (unpublished results, author's laboratory). Serafini et al. (46) have reported a sensitivity of 100% with this diagnostic approach in patients with pelvic and abdominal infection involving the female genital tract.

Serial ^{111}In-IgG imaging in patients with intraabdominal infection treated with antibiotic and/or drainage has been particularly revealing. Persistently positive scans after stopping therapy have been associated with poor clinical responses—either prompt relapse with cessation of antibiotics or evidence of continuing focal inflammation. In contrast, improvement on serial images has been associated with continued clinical well-being after stopping antimicrobial therapy (1,26) (Fig. 61.4).

Vascular Infections

A traditional diagnostic problem of growing importance is the inability of conventional imaging procedures to diagnose cardio-

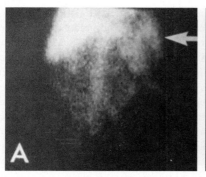
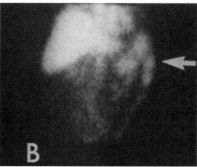
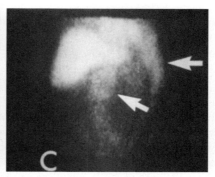

FIGURE 61.3. ^{111}In-IgG images acquired at 1-week intervals in a patient who had a transverse colectomy and then drainage of a left subphrenic abscess several weeks earlier. The patient remained febrile, and ultrasound and computed tomography (CT) were negative at the times of the first two studies; however, the IgG study revealed increasing inflammation in the left upper quadrant. At the time of the third IgG study, ultrasound and CT were also positive. At surgery, more than 1,000 cc of pus were removed from the two sites. In this patient with surgically altered anatomy, IgG imaging was more accurate than the conventional techniques.

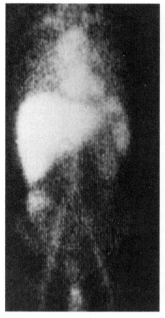
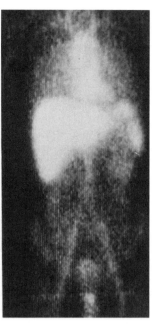

FIGURE 61.4. ¹¹¹In-IgG images obtained 3 weeks apart in a patient with Crohn's disease and fever, pain below the liver, and an uninterpretable computed tomography scan. At the time of the first scan (*left*) the patient was afebrile after 3 weeks of antibiotic therapy; however, IgG imaging revealed residual inflammation below the liver. When antibiotics were discontinued, the patient's symptoms promptly returned. The second scan (*right*), at the end of a second course of antibiotics, indicated that the inflammation had resolved and the patient did well when antibiotic therapy was stopped.

vascular infection. With the increasing numbers of individuals with vascular prostheses, the possibility of microbial seeding, either in the perioperative period or as a result of a transient bacteremia from another source, is becoming an increasingly common diagnostic problem.

Studies in more than 40 patients with suspected vascular graft infection have revealed a sensitivity of greater than 90% and a specificity approaching 100% (Fig. 61.5). The one group in which false-negative results have been obtained consistently is patients with aortoduodenal fistulas. Thus far, however, all pa-

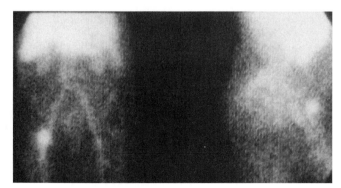

FIGURE 61.5. Anterior and right lateral ¹¹¹In-IgG images demonstrating focal infection and mycotic aneurysm at the site of a femoral-popliteal graft anastomosis. Imaging was performed 6 hours after injection of the reagent.

tients studied with this diagnosis were imaged when they were symptom free on antibiotics and, thus, had lesser amounts of inflammation (47).

Two diagnostic problems for which IgG imaging has been particularly useful are the definition of extent of infection and the differentiation of infection from hematoma in patients with atherosclerotic aneurysms who present with fever. In the first group, it has been possible to determine if one or both limbs of an aortobifemoral graft are involved in the process. This information has been extremely useful to surgeons in planning vascular repair. The ability to perform serial imaging over 72 hours with ¹¹¹In-IgG has proven to be useful in patients with evolving atherosclerotic aneurysms, in whom, because of a fever and/or a moderate leukocytosis, the possibility of a mycotic aneurysm is suspected. Although patients with true infection almost always had positive images by 24 hours postinjection, those with sterile processes, but with the leakage of blood into the surrounding tissues (which elicits a low-grade inflammatory response), had negative studies during the first 36 to 48 hours postinjection. Between 48 and 72 hours postinjection, low levels of accumulation of radiolabeled IgG have been observed. Although in theory infection with a relatively nonvirulent organism could result in a similar pattern, most infections of this type are caused by virulent organisms such as *S. aureus* or *Salmonella* species.

Because of the nature of the pathology of endocarditis (microorganisms seeding a platelet-fibrin thrombus on the surface of a heart valve, with little inflammatory infiltrate), it is not surprising that inflammation imaging with ¹¹¹In-IgG has not been useful for detecting vegetations. Although there is reason to believe that this approach could detect some cases in which infection has extended into the myocardium, echocardiography, particularly by the transesophageal approach, remains the diagnostic procedure of choice.

Bone and Joint Infections

Studies by our group (1), and others (48,49) have clearly shown that ¹¹¹In-IgG imaging is a sensitive technique for detecting focal inflammation of the skeletal system. In studies of more than 100 patients with suspected infection, focal accumulation of ¹¹¹In-IgG was detected in 69 of 71 patients with proven infection (48,49). In seven patients with positive studies who were found to be free of infection, other forms of inflammation were identified. In another study, true positive results were obtained in 14 of 14 patients studied (46).

¹¹¹In-IgG has been particularly useful in the evaluation of patients with possible infections of joint prostheses (1,17,50). In 40 patients suspected of having infected total hip or total knee prostheses, Oyen et al. (50) reported a 93% sensitivity and 88% specificity for infection and 100% specificity for inflammation. We have made similar observations in a smaller group of patients. Particularly noteworthy has been the utility of serial studies in the management of patients with prosthetic joint infections. As illustrated by the images shown in Fig. 61.6, an important clinical issue in these patients is long-term management. In this patient, *E. coli* infection of a hip prosthesis was diagnosed, the prosthesis was removed, and aggressive antibiotic therapy begun. The hope was to eradicate the infection and then

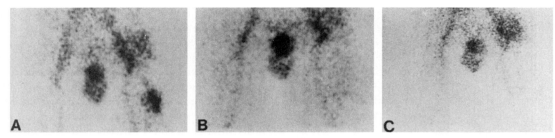

FIGURE 61.6. Serial ^{111}In-IgG images performed in a patient with an infected left hip prosthesis. Each time residual infection was found at the site of positive findings on the scan. Eventually, a negative scan was obtained, and reconstruction of the hip joint was successful.

reconstruct the hip. Over 3 years, seven ^{111}In-IgG studies were performed at times when the patient was considered to be clinically free of infection. On six of these occasions, focal infection, undiagnosable by routine hip joint aspiration or conventional radiography, was demonstrated with ^{111}In-IgG and confirmed by scan guided drainage procedures. Finally, a negative study was obtained, and the hip was reconstructed. Over the following 4 years, the patient had a normally functioning total hip prosthesis that was free of infection. Although this is the most dramatic example of this phenomenon, we have accumulated several such cases in which serial IgG studies for proof of cure were helpful in patient management.

Imaging with ^{111}In-IgG and ^{111}In-white blood cells (WBCs) was compared prospectively in 35 patients with suspected focal sites of subacute infection (51). Clinical, roentgenologic, and microbiologic findings were considered to be proof of the presence of infection or inflammation. In this group of patients, ^{111}In-IgG scintigraphy performed significantly better than ^{111}In-WBCs, especially in infections of the locomotor system but also in various soft tissue infections. Both techniques showed disappointing results in patients with disseminated *Yersinia* infection and in some patients with tuberculosis. Sensitivity and specificity was 74% and 100% for ^{111}In-IgG and 52% and 78% for ^{111}In-WBCs. Figure 61.7 shows representative images of a patient with a septic knee joint who was imaged at 18 hours after being coinjected with ^{99m}Tc-IgG and ^{111}In-labeled leukocytes. These results illustrate that, although the distributions of IgG and WBCs at the site of infection are similar, the quality of the IgG images is superior.

In another study, ^{111}In-IgG scintigraphy was compared with plain x-ray films and conventional bone scans in 16 diabetic patients with foot ulcers, gangrene, or painful Charcot joints (52). The results were verified by histologic examination of surgical specimens or long-term clinical follow-up. On bone scans, all seven osteomyelitic foci were detected. However, 19 additional foci not resulting from osteomyelitis were seen. The absence of true-negative bone scans in this study resulted in a specificity of 0%. On plain x-ray films, four of seven osteomyelitis foci were detected. ^{111}In-IgG scintigraphy detected 6/7 foci (sensitivity 57% and 86%, respectively). Plain x-ray films correctly ruled out osteomyelitis in 15/19 lesions, ^{111}In-IgG scintigraphy in 16 of 19 (specificity 79% and 84%, respectively). All imaging procedures yielded false-positive results in penetrating ulcers over the calcaneus in two patients and in one patient with

a Charcot joint. A false-negative ^{111}In-IgG study was observed in a patient with severe arterial angiopathy. These results demonstrate that ^{111}In-IgG scintigraphy can contribute to adequate evaluation of osteomyelitis in diabetic foot complications because it improves specificity when compared with bone scan and radiographic findings and improves sensitivity in comparison to plain x-ray films.

In a large clinical study ^{111}In-IgG was evaluated in 226 patients with 232 possible foci of infection or inflammation (53). Imaging was performed 4, 24, and 48 hours postinjection, and the results were verified by culture (61%) and long-term clinical and x-ray follow-up (39%). All infected total hip arthroplasties (THAs) and total knee arthroplasties, focal osteomyelitis, diabetic foot infections, septic arthritis, and soft tissue infections were detected (61 foci). Only one patient with early, low-grade spondylodiscitis was falsely negative. Because ^{111}In-IgG scintigraphy cannot discriminate between infection and sterile inflammation, careful interpretation is necessary (specificity for inflammation 100%, specificity for infection of 77%). These results indicate that ^{111}In-IgG imaging is a very sensitive tool for detec-

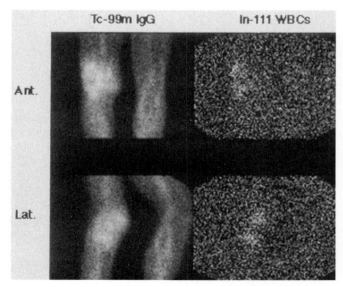

FIGURE 61.7. Anterior and lateral ^{99m}Tc-IgG and ^{111}In-white blood cell (WBC) images of at patient with a septic knee joint. Although the distributions of IgG and WBCs at the site of infection are similar, the quality of the IgG images are superior.

tion of infectious bone and joint disease. When uptake patterns that are characteristic for sterile inflammation are excluded, infection can be ruled out with a very high degree of certainty.

Preliminary studies (54,55) have suggested that IgG imaging may be useful in the evaluation of patients with inflammatory arthritis. In these patients, the issue is not usually a question of initial diagnosis, but the possibility that serial studies could provide an objective basis for directing therapy, with certain drugs being more effective for pain relief than as disease-modifying therapy. The latter agents are usually more toxic, so the more objective and quantifiable the evaluation, the better this type of therapy can be used.

Pulmonary Infections

In most patients with suspected pulmonary infection, conventional chest radiography is appropriate for assessing the presence and extent of disease. However, in some cases, such as patients with acquired immunodeficiency syndrome (AIDS), the chest x-ray film can be negative in the face of clinically significant infection, particularly that resulting from *P. carinii*. In these patients, ^{67}Ga citrate imaging has proven to be useful for detecting occult infection (55). Using an animal model of *Pneumocystis* infection, Fishman et al. (56) reported that ^{111}In-IgG is superior to ^{67}Ga citrate for detecting primary *Pneumocystis* infection and for diagnosing superinfection resulting from other fungal species and *P. aeruginosa*.

Several clinical studies have evaluated the efficacy of ^{111}In-IgG imaging in patients with human immunodeficiency virus (HIV) infection. In one study, 33 patients suspected of having lung infections, most of whom also had HIV infection, and three patients with HIV infection and diarrhea without lung disease were imaged with ^{111}In-IgG (57). Anterior and posterior lung images were acquired in the upright position were obtained within 24 hours after administration of ^{111}In-IgG. Of 29 patients suspected of having *P. carinii* pneumonia (PCP), diagnosis was confirmed by bronchoalveolar lavage in 18. Diffusely increased uptake of IgG in the lung was observed in 17 of 18 patients who had PCP, and normal uptake was observed in 10 of 11 patients without PCP. Two patients with bacterial lung infections had focal accumulation of IgG, whereas two patients with minor radiographic abnormalities had normal uptake. Normal lung uptake also occurred in 2/3 HIV-positive patients who had diarrhea but no lung disease. In another study, IgG was compared with ^{67}Ga citrate in HIV-positive patients with fever (58). Twenty-five studies performed using [67]Ga- and ^{99m}Tc-IgG were compared with a second group of 25 studies using ^{111}In-IgG in HIV-positive patients presenting with fever without localizing signs or symptoms. ^{111}In-IgG identified 20 of 22 sites of infection and also accumulated in 5 sites without infection (accuracy = 90%). This was significantly more accurate (*p* <0.05) than ^{67}Ga, which identified 19 of 20 sites of infection but accumulated in 18 sites without infection (accuracy = 74%), and ^{99m}Tc-IgG, which identified infection in 11 of 20 sites but accumulated in 8 sites without infection (accuracy = 77%). In a pilot study of 5 patients with AIDS and PCP, imaging with ^{111}In-IgG was performed before and after therapy (59). Lung uptake of ^{111}In-IgG, measured as a lung/heart ratio, was

calculated in both the pretherapy and posttherapy studies. In all five patients the lung/heart ratio of ^{111}In-IgG was reduced after treatment. The mean reduction in heart/lung ratio was 27%. If these results are confirmed by a larger study, ^{111}In-IgG could become a useful method for monitoring the response of PCP to therapy in patients with AIDS. In a relatively large prospective study, ^{111}In-IgG imaging was compared with chest radiography for identification of pulmonary infection in HIV patients (60). Sixty-three studies were performed in 57 patients with suspected chest infection or fever of unknown origin (FUO). The results of the two imaging modalities were compared with microbiologic or cytologic diagnosis. In 40 patients with confirmed pulmonary infection, 25 were correctly identified with chest radiography (sensitivity 62%), whereas 39 were identified with ^{111}In-IgG (sensitivity 97%). In patients without infection, chest radiography was abnormal in 13 (specificity 43%), whereas ^{111}In-IgG imaging was abnormal in only 1 case (specificity 95%). Overall ^{111}In-IgG correctly identified the presence or absence of active lung infection in 61 of 63 cases (accuracy 93%) in contrast to chest radiography that identified 35 of 63 cases (accuracy 55%).

In addition to detecting *Pneumocystis* infection in AIDS and organ transplant patients (1,17,46), ^{111}In-IgG has also proven useful in the detection of *Aspergillus fumigatus*, bacterial, or protozoan infections in severely granulocytopenic patients (34). What is less clear is the utility of IgG imaging in the evaluation of the patient with possible tuberculosis, because a significant number of false-negative results have been reported. It is possible that as long as there is a significant acute inflammatory component to the process, IgG imaging will be effective; however, for more chronic granulomatous processes, the approach may be too insensitive. Clearly more data are needed on this point.

In normal hosts, ^{111}In-IgG has been useful in detecting unsuspected pulmonary infections. For example, in a patient referred for study because of 6 weeks of fever after placement of a mandibular prosthesis, unsuspected pneumonia that was subsequently shown to be due to *Mycoplasma pneumoniae* was detected (Fig. 61.8). Thus, total body imaging can be useful in the evaluation of patients with fevers of diverse etiologies.

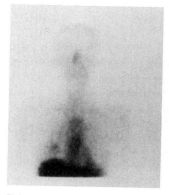 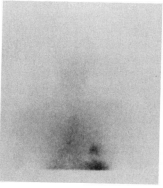

FIGURE 61.8. Anterior and posterior ^{111}In-IgG images in a patient with fever who had undergone reconstructive jaw surgery 6 weeks previously. The patient was referred for evaluation of the jaw. Imaging of the head and chest reveals no evidence of inflammation of the jaw but a clear focus of abnormal IgG accumulation in the right lower lung field, which is confirmed on chest x-ray film.

Detection of Infection in Immunocompromised Patients

Previous studies with animal models demonstrated that pretreatment with steroids, cyclophosphamide (including doses that induce severe neutropenia), or indomethacin does not interfere with the efficacy of IgG imaging (46). In an important preliminary study, Oyen et al. (34) reported that both fungal and bacterial infection, often undiagnosed with conventional techniques, could be diagnosed in febrile, granulocytopenic patients. In addition, we have observed that perforating sigmoid diverticulitis could be diagnosed in a highly immunosuppressed liver transplant patient (Fig. 61.9). Thus, IgG imaging holds promise for the early diagnosis of infection in immunocompromised individuals. Because early diagnosis is essential for effective therapy of these patient groups, a high priority should be given to getting more experience in this area.

Fever of Unknown Origin

Despite application of all known imaging techniques, localization of sites of infection in patients with FUO remains an important and largely unresolved clinical problem. In an early study, 24 patients with FUO who fulfilled the criteria of temperature of greater than or equal to 38.3°C for at least 3 weeks and no diagnosis during 1 week of hospital admission were imaged with ^{111}In-IgG (61). In 9 patients (38%), positive IgG images led to the final diagnosis, whereas in 4 patients (17%), the scintigraphic findings were not helpful. In the 11(45%) patients with negative scans, extensive diagnostic work-up failed to reveal a focal site of infection. Overall sensitivity and specificity of ^{111}In-IgG scintigraphy were 81% and 69%, respectively. In a larger study, 58 patients with FUO were imaged with ^{111}In-IgG (62). In 23 patients without potentially diagnostic clues (PDCs) or only misleading PDCs, the technique was used as a screening procedure. In 35 patients with PDCs pointing at local inflammation, the technique was used when indicated. After diagnostic work-up, infections were found in 17 patients (29%), neoplasms in 6 (10%), noninfectious inflammatory diseases in 14 (24%), miscellaneous disorders in 3 (5%), and no diagnosis in 18 (31%). ^{111}In-IgG imaging was helpful in the diagnostic process for patients with PDCs at local inflammation only; diagnostic yield was 26%. Infection was found in only 10/41 patients with negative scans. These infections were nonfocal or located in the heart, liver region, or urinary tract where physiologic tracer accumulation obscures possible pathologic uptake. The overall sensitivity and specificity was 60% and 83%, respectively. In patients without PDCs for local inflammation, the diagnostic yield of the technique was low because no focal inflammation was observed. In patients with PDCs at local inflammation, ^{111}In-IgG was helpful in the diagnostic process in 25% of the patients. Overall, diagnostic yield was comparable with that of most other scintigraphic techniques used for evaluating patients with FUO.

SUMMARY

The serendipitous discovery that radiolabeled nonspecific IgG accumulates at a site of focal inflammation has led to the development of a new radiopharmaceutical for infection and inflammation imaging. ^{111}In-IgG has been extensively studied in humans with focal infection and has been shown to be safe and effective. It has been especially useful in the evaluation of patients with possible abdominal and skeletal infection, and the ability to perform serial imaging has been important for evaluating proof of cure. Preliminary data suggest that this approach may be particularly useful in immunocompromised patients and may find a role in the quantitative assessment of patients with noninfectious inflammatory processes such as rheumatoid arthritis and inflammatory bowel disease. A new method of labeling IgG with technetium, the HYNIC derivative, holds promise for routine clinical imaging by using a more practical radionuclide. However, caution must be directed against total substitution, because processes such as suspected vascular or skeletal prosthesis infection may require the longer half-life of ^{111}In for satisfactory diagnosis.

When the results obtained with radiolabeled IgG are compared with the specifications for an ideal radiopharmaceutical for inflammation imaging, most of the requirements are met. The major weakness of this approach is that even with the ^{99m}Tc-labeled IgG, a minimum of 6 to 12 hours is necessary for a study to become positive. This delay is not acceptable in the evaluation of acutely evolving processes. Development of other radiopharmaceuticals for this purpose remains to be accomplished.

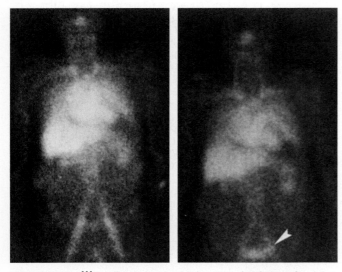

FIGURE 61.9. ^{111}In-IgG images acquired at 18 and 48 hours after injection in a highly immunosuppressed liver transplant patient with *Pneumocystis carinii* pneumonia. At 18 hours, bilateral pneumonia was clearly visualized, and the abdomen was negative. Approximately 4 hours later, the patient developed fever and scrotal pain. Repeat imaging at 48 hours revealed a new focus of pelvic inflammation. At surgery, acute diverticulitis with a perforation adjoining the base of the bladder was identified.

REFERENCES

1. Rubin RH, Fischman AJ, Callahan RJ et al. ^{111}In-labeled nonspecific immunoglobulin scanning in the detection of focal infection. *N Engl J Med* 1989;321:935–940.

2. Simon GL, Geelhoed GW. Diagnosis of intra-abdominal abscesses: a review. *Am Surg* 1985;51:431–436.

3. Hau T, Haaga JR, Aeder MI. Pathophysiology, diagnosis, and treatment of abdominal abscesses. *Curr Probl Surg* 1984;21:1–82.

4. Gerzof SG, Johnson WC. Radiologic aspects of diagnosis and treatment of abdominal abscesses. *Surg Clin North Am* 1984;64:53–65.

5. Mueller Pr, Simeone JF. Intra-abdominal abscesses: diagnosis by sonography and computed tomography. *Radiol Clin North Am* 1983;21:425–443.

6. Feldberg MA, Koehler PR, van Waes PF. Psoas compartment disease studied by computed tomography: analysis of 50 cases and subject review. *Radiology* 1983;148:505–512.

7. Gerzon SG, Oates ME. Imaging techniques for infection in the surgical patient. *Surg Clin North Am* 1988;68:147–165.

8. Littenberg RL, Taketa RM, Alazraki NR et al. Gallium-67 for localization of septic lesions. *Ann Intern Med* 1973;79:403–406.

9. Sfakianakis GN, Al-Sheikh W, Heal A et al. Comparison of scintigraphy with In-111 leukocytes and Ga-67 in the diagnosis of occult sepsis. *J Nucl Med* 1982;23:618–626.

10. McNeil BJ, Sanders R, Alderson PO et al. A prospective study of computed tomography, ultrasound, and gallium imaging in patients with fever. *Radiology* 1981;139:647–653.

11. Biello DR, Levitt RG, Melson GL. The roles of gallium-67 scintigraphy, ultrasonography, and computed tomography in the detection of abdominal abscesses. *Semin Nucl Med* 1979;9:58–65.

12. Knochel JQ, Koehler PR, Lee TG et al. Diagnosis of abdominal abscesses with computed tomography, ultrasound, and ^{111}In leukocyte scans. *Radiology* 1980;137:425–432.

13. Carroll B, Silverman PM, Goodwin DA et al. Ultrasonography and indium-111 white blood cell scanning for the detection of infra-abdominal abscesses. *Radiology* 1981;140:155–160.

14. Thakur ML. Cell labeling: achievements, challenges, and prospects. *J Nucl Med* 1981;22:1011–1014.

15. Lawrence PF, Dries DJ, Alazraki N et al. Indium-111-labeled leukocyte scanning for detection of prosthetic vascular graft infection. *J Vasc Surg* 1985;2:165–173.

16. Moragas M, Lomena F, Herranz R et al. ^{99m}Tc-HMPAO leukocyte scintigraphy in the diagnosis of bone infection. *Nucl Med Commun* 1991;12:417–427.

17. Oyen WJG, Claessens RAMG, van der Meer JWM et al. Indium-111-labeled human nonspecific immunoglobulin G: a new radiopharmaceutical for imaging infectious and inflammatory foci. *Clin Infect Dis* 1992;14:1110–1118.

18. Rubin RH. In search of the hot appendix—a clinician's view of inflammation imaging [Editorial]. *J Nucl Med* 1990;31:316–318.

19. Rubin RH, Young LS, Hansen WP et al. Specific and nonspecific imaging of localized Fisher immunotype 1 *Pseudomonas aeruginosa* infection with radiolabeled monoclonal antibody. *J Nucl Med* 1988;29:651–656.

20. Lind P, Langsteger W, Kotringer P et al. Immunoscintigraphy of inflammatory processes with a technetium-99m-labeled monoclonal antigranulocyte antibody (MAb BW 250/183). *J Nucl Med* 1990;31:417–423.

21. Jacobs A, De Geeter F, Zygas P et al. Immunoscintigraphy (ISG) with a Tc-99m-labeled monoclonal antigranulocyte antibody in patients with suspected inflammatory disease. *J Nucl Med* 1991;32:1002(abst).

22. Becker W, Saptogino A, Wolf F. Diagnostic accuracy of Tc-99m-granulocyte antibody scan in inflammatory or infectious diseases. *J Nucl Med* 1991;32:1002(abst).

23. Segarra I, Roca M, Baliellas C et al. Granulocyte-specific monoclonal antibody technetium-99m-BW 250/183 and indium-111 oxine-labeled leukocyte scintigraphy in inflammatory bowel disease. *Eur J Nucl Med* 1991;18:715–719.

24. Perkins AC, Frier M, Mahida YR et al. ^{99m}Tc-antigranulocyte antibody in the detection of inflammation in inflammatory bowel disease. *Nucl Med Commun* 1991;12:263(abst).

25. Rubin RH, Fischman AJ, Needleman M et al. Radiolabeled, nonspecific polyclonal human immunoglobulin in the detection of focal inflammation by scintigraphy: comparison with gallium-67 citrate and technetium-99m-labeled albumin. *J Nucl Med* 1989;30:385–389.

26. Fischman AJ, Rubin RH, Khaw BA et al. Detection of acute inflammation with ^{111}In-labeled nonspecific polyclonal IgG. *Semin Nucl Med* 1988;18:335–344.

27. Perenboom RM, Oyen WJ, van Schijndel AC et al. Serial indium-111-labelled IgG biodistribution in rat Pneumocystis carinii pneumonia: a tool to monitor the course and severity of the infection. *Eur J Nucl Med* 1995;22:1129–1132.

28. Breedveld FC, van Kroonenburgh MJPG, Camps JAJ et al. Imaging of inflammatory arthritis with technetium-99m-labeled IgG. *J Nucl Med* 1989;30:2017–2021.

29. Fischman AJ, Rubin RH, White JA et al. Localization of Fc and Fab fragments of nonspecific polyclonal IgG at focal sites of inflammation. *J Nucl Med* 1990;31:1199–1205.

30. Rubin RH, Nedelman M, Wilkinson R et al. Effect of anti-inflammatory agents in radiolabeled immunoglobulin scans for focal inflammation. *J Nucl Med* 1987;28:695.

31. Fischman AJ, Fucello AJ, Pellegrino-Gensey JL et al. Effect of carbohydrate modification on the localization of human polyclonal IgG at focal sites of bacterial infection. *J Nucl Med* 1992;33:1378–1382.

32. Morrel EM, Tompkins RG, Fischman AJ et al. Autoradiographic method for quantitation of radiolabeled proteins in tissues using indium-111. *J Nucl Med* 1989;30:1538–1545.

33. Oyen WJ, Claessens RA, van der Meer JW et al. Biodistribution and kinetics of radiolabeled proteins in rats with focal infection. *J Nucl Med* 1992;33:388–394.

34. Oyen WJG, Claessens RAMJ, Raemaekers JMM et al. Diagnosing infection in febrile granulocytopenic patients with indium-111 labeled human IgG. *J Clin Oncol* 1992;10:61–68.

35. Juweid M, Strauss HW, Yaoito H et al. Accumulation of immunoglobulin G at focal sites of infection. *Eur J Nucl Med* 1992;19:159–165.

36. Jasin HE. Oxidative cross-linking of immune complexes by human polymorphonuclear leukocytes. *J Clin Invest* 1988;81:6–15.

37. Fritzberg AR, Abrams PL, Beaumier PL et al. Specific and stable labeling of antibodies with technetium-99m with a diamide dithiolate chelating agent. *Proc Natl Acad Sci U S A* 1988;85:4025–4029.

38. Childs RL, Hnatowich DJ. Optimum conditions for labeling of DTPA-coupled antibodies with technetium-99m. *J Nucl Med* 1985;26:293–299.

39. Abrams MJ, Juweid M, tenKate CI et al. ^{99m}Tc human polyclonal IgG radiolabeled via the hydrazino nicotinamide derivative for imaging focal sites of infection in rats. *J Nucl Med* 1990;31:2022–2028.

40. Barrow SA, Graham W, Jyawook S et al. Localization of ^{111}In-IgG, ^{99m}Tc-IgG, ^{111}In-labeled white blood cells at sites of acute bacterial infection in rabbits. *J Nucl Med* 1993;34:1975–1979.

41. Fischman AJ, Solomon HIT, Babich JW et al. Imaging of focal sites of inflammation in Rhesus monkeys with ^{99m}Tc-labeled human polyclonal IgG. *Int J Nucl Med Biol* 1994;21:111–116.

42. Callahan RJ, Ahmad M, Hauser MM et al. Normal biodistribution and radiation dosimetry estimates for Tc-99m polyclonal human IgG. *J Nucl Med* 1991;32:1099(abst).

43. Buijs WC, Oyen WJ, Dams ET et al. Dynamic distribution and dosimetric evaluation of human non-specific immunoglobulin G labelled with ^{111}In or ^{99m}Tc. *Nucl Med Commun* 1998;19:743–751.

44. Dams ET, Reijnen MM, Oyen WJ et al. Imaging experimental intraabdominal abscesses with ^{99m}Tc-PEG liposomes and ^{99m}Tc-HYNIC IgG. *Ann Surg* 1999;229:551–557.

45. Dams ET, Oyen WJ, Boerman OC et al. Technetium-99m labeled to human immunoglobulin G through the nicotinyl hydrazine derivative: a clinical study. *J Nucl Med* 1998;39:119–124.

46. Serafini AN, Garty I, Vargas-Cuba R et al. Clinical evaluation of a scintigraphic method for diagnosing inflammations/infections using indium-111-labeled nonspecific human IgG. *J Nucl Med* 1991;32:2227–2232.

47. LaMuraglia GM, Fischman AJ, Strauss HW et al. Utility of the indium-111-labeled human immunoglobulin G scan for the detection of focal vascular graft infection. *J Vasc Surg* 1989;10:20–27.

48. Oyen WJG, Claessens RAMJ, van Horn JR et al. Scintigraphic detection of bone and joint infections with indium-111-labeled nonspecific polyclonal human immunoglobulin G. *J Nucl Med* 1990;31:403–412.

49. Oyen WJG, van Horn JR, Claessens RAMJ et al. Diagnosis of bone,

joint and joint prosthesis infections with indium-111-labeled nonspecific human immunoglobulin G scintigraphy. *Radiology* 1992;182: 195–199.

50. Oyen WJG, van Horn JR, Claessens RAMJ et al. Diagnosing prosthetic joint infections. *J Nucl Med* 1991;32:2195–2196.

51. Oyen WJ, Claessens RA, van der Meer JW et al. Detection of subacute infectious foci with indium-111-labeled autologous leukocytes and indium-111-labeled human nonspecific immunoglobulin G: a prospective comparative study. *J Nucl Med* 1991;32:1854–1860.

52. Oyen WJ, Netten PM, Lemmens JA et al. Evaluation of infectious diabetic foot complications with indium-111-labeled human nonspecific immunoglobulin G. *J Nucl Med* 1992;33:1330–1336.

53. Nijhof MW, Oyen WJ, van Kampen A et al. Evaluation of infections of the locomotor system with indium-111-labeled human IgG scintigraphy. *J Nucl Med* 1997;38:1300–1305.

54. van der Lubbe PAHM, Arndt JW, Calame W et al. Measurement of synovial inflammation in rheumatoid arthritis with technetium-99m-labeled human polyclonal immunoglobulin G. *Eur J Nucl Med* 1991; 18:119–123.

55. Rubin RH, Greene R. Etiology and management of the compromised patient with fever and pulmonary infiltrates. In: Rubin RH, Young LG, eds. *Clinical approach to infection in the compromised host,* 3rd ed. New York: Plenum Medical Book, 1994.

56. Fishman JA, Strauss HW, Fischman AJ et al. Imaging of *Pneumocystis carinii* pneumonia with ^{111}In-labeled nonspecific polyclonal IgG: an experimental study in rats. *Nucl Med Commun* 1991;12:175–187.

57. Khalkhali I, Mena I, Rauh DA et al. 111-indium-DTPA-IgG lung imaging in patients with pulmonary and HIV infection. *Chest* 1995; 107:1336–1341.

58. Buscombe JR, Oyen WJ, Corstens FH et al. Localization of infection in HIV antibody positive patients with fever. Comparison of the efficacy of Ga-67 citrate and radiolabeled human IgG. *Clin Nucl Med* 1995;20:334–339.

59. Buscombe JR, Khalkhali I, Mason GR et al. Indium-111 labelled pooled human immunoglobulin imaging to monitor the efficacy of specific therapy for Pneumocystis carinii pneumonia. *Eur J Nucl Med* 1994;21:1148–1150.

60. Buscombe JR, Oyen WJ, Corstens FH et al. A comparison of ^{111}In-HIG scintigraphy and chest radiology in the identification of pulmonary infection in patients with HIV infection. *Nucl Med Commun* 1995;16:327–335.

61. de Kleijn EM, Oyen WJ, Claessens RA et al. Utility of scintigraphic methods in patients with fever of unknown origin. *Arch Intern Med* 1995;155:1989–1994.

62. de Kleijn EM, Oyen WJ, Corstens FH et al. Utility of indium-111-labeled polyclonal immunoglobulin G scintigraphy in fever of unknown origin. The Netherlands FUO Imaging Group. *J Nucl Med* 1997;38:484–489.

INDEX

Page numbers in *italics* denote figures; those followed by "t" denote tables.

A

Abdomen
  infections of
    abscesses, 1206–1208, 1207, *1206, 1209*
    cellulitis, 1207–1208
    gallium-67 scan of, 1206–1210, *1207–1211*
    peritonitis, 1207–1208, *1210*
    technetium-99m HMPAO—labeled leukocyte study of, 1230
  tumors of, gallium-67 scan of, 925–926
Ablation
  defined, 664
  with radioiodine, in thyroid cancer treatment, 664–665
    ancillary benefits from, 664
    complications of, 665
    fixed millicurie amount of, 664
    indications for, 664
    recommendations related to, 664–665
Abscess(es)
  abdominal, 1206–1208, 1207, *1206, 1209*
  indium-111—labeled leukocyte scans for, 1222–1224, 1224t
  intrascrotal, in children, 1106
  liver, gallium-67 scan of, 1206, *1206*
  liver transplantation and, 1077, 1079
  in pouch of Douglas, 1206, *1207*
  renal, 891
  testicular, in children, 1106
  tuberculous, *438*
Absorbed dose, defined, 133
Absorptiometry
  dual x-ray, in bone density measurements, 699, *699–701*
  dual-energy x-ray, peripheral, in bone density measurements, 701, *703, 704, 704*
Absorption, photoelectric, 17–18, *17, 18*
Abuse
  cocaine, PET in, 799–800
  substance, RCBF SPECT in, 764–765
Accelerator(s), 117–121
  particle
    compounding process and procedure verification in, 120
    quality control measures for, 120–121, *120*
Accident(s), radiation, 159–160
Accuracy, statistical, 14
ACE inhibitors. *See* Angiotensin converting enzyme (ACE) inhibitor(s)
Achalasia, esophageal motility in, 489, *490*
Achilles tendonitis, 466
Acid-peptic diseases, gastric emptying in, 496–497

Acquired immunodeficiency syndrome (AIDS)
  gallium-67 scan of, 1214–1215
  RCBF SPECT in, 775–777, *776*
  scintigraphic studies of, 404–405, 405, 404
Acute focal bacterial nephritis, gallium-67 scan of, *1215*
Acute radiation syndromes, 193
Acute tubular necrosis (ATN), 891, *892*
  renal transplantation and, 1037, 1038, 1041–1042, 1044
Adamantinoma (ameloblastoma), 415
ADD. *See* Attention deficit disorder (ADD)
Adductor avulsion fracture, 469
Adenoma(s), autonomous, imaging of, 624
Adenosine, FPRNA and, 261
Adrenal carcinoma, in children, 1133
Adrenal cortex, 715–723
  imaging of, radiopharmaceuticals in, 715–716, 716t
  iodine-131—labeled 19-iodocholesterol study of, 715
  iodine-131—labeled 6-iodomethyl-19-norcholesterol (NP-59) study of, 715–723
    ACTH-stimulated scans in, 718
    clinical applications of, 718–723, 718t–720t, *719–723*, 723t
    in Cushing's syndrome, 719–720, 719t, 721, 720
    dose and route of administration, 717–718
    dosimetry in, 716, 717t
    drugs interfering with uptake of, 715–716, 716t
    gonadal hyperfunction in, 721–722
    imaging sequence in, 718
    incidentally discovered adrenal mass in, 722–723, 723, 722, 723t
    interpretation of, 718
    patient preparation for, 717
    in primary aldosteronism, 720–722, 720t, *721*
    suppression scans in, 718
    technique of, 717–718
    views obtained in, 718
Adrenal disorders, imaging of, radiopharmaceuticals in, 112–113
Adrenal gland, tumors of, in children, 1130, *1132–1136*, 1133
Adrenal medulla, imaging of, 723–727
  MIBG in, 723–727
    clinical applications of, 724–727, *725–728*
    dosimetry of, 724

interpretation of, 724
    technique of, 724
    radiopharmaceuticals in, 723–724
Adult respiratory distress syndrome (ARDS), scintigraphic studies of, 403
Aerosol(s), radioactive, 150–151
Affective disorders, RCBF SPECT in, 771–772, 774–775, 775, 774
Affinity, defined, 822
Afterload, defined, 223
Afterload-reducing drugs, 229
Aging, of brain, 783–784, *784*
Agreement states, 138
AIDS. *See* Acquired immunodeficiency syndrome (AIDS)
AIDS dementia, PET in, 798–799
Air kerma, 134
Akinesia, in ERNA assessment of left ventricular function, 251
Albumin, technetium-99m, leukocyte-labeling with, 1228
Alcoholism
  PET in, 799
  research for, neurotransmission SPECT in, 829, 831
Aldosteronism, primary, iodine-131—labeled 6-iodomethyl-19-norcholesterol (NP-59) study of, 720–722, 720t, *721*
Allograft vasculopathy, cardiac transplantation and, 1063–1065, *1063, 1064, 1064t*
α decay, 7, *7*, 7t, 10t
Alternate R wave gating, in ERNA assessment of left ventricular function, 242
Alveolar-capillary membrane permeability, scintigraphic studies of, 383–386, *385*
Alzheimer's disease (AD)
  PET in, 784–788, *785, 786*
  RCBF SPECT in, 767–771, *768–773*
Ameloblastoma, 415
Aminogluthemide, effects on thyroid hormone levels and function, 599t, 600
Amiodarone
  effects on thyroid hormone levels and function, 599t, 600
  thyrotoxicosis due to, 632, *632*
Amplitude images, in ERNA assessment of left ventricular function, 247–248, *247*
Anemia
  aplastic, bone marrow scintigraphy in, 578, *579*

1245